Mayes'
Midwifery

Senior Content Strategist: *Alison Taylor*
Content Development Specialist: *Veronika Watkins*
Project Manager: *Louisa Talbott*
Designer: *Christian Bilbow*
Illustration Manager: *Karen Giacomucci*
Illustrator: *Richard Tibbitts*

Mayes'
Midwifery

FIFTEENTH EDITION

Edited by

Sue Macdonald

FRCM (Hons) MSc PGCEA ADM RM RN ILTM FETC

Midwife Consultant
Formerly Education and Research Manager and Lead
Midwife for Education, Royal College of Midwives,
London, UK

Gail Johnson

MA DPSM PGDip Adult Education RM RN

Education Advisor, Royal College of Midwives,
London, UK

Foreword by
Cathy Warwick

CBE

Professor, Chief Executive Officer of the Royal College
of Midwives, London, UK

ELSEVIER

Edinburgh   London   New York   Oxford   Philadelphia   St Louis   Sydney   Toronto   2017

ELSEVIER

Twelfth edition 1997
Thirteenth edition 2004
Fourteenth edition 2011
Fifteenth edition 2017

ISBN 978-0-7020-6211-7
eISBN 978-0-7020-6336-7

Notice

Printed in Scotland

Last digit is the print number: 9 8 7 6 5

Contents

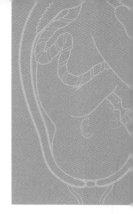

Contents

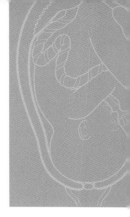

Contributors

Belinda Ackerman MA PGDip PGCEA ADM HV RM RN
Supervisor of Midwives, Women's Services,
Guy's and St Thomas' NHS Foundation Trust, London, UK
Chapter 3 Regulation of midwives

Luisa Acosta BSc (Hons) MSc PG(HE)Dip
Senior Midwifery Lecturer/Admissions Co-ordinator,
College of Nursing, Midwifery and Healthcare, University
of West London, London, UK
*Chapter 67 Complications related to the third stage of
labour*

Andrea Aras-Payne MA PGDip BSc (Hons) RM
Senior Lecturer in Midwifery, College of Nursing Midwifery
and Healthcare, University of West London, London, UK
*Chapter 67 Complications related to the third stage
of labour*

Debbie Barber BSc (Hons) MSc PGDE PGCMU PGD
Women's Health Dip Counselling RGN NT NMP
Advanced Nurse Practitioner, Women's Health, Oxford
University Hospitals; Associate Lecturer, Oxford Brookes
University, Oxford, UK
Chapter 28 Infertility and assisted conception

Tracey Barnfather RM RN ADM PGCEA MSc SFHEA
Principal Lecturer – Lead Midwife for Education, University
of Northampton, Northampton, UK
Chapter 61 Rhythmic variations of labour

Cecelia M. Bartholomew MSc BSc (Hons) RM RN PgDip
Teaching and Learning HEA fellow
Senior Lecturer in Midwifery, University of West London,
London, UK
*Chapter 38 Supporting choices in reducing pain
and fear during labour*
Chapter 52 Nausea and vomiting in pregnancy

Sam Bassett DHC MA BSc (Hons) DipHe Mid RGN PGSHSCE
Lecturer in Midwifery and Women's Health, Florence
Nightingale Faculty of Nursing and Midwifery, King's
College London, London, UK
Chapter 59 Obstetric interventions

Joanne Bates MEd PGDE for teachers of nurses and
midwives RN RM ONC Graduate Certificate in Women's Health
Senior Lecturer, Midwifery, Child and Reproductive
Health, University of Chester, Chester, UK
Chapter 55 Sexually transmitted diseases

Kuldip Kaur Bharj OBE PhD MSc BSc (Hons) MTD DN HSM
Cert RM RN RSA Counselling
Associate Professor, School of Healthcare, The University
of Leeds, Leeds, UK
*Chapter 32 Confirming pregnancy and care of the pregnant
woman*

Debra Bick RM BA MMedSci PhD
Professor, Florence Nightingale Faculty of Nursing and
Midwifery, King's College London, London, UK
Chapter 41 Content and organization of postnatal care

Judy Bothamley MA PGCEA ADM RM RCN
Senior Lecturer Midwifery, College of Nursing, Midwifery
and Healthcare, University of West London, London, UK
Chapter 54 Hypertensive and medical disorders in pregnancy

Maureen Boyle RN RM ADM PGCEA MSc
Senior Lecturer (Midwifery), College of Nursing, Midwifery
and Health Care, University of West London, London, UK
Chapter 33 Antenatal investigations
*Chapter 54 Hypertensive and medical disorders in
pregnancy*

Gwendolen Bradshaw EdD MA PGCEA ADM RM RN
Pro-Vice-Chancellor, Learning, Teaching and Quality,
University of Bradford, Bradford, West Yorkshire, UK
Chapter 14 National Health Service policy and midwifery

Alison Brodrick RGN RM MSc Midwifery
Consultant Midwife, Sheffield Teaching Hospitals NHS
Trust, Sheffield, UK
Chapter 60 Induction of labour and prolonged pregnancy
Chapter 63 Obstructed labour and uterine rupture

Gill Brook MCSP (DSA) CSP MSc
Independent Women's Health Physiotherapy, Otley, West
Yorkshire, UK
President of the International Organization of Physical
Therapists in Women's Health
*Chapter 22 Physical preparation for childbirth and beyond,
and the role of physiotherapy*

Melanie Brook-Read MSc PgDipEd RM SRN FHEA
Senior Lecturer Midwifery, Department of Healthcare
Practice, University of Bedfordshire, Luton, UK
Chapter 20 Preconception care

Barbara Burden RN RM ADM PGCEA MSc Social Research
MBA(HEM) PhD SFHEA
Head of School of Healthcare Practice and NMC Lead
Midwife for Education/CQC Professional Advisor,
University of Bedfordshire, Faculty of Health and Social
Sciences, Aylesbury, UK
Chapter 15 Legal frameworks for the care of the child
Chapter 20 Preconception care
Chapter 24 Anatomy of male and female reproduction
Chapter 30 The fetal skull

Anna Byrom BSc (Hons) Midwifery PGCert Health and Social
Care Education
Senior Midwifery Lecturer, School of Community Health,
Midwifery and Sexual Health, University of Central
Lancashire, Preston, UK
*Chapter 34 Choice, childbearing and maternity care:
the choice agenda and place of birth*

Sheena Byrom OBE Ed D honoris causa RM MA HFRCM
Independent Midwife Consultant, Whalley, UK
*Chapter 34 Choice, childbearing and maternity care:
the choice agenda and place of birth*

Sarah Church PhD MSc RGN RM PGDipEd PGCert (Research
Supervision)
Associate Professor in Midwifery, School of Health and
Social Care, London South Bank University and Bart's
Health NHS Trust, London, UK
Chapter 61 Rhythmic variations of labour

Terri Coates MSc RN RM ADM Dip Ed
Freelance Midwifery Advisor
Clinical Midwife, Salisbury NHS Trust, Salisbury, UK
Chapter 62 Malpositions and malpresentations
Chapter 64 Shoulder dystocia

Glenys Connolly MSc ANNP RSCN RGN Biomedical Science
Derriford Hospital, Plymouth NHS Trust, Plymouth, UK
Chapter 48 Neonatal infection
*Chapter 49 Congenital anomalies, neonatal surgery and pain
management*
Chapter 50 Metabolic and endocrine disorders

Lesley Daniels MABSc (Hons) MTD RM
Lecturer in Midwifery, University of Leeds, Leeds, UK
*Chapter 32 Confirming pregnancy and care of the
pregnant woman*

Frances Day-Stirk MHM ADM DN(Lon) RM RN FRCM (Hons)
Former Director of LRPD Royal College of Midwives
(RCM), UK
Former President ICM
Chapter 1 The global midwife

Jane Denton CBE FRCN RGM RM
The Multiple Births Foundation, Queen Charlotte's and
Chelsea Hospital, London, UK
Chapter 57 Multiple pregnancy

Bernie Divall PhD MA RM
Research Fellow in Maternity Care, School of Health
Sciences, University of Nottingham, Nottingham, UK
Chapter 7 Leadership and management in midwifery

Jean Donnison BA(Oxon) PhD
Formerly Senior Lecturer, Department of Social Policy and
Administration, University of East London, London, UK
*Chapter 2 A history of the midwifery profession in the
United Kingdom*

Lesley Dornan PhD BSc (Hons) RN SCPHN
Health Visitor Researcher, Maternal Fetal and Infant
Research Centre, Ulster University, Jordanstown,
Newtownabbey, Co Antrim, N Ireland, UK
*Chapter 6 Evidence-based practice and research for
practice*

Soo Downe OBE BA (Hons) MSc PhD RM
Professor of Midwifery Studies, School of Health,
University of Central Lancashire, Preston, UK
Chapter 37 Care in the second stage of labour

Jacqueline Dunkley-Bent OBE DHC MSc PGCEA
ADM RM RN
Head of Maternity, Children and Young People for NHS
England, Nursing Directorate, London, UK
Chapter 19 Health promotion and education

Francesca Entwistle MRes PGCEA ADM RN RM
Professional Officer – Policy and Advocacy, National
Infant Feeding Network Co-ordinator (NIFN),
UNICEF UK Baby Friendly Initiative, London, UK
Visiting Lecturer – Midwifery, Department of Allied Health
Professionals and Midwifery, University of Hertfordshire,
Hatfield, UK
Chapter 44 Infant feeding and relationship building

Anna Gaudion BSc MA
Researcher/Designer, The Polyanna Project, London, UK
Chapter 23 Vulnerable women

Kathryn Gutteridge RGN RM MSc Dip Counselling and
Psychotherapy
Consultant Midwife and Clinical Lead for Normality,
Maternity and Perinatal Medicine, Sandwell and West
Birmingham Hospitals NHS Trust, Birmingham, UK
Chapter 69 Maternal mental health and psychological issues

Jenny Hall EdD MSc RM ADM PGDip(HE) SFHEA
Senior Midwifery Lecturer, Faculty of Health and Social
Sciences, Bournemouth University, Bournemouth, UK
Chapter 27 Fertility and its control

Tina Harris PhD BSc (Hons) RM ADM
Lead Midwife for Education, Faculty Head of Research
Students and Principal Lecturer, School of Nursing and
Midwifery, Faculty of Health and Life Sciences, De
Montfort University, Leicester, UK
Chapter 39 Care in the third stage of labour

Sima Hay RN RM MSc PGCAP
Senior Lecturer, Department of Midwifery, School of Allied
Health, Midwifery and Social Care, Kingston and St George's
Faculty of Health, Social Care and Education, London, UK
Chapter 58 Preterm labour

Simon Hettle BSc (Hons) PhD CSci FIBMS FHEA
Lecturer In Biomedical Sciences, School of Science and
Sport, University of the West of Scotland, Paisley, UK
Chapter 26 Genetics

Caroline Hollins Martin PhD MPhil BSc PGCE ADM RM
RGN MBPsS
Professor, School of Health and Social Care, Edinburgh
Napier University, Edinburgh, UK
Chapter 21 Education for parenthood

Claire Homeyard BSc (Hons) MSc
Consultant Midwife (Public Health), Barking, Havering and
Redbridge University Hospitals NHS Trust, London, UK
Chapter 23 Vulnerable women

Caroline Hunter RM BA (Hons) MSc FHEA
Midwifery Tutor, Florence Nightingale Faculty of Nursing
and Midwifery, King's College London, London, UK
Chapter 41 Content and organization of postnatal care

Amanda Hutcherson Dip HE Mid RM MA Midwifery Practice
MA Academic Practice
Midwifery/Mentorship Lecturer, School of Health Sciences,
City, University of London, London, UK
Chapter 53 Bleeding in pregnancy

Karen Jackson BSc (Hons) MPhil
Division of Midwifery, University of Nottingham,
Nottingham, UK
Chapter 13 Sexuality

Karen Jewell RM MSc
Nursing Officer for Maternity and Early Years, Welsh
Government, Cardiff, UK
Chapter 17 Nutrition

Gail Johnson MA DPSM PGDip Adult Education RM RN
Education Advisor at the Royal College of Midwives,
London, UK
Chapter 8 An introduction to ethics and midwifery practice
Chapter 51 Stillbirth and sudden infant death syndrome
Chapter 70 Midwifery for the future … where next?

Julie Jomeen PhD MA PGCHE RM RGN
Professor of Midwifery, Faculty of Health and Social Care,
University of Hull, Hull, UK
Chapter 12 Psychological context of childbirth

Lyn Jones RMN RGN RM MSc Midwifery and Women's
Health
Senior Lecturer Midwifery, Anglia Ruskin University,
Cambridge, UK
Chapter 65 Presentation and prolapse of the umbilical cord

Sue Jordan MBBCh PhD
Professor of Medicines Management and Health Services
Research, Department of Nursing, Swansea University,
Swansea, UK
Chapter 10 Pharmacology and the midwife

Sue Macdonald MSc PGCEA ADM RM RN FETC
FRCM (Hons)
Midwife Consultant, formerly Education and Research
Manager and Lead Midwife for Education, Royal College
of Midwives, London, UK
*Chapter 2 A history of the midwifery profession in the United
Kingdom*
Chapter 5 The midwife as a lifelong learner
Chapter 10 Pharmacology and the midwife
Chapter 70 Midwifery for the future … where next?

Alison Macfarlane BA DipStat CStat MFPH
Professor of Perinatal Health, Centre for Maternal and
Child Health Research, School of Health Sciences, City,
University of London, London, UK
Chapter 16 Epidemiology

Contributors

Mary McNabb BSc (Hons) BA (Hons) MSc PGCEA ADM RN RM
Scientific Advisor, Childbirth Essentials, Banbury, Oxfordshire, UK
Chapter 25 Female reproductive physiology: timed interactions between hypothalamus, anterior pituitary and ovaries
Chapter 29 Fertilization, embryo formation and feto-placental development
Chapter 31 Maternal neurohormonal and systemic adaptations to feto-placental development
Chapter 35 Physiological changes from late pregnancy until the onset of lactation: from nesting to suckling-lactation and parental-infant attachment

Stephanie Michaelides PGCEA ADM RM RN
Programme Leader Graduate/Post Graduate Certificate In Neonatal Care, School of Health and Education, Middlesex University, London, UK
Chapter 42 Physiology, assessment and care of the newborn
Chapter 43 Thermoregulation
Chapter 47 Neonatal jaundice

Wendy O'Brien RM MSc PGCEA
Clinical Placement Facilitator, Imperial Healthcare NHS Trust, London, UK
Chapter 57 Multiple pregnancy

Irena Papadopoulos PhD MA(Ed) BA RN RM FHEA
Professor and Head, Research Centre for Transcultural Studies in Health, Mental Health, Social Work and Integrative Medicine, Middlesex University, London, UK
Chapter 11 Sociocultural and spiritual context of childbearing

Vivien Perry MA BSc (Hons) PgCert Ed RM RGN
Senior Lecturer, Department of Nursing, Midwifery and Health, Northumbria University, Newcastle, UK
Chapter 24 Anatomy of male and female reproduction

Julia Petty BSc (Hons) MSc MA PGCE FHEA RGN/RSCN
Senior Lecturer In Children's Nursing, School of Health and Social Work, University of Hertfordshire, Hatfield, UK
Chapter 45 The preterm baby and the small baby
Chapter 46 Respiratory and cardiac disorders

Michael Preston-Shoot BA (Hons) PhD PGDipSW PGDipPsychot
Professor Emeritus (Social Work), University of Bedfordshire, Luton, UK
Chapter 15 Legal frameworks for the care of the child

Jean Rankin PhD M Medical Science PGCert LTHE BSc (Hons) RN RM RSCN
Professor, Health, Nursing and Midwifery, University of the West of Scotland, Paisley, UK
Chapter 26 Genetics

Jessica Read RN RM BSc (Hons) MSc
LSA Midwifery Officer for London, NHS England, London, UK
Chapter 4 Clinical governance and the midwife

Lindsey Rose BSc (Hons) Midwifery RM MSc Licensed Acupuncturist FHEA
Senior Lecturer in Midwifery, Anglia Ruskin University, Cambridge, UK
Chapter 56 Abnormalities of the genital tract

Marlene Sinclair PhD MEd PG/Dip RM RN RNT BSc (Hons)
Professor, Maternal Fetal and Infant Research Centre, Ulster University, Jordanstown, Newtownabbey, Co Antrim, N. Ireland, UK
Chapter 6 Evidence-based practice and research for practice

Mary Steen RGN RM DipClinHyp PGCRM PGDipHE MCGI PhD
Professor of Midwifery, School of Nursing and Midwifery, University of South Australia, Adelaide, South Australia, Australia
Chapter 66 Maternal morbidity following childbirth

Andrew Symon MA (Hons) PhD RM
Mother and Infant Research Unit, University of Dundee, Dundee, UK
Chapter 9 The law and the midwife

Denise Tiran MSc RM ADM PGCEA
Educational Director, Expectancy
Visiting Lecturer, University of Greenwich, London, UK
Chapter 18 Complementary therapies and natural remedies in pregnancy and birth: responsibilities of midwives

Cheryl Titherly BSc Anthropology MA Anthropology and Sociology
Improving Bereavement Care Manager, Sands, London, UK
Chapter 68 Pregnancy loss and the death of a baby: grief and bereavement care

Denis Walsh MA PhD DPSM RM
Associate Professor in Midwifery, School of Health Sciences, University of Nottingham, Nottingham, UK
Chapter 36 Care in the first stage of labour

Amanda Willetts DipHE BSc (Hons) MSc PG CAP FHEA RM RN
Senior Lecturer, Midwifery, Healthcare Practice, University of Bedfordshire, Luton, UK
Chapter 30 The fetal skull

Angie Wilson PhD BSc (Hons) Health Studies SRN SCM ADM PGCEA MTD CPS
Independent Midwife Teacher and Specialist Midwife-Perineal Care, Royal Surrey County Hospital, Guildford, UK
Chapter 40 The pelvic floor

Foreword

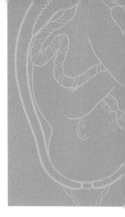

I am delighted to write the Foreword for the fifteenth edition of *Mayes' Midwifery*. It seems no time at all since I was writing for the fourteenth edition. In fact, that was seven years ago. How time flies! Whilst the fundamentals underpinning midwifery practice will always remain much the same, the political and social context in which midwives throughout the world practice changes rapidly, as does the evidence which underpins all of a midwife's decision making. This revised and updated edition of *Mayes' Midwifery* is a highly valuable resource and will be welcomed in the UK and around the world.

We now live in a world where access to knowledge and information is, for many of us, very easy. All we need to do is switch a computer on and off we go. That, however, is not true for every midwife. Globally many will either have no access or very poor access to electronic information sources. For them a comprehensive textbook is vital. But even for those who have easy internet access, *Mayes' Midwifery* is of huge importance. Its multi-author/multi-expert approach and its range of subject matter make it a crucial reference point. It ensures midwives can keep up to date with a very wide range of issues, quickly check the latest evidence and opinion, and be pointed towards further reading and information should this be of interest and importance to them. As midwives increasingly undergo formal revalidation to stay on their professional register, the reflective activities will be very much appreciated.

One of the things that I really value about *Mayes' Midwifery* is that it is far more than just a clinical textbook.

How midwives practice is significantly affected by the social and political context of birth. The health system midwives work in will enhance or inhibit midwifery practice, as will critical issues such as regulation and governance and, very importantly, the law of the land. Once again *Mayes' Midwifery* explores these issues. The chapters on these topics help midwives to understand the importance not just of high-quality day-to-day clinical practice but of engagement with the wider issues which may influence how they undertake their role and the ability of women to be informed partners in their care.

In my Foreword for the previous edition I talked of two challenges; economic uncertainty and the balancing act midwives have to undertake if they are to manage risk and uncertainty whilst also personalising care and meeting the needs of individuals. Neither of these two challenges has gone away and what I said then remains true today. That is, that if midwives are to play their part in meeting these two challenges, it is critical that there is an educated, thoughtful and flexible workforce that is prepared to consider its practice to ensure that it delivers the very highest quality of service to women, achieves the best outcomes for mothers and babies, and makes effective use of limited resources.

With its wide range of topics and expert authors I have no doubt that *Mayes' Midwifery* will help midwives and the midwifery profession achieve that position.

Professor Cathy Warwick, CBE

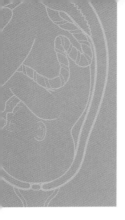

Preface

We were delighted and honoured to be invited to edit the fifteenth edition of *Mayes' Midwifery*. Since its birth in 1937 this textbook has been held in great esteem by students and midwives, becoming one of the leading midwifery textbooks nationally and internationally. During its lifetime it has developed from a single author text, through to a multi-authored, evidence-based and research-supported book, reflecting contemporary midwifery theory, practice and education. Editing such a textbook is both a challenge and a delight, with the aim of ensuring that all of the resources and knowledge are available, that the book is well structured and well supported by the evidence chosen and, above all, helps readers not only find the answers, but also begin to frame the questions that they will need to ask as qualified, competent and confident practitioners.

The need to offer more resources came with the fourteenth edition; authors and editors met the challenge to provide a range of additional materials including video clips, multiple choice quizzes for self-evaluation, and practice tools that readers could access online. For this new edition those resources, which continue to be useful, have been reviewed, updated and supplemented to maximize their usefulness. Thus users will find an extended range of supportive information, including new tools, checklists and assessment forms which can form part of the reader's personal 'knowledge and practice toolkit' in future work.

We believe that this textbook offers opportunities for the reader to consider how theories may be applied in practice and encourages them to question their practice. Some tools will help focus the practitioner on asking women about their experiences, helping to make the maternity service physically and psychologically safer and more user-friendly.

This textbook and online resources are designed for student as well as qualified midwives, and we believe that it is important to design a text that will assist students in their introduction into midwifery, and take them through their education programme to qualification and beyond. We also wanted to ensure that the book and resources would be relevant and useful for the registered midwife, whatever their sphere of practice, be it clinical, management or education.

The text has been informed by recent changes in practice, by national and international health and maternity care policy, by previous readers' evaluations and, of course, by the expert authors who have worked so hard to make this edition exciting and relevant to midwives.

The aim has been to provide extensive research- and evidence-based knowledge and information to support contemporary midwifery practice, in its myriad settings. This edition reflects the nature of midwifery today, and the needs of those who work globally, from highly technical settings to those with minimal facilities. Ultimately, this should facilitate the knowledge, confidence and competence of the midwives, and improve care to women, babies and their families.

The structure of the text takes the reader through the foundations of midwifery, from the pre-pregnancy period through to postnatal care, and care of the newborn. The book and web resource continue to have a strong physiological foundation. There are chapters focusing on maternal, fetal and neonatal physiology, while others, such as the chapters dealing with care in labour and the care of the newborn, weave physiology into applied practice. All chapters are fully referenced and well supported by research and evidence. Different approaches and perspectives appear throughout the text, making it an interesting and challenging resource for all of those interested in women's health and childbirth – both qualified and student readers.

The overall design of the chapters has been retained and further developed. Each chapter begins with learning outcomes, and includes reflective activities which will assist the reader in thinking about the content in practice terms and in applying learning locally. Each chapter concludes with key points to highlight the most important parts. Figures, diagrams and illustrations have been reviewed, updated, and increased, and colour has been added, providing a strong visual impact.

It is said that if you want something done, ask a busy person. This rang true to us as editors, and we were extremely fortunate in having such an excellent team of authors, all experts in their field, who approached the task of writing their chapter and the supporting work with complete commitment, energy and great creativity. Many took a fresh approach, introducing new thinking and new ideas, which has made the task a real labour of love, and we hope the result will be useful, interesting and challenging to the reader. As well as midwives, we have welcomed the work of other academics, including those from nursing, social work, physiology, social policy, epidemiology and pharmacology; truly a multidisciplinary and interdisciplinary authorship team!

The concept described by François de la Rochefoucauld in the 17th century that 'the only thing constant in life is change' continues to underpin the book and its accompanying online resources. This is illustrated by the stream of policy drivers, national and international reports and, above all, the changing needs of women and their families. Life has become more complex and thus maternity care has had to adapt and develop. Students and qualified midwives need knowledge, tools and resources that will support them in working with these changes, enable them to be proactive rather than reactive, and able to provide high quality, evidence-based, culturally sensitive and, above all, kind and compassionate care to the woman and her family.

Since the last edition a range of initiatives and policy drivers have emerged, and readers will note that the implications of these have been included in the appropriate chapters. An example is the *Lancet* midwifery series (Renfrew et al., 2014, ten Hoope-Bender et al., 2014); an international systematic examination of global midwifery. This is set to be a major influence on the ethos and provision of care to the mother and baby in the future, placing them firmly in the centre of care, with midwifery acting as the critical link between them and the services and resources that they need. This series included a quality framework for planning workforce development and resource allocation which may be used in service and curricula development. The England Review into maternity services (Cumberledge, 2016), and the recent Scottish Review and five year plan for maternity and neonatal care (Grant, 2017) will also shape the way that midwives work, and the way that women and babies receive care.

Attention has been placed not only on the physical safety of the woman and her baby, but also their psychological well being, and the importance of kindness and compassion is now highlighted both for women and their families, and for health professionals themselves (Byrom and Downe, 2015). As midwives we need to be alert, open and questioning and, above all, we must listen to the woman's experience and perspectives and that of her family, while using research and national reviews (National Childbirth Trust (NCT) and National Federation of Women's Institutes (WI), 2017, Redshaw, 2015) and opportunities to reflect with women for whom we have provided care.

The international midwifery and maternity care scene is also shifting, and this is reflected particularly in Chapter 1, and throughout other chapters, as the Millennium Development Goals (MDGs) have been superseded by the Sustainable Development Goals (SDGs), and the need to reduce maternal and perinatal mortality and morbidity, and improve the health of women and children world wide. Midwives need to be equipped for their global role and readers will note that though the textbook is based upon UK midwifery and maternity services, care has been taken to consider the international context and include good practice examples from other countries. Much of the evidence and research has been drawn from across the globe.

We have worked hard to ensure that this edition is women- and baby-centred, and to meet the needs of students and midwives in their roles caring for women, their babies and families.

We hope that the textbook will raise many questions, stimulate debate and encourage a spirit of enquiry. We see it as a stepping stone for readers to explore beyond its pages and to look at new evidence and the care we give as our knowledge expands, bearing in mind that evidence includes women's and midwives' experiences, as well as formal research.

We hope you enjoy using the fifteenth edition of *Mayes' Midwifery*. If you have any comments about the book we would be delighted to hear from you.

Sue Macdonald and Gail Johnson
London, Spring 2017

References

Byrom S, Downe S: *The roar behind the silence: why kindness, compassion and respect matter in maternity care*, Pinter & Martin, London, 2015.

Cumberledge B: *National Maternity Review: BETTER BIRTHS Improving outcomes of maternity services in England A Five Year Forward View for maternity care*, London and online, NHS England, 2016.

Grant J: *The Best Start A Five-Year Forward Plan for Maternity and Neonatal Care in Scotland*, Edinburgh, Scottish Government, 2017.

National Childbirth Trust (NCT) & National Federation of Women's Institutes (WI): *Support Overdue: Womens experiences of maternity services 2017*. National Childbirth Trust (NCT) and National Federation of Women's Institutes (WI), London, 2017.

Redshaw HJ: *Safely delivered: a national survey of women's experience of maternity care 2014*, Oxford and online, National Perinatal Epidemiology Unit, University of Oxford, 2015.

Renfrew MJ, Mcfadden A, Bastos MH, et al: Midwifery and quality care: findings from a new evidence-informed framework for maternal and newborn care, *Lancet* 384:1129–1145, 2014.

ten Hoope-Bender P, de Bernis L, Campbell J, et al: Improvement of maternal and newborn health through midwifery, *Lancet* 384:1226–1235, 2014.

Acknowledgements

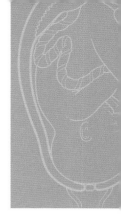

This book would not have been possible without the brilliant contributions of every one of the authors, all busy expert practitioners, who have worked so incredibly hard both on the book and the online material, coping with the deadlines and thinking creatively to make the content alive and contemporary for the reader.

We must also sincerely thank the many contributors to previous editions, whose fantastic work laid the foundations for the development of this fifteenth edition. Without the input from so many expert authors who have been concerned to ensure current evidence for practice, this edition would not have achieved its current quality. Previous contributors include: Maria Barrell, Carol Bates, Christine A Bewley, Jane Bott, Margaret Brock, Joan Cameron, Tandy Deane-Gray, Bridgit Dimond, Kathryn Eglinton, Liz Gale, Anne-Marie Henshaw, Tina Heptinstall, Patricia Jackson, Patricia Jones, Shirley R Jones, Tara Kaufmann, Chris Kettle, Paul Lewis, Patricia Lindsay, Gaynor D MacLean, Pat McGeowan, Stephanie Meakin, Carol Paeglis, Maria Simons, Mary Sidebotham, Susan Sapseed, Lynne T Spencer, Jenni Thomas, Rosemary Towse, Nicola Wales, Theresa Walsh, Margaret Yerby.

Jean Donnison's chapter on the history of midwifery remains a seminal text and it is with great sadness that we report that she passed away earlier this year.

Very special acknowledgement goes to Julia Magill-Cuerden, editor of the fourteenth edition.

We would also like to thank our colleagues and the Royal College of Midwives for their support through the whole gestation of the book.

As always, however, it is our friends and families who have had less of our time and attention, and who have been unfailingly supportive and generous in enabling us both to live transfixed by computers, websites and mountains of proofs. A special thank you goes to Alison Macdonald for providing support, particular expert advice and information, and to Paddy O'Connor for his great support and patience.

Alison Taylor and Veronika Watkins at Elsevier have seen this edition through from its conception and have provided us with guidance and support through the pregnancy and birth of the text and online platforms. Our sincere thanks go to them for their continued support, along with Louisa Talbott and other colleagues at Elsevier.

Finally our thanks go to the midwives and student midwives who are the present and future of the midwifery profession, and to their commitment to provide the best care to women, babies and their families, now and in the future.

Sue Macdonald
Gail Johnson

Part One

The midwife in context

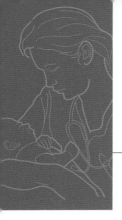

Chapter 1

The global midwife

Frances Day-Stirk

Learning Outcomes ?

After reading this chapter you will be able to:

- gain insight into the critical issues affecting maternal and newborn health globally
- consider the Sustainable Development Goals (SDGs), Global Strategy Women's, Children's and Adolescent's Health (GS2) and other global mandates and reflect on their significance to your area of practice
- identify the major causes of maternal and newborn death, explain historical and geographical perspectives and explore predisposing factors
- be aware of the range of international agencies and what their roles are
- reflect on the place of the midwife in the global context
- apply this knowledge in day-to-day practice within the area in which you work

INTRODUCTION

Midwives worldwide share a common aim to provide safe, quality, effective care for childbearing women and the newborn. Yet the overwhelming majority of maternal and newborn deaths occur in low- and middle-income countries (LMICs) and could easily be prevented by having better access to professional midwives, equipped and resourced within functional health systems. Midwives face different challenges according to the impact of globalization, migration, the country's status (low, middle or high income) and whether its health system is functional. Equally, perspectives on the role of the midwife in sexual, reproductive, maternal and newborn health (SRMNH) will be different depending on the country of practice,

whether low, middle or high income and whether located in the North or South (World Health Organization (WHO) 2015a).

Midwives and their role in the survival of pregnant and childbearing women and their newborns have been increasingly recognized, no more so than in the latter years leading up to 2015 and the end of the Millennium Development Goals (MDGs) (see Fig. 1.1). Yet countless women still experience childbirth without a midwife, fraught with fear and danger.

Three of the eight MDGs are health related: MDG 4 – to reduce child mortality, MDG5 – to improve maternal health and MDG 6 – to combat human immunodeficiency virus (HIV) infection and acquired immunodeficiency syndrome (AIDS), malaria and other diseases. MDG 5, the goal for which the least progress was made and that was not met, included two targets: MDG 5A – to reduce maternal mortality by 75% from the 1990 maternal mortality ratio (MMR), and MDG 5B – to achieve universal access to reproductive health by 2015.

Initiatives such as the United Nations (UN) Secretary-General's Global Strategy for Women's and Children's Health (Ki-moon 2010), the Every Woman Every Child movement (United Nations Foundation (UNF) 2016) and the Commission on Information and Accountability (COIA 2014), which stimulated 'global reporting, oversight, and accountability on women's and children's health', emerged in support of the MDGs (WHO 2015a).

The number of maternal deaths declined by 43% globally from approximately 532,000 in 1990 to an estimated 289,000 women per year in 2013. The MMR fell by approximately 44%, short of the MDG 5A target to reduce the MMR by 75%. The approximate global lifetime risk of maternal death fell from 1 in 73 to 1 in 180 (WHO 2015a).

Improvement in maternal and newborn health challenges is not only the role of health professionals,

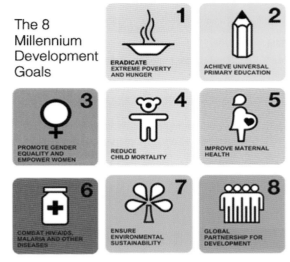

The 8 Millennium Development Goals

Figure 1.1 The Eight Millennium Development Goals. (United Nations Millennium Development Goals, Brazil.)

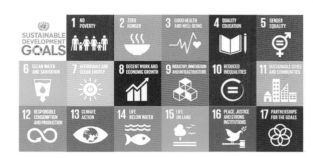

Figure 1.2 Sustainable Development Goals. (United Nations Social Development Network http://unsdn.org/get-involved.)

healthcare professional associations and health systems, but also other technical experts in infrastructure, including roads, transport, telecommunications, water and sanitation engineers. It takes engagement of all, including with communities, mobilizing community and political will. Humanitarian and conflict situations, post-conflict disease, pandemics (e.g. Ebola) and disaster lead to the breakdown of health systems, which significantly impedes the progress of maternal and newborn mortality reduction.

GLOBAL CHALLENGES FOR MIDWIFERY IN THE 2030 ERA

In a world described as being more 'volatile, uncertain, complex and ambiguous than before', with a global all-time high of young people (1.8 billion between the ages of 10 and 24 in 2015 and nearly 2.0 billion projected by 2030), 2016 began the start of a new agenda for the next 15 years (WHO 2015b).

The adoption of the SDGs and the launch of the GS2 at the UN General Assembly in September 2015 built on the lessons of the MDGs and set the 2030 agenda for *all* countries in *all* regions of the world (see Fig. 1.2).

Ending preventable maternal and newborn death

In support of the Every Woman Every Child movement, GS2 is based on new evidence around effective investments

and action, such as Every Newborn: An Action Plan to End Preventable Deaths (UNF 2016), with its ambitious vision of no preventable deaths of newborns and no stillbirths, and Ending Preventable Maternal Mortality (EPMM) (WHO 2015c), from which the global targets derived align closely with the SDGs (see Box 1.1).

The EPMM focus and targets aim to ensure that women, children and adolescents *survive, thrive, and transform*. The EPMM calls for a shift from a system focused on emergency care for a minority of women to wellness-focused care for all. *The Lancet Special Series on Midwifery* (Renfrew et al 2014) concurs with this approach. Promotion of normal reproductive processes with first-line management of complications and access to back-up emergency treatment when needed acknowledges that health outcomes for mothers and their newborns and children are inextricably linked; it also highlights the vital importance of protecting and supporting the mother–baby relationship. This dovetails with the midwifery philosophy and social model of care and midwives' scope of practice, remit and equal responsibility for mothers and newborns.

The SDGs are different from the MDGs, with 17 goals and 169 indicators, including one health-specific goal, 'ensure healthy lives and promote well-being for all at all ages', and 13 targets. The SDGs create a broader, new, transformative agenda, established for maternal health towards ending preventable maternal mortality and calls for acceleration of current progress to achieve the global MMRs and other targets (WHO 2015b).

SDG 3, 'ensure healthy lives and promote well-being for all at all ages', which encompasses ending maternal mortality, ending preventable newborn and child deaths and ensuring universal access to sexual and reproductive healthcare services, and SDG 5, 'achieve gender equality and empower all women and girls', are of particular importance to midwifery. In combination with GS2

Box 1.1 Every Newborn Action Plan (ENAP) and Ending Preventable Maternal Mortality (EPMM)

ENAP

Goal: To improve newborn health and prevent stillbirths by 2035
Call to action: Stakeholders to take specific actions to improve access to and quality of healthcare for women and newborns within the continuum of care.
Strategies:
1. Strengthen and invest in care during labour, birth and the first day and week of life.
2. Improve the quality of maternal and newborn care.
3. Reach every woman and newborn to reduce inequities.
4. Harness the power of parents, families, and communities.
5. Count every newborn through measurement, programme-tracking and accountability.

EPMM

Goal: To end preventable maternal deaths
Objectives:
1. Address inequities in access to and quality of sexual, reproductive, maternal and newborn healthcare
2. Ensure universal health coverage for comprehensive sexual, reproductive, maternal and newborn healthcare
3. Address all causes of maternal mortality, reproductive and maternal morbidities and related disabilities
4. Strengthen heath systems to respond to the needs and priorities of women and girls
5. Ensure accountability to improve quality of care and equity

---

Reflective activity 1.1

Think about your area of practice, the women receiving care and the elements of Table 1.1 and consider the following:
- What is the maternal mortality ratio (MMR)?
- How does the target neonatal mortality ratio (NMR) compare?
- What percentage of service users are adolescents?
- How many women experience domestic violence?
- Do any women with female genital mutilation (FGM) use your service?
- Can you see evidence of noncommunicable diseases (NCDs) in your client group?
- What do you understand by the term *financial risk protection*?

Box 1.2 Definitions of low-, middle- and high-income countries

The World Bank defines low-, middle- and high-income countries as follows:
Low-income countries – those with a gross national income (GNI) per capita of $1045 or less in 2014
Middle-income countries – those with a GNI per capita of more than $1045 but less than $12,736
High-income countries – those with a GNI per capita of $12,736 or more
Lower-middle-income and upper-middle-income countries are separated at a GNI per capita of $4125.

Source: World Bank 2016

---

targets, the single health-related SDG presents a powerful case for change and opportunities for midwives and midwifery (see Table 1.1).

GENDER, INEQUALITY AND INEQUITY

Gender inequality damages the physical and mental health of millions of girls and women across the globe, and gender relations of power constitute the root causes of gender inequality and are among the most influential of the social determinants of health (Sen and Ostling 2007). Nowhere is this more obvious than in maternal, newborn and child health, with persistent gender-based inequalities (UN 2013); the inability of women, whether in governments or households, to make decisions to seek healthcare;

and the unequal status of women and men being major barriers (Save the Children 2011; see also chapter website resources).

It has been emphasized that one of the most striking measurable contrasts between high-, middle-, and low-income countries (HMICs) becomes evident when maternal mortality ratios are compared (see Box 1.2).

Adolescent health issues such as early marriage, gender-based violence, female genital mutilation (FGM), lack of access to education, and availability of adolescent-friendly services all influence maternal and neonatal health. Developing regions still accounted for approximately 99% of the global maternal deaths in 2015, although all MDG regions of the world have experienced considerable reductions in maternal mortality (WHO 2015b) (see Table 1.2).

Table 1.1 Survive – Thrive – Transform targets of the GS2 mapped to specific Sustainable Development Goal (SDG) targets

SURVIVE (to end preventable death)	THRIVE (to realize the highest attainable standard of health)	TRANSFORM (to achieve transformative and sustainable change)
Reduce global maternal mortality to less than **70** per 100,000 live births (SDG 3.1)	End all forms of malnutrition and address the nutritional needs of adolescent girls, pregnant and lactating women and children (SDG 5.2)	Eradicate extreme poverty (SDG 1.1)
Reduce newborn mortality to at least as low as **12** per 1000 live births in every country (SDG 3.2)	Ensure universal access to sexual and reproductive healthcare services (including for family planning) and rights (SDGs 3.7 and 5.6)	Ensure that all girls and boys complete free, equitable and good-quality secondary education (SDG 4.1)
Reduce under-5 mortality to at least as low as **25** per 1000 live births in every country (SDG 3.2)	Ensure that all girls and boys have access to good-quality early childhood development (SDG 4.2)	Eliminate all harmful practices and all discrimination and violence against women and girls (SDGs 5.2 and 5.3)
End epidemics of HIV, tuberculosis, malaria, neglected tropical diseases and other communicable diseases (SDG 3.3)	Substantially reduce pollution-related deaths and illnesses (SDG 3.9)	Achieve universal and equitable access to safe and affordable drinking water and to adequate sanitation and hygiene (SDGs 6.1 and 6.2)
Achieve universal access to sexual and reproductive health and reproductive rights (SDG 3.7/5.6); ensure at least 75% of demand for family planning is satisfied with modern contraceptives Reduce by one-third premature mortality from noncommunicable diseases (NCDs) and promote mental health and well-being (SDG 3.6)	Achieve universal health coverage, including financial risk protection, and access to quality essential services, medicines and vaccines (SDG 3.8)	Enhance scientific research, upgrade technological capabilities and encourage innovation (SDG 8.2) Provide legal identity for all, including birth registration (SDG 16.9) Enhance the global partnership for sustainable development (SDG 17.16)

MATERNAL MORTALITY AND MORBIDITY

The 2015 estimates on maternal mortality confirm that the highest figures are in sub-Saharan Africa, at approximately 66%, followed by southern Asia (33%). Nigeria and India accounted for over one-third of all global maternal deaths in 2015, 19% and 15%, respectively. The least maternal deaths, in the developing regions, occurred in Oceania (WHO 2015a). The estimated lifetime risk of maternal mortality in high-income countries is 1 in 3300 in comparison with 1 in 41 in low-income countries. Sierra Leone and Chad share the highest estimated lifetime risk of maternal mortality, with an approximate risk of 1 in 17 and 1 in 18, respectively (WHO 2015b). WHO estimates that countries will need to reduce their MMRs by at least 7.5% each year, between 2016 and 2030, to achieve this global goal (WHO 2015b).

Causes of maternal death

Five main causes account for 75% of maternal deaths worldwide: *haemorrhage, hypertensive disorders, infection, obstructed labour and unsafe abortion* (Say et al 2014). In 2003–2009, 73% of all maternal deaths were a result of direct obstetric causes, and 27.5% were a result of indirect causes (Say et al 2014). The remainder were caused by, or associated with, pre-existing medical conditions, such as diabetes, malaria, HIV and obesity (28%) (WHO 2014) and AIDS-related indirect causes (1.6%) during pregnancy (WHO 2015a) (see Figs 1.3 and 1.4).

There are many contrasts and numerous inequalities, with the MMR in developing regions being roughly 20 times higher than that of developed regions. Sub-Saharan Africa has a very high MMR (Save the Children 2015); three regions – Oceania, southern Asia and South East Asia – have moderate MMRs. The remaining five regions have low MMRs (WHO 2015a). It is noted that the greatest

Table 1.2 Causes of maternal death by Millennium Development Goal (MDG) regions

Region	Abortion	Embolism	Haemorrhage	Hypertension	Sepsis	Other direct causes	Indirect causes
Worldwide	193,000	78,000	661,000	343,000	261,000	235,000	672,000
	−7.90%	−3.20%	−27.10%	−14%	−10.70%	−9.60%	−27.50%
Developed regions	1100	2000	2400	1900	690	2900	3600
Developing Regions	192,000	76,000	659,000	341,000	26,000	232,000	668,000
Northern Africa	490	720	8300	3800	1300	3800	4000
Sub-Saharan Africa	125,000	27,000	321,000	209,000	134,000	119,000	375,000
Eastern Asia	420	6500	20,000	5900	1500	8000	14,000
Southern Asia	47,000	17,000	238,000	80,000	107,000	65,000	229,000
South-East Asia	11,000	18,000	44,000	21,000	8100	20,000	25,000
Western Asia	860	2600	8900	3900	1400	4500	6700
Caucasus and Central Asia	250	590	1200	790	460	910	1200
Latin America and Caribbean	6900	2300	16,000	15,000	5800	10,000	13,000
Oceania	290	610	1200	560	200	510	710

Source: WHO 2015b

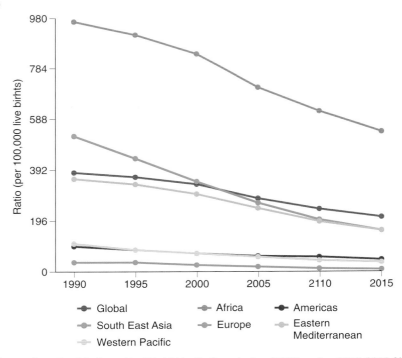

Figure 1.3 Maternal mortality ratio globally and by World Health Organization (WHO) region 1990–2015 (WHO 2016d).

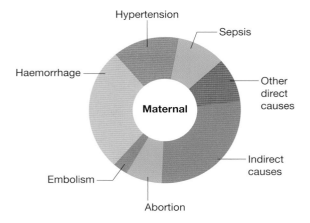

- Haemorrhage (27.1%)
- Hypertensive disorders (14.0%)
- Sepsis (10.7%)
- Abortion (7.9%)
- Embolism (3.2%)
- Other direct causes (9.6%)

Figure 1.4 Global major causes of maternal mortality. (Reprinted with permission from Say et al, 2014.)

disparity across regions is found in the *lifetime risk of maternal death* (Save the Children 2015) (see Table 1.3).

One global initiative to eliminate *preventable maternal mortality* is the Maternal Death Surveillance Response (MSDR), a continuous surveillance system to count every maternal death and inform public health action (WHO 2013). (See WHO Maternal Mortality Fact Sheet in the chapter Resources and Additional Reading section.)

In the UK, the MMR decreased significantly between 2009 and 2012 and between 2011 and 2013; although maternal mortality from direct causes continues to decline, maternal mortality from indirect causes remains high. (See Ch. 16.) The leading cause of direct maternal death is thrombosis and thromboembolism, and for indirect maternal deaths the cause is cardiac disease. Importantly, approximately 25% of maternal deaths between 6 weeks and 1 year after the end of pregnancy are attributed to psychiatric causes (Knight et al 2015). Definitions of maternal death can be found in the Confidential Enquiry into Maternal and Child Health (CEMACH 2007) document and in the chapter website resources.

Predisposing factors

Maternal death is influenced by numerous factors. The reasons why women die have been described as 'many and layered' (Abouzahr and Royston 1991); some of the obstacles and key issues are illustrated in the video *Why Did Mrs X Die?* (WHO 2010b, 2016a) and in *Dead Women Talking* (Subha and Khanna 2014) (see the case study in Box 1.3). These layers include *social, cultural,* and *political* factors, gender inequity, child marriage, gender-based violence and access to contraception (see Boxes 1.4 and 1.5).

Reflective activity 1.2 ✕

Consider the elements of the case study in Box 1.3.
- What do you see as the key factors, and how do you think midwives could make a difference?

Approximately 220 million women have no access to modern contraception, yet evidence suggests that access to contraception can reduce maternal deaths by at least 30% and has wider benefits, for example, 'improving maternal and child health and survival, increasing economic wellbeing of individuals, families, communities, and nations, fostering environmental sustainability, and empowering women' (Fabic et al 2014). It is further noted that none of the SDGs can be achieved without family planning (Fabic et al 2014); thus, investment in reproductive health, particularly family planning, is advocated (Singh et al 2009) and campaigned for (*Family Planning 2020*; WHO 2015b).

Maternal morbidity

Morbidity, described as the base of an iceberg, is less easily measureable. For every woman who dies of pregnancy-related causes, 20 or 30 others experience acute or chronic morbidity, often with permanent health problems that affect their normal functioning: physical, mental or sexual health; functionality in certain domains (e.g. cognition, mobility, participation in society); body image; and social and economic status. The burden of maternal morbidity – similar to that of maternal mortality – is estimated to be highest in LMICs, particularly for the poorest women (Firoz et al 2013).

Mothers with pre-existing medical conditions are at higher risk of serious complications and morbidity. Global assessments of maternal morbidities or disabilities are estimated to affect 15 to 20 million women (15%) world-wide each year. These are directly or indirectly related to obstetric events and include conditions such as uterine prolapse, stress incontinence, hypertension, haemorrhoids, perineal tears, urinary tract infections, severe anaemia, depression, obstetric fistula and ectopic pregnancy (Koblinsky et al 2012).

The term *severe acute maternal morbidity* (SAMM) has several definitions and includes the concept of a 'near miss' and situations where pregnancy-related complications lead to life-threatening organ dysfunction. *Near miss* and *severe acute maternal morbidity* are terms used in reference to a severe, life-threatening obstetric complication.

Box 1.3 Case study

Urmilla was a 32-year-old migrant worker with a past history of tuberculosis (TB). Of her previous three births, one was born at the construction site where she worked and the other two at home. In her fourth pregnancy she had one antenatal visit at a primary healthcare (PHC) center, where she was given a tetanus toxoid injection and 10 iron folate tablets. No haemoglobin or blood pressure (BP) was done. She subsequently developed severe breathlessness, and after seeking care at seven different facilities over 5 days, her family gave up and took her home, where she died.

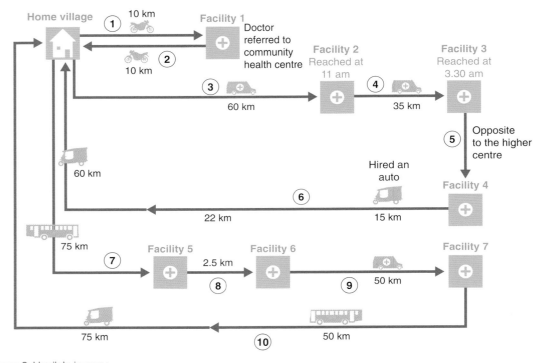

Figure 9 Urmila's journey.

Source: Subha and Khanna 2014

Box 1.4 Predisposing factors for maternal mortality

- **Child marriage** – A 10% reduction in child marriage could contribute to a 70% reduction in a country's maternal mortality rate and a 3% decrease in infant mortality rates.
- **Gender-based violence** – Among women, 1 in 3 have experienced physical or sexual violence, mostly perpetrated by an intimate partner. In addition to physical and emotional trauma, abused women suffer higher rates of depression, alcohol abuse, sexually transmitted infections and more.
- **Female genital mutilation** – In 29 countries in Africa and the Middle East where the practice is prevalent, 133 million girls and women have experienced female genital mutilation (FGM). In addition to trauma, FGM can cause infection, infertility and even death.

Source: UN Commission on the Status of Women (CSW) 2016

Table 1.3 Global lifetime risk of maternal mortality

Regions	Maternal mortality rate (MMR)	Range of uncertainty		Number of maternal deaths	Lifetime risk of maternal death (1 per)
		Lower estimates	Upper estimates		
World	210	160	250	289,000	190
Developed regions	16	12	23	2300	3700
Developing regions	230	180	320	28,500	160
Northern Africa	69	47	110	2700	500
Sub-Saharan Africa	510	380	730	17,900	38
Eastern Asia	33	21	54	6400	1800
Eastern Asia excluding China	54	35	97	480	1200
Southern Asia	190	130	250	69,000	200
Southern Asia excluding India	170	110	270	19,000	210
South East Asia	140	98	210	16,000	310
Western Asia	74	50	120	3600	450
Caucasus and Central Asia	39	31	53	690	920
Latin America and the Caribbean	85	66	120	9300	520
Latin America	77	59	110	7900	570
Caribbean	190	130	310	1400	220
Oceania	190	100	380	510	140

Source: WHO 2015b

The definition of a near miss is 'a woman who nearly died but survived a complication that occurred during pregnancy, childbirth or within 42 days of termination of pregnancy' (WHO 2011). Complications include severe obstetric haemorrhage, eclampsia, sepsis, pulmonary embolism, heart failure, malaria, amniotic fluid embolism, ruptured uterus or ectopic pregnancy and obstetric fistulae. Other morbidities include anaemia, infertility and depression.

NEWBORN MORTALITY

Significant progress has been made globally in the reduction of deaths of children under 5, yet this is *not* the case for newborn mortality (Unicef 2015); declines in the neonatal mortality rate (NMR) have been slower. Approximately 3 million babies die in the newborn period, and 2.6 million babies are stillborn each year. Newborn deaths currently account for 44% of all deaths among the under-5 age group, and 1% of the world's newborn deaths occur in industrialized countries, with the United States having the most first-day deaths (United Nations Inter-agency Group for Child Mortality Estimation (UN IGME) 2015; WHO 2015b). The causes of newborn deaths are shown in Figure 1.5. It is worth noting that newborns without mothers (i.e. the children of mothers who have died in childbirth) are 3 to 10 times more likely to die than those with mothers.

As with maternal deaths, the greatest number of newborn deaths occur in LMICs, with two-thirds found in 10 countries within the Africa and Asia-Pacific regions. The 'top 10' countries with the highest number of maternal and child deaths, and few or no midwives, are as follows (in rank order): India, Nigeria, Pakistan, China, Democratic Republic of the Congo

Box 1.5 Some key facts

- Every day, 16,000 children die, mostly from preventable or treatable causes.
- The births of nearly 230 million children under age 5 worldwide (about 1 in 3) have never been officially recorded, depriving them of their right to a name and nationality.
- The number of people who lack access to improved sanitation is 2.4 billion, including 946 million who are forced to resort to open defecation for lack of other options.
- Out of an estimated 35 million people living with HIV, over 2 million are 10 to 19 years old, and 56% of them are girls.
- Globally, about one-third of women aged 20 to 24 were child brides.
- Every 10 minutes, somewhere in the world, an adolescent girl dies as a result of violence.
- Nearly 50% of all deaths in children under age 5 are attributable to undernutrition.

Source: Unicef 2016

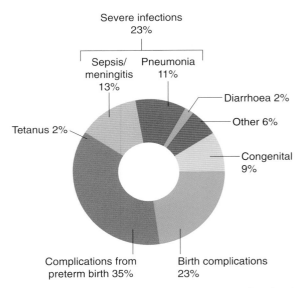

Figure 1.5 Global causes of newborn mortality. (Reprinted with permission from Elsevier, The Lancet, 2000, Volume 379, No. 9832, pp 2151–2161, Li Liu, et al. Global, Regional and National Causes of Child Mortality: An Updated Systematic Analysis for 2010 with Time Trends Since 2000.)

(DRC), Ethiopia, Bangladesh, Indonesia, Afghanistan and Tanzania (Save the Children 2013) (see Fig. 1.6).

INEQUITIES ASSOCIATED WITH BEING A MOTHER

'The world focuses on maternal health because saving women stimulates the economy, bolsters communities and strengthens families. Women's unpaid work equals about one third of world GDP [gross domestic product]; when a woman dies, children's risk of dying within two years increases tenfold'.

(Arulkumaran et al 2012)

The experience of childbearing can be vastly different depending on the country of residence. The Mothers' Index (Save the Children 2015) ranks the top 10 and bottom 10 countries in which to have a baby. Comparison of the data in Tables 1.4a (top 10) and 1.4b (bottom 10) provides a vivid insight into major factors affecting women in the 21st century (Save the Children 2015). The highest numbers of women and infants who die are in India and Nigeria, with the 10 countries listed previously contributing to the majority of global maternal and neonatal deaths (Table 1.5).

Survival of women at risk is extremely precarious in conflict-ridden and politically fragile countries where health services are inaccessible, inadequate or nonexistent. The *accessibility, availability, acceptability and quality* (AAAQ) of

services is an issue for women in many LMICs, with disparities being greatest in low-income countries (WHO 2015b).

The AAAQ human rights–based framework (United Nations Population Fund (UNFPA 2014) identifies these four AAAQ elements of healthcare facilities, goods and services as essential aspects of the right to health, and it is recommended to assess effective coverage for sexual, reproductive, maternal and newborn health (see Fig. 1.7). This approach to promoting health is guided by the key principles of availability, accessibility, acceptability and quality of facilities and services; participation; equality and nondiscrimination; and accountability.

Reflective activity 1.3

Although the State of the World's Midwifery (SoWMY) report (UNFPA 2014) is based on data from the 73 countries with the highest burden of maternal and newborn morality, reflect on midwifery services in your country within this framework.

- Are your services available, accessible, acceptable and of quality?
- Are your services woman-centred?
- Are your services equitable and nondiscriminatory?
- Are the concepts of professional teams and enabling environments understood?

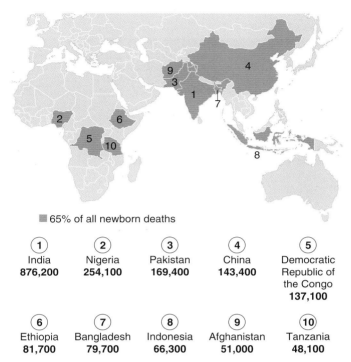

■ 65% of all newborn deaths

(1)	**(2)**	**(3)**	**(4)**	**(5)**
India	Nigeria	Pakistan	China	Democratic Republic of the Congo
876,200	**254,100**	**169,400**	**143,400**	**137,100**

(6)	**(7)**	**(8)**	**(9)**	**(10)**
Ethiopia	Bangladesh	Indonesia	Afghanistan	Tanzania
81,700	**79,700**	**66,300**	**51,000**	**48,100**

Figure 1.6 Ten countries with the most newborn deaths. (Save the Children (2013) Surviving the First Day: State of the world's mothers, A report by Save the Children on the situation facing world's mothers Save the Children UK and USA.)

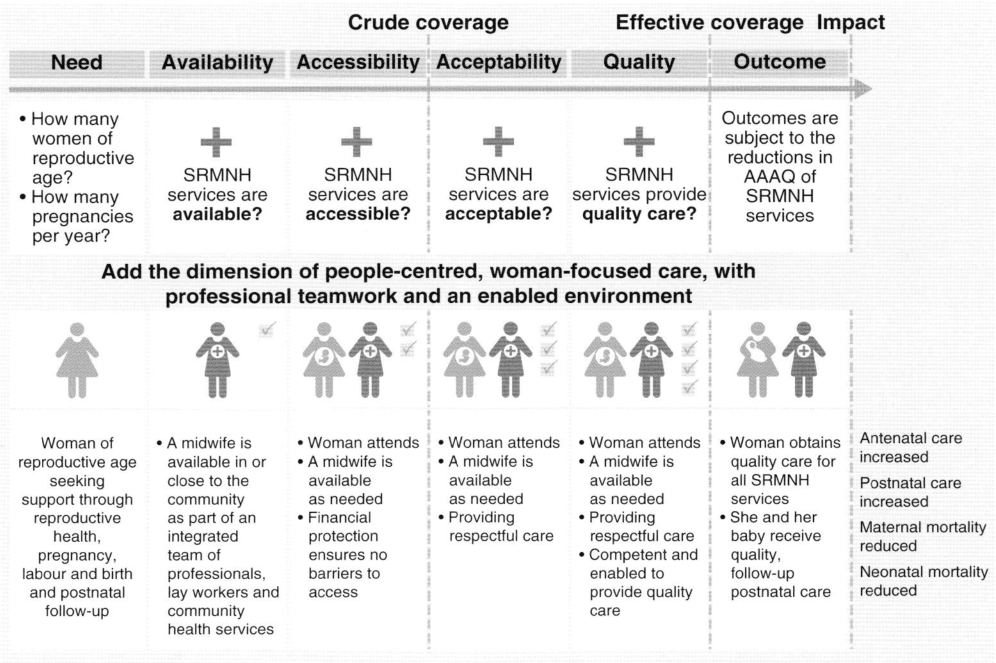

	Crude coverage			Effective coverage	Impact
Need	**Availability**	**Accessibility**	**Acceptability**	**Quality**	**Outcome**
• How many women of reproductive age? • How many pregnancies per year?	SRMNH services are **available?**	SRMNH services are **accessible?**	SRMNH services are **acceptable?**	SRMNH services provide **quality care?**	Outcomes are subject to the reductions in AAAQ of SRMNH services

Add the dimension of people-centred, woman-focused care, with professional teamwork and an enabled environment

Woman of reproductive age seeking support through reproductive health, pregnancy, labour and birth and postnatal follow-up	• A midwife is available in or close to the community as part of an integrated team of professionals, lay workers and community health services	• Woman attends • A midwife is available as needed • Financial protection ensures no barriers to access	• Woman attends • A midwife is available as needed • Providing respectful care	• Woman attends • A midwife is available as needed • Providing respectful care • Competent and enabled to provide quality care	• Woman obtains quality care for all SRMNH services • She and her baby receive quality, follow-up postnatal care	Antenatal care increased Postnatal care increased Maternal mortality reduced Neonatal mortality reduced

Figure 1.7 Availability, accessibility, acceptability and quality (AAAQ) SRMNH, sexual, reproductive, maternal and newborn health. (Used with permission from Jim Campbell, ICS Integrare. Adapted from Campbell et al, 2013 [25] Colston, 2011 [22].)

Table 1.4a Top 10 best places to be a mother

Mothers' Index Country Ranking*		Maternal Health	Children's Well-being	Educational Status	Economic Status	Political Status
Rank out of 179 countries	Country	Lifetime risk of maternal death (2015)	Under-5 mortality rate (per 100,000 live births)	Expected number of years of formal schooling	Gross national income per capita (current US$)	Participation of women in national government (% seats held by women)*
1	Norway	14,900	2.8	17.5	102,610	39.6
2	Finland	15,100	2.6	17.1	48,820	42.5
3	Iceland	11,500	2.1	19.0	46,400	41.3
4	Denmark	12,000	3.5	18.7	61,680	38.0
5	Sweden	13,600	4.2	15.8	61,760	43.6
6	Netherlands	10,700	4.0	17.9	51,060	36.9
7	Spain	15,100	4.2	17.3	29,920	38.0
8	Germany	11,000	3.9	16.5	47,270	36.9
9	Australia	9,000	4.0	20.2	65,390	30.5
10	Belgium	8,700	4.4	16.3	46,290	42.4
24	UK	6,900	4.6	16.2	41,680	23.5

Note: Skilled birth attendance is reported at > 99% in these countries
*Mothers Index rankings reflect a composite score derived from five different indicators related to maternal well-being: maternal health, children's well-being, educational status, economic status and political status

Source: Data compiled from Save the Children 2015, pp. 60–64

Table 1.5a World Health Statistics*

Maternal Mortality Rate (MMR)			Neonatal Mortality Rate (NMR)	Total Fertility Rate (TFR)	
Mother's Index Rank** (out of 179 countries)	Country	MMR (2013)** (per 100,000 live births)	(NMR) (2013)** (per 1000 live births)	TFR (women)	Number of pregnant adolescent girls aged 15–19 yrs (per 1000)
1	Norway	9	1.6	1.9	7
2	Finland	4	1.3	1.9	8
3	Iceland	4	0.9	2.1	11
4	Denmark	5	2.4	1.9	5
5	Sweden	4	1.6	1.9	6
6	Netherlands	6	2.6	1.8	5
7	Spain	4	2.6	1.5	10
8	Germany	7	2.2	1.4	8
9	Australia	6	2.4	1.9	15
10	Belgium	6	2.3	1.9	9

*From WHO 2016c
**From Save the Children 2015, pp. 60–64

Table 1.4b The 10 worst countries to be a mother

Mothers' Index Country Ranking*		Maternal Health	Children's Well-being	Educational Status	Economic Status	Political Status
Rank out of 179 countries	Country	Lifetime risk of maternal death (2015)	Under-5 mortality rate (per 100,000 live births)	Expected number of years of formal schooling	Gross national income per capita (current US$)	Participation of women in national government (% seats held by women)*
169	Haiti	80	72.8	7.6	8.10	3.5
	Sierra Leone	21	160.16	11.2	660	12.4
171	Guinea-Bissau	36	123.9	9.0	590	13.7
172	Chad	15	147.5	7.4	1030	14.9
173	Cote d'Ivoire	29	100.00	8.9	1450	9.2
174	Gambia	39	73.8	8.8	500	9.4
175	Niger	20	104.2	5.4	400	13.3
176	Mali	26	122.7	8.4	670	9.5
177	Central African Republic	27	139.2	7.2	320	12.5
178	Democratic Republic of the Congo	23	118.5	9.7	430	8.2

*Mothers Index rankings reflect a composite score derived from five different indicators related to maternal well-being: maternal health, children's well-being, educational status, economic status and political status

Source: Data compiled from Save the Children 2015, pp. 60–64

Table 1.5b World Health Statistics*

Rank** (out of 179 countries)	Country	Maternal Mortality Rate (MMR) MMR (2013)** (per 100,000 live births)	Neonatal Mortality Rate (NMR) NMR (2013)** (per 1000 live births)	Total Fertility Rate (TFR) TFR (women)	Number of pregnant adolescent girls aged 15–19 yrs (per 1000)
169	Haiti	380	24.9	3.1	65
	Sierra Leone	1100	44.3	4.7	125
171	Guinea-Bissau	560	44	4.9	137
172	Chad	980	39.8	6.3	203
173	Cote d'Ivoire	720	37.5	4.9	125
174	Gambia	430	28.1	5.8	88
175	Niger	630	27.5	7.6	206
176	Mali	550	40.2	6.8	172
177	Central African Republic	880	43	4.4	229
178	DR Congo	730	38.2	5.9	135
179	Somalia	850	46.2	6.6	—

*From WHO 2016c
**From Save the Children 2015, pp. 60–64

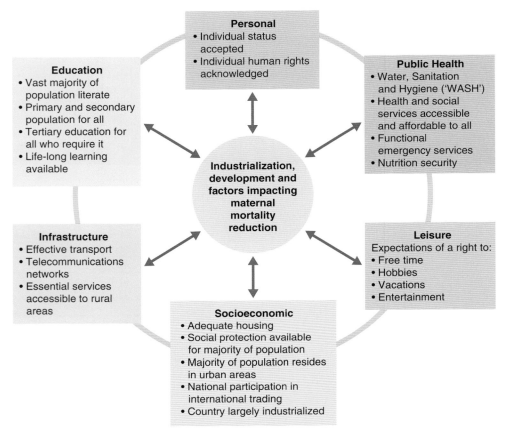

Personal
- Individual status accepted
- Individual human rights acknowledged

Education
- Vast majority of population literate
- Primary and secondary population for all
- Tertiary education for all who require it
- Life-long learning available

Public Health
- Water, Sanitation and Hygiene ('WASH')
- Health and social services accessible and affordable to all
- Functional emergency services
- Nutrition security

Industrialization, development and factors impacting maternal mortality reduction

Infrastructure
- Effective transport
- Telecommunications networks
- Essential services accessible to rural areas

Leisure
Expectations of a right to:
- Free time
- Hobbies
- Vacations
- Entertainment

Socioeconomic
- Adequate housing
- Social protection available for majority of population
- Majority of population resides in urban areas
- National participation in international trading
- Country largely industrialized

Figure 1.8 Industrialization and mortality.

As the Lancet Commission on Women and Health (Langer et al 2015) notes, 'worldwide priorities in women's health have changed from a narrow focus on maternal and child health to the broader framework of sexual and reproductive health, encompassing concept of women's health, which is founded on a life-course approach'. The commission recognizes the contribution of women – when they are healthy, enabled, empowered and valued by their societies – to families, communities and sustainable development (Langer et al 2015). The four key recommendations made – to value women, compensate women, count women and be accountable to women – can be applied to midwives, as recipients and providers of care, who comprise 99% of the workforce (see chapter website resources).

THE IMPACT OF MODERNIZATION AND DEVELOPMENT

The process of modernization and development is inextricably linked with numerous health issues. As countries develop, childbirth becomes safer. This is a complex issue, and the reader would do well to explore it further (see Fig 1.8). Progress to modernity tends to be inversely related to the lifetime risk of dying in childbirth. See the chapter website section for more links and information.

COVERAGE AND SKILLED ATTENDANCE AT BIRTH

The term *skilled birth attendant* (SBA) refers exclusively to an accredited health professional – midwife, doctor or nurse – who has been 'educated and trained to proficiency' with the skills to 'manage normal pregnancies and diagnose, manage or refer complications' (WHO 2004). *Traditional birth attendants* (TBAs) are *not* included in the definition; however, many LMICs have not applied this definition as they introduce new cadres to provide maternal and neonatal health (MNH) care to their populations. Employment of SBAs is regarded as a reproductive health indicator (WHO 2015b) and as such is considered a proxy for the provision of healthcare by a professional who is competent to provide care throughout the continuum of pregnancy, childbirth and the postnatal period. Global standards for midwifery competencies, education and regulation have been defined (International Confederation of Midwives (ICM) 2013). The development of human resources for health, in particular SBAs, is a challenge; 73 countries produce 78% of the world's annual births and carry the global burden of maternal and newborn mortality and stillbirths, yet these countries have less than 42% of the world's midwives, nurses and physicians (see Fig. 1.9).

The Global Strategy on Human Resources for Health (WHO 2016b) provides essential guidance to global, regional and country partners 'to address health workforce challenges to progress towards Universal Health Coverage' and to 'improve health outcomes related to the SDGs'.

Socioeconomic factors

Although a key indicator in reducing MMRs, employment of SBAs is not the only determinant; socioeconomic status and demographic indicators have affected and continue to affect the likelihood that women will receive skilled care during childbirth. Globally, the richest 20% of women are 2.7 times more likely than the poorest 20% to be attended by a skilled professional during childbirth, and for mothers and infants, the risk of dying during or shortly after birth is 20 to 50% higher for the poorest 20% of households than for the richest quintile. For women in LMICs, the lifetime risk of maternal death is more than 300 times greater than for women in an industrialized country (Unicef 2009; Fig. 1.10).

Socioeconomic factors also prevent women from receiving or seeking care during pregnancy and childbirth: poverty, distance, lack of information, inadequate services and cultural practices all influence the ability to seek and receive care. 'A woman's socioeconomic health and nutritional status, including HIV and anaemia, underlie these causes, along with societal factors such as poverty, inequity, women's low status and *attitudes* towards women and their needs' (Unicef 2009).

Inequalities in reproductive, maternal, newborn, child and adolescent health (RMNCAH) still exist across LMICs – with gaps in coverage between the richest and poorest, the

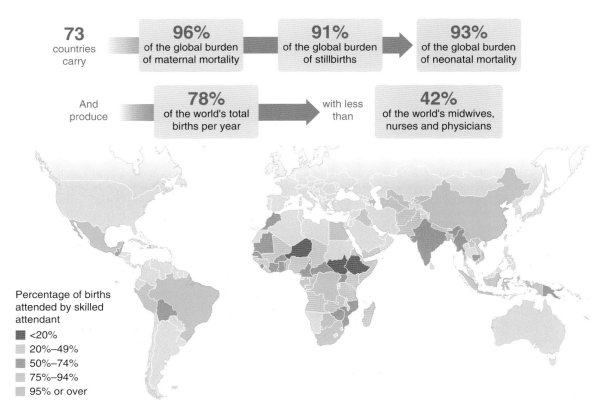

Figure 1.9 Global coverage by skilled birth attendant (UNFPA 2014).

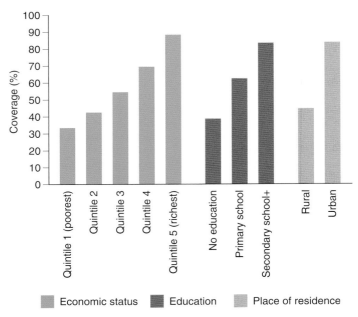

Figure 1.10 Skilled birth attendance by dimensions of inequity (WHO 2015b).

most and least educated, and urban and rural areas – when reported against births attended by skilled health personnel and by antenatal care coverage (Fig. 1.10). Two examples of the persistent rural–urban gap are access to reproductive health services and clean drinking water (WHO 2015d). An 80% difference in employment of SBAs between the richest and poorest countries was noted by WHO (2015a). In addition, almost 80% of all deaths related to noncommunicable diseases (NCDs) in 2008 occurred in LMICs, and most premature deaths in these countries are caused by infectious diseases, maternal and perinatal conditions and nutritional deficiencies (Partnership for Maternal, Newborn and Child Health (PMNCH) 2011).

Reflective activity 1.4

- Do the social determinants of health matter in your area of work?
- Consider the impact of whether the midwife is working in Cornwall or Cameroon – what disparities might be present?
- Are these socioeconomic issues pertinent to migrant and refugee women in your care?

INTERNATIONAL ORGANIZATIONS

International organizations comprise governmental, intergovernmental and non-governmental organizations (NGOs). Voluntary organizations, both faith-based and secular; civil society organizations; and healthcare professional associations are all involved in RMNCAH, and some are involved with SRMNCAH. Currently there is a focus on rebalancing the donor and recipient dependency of the previous decade, official development assistance (ODA) reduction and domestic financing generated to support health systems. This comes with the expectation that economic growth of LMICs will enable most costs to be covered from domestic sources, with acknowledgement that some countries will continue to need external assistance (Jamison et al 2013). In 2015, the Global Financing Facility (GFF) (World Bank 2015), a country-driven financing partnership, was established in support of the UN Secretary-General's Every Woman Every Child global strategy.

The reader might find it instructive to consider the role of governments and international NGOs in the context of poverty relief and debt repayment. (View the video *A New Era for Every Woman, Every Child*; see chapter website resources.)

Not all initiatives are government led; some are led by major actors in international developments in SRMNCAH

Table 1.6 International organizations

International organizations (UN agencies):
UNFPA
Unicef
WHO
The World Bank
UN Women
UNAIDS

Global partnerships:
Partnership for Maternal Newborn and Child Health
   (PMNCH)
Global Health Workforce Alliance (GHWA) 2006–2016, now
Global Health Workforce Network (a network of
   stakeholders)

Midwifery organizations:
International Confederation of Midwives (ICM)
European Midwives Association (EMA)

*Civil society organizations and non-governmental
organizations (NGOs):*
International Planned Parenthood Federation (IPPF)
Médecins Sans Frontières/Doctors Without Borders (MSF)
Save the Children
Voluntary Service Overseas (VSO)
WaterAid
Women and Health Alliance International (WAHA)
White Ribbon Alliance (WRA)

Faith-based organizations:
World Vision
World YWCA

Networks:
Action for Global Health
The Guardian Professional Development Network
Health Information for All (HIFA)
Healthy Newborn Network (HNN)
World Alliance for Breastfeeding Action (WABA)

Note: See website resources for more information.

Box 1.6 The Lancet Series on Midwifery

- What is midwifery? How does it work?
- What impact does it have on the survival, health and well-being of mothers and babies?
- What health system conditions are needed for it to work effectively?
- What is the role of midwives in quality maternal and newborn care globally?

Source: The Lancet Series on Midwifery 2014

temperature-controlled environments from manufacturer to storage and delivery to the end user. This is a challenge for many LMICs (The Guardian Online 2013), and one public–private partnership has provided a solution (Berry 2013, Goodier 2015; see chapter website resources).

THE PLACE OF THE MIDWIFE IN THE GLOBAL CONTEXT

In the 21st century the world is increasingly described as a global village. Globalization is important because the impact is not limited to world business, commerce or politics. In recent decades globalization has gathered significant pace with the advent of high-speed travel, the Internet and social media expediting communication, travel and news. Globalization has affected economic and human resources for health, healthcare and health systems. It affects sexual, reproductive, maternal and newborn health, midwives and midwifery. Increased awareness may assist in the global battle to combat the constant dangers and death associated with giving birth in the LMICs of the world. Many converging global initiatives and reports recognize midwives as central to the SRMNH workforce, to quality of care and to the prevention of maternal and newborn mortality (ICM 2013). Equally compelling, and growing, evidence indicates that midwives make a difference (UNFPA 2014; *The Lancet Series on Midwifery* 2014).

The most comprehensive research on midwifery, *The Lancet Series on Midwifery* (2014) aimed to identify the contribution of midwifery in tackling such issues as unacceptable rates of mortality and morbidity, high rates of unnecessary interventions, inequalities in care and outcomes, longer-term psychosocial and cost-effectiveness outcomes that are often overlooked, disrespect and abuse of women within the health system, and a wide range of health system problems and responses for HMICs and answer the core questions shown in Box 1.6.

Midwives, educated and regulated to international standards, are identified as an essential link in the

(see Table 1.6). In addition, there are a variety of resources, including international journals and twinning of organizations, that provide rich resources in both cases (see chapter website resources).

Schemes to improve health include various initiatives to reduce the impact of malaria, sexually transmitted diseases (STDs) and tetanus in neonates and to ensure that essential medicines, such as vaccines that need to be stored within a narrow temperature range, reach those who need them in a stable condition. This is known as the *cold chain*, and is vital to vaccine supply chains, which need continuum of care, able to provide 87% of the essential care needed for women and newborns (PMNCH 2012) and the full scope of midwifery as defined in *The Lancet Series on Midwifery*. The research identified 56 outcomes improved by midwifery care and midwifery, which were associated with more positive outcomes and cost savings when provided by midwives who were educated, trained, regulated and integrated in the health system, with effective teamwork (*The Lancet Series on Midwifery* 2014). Midwifery service along with family planning and interventions for maternal and newborn health could avert a total of 83% of all maternal deaths, stillbirths and neonatal deaths, illustrating that midwifery care has the greatest effect when provided within a functional health system with effective referral and transfer mechanisms to specialist care (Homer et al 2014).

A quality maternal and newborn care (QMNC) framework (Renfrew et al 2014), designed with the needs of women and their newborn infants at its centre, can be used and tested in a range of contexts, for example, planning, education and monitoring (see chapter website resources).

Reflective activity 1.5

Read Paper 1 in *The Lancet Series on Midwifery*, then consider the following:
- What is the definition of midwifery?
- What are the 56 outcomes improved by midwifery care?
- What impact do these outcomes have on MMRs and NMRs, and how do these relate to your own practice?

Global mobility of health professionals, particularly from East to West, is a 'growing phenomenon, impacting the health systems of receiving, transit, and sending countries', limiting countries' ability to provide high-quality care to women and children (Unicef and WHO 2015).

One study found that 18% of physicians and 11% of nurses working in Organisation for Economic Co-operation and Development (OECD) nations are found to be foreign born, and international migration of health workers to OECD nations is increasing (OECD 2007). Midwives, like other health professionals, are likely to be among them. There is an ethical dilemma associated with the 'brain drain', in that it depletes the resources of LMICs struggling with massive health issues to supplement relative shortages in the wealthier Western hemisphere, which is pitted against the right of individuals to improve their own career prospects and lift their families out of poverty.

Migration also occurs from South to South, within countries from rural to urban and out of the profession. Factors that push people away from their home countries

Table 1.7 Push–pull factors

Push factors	Pull factors
Unemployment	Targeted recruitment opportunities for employment
Lack of services; poor public health systems and amenities	Better services provision
Poor safety and securities	Safer environment
High crime rates	Lower crime rates
Drought and crop failure	Fertile land and food security
Environmental flooding; earthquakes	Less risk of natural disasters
Poverty	More affluent society
Conflict; political and religious persecution	Political security; stable, quality life
No career progression	Career and education opportunities
Low wages; poor and unstable working environments	Greater economic opportunities

and pull them towards another are referred to as *push–pull* factors, which can be economic, social, political, security related and environmental (see Table 1.7).

Migration can positively affect development when the right set of policies are in place, although the emigration of highly skilled health professionals can have considerable negative effects. Efforts have been made to address the issue of richer countries recruiting from LMICs with health personnel deficits, with high-income countries (HICs), for example, the UK, developing guidance (UK Department of Health 2004), WHO's development of Global Code of Practice on the International Recruitment of Health Personnel (WHO 2010a), and other efforts attempting to turn the 'brain drain' into 'brain gain' (Global Health Workforce Alliance (GHWA) 2015). The SDGs also include various targets related to health worker 'brain drain' from LMICs (WHO 2015b). But migration is not the only issue affecting, for example, the African health worker crisis; five key challenges – production, underutilization, distribution, performance and financing – have been identified (Soucat et al 2013). Thus, each country must review its recruitment, retention and remuneration policies to address migration out of the profession, South–South migration and migration to the private sector or NGOs.

Reflective activity 1.6 ✕✕

Think about the concept of *skilled attendance during childbirth* and consider the following questions:

- How would you define *skilled*?
- How is SBA defined by WHO? How is the midwife defined by the ICM?
- What national and local policies aim to ensure skilled attendance for every woman in your area of practice?
- What issues need to be addressed to ensure that midwives in your country acquire, retain and can utilize the clinical skills that you consider critical to promoting safe childbirth?

IMPORTANT CONSIDERATIONS FOR MIDWIVES INTENDING TO WORK OVERSEAS

In the context of reducing maternal mortality (SDG 3.1) and newborn mortality (SDG 3.2) worldwide, midwives may find that they are increasingly in demand for short-term or long-term assignments in LMICs burdened by these critical issues. Some may also travel to other HICs for study tours or personal professional advancement. Midwives practising in any country other than that in which they were educated must adapt to vastly differing situations.

Midwives who have been educated in HICs intending to work in LMICs need to have considerable experience and be conversant with relevant and current evidence-based practice. It can be helpful to acquire some advanced clinical skills where practicable (e.g. vacuum extraction, suturing cervical and vaginal tears, manual removal of placenta and intra-uterine contraceptive device insertion). UK regulations may restrict midwives from acquiring some of these skills, but policy and tradition can often be overcome in consultation with obstetricians and supervisors of midwives willing to arrange suitable learning opportunities. A short course in tropical medicine and health can be valuable, as can discussions with persons experienced in the intended country of practice. Invaluable information and advice can be sought from the Royal College of Midwives (RCM 2016), Voluntary Services Overseas (VSO 2016), Médecins Sans Frontières (MSF 2016) and other organizations (see chapter website resources).

National authorities determine their own country's health priorities and plans. Increasingly, needs are expressed for midwives with expertise in education or management. It is essential that all midwives be clinically competent and able and willing to adapt to local needs. Respect for different cultures and religions is crucial, and a second language or a willingness to learn one is an asset. It is important for expatriate workers to realize that they will *never* have full knowledge, understanding or appreciation of many aspects of their host countries. They must appreciate that change must come from *within* a country, and that external 'experts' can best help colleagues by being culturally competent: demonstrating appropriate knowledge, skills and attitudes. Midwives practising in cross-cultural situations need an acute sense of awareness, an attitude of humility and a willingness to learn. In low-income countries (LICs), they need to be able to empathize with colleagues working in very different situations, exercise patience and cope with extremely limited resources, including less accessibility to information and resources that are often taken for granted.

Midwives who have been educated in LMICs intending to work or study in HICs will find more advanced technology in use than they experienced at home. There may be more emphasis on informed choice for women and partnership in care. They may be migrating to a society that is very litigation conscious and will therefore find that medico-legal issues affect midwifery and medical practice. Midwives therefore need a good understanding of current issues and popular demands, and they may benefit from an orientation programme. Midwives must constantly update their knowledge and practice by critically evaluating research, for example, considering the benefits and hazards associated with both technology and freedom of choice. In returning to LMICs, local midwives, as with all expatriates, need to evaluate new practices in the light of local situations, available resources and national priorities before attempting transfer of knowledge and practice from one country to another.

Midwives who have practised in countries where resources are scarce may be skilled at improvising and can sometimes share innovations with colleagues who face different, although significant, resource limitations. Midwives who have practised in regions remote from medical services can share their experience of complications rarely seen in the West. It is salutary for all midwives to appreciate the consequences of delayed referral and intervention: the reality of, for example, obstructed labour and ruptured uterus, and the frightening speed with which septicaemia can occur. Such complications will, of course, result in maternal death anywhere in the world without appropriate skills and resources for intervention.

CONCLUSION

Issues relating to global midwifery have become an essential component of the body of knowledge possessed by midwives working in the West (*The Lancet Series on Midwifery* 2014). In all countries, preventable maternal and newborn mortality continues to receive attention with the adoption of SDGs (Table 1.1). Safety must be at the heart of every midwife's practice, and although tragedies associated with childbirth are not observed on a great scale in the West, experiences from the high-burden countries provide salutary lessons about fundamentals of midwifery care. Assertions along the lines of 'that could never happen here' must find evidence in reality. Safety needs to continue to be a priority in every country, including the UK. Historically, midwives have played a critical part in maternal and neonatal health, and the concept of promoting maternal and neonatal health remains within the midwife's remit. Midwives, globally, make their profession what it is today and what it will be tomorrow. This warrants critical evaluation and constant reappraisal of professional issues, including midwifery curricula, essential competencies, standards of practice, protocol and policy, professional politics and practice ethics. These must reflect safety as a priority. Other issues, although important, will always be secondary.

Midwives represent a large part of the solution to this dilemma. The global midwife holds the key to a chance of life instead of death for the world's childbearing women (see Box 1.7). Obstetric and paediatric colleagues form essential links in the life-saving change that can bring hope to the women, families and communities in the most desperate need. The right to live is the most fundamental human right, and midwives across the globe need to meet the challenge of the 2030 agenda

---

Box 1.7 Actions to achieve global target for reducing maternal deaths to 70/100,000 live births by 2030

- Political will and commitment
- Improved access to quality of care before, during and after childbirth
- Contraception and safe abortion services
- Strong health systems with educated health workers and essential medicines
- Health and well-being; nutrition, education, water, sanitation and hygiene
- Accountability: every death counted and its cause recorded
- Efforts to reach everyone, everywhere

Source: WHO 2015b

---

with superlative skills, infinite commitment and an enduring determination.

'I found – and it was not a finding I had expected – that whenever [there was] a system of maternal care… based on … trained and respected midwives… maternal mortality was at its lowest. I cannot think of an exception to that rule.'

(Loudon 1992)

Key Points

- MMRs vary enormously across the globe, with large discrepancies between HICs and LMICs – hence the rationale for activities directed at ending preventable maternal and newborn deaths.
- Midwives have a key role in achieving the SDGs.
- There are five major causes of maternal death worldwide, predisposed by numerous factors. WHO estimates that most of these deaths are preventable. Promoting safer childbirth embraces health, education, socioeconomic and political issues.
- Skilled attendance during childbirth is a key indicator for reproductive, maternal, newborn, child and adolescent health (RMNCAH).
- Numerous organizations exist that give priority to promoting maternal and child health.

- Migration of skilled health workers severely compromises critical human resources in many developing countries where maternal and newborn mortality remain high.
- Historical experience of MMR reduction in some Western countries offers inspiration in world regions where risks associated with childbirth remain as high in the 21st century as they were in the West more than a century ago.
- Internationally, high female literacy rates, low total fertility rates and large urban population ratios have been associated with MMR reduction.
- A midwife intending to work internationally needs special preparation, but considering her role as a global midwife should enrich personal professional development wherever she chooses to practice.

References

Abouzahr C, Royston E: *Maternal mortality: a global factbook*, Geneva, World Health Organization, 1991.

Arulkumaran S, Hediger V, Manzoor A, et al on behalf of Maternal Health Working Group 2012: *Saving mother's lives: transforming strategy into action*. Report of the Maternal Health Working Group 2012, Global Health Policy Summit Report 2012 (website). www.imperial.ac.uk/media/imperial-college/institute-of-global-health-innovation/public/Mothers-lives.pdf. 2012.

Berry S: *It's the value chain, stupid!* (website). www.colalife.org/2013/03/03/its-the-value-chain-stupid. 2013.

Commission on Information and Accountability for Women's and Children's Health (COIA): *Implementing the commission on information and accountability recommendations* (website). http://www.who.int/life-course/publications/accountability-progress-report-2015/en/. 2014.

Confidential Enquiry into Maternal and Child Health (CEMACH): *Saving mothers' lives: reviewing maternal deaths to make motherhood safer – 2003–2005*. Seventh Report of the Confidential Enquiries into Maternal Deaths in the United Kingdom, 2007.

Fabic MS, Yoonjoung Choi Y, Bongaarts J, et al: *Meeting demand for family planning within a generation: the post-2015 agenda* (website). www.thelancet.com. 2014.

Family Planning 2020 (website). www.familyplanning2020.org/about. 2015.

Firoz T, Chou D, von Dadelszen P, et al for the Maternal Morbidity Working Group: *Measuring maternal health: focus on maternal morbidity* (website). http://www.who.int/bulletin/volumes/91/10/13-117564/en/. 2013.

The Guardian Online: *Online debate briefing – getting medicines to the poor: solving the logistics challenge* (website). https://www.theguardian.com/global-development-professionals-network/2013/jul/11/global-healthcare-supply-chain-challenge. 2013.

Global Health Workforce Alliance (GHWA): *2015 health workforce migration: the brain drain to brain gain – supporting the WHO Code of Practice on the recruitment of health personnel* (website). www.who.int/workforcealliance/brain-drain_brain-gain/en/. 2015.

Goodier R: *What startups and governments can learn from Coca-Cola* (website). www.engineeringforchange.org/what-startups-and-governments-can-learn-from-coca-cola/. 2015.

Homer CSE, Friberg IK, Dias MAB, et al: The projected effect of scaling up midwifery, *Lancet* 384(9948):1146–1157, 2014.

International Confederation of Midwives (ICM): *Global standards, competencies and tools* (website). http://internationalmidwives.org/core-documents. 2013.

Jamison DT, Summers LH, Alleye G, et al: *Global health 2035 – a world converging within a generation*. Lancet Commission (website). http://dcp-3.org/sites/default/files/resources/Global%20Health%202035%20Report.pdf. 2013.

Ki-moon B: *Global strategy for women's and children's health. Every woman every child* (website). http://www.everywomaneverychild.org/global-strategy/. 2010.

Knight MTD, Kenyon S, Shakespeare J, et al on behalf of MBRRACE-UK, editors: *Saving lives, improving mothers' care - surveillance of maternal deaths in the UK 2011–13 and lessons learned to inform maternity care from the UK and Ireland. Confidential Enquiries into Maternal Deaths and Morbidity 2009–13*, Oxford, National Perinatal Epidemiology Unit (NPEU), University of Oxford, 2015.

Koblinsky M, Chowdhury ME, Moran A, et al: Maternal morbidity and disability and their consequences: neglected agenda in maternal health, *J Health Popul Nutr* 30(2):124–130, 2012.

The Lancet Series on Midwifery (website). www.thelancet.com/series/midwifery. 2014.

Langer A, Meleis A, Knaul FM, et al: The Lancet Commission on Women and Health: the key for sustainable development, *Lancet* 386(9999):1165–1210, 2015.

Liu L, Johnson HL, Cousens S, et al: Global, regional and national causes of child mortality: an updated systematic analysis for 2010 with time trends since 2000, *Lancet* 379(9832):2151–2161, 2012.

Loudon I: *Death in childbirth: an international study of maternal care and maternal mortality 1800–1950*, Oxford, Clarendon Press, 1992.

Médecins Sans Frontières (MSF): *Working overseas* (website). www.msf.org.uk/work-overseas.

Organisation for Economic Co-operation and Development (OECD): *Immigrant Health workers in OECD countries in the broader context of highly skilled migration. Part III in International migration outlook 2007*, Paris, OECD, pp 161–228, 2007.

Partnership for Maternal, Newborn and Child Health (PMNCH): *PMNCH knowledge summaries: #15 – non-communicable diseases* (website). http://www.who.int/pmnch/topics/maternal/knowledge_summaries_15_noncommunicable_diseases/en/. 2011.

Partnership for Maternal, Newborn and Child Health (PMNCH): *Essential interventions, commodities and guidelines for reproductive, maternal, newborn and child health – a global review of the key interventions related to reproductive, maternal, newborn and child health* (website). www.who.int/pmnch/knowledge/publications/201112_essential_interventions/en/. 2012.

Renfrew MJ, McFadden A, Bastos MH, et al: Midwifery and quality care: findings from a new evidence-informed framework for maternal and newborn care, *Lancet* 384(9948):1129–1145, 2014.

Royal College of Midwives (RCM): *Overseas midwifery placements – planning your elective* (website). www.rcm.org.uk/content/overseas-midwifery-placements-planning-your-elective. 2016.

Save the Children: *An equal start – why gender equality matters for child survival and maternal health*, London, Save the Children, 2011.

Save the Children: *Surviving the first day: state of the world's mothers. A report by Save the Children on the situation facing world's mothers*, London, Save the Children, 2013.

Save the Children: *The urban disadvantage: state of the world's mothers report 2015* (website). http://resourcecentre.savethechildren.se/library/state-worlds-mothers-2015-urban-disadvantage. 2015.

Say L, Chou D, Gemmill A, et al: Global causes of maternal death: a WHO systematic analysis, *Lancet Glob Health* 2(6):e323–e333, 2014.

Sen G, Östling P: *Unequal, unfair, ineffective and inefficient – gender inequity in health: why it exists and how we can change it.* Final report to the WHO Commission on Social Determinants of Health (website). www.who.int/social_determinants/resources/csdh_media/wgekn_final_report_07.pdf?ua=1. 2007.

Singh S, Darroch JE, Ashford LS, Vlassoff M: *Adding it up: the costs and benefits of investing in family planning and maternal and newborn health*, New York, Guttmacher Institute and United Nations Population Fund, 2009.

Smile to the Future (website). http://smiletothefuture.org/millenium developmentgoals/.

Soucat A, Scheffler R, Ghebreyesus T, editors: *The labour market for health workers in Africa: a new look at the crisis*, Washington, DC, World Bank, 2013.

Subha Sri B, Khanna R: *Dead women talking: a civil society report on maternal deaths in India.* Jan Swasthya Abhiyan Commonhealth Coalition for Maternal-Neonatal Health and Safe Abortion (website). www.commonhealth.in/Dead%20Women%20Talking%20full%20report%20final.pdf. 2014.

UK Department of Health: *Code of practice for the international recruitment of healthcare professionals* (website). http://webarchive.nationalarchives.gov.uk/20081027092128/dh.gov.uk/en/publicationsandstatistics/publications/publicationspolicyandguidance/dh_4097730. 2004.

Unicef: *The state of the world's children, maternal and newborn health* (website). www.unicef.org/sowc09/docs/SOWC09-FullReport-EN.pdfUnicef. 2009.

Unicef: *The neonatal period is the most vulnerable time for a child* (website). http://data.unicef.org/child-mortality/neonatal.html#sthash.MOdYrrQx.zOBBO3pb.dpuf. 2015.

Unicef: *Statistics* (website). www.unicef.org/statistics/. 2016.

Unicef and WHO, compiled by Requejo J, Bryce J, Barros AJD, et al: *Countdown to 2015 and beyond: fulfilling the health agenda for women and children* (website). www.countdown2015mnch.org. 2015.

United Nations: *The Millennium Development Goals report 2013* (website). www.un.org/millenniumgoals/pdf/report-2013/mdg-report-2013-english.pdf. 2013.

United Nations Commission on the Status of Women (CSW): *Every woman every child.* Fact Sheet for Commission on the Status of Women (CSW 60) (website). www.unwomen.org/en/csw. 2016.

United Nations Foundation (UNF): *Every woman every child* (website). www.everywomaneverychild.org. 2016.

United Nations Inter-agency Group for Child Mortality Estimation (UN IGME): *Levels and trends in child mortality: report 2015* (website). http://data.unicef.org/child-mortality/neonatal.html#sthash.MOdYrrQx.dpuf. 2015.

United Nations Population Fund (UNFPA): *The state of the world's midwifery 2014: a universal pathway. A woman's right to health*, New York, UNFPA, 2014.

Voluntary Services Overseas (VSO): *Becoming a volunteer* (website). www.vsointernational.org/volunteer/professional/types-of-volunteer-job/health/midwives. 2016.

World Bank: *Global financing facility in support of Every Woman Every Child* (website). http://www.worldbank.org/en/news/speech/2015/07/13/global-financing-facility-woman-child. 2015.

World Bank: *Country and lending groups* (website). http://data.worldbank.org/about/country-and-lending-groups. 2016.

World Health Organization (WHO): *Making pregnancy safer: the critical role of the skilled attendant*, Geneva, WHO. A joint statement by WHO, ICM and FIGO, 2004.

World Health Organization (WHO): *The WHO global code of practice on the international recruitment of health personnel*, Geneva, WHO, 2010a.

World Health Organization (WHO): *Why did Mrs X die? Multimedia centre* (website). http://www.who.int/maternal_child_adolescent/multimedia/en/. 2010b.

World Health Organization (WHO): *Evaluating the quality of care for severe pregnancy complications: the WHO near-miss approach for maternal health*, Geneva, WHO, 2011.

World Health Organization (WHO): *Maternal death surveillance and response: technical guidance. Information for action to prevent maternal death* (website). www.who.int/maternal_child_adolescent/documents/maternal_death_surveillance/en/. 2013.

World Health Organization (WHO): *Every newborn: an action plan to end preventable deaths* (website). www.everynewborn.org/every-newborn-action-plan/. 2014.

World Health Organization (WHO): *Trends in maternal mortality: 1990 to 2015.* Estimates by WHO, Unicef; UNFPA, World Bank Group and the United Nations Population Division (website). www.who.int/reproductivehealth/publications/monitoring/maternal-mortality-2015/en/. 2015a.

World Health Organization (WHO): *Health in 2015: from MDGs, Millennium Development Goals to SDGs, Sustainable Development Goals* (website). http://apps.who.int/iris/bitstream/10665/200009/1/9789241565110_eng.pdf?ua=1. 2015b.

World Health Organization (WHO): *Strategies towards ending preventable maternal mortality (EPMM)*, Geneva, WHO, 2015c.

World Health Organization (WHO): *State of inequality: reproductive, maternal, newborn and child health* (website). www.who.int/gho/health_equity/report_2015/en. 2015d.

World Health Organization (WHO): *Why did Mrs X die retold* (website). www.who.int/maternal_child_adolescent/multimedia/en/. 2016a.

World Health Organization (WHO): *Global strategy on human resources for health: Workforce 2030.* Draft 1.0 submitted to the

Executive Board (138th Session) (website). www.who.int/hrh/resources/globstrathrh-2030/en/. 2016b.

World Health Organization (WHO): *World health statistics 2015* (website).

http://apps.who.int/iris/bitstream/10665/170250/1/9789240694439_eng.pdf. 2016c.

World Health Organization (WHO): *Global Health Observatory (GHO) data* (website). www.who.int/gho/

maternal_health/mortality/maternal/en/index1.html. 2016d.

Resources and additional reading

Healthy Newborn Network: healthynewbornnetwork.org

Website includes a range of useful resources and information.

International Confederation of Midwives (ICM): www.internationalmidwives.org

Website includes information on the countries in the confederation, global standards and competencies in education and practice; core documents for regulation, association and education; and other resources.

The Lancet Series on Midwifery: www.thelancet.com/series/midwifery

Published in 2014, this series is a wide-ranging, evidence-based resource examining international midwifery that reviews clinical, policy and health system perspectives.

United Nations Foundation (UNF) – *Every Woman Every Child 2016*: www.everywomaneverychild.org

World Health Organization (WHO) – *Maternal Death Surveillance and Response: Technical Guidance.*

Information for Action to Prevent Maternal Death: www.who.int/maternal_child_adolescent/documents/maternal_death_surveillance/en/

World Health Organization (WHO) – *Maternal Mortality Fact Sheet No. 348, Updated November 2015*: www.who.int/mediacentre/factsheets/fs348/en/)

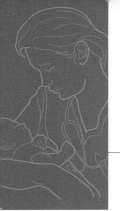

Chapter 2

A history of the midwifery profession in the United Kingdom

Dr Jean Donnison and Sue Macdonald

Learning Outcomes ?

After reading this chapter, you will be able to:

- appreciate the significance of socioeconomic factors in the development of an occupation such as midwifery
- understand the extent to which ruling ideas about women's abilities and social status have affected the occupation of midwife in the UK
- understand the innate power of healthy women, except in a small minority of cases, to give birth safely without intervention
- appreciate the importance of clarity and rigour in the use of concepts like 'normality' and 'risk'
- appreciate the context of the history of midwives in the UK
- have a clear understanding of the need for persistence, patience, pugnacity and organization among midwives in the continuance of midwifery professionals as guardians of normal childbirth

THE OFFICE OF MIDWIFE: A FEMALE DOMAIN

The office of midwife is a truly ancient calling. Sculptures of midwives attending birth date back at least 8000 years, and the Egyptian fertility goddess Hat-hor was frequently portrayed in this role. Midwives appear, too, in the Old Testament; the quick-witted Shiprah and Puah outmanoeuvre the Pharaoh, and the birth of Tamar's twins testifies to the midwife's resourcefulness and skill.

Until early modern times, childbirth was considered a female province, of which women alone had special understanding. No word existed in any language to signify a *male* birth attendant, and when these appeared in the late 16th century, new terms had to be created. The Anglo-Saxon *midwife*, meaning 'with-woman', denotes the office of *being with* the woman during labour and birth. Other titles, such as the Old French *leveuse* and the German *hebamme*, imply her function of *receiving the child*. The later French term *sage-femme* ('wise woman') implies wider concerns, and indeed, midwives were commonly consulted on matters of fertility, female ailments and care of the newborn.

Occasionally, when instruments were necessary to extract the child, a man might be called in. Traditionally, the use of instruments belonged to surgeons, who, with the increasing exclusion of women from medicine and surgery since the 1300s, were overwhelmingly male. Yet the surgeon's scope was limited. Using hooks and knives, he might extract piecemeal an infant presumed dead or, hoping to save its life, swiftly perform a caesarean section (CS) on the newly dead mother. Hence a man's advent into the birth chamber generally presaged the death of mother or child, possibly both. Where surgeons were unavailable, however, midwives themselves might undertake such operations. In wealthy households, a physician (usually a university-educated practitioner of internal medicine), whose midwifery knowledge came from classical writings rather than practical experience, might be called to prescribe medicines judged necessary for mother or child.

What manner of women were midwives?

'A midwife's skill lay in her ability to manage the mother and the birthing chamber, and this was closely linked to her social identity'.

(Thomas 2009)

Little is known about individual European midwives before the 16th century. As in later eras, they were married women or widows, generally of middle age or older. Most would have previously given birth; until the late 1700s this experience, except for daughters following their mothers into the work, was usually considered essential. The few formally educated midwives generally came from the artisan class or lower gentry. Such women invested time and money in several years of apprenticeship to a senior midwife, and by the 17th century, most would be literate. These midwives were commonly found in towns, where there was sufficient prosperity to make their apprenticeship outlays worthwhile. Most would start by practising among the poor, possibly acquiring a more affluent clientele as their reputations grew. Town midwives engaged by country nobility or gentry would arrive well before the birth and stay several days or weeks afterwards, being recompensed accordingly. Attendance on royalty was the greatest prize. In 1469, Margaret Cobb, midwife to Edward IV's queen, received, in addition to her fee, a life pension of £10 per year, as did Alice Massey, who attended Elizabeth of York in 1503. Mme Peronne, who in 1630 travelled from France to attend Charles I's French queen, was paid £300, with £100 for her expenses.

These midwives, however, were a minority. Inevitably the rest attended only the poor (the majority of the population), many living in rural, perhaps isolated, places. Such women would learn their midwifery through their own and their neighbours' birthing experiences, undertaking the work by virtue of their seniority or the large number of children they had borne (McMath 1694; Siegemundin 1690). Their work might entail travelling long distances on foot to outlying habitations, for a few pence or a small payment in kind. Many such women took up the work from necessity, eking out a poor living with nursing of the sick and laying out of the dead, as did their successors up through the early 20th century.

Midwifery knowledge

Before the 16th century, most midwifery knowledge, like knowledge in other fields, would be transmitted by word of mouth, by example from midwife to apprentice and, in some cases, from mother to daughter (Allotey 2011a). Some practice was based on superstition and the available evidence/information of the day (Allotey 2011b). The first midwifery manual printed in English appeared in 1540 – *The Byrth of Mankynde* (Jonas 1540), translated via Latin from a 1513 German work by Eucharius Roesslin, the city physician of Wurms. Drawn largely from ancient and mediaeval texts, the *Byrth* included many of their errors, thus demonstrating the ignorance of practical midwifery common among physicians in that age. Yet it contained much good sense on the care of the labouring woman, together with directions for managing abnormal cases,

including delivery of the infant by the feet, instrumental removal of the dead fetus and CS on the dead mother. However, although addressed to pregnant women and midwives, the work could only benefit the literate minority who could afford to buy it.

'In the straw'

Generally, birth took place at home, with poorer women typically delivering in the communal room, in front of the fire; the floor was covered with straw, which would later be burnt. Usually the birth chamber was darkened, with the windows and doors sealed, and a fire was lit and kept burning for several days. These precautions were taken lest the woman took 'cold' (developed the possibly lethal 'childbed fever') and, in more superstitious households, for fear that malevolent spirits might gain entrance, harming mother or infant (Gélis 1996: 97, Thomas 1973: 728–732). Care was taken, too, that the placenta (afterbirth) and its attachments (all credited with powerful magical properties) were disposed of safely, lest they be used in spells to harm the family. These beliefs were still current in remote parts of Europe in the early 20th century.

To hasten matters on in early labour the parturient would periodically be encouraged to walk, supported by two sturdy women, her strength sustained by warm broth or spicy drinks. The midwife, sharing the universal and time-honoured belief that the *child* provided the motive power for its birth, would follow ancient practice in greasing and stretching the woman's genitalia and dilating the cervix to 'help' the infant emerge. Hence the 'ideal' midwife possessed, along with appropriate qualities of character, small hands with long, tapering fingers (Temkin 1956).

The second stage of labour usually took place, as it had for millennia, with the woman in an upright or semi-upright position (Kuntner 1988). In rich households a birth chair might be used, but more commonly the parturient was held on a woman's lap. Some women knelt or stood, leaning against a support; some adopted a half-sitting, half-lying posture, with a solid object to push their feet against during contractions, whereas others delivered on all fours (Blenkinsop 1863: 8, 10, 73; Gélis 1996: 21–36). As labour progressed, the woman would instinctively change position, 'as shall seeme commodious and necessarye to the partie', as the *Byrth* put it, urging the midwife to comfort her with refreshments and encourage her with 'swete wurdes' (see Fig. 2.1). Following delivery, the mother would be put to bed to 'lie in' – rich women for up to a month, the poor for days at most. The infant would be washed and then swaddled to 'straighten' its limbs, and if circumstances permitted, an all-woman celebration of this female life event would ensue.

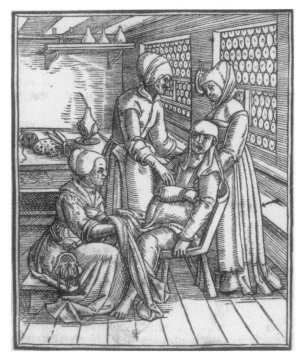

Figure 2.1 Midwife attending a labouring woman seated on a birth chair. Two women hold her shoulders firmly while the midwife carries on with her work. The midwife's sponge, with scissors and thread for cutting and tying the cord, lie in readiness by the rear wall. (From Rueff, Jacobus: Ein schön lustig Trost-büchle von den Empfengknussen und Geburten der Menschen, Zurich, 1554 (Courtesy of Wellcome Library, London.))

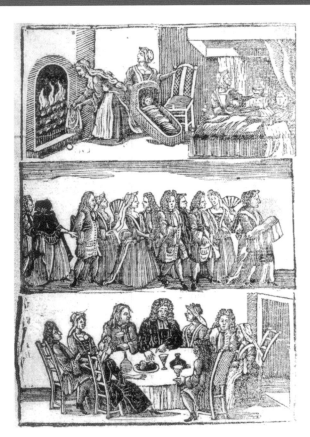

Figure 2.2 Frontispiece from Jane Sharp's *Compleat Midwife's Companion*, 1724, showing the midwife handing the mother a bowl of broth following the birth; later, infant in arms, she heads the christening procession to the church, subsequently appearing as a guest at the christening feast, where she will receive substantial tips from the assembled company. The mother is not present, being still in seclusion in the lying-in room until her churching some weeks later. (Courtesy of Wellcome Library, London.)

THE MIDWIFE, THE CHURCH AND THE LAW

The midwife's duties did not end with the birth, however. In pre-Reformation times, she also carried heavy responsibility for the salvation of the infant's soul, being required to take weak newborns directly to the priest for baptism. If the infant's death seemed imminent, she would perform the ceremony herself, taking care to use only the Church's prescribed words. If the woman died undelivered, the midwife was immediately to open the woman's body, and if the infant were alive, to baptise it. Stillborn infants, in their unhallowed state unfit for Christian burial, she was to bury in unconsecrated ground, safely and secretly, where neither man nor beast would find them.

If the birth was successful, baptism would generally take place within a week of birth, and the midwife, infant in arms, headed the procession to the church, the mother remaining in seclusion until she had been 'churched'. The

midwife enjoyed an honoured place at post-christening celebrations and in prosperous households would be liberally tipped by family and friends (see Fig. 2.2). Later, after the lying-in period, she would accompany the mother to her 'churching' – originally a 'purification' ceremony, but under Protestantism merely one of maternal thanksgiving.

The midwife also had an important role in legal matters. Where a woman condemned to death pleaded pregnancy in the hope of postponing or mitigating punishment, a panel of midwives would be summoned to examine her, although some post-execution dissections demonstrated these examinations' unreliability (Pechey 1696: 55–56). Midwife panels were also called to examine unmarried women alleging rape, women accused of aborting them-selves or of concealing the birth (and possible murder) of an unwanted infant, or to determine the alleged prematurity of infants born within less than 9 months of marriage. Midwives attending an unmarried woman were also expected to make her name the father, lest he escape the Church's punishment for fornication and his responsibility to the parish for the child's upkeep. A midwives' 'oath' from 1564, from Eleanor Pead, licensed by the Archbishop of Canterbury (Secara 2013), included a commitment to 'be ready to help poor as well as rich women in labour', to not allow substitution of another baby and to protect mother and baby (see chapter website resources). Use of this oath was thought to be led by a Church initiative to address the problem of illegitimacy, but also highlighted the process of baptism (Licence 2013).

Governing the midwife

In view of these religious and legal duties, the midwife's character and religious orthodoxy were inevitably of concern to the Church. In 1481, Agnes Marshall of Emeswell, Yorkshire, was 'presented' at the Bishop's court not because she lacked skill in midwifery, but because she used (pagan) 'incantations' to 'help' the labour. Midwives were suspect, too, because of their access to stillborn babies, allegedly used in devil worship. In 1415, a successful Parisian midwife, Perette, was turned in the pillory and banned from practice for supplying a tiny fetus used, unbeknownst to her, in sorcery. On account of her great skill, however, she was restored to practice by order of the king.

Probably the first system of compulsory midwife licensing in Europe was instituted in the city of Regensberg in Bavaria in 1452, a system gradually emulated in other European cities. Applicants for a licence were commonly examined by a panel of physicians, who, with lack of experience in practical midwifery, based their examination on classical texts. Generally, midwives were required to send for a physician or surgeon in difficult cases, and in Strasbourg, midwives were prohibited from using hooks or sharp instruments, with threat of corporal punishment for such use. Many cities appointed midwives to serve the poor, supplementing their remuneration with payment in kind and providing financial aid in old age or disability (Gélis 1988: 25; Wiesener 1993: 78–84).

In England, the first arrangements for formal control of midwives were made under the 1512 act for regulating physicians and surgeons. The act's aim was to limit unskilled practice and prevent the use of 'sorcery' and 'witchcraft' in medicine. It therefore provided for Church courts to license practitioners able to produce testimony to their skill and religious orthodoxy, and to prosecute the rest. A midwife applying for a licence would normally bring to the court a reference from the local parson, together with 'six honest matrons' she had delivered, to testify in person to her competence. There was, however, no *formal* examination on this point as existed under some continental schemes.

Successful applicants swore a long and detailed oath, promising 'faithfully and diligently' to help childbearing women, to serve 'as well poor as rich', not to charge more than the family could afford and not to divulge private matters. They swore not to use 'sorcery' to shorten labour, to use only prescribed words when performing emergency baptism and to bury as directed all stillborn children. They undertook not to procure abortion nor connive at child destruction, false attribution of paternity or substitution of infants. Neither were they to allow any woman to be delivered secretly, and always, if possible, they were to see that lights were available and 'two or three honest women' present, a requirement clearly aimed at preventing the speedy suffocation of an unwanted child.

ADVENT OF THE MAN-MIDWIFE

Around the mid-16th century came other changes laden with import for midwives, as surgeons, inspired by the new Renaissance spirit of enquiry, turned their attention to the anatomy of childbirth. Outstanding in this field was the French barber-surgeon Ambroise Paré (1510–1590), notable for his description in his 1549 *Briefve Collection* of the use of podalic version in malpresentation cases. The success of men like Paré was to encourage the extension of male attendance from 'extraordinary' to routine cases. This development gradually spread throughout Europe, being recognized around 1600 in Britain with the new term *man-midwife*, and in France that of *accoucheur*.

The centrality of anatomical knowledge to good midwifery was well understood by leading practitioners, both men and women. In 1671, the London midwife Jane Sharp began the *Midwives Book* by deploring 'the many Miseries' women endured at the hands of midwives who practised 'without any skill in Anatomy … merely for Lucres sake' (Sharp 1671; Allotey 2011a). Her contemporary, the Derbyshire man-midwife Willughby, concurred, finding that many country midwives could not manage malpresentations; however, Willughby also condemned inexperienced young surgeons and ill-prepared apothecaries, whose 'fatal bunglings' deserved the branding iron or the hangman's noose.

Maternal mortality

Given the general lack of statistics at that time, the extent of contemporary maternal mortality (calculated as death at or within the month after the birth) is impossible to discover. However, in his 1662 study of the London Bills of Mortality, John Graunt estimated maternal mortality in

London at about 15 per 1000 births. Those dying from the 'hardness' of their labour, as distinct from other causes, he put at *less than 1 in 200* (5 per 1000). Significantly, along with other authorities, Graunt believed that poor, hard-working countrywomen did best in childbirth. The celebrated Dr Harvey went further. Challenging the general practice of dilating the parturient's vulva and os uteri, he argued that women delivering unattended fared best because Nature, escaping the midwife's interventions, was allowed, unhindered, to take her course. His friend Willughby confessed himself converted to this view, condemning interference as always harmful in all but abnormal cases.

Interestingly, Willughby also links such interference with the woman 'taking cold' (Blenkinsop 1863: 6), a likely reference to 'puerperal' fever, not so named, but recognized under 'fevers' and 'agues' occurring after childbearing. Following ancient humoral theory, the condition was ascribed to an imbalance in bodily 'humours' (Jonas 1540: xxxiii; Sharp 1671: 243–250) and was probably then, as later, the chief single cause of maternal death. Not until the late 18th century was it publicly proposed that this deadly malady might be carried to the woman on the attendants' clothing or unwashed hands (Gordon 1795: 98–99), a view not completely accepted, even in medical circles, until the 1940s.

Midwives under threat

When urging midwives to study anatomy, Jane Sharp had recognized that women's exclusion from the universities and 'schools of learning', where this subject was taught, disadvantaged them compared to men. Girls were barred, too, from grammar schools, which taught Latin, knowledge of which was the mark of an educated person, the language still used for many medical texts. Leading male practitioners therefore enjoyed higher social status than midwives, however successful. Although in 1762 Mrs Draper delivered the future George IV, with Dr Hunter and the surgeon Caesar Hawkins waiting elsewhere, Hunter's diary makes their relative ranking clear (Stark 1908). Moreover, the distinction of great 18th-century practitioners like Manningham, Ould, Hunter and Smellie was to reflect credit on every man-midwife, deserved or not.

However, it was probably the general introduction in the 1720s of the midwifery forceps that precipitated the rapid acceleration of the existing trend. The forceps enabled the delivery of live infants where previously child or mother might have been lost, and the shortening of tedious labour. Because custom discouraged use of instruments by midwives, this development further enhanced the position of men and many surgeon-apothecaries; taking up midwifery, they became general practitioners in fact if not yet in name. Some men-midwives, too, saw childbirth as a *mechanical* process and themselves, with

their right to use instruments, as better suited to preside over it. Indeed, for many, the educated male practitioner represented the new enlightened age, whereas midwives, whose ranks included many ignorant, illiterate and superstitious women, appeared relics of a benighted past.

Keenly aware of the threat to their livelihood, midwives fought back, supported in books and pamphlets by both medical and lay sympathizers. For reasons of modesty, these argued, many women would not send for a man, nor would their husbands allow it. Many could not afford men's fees, and male assistance, especially in the country, was commonly unavailable. Men-midwives, it was contended, resorted to unnecessary use of instruments in order to save their time and increase their fees, and were thus responsible for increased maternal and infant mortality. Furthermore, they exaggerated the dangers of childbirth, frightening women into believing that extraordinary measures, and therefore male attendance, were more necessary than they actually were. Also, by insisting on being called to every 'trifling' difficulty, men were reducing midwives to 'mere nurses' while taking every opportunity to denigrate their competence and blame them, however unjustly, for any mishap, even those of their own cause (see Fig. 2.3).

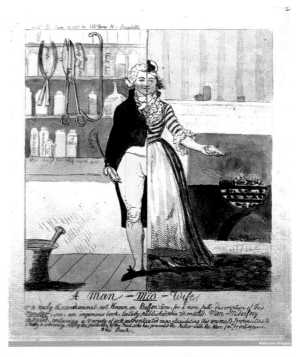

Figure 2.3 The *Man-Midwife* (1793). Behind the man-midwife are his instruments and potions, which, it was alleged, he used for nefarious purposes, contrasting starkly with the woman-midwife – homely and nurturing, holding a pap boat for infant feeding. (Courtesy of Wellcome Library, London.)

Lying-in hospitals and 'out-door' charities

One champion of the midwives' cause was the London surgeon John Douglas. Writing in 1736 to rebut men-midwives' claims that difficult births were beyond female capacities, he instanced the career of Mme du Tetre, who was the head midwife at the great Paris hospital Hôtel-Dieu. Douglas maintained that if English midwives had the same opportunities as Frenchwomen (the Hôtel-Dieu had trained midwives since 1631), they could reach equally high standards. British counterparts of such hospitals had been abolished in Henry VIII's dissolution of the monasteries, and Douglas, seeing lying-in hospitals as essential to improved midwife instruction, demanded their establishment in all the principal English cities. The first such permanent foundation, however, was the Dublin 'Rotunda', established in 1745. Two lying-in wards were created in the Middlesex Hospital in 1747, and four (tiny) lying-in hospitals opened in London shortly afterwards. Similar institutions appeared in major provincial cities as the century progressed.

These hospitals, like others founded at the time, were charitable institutions, funded by the subscriptions of the wealthy for the benefit of the poor (in this case 'respectable' poor married women) and run by voluntary lay boards. Hospitals were a mixed blessing for the women attending them. Outbreaks of puerperal fever, a regular feature until the adoption of antiseptic practice in the late 19th century (and occurring sporadically even in the 1930s), boosted death rates and necessitated closure for weeks on end. Safer and cheaper were 'out-door' charities, such as the Royal Maternity Charity, London (founded 1757). These provided poor women with midwife attendance at home and with designated medical assistance as necessary, and they probably trained far more midwives than the tiny hospitals. There was, however, no move in England from government, central or local, on this vital matter of midwife instruction. By this time, Bishops' licensing – which, although no great guarantee of skill, and never properly enforced, had given the licensed midwife some status – was generally defunct.

Continental comparisons

Meanwhile, on the Continent, state control in matters perceived to be in the public interest, including midwife instruction and regulation, grew ever stronger. Many German towns had midwife schools and 'midwife-masters' to teach midwives. In 1759, the French king sent the eminent midwife Mme du Coudray around the country to lecture to midwives and surgeons and to found lying-in hospitals. Educated English midwives, realizing that lack of official instruction and regulation at home was hastening the midwife's decline, called vainly for

Continental-style systems in England. Scotland, where Continental influence was stronger, was different. In 1694, the Edinburgh Town Council had established a system of midwife regulation, and in 1726, the council appointed an honorary professor of midwifery, Joseph Gibson, for their instruction. In 1740, the Glasgow Faculty of Physicians and Surgeons instituted a similar system for the city and surrounding counties, which, like Edinburgh's, appears to have operated throughout the century.

'Towards a complete new system of midwifery'

By the mid-18th century, male practitioners, disdaining the familiar designation *man-midwife*, began to adopt the French term *accoucheur*, which conveyed greater status. Their approaches to delivery varied, however. Some still dilated the cervix and the labia vulvae, practices continuing among the more ignorant at the century's close (Clarke 1793: 21). Some extracted the placenta immediately after delivery by introducing the hand into the uterus, whereas others roundly condemned this (Smellie 1752–64: 238–239). The general trend, however, was towards less intervention. This development stemmed from the new realization that it was not exertions by the child but uterine muscular action that provided the necessary expulsive force (Smellie 1752–64: 202). Significantly, Smellie (now regarded as the 'father of British obstetrics') concluded from his vast experience that out of 1000 parturients, 990 would be safely delivered 'without any other than common assistance' (Smellie 1752–64: 195–196).

Although ambulation in the first stage was still encouraged, women's freedom to choose their delivery position was gradually being curtailed. Earlier authorities, male and female, had encouraged women to adopt the position most comfortable to them as facilitating the best outcome for mother and infant. Smellie underlined the advantages of upright positions in furthering labour, partly through gravity and partly through the 'equalisation of the uterine force', recommending them for 'tedious labours' (Smellie 1752–64: 202). Yet, along with other authorities, Smellie generally advised delivery in bed (half-sitting, half-lying) for fear that otherwise the woman might take 'cold' and hence develop 'childbed fever' (Smellie 1752–64: 204). Others, like Dr John Burton of York, favoured the 'dorsal' and 'left lateral' positions as 'easiest for the Patient and most convenient for the Operator' (Burton 1751: 106–107). Indeed, sitting by the edge of the bed, his hand concealed under the sheet, was less tiring and less undignified for men hoping for recognition of their art as part of medicine proper than was crouching at the woman's knees on the midwife's low stool (see Fig. 2.4).

Recumbent delivery positions gradually became the norm for 'civilised' practice. Although delivery out of bed

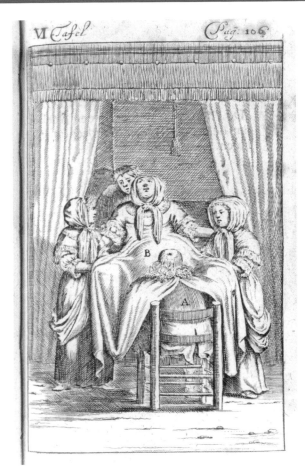

Figure 2.4 A man-midwife attends a birth in Holland. The parturient is now labouring in bed. Although in a semiupright position, she has lost some of the benefits of being fully upright, with her feet on the floor, in aiding her expulsive efforts. She holds on to her attendants' shoulders while they push against her feet to give her some base for her pushing. To protect the woman's modesty, the corners of a sheet are pinned around the man-midwife's neck so that he works blind, a situation that sometimes led to error. (From Janson S: *Korte en Bonding verbandeling, van de voortteelingen't Kinderbaren,* Amsterdam, 1711 (Courtesy of Wellcome Library, London.))

was to continue in rural areas into the 20th century, it was generally considered low class, if not inhumane. Significantly, the parturient's transfer to bed, together with her increasing designation as a 'patient' (a word originally used only to refer to the sick), indicated her transition from an active to a passive role in this important life event, and, implicitly, the growing medicalization of childbirth itself.

THE DECLINE OF THE MIDWIFE

By the early decades of the 19th century the midwife's situation had deteriorated still further. Growing prudery, largely the result of the Evangelical movement, had rendered reference to childbirth, and even the word *midwife*, taboo in polite society. Together with the male capture of the wealthier private practice and the growing reluctance of the middle classes to allow their women to work, this prudery meant that fewer educated women were entering midwifery, leaving many who wanted skilled assistance in childbirth forced to send for a man. Midwife supporters argued that midwives' instruction (where it existed) had not kept pace with men's, and increasingly calls arose for the better education of female practitioners to the highest professional standards, in midwifery and women's diseases. The medical response was predictable. Women were unfitted by nature for 'scientific mechanical employment' (which midwifery was), and they could never use obstetrical instruments with 'advantage or precision', even if presumptuous enough to try. Such remarks, together with allegations that midwives were generally abortionists, prompted one midwife supporter to remark that 'the greatest slanders against the moral and intellectual characters of women have been uttered by practitioners of man-midwifery'.

This animosity towards midwives arose partly from men-midwives' generally low status within the medical profession. Their specialty was not officially recognized as part of medicine, and no official qualification existed in England to distinguish men with midwifery training from those with none. Hence men seeking such qualifications were forced to go to Scotland or the Continent. For decades, leading accoucheurs had requested the English chartered medical corporations to establish such a qualification, but they had been repeatedly rebuffed. Many leading medical figures viewed attendance at childbirth as 'women's work' and below the dignity of professional men. In 1827, Sir Anthony Carlisle (later president of the Royal College of Surgeons) denounced man-midwifery as a 'dishonorable vocation', whose practitioners sought to turn a natural process into a 'surgical operation', acting from financial motives. It was 1852 before the College established its Midwifery Licence and 1888 before such qualification was required for admission to the Medical Register kept by the General Medical Council, the doctors' regulatory body established in 1859. Thenceforth midwifery was formally recognized in the UK as part of medicine.

Maternal mortality and the state

Beginning in 1839, maternal mortality statistics became available from the newly created Registrar-General's Office for Births, Marriages and Deaths. The office's statistical superintendent, Dr W Farr, deplored the high loss of maternal life represented by the estimated rate for 1841 of nearly 6 maternal deaths per 1000 live births. Looking wistfully at Continental legislation for midwife regulation, Farr concluded that comparable arrangements at home were ruled out by British suspicion of state direction combined with general prudery concerning childbirth. Yet with better-instructed midwives, Farr declared, the annual 3000 maternal deaths could be reduced by a third. That some midwives were incompetent was demonstrated in press reports of those who had pulled out the womb or torn the child's body from its head. Such disasters were paralleled, however, in accounts of ignorant male practitioners cutting out the womb or part of the intestines with scissors or a knife. Some of these men (graphically described in the *London Medical Gazette* in 1845 as 'disembowelling accoucheurs') were regularly qualified medical men, and others were chemists, but in neither case was instruction in midwifery required by law.

The end of the midwife?

The midwife's image had not been helped by Charles Dickens's caricature in *Martin Chuzzlewit* (1844) of the unsavoury Mrs Gamp, a poor widow who, like so many over the centuries, earned her living by practising midwifery, sick and 'monthly' nursing and laying out the dead. A blowsy, tippling, unscrupulous character, Mrs Gamp soon became the stereotypical midwife, illustrated by the caricature of a midwife going out to attend a birth, carrying a lantern and a bottle of spirituous liquor (see Fig. 2.5).

But although some medical men, along with Farr, advocated the replacement of such midwives by respectable, trained women, certain accoucheurs, seeking a male monopoly of midwifery (achieved in North America by the 1950s), were pressing for the midwife's total abolition. 'All midwives are a mistake', Tyler Smith told his students at the Hunterian Medical School in 1847, 'and it should be the aim of every obstetric practitioner to discourage their employment'. Furthermore, he stated that because of its origin, the word *midwifery* should no longer be used to describe male attendance on childbirth, being replaced by the new construct 'obstetrics'. Here Smith well understood that a term of Latin origin, even if derived actually from the Latin term for 'midwife' (*obstetrix*), had a snob value that would further elevate men above their female competitors. This substitution of *obstetrics* for *midwifery* in male practice was, however, not fully achieved until after World War II.

The Royal Maternity Charity and maternal mortality

Directly in Smith's line of fire was the 98-year-old Royal Maternity Charity. The Charity's employment of midwives,

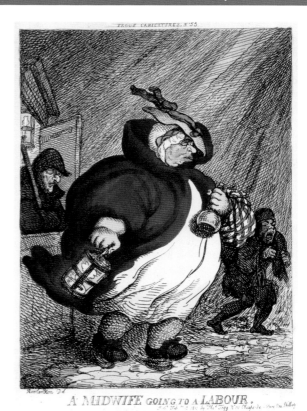

Figure 2.5 A caricature by Rowlandson (1811) of a midwife going to attend a labouring woman, equipped with a lantern and spirit bottle. (Courtesy of Wellcome Library, London.)

however well instructed, Smith contended, was 'degrading' to 'obstetrics' and harmful to its clients, who instead should be attended by 'educated' practitioners. Yet the Charity's statistics, published annually by the eminent medical men supervising its work, repeatedly disproved these allegations. Serving only poor women, many undernourished and living in unhealthy conditions, the Charity (and similar foundations) consistently demonstrated death rates of less than half the Registrar-General's current rates for England and Wales.

A further onslaught on such charities came in 1870 from the obstetrician Matthews Duncan in his *Mortality of Childbed*. Dismissing the charities' results as an impossibility because 'educated accoucheurs', in (affluent) private practice, lost five times as many women, Duncan postulated an 'irreducible minimum' of at least 8 per 1000, an admission suggesting that the rich might indeed fare worse in childbirth than the poor.

Despite this obvious inference, the anti-midwife faction had an answer. The cause of higher mortality among wealthier women lay not with their medical attendants but with their own 'artificial' way of life, which disabled them for parturition. *Increased* (medical) vigilance was therefore necessary in attending them, not less. The degree to which childbirth among the prosperous was progressively viewed as pathology was evident in Chavasse's 1842 *Advice to a Wife*. Although declaring childbirth a natural event, Chavasse required the 'pregnant female' to rest for 2 to 3 hours daily, and the post-parturient was to keep to a meagre diet, lying flat on her back for 10 to 14 days, lest she should faint, haemorrhage, or suffer a prolapsed womb (Chavasse 1878).

This invalidization of pregnancy and childbirth naturally implied more medical attention and higher fees, catching women in a double bind. Not only were they regarded as physically, intellectually and morally incapable of undertaking the ancient female duty of attendance on childbirth, but they were also increasingly seen as requiring male assistance to give birth at all.

THE MIDWIVES INSTITUTE, MIDWIFE REGISTRATION AND MATERNAL MORTALITY

Accepting this reality, in 1880 three educated midwives, together with Louisa Hubbard, a wealthy pioneer in women's employment, formed the Matrons Aid Society, later to become the Midwives Institute and ultimately the Royal College of Midwives (RCM) (Figs 2.6a and b). Even at its beginning, the importance of education and information for midwives was viewed as fundamental, with one of the first actions being to start a library and journal for midwives.

The Society's avowed aim was the improvement of midwife practice and, by implication, a reduction in maternal mortality. This was to be achieved through a registration act similar to other professional legislation, as was the rehabilitation of midwifery as a respectable profession for educated women. Realizing that general practitioners might view registered midwives as competitors for their better-paying cases, the Institute argued that midwives would attend only women too poor to pay doctors' fees and would not encroach on medical ground by acting in abnormal labour.

Yet what proportion of annual maternal mortality (still around 5 per 1000 live births) could be laid at the midwife's door? The obstetrician Dr Aveling, when pressing for midwife registration before the 1892 Commons' Select Committee, had implied that untrained midwives were responsible for most of the annual 3000 or so maternal deaths in England and Wales. Because there was as yet no notification of births, or any system of identifying the birth attendant, this was purely guesswork. Indeed, WC Grigg,

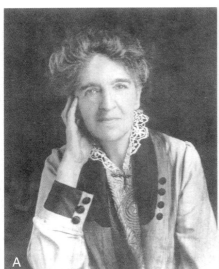 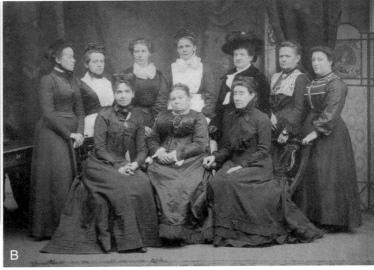

Figure 2.6 A, Rosalind Paget (1855–1948). Trained in nursing and midwifery, Miss Paget joined the Midwives Institute in 1886, in 1887 financing the establishment of the Institute's journal, *Nursing Notes*. Also prominent in the Queen's Nursing Institute, she was for 20 years its representative on the Central Midwives Board. (Courtesy of the Royal College of Midwives) **B,** Photograph of Rosalind Paget, honorary treasurer of the Royal College of Midwives; Mary Stephens, first midwife to appear on the Midwives Roll of the Central Midwives Board; and Paulina Fynes-Clinton, secretary of the RCM, with other unidentified but presumably prominent midwives who also campaigned for the registration and education of midwives. (Courtesy of the Royal College of Midwives.)

Physician to Queen Charlotte's Hospital, concluded in 1891 that more cases of 'injury and disaster' resulted from the imprudent use of forceps and turning by doctors than from the negligence and ignorance of midwives.

The Midwives Act of 1902

Despite continued strengthening of Continental midwife legislation, home governments, still heavily imbued with 'laissez-faire' ideology, declined to intervene. The Midwives Institute therefore began seeking friendly medical and parliamentary support for the promotion of a Private Member's Bill, a difficult task when women did not have the vote; there were no female members of parliament (MPs), and matters regarding childbirth were not discussed in polite circles. For 20 years, this handful of strong, but voteless women struggled against indifference and ridicule from an all-male Parliament and, latterly, bitter opposition from among general practitioners, their professional associations and the General Medical Council. Finally, however, possibly as a result of growing concern for the national welfare following revelations about the falling birth rate and poor health among Boer War volunteers, the first state registration measure in modern England for an all-female occupation became law. However, fierce medical opposition to registration had meant that the status of the new registered English midwife was much lower than that of her counterparts in leading Continental countries. Similar legislation for Scotland and Ireland (with the difference that new entrants must also be qualified nurses) followed in 1915 and 1918, respectively.

The Central Midwives Board

The act established a midwives' regulatory authority, the *Central Midwives Board (CMB)*, with responsibility for keeping a 'Roll' of 'certified' midwives. In recognition of midwives' general poverty, this regulatory machinery would be largely financed from public funds. Moreover, unlike doctors and chemists, midwives were not to be self-regulating. The bill's promoters, to keep their medical allies' support, had been forced to concede that the CMB should be in medical hands. The additional requirement of local government supervision through the agency of the (possibly hostile) Medical Officers of Health meant that at both national and local levels midwives would be regulated by a competing profession. There was a further burden: midwives, uniquely for a nationally regulated profession, were liable to erasure from the register (and subsequent loss of livelihood) for 'misconduct' in their *private*, in addition to their professional, lives.

In 1905, the first year of enrolment, over 22,308 midwives registered. Of these, less than half held relevant certificates of competence, with the remaining 12,521 registering as midwives in 'bona fide' practice. Five years'

grace was allowed for unregistered women to continue to practise, but after 1910 such activity became a criminal offence. For new entrants to the profession, 3 months' approved training was required before taking the CMB's examination (doubled to 6 months in 1916 for non-nurse-trained applicants, in 1926 to 1 year, and in 1938 to 2 years). The CMB's rules limited midwives to attendance at natural labour (which included twin and breech deliveries) and required them to send for a doctor in difficult cases. Significantly, it forbade them to lay out the dead, traditionally an important part of poorer midwives' work. Detailed directions also governed their daily practice, extending to their clothing, their equipment and their record-keeping; breaches of the rules could be punished by erasure from the Roll.

'Certified Midwife'

Despite these restrictions on midwives' independence, the act worked gradually to raise the occupation's status, consequently preventing the disappearance from the UK (in contrast with North America, where this was virtually achieved) of this ancient female calling. The requirement of hospital training and examination for new entrants, however, brought changes in the occupation's social composition as younger, single women entered its ranks. Meanwhile, the poorer, older, working-class women who had for centuries delivered their neighbours were prevented by the cost of training, books and examination fees from becoming registered midwives, being allowed to act as maternity nurses only (Leap and Hunter 1993: 44–47).

As always, life could be very arduous for midwives attending women at home. This was especially so in the country, where long distances would be travelled in all weather, on foot or by bicycle, possibly through difficult terrain. Fees were low (possibly 30 shillings to £2 per case) and generally paid in instalments during the pregnancy, although some payment might be in kind. In 1929, a few midwives with extensive practices were found to be earning over £275 annually, but many, even though practising full time, earned only £90–£100. Salaries for nursing association work in rural areas could also be low, the life very lonely and hardly supportable without private means. Hours worked could be very long, with some midwives delivering 90 to 100 women per year. A Portsmouth midwife recalled how, when in independent practice, she once went without sleep for 4 days while single-handedly conducting seven deliveries, one of a $12\frac{1}{2}$-lb baby, finally going home to sleep the clock around twice (Leap and Hunter 1993: 50–56, 63–68).

Domiciliary midwife practice appears to have followed guidelines laid down in contemporary obstetricians' textbooks. Although allowed by the CMB to give mild analgesics (only doctors were allowed to give chloroform), some midwives employed warm baths and back-rubbing to ease

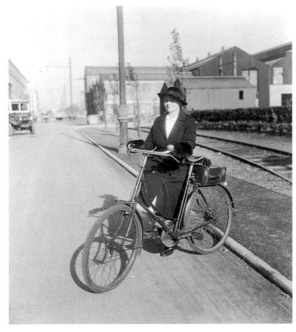

Figure 2.7 Midwife transporting analgesic gas-air machine by bicycle, circa 1937–1938, from the National Birthday Trust Fund Papers. (Courtesy of Wellcome Library, London.)

pain. It was not until the 1940s that the self-operated *Minnit inhalation analgesic apparatus* became available in portable form for carriage on the midwife's bicycle (see Fig. 2.7). In difficult cases midwives were required to send for medical help, but if this were delayed, they would have to manage the emergency themselves, and if the doctor were inexperienced, they might help him put on the forceps (Leap and Hunter 1993: 56–58, 176–178). Midwife–doctor relations varied, but, as in earlier centuries, some doctors sought to blame midwives for their own incompetence (Leap and Hunter 1993: 56–58).

After delivery, the mother was to lie flat for at least a day and to stay in bed for 10 to 14 days, for fear of uterine prolapse (Leap and Hunter 1993: 143, 164–171, 179). As tradition prescribed, she was kept, officially at least, on a meagre diet, a regimen that, as contemporary midwifery manuals show, only began to change in the 1950s.

The continuing problem of maternal mortality

After the 1902 act was passed, it was expected that maternal mortality would fall as untrained midwives, known to be reluctant to send for medical help in difficult cases, were gradually replaced by their formally trained successors. Instead, the rate remained puzzlingly stable. Worse still,

from 1928 it showed a significant rise, climbing to exceed 4 per 1000 live births in 1930. Interestingly, enquiries by the Ministry of Health showed that maternal mortality was lower among the poor, many of whom had poor health and lived in insanitary conditions, than among the better-off, who generally had medical attendance. Allegations of fatal abuse of instruments had followed male practitioners for over two centuries. Even in this era, reported an editorial in *The Lancet* (Anon 1929), many general practitioners (GPs) confessed to routinely using instruments solely to save time, maintaining that they could not afford to do otherwise. Another factor, contended Eardley Holland, president of the new College of Obstetricians and Gynaecologists, was the increasing tendency among GPs, despite warnings from leading obstetrics teachers, to view childbirth as pathology; consequently, they widened their indications for intervention, with catastrophic results (Holland 1935). Significantly, charitable and municipal outdoor midwife services for the poor consistently returned a maternal death rate of half the Registrar-General's national figure and lower than rates in more affluent areas where medical attendance predominated.

State midwifery

With continuing worries about the falling birth rate and high maternal mortality, Parliament's response was the 1936 Midwives Act. This required County Councils and County Borough Councils to provide for a whole-time midwife service adequate to local needs and free or at reduced cost to poorer women. From this point, the majority of midwives became salaried, uniformed, pensioned professionals, with paid leave, offering a more complete service and receiving official recognition of their contribution to the national well-being of women (see Fig. 2.8). Many of those not selected for the new service were bought out of their practices, and those considered unfit compulsorily retired. Further, unregistered women were no longer permitted to act as maternity nurses. The act passed without adverse comment from the medical press, probably because of GPs' improved financial security (largely a consequence of the 1911 National Insurance panel system), and GPs were now content to leave 'cheap midwifery' to the midwife. However, although municipal midwives were better off, interrupted nights followed by a full working day remained a feature of domiciliary practice.

THE NATIONAL HEALTH SERVICE, MATERNITY CARE AND THE MIDWIFE

Twelve years later, in 1948, under the free and comprehensive National Health Service (NHS) established by the

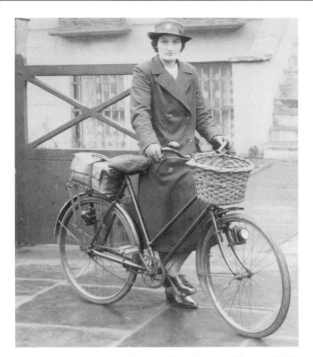

Figure 2.8 A London County Council domiciliary midwife prepares to go on a call. (Used with permission from RCM/RCOG archives, Royal College of Midwives (RCM).)

1945 Labour government as part of the new welfare state, midwife, GP and hospital services were provided free to all, irrespective of income. A great expansion of professional education also took place, and, at last, midwife training was free. Yet continuing prejudice was directed against non-nurse midwives. Indeed, the upper-middle-class ladies who had led the Midwives' Institute to victory had come into midwifery *from nursing*, already made 'respectable' by Florence Nightingale and others. By being nurses first, they had cast a cloak of respectability over midwifery and established an ethos that was to prevail for over 80 years. Midwives lacking the sanitizing badge of a nurse qualification were treated as if carrying the lingering taint of 'Mrs Gamp', and although many such midwives had more midwifery experience than those holding nurse qualifications, midwifery promotion invariably went to the latter (Radford and Thompson 1988). Furthermore, the Scottish and Irish registration acts had required all midwife pupils to be qualified nurses, and over time, English 'direct-entry' midwifery courses were officially discouraged, until by 1980 only one such school remained. Yet many nurses qualifying in midwifery never practised it, whereas the great majority of direct-entry midwives stayed in the work.

Place of birth

By the 1950s, the long-sought fall in maternal mortality had arrived. *Sulphonamide drugs* had appeared in 1936, followed a decade later by antibiotics. Together with stricter attention to asepsis and antisepsis in delivery and puerperium, these drugs had virtually eliminated puerperal sepsis, in 1930 still responsible for around 40% of maternal deaths. By 1945, the 1931–1935 statistic of 4 deaths per 1000 live births had been halved and by 1950 halved again. A crucial factor in this continued decline, however, as McKeown (1976) noted in relation to other health problems, was the generally improved standard of living, resulting, in particular, in a dramatic reduction in rachitic pelves and anaemia (Worth 2002).

Despite these advances and the excellent results consistently achieved by domiciliary midwives, the trend to (more expensive) hospital delivery was officially encouraged, on obstetricians' advice, as being safer for mother and baby in *all* cases, a view later challenged by independent statistical analysis (Tew 1978). By 1958, 64% of births took place in hospital, many in general practitioner units (GPUs), smaller and more local than consultant-led units (CUs). With estimated maternal mortality rates (now more widely defined as deaths from causes attributed to pregnancy and childbirth per 1000 total live and still-births) as low as 0.18 for England and Wales in 1968 (Department of Health and Social Security (DHSS) 1975: Table 1.3) and 0.14 for 1969 in Scotland (Macfarlane et al 2000: Tables A 3.3.2, A 10.2.1), attention had turned increasingly to *perinatal mortality*. Defined as stillbirth and infant death within the first week, and standing at over 23 per 1000 births, this was higher in low-income groups (where maternal health was poorer) than among the better-off.

In 1970, the Health Department's Maternity Advisory Committee, chaired by Sir John Peel, president of the Royal College of Obstetricians and Gynaecologists (RCOG), presented its recommendations for remedial measures (DHSS 1970). These were based (unscientifically, in the absence of impartial statistical analysis) on the facile but erroneous equation between the falling perinatal mortality rate (PMR) and increasing hospitalization. Ignoring substantial GP and midwife opinion to the contrary, the Committee recommended the transfer of home midwifery services to hospital control, effected in 1974 with their removal from elected local councils to the new unelected, hospital-dominated area health authorities. Hospital delivery was now over 80%, and expecting this soon to reach 100%, the Committee pronounced 'academic' any discussion of the scheme's advantages or disadvantages. The consultant-led 'obstetric team' (to include GPs and midwives) should therefore undertake the 'education' of the community on the 'benefits' of the reorganization (DHSS 1970).

Most obvious were the benefits to obstetricians' status and career prospects, with increased resources directed to CUs at the expense of home midwifery and GPUs. Equally clear were the drawbacks for midwives and mothers. Midwives, who had successfully looked after women throughout pregnancy, labour and puerperium, enjoying independence and variety in their duties and receiving recognition and respect from their communities, were forced into the impersonal and separated hospital ward to work under the direction of the obstetrician or restricted to community postnatal care. Women's choice of place of delivery under the NHS was also disappearing. Many had preferred the familiarity of home, with the attention of a known midwife; others had chosen the local GPUs, again with attendants known to them. Increasingly, however, women were to be compelled, possibly with children in tow, to make time-consuming visits to the large central district hospital for antenatal care and to deliver in stark, impersonal surroundings among strangers. In many areas, women insisting on home birth or other non-interventionist care made private arrangements with a midwife or doctor at their own expense.

Pathways to abnormality: the 'new obstetrics'

Perinatal mortality was considered further by the 1980 Commons' Social Services Committee (the Short Committee). Despite hospital births now standing at 98% and preferential allocation of medical resources to less favoured regions, the gap between perinatal mortality rates for wealthier areas compared to poorer areas had widened. Although admitting that some procedures employed in intrapartum care had never been scientifically evaluated, the Committee nevertheless accepted its medical advisers' view that it was 'reasonable' to believe that 'professional' intervention could substantially lower the PMR. It therefore recommended further increases in consultant obstetrician posts with even greater concentration of births in large CUs and further restriction of home birth. Furthermore, wholly accepting the view of childbirth as pathology, its report demanded that its routine management be on the same basis as acute illness, in conditions of 'intensive care' (DHSS 1980).

This was already the case in many CUs. Here, older obstetricians' 'watchful expectancy' in normal birth had been superseded by the current North American doctrine of 'active management' followed in other countries, including Ireland (O'Driscoll and Meagher 1986). The synthesis in the late 1950s of *oxytocin* as Syntocinon provided a more reliable means of induction of labour. Hitherto, induction had generally been employed only for fetal post-maturity and maternal pre-eclampsia; thenceforth, however, its use escalated, rising from 13% in 1958 to nearly 40% in 1974, and to 75% with some consultants.

Significantly fewer births took place on weekends or public holidays. Syntocinon could also be used to accelerate labour already ongoing and to shorten it to conform to new restricted definitions of 'normal labour' derived from the arithmetical averages of the new 'partograms', rather than the limits of healthy experience.

Yet none of these procedures, observed critics, was wholly benign. Instead they led to a 'cascade of interventions' as obstetricians, many apparently still infected with the ancient Aristotelian notion of the female body as defective (Barnes 1984: 1144) and hence requiring correction, persuaded themselves that techniques helpful in abnormal labour would assuredly benefit *all* cases. No birth therefore could be viewed as normal except in retrospect. Indeed, with multiple interventions, fewer births actually were normal. Syntocinon infusions and the use of continuous electronic fetal monitoring (which carries a high false-positive rate and is associated with higher CS rates) both inhibited mobility, for centuries valued as facilitating labour. Contractions were more violent and more painful than in natural labour, with greater risk of uterine rupture.

Enhanced pain required stronger pain relief, progressively supplied with new drugs and lumbar epidural analgesia. Epidurals may diminish uterine activity and reduce women's mobility during labour, tending to hinder the natural rotation and descent of the fetus, and inhibit the urge to push, thus prolonging labour, with the risk also of maternal circulatory collapse. More malpresentations and forceps deliveries resulted, with attendant risk to the child and the discomfort of episiotomy, with possible lasting adverse sequelae for the mother (Wagner 2001). If the epidural were mismanaged, permanent paralysis, coma or even death could ensue (May 1994). Episiotomy became routine, mistakenly justified as preventing serious perineal tears and pelvic floor damage; by 1980, episiotomies were being used on average in 52% of cases in England and Wales (Tew 1995: 165). The dorsal position (the legs possibly raised in stirrups) replaced the left lateral position for birth, becoming the standard delivery position. Although it was known to be more painful for the woman and problematic for the fetus, it was praised in a leading midwives' manual as more 'comfortable' and as facilitating pushing efforts (Myles 1981: 309).

Moreover, as 'failure to progress' (defined by the strict timetables routinely now governing labour) increasingly resulted in CS, rates for this major operation rose rapidly. This fact alone led to further intervention – the prohibition or restriction of nutrition to *every* parturient to fit her for general anaesthesia in case a caesarean should be required. Clearly such debilitating deprivation at a time when women need all their physical and mental strength is itself likely to contribute to 'failure to progress'. This deprivation is now contraindicated (National Institute for Health and Care Excellence (NICE) 2014) but was still imposed in some UK hospitals (NICE 2007: 18). Growing use of analgesic drugs, too, had consequences for the baby. Crossing the placenta, these have a depressing effect on the fetus, which may result in protracted difficulties in breathing and sucking, necessitating time in the (expensive) neonatal care unit.

Responses of the midwifery profession

Although the Peel and Short Committees had both recommended that full use should be made of midwives' expertise, their actual recommendations pointed in the opposite direction. The disappearance of home midwifery and increased medicalization of hospital birth meant that midwives, officially excluded by the 1902 act from attending abnormal labour, were now losing their role as guardians of normal birth. Midwifery skills were devalued in favour of interventionist methods that midwives themselves, many unwillingly, and against their professional judgement, were required to adopt (Reid 2002). Moreover, experienced midwives were increasingly required to defer to *senior house officers* who, despite their designation, were junior doctors doing their 6 months' obstetric training. Further, hospital midwives' work was increasingly compartmentalized into antenatal, intrapartum or postnatal care, with some midwives seldom delivering a baby and practically none following a pregnant woman throughout pregnancy to labour and delivery.

For domiciliary midwives whose long years of low pay and broken nights had nonetheless given them the immense satisfaction of birthing women successfully in their own homes, the condemnation of home midwifery, despite excellent safety records, as 'unsafe' was tantamount to the negation of their life's work. For many, the experience was traumatic, and retirement could not come too soon (Allison 1996: ix–x). Others tolerated the transfer to hospital as bringing shorter, more convenient hours, less responsibility and improved career opportunities. At this time, the RCM did not seriously oppose this transformation of the midwife's work. Overcome by the confidence with which obstetricians (generally male and of superior educational and social status) put their case to the government, the RCM appeared to acquiesce as the ancient office of midwife was increasingly eroded and its own avowed purpose, 'the advancement of the art and science of midwifery', effectively abandoned. Signalling its acceptance of the total hospitalization of birth in 1974, it abolished its long-standing Domiciliary Midwives Council. Some leading midwives expressed regret at these changes; others espoused them whole-heartedly, seeing reliance on technology as increasing midwives' status, rather than, in fact, reducing it. There was no sympathy for midwives seeking to undertake home delivery; women desiring this, or intervention-free hospital care, were to be bullied into acceptance of what was now NHS policy.

Especially striking was the turnabout demonstrated in the 1975, 1981 and 1987 editions of Margaret Myles's *Textbook for Midwives,* a standard work used in many midwifery schools since 1953. Hitherto, Myles, herself a midwife, had spoken of home as the 'ideal' place of delivery, affirming nature's power in the vast majority of cases to complete unaided childbirth successfully and warning against the dangers of 'meddlesome midwifery'. Yet later editions dismissed the older philosophy of 'watchful expectancy' in labour as 'negative', applauding instead the 'modern concept' of 'active management', with its 'planned positive approach'. The management of 'normal' labour now included routine interventions, justified as ensuring greater maternal and fetal safety, and psychophysical methods of pain management were dismissed in favour of drugs. Midwives must accept 'modern ideas', it advised, working to secure the compliance of the 'misinformed' minority of expectant mothers who demanded intervention-free birth and 'outmoded' continuity of carer. Hospital delivery was strongly advocated; indeed, for a midwife to take sole charge of a woman, depriving her of the 'scientific expert care' of the 'obstetric team', would be a retrograde step. Midwives should relish their new, more fulfilling role as technically qualified members of the medically controlled 'team' (as 'mini-obstetricians' is implied) rather than seeing themselves as clinically independent practitioners as sanctioned by the pervious acts. Not all midwives approved of these developments. Some, including the *Association of Radical Midwives (ARM),* decided to fight the trend from within the NHS; others left the service to practise privately as independent practitioners, offering home delivery and choice of birth positions.

User protest and the 'Active Childbirth' movement

Protests came, too, from among childbearing women themselves, their complaints supported by healthcare user organizations forming part of the post-war consumer movement. Among these were the National Childbirth Trust (NCT) and the increasingly assertive Association for Improvements in the Maternity Services (AIMS). AIMS demanded more sympathetic maternity care, including choice of home birth, of intervention-free care and of birthing positions, ideas generally dismissed in medical circles as the fads of a misguided middle-class minority. Such women, wrote one obstetrician, were too ignorant or selfish to accept their role as 'patients', even for their infants' safety. Clearly viewing the womb as a railway engine, he censured complainants for 'dictating their treatment', thus relegating professionals 'from the signal-box to the footplate' (namely, from their *rightful position of controlling labour* to one of merely *observing* it). Moreover, despite radiological evidence that squatting during the second stage enlarged the pelvic outlet by almost 30% compared to the generally used supine position (Russell 1982), upright delivery was condemned as too 'primitive' (outdated) or too 'innovative' (untested). Furthermore, the 'bizarre' positions 'professionals' would have to adopt would adversely affect their 'sense of security' in their work. This was a time of huge change and media and public interest in the quality of maternity care, which included a protest at a major London teaching hospital calling for choice in birthing position; increased interest in the work of birth possibilities as espoused by Michel Odent (suggesting upright and water births) (Odent 1976); and interest in the possible effects of a tranquil birth as demonstrated by Leboyer, both on television and in print (Leboyer 2011). Women were excited and enthused by these initiatives, which were supported by increased research and evidence validating active and upright birth and the value of a humane birthing environment. Midwives themselves began to be interested in this movement, more labour wards and delivery units were humanized and midwives began to use these strategies in their practice.

FURTHER LEGISLATIVE FRAMEWORKS: NURSES, MIDWIVES AND HEALTH VISITORS ACT OF 1979, NURSING AND MIDWIFERY ORDER 2001 AND BEYOND …

Meanwhile, midwives faced other problems following the implementation in 1983 of the government-sponsored Nurses, Midwives and Health Visitors Act of 1979. This replaced the different regulatory machinery for these three professions in England, Wales, Scotland and Northern Ireland with one umbrella organization, the United Kingdom Central Council (UKCC). Following representations to government by a reinvigorated RCM, the midwife's distinctive nature was recognized with the establishment of a statutory *Standing Midwifery Committee* to consider all 'matters relating to midwifery'. However, because the Committee was subordinate to the nurse-dominated UKCC, midwives were no more a self-regulating profession than they had been under the CMB.

Nurses' lack of empathy for midwifery matters was especially manifest in *Project 2000*, the UKCC's 1986 proposal for combining the basic education of the three professions into a 2-year nursing programme followed by 1 year's specialization, with midwifery as one of the 'specialties'. Midwifery education for students taking such courses would thus be reduced to 1 year of actual midwifery knowledge. Opposing this strongly, the RCM argued that midwives' clinical responsibilities clearly distinguished them from nurses, and that to cut midwife education would demote midwifery to a branch of nursing (RCM 1986). Moreover, the proposal contravened the 1980 European Union (EU) directives that laid down requirements for UK midwives wishing to practise in European Commission (EC) countries, where midwives, as in former times, had longer midwifery training and generally were not nurses. Faced with this reality, the Council yielded.

An interesting turnabout then took place. Direct-entry midwifery courses, instead of being phased out, were to be expanded and given higher status, thus reversing a century-old trend and preventing official downgrading of midwifery to obstetric nursing. Direct-entry courses now outnumber the shortened ones (see Ch. 5). It is also of note that the midwifery programmes achieved degree status ahead of the nursing profession.

The UKCC remained in place, with some modifications, until 2002, when the Nursing and Midwifery Order of 2001 came into being, establishing the *Nursing and Midwifery Council (NMC)*, which was tasked with maintaining a register, setting standards of education and practice and investigating allegations of poor practice (see Ch. 3). At this point the UKCC ceased to exist, and the National Boards – England, Wales, Scotland and Northern Ireland – were abolished. NHS Scotland, Healthcare Inspectorate Wales and Northern Ireland Practice and Education Council (NIPEC) took some of the roles formally undertaken by the National Boards.

From a midwifery perspective, the NMC retained the *midwifery committee*, a small number of senior midwives who are tasked with advising the NMC on 'any matters affecting midwifery', including professional and policy developments and prospective or actual changes in statutory regulation, and this includes education, practice and supervision (see Chs 3 and 4).

In September 2015, following a review informed by the Kirkup (2015) report and a report commissioned by the NMC (Baird et al 2015) evaluating supervision, the decision was taken to separate supervision from legislation. This has had a mixed reception, raising concern on the possible effect on the care of women and babies and the support of midwives, as expressed by Kirby (2015), who stated that the 'dismantling of statutory supervision would leave a void that will impact on midwives, women and maternity services' (see Ch. 3).

Finding a new voice

A further sign of a more vigorous, enterprising stance among midwives was demonstrated by the 1989 edition of *Myles' Textbook*, now under new authorship (Bennett and Brown 1989). The new edition contrasted sharply with previous ones, with referencing and research included, and in an entirely new departure for a midwifery manual, it emphasized the midwife's duty to accommodate, where feasible, women's choice of labour and delivery positions, forms of pain relief and so on. It also noted that midwives should also strive to make this normal but critical life event as happy as possible for mother, partner and family. Significantly, the corresponding edition of *Mayes' Midwifery*, the other standard textbook in the field, contained a similar approach, focusing on lifelong learning, research and evidence. Further noteworthy professional developments arising from the ranks were the foundation in 1986 of MIDIRS, a midwife-run quarterly critical digest of recent literature and research in maternity care. This, together with the arrival in 1993 of the *British Journal of Midwifery*, *'Midwifery'* and *Evidence Based Midwifery*, has provided a strong midwifery-led research and evidence base for students and qualified midwives to utilize. The increasing activity in research has also strengthened the profession's voice, especially with the rise of midwifery-led research and research questions focusing on issues of concern to women and midwives coming to the fore (Baxter 2007; Devane et al 2010; Downe et al 2001; Lavender et al 2006; Sandall et al 2015).

'Choice, continuity and control'

In 1991, on the initiative of Audrey Wise, MP, who wished to know why young women she knew were finding childbirth so traumatic, maternity services were again studied, this time by the Commons' Health Committee (Chairman Nicholas Winterton, MP). Unlike previous enquiries appointed by the Health Department, the Committee did not start from the negative standpoint of childbirth as an inevitably hazardous enterprise needing medical management, but as a normal physiological function that healthy women could generally perform successfully unaided. For the first time, too, midwives were included among the advisers, and submissions, written and oral, were invited from service users and providers. Again unlike previous Committee recommendations, Winterton placed more credence on impartial statistical analyses than on the unproven assertions of obstetricians.

Moreover, because evidence on safety did not support the policy of 100% consultant unit (CU) delivery, the Committee argued for wider choice of place of birth (House of Commons Health Committee (HCHC) 1992: xlviii). GPUs, rural or urban, offered a compromise between home birth and delivery in a CU, and it was recommended that their closure on presumptive grounds of safety or cost should be abandoned forthwith (HCHC 1992: lxv). Taking maternal satisfaction with maternity services as its criterion of success, the Committee condemned the current professional choice of the PMR as the sole yardstick of the performance of maternity services, arguing rather for these to be audited in terms of *maternal morbidity* (HCHC 1992: lxii).

The Committee observed that, like other medical specialties, obstetrics had been subject to fashion, with procedures introduced merely because they were available and used routinely without consideration of possible adverse maternal consequences (HCHC 1992: xlviii–xlix). Women should therefore be given the option of refusing interventions, including induction, electronic fetal monitoring, epidurals and episiotomies, rather than having to undergo them as routine (HCHC 1992: xxiii). They should also be enabled to feel in control of their labour, to adopt positions of choice (HCHC 1992: lxix) and to be attended throughout labour by the same midwife. The Committee summed up its philosophy under the tenets, *'choice, continuity and control'*. Significantly, it concluded that essential to the development of the more user-friendly maternity services was a reassessment of the midwife's role. Calling for the restoration of midwives' former clinical responsibilities, the Committee condemned the current use of midwives as 'a scandalous waste of money' (HCHC 1992: lxxxi).

The government's response, *'Changing Childbirth'* (Department of Health (DH) 1993), accepted Winterton's philosophy of 'woman-centred' care, suggesting 5-year targets towards the implementation of its recommendations. However, this document was merely consultative and lacked the 'teeth' and funding necessary to enforce any widespread change. Women seeking home birth still reported GPs threatening to strike them off their NHS lists, and many health authorities refused them on grounds of midwife shortages. Where they existed, midwife-run units, despite their recorded low intervention rates and increased maternal satisfaction, remained on sufferance, with health authorities resenting the expense of maintaining these 'experiments' in addition to their ordinary hospital establishments (Lee 2001).

Whose choice in childbirth?

Responding to *Changing Childbirth*, the RCOG qualified its acceptance of the ideal of 'woman-oriented care', invoking considerations of 'safety', a veiled justification of current interventionist practice. Significantly, it also argued for 'equal attention' to be paid to the welfare of the fetus, *'the other important person'* in the case (RCOG 1993). For centuries, English law had not recognized the unborn child as a 'person' (the principle underlying current abortion law). Yet in 1992, obstetricians from a London hospital had obtained a court order for a forced caesarean on a mother refusing her consent on religious grounds. Similar orders followed, all granted *without* maternal representation in court, until in May 1998 the Appeal Court ruled illegal the forcible invasion of a competent adult's body, even if a woman's life *or* that of her fetus depended on it. The fetus was *not* a separate person from its mother, and its medical needs could not override her rights to self-determination. Notwithstanding this definitive judgement, some obstetricians persist in a curious doublethink. This allows them to view the aborted fetus (up to term if 'handicapped') as a *non-person*, but to describe the fetus of the pregnant mother who may resist intervention as a 'patient', thus, illogically and incorrectly, endowing it with *full-person* status with rights equal to, or overriding, those of the mother (Royal Society of Medicine 2002).

Apart from the Appeal Court's clear-cut confirmation of the parturient's legal autonomy, the opportunity for true user choice is questionable. For true choice to be exercised, full and unbiased information on available options is essential (see Ch. 34). However, an assessment of hospital antenatal information-giving showed that in some units choice was limited. In effect, women were steered towards acceptance of obstetrician-determined technological intervention through information that minimized its risks and exaggerated the potential harm of doing without (Stapleton et al 2002).

Moreover, intervention was actually coming to be represented as part of normal birth. A 2001 study in the Trent region demonstrated that in over 60% of the 956 deliveries recorded as 'normal' or 'spontaneous' (that is, excluding instrumental or CS deliveries), interventions had occurred. These included amniotomy, induction and/or augmentation of labour, episiotomy and epidural anaesthesia. In about a third, induction or augmentation of labour had taken place, and 89% of amniotomies were performed before the cervix was fully dilated (Downe 2001; Downe et al 2001).

A more recent study indicated although there may be structures and programmes in place to support choice of birth place, the majority of women in the UK continue to give birth in a hospital environment, and this may be influenced firstly by practitioners making assumptions that women need to give birth in hospitals and secondly by a lack of reflection in those practitioners (Houghton et al 2008). A study by Grigg et al (2015) in New Zealand identified some of the complexities in this choice and highlighted the importance of women themselves having confidence in their ability to give birth in a smaller, midwife-led birth unit (see Ch. 34).

Childbirth a 'surgical operation'?

Given this high level of intervention, it was unsurprising that the 2001 Scottish Expert Advisory Group (Scottish Programme for Clinical Effectiveness in Reproductive Health (SPCERH) 2001) reported that Scotland's caesarean section rate (CSR) approached 20%, and the National Sentinel Audit revealed even higher rates in England, Wales and Northern Ireland. Moreover, remarkable variations in CSRs existed between regions and between hospitals. These disparities were inexplicable by reference to case mix, as were variations in CS percentages ascribed to different primary indications, clearly demonstrating the

absence of any agreed objective criteria of 'need'. Disturbingly, although half the obstetricians responding to the enquiry considered existing rates too high, 21% did not. Furthermore, in private hospitals, where obstetricians are paid by item-of-service, much larger fees are paid for this invasive procedure than for the oversight of vaginal delivery. Here, the CSR has been much higher, in some over 40% (Churchill et al 2006: 54). Yet the 1985 Consensus Conference of the World Health Organization (WHO) concluded that no improvement in outcomes could be expected from a CSR exceeding 10% to 15%, a rate maintained by Holland and the Scandinavian countries, which have some of the world's lowest maternal and perinatal mortality rates (Wagner 2000). Nor, declared Wagner, WHO's former director of Women's and Children's Health, was there any evidence for obstetricians' claims that CS reduced perinatal mortality (Wagner 2000).

Although the direct financial inducements that may influence obstetricians' CS decisions in private hospitals do not apply in the NHS, the system of *payment by results* (PBR), introduced in England in 2004, created perverse incentives for hospital trusts to favour elective CS (Baldwin et al 2007). Other factors include 'daylight obstetrics' to suit the obstetrician's convenience (Brown 1996; Gans et al 2007), fear of litigation and repeat CS (around 14% of the total (Churchill et al 2006: 88)), thus further augmenting the CSR. Another element in the rise in CS is the 7% or so of cases recorded by obstetricians as responses to 'maternal request'. Some women requesting CS are motivated by previous negative experience of vaginal birth; others are possessed by a general fear of childbirth generated by today's culture, especially by TV (Baxter 2007; Gould 2007). Some have been persuaded that CS is safer for the baby (NICE 2004; Weaver and Statham 2005), an opinion the 2001 Sentinel Audit found was held by half of its obstetrician respondents. The Sentinel Audit also found that obstetricians probably underestimated how many of women's decision to choose CS were in fact influenced by the advice they themselves had given. Obstetricians may also argue that they have no time to give women full and unbiased information on what is known about CS (Wagner 2000), and, as women's testimony demonstrates, some obstetricians believe that women do not need this knowledge (Barbieri 2006).

Certainly, research suggests that a significant proportion of women who have had CS did not understand the reason for it (Baldwin et al 2007; Baxter 2007), and some complain that they have been brow-beaten into having caesareans they did not want (Weaver and Statham 2005). AIMS reported that its representatives are contacted almost daily by women desperate to avoid a caesarean (Beech 2006). Constituting 24% or so of all births for 2005–2006, CS deliveries accounted for over 40% of delivery spending, at a cost of £2 billion a year to the NHS (NHS Institute for Innovation and Improvement 2006).

However, it seems the tide may be turning, with the most recent NICE recommendations emphasizing the need to consider CS for women who request this and highlighting the importance of the woman having a full discussion of her options, risks and benefits, which might include perinatal mental health support (NICE 2011).

Governmental views

The financial burden on the NHS was initially noted in the NICE 2004 CS guidelines, in the hope of reducing the ever-rising CSR (Scotland had similar guidelines). This has now been superseded by the NICE 2011 guidelines. Risks to mother and infant of both methods of delivery were compared, and CS is now discouraged where any supposed benefits over vaginal delivery are uncertain, and maternal request for CS is not automatically considered adequate grounds at this time. Although many obstetricians regard the CSR as too high, others celebrate its increase, and the guidelines ('this edict') came under immediate attack from two London obstetricians. Invoking the Winterton principle of 'choice in childbirth', they declared CS the safest method of delivery for the mother and (especially) the baby, insisting that 'most' obstetricians shared this view (Fisk and Paterson-Brown 2004).

Yet repeatedly the International Federation of Gynaecology and Obstetrics (FIGO) has declared normal vaginal delivery to be safer both in the short and long term for both mother and child, and that CS for non-medical reasons is ethically unjustified (FIGO 1999, 2003, 2008). Significantly, also, in 2002 the leading private health insurance firm AXA-PPP ceased paying for CS because it was becoming increasingly difficult for the company to distinguish between medically necessary CS cases and those that were a matter of personal choice (British Broadcasting Company (BBC) 2002).

FIGO's stance on the overall greater safety of vaginal over caesarean delivery is supported by the recent multicentre prospective cohort study (part of a WHO global survey) of 97,095 births. The study concluded that the increased CSR at an institutional level over recent years was not associated with any clear overall benefit for mother or baby, but linked it with greater morbidity for both (Villar et al 2007). A further study demonstrated that for those who had previously had a CS, low-risk women had a lower risk of maternal complications or perinatal mortality compared to high-risk women (Kaboré et al 2015).

Other negative effects may include emergency hysterectomy, reduced fertility, an increased rate of unexplained stillbirths, iatrogenic prematurity, fetal laceration, perforation of the maternal bowel and sepsis of the genital tract (Langdana et al 2001; Robinson 2004/5; Smith et al 1997, 2003a, 2003b; Wagner 2000). Indeed, two female London obstetricians propose that, in the absence of medical indications, CS should be performed only with a confirmatory second opinion (Bewley and Cockburn 2002).

'Choice, continuity and control'? From Winterton, to maternity matters to better births and beyond

One recent NICE publication had echoes of Winterton's tenets of choice, continuity and control, offering 'best practice advice' on the care of healthy labouring women and their babies (NICE 2014). These guidelines promote control, respect and compassion, highlighting the need for choice for the woman, based on good, evidence-based information. This includes being given explicit information and choice on place of birth, whether at home (Fig. 2.9), in the birth centre or hospital, and provision of one-to-one care. If all was progressing well, clinical interventions should be neither offered nor advised. The *Birth*

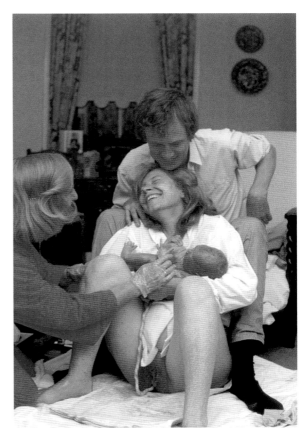

Figure 2.9 A modern home birth. (Sally and Richard Greenhill Photographic Library.)

Place Choices study was the first major study to investigate place of birth and safety (Birthplace in England Collaborative Group 2011a). The study's evidence suggested that birth is 'generally very safe', and birth centres and midwifery-led units provide a safe and beneficial choice for women and their babies. For second and subsequent pregnancies, the risk of interventions and need for CS were found to be lower for those booked into a birth centre. For first-time mothers, a planned home birth was found to carry a higher risk of a perinatal event, and for those first-time mothers giving birth in a birth centre or midwifery-led unit, there were higher risks of transfer during labour or after birth (Birthplace in England Collaborative Group 2011b).

However, the home-birth rate in England and Wales decreased slightly to 2.3% in 2013, compared to 2.4% in 2011 (Office for National Statistics 2014) (1.38% in Scotland and 0.28% in Northern Ireland). This may be because of active discouragement by practitioners who may have a lack of experience with, or confidence in, the process (Edwards 2005, 2008). It is also possible that a shortage of midwives may affect whether a home birth can be facilitated (RCM 2015a). Another birth choice is the midwife-led units, which currently support 4% to 5% of total births (Dodwell 2013). These birth units have increased slightly in number, although some have closed, and, despite their consistently good results (Rowbotham and Hunt 2006), government support for such centres is condemned by some obstetricians as a 'cheese-paring' move to substitute an 'inferior' service for that of the obstetrician-led CU (Carlisle 2007) and by some media as inherently dangerous (Sarler 2012).

It is encouraging that women's own views of their birth experiences, which were recorded by the Healthcare Commission's (HCC's) nationwide survey of 26,000 respondents giving birth early in 2007 (HCC 2007, 2008), and then more recently in 2013, are improving. However, the 2015 survey identified areas requiring further development (Care Quality Commission (CQC) 2015). Many women felt more supported, and they valued continuity and being listened to by the midwife. However, some women reported a lack of consistent information, and one in five felt that their concerns during labour were not taken seriously. This was supported by an NPEU report (Redshaw and Henderson 2015), which also highlighted that more women were aware of options for birth place, although 33% reported that they were only provided with one choice.

There were few differences between the 2008 and 2015 CQC reports in terms of position adopted during labour and birth, with few adopting alternative positions. A surprising 19% of women who had a normal birth did so with their legs in stirrups (CQC 2015), and 71% of women were able to move around most of the time during labour, to be comfortable. Of those birthing vaginally, 13% gave birth standing, squatting or kneeling; 18% sitting up in bed; 5% on their sides; and 32% lying flat/supported with pillows, the latter a position condemned by leading obstetricians over 15 years ago (Steer and Flint 1999). Unfortunately, 27% reported being left alone at a time of anxiety to them (Steer and Flint 1999), which indicates that although there has been some progress, there are still areas of concern.

A recent wide-ranging review in England was commissioned by the NHS Chief Executive, led by Baroness Cumberledge (Cumberledge 2016). The terms of reference were to 'review the UK and international evidence and make recommendations on safe and efficient models of maternity service, including midwife led units'. This was in the context of the events at Morecombe Bay, and thus safety and quality underpinned the work.

The review sought views from professionals, the public, users of the service and others over the period of 1 year, gathering information and views from all over England. This resulted in a visionary document and recommendations for ensuring choice and safety for women, including continuity of care. The media headlines were that women will hold the funding for their care. This might be seen as an updated 'Changing Childbirth', and many of the messages are similar. However, the NHS have responded with the Maternity Transformation Programme (NHS 2016) which appears to be actioning many aspects of Better Births, though it is presently too soon to evaluate what effect this might have on women and babies and midwives and their practice.

Rise of the birth centre/midwifery-led units

Increasingly, other options are becoming available to childbearing women, including more choice about home birth, midwifery-led units (MLUs) and birth centres (Redshaw and Henderson 2015; NICE 2014). The development of birth centres and MLUs, especially in England and Wales, has partly been led by service reconfigurations – for example, where services have been centralized in one larger centralized medical unit (CMU), an MLU has been set up alongside or in a previous smaller maternity unit. This has often been accompanied by vociferous local and national media reports opposed to 'downgrading' of maternity units, viewing the loss of consultant cover as a major disadvantage. This is often played out in the media, which portrays a "battle" to maintain maternity services within one region and consolidation of obstetrics into one unit and the development of MLUs only in another being promoted as unfair and unsafe (BBC 2013, 2015). Even the RCM, which supports MLUs and birth centres, has used similar terms for these changes (Dabrowski 2013). This inevitably gives the impression that midwife-led service is a lesser service for women and their babies in terms of quality and safety, and this is promulgated by those who are most affected by the change. Women's own expectations and wishes are also important. The women who are having babies now have grown up in a culture where hospital birth is the norm, and their lack of experience and knowledge of alternatives makes a birth centre, MLU, or home birth seem a radical choice.

However, as amalgamated units get larger, and more impersonal, there is the potential to move to 'conveyer-belt care' (Allotey et al 2012), perhaps making MLUs and birth centres more attractive choices. Approximately 1.8% to 4% of births take place in MLUs and birth centres, and there are significant regional variations, with the southwest and Wales having the highest proportions (Dodwell 2013). Just as these initiatives offer a more 'homely' atmosphere, better continuity of care for women and their families, less interventions and more satisfaction, they also offer midwives a better experience, with more autonomy of practice, continuity of care and relationship (Sandall et al 2015). However, as some birth centres and MLUs open, others close (Beech 2012; Dodwell 2013) – often because of financial constraints – again reducing women's and midwives' choices.

Risk, practices and research

Underpinning the much-used obstetricians' dictum that no birth is normal until it is over is the now ubiquitous concept of 'risk'. That certain risks exist in pregnancy and childbirth has always been known, the most serious of which are generally readily recognizable by expert clinicians. Yet difficulties in risk-factor definition and quantification render risk-scoring 'systems' highly suspect, and their predictive values, positive and negative, have proved poor (Enkin et al 2000: 49–51; Tew 1995: 110–111, 256–268, 330–338).

The medical preoccupation with risk can leave midwives, the supposed guardians of normal birth (intervention-free birth), isolated and their experience and expertise undermined. Nowadays, except when they attend home births or work in freestanding midwife-led birth centres, the practice of midwives is generally governed or at least heavily influenced by largely obstetrician-determined protocols. These include tools and approaches that may have been adopted on the basis of limited research and evidence. One example is the partogram (see Chs 36 and 37), which is used to plot the progress of the woman and the fetus throughout labour. A survey by Lavender et al (2008) found that most do not define the start of active labour. The rate of progress, too, was usually not reported, and when it was, some units specified 'normal' progress as cervical dilation of 0.5 cm an hour, others as 1 cm an hour, and others as *twice* as much. Interestingly, only seven units used a different partogram for multiparous and primiparous women. A Cochrane review suggested that there was limited evidence to support the routine use of partograms (Lavender et al 2013) for 'standard labour management and care'. However, partograms are still in use, and it appears that tools such as the partogram are 'entrenched' in the system (Lavender et al 2008). Such situations, however, are not new. In former times, childbearing women and their infants suffered from the currently accepted medical interventions and prescriptions, also presented as vital to their well-being and equally based on the false premise that nature *routinely* needs help, control and correction. Among many such discarded 'best' medical practices have been 'prophylactic' blood-letting in pregnancy, labour and miscarriage; routine purging of newborns and substitution of indigestible artificial foods for the 'harmful' colostrum; and for post-parturient women, the mandatory semi-starvation diet and prolonged bed rest, the latter, indeed, persisting until after World War II (Donnison 2007).

This example illustrates the changing landscape of midwifery practice and the potential for change towards more individualized, evidence-based care.

Increasingly, practice is being guided by research and evidence (see Ch. 6), and midwives themselves have taken a strong role in leading research. From a period in which midwives had few resources, including access to and standards of education, this has been a significant achievement, and it may go some way toward equalizing the relationships between professional groups.

Reflective activity 2.1

Which features of midwifery practice of former times do you think would be valuable in contemporary midwifery practice?

MIDWIFERY – NOW AND IN THE FUTURE

As already stated, the future of midwives proper (as opposed to those acting under medical direction in interventionist birth, in fact, as maternity nurses) is bound up with normal birth. However, except for births at home or in MLUs, normal births (defined as births without induction, caesarean, instrumental delivery or episiotomy but including epidurals and other anaesthetics) are becoming the minority, being around 45% in England, 35% in Scotland and Northern Ireland and 48% in Wales (RCM 2015b).

Some women planning home birth view NHS midwives as too controlling, hiring instead independent self-employed midwives; others decide to give birth on their own (Cooper and Clarke 2008; Walsh 2008). The recent cases of 'free birth' – where a woman chooses to give birth unattended – suggest that some women may not find an attendant a comfort, or indeed may believe that an attendant would hamper the childbirth experience. This focus on the quality of experience is perhaps at odds with parts of the world where women do not have the choice of a midwife or a trained birth attendant to support and care for them during pregnancy and childbirth, and where both pregnancy and childbirth carry significant morbidity and mortality (WHO 2014). Moreover, as in Willughby's day, some women hide their pregnancies, giving birth silently in secret, leaving the child to be found by strangers. Lest any doubt the continuing and awesome power of Nature, they need only recall Sophia Pedro, who in March 2000, after 4 days in a tree surrounded by the swirling floodwaters of the Limpopo River, gave birth there to a healthy daughter before her helicopter rescue (Daniel 2008; NPR News 2000).

In recent years, the government has demonstrated an unprecedented interest in NHS maternity care services, publishing evidence-based guidelines for practitioners and sponsoring research into user opinion, the latter giving rise to *Maternity Matters* (DH 2007). This proposed that by the end of 2009, pregnant women should be able to refer themselves to a midwife or GP, as preferred; to choose birth at home or a birth centre rather than hospital; and to receive individual midwife attendance throughout labour and birth. Yet allocation of NHS funds still favours interventionist over non-interventionist care (O'Sullivan and Tyler 2007), contributing to the persistent midwife shortages hampering provision of midwife attendance in the home and continuity of care in hospital. The future may hold more optimistic approaches should the maternity review recommendations be fully implemented (Cumberledge 2016).

Although many midwives are devoted to their calling, long hours (some possibly unpaid) and insufficient staffing result in a constant drain of registered midwives from the workforce. Additionally, many are disillusioned by the gulf between their aspirations to be *true* midwives, or 'with women', and the hurried reality of care ruled by medical direction and managerial imperative (Ball et al 2006; Curtis et al 2006; Kirkham 2007). Unsurprisingly, critics argued that the goals of *Maternity Matters* were unlikely to be realized in time for the target date (ARM 2007; Clift-Matthews 2009), and a recent National Audit Office (NAO) report confirmed that indeed the goals had not been met, and the NAO did not have a strategy to measure progress against its stated aims (NAO 2013).

Reflective activity 2.2   ＞＜

What do you see as the recurring themes throughout this history of midwives and maternity care?

CONCLUSION

Ahead of the pioneers of the tiny Midwives Institute stretched a long, hard road, before, in 1902, they achieved their aim of a midwives' registration act. Equally onerous was their successors' struggle for the acceptance of midwifery as a profession, only achieved with the Institute's official elevation in 1941 to a 'College' and the granting of a Royal Charter in 1947. Since then, however, the centralization of maternity care in hospitals and the development of the 'new obstetrics' have affected the rate of normal birth and influenced the art of midwifery itself. Although recent government support for midwife-conducted birth has encouraged the RCM to speak of a 'renaissance' in midwifery (Davis 2005), this rebirth will not come of itself. First and foremost, it requires the active and enthusiastic leadership of an RCM committed to the purpose stated in its Royal Charter, namely, the furtherance of the 'art and science of midwifery'. Second, it will need, through cooperation with user groups and wider women's organizations, to make allies of the women it aims to serve (Savage 2007: 176). Third, if its 'campaign' for normal birth – now the *Better Births Initiative* (RCM 2015b) – is to succeed, the RCM, like its Victorian founders, must continue to use the sophisticated political skills and combative determination necessary to hand down to posterity, as they did, the ancient office of midwife.

This will be assisted by the midwifery leaders of this generation – in all spheres of midwifery. These midwives are vocal and passionate, and they need to continue to raise the midwifery voice to the highest level – whether through their research, education practice and management roles or through social media.

What remains positive, both to those entering and those already within the profession, is that recruitment into midwifery remains strong in the UK and other countries where it is practiced. In the UK this may be partly attributable to the success of TV dramas such as *Call the Midwife* or of 'fly on the wall' documentaries following student midwives, midwives and women. It is likely also that women, and men, are attracted to a role that is as ancient as time, constantly changing and challenging, but offering the privilege to support a woman and her family through the unique transition of pregnancy labour and puerperium to new parenthood, and the new baby to independent life.

Key Points

When considering the history of midwives and of midwifery, we need to recognize the following:

- Until relatively recently, much of the text of the medical field was written by male practitioners, members of a dominant and rival group, many of whom, confident in their male superiority, looked forward to the total abolition of the midwife.

- Many of the medical writers displayed a clear misogynistic prejudice, or at best a belittling condescension towards midwives, however skilled they were, and in fact towards childbearing women themselves.

- Lessons from the past have real relevance for the present organization of maternity care and, indeed, for that of the future as well.

References

Unless otherwise referenced, material in this chapter is taken from Jean Donnison, Midwives and medical men: a history of the struggle for the control of childbirth, London, Historical Publications, 1988.

Allison J: *Delivered at home*, London, Chapman and Hall, 1996.

Allotey J: English midwives' responses to the medicalisation of childbirth (1671–1795), *Midwifery* 27(4):532–538, 2011a.

Allotey J: Writing midwives' history: problems and pitfalls, *Midwifery* 27(2):131–137, 2011b.

Allotey J, Nuttall A, Lynch M, et al: Mothers and midwives 1952–2012, *MIDIRS* 22(2):143–150, 2012.

Anon: Editorial, *Lancet* 1:507, 1929.

Association of Radical Midwives (ARM): *Maternity Matters* report – ARM's response, *Midwifery Matters* 113, 2007.

Baird B, Murray R, Seale B, et al: *Kings Fund Report commissioned by the NMC: Midwifery regulation in the United Kingdom Midwifery regulation in the United Kingdom*, London, Kings Fund, 2015.

Baldwin J, Brodrick A, Mason N, et al: Focus on normal birth and reducing caesarean section rates, *MIDIRS Midwifery Digest* 17(2):279, 2007.

Ball L, Curtis P, Kirkham M: Management and morale: challenges in contemporary maternity care, *Br J Midwifery* 14(2):100–103, 2006.

Barbieri A: Yes, we need to know, *The Guardian* 31, September 11, 2006.

Barnes J, editor: *The complete works of Aristotle: the revised Oxford translation* (vol 1), Bollingen Series, LXXI, 2, Princeton, Princeton University Press, p 1114, 1984.

Baxter J: Do women understand the reasons given for their caesarean sections?, *Br J Midwifery* 15(9):536, 2007.

Beech B: Defining and recording normal birth, *AIMS J* 18(4):3–4, 2006.

Beech B: Birth centre closures, *AIMS J* 24(2):13, 2012.

Bennett VR, Brown LK: *Myles textbook for midwives*, 11th edn, London, Churchill Livingstone, 1989.

Bewley S, Cockburn J: The unfacts of 'request' caesarean section, *Br J Obstet Gynaecol* 109(6):597–605, 2002.

Birthplace in England Collaborative Group: *Birth place choices study* (website). www.npeu.ox.ac.uk/birthplace/birthplace-choices-project. 2011a.

Birthplace in England Collaborative Group, et al: Perinatal and maternal outcomes by planned place of birth for healthy women with low risk pregnancies: the Birthplace in England national prospective cohort study, *Br Med J* 343, 2011b.

Blenkinsop H, editor: *Observations in midwifery by Percival Willughby*, Warwick, 1863.

British Broadcasting Corporation (BBC): *Health news* (website). http//news.bbc.co.uk/1/hi/health/2391843.stm. 2002.

British Broadcasting Corporation (BBC): *Eastbourne Maternity Services downgrade plans* (website). http://www.bbc.co.uk/news/uk-england-sussex-21660925. 2013.

British Broadcasting Corporation (BBC): *Glan Clwyd maternity temporary downgrade 'preferred option'* (website). http://www.bbc.co.uk/news/uk-wales-33869531. 2015.

Brown HS: Physician demand for leisure: implications for cesarean section rates, *J Health Econ* 15(2):233–242, 1996.

Burton J: *An essay towards a complete new system of midwifery*, London, James Hodges, 1751.

Care Quality Commission (CQC): *National findings from the 2013 survey of women's experiences of maternity care* (website). www.cqc.org.uk/sites/default/files/documents/maternity_report_for_publication.pdf. 2015.

Carlisle D: Safe in their hands?, *MIDIRS Midwifery Digest* 17(2):288, 2007.

Chavasse HP: *Chavasse's advice to a wife on the management of her own health and on the treatment of some of the complaints incidental to pregnancy, labor, and suckling*, 13th edn, London, Churchill, 1878.

Churchill H, Savage W, Francome C: *Caesarean birth in Britain: a book for health professionals and parents*, Enfield, Middlesex University Press, 2006.

Clarke J: *Practical essays on the management of pregnancy and labour*, London, J. Johnson, 1793.

Clift-Matthews V: Assessing progress in Maternity Matters, *Br J Midwifery* 12(1):4, 2009.

Cooper T, Clarke P: Home alone: a concerning trend?, *Midwives* (June–July):34–35, (August–September):34–35, 2008.

Cumberledge B chair: *National maternity review: Better Births improving outcomes of maternity services in England a five year forward view for maternity care*, London, NHS England, 2016.

Curtis P, Ball L, Kirkham M: Why do midwives leave? (Not) being the kind of midwife you want to be, *Br J Midwifery* 14(1):27–31, 2006.

Dabrowski R: *Call to save maternity services* (website). http://rcm .redactive.co.uk/midwives/news/call -to-save-maternity-services/#sthash .6jUqYQqn.dpuf. 2013.

Daniel L: There's no place like home, *Br J Midwifery* 16(12):819, 2008.

Davis K: Leading the midwifery renaissance, General Secretary's address to the RCM Annual Conference, Harrogate, *Midwives* 8(6):264–268, 2005.

Department of Health (DH): *Changing childbirth: report of the Expert Maternity Group*, London, 1993, HMSO.

Department of Health (DH): *Maternity matters: choice, access and continuity of care in a safe service*, London, DH, 2007.

Department of Health and Social Security (DHSS): *Report of the sub-committee on domiciliary and maternity bed needs [Peel Report]*, London, HMSO, 1970.

Department of Health and Social Security (DHSS): *Report on confidential enquiries into maternal deaths in England and Wales for 1970–1972*, Reports on Health and Social Subjects, No. 11, London, HMSO. Table 1.3. 1975.

Department of Health and Social Security (DHHS): *The second report from the Social Services Committee on perinatal and neonatal mortality [Short Report]*, London, HMSO, 1980.

Devane DBM, Begley C, Clarke M, et al: *Socio-economic value of the midwife: a systematic review, meta-analysis, meta-synthesis and economic analysis of midwife-led models of care*, London, Royal College of Midwives, 2010.

Dodwell M, on behalf of BirthChoiceUK for the Royal College of Midwives: *Trends in Free standing midwife-led units in England and Wales*, London, BirthChoiceUK, 2013.

Donnison J: *Midwives and medical men: a history of the struggle for the control of childbirth*, London, Historical Publications, 1988.

Donnison J: Sworn midwife: Mistress Katherine Manley of Whitby, her work and world, *MIDIRS* 17(1): 25–34, 2007.

Downe S: Active birth, active management, *RCM Midwives J* 4(7):228–230, 2001.

Downe S, McCormick C, Beech BL: Labour interventions associated with normal birth, *Br J Midwifery* 9(10):602–606, 2001.

Edwards N: *Birthing autonomy: women's experiences of planning home births*, Abingdon, Routledge, 2005.

Edwards N: Negotiating a normal birth, *AIMS J* 20(3):3–8, 2008.

Enkin M, Keirse MJNC, Neilson J, et al: *A guide to effective care in pregnancy and childbirth*, Oxford, OUP, 2000.

Fisk N, Paterson Brown S: The doctor's tale, *The Observer* 18:May 2, 2004.

Gans JS, Leigh A, Varganova E: *Minding the shop: the case of obstetrics conferences*, Centre for Economics Policy Research Discussion Paper 55, Australian National University, 2007.

Gélis J: *La sage-femme ou le médecin: une nouvelle conception de la vie*, Paris, Fayard, 1988.

Gélis J: *History of childbirth* (trans. Morris R), Cambridge, Polity Press, 1996.

Gordon A: *A treatise on the epidemic puerperal fever of Aberdeen*, London, 1795.

Gould D: Rising caesarean rates: the power of mass suggestion, *Br J Midwifery* 15(7):398, 2007.

Grigg CP, Tracy SK, Schmied V, et al: Women's birthplace decision-making, the role of confidence: part of the Evaluating Maternity Units study, *New Zealand Midwifery* 31(6):597–605, 2015.

Healthcare Commission (HCC): *Women's experiences of maternity care in the NHS in England: key findings from a survey of NHS trusts carried out in 2007*, London, HCC, 2007.

Healthcare Commission (HCC): *Towards better births: a review of maternity services in England*, London, Commission for Healthcare Audit and Inspection, 2008.

Holland E: *Lancet* 1:936, 1935.

Houghton G, Bedwell C, Forsey M, et al: Factors influencing choice in birth place – an exploration of the views of women, their partners and professionals, *Evidence Based Midwifery* 6(2):59–64, 2008.

House of Commons Health Committee (chaired by Winterton N) (HCHC):

Second report: maternity services (vol 1), London, HMSO, 1992.

International Federation of Gynaecology and Obstetrics (FIGO): *Recommendations on ethical issues in obstetrics and gynaecology by the FIGO*, London, 1999, FIGO, Committee for the Ethical Aspects of Human Reproduction and Women's Health. 2003, 2008.

Jonas R: *The byrth of mankynde*, London, 1540.

Kaboré C, Chaillet N, Kouanda S, et al: Maternal and perinatal outcomes associated with a trial of labour after previous caesarean section in sub-Saharan countries, *Br J Obstet Gynaecol* 2015.

Kirby J: The future for midwifery without statutory supervision, Nursing and Midwifery Summit at Holywell Park, Loughborough, 6th February 2015. Presentation available online: http://studylib .net/doc/5554793/the-future-for -midwifery-without-statutory -supervision. 2015.

Kirkham M: Retention and return in the NHS in England, *Midwives* 10(5):224–226, 2007.

Kirkup B: *The report of the Morecambe Bay Investigation: an independent investigation into the management, delivery and outcomes of care provided by the maternity and neonatal services at the University Hospitals of Morecambe Bay NHS Foundation Trust from January 2004 to June 2013*, London, Stationery Office, 2015.

Kuntner L: *Die Gebährung der Frau: Schwangerschaft und Geburt aus geschichtlicher, völkerkundlicher und medizinischer Sicht*, Munich, Marseille Verlag, 1988.

Langdana M, Geary W, Haw D, et al: Peripartum hysterectomy in the 1990s: any new lessons?, *J Obstet Gynaecol* 21(2):121–123, 2001.

Lavender T, Alfrevic Z, Walkinshaw S: Effect of different action lines on birth outcomes: a randomized controlled trial, *Obstet Gynaecol* 108(2):295–302, 2006. [for authors' abstract, and MIDIRS' comments, see Caine D: *MIDIRS Midwifery Digest* 17(1):78–79].

Lavender T, Hart A, Smyth RM: Effect of partogram use on outcomes for women in spontaneous labour at term, *Cochrane Database Syst Rev* CD005461, 2013.

Lavender T, Tsekiri E, Baker L: Recording labour: a national survey of partogram use, *Br J Midwifery* 16(6):359–362, 2008.

Leap N, Hunter B: *The midwife's tale: an oral history from handywoman to professional midwife*, London, Scarlet Press, 1993.

Leboyer F: *Birth without violence*, London, Pinter & Martin Ltd, 2011. (1975).

Lee B: Big is policy: small is beautiful: the amalgamation of maternity units, *RCM Midwives J* 4(1):12–13, 2001.

Licence A: *Christopher Marlowe's family and the birth of modern English midwifery in Elizabethan Canterbury* (website). http://authorh erstorianparent.blogspot.co.uk/ 2013/06/christopher-marlowes -family-and-birth.html2013. 2013.

Macfarlane A, Mugford M, Henderson J: *Birth counts: statistics of pregnancy and childbirth*, London, HMSO, 2000.

May A: *Epidurals for childbirth*, Oxford, OUP, 1994.

McKeown T: *The role of medicine: dream, mirage or nemesis?*, Oxford, Blackwell, 1976.

McMath J: *The expert mid-wife: a treatise of the diseases of women with child and in childbed*, Edinburgh, 1694.

Myles M: *Textbook for midwives*, 8th edn, London, Churchill Livingstone, 1975.

Myles M: *Textbook for midwives*, 9th edn, London, Churchill Livingstone, 1981.

Myles M: *Textbook for midwives*, 10th edn, London, Churchill Livingstone, 1987.

National Audit Office: *Maternity services in England* (website). www.nao.org.uk/report/maternity-services-england/. 2013.

National Health Service, NHS England Maternity Transformation Programme. https://www.england .nhs.uk/mat-transformation/. 2016.

National Institute for Health and Care Excellence (NICE): *Caesarean section*, NICE Clinical Guideline 13, London, NICE, 2004.

National Institute for Health and Care Excellence (NICE): *Intrapartum care: care of healthy women and their babies during childbirth*, NICE Clinical Guideline CG190, London, NICE, 2007.

National Institute for Health and Care Excellence (NICE): *Caesarean section*, NICE Clinical Guideline CG132, London, NICE, 2011.

National Institute for Health and Care Excellence (NICE): *Intrapartum care: care of healthy women and their babies during childbirth*, NICE Clinical Guideline CG190, London, NICE, 2014.

NHS Institute for Innovation and Improvement: *Focus on caesarean section*, London, NHS III, 2006.

NPR News: Music cues: *Rosetta Pedro was born this week, out of a biblical swirl of flood waters*, NPR News Weekend Edition (website). www.npr.org/programs/ wesat/000304.floods.html. 2000.

Odent M: *Entering the world: the demedicalization of childbirth*, London, Marion Boyers London, 1976.

O'Driscoll K, Meagher D: *Active management of labour*, Kent, Balliere Tindall, 1986.

Office for National Statistics: *Statistical bulletin: Births in England and Wales by characteristics of birth 2: 2013* (website). www.ons.gov.uk/ peoplepopulationandcommunity/ birthsdeathsandmarriages/livebirths/ bulletins/characteristicsofbirth2 /2014-11-172014. 2014.

O'Sullivan S, Tyler S: Payment by results: speaking in code, *RCM Midwives* 10(5):241, 2007.

Pechey J: *A general treatise of the diseases of maids, big-bellied women, child-bed women, and widows*, London, 1696.

Radford N, Thompson A: *Direct entry: a preparation for midwifery practice*, Guildford, University of Surrey, 1988.

Redshaw M, Henderson J: *Safely delivered: a national survey of women's experience of maternity care 2014*, National Perinatal Epidemiology Unit, University of Oxford (website). www.npeu.ox.ac .uk/maternity-surveys. 2015.

Reid L: Turning tradition into progress: moving midwifery forward, *RCM Midwives J* 5(8):250–254, 2002.

Robinson J: Why are more mothers dying?, *AIMS J* 16(4):1–5, 2004/5.

Rowbotham M, Hunt S: Birth centre closures: avoiding long-term costs for short-term savings?, *Br J Midwifery* 14(6):376–377, 2006.

Royal College of Midwives (RCM): *Project 2000: Comments of the Royal College of Midwives*, London, RCM, 1986.

Royal College of Midwives (RCM): *State of maternity services report 2015*, London, RCM, 2015a.

Royal College of Midwives (RCM) Normal Birth Campaign/Better Births Initiative: *Estimated proportion of normal births in the UK* (website). www.rcmnormalbirth.org.uk/home/ drawn from data from BirthChoiceUK. 2015b.

Royal College of Obstetrics and Gynaecology (RCOG): *Response to the report of the Expert Maternity Group: Changing childbirth*, London, RCOG, 1993.

Royal Society of Medicine: *The fetus as a patient*, Meeting of Obstetrics and Gynaecology Section Programme, November 11, 2002.

Russell JGB: The rationale of primitive delivery positions, *Br J Obstet Gynaecol* 89:712–715, 1982.

Sandall J, Soltani H, Gates S, et al: *Midwife-led continuity models versus other models of care for childbearing women*, Editorial Group: Cochrane Pregnancy and Childbirth Group (website). doi: 10.1002/14651858. CD004667.pub4. 2015.

Sarler C: Is the NHS's obsession with doctor-free births putting babies at risk?, *MailOnline* 21:44, 2012.

Savage W: *Birth and power: a Savage enquiry revisited*, London, Middlesex University Press, 2007.

Scottish Programme for Clinical Effectiveness in Reproductive Health (SPCERH): *Expert Advisory Group on Caesarean Section in Scotland: report and recommendations to the CMO* (website). www.healthcare improvementscotland.org/previous _resources/audit_report/scottish_ programme_for_clinica.aspx. 2001.

Secara MP: *Life in Elizabethan England: A midwife's oath 1567* (website). http://elizabethan.org/ compendium/88.html. 2013.

Sharp J: *The midwives book*, London, 1671.

Siegemundin J: *Die königliche Preussische und Chur-Brandenburgische Hof-Wehe-Mutter, Das ist, Ein höchstnötiger Unterricht von schweren und unrechtstehenden Geburthen*, Coln an der Spree, 1690.

Smellie W: *Treatise on the theory and practice of midwifery*, London, 1752–64.

Smith G, Pell J, Dobbie R: Caesarean section and risk of unexplained stillbirth, *Lancet* 362(9398):1779–1784, 2003a.

Smith G, Pell J, Dobbie R: Interpregnancy interval and risk of preterm birth and neonatal death: retrospective cohort study, *Br Med J* 327(7410):313–316, 2003b.

Smith JF, Hernandez C, Wax J: Fetal laceration at cesarean delivery, *Obstet Gynecol* 90(3):344–346, 1997.

Stapleton H, Kirkham M, Thomas G: Qualitative study of evidence based leaflets in maternity care, *Br Med J* 324(7338):639–643, 2002.

Stark JN: An obstetric diary of William Hunter 1762–1765, *Glasgow Med J* 70:167–177, 1908.

Steer P, Flint C: ABC of labour care: physiology and management of normal labour, *Br Med J* 318(7186):793–796, 1999.

Temkin O, editor: *Soranus' gynecology*, Baltimore, John Hopkins University Press, 1956.

Tew M: The case against hospital deliveries: the statistical evidence. In Kitzinger S, Davis J, editors: *The place of birth*, Oxford, OUP, 1978.

Tew M: *Safer childbirth? A critical history of maternity care*, London, Chapman and Hall, 1995.

Thomas K: *Religion and the decline of magic*, London, Penguin, 1973.

Thomas S: Early modern midwifery: splitting the profession, connecting the history, *J Soc Hist* 115–138, 2009.

Villar J, Carroli G, Zavaleta N, et al: World Health Organization 2005 global survey of Maternal and Perinatal Health Research Group: maternal and neonatal individual risks and benefits associated with caesarean delivery: multicentre prospective study, *Br Med J* 335(7628):1025, 2007.

Wagner M: Choosing caesarean section, *Lancet* 356(9242):1677–1680, 2000.

Wagner M: Fish can't see water: the need to humanize birth, *Int J Gynaecol Obstet* 75(Suppl 1):S25–S37, 2001.

Walsh D: Free-birthing and the midwifery services, *Br J Midwifery* 16(11):702, 2008.

Weaver J, Statham H: Wanting a caesarean: the decision-making process, *Br J Midwifery* 13(6):370–373, 2005.

Wiesener M: The midwives of South Germany and the public/private dichotomy. In Marland H, editor: *The art of midwifery: early modern midwives in Europe*, London, Routledge, 1993.

World Health Organization (WHO): *Maternal mortality, Fact Sheet 348* (website). www.who.int/mediacentre/factsheets/fs348/en/2014. 2014.

Worth J: District midwifery in the 1950s, *MIDIRS Midwifery Digest* 174–175, 2002.

Resources and additional reading

Martha Ballard's history: http://dohistory.org.
Shows how to piece together the past from the fragments that have survived. A case study of Martha Ballard's diary is used for examples.

Borsay A, editor: *Hunter B: Nursing and midwifery in Britain since 1700*, Basingstoke, Palgrave Macmillan, 2012.
A series of research-based essays that midwives interested in their history will find valuable.

McIntosh TA: *Social history of maternity and childbirth: key themes in maternity care*, New York, Routledge, 2012.
Using oral histories, women's memoirs, local health records and contemporary reports and papers, this book explores the experiences of women and families, and it includes the voices of women, midwives and doctors.

Thompson M: *The cry and the covenant*, New York, Doubleday, 1949.
This vivid and compelling novel is about Ignaz Semmelweis, an Austrian-Hungarian physician who recognized the causes of puerperal fever.

Chapter 3

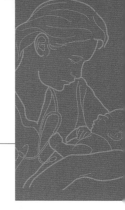

Regulation of midwives

Belinda Ackerman

Learning Outcomes ?

After reading this chapter, you will be able to:

- understand the purpose and processes of midwifery regulation
- be familiar with the role and functions of the UK Nursing and Midwifery Council (NMC)
- be conversant with the NMC codes, standards and guidelines
- have a working knowledge of the requirement for 3-year revalidation
- be aware of the revised role of the supervisor of midwives
- appreciate the changes in commissioning for midwifery education
- be conversant with regulation of independent midwives/midwives undertaking private practice

SUMMARY OF THE HISTORY OF LEGISLATION REGULATING THE MIDWIFERY PROFESSION

As illustrated in Table 3.1, since the first Midwives Act of 1902, there has been a series of further acts, amendments, orders and white papers that have affected midwifery and maternity care.

The history of statutory supervision of midwives is separately illustrated in Table 3.2, from its inception in 1902 to its planned disestablishment in April 2017.

Reflective activity 3.1 ><

Check the Department of Health website (Gov.UK) and find the legislation that currently regulates midwives in the UK (www.legislation.gov.uk).

Also see the NMC website at www.nmc.org.uk/about -us/our-legal-framework/our-legislation/.

INTRODUCTION

This chapter provides an overview of midwifery regulation, including its history, the demise of the UK Nursing and Midwifery Council (NMC) Midwifery Committee, statutory supervision of midwives and separate rules for midwives. It addresses the introduction of 3-year revalidation as a means of maintaining professional competence.

It is important that midwives are familiar with the fundamentals of regulation to be aware of the framework within which they are required to practice and to ensure the safety and quality of care given to women and their babies.

WHY DO WE HAVE REGULATION?

Midwives are regulated by the NMC to ensure public protection through initial and continuing registration and standard setting for education and practice. Quality assurance is maintained through the NMC fitness-to-practice process.

Core functions of the NMC

The primary function of the NMC is as a regulator of the professions, thereby safeguarding the public through the following activities:

1. Establishing and maintaining a register of all nurses, midwives and health visitors

2. Setting standards for the education and practice of all nurses, midwives and health visitors

3. Regulating fitness to practise, conduct and performance through rules and codes

The Council has the power to remove a person from the Register, thus preventing the individual from practising as a nurse, midwife or health visitor. It also has a statutory duty to inform and educate registrants and to inform the public about its work.

Membership

The Council consists of 14 members (seven registrants and seven lay members) appointed by the Appointments Commission on behalf of the Privy Council (see www.legislation.gov.uk/uksi/2008/2553/pdfs/uksi_20082553_en.pdf).

Table 3.1 Summary of the history of legislation regulating the midwifery profession

Reports and Legislation	Date	Purpose
The Midwives Act (the first act)	1902	Established a statutory body for midwives, the Central Midwives' Board for England and Wales (CMB), prescribed its constitution and laid down statutory powers. This act was amended in 1918, 1926, 1934, 1936 and 1950.
The Midwives Act	1951	Consolidated all previous acts.
Nurses, Midwives and Health Visitors Act	1979	For the purposes of regulation, midwives were amalgamated with other professional groups for the first time in their history under the United Kingdom Central Council (UKCC) and four country boards (England, Wales, Scotland and Northern Ireland). It established a Register of the three professions, containing 15 parts, to include the different specialities of nursing. Midwives are registered on Part 10. A separate Midwifery Committee was set up in statute following protests from the Royal College of Midwives (RCM) and Association of Radical Midwives (ARM) that midwives would be overruled by nurses (Jowitt and Kargar 1997). The act was amended in 1992
Nurses, Midwives and Health Visitors Act	1997	Consolidation of the 1979 and 1992 acts, incorporating all the reforms.
Health Act	1999	The current legislation for midwives drawn up under Section 62(9) of the Health Act 1999 (Department of Health [DH] 1999) sets out the Order for the establishment of the Nursing and Midwifery Council (NMC). It repealed the 1997 Nurses, Midwives and Health Visitors Act and replaced primary legislation with a statutory instrument by 'Order'.
Modernising Regulation in the Health Professions	2001	This National Health Services (NHS) consultation document set out the NHS Plan (DH 2000). It proposed the establishment of a *UK Council of Health Regulators* to act as a forum and coordinate complaints from all the professions and their regulatory bodies. This Council would be independent of the state and accountable to Parliament, as would all the professional regulatory bodies, through the new Council. It would have the power to require changes to the regulatory framework. It would not have the power to take over or intervene in individual fitness-to-practise cases (DH 2001).
Nursing and Midwifery Order	2001	The Orders to establish the Nursing and Midwifery Council were set out in draft and laid before Parliament in October 2001 for approval under Section 62(9) of the Health Act 1999. The Nursing and Midwifery Order 2001 came into force and the UK Nursing and Midwifery Council commenced office on 1 April 2002 under Statutory Instrument 2002 No. 253 (DH 2002a). The NMC became directly responsible to the independent Privy Council rather than the Secretary of State, thus removing a possible source of bias as the main employer of nurses and midwives.

Table 3.1 Summary of the history of legislation regulating the midwifery profession—cont'd

Reports and Legislation	Date	Purpose
National Health Service and Health Care Professions Act	2002	This act set up the Council for Healthcare Regulatory Excellence (CHRE), a UK health regulatory body (DH 2002b).
Trust, Assurance and Safety – The Regulation of Health Professionals in the 21st Century	2007	This white paper set out a major reform of the UK health professions following two reviews of professional regulation, *The Regulation of Non-medical Healthcare Professions* (DH 2006a) and *Good Doctors, Safer Patients* (DH 2006b), and recommendations of the Fifth Report of the Shipman Inquiry (HM Government 2004) and of the Ayling, Neale and Kerr/Haslam Inquiries (HM Government 2007a, 2007b). It changed several areas: • The Council structure of all professional regulators to parity of membership between lay and professional members • Independent appointment of professional members • The criminal standard of proof to the civil standard of proof • Improvement of fitness to practise through standards *(doctors to revalidate every 5 years)* and requiring greater accountability to Parliament (DH 2007)
Health and Social Care Act	2008	This extended the CHRE's (2008) powers to include reviewing fitness to practise where health is an issue and set up the *Care Quality Commission (CQC)* (DH 2008a).
Health and Social Care Act	2012	Section 222 set up the Professional Standards Authority for Health and Social Care (previously known as the Council for Healthcare Regulatory Excellence (CHRE)). This body oversees statutory bodies that regulate UK healthcare and social care professionals. It assesses their performance, conducts audits, scrutinizes their decisions and reports to Parliament (DH 2012).
The Nursing and Midwifery (Amendment) Order	2008	This updated the size and membership of the NMC Council and the Midwifery Committee and Practice Committees (see Box 3.1); it came into force in January 2009 (DH 2008b).
The Nursing and Midwifery (Amendment) Order	2014	Made changes regarding the disclosure of a midwife's indemnity insurance arrangements for the purposes of verifying insurance held. All midwives working privately or independently are required to arrange their own indemnity insurance before submission of their annual 'Intention to Practice' (ItP) and confirm before re-registration with the NMC every 3 years (DH 2014).
The Nursing and Midwifery Council Rules – Order of Council No. 52	2015	Relates to fitness to practice, fraud and indemnity insurance. This updated the previous 2004 Order (see www.legislation.gov.uk/uksi/2015/52/schedule/made).

HOW DOES THE NMC WORK?

The NMC has set up a series of statutory committees to carry out its role and functions, as described in the following sections.

1. Midwifery Committee

The Midwifery Committee, which will be abolished in April 2017, provides advice on 'any matter affecting midwifery practice'. It operates under the NMC Standing Orders 2009 (NMC 2010a).

2. Investigating Committee

Panels of the Investigating Committee (see Fig. 3.1) are responsible for considering any allegations of 'unfitness to practise' referred to the NMC.

A registered medical practitioner will be present if the registrant's health is in question. These deliberations take place in private, and the panel decides whether there is a case to answer. If there is, referral is made to the Health Committee or the Conduct and Competence Committee (Department of Health (DH) 2002a). The panel may refer immediately to an Interim Orders hearing if the registrant is thought to be an immediate threat to the public. The panel can then impose the following orders:

a. An *interim suspension* order – registration is suspended. This prevents registrants from working during investigation of the case. This can be imposed for up to 18 months but must be reviewed after 6 months and thereafter every 3 months. This would be used in cases such as rape, to protect the public.

b. An *interim conditions of practice* order – an alternative to postponing judgement in which the registrant agrees to be bound by a set of agreed conditions. It can be revoked, modified or replaced with a different order according to circumstances.

In addition, a 'removal' from the Register can be authorized by the Investigating Committee to correct an incorrect or fraudulent entry (NMC 2008a).

3. Health Committee

The Health Committee's role is to consider 'any allegation referred to it by the Investigating Committee or the Conduct and Competence Committee and any

application for restoration referred by the Registrar' (DH 2002a).

4. Conduct and Competence Committee

The Conduct and Competence Committee's role is to consider any allegations referred to it by the Investigating Committee or the Health Committee. Hearings are held in public, but parts of the case may be held in private to protect the identity of the person or confidential medical evidence (NMC 2008a). A panel must consist of at least three people, and it must include a layperson and a *due regard* (that is, someone from the same specialty as the professional being investigated).

Conduct and Competence Committee and Health Committee Panels' sanctions

The Conduct and Competence Committee and the Health Committee establish, in cases referred to them, whether fitness to practise is impaired by any of the following:

- misconduct
- lack of competence
- a criminal offence
- mental or physical health
- a determination by a UK health professions body that fitness to practise is impaired (NMC 2008a)

All decisions are based on evidence presented at the hearing of the case. The panel will only hear information about the previous history of the 'respondent' and any evidence in mitigation before making a final decision (NMC 2010b).

The range of powers it holds in relation to sanctions include various orders. The panel either decides to take *no further action* or makes one of the following orders to the Registrar:

a. *striking-off order* – this removes the registrant's name from the Register for a minimum of 5 years; it prevents individuals from employment requiring registration and will probably be implemented for cases of misconduct.

b. *suspension order* – this incurs a suspension not exceeding 1 year; this sanction usually applies in cases of lack of competence (LOC) or poor health.

c. *conditions-of-practice order* – this incurs a suspension not exceeding 3 years; it also usually applies in cases of LOC and poor health.

d. *caution order* – for not less than 1 year and not more than 5 years, the practitioner works normally and the caution remains on the Register entry for the prescribed period. Future employers will be alerted to the caution and will be informed as to why it was imposed.

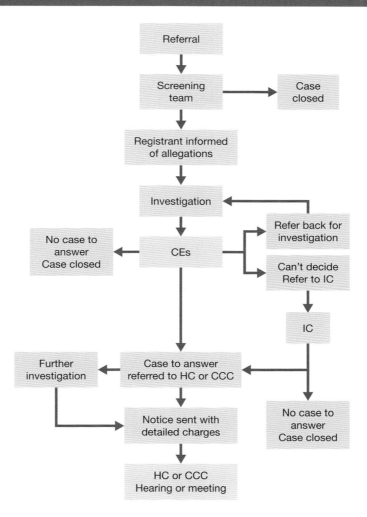

CE= Case Examiner
HC = Health Committee
IC = Investigating Committee
CCC = Conduct and Competence Committee

Figure 3.1 Flowchart regarding allegations of unfitness-to-practise process map. (With kind permission from the Nursing and Midwifery Council (NMC) June 2016.)

Once a decision has been made, the registrant can make an appeal, and this has to be done within 28 days of a committee's decision.

Restoration to the Register of practitioners who have been struck off

An application may be made before the end of 5 years, or in any period of 12 months in which an application for restoration to the Register has already been made, by the person who has been struck off. The application for restoration to the Register is made via the Registrar and is forwarded to the relevant committee that made the striking-off order. If the Committee is satisfied that the registrant has achieved the additional education, training or experience required, then the registration fee is paid and the practitioner can be restored to the Register.

If an application is unsuccessful, an appeal may be made within 28 days of the decision date. If a second or subsequent application is made while a striking-off order is in force and is rendered unsuccessful, the committee may direct that the person be suspended indefinitely (DH 2002a).

Other requirements

The NMC is required to appoint legal assessors, medical assessors and registrant assessors to advise the Council or its committees as appropriate.

Civil standard of proof

The *civil standard of proof* was brought into force on 16 October 2008 following the DH White Paper (DH 2007) and Health and Social Care Act 2008 (Commencement No. 3) Order 2008 (SI 2008/2717 (C. 120)) (DH 2008a). All NMC hearings have used this standard since 3 November 2008. This means that evidence is based on the 'balance of probabilities' rather than the previously used 'criminal standard of proof', where facts needed to be proved 'beyond reasonable doubt'.

Non-statutory NMC committees

The following non-statutory committees carry out the remaining roles and functions of the NMC.

1. Appointments Board

The Appointments board deals with the appointment, development and appraisal of Fitness to Practice panellists and the processing of applicants for non-Council membership of committees and local supervising authority (LSA) reviewers. It ensures relevant academic and/or clinical expertise on a committee and also advises Council on removal of panellists from office.

2. Audit, Risk and Assurance Committee

The Audit, Risk and Assurance Committee ensures that the business of the Council is conducted with integrity and probity. It agrees on procedures for internal and external auditing arrangements and management of risk. It also ensures that the quality and standards for education and training are being met and provides approval of training institutions and programmes by monitoring the UK Quality Assurance framework contract.

3. Business Planning and Governance Committee

Business Planning and Governance Committee advises the Council on all matters relating to the management of resources and the maintenance of good governance standards throughout the NMC. It appoints members to the Council, recommends any amendments to the Standing Orders or code of conduct for members, and oversees the development, performance and appraisal of Council members (NMC 2010c).

4. Fitness to Practise Committee

Fitness to Practise Committee is a strategic committee separate from the three practice committees. It advises the Council on matters related to standards, conduct, performance and ethics expected of registrants (and students who are prospective registrants). It also advises on the requirements as to good character and good health expected of registrants and ensures protection of the public where fitness to practise is impaired (NMC 2004, 2009a).

5. Professional Practice and Registration Committee

The Professional Practice and Registration Committee advises on all matters relating to nursing and community public health nursing, such as standards of education and training and practice guidance (midwifery standards and guidance will continue to be dealt with by the Midwifery Committee until they are disestablished by April 2017).

In addition, it advises on all aspects of registration and renewal of registration (NMC 2010d).

FUNCTIONS OF THE NMC

Function 1: The Register

The Register is divided into parts determined by the Privy Council. There are currently three parts to the Register (DH 2004):

1. Nurses
2. Midwives
3. Specialist community public health nurses (health visitors)

The Council determines the registration fee to be charged and coordinates the initial registration process and renewal to the Register. Visiting European Union (EU) nurses or midwives are deemed registered and can practise in the UK subject to knowledge of English and comparable qualifications (see NMC 2016).

Function 2: Setting standards for education and practice

Pre-registration midwifery education

The NMC is charged with establishing the **pre-registration** standards of education and training, including requirements for good health and character. It ensures that the standards of education programmes remain high through the network of lead midwives for education (LMEs) (NMC 2015a).

The length of the programmes is set at a **minimum** of 3 years (156 weeks) and 18 months (78 weeks) for registered nurses (shortened programme).

The NMC set competencies required by students to achieve the standards, which are divided into four domains:

- Effective midwifery practice
- Professional and ethical practice
- Developing the individual midwife and others
- Achieving quality care through evaluation and research

Essential skills clusters, including communication, initial consultation between the woman and midwife, normal labour and birth, initiation and continuance of breastfeeding and medicines management, are also required (NMC 2009c).

Declaration of good health and good character of each midwifery student must be made by the LME at the education institution on successful completion of the programme 'in order to satisfy the Registrar that an applicant is capable of safe and effective practice as a nurse or midwife' per Article 5(2)(b) of the Nursing and Midwifery Order of 2001 (NMC 2008c).

Time limits for completion of midwifery programmes have since been removed by the NMC (NMC 2015b).

Standards for Competence for Registered Midwives

The NMC published a comprehensive booklet that sets out the standards already agreed on for pre-registration midwifery (NMC 2015c).

Function 3: Regulating Fitness to Practise, Conduct and Performance

Function 3 is supported by the NMC rules, standards and advice publications set out by the NMC practice committees (see Box 3.1). In midwifery, audit and monitoring of compliance is carried out by the local supervising authorities and supervisors of midwives until the planned demise of the Midwifery Committee in April 2017 (NMC 2009d; DH 2016).

The practice committees ensure that non-compliance with the rules and standards is reviewed and individual cases are investigated.

GETTING REGISTERED

Once a student midwife has successfully completed a programme of midwifery education at an NMC-approved higher education institution (HEI), she or he is eligible to register as a midwife and commence practice (NMC

Box 3.1 Committee structure of the Nursing and Midwifery Council

Four statutory committees:
1. Midwifery Committee (to be removed by April 2017)
2. Investigating Committee*
3. Health Committee*
4. Conduct and Competence Committee*

Five non-statutory committees:
1. Appointments Board
2. Audit, Risk and Assurance
3. Business, Planning and Governance
4. Fitness to Practise
5. Professional Practice and Registration

*The Investigating, Health and Conduct and Competence Committees consist of pools of panellists and never meet.

2016). This requires an application from the student. At the same time, the university will inform the NMC that the student has successfully completed all theoretical and practical components and will include in the submission a *declaration of good character.* Until the registration is confirmed, the student **cannot** practice as a midwife.

STAYING REGISTERED

Once registered, to remain on the Register, all practitioners must pay an annual registration fee to the NMC. They are also required to demonstrate that they are safe and effective practitioners by revalidating their registration every 3 years (NMC 2015d) (see also Ch. 5).

NMC REVALIDATION FOR NURSES AND MIDWIVES

Revalidation is a process for nurses and midwives to complete every 3 years before each registration renewal. It utilizes the NMC Code 2015 as the guide for registrants to demonstrate that their practice is up to date. Failure to comply with this requirement will result in removal from the Register.

The requirements for revalidation include the following:

- 450 practice hours (or 900 if revalidating as both a nurse and midwife)
- 35 hours of continuing professional development (CPD), including 20 hours of participatory learning

- Five pieces of practice-related feedback
- Five written reflective accounts
- Reflective discussion
- Health and character declaration
- Professional indemnity arrangements
- Confirmation (NMC 2015d)

Revalidation is not an assessment of fitness to practise; fitness will continue to be reviewed via the NMC Fitness to Practise Committee following any concerns reported by an employer or member of the public. It is to ensure practitioners are aware of the Code and to raise professional standards.

'Peer review (rather than clinical supervision) will be necessary for those midwives in leadership and education roles, for example, and not in clinical practice. Such midwives are legitimately practising midwifery and are also registered with and regulated by the NMC' (NHS England 2016) (see Ch. 5).

Revalidation replaces the previous requirements for post-registration education and practice (PREP) every 3 years (NMC 2011) and the annual update in which midwives meet with a supervisor of midwives (NMC 2015d).

Continued competence

In addition to the 3-year NMC revalidation that every midwife and nurse must complete (see previous discussion), all practitioners must comply with the NMC Code (NMC 2015e) and other NMC guidance and standards.

A synopsis of the NMC rules, codes and guidance relating to midwives follows (see www.nmc-uk.org).

The Code – for nurses and midwives (NMC 2015e)

These standards must be upheld by all nurses and midwives who appear on the NMC Register. Practitioners will be required to produce evidence of practice validating their upholding of these standards for their 3-year revalidation.

Four key elements are included, as follows:

1. *Prioritize people* – requests practitioners to treat people with dignity and respect and to pay attention to their social and psychological needs along with their physical needs. To ensure privacy and confidentiality, consent must be granted before procedures, and care providers must acknowledge the patient's right to refuse treatment.

2. *Practise effectively* – requires the practitioner to keep up to date, communicate and document clearly and ensure accountability when delegating tasks. In addition, independent midwives must have

indemnity insurance; this is the first time that the NMC has made insurance a requirement for practice. Indemnity insurance is now required for all midwives (and nurses) who are practising in a 'private' or independent capacity. This includes midwives who set up private antenatal classes, give online advice to pregnant women or carry out private postnatal visits. However, if midwives are employed via the NHS or an agency, the indemnity insurance will be provided by the employer.

3. *Preserve safety* – requires the nurse/midwife to take action in an emergency, refer if outside the practitioners' level of capability, escalate concerns, protect vulnerable patients from harm and administer or prescribe medicines as required.

4. *Promote professionalism and trust* – requires the nurse/midwife to act with integrity and as a role model for others. The practitioner will not accept gifts, will cooperate with audits and investigations, will declare any criminal convictions and will provide leadership.

Raising Concerns: Guidance for Nurses and Midwives (NMC 2015f)

This guidance states that a concern should be raised in a timely manner to safeguard the public. Examples include issues of danger or risk to health and safety; issues regarding care delivery; issues relating to the environment of care, such as staffing problems; issues related to the health of a colleague; and issues related to misuse or unavailability of medical equipment. The guidance suggests contacting a Supervisor of Midwives, mentor or university tutor, and relevant contact organizations are listed.

Guidance on the Professional Duty of Candour (NMC 2015g)

The *Guidance on the Professional Duty of Candour*, developed jointly with the General Medical Council (GMC), describes the requirement for nurses and midwives to be open and honest with the people within their care and to report near misses within their organizations. This guidance was published as a direct result of the recommendations of the Morecambe Bay investigation (Kirkup 2015).

Advice and Information for Employers of Nurses and Midwives (NMC 2015h)

Responsibilities as an employer and recognition of misconduct, lack of competence, bad character and poor health, and how to investigate issues and refer them to the NMC, are discussed in this guidance.

Midwives Rules and Standards (NMC 2012)

The *Midwives Rules and Standards*, to be abolished by April 2017, cover the following key areas:

Part 2: Requirements for practice – notification of intention to practice; notifications by local supervising authority

Part 3: Obligations and scope of practice – scope of practice; storage of records

Part 4: Supervision and reporting – LSA responsibilities for supervision of midwives; publication of LSA procedures; visits and inspections; exercise by an LSA of its functions; LSA reports

Part 5: Action by the LSA – suspension from practice by an LSA

Standards for Medicines Management (NMC 2008d)

Twenty-six standards are listed under the following sections: supply and administration; dispensing; storage and transportation; practice of administration; delegation; disposal; unlicensed medicines; complementary and alternative therapies; managing adverse events; and controlled drugs. A CD-ROM is also provided that includes the relevant legislation.

SUPERVISION OF MIDWIVES

The demise of *statutory* supervision of midwives is scheduled to take place in 2017 via Section 60 of the Nursing and Midwifery Order. It will be replaced by *clinical* supervision or peer review for nonclinical midwives and will continue to provide a service to women (DH 2016).

What is the purpose of a supervisor of midwives?

The supervisor of midwives (SOM) provides professional leadership guidance and support to midwives in their provision of a high standard of care to women and their babies. SOMs contribute to risk management and clinical governance within the NHS and provide support for parents regarding choice for place of birth, concerns regarding midwifery care and maintenance of safety, for example, at a home birth (DH 2016; NMC 2009e, 2012, 2014f). The midwife has a duty of care to the woman and a contractual duty to the employer, and she may need to seek advice from her supervisor should any conflict arise.

Every midwife should have a named supervisor of her or his choosing. Supervisors have a responsibility to provide support to all midwives outside the NHS, including the private sector, HEIs, prisons, independent midwives and general practice midwives (DH 2016; NMC 2012, 2015i). The ratio of supervisors to midwives should not normally exceed 1:15 (Rule 9, NMC 2012).

History of statutory supervision of midwives

The purpose of statutory supervision of midwives is protection of the public and promotion of safe standards of midwifery practice (NMC 2015i).

After 114 years of statutory supervision of midwives, the Secretary of State for Health in England announced on 16 July 2015 that the government was to remove statutory supervision of midwives from regulatory legislation through changes to Section 60 of the Nursing and Midwifery Order (Hunt 2015). This effectively removes the power of a midwifery supervisor to investigate cases so that the NMC can undertake all investigations of midwives directly, bringing midwives in line with nurses.

The changes will not affect the protected title of 'midwife', and only a midwife or medical practitioner may attend a woman in childbirth (NMC 2015j).

Education and training for supervisors of midwives

In 1978, the CMB introduced courses of instruction for supervisors. These courses later became mandatory (United Kingdom Central Council (UKCC) 1986).

A formal training package, 'Preparation for Supervisors of Midwives', was first developed at diploma level in 1992 by the English National Board (ENB 1992). Programmes of education are now delivered by HEIs and approved and monitored annually by the NMC.

The current UK standards for the preparation and practice of SOMs were updated by the NMC in 2014 (NMC 2014e).

The future education for *clinical* supervisors of midwives is under discussion within the UK working group on changes to midwifery supervision (DH 2016).

The local supervising authority midwifery officer

The Nursing and Midwifery Council sets the rules and standards for the functions of the local supervising authorities (NMC 2012, 2015m). Each LSA appoints a practising midwife, known as the local supervising authority midwifery officer (LSAMO), who has responsibility for carrying out the statutory authority functions in all midwifery services, whether NHS or independent.

The NMC sets standards for statutory supervision of midwives and delegates the LSA to complete an annual audit of the standards of midwifery practice locally. This includes receipt of the annual intention-to-practise data from supervisors, evidence of liaison with services users, engagement with HEIs and any investigations of misconduct or lack of competence undertaken.

The LSAMO is responsible for suspension of midwives from practise, ensuring a full investigation is carried out and advising the investigating SOM if a period of supervised practise is required (NMC 2012).

An annual report is submitted to the NMC about the standards, local activities, good practise and trends affecting the maternity service within its area (NMC 2012).

The NMC reviews the LSA profiles annually using a risk-assessment approach (NMC 2012). Based on this, a decision is made to carry out a formal review of selected LSAs to verify that they are meeting the standards, and a panel is appointed by the NMC Appointments Board.

The Midwives Rules (NMC 2012), LSAs, LSAMOs and SOMs will be removed from statutory regulations by April 2017.

Reflective activity 3.3

Are you up to date with the changes to statutory supervision? Visit the relevant NHS UK country website to catch up.

Table 3.2 Summary of key legislation, reports and statements setting up and removing statutory supervision of midwives

Reports and Legislation	Date	Purpose
Midwives Act	1902	Set up the Central Midwives Board (CMB) and statutory supervision of midwives by medical and non-medical practitioners. The task was delegated to local supervising authorities (LSAs), then under the control of county councils and county borough councils, until 1973 when they came within the National Health Service (NHS).
Midwives Act	1936	Empowered the CMB to make rules relating to the qualifications of medical and non-medical supervisors of midwives.
NHS Reorganisation Act	1973	Nominated regional health authorities as LSAs. The delegation of duties to supervisors of midwives was nominated by district health authorities.
Statutory Instrument (SI) No. 1850	1977	Eradicated the role of 'medical supervisor' and removed the words 'non-medical' from the title of supervisor.
Nursing and Midwifery Order 2001	2001	Set out the responsibility of the LSA for the function of statutory supervision of midwives (DH 2002b).
Nursing and Midwifery Council (NMC) – Midwives Rules	2012	Statutory supervision of midwives is enshrined in the Midwives Rules and Standards (NMC 2012).
Parliamentary and Health Service Ombudsman (PHSO) 2013; Midwifery Supervision and Regulation: Recommendations for Change	2013	PHSO report recommending that 'midwifery supervision and regulation should be separated' and that 'the NMC should be in direct control of regulatory activity'. This was as a direct result of the completion of investigations into complaints from three families regarding a maternal death, a stillbirth and two neonatal deaths. Midwifery supervisors had failed to carry out effective investigations or identify poor midwifery practice and were not prompted by the LSA midwifery officer (LSAMO) at the time. Subsequently, the families were unable to mourn their losses (PHSO 2013).
NMC – Statement	2014	Announcement by the NMC of an immediate review of midwifery regulation. The NMC commissioned the King's Fund to carry out the review and report back by the end of the year (NMC 2014a).

Table 3.2 Summary of key legislation, reports and statements setting up and removing statutory supervision of midwives—cont'd

Reports and Legislation	Date	Purpose
NMC – Extraordinary LSA Review of Princess Elizabeth Hospital in Guernsey	2014	Review following reports of escalating concerns about supervision of midwives and clinical midwifery practice in Guernsey. The NMC found that the LSA was 'not compliant with the Midwives Rules and Standards', and therefore supervisors of midwives were not fit to carry out their duties and the public was placed at risk. All of the supervisors were suspended, and LSA functions were transferred to Jersey (NMC 2014b).
NMC – Response to Extraordinary Review	2014	NMC response confirming representatives were working with the LSA and Guernsey's Health and Social Services Department to make improvements to protect patients and the public (NMC 2014c).
NMC – Better Legislation for Better Regulation: The Case for Legislative Reform	2014	NMC request for changes to the way legislation reform is carried out by Parliament (NMC 2014d).
Midwifery Regulation in the United Kingdom – King's Fund Report	2014	King's Fund review of UK midwifery regulation that echoed the PHSO's recommendation that statutory supervision of midwives should be removed (Baird et al 2014).
NMC – Council meeting	2015	On 28 January 2015, the NMC made the decision to remove statutory supervision of midwives from regulation during a tabled agenda item at its Council meeting (NMC 2015k).
The LSA Midwifery Officers (LSAMO) Forum UK	2015	LSAMO statement vowing to work with stakeholders to maintain a service for women (LSAMO Forum UK 2015a).
The Royal College of Midwives (RCM) – statement	2015	The RCM recommended that non-regulatory aspects of supervision be retained to support revalidation. It also recommended that the replacement should include leadership and advocacy for midwives and 24-hour access to advice, ensuring concerns from midwives and women regarding choice of maternity provision are raised via clinical governance processes (RCM 2015).
The Report of the Morecambe Bay Investigation	2015	Report was commissioned by the Secretary of State for Health to examine the concerns raised by the occurrence of serious incidents in maternity services provided by what became the University Hospitals of Morecambe Bay NHS Foundation Trust (i.e. the investigation of 16 neonatal deaths and 3 maternal deaths). Concerns were raised regarding 11 neonatal deaths and 1 maternal death. Relatives of those harmed expressed concern over the incidents, over why they happened and over the responses to them by the Trust, the supervisors of midwives and by the wider National Health Service (NHS), including regulatory and other bodies. Forty-four recommendations were made for the Trust and the wider NHS, including noting the failure of the LSA to detect problems. It recommended an urgent response to the findings of the King's Fund review of midwifery regulation. *This appeared to be an overt suggestion for accepting the removal of statutory supervision of midwives and streamlining investigations directly under the NMC* (Kirkup 2015).
NHS England (NHSE) – response	2015	NHSE responded by making clear its shock and sadness for the occurrence of such tragic events, stating that the NHSE would implement a system-wide response in due course (NHSE 2015a).

Continued

Table 3.2 Summary of key legislation, reports and statements setting up and removing statutory supervision of midwives—cont'd

Reports and Legislation	Date	Purpose
Secretary of State for Health – statement	2015	In July 2015 the Secretary of State for Health made an announcement to improve 'safety' following the Morecambe Bay investigation report (Hunt 2015). Key points included the planned removal of statutory supervision in the UK 'moving to a model of professional supervision similar to that of other health professionals' and 'a full-scale review into current maternity services and provision across the country led by Baroness Cumberlege' (NHSE 2015b).
NMC – statement	2015	The NMC responded (NMC 2015l). A working group was set up including a number of stakeholders to discuss the way forward. This included the chief nurses of the four UK countries, a UK LSA representative, the RCM and the Royal College of Nursing (RCN).
LSA – proposals	2015	The LSA proposed a model for the provision of professional leadership support and advocacy in England, which was incorporated into the working group discussion (LSAMO Forum UK 2015b).
Department of Health (DH) – proposals for changing the system of midwifery supervision in the UK	2016	These proposals outlined changes to the statutory supervision of midwives to be introduced in 2017. An over-arching model of clinical midwifery supervision is recommended to replace the current statutory model, with peer review for those who work in nonclinical settings. Chief nursing officers, government midwifery officers, LSMAO and RCM officers from the four UK countries will propose a working model to take the new arrangements forward (DH 2016).

Midwifery Education

Midwifery education in England is currently commissioned from the HEIs by Health Education England (HEE), which took over this responsibility from Strategic Health Authorities in 2013. The other three countries coordinate their education programmes separately but maintain links with HEE.

HHE was originally established as a Special Health Authority in 2012 (HEE 2012). It then became a nondepartmental public body (NDPB), as of 1 April 2015, under the provisions of the Care Act of 2014 (HEE 2015a).

HEE has five key functions:

1. Providing national leadership on planning and developing the healthcare and public health workforce

2. Promoting high-quality education and training that is responsive to the changing needs of patients and local communities, including responsibility for the delivery of key national functions such as medical trainee recruitment

3. Ensuring security of the supply of the health and public health workforce, which can mean working with partners to deliver targeted recruitment initiatives, such as Return to Practise (RTP), the campaign to bring qualified nurses back into the NHS

4. Supporting the development and managing the performance of its 13 Local Education and Training Boards (LETBs), committees of the HEE Board that ensure that local decisions, local issues and local conditions are core to commissioning

5. Allocating and accounting for NHS education and training resources and the outcomes achieved (HEE 2015b)

The 13 LETBs across England have been responsible for the training and education of NHS staff, both clinical and nonclinical, within their areas (e.g. doctors, nurses, midwives, health visitors and physiotherapists) since 2013.

LETB boards are made up of representatives from local providers of NHS services and cover the whole of England.

HEE's role is to improve the quality of care delivered to patients by focusing on the education, training and development of current and future healthcare staff. With employers and professionals as part of their governing bodies, the LETBs plan to improve the quality of education and training outcomes to meet the needs of patients, the public and service providers in their areas (HEE 2015c).

See Figure 3.2 for the structure of HEE in relation to the Department of Health.

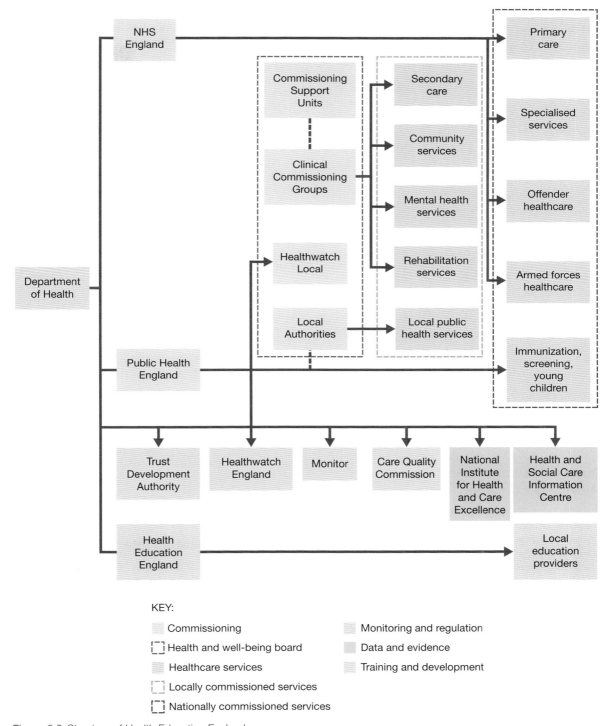

KEY:

Commissioning

[ ] Health and well-being board

Healthcare services

[ ] Locally commissioned services

[ ] Nationally commissioned services

Monitoring and regulation

Data and evidence

Training and development

Figure 3.2 Structure of Health Education England.

Pre-registration midwifery standards and fitness to practise

Standards for pre-registration midwifery education are agreed upon and produced by the NMC. The current standards were published in 2009 (NMC 2009c).

A minimum academic level of a degree for midwifery programmes was recommended by the Midwifery Committee (NMC 2007). Other recommendations were as follows:

- Practise-to-theory ratio – no less than 50% practise and no less than 40% theory
- Clinical practise to be included as part of the academic award and therefore graded
- Students to take on a small caseload of women to provide antenatal, intrapartum and postnatal care during their training

Supporting birthing women in a variety of settings, such as home births and birth centres, was also recommended (NMC 2007).

The second edition of standards to support learning and assessment in practise was published in 2008 (NMC 2008b). This edition includes recommendations that students are to be supported and assessed by mentors who have met the additional sign-off criteria. Sign-off mentors are now to make the final assessment of practise and confirm that the required proficiencies for practise have been achieved (NMC 2008b). A triennial review of mentors and practise teachers is required to be maintained on a local register, and all mentors must have completed an NMC-approved mentorship or teacher preparation programme (NMC 2009a, 2009b).

Quality Assurance for Midwifery Education

The NMC provides approval to HEIs to run nursing and midwifery education programmes. As a result of this, each Approved Educational Institution (AEI) employs and delegates day-to-day running of midwifery programmes to a Lead Midwife for Education (LME).

LMEs are senior experienced practising midwife teachers and are responsible for the quality, development, delivery and management of midwifery education programmes.

LMEs play a key role in informing the NMC regarding whether student midwives are competent to take on the role of a midwife at the end of their training (NMC 2015a).

All LMEs are members of the NMC's UK-wide Strategic Reference Group and provide advice to the NMC Midwifery Committee.

The NMC appoints 'quality assurance reviewers or visitors' to visit institutions and report back on the nature and quality of the instruction given, including facilities provided. The NMC visitors are trained for their role and are midwives drawn from the profession. Visitors are not allowed to be NMC employees or employees of the universities being visited or anyone who has a close connection with the university through, for example, lecturing. Visitors are required to complete a report summarizing the information gained and are reimbursed by the NMC for expenses incurred. If the Council is of the opinion that the standards established under Article 15(1) are not met, it may refuse to approve, or withdraw approval from, the particular institution (NMC 2013; DH 2002b); in such a case, the university is unable to continue to teach students undertaking professional programmes until approval is reinstated.

Institutions are required to provide information to the Council about all the programmes they offer for registration to the different parts of the Register.

Funding for Midwifery Students

Beginning on 1 August 2017, new nursing, midwifery and allied health students will no longer receive NHS bursaries. Instead, they will have access to the same student loan system as other students (DH 2015). The benefits as described by the DH are as follows:

- More nurses, midwives and allied health professionals for the NHS
- A better funding system for health students in England
- A sustainable model for universities

A 25% increase in the student loan for living costs for health students is planned. In addition, students who have previously studied for a degree would normally not be able to take out another loan, but exceptions to this rule will be made in the case of health students to maintain the numbers required by the NHS (DH 2015).

Midwifery education internationally

Global Standards for Midwifery Education were published by the International Confederation of Midwives (ICM) in 2010, then amended in 2013, to benchmark the preparation of midwives and raise the standards of maternity care to women across the world (see also Chs 1 and 5).

According to the ICM, it is anticipated that these global standards for midwifery education will be used by governments, policymakers, ministries of health and education, and healthcare systems in addition to midwives and midwifery associations. The shared goal is that competent midwives will be prepared and available to meet the health needs of the population, particularly those of women and childbearing families (ICM 2010).

Reflective activity 3.4

Visit the DH website at www.gov.uk and the NMC website at www.nmc-org.uk to get up to date information on current midwifery education provisions, standards and funding.

CONCLUSION

Midwifery legislation has provided over 100 years of statutory supervision, and protection of the public has been upheld through its quality and standards. The number of midwifery registrants referred to the regulating body for professional misconduct has remained very small. This demonstrates a mature, forward-thinking approach to continuing professional development and a proactive way of reducing harm to the public from misconduct, incompetence and poor practice.

Midwives have always worked closely with the users of the service throughout their history and continue to maintain standards and safety through multi-disciplinary work with women and their families.

Local risk-management arrangements will continue to be employer led, whereas the statutory requirement for SOMs to carry out investigations of serious incidents involving midwives will cease in 2017 following removal of regulations for the statutory supervision of midwives under Section 60 of the Order. All investigations of midwives' practice will be carried out directly by the NMC in the future.

Finally, the removal of the NMC Midwifery Committee and the Midwives Rules and Standards in 2017 will leave barely a trace of difference between the regulation of the midwifery and nursing professions. Midwives will need to remain alert to the possible removal of the title 'midwife' in the future and the consignment of the midwifery profession to the history books.

Key Points

* The statutory framework has continued, and will continue, to provide safety of practise for women and their babies and families.
* Midwives must be knowledgeable about the statutory and legal framework within which they practise and be aware of the upcoming and ongoing changes.
* Midwives should have a working knowledge of the NMC Code to maintain standards.
* Midwives must continue to work with women and their families to maintain quality and safety in their practise.

References

Baird B, Murray R, Seale B, et al: *Midwifery regulation in the UK 2013*. Report of King's Fund (website). www.nmc.org.uk/globalassets/sitedocuments/councilpapersanddocuments/council-2015/kings-fund-review.pdf. 2014.

Council for Healthcare Regulatory Excellence (CHRE): *Special report to the Minister of State for Health on the Nursing and Midwifery Council*, London, CHRE, 2008.

Department of Health (DH): *Health Act 1999*, London, Stationery Office, 1999.

Department of Health (DH): *The NHS plan. A plan for investment. A plan for reform*. CM 4818-4811, London, Stationery Office, 2000.

Department of Health (DH): *Modernising regulation in the health professions*. NHS consultation document (website). www.doh.gov.uk/modernisingregulation. 2001.

Department of Health (DH): *Nursing and Midwifery Order 2001, Statutory Instrument 2002, No. 253*, London, Stationery Office, 2002a.

Department of Health (DH): *NHS Reform and Health Care Professions Act 2002* (website). www.legislation.gov.uk/ukpga/2002/17/part/2/crossheading/the-council-for-the-regulation-of-health-care-professionals. 2002b.

Department of Health (DH): *Nurses and Midwives (Parts of and entries in the Register) Order of Council 2004, Statutory Instrument No. 175, Article 4* (website). www.legislation.gov.uk/uksi/2004/1765/article/2/made. 2004.

Department of Health (DH): *The regulation of non-medical healthcare professions: a review by the Department of Health*, London, Stationery Office, 2006a.

Department of Health (DH): *Good doctors, safer patients: proposals to strengthen the system to assure and improve the performance of doctors and to protect the safety of patients, a report by the Chief Medical Officer*, London, Stationery Office, 2006b.

Department of Health (DH): *Trust, assurance and safety – the regulation of health professionals in the 21st century*. CM 7013, London, Stationery Office, 2007.

Department of Health (DH): *The Health and Social Care Act*, London, Stationery Office, 2008a.

Department of Health (DH): *The Nursing and Midwifery Council (Constitution) Order 2008, No. 2553*, London, Stationery Office, 2008b.

Department of Health (DH): *Health and Social Care Act 2012* (website). www.legislation.gov.uk/ukpga/2012/7/section/222. 2012.

Department of Health (DH): *Nursing and Midwifery (Amendment) Order 2014* (website). www.legislation.gov.uk/uksi/2014/3272/note/made. 2014.

Department of Health (DH): *NHS Bursary Reform. Policy paper* (website). www.gov.uk/government/publications/nhs-bursary-reform/nhs-bursary-reform. 2015.

Department of Health (DH): *Proposals for changing the system of midwifery supervision in the UK* (website). https://www.gov.uk/government/publications/changes-to-midwife-supervision-in-the-uk. 2016.

English National Board (ENB): *Preparation of supervisors of midwives – an open learning programme*, London, ENB, 1992.

Health Education England (HEE): *Introducing Health Education England* (website). www.nwacademy.nhs.uk/sites/default/files/introducing-health-education-england-accessible-version.pdf. 2012.

Health Education England (HEE): *Health Education England (Special Health Authority) annual report and accounts 2014/15* (website). http://hee.nhs.uk/wp-content/blogs.dir/321/files/2015/07/Annual-Report_HR_web-without-signatures.pdf. 2015a.

Health Education England (HEE): *About Health Education England HEE* (website). https://hee.nhs.uk/about/. 2015b.

Health Education England (HEE): *Framework 15: A Health Education England strategic framework 2014–2029* (website). hee.nhs.uk/wp-content/uploads/sites/321/2014/06/HEE_StrategicFramework15_final.pdf. 2015c.

HM Government: *The Shipman Inquiry – safeguarding patients: lessons from the past, proposals for the future*, London, 2004, Stationery Office.

HM Government: *Safeguarding patients: the government's response to the recommendations of Shipman Inquiry's Fifth Report and to the recommendations of the Ayling, Neale and Kerr/Haslam Inquiries*, London, Stationery Office, 2007a.

HM Government: *Learning from tragedy, keeping patients safe*. CM7014, London, Stationery Office, 2007b.

Hunt J: *Jeremy Hunt announces new measures to improve safety across NHS. Press statement* (website). www.gov.uk/government/news/jeremy-hunt-announces-new-measures-to-improve-safety-across-nhs. 2015.

International Confederation of Midwives (ICM): *Global standards for midwifery education 2010* (amended 2013) (website). www.internationalmidwives.org/assets/uploads/documents/CoreDocuments/ICM%20Standards%20Guidelines_ammended2013.pdf. 2010.

Jowitt M, Kargar I: *Radical midwifery. Celebrating 21 years of ARM*, Lancashire, Association of Radical Midwives, 1997.

Kirkup B: *The report of the Morecambe Bay investigation* (website). www.gov.uk/government/uploads/system/uploads/attachment_data/file/408480/47487_MBI_Accessible_v0.1.pdf. 2015.

Local Supervising Authority Midwifery Officers (LSAMO) Forum UK: *Website statement* (website). www.lsamoforumuk.scot.nhs.uk/media/21573/lsamo_forum_uk_statement_for_website_290115.pdf. 2015a.

Local Supervising Authority Midwifery Officers (LSAMO) Forum UK: *Proposed model for professional leadership, support and advocacy* (website). www.lsamoforumuk.scot.nhs.uk/news/proposed-model-for-supervision-in-england.aspx. 2015b.

National Health Service England (NHSE): *Joint statement in response to the independent investigation into maternal and neonatal deaths at university Hospitals Morecambe Bay* (website). www.england.nhs.uk/2015/03/03/morecambe-bay/. 2015a.

National Health Service England (NHSE): *NHS England announces national review of maternity care* (website). www.england.nhs.uk/2015/03/03/maternity-care/. 2015b.

Nursing and Midwifery Council (NMC): *Rule 9(3) (Fitness to Practise) Rules Order of Council*, London, NMC, 2004.

Nursing and Midwifery Council (NMC): *Review of pre-registration midwifery education-decisions made by the Midwifery Committee*. Circular 14/2007, London, NMC, 2007.

Nursing and Midwifery Council (NMC): *Fitness to practise annual report 2007–2008*, London, NMC, 2008a.

Nursing and Midwifery Council (NMC): *Standards to support learning and assessment in practice*, ed 2, London, NMC, 2008b.

Nursing and Midwifery Council (NMC): *Good health and good character: guidance for educational institutions*, London, NMC, 2008c.

Nursing and Midwifery Council (NMC): *Standards for medicines management* (website). www.nmc.org.uk/standards/additional-standards/standards-for-medicines-management/. 2008d.

Nursing and Midwifery Council (NMC): *Operational guidance for sharing fitness to practise information*, London, NMC, 2009a.

Nursing and Midwifery Council (NMC): *Additional information to support implementation of NMC standards to support learning and assessment in practice*, London, NMC, 2009b.

Nursing and Midwifery Council (NMC): *Standards for pre-registration midwifery education* (website). www.nmc.org.uk/standards/additional-standards/standards-for-pre-registration-midwifery-education/. 2009c.

Nursing and Midwifery Council (NMC): *NMC framework for reviewing local supervising authorities*, London, NMC, 2009d.

Nursing and Midwifery Council (NMC): *Supervisors of Midwives: How they can help you. Leaflet for parents* (website). www.nmc.org.uk/globalassets/sitedocuments/midwifery-reports/nmc-supervisor-of-midwives-how-they-can-help-you.pdf. 2009e.

Nursing and Midwifery Council (NMC): *NMC Standing Orders 2009*, London, NMC, 2010a.

Nursing and Midwifery Council (NMC): *Conduct and Competence Committee* (website). www.nmc.org.uk/concerns-nurses-midwives/hearings-and-outcomes/our-panels-case-examiners/conduct-and-competence-committee/. 2010b.

Nursing and Midwifery Council (NMC): *Business Planning and Governance Committee*, London, NMC, 2010c.

Nursing and Midwifery Council (NMC): *Professional Practice and Registration Committee*, London, NMC, 2010d.

Nursing and Midwifery Council (NMC): *The PREP handbook* (website). www.nmc.org.uk/

standards/additional-standards/prep-handbook/. 2011.

Nursing and Midwifery Council (NMC): *Midwives rules and standards* (website). www.nmc.org.uk/standards/additional-standards/midwives-rules-and-standards/. 2012.

Nursing and Midwifery Council (NMC): *Quality assurance framework 2013* (updated August 2015) (website). www.nmc.org.uk/globalassets/sitedocuments/edandqa/nmc-quality-assurance-framework.pdf. 2013.

Nursing and Midwifery Council (NMC): *Immediate review of midwifery legislation* (website). www.nmc.org.uk/news/news-and-updates/review-of-midwifery-regulation/. 2014a.

Nursing and Midwifery Council (NMC): *Extraordinary LSA review – Princess Elizabeth Hospital, Health & Social Services Department & additional evidence, Guernsey 01-01* (website). www.nmc.org.uk/globalassets/sitedocuments/midwiferyextraordinaryreviewreports/extraordinary_review-lsa_south_west_guernsey__01-03-oct_14.pdf. 2014b.

[For additional evidence to the Guernsey report, see www.nmc.org.uk/globalassets/sitedocuments/midwiferyextraordinaryreviewreports/summary-of-additional-evidence_peh_guernsey.pdf. Annexe to the Guernsey Report: www.nmc.org.uk/globalassets/sitedocuments/midwiferyextraordinaryreviewreports/information-provided-following-the-extraordinary-lsa-review.pdf.].

Nursing and Midwifery Council (NMC): *Serious concerns with maternity services in Guernsey* (website). www.nmc.org.uk/news/news-and-updates/serious-concerns-with-maternity-services-in-guernsey/. 2014c.

Nursing and Midwifery Council (NMC): *Better legislation for better regulation: the case for legislative reform* (website). www.nmc.org.uk/globalassets/sitedocuments/press/better-legislation-for-better-regulation-the-nmcs-case-for-legislative-reform.pdf. 2014d.

Nursing and Midwifery Council (NMC): *Standards for the preparation of supervisors of midwives* (website). www.nmc.org.uk/standards/

additional-standards/Standards-preparation-supervisors-midwives/. 2014e.

Nursing and Midwifery Council (NMC): *Supervision of midwives: an NMC factsheet* (website). www.nmc.org.uk/globalassets/sitedocuments/factsheets/nmc-factsheet-supervision-of-midwives.pdf. 2014f.

Nursing and Midwifery Council (NMC): *The role of lead midwives for education* (website). www.nmc.org.uk/education/lead-midwifery-educators/the-role-of-lead-midwives-for-education/. 2015a.

Nursing and Midwifery Council (NMC): *Maximum time limits to complete education programmes removed* (website). www.nmc.org.uk/news/news-and-updates/maximum-time-limits-to-complete-education-programmes-removed/. 2015b.

Nursing and Midwifery Council (NMC): *Standards of competence for registered midwives* (website). www.nmc.org.uk/globalassets/sitedocuments/standards/standards-for-competence-for-registered-midwives.pdf. 2015c.

Nursing and Midwifery Council (NMC): *NMC revalidation for nurses and midwives* (website). www.nmc.org.uk/standards/revalidation/what-is-revalidation/ and www.nmc.org.uk/globalassets/sitedocuments/revalidation/how-to-revalidate-print-friendly-version.pdf. 2015d.

Nursing and Midwifery Council (NMC): *The Code NMC* (website). www.nmc.org.uk/standards/code/. 2015e.

Nursing and Midwifery Council (NMC): *Raising concerns: guidance for nurses and midwives* (website). www.nmc.org.uk/standards/guidance/raising-concerns-guidance-for-nurses-and-midwives/. 2015f.

Nursing and Midwifery Council (NMC): *Guidance on the professional duty of candour* (website). www.nmc.org.uk/standards/guidance/the-professional-duty-of-candour/. 2015g.

Nursing and Midwifery Council (NMC): *Advice and information for employers of nurses and midwives* (website). www.nmc.org.uk/globalassets/sitedocuments/ftp_information/advice-for-employers-15-october-2015.pdf. 2015h.

Nursing and Midwifery Council (NMC): *How midwifery regulation works; Supervision arrangements and the midwifery part of the register* (website). www.nmc.org.uk/standards/what-to-expect-from-a-nurse-or-midwife/how-midwives-are-regulated/how-midwifery-regulation-works/. 2015i.

Nursing and Midwifery Council (NMC): *Fact sheet: Modernising midwifery regulation: protected title, function and midwifery scope of practice* (website). www.nmc.org.uk/globalassets/sitedocuments/factsheets/midwifery-final-to-publish-9-november.pdf. 2015j.

Nursing and Midwifery Council (NMC): *Nursing and midwifery regulator calls for supervision to be removed from its legislation* (website). www.nmc.org.uk/news/news-and-updates/nursing-and-midwifery-regulator-calls-for-supervision-to-be-removed-from-its-legislation/. 2015k.

Nursing and Midwifery Council (NMC): *NMC response to Secretary of State's statement* (website). www.nmc.org.uk/news/news-and-updates/nmc-response-to-secretary-of-states-statement-on-midwifery-supervision/. 2015l.

Nursing and Midwifery Council (NMC): *LSAMOs: their role and how to contact them* (website). www.nmc.org.uk/standards/what-to-expect-from-a-nurse-or-midwife/how-midwives-are-regulated/lsamos/. 2015m.

Nursing and Midwifery Council (NMC): *Registering as a nurse or midwife in the UK – for applicants trained in the EU or EEA* (valid from January 2016) (website). www.nmc.org.uk/globalassets/sitedocuments/registration/registering-as-a-nurse-or-midwife-in-the-uk-for-applicants-trained-in-eea-jan2016.pdf. 2016.

Parliamentary and Health Service Ombudsman (PHSO): *Midwifery supervision and regulation: recommendations for change* (website). www.ombudsman.org.uk/reports-and-consultations/reports/health/midwifery-supervision-and-regulation-recommendations-for-change. 2013.

Royal College of Midwives (RCM) (Gillman LJ, editor): *Re-framing midwifery supervision: a discussion*

paper (website). https://www.rcm
.org.uk/sites/default/files/Re-framing
%20supervision%20-paper
%20for%20discussion%20final%20
23%203%202015.pdf. 2015.

United Kingdom Central Council for
Nursing, Midwifery and Health
Visiting (UKCC): *Midwives rules*,
London, UKCC, 1986.

Resources and additional reading

International Confederation of
Midwives (ICM): www.international
midwives.org.
*Excellent resource including information
on global standards, definition of the
midwife and country-specific
information and links.*
Nursing and Midwifery Council
(NMC): www.nmc.org.uk.
*Wide range of information, including
guidelines, the Code, standards and
up to date information relevant to
practice. It is useful to be aware of the
most up to date publications and policy,
and it is possible to get e-mail alerts
and electronic newsletters from the
NMC.*
Training nurses and midwives:
www.nmc.org.uk/globalassets/
sitedocuments/nmc-publications/
educators-leaflet.pdf.

Standards for midwifery education:
www.nmc.org.uk/globalassets/
sitedocuments/standards/nmc-
standards-for-preregistration-
midwifery-education.pdf.
Maintaining registration: www.nmc.org
.uk/registration/staying-on-the
-register/paying-your-fee/.
Indemnity insurance: www.nmc.org.uk/
registration/staying-on-the
-register/professional
-indemnity-arrangement/.
Student funding: www.gov.uk/
government/publications/nhs-
bursary-reform/nhs-bursary-reform.
Royal College of Midwives: www.rcm
.org.uk.

*Provides information on regulation,
education, policy and news. Also offers
the electronic learning programme,
which includes a module on validation.
The eLearning materials themselves are
suitable to complete for revalidation
purposes.*
See NHS England Website for
information regarding the
replacement of Statutory
Supervision of Midwives in
England. https://www.england.nhs.
uk/2016/10/shaping-midwifery/.
UK plans for replacement of Statutory
Supervision of Midwives will be
available on: https://www.gov.uk/
government/publications/changes-to
-midwife-supervision-in-the-uk.

Chapter 4

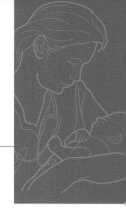

Clinical governance and the midwife

Jessica Read

Learning Outcomes ?

After reading this chapter, you will be able to:

- have a thorough understanding of clinical governance in the UK National Health Service (NHS) and be able to apply that understanding to midwifery
- describe a governance framework within the National Health Service
- discuss the core elements of clinical governance that support the delivery of safe and effective maternity care
- describe the midwife's responsibilities in relation to clinical governance

CLINICAL GOVERNANCE: A DEFINITION

Clinical governance is described as a systematic approach to maintaining and improving the quality of patient care within a health system such as the National Health Service (NHS).

Clinical governance in healthcare was prioritized following the Bristol Heart scandal in 1995 (Kennedy 2001) and the Shipman Inquiry, which commenced in 1998 (Smith 2002). The concept of clinical governance was seen to be a support to clinicians and providers as a means to ensure the delivery of safe effective care while taking into consideration the service user's experience. Clinical governance in the NHS was initially defined in 1998 by Scally and Donaldson (p. 61) as being:

'A framework through which NHS organisations are accountable for continually improving the quality of their services and safeguarding high standards of care by creating an environment in which excellence in clinical care will flourish'.

In 2008, the Department of Health (DH) published the *High-Quality Care for All: NHS Next Stage Review – Final Report*, which describes the definition of high-quality care in the NHS as being safe and effective and resulting in a positive patient experience (DH 2008).

These attributes are articulated in the Health and Social Care Act of 2012, which describes the Secretary of State's duty in improving the quality of health services provided to individuals and in securing continuous improvement in the outcomes achieved through the provision of services. The act states that the following three aspects must be demonstrated by services in relation to outcomes:

1. The effectiveness of the services
2. The safety of the services
3. The quality of the experience undergone by patients (Health and Social Care Act 2012, Part 1, 2)

NHS GOVERNANCE SYSTEMS

The NHS Outcomes Framework was developed in 2010 for the NHS in England and sits at the heart of the health and care system. The NHS Outcomes Framework undertakes the following functions:

1. Provides a national overview of how well the NHS is performing
2. Is the primary accountability mechanism, in conjunction with the mandate, between the Secretary of State for Health and NHS England
3. Improves quality throughout the NHS by encouraging a change in culture and behaviour focused on health outcomes, not process

The NHS Outcomes Framework is updated annually to ensure the framework reflects the contemporary landscape

67

of the health and care system; it is a dynamic tool that can be used to address the many challenges that the system faces.

The NHS Outcomes Framework is a set of 68 indicators organized into five domains (see below); these indicators measure performance in the health and care system at a national level. The framework is intended to provide a focus for accountability and improvement (DH 2014).

Domain 1:
Preventing people from dying prematurely

Domain 2:
Enhancing quality of life for people
with long-term conditions

Domain 3:
Helping people to recover from episodes of ill
health or following injury

Domain 4:
Ensuring that people have a positive experience of care

Domain 5:
Treating and caring for people in a safe environment
and protecting them from avoidable harm

Reflective activity 4.1   ✕❮

Consider which of the five domains apply to maternity services, and reflect on how midwives can affect those domains.

Clinical governance frameworks vary across the UK; however, the three key aspects of governance articulated in the Health and Social Care Act of 2012 underpin them all. Scotland published its Health Care Quality Strategy for NHS Scotland in May 2010 (Scottish Government 2010), which identifies three healthcare quality ambitions:

1. To support the delivery of person-centred care to the people of Scotland

2. To support the delivery of safe care to the people of Scotland

3. To support the delivery of effective care to the people of Scotland

The strategy for Scotland outlines 12 national quality outcome measures, which are similar to the NHS Outcomes Framework outlined previously. One of Scotland's

healthcare quality standards incorporates clinical governance and risk management; this standard will be used to measure the effectiveness of organizations in achieving the goals of the quality outcomes measures.

The Welsh government has produced Health and Care Standards that are structured along seven themes developed through engagement with patients, clinicians and stakeholders and identified as the priority areas for the NHS to be measured against (NHS Wales 2015). The Welsh government has aligned the Health and Care Standards to the NHS Outcomes Framework and the NHS Delivery Framework. The seven themes collectively describe how a service provides high-quality, safe and reliable care, centred on the person. Person-centred care is positioned in the centre, and the dependence on good governance, leadership and accountability surrounds the central theme.

In 2010, the Department of Health, Social Services and Public Safety in Northern Ireland (DHSSPSNI 2011) produced a 10-year strategy to protect and improve quality in healthcare and social care in Northern Ireland. The three key components the strategy focuses on are the same as those in all other UK countries: safety, effectiveness and patient and client focus. The DHSSPSNI also produced a set of quality standards that are used by the Regulation and Quality Improvement Authority (RQIA) to assess the quality of care delivery in Northern Ireland. This organization has a similar role to that provided by the Care Quality Commission (CQC) in England.

Every healthcare organization's board has a responsibility to oversee the quality of care being delivered throughout the organization and to seek assurance that high-quality care is resulting in good outcomes being achieved (National Quality Board 2011).

The following aspects are incorporated into the clinical governance framework at organizational level and represent the board's responsibility:

- Ensure that the essential standards of quality and safety are being met.

- Ensure that the organization is striving towards continuous quality improvement.

- Ensure that each staff member who has direct or indirect contact with patients is suitably qualified, motivated and enabled to deliver effective, safe patient-focused care.

International governance

Both the World Health Organization (WHO) and the Council of Europe highlight good governance in healthcare as being central to enhancing performance in healthcare delivery (WHO 2015). WHO recognizes that equitable access to quality integrated healthcare services for mothers and families is integral to the delivery of the

United Nations (2015) Millennium Development Goals (MDGs), specifically, MDG 4 (reducing child mortality) and MDG 5 (improving maternal health).

To gain understanding of healthcare governance throughout Europe, it is important to understand the complexity of the landscape in regard to decision making, which must incorporate both national- and institutional-level decision making for the predominantly publicly owned hospitals. National policymakers in Europe have focused on improving the quality and efficiency of their public services by adopting private-sector governance principles and strategies (Health Services Research Network 2013).

There is variation across Europe, with Germany, for example, having an emphasis on legal liability to individual patients and professional self-regulation; Germany has not extended its system to other forms of accountability as delivered by clinical governance in the UK. Spain has a life expectancy at birth that is ranked fourth worldwide, with mortality rates for the major causes of death among the lowest in Europe; however, there is significant variation across the country (Health Services Research Network 2013).

In Eastern Europe, the devolution of hospital responsibilities from central to local government has led (in the absence of effective control mechanisms) to an accountability vacuum in the region. Local authorities are charged with overseeing the public hospitals but have only limited defined responsibilities for governance, particularly with respect to accountability for the quality and safety of patient care delivered by the hospitals. In Eastern Europe, perhaps comforted by lower levels of litigation and regulation, hospitals have been less regimented than in, for example, North America; however, increasing legal liability for the safety of staff and patients along with increasing public expectations and increasing pressure for standardization between countries are demanding more transparency and accountability (Shaw et al 2009).

LEARNING FROM CLINICAL INCIDENTS: HUMAN FACTORS SCIENCE

Learning from clinical incidents requires an understanding of human factors and how the science of human factors interplays with professional behaviour and performance.

Human factors can be defined as follows:

'Huass all those factors that can influence people and their behavior. In a work context, human factors are the environmental, organisational and job factors, and individual characteristics which influence behavior at work'.

(Clinical Human Factors Group 2015)

Healthcare professionals are human beings, and like all human beings, they make mistakes in both their personal and professional lives. The effects of these mistakes are often nonexistent, minor or merely inconvenient. However, in healthcare there is always the underlying chance that the consequences could be catastrophic. There are many factors that interplay with one another within the clinical context during a high-risk situation, both positively and negatively. If there is a situation when all the negative factors are aligned, this increases the risk of human error, which can result in a clinical incident.

James Reason (1990) describes the Swiss cheese model of organizational accidents. This model hypothesizes that in any system there are many levels of defence. Each of these levels of defence has little 'holes' in it that are caused by poor system design, senior management decision making, out-of-date guidelines, lack of training, limited resources and so forth. These holes are known as 'latent conditions'.

If latent conditions become aligned over increasing levels of defence, they create a window of opportunity for a patient safety incident to occur. This is depicted by the arrow breaching all levels of defence (Fig. 4.1).

The Code (Nursing and Midwifery Council (NMC) 2015b) defines the nurse's and midwife's responsibility in identifying any potential for harm associated with practice. The Code stipulates that the midwife must:

'Take account of current evidence, knowledge and developments in reducing mistakes and the effect of them and the impact of human factors and systems failures'.

(NMC 2015b: 19.2)

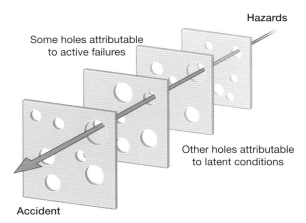

Figure 4.1 Swiss cheese model. (Reproduced from Human error: models and management, James Reason, BMJ 2000, with permission from BMJ Publishing Group Ltd.)

THE IMPACT OF PUBLIC INQUIRY ON CLINICAL GOVERNANCE IN THE UK

The importance of understanding the impact of human factors in healthcare was highlighted in two major public inquiries and a national report on patient safety in the NHS.

The Francis Report

Concerns were raised about levels of mortality and the standard of care delivered at the Mid-Staffordshire NHS Foundation Trust, which resulted in an investigation undertaken by the Healthcare Commission (HCC) in 2009. The published report by the HCC was highly critical and led to a public inquiry being requested by the Secretary of State (Francis 2010). The independent inquiry was chaired by Robert Francis QC, and the report was published in 2010. The report highlighted concerns and failings that went beyond the Trust itself and implicated the regulatory bodies, commissioners and the wider systems of management and oversight both locally and nationally. In June 2010, a full public inquiry was ordered and chaired by Robert Francis QC. The report was published in 2013 (Francis 2013), setting out an analysis of what went wrong and asking questions about the culture of the NHS as a whole (Thorlby et al 2014).

Five main themes were articulated by Francis, and the corresponding actions that needed to be taken were identified (Table 4.1).

In 2014, Thorlby et al published a report commissioned by the Nuffield Trust titled *The Francis Report: One Year On*. The report concluded that there was a concerning continuance of 'somewhat oppressive reactions' (p. 5) to reports of difficulties in meeting financial and other corporate requirements. This alludes to the inevitable tension between finance and quality that continues to persist within healthcare organizations.

The Berwick Report

In 2013, following the events at Mid-Staffordshire, the National Advisory Group on the Safety of Patients asked Don Berwick from the Institute of Healthcare Improvement to lead an advisory group to review the safety of patients in the NHS. Berwick published the report in August 2013: *A Promise to Learn – A Commitment to Act*.

The five themes identified by Francis continue through the Berwick Report, with additional focus on the following:

- Blame culture within the NHS – in the vast majority of cases it is systems issues and constraints that lead to patient safety problems.
- Incorrect priorities cause harm – the central focus must be on the patients.

- Clear warning signs must be heeded, especially from patients and carers.
- 'Fear is toxic to both safety and improvement' (p. 4).
- Use quantitative targets with caution; don't displace the primary goal of better care.
- Expect and insist on transparency.

Place the quality of patient care, especially patient safety, above all aims.

Engage, empower, and hear patients and carers at all times.

Foster whole-heartedly the growth and development of all staff, including their ability and support to improve the processes in which they work.

Embrace transparency unequivocally and everywhere, in the service of accountability, trust, and the growth of knowledge.

(Berwick 2013: 4)

The Kirkup Inquiry

Serious concerns were raised regarding the maternity services operating under the University Hospitals of Morecambe Bay NHS Foundation Trust during the period of January 2004 through June 2013. This included the deaths of mothers and babies and the lack of an appropriate response by the Trust and the wider NHS. Dr Bill Kirkup CBE was asked to chair a public inquiry, and his report was published in March 2015 (Kirkup 2015).

Unlike the Francis Report and the Berwick Report, the Kirkup Report is purely about maternity care. Kirkup acknowledges that the majority of women using maternity services are not ill but going through normal physiological changes of pregnancy that should culminate in two healthy individuals. Kirkup maintains that the safety of maternity care 'depends crucially on maintaining vigilance for early warning of any departure from normality and on taking the right, timely action when it is detected' (Kirkup 2015: 183).

The public inquiry found that in Morecambe Bay there was an inexcusable repeated failure to examine adverse events properly, and there was a lack of openness and honesty with families, both of which led to a lack of organizational learning and reoccurrence of mistakes and errors.

The Kirkup Report makes 44 recommendations, the themes of which correlate with those of both the Francis Report and the Berwick Report. The Kirkup Report highlights the challenges of providing healthcare in rural and isolated areas, which are difficult to recruit to, and recommends that the NHS should review the safe provision of services in these areas. The Kirkup Report also recommends that clear and unambiguous standards should be drawn up for the reporting and investigation of serious incidents in maternity.

Table 4.1 Five main themes from the Francis Report

Main Themes	Explanation	Action Taken
Fundamental standards	At the time, quality standards were unclear in terms of their objectives and the regulation of standards. Boards should publish comprehensive reports in relation to compliance with standards. Management of complaints must be robust and efficient, with attention given to detailed and timely sharing of information regarding complaints.	Clear standards set by Department of Health (DH), including set of 'fundamental standards' published by DH in November 2014, and assessed by the Care Quality Commission (CQC). Standards also set by regulatory bodies of the Nursing and Midwifery Council (NMC) and General Medical Council (GMC). • The Code (NMC 2015b) • Midwives Rules and Standards (NMC 2012) Maternity Services Review established in England 2015; part of the review is to look at a national standard for complaints management.
Openness, transparency and candour	A defensive culture existed, with a lack of openness with patients, the public and external agencies. Leadership lacked insight and awareness of the reality in the clinical areas.	Organizations cite 'candour' as a requirement in governance strategies. NMC and GMC produced *Openness and Honesty When Things Go Wrong: The Professional Duty of Candour* (NMC and GMC 2015).
Nursing standards	An inadequate standard of nursing was identified at Mid-Staffordshire, with poor leadership, recruitment and training. Cuts had been made to the nursing workforce.	National Institute of Health and Care Excellence published guidelines for safe staffing levels in 2015 (NICE 2015b).
Patient-centred leadership	Poor-quality leadership across all levels was highlighted. Wrong objectives were set at the cost of patient care; the focus was on self-promotion rather than analysis of the situation and openness.	National Health Service (NHS) Leadership Academy established to provide leadership courses at all levels. CQC to assess 'well-led services' during inspections from 2015.
Information	There were no systems in place to accurately collect real-time information about the performance of services against the standards required.	Clinical dashboards with ratings of red, amber, green (RAG) are utilized at local and regional levels; reviewed and monitored regularly.

THE PILLARS OF HEALTHCARE GOVERNANCE

There are a number of essential aspects of clinical governance, which together become catalysts to drive quality improvement (Fig. 4.2).

Quality improvement is defined as

'the combined and unceasing efforts of everyone – healthcare professionals, patients and their families, researchers, payers, planners and educators to make the changes that will lead to better patient outcomes

(health), better service performance (care) and better professional development'.

(Batalden et al 2007 p. 2)

Midwives have an important role to play in improving quality in healthcare, and this can be seen throughout the seven themes discussed next.

Staff training and revalidation

One of the key principles of clinical governance is to ensure that organizations and healthcare professionals

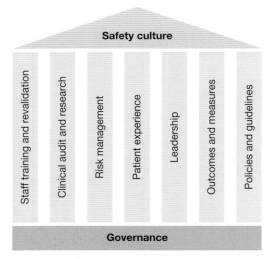

Figure 4.2 The pillars of healthcare governance.

remain up to date within their speciality and scope of practice. Every member of the public should be assured that a midwife they come into contact with has the correct knowledge, skills and competency to undertake the role efficiently and effectively (McSherry and Haddock 1999). Organizations have a responsibility to ensure that the midwives they employ are provided with regular mandatory training to remain updated and able to fulfil the roles they are employed to fulfil. Individual midwives have a responsibility to ensure that they meet the statutory requirements of the NMC.

The Midwives Act of 1902 established the legal framework for the regulation of midwives' practice, and supervision of midwives became the means of scrutinizing that practice. During the last decade supervision of midwives has been seen as supportive and proactive in ensuring that the public is protected from poor practice. Every practising midwife is allocated a named supervisor of midwives (SOM) who will meet with the midwife at least annually to ensure that the midwife is meeting the NMC post-registration education and practice (PREP) standards. The SOM also provides supportive development for the midwife when learning needs are identified and will investigate incidents where midwifery practice has been called into question. SOMs are appointed to the role by the local supervising authority (LSA); the role of the SOM is impartial to the employing organization and is accountable to the LSA.

The NMC launched revalidation for nurses and midwives in April 2016, and all nurses and midwives on the NMC Register will be required to revalidate every 3 years.

As a result of the Kings Fund review of midwifery regulation (Baird et al 2015), the NMC made the policy decision that the additional layer of regulation currently in place for midwives and the extended role for the NMC over statutory supervision should end. The intention is that revalidation will replace the supervisory role for midwives in ensuring that midwives meet the required standards and the Code (NMC 2015a) (see also Ch. 3).

Clinical audit and research

Clinical audit is how organizations refine clinical practice as a result of the measurement of performance against agreed standards; it is seen as a cyclical process for improving clinical care. Audit is used to evaluate the effectiveness and quality of care. Areas of poor practice or potential risk are highlighted so that standards can be reviewed to ensure that preventative measures are taken. Clinical audit and research are integral to the provision of high-quality, well-governed care because they both have a role to play in delivering evidence-based, safe maternity care.

CASE STUDY

A maternity service acknowledged a high number of incidents where babies had been 'born before arrival/attendance' (BBA). The service undertook an audit of those incidents and found that one of the contributory factors was the quality of advice given to women who phoned the unit when in labour. The service established a telephone assessment document that enabled the midwife to take a full picture of the woman's situation and be directed to the correct advice to give. Following implementation of the telephone assessment document, a further audit was undertaken, and the number of BBAs had declined.

To ensure high-quality care in midwifery practice, it is essential that care is based on the most recent and best scientific evidence. Midwives have a role in identifying areas of clinical practice that would benefit from further inquiry and research. McSherry and Haddock (1999) identify the following processes from literature that define the means by which to execute evidence-based care:

- Formulate clear clinical questions that, when answered, will result in a measurable improvement in midwifery care.
- Identify the most relevant evidence and literature from all sources.
- Critically appraise the evidence.
- Implement and incorporate relevant findings into practice.
- Continue to measure performance against expected outcomes or against peers.

An organization that has developed, integrated systems of audit and research will be enabled to maintain high-quality clinical care. Midwives have a responsibility to identify elements of practice that would benefit from auditing to ensure evidence-based practice is implemented.

Reflective activity 4.2

Within your healthcare organization, identify a recent clinical audit within the maternity service that has been undertaken. Explore how the clinical audit has improved midwifery care.

Risk management

Risk management in healthcare is a systematic process that reviews a whole spectrum of things that could go wrong. This includes risks to patients, midwives and other healthcare professionals and risks to the organization.

Healthcare providers across the world are increasingly expected to adopt a risk-management approach towards reducing harm to patients. In the UK the impetus for this approach came from the Department of Health expert report *An Organisation with a Memory* (DH 2000), which emphasized the need for organizations to learn from clinical error. A major step was taken with the establishment of the National Patient Safety Agency in 2001, and in 2015 the Department of Health announced plans for 'NHS Improvement,' a body that will incorporate patient safety into its strategic remit. In the United States, New Zealand and other countries, various governmental and non-governmental bodies have led the way in setting standards, establishing training courses and initiating research around patient safety.

The Royal College of Obstetricians and Gynaecologists (RCOG 2009) articulated four basic questions that are addressed by risk management, as summarized in Table 4.2.

There are a range of different means by which maternity services identify risk, including electronic notification systems. Risks can be identified through a variety of

Table 4.2 Basic questions addressed by risk management

What could go wrong?	Risk identification
What are the chances of it going wrong, and what would be the effects?	Risk analysis and evaluation
What can we do to minimize the chance of this happening or to mitigate damage when it has gone wrong?	Risk treatment; cost of prevention compared to the cost of getting it wrong
What can we learn from things that have gone wrong?	Risk control; sharing and learning

sources, which include internal (incident reporting) and external sources (patient complaints). National standards, local guidance and organizational protocols are used to benchmark practice. Midwives are responsible for identifying incidents and taking steps to reduce the level of harm to women and their families (NMC 2015b: 19.1).

Investigation of clinical incidents is utilized to identify contributory factors that have resulted in harm to the woman or baby. It is important that human factors are considered when undertaking a root-cause analysis of a clinical incident.

Identification of themes from clinical incidents is important, and groups of similar incidents can be investigated together. Recommendations for healthcare professionals and the organization come out of risk-management investigations, and it is important that the actions are logged and recorded when completed.

An element of risk management is to maintain a risk register. Organizations record significant risks on a risk register, which is reviewed regularly and can be escalated from a departmental risk register to a register for the entire healthcare organization. Ultimately, the organization's board is responsible for monitoring those risks on the organization's risk register.

Reflective activity 4.3

Access your organization's maternity risk register to review the risks that have been identified. Reflect on whether the risks have been suitably controlled in your organization.

Patient experience

The quality of the experience undergone by patients is one of the three key aspects articulated in the Health and Social Care Act (2002) that is integral to improving outcomes. Emerging evidence demonstrates that healthcare organizations with a strong emphasis on providing high-quality patient experience have found that it is linked to improving health outcomes (The Health Foundation, 2013).

Across the UK there are a number of relative policy documents, drivers, incentives and sanctions that make improving patient experience an imperative, and a useful place to start is the NHS Constitution. The NHS Constitution was created to protect NHS England and ensure that it will always do the things it was set up to do in 1948 – to provide high-quality healthcare that is free and for everyone. The Constitution establishes the principles and values of high-quality healthcare and sets out the rights to which patients are entitled. The NHS constitution focuses on the provision of high-quality care that is safe, effective and focused on patient experience (DH 2012). Wales, Scotland and Northern Ireland all have strategies for maternity care that encompass the importance of improving women's experience. Healthcare Inspectorate organizations (CQC, Health Inspectorate Wales, Health Improvement Scotland, Northern Ireland Practice and Education Council for Nursing and Midwifery) review woman-centred care systems during service inspections; this includes reviewing women's feedback and complaint systems and responses.

It is important that women are assured that their feedback is heard and acted on where appropriate and that themes are identified. It is also important that positive feedback is shared with midwives and other healthcare professionals. The involvement of service users in the planning, management and delivery of maternity services assists with the promotion of openness and public engagement.

Management of complaints also comes under the patient experience umbrella; it is important that maternity services have a clear pathway that is simple for women and their families to access should they choose to raise concerns about their care. Complaints should be investigated thoroughly and responded to within clear timeframes; actions need to be taken accordingly. Since the publication of the Francis Report (Francis 2013), there has been an emphasis on each health professional's 'duty of candour' and a requirement for transparency and openness involving service users in all aspects of the investigation process. The NMC Code states clearly that it is the role of the midwife to:

'Be open and candid with all service users about all aspects of care and treatment, including when any mistakes or harm have taken place'.

(NMC 2015b)

Being open and candid includes taking the time to visit a woman and her family who have had a difficult experience, especially if the midwife has cared for the family. Many maternity services offer debriefing opportunities

for women and their families, which results in preventative actions being taken to improve outcomes for all women.

Reflective activity 4.4

Reflect on an experience you have had when a woman has articulated concerns regarding her care. What were your actions, and what, if anything, would you do differently now? Refer to the NMC and GMC publication *Openness and Honesty When Things Go Wrong: The Professional Duty of Candour* (2015).

Leadership

It is important to acknowledge the role that strong, effective midwifery leadership has to play within the clinical governance framework. The Royal College of Midwives (RCM) and Midwifery Leadership Competency Framework (RCM and NHS Leadership Academy 2012) articulates how every midwife has a role to play in improving services for women and their families. The RCM competency framework (based on the NHS Leadership Academy Framework) describes the following attributes that midwives require to deliver the governance framework:

1. **Midwives show leadership by ensuring patient safety:** assess and manage the risk of patients while balancing economic considerations with the priority of patient safety.

2. **Midwives show leadership by critically evaluating:** think analytically to identify where service improvements can be made, working individually or as part of a team.

3. **Midwives show leadership by encouraging improvement and innovation:** create a climate of continuous service improvement.

4. **Midwives show leadership by facilitating transformation:** contribute to the change processes that lead to improvements in healthcare.

Every midwife has a role to play in providing leadership to make sure that women's health and well-being are protected at all times to improve their experiences of the healthcare system (NMC 2015b).

Reflective activity 4.5

What service improvement would you like to see in your organization? Describe the change you would like to see and articulate the improvements to women and their families that will be facilitated through this change.

Outcomes and measures

It is very important that healthcare organizations measure quality improvement in healthcare; measurement should underpin all of the pillars of governance mentioned previously. Healthcare organizations should ensure that they have the capability internally to undertake analysis, benchmarking and the presentation of metrics, which enable organizations to identify areas for improvement and those areas achieving high-quality care.

In January 2008, the RCOG published the Good Practice Guideline *Maternity Dashboard Clinical Performance and Governance Score Card*. The purpose of this guidance is to urge all maternity units to consider the use of a maternity dashboard to plan and improve their maternity services. The dashboard serves as a clinical performance and governance score card to monitor the implementation of the principles of clinical governance within the service and is intended to help identify patient safety issues in advance so that timely and appropriate action can be instituted to ensure woman-centred, high-quality, safe maternity care (RCOG 2008).

Maternity Services throughout the UK have modified the Maternity Dashboard to provide localized contemporary information about resources, including clinical activity, clinical incidents and user views, thus enabling early identification of risk where goals are not met and initiating timely action to avoid patient safety incidents and improve clinical care.

A traffic light system is often utilized to indicate the level of risk pertaining to each indicator:

Green: The goal is met.

Amber: The goal is not met. Action is required to avoid entering the red zone.

Red: The goal is not met, and the upper threshold is breached. Urgent action is needed from the highest level to maintain safety and to restore quality.

Four broad themes are generally covered within a maternity dashboard: clinical activity (birth rate); workforce (midwife-to-birth ratio); clinical outcomes (admissions to Intensive therapy unit); risk incidents, complaints and user surveys (number of complaints). Where there is a deviation from expected performance, it indicates that action should be taken.

Midwives need to be cognizant of the outcome metrics used within their own organizations and contribute to improvement programmes that facilitate high-quality care for women and their families.

Reflective activity 4.6

Find out what the normal birth rate and caesarean section rate are in your healthcare organization. How are clinical outcomes measured, and what actions are being taken to improve those outcomes within your organization?

Policies and guidelines

Clinical guidelines, policies and protocols that are evidence based contribute to clinical governance systems by eliminating variations in practice. Healthcare systems throughout the world have been influenced by the move towards evidence-based healthcare. Evidence-based practice is defined as practice that occurs through the integration of clinical expertise with the best available external evidence from systematic research (McSherry and Haddock 1999).

The National Institute for Clinical Excellence (NICE), now called the National Institute for Health and Care Excellence, was established in 1999 to reduce variation in the availability and quality of NHS treatments and care. In 2005, NICE began developing public health guidance to help prevent ill health and promote healthier lifestyles. In April 2013, NICE was established in primary legislation and became a non-departmental public body as set out in the Health and Social Care Act of 2012. At this time NICE took on responsibility for developing evidence-based guidance and quality standards in health and social care.

NICE guidance officially applies to England only; however, NICE has agreements to provide certain products and services to Wales, Scotland and Northern Ireland. Decisions on how NICE guidance applies in these countries are made by the devolved administrations (NICE 2015a).

NICE has produced a number of guidelines relating to maternity care, including those in the areas of smoking cessation, staffing levels in maternity care, antenatal care, intrapartum care and postnatal care, for example (NICE 2015b). The RCOG also produces evidence-based guidance, referred to as 'Green-top Guidelines', and is a NICE-accredited organization.

Midwives must ensure that the advice and guidance they give to women is evidence based and established within local and national guidelines. Women need to be equipped with contemporary information to enable them to make informed decisions about their care, and midwives have a key role to play in this.

Reflective activity 4.7

What is the most recent piece of evidence-based research relating to maternity care you have read, and how has it influenced midwifery practice?

CONCLUSION

Clinical governance provides a systematic approach to the delivery of safe, effective and high-quality care.

The woman's journey through the maternity pathway provides the opportunity for the midwife to ensure that the care given is of the highest quality, within the safest environment and incorporates the woman's own preferences and choices of care. All maternity healthcare providers have a responsibility to offer a well-led service, which encompasses high-quality clinical governance systems. The midwife whose practice is woman focused, evidence based and validated will work collaboratively with her peers and the multiprofessional team to have a positive effect on both short- and long-term health and the wider well-being of women, babies and their families.

Key Points

- All midwives should be able to describe the key elements of the clinical governance framework and ensure that they contribute to the delivery of safe, effective, woman-focused care.
- Midwives need to be aware of their own responsibility with regard to revalidation and maintaining their midwifery registration by delivering evidence-based midwifery care.
- Midwives need to be able to innovate and implement strategies to improve midwifery care within a context of financial restraint.
- Political awareness is key to understanding priorities in healthcare and ensuring that maternity care is high on the agenda.

- Understanding the importance of the interplay of human factors within clinical incidents will facilitate a robust discussion and analysis of the root cause.
- Midwives have an important role to play in research, audit processes, training, outcomes measurement and implementation of evidence-based guidelines.
- The care midwives give must respond to women's feedback and changes in evidence-based guidelines and research.
- Women must be given the opportunity to articulate their preferences for care and to contribute to the delivery of maternity care.

References

Batalden P, Davidoff F: What is 'quality improvement' and how can it transform healthcare? http://quality safety.bmj.com.

Baird B, Murray R, Seale B, et al: Midwifery regulation in the United Kingdom. Kings Fund Report commissioned by the NMC, London, Kings Fund, 2015.

Berwick D chair: 'A promise to learn – a commitment to act'; improving the safety of patients in England, London, National Advisory Group on the Safety of Patients in England, 2013.

Clinical Human Factors Group: Human factors theory (website). http://chfg.org/resource/human-factors-theory. 2015.

Department of Health (DH): An organisation with a memory. Report of an expert group on learning from adverse incidents in the NHS. Chaired by the Chief Medical Officer, London, Stationery Office, 2000.

Department of Health (DH): High-quality care for all: NHS next stage review final report (website).

www.dh.gov.uk/prod_consum_dh/groups/dh_digitalassets/@dh/@en/documents/digitalasset/dh_085828.pdf. 2008.

Department of Health (DH): NHS Constitution for England (website). www.gov.uk/government/publications/the-nhs-constitution-for-england. 2012.

Department of Health (DH): The NHS Outcomes Framework 2015/16 (website). http://nhsout comesframework@dh.gsi.gov.uk. 2014.

Department of Health, Social Services and Public Safety Northern Ireland: Quality 2020: A 10-year strategy to protect and improve quality in health and social care in Northern Ireland (website). www.dhsspsni.gov.uk. 2011.

Francis R chair: Independent inquiry into care provided by Mid Staffordshire NHS Foundation Trust: January 2005–March 2009 (vol 1), London, Stationery Office, 2010.

Francis R chair: Report of the Mid Staffordshire NHS Foundation Trust

public inquiry, London, Stationery Office, 2013.

Health Foundation, The; The Evidence center: No 18. Measuring Patient Experience. June 2013.

Health and Social Care Act 2012, Part 1, 2 (website). www.legislation.gov.uk/ukpga/2012/7/contents/enacted. 2012.

Health Services Research Network: Lessons from Europe. Provider governance' briefing. Issue 11 (website). www.nhsconfed.org/publications. 2013.

Kennedy I chair: The report of the public inquiry into the children's heart surgery on the Bristol Royal Infirmary 1984–1995: learning from Bristol. Department of Health (website). http://webarchive.national archives.gov.uk/+/www.dh.gov.uk/en/Publicationsandstatistics/Publications/Publications PolicyAndGuidance/DH_4005620. 2001.

Kirkup B: The report of the Morecambe Bay Investigation (website). www.gov.uk/government/publications. 2015.

McSherry R, Haddock J: Evidence-based health care: its place within clinical governance, *Br J Nurs* 8(2):113–117, 1999.

National Institute for Health and Care Excellence (NICE): *Who we are* (website). www.nice.org.uk/about/who-we-are. 2015a.

National Institute for Health and Care Excellence (NICE): *Safe midwifery staffing for maternity settings* (website). www.nice.org.uk/guidance/ng4. 2015b.

NHS Wales: *Governance e-manual* (website). www.wales.nhs.uk/governance-emanual/standards-for-health-services-in-wales-s. 2015.

Nursing and Midwifery Council (NMC): *Midwives rules and standards* (website). www.nmc.org.uk/standards/additional-standards/midwives-rules-and-standards/. 2012.

National Quality Board: *'Quality Governance in the NHS – a guide for provider boards* (website). www.gov.uk/government/uploads/system/uploads/attachment_data/file/216321/dh_125239.pdf. 2011.

Nursing and Midwifery Council (NMC): *Revalidation: what*

revalidation is* (website). www.nmc.org.uk. 2015a.

Nursing and Midwifery Council (NMC): *The Code* (website). www.nmc-uk.org/code. 2015b.

Nursing and Midwifery Council (NMC) and General Medical Council (GMC): *Openness and honesty when things go wrong: the professional duty of candour* (website). www.nmc-uk.org and www.gmc-uk.org. 2015.

Reason J: *Human Error*. Cambridge University Press. October 1990.

Royal College of Midwives (RCM) and NHS Leadership Academy: *Midwifery leadership competency framework*, London, RCM Trust, 2012.

Royal College of Obstetricians and Gynaecologists (RCOG): *Maternity dashboard clinical performance and governance score card*. Clinical Governance Advice No. 7, London, RCOG, 2008.

Royal College of Obstetricians and Gynaecologists (RCOG): *Improving patient safety: risk management for maternity and gynaecology*. Clinical Governance Advice No. 2, London, RCOG, 2009.

Scally G, Donaldson LJ: Clinical governance and the drive for quality

improvement in the new NHS in England, *Br Med J* 4:61–65, 1998.

Scottish Government: *The healthcare quality strategy for NHS Scotland* (website). www.gov.scot/resource/doc/311667/0098354.pdf. 2010.

Shaw C, Kutryba B, Crisp H, et al: Do European hospitals have quality and safety governance systems and structures in place?, *BMJ Qual Saf* 18:i51–i56, 2009.

Smith JDBE chair: *The Shipman inquiry. Report 1* (website). http://webarchive.nationalarchives.gov.uk/20090808154959/http://www.the-shipman-inquiry.org.uk/firstreport.asp. 2002.

Thorlby R, Smith J, Williams S, et al: *The Francis report: one year on. Nuffield Trust* (website). www.nuffieldtrust.org.uk. 2014.

United Nations: *Millennium goals* (website). www.un.org/millenniumgoals/. 2015.

World Health Organization (WHO): *New checklist for transparent, accurate and reliable health estimates* (website). www.who.int/en/. 2015.

Resources and additional reading

Monitor: *Applying for NHS Foundation Trust status: guide for applicants* (website). www.gov.uk/government/organisations/monitor. 2010.

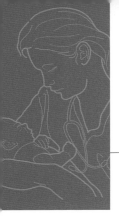

Chapter 5

The midwife as a lifelong learner

Sue Macdonald

Learning Outcomes ?

After reading this chapter, you will be able to:

- understand the development of pre- and post-registration education for midwives in the UK, including educational and academic structures

- determine your own learning style, and consider your education and development needs and how these might best be met

- support other students, practitioners, women and families in their learning and active reflection on their experiences

- develop a framework within which to effectively reflect on practice, and use this knowledge to guide future practice

- compile and develop a professional portfolio that demonstrates achievements, utilizes your learning needs and helps you plan your future development

- understand the requirements for initial registration, registration and revalidation

- fully utilize the clinical area, whether community or hospital based, as a learning environment, and facilitate the learning and development of those with whom you work

INTRODUCTION

One of the strengths of recent UK midwifery has been the control that midwives have of their education. This chapter includes an overview of the relevant history of midwifery education (see also Ch. 2), in the context of some of the policy and practice issues that have shaped and influenced the provision of pre- and post-registration education in the UK. To understand midwifery education in the UK now,

and to consider the future direction, it is helpful to appreciate some of the influencing factors and history of midwifery. The history of midwifery education has been shaped by politics, professional aspirations and professional rivalries, and the reader may consider whether these drivers might still exist, albeit in different formats.

Education and learning are also explored in a broader sense, including the concept of lifelong learning, current developments in education that affect student midwives, midwives and midwifery courses, and continuing professional development.

MIDWIFERY EDUCATION – FROM APPRENTICESHIP TO REFLECTIVE PRACTICE

Before the 1902 Midwives Act, midwives usually learned their craft from another experienced midwife. Practice was therefore varied because midwives usually had limited access to textbooks and to formal research. The body of available knowledge was small. This is in huge contrast to midwifery practice today, where there is a plethora of textbooks, manuals, journals and policies accessible to students and qualified midwives. Access to information is not universal – some lower-resource countries have limited journals and textbooks, although with greater use of the Internet, increasingly midwives are able to access more information and research (Health Education for All (HIFA) 2015; Jenkins 2014).

The corresponding growth in knowledge, research and practice development means that the information that is learned during pre-registration programmes before being registered as a midwife will not be sufficient for the midwife's whole career; often, as new research emerges, some practices actually need to cease.

Midwifery traditionally emerged from this apprenticeship model of education (Leap and Hunter 1993; Finnerty et al 2013). Midwives were usually older women, with their own experience of pregnancy and childbirth, who would literally 'learn by Nellie' by accompanying a midwife in her daily work. The 'education' of midwives, therefore, differed in the quality of experience to which a learner midwife was exposed and was limited by the difficulty of accessing the scientific information that would have been available to their male counterparts (Donnison 1988; see also Ch. 2). Education and practice reflected the society of the time, often guided by superstition, custom and practice, while also being influenced by the social standing of the midwife (Thomas 2009).

Many years of campaigning by the Midwives Institute (later to become the Royal College of Midwives (RCM)) and its redoubtable members, including Rosalind Paget and Louisa Hubbard, supported by a small number of powerful politicians, achieved the Midwives Act of 1902. The primary purpose of the legislation (which covered England and Wales) was to *safeguard the public* from the practices of uneducated and untrained women who assisted those who were too poor to pay for medical care during childbirth. Midwives were among the first to achieve professional regulation and were set on the pathway to standardized education, training and practice. Other parts of the UK attained registration of midwifery practice at a later date: Scotland in 1915 and Ireland in 1918. The Nurses Registration Act (1919) set up the General Nursing Council and introduced nursing training and standards along similar lines to those of midwives (see also Ch. 2).

The Central Midwives' Board (CMB), established by the 1902 act, was charged by government with responsibility for training midwives and conducting their examinations. The educational programmes developed accordingly, as shown in Table 5.1 and Fig. 5.1.

As illustrated in Table 5.1, the length of the midwife's training course, content and assessments increased gradually as knowledge of the physiology and management of pregnancy and childbirth increased, and the needs of women and babies changed. The regulatory bodies responsible for midwifery education also changed within this time (see Chs 2 and 3) from the CMB to the United

Table 5.1 The development of midwifery education courses in the UK

Year	Awarding Body	Length of Course	Examination	Award (Level)	Comments
Late 19th century	London Obstetrical Society	3 months	None formal	Certificate of proficiency	Small number of students led to negligible impact on practice
1902–1915	Central Midwives Board (CMB)	3 months	3-hour written examination 15-minute viva conducted by an obstetrician	Certificate	Focus on labour and postnatal care
1916	CMB	6 months (2-month exemption for nurses)		Certificate	
1926	CMB	1 year for non-nurses			
1938	CMB	Part 1: 12 months for non-nurses (hospital based); 6 months for nurses Part 2: 6 months for all (district and community experience)	Practical assessment and submission of set number of case histories	Certificate	Midwifery and obstetric theory and hospital-based practice Clinical experience based in community and some lectures from the local Medical Officer of Health
1968	CMB	1 year for nurses 2 years for direct entrants	Two 3-hour written examinations Viva voce	Certificate	Normal midwifery and complicated obstetrics and neonatal care

Continued

Table 5.1 The development of midwifery education courses in the UK—cont'd

Year	Awarding Body	Length of Course	Examination	Award (Level)	Comments
1980	CMB	18 months for nurses 3 years for direct entrants Education based in schools/maternity unit	Two 3-hour written examinations Viva voce	Certificate	Normal midwifery and complicated obstetrics and neonatal care + new technologies (i.e. Cardiotocographs (CTGs), inductions, etc.) – some doctors' lectures
1990s	United Kingdom Central Council for Nursing and Midwifery (UKCC) National Boards – registration Colleges/universities – academic qualification	18 months for nurses 3 years for direct entrants Education based in colleges	Development of continuous assessment processes and devolvement of assessment	Diploma of Higher Education (DipHE) degrees in midwifery	Increased focus on psychology, sociology, physiology and social policy
2000s	Nursing and Midwifery Council (NMC) – registration Universities – academic qualification	18 months for nurses 3 years for direct entrants Some variation in programmes (i.e. 20 months for nurses and 4 years for degree) Based in university	Continuous assessment theory and practice Use of mentors as assessors in the clinical area Midwifery lecturers' moderation	All programmes at university degree level – BSc/BA (Hons)	Most programmes in modular form Credit accumulation and transfer possible Minimum 50% practice Grading of clinical practice Increased emphasis on importance of knowledge and skills in normal practice

Kingdom Central Council (UKCC) for Nursing and Midwifery and associated country boards to today's Nursing and Midwifery Council (NMC).

By the late 1980s, there was increasing concern within the profession about both the direction midwifery education was taking and reduced recruitment into midwifery. By 1988, only one school in England offered a 'direct-entry' programme for non-nurses to become midwives, although it was believed that this route could be more cost-effective and a more health-focused way of training midwives.

Acting on the findings of a study funded by the English National Board (ENB) and Department of Health (DH) (Radford and Thompson 1988), the Department of Health supported seven pilot schools to develop direct-entry programmes in England, generally at DipHE level, linked to higher education institutions (HEIs). The success of these programmes was such that by 2011, the ratio of direct entrants to shortened programme had reversed, so that the majority of midwives are now direct entrants (Dunkley and Haider 2011 for the Centre for Workforce Intelligence). Although there remains debate about whether the shortened course

for nurses should be retained, this route is still supported by midwives, and its retention was recommended by the UKCC Commission for Education (1999) and is currently supported by commissioners (see chapter website resources).

Moving into higher education

The last 30 years have been a time of tremendous change, from a scenario where midwifery education was provided locally, managed by heads of midwifery in hospitals, funded from the maternity care budget, to being absorbed into schools of nursing and midwifery, then colleges of health and/or nursing, and the final move into universities, with more complex funding streams controlled through strategic health authorities.

Project 2000 (UKCC 1986) recommended that nursing and midwifery education have an 18-month shared core, followed by an 18-month 'branch' in midwifery, children's nursing, mental health, acute care or learning disabilities; that students be supernumerary, and courses be offered in *higher education (HE)* at *diploma or degree* level. Midwives overwhelmingly rejected this model for midwifery education, choosing to retain the direct-entry route or 18-month programme, generally keeping control over their curriculum, although midwifery education moved, like nursing, into higher education. It is possible that this rejection avoided some of the problems experienced in nursing as described in the Peach Report (UKCC Commission for Education 1999).

It has been suggested that the move into HE, which coincided with Project 2000 development, affected the student experience and the development of clinical expertise and confidence. Contributory factors were larger class sizes and the geographical move from hospitals and clinical areas (Bower 2002). Although some midwives worked closely with their nursing colleagues to the extent of sharing elements of their programmes, many others retained their midwifery identity, preferring to develop shared learning between the direct-entry and 18-month midwifery routes (Eraut et al 1995).

For students and teachers the move into HE brought both benefits and disadvantages. Student groups are larger, and students have access to an academic environment and the opportunity to mix with other students. Teachers have had to cope with the physical move out to the universities, and have faced the challenge of bridging the gap between clinical and academic learning. Although midwife teachers are able to work with academics from other disciplines, they do have a long history of being prepared for their role as teachers, whereas some academics are experts in their field but may not hold a teaching qualification.

The RCM Education Strategy (RCM 2003) highlighted actions to redress the balance and align education more closely with clinical practice. Some recommendations, such as the development of a national midwifery curriculum, are straightforward, especially given the development of a national curriculum in children's education. Others, including the recommendation that students undertake at least five home births and two births within a birth centre setting, complete at least two experiences of physiological third stage and have experience in a variety of settings, are more challenging. Utilizing the strategy could assist students and midwives to move clinical practice towards normality and community settings.

> *'There may be midwives who seek the academic ivory towers, but there are also a significant number of midwives locked in the turret'!*
>
> (RCM 2003: 9)

This strategy also recommends that educationalists spend a minimum of 20% of their time within the clinical area, and that clinical managers seek to find a space for educators and work to mitigate negative effects of geographical separation. The *MINT Project* investigating the role of the midwife teacher demonstrated the 'added value' of midwife teachers in assisting student learning, and it also highlighted the importance of being visible in the clinical arena (Fraser et al 2013) (see chapter website resources).

Regional shortages of midwives and the demographic picture of an 'aging population' indicate that there is a demographic 'time bomb' (Centre for Workforce Intelligence (CfWI) 2012; RCM 2015) approaching all midwifery spheres of practice, and this is reflected in each of the four countries. There is also an international issue, with an estimated global shortage of approximately 350,000 midwives (Save the Children Fund 2011). In the UK, it is estimated that the midwifery workforce needs an additional 2600 midwives (RCM 2015). Addressing this requires both better retention of midwives and more students in training. The difficulty in increasing student numbers is that every student needs sufficient quality clinical experience, and all students must be supervised and mentored by a qualified and experienced midwife. In addition, students need talented, skilled and experienced midwife teachers within the academic and clinical environments, and suitably qualified midwives must be recruited to undertake this role.

In teaching, the development of different roles, such as practice facilitator, clinical facilitator and practice development midwives, may, in part, replace the traditional role of the midwife teacher, but it removes a potentially valuable resource from students and qualified staff. Midwife teachers need to be highly experienced in clinical practice and thoroughly grounded in the theory of advanced midwifery, enhanced by knowledge of the principles and practice of the education of adults. Midwives, and midwife teachers especially, need to be strong, confident people, able to challenge and question both in academic and clinical settings, and be committed to high-quality, evidence-based practice, with good leadership, communication and caring skills (Byrom and Downe 2010). This level of knowledge and skills is a significant investment and makes the educationalist a key member of the maternity services, if fully involved and utilized.

Diplomas, degrees and scholarship

Two programmes are available to the person wishing to enter midwifery in the UK: either a 3-year direct-entry programme or an 18-month shortened programme for those who have completed an adult nursing qualification. Both are now at the degree level. There are slight variations in the length of the programme, as some universities provide an additional 2 to 4 months for students to gain confidence and competence in a preceptored component of a programme. Figure 5.2 illustrates the educational system in the UK, which has been influenced by developments in European universities, although there are slight difference between this and the Scottish system.

Courses are designed around the key competencies and clinical experience as laid down by the EC Midwives

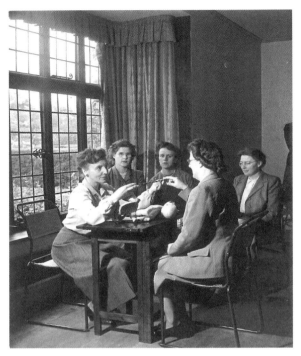

Figure 5.1 Midwifery education in the 1950s. (Courtesy of the Royal College of Midwives.)

Directives (EC 1983, 2005), the Nursing and Midwifery Council (NMC) proficiencies (NMC 2009a, 2009b) and clinical assessment (NMC 2008). In addition, increasingly, the International Confederation of Midwives (ICM) *global standards and essential midwifery competencies* (ICM 2013a, 2013b) are informing curricula, and this will increasingly help provide midwives with more international perspectives and understanding (see Ch. 1).

Clinical practice is a crucial part of the programme and includes students working a variety of shifts (including weekends and night shifts). Courses include 'self-directed study time' and a variety of different learning and teaching methods to enhance learning. Students are often mature people, sometimes on their second or third career, and possibly the family breadwinner, with different stressors from those of traditional university students.

There is often debate in the media and among professionals about practitioners (nurses and midwives) being too highly educated – 'too posh to wash', 'too clever to care' – centred on whether qualifications make the practitioner better (Bower 2002; Gill 2004; Scott 2004; Willis Commission 2012). Certainly research into the qualities of a good midwife has tended to highlight the importance of people skills, communication, caring and compassion rather than academic qualifications (Nicholls

and Webb 2006; Byrom and Downe 2010). Halldorsdottir and Karlsdottir (2011) suggest the need for professional wisdom, alongside the responsibility to be developing personally and professionally. However, increasingly, as service needs change, and women's and babies' needs become more complex, graduate skills have become important in helping midwives manage the knowledge, research and evidence to provide the highest possible standards of care. Initial debate was about whether graduate practitioners stayed in the profession and whether they were as clinically competent and confident. Research evidence suggests that this preparation does not adversely affect the clinical competence and skills of the practitioners (Bircumshaw and Chapman 1988), who demonstrate the ability to problem solve and have a similar level of competence as their diplomate colleagues (Bartlett et al 2000; While et al 1998), and they are more likely to be motivated to undertake continuing professional education (CPE) than are diplomates (Dolphin 1983). The Willis Commission explored the future of nursing education and looked at the need to 'create and maintain a workforce of competent, compassionate nurses to deliver future health and social care services'. This report supported graduate education as crucial for the future healthcare requirements, balancing critical thinking, research and the need for compassion and caring professionalism, and graduate education was seen as having applicability to midwifery (Willis Commission 2012).

As members of a graduate profession, midwives need analytical and reflective thinking in support of their practical skills. Although the academic requirements may discourage some people from pursuing midwifery, strategies are in place to provide additional academic and pastoral support for people with nontraditional qualifications. At present, students do not normally get any time taken from their course requirements even if they have completed previous degree studies, and this is ruled by the EU Midwifery directives (EC 1983, 2005).

Once the midwifery education programme is completed, the individual can then apply for registration with the NMC, having achieved the academic and practical requirements and been confirmed as being of good character. Following initial registration, the midwife needs to renew registration each year and comply with practice requirements.

Practitioners who have completed midwifery programmes in the past, or who have completed a diploma, can apply to 'top up' to the BSc (Hons) level if required. Most universities stipulate a total of 360 credits to gain an honours degree – usually consisting of 120 credits at each of the levels of four, five and six (previously one, two and three) (Fig. 5.3).

The RCM education strategy (2003) proposed a continuum of midwifery, from a 'pre-midwifery' programme, through pre-registration education and training, to different pathways of consultant midwife, educationalist or manager, always with a firm foundation of clinical practice.

Typical higher education qualifications awarded by degree-awarding bodies within each level	FHEQ FHEQ level	FQHEIS SCQF level	Corresponding QFEHEA cycle
Doctoral degrees (e.g. PhD/DPhil, EdD, DBA, DClinPsy)	8	12	Third cycle (end of cycle) qualifications
Master's degrees (e.g. MPhil, MLitt, MRes, MA, MSc)	7	11	Second cycle (end of cycle) qualifications
Integrated master's degrees (e.g. MEng, MChem, MPhys, MPharm)			
Primary qualifications (or first degrees) in medicine, dentistry and veterinary science (e.g. MB ChB, MB BS, BM BS; BDS; BVSc, BVMS)			
Postgraduate diplomas			
Postgraduate Certificate in Education (PGCE)/Postgraduate Diploma in Education (PGDE)			
Postgraduate certificates			
Bachelor's degrees with honours (e.g. BA/BSc Hons)	6	10	First cycle (end of cycle) qualifications
Bachelor's degrees			
Professional Graduate Certificate in Education (PGCE) in England, Wales and Northern Ireland		9	
Graduate diplomas			
Graduate certificates			
Foundation degrees (e.g. FdA, FdSc)	5	NA	Short cycle (within or linked to the first cycle) qualifications
Diplomas of Higher Education (DipHE)		8	
Higher National Diplomas (HND) awarded by degree-awarding bodies in England, Wales and Northern Ireland under licence from Pearson		NA	
Higher National Certificates (HNC) awarded by degree-awarding bodies in England, Wales and Northern Ireland under licence from Pearson	4	NA	
Certificates of Higher Education (CertHE)		7	

Figure 5.2 Examples of the typical higher education qualifications at levels of the Frameworks for Higher Education Qualifications of UK Degree-Awarding Bodies and their corresponding cycle in the Framework for Qualifications of the European Higher Education Area (FQ-EHEA). For more information, see the chapter website resources. (Adapted from Quality Assurance Agency for Higher Education (QAA) 2014a, 2014b.)

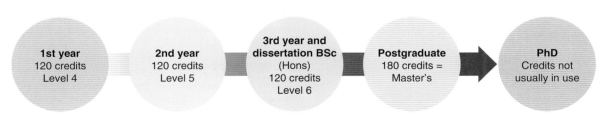

Figure 5.3 Credit accumulation.

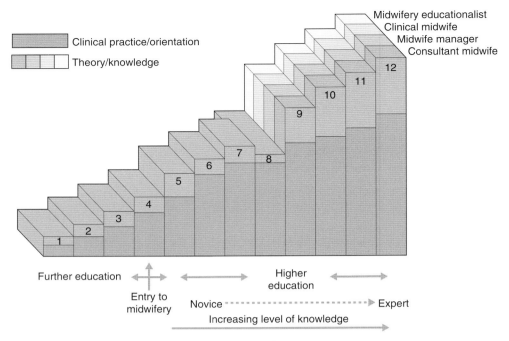

Figure 5.4 The professional escalator for midwives. (RCM 2003: 4.)

The process of moving along the continuum of midwifery illustrates that practitioners often start at different points and have enormous potential for professional and personal growth, and reiterates the commitment to continuing professional education (see Fig. 5.4).

THE COST OF EDUCATION

The cost of midwifery education can be roughly divided into two functions: the cost of the education programme, its commissioning and delivery, and the support provided to pre- and post-registration students undertaking the programme.

At present all programmes are provided by universities, although it has been suggested that this could reverse (McIntosh 2016).

Commissioning Education

In the UK the Departments of Health (England, Wales, Northern Ireland and Scotland) are responsible for educating, training and developing the UK healthcare workforce. And although there are other significant funding streams, this was in the region of £5.5 billion in 2012 (Universities UK 2012).

Each country has a different mechanism and structure for managing the process of ensuring that there are sufficient student places agreed upon to balance the workforce within the UK (see chapter website resources). The basic principles are that there is a process for assessing the clinical needs of health services, with a direct feedback mechanism to the commissioning body. In England this is the Local Education and Training Boards (LETBs) informing Health Education England (HEE); in Scotland, NHS Education for Scotland; in Northern Ireland, the Department of Health, Social Services and Public Safety (DHSSPS); and in Wales, the Welsh Assembly through to the Local Health Boards. Places can then be agreed upon among the local health services, which can provide the clinical placements, and the university that provides the education programme. It is always important to ensure that the numbers of students are calibrated with the experience and supervision available, and therefore communication between service providers and education providers is critical.

Student support

Before 2017 students had bursaries/grants to support their studies (see chapter website resources). Recent changes mean that health-based students will follow a structure similar to that of mainstream academic students

(HM Treasury 2015). Some universities also offer hardship grants that may be accessed.

LIFELONG LEARNING

Lifelong learning is understanding that the initial education programme (pre-registration midwifery) is a starting point for future practice, with the clinical area being a place of learning and development, and a commitment to continuing to learn (see chapter website resources). This approach encourages a dynamic and enriching process in which midwives think about and reflect on their practice, learn from each experience (good and bad), refine and improve their knowledge and skills and impart this philosophy to their clients and students. This creative and positive approach, where the health service is a learning organization, able to learn and develop from positive events and mistakes, can provide high-quality service to women, babies and families.

In reality, this must be more than 'paying lip service'. The pace of change and of the development of knowledge mean that midwives must continually be updating their knowledge and skills to provide a safe and effective level of care.

Lifelong learning in practice

It can be daunting thinking about the difficulties of keeping up to date and meeting the requirements for revalidation. There are many journals, texts and activities, and practice life is busy. It is useful, therefore, to think about how to keep up to date and to plan out the most practical and interesting ways of achieving this goal (see Table 5.2).

The continuing professional development plan (CPD) plan in Table 5.2 may appear to be idealistic – but it is important to have an individual plan, taking into consideration forward planning of external events and activities and balancing home and workload needs. There are also opportunities for 'learning as you go', in which if a new condition/problem arises in practice, then the person can make time to look up the issue and update his or her knowledge. This enables real and applied learning to occur and knowledge gained be better remembered.

Most students and midwives enjoy attending study days and conferences, which can be a useful means of learning new research and practice development. But even more precious is the learning that occurs from meeting practitioners from other parts of the country/countries or with different expertise and experience. Again, the most important thing is to record the learning and to consider how this can be added to practice, and this needs to include discussion with colleagues.

Table 5.2 Suggestion for a continuing professional development (CPD) plan	
Daily	Review – was there anything that you met in your practice that you need to update or look up? If you have time, look up the information. If insufficient time, write it down in your CPD notebook so you can include it in your weekly activity. If you attended a study day/conference or learning activity, try to complete your CPD record that evening, or jot down notes so that you can complete it later.
Weekly	Allocate 1 hour in the week to reflect back on the week: • Were there any instances where you did not know the answer to a question or what the current research was indicating for an area of care? • Check your CPD notebook for anything you have noted. • Was there an episode that would be useful to reflect on for your portfolio (see section on reflection)? Check your journals, aiming to read one article a week. Is your portfolio up to date?
Every month	Check that your portfolio is up to date. Check whether there are any study days that will add to your practice and discuss with your manager/supervisor as to whether you can attend. Select a learning module/learning activity online. This could be the RCM e-learning menu, for example, or you could access a YouTube lecture/video. Record what activity you complete. You should also reflect on the activity and consider what it will add to your practice as a midwife.
Every year	Select a conference that will contribute to your practice, and discuss with your colleagues and supervisor of midwives whether it is possible to attend.

Reflective activity 5.1   ＞＜

Using the suggestions in Table 5.2, design your own personal CPD plan on one sheet of A4 paper. Think about including activities that you will enjoy, but also ones in which you need to develop your knowledge and skills – even better if you can combine the two.

AFTER QUALIFICATION AND REGISTRATION: CONTINUING PROFESSIONAL DEVELOPMENT

Continuing professional development/education (CPD/E) forms a crucial and enduring part of the midwife's role, and has been part of midwifery practice since the *1936 Midwives Act*, requiring midwives to undertake periodic refreshment to be able to continue practising. The *Post-Registration Education and Practice* (PREP) Project (UKCC 1990) brought these principles to nursing and health visiting, requiring practitioners to complete 5 days every 3 years with a professional portfolio illustrating self-assessment, development plan and reflective activities.

The PREP standard previously required that practitioners complete a minimum of 450 hours of practice and 35 hours of study during the 3 years before renewal of registration, and those holding dual qualifications were required to demonstrate 900 hours of practice in nursing *and* midwifery (NMC 2011). This was to be recorded in a professional portfolio, the elements of which were to be shared with the practitioner's supervisor of midwives.

Revalidation

After some years of following the PREP requirements and keeping professional portfolios, the process has been developed further to *revalidation* (NMC 2015a). The NMC has set out the requirements that the midwife needs to maintain registration with the NMC, demonstrating the practitioner's ability to 'practise safely and effectively', and builds on systems already in place. At the centre is the Code for Nurses, Midwives and Health Visitors (NMC 2015b) and the desire to embed professional standards and behaviour throughout the midwife's career (see chapter website resources). The midwife is still required to keep a portfolio, and this is to be used with the '*confirmer*', who may be the practitioner's manager or another registrant (stipulated *not* to be a friend). Initially the supervisor of midwives would be an appropriate 'confirmer' (see Boxes 5.1 and 5.2).

There is a strong element of self-certification in the revalidation process, and this requires practitioners to be honest about their activities. Failure to do so, or making fraudulent submissions, puts the practitioner's registration at risk (see Chs 3 and 4). A small number of registrants' submissions will be scrutinized by the NMC to ensure quality and consistency (NMC 2015a).

The Professional Portfolio

As part of their revalidation, nurses and midwives need to maintain records of their practice, learning and development activity for re-registration purposes. A practical means of doing this is through maintaining a portfolio or profile, and this is recommended. This is a personal document, which does not belong to the NMC or to the nurse's or midwife's employer (NMC 2015a).

Developing a professional 'profile' (or portfolio) has resulted in structured approaches to recording learning and development. It is important to consider the 'shape' of the portfolio – moving from a view of a portfolio as a collection of certificates from different study days to a more dynamic tool allowing the practitioner to record activities, reflect on practice and consider learning and development in the past, present and future, as a development plan. The latter approach includes a curriculum vitae (CV), and one way of seeing the portfolio is to think of it as a *dynamic CV*.

There are several guidance publications available to guide portfolio development (NMC 2008, 2015a; RCM 2000, 2016). The practitioner can choose to use a commercially produced portfolio, self-designed portfolio, loose-leaf binder, computer, or tablet and mobile telephone to record learning and experience (see Fig. 5.5 and

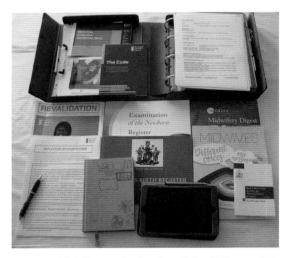

Figure 5.5 Midwifery professional portfolio. (With permission from the Royal College of Midwives and MIDIRS.)

Box 5.1 Checklist of requirements and supporting evidence for revalidation (NMC 2015) (By kind permission of the Nursing and Midwifery Council (NMC) 2015)

These are all of the requirements that you must meet in order to complete your revalidation and renew your registration every 3 years with the NMC.

Requirements	Supporting evidence
450 practice hours or 900 hours if revalidating as both nurse and midwife	Maintain a record of practice hours you have completed, including: • dates of practice; • the number of hours you undertook; • name, address and postcode of the organization; • scope of practice (see tip box on page 8); • work setting (see tip box on page 8); • a description of the work you undertook, and • evidence of those practice hours (such as timesheets, role profiles or job specifications).
35 hours of continuing professional development (of which 20 must be participatory)	Maintain accurate and verifiable records of your continuing professional development (CPD) activities, including: • the CPD method (examples of CPD method are self-learning, online learning, course); • a brief description of the topic and how it relates to your practice; • dates the CPD activity was undertaken; • the number of hours and participatory hours; • identification of the part of the Code most relevant to the CPD and evidence of the CPD activity (Guidance Sheet 3 provides examples of the kind of evidence you can record, see pages 44–45).
Five pieces of practice-related feedback	Notes of the content of the feedback and how you used it to improve your practice. This will be helpful for you to use when you are preparing your reflective accounts. Make sure your notes do not include any personal data (see Guidance Sheet 1 on pages 39–41).
Five written reflective accounts	Five written reflective accounts that explain what you learned from your CPD activity and/or feedback and/or an event or experience in your practice, how you changed or improved your work as a result and how this is relevant to the Code. You must use the NMC form on page 46, and make sure your accounts do not include any personal data (see Guidance sheet 1).
Reflective discussion	A reflective discussion form that includes the name and NMC Pin number of the NMC-registered nurse or midwife with whom you had the discussion and the date of the discussion. You must use the NMC form on page 47, and make sure the discussion summary section does not contain any personal data (see Guidance sheet 1).
Health and character	You will make these declarations as part of your online revalidation application.
Professional indemnity arrangement	Provide evidence to demonstrate that you have an appropriate indemnity arrangement in place. Identify whether your indemnity arrangement is through your employer, membership of a professional body or through a private insurance arrangement. If your indemnity arrangement is provided through membership of a professional body or a private insurance arrangement, you will need to record the name of the professional body or provider.
Confirmation	Include a confirmation form signed by your confirmer. You must use the NMC form on pages 48–50 (NMC 2015a).

Source: NMC 2015

It is important to be aware that this guidance may be subject to change. Readers should check the NMC revalidation microsite for any changes or additional information (see further resources).

Box 5.2 Process of revalidation

- Complete pre-registration programme
- Qualification as a midwife
  - Registration with the NMC
  - Complete initial Intention to Practice Form
  - Declaration of good character submitted by Lead Midwife for Education
- Each year:
  - Complete Intention to Practice Form (March)
  - Have an appraisal (can put this in the portfolio)
  - Complete portfolio and keep this up to date; portfolio includes:
    - Reflective accounts
    - Practice feedback
    - Peer review
    - Annual review with supervisor of midwives
- Every 3 years (within a 60-day period):
  - Compile portfolio; portfolio includes:
    - Five reflective accounts
    - Account of reflective discussion with colleague
    - Five pieces of evidence of practice feedback
  - Confirm that you are in good health and are of good character (declare any criminal convictions or charges that you may have against you or pending)
  - Confirm indemnity arrangements are in place
  - Complete validation requirements (see Fig. 5.1 and NMC 2015a)
  - Seek confirmer and have requirements confirmed
  - Submit confirmation to the NMC
- Receive confirmation that revalidation is received, processed and successful

---

Box 5.3 Recording continuing education/development

You need to include:
- Date, time and place of learning activity
- Where learning took place
- Conference centre/ward or community area/library
- A review of your current role
- *The learning activity:*
  - Why did you choose the particular topic/activity?
  - How did you plan this activity?
  - How many hours did you study/work?
  - Briefly describe the learning activity (i.e. reading a relevant clinical article; attending a course; observing practice)
  - Were there any disappointments or difficulties you had to face?
  - What was the best part of the learning for you?
- *Learning outcomes:*
  - What were the key aspects of the learning for you?
  - How will you put this into practice?
  - What sort of learning plans do you have for the future?

If a literature search or reading activity is used as an updating activity, rigour needs to be used to ensure that the work is focused and applied to the individual's practice. This makes **active reading** critical (see chapter website resources).

Reflective activity 5.2

After your next study day, spend some time afterwards thinking about it. What were the key elements of the day for you? Were there any keynote speakers who had an effect on you? Did you learn anything new? If not, why not?

Write down any new learning – perhaps using the framework in Box 5.3, or access an NMC template at http://revalidation.nmc.org.uk/download-resources/forms-and-templates/

Record at least **one thing** that you learned that you could bring into practice.

---

see chapter website resources). Part of the revalidation document includes templates for use in the portfolio, and some of these are available on the NMC site, including a reflective accounts form, reflective discussion form and practice log template (NMC 2015a).

Updating activities can include attending study days and conferences, working in different practice areas or private study, such as structured reading or undertaking a literature review. The important element is identifying the **learning** resulting from the activity, maximizing its effect (see Box 5.3). It is also important to have some 'participative activities' – which might be holding discussion groups with other practitioners or attending a resuscitation workshop, or could include learning new skills under the mentorship of a colleague (NMC 2015a; RCM 2015).

FUTURE DEVELOPMENTS: DEGREES, MASTERS AND PHD/APEL/APL

Midwives wishing to develop their knowledge and skills now have more choices than ever before. A decade or two ago, diplomas were the highest qualification available for the majority of practitioners, and a midwife wanting a master's degree had to settle for a master's degree in social science, psychology, nursing or education. Now, universities offer degree studies from the bachelor's to the master's level in midwifery studies or science.

A growing number of midwives are undertaking doctoral studies (PhD) and/or clinical doctorates (DClinPrac). Figure 5.2 illustrates the academic hierarchy, with the Master of Philosophy (MPhil) and PhD considered the pinnacle of study, requiring the practitioner to learn the knowledge and skills of research and apply them to a research project, thus generating original knowledge. As the number of midwives holding these higher degrees grows, the status of, and internal belief in, midwifery will increase, although it will be important to ensure that at the heart of what is studied is knowledge pertinent and applicable to midwives, midwifery and, above all, to women and their babies.

Work-based learning (WBL) may include elements of *accreditation of prior learning* (APL) or *accreditation of prior experiential learning* (APEL). This can involve guided study within the clinical area, practical sessions or activity. Some programmes include work-based learning to denote the practical part of the course, either self-assessed or under the supervision of the course tutor or suitably qualified colleagues. Students are provided with a workbook or logbook, and this forms part of the reflection and recording necessary for demonstrating their progress.

WBL is sometimes viewed as a way of providing practitioners with learning experience, without 'losing them' while they go elsewhere for study. It enables learning to be applied and placed firmly within the practitioner's own workplace, and it can contribute to the concept of the learning organization (ENB 1995). A learning organization is a dynamic one that can adapt and change as required and that enables its workers to participate at all levels in the organization (ENB 1995; Jarvis 1992; Marsick 1987; Boud et al 2005) (see chapter website resources). This requires a cultural and psychological shift in ensuring that there are appropriate opportunities for utilizing the principles of experiential learning and providing adequate opportunities for review and reflection.

APEL and APL present exciting possibilities for midwives and are used as a means to validate and add value to clinical practice. It is necessary to enrol in a university or further education college and formally apply to have academic credit applied to clinical practice and learning in that practice. Time must be spent in preparing a professional portfolio documenting clinical activities, including evidence of critical reflection and a 'claim' for the academic credits appropriate to the clinical learning and development achieved.

COMPUTERS, E-LEARNING AND THE NET

The development of computer-assisted learning and the growth of the Internet have revolutionized learning and information retrieval and further shortened the 5-year 'sell-by date' of knowledge. Midwives need to become comfortable using computers and retrieving information through varied databases (see Ch. 6). Courses and programmes such as the *European Computer Driving Licence* (ECDL) have been used to direct learning computer skills, including word processing and spreadsheet utilization (Jacob 1999; European Computer Driving Licence Foundation 2016).

Increasingly, modules and programmes of learning are available in electronic form (Jordan 1999; RCM 2016) (see chapter website resources) and *WebCT* (web course tools), and *massive online open courses* (MOOC) (see following discussion) are being developed to support different facets of learning, offering notice boards, chat rooms and a range of guided learning facilities. Research suggests that students like the variety this offers, although the development of electronic packages is time hungry (Wilson and Mires 1998), and that students need different skills to work with e-learning (Valaitis et al 2005). The way in which learning takes place using e-learning and Internet tools is different – even verging on the chaotic as the learner 'surfs' into different sites (Savin-Baden and Wilkie 2006), sometimes at considerable speed. There may be an influence on attention span.

The Internet also offers other activities, such as social networking possibilities, including *Facebook*, *Twitter*, and *YouTube*, which provide links with others, and access to PowerPoint presentations and video clips that can assist understanding of theory such as physiology (see chapter website resources). These social networking activities are being integrated into some programmes, and research suggests that they may support additional learning and provide a good platform for students to interact and share learning (Smith and Lambert 2014). However, it is crucial that students and midwives understand the limitations, risks and etiquette of social media and ensure that they are clear on aspects of safety and identity and their professional responsibilities, which include confidentiality (NMC 2015c).

There are a variety of useful resources online for midwives and other practitioners, including the following:

- NHS Library and Knowledge Service (NKS) (now under the Health Education England umbrella) – https://hee.nhs.uk/our-work/research-learning -innovation/library-knowledge-services: This resource covers clinical practice, healthcare, social care, and public health, providing a website of portals into databases and evidence-based resources, for patients, public, clinicians, managers and public health professionals (NHS 2010).

- National Institute for Health and Care Excellence (NICE) – www.nice.org.uk: The NICE site offers a huge range of quality standards, clinical guidelines, standards and indicators and Evidence series.

- Scottish Intercollegiate Guidelines Group (SIGN) – www.sign.ac.uk: This site also offers a range of useful resources, standards and guidelines.

- Health Protection Agency – www.gov.uk/topic/health-protection: This is an excellent resource with accessible information, well indexed and illustrated … from acetylene to zoonoses, this site enables the user to access further information on many topics.

- International Confederation of Midwives (ICM) – http://www.internationalmidwives.org

See the textbook website for other resources.

LEARNING AND DEVELOPMENT

By the time students and qualified midwives have begun studying, they have already had positive and negative experiences of educational activities. These include experiences of rote learning, tests and examinations, and inevitably some failures. Often, early negative experiences can colour people's approach to learning and to their self-image.

There are many different models and theories around learning styles, and several questionnaires and quizzes are available that can be used to identify a person's learning style. One is that proposed by Honey and Mumford (1992, 2000), based on work by Kolb (2014), which suggested that people fit into one of four main groups:

- *Pragmatist* – practical and keen to try out new ideas.

- *Reflector* – prefers to observe, think and gather information before making a judgement.

- *Theorist* – likes to tease out and think through information in a systematic way.

- *Activist* – likes to be active and moves straight into experimentation on learning something new.

Although this work is not new, it is still in use and relevant to midwifery education. One study identified that teaching reflection included a model incorporating surface, impersonal to deep personal, then surface personal and deep personal approaches (Miller et al 1994) (see chapter website for more information).

LEARNING

The complex nature of learning has been explored extensively (Bloom 1956; Boud et al 1988; Bruner 1977; Freire 1972; Jarvis 2010; Mezirow 1981). The sheer breadth and depth of previous work within this area precludes more than an overview within this chapter.

There are many approaches: behaviourist, humanistic, the cultural environs, cognitive, through the spectrum to radical and emancipatory learning and education. Most of the earlier experiments and research into learning in humans were based on experiments with animals – even birds. Only during the development of 'progressive' education did research into human learning begin to be carried out. When looking at children's and adult education broadly, there is evidence of a complex interplay of many of these different theories and approaches, and, indeed, in most situations, experience and how learning is approached are similarly complex.

Some learning theories, such as *conditioning*, can be applied to simple learning and are relevant in many situations – for example, how individuals learn fear and develop phobias, as discussed in Box 5.4, and how these might be diminished.

Box 5.4 Learning fear – applied to midwifery

Vaginal examination (VE) during labour
The woman is anxious. This may be based on previous experience of VEs – perhaps when having a smear test, or may be a deeper fear from abuse. Midwife perhaps does not realize the woman's anxiety:

VE acutely painful (unconditioned stimulus) → pain/fear (unconditioned response)

Suggestion that VE is required (conditioned stimulus) + VE painful (unconditioned stimulus) → pain/fear (unconditioned response)

Suggestion that VE is required (conditioned stimulus) → fear (conditioned response)

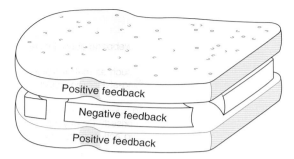

Figure 5.6 The 'Skinner sandwich'.

The example in Box 5.4 illustrates that fear and anxiety can be developed from one or two negative experiences of delivery, leading to negative feelings at the thought of the examination or even the sight of the midwife preparing the pack. This theory was reinforced by work by Dick-Read (1986), who advocated that those supporting women in childbirth needed to address the *fear–tension–pain cycle,* and this knowledge should inform the midwife's support and education approach. This means providing a safe environment for the woman, sensitively identifying her previous experiences, fears and anxieties, and then planning how best to aid understanding and learning (see also Ch. 21).

Behaviourist learning translates to providing feedback to the person learning – which might be yourself, the student you are working with or the woman and family. Praise and criticism are substituted for food or electric shocks as used in behaviourist experiments, remembering that *positive* rewards are more effective than negative reactions (see Fig. 5.6).

Positive feedback is provided first: 'You did really well …' followed by the negative criticism: '____ needed to be done differently because …' and the feedback is completed with another positive comment: 'This was really an excellent approach'. The person is then left with a clear idea of what needs to be improved, but is not swamped by thinking that nothing that was done was right or well.

Trial-and-error learning can be understood by knowing that the theory suggests that the individual may try out different approaches to solve a problem and then use that solution when faced with the same or a similar problem in the future (see chapter website resources).

Cognitive Gestalt theory is yet another approach. *Gestalt* means 'pattern, shape or form', and describes the individual's need to make sense of what is being seen and learned and put this into a 'whole'. This problem-solving aptitude helps the individual gain insight into learning – the 'Aha' experience. Gestalt includes concepts such as insightful learning, the nature-versus-nurture debate and field theory.

The individual's natural tendency to seek understanding needs to be supported, although some gaps in knowledge may act as an impetus for learning. In teaching, this can be used to help make sense of what is being learned – perhaps planning a learning activity in which some information is provided and some not, so that the learner is encouraged to develop *closure* in composing the whole problem and gets the experience of elements of *discovery learning*. Gestalt provided the tools for discovery learning and for the spiral curriculum that was taken forward by Gagne, in which new learning is linked with existing information and built upon further.

Another development in education came with Bloom's *taxonomy of learning*, which includes three *domains* or categories of educational activities: *cognitive (mental skill)*, *affective (growth in feelings)*, and *psychomotor (practical and physical skills)*. Although these were developed many years ago, the domains are still used to set learning objectives and in academic assessment (see Table 5.3). The taxonomy did not include the psychomotor domain; therefore, the experience of working with practical skills was limited (Bloom 1956), which echoes the difficulty experienced in healthcare settings of appropriately identifying and assessing practical skills and abilities.

The spiral curriculum, used extensively in education, is a way of structuring a course in which knowledge is provided in increasing depth as the programme continues.

The idea that 'teaching is a superb way of learning' (Bruner 1977: 88) is basically saying that to teach something, you have to understand it fully; and the idea that '[the] teacher is not only a communicator but a model' (Eraut 1994: 90) sums up the role of the teacher as role model. These are useful concepts for midwives to think about in their day-to-day lives, in their own learning and in teaching women and students.

There are other theories, such as the Index of Learning Styles™, which was developed by Felder and Soloman in the late 1980s, based on a learning styles model developed by Felder and Silverman. This is based on preferences that are said to be on a continuum, with, for example, sensory and intuition being two opposite styles (see chapter website resources for more information)

The *humanist theorists* Carl Rogers and Malcolm Knowles are probably the most influential adult education theorists in relation to midwifery. Rogers proposed that students be given intellectual freedom, allowing them to direct their own studies (Rogers 1969; Rogers and Freiberg 1994). This manifested in midwifery education in the form of self-directed sessions and negotiated programmes. The freedom concept cannot be wholly subscribed to, given the limited training time in which to learn and to be assessed as competent in certain skills to be deemed safe to practise (EC 1980, 2005; NMC 2008, 2015a; ICM 2013a, 2013b).

Knowles believed that the education of adults required a different approach to that of children, suggesting that

Table 5.3 Taxonomy of educational objectives within the cognitive domain

Competence	Skills	Descriptive terms used
Knowledge: • of specifics • of terminology • of specific facts • of theories and structure	• Observation and recall of information – facts or theories • Knowledge of dates, events, places • Knowledge of major ideas • Mastery of subject matter	List, define, tell, describe, identify, show, label, collect, examine, tabulate, quote, name, who, when, where, etc. Example: *The student will list the major landmarks of the pelvis and fetal skull.*
Comprehension: • understanding (lowest level) • translation • interpretation • extrapolation	• Understanding information • Grasp meaning • Translate knowledge into new context • Interpret facts, compare, contrast • Order, group, infer causes • Predict consequences	Summarize, describe, interpret, contrast, predict, associate, distinguish, estimate, differentiate, discuss, extend Example: *The student will describe the significance of the major landmarks of the pelvis and fetal skull.*
Application	• Use information • Use methods, concepts, theories in new situations • Solve problems using required skills or knowledge • Ability to predict possible effects of a change	Apply, demonstrate, calculate, complete, illustrate, show, solve, examine, modify, relate, change, classify, experiment, discover Example: *The student will demonstrate the mechanism of labour, describing the interaction of the fetal skull with the pelvis, and be able to teach students and women the basic principles.*
Analysis of: • elements • relationships • organizational principles	• Seeing patterns • Organization of parts • Recognition of hidden meanings • Identification of components	Analyse, separate, order, explain, connect, classify, arrange, divide, compare, select, explain, infer Example: *The student will be able to discuss the greater significance of different variations of shapes and sizes of pelves and the effect on the mechanism of labour and outcomes. She may question the sources of this knowledge.*
Synthesis – production of a • unique communication • plan or proposed set of operations • set of abstract relations	• Use old ideas to create new ones • Generalize from given facts • Relate knowledge from several areas • Predict, draw conclusions	Combine, integrate, modify, rearrange, substitute, plan, create, design, invent, what if …, compose, formulate, prepare, generalize, rewrite Example: *The student will be able to assess pelvic capacity and identify women who may have assisted labour difficulties. She may consider the effect of posture and mobilization and link research to this aspect of midwifery.*
Evaluation: • making judgements using internal and external evidence and criteria	• Compare and discriminate between ideas • Assess value of theories, presentations • Make choices based on reasoned argument • Verify value of evidence, recognize subjectivity	Assess, decide, rank, grade, test, measure, recommend, convince, select, judge, explain, discriminate, support, conclude, compare, summarize Example: *The student is able to merge her knowledge of anatomy and physiology with the research from major studies, and also the evidence of her own practice, to provide the woman with unbiased choices and to aid her own process of problem solving and decision making.*

Adapted from Bloom (1956) and Bloom et al (1964)

pedagogy – the science of teaching – was no longer appropriate. He analysed this concept, which he initially viewed as appropriate only for children, and presented a new word: *andragogy*, the art and science of helping adults learn (Knowles 1973, 1980; Knowles et al 2015) (see Table 5.4).

Andragogy was seen as a polar opposite to *pedagogy*, and it was presumed that it was inappropriate to use pedagogy for a group of adult learners (Knowles 1973). Later, he suggested that *andragogy* and *pedagogy* could be viewed as two 'extremes on a spectrum', used according to the needs of the student group of the time (Knowles 1980; Knowles et al 2015). This theory has been criticized for assuming that adults are more self-directing than children

(Tennant 1986), that adults differ from children in their 'reservoir' of experience (Jarvis 2010) and that motivation and readiness to learn are different between the two groups (Tennant 1986).

Andragogy was adopted almost completely by midwifery, and by nursing and other education involving adults, although some aspects do conflict with the current directive to be cost-effective, reduce teacher–student contact time, and increase the student–teacher ratio. In addition, there has been little recent literature/research exploring education theory within midwifery, although there is increasing interest in andragogy within other professions, including tourism, management and law.

Table 5.4 Comparisons of pedagogy and andragogy

	Pedagogy	Andragogy
Definition	Educating children in a didactic fashion – to lead	The art and science of helping adults learn
Learner	• The learner is dependent on the teacher for the direction, content and means of learning. • The learner's learning is assessed by the teacher.	• The learner has a deep need to be self-directing. • The learner is responsible for his or her own learning, but may be occasionally dependent – this is the learner's choice. • The learner is able to self-evaluate/assess.
Learner's previous experience	• Previous experience is limited. • Previous experience is of little worth. • The experience of the teacher is most important.	• Previous experience is a rich reservoir of resources for learning. • Previous experience can be used by self and as a group.
Learner's readiness to learn	• Determined by society or by the institution. • Set curriculum.	• When the individual feels ready – 'need to know'. • May be affected by a life change. • Desire to learn a new set of skills and knowledge to change role.
Learner's orientation to learning	• Subject oriented. • Topics structured in a prescribed order.	• Problem solving. • Needs to be relevant to real life issues. • Developing full potential.
Teacher	• The teacher holds the knowledge. • The teacher is in control of what and how learning takes place.	• The teacher is a co-learner. • The teacher is a facilitator of learning experiences rather than teacher.
Motivation	• Generally externally driven. • Focused on grades and achievements. • Must complete set programme.	• Not so focused on grades. • More on professional/personal development.
Practical implications	There is a fixed set of knowledge to be learned, although with time and societal changes, this fixed set is altered. Teaching is didactic, which may reduce ability to apply learning in different context.	Variety of teaching and learning approaches. Need self-directed opportunities. Co-learning approaches. Problem-based enquiry. Need to review previous experience (may prevent further learning). Need to explicitly value previous experience.

In addition to philosophical differences, andragogic approaches require different classroom settings – desks and chairs arranged in semicircles or circles; more experiential learning; negotiated sessions where students set the agenda; and an increase in self-directed provision (Leigh et al 2015).

Teachers (who become facilitators) use Knowles's assumptions and processes in the delivery of sessions and in designing programmes of learning that incorporates a process model (as in Fig. 5.7), in which the starting point is an environment conducive to learning, and the end point is an evaluation of the learning that has taken place and identification of the next step required. Although environmental factors may encourage learning, McIntosh et al's (2013) national study indicated a dissonance for student midwives who were anxious and sought a 'finite' body of knowledge and found andragogic methods at odds with their quest to be competent and confident as they completed their programme.

From andragogy to reflection

Another influential stream of theory emerged from Kolb's (2014) development of experiential learning, which included reflection as the crucial link between experience and learning (Fig. 5.8). This was also incorporated into midwifery education – through increased use of experiential learning and reflection – and reflective practice has become an important component of the midwife's daily work (Box 5.5).

Kolb's work proposed that people fit into one of four main groups having a matching learning style, linked closely with the experiential learning cycle. Individuals

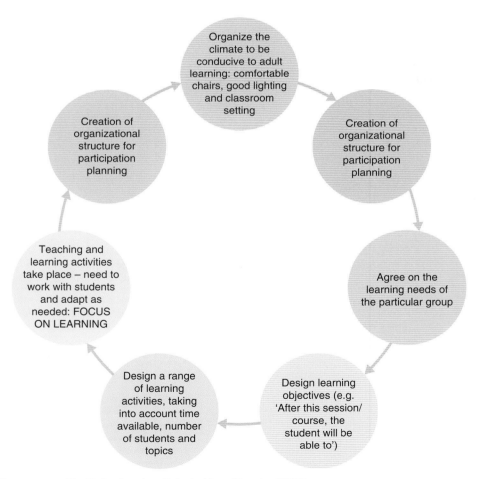

Figure 5.7 The process of facilitating learning. (Adapted from Knowles 1973.)

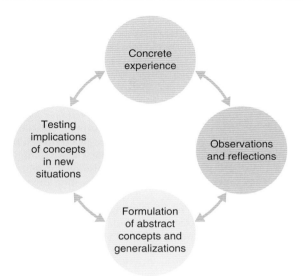

Figure 5.8 The Lewinian experiential model. (Kolb 1984: 21.)

Box 5.5 Practical illustration of reflective cycle

Normally, the cycle starts with the experience (at a concrete level) as something tangible to the senses of the individual. This might be the experience of a practical event, such as witnessing a normal birth. It might be that this delivery is a student's first experience of witnessing a birth, and the woman in labour may react as some labouring women do, by being quite noisy, but as she enters transition becomes centred on herself.

The baby is born, and it is a huge emotional experience. The student notes that the baby looks pink but has blue extremities. She observes and reflects as she is part of this experience. The result is a sorting out in her own mind of the practical experience and her previous knowledge plus her 'classroom knowledge', and she begins to add to her personal knowledge bank. Each component of the experience may be processed separately according to her knowledge. If we look at one aspect, say the colour of the baby, she may make sense of it by thinking that this is the way babies are, and initially this simple acceptance might serve as a temporary working knowledge. Taking this to the next step of the cycle, she will then perhaps be expecting a pink baby with blue extremities at the next birth.

However, as she becomes more experienced and, hopefully, begins to learn more about neonatal physiology, she will appreciate that this is a visual illustration of the transitional effects of birth. She will also begin to understand the individuality of the experience, for the mother, midwife and, indeed, the baby.

---

make their choice depending on their personalities, educational preparation, chosen career or role function at the time (Kolb 2014) (see chapter website resources).

Kolb viewed learning as a dynamic and fluid process, in which the experience and outcome are different for each person, and emphasized that, rather than being an empty vessel to be filled, the student enters learning with a range of learning and experience, and needs to 'relearn' rather than learn 'from scratch'. The teacher therefore assists individuals to modify or dispose of old ideas and change their belief system (see chapter website resources).

Experiential learning is an important tool in developing learning, especially in a practical profession like midwifery, in which more effective interaction with the concepts being taught is achieved as the person is encouraged to a lesser or greater degree to actually sense what the concept would feel like. An example in midwifery would be students learning how to give 'bad news' to women and their families. This could be achieved by practising in a classroom setting what it feels like from the perspective of the mother and midwife and determining what words, body language or strategies are most caring and effective. A crucial part of this exercise is the debriefing and reflective phase that follows, during which all participants can present their perspective and explore events and strategies together.

This type of learning is not always as easy as it might appear. To tell individuals just 'to act it out' does not provide enough guidance, and this approach may result in limited learning or, in the worst-case scenario, entering uncharted and unsupported territory.

If the midwife uses role play, either with student midwives or with women (such as during antenatal education), it is important to have a careful structure for the session, which includes clear objectives, defined roles and a reflective component, and often a short 'cooling down' exercise at the end to bring participants back to reality – which can be helpful following very emotional role play (see chapter website resources). There are some interesting variations, such as online role play (Warland and Smith 2012).

Reflection and reflective practice

The Reflective Practitioner (Schon 1983) began by describing a crisis of the professions, popularizing reflection. Reflection was discussed by Aristotle, and later by Dewey (1933). Schon brought it to the attention of professions, including nursing, midwifery and social work. This book espoused intuition and a more qualitative approach to problem-solving in practice, providing a means of understanding how practitioners make sense of and add to their repertoire of knowledge. Becoming a reflective practitioner has since become an ideal to which many practitioners aspire (Brockbank and McGill 1998; Driscoll 1994).

Schon's work describes a practitioner who chooses to utilize a technical rationality model and work logically to address the problems of the 'high, hard ground where practitioners can make effective use of research-based theory and technique' or, alternatively, take a more intuitive path through the 'swampy lowland where situations are confused "messes" incapable of technical solutions' (Schon 1983: 42). Schon suggested that clients were more likely to have the sort of problems that required the more creative and holistic approach, and, in a period of time when nursing and midwifery, in common with other emerging professions, wished to develop their professional standing, this supported the more feminine, tacit nature of clinical practice.

Certainly, clients often present with complex combinations of risk factors, clinical issues and psychosocial problems, presenting a profile more akin to the 'swampy lowlands' than those high hard grounds, and therefore this viewpoint is seductive. Although Schon described several 'exemplars' of teachers working with students to develop reflective practice, there was not really a clear tool available to assist a practitioner in developing the skills. Since that time, however, several other writers have published tools and frameworks to guide reflection. There have been some question about the interpretation of Schon's reflection in action and 'on-the-spot experimenting' by educationalists, with a suggestion that practitioners should understand that there may be different reflective mechanisms at play (Comer 2016).

It is often helpful to try out some of the many reflective tools to explore whether they can assist in making sense of experiences and help develop learning (see Box 5.6). This triggers questions to facilitate thinking about an experience or an area of practice and develop it into learning (Atkins and Murphy 1993; Benner 1984; Driscoll 1994; Johns 1995). This includes *critical incident analysis* (see chapter website resources), a term for analysis of an incident during which something went wrong, a crisis or a situation recorded for risk-management purposes, or an event that had special resonance for the individual; it is also used in research and increasingly in the field of reflective practice to denote a variety of situations. Many universities use reflective journals or reflective accounts to assist students in developing their knowledge and skills (Bedwell et al 2012; Ekelin et al 2016; Collington 2009), and this provides an opportunity to develop personal reflective and assessment skills and confidence (Macdonald 2014).

Reflective practice can be a potent model for the practitioner to audit day-to-day practice, to continue learning and development from the complex digestion and assimilation of theory and practice and to challenge assumptions (James 2009; Loughran 2012). It is also suggested that utilizing productive reflection with individuals is fundamental to the development of a dynamic learning organization (Boud

et al 2005). An interesting tool is the *debrief tool* (see Box 5.7), which is described as a mixture of reflecting and teaching; it mirrors Kolb's cycle and focuses on elements such as the 'gut feeling' that is experienced by some practitioners (Allan 2011). In addition, Power (2015) highlights the need for a more two-dimensional approach that allows for intuition within decision making and practice.

Reflection is not without problems and requires significant time and energy investment, plus support (Macdonald 2002). It is seldom highlighted that reflection can be difficult, which means that many people will avoid thinking beyond the most obvious. It may also be uncomfortable as areas of practice are revisited – some long forgotten and some more enduring. Reflection needs therefore to carry something of a 'health warning' and an understanding that it is not always possible, or indeed practical, to reflect on all areas of practice all of the time (see chapter website resources).

There is some evidence that just thinking about the individual's philosophy generates some reflection (Kottkamp 1990) (see website for reflective activity). This is a useful means of articulating what is personally believed in as a midwife and sharing this with colleagues. It is important to acknowledge at this point that reflection is an individual activity, and it is not possible to reflect for another person.

Reflective activity 5.4

Use the tool in Box 5.6 to reflect on an aspect of your practice. Choose an everyday event such as a 'booking interview', an antenatal examination or an examination of a newborn.

You may wish to do this with a peer or write it down as a reflective piece for your professional portfolio.

Reflection for you … and others

Others in the maternity service will be learners who will need to be assisted through the reflective cycle to make sense of their experiences. Student midwives usually have a clinical record and a clinical assessment tool in which they may be required to illustrate some critical reflection on their practice. They will therefore value working with midwives who are familiar with the terminology, and they will also find it helpful to have a chance to reflect on different experiences and issues in practice. Sharing reflective incident analysis can be interesting and bring different perspectives, serving as an illustration to the student of how practitioners utilize reflection in day-to-day practice.

Perhaps most fundamentally, women themselves need to reflect. It is clearly not practical to ask women to complete pages of reflective accounts of their experiences,

Box 5.6 A reflective model

Before the event/experience

- How did you prepare for the incident/experience? Were you prepared?
- Is this an issue that you have considered/thought about recently? Why?
- What was in your mind before the event?
- Did you have any worries/concerns about it? How did you address them?

The incident/experience

Describe what happened (no analysis at this stage):

- Who said/did what?
- Record the 'where' and 'how'
- Were you feeling:
  - discomfort?
  - troubled?
  - very positive?
- What other aspects affected your handling of the situation (i.e. busyness of ward/community, other stressors)?
- What knowledge did you use (was this from textbook/research or from colleagues/routine practice)?

Analysis stage

- What were you trying to achieve?
- Why did you respond to the situation/event in the way you did?
- What was the outcome for:
  - you?
  - the woman and baby?
  - your colleagues?
  - your student?
- How did others feel about what happened:
  - the woman and baby?
  - your colleagues?
  - your student?
- And how do you know:
  - from assessing body language/posture?
  - from what was said to you?
- Was this similar to previous responses from other similar situations/events?
- What were the main thoughts/concerns in your mind at the time?
- Thinking about the knowledge you were using, was it based on:
  - training/text book?
  - research?
  - evidence?
  - your assumptions?

- Were there any tensions or difficulties that arose from the knowledge you were using?
- Was this knowledge appropriate to the situation, and were you conscious of any gaps in your knowledge?

The 'what if' stage – alternatives and choices

- How could you have dealt with this differently?
- Would this have changed what happened – and how?
- Were you in a position to actually influence this?
- Would you do the same things if this situation happened again?
  - If so, why?
  - If not, why not?

Plan of action

- What did you learn from this – good and bad? (Don't forget your personal Skinner sandwich.)
- What element of practice, or what you did, did you feel was special and needs to be celebrated?
- Will you use this in your future practice?
- How will you share this with colleagues?
- If you do not want to share with your colleagues, why not? What does that tell you, and how do you deal with it?
- What do you need to update yourself on or find out next:
  - theory?
  - practical skills?
  - research?
- What is your personal calendar for this – tonight, tomorrow or next week?
- If you are not sure of what you have to learn, whom will you use to help you find out, and why:
  - supervisor of midwives?
  - link teacher?
  - consultant midwife?
  - doctor?
  - colleague?

Evaluation

- When will you review this reflection?
- With whom will you share this (supervisor/mentor or colleague)?

Perspective – suspended judgement

- At this point, what are your views on this event/experience?
- How have you incorporated this into your personal knowledge store?

Box 5.7 The DEBRIEF model

Describe events as factually as possible

Evaluate what went well/to change next time

Banish emotions/beliefs/assumptions that cloud
    judgement and development

Review and analyse in light of previous experience
    (pattern recognition)

Identify lessons learned

Establish follow-up actions

Feedback on actions

©Hayley Allan 2009 (Allan 2011)

Box 5.8 Trigger questions for assisting the
woman to reflect

- Having 'booked' to have your baby here, how did you
  feel when you first met your midwives?
  - Do you feel that account was taken of your
    individual needs (antenatal, labour and/or
    postnatal)?
- How do you feel the labour and birth were for you?
  - Were they how you thought they would be?
  - Was anything missing for you?
  - How do you feel in yourself about the birth?
- Did you feel you had sufficient information and
  support about becoming a mother (postnatal)?

---

although some women may find this beneficial, especially those who are familiar with keeping a daily journal or blog. It is, however, good practice to review aspects of the woman's experience with her, at a point where she has had time to consider events and has begun to question what happened and why. The midwife can give the woman a unique opportunity for reflection on the whole continuum of pregnancy and childbirth. In reflecting with women, it is important to remember that, as in all reflections, she has to *reflect on her own experience*. Some trigger questions (Box 5.8) and a focus on her as the key player can be helpful, just providing information and clarification when asked to do so. Counselling skills (i.e. learning *not* to be quick to give a neatly packaged answer) are really helpful at this stage.

Issues around debriefing may need more skilled support, and it is not unusual during the 'routine' reflections to identify a woman who may require additional counselling support and/or special referral. It is also important to appreciate that sometimes when the woman returns to the

service with her next pregnancy, she may need to reflect on her previous experience, should there be any unresolved issues for her.

NEW APPROACHES IN EDUCATION

Midwifery education links with other professions in interprofessional education, which can aid multidisciplinary collaboration and understanding. Examples of this include the Practical Obstetric Multi-Professional Training (PROMPT) Advanced Life Support in Obstetrics (ALSO) and Neonatal Life Support (NLS) courses. Some preregistration courses include interprofessional components in an effort to improve learning and work skills. Midwifery education has developed several approaches, including problem and *inquiry-based learning*, which is congruent with adult learning philosophy and enables students to develop higher-level problem-solving and critical skills (McCourt and Thomas 2001; McNiven et al 2002; Savin-Baden and Wilkie 2006). Other new approaches to learning include the following:

Enquiry-based learning (EBL) curriculum: Midwifery
    lecturers usually provide a 'trigger' activity, following
    which students work in small groups to develop
    questions and learning sessions. The teacher then
    monitors progress to ensure that the learning
    outcomes for the programme are achieved. Evaluation
    suggests that students enjoy this approach, build
    good working relationships with their peers and
    develop their knowledge and critical thinking skills.
    However, some students reported that they needed
    further guidance and input to 'know what they
    needed to know' (Snow and Torney 2015). Tully
    (2010) found that some students' motivation in
    preparing and presenting work was less than for an
    assessed piece of work, and this led to some
    interstudent dissatisfaction. She also found that some
    facilitators seemed more engaged than others, and
    this also affected the student learning experience,
    which suggested that teachers themselves need a
    process of preparation and support in their role
    (Peace 2012; Tully 2010). Peace (2012) found that
    both students and teachers found EBL effective and
    developmental, although highlighting the importance
    of the facilitator's role in guiding the students, and
    also strongly suggested that EBL should be one, but
    not the *only*, way in which students learn.

Phenomenon learning: Another interesting
    development in general education that may transmit
    to midwifery is *phenomenon learning*, a variant on
    self-direction and enquiry-based learning in which
    students are encouraged to broaden their learning,
    look at a phenomenon or scenario, search for gaps in

their knowledge and then research and develop knowledge – working individually or together to create dynamic content (Zhukov 2015). This is being pioneered in schools in Finland, and it is thought to be potentially revolutionary in learning and teaching – seen as individualizing the process of learning and also as enabling a more dynamic approach (Iyer 2015).

Academic gaming: An important aspect of learning that has been incorporated into some programmes, and that students and midwives may consider for presenting sessions, is making learning enjoyable, and this can include the use of quizzes, games and what may be seen as 'fun' activities (Baid and Lambert 2010; see also Ch. 21).

Creative learning: Other tools that have been investigated include the use of mind maps in helping student focus more creatively on their work (Noonan 2013).

Flipped learning/the flipped classroom: This is a way of altering the dynamics of learning. Students learn new content by watching video lectures or accessing podcasts at home and then attend classes, where they work together through exercises and group activities. This ensures that teachers can establish that students understand their learning. This was developed in the United States in high school education, and the method has demonstrated increased student engagement, better assessment results and better discipline (Hanadan et al 2013). It has been applied to other education arenas, including nursing (Simpson and Richards 2015; Alexandre and Wright 2013), medical, legal and librarian education. If adopted in midwifery, it would require planning and increased resources because teachers would need to provide a suite of online materials, video footage and worksheets before classroom sessions, which might also need to be realigned for more interactive work. However, this approach might suit midwifery education in terms of providing an opportunity for students to learn the theory at their own pace and use the classroom sessions to enhance their learning and consider practice applications.

Electronic learning (e-learning): This method emerged as computers were used increasingly in other areas, and it has been incorporated into university programmes for students at pre- and post-graduate levels (Clarke 2009). It is sometimes assumed that this is a more cost-effective use of resources and a good way of reaching greater numbers of students; however, the development of high-quality, interactive and appropriate materials can be time consuming and costly. In countries like Australia with a rich history of distance learning, some successful models, such as the *virtual clinic,* have been developed (Phillips et al 2013). The UK's RCM has a lively and growing menu of modules available to its members (see chapter website resources), and these have proved popular and are well evaluated (Macdonald et al 2011; Hunter et al 2014). The principles of good electronic learning are that it should be tailored to the particular profession and individual needs (Gould et al 2014), be interactive and engaging and be accessible for the user.

Massive open online courses (MOOCs): These are programmes that are designed to be accessed online by large numbers of learners, over a very large geographical area, often several countries. These are usually focused on learning, rather than qualification/credits, and can provide an interesting and original learning opportunity.

Experiential learning: This includes practical learning (i.e. clinical placements) practical skills activities, role play and indeed any learning activity that encourages the student or midwife to closely consider the learning from a practical and personal viewpoint. Experiences such as holding a small caseload alongside the mentor (Rawson 2011), continuity of care (Browne et al 2014), student-run clinics (Marsh et al 2015), a Virtual Maternity Clinic (Phillips et al 2013) and objective structured clinical assessments (OSCEs) (Einion 2013) can all provide students with stimulating and engaging ways of learning and developing cognitive and practical skills, and they therefore hold significant potential for students, women and their babies. As discussed previously, the key to successful experiential learning lies within the application, discussion and reflection, which need to be planned for.

MENTORSHIP AND THE MIDWIFE AS A ROLE MODEL

An important part of developing learning and practice is through interaction with others, and role modelling (Kenyon et al 2015) is a powerful way in which humans learn physical, communication and caring skills. Role modelling allows absorption of the culture of the service (Hindley 1999), which may be negative as well as positive learning (Kirkham 1999), and different parts of the service may have a varying approach to mentoring (Kroll et al 2009). This may also lead to tensions for students when mentors are not practising in an evidence-based way or contradict what students are being taught in university (Armstrong 2010).

Box 5.9 The student learns …

Midwife X sees Mrs Rooson, who is 32 weeks pregnant, with student midwife A. On examining Mrs Rooson, the midwife feels that the fetus is not growing perhaps as fast as she would expect. She asks Mrs Rooson about her nutrition patterns and whether she smokes, drinks alcohol and so forth. She provides the appropriate advice, but decides to ask Mrs Rooson to attend antenatal clinic the following week. She therefore makes the appointment and records this in the notes.

Student A works in the clinic a couple of weeks later, and is encouraged by midwife Y to undertake the examination and the 'talking' under her supervision. Mrs Sim is 32 weeks pregnant, and her observations are all within normal parameters – her fetus is growing well. Student midwife A makes an appointment for the following week.

Midwife Y is completely confused – surely this is not what they teach in the university these days! She challenges the student, and is actually a little sharp with her.

As a practitioner, it is important to be aware that actions, attitudes and demeanour may be observed and perceived in different ways by students, other practitioners, women and their families and friends. Students, especially, are observant of their mentors and may emulate their attitudes, although they tend to prefer the woman-centred and flexible rather than prescriptive approach (Bluff 2002). It is crucial that practitioners share the way decisions and judgements are made with junior colleagues – demonstrating how the very complex process that takes place during the woman's care in the context of the service can be learned (see Box 5.9).

Not to share this process robs the student and practitioner of a valuable learning experience. This process of talking through what is being done and why – almost like reflecting 'on your feet', which Loughran describes – can help students understand the thought processes an experienced practitioner has, and it illustrates the complexities of those processes (Loughran 1996, 2000, 2012).

Students learn theory (and practical skills) in the university setting, and the real-world practice is learned from their mentors in their placements (see chapter website resources). This requires close links and good communication between the academic and clinical areas, to identify outdated practice and ensure students are learning best practice based on evidence and research.

CONCLUSION

Midwifery education has been a dynamic area and one of change to meet the increased information and knowledge available and to support women and their families. What the future holds may be uncertain, but midwives themselves need to be aware of the importance of who controls the content, design, delivery and evaluation of the curriculum. Any education and preparation for midwives must prepare them for a varied career and the ability to work in a fast-paced, constantly changing environment, with the mother and baby placed at the centre of care.

It is crucial for midwives to understand midwifery education, as students, as preceptors and mentors, to understand their own learning patterns, and to be willing to review their own learning history. This all assists in planning education and development activities and, more importantly, in analysing the learning and development needs of the women with whom they are working and the students for whom they are responsible. The good teacher should be able to plan and assess learning, and this includes an analysis – even unlearning – of things that have been learned before or unpicking and addressing assumptions that others may have about learning, or about the whole experience of pregnancy, childbirth and motherhood.

An important part of practice is to have a framework and tools that can assist in critically reflecting on and assessing the effects of that practice. However, this requires the skills described many years ago of open-mindedness, wholeheartedness and responsibility (Dewey 1933). This does carry a health warning, in that truly reflecting on practice brings new challenges and perspectives, which may not always be comfortable.

This chapter reviews the multifaceted nature of learning, education and development. As midwifery faces new challenges and different ways of working, it is paramount that midwives continue to learn and develop. To do so well will certainly benefit the profession and the individual midwife both professionally and personally. Most importantly of all, it will benefit the care provided to women, their babies and families, and thus society as a whole.

Key Points

- An understanding of the structure of general education and professional education pathways is useful in viewing the opportunities that are available to those in the healthcare setting.
- Midwives should be aware of the impact of learning on themselves, their colleagues, students and the women with whom they work.
- An understanding of learning theory assists midwives in their professional and personal development and enables them to facilitate the learning of others.
- CPD is a fundamental part of the midwife's personal 'toolbox', and an effective portfolio and personal CPD

plan can assist in ensuring a systematic and ongoing updating process.

- Understanding and using the principles of reflection enables the midwife to consider and improve his or her practice, assists students to develop their reflective skills and provides an opportunity for the woman to reflect on her pregnancy and childbirth experience.
- The clinical area is a learning environment for midwives, students and women and families.
- There are a wide variety of educational and development opportunities available to practitioners, often accessible locally.

References

Alexandre MS, Wright RR: Flipping the classroom for student engagement, *Int J Nurs Care* 1(2):100–103, 2013.

Allan H: *Debrief: a reflective tool for workplace based learning* (website). www.kcl.ac.uk/lsm/research/divisions/meded/teachers/resources/debrief.pdf. 2011.

Armstrong N: Clinical mentors' influence on student midwives' clinical practice, *Br J Midwifery* 18(2):114–117, 119–123, 2010.

Atkins S, Murphy M: Reflection: a review of the literature, *J Adv Nurs* 18:1188–1192, 1993.

Baid H, Lambert N: Enjoyable learning: the role of humour, games, and fun activities in nursing and midwifery education, *Nurse Educ Today* 30(6):548–552, 2010.

Bartlett HP, Simonite V, Westcott E, et al: A comparison of the nursing competence of graduates and diplomates from UK nursing programmes, *J Clin Nurs* 9(3):369–379, 2000.

Bedwell C, McGowan L, Lavender T: Using diaries to explore midwives' experiences in intrapartum care: an evaluation of the method in a phenomenological study, *Midwifery* 28:150–155, 2012.

Benner P: *From novice to expert: excellence and power in clinical nursing practice*, California, Addison-Wesley, 1984.

Bircumshaw D, Chapman CM: A follow-up of the graduates of the 3-year post-registration bachelor of nursing degree course in the University of Wales, *J Adv Nurs* 13(4):520–524, 1988.

Bloom BS, editor: *A taxonomy of educational objectives. Handbook I: Cognitive domain*, New York, David McKay, 1956.

Bloom BS, Engelhart MD, Furst EJ, et al, editors: *A taxonomy of educational objectives. Handbook II: Cognitive domain*, New York, David McKay, 1964.

Bluff R: *The midwife as role model. International Confederation of Midwives. Midwives and Women Working Together for the Family of the World*, ICM proceedings Vienna, The Hague, International Confederation of Midwives, 2002.

Boud D, Cressey P, Docherty P: *Productive reflection at work: learning for changing organizations*, New York, Routledge, 2005.

Boud D, Keogh R, Walker D, editors: *Reflection: turning experience into learning*, London, Kogan Page, 1988.

Bower H: Educating the midwife. In Mander RF, Fleming V, editors: *Failure to progress: the contraction of the midwifery profession*, London, Routledge, Taylor and Francis, 2002.

Brockbank A, McGill I: *Facilitating reflective learning in higher education*, Buckingham, Society for Research into Higher Education and Open University Press, 1998.

Browne J, Haora P, Taylor J, et al: Continuity of care' experiences in midwifery education: perspectives from diverse stakeholders, *Nurse Educ Pract* 14(5):573–578, 2014.

Bruner J: *The process of education*, Cambridge, Massachusetts, Harvard University Press, 1977.

Byrom S, Downe S: 'She sort of shines': midwives' accounts of 'good' midwifery and 'good' leadership, *Midwifery* 26(1):126–132, 2010.

Centre for Workforce Intelligence (CfWI): *Workforce risks and opportunities: midwives education commissioning risks summary*, London, CfWI, 2012.

Clarke EC: Introduction of E-learning into the pre-registration midwifery curriculum, *Br J Midwifery* 7(7):2009.

Collington V: Reflection in midwifery education and practice: an exploratory analysis, *Evidence Based Midwifery* 4(3):76–82, 2009.

Comer M: Rethinking reflection-in-action: what did Schön really mean?, *Nurse Educ Today* 36:4–6, 2016.

Dewey J: *How we think*, London, DC Heath, 1933 (reprinted 1960).

Dick-Read G: *Childbirth without fear: the original approach to natural childbirth*, New York, Harper & Row, 1986.

Dolphin N: Why do nurses come into continuing education programs?, *J Contin Educ Nurs* 14(4):8–16, 1983.

Donnison J: *Midwives and medical men,* London, Heinemann, 1988.

Driscoll J: Reflective practice for practise, *Sr Nurse* 13(7):47–50, 1994.

Dunkley L, Haider S: Centre for Workforce Intelligence (CWI) Nursing & Midwifery. Workforce Risks and Opportunities. 2011 CWI.

EC Directive 2005/36/EC of the European Parliament and of the Council of 7 September 2005 on the recognition of professional qualifications, Article 40 (website). http://ec.europa.eu/internal_market/qualifications/future_en.htm. [See Section 6(40) at http://eur-lex.europa.eu/legal-content/EN/TXT/?uri=CELEX:02005L0036-20140117.]. 2005.

EC Directive 80/155/EEC, Article 4. Brussels, European Economic Community, 1980.

Einion A: OSCE assessment for emergency scenarios in midwifery education: a reflection and evaluation, *British Journal of Midwifery* 21(12):2013.

Ekelin M, Kvist LJ, Persson EK: Midwifery competence: Content in midwifery students' daily written reflections on clinical practice, *Midwifery* 32:7–13, 2016.

English National Board for Nursing, Midwifery and Health Visiting (ENB): *Creating lifelong learners: partnerships for care,* London, ENB, 1995.

Eraut M: *Developing professional knowledge and competence,* London, Falmer Press, 1994.

Eraut MA, Alderton J, Boylan A, et al: *Learning the use of scientific knowledge in nursing and midwifery education,* London, ENB, 1995.

European Computer Driving Licence Foundation: *Home page* (website). www.ecdl.org. 2016.

Felder RM, Soloman BA: *Index of learning styles* (website). www.ncsu.edu/felder-public/ILSpage.html. n.d.

Finnerty G, Bosanquet A, Aubrey D: Charting the history of midwifery education, *Pract Midwife* 16(8):23–25, 2013.

Fraser DM, Avis M, Mallik M: The MINT Project—An evaluation of the impact of midwife teachers on the outcomes of pre-registration midwifery education in the UK, *Midwifery* 29(1):86–94, 2013.

Freire P: *Pedagogy of the oppressed,* Harmondsworth, Penguin, 1972.

Gill C: *Too clever to care? Daily Mail* (website). www.dailymail.co.uk/health/article-259386/Too-clever-care.html#ixzz3yArKIzaN. 2004.

Gould D, Papadopoulos I, Daniel K: Tutors' opinions of suitability of online learning programmes in continuing professional development for midwives, *Nurse Educ Today* 34(4):613–618, 2014.

Halldorsdottir S, Karlsdottir SI: The primacy of the good midwife in midwifery services: an evolving theory of professionalism in midwifery, *Scand J Caring Sci* 25:806–817, 2011.

Hanadan N, McKnight PE, McNight K, et al: *A review of flipped learning. Flipped Learning Network/Pearson and George Mason University USA* (website). www.flippedlearning.org/review. 2013.

Health Information for All (HIFA): *Meeting the information needs of nurses and midwives* (website). www.hifa2015.org/nursesandmidwives/. 2015.

Hindley C: An assessment of clinical competency on an undergraduate midwifery programme: midwives' and students' experiences, *J Clin Excell* 1(3):157–162, 1999.

HM Treasury: *Spending review and Autumn statement 2015: Key announcements* (website). www.gov.uk/government/news/spending-review-and-autumn-statement-2015-key-announcements. 2015.

Honey P, Mumford A: *The manual of learning styles,* Maidenhead, Peter Honey Publications, 1992.

Honey P, Mumford A: *The Learning Styles Questionnaire: 80-item version,* Maidenhead, Peter Honey Publications, 2000.

Hunter L, Johnson G, Hall J: Online improvements: the RCM i-learn and i-folio have proved very successful as a means of learning and recording educational…, *Midwives Magazine* 17(3):2014.

International Confederation of Midwives (ICM): *ICM global standards for midwifery education (2010).* Amended 2013 (website). www.internationalmidwives.org. 2013a.

International Confederation of Midwives (ICM): *ICM essential competencies for basic midwifery practice (2010).* Amended 2013 (website). www.internationalmidwives.org. 2013b.

Iyer H: *EdTech meets phenomenon based learning* (website). edtechreview.in/trends-insights/trends/1981edtech-meets-phenomenon-based-learning. 2015.

Jacob S: Union learning fund supporting information technology training, *RCM Midwives J* 2(8):254, 1999.

James J: Using a reflective model to aid professional development: reactions and responsibilities in management of a major postpartum haemorrhage, *MIDIRS Midwifery Digest* 19(4):534–539, 2009.

Jarvis P: Quality in practice: the role of education, *Nurse Educ Today* 12(3):3–10, 1992.

Jarvis P: *Adult education and lifelong learning: theory and practice,* New York, Routledge, 2010.

Jenkins E: *An ethnographic exploration of labour ward midwives' accessing and using of information for practice.* Florence Nightingale Scholars Report (website). www.florence-nightingale-foundation.org.uk/content/page/352/2014. 2014.

Johns C: Framing learning through reflection within Carpers's fundamental ways of knowing in nursing, *J Adv Nurs* 22:226–234, 1995.

Jordan G: The use of communications and information technologies (C&ITS) as a tool for continuing professional development (CPD): a case study, *CTI Nurs Midwifery Newsl* 4(3):5–6, 1999.

Kenyon C, Hogarth S, Marshall J: Midwifery basics: mentorship 6. Challenges of mentorship, *Pract Midwife* 18(3):36–40, 2015.

Kirkham M: The culture of midwifery in the National Health Service in England, *J Adv Nurs* 30(3):732–739, 1999.

Knowles MS: *The adult learner: a neglected species,* Houston, Gulf Publishing, 1973.

Knowles MS: *The modern practice of adult education: from pedagogy to andragogy,* revised ed, Chicago, Association Press, 1980.

Knowles MS, Holton EF, Richard A, et al: *The adult learner: The definitive classic in adult education and human resource development*, London, Routledge, 2015.

Kolb DA: *Experiential learning: experience as the source of learning and development* (updated from 1984 ed.), Upper Saddle River (NJ), Pearson, 2014.

Kottkamp RB: Means for facilitating reflection, *Educ Urban Soc* 22(2):182–203, 1990.

Kroll D, Ahmed S, Lyne M: Student midwives' experiences of hospital-based postnatal care, *Br J Midwifery* 17(11):690–697, 2009.

Leap N, Hunter B: *The midwife's tale*, London, Scarlet Press, 1993.

Leigh K, Whitted K, Hamilton B: Integration of andragogy into preceptorship, *MPAEA J Adult Educ* 44(1):9–17, 2015.

Loughran J: *Developing reflective practice: learning about teaching and learning through modelling*, London, Falmer Press, 1996.

Loughran J: *Effective reflective practice. Making a difference through reflective practice: values and actions*, Worcester, Reflective Practice Conference, University College, pp 38–44, July 2000.

Loughran J: *What expert teachers do*, New York, Routledge, 2012.

Macdonald SE: Reflecting on reflection. *ICM 26th Triennial Congress Vienna*, pp. 1–19, April 2002.

Macdonald SE: *How to keep a reflective journal*, Midwives Magazine (website). www.rcm.org.uk/news-views-and-analysis/analysis/how-to-keep-a-reflective-journal. 2014.

Macdonald SE, Johnson G, Linay D, et al: Learning is just a click away, *Midwives* 14(1):34–35, 2011.

Marsh W, Colbourne DM, Way S, et al: Would a student midwife run postnatal clinic make a valuable addition to midwifery education in the UK? A systematic review, *Nurse Educ Today* 35(3):480, 2015.

Marsick VJ, editor: *Learning in the workplace*, London, Croom Helm, 1987.

McCourt C, Thomas BG: Evaluation of a problem-based curriculum in midwifery, *Midwifery* 17(4):323–331, 2001.

McIntosh T: Are we facing the end of midwifery education in England as we know it?, *MIDIRS Midwifery Digest* 26(1):5–10, 2016.

McIntosh T, Fraser DM, Stephen N, et al: Final year students' perceptions of learning to be a midwife in six British universities, *Nurse Educ Today* 33(10):1179–1183, 2013.

McNiven P, Kaufman K, McDonald H: A problem-based learning approach to midwifery, *Br J Midwifery* 10(12):751–755, 2002.

Mezirow J: A critical theory of adult learning and education, *Adult Educ* 32(1):3–24, 1981.

Miller C, Tomlinson A, Jones M: *Learning styles and facilitating reflection*, London, English National Board, 1994.

National Health Service (NHS): *The National Knowledge Service* (website). www.nks.nhs.uk. 2010.

Nicholls L, Webb C: What makes a good midwife? An integrative review of methodologically-diverse research, *J Adv Nurs* 56(4):414–429, 2006.

Noonan M: Mind maps: Enhancing midwifery education, *Nurse Educ Today* 33(8):847, 2013.

Nurses' Registration Act, London, HMSO, 1991.

Nursing and Midwifery Council (NMC): *Standards to support learning and assessment in practice: Preparation for mentors, practice teachers and teachers*, London, NMC, 2008.

Nursing and Midwifery Council (NMC): *Standards for pre-registration midwifery education*, London, NMC, 2009a.

Nursing and Midwifery Council (NMC): *Standards of competence for registered midwives*, London, NMC, 2009b.

Nursing and Midwifery Council (NMC): *The PREP handbook*, London, NMC, 2011.

Nursing and Midwifery Council (NMC): *Revalidation: how to revalidate with the NMC*, London, NMC, 2015a.

Nursing and Midwifery Council (NMC): *The Code: professional standards of practice and behaviour for nurses and midwives*, London, NMC, 2015b.

Nursing and Midwifery Council (NMC): *Social networking guidance*, London, NMC, 2015c.

Peace M: Enquiry-based learning in midwifery: the lecturer's experience, *Br J Midwifery* 20(5):361–368, 2012.

Phillips D, Duke M, Nagle C, et al: Karantzas G: The Virtual Maternity Clinic: a teaching and learning innovation for midwifery education, *Nurse Educ Today* 33(10):1224–1229, 2013.

Power A: Contemporary midwifery practice: Art, science or both?, *Br J Midwifery* 23(9):654–657, 2015.

Quality Assurance Agency for Higher Education (QAA): *Midwifery benchmarks standards* (website). http://www.qaa.ac.uk/en/Publications/Documents/Subject-benchmark-statement-Health-care-programmes---Midwifery.pdf. 2014a.

Quality Assurance Agency for Higher Education (QAA): *Frameworks for Higher education qualifications of UK degree-awarding bodies and their corresponding cycle in the Framework for Qualifications of the European Higher Education Area (FQ-EHEA). The framework for higher education qualifications in England, Wales and Northern Ireland*, London, 2014, QAA. 2014b.

Radford N, Thompson A: *Direct entry – a preparation for midwifery practice*, Guildford, University of Surrey, 1988.

Rawson S: A qualitative study exploring student midwives' experiences of carrying a caseload as part of their midwifery education in England, *Midwifery* 27(6):786–792, 2011.

Rogers CR: *Freedom to learn: a view of what education might become*, Columbus (OH), Charles E Merrill Publishing, 1969.

Rogers CR, Freiberg JM: *Freedom to learn*, 3rd edn, London, Prentice Hall, 1994.

Royal College of Midwives (RCM): *Portfolio development series*, London, RCM, 2000.

Royal College of Midwives (RCM): *Valuing practice: a springboard for midwifery education*, London, RCM, 2003.

Royal College of Midwives (RCM): *State of maternity services report 2015* (website). www.rcm.org.uk/sites/default/files/RCM%20State%20of%20Maternity%20Services%20Report%202015.pdf. 2015.

Royal College of Midwives (RCM): *RCM I-Learn Learning Suite* (website). www.rcm.org.uk. 2016.

Save the Children: Missing midwives. *Save the Children Fund UK* (website).

www.savethechildren.org.uk/
sites/default/files/docs/Missing
_Midwives_1.pdf. 2011.

Savin-Baden M, Wilkie K: *Problem based
learning on line*, Milton Keynes,
Open University, 2006.

Schon DA: *The reflective practitioner:
how professionals think in action*,
New York, Basic Books, 1983.

Scott H: Are nurses 'too clever to care'
and 'too posh to wash'?, *British
Journal of Nursing* 13(10):581, 2004.

Simpson V, Richards E: Flipping the
classroom to teach population
health: Increasing the relevance,
Nurse Education in Practice
15(3):162–167, 2015.

Smith T, Lambert R: A systematic
review investigating the use of
Twitter and Facebook in university-
based healthcare education, *Health
Education* 114(5):347–366, 2014.

Snow S, Torney L: An evaluation of the
first year of an enquiry-based
learning midwifery curriculum,
British Journal of Midwifery
23(12):2015.

Tennant M: An evaluation of Knowles'
theory of adult education,

*International Journal of Lifelong
Education* 5(2):113–122, 1986.

Thomas SS: Early modern midwifery:
splitting the profession, connecting
the history, *Journal of Social History*
115–138, 2009.

Tully SL: Student midwives' satisfaction
with enquiry-based learning, *British
Journal of Midwifery* 18(4):254–258,
2010.

UKCC Commission for Education:
Fitness for practice, London, UKCC,
1999.

United Kingdom Central Council
(UKCC): *Project 2000: a new
preparation for practice*, London,
UKCC, 1986.

United Kingdom Central Council
(UKCC): *The report of the Post-
Registration and Practice Project
(PREPP)*, London, UKCC, 1990.

Universities UK: *A picture of health and
education higher education – a core
strategic asset to the UK* (website).
www.universitiesuk.ac.uk. 2012.

Valaitis RK, Sword WA, Jones B, et al:
Problem based learning online:
perceptions of health science
students, *Advances in Health Sciences*

Education: Theory and Practice
10(3):231–252, 2005.

Warland J, Smith M: Using online
roleplay in undergraduate midwifery
education: a case-study, *Nurse
Education in Practice* 12(5):279–283,
2012.

While AEF, Fitzpatrick JM, Roberts JD: An
exploratory study of similarities and
differences between senior students
from different pre-registration nurse
education courses, *Nurse Education
Today* 18(3):190–198, 1998.

Willis Commission on Nursing
Education (chaired by Lord Willis of
Knaresborough): *Quality with
compassion: the future of nursing
education*. Report of the Willis
Commission on Nursing Education,
London, RCN, 2012.

Wilson TM, Mires G: Teacher versus the
computer for instruction: a study,
British Journal of Midwifery
6(10):655–658, 1998.

Zhukov T: *Phenomenon-based learning:
what is PBL?* (website).
www.noodle.com/articles/
phenomenon-based-learning-what-
is-pbl. 2015.

Resources and additional reading

Health Information for All (HIFA):
www.hifa2015.org/
nursesandmidwives/.
*This is a free resource for which you can
register. The HIFA resource provides
information for nurses and midwives in
developing countries. HIFA's common
goal is: 'A world where every nurse and
every midwife will have access to the
information they need to learn, to
diagnose, to provide appropriate care
and treatment, and to save lives'.*
International Confederation of
Midwives (ICM)
The ICM dissemination pack: http://
www.internationalmidwives.org/
assets/uploads/documents/
Dissemination/140508%20
Dissemination%20ICM%20V06.pdf.

Global Standards for Midwifery
Education (2010) (amended 2013):
http://www.international
midwives.org/what-we-do/
global-standards-competencies
-and-tools.html.
*The ICM is a useful resource for midwives
to access the global standards and
competencies, and also became familiar
with midwives in other countries, and
what their education, training and
practice is.*
Midwives Information and Resource
Service (MIDIRS) https://www
.midirs.org.
*This is a not-for-profit educational charity
providing effective information
resources for midwives, student
midwives and others interested in
midwifery and maternity care. Access is
via subscription, and provides
information on a quarterly basis, plus
online access. It also has a Twitter and
Facebook presence.*

Nursing and Midwifery Council (NMC)
*The NMC web-site https://
www.nmc.org.uk has the current
professional guidance and documents
which direct practice, and also includes
guidance when there is new research,
or media stories that might affect
midwifery and nursing practice. There
is a separate revaluation microsite
(http://revalidation.nmc.org.uk),
which includes full information and
guidance on revalidation, and includes
a range of useful templates that can be
used to record CPD activity, and also
includes the specific guidelines: https://
www.nmc.org.uk/globalassets/
sitedocuments/revalidation/
how-to-revalidate-booklet.pdf.*

Race P: *The lecturer's toolkit: A practical guide to assessment, learning and teaching*, New York, Routledge, 2014.

Really helpful textbook that provides practical and useful tools for helping plan teaching and assessment activities. Useful for teachers and for midwives undertaking teaching activities.

Royal College of Midwives (RCM): www.rcm.org.uk.

The RCM has an excellent website offering access to a range of useful materials, including practice papers, news, research reviews and events. Members (UK and international) have access to further menus of information. Electronic Learning RCM i-learn and i-folio has a wide range of CPD modules, including an excellent module on revalidation ('All you need to know about revalidation'), which includes guidance about this process and has a helpful video clip taking the participant through the whole process. Midwives, if registered, have their own electronic portfolio online (i-folio).

Willis Commission on Nursing Education (chaired by Lord Willis of Knaresborough): *Quality with compassion: the future of nursing education*. Report of the Willis Commission on Nursing Education, London, 2012, RCN. and online at: www.rcn.org.uk/williscommission.

Although this commission was focusing on the education of nurses in the UK, this resource provides information on the challenges facing a similar profession, and many of the recommendations will be as relevant to midwifery.

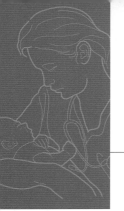

Chapter 6

Evidence-based practice and research for practice

Professor Marlene Sinclair and Dr Lesley Dornan

Learning Outcomes ?

After reading this chapter, you will be able to:

- define and understand the role of evidence and midwifery research in practice
- understand hierarchies and frameworks used to critically appraise research
- be aware of the different sources of evidence and research that inform midwifery practice
- read and review research papers and reports critically
- know and understand the challenges of implementing evidence into practice
- use research evidence for everyday practice

INTRODUCTION

Modern maternity services are expected to deliver care that is clinically effective, high in quality and meaningful to the recipients (Nursing and Midwifery Council (NMC) 2015; Kings Fund 2008). Key factors that underpin excellent care include knowing the person's medical and social history and the judicious use of optimal evidence. In midwifery practice, this requires shared decision making informed by robust research evidence, data from the woman's personal profile and professional expertise.

An *evidence-based approach* is recognized throughout the disciplines as a key skill within the current healthcare climate. Across the world, healthcare professionals are operating in different contexts, from high-tech Western settings to isolated rural regions. Regardless of the culture or setting, education and the transfer of knowledge are critical components of effective care. However, there is an increasing awareness of both the value and complications of integrating evidence into 'routine everyday practice' as learning takes place in many different ways. Experiential learning is a core element of nursing and midwifery practice, but the ability of the midwife to be able to identify a clinical problem, search for evidence to address it, appraise the evidence and find ways to implement and evaluate it can, on occasions, appear challenging. Arguably, gaining knowledge and understanding of the research process through exposure to reading and appraising evidence-based papers enables the midwife to embrace and understand theoretical aspects of research and provide more evidence-informed practice (Schneider et al 2013). However, it is important to note that although evidence-based practice is taking root in professional practice, it is hoped that earlier research by Gerrish (2010) exposing a lack of critical appraisal skill in nurses (and, by extension, midwives) has now been addressed in the new undergraduate midwifery programmes, textbooks such as this one and continuing professional development courses.

The purpose of this chapter is to examine the role of evidence and midwifery research in practice. It includes opportunities for readers to reflect on their practice, engage in challenging activities and explore new resources that will enhance their personal skill set, whether studying at BSc, MSc or PhD level.

Many excellent resources and activities are included in this chapter and the chapter's website resources that will provide an in-depth understanding to meet a variety of needs at all academic levels and, just as importantly, will help readers to be able to apply this understanding to everyday clinical practice. This is in the context that readers of this text include student and qualified midwives who will have different career trajectories, including clinical research, teaching, management and direct clinical practice.

All of the links to URLs have been checked and confirmed as being live and available in January 2016.

DEFINING RESEARCH AND 'MIDWIFERY' RESEARCH

Research is a 'systematic, rigorous investigation which aims to address specific questions about human caring through the steps of the scientific process' (LoBiondo-Wood and Haber 2014: 2). There are many different types of research, and these can be categorized into two broad research approaches. These are inductive and deductive approaches. Deductive research generally begins with a broad idea or theory and arrives at a more specific point (i.e. a top-down approach), whereas inductive research often moves from specific observations to broader theories, adopting a more exploratory approach and sometimes called a bottom-up approach (Trochim 2006). Through this process paradigms are constructed that influence the way the topic or phenomenon is being studied and the designs and methods that may be selected and implemented (Parahoo 2006). Research may include quantitative methods, such as questionnaires; qualitative methods, such as observations, case studies and interviews; or a mixed-methods approach that combines these methods. However, research does not take place in a vacuum but rather is influenced by the context of the topic of interest, the existing knowledge surrounding the topic and the relationship that exists between the theory and the research (Bryman 2012).

Bryar and Sinclair (2011) suggest that midwifery practice incorporates a range of theories from multiple disciplines, including physiology, psychology and sociological theories. Midwifery research has been defined as:

'A rigorous process of inquiry that aims to provide knowledge of and insights into the efficacy and effectiveness of midwifery practice; its effects on women, babies, parents, family, culture and society. It includes research on the education and training of midwives, developing and testing midwifery theory, multidisciplinary team working, the use of information and communication technologies, the organisation and delivery of maternity services, and employment conditions and terms affecting midwives' working lives'.

(Sinclair 2010a)

An interpretation of evidence in practice

There are many definitions of evidence, ranging from the broad concept of an available body of facts or information indicating whether a belief or proposition is true or valid, to the identification of something that suggests truth. One of the most widely known definitions of evidence-based practice within healthcare is as follows:

'Evidence-based medicine is the integration of best research evidence with clinical expertise and patient values'.

(Sackett et al 2000: 1)

A comprehensive definition of evidence-based nursing can be attributed to Ingersoll (2000: 151):

'the conscientious, explicit and judicious use of theory-derived, research-based information in making decisions about care delivery to individuals or groups of patients and in consideration of individual needs and preferences'.

Cluett, a midwife from the United States, states that evidence-based practice is:

'A philosophy and a process. It is logical, sensible and scientific; there are frameworks and processes that meet a need for 'certainty' and structure in many professionals and consumers alike'.

(Cluett 2006: 52)

This means integrating clinical expertise and practices, person-focused values, expectations and wishes and the best available research together to inform and improve care. Simply stated, the aim of evidence-based practice is doing the right thing, at the right time, for the right person to ensure quality of care for the individual (Cluett 2006).

Reflective activity 6.1

Think about the definitions of evidence-based practice. Which definition best describes evidence-based practice for you? You may want to also do a simple Google search for the term, although this is likely to result in a huge number of hits. You may find it helpful to look at the activities in the chapter website resources (LoBiondo-Wood and Haber 2014).

The implementation and influence of evidence-based practice has grown significantly during the last 20 years, affecting most areas of healthcare, including midwifery, nursing, public health, dentistry and mental health and the more distant fields such as social work, probation and education. However, the approach is not without its challenges. There are both strengths and weaknesses to evidence-based practice, and we prefer to categorize these as 'challenges'. Advocates of the approach argue that it is an effective way of achieving best practice and the most effective use of resources. The NMC (2015) makes its position clear and states that midwifery practice *must* be based on the best available evidence. However, it may lead to resource implications and a lack of professional autonomy. 'Evidence-based practice' is a commonly used phrase in clinical practice and academia, and it underpins all of our professional practice. Regardless of the pros and cons, it requires midwives to be advocates to ensure adoption, adaptation (where appropriate) and integration into everyday practice to facilitate implementation.

Reflective activity 6.2

What are the benefits and limitations of evidence-based practice for midwives and women?

Why does the attitude of the midwife towards evidence-based practice matter?

Tip for MSc researchers: If you want to measure attitudes towards evidence-based practice for a research project, you will find the paper by Aarons et al (2012) very useful.

Tip for doctoral midwives: If you want to explore debates on evidence-based practice, read the online paper by Hammersley (2005).

Other references that will be useful include Sinclair (2010b).

EVIDENCE-BASED PRACTICE IN NURSING AND MIDWIFERY

Midwives and nurses are on the frontline of the delivery of care, addressing the changing demographic trends and patterns of diseases and managing the complexities of the context and availability of resources in the settings in which they work. They are also central to the impact of the World Health Organization (WHO) Health Goals and the delivery of services to improve the health and well-being of populations, including mothers and infants, within the priorities of *Health 2020* (WHO 2013).

Evidence-based practice is now recognized as a key professional responsibility for nurses and midwives. The nursing and midwifery statutory and regulatory guidelines emphasize that nurses and midwives are required to deliver care based on the best available evidence or best practice, which means a continual updating and awareness of the changes in the evidence and practices, which are concurrent (NMC 2015). Being aware of the current research and the need for change within practice requires a level of critical analysis and a desire to improve practice. However, there is still a gap between research and practice, and many practitioners rely on training and experience, advice from peers and opinions to inform decision making (Rolfe et al 2008; Whall et al 2006; Trinder 2000).

Evidence-based practice is about 'curiosity and knowledge; understanding knowledge, where it has come from, how it was formed and the ability to decide whether it is reliable and valuable or not' (Farley et al 2009). However, with the volume of evidence now available, the rapidly

growing body of research and the everyday challenges of the workload, information-seeking behaviours need to be taught in a systematic and efficient manner.

How does evidence influence our practice?

Practice evolves from different sources, including research, experience and the adaptation of routines, depending on the context and the people involved. Habits can often be included in professional practices and can be influenced by the knowledge and experiences accumulated over a long period of time, and in spite of best evidence, change in practice is difficult to achieve. Examining and implementing evidence-based practice should challenge the practitioner to look at everyday routines and the standardized care given with objectivity, so that practitioners are constantly striving towards optimal and evidence-based care.

Many factors affect the adoption and implementation of evidence into practice, including strongly held beliefs and attitudes of the individual midwife. These can be manifested in conflict with other health professionals (Kennedy et al 2012). The midwife operates as a member of a team, and evidence demonstrates the importance and value of assembling the multiprofessional team and bringing clinicians, educators and researchers together to explore issues, opinions and barriers before engaging in plans to implement evidence into practice (Spiby et al 2006).

Reflective activity 6.3

Think about your practice. Is there evidence to support the effectiveness of your routine antenatal care regimes?

Action: Search for evidence to support the use of antibiotics for mothers and babies following a birth where there has been a 'spike' in temperature during labour.

Tip: For midwifery researchers interested in theory with illustrated clinical examples, critically review the paper by Whall et al (2006).

Evidence types and implementation

Synthesizing research is both an art and a science. Evidence generation requires adherence to basic principles of asking the question, searching systematically for the answers and critically appraising the evidence gathered.

Examining a topic from multiple angles can allow for a deeper understanding of the different facets within the subject but can also lead to an avalanche of information and the need for evidence-based policies and guidelines to steer practitioners and the public in the best direction possible to achieve optimal health and well-being. Data needs to be interpreted, filtered and synthesized to facilitate knowledge transfer and changes in practice. For example, a search conducted to obtain best evidence on the benefits of breastfeeding (see chapter website resources for the search strategy) will produce a large number of papers, including small qualitative studies, large randomized controlled studies (RCTs) and Cochrane systematic reviews.

However, in widely researched areas there are often seminal papers that are available and can be valuable to give a broad understanding of the current evidence. In the area of the benefits of breastfeeding, for example, seminal papers include those by Ip et al (2007), Kramer and Kakuma (2007, 2012), Horta and Victora (2013) and Horta et al (2007) examining the effects of breastfeeding on immunity, infection, obesity and maternal health. These reviews have already had a significant influence on global and national breastfeeding policies, leading to the introduction of the breastfeeding policy recommending exclusive breastfeeding for 6 months (WHO 2015). The impact of evidence on the benefits of breastfeeding have already been incorporated into both national and local policies and have fuelled the global acceptance of the UNICEF Baby-Friendly Initiative (BFI) as the gold standard approach to be adopted by midwifery educators, managers and clinicians (see Ch. 44). Research evidence is a powerful tool for change! The research pool of knowledge is growing continuously, and more recent systematic reviews were completed in 2015 supporting breastfeeding as a protector for newborns and children from otitis media and obesity (Bowatte et al 2015; Chowdhury et al 2015; Horta et al 2015). It is important to recognize that new research still needs to be absorbed and integrated within existing frameworks, policies and guidance if it is to be valuable to midwives and women. Easily interpreted and applied principles for quality assurance of the evidence need to be developed at the local level by midwives in practice. Setting up journal clubs at the clinical level is a worthwhile activity that the first author established in 1989 to support midwifery research in the Lagan Valley Hospital in Northern Ireland. This was a multiprofessional grouping, and staff generated clinical issues that were causing staff to act in a variety of ways depending on their experience – for example, managing constipation in the antenatal period for mothers with placenta praevia and in the postnatal period for women who were breastfeeding, suffered with haemorrhoids or experienced an instrumental delivery. At the journal meeting, the pharmacist provided advice to the obstetricians, dietitian, physio and the midwives. This was a long time ago, but the principle of searching for the papers to bring staff together to develop a working plan is still viable and useful because we must seek consensus for change at the clinical level and involve the multidisciplinary team. At that time, we did not have critical appraisal tools, but we did have a hunger to do what was best for the woman. Today, we have moved to a new level and work with the consumer in a very focused manner through the Midwifery Services Liaison Committees (MSLCs), and their input into our research, our policies and our practices is almost mandatory – but more importantly, their contribution is exceptionally valuable. This sort of model can lead to a genuine partnership between the maternity services and women and families.

Returning to the midwife in practice, it is important for us to know that the research underpinning a change in practice reaches the quality threshold for robust research. We need to ask simple questions:

- Is the research question clearly stated?
- Did the researchers provide a synthesis or summary of the literature?
- Did they select an appropriate design to answer the question?
- How did they select the sample?
- Did they have a large enough sample to have confidence in the results presented?
- Did they verify their data analyses and interpretation with a sample of the participants' sample, and do they provide easily understood statistics?

The exercise in Reflective activity 6.4 should demonstrate that evidence itself (no matter how robust) cannot change human behaviour on its own. People are complex and influenced by knowledge, social norms, life experience, genetics, environmental factors and so forth, all of which affect motivation towards the achievement of

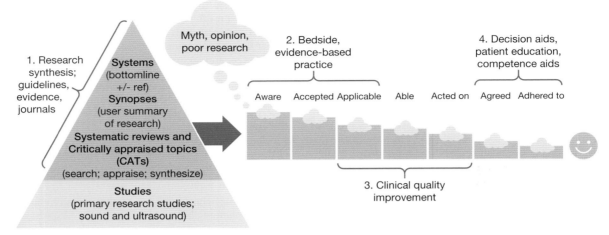

Figure 6.1 Research-to-practice pipeline. (Reproduced from Glasziou P, Haynes B. The paths from research to improved health outcomes, Evidence-Based Medicine 2005; 10:4-7 http://ebm.bmj.com/content/10/1/4.2.full.pdf+html EBM Volume 10 February 2005, with permission from BMJ Publishing Group Ltd.)

personal goals. Michie et al (2011) argue that evidence on its own is insufficient and requires local application, appropriate skills, understanding of the context and the engagement of key stakeholders. However, this is further complicated by human decision making. It is true that choice may free the mind and choice may shackle the behaviour! However, to choose effectively, it is crucial to have the best evidence possible to enable a truly informed choice to be made, and that is why the conduct of systematic and rigorous research is necessary. Michie et al (2011) published an excellent paper on the behaviour change wheel demonstrating how behaviour change occurs and the importance of three necessary prerequisites for a successful outcome: *capability, motivation* and *opportunity.*

However, establishing what counts as credible evidence is challenging, and there are numerous frameworks to facilitate the classification of the different types of studies and the levels of evidence. Broadly speaking, they have similar approaches to grading the evidence with a pyramidal structure that has systematic reviews at the pinnacle, followed by RCTs with definitive results, cohort studies, case-control studies, cross-sectional surveys and expert opinion (see Fig. 6.2).

A hierarchy of evidence is simply a grading system in which the levels of hierarchy reflect the study design (Munro and Spiby 2010). It offers a structured, logical approach to identifying, analysing, and implementing research. When examining the different types of studies, it is important to note that within the wide variety of methods come alternative risks of bias that may influence the outcomes.

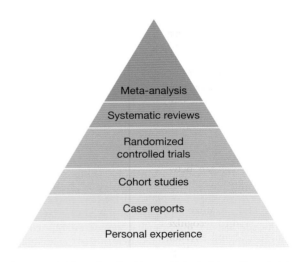

Figure 6.2 Hierarchy of evidence. (Adapted from Greenhalgh, T., (2006). How to Read a Paper: The Basics of Evidence-Based Medicine. fifth ed. Wiley and Sons, West Sussex, United Kingdom.)

There is a diverse range of organizations that are known to offer or recommend high-quality research standards, and these are an excellent place to begin searching. Examples of these are the *Cochrane Collaboration, National Institute of Health and Care Excellence* and the *Royal College of Obstetricians and Gynaecologists.* Details of these resources can be found in the reading list at the end of this chapter. The Royal College of Midwives (RCM) has a library based within the Royal College of Obstetricians and Gynaecologists (RCOG) library in London. RCM members are welcome to benefit from this service, and there is also a wide range of resources and support online in the form of midwifery journals, CPD opportunities and electronic learning (RCOG 2015; RCM 2016). Searching these resources for systematic reviews or guidelines in the topic being investigated will offer some indication of the priority being allocated to the topic and the volume of evidence available.

PROCESS STEPS TO IMPROVE PRACTICE

Implementing evidence into practice can be a rewarding and worthwhile process that should improve care and practice. Decision making plays a significant role in the daily life of a midwife, but it is important to examine the processes by which those decisions are made.

Reflective activity 6.5

Think about your individual thinking processes when faced with a choice of treatments/management for a clinical situation—for example, if a woman asks you for advice on place of birth.

- What helps you in making a decision regarding care/management, and how do you justify that decision?
- Do you have sufficient access to evidence in your day-to-day practice?

Bridging the gap between research and practice also requires a number of key skills to be able implement the required changes into practice. These include the ability to search and organize the literature, critically appraise research studies, recognize the value of the research in the clinical field and envision and achieve a realistic implementation of the findings. Finally, reflection throughout the process is crucial to learning what may or may not work within the range of clinical settings and to enable us to learn each time from the process. Although this may appear challenging, in practice, midwives use many of these skills on a daily basis in other areas of their work.

There are a series of steps that, when implemented, can help to cultivate a systematic process and maintain accountability, especially if working as part of a team to improve practice and these are standardized across the disciplines. These steps are as follows:

- **Ask** the question. Decide which question you would like to ask and write it in a clear and focused way. Information needs from practice are converted into

Table 6.1 PICO format

P	Patient, problem or population	Who is the patient/client or group, and what characteristics does the patient/client or group have?
I	Intervention	What is the main intervention being considered?
C	Comparison	Is there a control group or comparative element in the treatment/management options?
O	Outcome	What are the measures, effects or improvements that are being looked for?

focused, structured questions using a framework such as *PICO* (see Table 6.1).

- **Acquire** the best evidence available possible from the current literature. A framework such as PICO enables a search of the literature in a structured format.
- **Appraise** the evidence for credibility and reliability.
- **Apply** the evidence in your setting through an active and collaborative decision-making process and clinical expertise with all the affected individuals and groups.
- **Assess** the outcome through reflection, audit or peer assessment and disseminate the results (adapted from Fleming 1998).

Asking the question

A practitioner's initial exposure to clinical practice and information-seeking behaviour as a student are foundational to successful integration and the assimilation of best evidence into everyday practice. An evidence-based question invariably starts with a patient or an area of clinical practice. Frequently it can occur through meeting a clinical problem or question that arises during the activities in everyday routine practice. It may occur when faced with providing care for a woman with a rare genetic disorder, for example, or in response to an enquiry about the medication levels of maternal drugs transferred in breastmilk to the infant. Establishing the question that the practitioner would like to answer is an important first step in the evidence-based process. A well-designed question allows for a systematic approach to finding the evidence. One method of doing this is through implementing the PICO framework, particularly in clinical and therapy investigations (Huang et al 2006). This includes the following:

1. Who/what is the **patient/population/problem** you wish to study?

Table 6.2 Implementation of the PICO framework in a narrative review of the benefits of breastfeeding

PICO Framework	
Population/patient/problem	Breastfeeding mothers
Intervention/**exposure**	Benefits of breastfeeding
Main comparison	Partial/nonbreastfeeding mothers
Main outcome/**measure**	Effects of breastfeeding on infant and maternal health as evidenced in systematic reviews on benefits of breastfeeding
Dornan 2015	

Table 6.3 Additional frameworks for qualitative research

SPIDER	SPICE	PICO
Setting	Sample	Population
Perspective	PI phenomenon	Intervention
Intervention	Design	Comparison
Comparison	Evaluation	Outcome
Evaluation	Research type	

2. Which **intervention/prognostic factor or exposure** do you want to examine?

3. What is the main **comparison/alternative** you can use in the process?

4. What is the **outcome/measurement** you would like to achieve?

When thinking of and formulating the question, it is helpful to be as specific as possible, while remaining flexible, because it often takes several tries before the question may be finalized. This is a normal part of the process, particularly when the volume of literature is wide or the question is complex.

If the question is complex, breaking it down into different components may also help to decide which area requires the priority. An example of a PICO framework implemented during a narrative review on the benefits of breastfeeding is included in Table 6.2.

This review was further broken down into more components, including obesity, allergies and maternal health, to manage the volume of information available.

The chapter website offers further information on the use of PICO for quantitative questions and PICO, SPIDER and SPICE for qualitative questions. You can also read a comparative paper, "PICO, PICOS and SPIDER: A Comparison Study of Specificity and Sensitivity in Three Search Tools for Qualitative Systematic Reviews" online at www.ncbi.nlm.nih.gov/pmc/articles/PMC4310146/.

A summary of the differences between the SPIDER, SPICE and PICO frameworks is provided in Table 6.3.

Finding the evidence

A well-framed question can lead to a well-designed search strategy. Although not all terms might be used in a search strategy once the population and problem/phenomenon have been selected, this will assist in the design of the search strategy. Defining the search terms may feel arduous, but they are an important element in the process because the search terms are key in selecting and identifying relevant articles that may need to be included in the review of the topic. Equally important is the selection of the *types* of reviews or studies required, in addition to a clear understanding of how to search effectively. If there is a large volume of papers, it may be helpful to limit the time frame of the search (e.g. the last 10 years). However, in any search, it is important to be sensitive to the inclusion of key research papers because these are often seminal works that can be missed in the shortened literature review. There is no prescription for this, but any midwife undertaking this process as a formal requirement, such as for master's degree and especially doctoral studies, would need to be able to support the 'cutoff points' with a nonrefutable argument.

Once the search terms have been established, the next step in the process of acquiring the evidence is to decide which databases will be the most relevant to the search. Databases such as *MEDLINE, CINAHL, EMBASE* and *ProQuest* all have a wide range of similar papers; however, if the question includes topics outside the biomedical fields, it may be worth considering other databases, such as Web of Science or PsycINFO, to ensure the inclusion of key texts. Including more than one database will allow access to a breadth of studies that may inform the context or question more effectively. An important consideration in this process is how much access to databases within the university or organization is available (see chapter website resources for details on searching medical databases and the PICO framework).

Critical appraisal

Critical appraisal is defined as using a systematic process to identify the strengths and weaknesses of a research article or report to assess its usefulness and the applicability of the findings, which includes an evaluation of the appropriateness of the research design in answering the research question and an assessment of the methodological features (Young and Solomon 2009).

The nursing literature suggests that a lack of knowledge about research and a sense of discomfort with research terminology are primary reasons for a lack of evidence-based practice being implemented within the clinical setting (Hines et al 2015). The concept of having a framework of skills to examine the literature, which includes searching skills (as highlighted previously), the ability to read and critically appraise the identified literature, critical thought capacity and an awareness of ethical issues, has been advocated (Moule and Goodman 2013). However, these are skills that develop with experience. The first step in the process may be to examine the abstracts of all the identified articles to establish whether they fit the searching criteria. Often during database searches, articles are selected because a word or phrase has been recognized, but the focus of the study may not be relevant to the chosen topic.

Once all the articles have been selected, it may be helpful to use a categorization process to establish whether the articles are relevant to the specific clinical question. Although many systematic reviews are written by academic institutions or clinical collaborations, there are occasions when reviews may be published by advocacy groups or authors who may have a specific interest in the review. One of the fundamental skills of appraising the evidence is identifying potential bias or flaws within the reviews or studies. Another element to consider is the role and collaborations of the author(s).

Critical appraisal tools enable readers to make sense of the evidence and give guidelines to follow when examining it. There are a number of helpful guidelines to assist in these processes, including the Critical Appraisal Skills Programme (CASP) guidelines (Public Health Resource Unit 2008), Cochrane Guidelines, Quality of Reporting Meta-Analyses (QUORUM) (Moher et al 1999) and the Measurement Tool to Assess Systematic Reviews (AMSTAR) framework (Shea et al 2007). The Scottish Intercollegiate Guidelines Network (SIGN) critical appraisal resources are also helpful and include a variety of resources depending on the type of study being examined. Alternatively, the PICO framework can also be applied to critically analyse studies (Schardt et al 2007). Details of these can be found in the reading list and on the chapter website. Identifying and focusing on the highest-standard studies can help to manage the volume of information that is now available within the research field. In summary, when critically appraising the evidence, the reader needs to examine the results for:

- Level of evidence
- Reliability

- Evidence of bias
- Application to practice (Melnyk et al 2010)

Critical appraisal allows health professionals to use research evidence reliably and effectively and is intended to enhance healthcare professionals' skill in determining whether the research is free from bias and also relevant to their clinical practice and patients (Mhasker et al 2009). The hierarchy-of-evidence pyramid is also an important tool for reference and a guide to classification of different types of evidence (see Fig. 6.2).

However, despite the volume of resources available to aid the process of literary appraisal, there is no one single framework that is considered superior. In fact, it is important to bear in mind that even when using these frameworks and models for classification, there is still a level of clinical judgement and an evolving of both the practitioner's skills and the available research that must occur.

Discussion of the findings with other colleagues may help to clarify points of conflicts or interest during the analysis process. Appraisal of the evidence may not give a consistent picture, so it is valuable to use clinical expertise and judgement to critique and synthesize the findings before piloting and evaluating the practice (Cullen 2015).

New developments are constantly challenging the research community, and following global requests for improved access to review protocols, PROSPERO, a prospective register for systematic review protocols, has been developed (see www.crd.york.ac.uk/prospero/) and is now live and fully functioning. This international prospective register is an important database for midwifery researchers to know about and to ensure they register their protocols.

Reflective activity 6.6

Download the critical appraisal tools from the CASP website and apply them to a selection of research papers and a guideline:

http://www.casp-uk.net/#!casp-tools-checklists/c18f8

http://www.biomedcentral.com/content/
supplementary/2046–4053-3-139-S8.pdf

Practice Tip: It is helpful to work as part of a group if you are still building your skill set. Shared learning can be effective and supportive.

Applying the evidence in practice

Once the evidence has been collected and analysed, the next step is applying the evidence into practice. Understanding the role of evidence in everyday practice and having the freedom and support to apply the evidence are both key preludes to a successful outcome. Practical reasons, such as a lack of time and financial resources, the organizational culture and openness to change within the clinical setting, in addition to the relevancy and priority of the issue, all play a part in how successful the application to practice may be (Hunter 2013). Questions that are asked at this stage include:

- Is the study question relevant to the area of interest?
- Do the findings offer new insight or information?
- Is it practical to adapt or apply the findings in the clinical setting?

Planning for implementation of change and the dissemination of new knowledge should ideally be an integral part of an evidence-based midwifery approach. Good communication is a significant part of this. Being part of a team (as mentioned earlier) may allow a sense of ownership within the unit or staff and give a stronger voice for change if it is required. Implementing change through evidence-based practice can be complex, and having a strong support base and team may make the difference between success and failure.

Reflective activity 6.7 ><

Think of ways that you would implement the findings of your research into practice. What steps would you take?

Tip: For midwifery researchers searching for theoretical literature to make sense of implementation theories, models and frameworks, access the following article by Nielsen (2015): www.implementationscience.com/content/pdf/s13012–015–0242–0.pdf.

Clinical inquiry is an essential skill for all leaders and clinicians, and finding innovative solutions is an integral part of the troubleshooting and correction that helps to facilitate long-term, sustained changes in evidence-based practice (Cullen 2015). Implementing real and sustained change often will require small steps forward because progress occurs not only from big leaps forward but also from hundreds of small steps (Isaacson 2014).

Examining any current guidelines related to the clinical/research question is a good first step in the implementation process. Are there any guidelines available, and if so, are they in line with the current evidence? For example, the first step in the implementation of a project may be the design and/or updating of current clinical guidelines. The next step may then be evaluating to what extent those guidelines are already effective. This can occasionally create a barrier among staff members, particularly if the guidelines are not being followed. For instance, the breastfeeding guidelines within the Baby Friendly Initiative advise that all women should be encouraged to breastfeed their infants within 1½ hours of birth, but this may not be universally implemented (UNICEF 2015). Once again, building a sense of ownership and communication skills is critical in this process to allow staff to express their opinions.

There are a number of evidence-based implementation models that may help to give a structured approach to this stage of the process. These include the EBP Implementation Guide (Cullen and Adams 2012) and the Implementation of Change Model (Grol et al 2013). Alternatively, further reading on making sense of the theories, models and frameworks can be found in the reading list. Another important resource to be aware of, relating to patient safety, is the Agency for Healthcare Research and Quality (AHRQ). This organization provides a patient safety research portfolio for healthcare delivery that was developed by the dissemination subcommittee of the AHRQ Patient Safety Research Coordinating Committee. It has produced information detailing three major stages required for knowledge transfer from the research field to the person receiving care, as follows:

- Knowledge creation and distillation
- Diffusion and dissemination
- Organizational adoption and implementation

Assessing the outcomes and dissemination of the results

The outcomes of evidence-based practice can be effective and wide ranging. The assessment of the findings and the dissemination of the results require reflection by the health professional, peer assessment from the team and, on occasion, feedback from patients and users of the service. The dissemination of the results often is assisted through the interactions of the practitioner, the value and characteristics of the topic, the intended population that will benefit from it and the context, which will ultimately decide the rate and extent of the adoption of the changes (Rogers 2003; Greenhalgh et al 2004; Titler 2008). Evaluating the implementation of the results allows practitioners to identify changes within the practices and whether these have been of benefit or not. Monitoring the effect of an evidence-based practice on healthcare quality can help practitioners to analyse flaws in the implementation and evaluate which patients would benefit most from the changes (Melnyk et al 2010).

The assessment process may involve working not only with midwifery colleagues but also other multidisciplinary team members and patients to establish whether the changes in practice have actually affected patient care. Highlighting the value and compatibility of the suggested changes can go a long way towards a successful outcome.

Research Excellence Framework

Universities in the UK are allocated about £2 billion per year from the higher education funding bodies to contribute to 'economic prosperity, national well-being and the expansion and dissemination of knowledge' (Research

Excellence Framework (REF) 2014: 3). The purpose of the research assessment exercise was and is to assess the quality and impact of all UK research and to allocate funding based on excellence. Midwifery research was returned under unit of assessment 3: Allied Health Professions, Dentistry, Nursing and Pharmacy. To see the results, visit http://results.ref.ac.uk/Results/ByUoa/3.

Two midwifery professors were nominated to sit on the committee: Professor Billie Hunter from Cardiff and Professor Marlene Sinclair from Ulster. In the next REF round (2021) it will be critical that midwifery research be more visible and for the search term 'midwifery research' to be a MEsh heading in key databases. If the evidence for midwifery has a recognized growing body of knowledge through enhanced, open-access, high-quality publications, strategic research positions and research excellence profiles, there will be more power to request that the next REF unit of assessment has midwifery in the title. This will allow practitioners to access relevant contributions to knowledge more effectively and apply them to practice with a goal to improve maternity care.

CONCLUSION

Midwives need to become connoisseurs of evidence-based midwifery practice. We all need to develop more finely tuned skills in asking answerable questions, searching the literature effectively, using theory to underpin our research, critically appraising the evidence and knowing how to implement it in practice through collaboration with peers, medical colleagues and, most importantly, the women we serve.

Key Points

- Evidence may be gleaned from personal experience, expert knowledge, research and systematic investigation.
- Midwives need to be skilled in searching, accessing and appraising research and evidence to improve their practice, to share knowledge with colleagues and with women and families and to enable more effective decision making.
- Midwives need to develop their skills in understanding and using research in day-to-day practice.
- Effective use of evidence and research will contribute to quality of care for mothers, their babies and families.
- There are a number of useful tools and strategies for practitioners to read and utilize research systematically and critically.

References

Aarons GA, Cafri G, Lugo L, et al: Expanding the domains of attitudes towards evidence-based practice: the Evidence Based Practice Attitude Scale-50, *Adm Policy Ment Health* 39(5):331–340, 2012.

Bowatte G, Tham R, Allen KJ, et al: Breastfeeding and childhood acute otitis media: a systematic review and meta-analysis, *Acta Paediatr* 104(Suppl 467):S3–S13, 2015.

Bryar R, Sinclair M: *Theory of midwifery practice*, New York, Palgrave McMillan, 2011.

Bryman A: *Social research methods*, 4th edn, New York, Oxford University Press, 2012.

Chowdhury R, Sinha B, Sankar MJ, et al: Breastfeeding and maternal health outcomes: a systematic review and meta-analysis, *Acta Paediatrica* 104(Suppl 467):S96–S113, 2015.

Cluett ER: Evidence-based practice. In Cluett ER, Bluff R, editors: *Principles and practice of research in midwifery*, Edinburgh, Churchill Livingstone/Elsevier, pp 33–56, 2006.

Cullen L: Evidence into practice: awakening the innovator in every nurse, *J Perianesth Nurs* 30(5):430–435, 2015.

Cullen L, Adams SL: Planning for implementation of evidence based practice, *J Nurs Adm* 42:222–230, 2012.

Dornan L: Adapting a motivational instructional model to identify and analyse Thai cultural influences on breastfeeding behaviour. Thesis. Ulster University. 2015.

Farley AJ, Feaster D, Scapmire TJ, et al: The challenges of implementing evidence based practice: ethical considerations in practice, education, policy and research, *Soc Work Soc Int Online J* 7(2):2009.

www.socwork.net/sws/article/view/76/335.

Fleming K: Asking answerable questions, *Evid Based Nurs* 1:36–37, 1998.

Gerrish K: Evidence-based practice. In Gerrish K, Lacey A, editors: *The research process in nursing*, 6th edn, Chichester, Wiley Blackwell, pp 488–500, 2010.

Glasziou P, Haynes B: The paths from research to improved health outcomes, *Evid Based Med* 10:4–7. http://ebm.bmj.com/content/10/1/4.2.full.pdf+html. 2005.

Greenhalgh T: *How to read a paper: the basics of evidence-based medicine*, 5th edn, West Sussex, Wiley & Sons, 2006.

Greenhalgh T, Robert G, McFarlene F, et al: Diffusions of innovations in service organisations: systematic review and recommendations, *Milbank Q* 82(4):581–629, 2004.

Grol R, Wensing M, Eccles M, et al: *Improving patient care: the implementation of change in health care*, 2nd edn, West Sussex, Wiley & Sons, 2013.

Hammersley M: Is the evidence-based practice movement doing more good than harm? Reflections on Iain Chalmers' case for research-based policy making and practice, *Evid Policy* 1(1):85–100, 2005.

Hines R, Ramsbotham J, Coyer F: The effectiveness of interventions for improving the research literacy of nurses: a systematic review, *Worldviews Evid Based Nurs* 12(5):265–272, 2015.

Horta BL, Bahl R, Martines JC, et al: *Evidence on the long term effects of breastfeeding*, Geneva, World Health Organization, 2007.

Horta BL, de Mola CL, Victora CG: Long-term consequences of breastfeeding on cholesterol, obesity, systolic blood pressure and type 2 diabetes: a systematic review and meta-analysis, *Acta Paediatr* 104(Suppl 467):S30–S37, 2015.

Horta BL, Victora CG: *Long-term effects of breastfeeding: a systematic review*, Geneva, World Health Organization, 2013.

Huang X, Lin J, Demner-Fushman D: Evaluation of PICO as a knowledge representation for clinical questions, *AMIA Annu Symp Proc* 359–363, 2006.

Hunter B: Implementing research evidence into practice: some reflections on the challenges, *Evidence-Based Midwifery*. www.rcm.org.uk/learning-and-career/learning-and-research/ebm-articles/implementing-research-evidence-into-practice. (website). 2013.

Ingersoll G: Evidence-based nursing: what it is and isn't, *Nurs Outlook* 48:151–152, 2000.

Ip S, Chung M, Raman G, et al: Breastfeeding and maternal and health outcomes in developed countries, *Evid Rep Technol Assess* 153:1–186, 2007.

Isaacson W: *The innovators: how a group of hackers, geniuses and geeks created the digital revolution*, New York, Simon & Schuster, 2014.

Kennedy HP, Doig E, Hackley B, et al: "The midwifery two-step": a study on evidence-based midwifery practice, *J Midwifery Womens Health* 57:454–460, 2012.

Kings Fund: *Safe births: everybody's business* (website). www.kingsfund.org.uk/sites/files/kf/field/field_publication_file/safe-births-everybodys-business-onora-oneill-february-2008.pdf. 2008.

Kramer MS, Kakuma R: *The optimal duration of exclusive breastfeeding (review)* (website). http://apps.who.int/rhl/reviews/langs/CD003517.pdf. 2007.

Kramer MS, Kakuma R: Optimal duration of breastfeeding, *Cochrane Database Syst Rev* (8):CD003517, 2012.

LoBiondo-Wood G, Haber J: *Nursing research: methods and critical appraisal for evidence-based practice*, 8th edn, St. Louis (MO), Elsevier, 2014.

Melnyk BM, Fineout-Overholt E, Stillwell S, et al: *The seven steps of evidence-based practice* (website). www.nursingcenter.com/nursingcenter_redesign/media/EBP/AJNseries/SevenSteps.pdf. 2010.

Mhasker R, Emmanuel P, Mishra S, et al: Critical appraisal skills are essential to informed decision making, *Indian J Sex Transm Dis* 30(2):112–119, 2009.

Michie S, van Stralen M, West R: The behaviour change wheel: A new method for characterising and designing behaviour change interventions, *Implement Sci* 6:42, 2011.

Moher D, Cook DJ, Eastwood S, et al: Improving the quality of reports of meta-analyses of randomised controlled trials, *Lancet* 354(9193):1896–1900, 1999.

Moule P, Goodman M: *Nursing research: an introduction*, London, Sage, 2013.

Munroe J, Spiby H: The nature and use of evidence in midwifery care. In Spiby H, Munro J, editors: *Evidence-based midwifery care: applications in context*, Malaysia, Wiley, 2010.

Nilsen P: Making sense of implementation theories, models and frameworks, *Implement Sci* 10:53, 2015.

Nursing Midwifery Council: *The Code: standards of conduct, performance and ethics for nurses and midwives* (website). www.nmc.org.uk/globalassets/sitedocuments/standards/the-code-a4-20100406.pdf. 2015.

Parahoo K: *Nursing research: principles, processes and issues*, 2nd edn, New York, The Free Press, 2006.

Public Health Resource Unit: *Critical Appraisal Skills Programme (CASP)*, England, Public Health Resource Unit, 2008.

Research Excellence Framework: *Key facts* (website). http://www.ref.ac.uk/media/ref/content/pub/REF%20Brief%20Guide%202014.pdf. 2014.

Rogers EM: *Diffusion of innovations*, New York, The Free Press, 2003.

Rolfe G, Segrott J, Jordan S: Tensions and contradictions in nurses' perspectives of evidence based practice, *J Nurs Manag* 16:440–451, 2008.

Royal College of Midwives (RCM): *Royal College of Midwives (RCM) i-learn: electronic learning menu* (website). www.rcm.org.uk. 2016.

Royal College of Obstetricians and Gynaecologists (RCOG): *Library Services* (website). www.rcog.org.uk/en/guidelines-research-services/library-services/. 2015.

Sackett D, Strauss S, Richardson W, et al: *Evidence-based medicine: how to practice and teach EBM*, 2nd edn, Edinburgh, Churchill Livingstone, 2000.

Schardt C, Adams MB, Owens T, et al: Utilization of the PICO framework to improve searching PubMed for clinical questions, *BMC Med Inform Decis Mak* 7:16, 2007.

Schneider Z, Whitehead D, Biondo-Wood GL, et al: *Nursing and midwifery research: methods and appraisal for evidence based practice*, 4th edn, Australia, Mosby Elsevier, 2013.

Shea BJ, Grimshaw JM, Wells GA, et al: Development of AMSTAR: a measurement tool to assess the methodological quality of systematic reviews, *BMC Med Res Methodol* 15(7):10, 2007.

Sinclair M: *Definition of research in midwifery* (adapted from a definition in 2008). Doctoral Midwifery Research Society (website). www.doctoralmidwiferysociety.org/Research_Definition.aspx. 2010a.

Sinclair M: Midwifery in the context of new and developing technologies. In Kent B, McCormack B, editors: *Clinical context for evidence-based nursing practice*, New York, Wiley-Blackwell, 2010b.

Spiby H, McFadden A, Cranshaw S, et al: Evidence based midwifery network. 3rd national conference, *Br J Midwifery* 14(7):434, 2006.

Titler M: The evidence for evidence-based practice implementation. In Hughes RG, editor: *Patient safety and quality: an evidence-based handbook for nurses*, Rockville (MD), Agency for Healthcare Research and Quality, 2008.

Trinder L, Reynolds S: *Evidence-based practice: a critical appraisal*, Oxford, Blackwell Science, 2000.

Trochim MK: *Research methods knowledge base: deduction and induction* (website). www.social researchmethods.net/kb/dedind .php. 2006.

UNICEF: *The Baby Friendly Hospital Initiative* (website). www.unicef.org/ programme/breastfeeding/baby.htm. 2015.

Whall A, Sinclair M, Parahoo K: A philosophic analysis of evidence-based nursing: recurrent themes, metanarratives, and exemplar cases, *Nurs Outlook* 54(1):30–35, 2006.

World Health Organization (WHO): *Health 2020: A European policy framework and strategy for the 21st century*, Copenhagen, World Health Organization Regional Office for Europe, 2013.

World Health Organization (WHO): *Exclusive breastfeeding* (website). www.who.int/nutrition/topics/ exclusive_breastfeeding/en/. 2015.

Young JM, Soloman MJ: How to critically appraise an article, *Nat Clin Pract Gastroenterol Hepatol* 6(2):82–91, 2009.

Resources and additional reading

Please refer to the chapter website resources.

Critical Appraisal Skills Programme (CASP): *Making sense of the evidence* (website). www.casp-uk.net/#!casp-tools-checklists/c18f8. 2013.

Source of excellent tools for assessing articles and research reports.

Guyatt G, Tonelli M: *The role of experience in an evidence-based practice* (website). https:// themedicalroundtable.com/article/ role-experience-evidence-based-practice. 2012.

INVOLVE: *Resource centre* (website). www.invo.org.uk/resource-centre/. 2015.

LoBiondo-Wood G, Haber J: *Nursing research: methods and critical appraisal for evidence-based practice*, 8th edn, St. Louis (MO), Elsevier, 2014.

Melnyk BM, Fineout-Overholt E, Stillwell S, et al: *The seven steps of evidence-based practice* (website). www.nursingcenter.com/ nursingcenter_redesign/media/EBP/ AJNseries/SevenSteps.pdf. 2010.

Methley AM, Campbell S, Chew-Graham C, et al: *PICO, PICOS and SPIDER: a comparison study of specificity and sensitivity in three search tools for qualitative systematic reviews* (website). www.ncbi.nlm.nih .gov/pmc/articles/PMC4310146/. 2014.

Polit D, Beck CT: *Nursing research: generating and assessing evidence for nursing practice*, 8th edn, Philadelphia (PA), Wolters Kluwer, Lippincott Williams and Wilkins, 2008.

Royal College of Obstetricians and Gynaecologists: *Library Services* (website). www.rcog.org.uk/en/ guidelines-research-services/ library-services/. 2015.

Scottish Intercollegiate Network (SIGN): *Critical appraisal: notes and checklists* (website). www.sign.ac.uk/methodology/ checklists.html. 2014.

Spiby H, Munro J: *Evidence based midwifery: applications in context*, New York, Wiley-Blackwell, 2009.

Spring B: *Evidence-based behavioral practice: steps for evidence-based behavioral practice* (website). www.ebbp.org/steps.html. 2007.

University Library: *Evidence-based medicine: PICO* (website). http: //researchguides.uic.edu/c.php?g =252338&p=1683349. 2013.

YouTube videos:

Creating a good research question: www.youtube.com/ watch?v=89NonP_iZZo.

How to write a good research proposal: www.youtube.com/ watch?v=zJ8Vfx4721M.

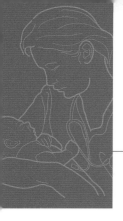

Chapter 7

Leadership and management in midwifery

Dr Bernie Divall

Learning Outcomes ?

After reading this chapter, you will be able to:

- understand the importance of developing strong and effective leadership within the midwifery profession
- consider how contemporary theories of leadership stress the value of developing leaders at every level of an organization
- understand how theories of leadership feed into the National Health Service (NHS) agenda of developing clinical leadership throughout the organization
- identify benefits and challenges of developing and enacting clinical leadership in the context of the NHS generally and midwifery specifically
- consider the place of management within a clinical leadership agenda, particularly in the context of contemporary NHS approaches
- reflect on your own beliefs, understanding and actions about leadership and management, as an individual and as a member of a distinctive professional group

INTRODUCTION

This chapter offers an introduction to theories of leadership and management, and then it contextualizes theoretical thinking within National Health Service (NHS) leadership, both past and present. The key debates arising from contemporary theory in leadership, particularly with reference to clinical leadership in the NHS, are addressed, and an explanation of why leadership and management are of particular importance to the midwifery profession is included. Although the main focus is on leadership and management within the UK NHS, the principles can be applied to any health service.

During the chapter, there are several opportunities for reflection on the subjects of leadership, management, career development and clinical credibility, through which individuals might consider their own potential career pathways in midwifery. Finally, some key resources for further reading and exploration of pertinent issues are included. There are also further resources and activities available on the textbook website.

WHY LEADERSHIP MATTERS TO MIDWIFERY

In 2007, the UK Department of Health (DH) published *Maternity Matters: Choice, Access and Continuity of Care in a Safe Service*, which highlighted the value of strong and effective leadership in the context of placing midwives at the centre of all women's care. A key statement within this document reads:

> *'It is imperative that organisations have good leadership, within an open and supportive culture which will provide the foundation for good maternity services that can fulfil the needs and expectations of women and their families. Organisations will need to consider the level of investment required to build and enhance leadership that will also support job satisfaction and staff morale'.*

(DH 2007: 24)

The DH also recognizes that a lack of representation by midwives at a senior level in some NHS trusts may have contributed to poor quality of care (DH 2009b: 32) and goes on to describe the development of leadership capabilities in the midwifery workforce as a high priority, suggesting that midwives should gain access to existing and new development opportunities in the NHS (DH

2009b: 33; Byrom and Kay 2011: 13). Similarly, *Midwifery 2020; Delivering Expectations* (DH 2010) and Scotland's *Refreshed Framework for Maternity Care* (Maternity Services Action Group (MSAG) 2011: 18) emphasize the importance of timely and appropriate development for midwives choosing leadership and management career options.

It is also important to consider that although it is crucial to have strong midwifery leadership at a strategic level, leadership ability must thread throughout the service. Not all midwives will seek to become heads of service, or team leaders, but all will need to have the following:

- Confidence to lead and manage clinical care, especially in an emergency;
- Understanding of their role in service delivery and the care of women;
- Courage to speak up about service improvement; and
- Awareness of their role in supporting colleagues at all levels.

Although midwifery was not specifically identified as problematic within the well-publicized Francis Report (2013), concerns have been raised about the profession in the aftermath of devastating events in other cases. Examples include the Healthcare Commission (HCC) investigations into a number of maternal deaths at Northwick Park Hospital (HCC 2006), which found that 'deficiencies in the management structures' and poor communication between midwives and obstetricians contributed to the poor quality of care women received. Similarly, another Healthcare Commission inquiry, this time based on several neonatal deaths and general public concern in relation to safety and quality of care at New Cross Hospital in Wolverhampton (HCC 2004), singled out leadership and management for criticism:

> *'The investigation… found problems around the leadership and management of the maternity services, team working and staffing. The leadership at all levels in the maternity services and in the women's and children's division, appears to have been weak and inconsistent for several years… The relationship between the Head of Midwifery, Clinical Director and Divisional Manager did not allow for effective leadership and management'.*
>
> (HCC 2004: 6)

Most recently, reports into the University Hospitals of Morecambe Bay maternity services (Kirkup 2015; Fielding et al 2010) and the most recent reports from the confidential enquiries into maternal deaths and morbidity (Knight et al on behalf of MBRRACE-UK, 2014, 2015) suggest devastating consequences associated with failures in leadership at all levels (Warwick 2015). The more recent MBRRACE report highlighted the need for clinical leadership in providing continuity and quality care for women

in identifying those with complex care issues and managing the care pathways for women who have developed complications requiring multiprofessional care (Knight et al 2015).

The management and leadership skills of all midwives are important at every level. All midwives need to be skilled in self-management and organizational skills, be able to manage junior staff and act as effective mentors and role models. This requires a high degree of emotional intelligence, confidence, ability to work within the team, clinical credibility and humility.

A further concern within the midwifery profession is the age profile of the senior workforce (DH 2010; HCC 2008). According to *Midwifery 2020* (DH 2010), 40% to 45% of those in the midwifery workforce are within 10 years of retirement; two-thirds are over age 40; and one-quarter are over age 50. The HCC has identified similar concerns (HCC 2008), adding that there is wide variation in the age of staff across maternity units and suggesting that some units are not paying sufficient attention to the looming problems associated with senior midwives retiring. These figures emphasize the importance of developing the next generation of midwifery leaders to further the vision of a midwifery voice at the strategic level, which Warwick (2015) believes is key to establishing the ideal of midwives at the centre of all care and working effectively alongside multidisciplinary colleagues.

Ralston (2005) agrees that, in any government vision of a patient-centred health service, midwives must be developed and supported to become future leaders. However, she argues that there has been little evidence of the encouragement of midwives with leadership potential, describing the NHS as an organization that rewards *conformity* rather than *innovation*. Although the development of leadership capabilities among midwives is seen as a high priority at the policy level (DH 2009b), Ralston (2005) believes the challenge lies in how midwives will be developed and equipped with the skills that will enable them to lead at clinical, organizational and national levels.

Reflective activity 7.1

In your local area, are you aware of any structured career development opportunities within maternity services? These might be at the individual level (e.g. within annual reviews with line managers or supervisors of midwives) or at the organizational level (e.g. Trust-based/hospital leadership development programmes, one-to-one coaching or informal learning opportunities).

Who do *you* think should take responsibility for developing the next generation of midwifery leaders?

Having established the importance of developing leadership and leaders in the midwifery profession, it is important to gain an overview of leadership theory in its contemporary context, within the NHS and beyond. At the end of the chapter, we then explore how this context affects existing and future midwifery leadership.

LEADERSHIP: TRADITIONAL AND CONTEMPORARY THINKING

A development of theory

The focus in past theories of leadership has typically been on individuals (Deckard 2010: 209), with these individual leaders conceptualized as active players in the process of leadership and followers portrayed as passive and reactive. In this conceptualization of leadership, there has been a clear definition of who the leaders and the followers are, and an associated power relationship has been seen to exist in the construction of formal hierarchies (Winkler 2010: 5).

Three key theories of leadership play into this conceptualization:

- The *trait theory* emerged from 'great man' thinking and attempted to define inborn characteristics, or traits, that resulted in effective leadership. However, problems arise when leaders exist who do not exhibit these traits, or when individuals who appear to have the necessary traits do not become effective leaders. A further criticism relates to the number of traits identified, with individuals struggling to demonstrate all of them.

- *Behavioural theories of leadership* (e.g. McGregor 1960; Blake and Mouton 1964) attempted to define behaviours associated with effective leadership. However, just as the trait approach failed to discover a universal set of characteristics, so the behavioural approach failed to identify a universal set of leadership behaviours.

- *Contingency or situational schools* of thought (e.g. Fiedler 1967; Hershey and Blanchard 1969) developed the idea of an interaction between a leader's traits and behaviours, plus the situation within which the leader was operating; thus, the effects of one variable on leadership would be contingent on others. This development in thinking allowed the possibility that leadership might be considered different in a range of situations, and the complexities of interactions between leaders and contextual influences could then be introduced. However, despite a consideration for the characteristics of followers and an evaluation of relevant situational concerns, the leader remains at the centre of the approach; leaders are appointed to an appropriate situation given their individual style

of leadership, or leaders are taught to exhibit different behaviours or a situation is altered to best match the existent leader.

Contemporary thinking in leadership theory

In recent years, there has been considerable rethinking within leadership theory, specifically a move away from the earlier focus on individual leaders, towards a more holistic approach (Avolio et al 2009). Leadership is now considered as less of a static set of skills and more a dynamic process of influence (Hartley and Benington 2011; Turnbull 2011). In this reconceptualization, the relational and contextual elements of leadership have been brought to the fore (Uhl-Bien 2006), with a greater emphasis on the interdependence between workers (Gronn 2002) and thus consideration of the potential for leadership at every level of an organization (Roebuck 2011) and recognition of a place for different types of leadership, such as formal and informal systems (Hartley and Benington 2011).

Fitzsimmons et al (2011) suggest several reasons for a move towards distributed patterns of leadership:

- Increased complexity and ambiguity in the workplace has resulted in a shift in the division of labour.

- Senior leaders might no longer alone have sufficient or relevant information to make effective changes.

- Knowledge workers have differing expectations and specialized expertise in the postindustrial era.

New conceptualizations of leadership include a critique of the individualistic focus of earlier thinking. In the era of the 'romance' of leadership, heroic and charismatic individuals were considered necessarily beneficial to organizations (Hartley and Benington 2011). However, this heroic model has more recently been described as an aberrant development (Gronn 2008), and even counter-productive (Grint and Holt 2011), given the unlikelihood of any individual having all the traits identified for effective leadership. A model of distributed leadership has been proposed as a response to these individualistic weaknesses, and as a means of tempering an inflated view of human agency (Gronn 2008), thus recognizing the significance of leaders' surrounding environments and organizational structures.

Distributed leadership

Distributed leadership has been defined as a situation where no single individual is required to perform all essential leadership tasks in an organization; rather, a set of people is required, between whom all necessary leadership tasks can be undertaken collectively. It may be that important decision making is shared by several group members, or that some functions of leadership might be allocated to individual members or that leadership functions are undertaken by different individuals at different times, according to organizational need (Yukl 1999).

Turnbull (2011) describes three central contentions associated with a distributed model of leadership:

1. That leadership involves multiple actors, with leadership roles being taken up formally and/or informally and shared by collaborative working, often across organizational boundaries;

2. That leadership can be distributed away from the top of an organization, with the potential for 'leaders at many levels', and new practices and innovations; and

3. That leadership is about more than attributes and leader–follower relationships; it also involves leadership practices and organizational structures.

In relation to the formation of collaborative relationships suggested by distributed leadership principles, Gronn (2002) suggests a continuum that ranges from spontaneous collaboration, through the gradual formation of partnerships over time, to institutionalized practices. Fletcher (2004) believes such an approach requires a paradigm shift in what it means to be a positional leader, including organizations moving from the need to control to understanding the value of learning, and individuals moving from a sense of self as leader to a sense of self-in-relation to others.

Although a distributed model of leadership has been widely embraced as a more appropriate and realistic approach than the individualistic, heroic model, it is not without its challenges. Organizations need to consider what degree or level of distributed leadership is required (Gronn 2008), and there have been suggestions that any transition to new models of practice within organizations can be challenging. There is a danger of paying insufficient attention to the emotional dynamics at play in shifts to alternative models of leadership, particularly within organizations that have tended towards hierarchical, managerial approaches (Fitzsimmons et al 2011).

The place of followers

Earlier leadership thinking has been accused of paying insufficient attention to the significance of *followership* (Grint and Holt 2011), but with the advent of distributed models of leadership, and following a 'tsunami of leaders gone wrong' (Bennis 2008: 4), interest in followers has grown. Where once followers might have been considered a homogenous mass, they have now been reconceptualized as 'the anvil of leadership' (Grint and Holt 2011). Studies have shown that followers' traits and characteristics influence relationships built between them and leaders

(Howell and Shamir 2005), and that followers' understanding of leaders affects the construction of leader identities (Meindl 1995; Meindl et al 1985). In some quarters, there have been suggestions that with the flattening of hierarchical structures in organizations, followership may be an outmoded concept altogether (Rost 1993). However, others counter that hierarchies are in fact alive and well, confirming the importance of considering followers in any leadership construction and enactment (Grint and Holt 2011).

Transactional and transformational leadership

Transactional, or *managerial*, leadership has its roots in the 'bottom line' (Bolden et al 2003: 15), with principles based on the need to get a job done and make a living. In this style of leadership, the focus tends to be on tactical issues, short-term goals and hard data, and working within systems that already exist (Covey 1992). There is recognition of positional power, with rewards exchanged between leader and followers when followers perform well and make good effort (Boseman 2008). However, although there are positive employee attitudes and behaviours associated with successful transactional leadership, there have been suggestions that followers in this scenario may deliver no greater performance than is expected and rewarded (Boseman 2008).

In an alternative view, Burns (1978) describes the concept of 'transforming' leadership, where there is a mutually stimulating relationship between leaders and followers. Through a process of engagement and motivation followers can become leaders, and leaders may become 'moral agents'. Bass (1990 and 1985) further develops this model, describing 'transformational' leadership, where a leader transforms followers through a number of key processes:

• Idealized behaviours – living one's ideals;

• Inspirational motivation – inspiring others;

• Intellectual stimulation – stimulating others;

• Individualized consideration – coaching and development opportunities; and

• Idealized attributes – respect, trust, faith. (Bass and Avolio 1994)

Through such processes, leaders act to increase awareness of what is right and important, raise motivational maturity and encourage followers to go beyond their self-interests for the good of the wider organization. Thus, followers are provided with a sense of purpose that goes beyond the simple exchange of rewards for effort provided, as seen in the transactional leadership model. In transformational leadership patterns, there is a sense of generalized proactivity: if leaders support the development, rather than just the performance, of followers, then they also optimize the development of the organization, because high-performing employees tend to build high-performing organizations (Bolden et al 2003: 16).

Transformational leadership has an intuitive appeal because it fits society's popular notion of what leadership means: the image of a leader 'out front, advocating change for others' (Northouse 2015: 191). However, there have been criticisms of this model because it may appear to advocate a return to an individualistic focus and trait-based theories of leadership (Deckard 2010: 209). Defending the model, Bass (1990) suggests that although there may be a tendency to emphasize charismatic characteristics of transformational leaders, these can be learned. Bass describes charisma in leadership in terms of energy, self-confidence, determination and verbal skills and suggests these can be taught, whereas Boseman (2008) believes charismatic qualities are just one element in the transformational leader's toolbox that need to be put to work alongside more follower-oriented behaviours.

Followers are highly significant within transformational models of leadership. Because the process of leadership incorporates the needs of both leader and follower, leadership emerges as an interaction between the two, rather than being the sole responsibility of the leader (Northouse 2015: 191). Further, when transformational leadership is successfully utilized in organizations, followers are more satisfied, more optimistic, less likely to leave the organization, more likely to trust the leader and more likely to put in greater effort with consequently higher performance levels (Boseman 2008).

Reflective activity 7.2

Think about these concepts of follower and leader. Where do you see yourself? What do you need from your managers/leaders to be able to trust and follow them?

Although transactional and transformational models of leadership have at times been described in opposing terms, transformational leadership should not be seen as a 'panacea' in organizations (Bass 1990). There are times when transactional leadership is considered entirely appropriate, for example, when organizations are functioning in a stable environment, and in these circumstances the model may foster good relationships between leaders and followers. Circumstances should dictate which model is used to best advantage in organizations, with recognition that both have their benefits and challenges (Deckard 2010: 212). As in contemporary leadership thinking more generally, emphasis is placed on adaptive, fluid processes of leadership rather than dichotomous models of thinking (Gronn 2008).

Reflective activity 7.3

Thinking about your workplace, do you consider there to be an emphasis on a transactional or a transformational model of leadership?

Do you believe these two approaches can work together?

LEADERSHIP AND MANAGEMENT IN THE NHS

It is useful to explore leadership in the NHS, as in any health service, to contextualize theoretical thinking. This can begin with a general consideration of the terms 'leadership' and 'management' as contested – but linked – concepts, and then a more focused description of NHS approaches to leadership, both past and present. This section describes the contemporary emphasis on clinical leadership, discussing the rationale, benefits and challenges of developing clinicians into formal leadership roles in the NHS.

Leadership and management: two sides of the same coin?

The leadership and management debate has been in progress for a good number of years. The main problem appears to be that leadership is an elusive concept (Bennis 1959), holding different meanings for different people. The result of this elusiveness has been a plethora of definitions and disagreements (Stogdill 1974: 259).

Many attempts have been made to distinguish between leadership and management. For example, Kotter (1990: 4–5) describes clear differences between the two:

- *Leadership* is establishing direction, aligning people, motivating and inspiring.

- *Management* is planning and budgeting, organizing and staffing, controlling and problem solving.

Similarly, much intellectual energy has gone into establishing definitions and conceptualizations of 'leaders' in contrast with 'managers' (e.g. Zaleznik 2004; Drucker 1955). However, there have been suggestions that a high degree of 'conceptual fuzziness' exists in deciphering meanings, and some studies have discovered a great deal of overlap between the two. Mintzberg (1989), for example, in a study of chief executives in the US, found that the leadership role was a subset of a broad range of management roles. Kotter (1990: 9), in spite of distinguishing between leadership and management, suggests there is an inherent danger in suggesting leadership is intrinsically 'good', whereas management is 'bad'. In the same way that transactional and transformational models of leadership are considered positive approaches under particular circumstances, the same may apply to leadership and management within organizations. The challenge lies in applying the appropriate model at any given time.

Reflective activity 7.4

Do *you* believe leadership and management are two separate things, or can they be seen as two sides of the same coin?

Where do you see an overlap between the two concepts? It might be helpful to think of people you have considered 'leaders' and those you might think of as 'managers' when exploring this question.

NHS leadership, past and present

In NHS leadership, there has been traditionally a focus on top management, rather than attending to the significance of leadership at all levels of the organization (NHS Confederation 2009). Such an approach, with a governance structure built on the principles of authority, control, tight performance management and accountability, makes the implementation of a purely transactional model of leadership almost inevitable (Millward and Bryan 2005). An emphasis on managerial leadership goes 'hand in hand with a set of seldom-questioned assumptions regarding the legitimacy and pervasiveness of hierarchy' (Edmonstone and Western 2002) and results in a view where middle and junior managers, and clinical professionals, are seen as dependent followers rather than as leaders in any sense. As a consequence of this approach, employees develop a tendency to operate as if the structure and culture of their organization are givens, and thus lose a sense of ownership in performing tasks (Millward and Bryan 2005). There have been suggestions that this hierarchical model, where leaders fail to offer the degree of discretion and participation required by staff, is a central part of the conflict in the agenda for a better health service: the need to ensure that staff remain accountable while simultaneously allowing their creativity and participation to flourish (Firth-Cozens and Mowbray 2001).

As seen in the wider organizational literature, it may be that both transactional and transformational styles of leadership are required within health services because of the amount of change regularly undertaken and the complexity of the organization (Edmonstone and Western 2002; Firth-Cozens and Mowbray 2001). Staff need an environment and structure in which they are able to both lead change and hold things stable (Alimo-Metcalfe and Alban-Metcalfe 2000), which suggests that a variety of styles and individuals may be suited to the many leadership requirements within the NHS. However, it should be noted that the 'largely remote managerial phenomenon' (Millward and Bryan 2005) seen in NHS leadership, in which decision making and influence happen at some distance from the frontline, has been roundly criticized in recent high-profile reports of systemic failures in patient care (e.g. Francis 2013). Meanwhile, a focus on leadership by clinicians in recent policy (DH 2015 and 2008) suggests recognition of the importance of incorporating elements of transformational principles in the NHS.

The rise of clinical leadership

Although transformational principles are evident in the encouragement of clinicians to become leaders in the NHS, other factors are also significant, including the challenges of managing financial constraints and increasing patient expectations (Storey and Holti 2013; Nicol 2012). A more cynical perspective might suggest that the dilution of distinctive professional values and cultural norms is a further motivation (Phillips and Byrne 2013; Storey and Holti 2013; Doolin 2002). However, hybrid clinician-managers are ideally placed to act as translators and mediators, bringing management norms into clinical practice (British Medical Association (BMA) 2012; Doolin 2002).

The benefits of clinical leadership – defined here as leadership for clinicians, by clinicians – have been described in terms of both patient and staff outcomes. For patients, there is an association with better care delivery (Phillips and Byrne 2013; Murphy et al 2009), and for staff, there is a greater degree of power and improved motivation (Fenton 2012; Murphy et al 2009), echoing the principles of transformational leadership as discussed earlier.

Reflective activity 7.5

Leaders, managers and midwives
Consider individuals at various levels of the midwifery profession, such as team leaders, ward managers, supervisors of midwives, heads of midwifery and consultant midwives.

Would you think of these individuals as leaders or as managers? Or simply as midwives?

Basing your thinking on what this chapter has addressed so far, what factors lead you to think of individuals in particular ways?

The *Next Stage Review* (DH 2008) clearly sets out a rationale for clinical leadership in the NHS. The report recognizes that change delivery is not simply related to incentives, policy and competition, but also requires high-quality leadership at every level, across local systems, and particularly by clinicians (NHS Confederation 2009; Oliver 2006). In relation to organizational performance, a number of benefits are associated with the implementation of clinical leadership. Looking at cultural differences between high- and low-performing healthcare organizations, Mannion et al (2005) found that leadership was of paramount importance, with strong and empowered clinical leaders forming an essential part of this picture when working as 'facilitators' rather than as 'enforcers'. In relation to effective change, Ham (2003) believes that well-developed systems of clinical leadership are key, particularly in the light of difficulties associated with general managers controlling medical work, and Oliver (2006) suggests that in recent years there has been formal recognition of the role that nurses and allied health professionals can play in effective change, and in the process become leaders within the organization. As Millward and Bryan (2005) point out, 80% of all healthcare is delivered by nurses and midwives, making the advent of clinical leadership in these professions an unsurprising development in the NHS vision.

Challenges in clinical leadership

Although clinical leadership has been widely welcomed in principle, a number of challenges have been described in relation to the complex nature of a hybrid clinical-managerial role (see Fig. 7.1). Clinicians may find a lack of role definition in formal leadership and management roles compared with their clinical work and an increase in pressure with little corresponding reward or recognition (Osborne 2011). A further challenge lies in attempting to maintain a clinical role while undertaking leadership and management tasks: time pressures and a lack of management skills or appropriate education (Storey and Holti 2013) can result in identity conflict, which in turn may lead to reduced job satisfaction and organizational commitment (Kippist and Fitzgerald 2009). On the other hand, moving away from clinical work altogether can result in a sense of loss (Divall 2015; Ham et al 2010).

In terms of challenges for clinical leaders at the group level of analysis, problems have been identified in both

interprofessional and intraprofessional relationships, and these relate to the complex history of interactions between professional groups and between clinicians and general managers (Dopson and Fitzgerald 2006). Studies of clinical leadership have found a tendency for clinical leaders to maintain a professional group identification in their leadership and management roles (Divall 2015; Ham et al 2010; Iedema et al 2004; Doolin 2002). These hybrid leaders see their professional identity, based on devotion to service, as superior to a management identity, based on politics and the 'bottom line' (Hotho 2008). At the same time, however, clinical leaders often face rejection by their own professional group because they are perceived to have moved to 'the dark side' (Divall 2015; Ham et al 2010). Hoff (1999) found a decrease in group cohesion associated with clinicians moving to managerial roles, and these individuals were faced with conflict, distrust, anger and resistance from members of their professional group.

Credibility is a key issue for clinical leaders, whose sense of loss in leaving clinical practice has been described in relation to both patient and colleague relationships. Meanwhile, a study by the British Medical Association (BMA) (BMA 2012) found that the main enabling factor in successful clinical leadership was peer support, provided by members of the professional group. Doolin (2002) found that validation of the hybrid clinical-managerial role occurred at individual and group levels: as individuals, clinical leaders' perception of the degree of control over their career choices was highly significant; but as members of a professional group, validation occurred through other members' acceptance of the leader's hybrid identity. Osborne (2011) found that clinicians held highly negative views of clinical leaders who did not have a clinical caseload.

Relationships with general managerial leaders are also considered part of the challenge for clinical leadership and can be described in terms of perceived differences between clinical and managerial foci. In terms of leadership, clinicians tend to have a microview focus on patients, client groups and services, whereas managerial leaders typically focus on the overall needs of the organization (Edmonstone 2005). Hybrid clinical leaders have to span these different sets of values, placing them at the intersection of the practice and business of health (Kippist and Fitzgerald 2009). Edmonstone (2005) relates this challenge to different leadership styles: whereas clinical leaders tend to subscribe to a 'reflective practice' or 'professional artistry' philosophy, where change is incremental, nonclinical leaders show more of a 'big bang' approach to change. If nonclinical leaders do not recognize clinical leaders' attachment to more shared and distributed models of leadership, Edmonstone believes there is a risk of widening the gulf between the two groups.

However, there have been suggestions that there may be benefits to sharing leadership between clinicians and

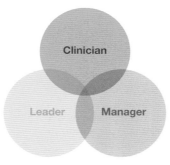

Figure 7.1 The hybrid clinical leader.

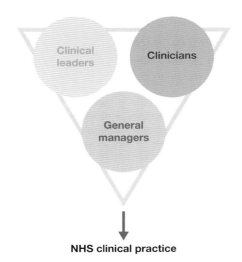

NHS clinical practice

Figure 7.2 Distributed leadership in the NHS.

nonclinicians in healthcare organizations (see Fig. 7.2). Ham et al (2010), for example, found that doctors were able to value working alongside nonclinical leaders, and Hoff (1999) found that clinical leaders with a strong professional group identification found little sense of division from general managers because they were perceived as a separate group doing a different job. Similarly, in the context of midwifery leadership, Divall (2015) found that although clinical leaders were keen to differentiate themselves from general managers, there was recognition of the value these nonclinical leaders brought to the NHS in terms of their own skills and expertise.

Reflective activity 7.6

Think about midwives who have moved to leadership and management roles and who no longer work clinically. Do you believe their understanding of life at 'the frontline' is compromised? What do you think can be done to support these midwives in their current roles, from the perspective of a clinician working alongside them?

Developing clinical leaders

The challenge for organizations lies in enabling and supporting the development and enactment of clinical leadership roles. A whole-organization approach is important if clinical leaders are to maintain a clinical presence, which, as described previously, is significant to both individual leaders and their professional groups. There have been suggestions that, currently, organizations place too much emphasis on the managerial aspects of clinical leadership roles (Fenton 2012).

Similarly, the development of clinical leadership careers has also received criticism. Various studies have identified deficiencies in this area; for example, development programmes have been poorly timed in terms of career trajectory (Phillips and Byrne 2013; BMA 2012; Osborne 2011), and opportunities for formal development have been delivered away from the clinical frontline and have involved teaching models of leadership rather than clinical realities (Phillips and Byrne 2013). Further, access to development has been highly variable (Ham et al 2010) and at times inadequate for the role of hybrid clinical-managerial leader (Iedema et al 2004; Hoff 1999). This inconsistent approach to development has been described as 'schizophrenic' on the part of the NHS (Storey and Holti 2013), with the organization saying it wants to develop clinical leadership careers, but then acting in direct opposition to this aim. Divall echoes this concern, finding that midwifery leaders returning from a leadership development programme felt they had little support within organizational structures in enacting new learning, or in continuing their professional development beyond the programme.

A talent management approach

In recent years, the NHS has introduced the concept of talent management into its leadership and career development agenda (NHS Employers 2009), an approach that is significant for its dual emphasis on individuals' career development and organizational succession planning (Yarnall 2009). A definition of talent management is provided by the Chartered Institute of Personnel and Development:

'The systematic attraction, identification, development, engagement/retention and deployment of those individuals with high potential who are of particular value to an organization'.

(Chartered Institute of Personnel and Development (CIPD) 2007: 3)

There has been significant debate in commentary on issues such as which members of staff should be managed as 'talent', with authors generally agreeing that a whole-organization approach is optimal (Cook and Macauley 2009; Stockley 2005), with senior and line managers and human resources departments ideally placed to take responsibility for developing individuals throughout the organization (CIPD 2007: 4). Central to the success of a talent management approach is the development of a 'talent culture' (Blass 2007: 10), which is dependent on all members of an organization understanding the importance of investing in a talent management strategy (Cook and Macauley 2009).

Within the NHS context, the *Next Stage Review* (DH 2008) was a key driver in embracing a talent management approach. The stresses on future requirements in the organization have been clearly stated, and they include demographic pressures such as an ageing senior workforce and an increasing recognition of the importance of a diverse workforce (NHS Employers 2009), embodied within the rise of clinical and distributed leadership ideals. Recent commitment to a talent management strategy in the NHS marks a departure from past approaches, which failed to systematically identify and nurture talent and leadership (DH 2009a: 4). This analysis is echoed in the experiences of clinical leaders throughout the NHS (Divall 2015; Phillips and Byrne 2013; BMA 2012; Ham et al 2010), where a generally unstructured approach to career development is reported, with little or no formal development before individuals take on clinical leadership roles.

Reflective activity 7.7

Are you able to think of yourself as 'talent'? Do you think a talent management approach to career development is a positive way of addressing both individual career aspirations and organizational needs?

When considering your own possible career path, do you think applying the principles of talent management might prove useful, and how might you discuss this with, for example, your line manager or supervisor of midwives?

IMPLICATIONS FOR MIDWIFERY LEADERSHIP

As described at the beginning of this chapter, midwifery leadership has received a great deal of attention over the past few years, echoing an increased focus on leadership more generally in the NHS. It is clear that current approaches to the development of clinical leadership careers are underpinned by ideas from transformational leadership. Leadership programmes available through the NHS Leadership Academy (www.leadershipacademy.nhs .uk) emphasize the importance of development for leadership at every level of the organization, and a strongly transformational approach is suggested in descriptions of these programmes.

However, as described previously, the experiences of clinical leaders in the NHS have not necessarily echoed these transformational and distributed leadership ideals, with development often having been offered relatively late in individuals' careers and with a number of challenges identified in the context of enacting hybrid clinical-managerial roles.

Within midwifery, little empirical research has been undertaken in the field of leadership. However, two recent studies (Divall 2015 and 2017, Byrom and Downe 2010)

illustrate the challenges facing leaders of the profession. In Byrom and Downe's (2010) study, which explored clinical midwives' perceptions of what makes a 'good' midwife and a 'good' leader, a number of attributes were identified in relation to leadership. Clinicians believed midwifery leaders need to be knowledgeable and credible at clinical and strategic levels, in addition to confident and competent in their dealings with women and with midwifery staff. Clinicians also identified a number of attitudinal aspects of the 'good' leader, including approachability, empathy, supportiveness and friendliness, motivation and empowerment of others and the ability to lead by example. As the study authors suggest, such characteristics are the hallmark of transformational leadership, rather than the transactional approach so often associated with leadership in the NHS. These attributes can also be seen as those of an excellent clinician also.

In Divall's study of midwifery leaders, observation of midwifery-specific leadership development programmes and a series of narrative interviews were undertaken, and a number of challenges were identified. First, although midwifery leaders might believe they are acting as transformational leaders, representative of their professional group identity, they were equally aware that their credibility with clinical colleagues was detrimentally affected if they no longer held a clinical role (Divall 2015). Figure 7.3 illustrates the challenges faced by midwives moving to clinical leadership roles, in the context of the

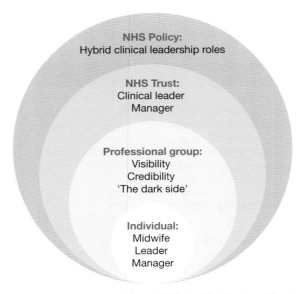

Figure 7.3 Challenges facing midwifery clinical leaders. (Divall, B., 2015. Negotiating competing discourses in narratives of midwifery leadership in the English NHS. Midwifery 31(1), 1060–1066.)

professional group and organizational discourses surrounding them. Second, although the leadership programmes they attended were very much based around transformational ideals, midwifery leaders struggled to enact this learning in their return to clinical life because they were working within an environment that was heavily influenced by the transactional mode of leadership so often criticized in NHS leadership literature (Divall).

These studies demonstrate a key concern in clinical leadership generally, and midwifery leadership specifically – that is, the importance of support for clinicians who move to formal leadership roles. Although strong midwifery leadership, associated with a clear philosophy of normality and one-to-one support, improves outcomes for women (Newburn 2003), a collaborative effort is required from all midwives if midwifery leadership is to be sustained and strengthened, and this effort includes supporting and coaching colleagues who aspire to leadership positions (Coggins 2005). Clearly, leadership matters to all midwives, just as it does to all clinicians in the NHS, and should be understood at the individual and professional group level:

'Introducing the principles supporting leadership skills throughout a student's training, as well as continued development when qualified, is essential if midwives are to take hold of their profession. Not all will choose to follow a career trajectory towards a clear leadership position such as Head of Midwifery, however, every midwife needs to grasp the principles if they are to understand the development of their profession. For some midwives, a greater understanding of leadership may help them to develop their future leadership potential'.

(Johnson 2012)

CONCLUSION

In this chapter, key concepts and challenges associated with leadership theory and practice are introduced. Contemporary theories of distributed patterns of leadership feed into the NHS agenda of developing clinical leaders to address key challenges facing the organization. The issues within midwifery leadership have been explored, and two recent studies that highlight challenges facing midwifery clinicians moving into leadership and management roles identified.

The reflective activities offered throughout this chapter are designed to support the ability to consider theoretical perspectives on leadership and management in the context of your own workplace and the contemporary NHS more generally.

Key Points

- Midwifery has been highlighted as an area of healthcare in need of strong, effective leadership.
- In the NHS, clinical leadership has been given high priority in the face of economic and patient care challenges.
- Leadership theory has evolved from leader-centric ideals to more distributed, collective, and transformational models. In principle, these are reflected in current NHS approaches to the development of clinical leaders.
- There are significant challenges facing individuals moving from clinical to leadership roles in the NHS, and these are seen within the midwifery profession.
- Midwives must work together as a cohesive professional group to support the establishment of operational and strategic leadership capacity.

Reflective activity 7.8

Thinking about your own role as a midwife or student midwife, and referring to the previous quote (Johnson 2012), do you think it is important to consider your potential as a leader in midwifery? Do you agree that every midwife is a leader at whatever level of the organizational hierarchy where she/he is working?

References

Alimo-Metcalfe B, Alban-Metcalfe R: Heaven can wait, *Health Serv J* 26–28, 2000.

Avolio B, Walumbwa F, Weber TJ: Leadership: current theories, research, and future directions, *Annu Rev Psychol* 60:421–449, 2009.

Bass BM: *Leadership and performance beyond expectations*, New York, Free Press, 1985.

Bass BM: From transactional to transformational leadership: learning to share the vision, *Organisational Dynamics* 18(3):19–31, 1990.

Bass BM, Avolio BJ: *Improving organisational performance through transformational leadership*, Thousand Oaks (CA), Sage, 1994.

Bennis W: Leadership theory and administrative behaviour, *Adm Sci Q* 4:259–301, 1959.

Bennis W: The art of followership: great followers create great leaders, *Leadership Excellence* 25(4):4, 2008.

Blake RR, Mouton JS: *The managerial grid*, Houston (TX), Gulf Publishing, 1964.

Blass E: *Talent management: maximising talent for business performance* (executive summary). Chartered Management Institute (website). www.ashridge.org.uk. 2007.

Bolden R, Gosling J, Marturano A, et al: *A review of leadership theory and competency frameworks* (website). www.leadership-studies.com. 2003.

Boseman G: Effective leadership in a changing world, *J Financ Serv Prof* 36–38, 2008.

British Medical Association (BMA): *Doctors' perspectives on clinical leadership* (website). www.bma.org.uk. 2012.

Burns JM: *Leadership*, New York, Harper & Row, 1978.

Byrom S, Downe S: 'She sort of shines': midwives' accounts of 'good' midwifery and 'good' leadership, *Midwifery* 26:126–137, 2010.

Byrom S, Kay L: Midwifery leadership: theory, practice and potential. In Downe S, Byrom S, Simpson L, editors: *Essential midwifery practice: leadership, expertise and collaborative working*, Oxford, Wiley-Blackwell, pp 7–22, 2011.

Chartered Institute of Personnel and Development (CIPD): *Research insight: talent management* (website). www.cipd.co.uk/NR/rdonlyres/B513502C-8F42-419C-818C-D3C12D87E0D3/0/talentmanage.pdf. 2007.

Coggins J: Strengthening midwifery leadership, *RCM Midwives* 8(7):310–313, 2005.

Cook S, Macaulay S: Talent management: key questions for learning and development, *Cranfield School of Management Training Journal* 37–41, (website): www.trainingjournal.com. 2009.

Covey S: *Principle centred leadership*, New York, Simon & Schuster, 1992.

Deckard GJ: Contemporary leadership theories. In Borkowski N, editor: *Organisational behaviour in health care*, Sudbury (MA), Jones and Bartlett, pp 209–230, 2010.

Department of Health (DH): *Maternity matters: choice, access and continuity of care in a safe service* (website). www.dh.gov.uk/prod_consum_dh/groups/dh_digitalassets/@dh/@endocuments/digitalasset/dh_074199.pdf. 2007.

Department of Health (DH): *High-quality care for all. NHS next stage review final report* (website). www.dh.gov.uk/prod_consum_dh/groups/dh_digitalassets/@dh/@en/documents/digitalass. 2008.

Department of Health (DH): *Inspiring leaders: leadership for quality* (website). www.dh.gov.uk/prod_consum_dh/groups/dh_digital assets/documents/digitalasset/dh_093407.pdfet/dh_085828.pdf. 2009a.

Department of Health (DH): *Delivering high-quality midwifery care: the priorities, opportunities and challenges for midwives* (website). www.dh.gov.uk/prod_consum_dh/groups/dh_digitalassets/documents/digital asset/dh_106064.pdf. 2009b.

Department of Health (DH): *Midwifery 2020: delivering expectations* (website). www.gov.uk/government/publications/midwifery-2020-delivering-expectations. 2010.

Department of Health (DH): *Better leadership for tomorrow: NHS leadership review* (website). www.gov.uk/government/publications/better-leadership-for-tomorrow-nhs-leadership-review. 2015.

Divall B: Negotiating competing discourses in narratives of midwifery leadership in the English NHS, *Midwifery* 31(1):1060–1066, 2015.

Divall B: *Bringing it back to work: the experiences of midwifery leaders undertaking a profession-specific leadership development programme in the English NHS*. 2017. In press.

Doolin B: Enterprise discourse, professional identity and the organisational control of hospital clinicians, *Organ Stud* 23(3):369–390, 2002.

Dopson S, Fitzgerald L: The role of the middle manager in the implementation of evidence-based health care, *J Nurs Manag* 14:43–51, 2006.

Drucker P: *The practice of management*, New York, Harper Collins, 1955.

Edmonstone J: What is clinical leadership development? In Edmonstone J, editor: *clinical leadership: a book of readings*, Chichester, Kingsham Press, pp 16–19, 2005.

Edmonstone J, Western J: Leadership development in health care: what do we know? *J Manag Med* 16(1):34–47, 2002.

Fenton K: *What is clinical leadership?* Nursing Times (website). www.nursingtimes.net/nursing-practice/leadership/what-is-clinical-leadership/5045399.article. 2012.

Fiedler FE: *A theory of leadership effectiveness*, New York, McGraw-Hill, 1967.

Fielding P, Richens Y, Calder A: *Review of maternity services in University Hospitals of Morecambe Bay NHS Trust* (website). www.morecambebayinquiry.co.uk/images/pdfs/fieldingreport.pdf. 2010.

Firth-Cozens J, Mowbray D: Leadership and the quality of care, *Qual Health Care* (Suppl II):S3–S7, 2001.

Fitzsimmons D, Turnbull James K, Denyer D: Alternative approaches for studying shared and distributed leadership, *Int J Manag Rev* 13:313–328, 2011.

Fletcher JK: The paradox of postheroic leadership: an essay on gender, power, and transformational change, *Leadership Quart* 15(5):647–661, 2004.

Francis R: *Report of the Mid-Staffordshire NHS Foundation Trust Public Inquiry* (website). www.midstaffspublic inquiry.com/report. 2013.

Grint K, Holt C: *Followership in the NHS. The King's Fund: commission on leadership and management in the NHS* (website). www.kingsfund.org.uk. 2011.

Gronn P: Distributed leadership as a unit of analysis, *Leadership Quart* 13:423–451, 2002.

Gronn P: The future of distributed leadership, *J Educ Admin* 46(2):141–158, 2008.

Ham C: Improving the performance of health services: the role of clinical leadership, *Lancet* 361:1978–1980, 2003.

Ham C, Clark J, Spurgeon P, et al: *Medical chief executives in the NHS: facilitators and barriers to their career progress*, Coventry, NHS Institute for Innovation and Improvement, 2010.

Hartley J, Benington J: *Recent trends in leadership: thinking and action in the public and voluntary service sectors*, London, The King's Fund, 2011.

Healthcare Commission (HCC): *Investigation of the maternity service provided by the Royal Wolverhampton Hospitals NHS Trust at New Cross Hospital*, London, Commission for Healthcare Audit and Inspection, 2004.

Healthcare Commission (HCC): *Investigation into 10 maternal deaths at, or following delivery at, Northwick Park Hospital, the North West London Hospitals NHS Trust, between April 2002 and April 2005*, London, Commission for Healthcare Audit and Inspection, 2006.

Healthcare Commission (HCC): *Towards better births: a review of maternity services in England* (website). http://webarchive.national archives.gov.uk/20120202152249/ www.nationalschool.gov.uk/policy hub/news_item/maternity_births _hc08.asp. 2008.

Hershey P, Blanchard KH: Life-cycle theory of leadership, *Train Dev J* 23:26–34, 1969.

Hoff TJ: The social organisation of physician-managers in a changing HMO, *Work Occup* 26(3):324–351, 1999.

Hotho S: Professional identity – product of structure, project of choice: linking changing

professional identity and changing professions, *J Organ Change Manag* 21(6):721–742, 2008.

Howell JM, Shamir B: The role of followers in charismatic leadership: relationships and their consequences, *Acad Manage Rev* 30:96–112, 2005.

Iedema R, Degeling P, Braithwaite J, et al: It's an interesting conversation I'm hearing': the doctor as manager, *Organ Stud* 25(15):15–33, 2004.

Johnson G: Leadership – what's that got to do with me? *Midwives* 15(3):52–53, 2012.

Kippist L, Fitzgerald A: Organisational professional conflict and hybrid clinician managers: the effects of dual roles in Australian health care organisations, *J Health Organ Manag* 23(6):642–655, 2009.

Kirkup B: *The report of the Morecambe Bay Investigation* (website). www.gov.uk/government/ publications/morecambe-bay -investigation-report. 2015.

Knight M, Kenyon S, Brocklehurst P, et al, on behalf of MBRRACEUK, editors: *Saving lives, improving mothers' care – lessons learned to inform future maternity care from the UK and Ireland Confidential Enquiries into Maternal Deaths and Morbidity 2009–12*, Oxford, University of Oxford National Perinatal Epidemiology Unit, 2014.

Knight MTD, Kenyon S, Shakespeare J, et al, on behalf of MBRRACE-UK, editors: *Saving lives, improving mothers' care – surveillance of maternal deaths in the UK 2011–13 and lessons learned to inform maternity care from the UK and Ireland Confidential Enquiries into Maternal Deaths and Morbidity 2009–13*, Oxford, University of Oxford National Perinatal Epidemiology Unit, 2015.

Kotter JP: *A force for change: how leadership differs from management*, New York, The Free Press, 1990.

Mannion R, Davies H, Marshall M: *Cultures for performance in health care: evidence on the relationship between organisational culture and performance in the NHS*, Maidenhead, Open University Press, 2005.

Maternity Services Action Group (MSAG): *A refreshed framework for maternity care in Scotland* (website).

www.gov.scot/Resource/ Doc/341632/0113609. 2011.

McGregor D: *The human side of enterprise*, New York, McGraw-Hill, 1960.

Meindl JR: The romance of leadership as a follower-centric theory, *Leadership Quart* 6(3):329–341, 1995.

Meindl JR, Ehrlich SB, Dukerich JM: The romance of leadership, *Adm Sci Q* 30:78–102, 1985.

Millward LJ, Bryan K: Clinical leadership in healthcare: a position statement, *Leadersh Health Serv* 18(2):13–25, 2005.

Mintzberg H: *Mintzberg on management: inside our strange world of organisations*, New York, The Free Press, 1989.

Murphy J, Quillinan B, Carolan M: Role of clinical nurse leadership in improving patient care, *Nurs Manage* 16(8):26–28, 2009.

Newburn M: Culture, control and the birth environment, *Pract Midwife* 6(8):20–25, 2003.

NHS Confederation: *Future of leadership paper 1: reforming leadership development…again* (website). www.nhsconfed.org/ Publications/Documents/ Debate%20paper%20%20 Future%20of%20leadership.pdf. 2009.

NHS Employers: *Talent for tough times: how to identify, attract and retain the talent you need*. Briefing 65 (website). www.nhsemployers.org/ Aboutus/Publications/Documents/ talent_for_tough_times-Briefing_65 .pdf. 2009.

Nicol ED: Improving clinical leadership and management in the NHS, *Journal of Healthcare Leadership* 2(4):59–69, 2012.

Northouse PG: *Leadership theory and practice*, 7th edn, Thousand Oaks, Sage, 2015.

Oliver S: Leadership in health care, *Musculoskeletal Care* 4(1):38–47, 2006.

Osborne JA: *How do they manage? A study of the realities of middle and front line management work in healthcare. Challenges facing healthcare managers: what past research reveals*. Cranfield Healthcare Management Group Research Briefing 6 (website). www.som .cranfield.ac.uk/som/dinamic -content/media. 2011.

Phillips N, Byrne G: Enhancing frontline clinical leadership in an acute hospital setting, *J Clin Nurs* 22:2625–2635, 2013.

Ralston R: Transformational leadership: leading the way for midwives in the 21st century, *RCM Midwives* 8(1):34–37, 2005.

Roebuck C: *Developing effective leadership in the NHS to maximise the quality of patient care: the need for urgent action. The King's Fund Commission on Leadership and Management in the NHS* (website). www.kingsfund.org.uk. 2011.

Rost JC: *Leadership for the twenty-first century*, Westport (CT), Praeger Publishers, 1993.

Stockley D: *Talent management concept – definition and explanation* (website). http://derekstockley.com .au/newsletters-o5/020-talent -management.html. 2005.

Stogdill RM: *Handbook of leadership: a survey of the literature*, New York, The Free Press, 1974.

Storey J, Holti R: *Possibilities and pitfalls for clinical leadership in improving service quality, innovation and productivity*. Final Report. NIHR Service Delivery and Organisation programme (website). www.netscc.ac.uk/hsdr/files/project/ SDO_FR_09-1001-22-V05.pdf. 2013.

Turnbull James K: *Leadership in context: lessons from new leadership theory and current leadership development practice*. The King's Fund (website). www.kingsfund.org. 2011.

Uhl-Bien M: Relational leadership theory: exploring the social processes of leadership and organising, *The Leadership Quarterly* 14(6):769–806, 2006.

Warwick C: *Leadership in maternity services*. The Health Foundation (website). patientsafety.health .org.uk/resources/leadership -maternity-services. 2015.

Winkler I: *Contemporary leadership theories: enhancing the understanding of the complexity, subjectivity and dynamic of leadership*, Berlin, Springer-Verlag, 2010.

Yarnall J: *Maximising the effectiveness of talent pools* (website). www.cipd.co.uk/NR/ rdonlyres/4EE379F3-4342-45C6 -A0A1-AB6D9C351940/0/centres09 _research_d.pdf. 2009.

Yukl G: An evaluation of conceptual weaknesses in transformational and charismatic leadership theories, *Leadership Quart* 10(2):285–306, 1999.

Yukl G: *Leadership in organisations*, 8th edn, London, Prentice Hall International, 2012.

Zaleznik A: Managers and leaders: are they different? *Harv Bus Rev* 82(1):74–81, 2004.

Resources and additional reading

For further reading around midwifery leadership, see (see also the chapter website):

Downe S, Byrom S, Simpson L: *Essential midwifery practice: leadership, expertise and collaborative working*, Oxford, Wiley-Blackwell, 2011.

For a range of resources around NHS leadership and its development, see:

The King's Fund: www.kingsfund .org.uk.

The NHS Leadership Academy: www.leadershipacademy.nhs.uk.

The Royal College of Midwives: www.rcm.org.uk.

The Royal College of Midwives (RCM) electronic learning (RCM i-learn) menu, which includes several modules on management and leadership: *Leadership* www.ilearn.rcm.org.uk/mod/book/ view.php?id=369&chapterid=863.

This programme includes a range of modules with excellent resources and activities, including a professional portfolio development opportunity.

The Royal College of Midwives (RCM) Midwifery Leadership Competency Model, developed with the NHS Modernisation Agency Leadership Centre: www.rcm.org.uk/sites/ default/files/MidwLead_ competencies.pdf.

Chapter 8

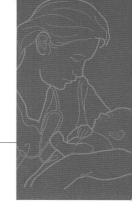

An introduction to ethics and midwifery practice

Gail Johnson

Learning Outcomes ?

After reading this chapter, you will be able to:

- understand the difference between morality and ethics
- appreciate the application of ethical theory to maternity practice
- recognize the importance of ethics in midwifery practice
- discuss ethical conflicts and dilemmas
- recognize the need to uphold the principle of women's autonomy in practice
- reflect on and appreciate your own ethical perspectives

INTRODUCTION

Ethics and ethical theory affect midwifery practice and maternity care on a daily basis, from allocation of resources to frontline delivery of care to women and babies.

Ethics is now recognized as a major part of midwifery education and practice; it permeates all professional relationships. Women are no longer passive recipients of care; they expect to be fully informed of all aspects of their care so that they, rather than the professionals, make informed decisions, thereby retaining their autonomy and control. Nonetheless, maternity, midwifery and service delivery are influenced and affected by professional and personal moral and ethical codes, which can bring challenges and dilemmas into practice. Knowledge of ethics and an understanding of how ethics influence individuals will enable midwives to be clearer on issues related to their practice and, in particular, on their role in empowering women.

WHAT IS ETHICS?

Often the words *ethics* and *morals* are used interchangeably, yet there are subtle differences between them, and how they influence individuals can manifest in different ways.

Ethical principles are sets of rules that guide conduct; they are externally driven within a social context, whereas *morals* can be viewed more as a personal, internally driven 'compass' in guiding the individual into doing what is right and avoiding what is wrong. People may follow an ethical principle because society says that they should but also from a personal belief that is internally driven. It is important to recognize that ethics and morals are also separate from the law, but a legal aspect may be in agreement with ethics and morals. For example, consider the law that sets out driving speed restrictions; most people will follow the law because of an understanding that the rationale behind the law is to reduce harm, not just to avoid being prosecuted. An understanding that the law is there to protect life comes within an ethical principle and is also likely to be supported by a personal moral belief that in failing to follow the law and ethics, harm could be done.

Thus, ethics is basically moral philosophy, or at least the vehicle by which moral philosophy is translated into practical, everyday situations. Within this chapter, ethics is explored within the concepts of how it relates to the 'rights and wrongs' or the 'ought and ought nots' of any situation and then considered in regard to midwifery practice and maternity services.

In everyday life, morality underpins our actions, particularly those that involve other people. It is translated into our thoughts and actions by principles and concepts, many of which were learnt in early childhood, such as truth telling. Individuals' personal ethics will also be shaped by their environment, schooling and media, for example. Within a community or culture, many of these beliefs will be the same, but it is important to appreciate that other perspectives may be different. Although people may interpret the moral codes differently, individuals will tend to be judged according to the code that is generally accepted by society, or a personal philosophy or what is accepted in civil law. Midwives and other health professionals need an understanding of ethical principles and their own personal perspective to enable them to give nonjudgement-based care.

There are numerous principles, concepts and doctrines, some of which are listed here. However, because ethics is a complex area, it is not possible to cover each principle in depth, and further reading is suggested at the end of the chapter.

- Beneficence
- Nonmaleficence
- Confidentiality
- Accountability
- Justice
- Autonomy
- Paternalism
- Consent
- Value of life
- Quality of life
- Sanctity of life
- Status of the fetus
- Acts and omissions
- Killing or letting die
- Ordinary or extraordinary means
- Double effect
- Truth telling

Moral theories

There are a number of theoretical models that help to describe moral theories – within this chapter, *utilitarian theory* and *deontology* will be explored and considered in relation to some of the issues in the previous list. It is helpful to keep in mind how the theories relate to 'right and wrongs', 'good and bad' and 'ought and ought not'.

Utilitarian theory – consequentialism

Consequentialism looks at the outcomes of actions and determines the right and wrong according to the outcome. That is, an act may be seen to be morally right if the outcome is deemed to be right. The origins of utility stem from Jeremy Bentham and John Stuart Mill in the early 18th and 19th centuries. Often the utilitarian

principle is described as doing the greatest good for the greatest number, an approach that promotes positive values for a greater number rather than a few. Beauchamp and Childress (2013) say that Bentham and Stuart Mill are often described as hedonistic utilitarians because they consider utility to be explored in relation to pleasure or happiness. Although the principle when applied to healthcare is not necessarily related to pleasure or happiness, it helps to consider that pleasure and happiness are positive values against which the principle can be measured, and the positive values can be viewed as benefits.

There are two forms of the theory: *act-utilitarianism* and *rule-utilitarianism*. The first is the purer form, which expects every potential action to be assessed according to its predicted outcomes in terms of benefit. The second form does not look directly at the actual benefit of each act; rather, it considers moral rules that are intended to ensure the greatest benefit, and each act is assessed as to its conformity to the rules.

Using in vitro fertilization (IVF) as an example, a technique initially researched in the concentration camps of the Second World War, it can be shown how these two schools of thought differ. Act-utilitarians would view the actions taken in light of the anticipated outcomes: many people today benefit from IVF; therefore, they may believe that this beneficial consequence justifies the research methods used. Rule-utilitarians, however, would want the benefit but would consider whether society would accept the means by which it was achieved. It is likely that they would want to find a more acceptable method of achieving the outcome.

Applying the utilitarian principle

Within the National Health Service (NHS) there are finite resources, and often a consequence-based approach can be applied to healthcare. This might mean that money is invested in a 'standardized' approach to care in an acute setting. For the majority of women this would be considered acceptable. However, if some women wanted care at home, this might not be possible. Nonetheless, the principle of utility means that the majority would have a positive experience, a 'greater happiness' than a smaller group who do not have their choices met. The decisions on how best to utilize limited resources frequently raises dilemmas in healthcare, and midwives may find that they are unable to support women in their pregnancy and birth choices.

Kantian theory – Deontology

Deontological, or nonconsequentialist, theory challenges the principle of utility. *Deontology*, from the Greek *deon*, means 'duty'. Deontologists believe that what is good in the world is brought about by people doing their duty. This principle is also referred to as Kantian philosophy from the work of Immanuel Kant, a German philosopher who lived in the late 1700s. Kant says that morality is grounded in reason and that people have "powers that motivate them morally" (Beauchamp and Childress 2013: 362). Kant believed that people demonstrated their moral worth by acting from a recognition of what is morally right. For example, a health hazard in the workplace is pointed out to staff by the employer – the moral obligation is to report the hazard to keep staff safe. If the employer highlights this to avoid being taken to court, then Kant would say there is no moral credit in the employer's action. At times it can seem that these theories are competing with one another as well as with utilitarianism. Kant developed *rational monism,* which he believed was how people already thought – that one's actions should be rational and stem from 'goodwill'; he believed in duty for its own sake – referred to as the *categorical imperative.* A deontological approach is based on acting in a morally good way, and the actions or inactions are decided on what is seen to be right at that time; that is, the individual does not need to look at the consequences of the action because it is the action per se which is either right or wrong. The categorical imperative is that the action should be based on reason and the moral acceptability of the act rather than carried out as a result of fear or coercion. Within Kantian theory, 'one must act to treat every person as an end and never a means to an end' (Beauchamp and Childress 2013: 363). This means that each person must be treated as an individual and not for personal gain. However, if a person chooses to allow himself or herself to be used for the benefit of another, that is acceptable if the choice is made by free will; a challenge with this, of course, involves differing understandings of the meaning of free will and how decisions are freely made.

Applying Kantian theory

Consider a duty-based principle when a sick baby is admitted to a neonatal intensive care unit. The baby is clearly distressed and appears to be in pain, and the medical team wants to administer analgesia. However, there is concern that in giving analgesia, the baby is likely to be further compromised and may die of respiratory failure. From a duty principle, the main aim would be to relieve suffering through giving analgesia, and in this instance the potential outcome of the baby's condition deteriorating would not be considered as part of the act.

Moral conflict

The previous example highlights a moral conflict that could readily arise in practice. There can be conflict between parents, between parents and professionals, and between professionals. A moral conflict could be considered to be a show of strength within a moral principle – for instance, the autonomy of the woman versus service provision that limits choice or, fortunately, less commonly, in life-and-death situations.

Reflective activity 8.1

Reflect on the service provision in your area of practice. Do you feel that resources are spent appropriately? Where is the greatest investment? Does it reflect the needs of the local population?

Given the finite resources available in healthcare, how can women be offered a choice throughout pregnancy and birth?

Talk to the head of service in your organization about how decisions around service provision are made.

Moral dilemma

When examination of an apparent conflict between principles indicates two or more options, none of which is morally ideal, then this is a dilemma, such as that presented in Case Study 8.1.

CASE STUDY 8.1

Amanda presents in her third pregnancy with a small antepartum haemorrhage; she appears to be in established labour and does not appear to be compromised by the blood loss. All of her pregnancy observations have been within normal limits, and she has been well previously. Amanda tells you that she is a Jehovah's Witness and that she will not accept a blood transfusion.

On further examination it becomes apparent that the fetus is becoming distressed, and it seems that the bleeding is from a ruptured vessel from a vasa previa. The baby is delivered by emergency caesarean section and is transferred to neonatal intensive care with an Hb of 8 g/dL. The neonatologist recommends a blood transfusion for the baby.

How are dilemmas solved?

The situation in Case Study 8.1 is clearly contrived; however, it reflects a dilemma that could, and indeed does, arise in practice. The woman is unlikely to consent to her baby having a blood transfusion even though it would improve the baby's condition.

A midwife needs to set aside personal feelings and beliefs – to do this it is important to have previously considered their own personal perspective so that the midwife can be non-judgemental to the family.

The Code of the Nursing and Midwifery Council (NMC 2015) clearly states the professional's duty to the woman and her baby. Section 1 states 'Treat people as individuals and uphold their dignity'. Box 8.1 notes other principles that professionals must uphold.

> **Box 8.1** Aspects of the NMC Code (2015)
>
> 1.3 Avoid making assumptions and recognize diversity and individual choice
>
> 1.5 Respect and uphold people's human rights
>
> 2.3 Encourage and empower people to share decisions about their treatment and care
>
> 2.4 Respect the level to which people receiving care want to be involved in decisions about their own health, well-being and care
>
> 2.5 Respect, support and document a person's right to accept or refuse care and treatment

Midwives are encouraged to be guided by their professional code even though at times the decisions and dilemmas they face may be hard to understand. For example, in Case Study 8.1, the professionals are seeking consent for the baby; there may be occasions where the parents' right to make decisions is overruled.

Traditionally in British law the child's welfare is paramount. Parents have a right and a duty to give *proxy consent* for a child. However, the parents' rights to consent are not absolute, and actions must be in the child's best interest; the court ultimately has overriding control (Woolley 2005).

If a duty-based theory is considered, the professional approach would be to act to improve the health of the baby by giving a blood transfusion. Within the deontological perspective, the person is the end and not a means to an end – therefore, the baby needs to be treated as an individual and not an extension of the mother.

Conversely, the utilitarian approach advises that the decision is based on the consequences of the action. If the baby in the previous scenario is given a blood transfusion, for example, the parents may reject the child as a result of the treatment. In the future, the parents may avoid contact with health services, potentially putting their lives and their children's lives at risk if they lack confidence in the service.

> **Reflective activity 8.2**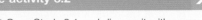
>
> Think about Case Study 8.1 and discuss it with some colleagues or your family.
>
> How does it make you feel? Do you think that you would be able to ignore your own moral compass to offer the family a nonjudgemental approach to their care?

A further challenge to ethical theory and deontology is *intuitionistic pluralism,* where it is believed that there are a number of moral rules that are of equal importance, leading to the possibility of rule conflict. David Ross (1877–1975) considered seven *prima facie* duties as constituting a framework (European Business Ethics Network Ireland (EBEN) 2011) that he felt was reasonable for people to abide by:

1. Duty of fidelity – involves keeping promises, being loyal and not deceiving
2. Duty of beneficence – the obligation to help others
3. Duty of nonmaleficence – not harming others; more stringent than the previous duty
4. Duty of justice – to ensure fair play
5. Duty of reparation – an obligation to make amends
6. Duty of gratitude – to repay in some way those who have helped us (owed to special people such as parents), also including loyalty
7. Duty of self-improvement

However, there is criticism of this framework because it fails to reconcile the conflict between duties and because it is considered arbitrary (EBEN 2011).

Because these duties are equal in importance, it is still possible for conflict to arise between them. However, there is a system that can assist in such a conflict – *casuistry;* this system allows for the duties to be prioritized according to the circumstances.

The NHS is generally essentially utilitarian, whereas midwifery, medicine and other similar disciplines tend towards a deontological approach. In fact, the duty with which midwives are most familiar – the duty of care – would appear to encompass at least the first four of the duties in Ross's list. This deontological approach is certainly apparent in the text of the NMC Code (NMC 2015).

To assist understanding of the different focus of utilitarianism and deontology when faced with a dilemma, reflect on the following situation.

> **Reflective activity 8.3**
>
> Consider a situation where, antenatally, a woman declined screening for Down syndrome (DS). However, at a busy clinic the phlebotomist took blood samples used for DS testing.
>
> When the results are returned, they indicate that the woman has a high risk for having a child with DS.
>
> What would your actions be in this scenario? Consider the ethical theories and identify which you relate to in your response.

The duty of care

As health professionals, midwives have a duty of care to those persons who could be affected by their actions or omissions. In midwifery, it is important to note that 'persons' relates directly to the woman and neonate. (Legally, the fetus is not yet a 'person'; see more on 'personhood' and 'potential life' in Harris (2001) in the further reading section). This duty of care would include at least the first four deontological duties listed earlier; failure in the duty of care would result in a civil law case for negligence (see also Ch. 9).

The duty of fidelity

The *duty of fidelity* requires professionals to be open and honest with women and their families; this suggests, therefore, that promises should not be made if they cannot be kept and that truth telling is paramount. Considering the previous example in which blood samples were taken for DS testing, if the practitioners involved were to withhold the truth from the woman, then they would be failing in their duty of fidelity, however good their motives might be.

The duty of beneficence

The *duty of beneficence* creates the obligation to help women. This is a positive duty that covers numerous activities, ranging from the various ways of helping to make them comfortable, to the educational aspects of caring for their babies.

The duty of nonmaleficence

The *duty of nonmaleficence* is a negative duty – to do no harm. On the surface, this would suggest that conducting unpleasant or painful procedures may breach this duty; this would be the case if the intention were to cause harm. If the intention is to eventually benefit the woman and, knowing that she might experience pain or discomfort, she is in agreement, then there is no breach in duty. Administration of analgesic injections, the siting of an epidural analgesic or urinary catheterization would fall under this category. This duty, although negative in its statement, can have a positive aspect: that of safety and protection from harm. This includes, among other things, consideration of the environment, observance of drug policies and adequate education and training of practitioners.

The duty of justice

The *duty of justice* requires that women are treated equally, without discrimination. For many people, the word *discrimination* is immediately associated with concepts such as race, skin colour or ethnic origin. Although it is essential that such concepts be considered, it is also important to be aware of the other forms of discrimination that can occur, such as between articulate and less articulate women. It is often easier to spend more time with the articulate women, giving as much information and as

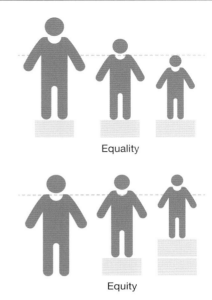

Equality

Equity

Figure 8.1 Comparing equality and equity.

much choice as possible, than it is with those who require greater explanations or who ask fewer questions. It could be argued that to consider and practise equality, professionals should aim to get all women to the same endpoint; this would then necessitate that more time be spent with the less articulate women. This is often referred to as a *level playing field* and refers to the need to treat people differently to get the same results.

PRINCIPLES

Knowledge of the underlying moral principles is important, if only to ensure that practitioners are 'talking the same language'. It is not possible, in one short chapter, to consider each of the major principles. However, a fundamental moral principle is that of autonomy because an understanding and observance of this principle should automatically lead professionals into the understanding and observance of many other principles.

Autonomy

Autonomy involves self-direction, self-governance and self-control of one's actions. It could be argued that it is impossible to be totally autonomous because society imposes certain rules, often sitting in judgement on the actions of individuals; in addition, professionals are required to adhere to a Code. However, there is a broad band of acceptability in most areas of life, at least in democratic societies, which gives individuals varying degrees of freedom of choice. What is expected of individuals is that their actions and decisions should be rational, that is, based on sound reasoning. These decisions should then be accepted, whether or not they match the views of others, such as midwives and doctors.

For women to make rational decisions about their care, it is imperative that they receive sufficient information at the level required by each individual. Many factors need to be considered—for example, the *environment* and the *language* used, with the avoidance of jargon and abbreviations. The *circumstances* in which a decision is required may vary – for example, whether there is time for contemplation or whether a fairly urgent situation is faced. Having given the information, it is also important for professionals to assess the woman's understanding of it. These points are of particular importance when midwives are caring for vulnerable and/or disadvantaged women.

After having determined that a woman has made an informed decision based on what she thinks is sound reasoning, that is, an autonomous decision, health professionals have no right to overrule that decision (Mental Capacity Act 2005; Griffith 2014). This principle is inextricably bound to informed consent: if the woman is autonomous, then nothing should be done to her without her prior consent; to do so would be to commit a *trespass against the person* (see Ch. 9). If her consent is being sought, then she is being considered to be autonomous; therefore, a situation should not arise where, on her refusal to consent to a procedure, professionals attempt to overrule her. There are two groups of people who might be deemed to not be autonomous and therefore unable to give consent. One group, previously briefly mentioned, includes children, but there is no longer a defined age; it depends on the circumstances and degree of rationality of the child (Children Acts 1989 and 2004). The other group includes those who are mentally incapacitated, either because of disability or by severe mental illness. With both groups, consent by proxy would be sought. There is also the possibility of temporary mental incompetence, for example, in cases of unconsciousness or possibly the effects of drugs or extreme fear, such as might occur during labour. In such cases, the professionals would be expected to act out of necessity, in the best interest of the woman, unless there was sound evidence that the woman would refuse consent if aware of the situation, such as a Jehovah's Witness carrying a card to identify his or her refusal of blood products.

The Mental Capacity Act of 2005 applies to all healthcare professionals. From a midwifery perspective, it places into primary law (statute) the position arrived at following decisions made in civil law in the 1980s and 1990s, with regard to certain 'enforced caesarean section' cases. Therefore, in both statutory and civil law, it is illegal to force any care or treatment on a woman, even for the sake of the fetus, if she is autonomous and her decision is fully informed. Only diagnosis of mental incapacity, by a psychiatrist, can overrule her decisions; even then, only treatment that is in her best interests, not those of her fetus or her family, can be undertaken. This principle applies also to young women under 16, except where refusal of treatment could result in the woman's death. It is important that all midwives familiarize themselves with this Act, particularly the following short sections, the last of which would cover 'living wills' and birth plans:

- The principles
- People who lack capacity
- Inability to make decisions
- Best interests
- Acts in connection with care or treatment
- Acts: limitations
- Advance decisions to refuse treatment: general
- Validity and applicability of advance decisions
- Effect of advance decisions

If women's autonomy is considered, then it is unlikely that the varying aspects of the duty of care would be breached. This would not remove situations of conflict and dilemma, but it would make decision making more straightforward, with all practitioners working from the same ground rules.

Using reflective practice can help, where midwives analyse and reflect upon their actions, particularly with regard to their observance of autonomy, then use the experience to formulate plans for their future decision making.

Reflective activity 8.4

Client autonomy
At the end of a shift, consider the clients for whom you cared. In each case, consider the following:

- Which aspects of her care did you discuss with her?
- Which aspects of her care did you *not* discuss with her?
- What information did you give her?
- What decisions did she make?
- What decisions did you make?
- Did you accept her decisions, or did you try to change them?
- What did you write in the records?
- Did you enable her to be autonomous?
- In light of this exercise, what will you do in similar circumstances in future?

Women's autonomy is a relatively new concept, especially given the medical model of midwifery and a paternalistic approach to care in the early years of the NHS. The autonomy of the midwife, however, is not new. Midwives have used the term *autonomous practitioner* for many years, particularly when trying to explain the difference between nurses and midwives. Unfortunately, however, this autonomy is not always evident in practice, particularly in the hospital setting. Midwives often plead that they are constrained by guidelines and policies within which they are expected to work. The opportunities to practise autonomously still need to be considered in light of what is best for the woman and how the midwife's practice sits within the professional code.

The aim is to appreciate the need to consider personal philosophies to help to understand the philosophies of others. An understanding of ethics will help midwives to make decisions in difficult circumstances, even if they do not choose directly to follow the theories outlined. The observance of ethical principles, especially autonomy, is the most direct route to assisting childbearing women to have the degree of choice and control that each individual feels is right for her. It also provides a starting point to explore some of the strategic challenges in maternity services around care provision: Who should get what care and where? What is the best use of resources, and where is the greater good?

Reflective activity 8.5

Midwife autonomy
Reflect on the care you gave to a woman who had requested care outside of the local/national guidelines— for example, a primigravida with a breech presentation requesting home birth or a woman with a history of postpartum haemorrhage requesting physiological management of the third stage.
   How did you discuss the care with the woman?
   Whom did you seek support from?
   How did you feel about supporting a woman who may have been making a decision you did not agree with?

Key Points

- Ethics is essential to professional midwifery practice.
- There are numerous ethical principles with which professionals should be familiar.
- Moral conflicts and dilemmas cannot be avoided in some cases; they can be disconcerting but must be resolved. Theories and principles are available to help resolve the dilemmas.
- Professional practise in the NHS requires both deontological and utilitarian consideration.
- The duty of care has an ethical basis and is not only a legal principle.
- Women's autonomy is an essential basis for good midwifery practice – it also enables midwife autonomy.

CONCLUSION

This chapter is only the beginning of exploring ethics and some of the ethical dilemmas faced in midwifery practice.

References

See also the chapter website resources.
Beauchamp TL, Childress JF: *Principles of biomedical ethics,* 7th edn, Oxford, Oxford University Press, 2013.
Children Act, www.legislation.gov.uk/ukpga/1989/41/contents. 1989.
Children Act 2004, London, HMSO, 2004.
European Business Ethics Network Ireland (EBEN):

Does integrity matter? EBEN Research Conference (website). https://ebeni.wordpress.com/decisions/frameworks/ross%E2%80%99s-prima-facie-duties-framework/. 2011.
Griffith R: Deprivation of liberty in midwifery – taking a case to court, *Br J Midwifery* 22(11):822–823, 2014.

Mental Capacity Act 2005, London, HMSO, 2005.
Nursing and Midwifery Council: *The Code: professional standards of practice and behaviour of conduct nurses and midwives,* London, NMC, 2015.
Woolley S: Children of Jehovah's Witnesses and adolescent Jehovah's Witnesses: what are their rights? *Arch Dis Child* 90:715–719, 2005.

Resources and additional reading

BBC: *Introduction to ethics*, http://www.bbc.co.uk/ethics/introduction/duty_1.shtml. 2016.

The BBC website provides an overview to ethical theory.

Beauchamp TL, Childress JF: *Principles of biomedical ethics*, 7th edn, Oxford, Oxford University Press, 2013.

This book is a good starting point for gaining depth of understanding of ethical theory beyond the narrow application to midwifery.

Ekland-Olson S: *Who lives, who dies, who decides? Abortion, neonatal care, assisted dying, and capital punishment*, 2nd edn, Oxford, Routledge, 2015.

This text addresses some very difficult issues and asks some challenging questions, but the format is easy to read, and it can help individuals clarify their own personal perspective.

Harris J: *The value of life; an introduction to medical ethics*, New York, Routledge, 1985.

Although this is now 30 years in print, it gives an excellent introduction to ethics and dilemmas in health care.

Harris J, editor: *Bioethics*, Oxford, Oxford University Press, 2001.

This book has chapters related to beginning-of-life and end-of-life issues, the value and quality of life, and professional ethics, all of which are important in midwifery.

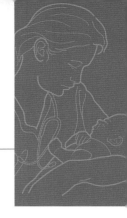

Chapter 9

The law and the midwife

Andrew Symon

Learning Outcomes ?

After reading this chapter, you will be able to:

- understand the language and sources of the law
- have an understanding of the UK legal framework
- understand how clinical competence is determined in law
- appreciate the essential role of consent and capacity in clinical practice
- understand how governments and health service employers try to minimize exposure to litigation through quality regulation

The law underpins a great deal of the work of a midwife. It establishes the practice framework, produces rules and regulations governing what can and cannot be done, and holds the midwife accountable for what is done or possibly not done. Many occupations have a legal framework, but midwifery is unique in some ways, for example, with regard to how supervision works (although this is under review – see discussion later in the chapter). Although the law may seem a distant feature of the working life of a midwife, it is always there, influencing what happens; and sometimes it takes centre stage.

This chapter includes an introduction to the courts and how laws are made. It examines how litigation is conducted in the UK and explores the key legislation that affects midwifery and the provision of maternity care services.

INTRODUCTION TO THE LAW: THE COURTS AND HOW LAWS ARE MADE

It is important to put the law into context and to appreciate that the likelihood of a midwife going to court in the course of employment is low; nonetheless, an understanding of the law will help to minimize risk. Therefore, it is important to have an understanding of the structure of the legal system to appreciate how it could affect midwifery practice.

The courts

The description of the court system in Figure 9.1 is not exhaustive – there are also coroners' courts in England and Wales and Fatal Accident Inquiries in Scotland, in addition to various employment, immigration and administrative tribunals that administer the law. Whereas some of these hearings adopt an *inquisitorial* approach that seeks to arrive at a common understanding, most UK courts proceed on an *adversarial* basis.

If a court's decision is appealed it can move to the next stage. Where European laws are concerned, this can be to the European Court of Justice, or, in human rights cases (see discussion later in the chapter), to the European Court of Human Rights.

Classification of the law

The *criminal* and *civil* law are different. A criminal offence is where a statute or the common law forbids a particular activity. Someone who allegedly breaks that law becomes the subject of criminal proceedings, with the prosecution required to establish guilt *beyond reasonable doubt*. If the accused pleads not guilty, a jury will hear the case and determine guilt or innocence.

Civil proceedings take place between individuals and organizations so that one party can obtain compensation or other remedy. This could include an injunction (interdict in Scotland) forbidding the other party to act in a particular way. In civil courts, the standard of proof is *on the balance of probabilities*. Juries sit in some civil legal

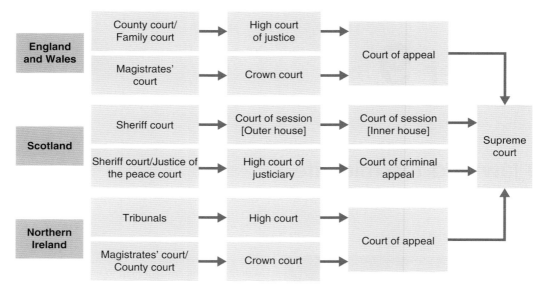

Figure 9.1 The courts.

hearings, but not in clinical negligence hearings, which are heard before one or more judges, depending on the level of the court in the court hierarchy.

An event could result in both criminal *and* civil proceedings. For example, touching someone without consent may be a trespass to the person (which is a civil matter) and constitute a criminal assault. In one rare obstetric case a doctor was both sued in the civil courts and prosecuted in the criminal courts for the same events (*R* v. *Bateman* 1925).

Another distinction is that between private and public law:

- *Private law,* which is part of the civil law, concerns matters between private individuals and others or between organizations and individuals.
- *Public law* concerns matters affecting the public. This comprises constitutional law, administrative law and the criminal law.

Some statutes may cover both areas. For instance, the Children Act 1989 has some sections that deal with matters of a private nature; others deal with public issues, such as local authorities' child protection responsibilities.

Sources of the law

The law recognized in the UK derives from two main sources:

- Legislation—acts of Parliament, statutory instruments and European Union (EU) regulations and directives
- Common law, which is formed from decisions made by courts in particular cases (see following discussion)

Legislation

Most UK legislation is enacted at Westminster, but within specified 'nonreserved' areas the Scottish parliament and Welsh and Northern Ireland assemblies can also pass legislation. Proposed laws always go through a series of review hearings, often in committee, before becoming law. As a member state of the EU the UK is obliged to ensure that EU directives and regulations are enforced; appeals can be made to the European Court of Justice. (See also the Human Rights Act section later in the chapter.)

An act of Parliament may delegate to ministers and certain others the power to enable detailed rules – known as *statutory instruments* or *secondary legislation* – to supplement a law that is about to be enacted. The Nursing and Midwifery Council (NMC) derives much of its powers this way.

Common law

Decisions by judges (and also by sheriffs in Scotland) create what is variously known as the *common law, case law* or *judge-made law.* The doctrine of *precedent* means that a court's decisions may be binding on courts below it in the court hierarchy. Thus, decisions of the Supreme Court (which in 2009 replaced the House of Lords in its judicial format as the highest UK court) are binding on those courts below it, but not on itself; and decisions of the Court of Appeal are binding on itself and those courts below it.

Precedent relies on a recognized system of reporting of judges' decisions, which ensures certainty over the facts of the case and what was stated. The decisions are recorded in law journals (e.g. the *All England Law Reports*) and identify the parties involved, the year the case was heard, and volume and page numbers of the relevant journal. For example, the citation *Bolam* v. *Friern Hospital Management Committee* (1957) 1 WLR 582 means that the case was reported in 1957, in the first volume of the *Weekly Law Reports* at page 582. The *Bolam* case is discussed later in the chapter. When cases go to appeal, each separate hearing will be listed, so the same case can have several citations – from a lower court as far as the Supreme Court. Legal cases that establish a precedent are cited until they are overturned.

Judges record the reasons for their decisions so similar cases will be treated in the same way. They may distinguish between the formal reasons (knowns as *ratio decidendi*: 'reasons for the decision'), and the more circumstantial reasons (known as *obiter dicta*: 'things said by the way'). Whereas the *ratio decidendi* are directly binding on lower courts, *obiter dicta* can be 'persuasive' in later cases. Judges may 'distinguish' a current case from previous cases and not follow them on the grounds that the facts are significantly different.

The Human Rights Act 1998

The UK is a signatory to the European Convention for the Protection of Human Rights and Fundamental Freedoms (1951). It is enforced through the European Court of Human Rights, based in Strasbourg. Since October 2000, under the terms of the Human Rights Act 1998, most of the European Convention articles which relate to public authorities or those exercising functions of a public nature are directly enforceable in the UK courts. Within healthcare, the following are particularly significant:

- *Article 2 – the right to life.* This may be used to justify the allocation of more resources. An unsuccessful attempt has been made to press for the continuation of treatment for a severely disabled baby (*A National Health Service Trust* v. *D Lloyd* 2000).

- *Article 3 – the right not to be tortured or subjected to inhuman or degrading treatment or punishment.* Shackling a woman in labour could be considered a breach of Article 3 (no such cases have been brought in Europe, although the practice is not unknown in the United States).

- *Article 5 – the right to liberty and security*

- *Article 6 – the right to a fair trial.* A French doctor successfully challenged his striking-off order on the grounds that the hearing had not been held in public (*Diennet* v. *France* 1996).

- *Article 8 – the right to respect of privacy and family life, and to physical integrity.* This was used in *Glass* v. *UK*

(2004) in the case of the withdrawal of life-sustaining treatment from a baby.

Under the Human Rights Act 1998, judges must refer back to Parliament any legislation that is considered incompatible with the rights set out in the European Convention. Parliament can then decide if that act should be changed. Further information, including guidance and the latest cases, can be obtained from the Ministry of Justice website (now located in www.gov.uk).

Reflective activity 9.1

Read through and consider Article 3 of the European Convention on Human Rights. In what circumstances could a pregnant woman claim that her rights under this article had been infringed?

The NMC Code, rules and other guidance

Midwifery, along with nursing and health visiting, is governed by a statutory system (i.e. one governed by law). This is covered in detail in Chapter 3. The Nurses, Midwives and Health Visitors Act 1979, amended in 1992, went through further changes following a review of the statutory bodies. This culminated in the Health Act (1999) and Health and Social Work Professions Order (2002). In 2002, the NMC replaced the United Kingdom Central Council (UKCC) as the statutory body. One of its duties is to produce guidance for practitioners. This includes the Code (NMC 2015a) (formerly the Code of Professional Conduct) and the Standards of Competence for Registered Midwives (2014), published in response to the Francis Report (see following discussion). Midwives are expected to comply with the Code and its other guidance, and they are expected to have copies of all the relevant NMC publications (available at www.nmc-uk.org/). Box 9.1 indicates

---

Box 9.1 Article 42 of the NMC Order 2001: Rules as to midwifery practice

The NMC shall:

1. Determine the circumstances in which and the procedure by means of which midwives may be suspended from practice.
2. Require midwives to give notice of their intention to practise to the local supervising authority for the area in which they intend to practise.
3. Require registered midwives to attend courses of instruction in accordance with the rules.

> **Box 9.2** Rule 5: Scope of practice
>
> A practising midwife who is responsible for providing care or advice to a woman or care to a baby during childbirth must do so in accordance with standards established and reviewed by the Council…
>
> Standard 2: You must make sure the needs of the woman and her baby are the primary focus of your practice…
>
> Standard 3: Except in an emergency, you must not provide any care, or undertake any treatment, that you have not been trained to give…
>
> Standard 4: In an emergency, or where a deviation from the norm, which is outside of your current scope of practice, becomes apparent in a woman or baby during childbirth, you must call such health or social care professionals as may reasonably be expected to have the necessary skills and experience to assist you in the provision of care.
>
> NMC (2012: 7)

the purpose of the Midwives Rules, which are set out under statutory instruments, and Box 9.2 sets out the midwife's responsibility and scope of practice. From 2017, these will be integrated within the Code (NMC 2015).

Supervision

Supervision is covered in depth in Chapter 3, but briefly to set the scene in its legal context, midwives are currently the only health professionals to have a statutory system of supervision. Appointed by the local supervising authority, a supervisor of midwives has clear statutory responsibilities in relation to the positive promotion of a high standard of midwifery practice and the protection of the public.

However, this situation is under review following the clinical failings noted in the Kirkup Report (2015). The Parliamentary and Health Service Ombudsman (PHSO) identified flaws in the system of public protection and recommended that the processes of midwifery supervision and regulation should be separated. This goes beyond specific action to be taken in a hospital that has been seen to fail, and requires legislation (currently at the early stages of planning). In time, midwifery supervision will no longer be part of the statutory framework, but the responsibility of employers. Supervision's role with regard to professional support, development and leadership will continue, but not under the same regulatory legislation. The projected timescale is for this process to be complete by the spring of 2017; from April 2017 the Midwives Rules and Standards (NMC 2012) will become obsolete.

LITIGATION

Litigation is the term used when one person or organization sues another person or organization. Within healthcare the focus of litigation is almost always on clinical and nonclinical negligence. Because of the way claims are handled, it is very difficult to be confident about the scale of such litigation in the UK. Most legal claims must be raised within 3 years (or within 3 years of individuals becoming aware that they may have grounds for a claim), but for 'baby' claims this rule effectively does not apply. Claims can be brought up to 25 years following the birth, and this limit has even been surpassed. Births that occurred many years ago may yet be the subject of claims raised many years from now. Some claims take many years to be resolved (for a host of reasons), making it difficult to state with certainty the 'success rate' of clinical claims.

NHS litigation is handled in England by the NHS Litigation Authority (NHSLA), in Scotland by the Clinical Negligence and Other Risks Indemnity Scheme, and in Wales by the Welsh risk pool. (See the section on NHS Indemnity Schemes later in this chapter.)

Claims range from the extremely serious to the comparatively trivial, but all must be investigated to see if they have any merit and to see whether they ought to be conceded or defended. The NHS Redress Act 2006, passed to establish an alternative route for securing compensation without necessitating action in the civil courts, has not stemmed the tide: the NHSLA (2015: 18) noted that it received over 11,000 new clinical negligence claims in 2014/2015, 'demonstrating a sustained high level of new claims'. The potential cost of claims can distort the picture: 'obstetrics' accounted for 10% of the 11,457 new NHSLA claims but 41% of their potential value. Costs related to birth injuries are high, typically because of the life-long care that may be required for a child suffering extensive neurological and other damage. The NHSLA stated that it paid out over £1.1 billion in 2014 (a third of it going to lawyers), with the payments sum predicted to rise significantly. Many different factors account for the cost of a claim; details about how these are generated can be found in the NHSLA annual reviews (available at www.nhsla.org).

NEGLIGENCE

What is negligence?

Negligence, the most common civil action, is when a claimant brings an action against a defendant alleging that there has been personal injury, death or damage or loss of property. Litigation is *adversarial*, in which one side challenges the other. The following discussion is necessarily truncated, given the space available. This and other medico-legal issues are covered in considerably more depth in several excellent textbooks, for example, Jackson (2010), Mason and Laurie (2013), Dimond (2013), and Herring (2014).

The legal systems in England and Scotland are distinct (at least until Scottish cases get to the Supreme Court), and there are differences in terminology: the law of wrongs is known in England as *tort*, but as *delict* in Scotland. The defendant is called a *defender,* and the claimant is called the *pursuer.* Having to repeat this every time a term is used gets cumbersome, so please accept the use of the English terms for the remainder of this chapter.

Compensation is sought for the loss that has occurred. To succeed, the claimant must show the following elements:

1. The defendant owed the person harmed a duty of care.
2. The defendant was in breach of that duty.
3. The breach of duty caused reasonably foreseeable harm.
4. The claimant has suffered harm recognized in law as compensable.

Rarely, the claimant may be able to claim that 'the thing speaks for itself' (known in law as *res ipsa loquitur*): there is no explanation for the damage other than a negligent act having taken place. The defendant is then required to explain how the events do not constitute negligence on his or her part.

Duty of care

The law recognizes that a duty of care will exist where one person can reasonably foresee that his or her actions and omissions could cause reasonably foreseeable harm to another. The legal precedent for this 'good neighbour' principle was established in a landmark case concerning a café owner and a customer:

> *'You must take reasonable care to avoid acts or omissions which you can reasonably foresee would be likely to injure your neighbour. Who then in law is my neighbour? The answer seems to be persons who are so closely and directly affected by my act that I ought reasonably to have them in contemplation as being so affected when I am directing my mind to the acts or omissions which are called in question'.*
>
> (*Donoghue* v. *Stevenson* 1932)

It is usually obvious in healthcare that a duty of care exists between practitioner and service user. For example, if a pregnant woman comes to the clinic or unit seeking maternity care, then the duty of care is presumed to exist. Where there is no existing professional–patient relationship the usual legal principle is that there is no duty

to perform a 'good Samaritan' act. Some argue there is an ethical obligation to do so, and indeed this was reflected in the 2002 version of the NMC Code, but this has not been included in the revised codes of 2008 and 2015.

In practical terms the duty of care issue is rarely problematic. If in the course of employment the midwife provides care to a pregnant woman or new mother, then that midwife owes her a duty of care. The baby, once born, is also owed this duty of care.

Breach of duty

The first step is to establish what happened. A potential claimant may seek legal advice, following which a request is made to see the relevant clinical records. Under the Data Protection Act 1998 (discussed later in the chapter) patients have the right to access information about themselves. Clear comprehensive documentation will be an important element in determining what took place. Witnesses of fact may be required to provide statements about the events. Having established what happened, it must be determined whether this met the requisite standard of care. The solicitor may instruct an expert witness to produce a report based on these various records. This report should apply a consideration of the standard of care. If negligence is not admitted straight away, a formal process of dispute then ensues in which the alleged facts and/or the legal liability are contested.

Almost all of this process takes place outside of a court setting. Only if the claim is impossible to decide one way or the other will it proceed to the court stage.

Determining the standard of care

In England the standard of care required by a professional is determined by the 'Bolam Test'. In *Bolam* the court laid down the following principle to determine the standard of care that should be followed:

> *'A doctor is not guilty of negligence if he has acted in accordance with a practice accepted as proper by a responsible body of medical men skilled in that particular art'.*
>
> (*Bolam* v. *Friern Hospital Management Committee* 1957)

The Bolam Test was later applied by the House of Lords in a case where negligence by an obstetrician in delivering a child by forceps was alleged:

> *'When you get a situation which involves the use of some special skill or competence, then the test as to whether there has been negligence or not … is the standard of the ordinary skilled man exercising and professing to have that special skill. If a surgeon failed to measure up to that in any respect (clinical judgement or otherwise) he had been negligent and should be so adjudged'.*
>
> (*Whitehouse* v. *Jordan* 1981)

143

In this case the House of Lords found that an error of judgement may or may not be negligence: it depends on the circumstances.

In Scotland the test is very slightly different; in *Hunter* v. *Hanley*, the judge stated:

'The true test for establishing negligence on the part of a doctor is whether he has been proven to be guilty of such failure as no doctor of ordinary skill would be guilty of if acting with ordinary care…'

(*Hunter* v. *Hanley* 1995)

Although the two definitions of medical negligence are not identical, and some believe the test for establishing negligence in Scotland is much harder, by and large the two judgements are considered to approach the question of clinical culpability in the same way. The question is not 'What would an expert midwife have done?' but 'What would an ordinary competent midwife have done?' Having established what happened (see previous discussion), the expert witnesses give evidence on whether this breached the standard of care. The Civil Procedure Rules state that:

'It is the duty of experts to help the court on matters within their expertise. This duty overrides any obligation to the person from whom experts have received instructions or by whom they are paid'.

These experts should be respected members of the profession who can advise on what constitutes competent care. They should not pass opinion on areas beyond their area of expertise; thus, a midwifery expert can be expected to comment on the care given by midwives, but not on what an obstetrician did, for example. This evidence is considered by the solicitors, who then negotiate with the other party to see whether the claim should be dropped, can be settled out of court or must proceed to a formal court hearing.

Although expert evidence is usually accorded great respect, judges can be critical of experts. In *Sardar* v. *NHS Commissioning Board*, the judge noted that the midwifery expert was 'nit picking' over the standards of record keeping (the events in question had been 24 years earlier), and he also labelled the obstetric expert's evidence as 'tortuous' and 'breathtaking', with his premises 'startling' (Symon 2014).

Very few claims end up going to court – almost all are resolved one way or the other at an earlier stage. Juries are not used in clinical negligence claims in the UK. The hearing (in a lower court) is before a single judge. Appeal cases are heard before a panel of judges.

Reflective activity 9.2   ⟫⟨

Consider any incident of which you are aware when harm occurred or nearly occurred to a woman or baby. What potential hearings could take place as a result of this harm, and what would have to be shown to secure a conviction/guilt/liability?

In a civil action, and in the light of the available evidence, the judge will decide whether the standard of care was breached. The standards at the time of the alleged negligence apply, not the standards at the time of the deliberations by the experts or judges. This is significant because many cases take several years to be raised, in which time standards may have changed. Reference is made to literature and procedures (e.g. local or national protocols), which are applied at the time of the alleged negligence to establish if a reasonable standard of care was followed.

Experts can of course differ. An expert acting for the claimant may state that the standard of care was breached by the defendant or its employees, whereas the defendant's expert might state that the defendant or its employees followed a reasonable standard of care. Where such disagreements arise, the House of Lords has laid down the following principle:

'It was not sufficient to establish negligence for the plaintiff (that is, claimant) to show that there was a body of competent professional opinion that considered the decision was wrong, if there was also a body of equally competent professional opinion that supported the decision as having been reasonable in the circumstances'.

(*Maynard* v. *W Midlands Regional Health Authority* 1985)

Each side could legitimately claim that its stance was reasonable, which then leaves a challenge of how to decide between a reasonable claim and a reasonable counterclaim. This was considered by the House of Lords in *Bolitho* v. *City and Hackney Health Authority*:

'The court had to be satisfied that the exponents of the body of opinion relied on can demonstrate that such opinion has a logical basis. … the judge…will need to be satisfied that, in forming their views, the experts … had reached a defensible conclusion on the matter'.

(*Bolitho* v. *City and Hackney Health Authority* 1997)

The upshot is that the Bolam Test has been amended: the medical reasoning used by either side must have a logic that a non-medical person can understand. Experts must be aware that baffling non-medical people with technical expertise is not helpful. The civil court proceedings rules set out the duties of experts and assessors, which include a duty to restrict expert evidence to that which is reasonably required to resolve the proceedings.

Which standards apply?

The growth of national protocols produced by organizations such NICE, the Care Quality Commission (CQC), the National Service Frameworks (NSF), the royal colleges (RCOG/RCM/RCA/RCPCH 2008) and the Scottish Intercollegiate Guidelines Network (SIGN) has seen local variations in practice diminish. Because these standards must be evidence based, they may increasingly be relied upon to demonstrate what a reasonably competent practitioner would do or know. Indeed, because they are available online, patients are able to use them to argue that inadequate care was provided in their case. To remain up to date, practitioners are expected to follow the results of relevant clinical effectiveness research.

In 2008, the four Royal Colleges – Midwives, Obstetricians and Gynaecologists, Anaesthetists, and Paediatrics and Child Health – demonstrated that they share the common goal of effective and acceptable clinical care by producing a single, comprehensive document setting out 30 standards for maternity care (available on the Royal College of Obstetricians and Gynaecologists (RCOG) website, www.rcog.org.uk).

Although guidelines may be used to determine issues of clinical negligence, they do not have the force of law. Practitioners can deviate from a guideline if the circumstances warrant this; guidelines cannot envisage every situation that may arise. If the midwife decides, in the light of the specific circumstances of a case, that a procedure or protocol or guideline is not appropriate, the midwife should ensure that the decision is documented fully. Practice must be seen to be justifiable against the guideline that others may assume represents the standard of the reasonable practitioner.

Effective communication is crucial in multidisciplinary teams. However, although an NHS employer's vicarious liability will apply for staff working in the course of their employment, the Court of Appeal stated in *Wilsher* that the courts do not recognize a concept of team liability. Each individual practitioner must ensure that his or her practice is in accordance with the approved standard of care. Professionals should not take instructions from another professional which they know would be contrary to the standard of care that their profession would require.

These standards ought to provide detailed evidence of what *should* have happened. Having established that the defendant owed a duty of care, but breached this duty, a claimant must now show that the substandard care caused an actual and reasonably foreseeable harm.

Causation

The claimant must establish (a) factual causation, (b) evidence that the type of harm that occurred was reasonably foreseeable and (c) that there was no intervening cause that breaks the chain of causation.

Factual causation

There may be a breach of the duty of care and harm but no link between them. In *Barnett* v. *Chelsea HMC* (1968), a casualty officer failed to examine a patient who presented with severe vomiting. The doctor had owed a duty of care; it was conceded that this was breached, but this claim failed because it was established that the man was suffering from arsenic poisoning and would have died even if reasonable care had been provided. There was no causal link between the doctor's breach of duty and the man's death.

The claimant has to establish this causative link. In *Wilsher* v. *Essex AHA* (1988), the claimants failed to establish that excess oxygen had caused the baby's retrolental fibroplasia. Excess oxygen was only one of five possible causative factors, and the House of Lords ordered a new hearing on the question of causation.

In a case where a baby suffered brain damage, a midwife was held to be negligent for failing to call a registrar an hour earlier than she did (*Khalid* v. *Barnet and Chase Farm Hospitals NHS Trust* 2007). The court held that this failure had led to the delay in proceeding to caesarean section. This constituted factual causation.

Reasonably foreseeable harm

Potential harm may not be within the defendant's reasonable contemplation, so that even though there is a breach of duty and there is harm, the defendant is not liable. This is because a negligent act may set off a 'chain reaction' of consequences and the courts have decided that there should be some limit on the defendant's liability. In other words, for compensation to be secured there must be a logical connection between negligence and harm. There should also be no intervening cause that breaks the chain of causation. For example, a community midwife may have arranged to transfer a labouring woman to the maternity unit because of concerns about serious fetal compromise. However, because of a road accident for which the midwife was not responsible, the woman suffered injuries, as a result of which the baby was stillborn. Although the fetus may have been compromised by the events of labour, and might have not survived in any case, the road accident would be seen as an intervening event that broke the chain of causation.

Harm

The claimant (or representative) must establish that he or she has suffered harm that the court recognizes as being subject to compensation. The main recognized areas of harm are personal injury, death and loss or damage to property. The courts have also ruled that nervous shock where an identifiable medical condition exists ('posttraumatic stress syndrome/disorder') can be the subject of compensation within strict limits of liability.

Vicarious and personal liability

Because an NHS employer will usually be vicariously liable for its employees' actions, it is unlikely that employees will be sued personally. To establish vicarious liability, the claimant must show the *employee* was *negligent* or was guilty of another wrong while acting in the *course of employment*. It is also possible for an employer to be sued directly for failing negligently to provide a service (*Bull* v. *Devon AHA* 1993).

Independent practitioners must accept personal and professional liability for their actions (as evidenced by the protracted dealings regarding indemnity insurance for independent midwives), but they may also be vicariously liable for the harm, caused during the course of employment, by anyone they employ. Employers are not liable for the acts of independent contractors (that is, self-employed persons who are working for them on a contract for services) unless they are at fault in selecting or instructing them.

An employer may challenge whether the actions were performed in the course of employment. For example, a midwife may have undertaken complementary therapy training. If she used these new skills while at work, without the express or implied agreement of the employer, and thereby caused harm, the employer might refuse to accept vicarious liability on the grounds that the employee was not acting in the course of employment.

Liability for students and unqualified assistants: supervision and delegation

Exactly the same principles apply to the delegation and supervision of tasks as to the carrying out of professional activities. Midwives must only delegate a task if they have good reason to be sure that the *delegatee* is reasonably competent and sufficiently experienced to undertake that activity safely (see NMC Code 2015, s.11, discussed later in the chapter). Midwives must also provide sufficient supervision to ensure that the delegated activity can be carried out reasonably safely. Should harm occur because an activity was carried out by a junior member of staff, student or assistant, it is **no defence** to argue that the harm occurred because that person did not have the ability, competence or experience to carry out that task reasonably safely (*Wilsher* v. *Essex AHA* 1986). Some midwifery duties, such as attendance at a birth, can never be delegated. Midwives are accountable for actions they delegate to others (NMC 2015a). To achieve this, you as a midwife must:

- Only delegate tasks and duties that are within the other person's scope of competence making sure that the delegatee fully understand your instructions;
- Make sure that everyone you delegate tasks to is adequately supervised and supported so they can provide safe and compassionate care; and
- Confirm that the outcome of any task you have delegated to someone else meets the required standard (NMC 2015a: 10).

Defences to an action

Practitioners against whom an allegation of negligence is made have several possible defences:

- Dispute the allegations.
- Deny that all the elements of negligence are established.
- Argue that there was contributory negligence.
- Argue exemption from liability.
- Argue that the claim is 'time-barred'.
- Argue that there was voluntary assumption of risk.

Dispute allegations

Many cases will be resolved entirely on what facts can be established. Clinical records should provide an accurate contemporaneous account of events, but this may be challenged by either party. Witnesses of fact could include the woman, her partner or other family member or visitor, or various members of staff. Recall becomes harder the longer the gap between a precise sequence of events and subsequently having to recall them. This is particularly acute in birth-related claims, which may take several years to be raised and to get to the stage of formal dispute. Staff may move, retire or die, or be otherwise uncontactable. In such claims the accuracy and level of detail provided by the clinical records is often the determining factor.

Deny that all the elements of negligence are established

A claim will fail if the defendant can show that any one of the required elements (duty of care, breach of this duty, ensuing causation and compensable harm) is absent.

Contributory negligence

If the claimant is partly to blame for the harm that has occurred, then the compensation payable might be reduced in proportion to the claimant's fault. The court, taking into account the claimant's physical and mental health and age, applies the Law Reform (Contributory Negligence) Act 1945 in determining what this proportion is. In extreme cases, if 100% contributory negligence is claimed, such a claim may be a complete defence.

A midwifery example of contributory negligence might be that of a labouring woman refusing to allow the midwife or doctor to conduct any examination or auscultation despite there being significant concerns about fetal well-being. In the event that the baby dies or is significantly compromised, it would be difficult for the woman to allege that it was the fault of staff that no close observation of fetal well-being had taken place.

Exemption from liability

It is possible in law for people to exempt themselves from liability for harm arising from their negligence, but the effects of the Unfair Contract Terms Act 1977 mean that this exemption only applies to loss or damage to property.

Box 9.3 Knowledge of the harm

The definition of knowledge for the purposes of the limitation of time is that a person must have knowledge of the following facts:

- that the injury in question was significant;
- that the injury was attributable in whole or in part to the act or omission that is alleged to constitute the negligence, nuisance or breach of duty; and
- the identity of the defendant.

A defendant cannot exclude liability from negligence which results in personal damage or death either by contract or by a notice. Therefore, a midwife could not agree with a woman that she would provide her with a pool for a water birth on the understanding that the mother would not hold the midwife (or the midwife's employer) liable for any negligence.

Limitation of time

The Limitation Act 1980 governs this. Actions for personal injury or death should normally be commenced within 3 years of the relevant date, or 3 years from the date on which the person had the necessary knowledge of the harm and the fact that it arose from the defendant's actions or omissions. Box 9.3 details what 'knowledge' of the harm entails.

The 3-year limit applies to the mother in obstetric litigation, but it only applies to the baby when he or she is 18 years old. A judge can extend the limitation period if it is just and equitable to do so.

These limitation rules influence the periods for which records must be retained. The Department of Health has specified minimum retention periods: 25 years after the last live birth for maternity records, and 8 years after treatment concluded (or death if this is sooner) for other records. One woman who suffered brain damage following heart surgery as a baby at the Bristol hospital (these events led to the Kennedy Report of 2001) received a seven-figure sum in compensation more than 20 years after the surgery (Rose 2008).

Voluntary assumption of risk

The defence of voluntary assumption of risk is unlikely to succeed in an action for professional negligence because professionals cannot contract out of liability where their negligence causes harm. Employers also have a duty to take reasonable care of the health and safety of employees (see following section on this topic). Where an employer fails in this duty, it cannot be argued successfully that an employee had accepted a risk of being harmed as an occupational hazard.

Compensation

Compensation is known as *quantum* (literally 'how much'). The general rule governing damages is that they should compensate the claimant for the loss he or she has suffered. The claimant should be restored, as far as possible, to the position he or she would have been in but for the negligent act. As noted earlier, birth-related claims account for a disproportionately high amount of the overall costs of clinical negligence compensation.

There are two kinds of damages. The term *special damages* refers to the actual financial losses between the time of the negligent act and the settlement. These include loss of earnings, purchase of special equipment or adaptations to the home and the costs of medical and nursing care. *General damages* constitute compensation for pain and suffering from the injury and loss of amenity (reduced enjoyment of life) plus future financial losses (e.g. loss of earnings and future expenses).

In some cases of negligence, liability might be accepted by the defendant, but there might be disagreement between the parties over the amount of compensation; or there may be agreement over the theoretical amount of compensation, but liability may be disputed.

DEVELOPMENTS IN THE CIVIL LAW

Concerns about the functioning of the civil legal system, and of clinical negligence litigation in particular, have led to reviews and reforms over the past 20 years. Lord Woolf's 1996 report on Civil Procedure Rules (CPR) recommended that the courts take an active role in case management, including control over the use of expert evidence. The principal objective was to ensure the system operated justly and at reasonable cost.

Lower value claims would be 'fast tracked', with a restriction on court time and the use of experts (court time is very expensive). For cases above a certain potential value the court would have wide powers to define the scope of expert evidence and prescribe the way in which experts should be used. Preaction protocols would encourage cooperation between the two parties to encourage a mutual resolution of the claim.

The purpose of the NHS Redress Scheme, established by the NHS Redress Act 2006, is to speed up the process of dispute resolution through a more proactive approach to claims. This includes explanation, apology where appropriate and an offer of compensation. It also aims to produce reports so that lessons are learned from mistakes and to move the NHS away from its 'blame culture'. Despite these attempts, and as noted earlier, the incidence of formal litigation has not fallen.

'No-fault compensation', which would remove the need to establish that a practitioner had breached the duty of care, was mooted in the 1990s as a possible solution to the 'litigation crisis'. Such schemes exist elsewhere, including New Zealand and the Nordic countries (Bismark and Paterson 2006; Hellbacher et al 2007). The Welsh Redress Scheme has considered introducing no-fault compensation, and a recommendation that this be considered in Scotland was also made to the Scottish government (Symon 2011). To date, the existing fault-based system continues to apply.

Conditional fees

Funding through the system of 'legal aid' is being phased out from personal injury litigation. A system of conditional fees has been introduced whereby the claimant is able to negotiate, with a solicitor, payment on a 'no win–no fee' basis. However, an unsuccessful claimant will have to pay the defendant's costs; insurance to meet these and other costs not covered by the agreement with the solicitor can be arranged. If agreed with, lawyers under the conditional fee agreement a successful party can claim enhanced fees from the unsuccessful party. The NHS Litigation Authority (NHSLA) reported that in 2014 one-third of its payments of £1.1 billion went to lawyers – most of that to claimants' lawyers.

NHS INDEMNITY SCHEMES

In 1995, the NHSLA was established in England to manage NHS litigation; this it does through the Clinical Negligence Scheme for Trusts (CNST). There are equivalent schemes in Scotland (CNORIS) and Wales (the Welsh Risk Pool). These schemes help to resolve disputes and claims between patients and the NHS, and they aim to keep legal actions out of court to keep costs down. They enable members to spread the risk of compensation payouts for negligence actions.

The NHSLA runs a National Clinical Assessment Service to help resolve concerns about the professional practice of UK-based doctors, dentists and pharmacists.

Because of the known risk associated with birth-related claims, the scheme aims to reduce risk by requiring its members to adhere to its generic risk management standards and its Maternity Clinical Risk Management Standards, which are updated annually and have three levels:

Level 1: The Trust is required to show that it has the required clinical risk management policies and procedures in place to provide a safe maternity service.

Level 2: The Trust must demonstrate that the policies and procedures are being implemented.

Level 3: The Trust must show that the process for managing risk is working across the entire maternity service, and that action plans are available and implemented where deficiencies are identified.

Maternity care varies; a small freestanding unit is a very different from an inner-city unit within a teaching hospital. Nevertheless, the same essential NHSLA risk management criteria apply:

- Organization of care: there is a risk management strategy with appropriate leadership ensuring that staffing levels are adequate, that records are maintained, that complaints and claims investigated and that staff are sufficiently educated and trained.

- Clinical care: essential and high-risk aspects are adequately covered; these include induction of labour, various aspects of intrapartum care, caesarean section, care of the severely ill woman and vaginal birth after caesarean section.

- High-risk conditions: these include (but are not limited to) pre-existing diabetes, severe pre-eclampsia, multiple pregnancy, obesity, operative vaginal birth, shoulder dystocia and postpartum haemorrhage.

- Communication: this relates especially to clinical appointments, information-giving, screening, clinical risk assessment, handover of care and ambulance transfer.

- Postnatal and newborn care: this includes detection of fetal abnormality, immediate newborn care, examination of the newborn, admission to the neonatal unit and bladder care.

These areas are reviewed in light of ongoing developments in risk assessment, and Trusts must demonstrate that they are proactively tackling these issues. There is a clear financial incentive to attain the higher levels: the higher the achieved level, the greater the discount on their contributions to the central fund.

The NHSLA oversees the CNST and also administers the scheme for meeting liabilities of health service bodies to third parties for loss, damage or injury arising out of the exercise of their functions. This covers claims by employees for work-related accidents and those by visitors for accidents on NHS premises.

CONSENT

Valid consent must be obtained before starting any treatment or physical investigation or providing personal care to a patient. This fundamental tenet of good legal and ethical practice reflects the right of individuals to determine what happens to their own bodies. Health professionals who disrespect this principle may be liable to civil legal action by the patient, action by their professional body and even criminal prosecution. Consent is an ongoing process, not a 'one-off'. A mentally competent patient can withdraw consent at any time, even during a procedure.

Although attention often focuses on the signing of consent forms before specific treatment, the law makes no absolute distinction between written and oral consent; what matters is that the consent is valid. Consent may also be implied: a pregnant woman who climbs up on an examination couch in the antenatal clinic and exposes her abdomen may not say that she is consenting to an examination, but she is implying it.

Nevertheless, where procedures entail risk, and where there is the possibility of a dispute over whether consent was given, it is advisable to obtain written consent because it is then easier to establish in a court of law that consent was given. It is, of course, open to challenge that the consent was withdrawn at some later stage, so it might not be definitive proof.

There are two distinct aspects of the law relating to consent to treatment: the actual giving of consent by the patient, which acts as a defence to an action for trespass to the person, and the practitioner's duty to give information to the patient before obtaining consent. The absence of consent could result in the patient suing for trespass to the person. The failure to provide sufficient relevant information could result in an action for negligence. These two different legal actions will be considered separately.

Trespass to the person

Trespass to the person can be a criminal action, in which case it is known as *assault,* or a civil wrong, which is known as *battery.* Although 'battery' sounds like serious harm has been caused, this is not the case here. Merely touching someone without his or her consent can be considered battery. A civil action under this heading does not have to show that physical harm was caused. Compensation can be awarded for the indignity of being treated without valid consent: 'it is the violation of the patient's right to make an informed choice which is being compensated' (Jackson 2010: 174) rather than a physical or emotional harm.

This is in contrast with an action for negligence, in which the victim must show that harm has resulted from the breach of duty of care. *Re B: adult – refusal of medical treatment* (2002) concerned a woman who was paralysed and refusing life-sustaining treatment; her fundamental right to refuse treatment was upheld by the court (the hearing took place at her bedside), and she was awarded notional damages for the technical assault that staff had perpetrated on her in carrying out care.

Reflective activity 9.3

Think about the activities that you undertake in relation to women in your care, and note the extent to which you obtain written, verbal or nonverbal consent. Is it possible that you need to consider making any changes to your practice so that the issue of consent is clearer?

Defences to an action for trespass to the person

The main defence to an action for trespass to the person is that a mentally competent person gave consent. In addition, there are two other defences in law:

1. Statutory authorization – for example, under the Mental Health Act 1983 (as amended by the Mental Health Act 2007)

2. The act was performed in the best interests of a mentally incapacitated person under the provisions of the Mental Capacity Act 2005 (or Adults with Incapacity Act 2000 in Scotland) (see following discussion).

Consent and negligence

Part of the duty of care requires the professional to inform a patient about any significant risks of substantial harm associated with the treatment. If the risk has not been properly explained, and the harm then occurs, the patient could then bring an action in negligence, claiming that had she known of this possibility she would not have agreed to the treatment. To succeed, she would have to show that:

- There was a duty of care to give specific information;

- The defendant failed to give this information and in so doing was therefore in breach of the reasonable standard of care that should have been provided;

- Because of this failure to inform, the patient agreed to the treatment; and

- The patient subsequently suffered the harm.

How much information needs to be given? It could be asked what a reasonable or prudent patient would expect to be told about potential risks of a treatment or therapy, but there may be particular circumstances in which an individual would want to know more or less than this. The leading case for many years was that of *Sidaway* v. *Bethlem Royal Hospital Governors* (1985) where the House of Lords stated that the professional should provide information to the patient according to the Bolam Test. In other words, 'What would a reasonable professional say under the circumstances?' This focuses on the giving of information rather than evaluating what has been understood by the person receiving the information.

A recent case has challenged – some would say overturned – the *Sidaway* ruling that the Bolam Test could be used to assess whether the practitioner's information-giving was sufficient or not (*Montgomery* v. *Lanarkshire HB* 2015). In Montgomery a woman argued that she should have been warned of the possibility of shoulder dystocia (Symon 2015). The Supreme Court noted that a growing case law in the UK and across Europe (based on the

Human Rights Act 1998 and the European Convention on Human Rights) emphasizes patients' rights to be kept informed. The bottom line is that practitioners must give relevant material information to patients/service users about risks and potential benefits, and it is up to them to decide whether or not they agree to a proposed course of action. The days of a professional deciding what a patient should be told are gone, not least because modern technology offers many other ways for service users to access information.

Elements of consent

For consent to treatment to be valid, it must be given *voluntarily*, by an appropriately *informed* person (the patient or, where relevant, someone with parental responsibility for a patient) who has *capacity* to consent to the intervention in question.

Voluntarily

Consent must be given voluntarily and freely, without pressure or undue influence being exerted on the patient by partners, family members or health professionals.

Informed consent

Some argue that the term 'informed consent' is a tautology: if it is not informed it is not consent (Mason and Laurie 2013). However, there is some value in emphasizing the fact that there must be a significant degree of understanding for consent to be valid. This includes – in broad terms – the nature and purpose of the procedure, together with its likely risks.

To ensure that the patient understands the information, there are considerable advantages in providing written confirmation of the details (such as in a leaflet). This would also assist if there was any dispute over what information had been given, but is of course dependent on that person being able to read and understand the leaflet.

Capacity

There is a presumption (which can be rebutted if the evidence exists) that a person over 16 years has the requisite mental capacity to give consent. This position is reaffirmed under the Mental Capacity Act 2005 (see following discussion).

For those under the age of 16 it is possible to give consent if 'Fraser competence' is demonstrated. This doctrine arose from the *Gillick* case, in which a mother tried to stop her teenage daughter from being prescribed contraceptive advice or treatment without parental knowledge and consent. The case was appealed to the House of Lords, and it is Lord Fraser's description of the approach to be adopted by health professionals that has come to known as 'Fraser competence'. Essentially it means that the child, although under age 16, has sufficient understanding and

intelligence to enable him or her to appreciate fully what is involved in a proposed intervention. The consent to treatment would therefore be valid. In practice professionals may seek to involve the minor's parents or guardians, but this is not an absolute requirement if the minor has demonstrated this capacity to consent. In Scotland this approach is also given approval in the Age of Legal Capacity (Scotland) Act of 1991.

Mental Capacity Act 2005

The Mental Capacity Act of 2005 sets out the definition of mental capacity in England and Wales. In Scotland, the Adults with Incapacity Act 2000 applies.

First, it must be determined whether a person has an impairment of, or a disturbance in, the functioning of the mind or brain. Second, if so, does this impairment or disturbance cause an inability to make a specific decision? A woman is unable to make a decision for herself if she is unable to:

1. Understand the information relevant to the decision,

2. Retain that information,

3. Use or weigh up that information as part of the process of making the decision, or

4. Communicate her decision (whether by talking, using sign language or through any other means).

The existence of a mental illness will not automatically mean that a person is incapable of giving a valid refusal of treatment in her or his best interests. In the case of *Re C* (1994), a Broadmoor patient who was diagnosed with paranoid schizophrenia was still considered to have the capacity to refuse an almost certainly life-saving amputation of the leg. An injunction prevented any doctors from carrying out an amputation without his consent. The Mental Capacity Act 2005 now reflects this recognition of an adult patient's right to refuse treatment.

In a situation where it is established that a patient lacks the capacity to consent, treatment can proceed under this act provided it is in the best interests of that individual and is given according to the reasonable standard of the profession. In *Great Western Hospitals* v. *AA* (2014), a 'confused and disoriented' woman (AA) who had a history of substance and alcohol abuse and affective bipolar disorder underwent a caesarean section without her explicit consent. Psychiatric opinion was that she was psychotic, and the judge concluded that she was 'unable to comprehend any aspect of her treatment' at the time. In granting the hospital legal authority to proceed, it was stipulated that any treatment or restraint to prevent AA from absconding had to be given with 'the minimum necessary reasonable force', and that 'all reasonable steps are taken to minimize distress to AA and to maintain her greatest dignity'.

In emergency situations it is also permissible to give treatment without explicit consent. For example, if a woman who collapses following postpartum haemorrhage at home is admitted to the hospital in a state of shock, she can be lawfully examined and given any necessary life-saving procedures even though at that stage she was not able to provide consent to this. Time permitting, the act requires steps to be taken to determine what is in that person's best interests, and, in the absence of carers who could be consulted over this, the appointment of an independent mental capacity advocate where serious treatment is being considered.

If a patient *does have* mental capacity, this defence of acting in the patient's best interests does not apply. For example, a mentally competent woman who refuses blood or blood products cannot be given these to save her life should her condition become critical.

The Mental Capacity Act enables a mentally capacitated person to draw up an *advance decision*, under which they can refuse treatment at a future time, when they lack capacity. Where life-saving treatment is refused in advance, specific statutory provisions must be satisfied, including a written statement signed by the maker and signed by a witness, making it clear that a life-saving measure is being refused.

Refusal to consent

The landmark case of *Re MB* (1997) set the benchmark for considerations of refusal of treatment, in which the House of Lords found that:

'A competent woman, who has the capacity to decide, may, for religious reasons, other reasons, for irrational or rational reasons or for no reason at all, choose not to have medical intervention, even though the consequence may be the death or serious handicap of the child she bears, or her own death. In that event the courts do not have the jurisdiction to declare medical intervention lawful and the question of her own best interests, objectively considered, does not arise'.

(*Re MB (an adult – medical treatment)*,
per Butler-Sloss LJ)

A woman with a needle phobia had refused to have a venous line sited before a caesarean section; without the venous line, the operation could not go ahead.

There is no room to doubt the force of this House of Lords decision, which is binding on all lower courts: no means no. And yet this stage was reached because in several cases a woman's refusal of treatment had been disregarded. In *Re S* (1992), a court authorized a hospital to carry out a caesarean section on a woman who had objected on religious grounds. In this case 'S' had been in labour for 2 days, and the fetus was lying transverse and with an elbow prolapsing – clearly an obstructed labour.

The ethical imperative to respect autonomy may be challenged by such circumstances.

Such obstetric cases, particularly the ones in later pregnancy, are distinctive. Not only might practitioners argue that a certain treatment is in the woman's best interests (if only she knew it), but the claim is sometimes made – as it was in *Re S* – that fetal interests must also be considered. However, although emotionally appealing to many, this claim is not valid in UK law: the fetus is not a legal personality, and as such has no legal rights until born. It cannot be argued, therefore, that a caesarean section should be performed 'for the sake of the baby'.

Arguing that a caesarean should be performed in the mother's own interests is superficially a plausible argument if it is genuinely felt that the woman might die if the operation is not performed. However, Lady Butler-Sloss's argument is clear: as long as the woman is mentally competent, a refusal of treatment is absolute, regardless of the clinical consequences.

For those trying to override this refusal the obvious recourse is to try to establish that the woman is not mentally competent. In *St George's Healthcare NHS Trust* v. *S* (1998), a woman with pre-eclampsia was advised that she needed urgent hospital bed rest and an induced delivery. Without that treatment, the health and life of both herself and the unborn child were in real danger. She fully understood the potential risks but rejected the advice because she wanted a normal birth.

Those involved in her care arranged for her assessment under Section 2 of the Mental Health Act of 1983, and she was duly admitted to a psychiatric hospital. From there she was transferred, again against her will, to an obstetric unit. In view of her continuing adamant refusal to consent to treatment, the hospital trust made an application to perform a caesarean, but without S being represented at the hearing. The judge ruled that the caesarean section could proceed, dispensing with S's refusal of consent. The operation was performed, and S was then returned to the psychiatric hospital; 2 days later her detention under the Mental Health Act was ended.

The woman then sought judicial review of her detention, the High Court judgement and the caesarean section. The Court of Appeal held that she was not suffering from mental disorder of a nature or degree that warranted her detention in hospital for assessment. Further, the Mental Health Act of 1983 could not be deployed to detain an individual against her will merely because her thinking process was unusual, bizarre or irrational. Only if her capacity to consent was diminished could a woman, detained under the act for mental disorder, be forced into medical procedures unconnected with her psychiatric condition. Her transfer to the obstetrical unit was unlawful; in addition, the High Court judge should not have made the declaration without S being represented at the hearing.

What if someone wishes to leave hospital?

It is a principle of consent that a person who gives consent can also withdraw it at any time; therefore, if people wish to leave hospital contrary to clinical advice, they are free to go unless they lack the capacity to make a valid decision. Should they lack that capacity, the Mental Capacity Act of 2005 has been amended to include Deprivation of Liberty Safeguards (Griffith 2014).

Clearly, there are advantages in obtaining the patient's signature that the self-discharge or refusal to accept treatment was contrary to clinical advice. If patients refuse to sign a form that they are taking discharge contrary to clinical advice, that refusal must be accepted. It is advisable to ensure that another professional is a witness to this and for both professionals to record this carefully.

LAWS REGULATING PREGNANCY, BIRTH AND CHILDREN

Abortion Act of 1967 as amended

The provisions of the Abortion Act of 1967, set out in Box 9.4, including the requirement to have two registered medical practitioners, do not apply in an emergency when a registered medical practitioner is of the opinion, formed in good faith, that the termination is immediately necessary to save the life or to prevent grave permanent injury to the physical or mental health of the pregnant woman.

This act does not apply in Northern Ireland.

Registration of births and stillbirths; births under 24 weeks

The law requires that every birth is registered. This includes stillbirths occurring after 24 weeks gestation. Miscarriages before 24 completed weeks do not have to be registered, but the body must be disposed of respectfully, taking into consideration the wishes and feelings of the parents. Where a live birth is followed by a death (irrespective of gestation), both the birth and the death must be registered. If a baby is born alive and survives even for a brief time, the birth must be registered even if the gestation is less than 24 weeks. If the baby subsequently dies, then the death must be registered.

Human Fertilisation and Embryology Acts 1990, 1992 and 2008

The Human Fertilisation and Embryology Acts 1990, 1992 and 2008 provide a legal framework for infertility treatment and embryo growth and implanting. For example,

---

Box 9.4 Abortion Act 1967 Section 1 as amended by the Human Fertilisation and Embryology Act 1990

S 1(1) A person shall not be guilty of an offence under the law relating to abortion when a pregnancy is terminated by a registered medical practitioner if two registered medical practitioners are of the opinion, formed in good faith:

(a) that the pregnancy has not exceeded its 24th week and that the continuance of the pregnancy would involve risk, greater than if the pregnancy were terminated, of injury to the physical or mental health of the pregnant woman or any existing children of her family; or

(b) that the termination is necessary to prevent grave permanent injury to the physical or mental health of the pregnant woman; or

(c) that the continuance of the pregnancy would involve risk to the life of the pregnant woman, greater than if the pregnancy were terminated; or

(d) that there is a substantial risk that if the child were born it would suffer from such physical or mental abnormalities as to be seriously handicapped.

S 1(2) In determining whether the continuance of a pregnancy would involve such risk of injury to health as is mentioned in paragraph (a) or (b) of subsection (1) of this section, account may be taken of the woman's actual or reasonably foreseeable environment.

---

under the 2008 act the creation and use of all human embryos outside the body are subject to regulation. When providing fertility treatment clinics must take account of 'the welfare of the child', but no longer have to take account of the child's 'need for a father'. The Human Fertilisation and Embryology Authority is responsible for licensing and regulating centres and issuing a code of practice, and it has general responsibility for ensuring that the law is followed.

Criminal law and attendance at birth

A midwife could face criminal proceedings in respect of her work if she offends against the criminal laws, such as health and safety laws or road traffic acts. If she acts with gross recklessness or negligence in her professional practice, then she could face criminal proceedings. For example, an anaesthetist was found guilty for the death of a patient in theatre where he acted with such gross recklessness as to amount to the criminal offence of manslaughter (*R* v. *Adomako* 1995). Two junior doctors were also found guilty of 'gross negligence manslaughter' when they failed to identify that a patient who had undergone routine surgery was seriously ill (*R* v. *Misra*).

Section 16 of the 1997 Nurses, Midwives and Health Visitors Act made it a criminal offence for a person other than a registered midwife or a registered medical practitioner (or student of either) to attend a woman in childbirth except in an emergency or undergoing professional training as doctor or midwife. This is reenacted in Article 45 of the Nursing and Midwifery Order 2001.

Children Acts of 1989 and 2004

The Children Act 1989 and the Children (Scotland) Act 1995 set up a framework for the protection and care of children and established clear principles to guide decision making in relation to their care. This legislation is considered in Chapter 15.

Health and Social Care Act of 2008

The Health and Social Care Act of 2008 created the Care Quality Commission (CQC), which is the independent regulator of adult health and social care in England. It can monitor and inspect NHS Trusts and independent hospitals, general practitioner practices, care homes, dentists and ambulance services.

Public Services Reform (Scotland) Act of 2010

The Public Services Reform (Scotland) Act of 2010 established Healthcare Improvement Scotland (HIS) in 2011. Part of the NHS, HIS consists of the Healthcare Environment Inspectorate, the Scottish Health Council (which relates to public engagement), the Scottish Intercollegiate Guidelines Network (SIGN) (see previous section on breach of the standard of care), the Scottish Medicines Consortium (NICE has an equivalent role in England and Wales) and the Scottish Patient Safety Programme.

HEALTH AND SAFETY LAWS

The Health and Safety at Work Act of 1974, supplemented by many more recent statutory instruments, defines the management of health and safety in the workplace and specific duties relating to manual handling, protective clothing, and clinical waste disposal. Workplaces should have accessible health and safety policies outlining the respective rights and duties of employer and employee.

An employer has statutory duties enforceable by the Health and Safety Executive (HSE) in the criminal courts, in addition to duties under the common law (HSE 1995). Every employer must take reasonable care of the physical and mental health and safety of its employees. Employees also have a duty to take reasonable care of their own health and safety and that of those around them (whether colleagues or visitors). Certain employees may be designated as a health and safety representatives.

Every employer has a responsibility to carry out a risk assessment of dangers and hazards in the workplace. This covers manual handling and an assessment for hazardous substances under the Control of Substances Hazardous to Health Regulations (2002). Incidents involving injuries must be reported. Adverse incidents involving medical devices are reported to the Medicines and Healthcare Products Regulatory Agency (MHRA; www.mhra.gov.uk). Any warnings issued by the MHRA must be acted upon.

LEGAL ASPECTS OF RECORD KEEPING

Midwives have clear responsibilities to ensure that their documentation is kept properly per Rule 6 (NMC 2012). In addition, if they leave their post, there are specified duties for the transfer of their records. The Midwives' Standards stipulate that care relating to mother or baby must be kept securely for 25 years; this follows directives from the departments of health within the UK. Self-employed midwives must ensure that women can access their records; they must notify the woman if the records have to be transferred to the local supervising authority.

The Data Protection Act of 1998, whose duties are enforceable under criminal law, covers both computerized and manual records. It requires those who deal with personal records to register their storage and use of those records. Service users can access their clinical case records under the act. There are a few specified exceptions to this rule, for example, where it is believed that serious harm would be caused to the physical or mental health of the applicant or another, or where a third party (not being a health professional caring for the patient) who would be identified by the disclosure has requested not to be identified.

MEDICINES

The NMC has produced comprehensive guidance in relation to medicines management (NMC 2007). In addition, midwives have statutory powers in relation to the prescribing of medication (NMC 2006). Further instructions are set out in the rules: 'You must only supply and administer those medicines for which you have received training as to use, dosage and methods of administration and for which you are exempt', and in Section 18 of the Code (NMC 2015a). Please refer to Chapter 10 for specific laws and rules governing drugs and medicines.

COMPLAINTS

A new complaints system covering both health and social care was introduced in 2009. The procedure has two stages: local-level resolution of complaints where possible and, where this is not possible, independent review by the Health Service Ombudsman. Further details of the procedure can be obtained from the NHS Choices website (see 'How Do I Make a Complaint About an NHS Service?' at www.nhs.uk/). This is further supported by the joint publication of "Openness and Honesty When Things Go Wrong: The Professional Duty of Candour" guidance produced by the NMC and the General Medical Council (NMC 2015b). Appendix 2 of this document notes the statutory duty of candour that will be enacted across the UK (different provisions will apply in England, Scotland, Wales and Northern Ireland).

Negligent advice

To establish liability for negligence in giving advice, a claimant would have to show that she had relied upon the advice and in so doing had suffered reasonably foreseeable loss or harm. For example, providing a reference for a student or colleague can lead to liability to the new employer if the employer suffers harm from having relied on that reference (*Hedley Byrne* v. *Heller and Partners* 1963). The person about whom a reference is written may also try to show that the reference was written without reasonable care and that harm occurred to him or her because a potential employer relied on that reference (*Spring* v. *Guardian Assurance* 1994). Every care should therefore be taken to ensure that a reference is written accurately in the light of the facts available.

STATUTORY DUTIES

Statutory duties are placed upon the Secretaries of State for Health in England and in the devolved governments to provide a comprehensive service to meet all reasonable needs. These duties are in turn delegated to various NHS organizations. In England, Clinical Commissioning Groups (CCGs) have replaced Primary Care Trusts and Special Health Authorities. The NHS constitution for England lays down the objectives of the NHS, including the rights and responsibilities of those involved (patients as well as staff and health organizations). It defines rights of access to quality healthcare and details rights of redress.

The Welsh Assembly oversees NHS Wales' administering of seven Local Health Boards and three NHS Trusts. In Scotland, NHS Scotland oversees 15 geographical Health Boards and several special Health Boards (Healthcare Improvement Scotland, the Scottish Ambulance Service, etc.). The Northern Ireland Executive's Health Department is responsible for administering health and social care in the province (see Ch. 14).

THE DUTY OF QUALITY

Although several statutory bodies exist to monitor care and to promote good practice, their existence has not been enough to prevent some very poor examples of care.

The *Care Quality Commission* (CQC) is part of the English Department of Health and can inspect health systems across the whole of the NHS in England and Wales. In Scotland, the equivalent is the Care Inspectorate. In Wales, the Care and Social Services Inspectorate Wales fulfils a similar function; in Northern Ireland, the equivalent independent health and social care regulator is the Regulation and Quality Improvement Authority (RQIA).

Despite these organizations and processes being in place, several recent investigations and reviews have highlighted significant shortcomings in the NHS and in maternity care in particular.

Following the deaths of 10 women in childbirth between 2002 and 2005 in Northwick Park Hospital, a Healthcare Commission (2006) report noted that in nine cases there were care and treatment deficiencies. Two years later the Healthcare Commission (2008) reported that its several reviews into individual hospitals had led it to conclude that many of the maternity services problems were not simply the result of poor practitioners or even any one organization, but rather were systemic in origin. It noted significant weaknesses in maternity and neonatal services across England, with a shortage of doctors, midwives and basic medical facilities.

The King's Fund (2008) published an independent inquiry, noting that 'safe teams' ('the right staff in the right place at the right time") were the key to improving the safety of maternity services. Shared objectives, good communication, effective leadership, adequate staffing – the list of recommendations covered what may seem obvious ground. And yet the problems have not gone away.

In 2015, the Kirkup Report (2015) into serious failings at Morecambe Bay found that the maternity unit was dysfunctional. There were failings at almost every level – from the maternity unit itself to those charged with regulating and monitoring the Trust. Clinical care and staff relationships were poor, and staff skills and knowledge were deficient, with the midwives being criticized for pursuing normal childbirth 'at any cost'. These failures were associated with three maternal deaths and the deaths of 16 babies. The CQC, which was involved in the initial review of care at Morecambe Bay, was itself criticized for failing to act on its own findings. The fallout from its review has led to moves to separate the NMC's regulatory and statutory supervision functions (see the earlier supervision section and Chapter 3).

Maternity care is not alone in having problems. The Francis Report (Francis 2013) covered significant Trust-wide failings at the Mid Staffordshire Foundation Trust. Although noting that the Trust was liable for the failings, the report also noted that what had happened 'was also a national failure of the regulatory and supervisory system which should have secured the quality and safety of patient care' (Francis 2013: 9). This was an organizational failure: although individual practitioners make mistakes, the culture of their working environment can lead to a systemic propensity to make these mistakes. The report criticized the Trust's lack of openness to criticism, its lack of consideration for patients, its defensiveness, the fact that it was inward-looking and tended to secrecy, and that it had simply accepted poor standards. A key recommendation was to stress the duty of candour: staff have an obligation to speak up when they see things failing (Griffith 2015).

Almost all of this rather depressing litany of poor care should be avoidable if systems are robust and staff are well trained and motivated. How, then, are standards for individual practitioners to be encouraged? This loops back to the question of how the law investigates whether there has been a breach of the standard of care. The NMC, for its part, produced the Standards of Competence for Registered Midwives (NMC 2014) in response to the Francis Report to demonstrate that it was directing the minds of practitioners to safety and good communication.

Clinical governance and the duty of quality

The secretary of state for health in England has the power to prepare and publish statements of standards in relation to the provision of NHS care, which must be implemented by NHS organizations and are monitored by the CQC (Health and Social Care Act 2008, s. 45). Failures in this statutory duty could result in the removal of a board or the dismissal of its chief executive and chairman.

The National Institute of Health and Care Excellence (NICE), established in 1999, investigates medicines, and other treatments, and in the light of its research makes recommendations to the Department of Health on the clinical and cost effectiveness of such treatments.

See Box 9.5 for some of its maternity care guidance.

NICE guidelines should record the level of the evidence base for their recommendations, and they may be informative in determining the appropriate standard of care should an allegation of negligence be made (see earlier section on negligence).

Because they advocate a certain standard of care and service, the guidelines and recommendations made by NICE can also be used by practitioners to press for

---

Box 9.5 NICE maternity care guidance
Antenatal care (CB62) (2008)
Hypertension in pregnancy (CG107) (2010)
Pregnancy and complex social factors (CB110) (2010)
Caesarean section (CG132) (2011)
Multiple pregnancy (CG129) (2011)
Antenatal and postnatal mental health (CG192) (2014)
These and other relevant guidelines relating to midwifery services are available on the NICE website (www.nice.org.uk).

---

additional resources if they are aware that the standards of care and services provided in their units are lower than those nationally recommended.

FUTURE CHANGES

Recommendations for improvements to the maternity services are part of contemporary healthcare. Indeed, they have been so for many decades. Reviews are conducted, reports produced and targets set. Important reports over the years include *Changing Childbirth* (Department of Health 1993), the *Expert Group on Acute Maternity Services* (*EGAMS*; Scottish Executive 2003), *Maternity Matters* (Department of Health 2007), *Maternity Services in England* (National Audit Office 2013), *A Refreshed Framework for Maternity Services in Scotland* (Scottish Government 2011) and the *Welsh Government Maternity Strategy* (Welsh Government 2013). The Scottish government's current review of maternity services is due to report in 2016. The awareness that a healthy future for the country starts with healthy pregnancies now informs policy preparation. The aim always is to ensure that best practice is identified and, where possible, shared. The need for recommendations to have a sound evidence base is well recognized. Student midwives and qualified practitioners have a duty to stay up to date with changes that occur as a result of such reports.

MISCELLANEOUS LEGAL ISSUES OF RELEVANCE TO THE MIDWIFE

There are various miscellaneous issues relevant to midwives, such as care of property, vaccine damage and the rights of disabled children under the Congenital Disabilities (Civil Liability) Act 1976. Further information about these is given online.

CONCLUSION

This chapter covers a large area of law of considerable importance to midwifery practice. This is a very complex and dynamic area, and it is suggested that the reader should follow up this chapter by referring to some of the recommended texts and online sources. The current emphasis on human rights, the growth of litigation and the requirement that there must be sound professional practice all show the importance of midwives having an understanding of their practice's legal framework. It is essential, as in all other areas of their competence, that midwives keep up to date. In addition, it is clear from the many reports into the maternity services that there are individual and systemic failings. Some of the lessons outlined in this chapter may appear daunting, and it is an open question as to how the maternity services will be shaped in years to come. However, only by remaining up to date and, crucially, by continuing to care can the midwife ensure that his or her practice is optimal.

Key Points

- It is important that the midwife is aware of how laws, statutes and regulations are developed.
- An understanding of the rules and laws governing practice and healthcare can assist the practitioner in developing strategies and approaches that can improve care and prevent situations that might lead to litigation.
- It is crucial that midwives keep abreast of developments within the law.
- The principles of good communication and informed consent are key to quality of care and experience for clients and their relatives.

Acknowledgement

The author would like to acknowledge the significant contribution of Professor Brigid Dimond, the author of the equivalent chapter in the previous edition of this textbook, on which this chapter is based.

References

Bismark M, Paterson R: No-fault compensation in New Zealand: harmonizing injury compensation, provider accountability, and patient safety, *Health Aff* 25(1):278–283, 2006.

Department of Health: *Changing childbirth: report of the expert maternity group (the Cumberlege report)*, London, HMSO, 1993.

Department of Health: *Maternity matters: choice, access and continuity of care in a safe service*, London, DH, 2007.

Dimond B: *Legal aspects of midwifery*, 4th edn, London, Quay Books, 2013.

Francis R: *Report of the Mid Staffordshire Foundation Trust Public Inquiry – executive summary*, London, Stationary Office, 2013.

Griffith R: Deprivation of liberty in midwifery – taking a case to court, *Br J Midwifery* 22(11):822–823, 2014.

Griffith R: Midwives' duty of candour, *Br J Midwifery* 23(4):297–298, 2015.

Health and Safety Executive (HSE): *Reporting of injuries, diseases and dangerous occurrences regulations (RIDDOR)* (website). www.hse .gov.uk/pubns/indg453.htm. 1995.

Healthcare Commission: *Investigation into 10 maternal deaths at, or following delivery at, Northwick Park Hospital, North West London Hospitals NHS Trust, between April 2002 and April 2005*, London, Healthcare Commission, 2006.

Healthcare Commission: *Towards better births: a review of maternity services in England*, London, Stationery Office, 2008.

Hellbacher U, Espersson C, Johansson H: *Patient injury compensation for healthcare-related injuries*, Sweden, Patient Claims Panel, 2007.

Herring J: *Medical law and ethics*, 5th edn, Oxford, Oxford University Press, 2014.

Jackson E: *Medical law*, 2nd edn, Oxford, Oxford University Press, 2010.

Kennedy Report: *Bristol Royal Infirmary Inquiry–learning from Bristol: the report of the public inquiry into children's heart surgery at the Bristol Royal Infirmary 1984–1995*, Command paper Cm 5207, London, Stationery Office, 2001.

King's Fund: *Safe births: everybody's business. An independent inquiry into the safety of maternity services in England*, London, King's Fund, 2008.

Kirkup BC: *The report of the Morecambe Bay Investigation: an independent investigation into the management, delivery and outcomes of care provided by the maternity and neonatal services at the University Hospitals of Morecambe Bay NHS Foundation Trust from January 2004 to June 2013*, London, Stationery Office, 2015.

Mason JK, Laurie GT: *Law and medical ethics*, 9th edn, Oxford, Oxford University Press, 2013.

National Audit Office: *Maternity services in England*, London, NAO, 2013.

NHS Litigation Authority (NHSLA): *Annual report 2014/2015*, London, NHSLA, 2015.

Nursing and Midwifery Council (NMC): *Standards of proficiency for nurse and midwife prescribers*, London, NMC, 2006.

Nursing and Midwifery Council (NMC): *Standards for medicines management*, London, NMC, 2007.

Nursing and Midwifery Council (NMC): *Midwives rules and standards*, London, NMC, 2012.

Nursing and Midwifery Council (NMC): *Standards of competence for registered midwives*, London, NMC, 2014.

Nursing and Midwifery Council (NMC): *The Code: professional standards of practice and behaviour for nurses and midwives*, London, NMC, 2015a.

Nursing and Midwifery Council (NMC): *Openness and honesty when things go wrong: the professional duty of candour [Joint guidance with the General Medical Council on the professional duty of candour]* (website). www.nmc.org.uk/standards/guidance/the-professional-duty-of-candour/. 2015b.

Rose D: *Brain damaged woman is first successful case in Bristol baby scandal*, The Times 14 March, p. 11, 2008.

Royal College of Obstetrics and Gynaecology, Royal College of Midwives, Royal College of Anaesthetists & Royal College of Paediatrics and Child Health: *National standards for maternity care: Report of a working party*, London, RCOG, 2008.

Scottish Executive: *Expert Group on Acute Maternity Services [EGAMS]*, Edinburgh, Scottish Executive, 2003.

Scottish Government: *A refreshed framework for maternity services in Scotland*, Edinburgh, Scottish Government, 2011.

Symon A: No-fault compensation: back on the legislative agenda, *Br J Midwifery* 19(6):400–401, 2011.

Symon A: Expert witnesses under criticism, *Br J Midwifery* 2(9): 677–678, 2014.

Symon A: Landmark case on negligence and consent, *Br J Midwifery* 23(6):446–447, 2015.

Welsh Government: *Welsh government maternity strategy*, Cardiff, Welsh government, 2013.

Woolf, Lord: *Access to justice. Final Report by the Right Honourable the Lord Woolf, Master of the Rolls to the Lord Chancellor on the Civil Justice System in England and Wales*, London, HMSO, 1996.

Statutes, orders and regulations

The various statutes mentioned in this chapter can be found in the chapter online resources.

Legal cases

The key legal cases referred to in this chapter are given here. For the full list, please see the chapter online resources.

Barnett v. Chelsea Hospital Management Committee [1968] 1 All ER 1068.

Bolam v. Friern Hospital Management Committee [1957] 1 WLR 582.

Bolitho v. City and Hackney Health Authority (HA) [1997] 3 WLR 1151.

Donoghue v. Stevenson [1932] AC 562.

Hunter v. Hanley [1955] SC 200.

Montgomery v. Lanarkshire [2015] UKSC 11, on appeal from [2013] CSIH 3; [2010] CSIH 10.

Re C (Adult: Refusal of Medical Treatment) [1994] 1 All ER 819.

Re MB (Adult, Medical Treatment) [1997] 38 BMLR 175 CA.

Re S [1992] 3 WLR 806.

Sidaway v. Bethlem Royal Hospital Governors [1985] 1 All ER 643.

St George's Healthcare NHS Trust v. S [1998] 3 All ER 673.

Whitehouse v. Jordan [1981] 1 All ER 267.

Wilsher v. Essex Area Health Authority [1986] 3 All ER 801 CA, [1988] AC 1074 HL.

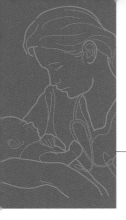

Chapter **10**

Pharmacology and the midwife

Professor Sue Jordan and Sue Macdonald

Learning Outcomes ?

After reading this chapter, you will be able to:
- appraise the potential benefits and harms of drugs administered in normal pregnancy, labour and the puerperium
- understand the actions of drugs commonly administered in childbirth
- use this knowledge to inform decisions on clinical monitoring, advice and advocacy
- understand the principles of safe dosage, storage and administration of medicines

Few women go through pregnancy, childbirth and the puerperium without receiving some form of medication. Ideally, all medicines' administration, management and monitoring would be based on the results of adequately sized randomized controlled trials with high response rates and representative samples, supported by large pharmacovigilance follow-up databases and service users' views (Jordan 2008; Jordan et al 2013). In practice, this 'gold standard' is rarely achieved in any discipline, and in midwifery there are additional ethical and practical difficulties, which are compounded when investigating the adverse reactions to prescribed medicines (Jordan 2010). Therefore, medication administration may be based on biological theories, observations, case reports or even 'custom and practice'.

THERAPEUTICS IN PREGNANCY AND CHILDBIRTH

Not all treatments are effective, and patients need to be monitored to detect nonresponse, particularly when antihypertensives, anticoagulants, antiemetics or analgesics are administered. Sometimes, underlying physiological problems may worsen, rendering a previously effective regimen useless; for example, as labour progresses, more analgesia may be required. More predictably, therapeutic failure may be induced by drug interactions – for example, if a patient with hypertension self-medicates with ibuprofen or another nonsteroidal anti-inflammatory drug (NSAID). Clinical response shows considerable individual variation, which is not always predictable, and idiosyncratic reactions can occur; for example, some women are unduly sensitive to oxytocin, and therefore infusions are commenced using very low doses.

Adverse reactions

An adverse drug reaction is any untoward and unintended response in a patient or investigational subject to a medicinal product that is related to any dose administered (International Conference on Harmonisation (ICH) 1996). Adverse drug reactions can be broadly divided into:
- dose-related and predictable,
- neither dose-related nor predictable, and
- transgenerational effects.

Dose-dependent adverse reactions

Dose-dependent adverse reactions are often the drug's main adverse effects. Because these are often significant and predictable, they are monitored. For example, without adequate monitoring, anticoagulants can cause bleeding, and insulin can cause hypoglycaemia.

Many drugs have more than one action, potentially causing diverse adverse reactions. For example, oxytocin acts on the oxytocic receptors of the uterus, but it also acts on the antidiuretic hormone (ADH) receptors in the nephrons and can cause water retention and fluid overload.

Adverse reactions unrelated to dose: hypersensitivity responses

Some of the most serious adverse events are unpredictable, *idiosyncratic, allergic* or *hypersensitivity* responses, which may occur in any situation with any drug at any dose: common offenders include antimicrobials (particularly intravenous), hormone preparations, dextrans, heparin, vaccines, blood products, iron injections and local anaesthetics. These adverse events are not related to known physiological actions of the drug, but they are initiated when drugs trigger the immune system of susceptible people. They include *anaphylaxis, drug rashes, bone marrow dysfunction* and *organ damage*.

A mild hypersensitivity reaction is usually a rash. Once this has occurred, and particularly if any itching was associated, the individual is likely to be sensitized and more likely to have an anaphylactic reaction at the next exposure. Where drugs have similar chemical structures, cross-allergies occur; for example, up to 10% of people allergic to *penicillins* will also be allergic to *cephalosporins*.

Transgenerational adverse reactions

Pregnancy, childbirth, breastfeeding or the developing infant may be affected.

DRUGS IN PREGNANCY

No drugs have been subjected to randomized controlled clinical trials for teratogenicity in human pregnancy; evidence is largely derived from observational studies, case reports of incidental exposure and animal studies; therefore, no drug has been demonstrated as 'safe'.

Approximately 5.2% of births and 4.5% of live births in Wales in 1998–2013 were associated with a congenital anomaly (Congenital Anomaly Register and Information Service for Wales (CARIS) 2014). The causes of about two-thirds of congenital anomalies remain unknown, and 2% to 3% are attributed to prescribed medicines (Niebyl 2008). Exposure of either parent to a medicinal product at any time during conception or pregnancy should be reported in association with congenital anomalies (ICH 1996).

Relatively few drugs are known to cause fetal malformations, but only drugs that have been used for many years in thousands of women with no evidence of harm can be designated 'generally regarded as safe'. No teratogenic drugs are harmful to the developing fetus in *all* cases. Estimates vary as to the incidence of congenital malformations: up to 30% with *warfarin*; up to 16% with *sodium valproate* (Aronson 2006). Some associations between prescribed medicines and congenital anomalies remain controversial; for example, although selective serotonin reuptake inhibitors (SSRIs) are prescribed to over 5% women in early pregnancy in the UK (Charlton et al

2014), only the most recent data indicates that the association with anomalies is unlikely to be attributable to maternal depression (Jordan et al 2016). Prescribed medicines may also affect fetal growth, birthweight, preterm delivery, childbirth, neonatal health (e.g. SSRIs (Jeffries et al 2011)) and childhood development (e.g. *valproic acid* (Bromley et al 2014)).

Fetus vulnerability is usually considered in stages (see chapter website resources also):

- *Preimplantation* (0–14 days): may result in death or no effect.
- *Cell division and implantation* (14–17 days): spontaneous abortion may follow exposure to some agents, such as cytotoxics.
- *Organ differentiation* (18–55 days): the crucial exposure period for teratogens, but the central nervous system (CNS), inner ear and palate continue developing after this.
- *Later stages of pregnancy:* the functioning, rather than the structure, of organs may be damaged throughout pregnancy by several drugs, including *alcohol, cocaine, insulin, furosemide* and *antithyroid agents*. Exposure to *valproic acid* (at a dose >800 mg) in pregnancy is associated with reduced cognitive performance, but it is recognized that *valproic acid* is sometimes the only way to control seizures (Bromley et al 2014).

Drug administration during pregnancy and breastfeeding is based on assessment of potential harms and benefits. Prescribing is likely to be restricted if drug exposure is known to result in a consistent pattern of similar anomalies or the incidence of congenital anomalies is above the rate in the population of 4% to 5%. The risks of fetal damage depend on several factors and the chemical composition of the drug:

- Stage of pregnancy
- Amount or dose of drug ingested
- Number of doses (e.g. a single dose may be less damaging than repeated exposure)
- Other agents to which mother and fetus are exposed
- Mother's nutritional status
- Genetic makeup of mother and fetus

This is complicated by epidemiological work linking congenital malformations, particularly cleft lip, cleft palate and congenital heart malformations, with adverse life events associated with severe maternal stress during the first trimester (Hansen et al 2000) and research linking stillbirth with high levels of psychological stress (Wisborg et al 2008).

Drugs in childbirth

Drugs given during childbirth may have long-term effects. Antibiotics may alter the microorganisms in the neonate's colon, which, in turn, might affect the regulation of the immune system, allowing development of allergy (Jordan et al 2008; Francinio 2014), but reduce the risk of infection following caesarean (Smaill and Grivell 2014). Also, drugs administered in labour may reduce the chances of breast-feeding (see following discussion on opioids).

Pharmacology in pregnancy and lactation

The actions and adverse reactions of any drug depend on the drug and its interactions with the body (*pharmacodynamics*) and on the concentration of the drug in the tissues, which is affected by how the drug is administered, absorbed, distributed and eliminated (*pharmacokinetics*). Following administration, drugs are absorbed and distributed to their sites of action before being removed from the body; if elimination is compromised, there is a risk of drug accumulation and toxicity in either the woman or the fetus/neonate.

Breastfed infants

Most drugs pass into breastmilk, but the concentrations are often too small to be harmful. Drugs that can be administered to neonates are usually suitable for nursing mothers, for example, *paracetamol*. For a few drugs, such as *fluoxetine, lithium* or *clozapine,* there are reports of serious adverse reactions in infants (Merlob and Schaefer 2015).

DRUG ADMINISTRATION AND ABSORPTION

Absorption makes the drug available for distribution. The extent to which a drug reaches its destination is its 'bio-availability' (Wilkinson 2001: 5) and depends on formulation and route of administration.

The formulation of a medicine refers to its physical and chemical composition and includes active ingredients and other chemicals present, the *excipients* or 'packing chemicals'. Excipients:

- Stabilize the active ingredient or modify its release.
- Are listed in the product information.
- May be responsible for adverse reactions; for example, sodium can be responsible for fluid retention and sugar for dental caries.
- May vary between brands; for example, brands of antiepileptic drugs, mood stabilizers or antipsychotics should not be regarded as interchangeable without advice from a pharmacist or consultant.

Routes of administration

Oral:

- Most convenient drug administration route.
- Presence of food, antacids or bulk laxatives in the stomach can affect drug absorption for up to 2 hours – for example, *amoxicillin, thyroxine, iron.*
- Administration with food is sometimes advantageous in smoothing the absorption profile – for example, *nifedipine, iron.*
- Drug molecules from the stomach or small intestine pass to the liver, where they are metabolized and detoxified before entering the systemic circulation. This reduces and delays absorption to a varying, and not always predictable, extent.

Intravenous administration:

- Employed when rapid, reliable and complete absorption is required.

Intramuscular injections:

- Rapidly deliver drugs to the bloodstream.
- Haemorrhage or shock may delay absorption and adverse reactions.

Subcutaneous injections:

- Slower absorption.

Sublingual or buccal administration:

- Bypasses the liver.
- Rapid, not necessarily predictable, action.
- Can be useful in emergencies, including recurrent seizures or hypoglycaemia.

Rectal route:

- Cultural considerations and practical difficulties.
- Useful for short-term drug administration, if other routes unavailable.
- Laxatives, antiemetics, analgesics and treatments for ulcerative colitis are sometimes administered this way.
- Drugs absorbed from the upper two-thirds of the rectum pass to the liver.
- Those absorbed from the lower region enter the general circulation – absorption unpredictable.

Topical applications:

- Examples, direct application to skin, eyes or ears.
- Systemic effects are reduced, but not abolished, and the same adverse drug reactions can occur.

Intrathecal (spinal) and epidural administration:

- Increases the proportion of drug reaching the central nervous system.

- Following intrathecal administration, drug diffuses into the epidural space before circulating (Eltzschig et al 2003). Appreciable quantities are absorbed into the epidural venous plexus and pass to the general circulation, the brain and the fetus.

- Headache, pruritus and fetal bradycardia (Collis et al 2008) and problems with catheter removal (Arkoosh et al 2008) may occur more commonly with intrathecal than epidural analgesia.

- Technical problems include: failure to flex the spine; kinking of lines; accidental removal of lines; dural puncture; need for reinsertion (Paech 1998).

- Complications include: puncture site tenderness for up to 7 days; dural puncture headache; intravascular injection; infection; epidural haematoma; abscess formation; accidental total spinal anaesthesia (Schrock and Harraway-Smith 2012). Around 4 in 1 million women suffer persistent neurological complications (Ruppen et al 2006).

Therapeutic range

Every drug has a therapeutic range for the concentration of drug in plasma and tissues: above this, toxic effects are more likely; below it, the drug is less likely to have the desired effect. For some drugs, the range is narrow, and the therapeutic concentration is close to the concentration at which side effects appear; for example, antiepileptic drugs, *warfarin, insulin, opioids*. For others, the therapeutic range is wide in most individuals, and there is a larger 'safety margin' between therapeutic and toxic dose. For example, in people not suffering from epilepsy, *penicillins* and *folic acid* are relatively safe, even in overdose.

For a medicine with a narrow therapeutic range, dose administration intervals are calculated to prevent more than twofold fluctuations in plasma concentrations. If strict adherence to dose intervals fails, both toxicity and therapeutic failure are likely. For example, where these drugs require administration twice each day, they should be given 12 hours apart (Wilkinson 2001). Where medicines must be given four times a day – that is, every 6 hours – this may involve disturbing sleep.

Drug distribution

Movement of drugs around the body is affected by drug properties (lipid solubility and binding), state of the circulation and other organs, pregnancy, breastfeeding and infancy. Highly lipid-soluble drugs rapidly pass into the brain, fetus and breastmilk. For example, *diamorphine* and *fentanyl* are distributed more rapidly than *morphine* – advantageous during emergency caesarean births.

Pregnancy

Most drugs are lipid soluble and cross the placenta during pregnancy, to varying extents, but not all are harmful.

Childbirth

The placenta is an ineffective barrier to the passage of drugs, and the blood–brain barrier is underdeveloped in the fetus. Permeability may be further increased during stress, labour and hypoxia. Drugs administered in labour may enter the fetus, and may cause adverse reactions in the neonate; for example, opioids, local anaesthetics or magnesium can induce respiratory depression.

Lactation

Most drugs pass into breastmilk (though concentrations are often too small to be harmful): the amount varies between women, during feeds, with the age of the infant and with use of a breast pump. The relative dose as a proportion of body weight received by the infant depends on the drug administered (for example, the dose of *lithium* is up to 80% of maternal dose) and the maturity of the infant's liver and kidneys (Merlob and Schaefer 2015).

Neonates

The body of the neonate contains a relatively high proportion of water and a low proportion of fat. Any lipid-soluble drugs are therefore distributed into a small volume. Thus, neonates, particularly premature babies, receive different drug doses from adults, even when body weight is taken into consideration.

Elimination or clearance of drugs

Route of elimination varies with individual drugs, but most are:

- Metabolized in the liver
- Excreted in the kidneys

A few drugs (such as *magnesium, lithium*) are eliminated unchanged, whereas others are extensively metabolized. Some metabolites are active, for example, those of *carbamazepine* and *opioids*, whereas others may cause adverse reactions, such as *norpethidine (normeperidine)*. Most drugs are excreted via the kidneys, although bile is also an important route of excretion, for example, for *oestrogens* and *corticosteroids*.

Drug metabolism

Most metabolism takes place in the liver, although the gastrointestinal tract and the central nervous system contain enzymes responsible for the metabolism of some drugs. Metabolism deals with and detoxifies foreign substances. Metabolism varies with:

- Genetic makeup/familial tendencies.
- Drug interactions: rate of metabolism and elimination may be increased or decreased by drugs, foods or herbal products.
- Pregnancy: elimination of some medicines (e.g. lamotrigine, SSRIs) increases in the first trimester, making them ineffective at usual doses. Women prescribed lamotrigine need specialist advice as early as possible to reduce the risk of therapeutic failure and seizures (Centre for Maternal and Child Enquiries (CMACE) 2011).

Drug excretion

Most drugs depend on the kidneys for excretion. Glomerular filtration rate (GFR) is usually considered the best overall measure of the kidneys' ability to eliminate drugs in health and disease (Levey et al 1999). It is the volume of fluid filtered into the nephrons every minute, that is, the sum of the volume of filtrate formed each minute in all the functioning nephrons in the kidneys. This represents about 20% of the plasma flowing through the kidneys. In normal pregnancy, the circulating volume expands by some 8 litres, and renal plasma flow and GFR rise by 30% to 50% in the second trimester and decline towards term. This increases the elimination of certain drugs (Loebstein et al 1997). Therefore, doses of ongoing therapeutic regimens may need to be increased, particularly antiepileptic drugs and low-molecular-weight heparins. By the fourth week of pregnancy, GFR has risen 20%; therefore, increased drug elimination and decreased drug effects may occur before the woman realizes she is pregnant (Perrone et al 1992).

If GFR falls, elimination of most drugs is impaired, causing accumulation and even toxicity. If GFR is below normal, as occurs in pre-eclampsia, most drugs are administered in reduced doses or at prolonged intervals. In seriously ill women, rapidly changing GFR may complicate administration of *magnesium sulphate*.

The kidneys of the fetus eliminate drugs slowly into the amniotic fluid, which is then ingested through the mouth, further reducing clearance. The GFR of the neonate is only 30% to 40% of adult values. Therefore, some drugs, such as *magnesium*, may accumulate following maternal administration. These neonates should be observed for signs of muscle weakness, including respiratory depression, for 48 hours after delivery. Some drugs, such as *lithium*, may accumulate during breastfeeding.

Pharmacodynamics

Most drugs work as a result of the physiochemical interactions between drug molecules and the recipient's molecules:

cell receptors, ion channels or enzymes. These chemical reactions may alter the way cells function, which in turn may lead to changes in the behaviour of tissues, organs and systems.

An agonist will bind to a receptor and alter its functioning. For example, *salbutamol*, prescribed for asthma or tocolysis, is a beta$_2$-agonist, and *pethidine* is an opioid agonist. Agonists usually augment the normal function of the receptors to which they bind. For example, *pethidine* stimulates the opioid receptors, increasing analgesia, sedation and constipation. Likewise, beta-agonists mimic some of the actions of the sympathetic nervous system, increasing heart rate, dilating bronchioles and relaxing the uterus.

An antagonist will bind to a receptor, blocking it and preventing the agonist reaching its site of action. For example, *naloxone* (*Narcan*) blocks the opioid receptors and reverses the actions of *pethidine, fentanyl or morphine,* reducing respiratory depression and sedation, but causing return of pain. Similarly, the beta-blockers (*propranolol, atenolol, labetalol*) block the actions of the sympathetic nervous system, slow and stabilize the heart rate and induce bronchoconstriction; they are contraindicated for people who suffer from asthma because of the risk of life-threatening narrowing of the airways (British Medical Association (BMA) and Royal Pharmaceutical Society of Great Britain (RPSGB) 2015: 101).

Most drugs act on more than one type of cell and therefore have multiple effects on the body. For example, nicotine acts on the central nervous system to 'calm the nerves', on the blood vessels to raise blood pressure and on the respiratory epithelium to cause irritation. Other drugs are relatively specific; for example, *penicillins* act almost exclusively on bacterial cell walls.

Where drugs act on the same or similar receptors, ion channels or enzymes have similar actions or adverse reactions; their actions are intensified if they are coadministered. For example, coadministration of two or more sedatives can cause respiratory depression.

The cells' receptors are continually being renewed by their protein-synthesizing machinery. When a drug is administered over a period of time, the cells or their receptors may adapt: the number of receptors available on the cell surface may change in response to the presence of drugs.

Tolerance or desensitization

The continued presence of an agonist may reduce the number of relevant receptors available. This desensitization or downregulation of receptors is believed to be responsible for the loss of response seen with continued use of *opiates, oxytocin* or *beta$_2$-agonists* (bronchodilators). For example, prolonged administration of *oxytocin* may render the uterine muscle unresponsive, leading to the uterus not contracting following delivery, increasing the risk of postpartum haemorrhage. In these circumstances, the uterus will not respond to *oxytocin* and other agents (e.g. *prostaglandins, ergometrine*) will be needed to combat the haemorrhage (Robinson et al 2003).

Supersensitivity

Conversely, the continued presence of an antagonist or blocking drug may increase the number of receptors. Therefore, if an antagonist is abruptly discontinued, the tissues may be unduly sensitive. For example, abrupt withdrawal of beta-blockers makes the myocardium unduly responsive to stress, which increases the risk of a heart attack.

DRUGS IN LABOUR

Analgesics

- Inhalational analgesia
- Opioids
- Local anaesthetics (see chapter website resources)

Many women request pharmacological pain relief during labour, and all analgesics have advantages and disadvantages.

Inhalational analgesia: nitrous oxide with oxygen (Entonox)

Widespread use of *nitrous oxide* for over a hundred years has established its relative safety (de Vasconcellos and Sneyd 2013). Nevertheless, administration requires close supervision. There is no evidence that *Entonox* affects the progress of labour or breastfeeding. Other methods of analgesia are more effective but are associated with more adverse reactions, both short and long term.

Inhalation analgesia is achieved by the use of an anaesthetic gas, nitrous oxide, in subanaesthetic concentrations. Concentrations of 50% nitrous oxide are needed for effective analgesia. If administered with air, rather than oxygen, hypoxia would ensue. Nitrous oxide is now administered as *Entonox*, using piped supplies or premixed cylinders of 50% nitrous oxide in 50% oxygen as a homogenous gas (BOC 2011). Nitrous oxide rapidly passes from the lungs to the circulation and brain. Analgesic effects of nitrous oxide are experienced some 25 to 35 seconds after administration, persisting for about 60 seconds after inhalation ceases. Therefore, women are advised to inhale at the beginning of a contraction, rather than wait for the pain to reach a crescendo.

Being lipid soluble, inhalation agents cross the placenta and enter adipose tissue. The concentration of nitrous oxide in the fetus reaches 80% of maternal values within 3 minutes of administration. Like all anaesthetic gases, it is rapidly eliminated through the lungs after delivery. This is an advantage over other analgesics, which depend on the immature liver and kidneys for removal. In both mother and neonate, it is estimated that the effects of *Entonox* have worn off after 2 to 3 minutes, although removal from tissues with low blood flow, such as fat, takes longer (Kennedy and Longnecker 1996).

When *Entonox* is inhaled, the women may overbreathe to maximize analgesia, risking the exhalation of too much carbon dioxide, lowering the concentration in the blood, and causing:

- Vasoconstriction of the placental bed and fetal hypoxia
- Maternal hypoventilation between contractions, leading to fetal hypoxia
- Cerebral vasoconstriction, causing dizziness
- Alkalosis, which may induce tetany

Therefore, women's respirations must be closely supervised during administration of *Entonox*.

Actions and adverse reactions

Anaesthetic gases gradually suppress the reticular activating system in the brainstem, producing four stages, or depths, of anaesthesia:

1. Analgesia
2. Delirium
3. Surgical anaesthesia
4. Depression of the vital centres of the medulla.

When *Entonox* is administered, the aim is to achieve analgesia – excessive administration may give the second stage of anaesthesia, characterized by 'lightheadedness', dizziness, nausea or 'laughing'. Sedation or confusion may occur, although nitrous oxide is insufficiently powerful to produce surgical anaesthesia when used alone. Neonates' respirations may be depressed. Prolonged exposure to nitrous oxide can inactivate vitamin B_{12} and may affect pregnancy, and exposure of theatre staff also needs to be monitored (BOC 2011; BMA and RPSGB 2015).

Interactions

The respiratory depressant action of opioids or other sedatives may be compounded by nitrous oxide, causing transient maternal hypoxia (Clyburn and Rosen 1993).

Cautions

Nitrous oxide is contraindicated where abnormal quantities of gas are trapped within the body, for example, in women with middle ear occlusion or sinus infections (BOC 2011). Nitrous oxide may also diffuse into air bubbles formed by epidural or intrathecal analgesia, hindering the spread of local anaesthetic (Sweetman et al 2007).

Nitrous oxide should not be administered to women whose level of consciousness is already impaired.

To avoid combustion risk, *Entonox* should not come into contact with oils, oil-based creams, alcohol gels or smoke (BOC 2011).

To reduce the risk of cross-infection, including hepatitis C, appropriate microbiological filters should be placed between the patient and the breathing system; supplying clean masks and mouthpieces is imperative, but may not be sufficient (Association of Anaesthetists of Great Britain and Ireland (AAGBI) 1996; Chilvers and Weisz 2000).

Opioids

The term *opioid* is used to describe any preparation acting on the body's opioid receptors, which normally respond to endorphins and enkephalins, the body's natural mood changers and analgesics. Thus, *morphine*®, *diamorphine*®, *pethidine*®, *meptazinol*®, *codeine*®, *buprenorphine*® *(Temgesic*®), *pentazocine*® *(Fortral*®), *fentanyl*® and its derivatives and the 'morphine antagonists' such as *naloxone*® *(Narcan*®) are all opioids.

Opioids are used in labour, preoperatively, intraoperatively, postoperatively and in intensive care, for analgesia, sedation and reduction of anxiety. Administration may be intramuscular, intravenous, epidural, intrathecal, oral, transdermal or buccal.

Opioids are rapidly transferred across the blood–brain barrier, the placenta and into colostrum. Transfer is more rapid and complete for the more lipophilic compounds, such as *diamorphine, fentanyl* and *fentanyl derivatives*. The fetus and neonate excrete opioids more slowly than adults because of the immaturity of their liver enzymes. The concentration of opioids will always be higher in the fetus than in the woman, in proportion to the dose administered. This delayed clearance allows accumulation in the central nervous system, which could be sufficient to produce subtle behavioural changes, such as depression of feeding reflexes (Jordan et al 2005).

Following a single intramuscular dose of *pethidine* to the mother, the fetus receives maximum exposure 2 to 3 hours later; therefore, respiratory depression in the neonate is most likely in babies born at this time. If birth occurs within 1 hour of *pethidine* administration, very little drug is transferred to the fetus. Should birth occur more than 6 hours after administration, much of the *pethidine* will have been transferred back to the mother, although the active metabolite, normeperidine, will remain in the neonatal tissues and is gradually excreted over several days. During this time the neonate's behaviour will be suboptimal (irritable and difficult to feed) (Crowell et al 1994).

Pethidine passes into breastmilk, which compounds early difficulties with feeding.

Epidural and intrathecal administration

Epidural administration entails injection into the fat in the narrow space between the dura mater and the bony canal.

Intrathecal administration involves placing the drug in the cerebrospinal fluid (CSF) by passing a very thin needle through the dura mater.

Opioids and local anaesthetics may be administered epidurally or intrathecally or in combination as combined spinal-epidural (CSE) analgesia. These are the most effective strategies for pain relief. Epidural or CSE analgesia is usually achieved and maintained with *bupivacaine* and *fentanyl*, with *diamorphine* reserved for urgent situations (NCC 2004).

Following epidural administration, drugs diffuse through the dura, where they act on the receptors in the spinal cord. Absorption is increased at delivery when the mother is spontaneously pushing, and 'top up' injections are usually avoided at this time.

Actions of opioids

Opioid receptor binding triggers changes within nerve or smooth muscle cells, usually inhibiting their activity and neurotransmitter release. Several classes of opioid receptors exist, and each opioid acts selectively.

In general, opioids (endogenous and pharmacological) depress the activity of target tissues and have a calming effect. They inhibit the hypothalamus and 'damp down' the level of activity in the autonomic nervous system, partly by reducing the stress response attributable to noradrenaline (norepinephrine). Sometimes, sedation, mental detachment or euphoria are the predominant effects, and the woman may be able to tolerate pain while still perceiving sensations.

Opioids regulate endocrine, gastrointestinal, autonomic and immune systems, and may trigger histamine release. They also act directly on the chemoreceptor trigger zone, which activates the vomiting centre, and interact with dopamine in the areas of the brain associated with 'reward'.

Adverse reactions

Opioids produce drowsiness, mental clouding and sometimes euphoria. They inhibit the vital centres in the brainstem of mother and neonate. Sedation is intensified with higher doses and intravenous administration. Administration of more than 100 micrograms of epidural *fentanyl* or more than 10 micrograms of intrathecal *fentanyl* or equivalent may sedate and depress the respirations of infants (Carvalho 2008), particularly if administered 1 to 4 hours before birth.

Respiratory depression

Opioids act directly on the respiratory centre to depress respiration. They reduce the sensitivity of the respiratory centre to carbon dioxide, thereby depressing the normal drive to respiration. Therefore, respiration fails to increase to meet the high metabolic demands of labour. Rate, depth and regularity of respirations are decreased, reducing alveolar ventilation and oxygenation. This effect is intensified if the woman becomes so sedated that she falls asleep. If the circulation is adequate, respiratory depression is maximal within 90 minutes of intramuscular administration. Following administration of normal doses of intrathecal or epidural opioids, maternal respiratory depression, apnoea and sedation may occur 30 minutes later or be delayed up to 16 hours (Clyburn and Rosen 1993).

Respiratory depression during labour may lead to:

- Retention of carbon dioxide and respiratory acidosis, in mother and fetus
- Hypoxia in mother and fetus, which causes fetal heart rate decelerations
- Acidosis in the fetus – increasing accumulation of *pethidine* and metabolites

In the neonate, measurements with fetal scalp electrodes indicate that transcutaneous oxygen tensions fall to 37% of baseline values 7 minutes after the intramuscular administration of 50 mg *pethidine* but recover within 15 minutes (Clyburn and Rosen 1993). Depression of the central nervous system reduces the neonate's reflexes, including the respiratory reflexes needed to cope with hypoxia and birth (Wagner 1993). Neonatal respiratory depression is occasionally sufficiently severe to warrant rapid reversal with *naloxone*.

Bradycardia

Opioids reduce the heart rate by direct action on the cardiovascular centres in the medulla, decreasing the activity of the sympathetic nervous system and reducing anxiety. In labour, this may contribute to a fall in blood pressure and a reduction in placental perfusion. The subsequent depression of the fetal heart rate and loss of fetal heart baseline variability may be interpreted as fetal distress, triggering medical interventions.

Some fetal bradycardia (<100 bpm) on administration of opioid analgesia by any route is normal, attributed to the transient release of oxytocin, causing a brief tetanic contraction of the uterus (Eberle and Norris 1996). Bradycardia lasting beyond 3 minutes may be a sign of metabolic stress (Arkoosh 1991) and cause for concern (National Collaborating Centre for Women's and Children's Health (NCC) 2014).

Hypotension

Opioids act on the cardiovascular centres, blood vessels and sympathetic nervous system to produce a fall in blood pressure, exaggerated on standing or sitting up, partly as a result of inhibition of the baroreceptor reflex. Any hypotension is likely to be exaggerated by the fetus compressing the maternal aorta and vena cava if the mother adopts the supine position.

When opioids are administered epidurally or intrathecally, hypotension is likely to occur within 30 minutes of administration. This may be accompanied by severe fetal bradycardia (Richardson 2000).

Thermoregulation

Opioids impair thermoregulation. Extra care needs to be taken to ensure that the neonate is kept warm.

Breastfeeding

Opioids administered in labour transfer into the fetus, impairing coordination and suckling (Jordan et al 2005). Women who have received high doses of analgesics in labour may need extra support over the first 1 to 3 days to support and establish breastfeeding (Jordan 2006).

Prolonged labour

The initial brief tetanic uterine contraction (Eberle and Norris 1996) is superseded by reduced contractility of uterine smooth muscle as a result of decreased release of oxytocin (Carter 2003). Opioids reduce both the uterine response to oxytocin and oxytocin release from the posterior pituitary (Thompson and Hillier 1994), diminishing uterine contractions (Carter 2003).

Retention of urine and dysuria

Opioids inhibit the smooth muscle of the bladder and the voiding reflex – a full bladder may inhibit uterine contractions both during labour and postpartum.

Gastrointestinal effects

Opioids inhibit the propulsive, peristaltic actions of the gut while increasing segmental, nonpropulsive contractions, particularly in the pyloric region of the stomach, the first part of the duodenum and the colon. Gastric stasis may cause nausea, vomiting, oesophageal reflux or inhalational pneumonia (BMA and RPSGB 2015). Opioids contribute to the constipation that commonly follows delivery and decrease gastrointestinal secretions, causing a dry mouth. Spasm of the biliary tract, producing pain on the right side of the abdomen, and gastrointestinal obstruction are rare adverse reactions.

Pruritus

Inhibition of peripheral nerves transmitting pain signals and histamine release may cause flushing, itching, 'nettle rash' and sweating, particularly following intrathecal administration (Simmons et al 2007; Kumar and Singh 2013).

Other potential problems

These include:

- Myoclonus
- Muscle rigidity
- Fluid imbalance

- Suppressed immune responses
- Bronchospasm
- Hallucinations

Cautions and contraindications

These include:

- Increased intracranial pressure (stroke, head injury): opioids may increase intracranial pressure and obscure vital signs/pupil reflexes.
- Decreased respiratory reserve, including obesity and kyphosis; contraindicated if carbon dioxide partial pressure is increased
- Pregnancy (long-term use) and breastfeeding
- Known allergy or dependence on opioids
- Renal insufficiency
- Neonates and premature babies require proportionately lower doses – fentanyl may cause jaundice.

Conditions that may be worsened include:

- Asthma
- Convulsive disorders (particularly *tramadol, pethidine*)
- Biliary colic, pancreatitis
- Conditions where there is a possibility of paralytic ileus
- Pre-existing hypotension – for example, as a result of haemorrhage
- Hypothyroidism or Addison's disease
- Acute alcohol intoxication
- Liver failure
- Phaeochromocytoma
- Myasthenia gravis

Interactions

Hypotension, sedation and respiratory depression may be intensified by alcohol, antihistamines, barbiturates, anaesthetics (nitrous oxide), benzodiazepines, metoclopramide, antipsychotics, tricyclic antidepressants, and other non-opioid sedatives. Protease inhibitors, cimetidine and, occasionally, ranitidine may have this effect. SSRIs may cause hypo- or hypertension.

Central nervous system toxicity may occur if *pethidine* or *fentanyl* are administered within 2 weeks of any *monoamine oxidase inhibitors* (MAOIs; including *moclobemide* and, possibly, *linezolid*) or *selegiline* or *rasagiline* (for Parkinson's).

Myoclonus is more likely with coadministration of *chlorpromazine, haloperidol, amitriptyline* and some *NSAIDs* (but not *diclofenac*).

Drying of secretions, and therefore need for mouth care, is intensified by coadministration of *hyoscine, cyclizine* or related drugs (see antiemetics).

Uterotonics

Uterotonics or oxytocics are used for induction and augmentation of labour, prevention and treatment of postpartum haemorrhage and control of bleeding resulting from incomplete abortion. The uterotonics used in the UK are:

- Prostaglandins
- Oxytocin
- Ergometrine
- Syntometrine – a combination of oxytocin and ergometrine

Prostaglandins

Prostaglandins are 'local hormones' and are used to stimulate uterine contractions.

- *Dinoprostone* (PGE_2), for cervical priming and induction of labour, is administered vaginally.
- *Carboprost* (15-methyl-$PGF_{2\alpha}$, synthetic derivative), for postpartum haemorrhage, is given by deep intramuscular injection.

Actions and adverse reactions

Prostaglandins act on distinct prostaglandin receptors, affect many systems and can occasionally cause adverse effects, including hypotension, bronchospasm, pyrexia, sensitization to pain, inflammation, glaucoma, tremor and diuresis. Hypertension may complicate administration of *carboprost*.

Following vaginal administration, the most important adverse reaction is uterine hyperstimulation. Uterine contractions may become abnormal and too intense, leading to pain, fetal compromise or even rupture of the uterus or cervix. Previous caesarean delivery or uterine surgery are contraindications (BMA and RPSGB 2015). Lower doses and, possibly, gel formulations of *dinoprostone* present less risk (NCC 2008).

Oxytocin

Oxytocin (Syntocinon) is manufactured to reproduce the structure and actions of the natural hormone. These actions include:

- Uterine contraction at term both by direct action on smooth muscle and by increased prostaglandin production
- Constriction of umbilical blood vessels
- Contraction of myoepithelial cells (milk ejection reflex)
- Development of bonding (Leng et al 2008)
- Attenuation of the stress response (Slattery and Neumann 2008)

- Sudden increase or decrease in blood pressure (particularly diastolic)
- Water retention

High-dose oxytocin can shorten prolonged labours (Blanch et al 1998; Sadler et al 2000), but can also increase the risk of uterine hyperstimulation and associated adverse infant outcomes (NCC 2014). Failure of induction necessitating emergency caesarean is more likely if the woman has a high body mass index or the baby is heavy (McEwan 2007).

Oxytocin is administered for:

- Induction of labour
- Augmentation or stimulation of delayed labour by intravenous infusion, to shorten first stage (NCC 2014)
- Prevention of postpartum haemorrhage, either by:
  - Intramuscular injection – alone, as recommended (Centre for Maternal and Child Enquiries (CMACE) 2011, NCC 2014) or combined with *ergometrine* – as *Syntometrine*
  - Slow intravenous injection or intravenous infusion for high-risk women or following caesarean delivery (CEMACH 2005)
- Treatment of postpartum haemorrhage by slow intravenous injection or infusion
- Incomplete, inevitable or missed abortion (BMA and RPSGB 2015)

Oxytocin acts within 1 to 4 minutes of intravenous administration; increased uterine contractions begin almost immediately, stabilize within 15 to 60 minutes of commencing intravenous infusion and last for 20 minutes after discontinuation. Oxytocin is removed by enzymes in the liver, spleen, ovaries and placenta. Estimates of half-life range from 1 to 20 minutes; pharmacological data indicates a value of 15 minutes (Gonser 1995).

Adverse reactions

Overstimulation of the uterus

When oxytocin is administered, the frequency and force of smooth muscle contractions are increased, intensifying the labour pain, more so than prostaglandins (NCC 2008). Women report that oxytocin-induced contractions are more painful than those of spontaneous labour. Augmentation of labour with oxytocin carries an inherent risk of uterine hyperstimulation: because some individuals are hypersensitive to oxytocin, infusion always entails risk of tetanic or spasmodic uterine contractions, however low the dose.

During uterine contraction, blood vessels are compressed, impairing delivery of oxygen to the uterus, placenta and fetus. Normally, oxygenation is restored during relaxation, preventing the accumulation of lactic acid. However, if the uterus is overstimulated and relaxation is too brief, fetal hypoxia and acidosis will follow. Uterine tetany or spasm may reduce uterine blood flow to a point where the fetus is asphyxiated.

Fluid retention

Oxytocin, particularly in high doses, mimics the actions of antidiuretic hormone, and without careful monitoring it may produce dangerous fluid retention. Any water retained passes, by osmosis, from plasma into tissue fluids, and thence into the cells, which swell. This causes confusion and disorientation, progressing to convulsions with or without oedema, raised jugular venous pressure and pulmonary oedema, which impairs breathing and oxygenation. The danger is greatest with administration of prolonged high doses of *oxytocin*, accompanied by infusions of large volumes of electrolyte-free or hypotonic fluids, such as 5% glucose (BMA and RPSGB 2015). In reported cases of water intoxication, more than 3.5 litres of fluid had been infused (Sweetman et al 2007).

Changes in blood pressure

In conjunction with its antidiuretic actions, oxytocin may induce vasoconstriction and hypertension, particularly in women with pre-eclampsia. In contrast, administration of large amounts of oxytocin may cause vasodilatation and a sudden profound fall in blood pressure. Vasodilatation complicates haemorrhage.

Postpartum haemorrhage

Protracted administration, particularly at high doses, may exhaust and desensitize the uterine muscle, leaving it unable to contract and respond to oxytocin, increasing postpartum haemorrhage risk. Observational studies have linked induction of labour with increased incidence of postpartum haemorrhage (Magann et al 2005).

Other adverse effects of oxytocin include nausea, hypersensitivity responses, and, possibly, reduced chances of breastfeeding (Jordan et al 2009; Out et al 1988; Rajan 1994; Wiklund et al 2009).

Breastfeeding

In view of the possible disruption to the delicate homeostatic balance at the sensitive transition period of parturition, the impact of exogenous oxytocin on breastfeeding success needs further research (Jordan et al 2009).

Cautions and scontraindications

Oxytocin is contraindicated in the following situations:

- The uterus is already contracting vigorously and/or labour has progressed well (Knight et al 2014)
- Fetal distress

- Vaginal birth not advised (e.g. presence of a mechanical obstruction to delivery and risk of uterine rupture)
- Oxytocin-induced uterine inertia
- Severe cardiovascular disease or pre-eclampsia, risk of disseminated intravascular coagulation (BMA and RPSGB 2015)

Cautions

- Oxytocin alone should not be used for induction of labour (NCC 2008).
- Potential disruption to fluid balance and blood pressure makes oxytocin unsuitable for women with pre-eclampsia, cardiovascular disease or those aged over 35 years (BMA and RPSGB 2015).
- 'Starved uterus': muscle contraction requires both glucose and oxygen. If either of these is not supplied to the contracting muscle, as a result of starvation or inadequate blood supply (most likely to arise in prolonged labour), the response to oxytocin will be inadequate, and dose increments will be ineffective (Clayworth 2000).

Interactions

- Prostaglandins, oestrogens: if more than one agent promoting uterine contractility is administered, uterine overstimulation is more likely. Six hours should elapse between prostaglandin and oxytocin administration for induction (BMA and RPSGB 2015).
- Vasoconstrictors, such as *ephedrine* or *adrenaline* used in caudal block, can induce hypertension (BMA and RPSGB 2015).
- Drugs predisposing to cardiac arrhythmia (long QTc syndrome) (Novartis 2015)
- Blood, plasma or metabisulphite will inactivate oxytocin if infused in the same intravenous giving set (Novartis 2015).

Ergometrine

Ergometrine, used alone, remains important in the management of acute postpartum or postabortion haemorrhage. With oxytocin in *Syntometrine* (comprising *ergometrine 500* micrograms plus 5 units *oxytocin*), it is widely used prophylactically for the active management of the third stage of labour.

When *Syntometrine* is administered:

- The almost immediate effects of oxytocin are followed by the slightly delayed and more sustained contractions induced by *ergometrine*.

- *Ergometrine* acts on the inner region of the myometrium, whereas oxytocin and prostaglandins act on the outer myometrium (de Groot et al 1998).

Onset of action is within 1 minute with intravenous administration and within 3 to 7 minutes with intramuscular administration. Duration of action is 3 to 8 hours. Excretion is via the kidneys.

Actions and adverse reactions

Actions on alpha$_1$ and serotonin receptors underlie the uterine and gut contractility brought about by *ergometrine*.

Contraction of the uterus

Ergometrine has a rapid stimulant effect on the uterus, particularly at term. There is a danger that the uterus will fail to relax between contractions, and *ergometrine* is never administered before the delivery of all fetuses. Retention of placental fragments may account for the reported association with increased problems with bleeding in the first 6 weeks postpartum (Begley 1990).

Vomiting and diarrhoea

Ergometrine mimics the actions of dopamine, and *Syntometrine* is more likely to cause nausea or vomiting than is oxytocin alone (McDonald et al 2004; Westhoff et al 2013). Mild or moderate diarrhoea may result from increased contractility of the gastrointestinal tract.

Vasoconstriction

Ergometrine acts on alpha$_1$ (noradrenergic) receptors in arterioles and veins to bring about vasoconstriction and venoconstriction. This raises total peripheral resistance, and may lead to:

- Cold hands and feet
- Hypertension
- Postpartum eclamptic fits
- Reflex bradycardia and reduced cardiac output
- Raised central venous pressure
- Cerebral vasoconstriction and sudden severe headache, tinnitus, dizziness, sweating, confusion, retinal detachment, cerebrovascular accident or seizures
- Coronary artery spasm and chest pain or palpitations
- Numbness, paraesthesia, pain, weakness or even gangrene in digits

Breastfeeding

Ergot alkaloids act on dopamine receptors to suppress prolactin production. One drug in this group, *bromocriptine*, is prescribed to manage galactorrhoea and, occasionally, to suppress lactation postpartum (Jordan et al 2009).

Cautions and contraindications

The vasoconstrictor properties of *ergometrine* make it unsuitable for women with pre-existing pulmonary, cardiac or vascular disorders – including pre-eclampsia, eclampsia, hypertension, migraine and Raynaud's phenomenon – or multiple pregnancy. If sepsis, renal or hepatic failure is present, sensitivity to *ergometrine* is increased. *Ergometrine* is contraindicated in the first and second stages of labour (BMA and RPSGB 2015).

Reflective activity 10.1

Go to the electronic Medicines Compendium at www.medicines.org.uk/emc/.
  Then look up ergometrine.

- Was the information new to you?
- Was the information easily accessible?
- How will you use this site in the future?

Drugs for third stage

Because of the differences in the side-effect profiles of the drugs, current guidelines (NCC 2014) suggest that *oxytocin* is the prophylactic drug of choice for the prevention of postpartum haemorrhage, and *ergometrine* should be used only if this is found to be ineffective, or in high-risk cases. *Oxytocin* is not currently licensed for intramuscular administration (BMA and RPSGB 2015), and intravenous access may be unavailable. Therefore, *Syntometrine* (*ergometrine 500* micrograms and 5 units *oxytocin*) by intramuscular injection is often administered for the routine management of the third stage. Use of this regimen necessitates the careful exclusion of women who should not receive *ergometrine*, for example, those with pre-eclampsia (Abalos 2009) or women who choose a physiological third stage.

Drugs for symptom relief

Drugs for symptom relief include:

- Antiemetics
  - Antihistamines
  - Dopamine (d_2) antagonists/blockers
- Control of gastric acidity
- Laxatives
- Analgesics
  - Nonsteroidal anti-inflammatory drugs (NSAIDs)
- Heparin
- Folic acid
- Vitamin K

For more specific and detailed information on these, see the chapter website resources.

Women prescribed medications for long-term conditions are usually referred to specialist care. Women with epilepsy or diabetes and rarer long-term conditions will need advice, and possibly medication changes, prior to conception. Some related UK guidelines are listed in the web material.

Preventive medicines

The midwife should also use every opportunity to emphasize health and well-being through advising about healthy diet and exercise because this may reduce the need for medications such as iron and some vitamins and minerals. It is also important to discuss spacing pregnancies and any need for contraception as early as 3 weeks postpartum for women not exclusively breastfeeding. UK guidelines are available from the National Institute for Health and Care Excellence (NICE 2014).

LEGAL ASPECTS

The principal statute regulating the use of medicines is the Medicines Act of 1968, which controls the sale and supply of medicines. Before a drug can be marketed in the UK, it must have a Marketing Authorization issued by the Secretary of State for Health. Drugs that have a manufacturing authorization are categorized into three types for the purpose of supply to the general public: *prescription only, pharmacy only* and *general sale*. Controlled drugs are prescription-only medicines that are further regulated by the Misuse of Drugs Act 1971. In health contexts, Misuse of Drugs Regulations 2001 categorizes controlled drugs into five numbered schedules, according to perceived risk of abuse (Griffith and Tengnah 2008). The most recent UK legislation includes the Human Medicines Regulations (2012) and the Human Medicines (Amendment) Regulations (2014), both of which were aimed at simplifying the legislation.

Registered midwives may supply and administer, on their own initiative, any of the substances that are specified in medicines legislation under midwives' exemptions (formerly referred to as 'standing orders'), provided it is in the course of their professional midwifery practice. They may do so without the need for a prescription or patient-specific direction (PSD) from a medical practitioner (NMC 2010a, 2011a and 2011b). Medicines that midwives may prescribe include *Anti D* (Rho) immunoglobulin, *ergometrine pethidine, lidocaine (lignocaine)* and *morphine*.

Some midwives have followed further education and training as midwife prescribers, and are permitted to 'prescribe any medicines for any medical condition within their competence, with the exception of some controlled drugs. They must however do this within their scope of practice and level of expertise and competence' (NMC 2006).

It is essential that midwives are aware of their statutory obligations around drug administration and are conversant with legislation governing drugs and medications. In administering medications, midwives must be knowledgeable regarding the storage, use, dosage, effect and methods of administration of any drug used (NMC 2012). This includes consideration that any equipment used is correct and properly maintained. Should the midwife be required to administer new drugs or use new equipment to administer medications, this must be under the direction of a medical practitioner (NMC 2012 and 2010a).

NMC standards are supported by NMC circulars that detail changes or clarify practice; for example, supply and administration via a Patient Group Directive cannot be delegated a to a student midwife. However, it is important that students are knowledgeable about the legal framework of medicines (NMC 2009), and therefore a later circular amended the guidance so that student midwives can administer medicines (except controlled drugs) supervised by a qualified midwife (NMC 2011a).

Midwives and controlled drugs

The legislation governing midwives and controlled drugs includes that the registered midwife can 'possess diamorphine, morphine, pethidine and pentazocine in her own right so far as is necessary for the practice of her profession' (NMC 2010b). Supplies of these drugs can be made on the authority of a midwife's supply order signed by the supervisor of midwives, or other appropriate medical officer (a doctor authorized in writing by the local supervising authority). The supervisor of midwives or other appropriate medical officer should be satisfied that locally agreed procedure is being followed before signing the supply order (that is that the amount being requested is appropriate, etc.). Midwife prescribing may be undertaken subject to the requirements set down by the NMC (2006, 2010b and 2012).

Once medicines are received – by midwives working in the community or independent midwives – they become the responsibility of the midwife. They should be stored safely and securely; if no longer required, they should be returned to the pharmacy or destroyed following set regulations (NMC 2006 and 2010b). Where it is necessary for midwives to keep medicines in their homes, the medicines should be placed in a secure, locked receptacle. If necessary, this should be provided by the employing body (NMC 2010b; NMC 2015).

Principles of administering medicines safely

The midwife needs to ensure that the medicine has been properly prescribed and documented on a medication sheet in line with local policy. The medication should be checked ideally by two qualified people, checking for the following:

- The right patient is being given:
  - The correct dose
  - The correct medication
  - The correct route of administration
  - At the correct time and date
- Also check the expiry date (if present on the packaging).

If the medication is being given for the first time, it is also important that the midwife establish whether the woman has any existing allergies to any medications. This requires that the midwife is conversant with the medicines used in her practice and knowledgeable about the normal dosage, route, interactions and adverse effects. It is also crucial that should the dosage be complex, the midwife is able to calculate the correct dosage. The midwife also needs to check with the woman to ensure that the right person is getting the right drug and to ensure that she understands the need for the medicine. If administering to a neonate, particular care is vital when calculating and checking doses, and two people should participate in the checking process.

Following administration, the midwife must record clearly that the drug has been administered and monitor the woman and infant for any adverse effects. If, for some reason, the medication is not administered, the reason for this should be documented clearly. In addition, any side effects must be reported and recorded (NMC 2015).

CONCLUSION

Drug administration may involve difficult decisions. These problems could be ameliorated by further research into the physiological changes associated with pregnancy, labour and the puerperium that may be responsible for either therapeutic failure or adverse drug reactions, including easily overlooked events, such as failure to breastfeed.

Acknowledgement

Thanks are due to Palgrave Macmillan for permission to adapt from Jordan S, *Pharmacology for Midwives* 2e, 2010.

Key points

- All drugs taken during pregnancy and childbirth may affect the woman, fetus or newborn.
- The midwife needs to ensure that the woman understands these potential effects and report any possible side effects to the health professional.
- Midwives must have contemporary knowledge about drugs, their interactions and possible adverse effects.

- Midwives must follow legal and practice guidelines and procedures for the safe storage, prescription and administration of medications.
- Pharmacists and drug information departments provide useful resources.

References

Abalos E: *Choice of uterotonic agents in the active management of the third stage of labour: RHL commentary (last revised: 2 March 2009). The WHO Reproductive Health Library*, Geneva, World Health Organization, 2009.

Arkoosh V: *Guidelines for regional anesthesia in obstetrics: viewpoint of an anesthesiologist in a tertiary care center* (website). www.anes.ccf.org:8080/soap/guideline.htm. 1991.

Arkoosh VA, Palmer CM, Yun EM, et al: A randomised, double-masked, multicenter comparison of the safety of continuous intrathecal labor analgesia using a 28-gauge catheter versus continuous epidural labor analgesia, *Anesthesiology* 108(2):286–298, 2008.

Aronson JK, editor: *Meyler's side effects of drugs: the international encyclopedia of adverse drug reactions and interaction*, London, Elsevier, 2006.

Association of Anaesthetists of Great Britain and Ireland (AAGBI): *A report received by Council of the Association of Anaesthetists on blood borne viruses and anaesthesia* (website). www.aagbi.org/publications/guidelines/archive/docs/hivinsert96.pdf. 1996.

Begley C: The effect of ergometrine on breast feeding, *Midwifery* 6(2):60–72, 1990.

Blanch G, Lavender T, Walkinshaw S, et al: Dysfunctional labour: a randomised trial, *Br J Obstet Gynaecol* 105(1):117–120, 1998.

BOC: *Entonox®: essential safety information. Summary of product characteristics*. BOC Healthcare, Manchester (website). http://www.boconline.co.uk/internet.lg.lg.gbr/en/images/entonox410_43539.pdf. 2011.

British Medical Association (BMA) and the Royal Pharmaceutical Society of Great Britain RPSGB), *British National Formulary* (BNF) 69 2015. BMJ Group, London, 2015.

Bromley R, Weston J, Adab N, et al: Treatment for epilepsy in pregnancy: neurodevelopmental outcomes in the child, *Cochrane Database Syst Rev* (10):CD010236, 2014.

Carter C: Developmental consequences of oxytocin, *Physiol Behav* 79(3):383–397, 2003.

Carvalho B: Respiratory depression after neuraxial opioids in the obstetric setting, *Anesth Analg* 107(3):956–961, 2008.

Centre for Maternal and Child Enquiries (CMACE): Saving mothers' lives: reviewing maternal deaths to make motherhood safer: 2006–2008, *BJOG* 118:1–203, 2011.

Charlton RA, Jordan S, Pierini A, et al: SSRI use before, during and after pregnancy: a population-based study in 6 European regions, *BJOG* 122(7):1010–1020, 2014.

Chilvers R, Weisz M: Entonox equipment as a potential source of cross-infection, *Anaesthesia* 55(2):176–179, 2000.

Clayworth S: The nurse's role during oxytocin administration, *MCN Am J Matern Child Nurs* 25(2):80–85, 2000.

Clyburn P, Rosen M: The effects of opioid and inhalational analgesia on the newborn. In Reynolds F, editor: *Effects on the baby of maternal analgesia and anaesthesia*, London, Saunders, pp 169–190, 1993.

Collis R, Harries S, Lewis E, et al: Regional analgesia for labour. In Clyburn P, Collis R, Harries S, et al,

editors: *Obstetric anaesthesia*, Oxford, Oxford University Press, pp 221–254, 2008.

Confidential Enquiries into Maternal and Child Health (CEMACH): *Why mothers die 2000–2002: the sixth report of the Confidential Enquiries into Maternal Deaths in the United Kingdom*, London, CEMACH, 2005.

Congenital Anomaly Register and Information Service for Wales (CARIS): *CARIS review 2014 including 1998–2013 data* (website). http://www2.nphs.wales.nhs.uk:8080/CARISDocs.nsf/85c507 56737f79ac80256f2700534ea3/1eab4fda6200532280257d8c004d 2541/$FILE/Caris%20review%20 %28Eng%29%20final.pdf. 2014.

Crowell MK, Hill P, Humenick S: Relationship between obstetric analgesia and time of effective breast feeding, *J Nurse Midwifery* 39(3):150–156, 1994.

De Groot AN, van Dongen PW, Vree TB, et al: Ergot alkaloids. Current status and review of clinical pharmacology and therapeutic use compared with other oxytocics in obstetrics and gynaecology, *Drugs* 56(4):523–535, 1998.

de Vasconcellos K, Sneyd JR: Nitrous oxide: are we still in equipoise? A qualitative review of current controversies, *Br J Anaesth* 111(6):877–885, 2013.

Eberle R, Norris M: Labour analgesia. A risk-benefit analysis, *Drug Saf* 14(4):239–251, 1996.

Eltzschig H, Lieberman E, Camann P, et al: Regional anesthesia and analgesia for labor and delivery, *N Engl J Med* 348(4):319–332, 2003.

Francinio M: Early development of the gut microbiota and immune health, *Pathogens* 3(3):769–790, 2014.

Gonser M: Labor induction and augmentation with oxytocin: pharmacokinetic considerations, *Arch Gynecol Obstet* 256(2):63–66, 1995.

Griffith RA, Tengnah CA: *Law and professional issues in nursing*, Exeter, Learning Matters, 2008.

Hansen D, Lou H, Olsen J: Serious life events and congenital malformations: a national study with complete follow-up, *Lancet* 356(9233):875–880, 2000.

Human Medicines Regulations (2012): *Statutory Instrument 2012 No. 1916*, London, TSO, 2012.

Human Medicines (Amendment) Regulations (2014): *Statutory Instrument 2014 No. 490*, London, TSO, 2014.

International Conference on Harmonisation (ICH): *ICH Harmonised Tripartite Guideline. Guideline for good clinical practice. E6 (R1)*, Marlow, Institute of Clinical Research, 1996.

Jeffries AL, Canadian Paediatric Society, Fetus & Newborn Committee: *Selective serotonin reuptake inhibitors in pregnancy and infant outcomes.* Position statement (website). www.cps.ca/en/documents/position/SSRI-infant-outcomes. 2011. [For abridged version, see *Paediatrics and Child Health* 16(9):562, 2011.].

Jordan S: Infant feeding and analgesia in labour: the evidence is accumulating, *Int Breastfeed J* 1:25, 2006.

Jordan S: *The prescription drug guide for nurses*, Maidenhead, Open University Press, 2008.

Jordan S: *Pharmacology for midwives: the evidence base for safe practice*, 2nd edn, Basingstoke, Palgrave/Macmillan, 2010.

Jordan S, Emery S, Bradshaw C, et al: The impact of intrapartum analgesia on infant feeding, *Br J Obstet Gynaecol* 112(7):927–934, 2005.

Jordan S, Storey M, Morgan G: Antibiotics and allergic disorders in childhood, *Open Nurs J* 2:48–57, 2008.

Jordan S, Emery S, Watkins A, et al: Associations of drugs routinely given in labour with breastfeeding at 48 hours: analysis of the Cardiff Births Survey, *Br J Obstet Gynaecol* 116(12):1622–1630, 2009.

Jordan S, Morris JK, Davies GI, et al: Selective Serotonin Reuptake Inhibitor (SSRI) antidepressants in pregnancy and congenital anomalies: analysis of linked databases in Wales, Norway and Funen, Denmark, 2016. Plos One accepted 7.10.16.

Jordan S, Watkins A, Storey M, et al: Volunteer bias in recruitment, retention, and blood sample donation in a randomised controlled trial involving mothers and their children at six months and two years: a longitudinal analysis, *PLoS One* 8(7):e67912, 2013.

Kennedy S, Longnecker D: History and principles of anaesthesiology. In Hardman J, Limbird L, Molinoff P, et al, editors: *The pharmacological basis of therapeutics*, 9th edn, New York, McGraw-Hill, pp 917–936, 1996.

Knight M, Kenyon S, Brocklehurst P, et al: on behalf of MBRRACE-UK, editor: *Saving lives, improving mothers' care – lessons learned to inform future maternity care from the UK and Ireland Confidential Enquiries into Maternal Deaths and Morbidity 2009–12*, Oxford, National Perinatal Epidemiology Unit, University of Oxford, 2014.

Kumar K, Singh S: Neuraxial opioid-induced pruritus: an update, *J Anaesthesiol Clin Pharmacol* 29(3):303–307, 2013.

Leng G, Meddle SL, Douglas AJ: Oxytocin and the maternal brain, *Curr Opin Pharmacol* 8(6):731–734, 2008.

Levey A, Bosch J, Lewis J, et al: A more accurate method to estimate glomerular filtration rate from serum creatinine: a new prediction equation, *Ann Intern Med* 130(6):461–470, 1999.

Loebstein R, Lalkin A, Koren G: Pharmacokinetic changes during pregnancy and their clinical relevance, *Clin Pharmacokinet* 33(5):328–343, 1997.

Magann EF, Evans S, Hutchinson M, et al: Postpartum hemorrhage after vaginal birth: an analysis of risk factors, *South Med J* 98(4):419–422, 2005.

McDonald SJ, Abbott JM, Higgins SP: Prophylactic ergometrine-oxytocin versus oxytocin for the third stage of labour, *Cochrane Database Syst Rev* (1):CD000201, 2004.

McEwan A: Induction of labour, *Obstet Gynaecol Reprod Med* 18(1):1–6, 2007.

Merlob P, Schaefer C: Specific drug therapies during lactation. Psychotropic drugs. In Schaefer C, Peters PW, Miller RK, editors: *Drugs during pregnancy and lactation: treatment options and risk assessment*, 3rd edn, London, Elsevier, pp 743–774, 2015.

National Collaborating Centre for Women's and Children's Health (NCC): *Caesarean section: clinical guideline*, London, RCOG, 2004.

National Collaborating Centre for Women's and Children's Health (NCC): *Induction of labour: clinical guideline*, London, RCOG, 2008.

National Collaborating Centre for Women's and Children's Health (NCC): *Intrapartum care: care of healthy women and their babies during childbirth. Clinical guideline 190*, London, NCC (commissioned by NICE) (website). http://www.nice.org.uk/guidance/cg190/evidence/cg190-intrapartum-care-full-guideline3. 2014.

National Institute for Health and Care Excellence (NICE): *NICE Guidelines: contraceptive services with a focus on young people up to the age of 25* (website). www.nice.org.uk/guidance/PH51. 2014.

Niebyl J: Teratology and drugs in pregnancy. *Global Library of Women's Medicine* (website). www.glowm.com/section_view/heading/Teratology%20and%20Drugs%20in%20Pregnancy/item/96#5191. 2008.

Novartis: *Syntocinon 5 IU/ml concentrate for solution for infusion. Summary of product characteristics*. Electronic Medicines Compendium (eMC). Datapharm Communications (website). www.medicines.org.uk/emc/medicine/30335. 2015.

Nursing and Midwifery Council (NMC): *Standards of proficiency for nurse and midwife prescribers* (website). www.nmc.org.uk/globalassets/sitedocuments/nmc-publications/nmc-standards-proficiency-nurse-and-midwife-prescribers.pdf. 2006.

Nursing and Midwifery Council (NMC): *Circular: supply and/or administration of medicine by student nurses and student midwives in* relation to Patient Group Directions (PGDs), London, NMC, 2009.

Nursing and Midwifery Council Circular: *Changes to Midwives Exemptions* (website). www.nmc-uk.org/Documents/circulars. 2010a.

Nursing and Midwifery Council (NMC): *Standards for medicines management*, London, NMC, 2010b. [Revision to 2008 version].

Nursing and Midwifery Council (NMC): *Circular: Changes to Midwives Exemptions* (website). www.nmc.org.uk/globalassets/sitedocuments/circulars/2011circulars/nmccircular07-2011-midwives-exemptions.pdf. 2011a.

Nursing and Midwifery Council (NMC): *Circular: Changes to Midwives Exemptions –annexes* (website). http://www.nmc.org.uk/globalassets/sitedocuments/circulars/2011circulars/nmccircular07-2011_midwives-exemptions-annexes.pdf. 2011b.

Nursing and Midwifery Council (NMC): *Midwives rules and standards 2012*, London, NMC, 2012.

Nursing and Midwifery Council (NMC): *The Code: professional standards of practice and behaviour for nurses and midwives* (website). www.nmc.org.uk/globalassets/sitedocuments/nmc-publications/revised-new-nmc-code.pdf 2015.

Out JJ, Vierhout ME, Wallenburg HC: Breast-feeding following spontaneous and induced labour, *Eur J Obstet Gynecol Reprod Biol* 29(4):275–279, 1988.

Paech M: New epidural techniques for labour analgesia: patient-controlled epidural analgesia and combined spinal-epidural analgesia, *Baillieres Clin Obstet Gynaecol* 12(3):377–395, 1998.

Perrone RD, Madias NE, Levey AS: Serum creatinine as an index of renal function: new insights into old concepts, *Clin Chem* 38(10):1933–1953, 1992.

Rajan L: The impact of obstetric procedures and analgesia/anaesthesia during labour and delivery on breast feeding, *Midwifery* 10(2):87–103, 1994.

Richardson M: Regional anesthesia for obstetrics, *Anesthesiol Clin North America* 18(2):383–406, 2000.

Robinson C, Schumann R, Zhang P, et al: Oxytocin-induced desensitization of the oxytocin receptor, *Am J Obstet Gynecol* 188(2):497–502, 2003.

Ruppen W, Derry S, McQuay H, et al: Incidence of epidural hematoma, infection, and neurologic injury in obstetric patients with epidural analgesia/anesthesia, *Anesthesiology* 105(2):394–399, 2006.

Sadler L, McCowan L, White H, et al: Pregnancy outcomes and cardiac complications in women with mechanical, bioprosthetic and homograft valves, *Br J Obstet Gynaecol* 107(2):245–253, 2000.

Schrock SD, Harraway-Smith C: Labor analgesia, *Am Fam Physician* 85(5):447–454, 2012.

Simmons SW, Cyna AM, Dennis AT, et al: Combined spinal-epidural versus epidural analgesia in labour, *Cochrane Database Syst Rev* (3):CD003401, 2007.

Slattery DA, Neumann ID: No stress please! Mechanisms of stress hyporesponsiveness of the maternal brain, *J Physiol* 586(2):377–385, 2008.

Smaill FM, Grivell RM: Antibiotic prophylaxis versus no prophylaxis for preventing infection after cesarean section, *Cochrane Database Syst Rev* (10):CD007482, 2014.

Sweetman SC, Blake P, McGlashan G, et al: *Martindale: the complete drug reference*, London, The Pharmaceutical Press, 2007.

Thompson A, Hillier V: A re-evaluation of the effect of pethidine on the length of labour, *J Adv Nurs* 19(3):448–456, 1994.

Wagner M: Research shows medication of pain is not safe, *MIDIRS Midwifery Digest* 3(3):307–309, 1993.

Westhoff G, Cotter AM, Tolosa JE: Prophylactic oxytocin for the third stage of labour to prevent postpartum haemorrhage, *Cochrane Database Syst Rev* (10):CD001808, 2013.

Wiklund I, Norman M, Uvnäs-Moberg K, et al: Epidural analgesia: breast-feeding success and related factors, *Midwifery* 25(2):e31–e38, 2009.

Wilkinson G: Pharmacokinetics. In Hardman J, Limbard L, Molinoff P, et al, editors: *Goodman & Gilman's: the pharmacological basis of therapeutics*, 10th edn, New York, McGraw-Hill, pp 3–30, 2001.

Wisborg K, Barklin A, Hedegaard M, et al: Psychological stress during pregnancy and stillbirth: prospective study, *Br J Obstet Gynaecol* 115(7):882–885, 2008.

Resources and additional reading

Please refer to the chapter website for more information on medications.

Davey L, Houghton D: *The midwife's pocket formulary*, 3rd edn, London, Churchill Livingstone, 2013.

A useful text for day-to-day referral.

Department of Health, Social Services and Public Safety (DHSSPS): *NIPEC midwives and medicines* (website). http://www.nipec.hscni.net/ work-and-projects/midwives-and -medicines/. 2014.

A useful resource specific for midwives working in Northern Ireland.

Human Medicines Regulations 2012: *Statutory Instrument 2012, No. 1916*, London, TSO, 2012.

Legislation supporting medicines.

Jordan S: *Pharmacology for midwives: the evidence base for safe practice*, 2nd edn, Basingstoke, Palgrave/ Macmillan, 2010.

A useful text with additional information regarding the evidence base for pharmacology.

Nursing and Midwifery Council (NMC): *Circular: Midwives Exemptions* (website). www.nmc .org.uk/globalassets/sitedocuments/ circulars/2011circulars/nmccircular 07-2011-midwives-exemptions.pdf. 2011.

Additional information regarding exemptions.

Nursing and Midwifery Council website: www.nmc.org.uk.

This is an excellent interactive learning resource for midwives that outlines the legislation and professional issues for midwives. It also includes some good activities and quizzes.

Royal College of Midwives – RCM I-learn Making Numbers Count in Practice module (website) www.rcm.org.uk.

This electronic learning module is about general numeracy skills and, more specifically, the application of numeracy in the workplace; it will assist in safe dosage calculation of medications.

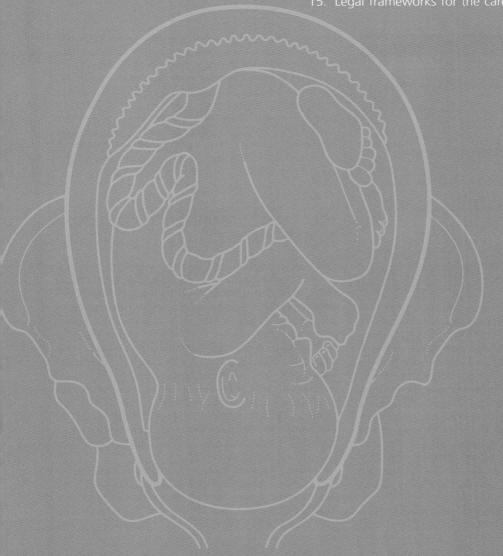

Part Two

Childbirth in context

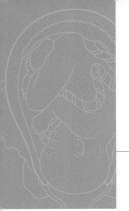

Chapter 11

Sociocultural and spiritual context of childbearing

Professor Irena Papadopoulos

Learning Outcomes

After reading this chapter, you will be able to:

- explain what cultural competence means and why it is important
- apply the principles of cultural competence to midwifery practice
- evaluate the ways in which midwives can develop positive, trusting relationships with women and their families
- discuss the role that spirituality plays during childbearing
- reflect on how religion and religious practices might influence practice

INTRODUCTION

Although pregnancy and childbirth are biological processes and universal events, they are also related to specific sociocultural factors that are socially created and given meaning. The diversity of language and understanding of pregnancy, childbirth, motherhood and fatherhood have varied over periods of time, across cultures, among women and men and between professional groups (Denny et al 2011; Davis-Floyd 2003; Squire 2009). Understanding these sociocultural factors has never been more important and relevant as it is currently. We are living in the era of superdiversity, described by Vertovec (2007) as the level and kind of complexity surpassing anything previously experienced in a particular society. In this chapter, the activities form an important part of the reader's understanding of culture and ethnicity.

Over the past 20 years, globally more people have moved from more places to more places; new and increasingly complex social formations have ensued, marked by dynamic interplays of variables such as country of origin, ethnicity, language, religious tradition, regional and local identities, cultural values and practices, new but specific social networks, legal statuses, needs for services and so on. The superdiversity phenomenon has inevitably produced new challenges for healthcare service providers and professionals, including the reproductive services, especially midwifery. Two of the many challenges are those related to *health inequalities* and *quality of care*. Both are linked to *cultural competence*.

CULTURAL COMPETENCE, CULTURE AND ETHNICITY

Papadopoulos (2006) defined cultural competence as the capacity to provide effective and compassionate healthcare taking into consideration people's cultural beliefs, behaviours and needs. Culturally competent care should be provided to all people who need it because all human beings are cultural beings. Culture is the shared way of life of a group of people that includes beliefs, values, ideas, language, communication, norms and visibly expressed forms such as customs, art, music, clothing, food and etiquette. Culture influences lifestyles, personal identity and relationships with others, both within and outside cultural groups. Everyone is influenced by the culture they were born and grown into and by the cultures they associate with, but individuals can also influence cultural changes, by varying degrees.

Ethnicity is closely associated with culture, but it is a more contested notion. However, just like culture, it is a fundamental factor in human life and human experience. The Greek historian Herodotus (c 480 BC) provided the following list of characteristics that defined the Greek ethnicity, which form the basis of current research and debate on ethnicity:

- Shared descent
- Shared language
- Shared sanctuaries and sacrifices (religion and religious rituals)
- Shared customs (Wikipedia 2016)

Reflective activity 11.1

- How would you define your own cultural and ethnic identity?
- Has your cultural/ethnic identity been ever challenged? Give an example and an account of how this made you feel.
- As a student midwife/qualified midwife, how do you feel when you care for a woman and her baby (either in the hospital or in her home) whose culture is very different to yours?
- Reflect on the benefits, challenges and possible negative aspects of living in a multicultural, multiethnic society.
- If you do not live in a multicultural, multiethnic society, choose a day (in the past or in the future), then choose three newspapers (mixture of national and local) that are available online and search for stories that include cultural/ethnic elements. Review how have these been reported in terms of benefits, challenges and negative aspects.

MIDWIVES AND CULTURAL COMPETENCE

In the UK, midwives are required by their professional regulating body, the Nursing and Midwifery Council (NMC 2015) to treat people as individuals and uphold their dignity. To achieve this, a midwife must treat people with kindness, respect and compassion; avoid making assumptions and recognize diversity and individual choice; respect and uphold people's human rights; listen to people and respond to their preferences and concerns; encourage and empower people to share decisions about their treatment and care; respect, support and document a person's right to accept or refuse care and treatment; and recognize when people are anxious or in distress and respond compassionately and politely.

In its policy document *Essential Competencies for Basic Midwifery Practice*, the International Confederation of Midwives (ICM 2013) describes seven key midwifery competencies required to provide quality care to the mother, baby and family. The document makes it very clear that unless midwives execute these competencies with cultural sensitivity, and through working in partnership with women and healthcare providers to overcome those cultural practices that harm women and babies and ignore their human rights, quality care will not be achieved.

This is underlined by the World Health Organization (2014) in its publication *Midwifery Educator Core Competencies*, which declares that neither quality nor equality can be achieved if midwifery educators are not educationally prepared according to the 8 domains and 19 competencies recommended in this document. Of particular note is competency No. 15 in domain No. 7 (Communication, leadership and advocacy), which requires educators to demonstrate cultural competence in course design and development, teaching and midwifery practice. The research evidence in this report states that midwifery educators must have knowledge of cultural diversity, identity and human rights and must understand the impact of power relations, racism and sexism. In terms of skills, midwifery educators must have the ability to recognize and describe multicultural, gender and experiential influences on teaching and learning, facilitate the provision of culturally appropriate care, encourage the expression and exchange of multicultural views, respect and protect human rights and speak up when there are violations of human rights. In addition, their behaviours should demonstrate cultural sensitivity in practice and when advocating change, and be accountable for their own actions and inactions in safeguarding human rights.

The Papadopoulos, Tilki and Taylor model of cultural competence

Having established what cultural competence is and why it is no longer an option but a fundamental requirement for midwifery education, practice and research, it is helpful to use a simple framework to hang on it, the declarations and assertions included in national and international policy documents such as those mentioned earlier. The *Papadopoulos, Tilki and Taylor model* (often referred to as the *PTT model*; Papadopoulos et al 1998) was originally designed for nursing in 1994 (Papadopoulos 2006). It soon became clear that other health disciplines were finding the simplicity and relevance of the model attractive and useful. It is suggested that its framework and underpinning values are also very compatible with midwifery. The framework (see Fig. 11.1) consists of four key constructs:

1. cultural awareness
2. cultural knowledge
3. cultural sensitivity
4. cultural competence

There are a few subconstructs that are recommended to be studied as a minimum and applied to the specific

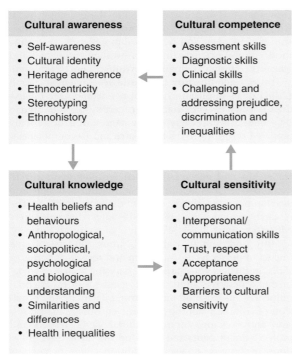

Cultural awareness	Cultural competence
• Self-awareness • Cultural identity • Heritage adherence • Ethnocentricity • Stereotyping • Ethnohistory	• Assessment skills • Diagnostic skills • Clinical skills • Challenging and addressing prejudice, discrimination and inequalities
Cultural knowledge	Cultural sensitivity
• Health beliefs and behaviours • Anthropological, sociopolitical, psychological and biological understanding • Similarities and differences • Health inequalities	• Compassion • Interpersonal/ communication skills • Trust, respect • Acceptance • Appropriateness • Barriers to cultural sensitivity

Figure 11.1 The Papadopoulos, Tilki and Taylor model for developing cultural competence.

professional practice. This framework is underpinned by the values of social justice, human rights, equality, human caring and transcultural ethics.

Cultural awareness

Cultural awareness is the degree of awareness people have about their own cultural background and cultural identity. This helps individuals to understand the importance of their cultural heritage and that of others and makes them appreciate the dangers of ethnocentricity. Cultural awareness is the first step to developing cultural competence and must therefore be supplemented by cultural knowledge.

Cultural knowledge

Cultural knowledge derives from a number of disciplines, such as anthropology, sociology, psychology, biology, midwifery, medicine and the arts, and can be gained in a number of ways, such as meaningful contact with people from different cultural/ethnic backgrounds, which can enhance knowledge about their health beliefs and behaviours and raise understanding around the problems they face. Through, for example, sociological

study, we learn about power, such as professional power and control, or make links between personal position and structural inequalities.

Cultural sensitivity

Cultural sensitivity entails the crucial development of compassion and appropriate interpersonal relationships with clients. An important element in achieving cultural sensitivity is how professionals view people in their care. Unless clients are considered as true partners, culturally sensitive care is not being achieved, and midwives and other healthcare professionals risk using their power in an oppressive way. Equal partnerships involve trust, acceptance and respect along with facilitation and negotiation.

Cultural competence

Cultural competence has already been defined earlier. But to expand on that definition, it is significant to mention that cultural competence is both a process and an output, and it results from the synthesis of knowledge and skills that are acquired during personal and professional lives and that are constantly being added to. The achievement of cultural competence requires the synthesis of previously gained awareness, knowledge and sensitivity and its application in the assessment of clients' needs, clinical diagnosis and other caring skills. A most important component of this stage is the ability to recognize and challenge racism and other forms of discrimination and oppressive practice.

Reflective activity 11.2

Think for a moment about your cultural identity. What does it mean?

Applying the PTT model: The story of Amal

To illustrate how this model can be used, a case study is presented to explore the key issues, as a means of reflecting on the issues, and to illustrate how application of the model might occur in practice.

Using as guidance the Papadopoulos, Tilki and Taylor model, reflect on Case Study 11.1.

Cultural awareness: The influence and relevance of cultural identity

You may start to think about your own cultural identity by considering your gender and your own ethnic and religious background. You will most probably conclude

CASE STUDY 11.1 The story of Amal

Amal is a 19-year-old Muslim Somali woman who has been admitted to the labour ward. She is accompanied by another Somali woman who claims she is her friend.

Amal speaks very little English, having arrived in the UK only 6 months ago. Her friend informs the midwife that Amal is an asylum seeker. She had not had antenatal care because she was too scared to go to the doctor to confirm the pregnancy and receive care. She does not have any family in this country, and she lives alone in a room provided by the government in a bed-and-breakfast hostel.

The midwife completes assessment of Amal's vital signs, then palpates her abdomen and establishes the presentation and position of the fetus; she notes that head is engaged, and the fetus has a normal heartbeat with good variability. Amal is having regular contractions lasting 30 to 60 seconds. The midwife explains to Amal through her friend that she needs to carry out a vaginal examination to establish how much the cervix is dilated. Amal appears scared but reluctantly consents to it. The midwife soon realizes that Amal has had female genital mutilation (FGM), and she will need to be deinfibulated to facilitate the birth. She communicates this to Amal through her friend. Amal understands that this needs to be done, but she requests that she is reinfibulated after the baby is born.

This is the first time that the midwife has had to deal with a case of FGM. To make sure she is following the correct practice, she calls the senior midwife, who confirms that reinfibulation is not permitted. Amal finds this very distressing and begins to cry. At the same time, the friend informs the midwife and Amal that she needs to leave to collect her children from school.

The midwife estimates that it may take Amal another 2 hours before she is ready to give birth, and therefore she encourages her to self-administer *entonox*. However, Amal remains very anxious and scared. Three hours later, she delivers a healthy baby girl by forceps.

that these factors are important in determining or defining who you are. Think about any cultural customs or religious rituals you observe or follow. You may also consider that these are important practices that remind you of your roots. Cultural identity is important to most people because this provides a sense of belonging to a group of people who have similar views on life and living and therefore have shared experiences. There is an unspoken understanding between the members of a cultural group. Increasingly, many people belong to more than one cultural group, which can be both a challenge and an advantage.

Amal would probably answer the questions in Reflective activity 11.2 the same way that you do. There are many aspects of Amal's care that need to be addressed in terms of her cultural identity. This might include particular practices around food and drink that she may need, particular religious ceremonies for herself and her baby, and clothing that may be required. Women have reported a lack of consideration from professionals for their personal cultural practices (Parker et al 2014). As one example, the practice of FGM in the cultural context will be explored.

The midwife might wonder how Amal can feel pride in a cultural practice such as FGM, which is now considered an abusive/unacceptable cultural custom perpetrated by her family and culture. Before judging Amal and her culture, it is important to try to understand her and the condition she finds herself in (see also Ch. 56).

Cultural knowledge

Regarding the practice of FGM, the first question that must be asked is 'Do I know enough about the cultural beliefs of Amal's culture, which allows/promotes the practice of FGM?'

Reflective activity 11.3

Think about your own knowledge of FGM – do you feel confident to care for and support a woman with FGM in your care?

Visit the following website to find out more: https://plan-uk.org/about/our-work/fgm

There is a plethora of information about all aspects of FGM that can be accessed online.

Real stories about young girls who have experienced FGM and the impact on their lives can be found on the 'Action-Aid' website, which also covers other issues, such as refugeedom and asylum seeking (see Reflective activity 11.4).

Reflective activity 11.4

Read some of the case studies found on the ActionAid site (https://www.actionaid.org.uk/blog/voices/2015/07/01/the-stories-behind-the-fgm-statistics) – were you surprised at what the women said?

Discovering the facts behind the myths will help when judging the culture and the people involved with compassion, without condoning this harmful practice. It is important to reflect on the role of the woman in those cultures and whether the mothers and grandmothers believe that FGM is a compassionate act, or whether they believe it to be an obligation that may derive from fear.

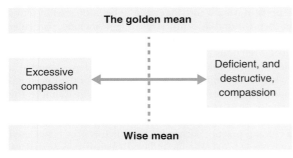

The golden mean

Excessive compassion ⟷ Deficient, and destructive, compassion

Wise mean

Figure 11.2 Aristotle's 'golden mean'.

Aristotle's golden mean and wise compassion

A relevant notion in the search of a way to make fair and informed judgements is to use what Aristotle (384 BC–322 BC), the Greek philosopher, called the 'golden mean'. He declared that this is the desirable middle between two extremes, one of excess and the other of deficiency (see Fig. 11.2).

Wise compassion is culturally competent compassion, which has been defined as the human quality of understanding the suffering of others and wanting to do something about it, using culturally appropriate and acceptable healthcare interventions that take into consideration both the patients' and the carers' cultural backgrounds and the context in which care is given (Papadopoulos 2011).

Cultural sensitivity: Developing therapeutic relationships

Amal is a young woman, an asylum seeker who is scared and alone, and to gain her trust and develop a therapeutic relationship, it will be important to communicate effectively with her.

Reflective activity 11.5

Think about how the midwife could best communicate and connect with Amal.

We know that Amal speaks very little English. As an asylum seeker, she is scared and confused about living in a new country and even more so in being in the very strange environment of a labour ward. Before the communication challenge is considered, it is useful to be reminded how international conventions define an 'asylum seeker' and what healthcare rights are provided under the UK legislation.

Asylum seekers and midwifery

An asylum seeker is someone who has fled his or her country of origin, applied for protection under the Geneva Convention (United Nations 1951) or Article 3 of the European Convention on Human Rights (torture) (European Court of Human Rights 2010), with the UK Border Agency at the Home Office, and is awaiting a decision regarding immigration status. This decision can take many months or even years. Although asylum seekers are entitled to primary and secondary healthcare without charge (Joels 2008), often they are not aware of this or can find it difficult to access (Mcleish 2002). Asylum seekers like Amal may have considerable health needs, including mental health needs – many will have witnessed or endured violence, rape and torture – and physical health needs such as poor nutrition from earlier deprivations (Kelley and Stevenson 2006). Pregnancy may be a result of rape by oppressors in their country of origin (Dunkley-Bent 2006) or from either consensual or forced intercourse while awaiting asylum. The House of Commons Select Committee on Health (2003) concluded that reasons why pregnant asylum seekers may not access care include the following: their future in the UK was uncertain; isolation from family and friends left them with no support; an inability to speak English. These same reasons increase their vulnerability, and this continues for both mother and child until a final decision is made on their right to remain in the UK.

The midwife may well wonder if Amal has been a victim of rape, if she is concerned about the outcome of her asylum application, or how she is going to cope with a baby. Perhaps some of these issues may also be going through Amal's mind as she lies in the labour ward, feeling both pain and fear. The key to getting the answers to these questions is *intercultural communication*.

Intercultural communication and the midwife

Intercultural communication is communication across cultures and social groups. It involves the understanding of language and other factors, such as cultural beliefs, values, customs, socioeconomic and religious backgrounds and nonverbal behaviours. The tone of voice, speed and pronunciation are all key elements of effective communication, as is the use of touch, personal space, hand gestures or eye contact, which can vary greatly between cultures. Because most professionals are not multilingual, the use of professional interpreters is commonplace in a number of developed countries.

Intercultural communication includes *nonjudgemental* and *active listening, clarification* and *summarising* in addition to *respecting others*. The issue of culture is a complex matter that influences the delivery of care and also how healthcare teams work together. Leininger

(1978) identified three potential strategies for communicating with people from diverse cultural groups; these are as follows:

- *Cultural preservation:* This refers to recognition of health practices specific to a culture, which may be helpful or harmful. It requires attention to artefacts that should be respected and considered when addressing the individual's health.

- *Cultural negotiation:* Negotiation between the healthcare professional, the service user and their significant other, if appropriate, to establish shared understanding and a way forward.

- *Cultural repatterning:* This relates to communication aimed at changing patterns of behaviour that are having a negative impact on the person's health.

In the case of Amal, it is clear that the midwife needs to involve a professional interpreter as soon as possible. Failing to do this will result in misunderstandings and will undermine any attempts to establishing a trusting relationship with Amal.

During labour the midwife will be giving a number of instructions to Amal that will help the normal progression from the first to second stage of labour and then birth. Amal needs to understand the instructions particularly because she has not had any contact with a midwife since becoming pregnant. Amal will be talking to the midwife, and unless the midwife has someone to interpret, she will not be able to respond or offer appropriate support to Amal. At some point after the birth the midwife will need to ask some very sensitive questions regarding the father of the baby and Amal's social circumstances, including support after transfer to the community after the birth.

Cultural competence: The challenge

The midwife caring for Amal should consider how she can provide culturally competent care to Amal. She should identify whether there are professional and/or organizational structures and practices that may exclude and/or discriminate against Amal. She needs to reflect upon how she may deal with or challenge any such practices/policies. Whatever the midwife considers, she should do this with wisdom and courage because she knows this is her duty and because indifference means accepting substandard, insensitive and unkind midwifery care.

Reflective activity 11.6

What key points would you need to know to help Amal maintain her cultural identity?

Based on the conclusion that Amal will consider her cultural identity to be important, the midwife becomes aware that Amal wishes to adhere to the cultural customs that have to do with FGM. Reflect on how the care should be customized to meet the needs of Amal.

Summary of the key points of the enacted midwifery care

- Knowing that reinfibulating Amal is not permitted, the midwife needs to appreciate and understand the impact that FGM would have had on Amal, particularly during her labour.

- The midwife offers culturally competent compassion to Amal by explaining the reasons why she cannot be reinfibulated and the support she can have in the postpartum period.

- Knowing that communication is crucial to Amal's safety and provision of support, the midwife requests the services of a professional interpreter. However, if this was delayed it could cause both Amal and the midwife unnecessary stress.

- Once Amal and her baby are safely in the postnatal ward, the midwife needs to scrutinize and challenge the protocol for requesting and getting the help of a professional interpreter without delays.

- When transferring care to the postnatal team, detailed and accurate care notes should clearly indicate that Amal is an asylum seeker who does not speak English and is living in bed-and-breakfast accommodation alone. She would need support services to be arranged before transfer to the community and when she is discharged to the care of the health visitor.

It can be concluded that if these key points are enacted, the midwife will be using wisdom and demonstrating culturally competent compassion even though this is the first time she has looked after a woman who required deinfibulation before giving birth. These key points act as a care/action plan and will help the professional team provide a high standard of culturally appropriate and sensitive care.

The example of Amal illustrates some of the cultural issues that may arise when the cultural background of the woman using midwifery services differs from that of the midwife providing care. The complexities of real-life situations are difficult to describe in full. In the case of Amal, apart from the midwife, there would be other health professionals involved, and because she had not come in contact with any health services before being admitted in labour, there will be many unknowns about any physical or mental health needs, the reasons for fleeing her country, any traumas she suffered during her migration journey and her views about the baby, particularly in terms of her age and religion.

FAMILY AND GENDER

Whereas anatomical and physiological differences between the sexes are biologically determined, gender may be described as the socially or culturally prescribed status of women and men in a society. The associated concepts of femininity and masculinity are similarly socially constructed and greatly affected by culture. In common with all social constructs, these expectations will vary between cultures and over time. Although related to it, gender is different from sexuality, which is a social construct of a biological drive. Although there are differences between the sexes, of which the ability to have children is a key one, it is the use of those differences as justification for ongoing inequalities between women and men that is challenged by feminist thinking (Squire 2009).

A society's expectation of gender roles reflects ongoing changes in women's lives and family life, yet despite these changes, gender inequalities persist and are most visible within career pathways and earning potential (Wild 2016). It has been demonstrated that by addressing these inequalities and reducing the gap, countries can gain significant positive economic and health benefits (World Economic Forum 2014).

Less visible are inequalities in the division of household chores and the responsibility of child care, particularly in some cultures that continue to be male orientated. In most developed nations, policy changes such as paternity leave and flexible working arrangements have resulted in more fathers taking up their parenting and home-care roles.

Despite some parents' attempts at avoiding traditional gendered differences in bringing up their children, the influence of society is pervasive. This is reflected in the media representation of gendered toys and the type of language used to talk to and about small children. Ideas about a person's gender roles and behaviour may be ascribed before birth. Rothman (1994) uses the phrase 'fetal sons and daughters' as she describes how women who know the sex of their child after amniocentesis describe fetal activity in a way that is gender stereotyped. The movements of the males were more often described as 'strong' and 'vigorous' and females were described as 'lively'. Gender stereotyping continues soon after birth because appearance and behaviour are gender related.

Families and their shapes are changing, although acceptance of these changes is being resisted by some cultural and religious groups. The definition of a family is of two parents with children, living in a unit together. In reality this is more complex and can include same-sex partners (male or female); single parents (often women), either by choice or loss of the partner by separation, divorce or death; and the 'traditional' nuclear family of one male and female with children. The children may biologically belong to one or both partners; may be adopted or fostered; or may be living in extended families, including those within 'blended' or 'reconstituted' families who may have step-brothers and step-sisters on both maternal and paternal sides. The term 'single parent' frequently conjures up images of young mothers and has often been used in a derogatory way within the media, particularly the tabloid press, for many years. Often cited as an indicator for antisocial behaviour among children and young people, its links to poverty, aspiration and employment prospects are ignored.

Midwives need to possess knowledge that family life and structure are not fixed or uniform. They themselves will come from a family, and this will have shaped their attitudes and beliefs about what a family is and can do. These attitudes and actions towards individuals are equally important. One example of this is lesbians and motherhood. Lesbians have some different needs than those of heterosexual women, but many have the same needs during pregnancy, in labour and during early motherhood. The primary tensions for lesbians lie in the values and attitudes of others (Brogan 1997), and midwives can make a significant difference to these mothers in terms of providing nonjudgemental support and care (Spidsberg and Sørlie 2012).

Although family is often assumed to be a place where individuals feel happy and safe, this is not the case for everyone. For example, 30% of abuse towards women starts or worsens in pregnancy (see Ch. 23). Midwives may also make an assumption that because a woman is married or lives with a partner or parents she is 'supported'. This may not be the experience for women whose partners are unsupportive because they feel ambivalent or unreceptive towards the woman's pregnancy and forthcoming child. Single mothers living alone may be well supported through family or friendships networks.

The midwife needs to find out the family pattern as early as possible and establish whether this means that the woman needs any additional support or referral to other agencies. This is usually asked at the initial interview with the woman (see Ch. 32), but it may be established at a later point, such as in Amal's case, when the woman presents late in the pregnancy, or in labour.

RELIGION AND SPIRITUALITY

As midwives have become increasingly aware of the sociocultural context of women's and men's lives, an understanding of each woman's religious and spiritual needs is equally important (Davies 2007; Hall and Taylor 2004; Pembroke and Pembroke 2008). Baldacchino (2010) believes that religion is commonly linked to spirituality. Evans and Mitchell (2014) state that, historically, spiritual care and religious care were one and the same. However, spirituality may or may not contain notions of religiosity.

Research by McSherry (2006) identified eight descriptors of spirituality:

- *Theistic:* belief in God or other deity
- *Religious:* belief in God and participating in certain religious practices
- *Language:* expression of spirituality
- *Cultural and sociopolitical ideologies:* spiritual attitudes and behaviours based on one's cultural and sociopolitical orientation
- *Phenomenological:* basing one's spirituality on lived experiences
- *Existential:* spirituality as a way for finding meaning and purpose in life
- *Quality of life:* included implicitly in definitions of spirituality
- *Mystical:* spirituality as a relationship between transcendent, interpersonal, transpersonal life after death

Religion usually refers to a system of faith and worship practices, shared by a group of people and an acknowledgement of the existence of a higher power or God.

Reflective activity 11.7

Reflect on whether religion and spirituality are linked to culture, and if so, how?

Crowther and Hall (2015) espouse that the childbirth experience for all involved is special, unique and spiritual in quality. Childbirth is deeply relational and spiritually meaningful, yet, they argue, spirituality remains on the peripheral of current discourse about childbirth.

Jesse et al (2007), in using the terms *religious faith* and *spirituality* interchangeably, describe how for some women spirituality is a significant resource in pregnancy. In their study on the relevance and meaning of spirituality for low-income African American and Caucasian women in the midwestern United States, around half of the respondents reported that spirituality had an important positive effect on their pregnancy. The women described how they felt guided, supported and protected by their faith; that it gave them strength and confidence; that their faith helped with difficult choices and enabled them to communicate with God.

Pembroke and Pembroke (2008: 324) explore the spirituality of midwifery care and consider that the 'capacity to respond loyally and authentically is at the heart of the spirituality of midwifery care'. These authors suggest that the midwife is a reassuring calm presence and is available for the woman not just to do practical things, but to be there, just for her, emotionally.

McHugh (2003) suggests that the 'sense of the spiritual' may be more readily achieved away from large obstetric units; home or birth centres are more appropriate places where the environment and culture embrace a more holistic approach, including a recognition of the spiritual dimensions of labour and birth. Nevertheless, although some physical hospital environments may not appear conducive to the 'sense of the spiritual', midwives can create an appropriate emotional environment in hospital settings through building meaningful, supportive relationships with women during the intense experience of labour and birth.

The challenges

Although, as noted, spiritual care is an integral part of midwifery care, numerous challenges remain and must be addressed to turn the rhetoric into reality. To start with, for a person like Amal, her religious and spiritual needs would most probably be responded to by the healthcare system (and the midwives) through providing facilities for prayer, by ensuring that she is given halal meals, by involving the local Muslim cleric should she request this and through other cultural and religious customs. It is important that midwives understand or have access to information about cultural customs associated with the various religions, but spirituality needs, associated or not associated with religion, are broader and deeper than customs and rituals. Crowther and Hall (2015) recommend the implementation of the following:

- Relevant training for midwives and other care staff
- An organizational culture that provides opportunities and encourages discussion and reflection around the spiritual needs of both the client and the carer
- Assessing and responding to spiritual needs beyond a tick-box exercise
- More research to unlock our understanding of the meaning, mystery and impact of spirituality during pregnancy and childbirth.

Reflective activity 11.8

How much do you know about the main religions you encounter in your practice?

Write down five key elements you are aware of about the following religions:

- Buddhism
- Christianity
- Hinduism
- Judaism
- Islam

Undertake an Internet search to check your understanding.

How do any of these religions affect pregnancy, birth, the puerperium and childcare?

It is also important to appreciate that although different religions will have particular practices around aspects of life, and indeed death, this does not mean that all people in that religion will carry out these practices. It is always useful to check with the woman as to her personal wishes around religious observance.

Prejudice

Prejudice, especially in terms of race and ethnicity, can be found in most large organizations, and it is critical that midwives address their personal prejudice and ensure that they treat all of their clients, and colleagues, with equity and respect. This would include challenging instances of bullying and safety for both women and families and their colleagues (Dietsch et al 2010).

CONCLUSION

The multicultural societies that many midwives and other healthcare workers operate in require that the services they provide be, at a minimum, culturally appropriate. There is no question in the 21st century that a human being is the composite of biological, psychological, sociocultural and spiritual elements, and that healthcare should be holistic, thus addressing the needs that arise from all the elements of a human being.

In midwifery, there has been a shifting of emphasis from dealing primarily with the biological needs to gradually understanding the interrelatedness of all elements and finding acceptable ways to address them. There is much to discover and learn, but it is hoped that this chapter has inspired the reader to begin a personal journey of discovery, the goal being the achievement of midwifery practice that responds to the essence of their clients' humanity, spirituality and cultural identity.

Key Points

- The construct of parenthood can be seen to be socially prescribed and controlled. Parenting is not a fixed role and changes with societal, cultural, ethical, political and economic influences.
- Cultural competence is complex, and the midwife has a key role in ensuring that the individual needs of women and families are met.
- Midwives must recognize the norms and values of different groups in society and strive to provide systems of care that are flexible to provide individualized care.

References

Baldacchino D: *Spiritual care: being in doing*, Malta, Preca Library, 2010.

Brogan M: *Healthcare for lesbians: attitudes and experiences, Nurs Stand* 11(45):39–42, 1997.

Crowther S, Hall J: Spirituality and spiritual care in and around childbirth, *Women Birth* 28: 173–178, 2015.

Davies L, editor: *The art and soul of midwifery: creativity in practice, education and research*, Oxford, Churchill Livingstone, 2007.

Davis-Floyd R: *Birth as an American rite of passage*, 2nd edn, California, University of California Press, 2003.

Denny E, Culley L, Papadopoulos I, et al: From womanhood to endometriosis: findings from focus groups with women from different ethnic groups, *Divers Equal Health Care* 8(3):167–180, 2011.

Dietsch E, et al: 'You can drop dead': midwives bullying women, *Women and Birth* 23(2):53–59, 2010.

Dunkley-Bent J: Reducing inequalities in childbirth: the midwife's role in public health. In Page L, McCandlish R, editors: *The new midwifery: science and sensitivity in practice*, 2nd edn, Philadelphia, Churchill Livingstone, 2006.

European Court of Human Rights, Council of Europe: *European Convention on Human Rights* (website). www.echr.coe.int/Documents/Convention_ENG.pdf. 2010.

Evans MR, Mitchell D: Exploring midwives' understanding of spiritual care and the role of the healthcare chaplain within a maternity unit, *Health and Social Care Chaplaincy* 2(1):2014.

Hall J, Taylor M: Birth and spirituality. In Downe S, editor: *Normal childhood: debate and the evidence*, Oxford, Churchill Livingstone, 2004.

House of Commons Select Committee on Health: *Eight report* (website). www.publications.parliament.uk/pa/cm200203/cmselect/cmhealth/696/69606.htm#a8. 2003.

International Confederation of Midwives: *Essential competencies for basic midwifery practice* (website). www.internationalmidwives.org/assets/uploads/documents/CoreDocuments/ICM%20Essential%20Competencies%20for%20Basic%20Midwifery%20Practice%202010,%20revised%202013.pdf. 2013.

Jesse DE, Schoneboom C, Blanchard A: The effect of faith or spirituality: a content analysis, *J Holist Nurs* 25(3):151–158, 2007.

Joels C: Impact of national policy on the health of people seeking asylum, *Nurs Stand* 22(31):35–40, 2008.

Kelley N, Stevenson J: *First do no harm: denying healthcare to people whose asylum claims have failed*, London, The Refugee Council, 2006.

Leininger M: *Transcultural nursing: concepts, theories, and practices*, New York, John Wiley and Sons, 1978.

McHugh N: Midwives of the soul: the spirituality of births, *Midwifery Matters* 97:4–5, 2003.

Mcleish J: *Mothers in exile: maternity experiences of asylum seekers in England*, London, Maternity Alliance, 2002.

McSherry W: The principal components model: a model for advancing spirituality and spiritual care within nursing and health care practice, *J Clin Nurs* 15:905–917, 2006.

Nursing and Midwifery Council: *The Code: professional standards of practice and behaviour for nurses and midwives* (website). www.nmc.org.uk/ globalassets/sitedocuments/nmc -publications/nmc-code.pdf. 2015.

Papadopoulos I: *Courage, compassion and cultural competence*. The 13th Anna Reynvaan Lecture, 19 May 2011, De Stadsschouwburg, Amsterdam City Theatre, Netherlands, 2011.

Papadopoulos I, editor: *Transcultural health and social care: development of culturally competent practitioners*, Edinburgh, Churchill Livingstone, Elsevier, 2006.

Papadopoulos I, Tilki M, Taylor G: *Transcultural care. A guide for health care professionals*, Dinton, Wilts, Quay Publications, 1998.

Parker S, McKinnon L, Kruske S: 'Choice, culture and confidence': key findings from the 2012 Having a Baby in Queensland Aboriginal and Torres Strait Islander Survey, *BMC Health Serv Res* 14(1):196, 2014.

Pembroke NF, Pembroke JJ: The spirituality of presence in midwifery care, *Midwifery* 24(3):321–327, 2008.

Rothman BK: *The tentative pregnancy: amniocentesis and the sexual politics of motherhood*, London, Pandora Press, 1994.

Spidsberg BD, Sørlie V: An expression of love – midwives' experiences in the encounter with lesbian women and their partners, *J Adv Nurs* 68(4):796–805, 2012.

Squire C, editor: *The social context of birth*, 2nd edn, Oxford, Radcliffe Medical Press, 2009.

United Nations. *Geneva Convention*, 1951.

Vertovec S: Super-diversity and its implications, *Ethn Racial Stud* 29(6):1024–1054, 2007.

Wikipedia: *Ethnic group* (website). https://en.wikipedia.org/wiki/Ethnic _group. 2016.

Wild S: *Equal PayPortal statistics on the European and UK* (website). www.equalpayportal.co.uk/ statistics/. 2016.

World Economic Forum: *The global gender gap index 2014: the case for gender equality* (website). http:// reports.weforum.org/global-gender- gap-report-2014/part-1/the-case-for- gender-equality/. 2014.

World Health Organization: *Midwifery educator core competencies* (website). http://www.who.int/hrh/nursing _midwifery/midwifery_educator _core_competencies.pdf. 2014.

Resources and additional reading

Information on FGM: www.plan-uk.org/ because-i-am-a-girl/female-genital- mutilation-fgm/?gclid=C On10rXA3ssCFQo6Gwodq8QMkg.

Real stories about young girls who had FGM done to them and the impact on their lives can be found on the ActionAid website, which also covers other issues such as refugeedom and asylum seeking: www.actionaid .org.uk/blog/voices/2015/07/01/ the-stories-behind-the-fgm-statistics.

International Confederation of Midwives (ICM): www.international midwives.org/assets/uploads/ documents/CoreDocuments/ ICM%20Essential%20 Competencies%20for%20Basic%20 Midwifery%20Practice%202010,%20 revised%202013.pdf.

The ICM standards reflect global practice and highlight essential skills.

Nursing and Midwifery Council (NMC): www.nmc.org.uk/globalassets/ sitedocuments/nmc-publications/ nmc-code.pdf.

The NMC Code sets the standards by which nurses and midwives must act. The NMC Code (2015) places people at the heart of care. Midwives need to have a sound understanding of the Code and how it relates to practice and the care provided.

The Royal College of Midwives (RCM): www.rcm.org.uk.

The RCM has a range of materials, including policy and news features and a useful electronic learning module (i-learn) on understanding asylum seekers and refugees. This module clarifies the differences between the groups and can help midwives understand and appreciate the needs of women seeking asylum or refuge.

World Health Organization (WHO): www.who.int/hrh/nursing_ midwifery/midwifery_educator_ core_competencies.pdf.

WHO Educator Core Competencies.

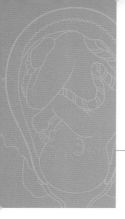

Chapter 12

Psychological context of childbirth

Julie Jomeen

Learning Outcomes

After reading this chapter, you will be able to:

- appreciate the psychological adjustments that affect a woman's experience of pregnancy, birth and early motherhood
- recognize the importance of normal and abnormal psychological adjustment
- appreciate the complexities of communication, and how this affects midwifery practice
- recognize that midwifery practice can be enhanced by understanding women's psychological context

INTRODUCTION

Psychological health is important with respect to how individuals function and adapt. Its relevance to childbearing women is clear when acknowledging the transition and adaptation that women go through in their journey from conception through to motherhood. Understanding the psychological context of a woman's pregnancy, birth and the postnatal period will help midwives to understand the complexity of a woman's experience and enable a more informed consideration of her emotional needs.

Remembering that the woman is situated within a social and cultural context, the woman's perception of herself within her context will inform and affect her maternity experience. Remember also that a midwife practices within a cultural context but that her individual experiences will lead her to have personal beliefs, which can potentially create tensions in practice. Midwives will bring their own

psychology and sociocultural influences to the maternity setting, and the challenge to midwives is to develop self-awareness and sensitivity to those influences and the related influence on women to develop a truly nonjudgemental, woman-centred approach. How midwives communicate and interact with women can have both momentous and enduring consequences.

Midwives are key to assuring the quality of women's experiences across the perinatal period and hence can be central to women's emotional health and well-being. Assessment of psychological health is now an integral part of the midwife's role. Psychological aspects of childbirth and perinatal mental illness (PMI) rose to prominence in the UK following the 2004 Confidential Enquiry in Maternal and Child Health (CEMACH 2004), when for the first time PMI was the largest cause of maternal deaths. This has remained a significant finding in subsequent reports (CEMACH 2007 and 2011), and the assessment of psychosocial health is of concern to practitioners globally (Darwin et al 2014).

Pregnancy, labour and the postnatal period are recognized as a period of physiological and psychological transition (Darvill et al 2010). The physiological effects, such as changing body shape, nausea and fatigue, are obvious, but psychological changes may not be as transparent to women or midwives. For most women the puerperium is a process of normal psychological adjustment to a major life event; for a smaller, yet significant, proportion, the adaptation will result in pathological changes (Raynor and England 2010). It is critical to avoid over-medicalization and potential stigmatization of women; hence, midwives need to be able make the distinction between normative psychological adjustment and emotional fluctuation across the perinatal period and an abnormal response that may result in a mental health problem.

PSYCHOLOGICAL ADJUSTMENT ACROSS THE PERINATAL PERIOD

Antenatal context

Pregnancy is a major life transition that significantly affects the physical, psychological and social realms of a woman's life. The journey to motherhood often requires women to address a changing body shape, shift in life focus and refocusing partner relationship and reevaluate life circumstances and future projections (Martin and Redshaw 2010). This transition results in a new conception of self, through a process of restructuring goals, behaviours and responsibilities (Barba and Selder 1995). The diverse changes that occur during pregnancy draw on and may strain a woman's psychosocial resources (Hamilton and Lobel 2008).

The prospect of becoming a mother and the associated necessary adaptations are psychologically challenging. Shaho (2010) demonstrates that physical symptom, and psychological feelings of uncertainty, doubt, regret, fear and anxiety may plague women, especially in the first trimester of pregnancy. These emotions and an absence of the anticipated elation associated with pregnancy can cause concern for expectant mothers (Modh et al 2011) and need to be acknowledged by midwives in a sensitive and supportive manner as generally normal and not pathologized.

Developing a maternal identity

Pregnancy sees the start of 'developing a maternal identity'. This complex, integrated process requires reflection on values and re-examination of relationships and identities (Hilfinger Messias and DeJoseph 2007) and involves physical, emotional, social and spiritual work (Modh et al 2011). The resulting maternal identity, however, is critical in supporting the transition to a parent responsible for the well-being of their children (Nakamura 2009). However, it may also require the relinquishment of women's own distinctiveness and aspirations. Managing a combination of roles in one's personal and professional lives has been shown to affect women's identity. In the course of pregnancy, expectant mothers may need to adapt to societal/familial expectations regarding the integration of motherhood with career and employment, in addition to adjusting their own attitudes and priorities in relation to work and family (Hilfinger Messias and DeJoseph 2007).

An expectant woman's transition is individual, and adaptation will differ among women (Lawson and Turriff-Jonasson 2006). It can be facilitated or inhibited by various factors, including cultural beliefs, life philosophy, support network availability, health and socioeconomic status and the woman's own personal expectations (Shaho 2010), all of which can influence psychological health, negatively or positively. The midwife's role is in recognising and acknowledging this process and supporting women when they appear to be finding the transition challenging.

Life circumstances can have a major influence on the pregnancy experience. Contexts such as ill-health (Tyer-Viola and Lopez 2014), domestic violence (Engnes et al. 2012), prior fetal loss (Côté-Arsenault et al 2006; Côté-Arsenault and Donato 2007), assisted conception (Lin et al 2013), the wrong time to have a baby (unplanned and/or unwanted pregnancy; Beck 2001) and age, either young (Spear 2001) or advanced (e.g. Yang et al 2007), can influence a woman's experience and pose a greater risk to the psychological health of women and their families. Identifying and assessing a woman's personal context can help midwives sketch out profiles of vulnerable women in particular; these profiles can then be considered when assessing a woman's needs across the perinatal period.

Body image

Pregnancy is a time of significant changes in weight and eating behaviour, and these changes may affect women's health and well-being. An altered body shape, diminished physical mobility and further physical changes, such as stretch marks, have been related to changes in self-concept (Chang et al 2010). Pregnant women experience varying levels of comfort with such changes (Birtwell et al 2015). Some women express increased body image satisfaction during the gestational period (Smith and Lavender, 2011) because the Western 'slim-body ideal' can be temporarily suspended (Johnson et al 2004). Body-image experiences may also be different across pregnancy (Johnson et al 2004), for example, women commonly express relief when the pregnancy becomes more obvious (Nash 2012).

Conflict has been identified between a woman's concerns regarding her own body image, versus concerns for the infant's well-being. Women express a desire for acceptance and support from those around them in this regard, particularly from their partners and peer group (Chang et al 2010), but this would also include midwives, who need to be mindful that dissatisfaction with body image during pregnancy has been linked to psychological distress (Lavender 2007) and a loss of self-confidence (Chang et al 2010).

Interpersonal relationships and social support

During pregnancy, intimate partner relationships have been found to evolve, undergoing an 'internal shift' as women's roles and expectations in relation to their significant other are renegotiated (Hilfinger Messias and DeJoseph, 2007). Patterns of communication alter and domestic responsibilities are redistributed in a process that is described as challenging, dynamic and complex (Hilfinger Messias and DeJoseph, 2007). For most couples the

187

intimate partner relationship improves during pregnancy (Schneider 2002). However, such a profound change can lead to relationship breakdown, especially if the bond was already fragile. It can also be in this context that domestic abuse can emerge for the first time or intensify, and midwives need to be observant for such signs (Raynor and England 2010).

In the woman's wider social circle, building, sustaining and/or reorganizing personal relationships is a part of the personal work of pregnancy (Hilfinger Messias and DeJoseph 2007), which may be most significant in a first pregnancy. Pregnancy often enables a woman to feel more connected to others, often most importantly to her own mother, who acts as an important source of support (Shaho 2010; Modh et al 2011) and also can provide a model from which to recreate positive childhood experiences. However, for some women it involves confronting perceived parental mistakes and poor parenting, which can be challenging and distressing (Raynor and England 2010).

The gestational period may also be experienced as a time of separation from others once regarded as close (Birtwell et al 2015) because of a disparity in life experiences. This may leave the women's sense of social identity somewhat challenged and her social networks diminished. Social isolation and inadequate social support have been consistently identified as significant psychosocial risk factors for PMI (Johnson et al 2012).

Responsibility to the baby

Expectant women feel that it is their duty to the protect the fetus, with the baby's health then a source of anxiety (Shaho 2010). Safekeeping of the fetus involves healthy habits and discontinuation of activities that could potentially cause harm (Hilfinger Messias and DeJoseph 2007; Birtwell et al 2015). Women are asked to make many decisions in pregnancy, which can test a sense of control and create anxieties, such as in Lucy's case (see web Case Scenario 12.1). Maternity choices are expected to be both safe and responsible, and women who make the 'wrong' societally perceived choice can be open to public disapproval and censure, with potentially negative psychological consequences (Jomeen 2010). A role of the midwife is to help a woman to make fully informed choice and, provided that is the case, to continue with nonjudgemental care.

The focus on choice and decision making aims to make women feel involved and empowered (see Ch. 34). This is, in part, a recognition that a negative perception of care during pregnancy and birth can have adverse effects on psychological well-being. When choices are fulfilled this can lead to high levels of satisfaction (Kirkham 2010), but midwives must be aware of potential negative consequences when choice cannot be fulfilled because of changing clinical contexts (Jomeen 2010); open communication and partnership in working with women are key in such cases.

Physical health and functioning

Physical functioning decreases during normal pregnancy; for example, more than 70% of pregnant women experience nausea and vomiting, and 28% report that symptoms create substantial lifestyle limitations and cause changes to usual activities, including family, social and work activities (Attard et al 2002). Women also report impairment through physical pregnancy symptoms and fatigue (Magee et al 2002), which affects women's ability to perform usual roles. Even in an uneventful pregnancy women have subtle changes that may detract from their quality of life. Quality of life has increasingly been shown to play a significant role in the psychological well-being of pregnant and postnatal women.

Current or previous mental health disorder

Pregnancy is a more vulnerable time for the origin of PMI than at other times in a woman's life. The risk of being admitted to hospital with a severe mental illness (SMI) following childbirth is significantly increased compared with the general population. New cases of SMI are more likely to occur in the postnatal rather than antenatal periods. However, for certain SMIs, such as severe depressive illnesses, schizophrenia and bipolar disorder, the risk of reoccurrence of relapse can be increased in pregnancy, particularly if medication is stopped (Joint Commissioning Panel for Mental Health 2012; see Ch. 69).

Summary of antenatal context

Pregnancy heralds a time of enormous change, socially, physically and emotionally. The numerous demands of pregnancy and the negotiation of all the changes create inevitable fluctuations of mood; women move between emotional highs and lows in addition to general ambivalence.

Reflective activity 12.1

Visit the website and read Case Study 12.2. Can you identify the issues that might be psychologically relevant in Sarah's pregnancy? Consider how significant these might be and how you would respond if you were to see Sarah at an antenatal appointment.

Midwives must be aware of and sensitive to the biophysical, social and personal adjustment that being pregnant creates for women (Raynor and England 2010). What is significant for psychological health is that the strongest predictors of postnatal depression (PND) and parenting stress are antenatal depression and anxiety, low self-esteem and stress related to child care (Beck 2001; Misri et al 2010). This demonstrates clearly how the emotional journey that begins antenatally can have potential consequences for the whole perinatal period (Alderdice et al 2013). It is essential for the midwife to be able to determine the difference between normal psychological adaptation to a life changing event and abnormal psychological adjustment that leads to psychological morbidity (see Ch. 69).

Labour and birth

The birth of a baby is a life-changing experience for women, and it can have a positive or negative influence on her psychological well-being. Raynor (2006) identifies a number of normative emotional responses to labour (Box 12.1).

Birth can be an experience that leaves a woman with positive memories, when her wishes and potential for empowerment were respected. Birth is an unknown for women, even for women who have previously given birth; each experience is unique, and women have to navigate and manage an excess of physical and emotional sensations and responses across the labour and birth period. Women reporting negative birth experiences describe feeling violated, vulnerable, excluded, cheated, frightened, undignified and depersonalized (Mercer et al 2012).

Sense of control

Perception of feeling in control has been related to positive psychological outcomes and a positive birth experience. Redshaw and colleagues (2007) identified four factors as important in supporting women's sense of control: continuity of carer, one-to-one care in labour, not being left alone for long periods and involvement in decision making. Some of these are difficult to achieve within some models of maternity care provision, and although they might be the 'gold standard', control can be related to how women perceive they were treated, and feeling 'cared about' and 'cared for' by caregivers was significantly and positively related to feelings of control (Jomeen 2010; Green and Baston 2003). The role of the midwife as effective communicator and caregiver is therefore clearly central. Maternal control can be facilitated in all birth settings and contexts when women feel informed and involved in decision making. Fulfilled birth choices are important for positive psychological outcomes; however, unfulfilled choices do not necessarily result in negative psychological consequences. Professionals' manner and communication can significantly affect women's feelings

of control of their birth experience (Salter 2009) and the ability to make informed decisions (Eliasson et al 2008). Choices made outside of the labouring context can sometimes be difficult to fulfil because of a changing clinical picture; in that context information should be sensitively discussed, and decision making should be shared and renegotiated as appropriate to the woman's cognitive and emotional state at the time (Jomeen 2010; Jefford and Jomeen 2015).

Conversely, loss of control can be significant in psychological terms. Low levels of perceived personal control have been shown to be related to the experience of post-traumatic stress symptoms following childbirth (Czarnocka and Slade 2000) and PND (Lemola et al 2007).

Traumatic birth

Experiencing childbirth as a traumatic event is a factor that has been highlighted as contributing to poorer psychological outcomes for mothers. Although prevalence is not entirely certain, up to 30% of women in the UK experience childbirth as a traumatic event, with many consequently going on to experience some form of anxiety, depression, or post-traumatic stress disorder (PTSD) following childbirth (Ayers 2014). In addition, some women may experience subclinical distress but not develop a subsequent psychological disorder (Elmir et al 2010).

The term *traumatic birth* is now used to include the notion that the birth experience per se, irrespective of physical injury or intervention, can be traumatic. Beck (2004) offers a definition for birth trauma centred round the mother's psychological rather than physical experience, as shown in Box 12.2.

Evidence indicates that one significant cause of a women's perception of birth as traumatic is the actions or inactions of caregivers, including midwives, which results in care being experienced as dehumanizing, disrespectful and uncaring (Elmir et al 2010). Women with traumatic delivery experiences often suggest that staff do not listen to them, fail to give clear information and explanations, are not respectful when they elect not to have examinations and interventions and fail to validate and recognize their fears during labour (McKenzie-McHarg et al 2014). Choice, information and involvement in decisions are potentially protective against a traumatic birth experience for women (Goodall et al 2009; also see

---

Box 12.1 Normative emotional responses to labour		
Excitement	Anxiety	Fear of pain
Anticipation	Fear of the unknown	Fear of birth
Relief	Fear of technology	
Sense of control	Fear of loss of control of bodily functions	
(Raynor 2006)		

Box 12.2 Definition of traumatic birth
'An event occurring during the labour and delivery process that involves actual or threatened serious injury or death to the mother or her infant. The birthing woman experiences intense fear, helplessness, loss of control, and horror' (Beck 2004: 28).

Ch. 38). Therefore, midwives need to understand that childbirth can be traumatic for women (Elmir et al 2010), acknowledge the role they may play in reducing the risk and recognize the signs of psychological trauma (Beck 2004).

There has been a recent acknowledgement that the psychological trauma can occur to others present at the birth. In particular, the woman's partner can have a psychological reaction to a traumatic birth (Ayers and Nicholls 2007), although this is not yet well understood. There is also evidence that staff witnessing traumatic childbirth have an increased risk of developing PTSD symptoms (Sheen et al 2014), meaning that midwives need to actively manage the boundary between recognizing and supporting women experiencing trauma and their own professional and personal resources.

As well as the short- and long-term mental health consequences, the significance of traumatic birth and its associated psychological outcomes may be in the future reproductive decisions women make, in particular those they make for subsequent births and the support required of midwives (see web Case Scenario 12.3). Despite the increasing knowledge of traumatic birth experiences, very few professional support services are available to help women after the event and before a subsequent birth (Thomson and Downe 2010). Fear of childbirth is both a consequence of (Elmir et al 2010) and a risk factor for Post Traumatic Stress Symptoms (PTSS) (Otley 2012). PTSS is the name given to the symptoms that can be experienced after a traumatic event but do not meet the diagnostic and statistical manual of mental disorders (American Psychiatric Association 2017) criteria for diagnosing PTSD. The jury is out in relation to debriefing following a traumatic birth. A less standardized 'postnatal discussion', in which a woman has the opportunity to evaluate the course of labour and birth, to ask questions and to voice her opinion to a trained professional, is recommended for women who wish to talk about their experiences (National Institute for Health and Care Excellence (NICE) 2014). Many women find it helpful in processing a negative birth experience, but research is ambiguous about its role in preventing PTSD or PND (McKenzie-McHarg et al 2014).

Fear of childbirth

Fear of childbirth as a consequence of traumatic birth or a negative birth experience occurs in multiparous women and is known as secondary fear of childbirth (tokophobia). However, fear of childbirth is actually more common in first-time expectant women. This fear is related to concerns about the baby but also anxiety about the unknown, a perceived lack of control and an inability to perceive the body as capable of giving birth safely. This can result in low expectations of positive outcomes and the ability to birth (Fenwick et al 2013). Primiparous women's perceptions are potentially influenced by media portrayals of childbirth, which catastrophize labour pain,

which increases the woman's sense of helplessness and fear of labour (Talbot 2012).

This has led in part to increased requests for an elective caesarean section (ECS), although other factors, such as convenience and body image, also underpin maternal requests for ECS. The midwifery role is in identifying and promoting strategies and behaviours to support women to consider vaginal birth and enhance self-efficacy but also to support the woman's choices where this is evidently beneficial to her psychological health. Goodin and Griffiths (2012) highlight that when the woman has severe tokophobia, denial of an ECS could lead to PTSD. Midwifery support for women with fear of childbirth who do choose to have a vaginal birth is also critical to a positive psychological experience (see Ch. 38 and web Case Scenario 12.3).

Mode of birth

Many women experience labour and birth with no problems, but a significant proportion of women will have an intervention such as a caesarean section (CS) or an instrumental delivery. The issues related to ECS were discussed earlier and may in some cases be psychologically protective. However, women who undergo a CS or an instrumental delivery have demonstrated higher levels of maternal grief, dissatisfaction and anxiety than women who have a spontaneous vaginal birth, with implications for self-efficacy, self-esteem and self-confidence (Raynor and England 2010). The promotion within midwifery of normality and the promotion of physiological birth as ideal must not lead to birth by CS being conceptualized as a failure. Language can be critical when discussing the reasons for an assisted delivery (Jomeen 2010), to avoid negative self-concept for women as they become new mothers. Midwives may also feel responsible and in need of support when a birth does not go as expected, and accessing the support mechanisms available is important to underpin continued professional confidence and positive communication with women.

High-risk women, such as those with a multiple pregnancy or medical risk factors, who may already be more psychologically vulnerable as a consequence, are more likely to end up with interventions during labour and birth. Technological interventions are premised on ensuring a safe outcome, yet the medicalized approach to managing women at high risk can often leave little space for consideration of psychosocial needs. The midwife's role here is to consider the psychological effects of a technologized birth and promote the women's sense of control through information-giving and good communication. Even within seemingly constrained circumstances, this will directly influence the degree of anxiety experienced and minimize emotional distress.

Summary of birth

There is a clear significance of the social and psychological dimensions of labour and birth for women's continuing journey into motherhood. Midwives must consider the emotional responses that women are likely to encounter at this time and the impact on the woman's psychological health and well-being. Awareness of psychological vulnerability offers caregivers the opportunity to enhance a woman's sense of control during labour and birth, resulting in positive psychological consequences.

Postnatal context

The preceding sections have identified many factors that, as part of a perinatal continuum, may influence a woman's psychological health in the postnatal period, not least her antenatal adaptation to impending motherhood and the events that happen in labour.

Physical recovery

The first 6 to 8 weeks after birth are a period of physical recovery alongside social and emotional adjustment, and women's mood status tends to be wide-ranging and unpredictable. New mothers are inevitably anxious, and it would be more concerning if they were not; women want to be competent mothers perceived as coping well. Many factors influence women's psychological health at this time; a woman's mood often reflects the baby's needs and patterns of crying, feeding and sleeping.

Lack of sleep is a major contributor to mood because sleep deprivation has a significant effect on human functioning; this includes cognitive and motor performance, but mood is the most significantly affected by sleep deprivation. Return to more normative sleep patterns is significant in resumption of normal daily functioning and activities, but for some women this will take months or even years. Profiles in terms of psychological well-being, for the majority of new mothers, will steadily improve over a period of 6 months as physical recovery from childbirth takes place (Spiteri et al 2013). Midwives can give reassurance to mothers in that regard, but should also encourage mothers to accept that recovery from birth is not immediate. It is important to remember that birth is a strenuous physical event; women now return home very quickly after birth and often associate that with an expectation that everything should be as it was before (see web Case Scenario 12.4). Midwives need to explain that activities should be built back up slowly, and rest should be taken whenever possible. In addition, encourage them to ask family and friends for practical support, especially in the early postnatal days, emphasizing that it is not a failure to not be able to do everything that was possible before. Without such advice and support women often feel pressure to return to 'normal' too soon, which can affect their sense of themselves as good mothers but also increases their exhaustion, leading to psychological vulnerability.

Other factors may contribute to distress, such as difficulty breastfeeding (Taylor and Johnson 2010), especially when women suffer physical effects such as mastitis or painful nipples. Midwives can contribute to maternal psychological well-being by giving practical support relating to feeding, again emphasizing that difficulties breastfeeding are normal and not a failure, building women's general confidence in their mothering skills (Marshall et al 2007).

Baby blues and postnatal depression

It is common for women to experience the 'baby blues' between 4 and 5 days postnatal. This fluctuation of emotions and low mood is transitory and should last no longer than 1 month. PND differs in that it can occur at any time up to 1 year postnatal and has a significant impact on the woman's recovery and transition to motherhood. It is estimated that up to 70% of mothers in the nonclinical population experience some negative emotional response in the days following childbirth, although incidence of PND is 10% to 15%. Over half of all mothers experience some form of psychological difficulty described as the baby blues (Royal College of Psychiatry 2015).

Oakley (2013) found that 40% to 50% of the women who had been labelled with PND were actually just reacting to the impact of exhaustion, sleep deprivation, experience of hospitalization and the shock of becoming a new mother, illustrating how normative adjustment can be mistaken as symptoms of mental illness. Midwives need to work carefully to differentiate between transient psychological difficulty and PND so they can make appropriate assessment and clinical decisions, but also to reassure women about the normality of their feelings.

Reflective activity 12.2

Consider the symptoms of baby blues and PND in Box 12.3. Identify the overlapping symptoms and think about what would lead you to be able to differentiate between them. Think about what action you might then take if you were concerned that it might be PND.

The reality of change

Although much adjustment has already begun in the antenatal period, including the definition of a maternal identity and renegotiation within the couple relationship, friendships and with family, the postnatal period signifies the reality of the situation.

This can be difficult when things are not as expected. Not all women will experience immediate overwhelming love for their baby, although most expect they will, and this can leave women feeling like bad mothers. Midwives can play a significant role in encouraging women to express these thoughts and in normalizing these feelings for women and thus help prevent increasing anxiety.

Box 12.3 Symptoms of baby blues and postnatal depression

Baby Blues

Transient low mood – peaks 4–5 days postnatally, usually disappears by 4 weeks

Women may experience:
- fatigue
- feeling overemotional, tearfulness
- mood swings
- low spirits
- anxiety
- forgetfulness and muddled thinking
- confusion
- headache
- insomnia irritability
- emotional lability

Does not usually require intervention

Postnatal Depression

Can occur at any time in the early or late postnatal period

Women may experience:
- an inability to experience pleasure
- depressed mood
- loss of interest or pleasure
- significant increases or decreases in appetite
- insomnia or hypersomnia
- psychomotor agitation or retardation
- fatigue or loss of energy
- feelings of worthlessness or guilt
- diminished concentration
- recurrent thoughts of suicide

Requires intervention at some level
Jomeen and Bateman (2014)

Some women will appear initially disinterested; this may be related to the birth experience or just general shock at the overwhelming sense of becoming a new mother (Jomeen 2010). For some women the baby will not meet the romanticized picture of their baby that was in their heads during pregnancy. This is usually transient, and adjustment usually occurs within a few days. If the situation is more enduring, then midwives need to explore the woman's feelings in more detail and undertake a more comprehensive psychological assessment. Women can sometimes be dissatisfied/disappointed with their role as a mother, although it is suggested that this can often stem from poor support rather than the role itself (Raynor and England 2010).

In the first few weeks, families need to make real-life adjustments to the way they live and manage their relationships, while undergoing changes on an individual level. Role conflicts and confusion are often a reality because of competing demands. Friendships become tested, and often existing friends, particularly those with no children, will drift away. Some friendships will be strengthened, and new relationships with other new parents are likely to be forged, but limited time to pursue other activities can leave some women feeling socially isolated (Raynor and England 2010). Existing family dynamics need to adjust, parents become grandparents and existing children have to adapt to a new baby, all of which can be emotionally taxing for women.

Midwives should remember that men are making the transition to fatherhood. Their own experiences of being fathered, their lifestyle and their non-father identities will all contribute to how they develop relationships within the new family structure. Like women, men are judged against a discourse of good and bad fathering, which is important when a healthy father–child relationship is as critical to positive child development as a mother–child relationship (Sethna et al 2015). Midwives should encourage father involvement because it contributes to the psychological and social well-being of both their children and partners. Men can be a source of strong psychological support, and active engagement with the father can help harness that support.

When a baby dies or is ill

For some parents the reality of parenthood will fail to transpire because of miscarriage, intra-uterine fetal loss, stillbirth, or neonatal death. This is clearly a profoundly distressing experience for women and their partners, and women's psychological status at this time is complex. Midwives need to be conversant with the various grief reactions and work to help parents through the stages of their grief, allowing opportunities to talk but also recognizing their limitations in this regard (see Chs 51 and 68).

When a baby is admitted to the neonatal intensive care unit (NICU) following birth, women and their partners can also experience a grief reaction. There is a sense of loss that things have not turned out as expected, and there is the trauma of initial separation. Midwives in the early postbirth period need to facilitate regular contact with the baby, and clear and regular explanations of the plan of care are critical to help parents make sense of what is happening. There is evidence that both fathers and mothers of preterm infants experience higher levels of anxiety and depression than parents of healthy, term infants (Lefkowitz et al 2010). Admission of the infant to the NICU presents the family with multiple stressors, such as disruption of family routines, concern for other children, fatigue and financial burden as a result of travelling to the hospital and loss of income (Howland 2007). However, good support and helping parents to understanding what has happened and why, alongside a formal diagnosis, if relevant, can be a critical factor in moderating anxiety levels (Jomeen and Martin 2012).

Assessing women's psychological health status

Individual women will demonstrate wide variation in their emotional status, from a minor transient experience, such as baby blues, to severe mental illness, such as puerperal psychosis. Practitioners will see women with an existing mental health disorder who become pregnant and women who develop mental illness when they have previously been well. In practice, assessment aims both to identify women with an existing mental health disorder and attempt to assess risk of future onset of a 'distress'/depression and anxiety. In the UK the NICE guidelines for antenatal and postpartum mental health (NICE 2014) give all healthcare professionals working with perinatal women a clearly defined remit for assessment of women's psychological health status. (See Ch. 69.)

Understanding the psychological context in which women become pregnant, give birth and enter motherhood helps midwives to identify women who might be at risk. Assessment of women's psychological health forms part of a broader psychosocial assessment, which aims to place assessment in the context of a woman's life circumstances, providing a holistic integrated, woman-centred approach. The administration of a standardized screening tool, such as those identified by NICE (2014), when coupled with discussing women's life situations may also make screening more acceptable to women and support disclosure (Brealey et al 2010). Identifying psychosocial risk factors can support healthcare professionals to sketch out profiles of vulnerability, profiles that can then be considered when assessing a woman's needs across the perinatal period and making appropriate and timely referrals for those women in need. Evidence from over several decades now identifies some fairly consistent psychosocial risk factors (Box 12.4).

Box 12.4 Psychosocial risk factors for PMI

Previous psychiatric disorder
Family history of serious mental ill-health
Social disadvantage and isolation
Poverty
Minority ethnic group
Asylum seekers and refugees
Late 'bookers' and nonattenders
Domestic violence and abuse, sexual abuse, trauma or childhood maltreatment
Substance misuse
Known to child protection services
Employment status
Physical ill health
Life events
Lack of support/social networks/quality of interpersonal relationships
The woman's attitude towards the pregnancy, including denial of pregnancy
The woman's experience of pregnancy/problems experienced by her, the fetus or the baby
The mother–baby relationship
Responsibilities as a carer for other children and young people or other adults

(CEMACH 2004, 2007 and 2011; NICE 2014)

Midwives are not counsellors or therapists; knowing when and where to refer women in need of specialist support is important. Access to specialist services is variable according to location (Jomeen and Martin 2014). Some areas will have clearly defined pathways and specialist perinatal mental health service provision or perinatal mental health midwives, yet none of this is universal. Referral back to the general practitioner may be the only route available in some areas. What is important is that midwives know when a woman's mental health is at risk, recognize that the care required is outside their scope of practice and know how a referral can be made.

Reflective activity 12.4 ✕

Consider whether you would know where and how to refer if you identified a woman with significant psychosocial risk factors/risk of perinatal mental illness.

MIDWIFE–WOMAN RELATIONSHIP

Understanding women's individual psychological context, challenges and resources in the journey to motherhood is

---

Reflective activity 12.3 ✕

When next taking an antenatal history from a woman, reflect on whether you gained a comprehensive and detailed history of the woman's psychosocial health. Did you use the questions recommended by NICE (2014)? Did you consider the woman's wider psychosocial context using the previously described checklist?

---

an important aspect of the midwifery role. Sensitive enquiry about the psychosocial aspects of women's lives can only be achieved through effective communication, which enables women to share anxieties, fears and worries, sometimes in situations when they are disadvantaged, either by pain or by circumstances that make disclosure difficult. It also helps women to cope with feelings and find words to express themselves. Supporting women to share those issues and feelings is essential so that appropriate care can be offered.

Most women review their experience and make the transition to motherhood smoothly, successfully dealing with their maternal emotions. How the midwife deals with emotion can have a significant impact on women. It is widely accepted that good communication between women, their partners and families is central to making them feel valued and enhancing well-being (Raynor and England 2010). Unfortunately, evidence persistently shows that communication with midwives is an area of dissatisfaction for women (Jomeen 2010; Jomeen and Redshaw 2013).

For some women, the relationship between themselves and the midwife may be critical. For women without an extended family network or friends that are socially isolated, a positive human relationship can have psychotherapeutic value. A sound relationship with the midwife will provide stability for the woman and reduce her experiences of anxiety or fear, enabling her to develop confidence in herself and experience a positive pregnancy and birth.

For a relationship to develop or establish, three components are required:

- Trust
- Respect
- Communication

Trust

Trust rests on common value, not necessarily on common viewpoints, but the midwife must have respect for the woman's values and priorities (Kirkham 2010). When a mother feels safe in her relationship with her midwife, a positive relationship is much more likely to develop because the mother feels acknowledged and valued. Advocacy goes hand in hand with trust, and this means that midwives need to trust and believe in a woman's ability to be pregnant, give birth and make decisions, so that the woman will believe in her own ability. This is in direct opposition to a midwife who exerts authority and offers choice but then proffers personal opinions either through her verbal or nonverbal communication or gatekeeps through the withholding of information. The notion of choice and the woman as an active decision maker then becomes compromised, which can have implications for women's psychological outcomes (Jomeen 2010).

A second aspect of trust is that if the midwife is confident in her own ability to provide care to a woman and her partner, they, in turn, will have confidence in the midwife. The woman will feel safe and as a consequence be prepared to tell her personal story, resulting in a woman-centred approach to care.

A third aspect of trust is compassion. It is a challenge for midwives to remain compassionate when they are working under pressure. The requirement for midwives to give the right emotional response to the clinical situations that emerge has been reported as challenging and stressful (Deery and Kirkham 2006 and 2007). Midwives develop their own strategies to deal with these pressures, including strategies to remain detached. Although this may enable midwives to cope, they inevitably create boundaries and distance from women. Where midwives conceal their own emotions, women experience them as uncaring, see no reason to confide in the midwife and respond by masking their own emotions (Deery and Kirkham 2007).

Respect

Respect for women is the foundation on which all meetings or interventions are built (Egan 2007). It is a way of seeing the woman as a unique individual and maintaining her dignity. The midwife needs to convey in her way of being that she will not cause any harm and that she is skilled, competent and confident in her practice. The midwife needs to convey that she will be the woman's advocate on her journey. This does not mean that the midwife should collude with requests or behaviours that are risky. Although colluding midwives often perceive themselves as advocates, they are failing to work in partnership with women and are in fact abdicating their professional responsibility (Jefford and Jomeen 2015). The midwife's role is to point out the risk in evidenced terms and allow the woman to make an informed decision, as is her right. This sometimes requires midwives to suspend personal judgements, but respecting women is to treat them as a true partner when providing care.

Communication

Communication, in its simplest form, is that one person speaks to another who hears and understands what is said and responds to the speaker (Fig. 12.1). However, this does not allow for the complexities surrounding human interaction (Box 12.5). Essentially, communication falls into two groups: verbal and nonverbal.

Making a first impression

Initiation of the relationship begins with early impressions; often this is through nonverbal communication. This can be negative or positive, but these early impressions are often the most significant and permanent. Once

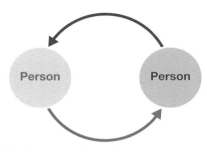

Figure 12.1 Communication cycle.

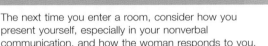

Box 12.5 Characteristics of communication

Verbal communication	Nonverbal communication
Uses speech to share thoughts, feelings and ideas	Uses all other ways to share thoughts, feelings and ideas
Affected by:	Facial expressions
Content	Touch
Tone of voice	Gestures
	Silence
	Posture
	Space
	See web Activity 12.2 for SOLER.

an impression has been formed, people look for evidence that reinforces their initial conclusions, so although first impressions (nonverbal or verbal) can be corrected, this requires a lot of emotional work on behalf of both parties and sometimes cannot be repaired (Raynor and England 2010).

Reflective activity 12.5 ><

The next time you enter a room, consider how you present yourself, especially in your nonverbal communication, and how the woman responds to you. Also consider her nonverbal communication – what is her body language telling you (Fig. 12.2)?

Building and/or maintaining a woman–midwife relationship

Relationships are not easy to build with everyone. Sometimes an emotional relationship is not possible; in those cases midwives need to ensure a professional relationship through which they provide good-quality care. Midwives are usually judged as "bad" because of their attitude, attributes and the lack of a relationship, rather than a failure to provide the physical aspects of care (Bharj and Chesney 2010). Good communication underpins women's assessments of a midwife's attributes; poor communication when described by

BODY
Her posture; is it upright and relaxed or crumpled and tense? Is her movement restricted? What gestures does she make?

EYES
Does she look at you with ease, or are her eyes downcast? Are her eyes staring or flitting about?

FACE
Does she look worried, biting her lips, frowning or smiling?

VOICE
Does she speak rapidly or slowly? High pitched? Quiet and/or mumbling? Struggle to find the right words?

PERSONAL SPACE
Does she need lots of personal space, or can you get physically close during conversations?

PHYSICALITY
Does she look prepared, is she caring for herself, does she look fit? Is she agitated or short of breath? Pupils dilated or constricted?

Figure 12.2 Reading a woman's body language.

women is consistently linked to the behaviours and characteristics that midwives display (Jomeen and Redshaw 2012; see Box 12.6).

Key concepts that underpin effective communication

Being heard is fundamental in any relationship (Kirkham 2010), yet listening is a difficult skill to develop because it takes time (Raynor and England 2010) and is about more than just letting someone talk. It involves the use of reflection and paraphrasing and demonstration of empathy, warmth and genuineness (see Table 12.1 for definitions).

Figure 12.3 illustrates some of the factors that might affect midwives' and women's ability to listen. The midwife

Box 12.6 Women's views of good and bad midwives

Good midwives

The attributes of a good midwife that are important to women include friendly, kind, smiling, caring, approachable, nonjudgemental, have time, are respectful, provide support and companionship and are good communicators (Nicholls and Webb 2006)

Good midwives establish rapport and create a relationship of a social nature (Bharj and Chesney 2010).

Bad midwives

Bad midwives are unhelpful, insensitive, abrupt, officious, fail to listen and lack concern (Nicholls and Webb 2006),

Bad midwives are disrespectful and insensitive, fail to respond to women's support needs and leave women feeling disempowered (Jomeen and Redshaw 2012).

Table 12.1 Activities involved in active listening

Reflection	The midwife, having listened to the woman, will repeat one or two words back to her to encourage what she is saying, rather like an echo (Egan 2007).
Paraphrasing	The midwife listens to the woman and then restates in her own words, demonstrating she has absorbed the information. This helps the woman to feel understood and, if the midwife has misunderstood, to correct her or him.
Questions	These can be closed, open, directive and multiple. Too many closed questions can make a woman feel vulnerable.
Empathy	This is the ability of the midwife to see the woman's inner world and communicate that back to the woman.
Genuineness	The midwife is her real self when working with the woman (Egan 2007).
Unconditional positive regard	This is the ability to see the woman as an individual unique person whose contribution is valued and valid.
Presence	Closeness in all domains; physical, psychological emotional and spiritual – it is 'being with' rather than 'doing to' and can be particularly valuable psychosocial support when words become redundant (Raynor and England 2010).

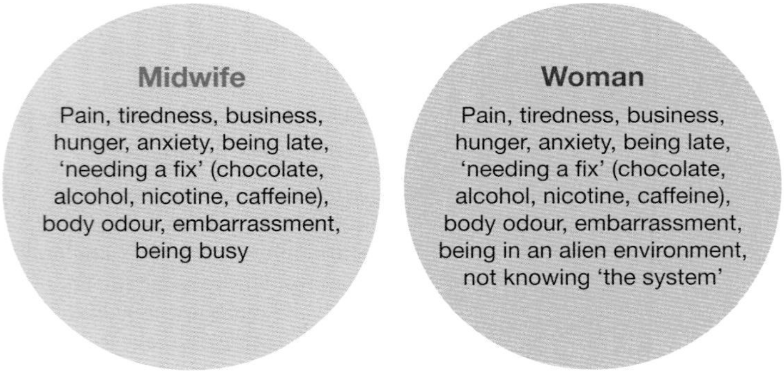

Midwife

Pain, tiredness, business, hunger, anxiety, being late, 'needing a fix' (chocolate, alcohol, nicotine, caffeine), body odour, embarrassment, being busy

Woman

Pain, tiredness, business, hunger, anxiety, being late, 'needing a fix' (chocolate, alcohol, nicotine, caffeine), body odour, embarrassment, being in an alien environment, not knowing 'the system'

Figure 12.3 Factors that might affect midwives' and women's ability to listen.

needs to concentrate on what the woman has to say and be present. The use of interpreters when a woman cannot speak English can pose challenges for midwives (see Ch. 23); midwives need to use support mechanisms available to enable effective communication to take place.

Summary

Midwives are not counsellors, but good midwife–women relationships are central to women's experiences of childbirth and are important to midwives as well. Poor communication can result in poor outcomes, so examining how well we communicate as midwives is essential to good care. The skills audit and checklist (website Tables 12.1 and 12.2) will help identify strengths and areas for improvement. Good relationships are built on trust, mutuality and empathy, which can be emotionally demanding, but when achieved they are immensely rewarding for both parties.

CONCLUSION

The perinatal period represents a period of immense physical and social change for women that requires significant emotional effort and is consequently characterized by fluctuating mood states and negative and positive emotions. Midwives must consider what is normative in emotional terms and how women cope with the challenges of pregnancy, recognizing that women's responses will inevitably be as individual as women themselves. Midwives are ideally placed to support women throughout the normative emotional adjustment of this period in women's lives but are equally well placed to identify the triggers that may signal psychological distress and initiate timely intervention.

Key Points

- Midwives need to recognize that a woman's individual psychological context will affect her journey through pregnancy, birth and the puerperium.
- Women can be supported in this journey by sensitive and holistic midwifery care that considers women's psychosocial needs as a fundamental aspect of care.
- Midwives must ensure they continually reflect on and refine their communication skills to enable them to effectively determine women's psychosocial needs.
- Midwives must be able to recognize the difference between normal and abnormal psychological adaptation across the perinatal period.
- Midwives must be aware of how their behaviour can influence women's experiences and their decision making.

References

Alderdice F, Ayers S, Darwin Z, et al: Measuring psychological health in the perinatal period: workshop consensus statement, 19 March 2013, *J Reprod Infant Psychol* 31:431–438, 2013.

American Psychiatric Association: *Diagnostic and statistical manual of mental disorders*, 5th edn, DSM. http://dsm.psychiatryonline.org/doi/book/10.1176/appi.books.9780890425596. 2017.

Attard CL, Kohli MA, Coleman S, et al: The burden of illness of severe nausea and vomiting of pregnancy in the United States, *Am J Obstet Gynecol* 186(5):222–227, 2002.

Ayers S: Fear of childbirth, postnatal post-traumatic stress disorder and midwifery care, *Midwifery* 30(7):145–148, 2014.

Ayers S, Nicholls K: Childbirth-related post-traumatic stress disorder in couples: a qualitative study, *Br J Health Psychol* 12(4):491–509, 2007.

Barba E, Selder F: Life transitions theory, *Nurs Leadersh Forum* 1:4–11, 1995.

Beck CT: Predictors of postpartum depression: an update, *Nurs Res* 50:275–285, 2001.

Beck CT: Birth trauma: in the eye of the beholder, *Nurs Res* 53(1):28–35, 2004.

Bharj KK, Chesney M: The midwife-mother relationship. In Kirkham M, editor: *The midwife-mother relationship*, Basingstoke, Palgrave Macmillan, pp 160–173, 2010.

Birtwell B, Hammond L, Puckering C: 'Me and my bump': an interpretative phenomenological analysis of the experiences of pregnancy for vulnerable women, *Clin Child Psychol Psychiatry* 20(2):218–228, 2015.

Brealey SD, Hewitt C, Green JM, et al: Screening for postnatal depression: is it acceptable to women and healthcare professionals? A systematic review and meta-synthesis, *J Reprod Infant Psychol* 28:328–344, 2010.

Chang S, Kenney NJ, Chao YY: Transformation in self-identity amongst Taiwanese women in late pregnancy: a qualitative study, *Int J Nurs Stud* 47(1):60–66, 2010.

Confidential Enquiry into Maternal and Child Health (CEMACH): *Why mothers die (2000–2002)*, London, RCOG, 2004.

Confidential Enquiry into Maternal and Child Health (CEMACH): *Saving mothers' lives: reviewing maternal deaths to make motherhood safer (2003–2005)*, London, RCOG, 2007.

Confidential Enquiry into Maternal and Child Health (CEMACH): Saving mothers' lives: reviewing maternal deaths 2006–2008, *Br J Obstet Gynaecol* 118(Suppl 1):1–203, 2011.

Côté-Arsenault D, Donato KL: Restrained expectations in late pregnancy following loss, *J Obstet Gynecol Neonatal Nurs* 3(6):550–557, 2007.

Côté-Arsenault D, Donato KL, Earl SS: Watching & worrying: early pregnancy after loss experiences, *MCN Am J Matern Child Nurs* 31(6):356–363, 2006.

Czarnocka AJ, Slade P: Prevalence and predictors of posttraumatic stress symptoms following childbirth, *Br J Clin Psychol* 39:35–51, 2000.

Darvill T, Skirton H, Farrand P: Psychological factors that impact on women's experiences of first-time motherhood: a qualitative study of the transition, *Midwifery* 26:357–366, 2010.

Darwin Z, McGowan L, Edozien LC: Antenatal mental health referrals: review of local clinical practice and pregnant women's experiences in England, *Midwifery* 31(3):e17–e22, 2014.

Deery R, Kirkham M: Supporting midwives to support women. In *The new midwifery: science and sensitivity in practice*, London, Elsevier Health Sciences, pp 125–140, 2006.

Deery R, Kirkham M: Drained and dumped on: the generation and accumulation of emotional toxic waste in community midwifery. In *Exploring the dirty side of women's health*, London, Routledge, pp 72–83, 2007.

Egan G: *The skilled helper: a problem-management and opportunity-development approach to helping*, 7th edn, California, Brooks/Cole, 2007.

Eliasson M, Kainz G, Von Post I: Uncaring midwives, *Nurs Ethics* 15(4):501–511, 2008.

Elmir R, Schmied V, Wilkes L, et al: Women's perceptions and experiences of a traumatic birth: a meta-ethnography, *J Adv Nurs* 66(10):2142–2153, 2010.

Engnes K, Lidén E, Lundgren I: Experiences of being exposed to intimate partner violence during pregnancy, *Int J Qual Stud Health Well-being* (website). www.ijqhw.net/index.php/qhw/article/view/11199. 2012.

Fenwick J, Gamble J, Creedy J, et al: Study protocol for reducing childbirth fear: a midwife-led psycho-education intervention, *BMC Pregnancy Childbirth* 13(1):190, 2013.

Goodall EK, McVittie C, Magill M: Birth choice following primary caesarean section: mothers' perceptions of the influence of health professionals on decision making, *J Reprod Infant Psychol* 27(1):4–14, 2009.

Goodin M, Griffiths M: Caesarean section on demand, *Obstet Gynaecol Reprod Med* 22(12):368–370, 2012.

Green J, Baston H: Feeling in control during labour: concepts, correlates and consequences, *Birth* 30(4):235–247, 2003.

Hamilton JG, Lobel M: Types, patterns, and predictors of coping with stress during pregnancy: examination of the Revised Prenatal Coping Inventory in a diverse sample, *J Psychosom Obstet Gynecol* 29(2):97–104, 2008.

Hilfinger Messias DK, Dejoseph JF: The personal work of a first pregnancy: transforming identities, relationships, and women's work, *Women Health* 45(4):41–64, 2007.

Howland LC: Preterm birth: Implications for family stress and coping, *Newborn Infant Nurs Rev* 7:14–19, 2007.

Jefford E, Jomeen J: Midwifery abdication. a finding from an interpretive study, *Int J Childbirth* 5:116–125, 2015.

Johnson M, Schmied V, Lupton SJ, et al: Measuring women's perinatal mental health risk, *Arch Womens Ment Health* 15:375–386, 2012.

Johnson S, Burrows A, Williamson I: 'Does my bump look big in this?' The meaning of bodily changes for first-time mothers-to-be, *J Health Psychol* 9(3):361–374, 2004.

Joint Commissioning Panel for Mental Health: *Guidance for commissioners of perinatal mental health services*, London, JCP, 2012.

Jomeen J: *Choice, control and contemporary childbirth. Understanding through women's experiences*, London, Radcliffe, 2010.

Jomeen J, Bateman L: Psychology applied to maternity care. In Lewis L, editor: *Fundamentals of midwifery*, London, Wiley, pp 61–82, 2014.

Jomeen J, Martin CR: Abnormalities in the baby. In Martin CR, editor: *Perinatal mental health: a clinical guide*, London, MK Update, pp 107–116, 2012.

Jomeen J, Martin CR: Developing specialist perinatal mental health services, *Pract Midwife* 17(3):18–21, 2014.

Jomeen J, Redshaw M: Ethnic minority women's experience of maternity services in England, *Ethn Health* 18:280–296, 2013.

Kirkham M: *The midwife-mother relationship*, 2nd edn, Basingstoke, Macmillan, 2010.

Lavender V: Body image: change, dissatisfaction and disturbance. In Price S, editor: *Mental health in pregnancy and childbirth*, Edinburgh, Churchill Livingstone, pp 123–146, 2007.

Lawson KL, Turriff-Jonasson SI: Maternal serum screening and psychosocial attachment to pregnancy, *J Psychosom Res* 60(4):371–378, 2006.

Lefkowitz DS, Baxt C, Evans JR: Prevalence and correlates of posttraumatic stress and postpartum depression in parents of infants in the neonatal intensive care unit (NICU), *J Clin Psychol Med Settings* 17:230–237, 2010.

Lemola S, Stadlmayr W, Grob A: Maternal adjustment five months after birth: the impact of the subjective experience of childbirth and emotional support from the partner, *J Reprod Infant Psychol* 25(3):190–202, 2007.

Lin YN, Tsai YC, Lai PH: The experience of Taiwanese women achieving post-infertility pregnancy through assisted reproductive treatment, *Fam J* 21(2):189–197, 2013.

Magee LA, Chandra K, Mazzotta P, et al: Development of a health related quality of life instrument for nausea and vomiting of pregnancy, *Am J Obstet Gynecol* 186(5):232–238, 2002.

Marshall JL, Godfrey M, Renfrew MJ: Being a 'good mother': managing breastfeeding and merging identities, *Soc Sci Med* 65:2147–2159, 2007.

Martin CR, Redshaw M: Psychological well-being in pregnancy: food for thought?, *J Reprod Infant Psychol* 28(4):325–327, 2010.

Mc-Kenzie-McHarg K, Ayers S, Ford E, et al: Post-traumatic stress disorder following childbirth: an update of current issues and recommendations, *J Reprod Infant Psychol* 33(3):219–237, 2014.

Mercer J, Green-Jervis C, Brannigan C: The legacy of a self-reported negative birth experience, *Br J Midwifery* 20(10):717–723, 2012.

Misri S, Kendrick K, Oberlander TF, et al: Antenatal depression and anxiety affect postpartum parenting stress: a longitudinal, prospective study, *Can J Psychiatry* 55(4):222–228, 2010.

Modh C, Lundgren I, Bergbom I: First time pregnant women's experiences in early pregnancy, *Int J Qual Stud Health Well-being* 6(2) (website). www.ncbi.nlm.nih.gov/pmc/articles/PMC3077216/pdf/QHW-6 s-5600.pdf. 2011.

Nakamura Y: Encouraging positive reactions to pregnancy in first-time mothers, *Br J Midwifery* 17(1):48–53, 2009.

Nash M: Weighty matters: negotiating 'fatness' and 'in-betweenness' in early pregnancy, *Fem Psychol* 22(3):307–323, 2012.

National Institute for Health and Clinical Excellence (NICE): *Antenatal and postnatal mental health: clinical management and service guidance*, London, NICE, 2014.

Nicholls L, Webb C: What makes a good midwife? An integrative review of methodologically-diverse research, *J Adv Nurs* 56(4):414–429, 2006.

Oakley A: *Women's experiences of childbirth in the 1970s in social science bites* (website). www.socialsciencebites.com. 2013.

Otley H: Fear of childbirth: understanding the causes, impact and treatment, *Br J Midwifery* 19(4) (website). www.baby-birth.com/articles/54-antenatal/321-fear-of-childbirth-understanding-the-causes-impact-and-treatment.html. 2012.

Raynor M: Social and psychological context of childbearing, *Womens Health Med* 32(2):64–67, 2006.

Raynor M, England C: *Psychology for midwives: pregnancy, childbirth and puerperium*, Maidenhead, Open University Press, 2010.

Redshaw M, Rowe R, Hockley C, et al: *Recorded delivery: a national survey of women's experiences of maternity care 2006*, Oxford, National Perinatal Epidemiology Unit, 2007.

Royal College of Psychiatry: *Postnatal depression* (website). www.rcpsych.ac.uk/healthadvice/problemsdisorders/postnataldepression.aspx. 2015.

Salter K: Beating the trauma of a bad birth experience, *Ment Health Today* 14–15, 2009.

Schneider Z: An Australian study of women's experiences of their first pregnancy, *Midwifery* 18(3):238–249, 2002.

Sethna V, Murray L, Netsi E, et al: Paternal depression in the postnatal period and early father-infant interactions, *Parent Sci Pract* 15:1–8, 2015.

Shaho R: Kurdish women's experiences and perceptions of their first pregnancy, *Br J Midwifery* 18(10):650–657, 2010.

Sheen K, Spiby H, Slade P: An integrative review of the impact of indirect trauma exposure in health professionals and potential issues of salience for midwives, *J Adv Nurs* 709(4):729–743, 2014.

Smith D, Lavender T: The maternity experience for women with a body mass index ≥ 30 kg/m2: a meta-synthesis, *BJOG* 118(7):779–789, 2011.

Spear HJ: Teenage pregnancy: 'Having a baby won't affect me that much', *Pediatr Nurs* 27(6):574–580, 2001.

Spiteri CM, Jomeen J, Martin CR: Reimagining the General Health Questionnaire as a measure of emotional wellbeing: a study of postpartum women in Malta, *Women Birth* 26(4):e105–e111, 2013.

Talbot R: Self-efficacy: women's experience of pain in labour, *Br J Midwifery* 20:317–321, 2012.

Taylor J, Johnson M: How women manage fatigue after childbirth, *Midwifery* 26:367–375, 2010.

Thomson G, Downe S: Changing the future to change the past: women's experiences of a positive birth following a traumatic birth experience, *J Reprod Infant Psychol* 28:102–112, 2010.

Tyer-Viola LA, Lopez RP: Pregnancy with chronic illness, *J Obstet Gynecol Neonatal Nurs* 43(1):25–37, 2014.

Yang Y, Peden-Mcalpine C, Chen C: A qualitative study of the experiences of Taiwanese women having their first baby after the age of 35 years, *Midwifery* 23(4):343–349, 2007.

Resources and additional reading

The Royal College of Midwives: *Maternal and Emotional wellbeing and Infant Development; a good practice guide for midwives.* https://www.rcm.org.uk/sites/default/files/Emotional%20Wellbeing_Guide_WEB.pdf. 2012.

This practice guide for midwives from the Royal College of Midwives raises awareness of the role of the midwife in supporting the woman through pregnancy and birth.

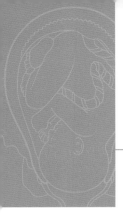

Chapter 13

Sexuality

Karen Jackson

Learning Outcomes

After reading this chapter, you will be able to:

- cite a basic definition of 'sexuality'
- outline the psychological, social and physiological implications of sex and sexuality during pregnancy, childbirth and afterwards
- describe the implications of pregnancy and childbirth for women who are survivors of sexual abuse, women who have undergone female genital mutilation and women who are lesbians
- list some of the factors that may affect sex and sexuality for women who are breastfeeding.

Reflective activity 13.1

While reading this chapter, think about the word *sexuality*. What does it mean? Write down a simple definition or words that you would associate with sexuality.

Did you find the task easy? If not, why do you think sexuality is difficult to define?

SEXUALITY

The word *sexuality* is scattered liberally throughout contemporary sexual health literature, but the text frequently fails to explore what sexuality actually means. The word itself did not come into being until the modern era, and many authors are reluctant to confine it to a simple definition. This may well be because sexuality is fundamentally dynamic. It has different meanings culturally, its definition changes throughout history, and individuals' feelings and values concerning their sexuality alter as they gain more life experience.

The World Health Organization (WHO 2006: 5) defines sexuality thus: '...a central aspect of being human throughout life encompasses sex, gender identities and roles, sexual orientation, eroticism, pleasure, intimacy and reproduction. Sexuality is experienced and expressed in thoughts, fantasies, desires, beliefs, attitudes, values, behaviours, practices, roles and relationships. While sexuality can include all of these dimensions, not all of them are always experienced or expressed. Sexuality is influenced by the interaction of biological, psychological, social, economic, political, cultural, legal, historical, religious and spiritual factors'. This definition alone demonstrates clearly that sexuality is more than overt sexual behaviour, encompassing the complete range of human experience (Pratt 2000). The Royal College of Nursing (RCN 2000, cited on contents page) states that sexuality is: 'an individual's self concept, shaped by their personality and expressed through a heterosexual, homosexual, bisexual or transsexual orientation'. This definition may reflect a Western culture's politically correct view of sexuality.

The word *sex* is usually employed to mean the act of having sex or to distinguish between the 'sexes' – that is, male or female. *Gender* is the name given to socially and culturally defined characteristics of the sexes – that is, masculinity and femininity.

SEX DURING PREGNANCY

Sex during pregnancy has historically been shrouded in myth, misconceptions and old wives' tales. The advice offered during traditional British antenatal care has been one of abstention, without any evidence to substantiate this stance.

During pregnancy, many couples are fearful of continuing their sexual relationship. They may feel that they may somehow provoke miscarriage, induce premature labour or damage the fetus; some men have expressed fear of breaking the 'bag of waters' (Kitzinger 1985). Couples can be reassured that this is not the case.

The overriding message from most well-conducted studies is that sex during pregnancy for the vast majority of women is safe and does not lead to any increase in complications (Kontoyannis et al 2012), although the male-superior position (Ekwo et al 1993) and a vagina colonized with specific microorganisms, for example *Trichomonas vaginalis* (Read and Klebanoff 1993), have both been associated with preterm birth. More studies are required in this area to provide definitive results. The National Institute for Health and Care Excellence (NICE 2014) antenatal care guidelines state that health professionals can inform healthy pregnant women that sexual intercourse during pregnancy is not known to be associated with any adverse outcomes.

There are a few definite or relative contraindications to different sexual practices or sexual intercourse during pregnancy. Forceful blowing of air into the vagina during oral sex is an absolute contraindication because this may lead to fatal air embolism (Aston 2005). The insertion of a foreign body into the vagina may cause damage to the internal structures and introduce infection (Walton 1994). Placenta praevia, vaginal bleeding, history of premature birth and rupture of membranes are often cited as clinical reasons to avoid sex during pregnancy (Aston 2005).

Although sex can be enjoyed by couples throughout the whole of pregnancy, other factors may play an important role. Change of body image (see chapter website resources), tiredness, breast changes, backache and frequency of micturition are some of the things that can affect a pregnant woman's sexuality (Aston 2005). There are many accounts that give a very negative view of sexuality and pregnancy. Kitzinger (1985 and 2012) acknowledges that some women have a distorted view of their bodies during pregnancy; they feel bigger than they really are and think that their partners must find them ugly, when in fact the partners often delight in pregnant women and find their physical changes exciting and beautiful.

Conversely, some women have a very positive body image during pregnancy. They feel incredibly attractive and womanly. It is viewed as the ultimate expression of femininity and an eminently powerful symbol of potency and fertility.

Physiological hormonal changes during pregnancy mean that oestrogen and progesterone act together to procure marked pelvic vasocongestion, which occurs as a result of increased vascularity and venous stasis. The results can mean a heightened manifestation of all aspects of sexual intercourse, including orgasm (Aston 2005). For some, this may be the first time that they experience orgasm (Walton 1994). For others, however, vasocongestion may predispose the woman to discomfort during sexual intercourse (Aston 2005).

It is often assumed that there is a linear decrease in sexual activity as pregnancy progresses, but for some women sexual activity may well increase during the second trimester. This may be because the disorders of pregnancy are subsiding and the woman is developing a sense of well-being. However, it is also well recognized that sex diminishes during the third trimester (Frohlich et al 1990), most probably because of the discomfort and mechanics of having sex with a greatly enlarged abdomen. Alternative positions to the missionary position, such as the man behind the woman or 'spooning', or the woman sitting or kneeling on top of the man, could be explored. Other nonpenetrative options such as self or mutual masturbation, oral sex, fondling or massage or purely kissing and cuddling may also be adopted (Walton 1994).

It is suggested that having sexual intercourse may be an alternative to other methods of induction, the theory being that sperm is rich in prostaglandins, thereby providing a stimulus for ripening the cervix. However, to date, this has been poorly evaluated, and more research is required in this area (Kavanagh et al 2001; Schaffir 2006; NHS Choices 2015).

Overall, keeping clear channels of communication open is the most important aspect of maintaining an intimate sexual or nonsexual relationship.

SEXUALITY AND LABOUR

Labour is usually synonymous with anxiety, discomfort and pain. It is not often viewed as being a 'sexual' experience. It is clear when reading literature in this area that for some women and their partners it can be an intensely pleasurable and sexual experience. The sounds a woman makes during contractions, the organs that are used in the process of childbirth and the overwhelming energies and powers that are at work during labour are all intimately related to sex and sexuality (Aston 2005; Gaskin 2002; Kitzinger 1985 and 2012; Williams 1996). Kitzinger (1985: 210) describes it thus: 'the most intensely sexual feeling a woman ever experiences, as strong as orgasm, even more compelling than orgasm'. In her book *Spiritual Midwifery*, Gaskin (2002) quotes a number of experiences of the sexual nature of childbirth. One woman recounts her birth experience with her husband: 'My rushes (contractions) hardly felt heavy at all, but I knew they must be because I was opening up. We just kept making out and rubbing each other. We got to places that we had forgotten we could get to… going through the birthing I felt his love very strong. It was like getting married all over again' (Gaskin 2002: 53). Rabuzzi (1994) cites examples of other couples' erotic experiences of labour. One husband of a woman having a home birth said: 'The birth was not only painless, but very pleasurable. We had never read about this aspect'. He goes on to describe the noises his wife made whilst the baby's head was crowning as being 'orgasmic' and ends with: "what a long way from the pain and agony of conventional myth' (Rabuzzi 1994: 120).

If labour can be such a sensual and gratifying experience, it may be a cultural or contextual aspect that makes it generally viewed negatively. It is suggested by some that the scientific and technological procedures have taken childbirth out of the hands of women and set it in the context of the powerful male-dominated institution of the hospital (Cosslett 1994; Williams 1996), where everything is controlled, the medical model's ultimate goal being 'safety', whatever the cost. In contrast, the natural childbirth discourse is focused on the power of the woman, which is more in evidence in home births (Cosslett 1994; Williams 1996). Midwives argue that 'safety' and 'satisfaction' are both achievable.

Nipple stimulation is known to produce oxytocin and therefore can be performed by the woman or her partner to attempt to initiate or augment labour naturally, although the safety of this in high-risk women has not been established (Kavanagh et al 2005). Privacy will of course be required if she wishes to try this activity.

WOMEN REQUIRING SPECIALIZED CARE

There are some groups of women who may need specialized care and attention during pregnancy, labour, childbirth and afterwards. Some are discussed in the following sections.

The women in the following list represent women whom you may well care for in clinical practice:

- Anne, a woman who is a survivor of sexual abuse
- Lydia, a pregnant lesbian
- Saadah, who underwent female genital mutilation as a child
- Katie, a woman who had chlamydia
- Bernie, a woman who is breastfeeding

What are the issues concerning sexuality for each of these woman?

It is important not to stereotype anyone; all women will probably have similar issues, but in addition, Anne from the previous list may have to deal with reactivated memories of the abuse; Lydia may have to deal with homophobia and sometimes hostile behaviour; Saadah may be terrified of labour and birth; Katie may face stigma and labelling of being promiscuous; Bernie may have conflict between being a nursing mother and a sexual being,

Survivors of sexual abuse

The prevalence rate for reported cases of childhood sexual abuse is around 24% for children in the UK (Radford et al 2011). The Council of Europe (2014) states that current data suggests that 1 in 5 children is a victim of some form of sexual violence. The incidence of sexual abuse is higher in females than in males. In a recent publication from the NSPCC (Jutte et al 2014), all four countries of the UK reported a clear rise in sexual abuse cases in children in the last year. They assert that this may be a result of high-profile sex abuse cases that have been in the media. It is clear, given the high prevalence of childhood sexual abuse, that midwives will, at some point, care for women who have survived sexual abuse. These women may or may not disclose such abuse to their carers.

Memories of abuse, even those that have been partially or wholly repressed, may be triggered by pregnancy and childbirth (Gutteridge 2009). The change in body image, submission to physical contact, and feelings of powerlessness are all factors that are likely to make the survivor regress back to times when she encountered similar susceptibilities.

In their qualitative research, Rhodes and Hutchinson (1994) found that women who have been previously sexually abused may display a range of behaviours, as follows:

- Extreme anxiety over intimate examinations,
- Needing to be in complete control,
- Dissociating themselves from the experience, or
- Being quite uninhibited, engaging freely in sexual banter.

Clearly, some of the styles exhibited by sexual abuse survivors may also be enacted by women who have not been abused; however, in the former group, the behaviour may appear extreme.

In a study by Garratt (2008), control has been identified as being of grave importance to women who have been sexually abused. Therefore, keeping women well informed, ensuring that they are central to the decision-making process and obtaining informed consent for all procedures are absolute requirements (Box 13.1).

Box 13.1 Practice points for sexual abuse survivors

Some practice points to consider when caring for survivors of sexual abuse are as follows:

- Use of effective and sensitive communication skills and information-giving by caregivers is essential.
- Ensure women are fully involved in decision making to support genuine informed consent.
- Respect privacy and dignity. Practitioners should be invited into the birthing environment, with the woman's consent.
- Consider place of birth – home birth, birthing units or midwife-led units may be a preferable option, where appropriate. Women must be supported to be in control, regardless of the birth environment.
- Be aware of the language used in labour, to avoid bringing back memories of abuse in the language used.
- Enable women to mobilize freely without restraints from equipment. This will prevent feelings of bondage where this might be an issue.
- If continuous monitoring is required, use of telemetry would assist with keeping mobile.
- Explain all procedures clearly and without medical jargon.
- Consider whether vaginal examinations (VEs) are necessary. If a VE is considered to be necessary, negotiate with the woman how best to do this (see following point). However, if a fully informed woman refuses, her wishes must be respected.
- Negotiate with the woman that if she wishes a procedure to stop, she can halt it at any point without question. This promotes empowerment and will make her feel more in control of the situation.
- Continue to communicate throughout the examination, as silent focus upon the genitalia can be reminiscent of the abuse.
- Suggest that the woman place her hand on the midwife's examining arm during the examination so that she can push the midwife's hand away, giving the woman control.

(Adapted from Garratt 2008; Marriott 2012)

It is also worthy of note that all individuals – husbands, partners, companions, midwives, sisters mothers – also bring with them to the birthing environment their own experiences and issues, which may include a history of sexual abuse.

Caring for the lesbian client

It is becoming more common for lesbian couples to fulfil the desire to become parents by using natural or artificial means. These couples will generally enter the maternity services for care and support during pregnancy and childbirth. It is therefore imperative that the needs of these clients are recognized. Many lesbian writers and researchers who have explored lesbian issues identify that lesbians encounter varying experiences, both positive and negative, during childbirth (Dahl et al 2013). As a group, lesbians are largely ignored and consequently become invisible in texts discussing women's health (Wilton 1996).

The rights of same-sex couples are protected in law (Equality Act 2010); it is illegal for anyone to be discriminated against because of sexual orientation. The Nursing and Midwifery Council (NMC 2015) also states that nurses and midwives must not discriminate for any reason. The Civil Partnership Act (2004) and the Marriage (Same Sex Couples) Act (2013) enabled same-sex couples to enjoy the same rights as heterosexual couples.

Midwives can do much to ensure that a lesbian's experience of pregnancy and childbirth is a positive and empowering one. They can attain this by being knowledgeable about lesbian sexuality, by using non-heterosexist language, by giving appropriate advice, by being nonjudgemental and by rejecting socially constructed stereotypes (Dahl et al 2013).

Paternal presence at the birth

Historically childbirth has been considered to be women's work, and male partners were not involved in or present at the births of their children, and this is still the case in many developing countries. In high-income, Western societies, there has been a cultural shift from men being virtually excluded from the birthing room to men being actively encouraged to attend the birth of their child. It is not known what effect paternal presence at birth has on the process of labour or on the subsequent relationship of the couple. It does appear, however, in some studies that the presence of a female companion such as a doula can have numerous positive effects on the outcome of labour (Kennell and Klaus 1991; Royal College of Midwives (RCM) et al 2016).

One dimension of paternal presence at birth that is rarely discussed is the possible adverse effects on subsequent sexual relationships. Some researchers have discovered that sexual dysfunction can sometimes be a sequelae of childbirth, such as in cases where the man or partner found the labour and birth experience traumatic and has subsequently stifled any sexual feelings for his wife/partner (Hanson et al 2009).

It is the midwife's responsibility to ensure that the couple realize the importance and enormity of the decision for the man 'to be there or not to be there'. They should be encouraged to discuss the issue openly, ideally antenatally, with the pros and cons clearly defined so that they can make an informed choice.

SEX AFTER CHILDBIRTH

As with sex during pregnancy, many social and cultural taboos surround the issue of sex after childbirth. The main issues appear to be fear of infection and trauma, but there is no evidence to support these possible complications provided that the sexual activity is considerate and gentle (Walton 1994; British Pregnancy Advisory Service (BPAS) 2014). The woman herself is therefore the best person to regulate when she is ready to resume sexual intercourse. In the past, there appeared to be an unwritten rule that women should abstain from sex until after the 6-week postnatal check, when the general practitioner (GP) could give her the 'all clear' to resume sexual relations. It was assumed that all would be well sexually after this period of time. The reality, however, is quite contrary. Limited research in this field demonstrates that childbirth causes high levels of sexual morbidity and states that this is not adequately addressed by health professionals (Abdool et al 2009; McDonald et al 2015).

There are also a number of areas related to sexuality and childbirth that appear to raise important issues for midwives and the women for whom they care. It is important that contraception is discussed with the woman soon after the birth; one of the reasons for this is that a woman's fertility can return quite soon after giving birth. In addition to this, fear of becoming pregnant can diminish desire for sex (BPAS 2014).

A reduced libido postnatally appears to be physiologically normal and usual, but if serious or long term, it may be an indication of underlying problems within the relationship, or it could be a symptom of postnatal depression. If this is the case, other professionals will need to be involved in giving specialized care and attention.

However, in the majority of cases, sexual problems following childbirth are directly linked to the pregnancy, the labour and birth or the baby. This being the case, midwives and other health professionals involved in childbirth are in a prime position to counsel, guide and support parents with sexual anxieties. Some of the more common reasons for breakdown in sexual relations may be related to negative body image or confusion over adopting the dual roles of mother and lover (see chapter website resources).

BREASTFEEDING AND SEXUALITY

The literature surrounding the effect of breastfeeding (see Ch. 44) on sexuality and sexual activity is confusing and largely conflicting. Some found a positive effect on sexual activity (Masters and Johnson 1966); some found a negative impact (Alder and Bancroft 1983); and yet others found that there was no effect on sexual interest (Reamy and White 1987).

A more recent review of the evidence further supports the hypothesis that breastfeeding reduces interest in sex (Abdool et al 2009). There are two assertions that may be derived from the conflicting evidence: firstly, that further well-conducted, comprehensive research is required in this field; and secondly, that no definitive conclusions can be drawn. Therefore, women's sexuality may be affected in any of the ways described, and each woman must be cared for, advised and counselled accordingly.

Breastfeeding, sexuality and sexual difficulties

As previously stated, Abdool et al (2009) found that overall during the early postnatal period, and particularly if the baby is being breastfed, many women report a significant decrease in libido, or a complete loss of interest in sex.

There may be several reasons why breastfeeding may interfere with sexual relations:

- The mother's requirements for intimacy are being met by the baby.
- She feels guilty and thrown into conflict about having sexual feelings while breastfeeding.
- High prolactin levels and low oestrogen levels may affect libido.
- Fatigue caused by regular feeding day and night may diminish libido.
- The partner's feelings of jealousy towards the baby may affect libido.
- Milk ejection during intercourse may cause concern.

Being sexually stimulated by a suckling baby can provoke feelings of confusion and guilt. The woman may feel that she is somehow abnormal or perverted (Bartlett 2005). It is hardly surprising that breastfeeding and sexual intercourse bring about such pleasurable feelings: these basic actions have evolved to secure the survival of the human race (Bartlett 2005). The woman should be reassured that breastfeeding is an immensely satisfying experience and one that should be relished.

If milk ejection during intercourse causes concern to the couple it can be minimized or alleviated by breastfeeding the baby or expressing milk before coitus. Some couples incorporate this phenomenon into their sexual play (Van Wert 1996); provided that both parties are happy with this, there is no physiological reason to discourage such an activity.

Vaginal dryness has been reported, particularly in breastfeeding mothers, possibly because of low oestrogen levels. An appropriate lubricating gel (water-based if used in conjunction with condoms) may be used to address this problem. This may be discussed in conjunction with family planning advice.

MENOPAUSE

Menopause is a time of immense change when a woman's fertility reduces, although she may continue to be fertile. A reduction in the fertility hormones, in particular oestrogen and progesterone, may cause bodily changes that may also affect a woman's sense of sexuality. Some find this a period of liberation, whereas others may experience a sense of loss of opportunities for fertility.

CONCLUSION

Sexuality does not cease simply because a woman is pregnant, in labour, giving birth or recovering from birth. The parameters of 'normality' in terms of sexuality are wide, varied and unique to each woman. Because the very essence of sexuality is embodied within childbirth, aspects of sexuality should be considered as an integral part of the care that women receive from midwives. A midwife should have the knowledge and skills to be able to advise, support, educate and counsel women appropriately, which includes acknowledging her limitations and referring to another health professional when necessary. For most women, the expert, sensitive care from the midwife will be all that is required.

Box 13.2 Further useful resources

Puberty and teenage pregnancy
  Please see the chapter website resources and Chapters 19, 23 and 32 for more information.

Female genital mutilation (FGM)
  Please see the chapter website resources and Chapter 56 for further information.

Sexually transmitted infections (STIs)
  Please see the chapter website resources and Chapter 55 for further information.

Perineal care
  Please see the chapter website resources and Chapter 40 for further information.

Key Points

- Sex during pregnancy is safe for the majority of women.
- Labour for some women can be an immensely satisfying, sensual or sexual experience.
- Sexuality should be an issue considered for all pregnant, labouring and postnatal women, but some women will require special care and attention: survivors of sexual abuse, lesbians, women who have undergone female genital mutilation, breastfeeding mothers.
- Sex following birth should initially be regulated by the woman, that is, when she feels ready.
- See Box 13.2 for further useful resources.

References

Abdool Z, Thakar R, Sultan A: Postpartum female sexual function, *Eur J Obstet Gynaecol Reprod Biol* 145(2):133–137, 2009.

Alder E, Bancroft J: Sexual behaviour of lactating women: a preliminary communication, *J Reprod Infant Psychol* 1(2):47–52, 1983.

Aston G: Sexuality during and after pregnancy. In Andrews G, editor: *Women's sexual health*, 3rd edn, London, Baillière Tindall, 2005.

Bartlett A: Maternal sexuality and breastfeeding, *Sex Educ* 5(1):67–77, 2005.

British Pregnancy Advisory Service (BPAS): *Sex and contraception after childbirth* (website). www.bpas.org/media/1187/sex-and-contraception-after-childbirth.pdf. 2014.

Civil Partnership Act: *An act to make provision for and in connection with civil partnership*. Act of parliament of the UK, 2004.

Cosslett T: *Women writing childbirth: modern discourses of motherhood*, Manchester, Manchester University Press, 1994.

Council of Europe: *One in five: the Council of Europe campaign to stop sexual violence against children* (website). www.coe.int/t/dg3/children/1in5/default_en.asp. 2014.

Dahl B, Fylkesnes A, Sørlie V, et al: Lesbian women's experiences with healthcare providers in the birthing context: a meta ethnography, *Midwifery* 29(6):674–681, 2013.

Ekwo E, Gosselink C, Woolson R, et al: Coitus late in pregnancy: risk of preterm rupture of amniotic sac membranes, *Am J Obstet Gynecol* 1(1):22–31, 1993.

Equality Act (Sexual Orientation) Regulations (website). http://legislation.gov.uk. 2010.

Frohlich E, Herz C, van der Merwe F, et al: Sexuality during pregnancy and early puerperium and its perception by the pregnant and puerperal woman, *J Psychosom Obstet Gynaecol* 11(1):73–79, 1990.

Garratt E: *The childbearing experiences of survivors of sexual abuse.* Unpublished PhD thesis, Sheffield Hallam University, 2008.

Gaskin I: *Spiritual midwifery*, 4th edn, Summertown, Book Publishing Company, 2002.

Gutteridge K: *MIDIRS*, 189(1):125–129, 2009.

Hanson S, Hunter L, Bormann J, et al: Paternal fears of childbirth: a literature review, *J Perinat Educ* 8(4):12–20, 2009.

Jutte S, Bentley H, Tallis D, et al: *How safe are our children? The most comprehensive overview of child protection in the UK*, London, NSPCC, 2014.

Kavanagh J, Kelly A, Thomas J: Sexual intercourse for cervical ripening and induction of labour, *Cochrane Database Syst Rev* (2):CD003093, 2001. (latest version published 2008).

Kavanagh J, Kelly AJ, Thomas J: Breast stimulation for cervical ripening and induction of labour, *Cochrane Database Syst Rev* (3):CD003392, 2005. (latest version published 2010).

Kennell J, Klaus M: Continuous emotional support during labor in a US hospital. A randomized controlled trial, *JAMA* 265(17):2197–2201, 1991.

Kitzinger S: *Women's experience of sex*, London, Penguin, 1985.

Kitzinger S: *Birth and Sex: the power and the passion*, Pinter and Martin, 2012.

Kontoyannis M, Katsestos C, Panagopoulos P: Sexual intercourse during pregnancy, *Health Sci J* 6(1):82–87, 2012.

Marriage (Same-Sex Couples) Act. *Marriage of same sex couples in England and Wales* (website). www.legislation.gov.uk/ukpga/2013/30/contents/enacted/data.htm. 2013.

Marriott S: Trauma: memories of childhood sexual abuse, *Pract Midwife*, 2012.

Masters W, Johnson V: *Human sexual response*, Boston, Little, Brown, 1966.

McDonald EA, Gartland D, Small R, et al: Dyspareunia and childbirth: a prospective cohort study, *Br J Obstet Gynaecol* 122:672–679, 2015.

NHS Choices: *Inducing labour* (website). www.nhs.uk/conditions/pregnancy-and-baby/pages/induction-labour.aspx. 2015.

National Institute for Clinical Excellence (NICE): *Antenatal care: routine care for the healthy pregnant woman*. Clinical guideline 6, London, NICE, 2008 (modified version December 2014).

Nursing and Midwifery Council (NMC): *The Code: professional standards of practice and behaviour for nurses and midwives*, London, NMC, 2015.

Pratt R: Sexual health and disease: an international perspective. In Wilson H, McAndrew S, editors: *Sexual health*, London, Baillière Tindall, 2000.

Rabuzzi K: *Mother with child*, Indiana, Indiana University Press, 1994.

Radford L, Corral S, Bradley C, et al: *Child abuse and neglect in the UK today*, London, NSPCC (website). www.nspcc.org.uk/childstudy, 2011.

Read J, Klebanoff M: Sexual intercourse during pregnancy and preterm delivery: effects of vaginal microorganisms, *Am J Obstet Gynecol* 168(2):514–519, 1993.

Reamy K, White S: Sexuality in the puerperium: a review, *Arch Sex Behav* 16(2):165–186, 1987.

Rhodes N, Hutchinson S: Labour experiences of childhood sexual abuse survivors, *Birth* 21(4):213–220, 1994.

Royal College of Midwives, Fatherhood Institute, Royal College of Obstetrics and Gynaecology, Department of Health: *Reaching out; involving fathers in maternity care* (website). www.rcm.org.uk/sites/default/files/Father's%20Guides%20A4_3_0.pdf. 2016.

Royal College of Nursing (RCN): *Sexuality and sexual health in nursing practice*, London, RCN, 2000.

Schaffir J: Sexual intercourse at term and the onset of labour, *Obstet Gynaecol* 107(6):1310–1314, 2006.

Van Wert W: When lovers become parents, *Mother* 81(Winter):58–61, 1996.

Walton I: *Sexuality and motherhood*, Cheshire, Books for Midwives, 1994.

Williams C: Midwives and sexuality: earth mother or coy maiden? In Frith L, editor: *Ethics and midwifery: issues in contemporary practice*, Oxford, Butterworth-Heinemann, 1996.

Wilton T: Caring for the lesbian client: homophobia and midwifery, *Br J Midwifery* 4(2):126–131, 1996.

World Health Organization (WHO): *Defining sexual health: report of a technical consultation on sexual health, 28–31 January 2002*, Geneva, WHO, 2006.

Chapter 14

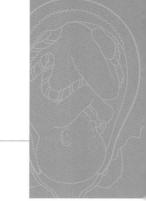

National Health Service policy and midwifery

Professor Gwendolen Bradshaw

Learning Outcomes ?

After reading this chapter, you will be able to:
- define health policy
- discuss the ways in which policy is made
- have contextual awareness of the role of the midwife within the complex system of health service delivery
- articulate the impact of policy for practitioners, mothers, babies and families of a perpetually evolving National Health Service (NHS)

INTRODUCTION

In the UK, all women are entitled to free healthcare, which includes maternity and newborn care. The majority of midwives are employed within the National Health Service (NHS), either directly or through models such as the one-to-one system (www.onetoonemidwives.org). Those employed within the NHS have their education and continuing professional education commissioned to ensure that care and services are competent, high quality and up to date.

It is therefore useful for midwives to understand the structure, workings and influence of the NHS, and how they individually and collectively can contribute to the development and delivery of the service.

This chapter explores the policy framework in which midwives in the UK practice. The principles of the political context and provision of maternity services within a health service may, however, be applied in any country.

THE POLICY CONTEXT

What are we talking about?

The NHS is an important edifice in British life. It emerged in 1942 from a Committee chaired by the economist William Beveridge who identified five 'Giant Evils' within 20th century Britain, namely *squalor, ignorance, want, idleness* and *disease*. After his investigation Beveridge proposed monumental reform to create an unprecedented network of social welfare agencies dedicated to meeting personal need (Beveridge 1942).

The creation of the NHS became part of this arrangement that has become so influential to British life. The NHS is among the biggest employers in the world, employing 1.4 million staff, rivalling the Chinese Peoples' Army and Indian Railways in size. Additionally, the NHS offers significant employment opportunities to women, as 80% of those employed by the NHS are women.

The UK has four different NHS systems, with England being the largest and most complex. All are funded primarily through general taxation. But since formalized political devolution to the Celtic countries in 1999, the four have diverged regarding their operational management. Each is autonomous, though for practical reasons some functions are performed routinely on behalf of the UK Department of Health for any one or all of the three other countries. For instance, the Human Fertilisation and Embryology Authority (HFEA) is the UK-wide independent regulator overseeing the use of gametes and embryos in fertility treatment and research.

The four systems are:

- The National Health Service England
- Health and Social Care in Northern Ireland

- NHS Scotland
- NHS Wales

Their commonality resides in the historic creation and articulation of their equity principles defined by their founder Aneurin Bevan (Foot 1999). Equity means fairness; being treated fairly at the point of clinical need is a cardinal quality of UK healthcare and these principles on which the NHS was founded in 1948 remain today. These underpin all the NHS does, rendering it unique internationally and something regarded widely as the envy of the world. Indeed the British NHS is frequently declared the best healthcare system by international comparison, as it is conducted by bodies of experts who rate its quality of care and its fairness superior to countries that spend far more on healthcare than does the UK (Commonwealth Fund 2014; Campbell and Watt 2014).

Its esteemed core principles comprise:

- universal access to a consistently high standard of care irrespective of where one lives
- services that are free at the point of delivery
- an inclusive range of services for all health needs from birth to death
- selection on the basis of clinical necessity that does not depend on the ability to pay (Enthoven 1991)

THE STRUCTURE OF THE NHS

The structure of the NHS is dynamic and changing, and had undergone a major reorganization in 2013. It is important to be aware that the NHS in Wales, Scotland and Northern Ireland are devolved, and work in slightly different ways compared with the NHS in England (NHS England 2014).

Reflective activity 14.1

Do you understand the structure of the NHS? See http://www.nhs.uk/NHSEngland/thenhs/about/Pages/nhsstructure.aspx and http://www.gov.scot/Topics/Health/About/Structure in Scotland, for an overall picture of the structure of the NHS in England and Scotland. You may also find it useful to read through the Kings Fund 'Alternative Guide to the NHS':

http://www.kingsfund.org.uk/projects/nhs-65/alternative-guide-new-nhs-england (Kings Fund 2015a)

The starting point

This discussion assumes midwives to have a fundamental understanding of healthcare provision and intends to enhance the capacity of the reader to assess and analyse the inner workings of health services in Britain. What follows is a brief, yet comprehensive, introduction to the study of the power relationships at work within health policy formulation and execution. It will convey both the substance as well as the process of policy making that has evolved from historic concerns for public health (Ham 2009, Ch. 2). This analysis employs a range of intellectual domains, drawing from the various literatures on medicine, philosophy, epidemiology, economics and organizational theory and behaviours. Policy makers develop eloquent and technically robust solutions to important health quandaries. Midwives understand fully 'midwifery specific' policies, yet little explanatory guidance is offered to those wishing to understand the broader origins of policy or its dynamics, despite their achieving a prominence that affects significantly their daily working lives. So it is these health policy mechanisms that matter to all and deserve attention within the formal taught curriculum that are discussed.

POLITICS AND POLICY

In the course of everyday language the terms 'politics' and 'policy' are often used interchangeably, as they can certainly be synergistic (Prabhat 2011). Yet politics is about gaining, sustaining and increasing power and control within any governed entity requiring direction, be that a nation, the NHS or an individual health service organization. In contrast, policies are statements of intent. They concern a prudent stance and a blueprint of how political decisions should be best executed. The two are intended to operate in tandem. Clearly the difference is blurred and at its haziest and in the interests of decisiveness, politics always overrules even the best policies when those governing believe a policy is not working or may threaten their own position of power.

What is health policy?

Health Policy is multifaceted. The United Nations' Universal Declaration of Human Rights (UDHR 1948) asserts that fundamental care is a right of all people stating:

'Everyone has the right to a standard of living adequate for the health and well-being of himself and of his family, including food, clothing, housing, medical care and necessary social services, and the right to security in the event of unemployment, illness, disability, widowhood, old age or other lack of livelihood in circumstances beyond his control'.

(UN, UDHR Article 25:1948)

This somewhat idealistic and aspirational definition provides a professional philosophy and a set of values that underlie the practice of midwifery and other caring professions. The components of health policy are thus eclectic and transcend a range of academic disciplines. Captured briefly these span:

Philosophy – this concerns fundamentally the right to life and the cultural, social and economic entitlement to a minimum standard of humanized health services that all individuals might expect (Todres et al 2007). It also embraces a massive spectrum of practical activity that addresses personal health, children's health, pharmaceutical policy, mental health and public and population well-being. Of interest to midwives are women's rights within health systems, ranging from privacy and dignity to their sexual and reproductive rights, immunization, breastfeeding policy and those policies related to disparities in maternal mortality.

Economics – health services in developed countries have surpassed their ability to afford all the care and treatment options that are available, and all need to manage scarcity (Jackson 2012). Health economics is a preoccupation within all societies needing to manage a degree of rationing. Health systems are individualistic in nature, have grown up in their own time and context and their outcomes are often difficult to compare. Most nations agree, however, on three cardinal intentions for spending their resources widely. These are:

- Equity – how can scarce resources be more fairly distributed?
- Effectiveness – is there reassurance that practising midwives use those techniques that are evidence-based and are proven to work best?
- Efficiency – how is the very greatest value for money secured? This relies on assigning financial value to a particular procedure and comparing its cost-benefits with alternative options.

Workforce – health services depend substantially on technology and drugs, but their most important asset is their workforce. The workforce also accounts for 75% of expenditure, so it is elusive to plan and manage (Trueland 2014). Having the right skill-mix at the right time is basic to good results for mothers and babies and for patients universally. This raises the interesting association between organizational structures, systems of finance and the personal behaviour of practitioners. In consequence, there is a maturing field bringing together the social and behavioural sciences to better understand the distinct contribution of individual midwives to the cost and quality of specific outcomes for mothers and babies (Cookson et al 2014).

Medical Research Policy – Therapeutic-oriented research is a self-evident prerequisite to sound diagnosis and clinical interventions, and evidence-based practice takes this from the traditionally perceived laboratory setting to the bedside. Here the accumulated skills of the midwife from her own learned experience integrate the best research evidence into effective clinical decision making while also considering both safety, satisfaction and the cost-benefits of particular interventions (Sandall et al 2013; Cookson et al 2014).

International Health Policy – Many governments have their health strategies embedded within their overall foreign policy to foster good international relations and improve health in poorer, vulnerable nations. The UK Department for International Development (DFID) epitomizes this. It has a plethora of ways of approaching the *United Nations (UN) Millennium Goals* in the eradication of poverty, hunger, the promotion of gender equality, improvement of maternal health, reducing neonatal and child mortality, combating HIV and AIDS, malaria and other tropical diseases and generating economic sustainability through partnerships with the developed world (Department for International Development (DfID) 2015; UN 2015).

Politics and Policy – The NHS in the UK is politicized and is invariably in the most prominent manifesto commitments of all parties expressed during general elections. It is important for politicians wishing to maintain favour with the electorate to not ignore it. All parties strive to emphasize the merits of their proposals over those of their competitors. The evidence that any particular party makes much difference to the performance of a health system or its outcomes is indeed conjectural. The debate between countries is important and what the similarities and differences between the UK countries mean overall.

The similarities all begin with the electorate, which is each person placing a vote. Once a Government is elected, its Prime Minister or First Minister elects a Cabinet of other high-ranking ministers that take collective responsibility for the nation's policy. Prominent within this is the Secretary of State for Health or Health Minister, who is invested with the power to manage the NHS in the particular country. How this is done depends on the individual national legislature, and the last 15 years have seen some stark internal differences in policies in the UK. England had pursued macho, quasi-market, privatizing strategies that have been characterized by performance management from above. This is described succinctly by the Kings Fund (Kings Fund 2015b and 2015c).

In Scotland, there has been more managerial passivity and less inclination for the constant reorganizations as seen in England; the more recent resurgence of nationalism has reinforced powerfully a rejection of privatized solutions. Wales has maintained its own pathways with a particular emphasis on health promotion and disease prevention through public health initiatives. The NHS differs in Northern Ireland significantly in that it provides both healthcare and social care (which is normally provided by local authorities in the other three countries). Outcome measures from the different systems remain difficult to compare.

Internationally comparable data is limited in scope and validity. Taking proxy measures of performance such as waiting times in Accident and Emergency (A&E) or cancer survival rates produces negligible outcome differences

209

between the home countries and is inconclusive. More resilient epidemiological data on the nature of sampled populations, age distribution, demography and socioeconomic status would be needed to draw more rigorous conclusions (Bevan and Mays 2014).

So although politicians' effect on population health might be marginal, it nevertheless influences the expectations of the electorate and is a source of pressure in the allocation of resources (Blunt 2015).

Who makes policy and how?

Health policy making is determined by concern for the public good that might range from a condition affecting a few, through to how best to provide population-wide services. Policy necessitates governments' use of power to both reassure the electorate and influence health outcomes positively. Any government's ideological and philosophical stance on health services is significant and its political influence in the legislature is important to it getting its own way. Governments with small parliamentary majorities rarely enact risky health legislation successfully. Nevertheless, governments do take account of a wide variety of interests in reaching their conclusions. So although it is political decisions that determine the allocation of crucial resources, it is their economic evaluation and perceived value for money that ultimately determines their implementation as policy. Understanding the politics of the policy process therefore is perhaps as important to innovation as understanding why a particular intervention enhances clinical outcomes or the overall public good (Buse et al 2012).

Politicians do not operate in a vacuum, especially so in democratically elected countries like the UK, and it can be seen there exists a constellation of pressures on ministers. These have been depicted briefly as follows:

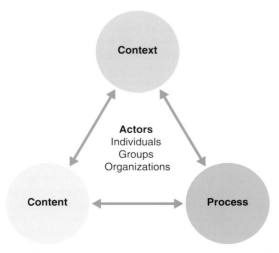

Figure 14.1 A policy analysis triangle (Walt and Gibson 1994).

DETERMINANTS OF HEALTHY POLICY

Policy (see Fig. 14.1) exists in a *context* and its *content*, though often predetermined, becomes modified through individual, group and organizational influences on the policy making *process*. So policy is accommodating, but even its best ministerial form becomes tempered and manipulated by a considerable range of influences. The dynamics of policy modification concern the following sources of pressure:

Ministers, civil servants and 'evidence-based policy'

In the UK, there are many sources of demand on governments. Historically the key navigational influence came from ministers, the Civil Service and the medical profession. This now is by no means the case and claims on the policy-making process are multitudinous. Policy is not just handed down in a linear fashion from Government. From their inception the ideas central to any subsequent policy are subject to a range of influences that cause their refashioning.

Health Ministers are responsible for managing one of the highest spending ministries of government. It can be seen that health secretaries in England who have been successful have gone on to achieve higher office while those less successful have not enjoyed the same professional successes (BBC 2003). Health secretaries have therefore a personal and career motivation to be initiators of successful change and in particular are tasked to produce 'evidence-based policies' that have a chance of success.

The prioritization and funding of NHS policy is determined by national economic priorities, by society's health needs and also through the application of reliable and valid research findings. Making use of existing data that is electorally convincing is something capitalized upon by politicians in recent years in their quest to convey that they know from research *'what works'*. Midwifery practitioners have also grasped this *evidence-based* philosophy as a means of advertising best practice, a bi-product of which is intended to enhance public confidence in them. But *'what works'* is not simply a matter of research findings. The interface between research evidence and the use of political power within health systems is always a consideration in determining the success of any particular policy. Judgement should thereby be reserved on the true bearing of research evidence on any particular health policy (Solesbury 2001).

A reasonable skepticism may be had concerning the real efficacy of *evidence-based* policy. It is alleged that politicians promulgate policies in the name of scientific evidence that often fail to have any value when they are implemented within the general population (Whyte 2013). The accusation is therefore that political imperatives can taint scientific findings and their implementation may be conducted within limited scientific understandings and economic reasoning. The call then is for discernment and balance in the assumptions and claims for what is truly *'evidence based'.*

Special advisers and media managers

The UK Government makes increasing use of special advisers and media managers who bring weighty pressure on health service policy presentation. They are legally employed, unelected political personnel with unswerving dedication to the Government of the day. They advise and, importantly, may influence access to ministers. They are inextricably joined to the public relations function of Government and work to portray favourably the nature and intent of government policy. The role of the media-management by Government must never be underestimated. Although special advisers and media managers do not make health policy per se, they shape its imaginative expression and the priority with which policy information becomes public knowledge.

They also emphasize the Prime Minister's particular interest in Health Policy, reflecting the way in which the Cabinet Office can at times overshadow individual government departments. In recent years it has become a norm that the Prime Minister makes important statements on NHS policies as a symbol of Government commitment to them rather than merely leaving this to the health secretary whose business it really is (House of Lords 2010). The permanent Civil Service is apolitical, yet its advice may be overridden by special advisers with strong political commitment to ministerial doctrine.

Think Tanks

These are organizations that research public policy. They tend to be nonprofit-making organizations, deriving their funding from Government, consultancy for commercial organizations or from campaign groups who hire their services. They can be influential drivers of health policy and have found favour with governments of all political persuasions. The *Fabian Society*, for example, founded in 1884 and affiliated to the Labour Party, influenced the shape of the original NHS. As a further example, the *Adam Smith Institute* was a principle source of free market thinking in the 1990s that has done much since to shape UK policy governing economic policy. In this century, the *Institute for Public Policy Research* moulded the policy of New Labour and its lasting legacy that sees increasing private involvement in the NHS. In addition, the *Centre for Social Justice*, created with the approval of the Conservative Government, exists to seek solutions to poverty and its consequences.

Think Tanks are therefore small, moderately financed organizations. Their aim is to influence the policy debate by analysing policy dilemmas. They receive political acceptance for their findings through cooperation with industry, banking, the media and ultimately politicians. Think Tanks have emerged generally as organizations producing *bona fide* research and consultancy. Whether this is conducted impartially without pursuing skewed findings in support of particular political agendas is the moot point concerning their influence on policy (Stone 2006).

The influence of academics

The articulation between Government and academics and hence policy formation takes two principal forms. Firstly, there is the effect of academic findings on policy formation. Unlike Think Tanks, traditional academics have greater difficulty in shaping policy. This is very much a function of the way they articulate and receive validation from their own scholarly community before their findings can be publicized. The form of communication to a scientific audience therefore is not necessarily that which articulates smoothly with politicians and policy makers. Converting technical information to something inclusive and comprehensible to a policy-making audience requires well-designed communication to convey palatably the potential of technical scientific findings to society at large (O'Brien 2011).

Secondly, academics have had governments endorse existing policy with their assumptions. An example of this was the work of the social democratic theorist Anthony Giddens, which was used by the UK Labour Party as a legitimate means to remove the inequitable aspects of capitalism, yet provide a form of ethical socialism that met social need (Giddens 1994). Giddens' academic work was thus used as a retrospective justification for what was to become the 'Third Way' adopted by the New Labour of Tony Blair.

Adverse events

Adverse events are unanticipated, untoward occurrences during care and treatment. The spectrum of things that can go wrong is as broad as are their causes. These are errors and mishaps, many of which are associated with accidental human miscalculation that may concern defective knowledge, skills and technical oversight. Consequently all NHS organizations have a risk strategy that enables them to deliver a large, constant volume of good quality care. Yet things do go wrong, with serious and damaging consequences for service users and their families, and some are almost predictable (DH 2000). So measures are in place to protect service users and clients and ensure that robust investigations are carried out when things do go awry. It is always intended to learn from serious incidents with the express intention to minimize the risk of the incident happening again in the future (NHS England 2015).

The NHS is not inherently negligent and adverse events arise more from systems failure than from individual error. Yet the service can always learn from its mistakes. It has historically harboured a *'blame culture'*, whereby the open reporting of things that do go wrong were often concealed with the energies of those investigating and were concentrated on finding scapegoats in preference to studying how accidental happenings might be prevented in the future (Fast 2010). This in turn had led to a dearth of information that could be usefully shared to prevent those things that will go amiss (Department of Health (DH) 2000). Greater transparency is now nurtured to systematically collect the necessary intelligence about harmful or potentially harmful incidents and to disseminate it more widely. The concept of reporting the *'near miss'* that is used within the aviation industry is also employed as a routine practice across the NHS in creating better patient safety.

Of interest in policy terms are those events that arise from organizational dysfunction through poor local policy, lack of safety awareness, poor communication, deficient record keeping and the inadequate resources that create a climate for error (NHS Commissioning Board 2013).

Landmark examples of organizational dysfunction exist. The Bristol Heart Scandal in the 1990s led to unnecessary high infant mortality after cardiac surgery, resulting from system failures culminating in surgeons and hospitals being required to publish more of their performance data. Harold Shipman, a British general practitioner (GP), became one of the world's most prolific killers between 1975 to 1998. His conviction resulted in death certification policies becoming reviewed and modified as a direct and indirect result of his crimes. The unauthorized removal of children's organs at Alder Hey Hospital between 1988 and 1995 led to the Human Tissue Act 2004, which overhauled legislation regarding the retention of body parts and saw creation of the Human Tissue Authority to regulate such matters.

Of interest especially to midwives is *The Report of the Morecambe Bay Investigation* (DH 2015). This recounts a chain of events originating with fundamental failures of clinical care in the maternity unit at Furness General Hospital, part of what became the University Hospitals of Morecambe Bay NHS Foundation Trust. This investigation discovered needless hurt to mothers and babies, including catastrophic and unnecessary deaths. Opportunities to prevent the sequence of failure within the dysfunctional unit were missed over a protracted period, resulting in the grave consequences that the report narrates.

Reflective activity 14.2

Look at the Morecambe Bay Investigation report. What factors do you think were the most significant in the management and service failures?

A highly politicized service

The political problems caused to governments by the NHS are inevitable. The Service holds a precious place in the imagination of the British people, and it serves to unite them. It has been claimed that its standing is comparable even to that of a religion and that it is this preciousness that suppresses much of the debate about it that is really required of it (Neuberger 1999; Sikora 2008; Murray 2015). It can be seen therefore that the overall condition of the NHS and the Government's standing with the public are closely intertwined. To be successful, politicians need to do well by their constituents regarding their NHS locally as well as nationally. Some would argue that it is politicians themselves who suggest that more health services produce better health, and it is politicians who raise public expectations (Seyd 2015).

This means usually that the NHS is so politicized to put it among the top three issues at any general election. The people thus believe what politicians tell them; that better services produce better health outcomes, which leads them to assume that medicine can always do something extraordinary. These romantic perceptions sometimes hinder the recognition that although organized medicine is clearly important to length and quality of life, its real achievements can be elevated to a point of exaggeration. What is evident is that the service is afflicted by delay and variable outcomes for clients and patients, and this fuels controversy and adds to its politicization (Toynbee 2015).

This basic political problem is double-edged; the demands made on services are infinite and will invariably exceed their supply. So the NHS is politicized by its image of having constant deficiency and debt. The reasons relate directly to its effectiveness. NHS access, unlike health systems where there are user charges, is unimpeded because it is free at the point of delivery so there are few disincentives for those who seek to use it. Hence the service cannot control demand and is inherently expensive to provide. The comprehensiveness of what is on offer means constant pressure for payment from its product suppliers, including the pharmaceutical industry. Its use of innovative technology and new clinical advances are usually more expensive than those they replace. The Government also fuels the politicization through a commitment to provide high quality of standards of care and treatment that are available readily wherever locally, so travelling many miles to receive specialist services is not commonplace but is a common occurrence elsewhere in the world.

After almost 70 years since its birth, the NHS can still be confirmed that three of its policy precepts on which the service was founded, namely, free access to services, their comprehensive range and their high quality, are alive and well and are still being pursued with vigour by all governments, irrespective of their political ideology

(Conservative Party 2015). Delivering these for all people all the time is an inevitable challenge facing all political administrations.

Policies on free services and comprehensiveness mean that the cheaper, less effective treatment options that could potentially threaten the quality of service might have to be used. The pursuit of the highest quality service that is universal and also free will similarly pose threats to the breadth of services that are on offer, threatening the availability to all who need them. This means that some services such as infertility treatment are not freely available universally to those who wish for it to be, resulting in some having to purchase it privately.

The NHS is the victim of its own success and because it is highly politicized, opposing politicians of any persuasion are always in a position to capitalize on its perceived deficiencies. Because the NHS has exceeded the ability to afford all the care and treatment that is available, it is not difficult to portray the NHS as an organization that is in a state of chronic crisis, and politicians in opposition profit from this to their advantage to the point of using the NHS in political debates (Swinford 2015).

Affording the NHS – the political football

The prominence of the NHS can result in it being used as a political football from which politicians demand more, irrespective of the certainty it can only be allocated a finite resource (Bailey 2015). All governments have recognized tacitly that meeting the most creditable of aims of the NHS are not always achievable in practice. Indeed its more perfectionist aspirations are at the heart of the funding problems confronted by any Government. It is agreed that the source of any NHS failings or deficiency can be traced to money, its insufficiency or its misuse, and these two factors are the permanent focus of the policy debate.

Some would argue that the NHS is the architect of its own troubles. The more staff it employs, the more investment in technology and drugs it makes, the better the quality of care it provides and the more work it does, the more it costs. So it is agreed that funding feeds the politicization of the service and makes it a challenging item to handle.

Causes of funding pressure

Controlling demand can only be achieved by making patients wait, and this has become a politically charged matter because people expect better. Expenditure pressures are nevertheless obvious. The 1.4 million NHS employees consume over 75% of its income. Its reserves are further pressurized by spending, generated by an escalating elderly population that will increase substantially over the next 30 years. The older people become, the more they tend to use the NHS, and this is exemplified by a year-on-year increase in the cost of their social care (Holt 2015).

Unavoidable pressure on funding arises also from the relentless rise of expensive new drugs and technology and the clamour for their availability from clinicians in all sectors. Historically, if new drugs or new equipment became available, both would be purchased with little questioning. Rigorous cost-benefit analyses of new technologies and drugs by the National Institute for Health and Care Excellence (NICE) is now the norm, with investment in only those items that are proven to be effective and that give value for money. This perceived rationing happens ruthlessly for products that might work for some but are not sufficient to warrant their overall licensing for all. This leaves Government vulnerable politically if it is seen to be denying to a particular patient, some treatment that, although available, is not thought to provide good value monetarily.

The persistent reorganizations of the health service and their negative budgetary consequences are another source of expenditure, especially so in England. But this is difficult to measure, and the effect of efficiency of persistent reorganizations is never measured, so whether they have been a good investment is questionable (Johnstone 2014).

Raising the revenue

The need to properly fund healthcare catches the public imagination on the assumption that therapeutic mediation is inexhaustible. Yet spending on clinical interventions is only a partial solution, given that the origins of ill health are also socioeconomic, behavioural and rooted more deeply in broader dysfunction within modern society. The corollary is that the Government should be spending more on health promotion, disease prevention, housing and Social Services. But ministers can prefer the eye-catching, high technological investments.

Governments strive continuously to make better use of existing money. This is meant to optimize resource allocation to get the maximum return for each pound spent. Efficiency savings and improved productivity are at the heart of policy, with providers being charged to reduce waste and to deliver more care each year from the same amount of money. On this basis, the more efficient managers are, the more difficult it becomes for them to be even more efficient in the future, trying to squeeze even better results from the same amount of cash (Kings Fund 2015b and 2015c). Yet despite a relentless approach to effectiveness and efficiency, the question about how to best raise more resources recurs.

Funding is now seen recurrently at the foundation of any debate about the NHS and all of its reconfiguration and reforms are predicated on its improved economic efficiency. In generating the necessary financial resources and enriching economic performance of the NHS, governments have several options:

General taxation: General taxation has provided the major funding source for the NHS and seems likely to do so for the foreseeable future, not least because changing to an alternative is untested and unpredictable. As a funding supply, it has much to commend it; it is cheap to collect and raises well over 80% of the cash required (Kings Fund 2015b). It draws from a broad constituency, mainly of those in employment whose taxable contribution is proportionate to their earnings and who arguably 'can afford' to pay income tax, so this makes it a fair means of revenue. It is also sufficiently adaptable such that its rate can be altered according to national needs.

Though general taxation is the prime source of revenue, it is nevertheless politically laden, and this determines the feasibility of manipulating its strategic use as a source of cash. The population generally does not vote to have their general taxation increased. So Government has the option to divert money from other items of public expenditure to the NHS from other spending Ministries, but this runs the risk of political unpopularity through depriving other areas of their resources. Similarly, there is a political hazard for any Government considering an increase in income tax and a commitment to avoid this is a pledge of all pre-election manifestos.

Earmarked health taxes: The National Insurance (NI) stamp was intended in 1948 to serve partly as an earmarked tax for the NHS, but there was no appreciation at the time of the demands that would eventually be made on it by the welfare benefits system. National Insurance, like General Taxation, is a compulsory deduction from those in work and is administratively convenient to collect. It too is contributed proportionately to earnings and is also relatively fair, meeting over 18% of the total NHS purse (Kings Fund 2015b).

The point about both General Taxation and National Insurance as sources of NHS income is that the person from whom payday deductions are made has no control of where *'their'* money is spent. This provokes a more enduring question about the introduction of a ring-fenced 'Health Tax'. Because the public might be willing to pay more towards a fund that is dedicated totally to healthcare, it is less certain whether they would be happy to pay more income tax that might be invested in a venture that may conflict with personal beliefs. The protagonists for a protected 'Health Fund' would argue that the NHS should have a dedicated resource that is outside the control of Government, which would shelter it from the financial fluctuations that have hindered its planned development during its history. The idea though could become unsustainable during economic recession when the Treasury needs every penny of public money at its disposal to sustain national economic viability.

Conserving a service providing universal coverage requires compulsory contributions, and this always raises questions of alternatives to the present system that we know to be reliable.

User charges: Unlike international comparators, the UK has a very low level of direct patient charges. This then is possibly a rich source of income. Two considerations prevail: those who support private payment and those against private payment (Maynard 2012; Campbell 2014; Haldenby and Corrie 2014). Supporters of more charges argue that paying privately for services confers personal choice and the expression of a preference that is not generally available when accessing routine state services. Those against charging create the political imagery that it undermines the motives of the welfare state. What is certain is that user charges suppress demand, best illustrated by the introduction of an almost privately run optician service in the UK that severely curtails the uptake of routine eye tests. A similar stifling of access to treatment results from a progressively privatized dental service. User charges are a serious disincentive because they are dependent on the ability to pay, not on clinical necessity. But they require an accompanying exemptions policy for the needy and therein resides a second major question concerning what charge would be appropriate. If the charge is too low it may be uneconomical to collect. If the charge is too high it might be similarly self-defeating and exclude those with treatable conditions that become unavoidably neglected. Or if too many people are exempt, the charge may be just not worthy of collection.

Periodically, discussion arises about broadening the spectrum of charges, including charges for general practitioner (GP) surgery consultation, GP home and 'out of hours' visits, A&E attendance, outpatient visits, hospital transportation and nonclinical 'hotel' services for an inpatient stay, such as payments for food and laundry. Extending patient charges could, however, further privatization and act as an inspiration to individuals to insure against those things that might otherwise become an unexpected, out-of-pocket expense. In reality, patient charging is unwieldy both politically and practically and, though threatening, it is a way to control demand; governments back down from the proposal if it seems politically damaging to their commitment to a largely free NHS.

Private medical insurance: There is worthy suspicion in England that the NHS is being prepared for privatization and that there are pros and cons to this eventuality (El-Gingihy 2015a and 2015b; The Week 2015; Kings Fund 2015d). But for this to happen, private insurance would have to be near universal.

Private insurance has historically made little financial contribution to the NHS because its benefits were largely spent on treatments in the private hospital sector. But the NHS is now the largest provider of private elective surgery that accounts for most of the activity conducted for the privately insured. Managers have realized that competition with private hospitals for elective work is worthwhile because it provides a funding stream in addition to that from the exchequer and earnings from private patients that have become a valued source of income generation.

The idea of a privatized NHS is mooted periodically. Its adoption has not happened because a large number of the population is uninsurable and insurance companies eschew risky subscribers, especially those with chronic debilitating and intractable conditions. Companies also have exclusions for expensive treatments and those conditions associated with risk of any kind, such as maternity care. In addition, those without means to sustain insurance premiums would require a substantial state NHS safety net to meet their needs, and the question arises whether this might make a remnant NHS become a second rate service (Kings Fund 2015d).

Advocates for the more wholesale introduction of private medical insurance argue that it reduces the drain of the NHS and the demand for public funding and results in less personal taxation. It is also claimed that privatization cuts waiting times and brings more personally tailored, consumer responsive care. Proponents argue private medicine introduces cost consciousness with insurance subscribers, unlike NHS users not overusing services that might otherwise increase their premium.

Critics hold that privatization is a mark of privilege in an unequal society where wealth buys preference that guarantees 'a place at the front of the queue' and overrides clinical importance. They also note its higher administrative costs and its market selectivity in only taking cases that make a profit. They are especially reproachful of it being parasitical on the NHS. The private sector does little in the way of pre-registration training for the major health professions and recruits its staff from the NHS. It similarly is heavily state-subsidized through its heavy reliance on NHS consultants. This dependence on NHS medical staff means that the doctoring quality of privatized care is no better than that of the NHS simply because the private sector relies on NHS spare consultant capacity.

CONCLUSION

The NHS affects every single person in the UK, and its policies embody principles that make the service even more cherished than the monarchy and the army (Katwala 2013).

From its birth in 1948 the NHS has wrestled with tough decisions concerning the judicious use of its scarce resources. It remains a service without precedent and continues as it began as part of the relief of the five giants of want, disease, squalor, ignorance and idleness. It has tried repeated reforms to better cope with financial constraints, and these will continue. Politicians demand radical amendments to make the system affordable, better at what it does and fairer to all, but they recognize always

this needs broad public support. The NHS represents a concept of fairness that comes from doing what it does freely and never judging those it treats solely on their spending capability. No Government is likely to design policies that undermine these fundamental objectives in the foreseeable future and must appreciate that effective policies rely also for their implementation on the goodwill and cooperation of NHS staff.

The NHS has a 'target-driven' culture as its way to secure a successful operation. This requires rigid labour demarcation with standardized, results-oriented procedures within a system of hierarchical managerial control. It is established in the management literature though, that when frontline staff are rigidly overseen and driven, that hierarchical management does not necessarily work (Walton 1985; Bevan 2010). Overmanaged staff who work under pressurized conditions do not properly control their own professional performance and, thus, experience disempowerment. An alternative suggests that frontline clinicians improve efficiency best by having ownership of the intended objectives of their particular organization. Rather than having change imposed on them from their superiors, their commitment is better secured by enabling them to lead the very transformation that policy makers and management require. This draws the distinction between 'compliance' and 'commitment' that has been simply explained as follows in Table 14.1 (Bevan 2010).

It can be seen from this comparative table that 'compliance' emphasizes rigid, managerially inflicted 'top down' performance targets whereas 'commitment' results in the sharing of collectively held goals and a generation of their ownership (Walton 1985). Management still has a decisive role in providing general direction, but the evidence suggests that a milieu that promotes openness and trust in frontline staff acts, motivates and stretches their aspirations and achieves key performance indicators at the same time (Leslie et al 2006). The operative word therefore is 'commitment' that is proven to deliver transformational change at both pace and volume in ways unachievable by the 'carrot and stick' approach demanded by 'compliance'.

Our conclusion therefore pursues the policy and managerial options for action that are available to midwives. This draws attention to the slippery and somewhat messy nature of health policy and provides confirmation that there is no 'right way' to proceed for those who make policy decisions. Someone else, and by no means only midwives and politicians in an opposing political party, can usually think of a better way to do things than the Government of the day.

Midwives therefore need the knowledgeable facility to interpret policy and provide explanations for its implementation at whatever level they function. This begins from the premise that a persistent conflict exists between the creation of health policy and its implementation. Government strategy makers have a central concern to act for the collective good. Yet this often creates tension for

Table 14.1 Compliance and commitment contrasted

From ..... Compliance goals	.....To Commitment goals
States a minimum performance standard that everyone must achieve	States a collective improvement goal that everyone can aspire to
Uses hierarchy, systems and standard procedures for coordination and control	Uses hierarchy, systems and standard procedures for coordination and control
Delivered through formal command and control structures	Delivered through voluntary connections and teams
Threat of penalties/sanctions/shame creates momentum for delivery	Commitment to a common purpose creates energy for delivery
Based on organizational accountability ("if I don't deliver this, I fail to meet my performance objectives")	Based on relational commitment ("If I don't deliver this, I let the group and its purpose down")

(Bevan 2010)

clinicians implementing policy to make it meet individual client need and choice within the resources that are available. Health services and the policies that govern them are a very public matter, yet, simultaneously, an individual and personal one. So though policy intends to be therapeutic, it can also be stressful for those midwifery professionals who have to put it into practice. This raises debate for midwives about the key principles on which the NHS was founded concerning the fundamental ingredients of social justice governing their ethos of practice.

Attention has been drawn to major dilemmas for health service organizations that are both current and enduring and will remain so irrespective of which Government is in office. This awareness arises knowing all midwives are busy people and their concerns for the clinical challenges in hand are their foremost concern. Yet achieving a broader grasp of where midwifery is located within the broader policy context is a critical quality in the qualified practitioner. This necessitates an expansive conceptual understanding and familiarity with policy at a local organization level and in the wider healthcare environment. Having policy 'knowhow' produces more shrewd and effective clinicians who have the ability to cope with both transition and transformation. 'Know how' illuminates who and what are the key drivers of change both internal and external to your

organization, and it is 'know how' that mobilizes support for midwifery innovation and service improvements.

It is easy for the midwife embroiled in the melee of everyday clinical pressures to become frustrated about the hectic work environment, the lack of staff and constant change. But there is absolutely no point in becoming frustrated about unfairness and injustice unless there is understanding of 'know how' the way things work – hence the importance of policy.

Those who successfully lead the midwifery profession attain the knowledgeable competence to identify the bigger problems and find workable ways of resolving them by not letting themselves be distracted by conflicts and criticism about what they do. They nurture the capacity to prioritize information, to effectively martial data and to discriminate on the relative explanatory value of the various evidence available to them. Having appraised the data, they systematically evaluate the alternative arguments before drawing conclusions.

Central to all these important intellectual processes returns to the significance for the midwife of knowing how things work. Midwives with organizational 'know how' possess a crucial characteristic – namely *political astuteness*. This quality sustains the ability to understand the diverse complexity of interest groups and power bases within health service organizations, the wider professional communities such as medicine and management and within the local health economy. The acquisition of *political astuteness* requires a perceptive comprehension of every dimension of policy debates. It requires effective judgements on policy that ultimately leads to more effective leadership of midwifery services wherever they exist. In short, the *politically astute* midwife by definition is a more effective leader, advocate and representative for maternal child and family healthcare than one who is not (DH 2014).

Key Points

- Since its inception, the NHS has been undergoing a process of constant change and development alongside society.
- The NHS affects everyone in the UK, and its principles and service are valued by the public.
- It began as part of the relief of the five giants of want, disease, squalor, ignorance and idleness.
- Midwives need to be knowledgeable about the structure and workings of the NHS at organizational and local levels.
- It is important for midwives to be politically aware of their part in the service and contribute to the growth and well-being of the organization to the service of women, babies and families.
- Midwives need to be alert to changes within the health service to innovate and change alongside the service.

References

Bailey C: *Calling time on the NHS as a political football. The debate* (website). www.politics.webershandwick.co.uk/calling-time-nhs-political-football. 2015.

Bevan G, Mays N: *The four health systems of the UK: how they compare?* (website). http://www.nuffieldtrust.org.uk/compare-UK-health. 2014.

Bevan H: *From compliance to commitment. NHS Institute for Innovation and Improvement, London* (website). www.institute.nhs.uk/nhsalert/articleofthemonth/fromcompliancetocommitment.html#sthash.IW5d9fOz.dpuf. 2010.

Beveridge W: *Social insurance and allied services* (website). www.bl.uk/onlinegallery/takingliberties/staritems/712bever idgereportpic.html. 1942.

Blunt I: *Fact or fiction: politicians make a difference to health service performance* (website). www.nuffieldtrust.org.uk/blog/fact-or-fiction-politicians-make-difference-health-system-performance?gclid=CNiA6-H1uccCFaPnwgodmuYCoQ. 2015.

British Broadcasting Corporation (BBC): *Dispute over Milburn Departure* (website). http://news.bbc.co.uk/1/hi/health/2984352.stm. 2003.

Buse K, Maya N, Walt G: *Making health policy (understanding public health)*, Maidenhead, England, Open University Press, McGraw Hill, 2012.

Campbell D: *NHS users should pay £10 a month, says former health minister* (website). www.theguardian.com/society/2014/mar/31/nhs-users-pay-membership-charge. 2014.

Campbell D, Watt N: *NHS comes top in healthcare survey* (website). www.theguardian.com/society/2014/jun/17/nhs-health. 2014.

Commonwealth Fund: *Mirror, mirror on the wall, 2014 update: how the US health care system compares internationally* (website). www.commonwealthfund.org/publications/fund-reports/2014/jun/mirror-mirror. 2014.

Conservative Party Manifesto: *Strong leadership. A clear economic plan. A brighter more secure future* (website). https://www.conservatives.com/manifesto. 2015.

Cookson G, Jones S, van Vlymen J, et al: *The cost-effectiveness of midwifery staffing and skill 4 mix on maternity outcomes* (website). www.nice.org.uk/guidance/NG4/documents/safe-midwifery-staffing-for-maternity-settings-economic-analysis-and-modelling-report2. 2014.

Department for International Development (DfID): *About us* (website). www.gov.uk/government/organisations/department-for-international-development/about. 2015.

Department of Health (DH): *Organisation with a memory. Report of an expert group on learning from adverse events in the NHS*, London, DH, 2000.

Department of Health (DH): *NHS five year forward view NHS England*, London, DH, 2014.

Department of Health (DH): *The report of the Morecambe Bay investigation* (website). www.gov.uk/government/uploads/system/uploads/attachment_data/file/408480/47487_MBI_Accessible_v0.1.pdf. 2015.

El-Gingihy Y: *How to dismantle the NHS in 10 easy steps* (website). www.zero-books.net/books/how-dismantle-nhs-10-easy-steps. 2015a.

El- Gingihy Y: *The NHS is on a one-way road to privatisation* (website). www.theguardian.com/healthcare-network/2015/oct/02/nhs-one-way-road-privatisation. 2015b.

Enthoven A: Internal market reform of the British National Health Service, *Health Aff* 10(3):60–70, 1991.

Fast NJ: *How to stop the blame game* (website). https://hbr.org/2010/05/how-to-stop-the-blame-game. 2010.

Foot M: *Aneurin Bevan 1887–1960*, London, Orion, 1999.

Anthony Giddens: *Beyond left and right: the future of radical politics*, Cambridge, England, UK, Polity Press, pp 71–72, 1994.

Haldenby A, Corrie C: *Can we ignore NHS charges any longer?* (website). www.kingsfund.org.uk/blog/2014/08/can-we-ignore-nhs-charges-any-longer. 2014.

Ham C: *Health policy in Britain*, 6th edn, Basingstoke, Palgrave Macmillan, 2009.

Holt A: *Why the rising cost of social care cannot be ignored* (website). www.bbc.co.uk/news/health-31001151. 2015.

House of Lords Select Committee on the Constitution, *4th Report of Session 2009–10* (website). www.publications.parliament.uk/pa/ld200910/ldselect/ldconst/30/30.pdf. 2010.

Jackson D: *Healthcare economics made easy*, Oxford, Scion, 2012.

Johnstone I: *Government's reorganisation of the NHS was its biggest 'mistake', say senior Tories* (website). www.independent.co.uk/news/uk/politics/government-s-reorganisation-of-the-nhs-was-its-biggest-mistake-say-senior-tories-9790247.html. 2014.

Katwala S: *The NHS: even more cherished than the monarchy and the army* (website). www.newstatesman.com/politics/2013/01/nhs-even-more-cherished-monarchy-and-army. 2013.

Kings Fund: *An alternative guide to the new NHS in England* (website). www.kingsfund.org.uk/projects/nhs-65/alternative-guide-new-nhs-england. 2015a.

Kings Fund: *How the NHS is funded* (website). www.kingsfund.org.uk/projects/nhs-in-a-nutshell/how-nhs-funded?gclid=CO-V2r7u1cgCFcHGGwodcJ4GeQ. 2015b.

Kings Fund: *Better value in the NHS* (website). www.kingsfund.org.uk/publications/better-value-nhs/summary?gclid=CO2aiaHa58gCFcafGwod8WUDPg. 2015c.

Kings Fund: *Is the NHS being privatised?* (website). www.kingsfund.org.uk/projects/verdict/nhs-being-privatised?gclid=COeU5Kf46cgCFckaGwodrOAM-Q. 2015d.

Leslie K, Loch M, Schaninger W: *Managing your organization by the evidence* (website). http://integral.ms/_Uploads/dbsAttachedFiles/95ManbyEv.pdf. 2006.

Maynard A: *Time for user charges in the NHS? Health policy insight: health management online analysis and intelligence* (website). www.healthpolicyinsight.com/?q=node/971. 2012.

Murray D: *Treat the NHS as a religion, and you give it the right to run your*

life (website). http://new.spectator
.co.uk/2015/06/doctors-orders/.
2015.

National Health Service (NHS)
Commissioning Board: *Serious
incident framework*, London,
Department of Health, 2013.

National Health Service (NHS) England
2014: *Understanding the new NHS
BMJ on behalf of NHS England*
(website). www.england.nhs.uk/
wp-content/uploads/2014/06/
simple-nhs-guide.pdf. 2014.

National Health Service (NHS)
England: *Serious incident framework*
(website). www.england.nhs.uk/
patientsafety/wp-content/uploads/
sites/32/2015/04/serious-incidnt
-framwrk-upd2.pdf. 2015.

Neuberger J: *The NHS as a theological
institution* (website).
www.ncbi.nlm.nih.gov/pmc/articles/
PMC1127078/. 1999.

O'Brien C: *Why academics should learn
how to influence government policy*
(website). www.theguardian.com/
higher-education-network/blog/
2011/jun/07/academics-learn
-influence-government-policy. 2011.

Prabhat S: *Differences between policy and
politics* (website). www.difference
between.net/miscellaneous/politics/
difference-between-policy-and
-politics/. 2011.

Sandall J, Soltani H, Gates S, et al:
*Midwife-led continuity models versus
other models of care for childbearing
women* (website). http://online
library.wiley.com/doi/10.1002/
14651858.CD004667.pub3/abstract.
2013.

Seyd B: *Expectation management: can
politicians win back political trust by*

limiting what the public expects of
them? (website). http://blogs
.lse.ac.uk/politicsandpolicy/
expectation-management-can
-politicians-win-back-political
-trust-by-limiting-what-the-public
-expects-of-them/. 2015.

Sikora K: *It sounds like heresy but we've
got to stop treating the NHS like a
national religion* (website).
www.dailymail.co.uk/health/article
-1030671/It-sounds-like-heresy-weve
-got-stop-treating-NHS-like-national
-religion.html#ixzz3pHqZIDMI.
2008.

Solesbury W: *Evidence-based policy:
whence it came and where it's going?*,
University of London, ESRC UK
Centre for Evidence Based Policy
and Practice, Queen Mary, 2001.

Stone D: Think tanks and policy
analysis. In Fischer Frank, Miller
Gerald J., Sidney Mara S., editors:
*Handbook of public policy analysis:
theory, methods, and politics*, New
York, Marcel Dekker Inc, 2006.

Swinford C: *Ed Milliband said he wanted
to 'weaponise' NHS in secret meeting
with BBC executives* (website).
www.telegraph.co.uk/news/
politics/ed-miliband/11338695/Ed
-Miliband-said-he-wanted-to
-weaponise-NHS-in-secret-meeting
-with-BBC-executives.html. 2015.

The Week: *Pros and cons of privatising
the NHS: could it ever work?*
(website). www.theweek.co.uk/nhs/
63360/pros-and-cons-of-privatising
-the-nhs-could-it-ever-work. 2015.

Todres L, Galvin K, Dahlberg K: *Life
world-led healthcare: revisiting a
humanising philosophy that integrates
emerging trends* (website). http://

link.springer.com/article/10.1007/
s11019-006-9012-8#page-1. 2007.

Toynbee P: *Yes, the NHS has been
weaponised, but it was the Tories who
primed the guns* (website).
www.theguardian.com/comment
isfree/2015/jan/29/nhs-weaponised-
tories-politicised-health-service.
2015.

Trueland J: *How to tackle the workforce
planning issue* (website). www.hsj
.co.uk/hsj-knowledge/downloads/
hsj-roundtable-how-to-tackle-the
-workforce-planning
-issue/5075138.fullarticle.
2014.

United Nations (UN): *The Universal
Declaration of Human Rights. Adopted
on 10 December 1948 by the General
Assembly of the United Nations*
(website). www.un.org/en/
documents/udhr/index.shtml#a25.
1948.

United Nations (UN): *UN development
goals – we can end poverty –
millennium goals beyond 2015*
(website). www.un.org/
millenniumgoals/bkgd.shtml.
2015.

Walt G, Gibson L: Reforming the health
system in developing countries: the
central role of policy analysis,
Health Policy Plan 9:353–370,
1994.

Walton R: *From control to commitment in
the workplace* (website). https://
hbr.org/1985/03/from-control-to
-commitment-in-the-workplace.
1985.

Whyte J: *Quack policy: abusing
science in the cause of paternalism*,
London, Institute of Economic
Affairs, 2013.

Resources and additional reading

The Kings Fund: *The New NHS*:
www.kingsfund.org.uk/sites/files/kf/
media/nhs-structure-2015.pdf
*Excellent source of information on how the
NHS is organized, funded and
regulated.*

The Nuffield Trust: http://www
.nuffieldtrust.org.uk/talks/
slideshows/new-structure
-nhs-england
*Good source for further information on the
NHS structure.*

The History of the NHS: http://
www.nhshistory.net
*This has key issues and milestones within
the NHS history compiled by Geoffrey
Rivett.*

Royal College of Midwives (RCM)
– website: https://www.rcm.org.uk
*This site has features that include regular
policy briefings from the RCM, CPD
events often including NHS issues, plus
consultations and news features.*

*There are also a range of relevant modules
in the 'i-learn' electronic learning
(e-learning) suite, which is free for
RCM members to access. These
modules include 'the Changing NHS';
and 'Understanding the Kirkup Report'.*

Chapter 15

Legal frameworks for the care of the child

Dr Barbara Burden and Professor Michael Preston-Shoot

Learning Outcomes ?

After reading this chapter, you will be able to:

- understand the legislative basis and key principles within the Children Act 1989; Children Act 2004 and other relevant legal rules, including the Human Rights Act 1998
- appreciate the range of resources available to support families in caring for their children
- assess the role and responsibilities of local authority and voluntary sector organizations in providing and monitoring services for children and families
- identify the particular needs of children with disabilities and those from different racial and cultural backgrounds
- evaluate the role and responsibilities of the midwife in assisting Councils with social service responsibilities to promote and safeguard the welfare of children in need and at risk
- realize the midwife's contribution to the assessment of children and families

Note: Please see the website for a list of all the Acts/Statutes referred to in this chapter.

INTRODUCTION

Safeguarding children and promoting their welfare is the responsibility of every health and social care professional. An increasing emphasis is placed on outcomes to be delivered through multiagency workings and information-sharing. Repeatedly, government documents continue to highlight the requirement for interagency and interprofessional workings and a whole system focus to safeguard and promote the well-being of children and young people (Laming 2009, HM Government 2015a, Munro 2011). Decisions about children's welfare and safety are complex, with high-profile deaths of children, such as Victoria Climbié and Baby P, raising criticisms and anxieties about professional decision making, leadership and management (Department of Health (DH) 2003, DH 2015a, Joint Area Review 2008, Office for Standards in Education, Children's Services and Skills (OFSTED) 2010). While the quality of children's services may be improving, criticisms remain of partnership arrangements, performance management, the involvement of young people in decision making, the use of assessment to identify need and track progress and communication to ensure the emergence of a comprehensive picture of a child's needs (OFSTED 2009; Statham and Aldgate 2003; Preston-Shoot 2014). There are also concerns about high thresholds limiting access to services (Eastman 2014) and lack of compliance by local authorities with regard to legal rules (Preston-Shoot 2010).

This chapter seeks to enable midwives in understanding the legislative framework and related policies, procedures and resources needed to carry out their role effectively and work together with parents and other professionals to ensure the well-being and safety of children. For the definition of the child, please see Box 15.1.

The legal rules highlighted herein are those for England and Wales, principally the Children Act 1989. Midwives working in Scotland should refer to the Children (Scotland) Act 1995 and those in Northern Ireland to the Children (Northern Ireland) Order 1995. Subsequent legislation shows an increasing differentiation between the four UK nations. While these differences reflect the different legal and judicial systems pertaining within the UK, all primary legislation relating to children contains provisions for emergency protection, accommodating children with parental consent, and care and supervision orders for those who have experienced or are likely to suffer significant harm. It emphasizes the importance of ascertaining and paying due regard to the child's wishes and feelings, the views of those with parental responsibility and others who are significant in the life of the child. There are mandates for information-sharing and multi-agency, interprofessional cooperation. Those midwives working outside the UK must familiarize themselves with the distinctive national legal rules for their country of residence. Those working in Europe must positively promote the rights contained within the European Convention on Human Rights and Fundamental Freedoms, which across the UK have been integrated into the national legal framework. The Articles contained within the United Nations Convention on the Rights of the Child (United Nations (UN) 1989) also provide strong principles for practice, the more so if a country has integrated them into national child care law (which in the main four countries of the UK have not).

The discussion in the following section may be linked to three scenarios that may be encountered by midwives (see Case Study 15.1 that follows and Web Scenarios 15.1 and 15.2, and a range of activities on the website suggested for learning). These all illustrate the complexity of issues that might face midwives in their day-to-day practice.

THE CHILDREN ACT 1989

The *Children Act 1989*, amplified by associated regulations and statutory guidance, covers legislation relating to aspects of care, upbringing and protection of children (Braye and Preston-Shoot 2009). This includes the welfare and protection of children in disputed divorce proceedings, children in need, children at risk, children with disabilities or special educational needs and those who need to live away from home (short-term or long-term), including children in hospital, boarding schools, residential homes and foster homes. These rules have been amended and supplemented by subsequent legislation, most notably the *Family Law Act 1996* (to protect victims of domestic violence), the *Children (Leaving Care) Act 2000* (duties regarding young people leaving care), the *Adoption and Children Act 2002* (reform of adoption law and changes to the Children Act 1989 provisions, for instance concerning parental responsibility, special

CASE STUDY 15.1 Gill

Gill, aged 28, has just given birth to a baby boy. Her 6-month-old child was removed from her previously because care was found to be inadequate. Gill has learning difficulties.

A pre-birth assessment, in which Gill cooperated, commenced when she notified her general practitioner (GP) of her pregnancy at 28 weeks gestation.

Initially Gill maintained that she was raped at a party and did not know the baby's father. She claimed that she had separated from Jack, the father of her first baby, a year ago. Jack has spent the last 4 months in prison for grievous bodily harm and has a reputation for violent behaviour. He was released from prison 2 days ago. Gill now states that Jack is the father of this baby. She is no longer willing to cooperate with the hospital or social services and is threatening to discharge herself. Jack is encouraging her in this process.

The paediatric consultant would like the baby to stay in the hospital for observation because antenatal care was poor, and the baby has a low birthweight. Gill's health also requires monitoring. She suffers from epilepsy and is extremely obese.

Consider the role and responsibilities of the midwife in situations like this:

* What might be your concerns?
* Who would you report your concerns to?
* What can you contribute to a pre-birth assessment?
* What would you be looking for in your contact with parents?
* How do you think parents could be supported to care for their baby while not putting the child at risk?

guardianship and advocacy), the *Children Act 2004* (specifying outcomes for children and requirements for interagency working), the *Children and Adoption Act 2006* (sanctions for disrupting contact between children and nonresident parents, and changes to family assistance orders), the *Children and Young Persons Act 2008* (amendments to children in need and emergency protection order provisions, and changes concerning accommodated children), the *Apprenticeships, Skills, Children and Learning Act 2009* and the *Children and Families Act 2014* (changes to adoption provisions and support for disabled children, and amendments to care proceedings and to Section 8 under the Children Act 1989).

Guidance and regulations produced by central government departments provide detailed information about how legislation should be implemented. When guidance is issued under Section 7, Local Authority Social Services Act 1970, it should be followed. One such guidance is *Working together to safeguard children* (HM Government 2015), which provides the blueprints for agencies to work

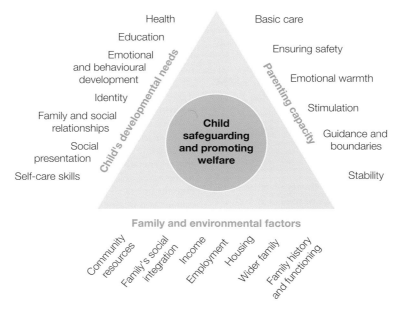

Figure 15.1 The assessment framework. (HM Government 2015 Working Together to Safeguard Children: A guide to interagency working to safeguard and promote the welfare of children, London, The Stationery Office.)

together with children (see Fig. 15.1). Guidance has also been issued to clarify how outcomes for children, detailed in the Children Act 2004, should be approached (Children's Workforce Development Council (CWDC) 2009; Department for Education and Skills (DfES) 2005).

The midwife has a universal and accepted role in working with pregnant mothers, newborn babies and their families and is in a unique position to comment on all aspects of the health and care of newborn babies (see case studies and reflective activities on website). This is in direct contrast to some other professionals, for example, social workers and police, who tend to be involved with families when there is cause for concern. In 2013, there were 698,512 live births in England and Wales (Office for National Statistics (ONS) 2014a), the majority in the presence of a midwife. In comparison there were 657,800 referrals to children's social care in England in 2013-14, 397,600 of which were classified as children in need, with 142,500 Section 47 enquires completed and 48,300 children on a child protection plan (Department for Education (DfE) 2014) (see chapter website resources and Reflective activity Web 15.2).

Key features of the Children Act 1989

The Children Act 1989 was formulated on key beliefs about children, young people, parents and the role of the State, which are given statutory recognition in the Act.

These include the following:

- There is a universal duty to promote and safeguard the welfare of the child.

- Children are best brought up within their family, and local authorities have a duty to give support to children and families to facilitate this, when it is safe and appropriate so to do.

- Even when children are separated from their families, they should maintain contact with them, except where this puts them at risk.

- The state should only intervene where it is in the child's best interests and legal measures are only taken as a last resort.

- Professionals should work in partnership with parents, where possible, involving them in the care of their children and decisions made about them.

- The wishes and feelings of children and young people should be sought (depending on their age and level of understanding), and taken into account when making decisions about their lives.

- The child's welfare should be the paramount consideration in court decisions.

- The race, religion, culture and language of a child should be taken into account in provision of any services.

The Act is clear. The paramount duty for everyone is to *safeguard and promote the welfare of children*. While other objectives, such as working in partnership with parents, are also highlighted, it is important to recognize that these practice principles do not overturn the paramount duty of the local authority to safeguard and promote the welfare of children (Braye and Preston-Shoot 2009; Brayne et al 2015).

CONTENT AND STRUCTURE OF THE CHILDREN ACT

Of particular interest to midwives are the parts of the 1989 Act that deal with the responsibilities of the Local Authority (LA) in providing support for children and families (Part III) and the protection of children (Part V).

Part 1 (Section 1): Welfare of the child

The Children Act 1989 begins with a statement that the child's welfare is the paramount issue to be taken into account in decisions made by a court in respect of children and young people (s1:1). The Act advocates avoiding delay in making decisions about a child's upbringing (s1:2) as it can prejudice the welfare of the child. Where the court is required to take action, the Act requires it to take account of the following *'welfare checklist'* (s1:3):

- the ascertainable wishes and feelings of the child concerned (subject to age and understanding)
- the child's physical, emotional and educational needs
- the likely effect on the child of having any changes in their circumstances
- age, sex, background and any characteristics the court considers relevant
- any harm which the child has suffered or is at risk of suffering
- how capable each of the parents and any other person in relation to whom the court considers the question to be relevant is in meeting the child's needs
- the range of powers available to the court

While this applies to only parts of the Act and relates specifically to decisions of the court, professionals are expected to take this checklist into account when making decisions about a child.

The Act also states (s1: 5) that courts can only make an order with respect to a child if this would be better for the child than not making an order. This is based on the principle that the State should intervene only in private and family life to the degree necessary. This conforms to Article 8 of the *European Convention on Human Rights*, with its principle of proportional intervention, incorporated into UK law by the *Human Rights Act 1998*.

Part 1 (Section 2): Parents and parental responsibility

The concept of *parental responsibility* is described in Sections 2, 3, 4 and 5. Parental responsibility is defined as: all the rights, duties, powers, responsibilities and authority, which by law a parent has in relation to the child and his property (Children Act 1989: S.3(1)).

This includes the responsibility to care for the child and promote and protect the child's moral, physical and emotional health. Although not specifically defined in the Act, this is generally considered to include decisions with respect to the name, religion and education of the child, the right to consent or not to medical treatment and adoption, to have contact and to arrange for the burial or cremation of a child.

Who has parental responsibility?

Having parental responsibility does not automatically equate with being the legal or biological parent of the child. For example, the birth mother automatically acquires parental responsibility at the moment of birth. However, the father does not have parental responsibility automatically unless he has been married to the mother. An unmarried father has parental responsibility if he is registered as the father on the child's birth certificate (an amendment in the Adoption and Children Act 2002), or if the birth mother or a court gives him parental responsibility. Other people may also acquire parental responsibility through decisions of the court, for example, grandparents, guardians, foster carers or the local authority. In these circumstances, parental responsibility can be shared among several people. The only circumstance in which a birth mother and married father would lose parental responsibility is when their child is adopted or a placement order is made, permitting adoption to be planned. If an unmarried birth father has been given parental responsibility, it can, in exceptional circumstances, be removed by a court. In divorce, both parents retain parental responsibility, even if it is decided that the child should live with one of the parents.

The issue of parenting and parental responsibility has become increasingly complicated with the advent of surrogacy and in vitro fertilization. For example, the woman who gives birth is the legal mother and has parental responsibility, whereas other adults may need to adopt the child to become the legal parents (see chapter website resources and Reflective activity Web 15.3).

SUPPORT FOR CHILDREN AND FAMILIES

The changing nature of the family

Practice with children and families needs to take account of the changing nature of family life. The UK has become an increasingly multicultural society, bringing a diversity of ideas with respect to different family structures and ways of life. This diversity has been recognized within the Children Act 1989. Firstly, the Act widened the concept of people who are important to children by allowing absent parents and other relatives to be consulted and involved in decisions about the care of children, and to apply, under Section 8, for a child arrangements order (regulating issues of residence and contact). Secondly, for the first time in English law, the diversity and multicultural context of families have been recognized and should be taken account of and respected (s1:3). The legal rules have been changed subsequently to recognize civil partnerships and same-gender marriages to extend to same-gender couples the right to adopt, to allow step-parents to acquire parental responsibility with the agreement of birth parents and to create the concept of special guardianship (Adoption and Children Act 2002).

Reflective activity 15.1

Find out where your local authority children's services department is. How has it organized its responsibilities to children?

What initiatives do you have in your area for helping vulnerable children and their families?

See if you can obtain a copy of the Children and Young People's Plan for your area. What are the key aims and objectives for your area?

Poverty and social exclusion

Sources of stress and disadvantage for children and families include poverty and accompanying social exclusion. The *Child Poverty Act 2010* sets out targets for ending child poverty by 2020. *A new approach to child poverty: tackling the causes of disadvantage and transforming families' lives* outlines the Government's strategy to tackle childhood poverty (HM Government 2011). In 2014, 1.5 million children were living in households where there was no adult in paid work (ONS 2014b), with the effect of poverty on their families being recognized as having a major effect on life chances, health, education and future employment (Naven and Egan 2013; Platt 2009).

Employment rights

Pregnant women and their partners can access a range of benefits to help combat social inequality caused by poverty. Under the *Employment Rights Act 1996*, women retain employment rights while they are pregnant and should not be discriminated against. This includes paid time off for antenatal appointments, protection from unfair treatment or dismissal, the right to maternity leave, maternity pay, redundancy payment and return to work after pregnancy (see Reflective activity Web 15.5). The Employment Act 2002 provides that every working father is entitled to paternity leave. The Children and Families Act 2014 makes provisions for both parents to have time off to attend clinic appointments before their baby's birth, to look after a newborn child, and to meet a child they intend to adopt and to attend meetings about the adoption.

Family support and the Children Act

Central and local government strategies have been designed to aid vulnerable children. For example, *Sure Start* targets children under four and their families within some of the most disadvantaged communities, addressing the health and well-being of children and families before and after birth. The aim has been to improve the health of children before entry to school to enhance their potential at school. The programmes provide access to family support, advice on nurturing, health services and early learning. Other initiatives include the concept of extended schools and the requirement on local authorities to ensure that they have sufficient children's centres to meet local need (Apprenticeships, Skills, Children and Learning Act 2009).

The Children Act 1989 places a duty on local authorities to target particular services to children defined as being *in need*.

Local authorities have a general duty to:

- safeguard and promote the welfare of children 'in need'

and

- promote the upbringing of such children by their families by providing a range and level of services appropriate to those children's needs (Children Act 1989: s.17(1)).

The aim of the duty to children in need within the Children Act is to target services to the most vulnerable, including those at risk, providing support to avoid the need for the state to seek statutory control. Service provision under Section 17 may be one means by which a local authority seeks to deliver good outcomes for children and young people, as defined in the Children Act 2004.

FAMILY SUPPORT SERVICES

Part 3 of the Children Act 1989, especially Section 17 and Schedule 2, outlines the provision of services for children in need. These services may be provided by the local authority and/or the voluntary and private sector. Such services include family centres, day nurseries, fostering, childminding or playgroups, and support within the home, such as family aides (see chapter website resources). The local authority may charge for these services, but any person in receipt of social benefits, such as income support or child tax credit, is exempt.

Children living away from home

The local authority has a duty to provide accommodation in a range of situations, including when children are *in need*, and there is no person who has parental responsibility for them; they are *lost* or *abandoned* or the person who has been caring for them is prevented from providing them with suitable accommodation or care. When the local authority accommodates children, they become *looked after* children.

Accommodation for young babies

Where there are concerns about a young baby, it is likely that the local authority would – unless there is very good reason against such – try to maintain the mother and child in their own home by provision of a family aide and/or home help. If this is not possible, efforts would be made to try to place mother and child together with foster carers who specifically work with mothers. There are still a small number of residential mother and baby homes, predominantly managed by the private and voluntary sector, which provide care, support and training for mothers with specialist needs, such as drug dependency. (For foster care and teenage pregnancy, please see chapter website resources.)

ADOPTION

Adoption is the dissolution of parental rights and duties, which are subsequently transferred to the new adoptive parent(s).

In some cases, midwives become involved with a mother who has decided to give up her child for adoption. In rare circumstances, the mother may decide that she does not want to care for the baby after birth. If this is the case, then midwives will be involved in planning with Councils with social service responsibilities or an adoption agency to manage this process (see chapter website resources).

CHILDREN WITH DISABILITIES

The Children Act 1989 (Section 17) recognizes children with disabilities as children **first** and includes them in the definition of children *in need*, enabling them to benefit from the same services as other children (see chapter website resources).

Midwives are at the frontline of working with parents who are expecting a child with disability or where a disability is diagnosed at birth. They need to be sensitive to how information is conveyed to parents and ensure openness and honesty. In many cases, this involves referral to fetal medicine centres or paediatric specialists.

An important principle in working with children with disabilities is to ensure that the views and wishes of the child are sought and not to make the assumption that this is not possible.

Disabled children are particularly vulnerable and face an increased risk of abuse in many settings. This may arise in part from social attitudes and special treatment, resulting in a child with a disability being more isolated, more dependent, having less control over their lives and bodies and being less able to communicate their abuse. The UN Convention for the Rights of the Child (**Article 23**) does stipulate that *A child with a disability has the right to live a full and decent life in conditions that promote dignity, independence and an active role in the community'*, and indeed tasks governments to ensure that this is facilitated through free care and assistance to children with disability.

Genital mutilation

The midwife must be alert to the possibility of some families wishing to have their child 'circumcised'. This might be from an awareness that the mother/family is from a culture where this practice is accepted and, in the case of female genital mutilation, if the mother herself has had this procedure. Occasionally, the mother may ask for information that might alert the midwife. Under the terms of the *Female Genital Mutilation Act 2003* and *Serious Crime Act 2015*, it is illegal to have this carried out abroad under the principle of 'extraterritoriality' (see Ch. 56 and chapter website resources). This is a sensitive and difficult situation, and seeking assistance from the Supervisor of Midwives and using the Government practice guidelines can be useful (HM Government 2014; DH 2015a; DH 2015b; Royal College of Midwives (RCM) 2015). Midwives have a mandatory duty to report if they believe that a female child is at risk in such cases and must initiate their local child protection process.

Male circumcision is most common among those of Jewish and Islamic faiths and includes the surgical removal of the foreskin from the child's penis. It is performed for either religious or medical reasons and is currently not illegal in this country. There has been considerable debate on whether nontherapeutic circumcision is right for a child, as it has been known to be undertaken without adequate anaesthesia or pain relief (BMA 2006).

THE PROTECTION OF CHILDREN

The effect of domestic violence on children and adolescents is becoming increasingly recognized and has been well researched (DH 2013; Hester et al 2006; Humphreys and Stanley 2015). In some circumstances, alcohol and drug misuse and mental illness may also adversely affect parents' abilities to care for their children (Forrester and Harwin 2011). Women's refuges have been established to provide a safe haven and to provide advice for women and their children, accessed through the Samaritans, the police or social services. The legal rules have been strengthened to recognize the effect of domestic violence. The Adoption and Children Act 2002 makes a child who is a victim of, or witness to, domestic oppression, a child in need. The Family Law Act 1996 allows a court to add an *exclusion order* to an *interim care order* or *emergency protection order* made under the Children Act 1989, with the objective of removing the perpetrator from the family home rather than the child. If this does not prove possible, then the child may be removed using a granted *emergency protection order* or *interim care order powers.*

Along with all other professionals and voluntary sector workers involved with children, midwives have a responsibility to be alert to the possibility of child abuse and to take appropriate action where indicated. Should a midwife have any concerns about a family, she should discuss this with her senior colleagues and others who may be involved in the care of the family. This involves discussion with a Supervisor of Midwives, senior colleague or doctor (Box 15.2).

Section 47 of the Children Act 1989 places a duty on any clinical commissioning group or NHS Trust to help a local authority in its inquiries in cases where there is reasonable cause to suspect that a child is suffering or is likely to suffer significant harm. It is important for midwives to recognize the roles and responsibilities of other professionals in working with children and access joint multidisciplinary training with respect to assessment and child protection. Where it is agreed, following a *strategy decision*, that a *Section 47 enquiry* should be instigated and the child may be at risk of significant harm, the midwife may become involved in a *child protection conference*. If the child is made the subject of a *child protection plan*, *core group meetings* and *review conferences* will follow.

Local Safeguarding Children Boards

Each clinical commissioning group is required to identify a senior nurse as designated senior professional to the Local Safeguarding Children Board (LSCB). Each NHS Trust must also identify a named nurse or midwife to lead on child protection matters (CWDC 2009).

The overall management of the cooperation between various agencies with respect to child protection in any

---

Box 15.2 Responsibilities of the senior midwife

Those who manage midwifery should ensure that:

- There are agreed arrangements to give the name and telephone number of the health visitor to the mother the first week after the birth.
- They provide professional advice and guidance to any midwife who is concerned about a child or who is involved where a child is suspected of being at risk or has been abused or neglected.
- There is an early response to information of a pregnancy in a family where there has been an identified concern. The concern should be shared with other professionals as appropriate.
- Where the mother is known to have abused drugs or alcohol during pregnancy, the risk factors are taken into account for the unborn child and any other children. Where a baby is born with fetal alcohol syndrome or has signs or symptoms of addiction to narcotics, a referral to social services should be made.
- Midwives and nurses in neonatal units are aware that infants separated from their mother at birth may be at greater risk of child abuse later in childhood. Their observations may be the first crucial step in alerting others to an 'at risk' situation.
- Midwives and nurses have an important part to play in promoting parent and child contact to ensure strong parent/child relationships and the development of good parenting skills. This is particularly important where there are problems, e.g. mental or physical illness and/or physical or learning disability.
- Where the midwife is notified of a child or young person under 18 who is pregnant, she should consider whether there is a child protection concern.
- The special needs of the mother and father are met, e.g. a parent(s) with a disability, including a learning disability, referring them to appropriate sources of support.

Adapted from DH 1997: 9–10

---

local authority is the responsibility of the Local Safeguarding Children Board (Children Act 2004; Local Safeguarding Children Board Regulations 2006; Apprenticeships, Skills, Children and Learning Act 2009). Each board has a representative at a senior management level from each of the relevant agencies. They have a responsibility to develop, audit and challenge local policies and procedures for interagency working and for the safeguarding and promotion of the welfare of children. They must ensure provision is made for training and raising awareness within the wider community, and for monitoring and evaluating the effectiveness of partner agencies, individually and collectively. They will publish an annual report.

They also conduct a serious case review of any particularly difficult cases that arise, or where a child dies as a result of abuse or neglect in their area.

Significant harm

Important in the assessment of risk is the concept of *significant harm*. If there is reasonable cause to suspect that a child is suffering or is likely to suffer significant harm, the local authority has a duty to make enquiries necessary to enable them to decide whether to take any action to safeguard or promote the child's welfare (Children Act 1989: s.47). This enquiry is commonly known as a *Section 47 investigation*.

Harm is defined in Section 31(9) and (10) of the Children Act as: *'ill treatment or impairment of health or development'*.

Ill treatment includes sexual abuse and other forms of ill treatment that are not necessarily physical (see Box 15.3). The decision as to whether the harm is *significant* is measured on a comparison with the health and development reasonably expected of a similar child. It will be informed by a comprehensive assessment (HM Government 2015) and takes into account legal advice. Assessments should be child-centred so that the effect of parenting capacity, family and environment on the child can be clearly identified and understood (HM Government 2006).

Working together to safeguard children (HM Government 2015) advises that abuse or neglect is caused by inflicting harm. While it is not within the remit of this chapter to provide detail of signs and symptoms of abuse, there are well-documented warning signs that may alert the midwife. Physical abuse includes hitting, shaking, throwing, poisoning, burning, scalding and suffocating (RCN 2014). Midwives need to be concerned about any bruising on a baby, particularly bruising around the face or on any soft tissues, bruising consistent with an implement being used to hit a child, finger-tip bruising or slap marks, black eyes or ears, bites, scald and burn marks anywhere on the body or a torn frenulum. Suspicion may be raised if parents delay seeking advice about injuries or if there are discrepancies between the parents' explanation and the actual injuries found.

The midwife may observe emotional abuse in terms of poor emotional bonding, possible rejection of the pregnancy and child, unrealistic expectations and/or demands of the child, constant criticism, unequal treatment or a child being made to feel worthless and unloved. Failing to meet a child's basic physical or psychological needs with respect to food, clothes and safety, failing to protect the child from harm and failing to ensure access to appropriate medical care or treatment may be examples of neglect. Failure to follow medical advice through pregnancy and postnatal care, the mental state of the mother, rough handling and a history of drug or alcohol abuse or domestic violence also give cause for concern.

The time immediately after birth is important in establishing a positive relationship between parent and baby. Prematurity, illness of either mother or child or other factors sometimes hinder this relationship. The midwife is a key figure in fostering a positive relationship, recognizing what is likely to support or hinder this.

While stress does not automatically lead to child abuse, it may make it more likely. Sources of stress for families include issues relating to finances, social exclusion (MacInnes et al 2014), domestic violence, mental illness of a parent and drug or alcohol abuse (Hughes and Owen 2009; Forrester and Harwin 2011).

While acknowledging that these factors do not necessarily lead to abuse or neglect, the potential or actual effect of these on a child needs to be assessed and action taken to support the child and family and ensuring the child's safety.

A midwife who is involved with a child where there is concern may be involved in a *strategy discussion* with other professionals to share information, determine a plan for Section 47 enquiries, and consider how to immediately safeguard the child and provide interim services and support. This includes consideration of how to take race and ethnicity into account, including use of interpreters; the needs of other children; decisions about what information should be shared with the family; and the role of the police where an offence may have been committed.

Box 15.3 Categories of abuse and neglect

Abuse and neglect are generally considered under the following categories:

- physical abuse
- emotional abuse
- sexual abuse
- neglect

  These are generally used as the basis for making children the subject of child protection plans.

ASSESSING CHILDREN 'IN NEED' AND THEIR FAMILIES

Working together to safeguard children (HM Government 2015) guidelines emphasize that promoting the welfare of children and safeguarding their needs are not separate activities. They aim to refocus attention on preventive work, together with producing a more holistic and inter-agency assessment focusing on strengths and needs

(Hart 2010; Hodson and Deery 2014). Assessment begins from the point of referral and emphasizes the corporate responsibility of local authority departments, the NHS and voluntary organizations in contributing to both the assessment and the provision of services to children in need. The assessment seeks to discriminate between different types and levels of need and is crucial to improving the success of services for children. Focus on an inter-agency approach starts as soon as there are concerns about a child's welfare, not just when there is concern about the child being at risk of significant harm.

The assessment must take account of current research to produce an approach that retains the child at the centre of three domains, which interact to affect the well-being and development of a child within the family (Aldgate and Statham 2001; HM Government 2015). These are:

(a) the child's developmental needs

(b) parenting capacity

(c) family and environmental factors (see Fig. 15.1).

Where families fail to cooperate with an assessment, and where it remains unclear if criteria are met for application for an emergency protection order, the local authority may apply for a child assessment order which, if granted by the court, requires parents to make the child available for assessment (see Reflective activity Web 15.6).

Midwives are well placed to comment on all three assessment domains, given their close and frequent contact with newborn babies and parents; their skills in assessment, observation and communication; and their knowledge of early childhood development and needs. In visiting the home, midwives see the mother, baby and family in their normal cultural context, and may become aware of the care, not only of newborn babies, but also of older children, lifestyles, home conditions, parenting and child or elder abuse. Midwives can identify vulnerable children and refer them to social services for assessment, contributing to the assessment, planning and intervention as required (DH 2015a and 2015b; Powell 2016; Watson and Rodwell 2014). The most common situations where midwives are involved in working with social workers with respect to children in need or at risk are pre-birth assessments and post-birth concerns.

Making a referral

Working together to safeguard children states that anyone who believes a child to be suffering or at risk of suffering significant harm should refer their concerns to children's social care departments (HM Government 2015).

Before making a referral, the midwife should discuss concerns with a manager or a Supervisor of Midwives and, unless this would place the child at increased risk, discuss concerns with the family and gain their agreement for the referral. The general practitioner (GP) should also be informed. In making the referral, it is important to be clear about the nature of the concerns and document these, referring only to known facts.

Consent and confidentiality

Personal information about children and families is subject to a duty of confidence and should not normally be shared without consent. However, the *Data Protection Act 1998* permits disclosure of confidential information if it is necessary to safeguard a child. Trusts have local policies regarding this. In circumstances where there are concerns about the child being at risk or suffering significant harm, the overriding duty is to safeguard the child. Information regarding data protection is available in *Information sharing: advice for practitioners providing safeguarding services* (HM Government 2015b). In keeping with the Human Rights Act 1998 and Article 8 of the European Convention, because the right to private and family life, disclosure of otherwise confidential information is permitted, providing it is done according to law and is proportional to the need identified to safeguard and promote the child's welfare. When safe to do so, midwives should practise openly and honestly with families about child protection concerns to ensure that this relationship is not compromised and involvement with both parents and child can continue (Hart 2010; Hodson and Deery 2014).

The midwife's role in assessment

Early identification, assessment and intervention associated with child protection cases are clearly outlined in the *Common Assessment Framework for Children and Young People: a guide for practitioners* (CWDC 2009). This detailed and comprehensive document outlines the role that practitioners play in the multiagency approach to safeguarding children. The Framework is described as 'a shared assessment and planning framework for use across all children's services and all local areas in England. It aims to help the early identification of children and young people's additional needs and promote coordinated service provision to meet them' (CWDC 2009: 8). All children considered at risk of significant harm must be referred directly to children's social services or the police, in keeping with Local Safeguarding Children Boards (LSCB) procedures (HM Government 2015).

Where a midwife refers a child, she should confirm this in writing within 48 hours using the *Common Assessment Framework* (see Box 15.4). In turn, the local authority should acknowledge the referral within one working day of receipt. The midwife may be asked to contribute to an assessment of whether a child is in need and, if so, the services which may be appropriate to promote the child's welfare and upbringing within the family (see chapter website resources). With respect to women who have been

---

Box 15.4 Common assessment framework

'The situations that might lead to a common assessment include where a practitioner has observed a significant change or worrying feature in a child's appearance, demeanour or behaviour; where a practitioner knows of a significant event in the child's life or where there are worries about the parents or carers or home; or where the child, parent or another practitioner has requested an assessment. A common assessment might be indicated if there are parental elements (e.g. parental substance abuse/misuse, domestic violence, or parental physical or mental health issues) that might impact on the child.'

(HM Government, 2006: 4)

---

referred, the midwife would be contacted for information about previous pregnancies, attitudes towards antenatal and self-care or home conditions, as part of the assessment (See Case Studies Web 15.1 and 15.2).

In circumstances requiring a more in-depth exploration, an assessment must be completed within 45 days (HM Government 2015). Depending on the degree of involvement, the midwife may be invited to provide information, specialist knowledge and advice and, in some cases, undertake specific assessments. The midwife is expected to contribute to the *plan* for providing support – *The Child in Need Plan*. However, it is important to note that it is not necessary to wait until the outcome of the assessment to begin to provide services.

Pre-birth assessment

Pre-birth assessments are undertaken when the local authority is concerned that the baby, when born, will be in need or be at risk of significant harm. The safety of the child is paramount, with the pre-birth assessment evaluating the needs of the child and whether support is possible to enable the family to succeed. Assessments include consideration of parenting skills, preparation for the baby, use of medical advice and guidance, and consideration of the family and environment (HM Government 2015). In these situations, the identified midwife works with social workers and other professionals in contributing to the assessment.

Particular issues that may trigger a referral to children's social care or a pre-birth assessment are:

- *a mother who has a learning disability or physical disability* that makes it difficult for her to care for her baby (note that disabled parents are also entitled to assessment and service provision under community care law, the responsibility for which will fall to adult social care departments)

- *consistent use of illegal drugs,* substances or alcohol by the mother or within the environment

- *a mother living with, or having frequent contact with, a violent partner* or Schedule 1 offender (a Schedule 1 offender is someone who has been convicted of serious physical or sexual offences, whether or not against children)

- *young and vulnerable mothers with no support mechanisms* – for example, this may be a girl who is herself 'in need', accommodated by the local authority or subject to a Care Order

- *concerns about the mental health of the mother* (or anyone else likely to have care of the child) and the effect of her ill health on the baby

- *extreme poverty or inadequate housing*

- *families where a child has previously been the subject of a child protection plan* or was removed from the home

- *where pregnancy is the result of rape*

The unborn baby can be made the subject of a child protection plan, but no further action can be taken until the child is born.

Post-birth assessment

It has been held that where a local authority wishes to take early action to protect a newly born baby from potentially inadequate parents, they cannot intervene before birth. However, they can intervene immediately after the birth and base this intervention on the mother's behaviour while pregnant, and the presumption that this would lead to the child being at risk of significant harm (Gilmore and Bainham 2013).

In cases where there is serious concern about the child, they may be made subject to an *Emergency Protection Order* and removed from the mother after birth. This should be preplanned to enable removal to take place as sensitively as possible. It can be a very traumatic time for all concerned, including professionals, and it is essential that those involved are supported throughout.

The Emergency Protection Order (EPO)

Where safe for children to do so, plans to protect a child should proceed in agreement with parents; however, some cases may require emergency action. The Children Act 1989 (Section 44) allows for an Emergency Protection Order (EPO) to be made if there is reasonable cause to believe that a child is likely to suffer significant harm if:

- the child is not removed to accommodation; or

- the child does not remain in the place in which he or she is being accommodated

An EPO can be made if access to a child is being denied as part of a Section 47 enquiry. It gives authority to remove a child or cause the child to remain in the protection of the local authority or National Society for the Prevention of Cruelty to Children (NSPCC) for a maximum of 8 days. Police also have powers to remove children to suitable accommodation or to prevent their removal from hospital or safe accommodation (Section 46).

In situations where parents are refusing to cooperate with Section 47, but there is not sufficient concern to justify an EPO, the local authority can apply for a child assessment order (Section 43). This order directs the parents or carer to cooperate with an assessment of the child.

With respect to young babies, an EPO may be applied for at birth if there are concerns that the parent will remove the child. Other examples may include a child who has been seriously injured by a parent who is refusing to allow access to the child or a parent who is threatening to remove the child from hospital. In line with the best interests of the child, the Family Law Act 1996 allows for a perpetrator to be removed from the home instead of the child through an *exclusion order* attached to an EPO or Interim Care Order.

The child protection conference

The child protection conference is the first meeting at which representatives of all agencies that have dealings with the child or the child's family get together to share and evaluate information and consider the level of risk to a child or children. The conference decides whether the child should be made the subject of a child protection plan and makes plans for the future. Councils with social service responsibilities, or, in some areas, the NSPCC, have responsibility for calling and arranging the conference. Conferences will be led by an independent Chair.

The midwife may attend a case conference to present and share information about the child and family and will be one of many professionals in attendance. Generally, there is a manager representing each agency that attends regularly, including a representative from health, education and the police. Other professionals include social workers and their managers, local authority solicitors, paediatricians, general practitioners, health visitors, housing officers, police, teachers, foster carers and anyone who may have a significant contribution to make to the assessment. Parents and/or carers are invited to attend but may be excluded if the independent conference chair deems their attendance would potentially jeopardize the welfare of the child (HM Government 2006; HM Government 2015). This sometimes places professionals in a situation where they feel unwilling to speak frankly in front of parents for fear of jeopardizing their relationship with them. However, it is good practice to share child

> **Box 15.5** Checklist of preparation for a child protection conference
>
> Who is the health representative attending?
> Where and at what time is the meeting to be held?
> Will the parents be present?
> Do I need a written report?
> Am I clear about the information to be presented? – Is my opinion based on facts?
> Have I written down notes for myself to assist in my contribution to the conference?
> What is my view of the child's developmental needs? – What is my evidence?
> What is my view of the parents' capacity to parent? – What is my evidence?
> What is my view of family support systems and resources? – What is my evidence?
> Have I taken into account the needs of the child as being the primary concern?
> What do I think needs to happen to promote the welfare of this child/these children?
> Is there anything I can contribute to this directly?
> Do I know of other resources/aids/assistance that may be helpful?

protection concerns openly so parents have an opportunity to respond (see Reflective activities Web 15.7–15.10 and 15.12.).

All discussions that take place within child protection conferences are confidential. Professionals involved in child protection have their duty of confidentiality to their client overridden by their duty to contribute to the protection of a child at risk. It is important for midwives to be adequately prepared for attendance at a conference. If the midwife is requested to attend a case conference, it is advisable to have a discussion with the Supervisor of Midwives. Box 15.5 provides a checklist of things to consider.

Child protection plan

If a child is made the subject of a plan, a *key worker* is appointed. The key worker is a social worker from either the local authority or NSPCC. They have responsibility for making sure the child protection plan is developed into a more detailed interagency plan, ensuring completion of the core assessment, putting the plan into effect and monitoring it.

A *core group* of professionals, composed of those who have direct contact with the child, is established to develop and implement the child protection plan in conjunction with the family. Members of the core group are jointly responsible for developing, implementing and monitoring the plan. A meeting of the group should take place within 10 working days of the initial conference.

The child protection plan identifies how the child can be protected, including completion of a core assessment, short- and long-term aims to reduce risk to the child and promote the child's welfare, clarity about who will do what and when, and ways of monitoring progress.

If the child is made the subject of a child protection plan, this certainly does not mean that all other work with the child and family ceases. They may also still be eligible to be considered as children 'in need' for whom a range of services may be provided.

Reflective activity 15.2

Find out who are the designated senior professional and named midwife and doctor in your area. Ensure that you have these details in your contact file/work diary.

Obtain a copy of the Local Safeguarding Children Board procedures in your area of practice. Consider what actions you would need to take should you be concerned about a baby in your practice.

CONCLUSION

The Children Act 1989, together with subsequent legislation, protects the rights of children, promoting their status within society. Midwives must be aware of the implications of the Act and apply them to their practice. Midwives are uniquely situated to identify risk factors and act as advocates for newborn babies and other children during

their professional practice. Detailed and contemporaneous records must be maintained throughout, as these may be required in assessments and child protection conferences (Nursing and Midwifery Council (NMC) 2015). Key amendments are constantly made to the Children Act and so it is important to keep up to date and access relevant websites and support organisations so that knowledge is current. Using the three case scenarios identified at the beginning of this chapter (two of which are available in the chapter website resources) will have helped you explore aspects of child care law in relation to midwifery practice, through exploration of supporting concepts, online materials, and professional and statutory documents. In all cases, it is important that the midwife liaises with the Supervisor of Midwives and with other professionals, thus perpetuating a multiagency approach to child support.

Key Points

- The key features of the Children Act 1989 include paramountcy, parental responsibility, promotion of upbringing within the family where safe to do so, provision of services and support to enable this, and protection of children at risk.
- Midwives need to know the context of working with vulnerable families and how this affects their practice.
- The role of the midwife is significant to interagency working, promoting the welfare of children defined by the Children Act as being *in need*, including those at risk of significant harm and requiring protection.
- The midwife plays a vital role in both pre-birth and post-birth assessments.

References

Adoption and Children Act 2002, London: The Stationery Office, http://www.legislation.gov.uk/ukpga/2002/38/contents. 2002.

Apprenticeships, Skills, Children and Learning Act 2009, London: The Stationery Office. 2009.

Aldgate J, Statham J: *The Children Act now: messages from research*, London, The Stationery Office, 2001.

Braye S, Preston-Shoot M: *Practising social work law*, 3rd edn, Basingstoke, Palgrave Macmillan, 2009.

Brayne H, Carr H, Goosey D: *Law for social workers*, 13th edn, Oxford, Oxford University Press, 2015.

British Medical Association (BMA): *The law and ethics of male circumcision*, London, BMA, 2006.

Children Act 1989 (sections where listed), London: The Stationery Office. (website) http://www.legislation.gov.uk/ukpga/1989/41/contents. 1989.

Children Act 2004 (sections where listed), London: The Stationery Office. (website) http://www.legislation.gov.uk/ukpga/2004/31/contents. 2004.

Children's Workforce Development Council (CWDC): *Common Assessment Framework for Children and Young People: practitioners' guide*, Leeds, CWDC, 2009.

Children's Workforce Development Council (CWDC): *The team around the child and the lead professional: a guide for practitioners*, London, CWDC, 2009.

Department for Education and Skills (DfES): *Statutory guidance on making arrangements to safeguard and promote the welfare of children under section 11 of the Children Act 2004*, London, DfES, 2005.

Department for Education (DfE): *Statistical first release: characteristics of children in need in England* (website). www.gov.uk/government/ uploads/system/uploads/ attachment_data/file/367877/ SFR43_2014_Main_Text.pdf. 2014.

Department of Health (DH): Child Protection guidance for senior nurses, health visitors, midwives and their managers, 3rd edn, London, The Stationery Office, 1997.

Department of Health (DH): *The Victoria Climbié inquiry: report of an inquiry by Lord Laming*, London, The Stationery Office, 2003.

Department of Health (DH): *Domestic violence and abuse – professional guidance*, London, DH, 2013.

Department of Health (DH): *What to do if you're worried a child is being abused – advice for practitioners*, London, DH, 2015a.

Department of Health (DH): *Female genital mutilation risk and safeguarding: guidance for professionals*, London, DH, 2015b.

Eastman A: *Enough is enough: a report on child protection and mental health services for children and young people*, London, The Centre for Social Justice, 2014.

Forrester D, Harwin J: *Parents who misuse drugs and alcohol: effective interventions in social work and child protection*, London, Wiley-Blackwell, 2011.

Gilmore S, Bainham A: *Children: the modern law*, 4th edn, Bristol, Jordan Publishing Ltd., p 4, 2013.

Hart D: Assessment before birth. In Horwath J, editor: *The child's world: the comprehensive guide to assessing children in need*, 2nd edn, London, Jessica Kingsley Publishers, Chapter 14, pp 229–240, 2010.

HM Government: *The Common Assessment Framework for Children and Young People: supporting tools* (website). www.dcsf.gov.uk/every childmatters/resources-and-practice/ IG00146/. 2006.

HM Government: *A new approach to child poverty: tackling the causes of disadvantage and transforming families' lives*, London, The Stationery Office, 2011.

HM Government: *Multi-Agency Practice Guidelines: female genital mutilation*, London, The Stationery Office, 2014.

HM Government: *Working Together to Safeguard Children: a guide to inter-agency working to safeguard and promote the welfare of children*, London, The Stationery Office, 2015a.

HM Government: *Information sharing: advice for practitioners providing safeguarding services to children, young people, parents and carers* (website). www.gov.uk/government/ publications. 2015b.

Hester M, Pearson C, Harwin N, et al: *Making an impact: children and domestic violence – a reader*, London, Jessica Kingsley Publishers, 2006.

Hodson A, Deery R: Protecting unborn babies: professional and ethical considerations for social work and midwifery, Chapter 10. In Jindal-Snape D, Hannah E, editors: *Exploring the dynamics of personal, professional and interprofessional ethics*, Bristol, Policy Press, pp 151–166, 2014.

Home Office: *Mandatory reporting of female genital mutilation – procedural information*, London, The Stationary Office, 2015.

Hughes L, Owen H: *Good practice in safeguarding children: working effectively in child protection*, London, Jessica Kingsley Publishers, 2009.

Humphreys C, Stanley N: *Domestic violence and protecting children: new thinking and approaches*, London, Jessica Kingsley Publishers, 2015.

Joint Area Review (OFSTED) Health Commission and HM Inspectorate of Constabulary): *Review of services for children and young people, with particular reference to safeguarding*, London, JAR, 2008.

Laming Report: *The protection of children in England: a progress report*, London, HMSO, 2009.

Local Safeguarding Children Board Regulations. London: The Stationery Office, 2006.

MacInnes T, Aldridge H, Bushe S, et al: *Monitoring poverty and social exclusion 2014*, York, Joseph Rowntree Foundation & New Policy Institute, 2014.

Munro E: *The Munro Review of Child Protection: final report – moving towards a child centred system*, London, The Stationery Office, 2011.

Nursing and Midwifery Council (NMC): *The Code: Professional standards of practice and behaviour for nurses and midwives*, London, NMC, 2015.

Naven L, Egan J: Poverty in Scotland: the role of nurses, *Prim Health Care* 23(5):16–22, 2013.

Office for National Statistics (ONS): *Births in England and Wales by characteristics of birth 2* (website). www.ons.gov.uk/ons/ dcp171778_384394.pdf. 2014a.

Office for National Statistics (ONS): *Largest fall in the percentage of workless households since comparable records began* (website). www.ons.gov.uk/ons/rel/lmac/ working-and-workless-house holds/2014/sty-working-and -workless-households-2014.html. 2014b.

Office for Standards in Education, Children's Services and Skills (OFSTED): *The Annual Report of Her Majesty's Chief Inspector of Education, Children's Services and Skills 2008/09*, London, The Stationery Office, 2009.

OFSTED: *Learning lessons from serious case reviews: interim report 2009–2010*, Manchester, OFSTED, 2010.

Platt L: *Ethnicity and child poverty, Research Report Number 576*, London, Department for Work and Pensions, 2009.

Powell C: *Safeguarding and child protection for nurses, midwives and health visitors: a practical guide*, 2nd edn, Buckingham, Open University Press, 2016.

Preston-Shoot M: On the evidence for viruses in social work systems: law, ethics and practice, *Eur J Soc Work* 13(4):1–18, 2010.

Preston-Shoot M: *Making good decisions: law for social work practice*, Basingstoke, Palgrave Macmillan, 2014.

Royal College of Midwives (RCM): *Position statement: female genital mutilation*, London, RCM, 2015.

Royal College of Nursing (RCN): *Safeguarding children and young people – every nurse's responsibility*, London, RCN, 2014.

Statham J, Aldgate J: From legislation to practice: learning from the Children Act 1989 research programme, *Child Soc* 17:149–156, 2003.

United Nations (UN): *United Nations Convention on the Rights of the Child (UNCRC)*, Geneva, UN, 1989.

Watson G, Rodwell S, editors: *Safeguarding and protecting children, young people and families: a guide for nurses and midwives*, London, Sage Publications Ltd., 2014.

Resources and additional reading

Department of Health (DH): *What to do if you're worried a child is being abused – advice for practitioners* (website). www.gov.uk/government/publications/what-to-do-if-youre-worried-a-child-is-being-abused–2. 2015a.
This guide is useful as a resource for practitioners in identifying actions should there be concerns about abuse.

Childrens Workforce Matters Common Assessment Framework
http://www.childrensworkforcematters.org.uk/workforce-matters/archive/common-assessment-framework/
This document provides midwives with information and supporting tools when using the Common Assessment Framework for children and young people. It gives examples of when to initiate a common assessment and how to do so, giving an example of its use with an unborn baby.

Every Child Matters: Change for Children programme.
www.everychildmatters.gov.uk
Information and publications relating to all aspects of the Every Child Matters: Change for Children programme.

National Society for the Prevention of Cruelty to Children.
https://www.nspcc.org.uk/fighting-for-childhood
An excellent resource for practitioners and for families.

United Nations International Children's Emergency Fund (Unicef)
http://www.unicef.org.uk/Unicef's-Work/
A good resource which includes Unicef UK and international information focused on children. This includes access to the United Nations Convention on the rights of the child (UNCRC) (http://www.unicef.org.uk/UNICEFs-Work/UN-Convention/)

Part Three

Public health, health promotion in the context of childbirth

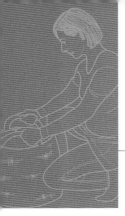

Chapter 16

Epidemiology

Professor Alison Macfarlane

Learning Outcomes ?

After reading this chapter, you will be able to:

- understand how the health of populations can be measured
- describe the main sources of routinely collected data for England, Wales, Scotland, Northern Ireland and the Republic of Ireland
- describe definitions of population-based rates of birth and death
- describe trends in the key statistics relevant to birth and maternity care
- understand the importance of interpreting data about maternity care in their socioeconomic context
- describe the main sources of data used for international comparisons and the factors to be taken into account when interpreting them.

INTRODUCTION

Epidemiology, the science of measuring the health of populations, had its origins in ancient Greece with Hippocrates' interest in the influence of the environment on health. Major developments took place in the late 19th century in investigations of outbreaks of communicable diseases, such as cholera. From the mid-20th century onward, its scope was extended to the investigation of patterns of chronic diseases, such as respiratory and cardiovascular conditions. Most recently, it has also been used to investigate variations in healthcare practice, such as the 'epidemic' of caesareans. It has been formally defined as follows:

The study of the occurrence and distribution of health related events, states and processes in specific populations, including the study of the determinants influencing such processes and the application of this knowledge to control relevant health problems'.

(Porta 2014: 95)

Epidemiology includes both use of data to describe trends and variations in rates of ill-health and mortality and also a set of study designs and analytical techniques. There is not room to describe these here, and readers are advised to consult epidemiology textbooks for further information (Bonita et al 2006; Bailey et al 2005; Stewart 2010). The aims of this chapter are to explain the definitions used in relation to birth and its outcome, to provide information on the sources of data collected routinely in the countries of Britain and Ireland, to discuss how to interpret the data and to give an overview of trends and variations in the key measures and ways in which they may be associated with social and environmental factors. This is important for planning both services for maternity care and also preventive services.

NOTIFYING AND REGISTERING BIRTHS

Birth and death registration and birth notification are the sources of the most complete data about births and deaths because they are required by law in the UK. Civil registration of live births, marriages and deaths started in 1837 in England and Wales, 1855 in Scotland and 1864 in Ireland. Organizations called *general register offices* were set up to process the registrations recorded by local registrars of births marriages and deaths and use the information in them to compile and publish statistics (Macfarlane and Mugford 2000).

In recent years, these functions have become separated. Box 16.1 shows the organizations responsible for overseeing

Box 16.1 Organizations responsible for civil registration and publication of statistics

Country or territory	Responsible for civil registration	Responsible for statistical publications
England and Wales	General Register Office, now part of HM Passport Office www.gro.gov.uk/gro/content/	Office for National Statistics www.ons.gov.uk/
Scotland	National Records of Scotland www.nrscotland.gov.uk/registration	National Records of Scotland www.nrscotland.gov.uk/statistics-and-data
Northern Ireland	General Register Office for Northern Ireland www.nidirect.gov.uk/contacts/contacts-az/general-register-office-northern-ireland	Northern Ireland Statistics and Research Agency www.nisra.gov.uk/
Isle of Man	The Civil Registry www.gov.im/registries/general/civilregistry/	Isle of Man Government
Guernsey	The Royal Court of Guernsey www.guernseyroyalcourt.gg/article/1637/Births-Marriages-and-Deaths	For birth statistics in Guernsey contact the Royal Court, Greffe Department on 01481 725277, or e-mail the Royal Court via its website.
Jersey	www.gov.je/pages/contacts.aspx?contactId=71	www.statesassembly.gov.je/AssemblyReports/2015/R.104-2015.pdf#search=birth
Irish Republic	Health Services Executive www.hse.ie/eng/services/list/1/bdm	Central Statistics Office www.cso.ie

civil registration and those from which statistics are available. Although detailed data is published for England and Wales, Scotland, Northern Ireland and the Irish Republic, birth and death data for the Crown Dependencies of the Isle of Man, Jersey and Guernsey is fairly limited and usually included in other official reports.

The legislation allows parents up to 42 days to register a birth, but at the beginning of the 20th century, there was concern that parents needed professional support and advice much sooner than that. This led to the *Notification of Births Act 1907*, the *Notification of Births (Extension) Act 1915* and legislation passed since then, under which midwives or other birth attendants have been required to notify a birth within 36 hours. Originally births were notified to the local Medical Officer of Health so that the child health and health visiting services were aware of the birth and could visit mothers and their newborn babies. In recent years the process has been changing and in ways that differ between the constituent countries of Britain and Ireland. The term *Britain*, or *Great Britain*, is used to describe England, Wales and Scotland; at the time of writing, the UK is made up of England, Wales, Scotland and Northern Ireland.

Since 2002, in England, Wales and the Isle of Man, notification has been linked to the allocation of National Health Service (NHS) numbers as soon as possible after birth. The initial interim system has now been replaced by a system that notifies births directly to the Personal Demographics Service maintained by NHS Digital, formerly the Health and Social Care Information Centre (HSCIC 2016).

If the maternity unit/service does not have a system that is compliant with the Personal Demographics Service,

midwives have to use a *Birth Notification Application* to notify the birth. Once the notification has been completed, the Personal Demographics Services passes on the notification information to the child health services, the NHS Newborn Hearing Screening Service and the Office for National Statistics (ONS). When parents go to register their babies' births, the local registrar will add details to their babies' records, which should already be in the system.

Scotland is in the process of implementing a *Community Health Index*, similar to the NHS Register in England and Wales, and information about newly registered births is usually passed to the Index. The way birth notification is handled varies between health boards. When a baby is born the maternity service is responsible for notifying the relevant board's child health administrative department so that a record can be created for the baby in the national child health information systems.

In Northern Ireland, parents registering a birth are given an Infant Registration Card (HS123) to register with the family doctor and obtain a medical card. In parallel with this, the Northern Ireland Maternity System (NIMATS) uploads birth notifications and associated information to the relevant child health system depending on where the mother lives in Northern Ireland. These data are also sent to general practitioners (GPs) and community midwives for use in follow-up visits.

In the Irish Republic, the four-part Birth Notification Form (BNF/01) should be completed by one or both of the parents to guarantee that correct and accurate information is registered. This form is given to mothers in the hospital and should be completed and returned to hospital staff before the mother is discharged. One copy of the form will be forwarded to the Registrar's Office to inform the Registrar that a birth has occurred, but to register it, one of the parents or another 'qualified informant' has to go to the local register office to sign the birth register. The second copy is sent to the Director of Public Health and Medicine, and the third is sent to the National Perinatal Reporting System, which uses the information to compile the annual Perinatal Statistics for Ireland. The fourth copy is kept by the hospital for its own records. Since 2014, this process has been overseen by the Healthcare Pricing Office of the Health Information and Quality Authority.

There are a few occasions when neither the parents nor another next of kin is available to register a birth. In these cases, it may be necessary for the midwife attending the birth to register it. The arrangements for doing this vary between the countries of Britain and Ireland. Details can be found on the websites listed in Box 16.1.

DEFINITIONS AND SOURCES OF DATA

The World Health Organization (WHO) sets out definitions of live birth and fetal deaths and makes recommendations about which births and fetal deaths should be registered and counted (WHO 2016a). These definitions are shown in Box 16.2. Individual countries have their own legislation, based to a greater or lesser extent on these definitions. The definitions in use in Britain and Ireland are shown in Box 16.3. Stillbirth registration was introduced in July 1927 in England and Wales, in 1939 in Scotland and 1961 in Northern Ireland, under which fetal deaths at 28 or more weeks gestation had to be

---

Box 16.2 World Health Organization definitions of live birth and fetal death

Live birth

Live birth is the complete expulsion or extraction from its mother of a product of conception, irrespective of the duration of the pregnancy, which, after such separation, breathes or shows any other evidence of life, such as beating of the heart, pulsation of the umbilical cord, or definite movement of voluntary muscles, whether or not the umbilical cord has been cut or the placenta is attached; each product of such a birth is considered liveborn.

Fetal death (deadborn fetus)

Fetal death is death prior to the complete expulsion or extraction from its mother of a product of conception, irrespective of the duration of pregnancy; the death is indicated by the fact that the fetus does not breathe or show any other evidence of life after such separation, such as beating of the heart, pulsation of the umbilical cord or definite movement of voluntary muscles.

Source: WHO 2016a

Box 16.3 Definitions of live and stillbirth used in the countries of the United Kingdom

	England and Wales	Scotland	Northern Ireland
Birth	'Birth means a live birth or a stillbirth'	'Birth includes a stillbirth'	'Birth means a live birth or a stillbirth'
Live birth	'Live birth means a child born alive'	No explicit definition	'Live birth means a child born alive'
Stillbirth	A stillborn child is 'A child which has issued forth from its mother after the 24th week of pregnancy and which did not at any time after being completely expelled from its mother breathe or show any other signs of life'	A stillborn child is 'A child which has issued forth from its mother after the 24th week of pregnancy and which did not at any time after being completely expelled from its mother breathe or show any other signs of life'	A stillbirth 'means the complete expulsion from its mother after the 24th week of pregnancy of a child which did not at any time after being completely expelled or extracted breath or show any other evidence of life'

Time within which event is required to be registered

Live birth	42 days	21 days	42 days
Death	5 days	8 days	5 days
Stillbirth	42 days	21 days	Up to 1 year

Source: Births and Deaths Registration Act, 1953, Registration of Births, Deaths and Marriages (Scotland) Act, 1965 and Births and Deaths Registration (Northern Ireland) Order, 1976, all as amended by the Stillbirth (Definition) Act, 1992.

registered as stillbirths. The limit was lowered to 24 weeks from October 1, 1992, onward (ONS 2016a).

In the Irish Republic, notification of late fetal deaths at 28 or more completed weeks gestation as stillbirths started in 1957, but the process was incomplete. Compulsory civil registration of stillbirths began in 1995 with a lower limit of 24 completed weeks gestation and a birthweight of 500 g. Unlike in many other countries, no lower gestational age limit is set for the registration of live births in the countries of Britain and Ireland.

Live birth and fertility rates

Different rates are used to monitor trends in births and their variance between geographical areas (ONS 2016b). These are defined in Box 16.4. The *crude birth rate* relates the numbers of births to the size of the population as a whole, whereas the *general fertility rate* relates them broadly to the population of childbearing age.

Trends in the general fertility rate for England and Wales are shown in Fig. 16.1. The apparent increase in the mid-19th century reflects a gradual increase in registration at a period when birth registration was not compulsory until further legislation was passed in 1874. Figure 16.1 also shows overall declines in birth rates from the 1880s to the 1940s, punctuated by peaks after the two world wars. A much more sustained 'baby boom' in the 1960s was followed by a fall in fertility rates, then a levelling off. This was followed by an increase since the turn of the century, which now appears to be ending.

The overall rates shown in Fig. 16.1 mask a considerable difference between age groups in their age-specific fertility rates in England and Wales. Rates among women aged 25 to 29 and 30 to 34 are well above the overall rate, and those for women aged under 20 or in their 40s are below it. Over the last 25 years of the 20th century, fertility rates for women in their 20s fell, whereas those for women in their 30s and 40s rose. The patterns have been more complex since the turn of the century. Up to about 2010, rates for women aged 25 to 29 rose steeply, with a much smaller rise among women aged 20 to 24. Since 2010, rates

---

Box 16.4 Definitions of birth and fertility rates

Crude birth rate

The number of live births in a year per 1000 mid-year population.

General fertility rate (GFR)

The number of live births per 1000 women aged 15 to 44 in the same population. Measure of current fertility levels.

Age-specific fertility rate (ASFR)

The number of live births to mothers of a particular age per 1000 women in that age group. Useful for comparing fertility of women at different ages or women of the same age in different populations.

Total fertility rate (TFR)

The TFR is the average number of live children a group of women would have if they experienced the age-specific fertility rates for the calendar year in question throughout their childbearing lifespan. National TFRs are derived by summing single-year ASFRs over all ages within the childbearing lifespan.

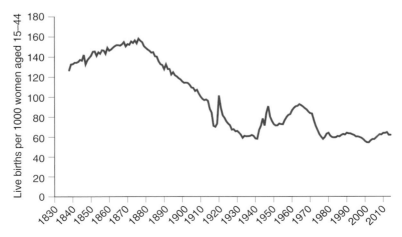

Figure 16.1 General fertility rate, England and Wales, 1838–2014. (Source: General Register Office, OPCS, Office for National Statistics.)

have been falling for all women under 35 years of age. By 2015, fertility rates for women aged 40 and over had risen above the rates for women under age 20 (ONS 2016c).

One way to summarize these trends and also make comparisons between countries is to use the total fertility rate, defined in Box 16.4.

The total fertility rate can be interpreted as the average family size if women were to experience the age-specific fertility rates for the current year throughout their child-bearing years. Total fertility rates for Britain and Ireland are compared in Fig. 16.2. As in Fig. 16.1, they show the 'baby boom' of the 1960s, the subsequent decline and levelling off of rates and the increase since the turn of the century followed by the slight decline since 2010. They also show that whereas both parts of Ireland had much higher fertility rates in the middle of the 20th century, there has been a relatively large decline to levels only slightly above those for England and Wales and for Scotland.

All of the countries discussed publish detailed tables of births and birth rates by local authority areas and social characteristics, often with accompanying maps and online tools. Because of differences in birth rates by age and the differences between age structures of populations, some rates are adjusted to allow for this, using procedures known as *standardization*. These are explained later in the chapter in the discussion of mortality.

Multiple births

Multiple birth rates are measured in terms of maternities, that is, pregnancies leading to one or more registrable births. The multiple pregnancy rate is the proportion of all maternities leading to two or more registrable births.

In the Irish Republic, only live births are included in multiple birth rates, and this was also the case in Scotland before 1960.

The trends in multiple births in Britain and Ireland are shown in Fig. 16.3. The reasons for the decline up to the mid-1970s were unclear at the time (*British Medical Journal* 1976). Certain factors have contributed to the increase in multiple birth rates since then. It is often assumed that this is simply a consequence of the use of ovarian stimulants from the late 1970s onward followed by the development and increasing use of assisted conception since the 1980s. This ignores another major factor, the rising age at childbirth. Spontaneous multiple birth rates are higher among women their 30s than among younger women and increase as women grow older. In addition, because older couples may be more likely to have more problems in conceiving, they are more likely to turn to assisted conception.

Data about assisted conception in clinics in the UK is collected by the Human Fertilisation and Embryology Authority (HFEA) as part of its monitoring role and are published on its website (HFEA 2016). These data relate to the outcomes of procedures in clinics in the UK. A project is under way to link them with NHS records, but they can include births outside the UK to women who used clinics in the UK. The data is compiled separately from data recorded at civil registration. If couples travel outside the UK for assisted conception, data about this will not be compiled by the HFEA.

After a rise in the rate of triplet and higher-order births in the mid-1990s, the HFEA and the Royal College of Obstetricians and Gynaecologists (RCOG) implemented policies to restrict the use of three or more embryos, and since 2009 the HFEA has set targets for clinics to reduce

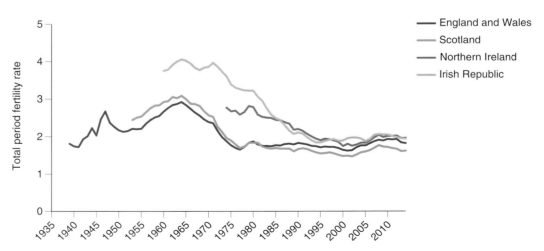

Figure 16.2 Total fertility rates, Britain and Ireland, 1938–2014. (Source: General Register Offices, Office for National Statistics, CSO Ireland.)

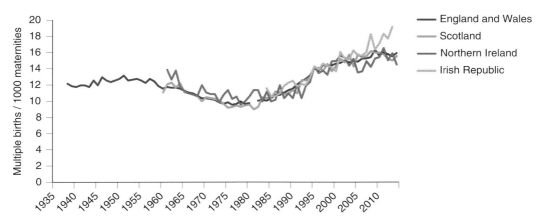

Figure 16.3 Multiple birth rates, Britain and Ireland, 1938–2014. (Source: General Register Offices, Office for National Statistics, CSO Ireland.)

their multiple live birth rates by encouraging the use of only one embryo in assisted conception. Although this has had an impact on multiple birth rates following assisted conception (HFEA 2015), because of the increasing use of assisted conception and the continuing rise in the age at childbirth, multiple maternity rates in the population as a whole have not decreased, as can be seen in Fig. 16.3.

Teenage conception rates

Birth rates underrepresent pregnancy rates because they do not include those cases where women miscarry spontaneously or pregnancies that end in induced abortion, and the proportions of pregnancies terminated are particularly high among teenagers. Pregnancies terminated in England, Wales or Scotland under the Abortion Act of 1967, amended by the Human Fertilisation and Embryology Act of 2008, should be notified to the relevant Chief Medical Officer (Department of Health (DH) 2016). Data about terminations in England and Wales is analysed and published by the Department of Health (DH 2016), and data about terminations in Scotland is published by the Information Service Division (ISD) Scotland (ISD 2016). If a woman is admitted to the hospital following a miscarriage, this is recorded in the relevant hospital statistics, but data about miscarriages is not presently brought together in a consistent way to produce comprehensive statistics.

Data from birth registration and abortion notifications is brought together to derive numbers of conceptions, defined as the numbers of maternities leading to one or more registrable live or stillbirths plus the numbers of induced abortions. These are expressed as rates per thousand women in the population and analysed by age, local authority area and other factors. The ONS and ISD Scotland websites have tables, maps and diagrams to show how conception rates vary between areas and their characteristics. They show, for example, that the more deprived areas have higher rates of teenage conception and that pregnant teenagers in more deprived areas are less likely to have terminations, although the gap has been narrowing over recent years.

Trends in teenage conception rates since 1969 in England and Wales are shown in Fig. 16.4, where they are compared with conception rates at all ages. Rates at all ages fell rapidly in the early 1970s – a time when access to contraception was becoming widely available free of charge under the NHS in 1974. Increases in the number of conceptions that occurred in 1976 to 1977, 1983, 1986 and 1995 to 1996 coincided with reports questioning the safety of oral contraceptives. These may have deterred the population as a whole and teenagers in particular from using them.

Since 2007, there have been major declines in teenage conception rates. A number of factors could have influenced this, including sex and relationship education programmes, improvements in the accessibility of contraceptives to young people and increased aspirations to participate in further and higher education.

In the past, teenage conception rates for Scotland were calculated in a different way from those for England and Wales. Scotland has now revised its methods and recalculated rates for previous years. As a result, conception rates can now be compared, as in Fig. 16.5. This figure shows that trends in Scotland and England have been similar since the early 1990s, although rates in England and Wales combined have tended to be higher.

The Abortion Act does not apply to women living outside England, Wales and Scotland. A small and declining number of terminations are undertaken in Northern Ireland under the case law that preceded the Abortion Act.

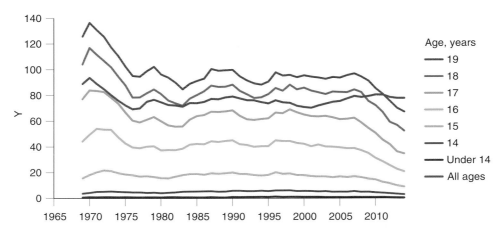

Figure 16.4 Teenage conception rates and all-ages conception rate, England and Wales, 1969–2014. (Source: Office for National Statistics.)

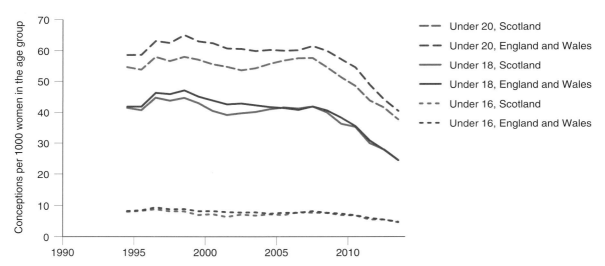

Figure 16.5 Teenage conception rates, England and Wales compared with Scotland, 1994–2013. (Source: Office for National Statistics and National Records of Scotland.)

Reports are published on the website of the Department of Health, Social Services and Public Safety (DHSSPS 2016). Much larger numbers of women resident in Northern Ireland travel to England and Wales for terminations, along with women from the Irish Republic, the Isle of Man, the Channel Isles and other countries, notably Malta and Poland, where legal abortion is not available. In addition, a small and declining number of women resident in Scotland have terminations in England and Wales. The annual abortion statistics reports for England and Wales include a table of numbers of abortions for 'non-residents', women whose address is outside England and Wales. Because some women who are residents of other countries give an address in England and Wales, this means that it is not possible to derive conception statistics for Northern Ireland or the Republic of Ireland.

Outcome of pregnancy

Many measures have been used to measure the outcome of pregnancy in relation to the clinical and social characteristics of mothers and babies and the care to which they have access. *Mortality,* the death of a mother or baby, is the longest-standing measure because there is a legal requirement to report deaths in high-income countries. This means that deaths are the most comprehensively reported events, although they are much less well reported in poorer countries, where rates are considerably higher. When registering a death, the next of kin has to produce a medical certificate of cause of death signed by a doctor or other clinician. The causes of death reported on the certificate are coded according to the International Classification of Diseases and tabulated according to other information, such as age, sex, country of birth and marital status recorded at death registration.

Morbidity, ill-health, is more common, and a range of outcome measures can be used. Specific illnesses or disabilities, such as asthma or cerebral palsy, can be used, but these are much more difficult to ascertain. People with the same condition can receive care in a range of hospital and general practice settings, but the information is not routinely brought together in a single place. Considerable developments in data linkage have taken place in Scotland, Wales and Northern Ireland, but attempts to link together information from hospital and general practice systems at a national level in England have met with resistance because of concerns about how the data were to be used.

In measuring morbidity, a distinction should be made between *prevalence*, which measures conditions people have over a period of time, such as heart and respiratory conditions, and *incidence*, which measures the occurrences of conditions such as communicable diseases from which people recover or die. These terms are defined in Box 16.5.

Physical measures of mothers and babies, such as blood pressure, height, weight and body mass index (BMI) of mothers and birthweights of babies can be regarded as proxy measures of morbidity and are commonly recorded in most clinical information systems. The extent to which they are recorded at a national level and the completeness of the data vary between and within countries. The same applies to composite measures such as Apgar scores.

Other data is recorded in situations where no clinicians are involved, most notably, self-reported morbidity. This is used in interviews and postal surveys, which may also be used to collect data about service users' views. Such questions, also used in the population censuses, ask respondents about their general health. Another standard question is whether respondents have a long-term health problem or disability and whether it affects their day-to-day activities. The ONS has more recently started to derive and publish broader measures of national well-being (ONS 2016d; Allin and Hand 2017).

MORTALITY

Death rates in general are used as broad measures of the extent of ill health, both nationally and internationally. This applies particularly in high-income countries where death registration is compulsory because death certificates are needed for legal purposes, so data is readily available. Death rates are commonly analysed in terms of other data collected at death registration, notably, age, sex, area of residence and clinical cause of death, to produce specific death rates for subgroups of the population. For example, the age-specific mortality rate per 1000 population for women aged 45 to 54 is derived by dividing the number of deaths of women aged 45 to 54 by the numbers of women aged 45 to 54 in the same population.

These data show that, as would be expected, death rates are higher in older age groups. As a consequence, comparisons between countries or areas within the same country may reflect differences in the age structure of the populations, as well as the extent of ill-health and the availability of effective healthcare. To enable more valid comparisons, death rates are adjusted to take account of differences in age distributions. The two ways of doing this, *direct* and *indirect standardization*, are explained in Box 16.6. In addition to tables of age-standardized rates, the ONS website has interactive maps showing changes over time in age-standardized death rates for local authority areas. It also uses the same approach to produce age-standardized fertility rates.

The two categories of mortality of greatest relevance to birth maternity care, deaths of mothers and babies, are analysed in fuller detail than death rates in general and also use some different approaches.

MATERNAL MORTALITY

Maternal deaths are now rare events in Britain and Ireland, as in other high-income countries. Definitions of maternal death are shown in Box 16.7.

Box 16.5 Incidence and prevalence

Morbidity
The presence of a disease or other condition in a population

Incidence
The number of new cases of a particular condition in a given population, expressed as a rate (e.g. the incidence of anencephaly per 1000 births to residents of England and Wales in 2008)

Prevalence
The proportion of the given population affected by a condition at a particular time in a given period (e.g. the prevalence of cerebral palsy among children aged 5 to 9 resident in England and Wales in 2008)

Box 16.6 Standardization

Direct standardization

Direct standardization takes the birth or death rate in each age group in the population of interest.

It multiplies this rate by the size of the population in the same age group in a reference 'standard population' to calculate the 'expected number of deaths' in the 'standard population'.

It then adds up the 'expected numbers of deaths' and divides the total by the size of the 'standard population' to produce directly standardized mortality rates.

The hypothetical 'European standard population' (ONS 2013) is usually used for this.

Indirect standardization

Indirect standardization involves calculating standardized mortality ratios (SMRs).

A 'reference standard population' is chosen and allocated an SMR of 100.

For each age group, the age-specific rates in the standard population are multiplied by the numbers of people in the same age group in the population of interest to calculate the 'expected number' of deaths in that group.

These 'expected numbers' are added up over all age groups in the population to be compared.

The actual numbers of deaths in this population are divided by the 'expected numbers' to derive the SMR.

Box 16.7 Definitions of maternal deaths

Pregnancy-related death

A pregnancy-related death (death occurring during pregnancy, childbirth and puerperium) is the death of a woman while pregnant or within 42 days of termination of pregnancy, irrespective of the cause of death (obstetric and non-obstetric).

Maternal death

A maternal death is the death of a woman while pregnant or within 42 days of termination of pregnancy, irrespective of the duration and the site of the pregnancy, from any cause related to or aggravated by the pregnancy or its management, but not from accidental or incidental causes.

Direct and indirect maternal deaths

Maternal deaths should be subdivided into two groups:

1. Direct obstetric deaths: those resulting from obstetric complications of the pregnant state (pregnancy, labour and puerperium), from interventions, omissions or incorrect treatment, or from a chain of events resulting from any of these.

2. Indirect obstetric deaths: those resulting from previous existing disease or disease that developed during pregnancy and that was not attributable to direct obstetric causes but that was aggravated by physiological effects of pregnancy.

Late maternal death

A late maternal death is the death of a woman from direct or indirect obstetric causes more than 42 days but less than 1 year after termination of pregnancy.

Maternal deaths are usually expressed as rates per 100,000 maternities. Figure 16.6 is an exception because it includes data for years before 1938 when the identification of multiple births at birth registration started. The rates are derived from numbers of maternal deaths based on death registration alone. These are mainly restricted to those where complications of pregnancy are explicitly mentioned on the death certificate and the deaths occurred within 42 days of the end of the woman's pregnancies.

Long-term trends in maternal mortality show a pattern different from adult mortality and infant mortality as a whole. Maternal mortality remained high in England and Wales up to the 1930s, as Fig. 16.6 shows, and the rate in Scotland rose, at a time when adult mortality overall was falling. From the mid-1930s onward, maternal mortality declined rapidly in England and Wales. The use of *prontosil*, an early sulphonamide drug, to treat puerperal sepsis is likely to have had an impact on maternal mortality. In parallel with this trend, a reduction in the severity of puerperal sepsis may have also contributed because the downward trend started before *prontosil* was introduced. A few years later, the introduction of blood transfusions led to reduction in mortality from severe haemorrhage. The availability of *penicillin* and changes in maternity services probably also contributed to the fall in mortality (Macfarlane and Mugford 2000; Macfarlane 2001 and 2004).

The high rate of maternal mortality in the 1920s was a cause of public concern, and this prompted a number of investigations, including in-depth enquiries into the causes of individual maternal deaths. Certificates of deaths that are an indirect consequence of pregnancy, for example, deaths from suicide, do not usually mention the pregnancy. Therefore, to gain a fuller picture of maternal mortality, additional data collection is needed, and the countries of the UK were at the forefront of developing in-depth enquiries into maternal death.

Confidential enquiries

The first such confidential enquiry into maternal deaths was set up in 1917 in Aberdeen, by Matthew Hay, the Medical Officer of Health. This led into an enquiry covering all of Scotland. In England and Wales, Janet Campbell, appointed in 1919 as Head of the Maternal and Child

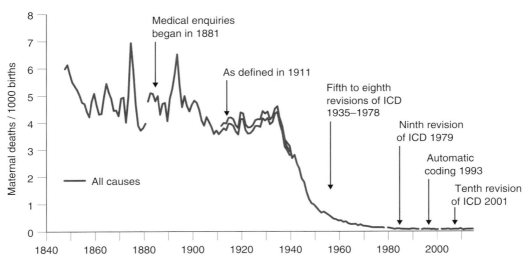

Figure 16.6 Maternal mortality, England and Wales, 1847–2014. ICD, International Classification of Diseases. (Source: General Register Office, OPCS and ONS mortality statistics.)

Welfare Division of the Ministry of Health, produced a series of reports on maternal mortality and then established enquiries into maternal deaths in England and Wales. Starting in 1928, local medical officers of health were asked to complete forms to report details of maternal deaths to the enquiry, and the information was reviewed by panels of clinical assessors. After the enquiry published its reports (Macfarlane 2001 and 2004), local medical officers of health were asked to continue completing and sending in the forms to the health ministries. Reports were published annually in the reports of the Chief Medical Officers for England and Wales. Similar systems were set up in Scotland and Northern Ireland (see also Ch. 2).

Despite the substantial fall in rates, maternal mortality was still a cause for concern in the early 1950s. The enquiries in England and Wales were reorganized in 1952, and the information was coordinated and analysed by the Ministry of Health and published in reports every 3 years. Similar systems were set up in Northern Ireland in 1956 and Scotland in 1965, although reports covered longer time periods because of the smaller numbers of deaths involved.

From 1985–1987 onward, the enquiries were brought together with a single report being published every 3 years for the UK as a whole, overseen and coordinated by its four health ministries. From 2000–2002 onwards, responsibility passed to the Centre for Maternal and Child Health (CEMACH), subsequently known as the Centre for Maternal and Child Enquiries (CMACE). After CMACE closed on March 31, 2011, there was a gap while the programme, which had become part of the Maternal, Newborn and Infant Clinical Review Programme, was reviewed. The contract was then awarded to the Mothers and Babies: Reducing Risk through Audits and Confidential Enquiries

across the UK (MBRRACE-UK) collaboration in June 2012 (Knight et al 2014). Reports are now published annually and have two components, described in the following sections.

Surveillance of maternal mortality

The first component is surveillance of trends in maternal mortality in Britain and Ireland. The first report in the new series, published in 2014, compared mortality in the period 2009–2012 with mortality in 2006–2008, which had been analysed in the last of the 3-year reports (Knight et al 2014). The next report extended this analysis to the years 2011–2013 (Knight et al 2015).

Figure 16.7 shows trends in direct and indirect maternal mortality since the enquiries were established on a UK basis in 1985–1987. Even when data for the 3 years is combined, the numbers of deaths is small, so the 95% control limits shown in Fig. 16.7 are wide. The data shows that from the late 1980s to 2006–2008, rates of direct maternal mortality remained at about the same level but showed signs of decline in 2009–2011, a trend that continued in subsequent years.

Thrombosis and thromboembolism were the leading causes of *direct maternal death* in 2009–2011, with the rate being twice as high as for the next most common causes, genital tract sepsis, haemorrhage and pre-eclampsia and eclampsia, followed by amniotic fluid embolism. Because the numbers of deaths are so low, it is almost impossible to detect year-to-year changes in mortality from specific conditions.

In contrast, rates of *indirect maternal death* appear to have risen since 1985–1987, but this is not a real increase

243

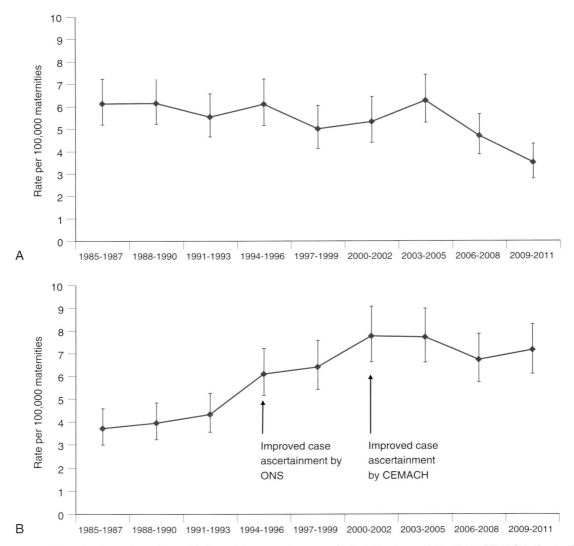

Figure 16.7 Mortality from direct (**A**) and indirect (**B**) maternal causes, United Kingdom, 1985–2011. CEMACH, Centre for Maternal and Child Health; ONS, Office for National Statistics. (Source: Confidential enquiries into maternal deaths.)

because it results from improvements in the ascertainment of these deaths. The first increase occurred in 1993 when the ONS started to computerize all the conditions mentioned on death certificates. Prior to that, only the underlying cause of death, coded manually, was included in computer records. This change considerably increased the identification of indirect maternal deaths.

It was also known from deaths reported directly to the enquiries that there were deaths where the pregnancy was not mentioned on the death certificate. To identify these, from 2000–2002 onward, the ONS has linked deaths of

women of childbearing age in England and Wales to birth registration records. This greatly increased the ascertainment of deaths from suicides, accidents and violence among women who had given birth and widened the scope of the enquiries to include mental health problems and domestic violence during and after pregnancy. Deaths in Scotland are now also linked in a similar way.

The leading cause of indirect maternal death in 2009–2011 was cardiac disease, followed by infections, notably influenza and pneumonia; neurological conditions, including epilepsy; and psychiatric causes. Influenza contributed more to mortality in this 3-year period than in subsequent years because of influenza epidemics in 2009 and 2010.

The much smaller numbers of coincidental deaths are not included in Fig. 16.7, which is also restricted to deaths within 42 days of the end of the pregnancy. When late maternal deaths after 42 days but less than 1 year after the end of the pregnancy are analysed, malignancy, psychiatric causes and cardiac conditions play an even more prominent role (Knight et al 2015).

Confidential reviews of maternal deaths

The other component of maternal death enquiries is in-depth review of each individual maternal death in the United Kingdom and Ireland. The Maternal Death Enquiry Ireland, established in 2009, publishes its own surveillance reports on deaths in the Republic of Ireland (Confidential Maternal Death Enquiry in Ireland 2015). Because of the very small numbers of deaths involved, the in-depth reviews are conducted and published alongside those of deaths in the UK to preserve anonymity and confidentiality.

The aim of the reviews is to identify ways of improving care to prevent death in the future. To undertake the reviews, demographic and clinical details are brought together with reports from units that provided care and from postmortems. The information is then anonymized and reviewed by multidisciplinary panels, whose remit is to establish whether any aspects of the woman's care were substandard and whether any substandard care might have contributed to the death.

The 3-year reports published in the past contained reviews of the full range of conditions and circumstances of maternal death. Each of the annual reports compiled by MBRRACE-UK focuses on a subset of the conditions in rotation.

Confidential enquiries into maternal morbidities

The confidential enquiry method has frequently been criticized for its lack of comparison between women who died and women who had the same conditions but did not die. If suitable data is available, it is possible to use techniques such as cohort studies or case-control studies to make comparisons and draw conclusions about how to improve care to prevent maternal death. The UK Obstetric Surveillance System (UKOSS), which started in 2005, collects data from multiple sources about rare conditions, including those that contribute to maternal death. It can therefore be used as a basis for comparisons with care given to women who died. A UKOSS study of women with severe sepsis was used in this way as part of the 2014 (Knight et al 2014) report, and reports on other causes of severe maternal morbidity will be included in reports from 2016 onward (Knight et al 2015).

STILLBIRTH AND INFANT MORTALITY RATES

In the mid-19th century when civil registration began, the term *infant mortality* was used fairly loosely, and it was not until later in the century that the concept and definition used today, shown in Box 16.8, was adopted, reflecting changes in the perception of childhood. Nevertheless, it was possible to use current definitions to derive the rates shown in Fig. 16.8.

As mentioned earlier, not all births were registered in the mid-19th century, and those that were not registered are likely to have been those where the baby died. This means that the infant mortality rates in the mid-19th century were likely to have been even higher than the data

---

Box 16.8 Definitions of stillbirth and infant mortality rates

Stillbirth rate $= \dfrac{\text{Stillbirths} \times 1000}{\text{Live births} + \text{stillbirths}}$

Perinatal mortality rate

$= \dfrac{(\text{Stillbirths} + \text{deaths at } 0{-}6 \text{ days after live birth}) \times 1000}{\text{Live births} + \text{stillbirths}}$

Early neonatal mortality rate

$= \dfrac{\text{Deaths at } 0{-}6 \text{ days after live birth} \times 1000}{\text{Live births}}$

Late neonatal mortality rate

$= \dfrac{\text{Deaths at } 7{-}27 \text{ days after live birth} \times 1000}{\text{Live births}}$

Neonatal mortality rate

$= \dfrac{\text{Deaths at } 0{-}27 \text{ days after live birth} \times 1000}{\text{Live births}}$

Postneonatal mortality rate

$= \dfrac{\text{Deaths at } 1{-}11 \text{ months after live birth} \times 1000}{\text{Live births}}$

Infant mortality rate

$= \dfrac{\text{Deaths under the age of 1 year after live birth} \times 1000}{\text{Live births}}$

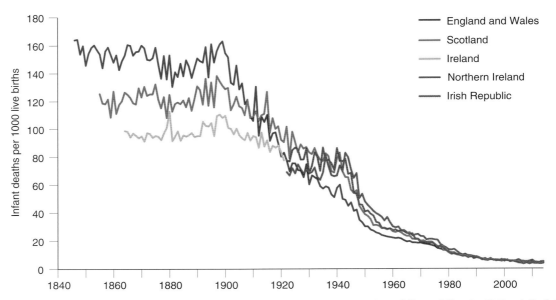

Figure 16.8 Infant mortality, Britain and Ireland, 1846–2014. (Source: General Register Offices, Office for National Statistics, CSO Ireland.)

in Fig. 16.8 suggests. After falling slightly in the late 1870s, the infant mortality rates rose until the turn of the century. In England and Wales, the rise was concentrated in urban areas, and the rates in rural areas remained stable (Tatham 1904). The fall in infant mortality throughout the 20th century was punctuated by peaks caused by epidemics of summer diarrhoea and influenza. The rates in England and Wales fell from 154.2 per 1000 live births in 1900 to 5.6 in 2000, and the rates in Scotland and Ireland fell to a similar extent.

Definitions of infant mortality and stillbirth rates are shown in Box 16.8. Data from civil registration of deaths is published on the same websites as for births, shown in Box 16.1. Although the term *neonatal* was not used for births in the first months after live birth until the 1930s, it became possible to subdivide infant deaths into neonatal and postneonatal deaths in England and Wales from 1905 onward. This showed that although neonatal mortality decreased fairly steadily throughout the 20th century, postneonatal mortality fell much more substantially, punctuated by the epidemic peaks shown in Fig. 16.8 (Macfarlane and Mugford 2000).

Trends in neonatal and postneonatal mortality from 1960 onward are compared in Figs 16.9a and b. As in Fig. 16.8, differences can be seen in the rates up to the mid-1970s, with England and Wales having the lowest rates, but these differences then narrow considerably. Neonatal mortality fell substantially in the late 1970s and early 1980s, whereas postneonatal mortality levelled off before falling substantially at the end of the 1980s. Much of the

decrease was a consequence of a fall in mortality attributed to *sudden infant death syndrome*. This preceded the government's 'Back to Sleep' campaign, mounted to decrease the numbers of such deaths by encouraging parents to lay babies on their backs (Macfarlane and Mugford 2000) (see also Ch. 51).

As mentioned earlier, stillbirths did not have to be registered until well into the 20th century. Figure 16.10 shows trends in England and Wales, along with perinatal mortality rates, derived by adding together numbers of stillbirths and neonatal deaths, as shown in Box 16.8.

This figure also shows how the change in inclusion criteria for stillbirth registration in 1992 increased the reported stillbirth and perinatal mortality rates. Unlike infant mortality rates, which showed a consistent downward trend, stillbirth rates levelled off in the late 1990s in England and Wales and even rose slightly in the early years of the 20th century before starting to fall again from 2011 onward.

Stillbirths and infant death rates are tabulated by sex, multiplicity, cause of death and parents' age, socioeconomic status, country of birth and area of residence in the reports published annually by the Office for National Statistics, National Records of Scotland, the Northern Ireland Statistics and Research Agency and the Central Statistics Office for Ireland.

Because of the considerably larger numbers of births and deaths in England and Wales combined compared with the other countries, much more detailed analyses are possible, for example, by birthweight and gestational age,

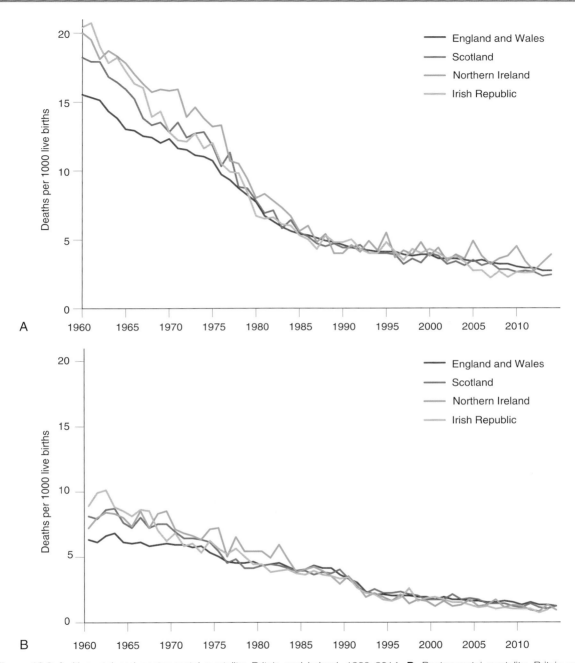

Figure 16.9 **A,** Neonatal and postneonatal mortality, Britain and Ireland, 1960–2014. **B,** Postneonatal mortality, Britain and Ireland, 1960–2014. (Source: General Register Offices, Office for National Statistics, CSO Ireland.)

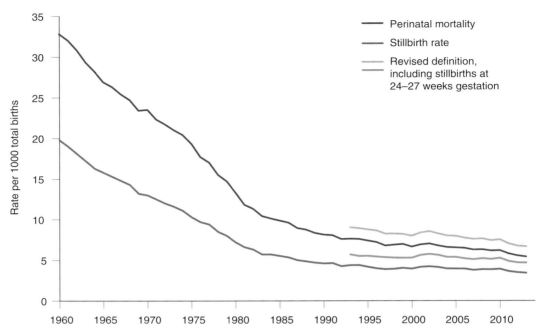

Figure 16.10 Stillbirth and perinatal mortality rates, England and Wales 1960–2014. (Office for National Statistics, Mortality statistics, Series DH3.)

defined in Boxes 16.9 and 16.10. Being born too soon or too small, in other words, preterm or of low birthweight, are key risk factors for stillbirth and infant death and are more common among babies born to more disadvantaged parents. These are also the babies among whom mortality rates are highest, as Fig. 16.11 shows.

Confidential enquiries into stillbirths and neonatal deaths

Beginning in the late 1970s, there were calls for confidential enquiries into perinatal deaths on similar lines to the maternal death enquiries. In response, a number of enquiries were set up at the local and regional levels in England and at the national level in Scotland and Wales. Reaction to a small rise in infant mortality in England and Wales in 1986 led eventually to the establishment in 1992 of the Confidential Enquiry into Stillbirths and Deaths in Infancy. This programme and its successors have been run on similar lines to the maternal deaths enquiries, but because of the much larger numbers of deaths involved, they have focused on a series of specific categories of stillbirth and neonatal death. Like the maternal deaths enquiries, they became a component of CEMACH then

---

Box 16.9 Definitions of birthweight

Birthweight is the first weight of the fetus or neonate obtained after birth. For live births, birthweight should preferably be measured within the first hour of life before significant postnatal weight loss has occurred. Although statistical tabulations include 500-g groupings for birthweight, weights should not be recorded in those groupings. The actual weight should be recorded to the degree of accuracy to which it is measured. The definitions of 'low', 'very low', and 'extremely low' birthweight do not constitute mutually exclusive categories. Below the set limits, they are all inclusive and therefore overlap (i.e. 'low' includes 'very low' and 'extremely low'; 'very low' includes 'extremely low').

Low birthweight

Less than 2500 g (up to and including 2499 g)

Very low birthweight

Less than 1500 g (up to and including 1499 g)

Extremely low birthweight

Less than 1000 g (up to and including 999 g)

Source: WHO 2016a

The duration of gestation is measured from the first day of the last normal menstrual period. Gestational age is expressed in completed days or completed weeks (e.g. events occurring 280 to 286 completed days after the onset of the last normal menstrual period are considered to have occurred at 40 weeks gestation).

Gestational age is frequently a source of confusion when calculations are based on menstrual dates. For the purposes of calculation of gestational age from the date of the first day of the last normal menstrual period and the date of delivery, it should be borne in mind that the first day is day 0 and not day 1; days 0 to 6 therefore correspond to 'completed week 0'; days 7 to 13 to 'completed week 1'; and the 40th week of actual gestation is synonymous with 'completed week 39'. Where the date of the last normal menstrual period is not available, gestational age should be based on the best clinical estimate.

To avoid misunderstanding, tabulations should indicate both weeks and days.

Preterm

Less than 37 completed weeks (less than 259 days) of gestation

Term

From 37 completed weeks to less than 42 completed weeks (259–293 days) of gestation

Postterm

42 completed weeks or more (294 days or more) of gestation

Source: WHO 2016a

CMACE and since June 2012 have been run by the MBRRACE-UK collaboration (Manktelow et al 2015a). The earlier enquiries covered deaths in England, Wales, Northern Ireland, the Isle of Man, Jersey and Guernsey, whereas Scotland continued with its own enquiry, but since 2013 Scotland has been included as well.

Stillbirths and neonatal deaths are notified to the enquiry by maternity units in parallel with civil registration by parents. Late fetal deaths at 22 and 23 weeks gestation are also notified in line with WHO's recommendation that fetal deaths and neonatal deaths from 22 weeks gestation should be included in statistics. This information is used to compile surveillance reports, which have been published from 2013 onward, and for in-depth enquiries into specific causes of stillbirth and neonatal death. An important focus of the surveillance has been to develop new methods of presenting stillbirth and neonatal mortality rates for local authority and other areas. The rates are stabilized to allow for the effects of chance variation as a result of small numbers and statistically adjusted for factors that are known to increase the risk of mortality. The rationale for this is discussed briefly in the following section, and the methods are described in MBRRACE-UK reports (Manktelow et al 2015a, 2015b, 2016). The aim is to identify those rates that are significantly above the UK average, suggesting that remedial action is needed.

Classifying causes of stillbirth and infant death

There are a number of differing ways of categorizing the conditions leading to stillbirth and infant death and a lack of consensus about which is the best. Any approach has to take account of conditions in both the mother and the baby and the type of information available. Numerous classifications have been developed over the years. A *pathophysiological* classification, which relied on information from postmortems, was developed by a pathologist, Jonathan Wigglesworth (Wigglesworth 1980). An earlier approach, developed in Aberdeen, classified conditions in mothers and babies separately and was revised in the 1980s and is widely used (Cole et al 1986; Hey et al 1986).

In Scotland and Northern Ireland, the underlying causes of registered stillbirths and infant deaths are coded to the codes and chapters of the International Classification of Diseases. In England and Wales, special stillbirth and neonatal death certificates, based on a perinatal death certificate proposed by WHO, are used. These have separate spaces to code conditions in mothers and babies. The ONS codes the conditions on the medical certificates according to the codes in the International Classification of Diseases and then groups them using a hierarchical classification system the ONS has developed, based on the Wigglesworth classification (Dattani and Rowan 2002; ONS 2016a). There was a discontinuity in 2014, when the ONS introduced new software for coding the causes of death, which led to an increase in the numbers of deaths attributed to infection (ONS 2016e). These differences make it difficult to derive stillbirth and infant mortality rates by cause for the UK as a whole.

The confidential enquiries have used different methods of classifying deaths. In Scotland, the separate obstetric and neonatal classification mentioned previously was used, whereas CESDI/CEMACH/CMACE used this along with an extended version of the Wigglesworth classification similar to that used by the ONS. In both cases, the classifications were revised to include more conditions contributing to stillbirths whose cause had previously been classified as unknown. MBRRACE-UK is using a new and different approach, the Causes of Death and Associated Conditions (CODAC) system, which uses a three-level hierarchical tree of coded causes of death (Manktelow et al 2015a).

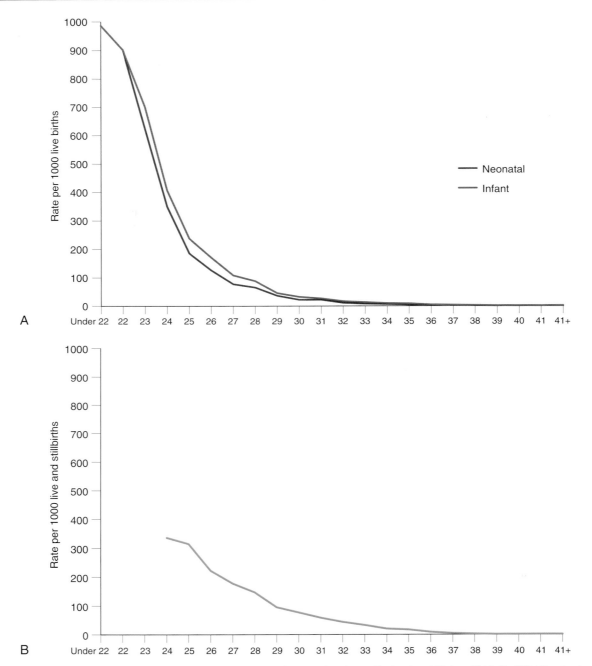

Figure 16.11 **A,** Stillbirth, neonatal and infant mortality rates by gestational age, England and Wales, 2013. **B,** Stillbirth rates by gestational age, England and Wales, 2013. (Source: Office for National Statistics.)

INTERPRETING DIFFERENCES IN THE OUTCOME OF PREGNANCY

Measures of the outcome of pregnancy, notably, stillbirth, neonatal and infant mortality rates, are frequently used within countries in comparisons between maternity units and between populations and internationally between countries as indicators of the quality of the care provided. Although this is an important factor, there are other crucial factors that can also contribute to reported differences in measures of outcome.

The first is differences in criteria for including births in statistics. This plays a major role in international comparisons. Although WHO makes recommendations about which births should be recognized and included in national statistics, countries vary in their legislation. For European countries, these have been documented in a series of European Perinatal Health Reports and articles by the *Euro-peristat group* (Euro-peristat 2013). The differences largely affect the lower cutoff point in terms of birthweight and gestational age. As Fig. 16.11 shows, these are the babies with the highest mortality rates, so this affects the comparability of statistics.

The extent to which reporting complies with the specified criteria can vary within countries and can affect comparisons within and between local areas. For example, legislation in Britain and Ireland does not specify a lower gestational age limit for registering a live birth, so there are local differences in the extent to which very preterm births are included (Smith et al 2013). This has implications for comparisons of overall rates of death. Even where reporting is consistent, many rates are based on relatively small numbers, so random variation can play a role, even at a national level. Figures 16.9a and b and 16.10 show year-to-year fluctuations in trends in rates at a national level for all countries apart from those for England and Wales combined, which are dominated by England, which has a much larger population. It plays a much larger role in local comparisons, where the numbers of stillbirths, neonatal and infant deaths are small. Various approaches have been used to take account of this. In the past, confidential enquiries and other analyses have used diagrams called *funnel plots*, which plot death rates against the numbers of births in the denominator, to give an indication of the extent to which differences are or are not compatible with random variation. MBRRACE-UK now uses a technique called stabilization to adjust for random variation (Manktelow et al 2015a).

After taking account of these factors, stillbirth and infant mortality rates, along with rates of preterm birth and low birthweight, vary considerably according to the socioeconomic status of the babies' parents and according to the social characteristics of the areas in which they live. This is discussed in the next section. MBRRACE uses a combination of standardization and statistical modelling to adjust rates, using sociodemographic variables that are recorded throughout the UK. These are the mother's age, the baby's sex, whether or not the babies are from a multiple birth and the socioeconomic characteristics of the area where the mother lives. For neonatal deaths, gestational age at birth is also used (Manktelow et al 2015a and 2015b).

Inequalities in the outcome of pregnancy

There are considerable demographic and socioeconomic differences in the outcome of pregnancy, and many of them are interrelated. As a result, many of the common measures are correlated with one another. In epidemiology, this is known as *confounding*. These differences can be explored in depth in specially designed surveys, but in routine data systems containing data about large numbers of births, a limited range of data items is recorded. Tabulations using these data items are included in annual publications of data for England and Wales, Scotland, Northern Ireland and the Republic of Ireland.

Mortality rates of babies and their mothers are highest for women aged under 20 and those aged 40 and over, but the ages at which women have children also vary according to their socioeconomic circumstances, with professional women tending to delay childbirth until they are in their 30s. In this age group, women are more likely to have multiple births, and mortality rates for babies from multiple births are higher overall than for babies from singleton births. This is because babies from multiple births are more likely to be born preterm, and therefore this group includes higher proportions of low-birthweight babies. Paradoxically, in some categories of low birthweight, babies from multiple births have lower mortality rates than singleton babies.

In general, there is a correlation between birthweight and mortality, but this does not apply to differences between boys and girls. Boys are, on average, heavier than girls but have higher mortality rates.

Parents' countries of birth

Parents' countries of birth are recorded at birth registration, and rising proportions of babies are born to parents who were themselves born outside the UK. In 2014, 27% of live births in England and Wales, 16% of live births in Scotland, and 13% of births in Northern Ireland were to mothers born outside the UK. Although stillbirth and infant mortality rates tend to be higher for babies of migrant women than for those born in the UK, this is not universally the case. People who have the resources to migrate may be some of the healthiest in their countries of origin, but they may settle initially in socially deprived areas where the host population is less healthy than the population as a whole. This is called the 'healthy migrant'

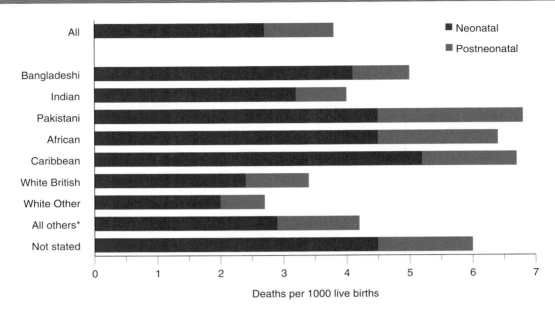

* Chinese, Other Asian, Other Black, Other and all Mixed groups

Figure 16.12 Infant mortality by baby's ethnicity, England and Wales, 2013. (Source: Office for National Statisics.)

effect, but in some cases, it wears off if the next generation adapts to unhealthy features of life in Britain and Ireland.

Ethnicity

By the 1980s, it was increasingly recognized that although data about country of birth yielded information about the health of migrants, the population born in the UK, including the offspring of migrants, was becoming diverse. Combined with this was a concern that people from non-white groups were experiencing disadvantage, and data was needed to monitor this. This led to the development of ethnicity classifications used initially in the 1991 census of population and then subsequently used to a greater or lesser extent in NHS and other data collection systems.

Ethnicity is designed to be self-reported, although many people from diverse backgrounds find it difficult to allocate themselves to the categories, and reporting is particularly likely to be problematic for people who do not speak fluent English. Ethnicity was not added to the data collected at birth registration, but the baby's ethnicity was included in the data set recorded in the birth notification in England and Wales. This is now linked to data recorded in the birth registration and used in published statistics. There are questions about whose ethnicity is recorded, given that newborn babies are too young to report themselves, but a data linkage exercise showed that their reported ethnicity appeared to be similar to their mothers' reported ethnicity. Each of the four countries of the UK defines its own ethnic question for the census. Although

they differ in detail, there is a common structure, which is shown in Fig. 16.12.

Although the ethnicity classification is said to be based on 'culture', it appears to be more closely related to skin colour and geography, based on the migration patterns up to the late 1980s when it was designed. Figure 16.12 shows differences in infant mortality between apparently similar groups of babies. Infant mortality for Pakistani babies, among whom there are high rates of lethal congenital anomalies, are much higher than those for Indian and Bangladeshi babies. The high infant mortality rate for Caribbean babies, most of whose mothers were born in the UK, is a consequence of the high rate of preterm birth in this group. Among the African babies, most of whose mothers were born outside the UK, there were similarly high rates of preterm birth and low birthweight among babies whose mothers had been born in West and Middle Africa (Datta-Nemdharry et al 2012). This wide range of rates also calls into question the common practice of grouping together non-white women and labelling them as 'black and minority ethnic' (BME).

Social class based on occupation

There are differences in socioeconomic status within the population as a whole and between and within parents' ethnic groups. In some countries, parents' level of education is used as a measure of socioeconomic position, but the tradition in the countries of the UK has been to use social class based on occupation. The original classification, the Registrar General's Social Classes, used in the 20th century

The National Statistics Socioeconomic Classification now used in the United Kingdom is as follows:

1. Higher managerial and professional occupations
   1.1 Large employers and higher management occupations
   1.2 Higher professional occupations
2. Lower managerial and professional occupations
3. Intermediate occupations
4. Small employers and own account workers
5. Lower supervisory and technical occupations
6. Semi-routine occupations
7. Routine occupations
8. Never worked and long-term unemployed
   Students, occupations not stated or inadequately described, and occupations not classifiable for other reasons are added as 'Not classified'.

Source: ONS 2010

Box 16.12 Indices of area deprivation

English Indices of Deprivation
www.gov.uk/government/statistics/
   english-indices-of-deprivation-2015
Welsh Index of Multiple Deprivation
https://statswales.gov.wales/Catalogue/Community-
   Safety-and-Social-Inclusion/Welsh-Index-of-Multiple-
   Deprivation/WIMD-2014
Scotland Indices of Multiple Deprivation
www.gov.scot/Topics/Statistics/SIMD
Northern Ireland Multiple Deprivation Measure
www.nisra.gov.uk/deprivation/archive/
   updateof2005measures/nimdm_2010_report.pdf
Children in Low-Income Families Local Measure
www.gov.uk/government/statistics/
   personal-tax-credits-children-in-low-income-families-
   local-measure
All-Island HP Deprivation Index
http://airo.maynoothuniversity.ie/mapping-resources/
   airo-census-mapping/national-viewers/
   all-island-deprivation-index

---

showed a strong gradient between social groups, but the National Statistics Socioeconomic Classification, adopted at the turn of the 21st century, shows a more complex picture (ONS 2010). Box 16.11 shows the version with eight 'analytical classes'. These classes can be aggregated or disaggregated into smaller or larger numbers of classes if the numbers in each category are small.

The social class differences in infant mortality shown in Fig. 16.13 do not follow a gradient, but there is a marked difference between the more disadvantaged social class groups and the others.

Area deprivation scores

Area deprivation scores are designed to measure inequalities between categories of individuals. To measure inequalities between small local geographical areas, going down to areas smaller than electoral wards, scores have been constructed based on a range of data about the population. These area deprivation scores, which have been constructed separately for each country of the UK and for Ireland, are listed in Box 16.12.

The index for England is based on indicators grouped into seven domains:

1. Income deprivation
2. Employment deprivation
3. Health deprivation and disability
4. Education, skills and training deprivation
5. Crime
6. Barriers to housing and services
7. Living environment deprivation

These are put together to form the overall index. The indices for the other countries are constructed on similar lines.

MBRRACE uses a special deprivation score, the Children in Low-Income Families Local Measure, derived by HM Revenue and Customs for measuring child poverty. It was selected because it is produced for all the countries of the UK.

CARE IN PREGNANCY AND AT BIRTH

Data about maternity care is collected separately in England, Wales, Scotland and Northern Ireland, and the differences between them make it virtually impossible to aggregate the data to derive statistics for the United Kingdom as a whole. In England, data about care at birth, including method of delivery, diagnostic codes and procedures undertaken in NHS hospitals is collected via the *Maternity Hospital Statistics* run by *NHS Digital*, formerly the Health and Social Care Information Centre. Data is published annually, by financial year. Figure 16.14 uses data from this source and shows the rise in caesarean section rates in England since the late 1980s. It also charts trends in operative delivery rates from 1955 to 1985 using data from an earlier system that covered both England and Wales.

A more recently introduced system, the *Maternity Services Dataset* collects a much wider range of data for England but is still very incomplete at the time of writing. In Wales, the maternity data in the *Patient Episode Database Wales* are very incomplete, so there is routine linkage with the

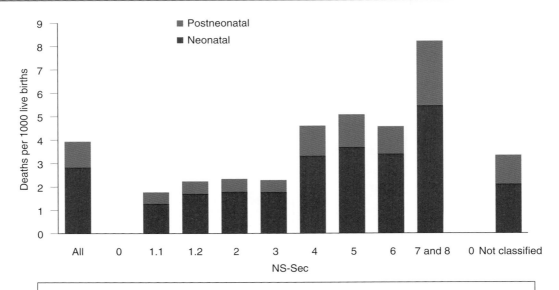

National Statistics Socioeconomic Classification (NS-SEC) analytic classes

1 Higher managerial and professional occupations

  1.1 Large employers and higher managerial occupations

  1.2 Higher professional occupations

2 Lower managerial and professional occupations

3 Intermediate occupations

4 Small employers and own-account workers

5 Lower supervisory and technical occupations

6 Semi-routine occupations

7 Routine occupations

8 Never worked and long-term unemployed students, occupations not stated or inadequately
  described and occupations not classifiable for other reasons are added as 'Not classified'.

Figure 16.13 Infant mortality rates by social class of most advantaged parent, babies born in England and Wales in 2013. (Source: ONS, Birth cohort infant mortality.)

National Community Child Health Database, which includes information about children's births.

ISD Scotland's annual publication *Births in Scottish Hospitals* contains a range of data about birth and the characteristics of mothers. For many years, Northern Ireland did not regularly publish data from its *NIMATS system,* but in 2016, the Northern Ireland Public Health Agency produced a publication bringing together data about birth and child health in Northern Ireland from several different sources (Northern Ireland Public Health Intelligence Unit 2016). In the Irish Republic, the annual volume of *Perinatal Statistics* is now published by the Health Information and Quality Authority.

INTERNATIONAL COMPARISONS

WHO has a Global Health Observatory that publishes an annual volume of World Health Statistics (WHO 2016b). Its website has a repository of data, graphical tools and descriptions of the methods. This and other websites with international data are shown in Box 16.13.

Unicef compiles statistics to monitor the health of children, including data about childbirth, and publishes a high-profile annual report, the *State of the World's Children.* *The Lancet* has published a series of global reports on a range of subjects, including maternal mortality, neonatal

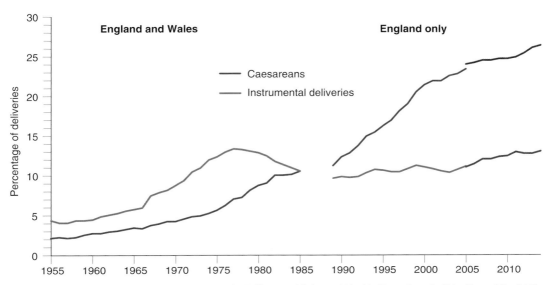

Figure 16.14 Operative delivery rates, 1955 to 2014–2015. (Source: Ministry of Health, Department of Health and Social Security, Welsh Office, Office of Population Censuses and Surveys, Maternity Hospital In-patient Enquiry and Health and Social Care Information Centre, Hospital Episode Statistics.)

Box 16.13 Key websites with international health statistics		
Organization	Website	Data available
World Health Organization	www.who.int/gho/en/	WHO Global Observatory data
Unicef	www.unicef.org/statistics/	Statistics and monitoring
Unicef	www.unicef.org/sowc/	State of the World's Children
Unicef	http://mics.unicef.org/	Reports of multiple indicator cluster surveys and downloadable data
DHS Program	http://dhsprogram.com/	Reports of demographic and health surveys and downloadable data
The Lancet	www.thelancet.com/series	Series on specific topics
OECD	https://data.oecd.org/health.htm	Data about health and care generally in partner countries
Eurostat	http://ec.europa.eu/eurostat/web/population-demography-migration-projections	Data on many subjects, including demography
Euro-peristat	www.europeristat.com	European perinatal health reports and in-depth articles

survival, stillbirth, preterm birth and midwifery (Renfrew et al 2015) (see also Ch. 1).

The Organization for Economic Cooperation and Development (OECD) includes data about health and healthcare in its 34 member countries, and these include data about caesarean section and immunization. Its annual publication shows wide variations between high-income countries (OECD 2015). Statistics for the countries of the European Union on a wide range of subjects are compiled and published by Eurostat and include data about populations and birth and death rates.

As mentioned earlier, international comparisons between can be problematic. Countries vary in their legislation that defines which births and deaths should be included in statistics and the extent to which their data collection systems are complete and comply with these criteria. This is the case even in high-income countries where data is derived from birth and death certificates and registration is relatively complete.

Differences within Europe have been documented in detail in a series of European Perinatal Health Reports and the papers and reports by the Euro-peristat collaboration, which aims to publish statistics on a comparable basis. These reports

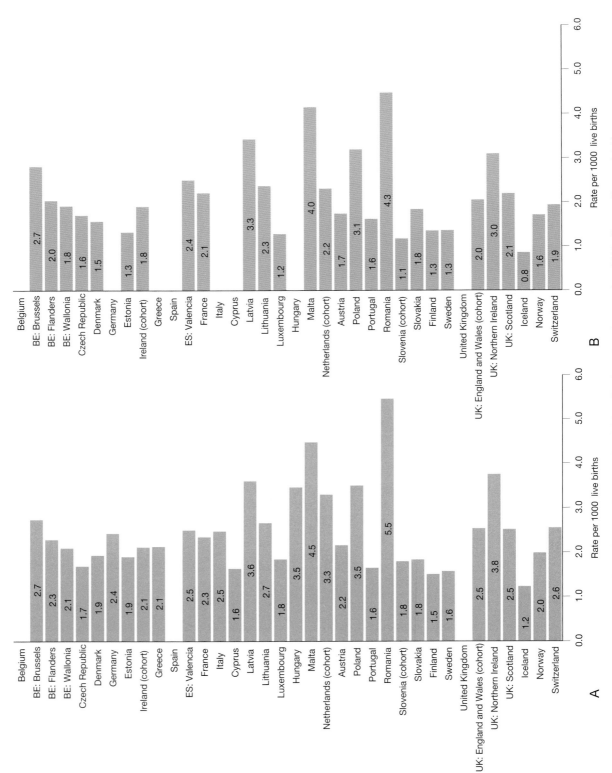

Figure 16.15 Neonatal mortality rates for all live births and live births **A**, at birth or **B**, after 24 weeks gestation, 2010. (Source: Euro-peristat.)

show, for example, that differences between the comparatively low rates of stillbirth and infant mortality are sensitive to differences in criteria for inclusion in statistics. Figure 16.15 shows comparisons of neonatal mortality rates for 2010 for countries participating in Euro-peristat using the countries' own criteria and then using a common cutoff of 24 weeks gestational age (Euro-peristat 2013).

In most middle- and low-income countries, birth and death registration are incomplete to a varying extent, although the situation is improving (*The Lancet* 2015). Because of this, data for many countries is estimated using surveys and other data sources. The most widely used surveys are the national *Demographic and Health Surveys* funded by USAID (Rutstein and Rojas 2006) and the *Multiple Indicator Cluster Surveys* funded by Unicef (2016). These surveys use common questionnaires to interview household members to collect information about topics such as fertility, use of contraception and women's and children's health.

Strategic development goals

Pregnancy-related deaths are a major cause of death worldwide. Reducing their numbers was one of the Millennium Development Goals and now forms part of Sustainable Development Goal 3 (United Nations n.d.) (see also Ch. 1). International comparisons are based on the maternal mortality ratio, the numbers of deaths per 100,000 live births. Data about maternal mortality is published by WHO (e.g. WHO 2015) and also appear in international publications from Unicef.

Trends in maternal mortality in UN regions, such as those shown in Fig. 16.16, show substantial decreases. On the other hand, none had met the goal of reducing the ratio by three-quarters between 1990 and 2015, and very wide differences between high- and low-income countries still persist (WHO 2015).

The estimated global ratio for 2015, 216 per 100,000 live births, was well above the new target of 70 per 100,000 live births set for 2030. Because of the incompleteness of birth and death registration, statistical methods have been developed to estimate these maternal death ratios (Wilmoth et al 2012). It was estimated that in 2015, only 1% of maternal deaths in the world took place in the European Region, 35% in the Americas and a further 3% in the Western Pacific Region. In contrast, an estimated 64% of maternal deaths took place in Africa.

The picture is similar for childhood mortality (Interagency Group for Child Mortality Estimation 2015). The key measure was the under-5 mortality rate, and it was estimated that 62 of the 195 countries for which data was available met the Millennium Development Goal (MDG) 4 target of a two-thirds reduction in the rate between 1990 and 2015. This included 24 low- and lower-middle-income countries. Infectious diseases and neonatal complications are responsible for the vast majority of under-5 deaths globally, and many of these are treatable with proven low-cost interventions. The Sustainable Development Goal (SDG) target on child survival is a rate of 25 or fewer deaths per 1000 live births by 2030, and further major reductions in rates are needed to achieve it (see also Ch. 1).

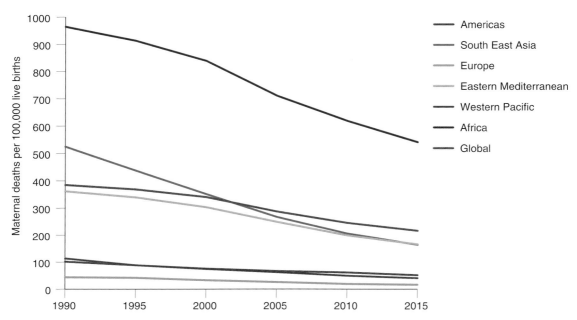

Figure 16.16 Maternal mortality ratio by UN region 1990–2015. (Source: World Health Organization.)

Use the data described in this chapter to find statistics for your country and your local area, in particular, find statistics on the following:

- Birth rates
- Teenage pregnancy rate and, if available, teenage conception rates
- Multiple birth rates
- Caesarean section rates
- Stillbirth rates
- Neonatal mortality rates

How do rates for your area compare with national rates?

Compare the nationally-produced data with data produced within your maternity unit. If they are different, why do you think this might have occurred?

Have these rates changed during the last few years? If so, think about your local area and why this might have happened and the extent to which it might have arisen from changes in the population.

Has this information been used to design services and, if so, how?

CONCLUSION

A list of the main websites containing the data for Britain and Ireland described in this chapter can be found in Box 16.14 and this is of considerable importance for the midwife. The chapter has aimed to point to the sources of key data about birth and its outcome, although it has been written at a time of considerable organizational and other changes. These mean that not only the websites but also the data found on them can change. It is important that the midwife is aware of these changes and can access the most current information.

The development of new methods of presenting data in maps and diagrams can greatly enhance our ability to understand data. Occasionally, however, superficially attractive graphics can be misleading, so it is important to read the small print and definitions to understand the data and what they can tell us about pregnancy, birth and maternity care in their social and economic context.

Box 16.14 Key websites containing data for Britain and Ireland

Organization	Website	Data available
England and Wales		
Office for National Statistics	www.ons.gov.uk	Birth and infant mortality statistics for England and Wales combined, census data and data on many other subjects
Department of Health	www.gov.uk/government/ collections/abortion-statistics-for-england-and-wales	Data about abortions in England and Wales
England		
NHS Digital, formerly the Health and Social Care Information Centre	www.hscic.gov.uk	Data about health and care
Public Health England	www.gov.uk/government/ organisations/public-health-england	Population-based data for public health
National Child and Maternal Health Intelligence Network	www.chimat.org.uk/ moving to gov.uk website	Now part of Public Health England
Wales		
Health in Wales	www.wales.nhs.uk/ statisticsanddata/sourcesofdata	Website commissioned by NHS Wales Informatics Service to act as a guide to data about health and care in Wales
StatsWales	https://statswales.gov.wales/ Catalogue/Health-and-Social-Care	Health and Social Care pages of general website containing official statistics for Wales
All Wales Perinatal Survey	https://awpsonline.uk/	Continuous surveillance of perinatal and infant mortality in the principality, funded by the Welsh government

Box 16.14 Key websites containing data for Britain and Ireland—cont'd

Organization	Website	Data available
Public Health Wales Observatory	www.wales.nhs.uk/sitesplus/922/page/84657	Pregnancy and childhood surveillance tool
Scotland		
National Records of Scotland	www.nrscotland.gov.uk/statistics-and-data	Birth and infant mortality statistics for Scotland, census data
ISD Scotland	www.isdscotland.org/Health-Topics/Maternity-and-births/	Pages with data about maternity care; part of much larger website with data on many aspects of health and care
Northern Ireland		
Northern Ireland Statistics and Research Agency	www.nisra.gov.uk/	Birth and infant mortality statistics for Northern Ireland, census data
Northern Ireland Public Health Agency	www.publichealth.hscni.net/	Responsible for NIMATS and child health system
United Kingdom as a whole		
Mothers and Babies: Reducing Risk through Audits and Confidential Enquiries across the UK (MBRRACE-UK)	www.npeu.ox.ac.uk/mbrrace-uk	Enquiries into maternal deaths and stillbirths and infant deaths in the United Kingdom
UK Obstetric Surveillance System	www.npeu.ox.ac.uk/ukoss	Audits of severe maternal morbidity
Health Quality Improvement Partnership	www.hqip.org.uk/national-programmes/a-z-of-clinical-outcome-review-programmes/cmace-reports/	Archive of confidential enquiry reports produced by CMACE and CEMACH
Human Fertilisation and Embryology Authority	www.hfea.gov.uk/	Data collected in its role as UK's independent regulator overseeing the use of gametes and embryos in fertility treatment and research
Republic of Ireland		
Central Statistics Office	www.cso.ie	Birth and infant mortality statistics for the Republic of Ireland, census data and data on many other topics
Health Information and Quality Authority	www.hiqa.ie/healthcare/health-information/data-collections/online-catalogue/national-perinatal-reporting-system	Responsible for National Perinatal Reporting System
Maternal Deaths Enquiry Ireland	www.ucc.ie/en/mde/	Enquiries into maternal deaths in Ireland

Key Points

- Midwives need to be conversant with the range of definitions used in relation to birth and its outcomes.
- A knowledge of national and local statistics published by national statistical organizations, including how they are compiled, where they can be found and how they should be interpreted, is essential in understanding the context of midwifery practice and the women using maternity services.
- Statistics have a key role in measuring the quality and extent of services provided and the sociodemographic characteristics of the local populations for whom they are provided.

- Confidential enquiries into maternal and perinatal mortality are important for informing improvements in clinical practice and reducing risks for mothers and their babies. They do this by highlighting shortcomings in practice and, along with evidence from systematic reviews of research, supporting the development of appropriate protocols and guidelines to prevent and manage high-risk situations in obstetrics and neonatal care.
- Midwives play a key role in the compilation of statistical data and in using and interpreting the data to inform practice. Therefore, they must be knowledgeable about the whole process and know where to find the most recently available local and national information.

References

Allin P, Hand DJ: New statistics for old? Measuring the wellbeing of the UK, *J Roy Stat Soc A* 180(1):1–22, 2017.

Bailey A, Vardulaki K, Langham J, et al: *Introduction to epidemiology*, Maidenhead, Open University Press, 2005.

Bonita R, Beaglehole R, Kjellström T: *Basic epidemiology*, World Health Organization (website). http://apps.who.int/iris/bitstream/10665/43541/1/9241547073_eng.pdf. 2006.

British Medical Journal: Editorial: Worldwide decline in dizygotic twinning, *Br Med J* 1(6025):1553, 1976.

Cole SK, Hey EN, Thomson AM: Classifying perinatal death: an obstetric approach, *Br J Obstet Gynaecol* 93(12):1204–1212, 1986.

Confidential Maternal Death Enquiry in Ireland: *Report for 2009–2012* (website). www.ucc.ie/en/media/research/maternaldeathenquiryireland/ConfidentialMaternalDeathEnquiryReport2009-12.pdf . 2015.

Datta-Nemdharry P, Dattani N, Macfarlane AJ: Birth outcomes for African and Caribbean babies in England and Wales: retrospective analysis of routinely collected data, *BMJ Open* 2:e001088, 2012.

Dattani N, Rowan S: Causes of neonatal deaths and stillbirths: a new hierarchical classification in ICD–10, *Health Stat Q* 15:16–22, 2002.

Department of Health (DH): *Abortion statistics 2015* (website). www.gov.uk/government/uploads/system/uploads/attachment_data/file/570040/Abortion_Statistics_2015_v3.pdf. 2016.

Department of Health, Social Services and Public Safety (DHSSPS): *Northern Ireland termination of pregnancy statistics, 2014/15* (website). www.health-ni.gov.uk/news/northern-ireland-termination-pregnancy-statistics-201415. 2016.

Euro-peristat: *European perinatal health report: The health and care of pregnant women and their babies in 2010* (website). www.europeristat.com, 2013.

Health and Social Care Information Centre (HSCIC): *Birth notification service (website)*. http://systems.hscic.gov.uk/demographics/births. 2016.

Hey EN, Lloyd DJ, Wigglesworth JS: Classifying perinatal death: fetal and neonatal factors, *Br J Obstet Gynaecol* 93(12):1213–1223, 1986.

Human Fertilisation and Embryology Authority (HFEA): *Improving outcomes for fertility patients: multiple births 2015* (website). www.hfea.gov.uk/docs/Multiple_Births_Report_2015.pdf. 2015.

Human Fertilisation and Embryology Authority (HFEA): *Fertility treatment 2014. Trends and figures* (website). www.hfea.gov.uk/docs/HFEA_Fertility_treatment_Trends_and_figures_2014.pdf. 2016.

Information Services Division, National Services Scotland (ISD Scotland): *Termination of pregnancy statistics year ending December 2015* (website). https://isdscotland.scot.nhs.uk/Health-Topics/Sexual-Health/Publications/2016-05-31/2016-05-31-Terminations-Report.pdf. 2016.

Inter-agency Group for Child Mortality Estimation: *Levels and trends in child mortality. Report 2015*. UNICEF (website). www.data.unicef.org/corecode/uploads/document6/uploaded_pdfs/corecode/IGME-report-2015-child-mortality-final_236.pdf. 2015.

Knight M, Kenyon S, Brocklehurst P, et al on behalf of MBRRACE-UK: *Saving Lives, improving mothers' care: lessons learned to inform future maternity care from the UK and Ireland Confidential Enquiries into Maternal Deaths and Morbidity 2009–2012*, Oxford, University of Oxford, 2014.

Knight M, Tuffnell D, Kenyon S, et al, editors: *Saving lives, improving mothers' care – surveillance of maternal deaths in the UK 2011–13 and lessons learned to inform maternity care from the UK and Ireland Confidential Enquiries into Maternal Deaths and Morbidity 2009–13*, Oxford, National Perinatal Epidemiology Unit, University of Oxford, 2015.

Macfarlane AJ: Enquiries into maternal deaths during the twentieth century. In National Institute for Clinical Excellence, Scottish Executive Health Department, Department of Health, Social Services and Public Safety, Northern Ireland, editor: *Why mothers die: the confidential enquiries into maternal deaths in the United Kingdom*, London, RCOG Press, 2001.

Macfarlane AJ: Confidential enquiries into maternal deaths: developments and trends from 1952 onwards. In *Confidential Enquiry into Maternal and Child Health. Why mothers die 2000-02: the sixth report of Confidential Enquiries into Maternal Deaths in the United Kingdom*, London, RCOG Press, 2004.

Macfarlane AJ, Mugford M: *Birth counts: statistics of pregnancy and childbirth*, vol 1, 2nd edn, London, The Stationery Office, 2000.

Manktelow BM, Smith LK, Evans TA, et al on behalf of the MBRRACE-UK Collaboration: *Perinatal Mortality Surveillance Report. UK perinatal deaths for births from January to December 2013*, Leicester, Infant Mortality and Morbidity Group, Department of Health Sciences, University of Leicester, 2015a.

Manktelow BM, Smith LK, Evans TA, et al on behalf of the MBRRACE-UK Collaboration: *MBRRACE-UK Perinatal Mortality Surveillance Report. UK perinatal death for births from January to December 2013 – supplementary report: UK Trusts and Health Boards*, Leicester, The Infant Mortality and Morbidity Studies Group, Department of Health Sciences, University of Leicester, 2015b.

Manktelow BN, Smith LK, Seaton SE, et al on behalf of the MBRRACE-UK Collaboration: *MBRRACE-UK Perinatal Mortality Surveillance Report. UK perinatal deaths for births from January to December 2014*, Leicester, The Infant Mortality and Morbidity Studies, Department of Health Sciences, University of Leicester, 2016.

Northern Ireland Public Health Intelligence Unit: *2016 Children's Health in Northern Ireland. A statistical profile of births using data from the Northern Ireland Child Health System, Northern Ireland Maternity System an Northern Ireland Statistics and Research Agency*, Belfast, Public Health Agency, 2016.

Office for National Statistics (ONS): *The National Statistics Socio-economic Classification (NS-SEC)* (website). www.ons.gov.uk/methodology/classificationsandstandards/otherclassifications/thenationalstatisticssocioeconomicclassificationnssecbasedonsoc. 2010.

Office for National Statistics (ONS): *Revised European standard population 2013 (2013 ESP)* (website). http://webarchive.nationalarchives.gov.uk/20160105160709/www.ons.gov.uk/ons/guide-method/user-guidance/health-and-life-events/revised-european-standard-population-2013--2013-esp-/index.html. 2013.

Office for National Statistics (ONS): *Vital Statistics Outputs Branch. User guide to child mortality statistics* (website). www.ons.gov.uk/peoplepopulationandcommunity/birthsdeathsandmarriages/deaths/methodologies/childmortalitystatisticsmetadata. 2016a.

Office for National Statistics (ONS): *Vital Statistics Outputs Branch. User guide to birth statistics* (website). www.ons.gov.uk/peoplepopulationandcommunity/birthsdeathsandmarriages/livebirths/methodologies/userguidetobirthstatistics. 2016b.

Office for National Statistics (ONS): *Vital Statistics Outputs Branch. Statistical bulletin: Births in England and Wales: 2015. Live births, stillbirths, and the intensity of childbearing measured by the total fertility rate* (website). www.ons.gov.uk/peoplepopulationandcommunity/birthsdeathsandmarriages/livebirths/bulletins/birthsummarytablesenglandandwales/2015. 2016c.

Office for National Statistics (ONS): *Well-being* (website). www.ons.gov.uk/peoplepopulationandcommunity/wellbeing. 2016d.

Office for National Statistics (ONS): *Impact of the implementation of IRIS software for ICD-10 cause of death coding on stillbirth and neonatal death statistics: England and Wales* (website). www.ons.gov.uk/peoplepopulationandcommunity/birthsdeathsandmarriages/deaths/bulletins/impactoftheimplementationofirissoftwareforicd10causeofdeathcodingonstillbirthandneonataldeathstatistics/englandandwales. 2016e.

Organization for Economic Cooperation and Development (OECD): *Health at a glance 2015: OECD indicators* (website). http://dx.doi.org/10.1787/health_glance-2015-en. 2015.

Porta M, editor: *A dictionary of epidemiology*, 6th edn, Edited for the International Epidemiological Association, New York, Oxford University Press, 2014.

Renfrew MJ, et al: Midwifery and quality care: findings from a new evidence-informed framework for maternal and newborn care, *The Lancet* 384(9948):1129–1145, 2015.

Rutstein SO, Rojas G: *Guide to DHS statistics* (website). http://dhsprogram.com/pubs/pdf/DHSG1/Guide_to_DHS_Statistics_29Oct2012_DHSG1.pdf. 2006.

Smith L, Draper ES, Manktelow BN, et al: Comparing regional infant death rates: the influence of preterm births <24 weeks of gestation, *Arch Dis Child Fetal Neonatal Ed* 98(2):F103–F107, 2013.

Stewart A: *Basic statistics and epidemiology*, 3rd edn, Cambridge, Radcliffe Publishing, 2010.

Tatham J: English mortality among infants under one year of age. In Interdepartmental Committee on Physical Deterioration, editor: *Report Cd 2175*, vol I, London, HMSO, 1904.

The Lancet: Counting births and deaths (website). www.thelancet.com/series/counting-births-and-deaths. 2015.

UNICEF: *The Multiple Indicator Cluster Surveys (MICS) 1995–2015: Monitoring the situation of children and women for 20 years* (website). http://mics.unicef.org/publications/reports-and-methodological-papers. 2016.

United Nations: *Sustainable Development Goal 3. Sustainable development knowledge platform* (website). https://sustainabledevelopment.un.org/?menu=1300. (not dated).

Wigglesworth JS: Monitoring perinatal mortality. A pathophysiological approach, *Lancet* 2:684–686, 1980.

Wilmoth JR, Mizoguchi N, Oestergaard MZ, et al: A new method for deriving global estimates of maternal mortality, *Stat Politics Policy* 3(2):2151–7509, 2012.

World Health Organization (WHO): *Trends in maternal mortality: 1990 to 2015. Estimates by WHO, UNICEF, UNFPA, World Bank Group and the United Nations Population Division* (website). http://apps.who.int/iris/bitstream/10665/194254/1/9789241565141_eng.pdf?ua=1. 2015.

World Health Organization (WHO): *International Statistical Classification of Diseases and Related Health Problems*, 10th Revision. Online version, 2016 edition (website). http://apps.who.int/classifications/icd10/browse/2016/en. 2016a.

World Health Organization (WHO): *WHO global observatory data* (website). www.who.int/gho/en/. 2016b.

Resources and additional reading

Please see the chapter boxes and the chapter website for further resources.

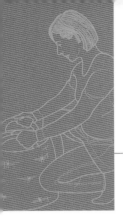

Chapter 17

Nutrition

Karen Jewell

Learning Outcomes   **?**

After reading this chapter, you will be able to:

- understand the basic principles of good maternal nutrition
- use a knowledge of nutrition to advise women about their diet during pregnancy
- appreciate the value of nutrition as a therapeutic intervention for specific conditions during pregnancy

WHAT IS NUTRITION?

Nutrition is the sum of the processes involved in taking in, utilizing and assimilating nutrients. Nutrients such as proteins, carbohydrates, fats, vitamins and minerals are necessary for development, growth, normal functioning and maintenance of life. As the body cannot produce them, they need to be obtained from a variety of food sources. Nutritional status is affected by the amount and quality of food eaten; the digestion, absorption and utilization of food nutrients; and biochemical individuality. In Westernized countries, eating enough food is not normally a problem. Many people, however, do not eat the correct balance of nutrients, which can lead to malnourishment and impaired health. In the UK, malnourishment occurs for reasons different to those in developing countries, where food is scarce. Food quality may be affected by nutrient-deficient soil in which crops are grown for human or livestock consumption or by the use of pesticides. The addition of chemical preservatives, colourings and flavourings to ready-prepared food and the addition of antibiotics to meat will also adversely influence nutrient absorption and utilization.

Digestion and absorption may be affected by general health or combinations of foods eaten. Conversely, impaired absorption of certain nutrients may be iatrogenic, for example, with specific drugs. Overindulgence in some foods can affect absorption of essential nutrients; for example, coffee and tea interfere with absorption of zinc and iron from food. Similarly, alcohol, cigarettes or recreational drug abuse, or environmental factors, including lead pollution, may lead to malnourishment through inadequate absorption and utilization of nutrients from food. Each person has unique nutritional requirements that alter according to age, gender, general health, activity level, genetic influences and stressors, including pregnancy. Some people need professional help to direct them towards the most appropriate diet.

ESSENTIAL NUTRIENTS AND FUNCTIONS

Proteins and amino acids

Required for:

- development of cells, enzymes, hormones, antibodies, haemoglobin
- buffers, helping to regulate acid–base balance
- controlling osmotic pressure between body fluids
- assisting in the transport of lipids as lipoproteins, and free fatty acids and bilirubin

Protein foods:

- meats, poultry, fish
- cheese, milk, eggs and other dairy produce
- beans, peas and other legumes
- corn, wheat products

- grains, seeds, nuts
- Brewer's yeast, soya

Proteins are digested by being broken down into amino acids and transported to the liver, where amino acid transferase enzymes convert them into a more usable form. Essential amino acids include leucine, lysine, methionine, cystine, phenylalanine and tryptophan; nonessential amino acids include alanine, glutamic acid, glycine and tyrosine. This process requires vitamin B_6; consequently, a high protein intake will require an increase in vitamin B_6 intake. Pregnant women have higher blood levels of tryptophan, an amino acid converted to serotonin, a calming and antidepressive agent.

Essential fatty acids

Required for:

- energy, heat insulation
- a healthy carrier for the fat-soluble vitamins that are needed for fetal development, particularly:
  - Vitamin D – regulates calcium and phosphate, which help keep bones and teeth healthy
  - Vitamin E – helps give cells their structure by supporting cell membranes
  - Vitamin K – aids blood clotting and also contributes to bone health
- Contain Omega 6 essential fatty acids
- Omega 3 Fatty acid:
  - development of brain, nervous system and retina
- High levels can lead to increased cholesterol and weight gain

Foods which contain monounsaturated fats:

- olive oil, Rapeseed oil/spread
- walnuts, almonds
- seeds e.g. linseed, pumpkin

Foods which contain polyunsaturated fats:

- sunflower, soya, corn, safflower oil/spread
- avocados
- peanuts

Foods which contain long chain Omega 3 fats

- salmon (fresh or canned)
- trout, mackerel
- tinned tuna
- sardines/pilchards
- animal fats: butter, lard, meat fat
- margarines and vegetable shortening

Fats are composed of triglycerides, which are broken down during digestion. Most fatty acids are synthesized by the body, with the exception of linoleic acid, linolenic acid and arachidonic acid, which must be obtained from food. Fatty acids are either monounsaturated or polyunsaturated. Unsaturated fatty acids are preferable to saturated ones, and polyunsaturated are the most favourable, as they are more readily converted into energy; however, a balance of each type is required for adequate nutrition.

Fatty acids depend on adequate intake of zinc, magnesium, selenium, and vitamins B_3, C and E. Fat requirements are slightly increased during pregnancy, for extra energy and to avoid protein calories being misused. Omega-3 fatty acids are essential for the developing fetus, particularly visual and cognitive functioning. They may prevent preterm labour, intra-uterine growth retardation, pre-eclampsia and postnatal depression (Cetin and Koletzko 2008; Innis and Friesen 2008).

Carbohydrates

Required for:

- energy supply for fetal growth
- regulation of gastrointestinal function
- balancing the growth of normal bacterial flora against undesirable flora

Carbohydrate foods:

- starches – potatoes, bread, cereals, pasta, rice, plantain, yam
- intrinsic sugars – fruit (fresh and dried), green vegetables
- extrinsic sugars – milk, fruit juice, honey, sugar, jams, biscuits, cakes

Carbohydrates are classified as sugars (mono and disaccharides) or starches and fibre (polysaccharides). They are the most easily digested nutrients, which can be stored and released as energy when required, preventing excessive oxidation of fats for energy. All carbohydrates are partly broken down in the mouth but mainly in the small intestine, to the simplest compound, glucose; excess glucose is converted into glycogen and stored by the liver. Carbohydrate intake should equate to approximately half of all food consumed. This may indicate a need to increase starches and fibre and decrease fats and proteins.

Vitamins and minerals

Vitamin A

Required for:

- growth and repair of cells
- fighting infection
- synthesis of ribonucleic acid (RNA)

- healthy eyes, especially night vision
- protein metabolism
- aids in detoxification processes
- as an antioxidant

Foods which contain Vitamin A:

- liver, kidneys
- fish oils
- eggs, dairy produce
- apricots, carrots, other yellow vegetables
- broccoli, parsley, green leafy vegetables

Deficiency of vitamin A may cause anaemias, blindness, skin disorders, tooth decay, allergies and gastrointestinal disorders. Absorption can be impeded by vitamin D deficiency, alcohol, coffee, mineral oil, nitrate fertilizers and strong, glaring sunlight. However, women should be discouraged from taking vitamin A supplements (more than 700 mg) or eating excessive amounts of vitamin A-containing foods, such as liver or liver products, during the first trimester, as birth defects have been reported (National Institute for Health and Clinical Excellence (NICE) 2008a).

Thiamin (vitamin B_1)

Required for:

- synthesis of acetylcholine within the cells
- maintenance of healthy nerves, cardiac muscle, digestive tissues
- digestion of carbohydrates

Foods which contain thiamin:

- whole grains
- nuts, seeds, such as sunflower
- Brewer's yeast
- fruit, green vegetables
- liver, kidneys
- fish
- eggs, milk

Thiamin absorption is impaired by stress, food additives, alcohol, coffee, excessive sugar consumption, overcooking vegetables and some antibiotics. Thiamin requirements increase during pregnancy and lactation. Long-term deficiency can lead to irritability, insomnia, weight loss, oedema, poor reflexes and impairment of the cardiovascular, nervous and gastrointestinal systems.

Riboflavin (vitamin B_2)

Required for:

- metabolism of fats, proteins, carbohydrates
- wound healing

- regulation of hormones
- growth and development of the fetus

Foods which contain vitamin B_2:

- foods which also contain thiamin (see list previously mentioned)

Absorption is adversely affected by antibiotics and the contraceptive pill. Deficiency may cause various external lesions, fatigue, personality disturbance, anaemia, digestive upset and hypertension.

Niacin (vitamin B_3)

Required for:

- conversion of food to energy
- metabolism of fats, proteins, carbohydrates
- regulation of hormonal and enzymal actions
- vasodilatation

Foods which contain vitamin B_2:

- liver, lean meat
- poultry
- fish
- grains
- yeast
- butter
- nuts

Absorption of niacin is antagonized by alcohol, stress, coffee, high carbohydrate intake, antibiotics and antitubercular drugs. Various skin and gastrointestinal disturbances may result from inadequate intake and headache, memory loss, insomnia and poor appetite. If a woman is deficient in vitamin B_6, her niacin needs will also increase.

Pyridoxine (vitamin B_6)

Required for:

- production of antibodies
- manufacture of erythrocytes
- enzyme reactions
- development of the nervous system
- healthy teeth and gums
- release of stored glycogen
- synthesis of proteins

Foods which contain pyridoxine:

- foods that contain other B vitamins
- bananas, grapefruit
- prunes, raisins

Absorption is affected by some drugs, including the contraceptive pill, cortisone and penicillamine. Pyridoxine requirements increase during pregnancy and lactation; insufficient intake triggers anaemia, neuritis, convulsions, depression, dermatitis and renal calculi.

Cobalamin (vitamin B₁₂)

Required for:
- bone marrow function and erythrocyte production
- nervous system development, including myelin formation
- development of RNA and DNA
- regulation of normal blood ascorbic acid levels
- carbohydrate metabolism

Foods which contain cobalamin:
- liver, kidney
- fish, shellfish

Absorption may be adversely affected by aspirin, the contraceptive pill, codeine, alcohol and nitrous oxide. Deficiency can result in pernicious anaemia, poor growth, memory loss, nervous disorders and ataxia. Although requirements do not increase significantly during pregnancy, certain women are at risk of deficiency, including vegetarians, epileptics and those with tapeworms. The risk of neural tube defects and that of neurological symptoms, including failure to thrive, irritability and poor milestone development, is increased in the infants of women with vitamin B₁₂ deficiency (Dror and Allen 2008; Ray et al 2007).

Folic acid

Required for:
- production of erythrocytes, in conjunction with B₁₂
- maintenance of the nervous system
- gastrointestinal tract functioning
- production of leucocytes
- production of choline and methionine
- development of the fetus

Foods which contain cobalamin:
- leafy green vegetables
- whole grains, nuts
- oranges
- broccoli
- tuna
- liver, kidney

The incidence of neural tube defects increases in women deficient in folic acid. In the woman, folic acid deficiency can lead to some anaemias, depression, nervousness, cell and tissue disruptions, and premature greying or loss of hair and may contribute to placental abruption (Nilsen et al 2008). Impaired absorption and utilization may occur if the woman is stressed, drinks alcohol, has recently discontinued the contraceptive pill, or is taking drugs such as aspirin, sulphonamides or anticonvulsants.

Vitamin C

Required for:
- cell, tissue, nerve, tooth and bone health
- wound healing
- metabolism of amino acids
- facilitation of iron absorption

Foods which contain vitamin C:
- all citrus fruits
- berries
- melons
- tomatoes
- potatoes
- parsley
- green vegetables (cooking destroys it)
- blackcurrants

Inadequate levels of vitamin C lead to infections, bruising, oedema, haemorrhage, anaemia, poor digestion, tooth and gum disease and scurvy. Some drugs, including aspirin, anticoagulants, antibiotics, diuretics, cortisone, the contraceptive pill and antidepressants, interfere with absorption, as can pollution, industrial toxins, and overcooking or poor storage of food sources. There is some suggestion that daily vitamin C supplementation may reduce the incidence of urinary tract infections in susceptible pregnant women (Ochoa-Brust et al 2007; Hickling and Nitti 2013).

Vitamin D

Required for:
- calcium absorption
- healthy bones and teeth
- renal, cardiac, nervous systems
- blood clotting

Foods which contain Vitamin D:
- fish liver oils
- liver
- Brewer's yeast
- tuna
- avocados
- cereals

The main source of vitamin D is from sunshine. Drugs such as laxatives and antacids inhibit absorption; therefore, women with constipation or heartburn should take care not to overuse them. The woman and fetus both require additional vitamin D to prevent skeletal malformations, rickets, osteoporosis, poor muscle tone, and reduced kidney and parathyroid gland function. Women predisposed to pre-eclampsia should be encouraged to increase their vitamin D intake because vitamin D deficiency may contribute to the disease (Hyppönen et al 2013). Pregnant women who restrict their consumption of milk, a source of vitamin D, protein, calcium and riboflavin, may be at greater risk of having babies of low birthweight (Mannion et al 2006) or who suffer hypocalcaemic convulsions (Camadoo et al 2007). The NICE guidelines on antenatal care (2008a) and maternal nutrition (2008b) advocate vitamin D supplementation for pregnant women with limited exposure to sunlight, such as long-stay antenatal inpatients or those who habitually cover the skin when outdoors. This recommendation also applies to women with a body mass index of 30 or higher, those who are breastfeeding and those who eat a diet low in foods containing vitamin D (NICE CG62 2008, PH11 2008).

Vitamin E

Required for:

- maintenance of erythrocytes
- major bodily functions, including reproduction
- retarding ageing
- helping the body to respond to stress

Foods which contain Vitamin E:

- whole grains
- eggs
- leafy greens, broccoli, cabbage
- avocados
- nuts
- liver, kidneys
- cold-pressed vegetable oils

Vitamin E is destroyed by food processing, rancid fats and oils and inorganic iron. Absorption is adversely affected by mineral oil, the contraceptive pill, chlorine and thyroid hormone. Requirements for vitamin E increase during pregnancy: what was originally called vitamin E is now known to be a group of compounds called tocopherols. In humans, deficiency may result in spontaneous abortion, preterm labour, stillbirth, anaemia, and muscular or cardiovascular diseases.

Calcium

Required for:

- formation of bones and teeth
- utilization of iron

- assisting coagulation
- regulation of cardiac rhythm

Foods which contain Calcium:

- milk and dairy products: yogurt, egg yolk
- sardines and salmon with bones
- green beans
- bone marrow
- tofu, soya beans

High-protein or high-phosphorus diets will antagonize calcium absorption, as will either excessive or inadequate physical activity, or stress. Drugs affecting calcium absorption or utilization include antacids, laxatives, diuretics and anticonvulsants. Deficiencies may lead to bone disorders, such as osteoporosis or osteoarthritis, dental problems, palpitations, hypertension, insomnia or muscle cramps. Routine calcium supplementation may be helpful in women at risk of pre-eclampsia or those who have an identified low level of calcium.

Zinc

Required for:

- cell development in the brain, thyroid gland, liver, kidneys, lungs, prostate gland
- skeletal growth, skin, hair, repair of body tissues, wound healing
- metabolism of proteins, carbohydrates and phosphorus
- facilitation of release of stored vitamin A

Foods which contain zinc:

- herrings, oysters, fish bones
- liver, red meat, meat bones
- eggs, milk
- nuts, whole grains
- mushrooms, leafy green vegetables
- paprika

Zinc requirements rise by approximately 30% during pregnancy to provide for the development of the fetal central nervous system, and by 40% in lactating women. Absorption is enhanced by adequate intakes of calcium, copper, vitamins A, B_6, B_{12} and C, and certain amino acids. Absorption and utilization are impaired by tea, coffee, alcohol, processed grains, iron tablets, the contraceptive pill, and by excess levels of phytates, found in bran and calcium. Jewish women may be deficient in zinc, owing to the presence of phytates in unleavened bread. Zinc neutralizes the toxic effects of cadmium, a contributory factor in hypertension; conversely, high levels of cadmium, found in cigarettes, some processed and canned foods, instant coffee and gelatine, inhibit the action of zinc.

Excessive sweating can cause a loss of up to 3 mg of zinc per day. Zinc is lost in the urine at times of stress and during increased diuresis, such as following high alcohol consumption.

Zinc deficiency can lead to retarded growth and mental development, delayed sexual maturity or sterility (semen contains large quantities of zinc). It may exacerbate gestational sickness and worsen the appearance of striae gravidarum. Women who are zinc deficient may have white spots on their fingernails, experience a metallic taste in the mouth and have a poor appetite. Maternal intake of less than 6 mg daily may lead to babies of low birthweight or prematurity and impaired immune systems (Mahomed et al 2007). Zinc antagonizes lead and cadmium, both of which may be found in higher than normal quantities in the bones of stillborn infants; by inference, therefore, adequate zinc levels may decrease the risk of stillbirth, caused solely by nutritional deficiencies.

Iron

Required for:

- manufacture of haemoglobin for oxygenation of the blood
- protein metabolism
- bone growth
- resistance to disease

Foods which contain iron:

- red meats, liver
- sardines, pilchards, sprats, whitebait, cockles
- eggs, especially the yolks
- wholemeal bread, chapatis, oatcakes
- cereals
- potatoes, parsley, chives, spinach
- dried fruits, nuts, cherries
- soya beans, red kidney beans, lentils, chickpeas

An inadequate iron level will lead to anaemia, fatigue, headache, palpitations and heartburn. Supplementation will be required to treat iron-deficiency anaemia. Dietary iron consumption will normally achieve sufficient serum levels, although a high zinc intake, tea, coffee, intestinal parasites, antacids and tetracycline will interfere with absorption. Women who consume adequate amounts of foods containing vitamins C, E, B_6, B_{12}, folic acid, calcium, copper and other trace elements will normally be able to utilize the iron from dietary intake efficiently. While there is no indication for routine iron supplementation in pregnancy (NICE 2008b), women who require additional iron should be advised to take tablets with orange juice (or other vitamin C-containing drink), which facilitates absorption of the iron, while overconsumption of tea hinders its absorption.

THE IMPORTANCE OF GOOD NUTRITION BEFORE AND DURING PREGNANCY

During pregnancy, the maternal diet must provide sufficient nutrients to meet the woman's usual requirements and those of the growing fetus and stores for use during the third trimester and lactation. A healthy, balanced diet for pregnancy is based on the five food groups in the Eatwell plate (Fig. 17.1) with additional supplements of folic acid during the first trimester and vitamin D if required throughout pregnancy.

The nutritional status of a woman before and during pregnancy influences:

- The growth and development of her fetus and forms the foundations for the child's later health
- The woman's own health, both in the short and long term

Nutrition and preconception

To ensure optimal development of the fetus, some changes to diet and lifestyle may be required even before conception. National UK guidance to women before conception (NICE 2012) recommends women planning pregnancy:

- take folic 400 micrograms daily (5 mg if body mass index (BMI) is of 30 kg/m^2 or more, or other risk factors), and once pregnant, to continue this until the 12th week of pregnancy
- not to take any herbal remedies
- not to exceed 10,000 IU of vitamin A (from supplementation), either before becoming pregnant or at any time during pregnancy.

Women who are trying to become pregnant are also advised in proposed 2016 guidance to stop drinking alcohol altogether (Department of Health (DH) 2016). Couples who are trying for a baby are also advised to stop smoking, as smoking (including passive smoking) may reduce the chances of conceiving and can harm the fetus. Infertility can be exacerbated by nutritional deficiencies (Chavarro et al 2007 and 2008), and dietary advice is a major component of preconceptional care, especially for medical conditions (Tieu et al 2008).

Body weight seems to be associated with fertility. If a woman who is obese (BMI >30 kg/m^2) or underweight (BMI <19 kg/m^2) is having problems conceiving, she should be advised that achieving a healthy body weight may increase her chances of conceiving. Ovulation is dependent on adipose tissue (fat) distribution, equal to at least 17% of a woman's total body weight; women who are anorexic are thus less likely to conceive and more likely to miscarry from vitamin and mineral imbalances. Obesity

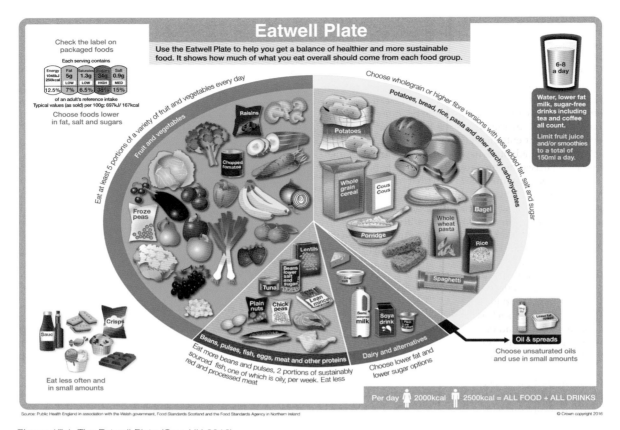

Figure 17.1 The Eatwell Plate (Gov, UK 2016).

can lead to potential health risks for the infant including neural tube defects, heart defects, cleft palate and/or cleft lip, anorectal atresia, hydrocephaly and limb reduction abnormalities. Increasing obesity is associated with a proportionally increased risk of adverse pregnancy outcomes, for example, an increased risk of impaired glucose tolerance, gestational diabetes, miscarriage, stillbirth and maternal death (NICE 2012).

Similarly, male infertility due to poor sperm production may be associated with nutritional deficiency, particularly folic acid, zinc and vitamin E_1 selenium, exacerbated by contemporary Western diets (Eskenazi et al 2005; West et al 2005).

A nutritional diet is high in beneficial nutrients, such as those that suppress the effects of toxicity caused by environmental pollution, and low in substances such as nicotine, tea, coffee, alcohol and drugs (Vujkovic et al 2007). The contraceptive pill interferes with the absorption of vitamin B_6 and zinc and should ideally be discontinued for at least 3 months preconception. Premenstrual syndrome, triggered by magnesium, zinc, vitamin B_6 and other vital nutrient deficiency, may affect conception. Women

who are deficient in essential fatty acids, zinc, manganese and vitamin E or who indulge in potentially toxic substances are also more susceptible to recurrent miscarriage (Bailey and Berry 2005; Ronnenberg et al 2007). Research by Konje et al (2008) on behalf of The Food Standards Agency advised to limit daily caffeine intake in pregnancy, ideally keeping this below 200 mg a day. This is roughly two mugs of coffee a day, although caffeine is also present in tea, chocolate, some soft drinks and certain medicines. Too much caffeine might result in a baby having a lower birthweight than it should, which can increase the risk of some health conditions for the baby in later life, or could possibly result in spontaneous miscarriage.

Nutrition and pregnancy

Healthy eating is important at any time, but particularly during pregnancy when women are supplying nutrients for themselves and their growing baby. After conception, in the first few weeks of pregnancy, the fetus relies on simple diffusion of oxygen and nutrients from the woman's blood. From about 12 weeks, the placenta controls the nutrient and oxygen supply to the fetus and the removal of waste products. Maternal supply of nutrients needs to accord with fetal demand to achieve healthy growth and development of the fetus, thus avoiding potential consequences for long-term health. Although the woman has some ability to adapt to ensure a supply of nutrients to the fetus, her dietary supply remains important. Interdependency between nutrients emphasizes the importance of dietary balance: for example, supply of micronutrients may alter the way in which macronutrients are utilized for energy.

Physiological adaptations of the woman in pregnancy include: increased absorption and decreased excretion of some nutrients, together with increased storage of nutrients in early pregnancy to meet the needs of the woman and fetus later in pregnancy and during lactation. Consequently, pregnant women only require higher amounts of some nutrients in their diet: thiamine, riboflavin, folate, vitamins A, C and D, calcium, selenium, iodine and omega 3 and 6 fatty acids.

Inadequate preconceptional and antenatal nutrition may have adverse fetal effects, increasing the risk of perinatal morbidity and mortality, low birthweight or preterm infants, birth defects such as neural tube defects (Carmichael et al 2007; Tamura and Picciano 2006) or maternal complications (Bodnar et al 2006). Impaired maternal nutrition can also adversely affect fetal disease programming, increasing the tendency for hypertension and cardiovascular disease in adult life (Plagemann et al 2008; Woods 2007).

Fetal undernutrition can occur in adolescent pregnancies because of competition between the young woman and the fetus for nutrients. Low birthweight and preterm birth are twice as common and neonatal mortality is almost three times higher in adolescent pregnancies compared to adult pregnancies (Wu et al 2004).

Nutritional advice in pregnancy

Midwifery advice about healthy eating during pregnancy can have long-term benefits for the whole family. Midwives should enable discussions of healthy eating throughout pregnancy, utilizing tools such as the Eatwell guide (Fig. 17.1) to motivate and encourage changes in lifestyle. Expectant women should be advised (NICE PH27 2010) to:

- Base every meal on starchy foods such as bread, potatoes, rice, pasta, chapatis, yams and breakfast cereal
- Eat as much fresh food as possible, with a minimum of five portions of fruit, vegetables and salad daily
- Choose foods rich in protein: lean meat, chicken, fish, eggs and pulses
- Eat more fibre rich foods: wholegrain breads and pasta, brown rice, wholegrain cereals, pulses, fruit and vegetables

- Eat plenty of dairy foods for calcium: milk, cheese and yogurts
- Make snacks nutritious: pita bread, yogurt, vegetable sticks, fruit
- Minimize salt intake and salty foods: do not add salt to food
- Get active and keep a healthy weight
- Drink plenty of water (recommended 1900 mL per day in pregnancy, British Diabetic Association (BDA) 2013)
- Eat breakfast

Regular meals with healthy snacks in between should be encouraged to avoid highs and lows in maternal blood glucose levels. There is evidence that maternal nutrition in pregnancy can influence fetal programming because of in utero physiological adaptations, as seen in the Dutch famine 1944-45 (Lumey 1998).

Some foods should be avoided during pregnancy, as acquired infections may affect fetal well-being and women should reduce or eliminate their consumption of the foods likely to harbour these pathogens (NICE PH11 2008). Examples include *Listeria monocytogenes*, found in nonpasteurized milk, soft cheeses, such as Brie and Camembert, blue-veined cheeses, meat and vegetable pâtés and uncooked or undercooked ready-prepared meals, while *Salmonella* infection can arise from eating raw or partially cooked meat or eggs or egg products, such as mayonnaise. Certain protein foods are potential infection sources for pregnant women, in particular, contaminated meat; advice regarding thorough cooking may prevent gastrointestinal disorders. Raw meat may be contaminated with *Listeria monocytogenes* or *Toxoplasma gondii*, so pregnant women should avoid raw or undercooked meat. *Listeria monocytogenes* may also be present in unpasteurized milk, including in soft cheeses.

Weight gain in pregnancy

NICE (PH27 2010) advised that dieting during pregnancy is not recommended, as it may harm the health of the unborn child. The amount of weight a woman may gain in pregnancy can vary a great deal. Only some of it is due to increased body fat – the fetus, placenta, amniotic fluid and increases in maternal blood and fluid volume all contribute.

Many pregnant women ask health professionals for advice on what constitutes appropriate weight gain during pregnancy. However, there are no evidence-based UK guidelines on recommended weight-gain ranges during pregnancy. The Institute of Medicine (2009) in America published revised weight gain recommendations for pregnancy (Box 17.1); these have met with controversial reactions from some professionals who believe that the weight gain targets are too high, especially for overweight and obese women. Also, these perceived high weight gain targets

Box 17.1	Institute of Medicine (2009) weight gain recommendations		
Prepregnancy weight category	BMI	Total recommended weight gain in pregnancy	Mean range (kg/week)
Underweight	<18.5	12.5–18 kg	1 (1–1.3)
Normal Weight	18.5–24.9	11.5–16 kg	1 (0.8–1)
Overweight	25–29.9	7–11.5 kg	0.6 (0.5–0.7)
Obese	30 and over	5–9 kg	0.5 (0.4–0.6)

do not address concerns regarding postpartum weight retention (Nehring et al 2011). In addition, concerns have been raised that the guidelines do not differentiate degrees of obesity, especially for morbidly obese women. However, these currently provide some guidance on weight gain in pregnancy.

Weight gain depends on maternal diet, activity, food availability and gestational factors, such as sickness or multiple pregnancies. In women within a normal BMI range at conception, a balanced diet usually results in full-term babies of adequate birthweight. Preconceptional, gestational and lactational nutrition affect the birthweight, well-being and long-term prognosis of infants, with effect on risk of maternal obesity in later life (Uauy et al 2008).

Obesity has become a significant issue in the Western world, with serious consequences for UK maternity services (Heslehurst et al 2007). Around a third to a half of pregnant women in the United States (US), UK and Australia are overweight or obese (Callaway et al 2006; Centre for Maternal and Child Enquiries (CMACE) 2010; American College of Obstetricians, Gynecologists (ACOG) 2013). Pregnancy is an important influence in the development of obesity in women (Mannan et al 2013). In Europe and the US, 20% to 40% of women gain more weight during pregnancy than is recommended (Thangaratinam et al 2010). A national 3-year study conducted by the Centre for Maternal and Child Enquiries (CMACE 2010) across Maternity units in the UK, found that 4.99% of women had a BMI greater than or equal to 35, 2.01% greater than or equal to 40 and 0.19% over 50. The stillbirth rate in this cohort was 8.6 per 1000 total births compared to 3.9 per 1000 in the general population. Many women retain weight gained over several pregnancies, and women with high weight gain during pregnancy tend to retain this weight in the longer term (Linne et al 2004). Obesity has been linked to an increased risk of complications during pregnancy and birth, including gestational diabetes mellitus (Scott-Pillai et al 2013), hypertension (Callaway et al 2007), increased emergency caesarean section rates and increased postpartum haemorrhage (Sebire et al 2001). There are also increased risks for the child, including preterm birth, admission to a neonatal unit, and birth defects (Scott-Pillai 2013). Healthcare costs are significantly higher in overweight and obese pregnant

women compared to normal weight women (Morgan et al 2014). Excess maternal weight gain during pregnancy is also associated with child obesity (Oken et al 2007).

Women who restrict their energy intake in pregnancy also cause concern. In societies where lack of food forcibly restricts energy intake, maternal metabolic adaptations enable energy production for fetal growth. However, care must be taken when advising immigrant women in Britain, such as those from the Indian subcontinent. Fasting during the month of Ramadan is one of the five pillars of Islam, although pregnant women are exempt if it poses a risk to their health. However, some Muslim women still choose to fast, despite the health implications. Midwives should be aware of this and inquire about plans for fasting, making plans to ensure the woman is safe.

Anorexia nervosa and bulimia nervosa are associated with poor pregnancy outcome, including subfertility, risk of miscarriage, obstetric complications, intra-uterine growth retardation and postnatal depression. Midwives should be alert to signs of possible eating disorders, particularly in women with a very low body mass index, those who appear to have poor body image and those who report prolonged hyperemesis gravidarum.

Reflective activity 17.1

Describe a balanced diet appropriate in pregnancy and give examples of meals for a day and the nutrients they contain.

NUTRITION AS A THERAPEUTIC INTERVENTION

Nausea and vomiting

Many women find that nausea is exacerbated by hypoglycaemia, especially if they are also tired. Advice can be given by the midwife to eat small, frequent meals of complex carbohydrate foods, such as bread, cereal or potatoes, but not those that are high in sugar or salt. Bananas are a good source of carbohydrate, and may also help prevent potassium deficiency. Sickness in pregnancy is worse for women lacking in vitamin B$_6$, magnesium and zinc. Women should be advised to eat foods rich in these substances or to take a good-quality supplement. Reducing the amount of dairy produce may also help, as may increasing the intake of citrus fruits or juices (Tiran 2004 and 2006). (See Ch. 52.)

Constipation

The midwife can advise women to increase their intake of high-fibre foods, but more importantly, they must increase their fluid intake to at least 2 litres of water daily. Tea consumption should be decreased. Tannin reduces peristalsis and inhibits the absorption of iron, which might result in the prescription of iron tablets; these, in turn, exacerbate constipation.

Women should eat five portions of fresh fruits and vegetables a day, unrefined carbohydrates, seeds, grains and pulses, such as beans (Derbyshire et al 2006). Bran should be *avoided*, unless there is a substantial increase in fluid intake, as it absorbs fluid from the intestines and makes the stool hard, increasing the severity of the constipation. Wheat and wheat products, such as bread and cereals, may increase bloating or abdominal discomfort, particularly if the problem was present before pregnancy, as it may be caused by mild wheat intolerance. Long-term use of laxatives should be discouraged, as they will not treat the cause of the problem and can often create other side effects. Vitamin C supplements may be necessary in some women. If iron tablets are prescribed for anaemia and found to exacerbate the problem, other sources of iron-containing foods should be advised. It may be necessary to suggest alternatives to medication, such as herbal liquid preparations, available from health food stores.

Heartburn and indigestion

The woman should be advised to eat small, frequent meals and avoid drinking with meals, but maintain a high fluid intake between meals. She should avoid foods that aggravate the condition, such as spicy or greasy foods, as well as coffee, tea, alcohol and cigarettes. Milk and milk products do not always help relieve the symptoms and may exacerbate them, as may sugar, sweet foods, wheat and bread. Excessive antacid use should be avoided, especially those containing aluminum, as this may be absorbed and cause mild toxicity.

Anaemia

Anaemia may be prevented, or the effects reduced, by encouraging the woman to eat foods rich in iron. Her diet should include fresh green leafy vegetables, such as cabbage, spinach, watercress, parsley, spring onions, chives, sprouted grains and seeds. Seaweeds, nettle tops and dandelion leaves are also good sources of iron. Dried prunes, raisins, figs and unsulphured apricots are helpful, as are blackcurrants, blackberries, cherries and loganberries. Wholegrain bread, oatcakes and chapatis should be eaten rather than highly refined carbohydrates. Pilchards, salmon, kippers and organic liver also provide iron. Bran should be avoided, as it inhibits the absorption of iron from foods. Tea and coffee, particularly when taken with meals, have similar effects. Fruits and vegetables that contain Vitamin C, that enhances the uptake of iron, include kiwi fruits, oranges, rosehips, potatoes, cauliflower, broccoli, Brussels sprouts and parsley. If iron supplements are prescribed, the woman should be advised to take them with a glass of orange juice and avoid drinking too much tea or coffee.

Candida albicans ('thrush')

Candida albicans yeast infection (see Ch. 55) is common in pregnancy and, if left untreated, can complicate delivery and may develop into a chronic condition. Women on antibiotics, especially those who have had recurrent infections or when antibiotics are required long term, are more susceptible to thrush. Zinc deficiency compromises the immune system, so infection is more likely, and any nutritional deficiencies should be corrected, initially with an increase in foods containing the relevant minerals and vitamins, or with supplements.

Refined carbohydrates and yeast-containing foods exacerbate the condition and facilitate multiplication of the *Candida* bacteria, so should be eliminated from the diet, especially white flour, white or brown sugar or any foods containing these. Similarly, foods containing yeast should be avoided, for example, bread, cheese, alcohol, yeast extract, frozen or concentrated orange juice, grapes, grape juice, unpeeled fruits, raisins, sultanas and B vitamin supplements (unless labelled as yeast-free). Food that is not absolutely fresh should not be consumed, whereas foods containing natural antifungal agents, such as garlic, fresh herbs, spices and fresh green leafy vegetables, can be eaten frequently.

CONCLUSION

Adequate nutrition during pregnancy and lactation is vital for good maternal and fetal health. The midwife is in an invaluable position to educate women, thereby influencing family nutrition and health from the beginning. This chapter has discussed the needs of normal women and no mention has been made of the special nutritional requirements of some women, for example, diabetics. Midwives should have a basic knowledge of the main dietary needs of women and be able to advise women accordingly. However, it is also important that midwives are able to identify women more at risk of poor nutrition, so that they can be referred to a specialist, nutritional therapist or dietician for appropriate information. It has not been possible here to provide more than a general introduction to the subject of nutrition, but further suggestions are on the website.

Key Points

- Good nutrition is essential both before and during pregnancy, for the woman and the fetus. The midwife has a vital role to play in educating parents about good family nutrition.
- There is a correlation between poor nutritional status and pathophysiological conditions in pregnancy. Nutrition can be used as a therapeutic tool to correct or treat some of these conditions.
- Midwives require a comprehensive understanding of what constitutes a balanced diet to advise women in their care accordingly.

References

American College of Obstetricians, Gynecologists (ACOG): Committee opinion no. 549: obesity in pregnancy, *Obstet Gynecol* 121(1):213–217, 2013.

Bailey LB, Berry RJ: Folic acid supplementation and the occurrence of congenital heart defects, orofacial clefts, multiple births, and miscarriage, *Am J Clin Nutr* 81(5):1213S–1217S, 2005.

Bodnar LM, Tang G, Ness RB, et al: Periconceptional multivitamin use reduces the risk of preeclampsia, *Am J Epidemiol* 164(5):470–477, 2006.

British Diabetic Association (BDA). *Fluid fact sheet* (website). www.bda.uk.com/foodfacts/fluid.pdf. 2013.

Callaway LK, McIntyre HD, O'Callaghan M, et al: The association of hypertensive disorders of pregnancy with weight gain over the subsequent 21 years: findings from a prospective cohort study, *Am J Epidemiol* 166(4):421–428, 2007.

Callaway LK, Prins JB, Chang AM, et al: The prevalence and impact of overweight and obesity in an Australian obstetric population, *Med J Aust* 184(2):56–59, 2006.

Camadoo L, Tibbott R, Isaza F: Maternal vitamin D deficiency associated with neonatal hypocalcaemic convulsions, *Nutr J* 6(9):23, 2007.

Carmichael SL, Yang W, Herring A, et al: Maternal food insecurity is associated with increased risk of certain birth defects, *J Nutr* 137(9):2087–2092, 2007.

Cetin I, Koletzko B: Long-chain omega-3 fatty acid supply in pregnancy and lactation, *Curr Opin Clin Nutr Metab Care* 11(3):297–302, 2008.

Chavarro JE, Rich-Edwards JW, Rosner BA, et al: Diet and lifestyle in the prevention of ovulatory disorder infertility, *Obstet Gynecol* 110(5):1050–1058, 2007.

Chavarro JE, Rich-Edwards JW, Rosner BA, et al: Use of multivitamins, intake of B vitamins, and risk of ovulatory infertility, *Fertil Steril* 89(3):668–676, 2008.

Centre for Maternal and Child Enquiries (CMACE): *Maternal obesity in the UK: Findings from a national project*, London, CMACE, 2010.

Department of Health (DH): *How to keep health risks from drinking alcohol to a low level: public consultation on proposed new guidelines*, 2016.

Derbyshire E, Davies J, Costarelli V, et al: Diet, physical inactivity and the prevalence of constipation throughout and after pregnancy, *Matern Child Nutr* 2(3):127–134, 2006.

Dror DK, Allen LH: Effect of vitamin B12 deficiency on neurodevelopment in infants: current knowledge and possible mechanisms, *Nutr Rev* 66(5):250–255, 2008.

Eatwell Plate. The Eatwell Guide Gov.uk 2016 (website). https://www.gov.uk/government/publications/the-eatwell-guide. 2016.

Eskenazi B, Kidd SA, Marks AR, et al: Antioxidant intake is associated with semen quality in healthy men, *Hum Reprod* 20(4):1006–1012, 2005.

Heslehurst N, Lang R, Rankin J, et al: Obesity in pregnancy: a study of the impact of maternal obesity on NHS maternity services, *BJOG* 114(3):334–342, 2007.

Hickling D, Nitti V: Management of recurrent urinary tract infection in healthy adult women, *Urology Rev Urol* 15(2), 2013.

Hypponen E, Cavadino A, Williams D, et al: Vitamin D and Pre-eclampsia: Original data systematic review and metal-analysis, eISSN 1421-9697 online. 2013.

Innis SM, Friesen RW: Essential n-3 fatty acids in pregnant women and early visual acuity maturation in term infants, *Am J Clin Nutr* 87(3):548–557, 2008.

Institute of Medicine (Subcommittees on Nutritional Status and Weight Gain During Pregnancy and Dietary Intake and Nutrient Supplements During Pregnancy, Committee on Nutritional Status During Pregnancy and Lactation, Food and Nutrition Board): *Nutrition during pregnancy: part I, weight Gain; part II, nutrient supplements*, Washington, DC, National Academy Press, 2009.

Konje JC, Cade JE: Maternal caffeine intake during pregnancy and risk of fetal growth restriction: a large prospective observational study, *BMJ* 337:a2332, 2008.

Linne Y, Dye L, Barkeling B, Rossner S: Long-term weight development in women: a 15-year follow-up of the effects of pregnancy, *Obes Res* 12(7):1166–1178, 2004.

Lumey LH: Reproductive outcome in women prenatally exposed to undernutrition: a review of findings from the Dutch famine birth cohort, *Proc Nutr Soc* 57:129–135, 1998.

Mahomed K, Bhutta Z, Middleton P: Zinc supplementation for improving pregnancy and infant outcome, *Cochrane Database Syst Rev* (2):CD000230, 2007.

Mannan M, Doi SAR, Mamun AA: Association between weight gain during pregnancy and postpartum weight retention and obesity: a bias-adjusted meta-analysis, *Nutr Rev* 71(6):343–352, 2013.

Mannion CA, Gray-Donald K, Koski KG: Association of low intake of milk and vitamin D during pregnancy with decreased birth weight, *Can Med Assoc J* 174(9):1273–1277, 2006.

Morgan KL, Rahman MA, Macey S, et al: Obesity in pregnancy: a retrospective prevalence-based study on health service utilisation and costs on the NHS, *BMJ Open* 4(2), 2014.

National Institute for Health and Clinical Excellence (NICE): *Public Health Guidance 11: maternal and child nutrition*, 2008a.

National Institute for Health and Clinical Excellence (NICE): *Clinical guideline 62: antenatal care – routine care for the healthy pregnant woman*, 2008b.

National Institute for Health and Clinical Excellence (NICE): *Public Health Guidance 27: weight management before, during and after pregnancy*, 2010.

National Institute for Health and Clinical Excellence (NICE): *Clinical knowledge summary: pre-conception advice and management*, 2012.

Nehring I, Schmoll S, Beyerlein A, et al: Gestational weight gain and long-term postpartum weight retention: a meta-analysis, *Am J Clin Nutr* 94(5):1225–1231, 2011.

Nilsen RM, Vollset SE, Rasmussen SA, et al: Folic acid and multivitamin supplement use and risk of placental abruption: a population-based registry study, *Am J Epidemiol* 167(7):867–874, 2008.

Ochoa-Brust GJ, Fernández AR, Villanueva-Ruiz GJ, et al: Daily intake of 100 mg ascorbic acid as urinary tract infection prophylactic agent during pregnancy, *Acta Obstet Gynecol Scand* 86(7):783–787, 2007.

Oken E, Taveras EM, Kleinman KP, et al: Gestational weight gain and child adiposity at age 3 years, *Am J Obstet Gynecol* 196(4):322. e1–e8, 2007.

Plagemann A, Harder T, Dudenhausen JW: The diabetic pregnancy, macrosomia, and perinatal nutritional programming, *Nestle Nutr Workshop Ser Pediatr Program* 61:91–102, 2008.

Ray JG, Wyatt PR, Thompson MD, et al: Vitamin B_{12} and the risk of neural tube defects in a folic-acid-fortified population, *Epidemiology* 18(3):362–366, 2007.

Ronnenberg AG, Venners SA, Xu X, et al: Preconception B-vitamin and homocysteine status, conception, and early pregnancy loss, *Am J Epidemiol* 166(3):304–312, 2007.

Scott-Pillai R, Spence D, Cardwell C, et al: The impact of body mass index on maternal and neonatal outcomes: a retrospective study in a UK obstetric population, 2004-2011, *BJOG* 120:932–939, 2013.

Sebire NJ, Jolly M, Harris JP, et al: Maternal obesity and pregnancy outcome: a study of 287,213 pregnancies in London, *Int J Obes Relat Metab Disord* 25(8):1175–1182, 2001.

Tamura T, Picciano MF: Folate and human reproduction, *Am J Clin Nutr* 83(5):993–1016, 2006.

Thangaratinam S, Jolly K: Obesity in pregnancy: a review of reviews on the effectiveness of interventions, *BJOG* 117:1309–1312, 2010.

Tieu J, Crowther CA, Middleton P: Dietary advice in pregnancy for preventing gestational diabetes mellitus, *Cochrane Database Syst Rev* (2):CD006674, 2008.

Tiran D: *Nausea and vomiting in pregnancy: an integrated approach to care*, London, Elsevier, 2004.

Tiran D: Nutritional approaches to nausea and vomiting in pregnancy, *RCM Midwives J* 9(9):350–352, 2006.

Uauy R, Kain J, Mericq V, et al: Nutrition, child growth, and chronic disease prevention, *Ann Med* 40(1):11–12, 2008.

Vujkovic M, Ocke MC, van der Spek PJ, et al: Maternal Western dietary patterns and the risk of developing a cleft lip with or without a cleft palate, *Obstet Gynecol* 110(2 Pt 1):378–384, 2007.

West MC, Anderson L, McClure N, et al: Dietary oestrogens and male fertility potential, *Hum Fertil (Camb)* 8(3):197–207, 2005.

Woods LL: Maternal nutrition and predisposition to later kidney disease, *Curr Drug Targets* 8(8):906–913, 2007.

Wu G, Bazer FW, Wallace JM, et al: Maternal nutrition and fetal development, *J Nutr* 134:2169–2172, 2004.

Resources and additional reading

NHS Choices http://www.nhs.uk/ conditions/pregnancy-and-baby/ pages/healthy-pregnancy-diet.aspx.

The British Nutrition Foundation has a range of resources for women and midwives. https://www.nutrition. org.uk/nutritionscience/life/ pregnancy-and-pre-conception.html.

The Eatwell Guide Gov.UK 2016 https://www.gov.uk/government/ publications/the-eatwell-guide.

The Royal College of Midwives (RCM) on line learning i-learn has a number of modules on diet, nutrition and weight management in pregnancy. www.rcm.org.uk.

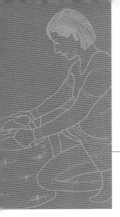

Chapter 18

Complementary therapies and natural remedies in pregnancy and birth: responsibilities of midwives

Denise Tiran

INTRODUCTION

Complementary and alternative medicine (CAM) comprises any form of healthcare, which sits outside the mainstream health modalities (medicine, midwifery, physiotherapy, etc.), and usually outside conventional health service provision. The focus of complementary and alternative medicine is 'holism' in which the client is viewed as a whole, taking into account their physical, mental and spiritual condition – often referred to as 'body-mind-spirit' medicine.

'CAM' is the term often used by medical practitioners who practise therapies such as acupuncture or homeopathy alongside their normal practice. 'Complementary therapies' incorporates strategies that can be used as an *adjunct to* conventional healthcare, whereas 'alternative therapies' are used *instead* of orthodox care, although this latter term is less frequently used now. A more commonly used term is 'integrative medicine', which implies that the therapies are integrated into conventional healthcare, as

seen in the clinical fields of oncology and palliative care. Any complementary therapies used for pregnant, labouring or newly birthed mothers should be *complementary* to standard maternity care, whether they are provided by independent practitioners or used by midwives within antenatal, intrapartum or postnatal care.

However, this term 'complementary therapies' is not simply a single 'add-on' to maternity care: there are *several hundred* different modalities, each with its own specialist knowledge, skills, mechanism of action, indications, precautions, contraindications and side effects. Complementary therapies may be manual techniques such as massage, osteopathy, chiropractic, reflexology or shiatsu; energy therapies, for example, acupuncture or homeopathy; or psychological therapies such as hypnosis. The term 'natural remedies' applies to any substances that are not commercially prepared drugs. This includes herbal medicines and aromatherapy oils, all of which act pharmacologically, and energy-based medicines, such as homeopathic and Bach flower remedies, plus the remedies made from indigenous plants used in Chinese medicine, Indian Ayurveda and other traditional forms of medicine. Nutritional supplements and herbal teas, which act pharmacologically, when intended for use as therapeutic agents, would also fit into this category.

Incidence of use of complementary therapies and natural remedies

During pregnancy, women demand more choices and wish to remain in control of their bodies at a time when they can feel very vulnerable. Increasingly, pregnant women request information and advice on natural ways to deal with the discomforts they experience, not least because they are warned that they should, wherever possible, avoid taking medication – sometimes even that which is prescribed by the doctor. Some women consult independent therapists before conception, then continue to use complementary therapies once pregnant, or they may self-administer natural remedies at home; some may wish to be accompanied in labour by an independent therapist or a doula or birth supporter who uses complementary therapies. Many pregnant women are now self-administering natural remedies, such as raspberry leaf tea, echinacea or homeopathic arnica, or using aromatherapy oils at home. However, many women do not appreciate that there are specified doses, indications, contraindications, precautions and possible side effects and interactions with drugs that apply to natural remedies, particularly herbal medicines that act pharmacologically.

In Westernized countries, the incidence of use of complementary therapies and natural remedies in pregnancy is estimated to be anything from 6% to 91% (Bishop et al 2011; Hall et al 2011; Babycentre 2011; Frawley et al 2014; Pallivalapila et al 2015). However, the lower figures may not reflect a true picture because the majority of studies focus on the self-administration of natural remedies, rather than complementary therapies for which women may have consulted qualified practitioners. This was illustrated in a large study (Kennedy et al 2013) across 23 countries in Europe, North and South America and Australia, which showed an average herbal medicine use of 28.9%, with wide variations between countries, the highest being 69% in Russia.

Use of natural remedies appears to increase, as pregnancy progresses and women prepare for birth (Bishop et al 2011), but declines postnatally (Birdee et al 2014), although many women turn to herbal remedies to aid lactation (Sim et al 2013). Only about half of women using complementary therapies or taking natural remedies inform their maternity care providers, possibly because they think it is not important or that midwives and doctors will be sceptical or angry (Strouss et al 2014). Most women appear to access the Internet, television and magazines or friends and family for information about complementary therapies and natural remedies rather than referring to health professionals (Strouss et al 2014).

The risks and benefits of complementary therapies and natural remedies in pregnancy and birth

Facilitating women to use complementary therapies safely empowers them and provides them with additional resources, which are not only therapeutically effective but also often relaxing and calming. Many therapies, particularly massage, aromatherapy, reflexology and acupuncture, are known to reduce stress hormones, such as cortisol, which has a direct physiological advantage in facilitating oxytocin output, thus contributing to a more efficient labour (Wu et al 2014; McVicar et al 2007). Given that many women continue to work almost for the entire

pregnancy, with all the demands of modern-day life, accessing complementary therapies may be one of the few ways in which they can have some time for themselves. In addition, women may feel that the midwife is too busy and overworked to have time to discuss the myriad worries and anxieties they may have, so perhaps they also turn to complementary therapies as an opportunity to off-load some of their concerns.

Women may also wish to access complementary therapies for the treatment of specific conditions, especially if they feel their symptoms are not validated by midwives or doctors. Examples include consulting an osteopath or chiropractor for the treatment of backache, rather than waiting for an appointment with the National Health Service (NHS) physiotherapist, or having acupuncture treatment for sickness, a problem with which women are often left to cope alone, or feel that their general practitioner dismisses it as normal without any regard for how it is affecting the woman and her family.

During labour, relaxation therapies such as hypnosis ("hypno-birthing") can help keep the woman calm; aromatherapy, shiatsu or acupuncture may aid contractions; and aromatherapy and reflexology can be useful to ease pain. In the early puerperium, various remedies may influence perineal healing, including lavender (Sheikhan et al 2012), homeopathic arnica (Oberbaum et al 2005), cinnamon cream (Mohammadi et al 2014) and aloe vera with calendula (Eghdampour et al 2013).

However, there is a common misconception that, because these therapies and remedies are 'natural', they are also 'safe' or at least, safer than drugs. This seems to be a particular problem in relation to natural remedies, most notably herbal teas and aromatherapy oils, and may be one of the reasons why women do not feel the need to inform midwives of their use. However, *no* natural substance or manual technique is completely safe: if a remedy or therapy has a therapeutic action, whether it is pharmacological, energy-based, psychological or some other mechanism, there will be specific indications for use, and significant contraindications and precautions. This author has received numerous anecdotal reports from midwives of women's inappropriate use of natural remedies, resulting in preterm labour, hypertonic uterine action and fetal distress. Midwives and other maternity professionals must also account for the multiethnic nature of today's society: many women from Asia, Africa and the Middle East use remedies sent from their home countries, most of which will be unfamiliar to UK maternity care providers.

Reflective activity 18.1

- Ask 10 women in your care whether or not they have used any complementary therapies or natural remedies, either before or during pregnancy.

Traditional Chinese medicine

Acupuncture is based on the principle that the body has energy channels running through it, transporting internal energy (called *Qi*) and linking one part of the body to another. These channels, called meridians, have been shown to exist anatomically (Hong et al 2007) and have focus points (acupuncture points or *tsubos*) along them where the energy is concentrated. When the body, mind and spirit are in optimum health, energy flows along the meridians unimpeded, but disorder, disease or – in the case of pregnancy – altered physiology may cause blockages (stagnation or deficiency) or overstimulation (excess) of energy at specific acupuncture points. Fine needles are inserted, or **acupressure** (thumb pressure) may be used, to rebalance the body's internal energy and facilitate a return to homeostasis.

Acupuncture and acupressure can be effective for fertility problems (Nandi et al 2014; Zheng et al 2014), sickness during pregnancy and post-caesarean (Noroozinia et al 2013; Lythgoe 2012; El-Deeb and Ahmadi 2011) and for pain relief in labour (Mucuk and Baser 2014; Vixner et al 2012). Djakovic et al (2015) suggest that acupuncture in the first and second stages of labour may facilitate better placental separation in the third stage, thereby reducing retained placenta and postpartum haemorrhage. Women who receive acupuncture during pregnancy generally perceive it as being beneficial in treating a wide range of conditions (Soliday and Hapke 2013).

Another element of Chinese medicine, **moxibustion**, involves the use of sticks of dried compressed mugwort (herb) used as a heat source to stimulate acupuncture points where energy is deficient. It is best known in maternity care for turning breech presentation to cephalic by focusing the heat source over an acupuncture point at the base of the little (fifth) toe nails. It is thought to be between 88% and 60% effective (Vas et al 2013; Manyande and Grabowska 2009), but may be even more so when combined with acupuncture (Smith and Betts 2014). Midwives in some units now offer moxibustion in dedicated 'breech clinics' (Weston and Grabowska 2012; personal communications with midwives). The procedure can be taught to the mother and her partner and performed at 34 to 35 weeks gestation for 30 minutes a day for 5 days.

It is, however, of concern that some women purchase moxa sticks to perform the procedure at home, often without informing their midwives. The contraindications for moxibustion are exactly the same as those for external cephalic version, *plus* hypertension and severe respiratory disease. If the woman has been told that it is inappropriate for her to have an external cephalic version, she should not do moxibustion. The moxa heat is known to increase blood pressure, so anyone with hypertension should avoid the procedure; the smoking sticks could also trigger asthma or hay fever attacks in susceptible women. Although some maternity units offer external cephalic version when there is a uterine scar from a previous caesarean section, women should be very strongly discouraged from using moxibustion in this situation. External cephalic version performed under controlled conditions in the hospital, where there are facilities to attend to any emergency that arises, is very different from doing a procedure at home, which is relatively new to Western obstetrics, not well understood and on which there is a need for further research.

Shiatsu is a modern Japanese form of **acupressure**, incorporating pressure and holding techniques combined with gentle stretching. Touch is used as a means of adjusting the internal energies of the body, treating and preventing energy imbalances. A study by midwives in Bristol (Ingram et al 2005) indicated that women who were taught self-administration of specific shiatsu points were more likely to labour spontaneously than those who did not use the techniques, although recent research by midwives in collaboration with this author refutes this (Gregson et al 2015). Shiatsu or acupressure techniques to stimulate contractions ease labour pain and anxiety and can be very effective (Moradi et al 2014; Akbarzadeh et al 2014).

Natural remedies

Aromatherapy, which is part of herbal medicine, is one of the most popular therapies used by pregnant women (Sibbritt et al 2014) and is increasingly being incorporated into midwifery practice. Concentrated essential oils extracted from plants contain chemical constituents with various physiological and psychological effects. Aromatherapy works through a combination of the chemistry, the aromatic effect of the essential oils on the brain and the method of administration. The most common method of administration is massage, but oils can also be added to water, for example, in the bath (but must not be added directly into the water in the birthing pool). The oils are also absorbed through inhalation, the chemicals being transported both to the systemic circulation via the respiratory tract, crossing to all organs – including via the placenta to the fetus and via the olfactory system to the limbic system, where they affect the mood and emotions. Importantly, if you can smell the aromas, you are inhaling the chemicals which will enter the circulation. Women using vaporizers at home should not use them for longer than 10 to 15 minutes at a time and *never* all night or for the duration of a labour, nor should they be used in the baby's room. Gastrointestinal (oral) use, pessaries and suppositories should not be used at all during pregnancy. The use of vaporizers in an institutional setting, such as the labour ward or birth centre, is unsafe and unethical and should be avoided.

Expectant mothers must be extremely cautious about using aromatherapy, as many oils are contraindicated during pregnancy, labour and breastfeeding. Although there is no definitive evidence of teratogenicity, the possible adverse effects on the fetus, pregnancy progress and maternal health are uncertain. Some oils raise the blood pressure, others lower it, particularly when inhaled directly (Schneider 2015; Yang et al 2014; Seol et al 2013); some potentiate the action of certain drugs – for example, lavender and clary sage oils are known to reduce blood pressure (Nagai et al 2014) so should not be used in conjunction with epidural anaesthesia. All oils contain antibacterial chemicals, some are also antiviral and/or antifungal, such as tea tree (Chen et al 2014; Chin and Cordell 2013; Mith et al 2014; Sienkiewicz et al 2014). Many oils are relaxing and some appear to have strong analgesic properties (Olapour et al 2013).

An oil of particular concern is clary sage, thought to aid uterine contractions (Burns et al 2000a and 2000b); women increasingly buy it to attempt to avoid labour induction or, alarmingly, use it in conjunction with prescribed oxytocics. Anecdotal reports suggest that women may use it as early as 30 weeks gestation, in some cases triggering preterm labour, and one incident is known to this author in which overzealous intrapartum use of clary sage may have contributed to stillbirth. Prolonged or repeated use of any oils may cause side effects including skin irritation, loss of concentration, lethargy, headaches or nausea.

Aromatherapy is *completely contraindicated* in babies less than 3 months of age because the skin is too sensitive for dermal application and the strong aromas may interfere with mother-baby interaction (Hugill 2015). Midwives should be mindful of the effects of aromatherapy on themselves (for example, when driving or making clinical decisions, especially in an emergency, or if they are pregnant) and on the woman, baby, relatives and other staff and visitors.

Conversely, aromatherapy is now used by many midwives, with good effect, notably in labour. Clary sage may aid pain relief and shorten labour (Kaviani et al 2014) and is being used by midwives in some units for post-dates pregnancy (Pauley and Percival 2014; Weston and Grabowska 2013). Lavender oil appears to aid wound healing after episiotomy (Marzouk et al 2014; Vakilian et al 2011) although midwives should be cautious about giving incorrect or incomplete information to women about this. In the largest ever aromatherapy study, Burns et al (2000a and 2000b) used essential oils and massage for 8085 labouring women in Oxford over a 9-year period, demonstrating decreased analgesia and oxytocic use and improved progress and maternal satisfaction. Although this study was not randomized or controlled, a subsequent trial (Burns et al 2007) also showed that randomization with a control group is an appropriate research method for the investigation of intrapartum aromatherapy.

Herbal medicine involves the therapeutic (medicinal) use of plants, including essential oils (aromatherapy) and herbal teas. Herbal remedies act pharmacologically: irrespective of the method of administration, they are absorbed into the body and act in exactly the same way as drugs. This poses the potential problem of interactions with other medications and the risks of side effects, which are usually related to taking too much or for too long a period. There is an immense body of research evidence to demonstrate this in relation to numerous herbal remedies in popular use. Many herbal preparations are contraindicated during pregnancy, as they may affect embryonic development, cause miscarriage or affect the mother's systemic well-being. Numerous herbal remedies, including ginger and other Chinese herbs, have strong anticoagulant effects and should never be taken by women on medications with a similar action, such as warfarin and aspirin (Tsai et al 2013; Tiran 2012). Women must use *extreme caution* with herbal remedies during pregnancy, and *all remedies* must be discontinued at least 2 weeks before elective caesarean section, mainly because of the commonly occurring anticoagulant effects (Nordeng et al 2011). Any woman with a medical condition or obstetric complication should avoid herbal remedies altogether, especially if she is taking conventional medication or experiences bleeding. If midwives are aware that a woman is taking any herbal remedies, she or he must record this information in the maternity notes.

One herb commonly used in pregnancy is raspberry leaf (tea or tablets). This is intended as a preparation for birth taken from about 32 weeks of pregnancy, and should *never be used at term* as a means of inducing labour, when it may cause uterine hypertonia and fetal distress (Jing Zheng et al 2010; Tiran 2010a). Evidence for its effectiveness is variable and largely inconclusive, but there is some suggestion that taking too much may *prolong* pregnancy and the first stage of labour rather than shortening it (Johnson et al 2009). Questions have been raised as to whether women need to take raspberry leaf at all (Holst et al 2009) because their bodies are physiologically designed to be pregnant and to give birth. Inadvertent, inappropriate or excessive use of raspberry leaf may interfere with the delicate balance of normal physiology and, as with other natural remedies, should be considered an intervention in the same way as medical interventions, such as syntocinon. Women with a medical condition, notably hypertension, or an obstetric complication such as antepartum haemorrhage or multiple pregnancies should not take raspberry leaf, nor should anyone with a uterine scar from a previous caesarean or if an elective caesarean section is planned for a medical or obstetric indication.

Reflective activity 18.2

- Keep a record of how often you are asked for information about raspberry leaf tea or the use of aromatherapy oils in pregnancy and labour, and consider how you respond to these queries.

Homeopathy involves the use of minute doses of substances, which, if given in their full dose, would actually cause the problems they are attempting to treat. Homeopathy does *not* work pharmacologically (i.e. chemically) but is a powerful energy medicine thought to be based on quantum physics. However, it should not be considered 'harmless' even though chemically there is very little of the original substance in the remedies. Remedies are individually prescribed according to the *precise* symptom picture, also taking into account the individual's personality and factors that exacerbate or inhibit the presenting symptoms. This means that several women with the same condition would not necessarily receive the same homeopathic remedy, because the manifestation of the condition may be different in each individual.

One popular remedy is arnica, used to combat bruising, trauma and shock (Oberbaum et al 2005; Seeley et al 2006). However, women should be aware of the correct dose (usually one 30C tablet three times daily for 3 days, then the remedy should be stopped). Taking too much or for too long can cause a 'reverse proving' in which symptoms appear that the remedy is designed to treat in this case, and severe systemic bruising can occur and has been witnessed on more than one occasion by this author.

Bach flower remedies are also a form of energy medicine, involving liquid preparations that are used to treat the emotional symptoms associated with disease and disorder. Rescue Remedy, the best known, is a combination of five from the full range of 38 remedies, useful for stress, panic and nervous tension, which may help women in the transition stage of labour or for those with a fear of needles. Because the remedies are preserved in brandy, they are contraindicated in anyone with alcohol intolerance or hepatic disease, but because only a few drops of the remedy are ingested, they are generally considered safe in pregnancy. There is limited research, but there is some suggestion that Bach flower remedies may relieve pain through psychophysiological effects (Howard 2007), although Ernst (2010) found no real difference between Bach flower remedies and placebo. The remedies are readily available in high street health stores and chemists, with widespread public advertising, so women may be familiar with these remedies before pregnancy.

Manual therapies

Massage is the applied use of touch. Touch impulses reach the brain more quickly than pain impulses; therefore, massage is useful for pain in labour (Silva Gallo et al 2013; Janssen et al 2012; Kimber et al 2008; McNabb et al 2006) and after caesarean (Abbaspoor et al 2014). Massage is known to reduce cortisol and other stress hormones, aiding relaxation (Stringer et al 2008; Field 2014) and reducing blood pressure (Liao et al 2014). It may also stimulate excretory processes; gentle clockwise abdominal massage can be effective in stimulating intestinal transit to treat constipation in the postpartum period.

Many midwives spontaneously use touch and massage, such as sacral pressure and lower back massage, for women during labour. Learning a few extra techniques can provide invaluable tools to help women and may, for example, enable the woman to endure the last part of the first stage and into transition without recourse to epidural anaesthesia. In units where aromatherapy is offered by midwives, women whose medical or obstetric condition precludes them from receiving essential oils can still enjoy the benefits of massage. However, massage should not be used over areas of the body with thrombosis or varicose veins; abdominal massage is contraindicated if the woman has an anteriorly situated placenta. A carrier or base oil is used to facilitate the massage; grapeseed is the most commonly used and is universally acceptable, whereas sweet almond oil has been associated with a higher incidence of preterm birth (Facchinetti et al 2012). Baby massage has also become increasingly popular and has been found to be of particular benefit for preterm babies (Diego et al 2014; Abdallah et al 2013), although care should be taken with the carrier oils used. Olive oil contains oleic acid, which has been found potentially to damage the skin barrier in adults, and it is recommended that olive oil is not used for baby massage (Danby et al 2013).

Osteopathy is a manual manipulative system that aims to restore and maintain balance within the body, particularly among the neural, muscular and skeletal systems and by examining and maintaining the biomechanical functioning of the body. It is particularly effective for the treatment of back pain in pregnancy but can be useful for other problems, for example, heartburn or carpal tunnel syndrome (Randall 2014). A similar therapy, chiropractic, is concerned with the relationship of the nervous system to the mechanical structure of the body, placing emphasis on the spinal joints and related muscles and ligaments. It is particularly appropriate for musculoskeletal conditions of pregnancy, especially symphysis pubis diastasis and sacroiliac joint pain (Alcantara et al 2015) and heartburn (Petersen 2012). It is also effective in treating infants with colic and hyperactivity disorder (Miller et al 2012; Alcantara and Davis 2010). Both osteopathy and chiropractic have been statutorily regulated since the mid-1990s and are no longer seen as complementary therapies but as professions supplementary to medicine.

Reflexology is based on the principle that the feet represent a map of to the rest of the body; by working on specific areas of the feet, other distal parts of the body can be treated. Reflexology is *not* simply foot massage, but a very powerful therapy which should be used with caution in pregnancy unless the practitioner has a thorough working knowledge of physiopathology (see Tiran 2010). In maternity care, reflexology may be useful for antenatal oedema (Coban and Sirin 2010; Mollart 2003) and dealing with backache, sickness and other antenatal disorders. It can ease labour pain, aid progress by stimulating contractions and treat retained placenta; postnatally reflexology can aid recovery, improve sleep and facilitate lactation (Li et al 2011; Tiran 2010).

Unfortunately, the evidence-base for reflexology in pregnancy and birth is limited; possibly because of the fact that there are so many different styles of reflexology, with different charts and techniques, so even within the profession, there are inconsistencies and dissent. The style that most closely aligns with midwifery practice is reflex zone therapy, devised by the German midwife, Hanne Marquardt (see Tiran 2010b and 2009). Where reflexology is implemented into midwifery care, it is essential to ensure that all those involved practise the same style within one unit to ensure consistency and safety and to enable clinical audits to be undertaken.

Hypnotherapy is the clinical use of deep relaxation to access the subconscious mind, often likened to daydreaming. It can be used to change behaviour, such as habitual and addictive behaviours or to reduce fears and phobias. There are mixed results from studies investigating whether hypnosis alters women's perceptions of labour pain and reduces analgesia use (Cyna et al 2013; Werner et al 2013a and 2013b; Madden et al 2012). Other effects may include shortening of the first stage of labour and improved Apgar scores in the baby (Landolt and Milling 2011).

More recently, Professor Soo Downe and colleagues (2015) undertook a large, randomized controlled trial of the use of self-hypnosis for birth preparation in 680 women in three NHS trusts. The primary object of the study was to explore the use of epidural use in women who had used self-hypnosis in preparation for birth. However, they found that, for those who attended two third-trimester group sessions of self-hypnosis training, followed by home use of a CD, the incidence of use of epidural anaesthesia in labour was not statistically different from that for women in the control group (27.9% compared to 30.3%), nor were there any real differences relating to experiences of pain in labour or clinical outcomes. However, there did appear to be some statistically significant subjective variations in women's expected versus actual anxiety and fear of labour and birth, which the team suggested requires further investigation. This study, called the SHIP (Self-Hypnosis in Pregnancy) trial, is the largest randomized controlled multicentre study undertaken in the UK to date. One limitation of the study was that approximately 10% of the women in the control group also reported using self-hypnosis after attending private preparation sessions.

There are many different styles of deep relaxation that have collectively been termed 'hypno-birthing', some of which are rather more formulaic than others. Occasionally, a midwife may be caring for a mother using a particular style of 'hypno-birthing' who requests to be left to labour without being touched, having vaginal examinations or even being spoken to; in some styles, the midwife is requested not to use the words 'contractions' or 'pain'. Also, unfortunately, the way in which some styles of self-hypnosis are taught can give the mother unrealistic expectations that her labour will progress normally, sometimes leading to a disappointing labour experience if progress deviates from normal. If the midwife is aware during pregnancy that a mother is attending 'hypno-birthing' classes or preparing to use self-hypnosis during labour, she should try to determine which style the mother is learning, and ask if there are any specific desires she has for her labour – this can be discussed when labour and birth planning is raised. There may also need to be some discussion about her expectations for the labour and birth.

Yoga involves learning a series of postures and positions, often in conjunction with meditation and breathing techniques, for relaxation and relief of symptoms. It encourages flexibility, suppleness and strength and is valuable for preparing for labour (Babbar et al 2015; Battle et al 2015; Sharma and Branscum 2015). There is also some suggestion that yoga may improve fetal growth and aid utero-fetal-placental circulation in women with high-risk pregnancy (Rakhshani et al 2015). Bershadsky et al (2014) demonstrated a reduction in cortisol and enhanced mood in women on the days they practised yoga during pregnancy. Kinser and Masho (2015) advocate the use of group yoga sessions for adolescent pregnant women who are stressed; similarly, Newham et al (2014) found that antenatal yoga can play a part in reducing women's anxieties about birth and preventing exacerbation of symptoms into depression.

MIDWIVES' RESPONSIBILITIES REGARDING COMPLEMENTARY THERAPIES AND PRACTICE

The midwife will increasingly come into contact with women who wish to self-administer natural remedies or who choose to consult independent therapists during pregnancy, or in preparation for labour. It is important to have a basic appreciation of the many different therapies to advise the woman about the use of complementary therapies and natural remedies, for example, understanding the difference between herbal and homeopathic medicines and their implications in relation to the progress of her pregnancy (see previous mention). The Nursing and Midwifery Council (NMC) *Standards for Medicines Management* (2010) emphasizes that women have the right to self-administer natural remedies but note that they may interact with other medications and with some laboratory tests. If a woman wishes to self-administer natural remedies, but the midwife is unfamiliar with the effects, indications, contraindications and side effects of a particular remedy, she should discuss this with the woman and, if necessary, consult an appropriately trained professional for advice. This may be a therapist who is trained, experienced and insured to work with pregnant women, or a midwife who has specialized in this area of extended midwifery practice.

It would be wise to enquire, when taking the initial 'booking history', whether the woman has used any natural remedies, in the same way as enquiring about the use of over-the-counter and recreational drugs. It may be necessary to be specific and to identify remedies such as aromatherapy oils, herbal, homeopathic or Bach flower remedies, because women do not always recognize that these are "natural remedies" or may feel that the midwife does not need to know. Not only does asking her specific questions implicitly give the woman 'permission' to discuss complementary therapies, but it will also alert the midwife to any potential problems which may arise, for example, the possibility of interactions with drugs or exacerbation of existing medical problems. As pregnancy progresses, women may ask the midwife about different remedies, notably in preparation for birth or, of course, they may choose not to confide in the midwife at all. The midwife should again question the woman carefully about her use of natural remedies and complementary therapies. It is essential that midwives maintain comprehensive and accurate records of any discussions they have with the woman on this subject. For example, it would not be enough to record that a woman had enquired about the use of raspberry leaf tea; the midwife should record in more detail what advice (if any) has been given, including when to commence taking it, the correct dose and frequency and how to recognize and what to do if side effects occur. If the midwife has not received adequate education on the subject or feels unable to advise the woman, this should also be recorded, together with any advice about where the expectant mother may be able to obtain the appropriate information, for example, a local complementary practitioner who is trained and insured to work with pregnant clients.

Occasionally, the midwife may care for a woman in late pregnancy who has been admitted with threatened preterm labour or fetal distress. If no obvious cause can be found, it would be wise to ask the woman if she has taken any natural remedies or herbal teas, used aromatherapy oils or had treatment from a complementary therapist. Self-administration is popular, but often women are unaware of the risks of inappropriate use, and there is a common misconception that, because these are natural substances, they therefore must be safe.

Furthermore, the increase in the number of women from overseas giving birth in the UK adds to the problems experienced by midwives when women choose to use traditional remedies that are often strongly embedded in their own cultures. Herbal remedies cause the most concern because they act pharmacologically and have the potential to interact with prescribed medications. There is a growing body of research evidence to show not only the benefits of herbal medicines but also the risks, although little is yet known of the potential teratogenic or abortifacient effects of many herbs. In this respect, research is almost impossible because ethical clearance to study unknown substances on women in early pregnancy would not be granted; knowledge of adverse effects is generally gathered from reports of adverse reactions and side effects experienced by individuals. There seems to be an almost universal practice in many countries around the world for women to use plant remedies aimed at preparing for birth, nourishing the fetus and strengthening the uterine muscle. Unfortunately, access to information and misinformation via the Internet has meant that Westerners make assumptions about the effectiveness of particular remedies and their application to pregnancy and childbirth. An example of this would be the common belief that herbal remedies, known potentially to cause miscarriage, will also aid labour onset, despite the physiological action of rejection in the first trimester being different from that of myometrial contraction and retraction that occurs in term labour.

Some women wish to self-administer natural remedies during labour, such as aromatherapy, essential oils or homeopathic or Bach flower remedies. They have the right to do so and should be facilitated in this wish where possible, but the midwife should record contemporaneously in the woman's notes and on the partogram when she administers a remedy to herself, even if the midwife is not familiar with its actions. If the midwife feels, at any time, that using the remedy may be detrimental to maternal or fetal health, the midwife must discuss the situation with the woman, and consult a relevant expert, if possible, to ascertain safety. If the labouring woman wishes to use herbal remedies that act pharmacologically and include essential oils, care needs to be taken regarding possible interactions with any other drugs she may require, for example, clary sage, which is thought to aid smooth muscle contraction, should not be used concomitantly with oxytocics, and lavender oil, which reduces blood pressure, should not be used with epidural anaesthesia. Conversely, homeopathic remedies do not act pharmacologically so will not interact with prescribed medications; however, they need to be used correctly to avoid triggering new symptoms in response to the initial dose, which can sometimes confuse the presenting clinical picture. Some women purchase special 'homeopathic kits for childbirth' which include brief instructions on self-use, but as labour progresses, she may be less able to make an objective decision regarding the most appropriate remedy, for what is, after all, a very dynamic and rapidly changing clinical situation. An example might be the woman who takes homeopathic remedies designed to aid contractions; she should discontinue taking these remedies once contractions have become established, as the original remedies are no longer needed and continuing to take them may disturb the physiological harmony of labour.

Women sometimes ask the midwife about visiting a private complementary therapist, perhaps for relaxation with reflexology, aromatherapy or massage or for the treatment of specific problems such as backache or symphysis pubis pain. The midwife must record any conversations regarding independent therapists, and the reasons the pregnant woman gives for consulting them. Practitioners of some therapies will have received adequate training to treat pregnant women safely. For example, osteopaths and chiropractors, whose professions are statutorily regulated in the same way as midwifery, will have completed a nationally regulated pre-registration training, which includes reproductive health; acupuncturists and medical herbalists will also have undertaken a 3 to 4 year training, often to degree level, during which they will have covered pregnancy and women's health. However, most therapies are not nationally regulated nor are the training programmes necessarily of the most appropriate academic calibre to prepare practitioners to treat pregnant women at the point of qualification. It is disconcerting that some therapists presume to treat expectant mothers without any relevant post-qualifying education (personal communications with therapists). Therefore, midwives should be wary of recommending specific therapies or therapists unless they can vouch for their credentials. The mother should be advised to ask directly about the therapist's training and experience in treating pregnant women and ensure that the therapist is in possession of personal professional indemnity insurance coverage for pregnancy (and birth, if appropriate) and has Disclosure and Barring clearance (DBS). Therapists who are registered with the Complementary and Natural Healthcare Council are NHS compliant and meet set standards of education, practice and insurance.

A contemporary trend of particular concern is that of women nearing term asking therapists to facilitate the onset of labour. This is often before the estimated delivery date and, most commonly, it appears to be reflexologists who are consulted (personal communications with pregnant women and therapists of numerous disciplines). Women should be advised that it would be inappropriate for a therapist to attempt to expedite labour before term and that *any* intervention, even those which are 'natural', could complicate maternal physiology and trigger the cascade of intervention that can occur with medical induction. On the other hand, if the woman progresses beyond her expected date and is being advised to follow an induction of labour protocol, this may be adequate

justification for receiving complementary therapies, although midwives and therapists should liaise to ensure safe care for the woman and her baby. It is unlikely that the therapist will make direct contact with the midwife or doctor, but may ask the woman to discuss with the midwife if it is acceptable to have the therapy. It is natural that the midwife may assume that the woman is to receive the therapy for relaxation, which is acceptable and may be very beneficial, but she should question the woman about her reasons for wanting treatment. If the woman wants to have labour induced naturally, the midwife should consider whether this is appropriate. Before 40 weeks gestation, complementary techniques with the specific aim of triggering labour contractions should not be used, although relaxation therapies may be beneficial in facilitating normal physiology by reducing cortisol and increasing oxytocin. Any woman with an obstetric or medical complication should not receive complementary therapy treatment to start labour unless this can be done by an appropriately trained midwife in an environment where facilities are available to deal with complications that may arise.

MIDWIVES' RESPONSIBILITIES REGARDING INDEPENDENT PRACTITIONERS

Some women choose to be accompanied by an independent practitioner so that they can receive complementary therapies during labour. This may be a qualified complementary therapist, or a doula who has acquired some skills in complementary therapies, but who may not always be adequately trained or insured to use them. The midwife remains accountable for the woman's care and has a duty to ensure that care is safe and in keeping with normal midwifery care. Ideally, the woman should be encouraged to inform her midwife when discussing her birth plans if she thinks she may want to have a therapist or doula with her during labour.

When caring for a woman in labour, the midwife should record in the notes and on the partogram when natural remedies are taken or treatments are administered by the therapist/doula. Some hospitals/maternity units require independent therapists/doulas to sign a disclaimer form stating that they acknowledge the midwife remains responsible for the woman's care, that they have independent indemnity insurance coverage and that, in the event of an emergency, they agree to discontinue complementary therapies and facilitate the midwife to manage the situation. As with other occasions, if the midwife believes complementary therapies are inappropriate, she should discuss this with the expectant mother and her therapist/doula, and record the outcome of any discussion.

MIDWIVES USING COMPLEMENTARY THERAPIES IN THEIR OWN PRACTICE

The *Code* (NMC 2015) requires midwives to respond to changing health needs of society, which should include being aware of the widespread use of complementary therapies and natural remedies. Midwives must ensure that any information or advice given on natural remedies to women is evidence-based where possible, and should be appropriately trained if they intend to use complementary therapies in their own practice. They must work within the limits of their training, competence, UK and European Union law, NMC guidance and other relevant policies, for example, health and safety regulations. It is essential to keep updated through regular continuing professional development in both midwifery and complementary therapies.

Many midwives now train in specific therapies, or aspects of complementary therapies, and are tasked with establishing services such as aromatherapy, 'hypno-birthing', acupuncture or reflexology in their unit, in order to develop low-risk birthing units, normalize birth and reduce soaring caesarean section rates. Complementary therapies are shown to reduce intervention, and consequently 'near miss' incidents and costs, and enhance maternal satisfaction (Kings' Fund 2009). Strategies such as aromatherapy, reflexology and massage lower stress hormone levels and facilitate oxytocin release, leading to improved labour progress and birth outcomes (McNabb et al 2006; Silva Gallo et al 2013; Field 2014). More recently, midwives have explored ways in which complementary therapies can help them deal with specific clinical conditions, especially those which cause difficulties for women or which have cost implications for the health service. In addition, the need to reduce interventions such as caesarean section, induction of labour and epidural anaesthesia, which not only pose risks to mothers and babies, but also take up increasingly limited resources, has fuelled considerable interest among midwives and obstetricians (Pauley and Percival 2014; Dhany et al 2012; Weston and Grabowska 2012 and 2013).

The National Institute for Health and Care Excellence (NICE) viewpoint

Unfortunately, midwives in some units may be thwarted in their desires to implement complementary therapies into their practice because of the guidelines published by the National Institute of Health and Care Excellence (NICE). Some units take these guidelines to mean 'policy' and comply more firmly with them than other maternity units. The 2014 revision of the 2008 guidelines on *Care of the Healthy Pregnant Woman* includes the recommendation that:

'pregnant women should be informed that few complementary therapies have been established as being safe and effective during pregnancy. Women should not assume that such therapies are safe and they should be used as little as possible during pregnancy'. (page 17)

This is neither true nor helpful, because women will resort to using complementary therapies and, in particular, taking natural remedies without informing midwives and maternity professionals of their use, a fact that can lead to problems of interactions with prescribed medications and may potentially interfere with a close and trusting relationship with caregivers. In addition, in the section on management of common symptoms in pregnancy, the guideline erroneously states that 'non-pharmacological ginger' should be advised for women with sickness in pregnancy. This statement is incorrect on two counts: firstly, ginger, when used as a therapeutic substance, should be taken as a tea made from ginger root, which definitely has a pharmacological action; secondly, there is considerable risk to some women of side effects, including heartburn and, more significantly, an anticoagulant effect, which means that ginger is not a safe nor universal remedy for nausea and vomiting (Tiran 2012). Furthermore, an additional suggestion to use P6 acupressure wristbands for sickness fails to acknowledge that this is also an element of complementary therapies, and that midwives and doctors need to be able to advise women how to position the wristbands accurately over the relevant acupuncture point. Similarly, in the section on backache, the guideline suggests that massage – a complementary therapy – may be helpful, yet this is not always appropriate for backaches experienced in pregnancy.

Of even more concern are the new recommendations in the intrapartum care guideline (NICE 2014), particularly in relation to pain relief. Recommendation 1.3.10 states categorically that, during the latent phase of labour, care providers should:

'not offer or advise aromatherapy, yoga or acupressure for pain relief …. (although) if a woman wants to use any of these techniques (midwives should) respect her wishes'.

In Section 1.8 on pain relief in established labour, the guideline recommends that if a woman wishes to receive massage that has been taught to birth partners, she should be supported in this choice, but 'do not offer acupuncture, acupressure or hypnosis' although, again, the woman should not be prevented from using these techniques should she wish to do so. It is interesting to note that the guideline also discourages the use of transcutaneous electrical nerve stimulation (TENS) and sterile water injections, which are standard components of care in many units.

However, if a midwife has permission to use complementary therapies and wishes to use them in her or his own practice, it is not necessary to be a fully qualified practitioner. It is *essential* to be able to apply the principles of the therapy to the reproductive physiopathology of individual mothers and to use that therapy within an institutional setting. For example, midwives could learn the chemistry, indications, contraindications and precautions, methods of administration and possible side effects of a selected number of aromatherapy essential oils for use in labour without needing to be fully qualified aromatherapists; however, they must also be able to relate the use of these oils to health and safety issues within the unit, such as not using a vaporizer with a naked flame to dispense aromas into the air because of the fire risks and, in fact, not using vaporizers of any kind in the unit, as this is not safe for all mothers or staff. It would also be acceptable to learn the technique of moxibustion to turn a breech-presenting fetus to cephalic without becoming a fully qualified practitioner of traditional Chinese medicine, but midwives would need to understand fully the mechanism of action, indications, contraindications and precautions of the technique, and have a comprehensive working knowledge of the conventional management of breech presentation.

It is certainly not acceptable for midwives to 'dabble' in complementary therapies, for not only are they jeopardizing the health of women and babies, they are also risking their own professional careers. Stewart et al (2014) found that approximately a third of maternity professionals, most commonly midwives, recommended complementary therapies or natural remedies to women, despite lack of firm evidence of safety. In addition, although some professionals were trained in one or more therapies, many inappropriately based their advice to women on personal use. A genuine desire to act as the woman's advocate by facilitating her use of complementary therapies has, unfortunately, led to numerous examples of midwives who overhear colleagues giving advice on natural remedies, advice which they assume is accurate. They then proceed to offer this advice to other women in their care, without adequate training or any real understanding of the pertinent issues. Common examples are raspberry leaf to aid labour, aromatherapy, including lavender and clary sage for labour or homeopathy, such as arnica, for episiotomy pain.

Sadly, in this day of frequent litigation, it is essential for midwives to acknowledge the risks of *any* clinical intervention and be able to justify their actions in case they are required to do so in a court of law. It is also vital to recognize that, just because complementary therapies are 'natural', this does not mean that they are always automatically safe. Obtaining informed consent and maintaining contemporaneous records is vital, as in all other aspects of care, and midwives must appreciate the limitations of their own professional practice. The NMC regulates the practice of nurses and midwives to protect the public but can only regulate midwives' use of complementary therapies when it relates to their *midwifery* practice. It is not possible for qualifications in different therapies to be added to an individual's entry on the NMC register.

When working in an employment situation, rather than as an independent practitioner, midwives wishing to implement complementary therapies within the unit will also need to develop and gain approval for the relevant guidelines and protocols. These should state clearly the rationale for incorporating the specific elements of complementary therapies into midwifery practice, supported by contemporary research or authoritative references. The guidelines should state which midwives are eligible to use the therapy, based on having acquired the relevant initial knowledge and skills and maintaining these via continuing professional development. They may also state which midwives should not use the therapy; for example, midwives who are pregnant or trying to conceive should not use uterotonic essential oils, such as clary sage, when caring for labouring women. The guidelines should also identify which women may receive the therapy and those for whom it is inappropriate. An example might be the establishment of a reflexology service within the delivery suite, from which women with medical or obstetric problems may need to be excluded. Other specific information regarding the use of a particular therapy may be included in a precise protocol, for example, moxibustion for breech presentation. If a midwife is appropriately trained in aspects of complementary therapies and has the permission of her employing authority to incorporate this into her practice, the Royal College of Midwives' and the Royal College of Nursing's personal professional indemnity insurance schemes provide suitable indemnity insurance coverage. However, the vicarious liability coverage of the employing authority will be invalidated unless the midwife has gained permission of the relevant authorities to use complementary therapies in her work. If the midwife chooses to practise independently as a therapist, she must arrange additional indemnity insurance coverage through one of the complementary therapy organizations.

CONCLUSION

Women increasingly turn to complementary therapies and natural remedies to expand their options during pregnancy, labour and the puerperium, for relaxation and for specific physiological discomforts. As the general public's use of complementary therapies has risen, so too has the possibility that pregnant women will ask their midwives about the use of complementary therapies or natural remedies. Midwives are in an invaluable position to facilitate women's wishes but must balance their enthusiasm for the benefits of complementary therapies with an appreciation of the potential safety issues, and recognize their own professional boundaries when advising women. While all midwives should have a basic understanding of the principles, the use of complementary therapies within midwifery is a specialist area of practice. In the same way as some midwives specialize in obstetric ultrasound scanning, parent education, or caring for women with high risk pregnancies, so too should complementary therapies be seen as a broad subject area which requires in-depth knowledge and skills. It is neither appropriate nor necessary for midwives at the point of registration to be able to practise specific complementary therapies, which should be seen as a post-registration specialism, but *all* midwives should have an overview of the subject area to work with women safely and appropriately.

Reflective activity 18.3

- Make a note of any situations in which a woman has used complementary therapies or has self-administered natural remedies during labour. How did your midwife-mentor deal with these episodes? Did any problems arise during the labour and, if so, to what extent do you think these difficulties may have been caused by the complementary therapies or natural remedies?

Key Points

- Ask women at 'booking' about their use of complementary therapies and natural remedies before and during pregnancy.
- During the third trimester, ask about the woman's intentions regarding preparation for birth and planned use of complementary therapies, natural remedies or being accompanied by an independent therapist or doula.
- Be alert to the possibility that women admitted for preterm labour and other complications may inadvertently have used or overused natural remedies, such as raspberry leaf tea or clary sage essential oil.
- When women are admitted in labour, enquire what they have used so far in terms of natural pain relief or means of accelerating contractions, and their intentions for the duration of the labour.
- Midwives wishing to implement complementary therapies in their own practice must be adequately and appropriately trained to do so, have the permission of their employing authority and work within local guidelines.

Summary of issues for midwives incorporating complementary therapies into their practice

- Education, training and continuing professional development – midwifery-specific
- Professional indemnity insurance/vicarious liability insurance of employer
- Disclosure and Barring Service clearance
- Acknowledge parameters of practice in relation to service obligations
- Consent, confidentiality and comprehensive, contemporaneous record keeping
- Advocacy for, and understanding of, the rights of the mother and fetus
- Communication and collaboration with colleagues
- Work in accordance with local clinical guidelines, national and international law
- Evaluation and audit of complementary therapy services provided within midwifery
- Evidence-based practice where possible

References

Abbaspoor Z, Akbari M, Najar S: Effect of foot and hand massage in post-cesarean section pain control: a randomized control trial, *Pain Manag Nurs* 15(1):132–136, 2014.

Abdallah B, Badr LK, Hawwari M: The efficacy of massage on short and long term outcomes in preterm infants, *Infant Behav Dev* 36(4):662–669, 2013.

Akbarzadeh M, Masoudi Z, Hadianfard MJ, et al: Comparison of the effects of maternal supportive care and acupressure (BL32 acupoint) on pregnant women's pain intensity and delivery outcome, *J Pregnancy* 129208, 2014.

Alcantara J, Alcantara JD, Alcantara J: The use of validated outcome measures in the chiropractic care of pregnant patients: a systematic review of the literature, *Complement Ther Clin Pract* S1744-3881(15)00005-5, 2015.

Alcantara J, Davis J: The chiropractic care of children with attention-deficit/hyperactivity disorder: a retrospective case series, *Explore (NY)* 6(3):173–182, 2010.

Babbar S, Chauhan SP: Exercise and yoga during pregnancy: a survey, *J Matern Fetal Neonatal Med* 28(4):431–435, 2015.

Babycentre.co.uk: *Survey on use of herbal remedies in pregnancy and childbirth* (website). www.midirs.org/development/midwiferyweb.nsf/news. 2011.

Battle CL, Uebelacker LA, Magee SR, et al: Potential for prenatal yoga to serve as an intervention to treat depression during pregnancy, *Womens Health Issues* 25(2):134–141, 2015.

Bershadsky S, Trumpfheller L, Kimble HB, et al: The effect of prenatal Hatha yoga on affect, cortisol and depressive symptoms, *Complement Ther Clin Pract* 20(2):106–113, 2014.

Birdee GS, Kemper KJ, Rothman R, et al: Use of complementary and alternative medicine during pregnancy and the postpartum period: an analysis of the National Health Interview Survey, *J Womens Health (Larchmt)* 23(10):824–829, 2014.

Bishop JL, Northstone K, Green JR, et al: The use of complementary and alternative medicine in pregnancy: data from the Avon Longitudinal Study of Parents and Children (ALSPAC), *Complement Ther Med* 19(6):303310, 2011.

Burns EE, Blamey C, Ersser SJ, et al: An investigation into the use of aromatherapy in intrapartum midwifery practice, *J Altern Complement Med* 6(2):141–147, 2000b.

Burns E, Blamey C, Ersser SJ, et al: The use of aromatherapy in intrapartum midwifery practice an observational study, *Complement Ther Nurs Midwifery* 6(1):33–34, 2000a.

Burns E, Zobbi V, Panzeri D, et al: Aromatherapy in childbirth: a pilot randomised controlled trial, *BJOG* 114(7):838–844, 2007.

Chen CC, Yan SH, Yen MY, et al: Investigations of kanuka and manuka essential oils for in vitro treatment of disease and cellular inflammation caused by infectious microorganisms, *J Microbiol Immunol Infect* S1684-1182(13)00246-6, 2014.

Chin KB, Cordell B: The effect of tea tree oil (*Melaleuca alternifolia*) on wound healing using a dressing model, *J Altern Complement Med* 19(12):942–945, 2013.

Coban A, Sirin A: Effect of foot massage to decrease physiological lower leg oedema in late pregnancy: a randomized controlled trial in Turkey, *Int J Nurs Pract* 16(5):454–460, 2010.

Cyna AM, Crowther CA, Robinson JS, et al: Hypnosis antenatal training for childbirth: a randomised controlled trial, *BJOG* 120(10):1248–1259, 2013.

Danby SG, Al Enezi T, Sultan A, et al: Effect of olive and sunflower seed oil on the adult skin barrier: implications for neonatal skin care, *Pediatr Dermatol* 30(1):42–50, 2013.

Dhany AL, Mitchell T, Foy C: Aromatherapy and massage intrapartum service impact on use of analgesia and anesthesia in women in labor: a retrospective case note analysis, *J Altern Complement Med* 18(10):932–938, 2012.

Diego MA, Field T, Hernandez-Reif M: Preterm infant weight gain is increased by massage therapy and exercise via different underlying mechanisms, *Early Hum Dev* 90(3):137140, 2014.

Djakovic I, Djakovic Z, Bilić N, et al: Third stage of labor and acupuncture, *Med Acupunct* 27(1):10–13, 2015.

Downe S, Finlayson K, Melvin C, et al: *Self-hypnosis for intrapartum pain management in pregnant nulliparous women: a randomised controlled trial of clinical effectiveness* (website). www.bjog.org, 2015.

Eghdampour F, Jahdie F, Kheyrkhah M, et al: The impact of aloe vera and calendula on perineal healing after episiotomy in primiparous women: a randomized clinical trial, *J Caring Sci* 2(4):279286, 2013.

El-Deeb AM, Ahmady MS: Effect of acupuncture on nausea and/or vomiting during and after cesarean section in comparison with ondansetron, *J Anesth* 25(5):698–703, 2011.

Ernst E: Bach flower remedies: a systematic review of randomised clinical trials, *Swiss Med Wkly* 140:w13079, 2010.

Facchinetti F, Pedrielli G, Benoni G, et al: Herbal supplements in pregnancy: unexpected results from a multicentre study, *Hum Reprod* 27(11):31613167, 2012.

Field T: Massage therapy research review, *Complement Ther Clin Pract* 20(4):224–229, 2014.

Frawley J, Adams J, Broom A, et al: Majority of women are influenced by non-professional information sources when deciding to consult a complementary and alternative medicine practitioner during pregnancy, *J Altern Complement Med* 20(7):571–577, 2014.

Gregson S, Tiran D, Absalom J, et al: Acupressure for inducing labour for nulliparous women with post-dates pregnancy, *Complement Ther Clin Pract* published online 15 August 2015.

Hall HG, Griffiths DL, McKenna LG: The use of complementary and alternative medicine by pregnant women: a literature review, *Midwifery* 27(6):817–824, 2011.

Holst L, Haavik S, Nordeng H: Raspberry leaf – should it be recommended to pregnant women? *Complement Ther Clin Pract* 15(4):204–208, 2009.

Hong S, Yoo JS, Hong JY, et al: Immunohistochemical and electron microscopic study of the meridian-like system on the surface of internal organs of rats, *Acupunct Electrothe Res* 32(3–4):195–210, 2007.

Howard J: Do Bach flower remedies have a role to play in pain control? A critical analysis investigating therapeutic value beyond the placebo effect, and the potential of Bach flower remedies as a psychological method of pain relief, *Complement Ther Clin Pract* 13(3):174183, 2007.

Hugill K: The senses of touch and olfaction in early mother-infant interaction, *Br J Midwifery* 23(4):238–243, 2015.

Ingram J, Domagala C, Yates S: The effects of shiatsu on post-term pregnancy, *Complement Ther Med* 13(1):11–15, 2005.

Janssen P, Shroff F, Jaspar P: Massage therapy and labor outcomes: a randomized controlled trial, *Int J Ther Massage Bodywork* 5(4):15–20, 2012.

Jing Zheng, Pistilli MJ, Holloway AC, et al: The effects of commercial preparations of red raspberry leaf on the contractility of the rat's uterus in vitro, *Reprod Sci* 17(5):494–501, 2010.

Johnson JR, Makaji E, Ho S, et al: Effect of maternal raspberry leaf consumption in rats on pregnancy outcome and the fertility of the female offspring, *Reprod Sci* 16(6):605609, 2009.

Kaviani M, Maghbool S, Azima S, et al: Comparison of the effect of aromatherapy with Jasminum officinale and Salvia officinale on pain severity and labor outcome in nulliparous women, *Iran J Nurs Midwifery Res* 19(6):666–672, 2014.

Kennedy DA, Lupatelli A, Koren G, et al: Herbal medicine use in pregnancy: results of a multinational study, *BMC Complement Altern Med* 13:355, 2013.

Kimber L, McNabb M, Mc Court C, et al: Massage or music for pain relief in labour: a pilot randomised placebo controlled trial, *Eur J Pain* 12(8):961–969, 2008.

Kings' Fund 2009 *Safer Births: everybody's business* http://www.kingsfund.org.uk/sites/files/kf/field/field_publication_file/safe-births-everybodys-business-onora-oneill-february-2008.pdf, 2009.

Kinser P, Masho S: "I just start crying for no reason": the experience of stress and depression in pregnant, urban, African-American adolescents and their perception of yoga as a management strategy, *Womens Health Issues* 25(2):142–184, 2015.

Landolt AS, Milling LS: The efficacy of hypnosis as an intervention for labor and delivery pain: a comprehensive methodological review, *Clin Psychol Rev* 31(6):1022–1031, 2011.

Li CY, Chen SC, Li CY, et al: Randomised controlled trial of the effectiveness of using foot reflexology to improve quality of sleep amongst Taiwanese postpartum women, *Midwifery* 27(2):181–186, 2011.

Liao IC, Chen SL, Wang MY, et al: Effects of massage on blood pressure in patients with hypertension and prehypertension: a meta-analysis of randomized controlled trials, *J Cardiovasc Nurs* 2014.

Lythgoe J: Acupuncture treatment for hyperemesis gravidarum, *Midwives* 15(2):28, 2012.

Madden K, Middleton P, Cyna AM, et al: Hypnosis for pain management during labour and childbirth, *Cochrane Database Syst Rev* (11):CD009356, 2012.

Manyande A, Grabowska C: Factors affecting the success of moxibustion in the management of a breech presentation as a preliminary treatment to external cephalic version, *Midwifery* 25(6):774–780, 2009.

Marzouk T, Barakat R, Ragab A, et al: Lavender-thymol as a new topical aromatherapy preparation for episiotomy: a randomised clinical trial, *J Obstet Gynaecol* 10:1–4, 2014.

McNabb MT, Kimber L, Haines A, et al: Does regular massage from late pregnancy to birth decrease maternal pain perception during labour and birth? – A feasibility study to investigate a programme of massage, controlled breathing and visualization, from 36 weeks of pregnancy until birth, *Complement Ther Clin Pract* 12(3):222–231, 2006.

McVicar AJ, Greenwood CR, Fewell F, et al: Evaluation of anxiety, salivary cortisol and melatonin secretion following reflexology treatment: a pilot study in healthy individuals, *Complement Ther Clin Pract* 13(3):137–145, 2007.

Mith H, Duré R, Delcenserie V, et al: Antimicrobial activities of commercial essential oils and their components against food-borne pathogens and food spoilage bacteria, *Food Sci Nutr* 2(4):403416, 2014.

Miller JE, Newell D, Bolton JE: Efficacy of chiropractic manual therapy on infant colic: a pragmatic single-blind, randomized controlled trial, *J Manipulative Physiol Ther* 35(8):600607, 2012.

Mohammadi A, Mohammad-Alizadeh-Charandabi S, Mirghafourvand M, et al: Effects of cinnamon on perineal pain and healing of episiotomy: a randomized placebo-controlled trial, *J Integr Med* 12(4):359–366, 2014.

Mollart L: Single-blind trial addressing the differential effects of two reflexology techniques versus rest, on ankle and foot oedema in late pregnancy, *Complement Ther Nurs Midwifery* 9(4):203–208, 2003.

Moradi Z, Akbarzadeh M, Moradi P, et al: The effect of acupressure at GB-21 and SP-6 acupoints on anxiety level and maternal-fetal attachment in primiparous women: a randomized controlled clinical trial, *Nurs Midwifery Stud* 3(3):e19948, 2014.

Mucuk S, Baser M: Effects of non-invasive electro-acupuncture on labour pain and duration, *J Clin Nurs* 23(11–12):1603–1610, 2014.

Nagai K, Niijima A, Horii Y, et al: Olfactory stimulatory with grapefruit and lavender oils change autonomic nerve activity and physiological function, *Auton Neurosci* 185:29–35, 2014.

Nandi A, Shah A, Gudi A, et al: Acupuncture in IVF: a review of current literature, *J Obstet Gynaecol* 34(7):555–561, 2014.

National Institute for Health and Care Excellence (NICE): *Antenatal care, Issued: March 2008 last modified: December 2014* (website). https://www.nice.org.uk/guidance/cg62/resources/antenatal-care-for-uncomplicated-pregnancies-975564597445, 2014.

National Institute for Health and Care Excellence (NICE): *Intrapartum care: care of healthy women and their babies during childbirth* (website). www.nice.org.uk/guidance/cg190/chapter/1-recommendations#place-of-birth, 2014.

Newham JJ, Wittkowski A, Hurley J, et al: Effects of antenatal yoga on maternal anxiety and depression: a randomized controlled trial, *Depress Anxiety* 31(8):631–640, 2014.

Nordeng H, Bayne K, Havnen GC, et al: Use of herbal drugs during pregnancy among 600 Norwegian women in relation to concurrent use of conventional drugs and pregnancy outcome, *Complement Ther Clin Pract* 17(3):147–151, 2011.

Noroozinia H, Mahoori A, Hasani E, et al: The effect of acupressure on nausea and vomiting after cesarean section under spinal anesthesia, *Acta Med Iran* 51(3):163–167, 2013.

Nursing and Midwifery Council (NMC): *Standards for Medicines Administration* (website). www.nmc.org.uk/globalassets/siteDocuments/NMC-Publications/NMC-Standards-for-medicines-management.pdf, 2010.

Nursing and Midwifery Council (NMC): *The code: professional standards of practice and behaviour for midwives and nurses*, NMC London, 2015.

Oberbaum M, Galoyan N, Lerner-Geva L, et al: The effect of the homeopathic remedies *Arnica montana* and *Bellis perennis* on mild postpartum bleeding-a randomized, double-blind, placebo-controlled study – preliminary results, *Complement Ther Med* 13(2):87–90, 2005.

Olapour A, Behaeen K, Akhondzadeh R, et al: The effect of inhalation of aromatherapy blend containing lavender essential oil on cesarean postoperative pain, *Anesth Pain Med* 3(1):203–207, 2013.

Pallivalapila AR, Stewart D, Shetty A, et al: Use of complementary and alternative medicines during the third trimester, *Obstet Gynecol* 125(1):204–211, 2015.

Pauley T, Percival R: *Reducing post-dates induction numbers with post-dates complementary therapy clinics* (website). http://www.magonline library.com/doi/full/10.12968/ bjom.2014.22.9.630, 2014.

Petersen C: A case study of chiropractic management of pregnancy-related heartburn with postulated fetal epigenome implications, *Explore (NY)* 8(5):304–308, 2012.

Rakhshani A, Nagarathna R, Mhaskar R, et al: Effects of yoga on utero-fetal-placental circulation in high-risk pregnancy: a randomized controlled trial, *Adv Prev Med* 373041, 2015.

Randall S: Osteopathy: helping pregnant women in pain, *Pract Midwife* 17(5):38–41, 2014.

Seeley BM, Denton AB, Ahn MS, et al: Effect of homeopathic *Arnica montana* on bruising in face-lifts: results of a randomized, double-blind, placebo-controlled clinical trial, *Arch Facial Plast Surg* 8(1):54–59, 2006.

Seol GH, Lee YH, Kang P, et al: Randomized controlled trial for *Salvia sclarea* or *Lavandula angustifolia*: differential effects on blood pressure in female patients with urinary incontinence undergoing urodynamic examination, *J Altern Complement Med* 19(7):664–670, 2013.

Sheikhan F, Jahdi F, Khoei EM, et al: Episiotomy pain relief: use of lavender oil essence in primiparous Iranian women, *Complement Ther Clin Pract* 18(1):66–70, 2012.

Schneider R: There is something in the air: testing the efficacy of a new olfactory stress relief method (AromaStick®), *Stress Health* 2015.

Sharma M, Branscum P: Yoga interventions in pregnancy: a qualitative review, *J Altern Complement Med* 21(4):208–216, 2015.

Sienkiewicz M, Głowacka A, Kowalczyk E, et al: The biological activities of cinnamon, geranium and lavender essential oils, *Molecules* 19(12):20929–20940, 2014.

Silva Gallo RB, Santana LS, Jorge Ferreira CH, et al: Massage reduced severity of pain during labour: a randomised trial, *J Physiother* 59(2):109–116, 2013.

Sibbritt DW, Catling CJ, Adams J, et al: The self-prescribed use of aromatherapy oils by pregnant women, *Women Birth* 27(1):4145, 2014.

Sim TF, Sherriff J, Hattingh HL, et al: The use of herbal medicines during breastfeeding: a population-based survey in Western Australia, *BMC Complement Altern Med* 13:317, 2013.

Smith CA, Betts D: The practice of acupuncture and moxibustion to promote cephalic version for women with a breech presentation: implications for clinical practice and research, *Complement Ther Med* 22(1):75–80, 2014.

Soliday E, Hapke P: Patient-reported benefits of acupuncture in pregnancy, *Complement Ther Clin Pract* 19(3):109–113, 2013.

Stewart D, Pallivalappila AR, Shetty A, et al: Healthcare professional views and experiences of complementary and alternative therapies in obstetric practice in North East Scotland: a prospective questionnaire survey, *BJOG* 121(8):10151019, 2014.

Stringer J, Swindell R, Dennis M: Massage in patients undergoing intensive chemotherapy reduces serum cortisol and prolactin, *Psychooncology* 17(10):10241031, 2008.

Strouss L, Mackley A, Guillen U, et al: Complementary and alternative medicine use in women during pregnancy: do their healthcare providers know? *BMC Complement Altern Med* 14:85, 2014.

Tiran D: Structural reflex zone therapy in pregnancy and childbirth: a new approach, *Complement Ther Clin Pract* 15(4):234–238, 2009.

Tiran D: Complementary therapies and the NMC, *Pract Midwife* 13(5):4–5, 2010a.

Tiran D: *Reflexology in pregnancy and childbirth*, Edinburgh, Churchill Livingstone, 2010b.

Tiran D: Ginger to reduce nausea and vomiting during pregnancy: evidence of effectiveness is not the same as proof of safety, *Complement Ther Clin Pract* 18(1):22–25, 2012.

Tsai HH, Lin HW, Lu YH, et al: A review of potential harmful interactions between anticoagulant/antiplatelet agents and Chinese herbal medicines, *PLoS One* 8(5):e64255, 2013.

Vakilian K, Atarha M, Bekhradi R, et al: Healing advantages of lavender essential oil during episiotomy recovery: a clinical trial, *Complement Ther Clin Pract* 17(1):50–53, 2011.

Vas J, Aranda-Regules JM, Modesto M, et al: Using moxibustion in primary healthcare to correct non-vertex presentation: a multicentre randomised controlled trial, *Acupunct Med* 31(1):31–38, 2013.

Vixner L, Mårtensson LB, Stener-Victorin E, Schytt E: Manual and electro-acupuncture for labour pain: study design of a longitudinal randomized controlled trial, *Evid Based Complement Alternat Med* 943198, 2012.

Werner A, Uldbjerg N, Zachariae R, et al: Effect of self-hypnosis on duration of labor and maternal and neonatal outcomes: a randomized controlled trial, *Acta Obstet Gynecol Scand* 92(7):816–823, 2013b.

Werner A, Uldbjerg N, Zachariae R, et al: Antenatal hypnosis training and childbirth experience: a randomized controlled trial, *Birth* 40(4):272–280, 2013a.

Weston M, Grabowska C: Complementary therapy for induction of labour, *Pract Midwife* 16(8):S16–S18, 2013.

Weston M, Grabowska C: Moxibustion to turn the breech, *Pract Midwife* 15(8):S3–S4, 2012.

Wu JJ, Cui Y, Yang YS, et al: Modulatory effects of aromatherapy massage intervention on electroencephalogram, psychological assessments, salivary cortisol and plasma brain-derived neurotrophic factor, *Complement Ther Med* 22(3):456–462, 2014.

Yang HJ, Kim KY, Kang P, et al: Effects of *Salvia sclarea* on chronic immobilization stress induced endothelial dysfunction in rats, *BMC Complement Altern Med* 14:396, 2014.

Zheng CH, Zhang J, Wu J, et al: The effect of transcutaneous electrical acupoint stimulation on pregnancy rates in women undergoing in vitro fertilization: a study protocol for a randomized controlled trial, *Trials* 15:162, 2014.

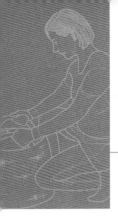

Chapter 19

Health promotion and education

Professor Jacqueline Dunkley-Bent

Learning Outcomes ?

After reading this chapter, you will be able to:

- appreciate the scope of health promotion in midwifery practice
- discuss the provision of health promotion within the context of inequalities in health and healthcare provision
- identify the emerging public health role of the midwife in the primary care setting
- consider ways in which public health issues may be integrated into day-to-day practice
- apply the principles of health promotion to enhance the health of the woman and her family

INTRODUCTION

Health promotion is an important and significant part of the midwife's role that has the potential to enhance health before conception, during the antenatal, intrapartum and postnatal periods and beyond. Understanding the meaning of health, health promotion and education will be explored within the context of pregnancy and childbirth. The potential for enhancing health gain for the woman and her family, by strengthening the health promotion role of the midwife will also be described, enabling readers to understand foundational principles for effectively progressing their health promotion work and wider public health role.

THE MEANING OF HEALTH

Health is a state of being to which most people aspire, yet a concept difficult to define, as personal meanings of health are enshrined in social structure, culture and beliefs.

In 1946, the World Health Organization (WHO) described health as a state of complete physical, mental and social well-being, not merely the absence of disease or infirmity (WHO 1946). This definition describes health as an ideal state of being that may be impossible to achieve, particularly when ideal states of health are subject to personal interpretation of health and illness. The woman who experiences nausea during pregnancy may describe herself as feeling ill, but nausea may not be defined as an illness unless hyperemesis develops, particularly if dietary intake supports healthy weight gain. Similarly, a complete state of social well-being is subjectively interpreted and, therefore, difficult to define.

Reflective activity 19.1

What does being healthy mean to you? Write down your personal definition of 'health'. What things affect how healthy you feel?

Constructs of health are influenced by an individual's attitudes and beliefs, culture, ethnicity, social class, religion, gender, poverty and economic status. It is crucial, therefore, that health professionals are aware of their own attitudes, beliefs and personal constructs of health before promoting the health of others.

Health should be viewed holistically and involve dimensions of health that are inextricably linked, namely as follows: physical, mental, emotional, societal, sexual and spiritual. If one dimension is negatively affected, this will have an effect on other dimensions.

MODELS OF HEALTH

Health models have been developed to try to explain why some individuals engage in healthy behaviours and others do not. The *Health Belief Model* (HBM) is one of the most frequently cited theoretical frameworks in the social cognitive literature (Guvenc et al 2011). This model was developed by Rosenstock (1966) as a model for health educators to explain why people would not participate in health education programmes or practices to detect or prevent disease. The model consists of four dimensions or '*constructs*':

* perceived susceptibility (to disease)
* perceived severity
* perceived barriers
* perceived benefits and cues to action

The model is used by combining the individuals' perceptions of constructs, which influence them to seek health advice or undertake the health advice provided (Becker et al 1977). The *locus of control* was developed by Rotter in 1966 to explore how people's beliefs about health and illness influence their actions. Locus of control refers to an individual's perception about the main causes of events in her or his life. The theory espouses that an individual has an internal or external locus of control. The belief that one can control one's own destiny is associated with having an internal locus of control. This individual believes that action taken equals consequence and seeks to manage and control life events, including health and illness (Wallston et al 1978). The individual who believes that one's destiny is controlled by external forces, including destiny, fate or bad luck, is associated with having an external locus of control. For wider reading, the reader is directed to the references.

REDUCING INEQUALITIES IN HEALTH

Understanding the social, cultural and economic context of health and illness increases the opportunity for health promotion to be meaningful and effective. Generally, premature mortality is influenced by deprivation and poverty. In England, people who live in areas of high deprivation are more likely to die on average 7 years earlier than people living in more affluent areas. Similarly, rates of mental illness and harm from alcohol, drugs and smoking are higher in areas where there is a high index of multiple deprivation (Fisher et al 2011). To have an understanding of global plans to improve health and tackle extreme poverty, promote gender equality, education and environmental sustainability, the reader should be familiar with the *Millennium Development Goals* (United Nations 2015) and more recently, the sustainable millennium goals that pledge a global commitment to tackle these issues by 2030 (Norheim et al 2015). Further information is available at the references and in Chapter 1.

In the UK, the National Health Service (NHS) was set up in 1948 to provide free medical care to the whole population and thereby achieve equality of access to health services for those in need. The aim was to eliminate or greatly reduce inequalities in health. Unsurprisingly, this single approach to improving the health of those worst off in society did not succeed.

In 2013 in the UK, pregnancies of women living in areas with the highest levels of social deprivation were over 50% more likely to end in stillbirth or neonatal death. However, the highest risk of extended perinatal mortality was associated with babies of black or black British and Asian or Asian British ethnicity, which suggests that inequalities in perinatal outcomes persist in the UK (Manktelow et al 2015). In contrast to the maternal deaths in the UK that have decreased from 11 per 100,000 women giving birth in 2006-2008 to 10 per 100,000 women giving birth in 2009-2012, maternal deaths from medical and psychiatric causes (indirect) have not reduced over the last 10 years (Knight et al 2015) (see Ch. 16).

The provision of health services cannot singularly solve inequality in health without addressing factors that influence ill health. Even when health improvements are made for all, inequalities continue to persist. Health inequalities are linked to wider determinants, including income, housing, education and other opportunities, which must be tackled so that health interventions can be effective (Office for National Statistics (ONS) 2014; Marmot 2010).

A commitment to improve healthcare for all

Over the last three decades, a plethora of policy documents and guidance focusing on tackling health inequalities have been published. The following documents present a helpful insight into health policy and guidance and its development:

* *The Black Report* (Black et al 1982)
* *Independent inquiry into inequalities in health* (Acheson 1998)
* *Saving lives: our healthier nation* (Department of Health (DH): 1999)
* *The NHS plan* (Secretary of State for Health 2000)
* *National Service Framework for Children, Young People and Maternity Services: Core Standards* (DH 2004)
* *Maternity matters: choice, access and continuity of care in a safe service* (DH 2007)
* *Health inequalities: progress and next steps* (DH 2008)
* *Fair Society, Healthy Lives* (Marmot et al 2010)
* *The Health and Social Care Act 2012*
* *The Public Health Outcomes Framework for England, 2013-2016* (DH 2012)

- *NHS England Five Year Forward View*
  (NHS England 2014)

The Marmot review (Marmot et al 2010), suggests that to reduce health inequalities, it will require action on six policy objectives outlined in Box 19.1.

Reflective activity 19.2

Reflect on what role central and local government, the NHS, the third and private sectors and community groups should play in reducing health inequalities.

WHAT IS HEALTH PROMOTION?

The World Health Organization defines health promotion as the process of enabling people to increase control over their health and improve it (WHO 1984). The process of

---

Box 19.1 Policy objectives to reduce health inequalities

Reducing health inequalities will require action on six policy objectives:

- Give every child the best start in life
- Enable all children, young people and adults to maximize their capabilities and have control over their lives
- Create fair employment and good working for all
- Ensure healthy standards of living for all
- Create and develop healthy and sustainable places and communities
- Strengthen the role and effect of ill health prevention

(Marmot et al 2010)

---

empowerment is key to the success of people taking control and should be integral to conversations that occur between the woman and the midwife.

Health promotion is likely to be successful if the most appropriate approach is used to promote health.

Health promotion approaches

A health promotion approach can be described as the vehicle used to achieve the desired aim. An example of this would be discussing with a mother the importance of vitamin K administration for her baby. The discussion would involve empowering the woman to make an informed decision about its use. The health promotion approach may vary according to the woman's needs, but invariably it would include a client-centred, educational approach.

Scriven (2010) identifies five health promotion approaches:

- medical or preventive
- behavioural change
- educational
- client-centred
- societal change

(see Box 19.2 for practice application).

A health promotion model

A model may be described as a conceptual framework for organizing and integrating information, offering causal links among a set of concepts believed to be related to a particular problem. There are several health promotion models that assist the practitioner in undertaking health promotion work. Here, only one model will be presented and explored in detail.

The health development model (Bauer et al 2006) in Fig. 19.1 shows that health development is an ongoing

---

Box 19.2 Health promotion in practice

Medical approach

Seeks to prevent and/or cure illness through medical intervention.

Example: the midwife may offer the woman who is nonimmune to rubella the vaccination in the postnatal period and contraceptive advice for a period of 3 months, or iron tablets for iron deficiency anaemia. Education and discussion should form part of this process. Didactic instruction should be avoided.

Behavioural change approach

Primary focus is on encouraging people to change their behaviour, which involves a change in attitude.

Example: dietary adjustment to include more fruits and vegetables. This may involve raising awareness through education, empowerment and decision making. Placing the woman at the centre of care is pivotal to the success of this approach. Also understanding the principles of behavioural change as shown in Box 19.3 is essential.

Educational approach

Provision of information, tailored to meet the individual needs of the client.

Example: this approach raises awareness through the provision of knowledge with the aim of validating current behaviour or changing behaviour that is injurious to health.

Box 19.2 Health promotion in practice—cont'd

Educational methods frequently used include group work, discussion and problem solving. Education can involve empowering conversations where the woman is empowered to make informed choices. Examples include: begin pelvic floor exercises, undertake perineal massage, stop smoking.

Client-centred approach

This places the client at the centre of an interaction that is based on an equal partnership between the client and the professional. Empowerment is integral to this approach where individuals are encouraged to utilize personal strength towards health gain.

Example: making an informed decision about the uptake of antenatal screening tests, making decisions about pain relief during labour and behavioural changes, including stopping drinking. These examples also require the education approach.

Societal change approach

Health promotion initiatives are focused on societal health and involve, for example, policy planning and political action.

Example: political and community action towards the prohibition of smoking in enclosed public spaces and workplaces and appropriate food labelling.

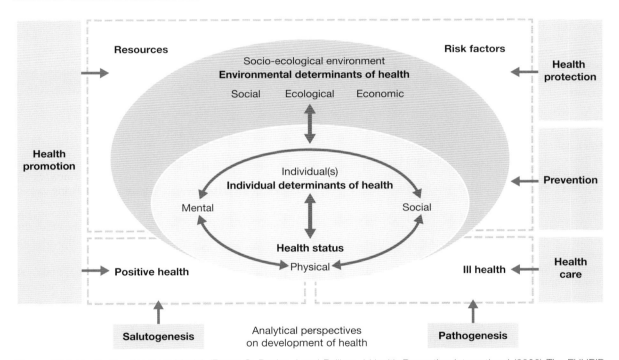

Figure 19.1 Health Development Model. (Bauer G, Davies J and Pelikan J Health Promotion International (2006) The EUHPID Health Development Model for the classification of public health indicators Vol 21 (2) pages 457-462 by permission of Oxford University Press.)

process and health promotion is intentional and planned. The model identifies three dimensions of health: physical, mental and social, and shows the interrelationship between health promotion and public health. The arrows pointing between these dimensions show that they are interdependent and interrelated. For example, exercising during pregnancy positively influences mental health and enables interaction and communication with others, thereby supporting social health.

This model shows the central role of *salutogenesis* and *pathogenesis*, which is integral within health and the health promotion process, illustrating that health development is an ongoing process, and health promotion is an intentional and planned approach aiming to sustain change within the health development process.

When using the model it is useful to note that the health of an individual is not created and lived in isolation but results from a dynamic ongoing relationship with the relevant socio-ecological environment, including the cultural dimension (Bauer et al 2006). The health promotion approach taken, therefore, must reflect this. The model also identifies that an individual's health status determines future health and can be used as a predictor of health; however, a targeted health promotion approach can improve the health potential of that individual. For example, a mother who smokes may be helped to stop smoking during pregnancy and, therefore, enhance her life potential and that of her baby.

The majority of studies that set out to establish the determinants of health and ill health are set within the *pathogenic paradigm* (Tones and Green 2004). *Pathogenesis* analyses how risk factors of individuals and their environment lead to ill health. Antonovsky (1996) proposed that an additional perspective should be adopted by health promotion practitioners, that of *salutogenesis*, which examines how resources in human life support development towards positive health. Bauer et al (2006) suggest that in real life, salutogenesis and pathogenesis are simultaneous, complementary and interacting real-life processes (see chapter website resources for case scenario 19.1).

Health promotion in the community

Antenatal and postnatal care is predominantly provided in the community, where care is accessible with opportunity for flexibility at the point of provision. Children's Centres provide a multiagency, multidisciplinary focus for healthcare provision, located in the heart of the community in deprived urban communities. The aim of a Children's Centre is to improve the health and well-being of children and their families by providing health and social care opportunities closer to their homes. They bring together childcare, health, family support and early education to improve access to services. It is commonplace for a midwife to provide maternity care in a Children's Centre within a multiagency, family-focused setting and is a model of care that continues to be supported by healthcare policy (National Health Service England (NHSE) 2014). With additional support from maternity services, midwives have the potential to develop further services in areas where they have the greatest reach, including, for example, supermarkets and leisure centres.

Healthcare provision in an environment outside of the hospital setting increases opportunities for developing equal partnerships between midwives and women – reducing the potential and sometimes held perception of medical dominance and power.

In England, plans to develop new care models will vertically integrate Primary and Acute Care Systems, helping women who use maternity services to have a greater choice over where and when they receive care (NHSE 2014).

Mental health promotion

Impaired mental health has a negative effect on emotional and physical health and reduces the individual's capacity to cope with everyday life activities. During the antenatal period, midwives routinely discuss mental health with the women and establish a history of pre-existing and current experiences. Timely support and referral to appropriate mental health support services is key in mitigating the progression of mental ill health. Specialist mental health services and allocation of the named midwife should coordinate a multidisciplinary care plan and postnatal follow-up. Women who miss appointments must have a bespoke care package that enables them to engage with health services. This approach may contribute to reducing further mortality in this area in the future, particularly as almost a quarter of women who died between 6 weeks and 1 year after pregnancy in 2009-2012 in the UK, died from mental-health related causes (Cantwell et al 2015), with variable levels of mental health support (see Ch. 69).

Reflective activity 19.2

Think about your midwifery practice over the past 2 months in terms of public health. How many public health activities have you been involved in?

Reading the next section may increase the number of activities identified.

Sexual health promotion

Addressing sexual health issues may contribute to the overall well-being of the woman and family; therefore, the midwife has an important role to play in this area of public health (see Ch. 55).

Influenza during pregnancy

Health education guidance regarding the influenza ('flu') vaccine should be provided to all women during early pregnancy and advice can be given at routine antenatal appointments. Influenza can cause pregnant women to become seriously ill, mainly as a result of changes to immune system are more prone to cause stillbirth, premature labour and low birthweight. The neonate will gain some protection if the mother is vaccinated in pregnancy. While there were no deaths from influenza in 2012 and 2013, predominantly because of a low level of influenza during this time, increasing immunization rates in pregnancy against seasonal influenza remains a public health priority (Knight et al 2015).

The midwife is ideally placed to provide health education about this important public health issue. Sharing the health gains should be integral to this discussion, including the protection that the vaccine provides during pregnancy for both the mother and fetus and postnatally until the baby is 6 months old (Kharbanda et al 2013; Nordin et al 2014; Centre for diseases control and prevention 2015).

For further information the reader is directed to the references.

Preconception care

Preconception care is described as the 'passport' to positive health during pregnancy. The aim of care is to optimize the chances of conception, ensure maintenance of a healthy pregnancy, and promote a healthy outcome for mother and baby (see Ch. 20).

Diet and nutrition

The midwife can provide effective health education in the area of diet and nutrition that may contribute to long-term healthy lifestyle changes (see Ch. 17). When discussing diet and nutrition, it is important to use a client-centred, empowerment approach supported by education. Behaviour change may also be necessary to promote immediate and long-term health. In an ever-changing healthcare climate where facts and knowledge change as new research emerges, the midwife must maintain current knowledge regarding diet and nutrition, as the woman and her family naturally look to the midwife for advice and guidance. Discussing a healthy diet and nutritional requirements during pregnancy are invaluable before and during the first trimester of pregnancy and, in particular, during embryogenesis.

Discussion should also include foods to avoid, for example, mould-ripened soft cheeses and soft blue-veined cheeses, as they are associated with miscarriage, still birth and the sick neonate because these cheeses may contain the *Listeria* bacterium.

Other items for discussion should include avoiding foods such as raw eggs, as they may contain the salmonella bacterium; unpasteurized milk, pâté, raw meat and cold meats and liver. Vitamin A supplementation should also be avoided and adequate vitamin D stores should be maintained during pregnancy and while breastfeeding. Caffeine consumption should also be reduced (Food Standards Agency 2015). Further information regarding diet and nutrition can be found in Chapter 17 and in the references.

Exercise during pregnancy

Exercise has many positive health benefits during pregnancy, including maintaining and improving fitness, mental well-being, improvement in cardiovascular function, reduction in excess weight gain, improvement in stamina and posture and maintenance of good muscle tone. While most people are aware of the benefits of exercise and sport, the midwife has a key role to play in supporting women to make wise exercise choices during pregnancy (see Ch. 22). When discussing the uptake and/or continuation of exercise during pregnancy, the client-centred, health promotion approach will enable an individualized approach, where the discussion is focused within the context of the woman's lived experience. It is important to adhere to safety principles during exercise and to enable physiological adjustment to take place, and midwives can use these to advise women (see chapter website resources for Web Case scenario 19.1). Women should avoid strenuous exercise to exhaustion, as this may cause blood flow diversion from the uterus, with resultant acute fetal hypoxia (De Oliveria et al 2012; Lewis 2014); 'jumpy, jerky' movements should also be avoided (NICE 2010; Lewis 2014).

Just as the maternal system copes with gradual respiratory and cardiac adjustments during pregnancy, the body also adjusts during exercise in a pregnancy identified as low risk. The woman who leads a sedentary lifestyle before pregnancy should be encouraged to undertake gentle exercise during pregnancy (NICE 2010); for example, walking, swimming and aquanatal exercise. Aquanatal is aerobic exercise in water for pregnant and postnatal women. The benefits of this type of exercise includes nonweight-bearing activity, hydrostatic pressure, buoyancy and upthrust. Additionally, the increased mobility experienced reduces strain on joints and may relieve backache. By encouraging women to take exercise at this point may have significant longer term health and well-being gains.

Tobacco use during pregnancy

Smoking is the largest single preventable cause of mortality and is responsible for reducing the female advantage in life expectancy (Lowry and Scammell 2013). It is a major cause of coronary heart disease, stroke, chronic bronchitis, and lung and other cancers, and is also associated with reduced fertility and early menopause in women (Essex et al 2014). In pregnancy, smoking is associated with low birthweight, preterm labour and perinatal death (Kuypers et al 2015). Other reports show an association between maternal smoking and wheeze during early childhood (Centre for diseases control and prevention 2015).

There has been a reduction in the number of women recorded as smoking at the time of delivery, with a fall from 15.1% in 2006-2007 to 12.7% in 2012-2013 (Action on Smoking and Health (ASH), Lowry and Scammell 2013).

Women from lower, unskilled occupations are five times more likely to smoke in pregnancy than those in professional roles. In England, teenagers are six times more likely to smoke than older mothers (ASH 2014).

Children who are exposed in the home to cigarette smoke are more likely to develop otitis media and asthma and have higher hospitalization rates for severe respiratory illness (ASH 2014). The commitment to reduce smoking during pregnancy is outlined in public health policy (DH 2012), which outlines a coordinated programme of work to reduce the proportion of women smoking during pregnancy.

Tobacco use: the midwife's role

Midwives play a key role in supporting pregnant smokers to quit. Timely identification and referral to stop smoking services is an integral part of the midwife's role. In more recent times, it is recommended that in addition to a discussion about the health benefits associated with stopping smoking during pregnancy, midwives should use carbon monoxide (CO) screening. The carbon monoxide test assesses exposure to tobacco smoke and should be used as a part of a motivational process to support women to stop smoking. When tobacco is burned and inhaled, CO is inhaled and absorbed into the bloodstream. Breath CO can be measured in a person's exhalation in parts per million of breath.

At the antenatal booking visit, the midwife should establish the woman's smoking status and, if she is a smoker, inform her about the risks of smoking to her unborn child and the effect of exposure to secondhand smoke (NICE 2013).

In preparation for undertaking the carbon monoxide test, the midwife must ask the woman if she or anyone in her household smokes. Establishing the smoking status of her partner is also required. The midwife should assess the woman's exposure to tobacco smoke through discussion and use of a CO test. The test will show the woman a measure of her smoking and her exposure to the smoke of others.

Before doing the test, establish that:

- the woman's smoking behaviour, for example, determine whether she is a light or infrequent smoker. This information will assist in interpreting the CO reading.

- the time the last cigarette was smoked and how many and at what times they were smoked. The midwife should be mindful of low early morning CO results, as levels fall overnight.

- for all women who smoke, or have stopped smoking within the last 2 weeks, to be referred to the NHS Stop Smoking Services. There is a risk of relapse for women who have recently stopped smoking; therefore, support from stop smoking services may be required. Women whose CO is 3 ppm or higher or should also be referred.

- women, who say they do not smoke but have a high CO reading of more than 10 ppm, be advised of the possibility of CO poisoning. They should be advised to call the free Health and Safety Executive gas safety advice line (NICE 2013).

The midwife should encourage the woman to use local NHS Stop Smoking Services and facilitate the referral. At subsequent antenatal appointments, the midwife should monitor the smoking status by using a carbon monoxide monitor if this is available in the practice area. If smoking cessation support is declined, there should be a discussion about the risks and benefits of nicotine replacement therapy (NRT), which is considered an option for some women and can be prescribed after consultation and counselling (NICE 2013). The effectiveness of NRT and its effect on the health of the fetus remains debatable (NICE 2013). The midwife should advise the woman that if NRT is the preferred option, the chances of successful quitting are still low if it is not accompanied by psychological support.

Supporting women to stop smoking during pregnancy requires a health promotion approach that is client-centred and the education, empowerment and behaviour change principles used. Ultimately, the midwife should empower the woman to make decisions about her own smoking behaviour. Approaches such as persuasion, cajoling and scaremongering, therefore, should be avoided, and it is important that the midwife aim for a supportive rather than judgemental approach.

Prochaska et al (1993) developed a behaviour change cycle to assist health professionals in identifying the readiness of clients to change their smoking behaviour (see Box 19.3).

Women who are highly dependent on tobacco may feel guilty and inadequate at not being able to give it up. The midwife must be encouraging and supportive and ready to offer help to women who express the desire to stop smoking, particularly if they are reluctant to attend smoking cessation counselling. Reducing the number of cigarettes smoked should generally be discouraged, but praised if this action is taken before contact with the midwife. While cutting down, people tend to drag on the cigarette more frequently than usual, inhale more deeply and smoke the cigarette as far to the end as is physically possible. The amount of noxious chemicals inhaled, therefore, may be the same as the dose inhaled before cutting down, when the nature of the smoking behaviour was casual.

Together with current knowledge of specialist support services available in the local area, the midwife can also offer health education leaflets, 'quit line' numbers and information about self-help groups, but leaflets should not be used as a replacement for discussion, personal support or sign-posting to other services and advice.

Damage limitation

Overwhelming evidence shows the association between secondhand smoke and sudden infant death syndrome (SIDS) (ASH 2014). Further evidence points towards the long-term effects of postnatal neonatal exposure, with associations made between secondhand smoke and heart disease, and increased risk of asthma attacks among those already affected (Del Ciampo and Del Ciampo 2014). An association has also been made between secondhand smoke breathed by the pregnant nonsmoker and increased maternal circulating absolute nucleated red blood cell

---

Box 19.3 The model of behaviour change in practice

Precontemplator

Not interested in stopping, has no intentions of stopping

What can I do?

- Present the risk factors and offer damage-limitation advice
- Refer for smoking cessation counselling

Contemplator

Is thinking about stopping, may have been thinking about stopping for several years

What can I do?

Encourage the woman to:

- attend smoking cessation counselling services
- explore reasons for wanting to stop; explore barriers to stopping
- discuss preparation needed to stop – this may involve removing all ashtrays and similar appliances
- consider triggers to smoking, e.g. telephone, coffee, after a meal, and think of an alternative strategy
- consider substitutes for habitual feelings, e.g. something in the mouth or hand
- consider substitutes if smoking is regularly used as a relaxer, or ice melter
- consider strategies that may help overcome the nicotine craving; think of times when the craving is strongest and consider strategies that may help overcome this

Ready for action

Ready to stop – may need help and support in doing so

What can I do?

Encourage the woman to:

- attend smoking cessation counselling services
- choose a time to give up when there are fewer triggers to smoke (e.g. stress)
- set a date to stop and stick to it (make plans for stopping as detailed in the contemplator section)

Relapse

Stopped smoking but has restarted

What can I do?

- Unsuccessful attempts to quit work towards successful quitting; the smoker may learn valuable lessons after each relapse episode, which may increase the chances of future success
- Encourage the woman to make a list of everything that went wrong, think of strategies that may reduce the likelihood of relapse
- Encourage her to attend smoking cessation counselling services

NB: Strategies must be client led and not prescribed by the midwife, whose role is primarily facilitating the discussion and offering support and guidance. The carbon monoxide monitor can be used in any of the behavioural change stages.

---

counts, which suggests there may be subtle negative effects on fetal oxygenation (Dollberg et al 2000).

The midwife has a responsibility to provide health information and education to women and their families to reduce the damage to the fetus/infant, without making the parents feel guilty. Through two-way communication with the woman and her partner, the midwife should establish the nature of the smoking behaviour and establish their readiness to change. If the woman is ready to stop smoking, the midwife should refer her for specialist support. However, if the woman is not ready to stop, damage limitation advice should be offered. This can involve exploring strategies for reducing the tobacco exposure to the neonate by suggesting that a smoke-free environment is created for the baby; that parents use another room to smoke – outside or near a window. Parents must be actively encouraged to explore strategies that best work for them rather than those prescribed by the midwife. This encourages ownership of plans made and ultimately ensures effectiveness.

Alcohol intake during pregnancy

Alcohol ingestion is a socially accepted behaviour that forms part of social interaction in the Western world (O'Keeffe et al 2015). Over the past 30 years, the number of women drinkers has increased more than that of men. Excessive alcohol intake is potentially lethal, affecting virtually every organ and system in the body, including the liver, gastrointestinal tract, and cardiovascular and neurological systems. It affects nutrition by suppressing the appetite and by altering the metabolism, mobilization and storage of nutrients (O'Keeffe et al 2015). Excessive or chronic alcohol abuse is associated with several vitamin and mineral deficiencies, including folic acid, vitamin B, magnesium and iron. Learning difficulties, loss of memory and other mental problems are associated with infants born to parents who have abused alcohol (Nykjaer et al 2014). Women's tolerance of alcohol is lower than that of men's because of differences in body size, absorption and metabolism. Women have a higher proportion of fat to water; therefore, alcohol becomes more concentrated in body fluids and damaging effects such as gastritis, pancreatitis, peptic ulcers and malnutrition are more likely to develop.

Drinking alcohol during pregnancy is both teratogenic and fetotoxic (NICE 2008) and excessive intake during pregnancy is associated with fetal alcohol syndrome and fetal alcohol spectrum disorder (see Ch. 49).

Safe measures of alcohol during pregnancy

Despite numerous research studies, to date there is no universally acceptable safe measure of alcohol consumption during pregnancy. In the US, alcohol consumption of any amount during pregnancy or for women considering a pregnancy is not recommended – advice consistently given since 1981 by the US Surgeon General's Office. Alcohol-containing products also carry a health warning.

In the UK, a range of options are available that allow some drinking during pregnancy. For example, the Royal College of Obstetrics and Gyynaecology (RCOG) advises that drinking alcohol during pregnancy and breastfeeding should be avoided, but small amounts of alcohol after the first trimester may not be harmful to the fetus. Current guidance states that women should not drink more than one or two units of alcohol once or twice per week (RCOG 2015).

Women should be informed that getting drunk or binge drinking during pregnancy (defined as more than 5 standard drinks or 7.5 UK units on a single occasion) may be harmful to the unborn baby. New Department of Health guidance released in 2016 stated clearly that:

> 'The Guidelines development group recommends that women who are pregnant or planning a pregnancy should be advised that the safest approach is not to drink alcohol at all. There is no scientific basis for setting a limit below which alcohol consumption will not harm the fetus'
>
> (DH 2016: 4)

See chapter website resources for additional information.

Antenatal screening

During the antenatal period, starting at the booking visit, questions relating to alcohol intake should be specific and focused enough to identify women who have a drinking problem. At the first antenatal visit, the midwife should ask the woman if she drinks alcohol. Common responses include 'no', 'yes', 'not really', or 'just socially'. Further enquiry must follow to establish clear meaning to ensure the appropriate health promotion approach is taken. There is a general trend towards underreporting, which will inhibit the identification of high-risk drinkers. Heavy drinkers may book late for maternity care and require

intensive counselling with referral to specialist agencies to help them reduce alcohol consumption. Highlighting teratogenic effects on the fetus forms part of health education, but midwives should be sensitive in ensuring that the information they provide is balanced and informed, and does not result in fear or guilt, as this may impede the woman's ability to reduce drinking levels.

A useful way of taking a drinking history is to ask specifically about the preceding 7 days. If alcohol has been consumed, the amount in units should be recorded and discussed with the woman.

The Alcohol Use Disorders Identification Test is a 10-question test developed by the World Health Organization (WHO) to determine whether a person may be at risk of drinking levels of alcohol that may be excessive (Saunders et al 1993). The test was designed to be used internationally, and evidence supports the tool as a screen for alcohol dependence and for less severe alcohol problems (Public Health England 2012). (See chapter website resources for access to the tool and the guidance for its use.)

Drugs in pregnancy

Pregnant women should be advised to take only those drugs that are prescribed by a doctor. It is important to explain to the woman the reasons for this and to establish whether she is taking any particular medications and record these. The British National Formulary (BMA and RPSGB 2015), also available online, offers an excellent guide on drugs contraindicated in pregnancy (see Ch. 10 and the recommended reading list for further information about drugs in pregnancy and drug misuse).

Domestic violence and abuse

Domestic violence poses a serious threat to women's health and may be emotional, sexual, physical or financial abuse and can result in homicide (WHO 2011). Another form of abuse is within the partner demonstrating controlling and coercive behaviour, which can result in all aspects of the woman's life being under the partner's direct control and influence (Home Office 2015). Approximately 1 million women a year experience at least one incident of domestic violence, equating to nearly 20,000 women a week (DH 2013). It is well established that violence towards women increases during pregnancy (Duxbury 2014). Reasons for this are numerous and may include feelings of overpossessiveness, jealousy and denial of the women having any other role than spouse. The perpetrator may feel jealous of the woman's ability to produce a child or see the fetus as an intruder. He or she may also become violent because of strained finances or reduced sexual activity (Duxbury 2014).

The perpetrator is usually the male partner or ex-partner, but domestic violence may occur in same-sex relationships or from other family members.

Abused women and abusers come from all cultural, educational, racial, religious and socioeconomic backgrounds. Disabled women are twice as likely to experience domestic violence than nondisabled women and a proportion of these may be pregnant at some point in their lives (DH 2014).

Female genital mutilation is also recognized as violence against girls and women (RCM 2010; WHO 2014) and more information can be found in Chapter 56.

Midwives must be able to recognize women at risk of violence and provide information and support, acting as a conduit to local resources, support networks and services (Box 19.4).

Risk to the woman and fetus

Domestic violence and abuse during pregnancy has been associated with adverse pregnancy outcomes, including low birthweight. They are at risk of having undetected complications that may lead to poor outcomes because they may be unable to attend for antenatal care. The physical and psychological risks to the woman and fetus are overwhelmingly high, and the fetus may be injured or may die during the pregnancy. Between 2009 and 2013 in the UK, 36 women were murdered during pregnancy or up to 1 year after giving birth (Knight et al 2015). There was no evidence that all of these women had been asked about a history of domestic abuse.

Risks to other family members

In households where there is domestic violence, the children within that household may be affected. They may observe the abuse or be injured directly or indirectly as a result of the abuse (Knight 2015). The fear experienced and the psychological consequences are immeasurable and may influence the child's emotional development. The child may also try to protect younger siblings or take on the role of prime carer.

The midwife's role

Because of the number of domestic violence cases that start or intensify during pregnancy, domestic abuse routine enquiry is now commonplace. Routine enquiry for domestic violence during pregnancy has been found to increase the rate of detection, enabling women who disclose domestic violence to seek help early (NICE 2008).

Women who disclose domestic violence should have a named midwife who will provide support and continuity for the woman throughout the antenatal, intrapartum and postnatal periods.

When violence is suspected, the best way to confirm suspicion is by direct questioning. However, the environment **must be assessed as safe** before questions being asked (Box 19.4).

Denial of abuse

The woman may choose to deny being abused, but awareness that help is available is useful to provide. For some women, however, pregnancy provides a unique opportunity for change and, therefore, disclosure of violence may be likely (NICE 2014). Common difficulties for routine enquiry include:

- finding an appropriate time to ask the question, particularly when the woman is not accompanied by her partner
- denial of abuse and subsequent nonattendance for antenatal care
- lack of supervision services for midwives who receive disclosure

In anticipation of some of these difficulties, many maternity services inform the woman via the booking

---

Box 19.4 Domestic abuse: raising the subject of domestic violence and abuse

To introduce the subject of violence you may choose to frame the question:

'As violence in the home is so common, we now ask about it routinely.'

Direct questions may include:

'Are you in a relationship with someone who hurts or threatens you'?

'Has someone hurt you'?

'Did someone cause these injuries to you'?

It is helpful to validate the response(s) you receive by saying:

'You are not alone'.

'You are not to blame for what is happening to you'.

'You do not deserve to be treated in this way'.

It is helpful to assess the woman's safety by asking:

'Is your partner here with you'?

'Where are the children'?

'Do you have any immediate worries'?

'Do you have a place of safety'?

Now, use your knowledge of domestic violence support, and be responsive to the woman's needs.

Know how to contact your local domestic violence agency and local independent domestic violence advisor.

Be familiar with the supportive leaflets, referral processes and safeguarding procedures.

Ensure that your documentation is in line with the principles of confidentiality defined by your organization.

(Adapted from DH 2014)

appointment letter that she will be required to see the midwife alone on at least one occasion during the pregnancy.

Fostering a safe, nurturing and private environment during antenatal visits, with the midwife expressing genuineness, positive regard, empathy and honesty, may empower the woman to seek help. Survivors of domestic violence often feel ashamed about being abused by their partner, have low self-esteem and have conflicting feelings about disclosure, including the repercussions of their actions. Very often, leaving the abuser is not considered a favourable option. Some women are financially and emotionally dependent on their abusers, who often have control over all domestic arrangements. Religious and cultural influences often encourage people to stay in abusive marriages where separation or divorce is considered unacceptable.

The midwife should understand the nature of domestic violence, be sensitive and alert for clues that may suggest abuse (see Box 19.5) and be aware of the effect of abuse on everyday life. When the woman and midwife are not in the company of the partner – for example, when showing the woman where the toilet is – an opportunity for the woman to disclose something about how she is feeling that may be indirectly related to the abuse-may occur. The midwife should be mindful that the woman may have multiple abusers who may be colluding; therefore, time alone with the woman must always be facilitated.

Although considered a viable approach, direct questioning is not the only option for obtaining information. Some midwives may be reluctant to acknowledge domestic violence or ask questions about it because of:

- fear of offending the woman
- fear of disclosure

- lack of knowledge of what action to take if this occurs
- feeling that it is a private matter and belief that it is not a part of their role
- they themselves have been or continue to be abused

In addition to providing information about domestic violence in booking information and handheld maternity notes, each maternity provider in the hospital or community should have current details about domestic violence units and the Women's Aid Federation, which provides a safe refuge for those who need it (see details in the chapter website resources). The Samaritans, Relate and Victim Support all offer support services to survivors of domestic violence. The healthcare environment should be designed to enable disclosure of domestic violence, including, for example, posters, fliers and flash cards that include details of relevant helplines (NICE 2014).

Employment and health

For the majority of women, work during pregnancy does not pose a threat to their health or that of their babies (NICE 2008). For some, it may be necessary to modify working practices to promote safety and comfort.

The pregnant woman should avoid heavy lifting. Seating for sedentary workers should be supportive to the back because of increased *lumbar lordosis*. Standing for long periods should be avoided and rest periods instituted because of the risk of development of varicosities. Smoky environments should be avoided because of the risks associated with passive smoking.

Some occupations may be hazardous to the health of the fetus and expectant mother, including exposure to

---

Box 19.5 Possible signs of domestic abuse in women

Frequent appointments for vague symptoms	Frequent missed appointments
Injuries inconsistent with explanation of cause	Multiple injuries at different stages of healing
Woman tries to hide injuries or minimize their extent	Patient appears frightened, overly anxious or depressed
Partner always attends unnecessarily	Woman is submissive or afraid to speak in front of her partner
Woman is reluctant to speak in front of partner	Partner is aggressive or dominant, talks for a woman or refuses to leave the room
Suicide attempts – particularly with Asian women	Poor or nonattendance at antenatal clinics
History of repeated miscarriages, terminations, stillbirths or preterm labour	Injuries to the breasts or abdomen
Repeat presentation with depression, anxiety, self-harm or psychosomatic symptoms	Recurring sexually transmitted infections or urinary tract infections
Non-compliance with treatment	Early self-discharge from hospital

None of these mentioned signs automatically indicates domestic abuse. But they should raise suspicion and prompt you to make every attempt to see the woman alone and in private to ask her whether she is being abused. Even if she chooses not to disclose her circumstance at this time, she will know you are aware of the issues, and she might choose to approach you at a later time. If you are going to ask a woman about domestic violence, always follow your Trust's or Health Authority's guidance or the suggestions, as provided in Box 19.4.

toxic chemicals (such as lead, pesticides, anaesthetic gases and radiation). Utilization of protective clothing in the home and the workplace, where appropriate, and adhering to safety parameters and work codes will minimize exposure to teratogenic hazards. This makes it important for the midwife to establish the woman's normal working environment, identify any potential hazards, and provide a conduit for further information should this be required (see chapter website resources).

Travel

The midwife has a responsibility to raise awareness about travel and health. The most basic but essential information can reduce the risk of harm to the woman, fetus and infant. Health education during the antenatal period should include the appropriate use of car seats and the correct application of seatbelts during pregnancy, including, for example, the correct positioning of the seatbelt above and below the uterus (NICE 2008).

Other travel advice given to pregnant women may need to include information about airline travel, particularly 'long haul' flights, when the risk of venous thrombosis is increased. Many airlines do not allow women to fly after 36 completed weeks of pregnancy because of the risk of labour starting. If women are at risk of preterm labour, they should not fly after 32 completed weeks gestation.

Some airlines require a letter from a midwife or doctor confirming the expected date of delivery and anticipated complications, if air travel takes place after 28 weeks gestation.

It also useful to be aware of any risks to health in parts of the world to which the woman may travel, and advise accordingly. NHS Scotland provides useful information to be considered (NHS Scotland 2017).

For further information regarding air travel and pregnancy, please access Air Travel and Pregnancy (RCOG 2013).

Public transport usually provides some seating allocated to pregnant and childbearing women, and some initiatives, such as the London Transport 'Baby on Board' badge, which enables women easy access to these courtesies.

Evaluation

Evaluation is the process by which criteria to determine the value of an idea or method is formulated. The aim of this is to demonstrate the success of the method based on designated aims and learning outcomes.

Without the use of appropriate evaluation tools, the potential to challenge the efficacy of midwifery health promotion is reduced. Evaluation is a worthwhile process and needs to be used to demonstrate the effect and outcome of interventions deemed to enhance health. Knowledge about the most suitable methods of evaluation

is essential not only to highlight the most effective health interventions but also to demonstrate their efficacy to key stakeholders who influence resource allocation. Midwives may use qualitative or quantitative methods of data collection to formulate evaluation results (see Ch. 6).

Health promotion evaluation can be extremely difficult for the midwife, particularly when assessing long-term success of a health intervention or behavioural change. Other areas that present challenges in terms of evaluation include awareness raising and empowerment.

Reflective activity 19.3

Consider the content of this chapter and the midwife's health promotion role. Collate a list of local and national referral agencies and support groups that are relevant to the areas mentioned. Continue to add to this list as you engage with more services and refresh the list if contacts close their services, or new services become available. This will become a useful resource in your daily practice in supporting women and families.

CONCLUSION

Health promotion is an integral part of the midwife's role, with many potential health-gain benefits for the childbearing population. Understanding the context of health and illness is a key factor in promoting health, and choosing the appropriate health promotion approach to achieve the desired aim is essential if the health promotion approach is to be effective. The midwife's scope of practice provides room for the public health role to be enhanced and community initiatives to be embraced. The midwife is a vital resource for health enhancement throughout pregnancy, birth, postnatal period and beyond. The current UK political health agenda recognizes the valuable contribution midwives make to the health of the nation. Evaluation of all health promotion activities will provide evidence of the effect of the midwife's work in terms of health gain.

Key Points

- The concept of health and the meaning of health promotion are fundamental to the role of the midwife.
- The midwife needs to be aware of her own attitudes, behaviours and understanding of health to promote the health of others.
- The midwife should expand his/her knowledge of women's health and screening to improve the health promotion approach.
- It is important to provide realistic and appropriate health promotion strategies, and develop a mechanism for evaluating their effectiveness.

References

Acheson D (Chair): *Independent inquiry into inequalities in health*, London, 1998, The Stationery Office (TSO).

Action on Smoking and Health (ASH): *Secondhand smoke: the impact on children 2014* (website). www.ash .org.uk/files/documents/ASH_596 .pdf. 2014.

Antonovsky A: The salutogenic model as a theory to guide health promotion, *Health Promot Int* 11(1):11–18, 1996.

Bauer G, Davies J, Pelikan J: The EUHPID Health Development Model for the classification of public health indicators, *Health Promot Int* 21(2):457–462, 2006.

Becker MH, Haefner DP, Kasl SV, et al: Selected psycho-social models and correlates of individual heath-related behaviours, *Med Care* 15(5):27–46, 1977.

Black D, Morris JN, Smith C, et al: *Inequalities in health: the Black Report*, Harmondsworth, 1982, Penguin.

British Medical Association (BMA), Royal Pharmaceutical Society of Great Britain (RPSGB): *British National Formulary*, ed 56, London, 2015, BMA.

Cantwell R, Knight M, Oates M, et al: On behalf of the MBRRACE-UK mental health chapter writing group. *Lessons on maternal mental health*. In Knight M, Tuffnell D, Kenyon S, et al, editors: *on behalf of MBRRACE-UK. Saving Lives, Improving Mothers' Care – Surveillance of maternal deaths in the UK 2011–2013 and lessons learned to inform maternity care from the UK and Ireland Confidential Enquiries into Maternal Deaths and Morbidity 2009–2013*, Oxford, 2015, National Perinatal Epidemiology Unit, University of Oxford, pp 22–41.

Centre for diseases control and prevention. *Seasonal Flu Vaccine Safety and Pregnant Women* (website). http://www.cdc.gov/flu/ protect/vaccine/qa_vacpregnant.htm. 2015.

De Oliveria A, Silva J, Tavares J, et al: Effect of a physical exercise programme during pregnancy on uteroplacental and fetal blood flow and fetal growth: a randomized controlled trial, *Obstet Gynecol* 120:302, 2012.

Del Ciampo L, Del Ciampo L: Passive smoking and children's health, *Health* 6(12):2014.

Department of Health (DH): *Saving lives: our healthier nation; a contract for health*, London, 1999, The Stationery Office (TSO).

Department of Health (DH): *National service framework for children, young people and maternity services: core standards*, London, 2004, DH.

Department of Health (DH): *Maternity matters: choice, access and continuity of care in a safe service*, London, 2007, DH.

Department of Health (DH): *Health inequalities: progress and the next steps*, London, 2008, DH.

Department of Health (DH): *Improving outcomes and supporting transparency part 1: a public health outcomes framework for England, 2013–2016*, 2012, DH.

Department of Health (DH): *The public health outcomes framework for England, 2013–2016*, 2012, DH.

Department of Health (DH): *Guidance for health professionals on domestic violence*, London, 2013, DH.

Department of Health (DH): *Visiting and school nursing programmes: supporting implementation of the new service model*. Domestic Violence and Abuse – Professional Guidance, DH, 2014.

Department of Health (DH): *2016 Alcohol Guidelines Review – report from the guidelines development group to the UK Chief Medical Officers*, 2016, DH. https://www.gov.uk/ government/uploads/system/ uploads/attachment_data/ file/489797/CMO_Alcohol_ Report.pdf.

Dollberg S, Fainaru O, Mimouni FB, et al: The effect of passive smoking in pregnancy on neonatal nucleated red blood cells, *Pediatrics* 106(3):E34, 2000.

Duxbury F: *Domestic violence and abuse, in ABC of domestic and sexual violence*. S. Bewley and J. Welch, Chichester, 2014, John Wiley & Sons Ltd, pp 9–16.

Essex H, Parrott S, Wu Qi, et al: *Cost-effectiveness of nicotine patches for smoking cessation in pregnancy: a placebo randomized controlled trial (SNAP)*. Nicotine and Tobacco

Research, 2014, Oxford University Press.

Fisher J, Cabral de Mello B, Patel V, et al: *Prevalence and determinants of common perinatal mental disorders in women in low- and lower-middle -income countries: a systematic review* (website). www.who.int/bulletin/ volumes/90/2/11-091850/en/. 2011.

Food Standards Agency (FSA): (website). www.food.gov.uk.

Guvenc G, Akyuza A, Ikel C: Health belief model scale for cervical cancer and Pap smear test: psychometric testing, *J Adv Nurs* 67(2):428–437, 2011.

Health and Social Care Act 2012 (website). www.legislation.gov.uk/ ukpga/2012/7/contents/enacted. 2002.

Home Office. *Serious Crime Act 2015 part 5 domestic abuse section 76.*

Kharbanda E, Vazquez-Benitez G, Lipkind H, et al: Vaccine safety datalink. 'Inactivated influenza vaccine during pregnancy and risks for adverse obstetric events, *Obstet Gynecol* 122(3):659–667, 2013.

Knight M, Tuffnell D, Kenyon S, et al, editors: *on behalf of MBRRACE-UK: Saving lives, improving mothers' care – surveillance of maternal deaths in the UK 2011–2013 and lessons learned to inform maternity care from the UK and Ireland confidential enquiries into maternal deaths and morbidity 2009–2013*, Oxford, 2015, National Perinatal Epidemiology Unit, University of Oxford.

Kuypers L, Xu X, Jankipersadsing S, et al: *DNA methylation mediates the effect of maternal smoking during pregnancy on birthweight of the offspring. International journal epidemiology* doi: 10.1093/ije/dyv048 (website). http://ije.oxfordjournals .org/. 2015.

Lewis E: Exercise in pregnancy, *Aust Fam Physician* 43(8):541–542, 2014.

Lowry C, Scammell K: *Smoking cessation in pregnancy – a call to action* (website). www.ash.org.uk/ pregnancy2013. 2013.

Manktelow BM, Smith LK, Evans TA, et al, on behalf of the MBRRACE-UK collaboration: *Perinatal mortality* surveillance report UK perinatal deaths for births from January to December 2013, Leicester, 2015, The Infant Mortality and Morbidity Group, Department of Health Sciences, University of Leicester.

Marmot M: Fair society, healthy lives. The Marmot review. Strategic review of health inequalities in england post-2010. The Marmot Review, London (website). http://www.instituteofhealthequity.org/projects/fair-society-healthy-lives-the-marmot-review. 2010.

Nykjaer C, Alwan N, Greenwood D, Cade J: Maternal alcohol intake prior to and during pregnancy and risk of adverse birth outcomes: evidence from a British cohort, *J Epidemiol Community Health* 68(6):542–549, 2014.

National Health Service (NHS) England (NHSE): *Five year forward view* (website). www.england.nhs.uk/wp-content/uploads/2014/10/5yfvweb.pdf. 2014.

NHS Scotland/Health Protection Scotland: *Fit for Travel: travel health information for people travelling abroad from the UK* (website). http://www.fitfortravel.scot.nhs.uk/home.aspx. 2017.

National Institute for Health and Care Excellence (NICE): *Antenatal care* (website). www.nice.org.uk/guidance/. 2008.

National Institute for Health and Care Excellence (NICE): *Weight management before, during and after pregnancy. Public health guideline* (website). nice.org.uk/guidance/ph27. 2010.

National Institute for Health and Care Excellence (NICE): *Smoking: smoking: acute, maternity and mental health services* (website). www.nice.org.uk/guidance. 2013.

National Institute for Health and Care Excellence (NICE): *Domestic violence and abuse: how health services, social care and the organisations they work with can respond effectively* (website). www.nice.org.uk/guidance/ph50. 2014.

Nordin J, Kharbanda E, Vazquez G, et al: Datalink, vaccine safety. 'Maternal influenza vaccine and risks for preterm or small for gestational age birth', *J Pediatr* 164(5):1051–1057, 2014.

Norheim O, Jha P, Philb D, et al: Avoiding 40% of the premature deaths in each country, 2010–30: review of national mortality trends to help quantify the UN Sustainable Development Goal for health, *Lancet* 385(9964):17–23, 2015.

Office for National Statistics (ONS): *Inequality in healthy life expectancy by area deprivation 2009–2011.* (website). www.ons.gov.uk/ons/rel. 2014.

O'Keeffe L, Kearney P, McCarthy F, et al: Prevalence and predictors of alcohol use during pregnancy: findings from international multicentre cohort studies, *BMJ Open* 5, 2015.

Prochaska J, Diclemente C, Norcross C: In search of how people change: applications to addictive behaviours, *Addiction Nursing Network* 5(1):3–16, 1993.

Public Health England 2012 AUDIT: *Alcohol use disorders identification test* (website). www.alcohollearning centre.org.uk/Topics/Browse/Brief Advice/?parent = 4444&child = 4896. 2012.

Rosenstock I: Why people use health services, *Milbank Mem Fund Q* 44(3):94–127, 1966.

Rotter JB: Generalized expectancies for internal versus external control of re-enforcement, *Psychol Monogr* 80(1):1–28, 1966.

Royal College of Obstetricians and Gynaecologists (RCOG): *Air travel and pregnancy* (website). www.rcog.org.uk/en/guidelines-research-services/guidelines/sip1/. 2013.

Royal College of Midwives (RCM): *Position statement violence against women and girls* (website). www.rcm.org.uk/violence-against-women-and-girls. 2010.

Royal College of Obstetricians and Gynaecologists (RCOG): Alcohol during pregnancy, *Pregnancy* (website). www.rcog.org.uk/. 2015.

Secretary of State for Health: *The NHS plan: a plan for investments. A plan for reform, Cm4818-1*, London, 2000, The Stationery Office (TSO).

Saunders J, Aasland O, Babor T, et al: Development of the Alcohol Use Disorders Identification Test (AUDIT): WHO collaborative project on early detection of persons with harmful alcohol consumption, *Addiction* 88:791–804, 1993.

Scriven A: *Promoting health a practical guide*, London, 2010, Elsevier.

Tones K, Green J: *Health promotion: planning and strategies*, London, 2004, Sage.

United Nations: *The Millennium Development Goals Report New York* (website). www.un.org/millennium goals/2015_MDG_Report/pdf/MDG%202015%20rev%20(July%201).pdf. 2015.

US Surgeon General Surgeon: *General's Advisory on Alcohol and Pregnancy* (website). http://come-over.to/FAS/SurgeonGeneral.htm. 1981.

Wallston K, Wallston B, DeVellis R: Development of the multidimensional health locus of control scales, *Health Educ Monogr* 6:161–170, 1978.

World Health Organization (WHO): *Constitution*, New York, 1946, WHO.

World Health Organization (WHO): *Health promotion: a discussion document on concepts and principle*, Geneva, 1984, WHO.

World Health Organization (WHO): *Intimate partner violence during pregnancy* (website). http://whqlibdoc.who.int/hq/2011/WHO. 2011.

World Health Organization (WHO): *Worldwide action needed to address hidden crisis of violence against women and girls* (website). www.who.int/mediacentre/news/releases/2014/violence-women-girls/en/. 2014.

Resources and additional reading

Please refer to the chapter website resources.

Salutogenesis – an introduction *by Bengt Lindström Professor of Health Promotion Nordic School of Public Health,* available at: http://www.ndphs.org///documents/2502/SALUTOGEN%20ESIS%20and%20NCDs.pdf.

Very good overview of salutogenesis and its potential for health promotion.

The American College of Obstetricians and Gynaecologists produce useful resources for women and families, including a 'Frequently Asked Questions' sheet:

Exercise during pregnancy: www.acog.org/-/media/For-Patients/faq119.pdf?dmc=1&ts=20160119T1138234385.2011.

https://www.rcog.org.uk/en/news/rcog-release-air-travel-and-pregnancy--all-you-need-to-know/.

Guidance from the UK Royal College of Obstetricians and Gynaecologists.

The midwifery public health contribution – https://www.gov.uk/government/…/**Midwifery**_strategy_visual_B.pdf.

Promoting *normality throughout labour and birth within a sensitive and safe birth.* **Midwifery** *public* **health** *actions throughout the maternity pathway. Useful diagram showing the varied role of the midwife in public health.*

Royal College of Midwives (RCM) – Midwives and Public Health – webpage, which includes new publications and news. https://www.rcm.org.uk/subject/public-health-and-health-promotion.

Chapter 20

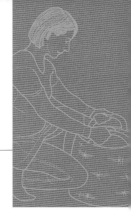

Preconception care

Melanie Brooke-Read and Barbara Burden

Learning Outcomes ?

By the end of this chapter, the reader should be able to:

- critique the key concepts of preconception care and screening
- apply professional judgement when advising, screening and developing a preconception plan of care for women and partners

INTRODUCTION

This chapter will consider contemporaneous health and well-being issues and reducible or reversible risks that can be identified before conception occurs, to enable midwives and other healthcare providers to assist women and their partners in achieving optimal outcomes for maternal and neonatal health.

Preconception care encompasses wide-ranging information, advice, screening and care provision for women and their partners before conception that focuses on optimizing maternal and neonatal health (Basatemur et al 2013). Importantly, preconception care should be valued as a continuum of support from healthcare providers rather than an isolated contact, to ensure that prospective parents are at the peak of their health potential at the point of conception and organogenesis (subsequent 17–56 days), when the potential for fetal abnormality is at its highest (Flower et al 2013). When pre-existing health concerns are present, preconception care should also involve specialist practitioners and coordinated care plans (Mothers and Babies: Reducing Risk through Audits and Confidential Enquiries across the UK (MBRRACE-UK) 2014).

Best practice would involve prospective parents seeking health advice and screening from appropriately trained health professionals in the 6 months before conception. Though some prospective parents will seek this, in reality few perceive the benefits of preconception health assessment and screening. It is in those pregnancies where the outcome is already compromised, that parents then seek to identify the risks that could have been prevented or minimized. Preconception care should focus on women and men who have potential for conception in any given context or circumstance, for example, a traditional relationship, same-sex relationship or parenting through surrogacy.

Developing public health and family-centred care is essential to the role of the midwife, with every health promotion activity, including elements of preconception information. In addition, this care must be included in routine health screening activities offered by other healthcare professionals through the use of literature and classes in schools, family planning or cervical screening sessions (Tuomainen et al 2013). Addressing the full range of preconception advice would not be feasible nor appropriate at each encounter; therefore, healthcare professionals must use their clinical acumen in providing targeted risk assessment, individualized screening and specific interventions as required. Additional written preconception and health promotion literature should be available in pregnancy testing kits, abortion centres, pharmacies and general practitioner (GP) surgeries, where women can be targeted post-termination or after a negative pregnancy test.

Lifestyle choices, relationship and reproductive sexual health education is embedded in the UK schools' curriculum, and healthcare professionals who visit or work in schools have an ideal opportunity to inform adolescents about planning for pregnancy and preparedness for parenting. Supportive health promotion literature should be readily available in school/college common rooms (Hill et al 2013).

PRECONCEPTION CARE CHALLENGES

From an idealistic perspective, every pregnancy would be well planned, with every infant conceived in an optimally healthy environment. The reality is that preconception care varies widely at all levels – local, national and international – generally reaching out to a small sector of the population (Knight et al 2014). The more motivated, articulate and informed individuals, or those who may have experienced a compromised pregnancy already, are likely to access preconception support and advice (Anderson, Norman and Middleton 2010). Women of reproductive age and men with the potential for adverse outcomes of pregnancy (such as those who smoke, have high alcohol or drug use, poor dietary habits or pre-existing infection or disease) should be perceived as a priority by midwives and other health professionals.

Competing priorities in healthcare may not place preconception care high on the public health agenda; however, midwives and healthcare professionals should acknowledge that the provision of appropriate, targeted preconception care has a direct effect on pregnancy and outcomes. See example Table 20.1: Example of targeted preconception care.

Preconception care has led to some significant health improvement outcomes. Notably, a reduction in neural tube defects since the recommendation of folic acid supplementation, particularly pre-pregnancy and during early embryonic development (organogenesis), and a reduction in congenital abnormalities associated with women with diabetic hyperglycaemia. Notwithstanding, the challenges moving onwards include breaking down existing barriers to preconception care, so that women marginalized because of low-income, culture, ethnicity, age, intellect or ill health can readily access this care when necessary.

Consider an opportunistic contact you have experienced with a woman in a healthcare setting other than midwifery.
   How could you have initiated a conversation about preconception health and well-being?
   What information would you prioritize and why?

AIMS AND OBJECTIVES OF PRECONCEPTION CARE AND INTERVENTIONS

Effective preconception care encompasses three fundamental elements: identification of risk, education and behavioural change, and interventions for optimal pregnancy

Table 20.1 A woman with epilepsy diagnosed in childhood

Preconception advice and care nationally and internationally recommended (Harden et al 2009; National Institute for Health and Clinical Excellence (NICE) 2012) *NICE Epilepsy guideline CG137*	
Preconception intervention	**Effect/benefit on planned pregnancy**
Review of potentially outdated treatment plan and referral to an epilepsy specialist	An opportunity to base care on best available evidence
Discussion with woman/couple to raise perception of epilepsy as a high-risk condition	More likely to access services and treatment and understand effects of drugs and seizures on pregnancy and fetus
Review of antiepileptic drug (AED) regimen	To limit the teratogenic effect of certain AEDs (avoiding sodium valproate, for example) and to use the lowest, effective dose possible
Inclusion of specialist epilepsy nurse/physician	Improved psychosocial outcomes; improved treatment compliance; reduced admissions due to seizures; better seizure control; more frequent clinical reviews. Prevention of associated deaths from seizures (drowning) (MBRRACE 2014)

Additional reading:
http://www.nice.org.uk
http://www.npeu.ox.ac.uk/mbrrace-uk

outcomes, which will be outlined later under these three significant themes. A noteworthy learning and educational resource is available to healthcare professionals on the National Institute for Health and Care Excellence (NICE) website, such as http://cks.nice.org.uk/preconception-advice-and-management. (See chapter website resources for additional links.)

The health and well-being of prospective parents, ensuring that their maximum health potential at the point of conception and throughout the organogenesis period, is the ultimate aim of preconception care.

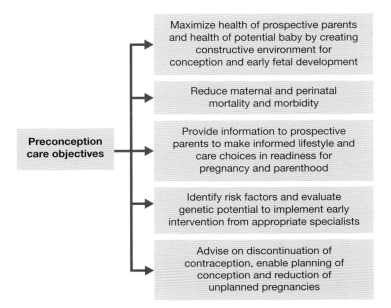

Figure 20.1   The objectives of preconception.

In the past, criticism was made of the predominantly clinical approach to preconception care, however attitudes and approaches are changing. Tuomainen et al (2013) recommend that a broader, inclusive collaboration between healthcare professionals, organizations, charities and social policy makers is needed, coupled with improving the potential for innovative marketing and social media exposure, to enhance the face-face, planned or opportunistic contacts, which women value. The objectives of preconception care are summarized in Fig. 20.1. Implementing an all-inclusive approach to preconception care offers significant opportunity to improve both maternal and child health outcomes. It is apparent that major clinical influencers in the UK such as the Royal College of Obstetricians and Gynaecologists (RCOG), National Institute for Health and Care Excellence (NICE), Scottish Intercollegiate Guidelines Network (SIGN), MBRRACE-UK, Royal College of Midwives (RCM) and National Screening Committee (NSC) continue to focus their attention on targeted preconception care in situations where risks have already been highlighted. The challenge in moving forward is to adopt a 'life-course perspective' approach to improving maternal and child outcomes By addressing the three overarching themes of significance, every midwife and healthcare practitioner can begin to influence change in delivering preconception care. These themes are as follows:

1. Identifying risk

2. Education/lifestyle

3. Interventions

1. Identification of risk

The preconception care assessment and reproductive awareness

When a woman and/or her partner present for preconception advice, the supporting professional should record a full and detailed health history from both potential partners and significant others, such as where genetic screening is indicated or in the case of surrogacy or ovum/sperm donation (Goldman et al 2014). Creating a therapeutic relationship where the healthcare professional can educate and counsel prospective parents is essential to achieving optimum health in readiness for pregnancy and beyond. Information obtained during this assessment will be crucial in creating an effective plan of care, providing a baseline for subsequent comparative tests and collaborating with other specialist practitioners where necessary.

Ideally, this discussion is undertaken in a private environment where confidentiality is maintained and enough time allowed for actively listening, offering advice and undertaking of any necessary screening tests. This is an ideal opportunity to educate through detailed explanation and to obtain informed consent, supported further with information literature and other resources. Couples should be given the opportunity for an individual private discussion, as they may have information they do not wish to disclose with their partner while present.

Couples should be given practical information on discontinuation of contraception and fertility awareness advice to assist them in planning and optimizing their chances of a successful pregnancy.

Risk assessment focuses on identification of conditions or pre-existing factors that could adversely affect a potential pregnancy in an attempt to assess the required interventions needed to reduce the severity of the complications. It should contain a detailed medical, psychological and social history, physical examination and health screening of both prospective parents where possible. A holistic approach to the preconception care assessment links the risk assessment to supportive health promotion activities, to ensure that care focuses on creating a healthy environment for the proposed conception and on clinical diagnostics and testing. Both the woman and her partner should be involved in sensitive discussion on, but not limited to, the following information.

Toxins and teratogens and infectious diseases

Preconception care includes identifying potential environmental toxin exposure in women and men along with avoidance advice (see Table 20.2). Commonly used pesticides are associated with increased risk of miscarriage, preterm birth, birth defects and learning disability (Sathyanarayana et al 2012). The preconception history must

Text continued on p. 310

Table 20.2 Toxins, teratogens and infectious diseases: preconception advice, care and further reading

Feature	Advice and information	Further information and resources
Employment	Advice appropriate to type/place of work Assess for potential occupational hazards for both men and women Access health and safety policies at work regarding identified preconception and pregnancy-related issues Avoidance of jobs that involve vibrating machinery, toxic substances, radiation, excessive cold/heat, heavy lifting, prolonged travelling times Discuss any concerns with employer	http://www.hse.gov.uk
Smoking	Reduces sperm count in men Both partners should stop smoking at least 4 months before conception. Cigarettes produce (among many toxins) carbon monoxide and nicotine, which reduce oxygen supply to the fetus and cause vasoconstriction of the spiral arterioles in the placenta Refer to support groups Avoid secondary smoke/smoky environments	NHS smoking helpline 0800 169 0169 http://www.nhs.uk/smokefree http://www.smokefree.nhs.uk/smoking-and-pregnancy/ App available: www.nhs.uk/app/nhs-quit-smoking/ http://www.quit.org.uk
Drugs (self-prescribed; prescribed; recreational/addictive; alternative therapies)	Increased risk of structural abnormalities during organogenesis, such as in the heart and great vessels, digestive system and musculoskeletal system Woman/partner may not wish to disclose information May need to cease medication, reduce intake or substitute with another less hazardous drug (i.e. heroin substituted by methadone)	http://www.actiononaddiction.org.uk/home.aspx

Table 20.2 Toxins, teratogens and infectious diseases: preconception advice, care and further reading—cont'd

Feature	Advice and information	Further information and resources
	Referral to specialist practitioners (Peake, Copp and Shaw 2013) Therapies that include herbal remedies require careful monitoring. Treatment should be prescribed by a registered therapist, so care is needed if self-prescribing (Hak et al 2013)	http://www.nlm.nih.gov http://grcct.org
Alcohol	Alcohol crosses the placenta and is toxic in early pregnancy. It can be metabolized by the fetal liver enzymes once matured sufficiently in the second half of pregnancy (Nykjaer et al 2014) Avoidance of binge drinking – particularly during organogenesis Decreases sperm count, sperm motility and causes sperm malformation (Goldman et al 2014) Is a testicular toxin with potential to cause subfertility, infertility and impotence	
Infectious diseases	Many common and less commonly known infectious diseases can have an adverse outcome on potential pregnancies. Some excellent Government resources for healthcare professionals are available – see web pages at right	https://www.gov.uk/government/uploads/system/uploads/attachment_data/file/266583/The_Green_book_front_cover_and_contents_page_December_2013.pdf https://www.gov.uk/health-protection/infectious-diseases
Chicken pox virus (varicella zoster VZ)	Most women who have had chicken pox develop lifelong immunity (up to 90% of the adult population, and this will protect their baby during pregnancy). There are no statistics highlighting loss of immunity; however, it is stated to be 'very rare' Test for VZ antibody; if not present, the woman can have varicella zoster immunoglobulin BUT AVOID pregnancy for 3 months after vaccination 1 : 3 women suffer spontaneous abortion after infection with VZ Occupational risk groups: school teachers, childcare workers and nursery nurses Avoid contact with infected others. If contact occurs and NOT immune, avoid conception/use contraception until end of incubation period	www.nhs.uk/conditions/chickenpox http://www.nhs.uk/Conditions/Chickenpox/
Cytomegalovirus (CMV)	CMV is a virus that lives within the salivary glands. Many adults will have contracted CMV but will be asymptomatic Spread via bodily fluids, mainly by the saliva and urine. It is transmitted through close contact (i.e. changing a baby's nappy, kissing, sexual activity) and rarely via an infected organ post-transplantation	

Continued

Table 20.2 Toxins, teratogens and infectious diseases: preconception advice, care and further reading—cont'd

Feature	Advice and information	Further information and resources
	CMV status is important information to couples who are or who may be seeking fertility treatment, such as ovum donation or embryo donation. All gamete donors should be screened for CMV Risk prevention or reduction, predominantly through good hygiene measures, including hand washing after changing nappies and before preparing meals, should be highly encouraged	http://www.hfea.gov.uk http://www.nhs.uk/Conditions/Cytomegalovirus/
Erythema infectiosum (Slapped Cheek disease or parvovirus)	Avoidance of children already with the disease (i.e. childcare workers/nursery nurses/teachers) Thought to be communicable 1 week before onset of symptoms and can cause hydrops fetalis or intra-uterine death if contracted in pregnancy (Nabae et al 2014)	
Group B *Streptococcus* (GBS)	25% of childbearing aged women have GBS in their vagina with no obvious symptoms Useful information if previously known GBS – screening in future pregnancy may be offered (though not routine yet) Advise women of the need for intravenous antibiotic prophylaxis in labour or after rupture of membranes to reduce transmission to their baby GBS is associated with maternal infection in pregnancy, late miscarriage or stillbirth, preterm delivery and neonatal meningitis	www.gbss.org.uk
Hepatitis B	Assess preconception hepatitis status Vaccinate before conception for at-risk groups (those with body piercing/tattoos) or high-risk groups such as those with history of IV drug use or sex worker Liver function tests may be advocated to assess severity of disease	http://nhs.uk/conditions/hepatitis-B/
HIV/AIDS	Steady maintenance of low viral load and high CD4 count before conception reduces risk of fetal/newborn transmission. CD4 count is a laboratory test that measures the number of CD4 T lymphocytes cells in a blood sample. In HIV, it is the most important laboratory indicator of how well the immune system is working (high count) and the strongest predictor of HIV progression (low count) Continued unprotected sex can result in an increased viral load	http://www.ght.org.uk

Table 20.2 Toxins, teratogens and infectious diseases: preconception advice, care and further reading—cont'd

Feature	Advice and information	Further information and resources
	Sperm washing and artificial insemination available in limited assisted conception units in the UK. The aim is to reduce the risk of HIV transmission by attempting to achieve pregnancy through insemination of sperm washed free of HIV rather than through unprotected intercourse Treatment with antiretroviral drugs, such as Zidovudine or Azidothymidine (AZT) Referral and close liaison with sexual health team	http://www.chelwest.nhs.uk/services/womens-health-services/assisted-conception-unit-acu/treatment-options/sperm-washing - sthash.OXCllrq2.dpuf http://www.bhiva.org
Listeriosis (*Listeria monocytogenes*)	A food-borne pathogen found in soil, water and other vegetation May be present in ready-prepared foods, meat pies, pâtés, unpasteurized cow's milk or goat's milk and soft cheeses (such as feta; camembert; brie; stilton). It can survive and multiply in refrigerators at temperatures of 6°C or above Can take 8 weeks for illness to emerge. Advise to avoid conception during this time Avoid contact with sheep during lambing and avoid handling silage Reheat all food to steaming point to kill pathogen Treat with antibiotic therapy	http://www.nhs.uk/Conditions/Listeriosis/
Mumps	From a male perspective, this must be considered because of associated infertility	
Rubella virus (German measles)	Avoid contact with infected persons for 7 days and 5 days after appearance of rash Determine status before conception – vaccinate, BUT delay pregnancy for 3 months afterwards High fetal risk if disease is contracted in first trimester	http://www.nhs.uk/Conditions/Rubella/Pages/Prevention.aspx
Tetanus (*Clostridium tetani*)	Spores found in soil, dust and animal gut/faeces Cases rare in UK because of successful childhood vaccination programme Vaccination recommended with tetanus immunoglobulin if wound injury is in contact with soil/animal faeces and immunity is unclear Protection during and washing after gardening/dusting	http://www.nathnac.org/travel/factsheets/tetanusinfo.htm http://www.nhs.uk/Conditions/Tetanus/Pages/Introduction.aspx

Continued

Table 20.2 Toxins, teratogens and infectious diseases: preconception advice, care and further reading—cont'd

Feature	Advice and information	Further information and resources
Toxoplasmosis *(Toxoplasma gondii)*	Parasitic infection with minimal risk to pregnancy if tested positive before conception; found in soil (Kovac and Briggs 2015) No risk to healthy women unless they are immunocompromised Because of soil contamination, women should be advised to wear gloves for emptying cat litter trays and washing hands carefully after gardening and after handling meat, fruit and vegetables Thorough cooking of meat and avoidance of raw or cured meats is recommended	
Tuberculosis (TB)	TB is caused by bacteria. It is airborne and infectious, transmitted when a sick patient coughs or sneezes	http://www.publications.parliament.uk/pa/ld201415/ldhansrd/text/141211-gc0002.htm
	Vaccination recommended before travel to high prevalence areas Seek GP's or specialist's advice if contact with infected person occurs If diagnosed with TB, then treatment before conception is recommended Consider targeted preconception advice and care to raise awareness in migrant groups (Public Health England 2015)	https://www.gov.uk/government/news/phe-and-nhs-england-launch-joint-115m-strategy-to-wipe-out-tb-in-the-uk

include identifying higher risk associated with living or working in an environment subject to pesticides, i.e. agriculture or other toxins such as phthalates (a type of plastic), lead (paint in older homes), mercury (contained in large fish, including mackerel and swordfish) and arsenic (exposure near waste management sites using incinerators).

Reflective activity 20.2

A couple owns and works on their large market garden supplying fruit and vegetables to large-chain supermarkets.
> What are the potential risk factors for this couple?
> What preconception advice would you offer?

2. Education and lifestyle

Prepregnancy health promotion and the public health role is a key part of maternity service provision. There were 74% of the mothers who died between 2009–2012, and 66% between 2011–2013 were shown to have pre-existing risk or disease and 27% in 2009–2012, and 30% in 2011–2013 were classified as obese. Obesity is also known to contribute to poor outcomes from other pregnancy complications (MBRRACE-UK 2014), and greater public awareness is needed.

Preconception care must include a detailed, holistic history with opportunity for health promotion and counselling about risk screening tests. Dependent on individual need and service availability, some of the following tests may be accessed if deemed necessary. Specialist support services are available through organizations such as Foresight (http://www.foresight-preconception.org.uk/).

Screening tests

These include:

- Physical examination to identify any medical or surgical conditions requiring referral to members of the multiprofessional team

- Blood pressure measurement

- Cardiac function

- Thyroid function

- Respiratory function
- Review of gastrointestinal activity
- Weight and body mass index (BMI)
- Sexual health status, i.e. vaginal, urethral or anal swabs
- Cervical smear
- Serum screening:
  - for haemoglobinopathies (Davies 2014)
  - full blood count
  - rubella status
  - tuberculosis status
- Assessment of vitamin, zinc and lead levels
- Hair analysis:
  - nutritional state
  - exposure to toxic metals
- Karyotyping/genomics (Dolan et al 2007)
- Urinalysis for protein, ketones, glucose and bacteriuria

Educational information

Results should be discussed with women and their partners in a timely manner, being cognizant of not overloading them with too much information at once. Verbal information conveyed should always be supported by evidence-based written material in the form of leaflets and patient information sheets and advising them about specific Internet-based resources. Referral to other members of the multidisciplinary team should also be considered once results of screening are known so that women and their partners can access specialist services in an attempt to reduce associated mortality and morbidity (Knight et al 2014 and 2015).

Aside from specific care pathways, it is important to offer more general education and advice to ensure an optimum pregnancy and neonatal outcome. These include sexual health; nutrition and exercise; dietary and vitamin supplements and dental care (Robertson et al 2015; Wyness 2014; O'Reilly and Reynolds 2013; Peake, Copp and Shawe 2013; Williamson and Wyness 2013).

Sexual health

The important discussion regarding safe sex should be conducted as opportunistically as possible. Safe sex discussion should include methods used to prevent transmission of sexually transmitted infections, safe sexual practices and recommendations for specific interventions when a risk is identified. Interventions include, but are not limited to, human papilloma virus (HPV) immunization and additional screening for sexually transmitted infections such as gonorrhea, syphilis, HIV and chlamydia.

Nutrition

An adequate diet at conception and during pregnancy is identified as a vitally important key factor in adult health, with associated links to illness such as coronary heart disease (Department of Health (DH) 2000). There is a direct relationship between nutritional intake, malnutrition and suboptimal nutrition in pregnancy and maternal and child health (Martin, Duxbury and Soltani 2014). Women with conditions requiring specific diets or nutritional requirements are referred or advised to seek specialist advice from a dietician. The aim is to ensure that women have a healthy BMI, sensible eating habits and suitable nutritional stores at the point of conception (Cuco et al 2006). Diet in pregnancy can be influenced by morning sickness, hyperemesis, pica (unusual or non-food cravings) and dislike of certain foods. Nutritional assessment is important because of the increase in malnutrition and the recognition that someone who is obese can also be malnourished.

BMI is still the recognized method of estimating nutritional status (see Ch. 32). A BMI of 20 or less is indicative that the individual is underweight, whereas a BMI of 30 or over is indicative of obesity. Obesity and resulting lack of essential nutrients influences organogenesis and fetal formation. Women should be advised to achieve a BMI between 21 and 29 before conception. Weight management should be supervised by a dietician or weight loss organization and, once a woman becomes pregnant, unsupervised dieting is not advised (Abayomi et al 2013). Consumer organizations exist to support weight management, and Slimming World (an organisation that focuses on encouraging lifestyle changes for the future health benefits of women, men and their families) have joined forces with the Royal College of Midwives (RCM) to support women and midwives in reducing obesity in childbearing women. The midwife should spend some time with women discussing healthy eating and be aware that a 'normal diet' can have different meanings for different people. Using resources such as the *'eatwell plate'* can be a helpful source of information on food groupings and healthy eating (National Health Service (NHS) Choices 2015).

Preconception care involves a discussion about women's eating habits, though there may be reluctance to disclose information. Women with eating disorders, such as anorexia or bulimia, have higher risks of miscarriage, infants born with low birthweights, obstetric complications and perinatal mental health problems and postnatal depression; therefore, referral to a specialist obstetrician or psychiatrist should be considered preconceptually. Many women report an improvement in their bulimic condition during pregnancy, with a third no longer suffering after childbirth (Easter et al 2011).

Women with pre-existing metabolic conditions, such as phenylketonuria, should be advised to maintain a diet low in phenylalanine when planning to become pregnant. This needs to be guided by a specialist dietician or physician.

Dietary supplements

Midwives and healthcare practitioners should advise women planning a pregnancy that vitamins and herbal or homeopathic products must be prescribed and monitored by a regulated practitioner. High doses of vitamin A, for example, found in foods high in retinoids such as liver and fish liver oil can cause fetal malformation in the first trimester of pregnancy. Women should always seek guidance if uncertainty exists. Common vitamins advised as part of preconception care include folic acid for all women, as it reduces the risk of the newborn presenting with spina bifida at birth. A dose of 0.4 mg of folic acid should be taken 2 to 3 months before conception until the first trimester is complete for women with no other risk factors. Women can also be advised to increase their consumption of leafy vegeatables and wholemeal foods. A higher dose of folic acid may be recommended for women with epilepsy, alcoholics, smokers and lactating women. For these women, a dose of 4 mg should be taken daily for 2 to 3 months before conception and continued until the end of the first trimester of pregnancy.

Many women do not meet the daily recommendation of 700 mg of calcium before conception. They should ensure an adequate intake of calcium in dairy produce and fish. Vitamin D supplementation is recommended for dark skinned women who have minimal exposure to sunlight (RCOG 2010; NICE 2008).

A haemoglobin assessment for anaemia is advised and, if detected, any obvious cause found should be treated before conception. A diet rich in iron from sources found in bread, pulses, red meat and green leafy vegetables should be encouraged.

A discussion regarding caffeine intake is important. Women should be advised that caffeine consumption can reduce implantation and reduce rates of conception by 27%.

Dental care

Poor oral health and significant dental caries carries a risk of preterm birth. Healthcare professionals, including dentists, should raise awareness of the need for good oral hygiene and prioritize dental treatments to ensure they are completed before conception. The increased blood volume during pregnancy increases blood supply to the gums and excessive bleeding could occur if dental surgery is performed.

3. Interventions for optimum pregnancy outcome

A well-coordinated, multiprofessional approach is strongly advised when women and their partners with a pre-existing medical condition present for preconception advice. This team needs to include midwives, specialist practitioners, obstetricians and physicians who have experience in managing their condition in pregnancy (Knight et al for MBRRACE 2014). Women who have any medical conditions, including rare disorders, need to be identified and reviewed before conception in order for appropriate advice and care to be provided (Knight et al for MBRRACE 2014).

Medical conditions

Most medical conditions, if managed effectively prepregnancy, then throughout organogenesis and the first trimester of pregnancy, result in sucessful outcome for mother and baby at birth (see Table 20.3).

Reflective activity 20.3

A 26-year-old woman, diagnosed with type 1 diabetes mellitus (T1DM), has experienced poor diabetic control for 4 years. Her Hb A$_{1c}$ a month ago was 10%. She attends her GP for a cervical smear test and says that she is considering starting a family soon.

Are you concerned? What preconception advice would you offer, and what plan of care should you recommend?

Table 20.3 Medical conditions: preconception care, advice and further resources

Asthma/ respiratory	Asthma is the most common of all respiratory diseases. Preconception advice from the Royal College of Physicians (2014) advises women to continue with asthma medication, which is deemed safe in pregnancy to reduce associated mortality. Pregnancy may have unpredictable effect on asthma (MBRRACE 2014).	http://www.patient.co.uk/doctor/ management-of -adult-asthma Royal College of Physicians (2014). *'Why asthma still kills. The National Review of Asthma Deaths (NRAD) Confidential Enquiry report'*. London.

Table 20.3 Medical conditions: preconception care, advice and further resources—cont'd

Autoimmune disorders	The most commonly known conditions are rheumatoid arthritis (RA) and systemic lupus erythematosus (SLE). Preconception review of medication is imperative, as some drugs (methotrexate and leflunomide) are teratogenic. Cautionary use of low-dose NSAIDs may be indicated. Up to 80% of women with RA find an improvement in their condition once pregnant. SLE is a multisystem, autoimmune disorder and a most common one in women of childbearing age. SLE has many risks, but the more stable the condition, the less adverse are the outcomes.	http://www.nhs.uk/Conditions/ Lupus/Pages/Introduction.aspx Arthritis Research UK at: http://www.arthritisresearchuk .org/arthritis-information/ conditions/lupus.aspx
Cancer	Women or their partners needing chemotherapy or other cancer-treating regimens, which will affect spermatogenesis or oogenesis, should seek advice on storing sperm and ova. Delay in conception may be advised if urgent cancer treatment is needed. Pregnancy after cancer treatments may be associated with higher risks, so specialist oncological advice is needed. Once a woman has recovered from cancer treatment, no clear guidelines exist about the length of time to wait before attempting to become pregnant (Grady 2006).	Anderson K, Norman RJ, Middleton P: Preconception lifestyle advice for people with subfertility. *Cochrane Database of Systematic Reviews*, 4:CD008189, 2010. See also Knight et al for MBRRACE http://www .hqip.org.uk/public/cms/253/ 625/19/366/Maternal%20 Mortality%20report%20 2015%20final%20version .pdf?realName = qpcvxZ.pdf
Cardiac disease	Careful pregnancy planning with cardiologist and neonatologist input. Preconception assessment of cardiac function. Anticoagulation therapy should be reviewed, as warfarin can cause embryonic abnormalities; heparin is a suitable substitution. Genetic counselling may be indicated, as some cardiac disorders can be inherited. The woman should be adequately prepared for the intensity of antenatal care if pregnancy is achieved.	https://www.bhf.org.uk The British Heart Foundation
Diabetes	Involve specialist practitioners, such as a lead midwife in diabetes, specialist dietician, endocrinologist or physician (McCorry et al 2012). Measure glycosylated haemoglobin (HbA_{1c}) 48 mmol/mol or 6.5% is the target for diabetic person. This test provides a useful gauge of longer term glucose control over the previous weeks or months. HbA_{1c} greater than 59 mmol/mol or 7.5% is more likely to result in hypoglycaemia. Poor diabetic control increases the risk of miscarriage, congenital malformations and abnormalities, preterm birth, pre-eclampsia, large for gestational age (LGA), caesarean delivery, shoulder dystocia and stillbirth (Abayomi et al 2013).	http://www.diabetes.co.uk http://www.nice.org.uk/guidance/ ng3/resources/diabetes-in-pregnancy-management-of-diabetes-and-its-complications-from-preconception-to-the-postnatal-period-51038446021 McCorry, N. K., Hughes, C., Spence, D., Holmes, V. A. and Harper, R. (2012), Pregnancy planning and diabetes: a qualitative exploration of women's attitudes toward preconception care. *Journal of Midwifery & Women's Health*, 57: 396–402.

Continued

Table 20.3 Medical conditions: preconception care, advice and further resources—cont'd

Epilepsy	Epilepsy is the most comonly known seizure disorder. 12 out of 14 women with epilepsy who died in childbirth between 2009–2012 were a direct result of seizure. The emphasis must be on preconception counselling. It is recommended that all women should have access to a nurse or midwife with additional expertise in epilepsy before the woman becomes pregnant. Early referral to specialist services/neurologist is recommended if pregnancy is contemplated. Early review of antiepileptic medication (AED) to use safest, but most effective combination to reduce the teratogenic effect leading to fetal malformations. (National Institute for Health and Clinical Excellence (NICE) 2012) Daily folic acid supplemetation is recommended with dose prescribed by GP or physician.	http://www.nice.org.uk/guidance/cg137 British Epilepsy Association: http://www.epilepsy.org.uk Helpline number 0808 800 5050
Hypertension	Preconception care should include retinopathy and renal function screening. Pre-existing hypertension may increase during pregnancy and pose risk to fetus (Knight 2013). Risk increases with the severity of the hypertension. Women with hypertension may develop a superimposed pre-eclampsia when pregnant, leading to further risks. The ultimate aim is for blood pressure control within the medical recommendations using minimal medication, as some are known to increase risk of fetal malformation, oligohydramnios, fetal growth restriction and, rarely, fetal death (NICE 2010).	https://www.nice.org.uk/guidance/cg107
Multiple sclerosis	Specialist advice regarding medication is important as certain drugs for MS can be teratogenic. Women may be advised to stop or change medication in the 3 months before conception. Multiple sclerosis (MS) does not appear to increase risk in pregnancy.	http://www.mssociety.org.uk/what-is-ms http://www.nhs.uk/Conditions/Multiple-sclerosis/Pages/Introduction.aspx
PKU	Phenylketonuria (PKU) is a monogenic, autosomal recessive inherited disorder that affects phenylalanine metabolism. Phenylalanine is primarily present in dairy and meat products. Phenylalanine levels should be maintained between 120–360 mmol/l by returning to a low-phenylalanine diet before conception and throughout the first trimester of pregnancy. Dietician referral is essential (Boocock and MacDonald 2013).	http://www.nspku.org The National Society for Phenylketonuria website is a valuable resource.
Thyroid disorders	Surveillance and maintaining a euthyroid (balanced) state before conception is advised. Hypothyroidism (low thyroxine levels) can cause dwarfism and intellectual impairment, whereas hyperthyroidism (high levels of thyroxine) can predispose to miscarriage, preterm birth, pre-eclampsia, placental abnormalities and low birthweight. Preconception advice is recommended with early specialist medical/endocrinology referral (Robson and Waugh 2013).	

CONCLUSION

'Healthy lifestyle; healthy parents; healthy baby'

The prevailing message to women and their partners when seeking preconception advice and care is that good health and well-being at preconception increases the likelihood of a healthy pregnancy and reduces maternal and neonatal mortality and morbidity. Knowledgeable midwives working directly together with other healthcare professionals are ideally positioned to deliver preconception care by paying special attention to promoting well-being, preventing ill health and meeting the changing health and care needs of people throughout these significant life stages.

Key Points

- The preconception period is the optimal time to help potential parents identify conditions, actions or lifestyle choices that might adversely affect pregnancy and fetal outcome and to help support them in making favourable changes.
- A critical period of early fetal development (17–56 days after conception) is when the early cell mass of conception becomes organized into three layers: *ectoderm, mesoderm* and *endoderm,* each responsible for different organs of body structures in the developing baby.
- Midwives need to be aware of the range of teratogens that may disturb embryonic or fetal development and cause miscarriage or result in a birth defect in the baby, and ensure that the woman and family are also informed of these.
- Women with pre-existing medical conditions or risk factors need to be encouraged to attend with their partners for preconception advice. A multiprofessional approach needs to be ensured, and the team should include midwives, specialist practitioners, obstetricians and physicians who have experience in managing their condition during pregnancy.

References

Abayomi J, Wood L, Spelman S, et al: The multidisciplinary management of type 2 and gestational diabetes in pregnancy, *Br J Midwifery* 21(4):236, 2013.

Anderson K, Norman RJ, Middleton P: Preconception lifestyle advice for people with subfertility, *Cochrane Database Syst Rev* (4):CD008189, 2010.

Basatemur E, Gardiner J, Williams C, et al: Maternal prepregnancy BMI and child cognition: a longitudinal cohort study, *Pediatrics* 131(1):56–63, *Academic Search Elite,* EBSCO*host,* 2013.

Boocock S, MacDonald A: Body mass index in adult patients with diet-treated phenylketonuria, *J Hum Nutr Diet* 26:1–6, Academic Search Elite, EBSCO*host,* 2013.

Cuco G, Fernandez-Ballart J, Sala J, et al: Dietary patterns and associated lifestyles in preconception, pregnancy and postpartum, *Eur J Clin Nutr* 60(3):364–371, 2006.

Davis B: Fertility and pregnancy in thalassaemia and sickle cell disease. The UK guidelines, *Thalassemia Reports* 4(3):63–67, Academic Search Elite, EBSCO*host,* 2014.

Department of Health (DH): *Coronary Heart Disease: National Service Framework for Coronary Heart Disease: Modern Standards and Service Models,* London, DH, 2000.

Dolan S, Biermann J, Damus K: Genomics for health in preconception and prenatal periods, *J Nurs Scholarsh* 39(1):4–9, 2007.

Easter A, Treasure J, Micali N: Fertility and prenatal attitudes towards pregnancy in women with eating disorders: results from the Avon Longitudinal Study of Parents and Children, *BJOG* 118(12):1491–1498, 2011.

Flower A, Shawe J, Stephenson J, et al: Pregnancy planning, smoking behaviour during pregnancy, and neonatal outcome: UK millennium cohort study, *BMC Pregnancy Childbirth* 13(1):1, Publisher Provided Full Text Searching File, EBSCO*host,* 2013.

Goldman MB, Thornton KL, Ryley D: A randomised clinical trial to determine optimal infertility treatment in older couples: the forty and over treatment trial (FORT- T), *Fertil Steril* 101:1574–1581, 2014.

Grady M: Preconception and the young cancer survivor, *Matern Child Health J* 10(5):s165–s168, 2006.

Hak E, Mulder B, Schuiling-Veninga C, et al: Use of acid-suppressive drugs in pregnancy and the risk of childhood asthma: bidirectional crossover study using the general practice research database, *Drug Saf* 36(11):1097–1104, MEDLINE with Full Text, EBSCO*host,* 2013.

Harden CL, Meador KJ, Pennell PB, et al: Practice parameter update: management issues for women with epilepsy–focus on pregnancy (an evidence-based review): teratogenesis and perinatal outcomes. Report of the Quality Standards Subcommittee and Therapeutics and Technology Subcommittee of the American Academy of Neurology and American Epilepsy Society, *Neurology* 50:1237–1246, 2009.

Hill S, Young D, Briley A, et al: Baby be smoke free: teenage smoking cessation pilot, *Br J Midwifery* 21(7):485, Publisher Provided Full Text Searching File, EBSCO*host*, 2013.

Kovac G, Briggs P: *Infections during pregnancy – varicella, herpes, cytomegalovirus, toxoplasma, listeria, group B streptococcus in Lectures in Obstetrics, Gynaecology and Women's Health*, Switzerland, Springer International, 2015.

Knight M: Sharper focus on uncomplicated pregnancy, *BMJ* 347(7935):9, Publisher Provided Full Text Searching File, EBSCO*host*, 2013.

Knight M, Kenyon S, Brocklehurst P, et al, editors: *On behalf of mothers and babies: reducing risk through audits and confidential enquiries across the UK (MBRRACE-UK). Saving lives, improving mothers' care – lessons learned to inform future maternity care from the UK and Ireland confidential enquiries into maternal deaths and morbidity 2009–2012*, Oxford, National Perinatal Epidemiology Unit, University of Oxford, 2014.

Martin S, Duxbury A, Soltani H: An overview of evidence on diet and physical activity based interventions for gestational weight management, *Evid Based Midwifery* 12(2):40, Publisher Provided Full Text Searching File, EBSCO*host*, 2014.

McCorry NK, Hughes C, Spence D, et al: Pregnancy planning and diabetes: a qualitative exploration of women's attitudes towards preconception care, *J Midwifery Womens Health* 57:396–402, 2012.

Nabae K, Satoh H, Nishiura H, et al: Estimating the risk of parvovirus B19 infection in blood donors and pregnant women in Japan, *PLoS One* 9(3):e92519, 2014.

National Health Service (NHS) Choices: *Live well: The eatwell plate* http://www.nhs.uk/Livewell/Good food/Pages/eatwell-plate.aspx. 2015.

National Institute for Health and Clinical Excellence (NICE): *Maternal and child nutrition NICE guidelines [PH11]* available online at: http://www.nice.org.uk/guidance/ph11/chapter/1-recommendations, 2008.

National Institute for Health and Clinical Excellence (NICE): *Hypertension in pregnancy: diagnosis and management NICE guidelines [CG107]* August NICE Manchester and online: http://www.nice.org.uk/guidance/cg107. 2010.

National Institute for Health and Clinical Excellence (NICE): Epilepsies: diagnosis and management *NICE guidelines [CG137]* NICE Manchester and online: http://www.nice.org.uk/guidance/cg137. 2012.

Nykjaer C, Alwan N, Greenwood D, et al: Maternal alcohol intake prior to and during pregnancy and risk of adverse birth outcomes: evidence from a British cohort, *J Epidemiol Community Health* 68(6):542, Publisher Provided Full Text Searching File, EBSCO*host*, 2014.

O'Reilly J, Reynolds R: The risk of maternal obesity to the long-term health of the offspring, *Clin Endocrinol (Oxf)* 78(1):9–16, Academic Search Elite, EBSCO*host*, 2013.

Peake J, Copp A, Shawe J: Knowledge and periconceptional use of folic acid for the prevention of neural tube defects in ethnic communities in the United Kingdom: systematic review and meta-analysis, *Birth Defects Res A Clin Mol Teratol* 97(7):444–451, MEDLINE, EBSCO*host*, 2013.

Robertson L, McStravick N, Ripley S, et al: Effectiveness of folic acid supplementation in pregnancy on reducing the risk of small-for-gestational age neonates: a population study, systematic review and meta-analysis, *BJOG* 122(4):478–490, MEDLINE, EBSCO*host*, 2015.

Robson S, Waugh J: *Medical disorders in pregnancy: a manual for midwives*, London, Wiley Blackwell, 2013.

Royal College of Obstetricians and Gynaecologists (RCOG), 2010: *Preconception vitamin D supplements (query bank)* (website). www.rcog.org.uk/en/guidelines-research-services/guidelines/preconception-vitamin-d-supplements--query-bank/. 2010.

Royal College of Physicians: *Why asthma still kills. The National Review of Asthma Deaths (NRAD) Confidential Enquiry Report*, London, 2014.

Sathyanarayana S, Braun J, Yolton K, et al: Bisphenol A and infant neonatal neurobehavior: Sathyanarayana et al. Respond, *Environ Health Perspect* 120(3):2012.

Tuomainen H, Cross-Bardell L, Bhoday M, et al: Opportunities and challenges for enhancing pre-conception health in primary care: qualitative study with women from ethnically diverse communities, *BMJ Open* 3:e002977, 2013.

Williamson C, Wyness L: Nutritional requirements in pregnancy and use of dietary supplements, *Community Pract* 86(8):44, Publisher Provided Full Text Searching File, EBSCO*host*, 2013.

Wyness L: Nutritional issues of vulnerable groups around pregnancy, *Br J Midwifery* 22(2):94, Publisher Provided Full Text Searching File, EBSCO*host*, 2014.

Resources and additional reading

Mothers and Babies: *Reducing Risk through Audits and Confidential Enquiries across the UK (MBRRACE-UK)* https://www.npeu .ox.ac.uk/mbrrace-uk/reports.

This website has links to the recent Confidential reports into maternal mortality, perinatal mortality and also birthplace research.

Robson S, Waugh J: *Medical disorders in pregnancy: a manual for midwives,* London, Wiley Blackwell, 2013.

An excellent text focusing on medical disorders.

World Health Organization (WHO): *Preconception care to reduce maternal and childhood mortality and morbidity. Meeting report and packages of interventions: WHO HQ, February 2012* Geneva and online: http:// www.who.int/maternal_child _adolescent/documents/concensus _preconception_care/en/. 2012.

This report reflects the proceedings from a meeting to develop global consensus on preconception care to reduce maternal and childhood mortality and morbidity. It provides packages of interventions in 13 domains, listing the health problems, problem behaviours and risk factors that contribute to maternal and childhood mortality and morbidity and evidence-based interventions to address them and mechanisms of delivering them.

Other websites

www.nice.org.uk
www.hse.gov.uk
www.nhs.uk
www.quit.org.uk
www.actiononaddiction.org.uk
www.nlm.nih.gov
www.grcct.org
www.gov.uk

www.hfea.gov.uk
www.gbss.org.uk
www.chelwest.nhs.uk
www.bhiva.org
www.nathnac.org
www.publications.parliament.uk
www.rcog.org.uk
www.eatwell.gov.uk

www.patient.co.uk
www.arthritisresearchuk.org
www.bhf.org.uk
www.diabetes.co.uk
www.epilepsy.org.uk
www.mssociety.org.uk
www.nspku.org

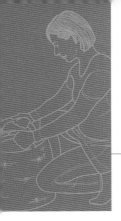

Chapter 21

Education for parenthood

Professor Caroline J Hollins Martin

Learning Outcomes ?

After reading this chapter, you will be able to:

- understand the importance of delivering parenthood education that empowers women and their partners to write personalized evidence-based birth plans
- critically appraise the importance of assessing needs of partners and preparing them for the role of birth partner and parenthood
- construct the potential content of a parenthood education curriculum and appreciate the value of having a national syllabus
- critically understand the importance of evaluating parenthood education delivered and assessing its relationship to consumer satisfaction
- write a lesson plan that includes a variety of engaging teaching methods

MEETING WOMEN'S NEEDS

In *Midwifery 2020 Delivering Expectations* (Department of Health (DH) 2010), the midwives' focus in delivering parenthood education involves preparing women and their partners for a positive experience of pregnancy, childbirth and early parenting. In relation to childbirth, women have been shown to value care that is personalized and coordinated by a midwife they know and trust, and they value being offered choices that take into account their individual needs, risks and circumstances (DH 2010). To uphold this philosophy, the midwife has responsibility for integrating a social model of maternity care in which the woman, as opposed to the organization, is placed at the centre of care.

EMPOWERING WOMEN

For a woman and her partner to be empowered to make choices about childbirth, they need to be given appropriate education to underpin their decision making (Hollins Martin 2008a). To achieve this purpose, the role of the midwife is to provide realistic, flexible and safe information, which will equip women to formulate an accurate landscape from which realistic aspirations can be constructed.

The importance of choice provision

Educating women for informed choice is an integral part of contemporary heath policy (DH 2007, 2010). Choice as a process requires implementation of reasoning and rational decision making, together with an assessment of risks, benefits and prioritization based on availability. A woman's choice is about her request for a personalized experience, and it is about assessing the risk involved. Although some women embrace education to empower themselves with information from which to make informed choices, one must concede that some decisions are underpinned by complex reasoning. The cognitive processes involved in making a choice are filtered through often complex belief systems, are at the mercy of availability, and may be limited by 'stumbling blocks' placed by midwives, obstetricians and even the women themselves (Hollins Martin and Bull 2006). Choices can also be influenced by hospital policy, hierarchical control and fear of consequences from challenging senior staff.

Choice provision is associated with *information provision* and empowerment with *control*, with both being important when a midwife considers what information to share with childbearing women. Information sharing is necessary if women are to be empowered to participate in decision making. Equipping a woman to make an appropriate choice involves the following aspects:

- Providing her with information about why some decisions are necessary

- Involving her in decisions about potential interventions

- Affording her the right to refuse a specific treatment

- Providing opportunity for her to choose from options that are actually available

Another main objective of education is to include information that equips the woman with enough information to effectively complete her 'birth plan', with potential content outlined in Table 21.1.

Table 21.1 The midwife's guide to birth planning

Maternity unit number Name	Address Phone number E-mail
Questions to ask the childbearing woman	Points for discussion
1. Where would you like to give birth?	Options available Advantages and disadvantages of having: Home birth Hospital birth Water birth etc.
2. What kind of birth would you like?	Differences between natural, augmented and induced labour Advantages and disadvantages of adopting different positions during the second stage of labour Differences between active and physiological third stage The purpose of episiotomy, instrumental delivery and caesarean section
3. What would you like the environment to be like?	Homeliness (e.g. music, lighting, bed, beanbags) Freedom to move, walk, change positions Own or hospital clothes Degree of privacy desired Who is to cut the cord The place of taking photographs
4. Do you want to be mobile during labour?	Advantages and disadvantages of ambulating during first stage of labour Interventions and their consequences: Cardiotocography (CTG) Epidural Intravenous (IV) infusion
5. Do you want/not want pain relief?	The benefits of endorphins as natural pain relief and their role in promoting bonding Natural methods of pain relief, for example: Water Transcutaneous electrical nerve stimulation (TENS) Ambulation Medical forms of pain relief, for example: Opiates Entonox Epidural The relationship of epidural to monitoring, IV infusion, catheterization and forceps

Table 21.1 The midwife's guide to birth planning—cont'd

6. Who would you like to be your birth partner?	The role of the birth partner The importance of partner choice Preparation available for the woman's selected birth partner
7. Do you wish the baby to 'room in' with you?	Initiation of feeding The importance of mother and baby interaction
8. Ask the childbearing woman to make a list of her choices in order of priority (put most important first).	
9. Explain that the birth plan is more likely to actualize when labour remains normal (unexpected situations may arise).	
10. Clarify that the birth plan requires presenting in a comprehensive manner and must hold a polite and pleasant tone.	
11. Provide the woman with an information pack (could be online) and a matching template for her birth plan.	
12. Make an appointment to review the birth plan and discuss its achievability.	

Source: Hollins Martin 2008a

REASONS FOR PARENTS ATTENDING PARENTHOOD EDUCATION CLASSES

Newburn et al (2011) reported that 97% of childbearing women who attend parenthood education classes do so because they desire to meet others in the same situation. Additional reasons include to prepare for breastfeeding (96%), to obtain evidence-based information (91%), to acquire information about pain relief (87%) and to learn about procedures such as induction, epidural, monitoring and assisted birth (86%). Over half said they wanted to prepare for a natural birth (57%) and that they wanted to find out more about non-invasive approaches for dealing with labour pain (Leap and Anderson 2008; Leap et al 2010) and physical positioning and movement. Newburn et al (2011) also asked both women and partners to consider their level of confidence in relation to birth prior to and following a parenthood education programme, with half feeling more confident about facing childbirth following course compared with 3% prior to preparation ($p = 0.01$). Boosted confidence was directly proportional to an increase in contact hours.

THE IMPORTANCE OF EDUCATING FATHERS FOR THE ROLE OF BIRTH PARTNER

Classes more often do not focus on the perspective of fathers, which can result in feelings of helplessness and isolation (Deave and Johnson 2007; World Health Organisation (WHO) 2007). The Fatherhood Institute (see fatherhoodinstitute.org) is a think tank that considers both mothers and fathers as earners and carers in equal capacity, and as such it places value on the attendance of fathers at education classes. Newburn et al (2011) highlight the importance of educating fathers for the role of birth partner and parenting. For this purpose, Hollins Martin (2008b) developed an instrument called the Birth Participation Scale (BPS) (see Box 21.1), which can be used for the following:

- To identify whether fathers genuinely wish to be present at the birth
- To ascertain fathers' concerns in relation to birth participation
- To individualize fathers' preparation to be a birth partner

Items on the BPS are scored using a 5-point Likert scale based on level of agreement with each statement (questionnaire and scoring grid are available on the chapter website resources). The possible range of scores is 25 to 125, with a score of 25 representing the most negative attitude towards birth participation and 125 the most positive. An example question follows:

(Q2) I feel well prepared for the role of birth partner.				
Strongly agree	Agree	Neither agree or disagree	Disagree	Strongly disagree
5	4	3	2	1

Scores are for illustration purposes.

Box 21.1 The birth participation scale (BPS)

1. I would like to be present at the birth of my baby.
2. I feel well prepared for the role of birth partner.
3. I will be present during the labour and birth for the sole reason that I want to be there.
4. I do not worry about becoming emotional during or after the birth.
5. Being present during the labour and birth does not alter my commitment to fatherhood.
6. I want to help during the labour and birth.
7. I feel that I am the best person to be with my partner during labour and delivery.
8. I will be present during the labour and delivery only because my partner expects me to be there.
9. I would prefer to stay only during the labour and leave for the birth.
10. I worry that I may become emotional when my baby is born.
11. I will be present only for the birth and not the labour.
12. The thought of being present at the birth makes me feel queasy.
13. I think I will be a good birth partner.
14. I want to help my partner with her breathing exercises and relaxation techniques.
15. I feel certain that if problems arise they will be taken care of by highly skilled professionals.
16. I know I can help both my partner and the midwives.
17. I would prefer not to be present during the labour and birth.
18. One of my fears is that I will be useless and get in the way.
19. I will leave support and relaxation techniques to the midwife.
20. It is not necessary for men to attend birth preparation classes.
21. Being present at the birth is the best start to fatherhood.
22. If I am present I don't want to help during the labour and birth.
23. I am scared that I just won't cope during the labour and birth.
24. It would be better if my partner's mother/sister/friend undertakes the role of birth partner.
25. If I am present during the labour and birth it is because I want to be.

To obtain a copy of the 10-Item BBS-R and marking grid, contact Prof Caroline J Hollins Martin (e-mail: c.hollinsmartin@napier.ac.uk).
Source: Hollins Martin 2008

What has been established is that childbirth is an emotionally demanding experience for fathers (Johansson et al 2012), with many wishing to attend the same antenatal classes as their partners. Some partners from ethnic minorities may prefer a separate class for religious or cultural reasons (Shia 2013). The midwife also needs to be aware of the differing needs of her clients, to include teenage mothers, men who are working with a surrogate and lesbian couples, all of whom require a nonjudgemental and supportive approach equal to that used with a heterosexual couple.

CONTENT OF PARENTHOOD EDUCATION PROGRAMMES

Health outcomes are strongly influenced by factors that operate in pregnancy and the first years of life, and hence pregnancy is a crucial time for establishing the underpinnings for the future health of the infant (DH 2009). Consequently, it is important to recognize that maternal health is a foundation for family well-being (Mensah and Kiernan 2010) and also an important predictor for child development (Waylen and Stewart-Brown 2010). Delivery of parenthood education can be via individual contact within the antenatal clinic, face-to-face group sessions, web-based platforms, use of iPods, YouTube clips and/or video clips that contain birth stories, animations, activities, and games. Such education has the following purposes:

- Advise on eating a healthy diet and avoidance of teratogenic substances
- Aid understanding of pregnancy physiology and its effects (e.g. discomforts, warning signs, nutrition, exercise etc.)
- Learn about labour (e.g. preparing for birth, prelabour signs, onset of labour, stages of labour)
- Illustrate potential places to labour and give birth (e.g. tour of facilities)
- Illustrate events through the use of real-life birth stories and films of births in a variety of settings (e.g. home, water, midwife-led unit, caesarean section, epidural etc.)

- Explain comfort techniques (e.g. breathing, relaxation, massage, visualization, focal points, hydrotherapy, labour and pushing positions)
- Demonstrate potential positions and movement for labour
- Educate the birth partner
- Teach pain relief techniques and methods of how to cope with pain
- Explain what happens following birth
- Teach infant care, safety and patterns of infant behaviour (e.g. feeding, crying, settling, sleeping, play routines)
- Discuss potential unexpected outcomes, variations of labour and obstetric complications
- Teach pre- and postnatal exercises and their potential benefits
- Describe services available in the community
- Engage siblings as part of preparation for the newcomer
- Debate potential changes in relationships
- Discuss the processes of mother–infant attachment
- Consider sensitive responsiveness to the infant (as well as practical baby care)
- Engage individuals with specialist teaching (e.g. teenagers, those who are having a planned caesarean section, single parents, those with medical diagnoses etc.)

Some parents may benefit from preparation for the changing relationship between partner and self (Deave and Johnson 2007). For ideas about what parents need to address in education for parenthood groups, see Box 21.2. New parents often find their established routines thrown into confusion and feel that they lack skills to cope (Wilkins 2006).

The Child Health Promotion Programme (CHPP; DH 2008a) asks that professionals empower parents by focusing on their strengths and promoting self-knowledge. Promoting parent–infant attachment involves encouraging both parents to be empathetic and sensitive in their responses to their infant, with this attunement leading to loved and loving individuals who are less at risk of becoming antisocial individuals. Such action considers the mental well-being of future generations, which is one of the goals of the Darzi report (DH 2008b). The Worldwide Alternatives to Violence (WAVE) Trust report (WAVE Trust 2005) summarizes the importance of this intervention and outlines brain development that can become impaired when parenting is inadequate.

The CHPP (DH 2008a) cites several programmes that meet both the needs of parents and government recommendations for promoting attachment, including First Steps in Parenting (Parr 1998; Parr and Joyce 2009). Undoubtedly the most important determinants of success of such programmes are the quality and skills of the practitioners who deliver them. Hence, it is imperative that midwives learn groupwork skills, understand how to facilitate learning rather than teach, and develop ability to communicate with sensitive responsiveness (Deane-Gray 2008), with this investment of practitioners making considerable difference when working with new parents (Douglas and Brennan 2004). Preparation of lesson plans that are effective and engaging is a challenge for any midwife, which increases the potential benefits of developing a large-scale syllabus that has been positively evaluated for its effectiveness. For suggested content of education classes, see Box 21.3.

The role of a core curriculum

One example of a core curriculum is that of Health Improvement Scotland (2011), which published a core syllabus for professional practice that supports education for pregnancy, birth and early parenthood. Key content, theoretical basis, evidence and target outcomes are clearly outlined in this document. This national curriculum is designed to help midwives deliver consistent education that respects and reflects upon individual requirements. In addition to physical and social dimensions, it also incorporates emotional dimensions and reflection. Outcomes of the Health Improvement Scotland (2011) curriculum are as follows:

1. Improve the health of childbearing women and their infants through the following:

   - Improving maternal nutrition
   - Reducing levels of smoking
   - Reducing alcohol consumption
   - Increasing exercise
   - Reducing the incidence of premature births
   - Increasing the incidence of healthier neonates

Box 21.2 What do parents need to address in education for parenthood groups?

- The psychological, social and emotional changes for themselves and their infants
- The changing relationship between the couple and incorporating their baby
- Self-knowledge and problem-solving skills
- Developing attachment and sensitive responsiveness to infants
- Practical aspects of baby care
- Postnatal issues

Box 21.3 Suggested content of education classes

Early pregnancy classes

- Explanation of informed and shared decision making
- Options and patterns of care
- Expected fetal movement patterns
- Tests that are offered and what they discover
- Tests and what they tell you
- Minor disorders of pregnancy and how to alleviate
- Community resources for parents
- Recognizing physical/psychological complications during the antenatal period

Parenthood education classes

- Selecting equipment for infant care
- Infant feeding
- Parental division of labour and working together
- Child-care options

Birth preparation classes

- Explanation of what 'normal' means
- Writing a 'birth plan'
- Implications of interventions and keeping of birth normal

- Analgesia (complementary and pharmaceutical)
- Hypothetical and real risks
- Mobility and potential positions for labour and birth
- Role of the birth partner
- Birth complications and how to cope should they arise
- Induction issues
- Tour of the delivery suite

Postnatal issues

- The transition to motherhood/fatherhood
- The growth of human love through attachment theory
- The importance of social support
- Parenting styles and working together
- Postnatal exercises
- How to recognize physical/psychological complications in the puerperium
- Managing the new infant and feeding
- Managing a discontented infant
- Contraception and reengaging in sexual relations with partner
- Sources of support and information for parents

2. Increase the number of normal births through the following:
   - Reducing intervention
   - Reducing the caesarean birth rate
3. Improve the health of new parents and their infants through the following:
   - Increasing breastfeeding rates
   - Promoting rapid emotional and physical recovery following birth
   - Reducing the incidence of perinatal depression (including that of the partner)
   - Increasing parents' resilience
   - Improving parent–infant attachment
   - Reducing relationship breakdown
   - Improving child protection
   - Creating stronger social networks

Parent education needs to include sessions on the transition to parenthood, relationship issues, preparation for new roles and responsibilities, parent–infant relationships and how to problem solve. Incorporating these psychosocial elements is associated with high consumer satisfaction (McMillan et al 2009).

The advantages of antenatal education for childbirth and the most suitable educational approaches for the midwife to take remains unclear. Prospective parents ordinarily seek out knowledge to help them with decision making, to develop skills, to deal with pain, to learn about postnatal care and breastfeeding and to cultivate parenting abilities. Gagnon and Sandall (2007) reviewed nine trials involving a total of 2284 women and found that there was lack of high-quality evidence to support the effectiveness of antenatal education. Hence, there is room for further research to investigate effective ways of helping women prepare for birth and parenthood. What is certain is that in terms of subject choice, an individualized approach is required to tailor education to meet personalized needs, and a creative approach towards delivering a variety of engaging teaching strategies.

Educating women for birth satisfaction?

Every woman constructs expectations of childbirth, with variation in appreciation of the concept (Hollins Martin and Fleming 2011; Hollins Martin et al 2012). Literature supports that birth satisfaction includes the following aspects:

- Having one's comfort considered
- Being listened to
- Receiving the type of pain relief requested
- Coping well during labour
- Feeling in control
- Being well prepared

- Receiving minimal obstetric injuries
- Achieving the desired style of delivery

Three overarching themes identified in the literature were found to influence levels of birth satisfaction (Hollins Martin and Fleming 2011; Hollins Martin et al 2012):

1. Quality of care provision
2. Personal attributes
3. Stress experienced during labour

To view questions from the valid and reliable 10-Item Birth Satisfaction Scale (BSS) (Hollins Martin and Martin 2014), see Box 21.4.

Overall education to prepare women to make decisions (Q3), reduce anxiety (Q4), feel in control (Q8) and reduce distress (Q9) during labour and childbirth is key to birth (questionnaire and scoring grid are available on the chapter website resources).

Box 21.4 Valid and reliable 10-item Birth Satisfaction Scale–Revised (10-item BSS-R) post-psychometric statistical testing

- Quality of care provision (Qs 3, 5, 6,10)
- Woman's personal attributes (Qs 4, 8)
- Stress experienced during labour (Qs 1, 2, 7, 9)
  1. I came through childbirth virtually unscathed.
  2. I thought my labour was excessively long.
  3. The delivery room staff encouraged me to make decisions about how I wanted my birth to progress.
  4. I felt very anxious during my labour and birth.
  5. I felt well supported by staff during my labour and birth.
  6. The staff communicated well with me during labour.
  7. I found giving birth a distressing experience.
  8. I felt out of control during my birth experience.
  9. I was not distressed at all during labour.
  10. The delivery room was clean and hygienic.

Participants respond on a 5-point Likert scale based on level of agreement/disagreement with each of the statements placed, with a possible range of scores between 10 and 50. A score of 10 on the 10-Item BSS-R represents the least 'birth satisfaction'; 50 represents the most.

- Strongly agree
- Agree
- Neither agree or disagree
- Disagree
- Strongly disagree

To obtain a copy of the 10-Item BBS-R and marking grid, contact Prof Caroline J Hollins Martin (e-mail: c.hollinsmartin@napier.ac.uk).
Source: Hollins Martin and Martin 2014

EFFECTIVE FACILITATION OF PARENTHOOD EDUCATION

Effective communication and supporting transitions are two areas of expertise required for working with children and families, as outlined in Every Child Matters (Department for Education and Skills (DfES) 2005). Interactive group-based parenting programmes have been evaluated as most effective, with parents appreciating sharing of experiences (Wilkins 2006). Such group discussions can enable parents to understand others, with an effective group being a strong source of nonstigmatizing support that increases confidence in self-capability.

The skill in preparing a lesson plan involves providing experiences that engage parents and their prior experience. Information presented needs to be contemporary, which may require a prior literature search and relevant discussion with colleagues and clinical peers to bridge the theory–practice gap. It is also important to reflect upon the session, incorporating an evaluation of both performance and achievement of group outcomes to validate what worked well and what requires further development upon repetition (Nolan 2002). Use of practical activities (e.g. group work, discussion, experiential activities) should keep the group active and assist with developing meaningful learning. It is also important to consider learners' needs. Maslow developed a theory of human needs that works from the bottom up (Maslow 1943; see Fig. 21.1).

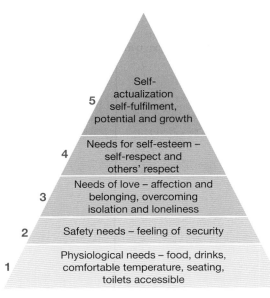

Figure 21.1 Maslow's (1943) hierarchy of needs.

First the midwife must ensure that clients' physiological needs are met in terms of warmth, drink, food and elimination of waste. Once these have been met, the next requirement is for them to feel safe, and so on, up to the top of the pyramid. Of course it is not the responsibility, nor is it possible, for the midwife to meet all of a childbearing woman's needs, but it is important to consider those that can be influenced.

Reflective activity 21.1

Formulate a lesson plan
Review what you have read so far, and plan out a session that covers the following areas:
1. Discuss preparation of the environment – for example, refreshments, comfortable seats, mats, music, props, heating, toilets.
2. Identify a topic relevant to your childbearing population – for example, 'Preparing for pain experienced during labour'.
3. Specify the overall aim of this session – for example, 'Coaching for pain experienced during labour'.
4. Identify learning objectives to address during this session – for example:
   - Discuss the physiology of pain.
   - Explain the role of endorphins and what inhibits their release.
   - Debate the advantages and disadvantages of the variety of natural and pharmaceutical pain relief methods available.
   - Consider the relationships between maternal movement/positions and pain experience.
   - Describe relationships between adrenalin release and oxytocin inhibition and potential effects on labour and the unborn baby.
   - Discuss and rehearse relaxation techniques.
5. Plan an assortment of interactive teaching methods to deliver decided learning outcomes.
6. Ask a childbearing woman to consider and flexibly complete the pain relief section of her birth plan.
7. Plan a means by which to evaluate the session.

For parents to approach tasks with confidence, it is essential that both the physical and psychological climates are comfortable. Within a receptive environment, midwives will be able to facilitate parents towards directing their own learning. The midwife's role is to negotiate and agree on the aims and objectives of the group prior to delivery. Using this flexible model, the midwife (facilitator) cannot claim full control and instead is a joint shareholder with the group. Enabling parents to lead discussion creates ownership that equips them to make the decisions that new parenthood brings.

Reflective activity 21.2

Reflecting after a session
Following a session, it is important for the facilitator to reflect, using questions such as these:
- How did the group perform in terms of energy, interest, involvement, reactions and responses?
- Use three words to describe your own feelings about the session delivered.
- Did any aspects of the session surprise you?
- Did any members of the group express a special need, interest, anxiety or concern?
- Would additional props or strategies have improved delivery of the session?
- Were there aspects of the venue that could be improved?

Adapt the lesson plan in response to what you have learned from your own and the attendees' evaluation.

ASPECTS OF THE GROUP TO CONSIDER

When organizing parenthood classes, it is important to consider the constitution and orientation of the group. The childbearing community is constructed of many individuals, to include traditional and reconstituted families, lesbian parents, teenagers (see bestbeginnings.org) and young and older parents. Education needs to be tailored to meet individual requests, and it is also important to understand that individuals will have developed their own patterns of absorbing and assimilating information. Such strategies will have been acquired in the home, at school, during adult education and in the workplace. In addition, experiencing feelings of warmth, having mutual respect and trust for one another, not being judged, finding a friend and knowing the environment and rules are essential aspects of delivering an education session. Each group member must benefit from group activities, acknowledging that they will have personal views, beliefs and responses. Empowering members to express themselves can be achieved through a variety of activities, which can include the following:

- Directing them towards self-directed learning
- Encouraging them to take personal responsibility for their learning
- Ensuring that what is taught sits comfortably with their prior experience, beliefs and cultural values
- Meeting, where possible, their personal needs and wants

Several styles of teaching and learning can be implemented to meet the varied needs of the group, as explained in the following sections. None of these is mutually exclusive.

Visual learning style

individuals who are visually oriented respond to pictures, demonstrations, models, videos and written words. they respond well to charts, diagrams and videos, and they are more likely to read referenced materials.

Auditory learning style

individuals with an auditory orientation respond to verbal discussion and like listening to people's experiences and stories. they respond well to verbal instruction and enjoy soundtracks, music and singing.

Kinesthetic learning style

individuals with a kinesthetic orientation respond to activities that engage all of their senses and involve the whole body, such as physical movement, role play, exercise, tours and demonstrations.

Although most people have a preferred learning style, they respond in varying degrees to all three. it is therefore important to consider all three when structuring a parenthood education session. if childbearing women are to be empowered to make choices about education methods, it is important that the midwife explores and discusses their wishes and feelings about potential options that are available to them. it is also important to provide practical and sensible information and to construct an accurate picture from which realistic hopes, fears and expectations can be formulated. holding a birth planning session can help childbearing women to assimilate their ambitions and desires for labour (see table 21.1). because desires differ, it is recommended that midwives audit birth satisfaction against women's birth plans (see box 21.1).

Be aware of your own needs

Midwives have their own personal needs, emotions, feelings, fears and anxieties. As people, midwives also can become stressed, upset and challenged from time to time. On occasion these aspects will interfere with their ability to deliver effective education. Acknowledging personal vulnerabilities is important, and through identification we can prepare strategies for resolution.

Facilitation of a new parenthood education group

You will have a set number of parenthood education sessions (e.g. 8–10). Flexibly agree with the group on the content of these scheduled meetings. During session 1, the warm-up phase may include finding out what the group wants to cover and what their expectations and fears might be. The group can be set 'homework' with activities such

---

> ### Reflective activity 21.3
>
> Write a list of topics that make you feel uncomfortable and consider how you can find resolution for each one on the list.
> In relation to a session you have found particularly stressful, consider the following:
> - What were your own response behaviors?
> - What were the group's response behaviors?
> - Identify particular stressors, and outline how you intend to deal with these stressors at a future session.

---

as accessing online learning resources. During the subsequent work phase, topics need to be structured by the midwife and agreed on by the group. The integration phase requires the inclusion of reflection on personal meaning and the integration of the understanding of the significance and usefulness of the session for the future. Remember to give time for the topic to sink in by repeating instructions several times, and allow silent phases for thinking.

Group activities

It is helpful to encourage group members to share ideas in pairs. For example, ask them to talk about pain they have experienced in their lives. After this activity, it is useful to invite a group discussion by initiating questions such as the following:

- What did you notice about your discussion together?
- What is your reaction to another's pain, such as a headache?
- What do you want to do if someone is crying?
- What does pain mean to you?
- What makes pain easier or seem more painful?
- What do you imagine labour is like for the baby?

Group size may influence the choice of activity, but dividing the group into smaller groups enables parents to work with different people.

Pictures

One strategy is to print a photograph from the Internet or from a magazine of a childbearing woman in pain during labour and ask group members to discuss their thoughts in relation to viewing this picture. In this case it is better to have a 'stock picture' because you need to be aware of copyright issues.

Quizzes

Lists of questions or cards with facts, feelings and myths can be utilized, with responses shared with other group members.

Stories, scenarios and case studies

Stories, scenarios and case studies can be presented. For instance, parts of the story can be distributed and parents asked to discuss circumstances (e.g. early labour beginning while out shopping together). Once the first part has been discussed, the next part of the story is given. Such activities can help parents consider realistic situations, test ideas and explore attitudes as to when and if they actually want pain relief.

Problem solving

- Realistic problems may be presented for small groups of parents to solve. Examples of topics follow:
  - You arrive at the delivery suite after labouring at home for 12 hours and are told you are in early labour. What do you do?
  - You enter the pool and find you do not like it. What do you do?
  - Your mother is with you during labour and says that this is just the beginning and you should have an epidural. What will you do?

This approach challenges and encourages self-direction, self-investigation and exploration of what resources are available.

'Wind-down' sessions

Couples can engage in a 'wind-down' of the session, giving them time together to discuss what they will take away from the session.

MODERN METHODS OF DELIVERING EDUCATION

There is need to acknowledge that for some women group education will not be acceptable or appropriate; these individuals may require one-to-one support and/or alternative creative sessions (e.g. media and web-based approaches). It is currently recommended that midwives provide personalized education that meets individual childbearing women's requests for choice, information, support and reassurance. Delivery of tailor-made education may be formal or informal, professional or peer-based, face-to-face or remote.

Traditionally, health education and support in pregnancy have focused on face-to-face midwife–woman contact, but it is now argued that more women access the Internet for information. Hence, midwives need to include this medium in their formal and informal education with women and families. There is a growing body of evidence showing that adults in the general population use social media to access health-related information, with use of digital and social media during pregnancy less well researched (Lima-Periera et al 2012). Fox (2011) found that among Internet users, 80% have accessed health information online, and as such online health resources are a significant source of health information.

The Maternity Services Survey 2013 (Care Quality Commission (CQC) 2013) reported that maternity service users perceive that information given is inconsistent, with a global parenthood education site perhaps the way forward. In addition, online education affords women greater flexibility in terms of time, given that they are not obliged to travel to classes to access information. Ability to seek out information on a midwife-patrolled site also provides opportunities for information exchange and peer support if discussion groups are established (Redshaw and Heikkila 2010). To prevent inaccuracies in this information sharing, it is imperative that midwives confirm the validity of all information given, check women's comprehension and elaborate on information upon request. The midwife should be aware of the most useful high-quality websites that women might find helpful, including the following:

- Tommy's charity (www.tommys.org)
- National Institute for Health and Care Excellence (www.nice.org.uk)
- Scottish Intercollegiate Guidelines Network (www.sign.ac.uk)
- WHICH Birth Choice (http://www.which.co.uk/birth -choice)

It is unlikely that a 'one-size-fits-all' approach to meeting information needs will be effective for all women, and hence delivery of parenthood education should take a variety of forms. Nonetheless, social networking sites (SNSs) are an area of significant and rapid growth, with 65% of online adults currently using them, compared with 8% in 2005. Young women aged 18 to 29 are the most frequent users, with engagement not significantly affected by race, ethnicity, household income, education level or location (Madden and Zickuhr 2011). In response, SNSs are an important growing medium for providing accurate pregnancy-related health information and parenthood education.

Evaluating experiences of childbirth

Midwives should embrace an attempt to appropriately prepare women for childbirth and parenting, which raises the importance of evaluation of the education delivered to elucidate whether learners considered what did or did not go well during labour and childbirth. Measuring women's experiences of childbirth can be achieved using the 10-Item Birth Satisfaction Scale–Revised (10-Item BSS-R) developed and validated by Hollins Martin and Martin (2014). Education for childbirth should include a problem-solving approach and explain how to identify and encourage

Reflective activity 21.4

Exploring the life cycles of groups

It is important for parenthood education facilitators to understand the *normal life cycle* of a group because this may be helpful towards understanding changing dynamics within an assembly of childbearing women/ couples across time. Although the following theories are relatively old, they are the underpinning of more modern theories of group dynamics (see Forsyth 2014). Access the Internet and read about one of the following:

1. Tuckman's (1965) Stages Model
   - Forming
   - Storming
   - Norming
   - Performing
   - Adjourning
2. Tubb's (1995) systems approach
   - Orientation
   - Conflict
   - Consensus
   - Closure
3. Fisher's (1970) theory of decision emergence in groups
   - Orientation
   - Conflict
   - Emergence
   - Reinforcement

   When you have facilitated a group, think about how group members worked together and whether any of the models in particular described how the members behaved as a group.

parents to take advantage of supportive networks within local communities (DH 2008a). During education classes, midwives and women ordinarily focus on physical aspects of pregnancy, with psychological components given somewhat reduced attention (Barnes and Balber 2007). Consequently, parents can become dissatisfied and complain that they were ill-prepared for the emotional impact of labour, birth and becoming a parent (Woollett and Parr 1997).

The facilitator can ask for feedback or simply ask couples to state a word that captures the session for them. Alternatively, the midwife can provide them with an evaluation form (see chapter website resources) that assesses satisfaction with the session. Evaluating the aims and objectives of the session and achievement will clarify the bigger picture of what was achieved during the session. It is also important to evaluate the environment. For example, did the attendee feel that the room was warm and inviting, that the seating plan was appropriate, and that enough and appropriate resources were utilized? Midwives can also evaluate from their perspective, through matching group learning with the planned aims and objectives of the session. Analysing such findings will enable a cycle of continual improvement to evolve.

CONCLUSION

This chapter suggests a few approaches that midwives can consider to deliver flexible and accommodating parenthood education. Whatever the method, education should promote parents' understanding of the physical, social and psychological experiences of childbirth and the transition to parenthood. Session content needs to include delicate areas, such as changes in relationships, attachment and sensitive responsiveness to the infant, in addition to the practicalities of childbirth and baby care. Also, promoting problem-solving and decision-making skills prepares parents to manage and develop coping skills, which in turn will promote self-knowledge and empowerment. The midwife must also ensure that parenthood education programmes integrate evidence-based knowledge, are focused on parent needs and are delivered with an empowering philosophy that equips women and partners for labour and their new role.

Key Points

- Midwives are in a privileged position to prepare parents for childbirth and their transition to early parenthood by providing education that can facilitate this more fully, particularly including addressing the needs of parents and promoting attachment in the parent–infant relationship.
- The government has given parenting a high priority, and this is congruent with the changing role of midwives in developing their public health role.
- Midwives need to develop their facilitation and group management skills to promote interaction and learning in groups.
- To create meaningful learning, midwives must teach parents how to access information, learn from a wide range of sources and develop their repertoire of life skills.

References

Barnes DL, Balber L: *The journey to parenthood: myths, reality and what really matters*, Oxford, Radcliffe, 2007.

Care Quality Commission (CQC): *National findings from the 2013 survey of women's experiences of maternity care* (website). www.cqc.org.uk/sites/default/files/documents/maternity_report_for_publication.pdf. 2013.

Deane-Gray T, Effective communication. In Peate I, Hamilton C, editors: *Becoming a midwife in the 21st century*, Sussex, John Wiley, 2008.

Deave T, Johnson D: *The needs of parents in pregnancy and early parenthood*, final report, Bristol, Centre for Child and Adolescent Health and University of Bristol, 2007.

Department for Education and Skills (DfES): *Common core of skills and knowledge for the children's workforce. Every child matters. Change for children*, London, HMSO, 2005.

Department of Health (DH): *Maternity matters: choice, access and continuity of care in a safe service*, London, HMSO, 2007.

Department of Health (DH): *The child health promotion programme, pregnancy and the first five years of life*, London, HMSO, 2008a.

Department of Health (DH): *High-quality care for all, NHS next stage review final report (Prof Lord Darzi report)*, London, HMSO, 2008b.

Department of Health (DH): *Healthy child programme: pregnancy and the first five years of life*, London, HMSO, 2009.

Department of Health (DH): *Midwifery 2020: delivering expectations*, London, HMSO, 2010.

Douglas H, Brennan A: Containment, reciprocity and behaviour management: preliminary evaluation of a brief early intervention (the Solihull approach) for families with infants and young children, *Infant Observation* 7(1):89–107, 2004.

Fisher BA: Decision emergence: phases in group decision making, *Speech Monogr* 37:53–66, 1970.

Forsyth DR: *Group dynamics*, 6th ed, Belmont (CA, 2014, Wadsworth.

Fox S: *The social life of health information: A project of the Pew Research Centre. California Health Care Foundation* (website). http://pewinternet.org/Reports/2011/Social-Life-of-Health-Info.aspx. 2011.

Gagnon AJ, Sandall J: Individual or group antenatal education for childbirth or parenthood, or both, *Cochrane Database Syst Rev* 18(3):CD002869, 2007.

Health Improvement Scotland: *Core syllabus for professional practice to support education for pregnancy, birth and early parenthood. NHS Health Scotland, Edinburgh* (website). www.healthcareimprovementscotland.org/programmes/reproductive,_maternal__child/parent_education/parent_education_syllabus.aspx. 2011.

Hollins Martin CJ: Birth planning for midwives and mothers, *Br J Midwifery* 16(9):583–587, 2008a.

Hollins Martin CJ: A tool to measure fathers' attitudes towards and needs in relation to birth participation, *Br J Midwifery* 16(7):432–437, 2008b.

Hollins Martin CJ, Bull P: What features of the maternity unit promote obedient behaviour from midwives? *Clin Effect Nurs* 952:e221–e231, 2006.

Hollins Martin CJ, Fleming V: The Birth Satisfaction Scale (BSS), *Int J Health Care Qual Assur* 24(2):124–135, 2011.

Hollins Martin CJ, Martin C: Development and psychometric properties of the Birth Satisfaction Scale-Revised (BSS-R), *Midwifery* 30:610–619, 2014.

Hollins Martin CJ, Snowden A, Martin CR: Concurrent analysis: validation of the domains within the Birth Satisfaction Scale, *J Reprod Infant Psychol* 30(3):247–260, 2012.

Johansson M, Rubertsson C, Radestad I, et al: Childbirth: an emotionally demanding experience for fathers, *Sex Reprod Healthc* 3:11–20, 2012.

Leap N, Anderson T: The role of pain in normal birth and the empowerment of women. In Downe S, editor: *Normal childbirth: evidence and debate*, 2nd ed, Edinburgh, Churchill Livingstone, pp 29–46, 2008.

Leap N, Dodwell M, Newburn M: Working with pain in labour: an overview of evidence, *New Digest* 49:22–26, 2010.

Lima-Pereira P, Bermudez-Tamayo C, Jasienska G: Use of the Internet as a source of health information amongst participants of antenatal classes, *J Clin Nurs* 21(3–4):322–330, 2012.

Madden M, Zickuhr K: *65% of online adults use social networking sites. Pew Internet & American Life Project* (website). http://pewinternet.org/Reports/2011/Social-Networking-Sites.aspx. 2011.

Maslow AH: A theory of human motivation, *Psychol Rev* 50(4):370–396, 1943.

McMillan AS, Barlow J, Redshaw M: *Birth and beyond: a review of the evidence about antenatal education* (website). www.dh.gov.uk/prod_consum_dh/groups/dhdigitalassets/@dh/@en/documents/digitalasset/dh_110371.pdf. 2009.

Mensah FK, Kiernan KE: Parents' mental health and children's cognitive and social development: families in England in the Millennium Cohort Study, *Soc Psychiatry Psychiatr Epidemiol* 45:1023–1035, 2010.

Newburn M, Muller C, Taylor S: *Preparing for birth and parenthood: report on first-time mothers and fathers attending NCT antenatal courses*, London, NCT, 2011.

Nolan M: Evaluating parent education. In Nolan M, editor: *Education and support for parenting: A guide for professionals*, London, Baillière Tindall, 2002.

Parr M: A new approach to parent education, *Br J Midwifery* 6(3):160–165, 1998.

Parr M, Joyce C: First steps in parenting: developing nurturing parenting skills in mothers and fathers in the pregnancy and postnatal period. In Barlow J, Svanberg P, editors: *Keeping the baby in mind. Infant mental health in practice*, London, Routledge, 2009.

Redshaw M, Heikkila K: *Delivered with care: a national survey of women's experience of maternity care 2010. National Perinatal Epidemiology Unit, University of Oxford* (website). www.npeu.ox.ac.uk/files/downloads/

reports/Maternity-Survey-Report-2010.pdf. 2010.

Shia N: An evaluation of male partners' perceptions of antenatal classes in a national health service hospital provision in London: implications for service, *J Perinat Educ* 22(1):30–38, 2013.

Tubbs SA: *Systems approach to small group interaction*, New York, McGraw Hill, 1995.

Tuckman BW: Developmental sequence in small groups, *Psychol Bull* 63:384–399, 1965.

Waylen A, Stewart-Brown S: Factors influencing parenting in early childhood: a prospective longitudinal study focusing on change, *Child Care Health Dev* 36:198–207, 2010.

Wilkins CA: Qualitative study exploring the support needs of first time mothers on their journey towards intuitive parenting, *Midwifery* 22(2):169–180, 2006.

Woollett A, Parr M: Psychological tasks for women and men in the transition to parenthood,
J Reprod Infant Psychol 15(2):159–183, 1997.

World Health Organization (WHO): *Fatherhood and health outcomes in Europe*, Copenhagen, WHO Regional Office for Europe, 2007.

Worldwide Alternatives to Violence (WAVE): *Trust: violence and what to do about it*, Surrey, Copenhagen, Wave Trust, 2005.

Resources and additional reading

Ahlden I, Ahlehagen S, Dahlgren LO, et al: Parents' expectations about participating in antenatal parenthood education classes, *J Perinat Educ* 21:11–17, 2012.

Bergstrom M, Kieler H, Waldenstrom U: A randomised controlled multicentre trial of women's and men's satisfaction with two models of antenatal education, *Midwifery* 27:e195–e200, 2011.

Bloomfield J, Rising SS: Centering parenting: an innovative dyad model for group mother-infant care, *J Midwifery Womens Health* 58:683–689, 2013.

Duncan L, Bardacke N: Mindfulness-based childbirth and parenting education: promoting family mindfulness during the perinatal period, *J Child Fam Stud* 19:190–202, 2010.

Howell M: Effective birth preparation: your practical guide to a better birth, Hants (UK), Intuition UN Ltd, 2009.

Shorey S, Chan SW, Chong YS, et al: Perceptions of primiparas on a postnatal psychoeducation programme: the process evaluation, *Midwifery* 31:155–163, 2015.

Svensson J, Barclay L, Cooke M: The concerns and interests of expectant and new parents: assessing learning needs, *J Perinat Educ* 15:18–27, 2006.

Svensson J, Barclay L, Cooke M: Effective antenatal education: strategies recommended by expectant and new parents, *J Perinat Educ* 17:33–42, 2008.

Useful websites:

Antenatal online: midwife led classes and pregnancy support.

http://www.antenatalonline.co.uk/.
This is a UK based resource for women and families, and has useful tools and videos for women.

Baby centre.

http://www.babycentre.co.uk/a536329/antenatal-classes.

NCT antenatal courses.

https://www.nct.org.uk/courses/antenatal?gclid=CJGzgrq_r9ACFYu4GwodVokELQ.

NHS choices: pregnancy and baby.

http://www.nhs.uk/Conditions/pregnancy-and-baby/Pages/antenatal-classes-pregnant.aspx.

NHS DH: Preparation for Birth and Beyond.

https://www.gov.uk/government.
A resource pack for leaders of community groups and activities.

Chapter 22

Physical preparation for childbirth and beyond, and the role of physiotherapy

Gill Brook

Learning Outcomes ?

After reading this chapter, you will be able to:

- have increased awareness of the effects of pregnancy, labour and the postnatal period on the musculoskeletal system
- understand the benefits of exercise during pregnancy and postnatally
- competently advise women in your care on appropriate exercise and strategies to minimize the symptoms of any musculoskeletal dysfunctions they are experiencing
- explain the role of physiotherapy in relation to women during childbearing and the history of the specialty
- know when and how to refer women in your care to a women's health physiotherapist, where available

INTRODUCTION

This chapter aims to equip midwifery students and midwives with the knowledge and skills required to understand issues such as exercise, good posture, relaxation techniques and effective physical preparation for pregnancy and childbirth, plus common musculoskeletal dysfunctions in pregnancy and postnatally. This will enable them to advise and support women in their care and recognize situations when referral to another professional is indicated. The author is a women's health physiotherapist and will refer to the role throughout, with further information on the specialty toward the end of the chapter.

EXERCISE AND SPORT DURING PREGNANCY

Pregnancy is a time when women are often receptive to health education messages. This can include the introduction of exercise as not just having short-term benefits during the pregnancy and childbirth period, but also holding long-term health gains. There is evidence that exercise during pregnancy can benefit both the woman and fetus (Royal College of Obstetricians and Gynaecologists (RCOG) 2006) and is harmful to neither, provided the pregnancy is uncomplicated and exercise is not contraindicated (ACOG 2015). Therefore, it is suggested that women should be encouraged to start, or continue with, appropriate exercise to derive the associated health benefits (National Institute for Health and Care Excellence (NICE) 2008 and 2010; RCOG 2006). These include a reduction in fatigue, varicosities and peripheral swelling; a lower incidence of insomnia, stress, anxiety and depression; and, possibly, weight-bearing exercise in pregnancy may result in a shorter labour and a decrease in delivery-related complications (RCOG 2006). Physical activity during pregnancy has also been shown to reduce gestational weight gain (Oteng-Ntim et al 2012; Thangaratinam et al 2012). In addition, NICE (2015) recommends that women with gestational diabetes engage in regular exercise (such as walking for 30 minutes after a meal) to improve blood glucose control. However, there is no conclusive evidence that exercise will prevent the onset of gestational diabetes in women (Han et al 2012; Stafne et al 2012).

Thangaratinam et al (2012) undertook a systematic review and meta-analysis of randomized controlled trials investigating the effect of three interventions during pregnancy – diet, physical activity and a mixed approach – on maternal weight and obstetric outcomes. They concluded that such interventions can reduce maternal gestational weight gain and improve outcomes for both mother and baby. The authors also identified trends towards a reduction in intrauterine death, birth trauma and hyperbilirubinaemia, and a 61% reduction in overall risk of shoulder dystocia, with all interventions compared with controls.

There appears to be some variation between what are considered absolute or relative contraindications to (aerobic) exercise in pregnancy (American College of Obstetricians and Gynecologists (ACOG) 2015) and conditions requiring medical supervision while undertaking exercise in pregnancy (RCOG 2006). Guidance produced by physiotherapists (Association of Chartered Physiotherapists in Women's Health (ACPWH) 2013a) suggests the contraindications and precautions indicated in Table 22.1.

The aim of exercise during pregnancy should be to maintain or moderately improve fitness levels (ACPWH 2013a) without trying to reach peak fitness or train for competition (RCOG 2006). It is impossible to go into any detail of different regimens within the constraints of this chapter, but the needs of different women will vary, based on whether they were a complete non-exerciser, non-regular exerciser, regular exerciser or elite athlete before conception (ACPWH 2013a). Women should be advised to monitor their level of effort during exercise to ensure that they are not overexerting themselves; if using a gym,

Table 22.1 Absolute contraindications and precautions to exercise in pregnancy

Absolute contraindication	Precaution
Serious cardiovascular, respiratory, renal or thyroid disease	Asthma Anaemia
Poorly controlled type 1 diabetes	Diabetes type 1 – but moderate exercise may be appropriate if the diabetes is well controlled. Discuss with diabetes consultant, general practitioner (GP) or nurse.
A known risk of premature labour with or without a history of risk of intrauterine growth retardation (IUGR) – seek specific medical guidance	History of miscarriage Reduced fetal movement
Cervical incompetence	
Hypertension/hypotension – should be discussed with the woman's doctor	Prepregnancy hypertension
Placenta praevia after 26 weeks gestation – should be discussed with the woman's doctor	Placenta praevia Vaginal bleeding
Sudden swelling of ankles, hands or face	
Acute infectious disease	
Severe rhesus isoimmunization	
	Extreme obesity
	Breech presentation
	Extreme underweight/very low body mass index (BMI)
	Heavy smoking
	Thyroid disease
	Pelvic girdle pain – seek an assessment from a specialist women's health physiotherapist
	Twins

Adapted from ACPWH 2013a, with permission to reproduce

they should seek advice from professional staff. Commonly described tools are the 'talk test' and Borg's scale of perceived exertion; while exercising, pregnant women should be able to carry on a conversation and perceive that their level of exertion is moderate, somewhat hard or hard (ACPWH 2013a).

Women should avoid overheating during exercise because a maternal core temperature over 39.2°C might be teratogenic in the first trimester (RCOG 2006). They can minimize this risk by drinking sufficient fluids during exercise and avoiding exercise in very hot conditions. Women must also know when to stop exercising and seek a medical opinion. Indications might include onset of abdominal pain; leakage of amniotic fluid; pelvic girdle pain and resultant difficulty with walking; vaginal bleeding; shortness of breath, dizziness, faintness, palpitations or tachycardia; persistent severe headache; calf pain; and absence of, or reduced, fetal movement (ACPWH 2013a).

Regular exercisers familiar with a particular activity or sport, such as walking, aerobics, swimming or dancing, can usually continue with it.

Those unaccustomed to exercise should be advised to wait until 13 weeks gestation before embarking on a new exercise regimen, which initially should be a low-impact and reduced-weight-bearing regimen (ACPWH 2013a), starting with 15 minutes of continuous exercise three times a week and gradually increasing to 30-minute sessions four times a week (RCOG 2006). Exercise in water, often referred to as *aquanatal exercise*, may offer a feeling of weightlessness and reduced jarring of the joints, possibly offering some relief from aches and pains, an increase in energy and better sleeping (Brook et al 2013).

Scuba diving is contraindicated during pregnancy because the fetus is not protected against decompression sickness and gas embolism. Physical exertion at an altitude over 6000 feet (1850 metres) is considered dangerous, and women should be warned that contact sports and pursuits that might result in a fall, such as horse riding, could result in fetal trauma (RCOG 2006; ACPWH 2013a). Recent guidance (ACOG 2015) also advises against 'Hot Yoga' and 'Hot Pilates'.

Readers are advised to access appropriate sources – for example, the ACPWH (2013a) – for further and updated evidence-based information before discussing recreational exercise with pregnant women in their care.

Reflective activity 22.1 ✕❮

What exercise groups or activities are available specifically for pregnant or postnatal women in your area? If possible, ask to attend one, or check whether any women you know have attended them, and assess their value. Do you think the content adheres to any evidence-based guidance that you have found? Record this information for future reference.

Muscle groups

Two muscle groups that are affected more than others by pregnancy and childbirth because of their position, structure and function are those of the pelvic floor and abdominal wall. The pelvic floor is described and illustrated elsewhere within this book (see Ch. 40), but it is also useful to understand the structure and function of the abdominal muscles (Fig. 22.1).

The abdominal muscles have various roles, including protection and support for the abdominal contents. More specifically, their main functions are flexion of the lumbar spine (*recti abdominis*), side flexion and rotation of the spine (external and internal obliques) and postural support (*transversus abdominis*, working with the pelvic floor muscles, multifidus and the diaphragm). The muscles also contribute to urination and defaecation (Brook et al 2013). As pregnancy progresses, the abdominal muscles are stretched considerably by the gravid uterus, causing the recti abdominis to become longer, wider and thinner (Coldron 2006). In addition, the *linea alba* (an area of connective tissue in the midline) may become wider and thinner (*divarication*) (see Fig. 22.2) or even split (*diastasis*), and this can persist postnatally (Coldron et al 2008). Midwives may notice this separation when examining women antenatally or in the postpartum period and should be alert to its possible effect because it may predispose some women to the low back or pelvic girdle symptoms described later in the chapter. No data related to the incidence of umbilical or para-umbilical hernia development is available, and there is debate about the suggestion that pregnancy is a significant aetiological factor in the development of such defects (Dabbas et al 2011). Although there is little information on the effect of pregnancy on the transversus abdominis (Brook et al 2013), its role along with the pelvic floor and other muscles – that is, support for the intra-abdominal organs, lower spine and pelvic girdle joints – is significant.

Many women's health physiotherapists will include pelvic floor muscle and abdominal exercises in any advice they give to pregnant women, whether it is in a parent education session, exercise class or during individual assessment of a musculoskeletal problem. Midwives may wish to do the same because this is an ideal time to improve women's knowledge of the importance of pelvic floor integrity.

Pelvic floor muscle exercises

Urinary incontinence is not rare in pregnancy, with recent data suggesting an incidence of 39.1% (Solans-Domènech et al 2010), although women may not share this information unless asked directly. There is evidence that pelvic floor muscle exercises during pregnancy can prevent and treat urinary incontinence (Mørkved and Bø

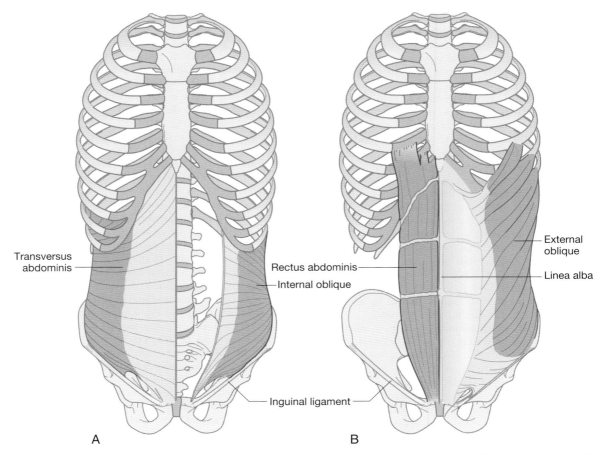

Figure 22.1 Muscles of the abdominal wall. **A,** Right rectus abdominis and left internal oblique muscles. **B,** Right rectus abdominis and left external oblique muscles. (Adapted from Palastanga et al 2006.)

2014) and reduce the likelihood of prolonged second stage labour (Salvesen and Mørkved 2004); evidence also indicates that they do not increase the risk of perineal lacerations, episiotomy, instrumental delivery or emergency caesarean section (Bø et al 2009). NICE (2008) has suggested that all pregnant women should be advised to undertake pelvic floor muscle exercise. Within the UK, the Chartered Society of Physiotherapy and Royal College of Midwives have jointly published an evidence-based advice leaflet on the subject for pregnant women (CSP and RCM 2013).

In non-pregnant women, research has suggested that a sizeable minority of women given verbal instructions on pelvic floor muscle exercises will not perform an optimum contraction (Bump et al 1991), and guidance on the management of urinary incontinence suggests that a digital assessment of the muscles should be undertaken before commencing a course of exercises (NICE 2013). It

might be considered prudent to avoid such an examination on pregnant women if there is a history of miscarriage or the woman has been advised to avoid sexual intercourse while pregnant. Also, vaginal examination would not be practical in many situations when a pregnant woman is being advised on pelvic floor muscle exercises (e.g. parent education sessions or exercise classes). In addition, healthcare professionals might not feel sufficiently skilled to undertake such an assessment, or it might fall outside their scope of practice. Therefore, it is important that physiotherapists, midwives and any other health professionals teaching pelvic floor muscle exercises give clear instructions. There are many different ways to do this, including the following example:

'Tighten the muscles around your back passage (as if trying to stop yourself breaking wind) and draw them up and forwards. At the same time tighten the muscles

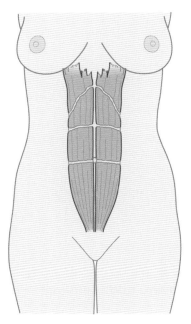
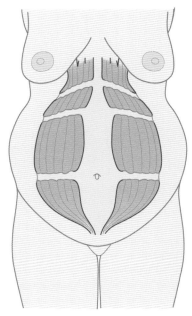
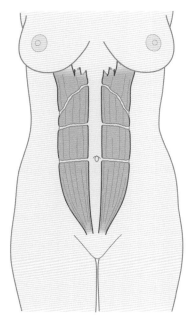

Rectis abdomins pre-pregnancy   Divarication/diastasis of   Persistent divarication postnatally
                                     recti abdominis during pregnancy

Figure 22.2 Diastasis recti.

around your front passage (as if to stop passing water). You should feel a "lift and squeeze" inside' (CSP and RCM 2013); the 'lift' analogy, i.e. closing the doors (squeeze) and moving upstairs (lift); the action of a vacuum cleaner. (Bø and Mørkved 2015)'

If women are not sure that they are contracting the muscles correctly, they could look at the perineum using a hand mirror and see if the area lifts away from the mirror as they squeeze. Alternatively, they could try to stop the dribble at the end of voiding but should not stop midstream because this may disturb normal neurological activity (Bø and Mørkved 2015) and affect emptying of the bladder.

Advice on how often to exercise and how many squeezes to undertake varies from author to author, but a recent review of evidence suggests building up to 8 to 12 near-maximum contractions three times a day. In addition, any women experiencing stress urinary incontinence should also squeeze before and during those activities that make them leak (e.g. coughing, sneezing, laughing and lifting; Bø 2015). A study of 23 pregnant women complaining of stress urinary incontinence (Miller et al 2008) showed they could reduce leakage by undertaking this anticipatory contraction, often referred to as 'the knack'. Women who experience urinary urgency or urgency urinary incontinence (leakage on their way to the toilet) might also benefit from contracting their muscles at this time.

Abdominal muscle exercises

Although many women have heard of pelvic floor muscles, far fewer will be aware of transversus abdominis and the other so-called 'core' abdominal muscles, although this is changing with recent interest in gym ball exercise, Pilates, and other regimens that focus on core stability. Professionals may prefer to use lay terms such as 'deep' or 'support' muscles.

Because the transversus abdominis lies deep under other muscle and soft tissue, it is difficult to feel or see, so, as with pelvic floor muscle exercises, clear instructions are necessary. One description is as follows:

'Place your hand on the lower part of your tummy under your bump. Breathe in through your nose. As you breathe out, gently draw in your lower tummy muscles. Your tummy should lift away from your hand, and towards your lower back. Now relax'.

(ACPWH 2013b)

As with pelvic floor muscle exercises, a review of the literature regarding exercise and pregnancy-related pelvic girdle pain (Vleeming et al 2008) suggests that researchers use a range of exercise regimens, but the Association of Chartered Physiotherapists in Women's Health (now known as Pelvic Obstetric and Gynaecological Physiotherapy (POGP)) suggests progression as able, starting with a contraction lasting 4 seconds and increasing to one lasting up to 10 seconds, with up to 10 repetitions (if achievable), repeated several times every day (ACPWH 2013b).

Low back and pelvic girdle pain

Many women experience low back or *pelvic girdle pain* during pregnancy (sometimes referred to in combination as lumbopelvic pain). Low back pain normally refers to pain of (lumbar) spinal origin, whereas pelvic girdle pain (PGP) originates in the symphysis pubis or sacroiliac joints (Brook et al 2013). Different authors report variations in prevalence, in no small part as a result of wide methodological differences, but there is evidence to suggest 20% is accurate for PGP (Vleeming et al 2008) and 50% to 70% for lumbopelvic pain (Brook et al 2013). There are many factors that make pregnant women prone to low back pain or PGP, including fatigue, increased joint mobility related to hormonally induced changes in collagen, pressure on pain-sensitive structures by remodelled collagen, weight gain with an associated change in posture and pressure from the growing fetus (Barton 2004a). Specific risk factors are probably a history of previous low back pain or trauma to the pelvis (Vleeming et al 2008), but in many cases there is no obvious explanation (POGP 2015a). Common signs and symptoms include difficulty walking (a waddling gait); clicking or grinding in the anterior or posterior pelvic joints; limited hip movements; difficulty with activities such as housework, sexual intercourse and lying in certain positions; and a limited ability to stay in any one position (be that standing, sitting or lying) for any prolonged period (POGP 2015a). Pain may occur in one or more of a variety of sites around the lower back, posterior or anterior pelvis, hips and groin. Common triggers include standing on one leg (e.g. climbing stairs, dressing) and straddling movements (e.g. getting in and out of the bath, turning in bed; POGP 2015a). Evidence-based guidance for the management of pregnancy-related PGP recommends exercise in pregnancy, physiotherapy, a pelvic belt for short periods, acupuncture, appropriate analgesia and specific stabilizing exercises postnatally (Vleeming et al 2008). It might also be appropriate to refer some affected women to an obstetrician, pain clinic, occupational therapist or social worker (POGP 2015a). Guidance on the management of backache during pregnancy (NICE 2008) suggests women should be advised that exercising in water, massage therapy, and group or individual back care classes might help to ease their symptoms.

Midwives are often the first health professional with whom pregnant women will discuss any PGP, and having excluded any other possible cause of the symptoms, such as urinary tract or other infection, Braxton Hicks or labour contractions or lumbar spine problems (which require a physiotherapy referral), the midwife needs to explain the condition, advise on analgesia and offer general advice such as that in Table 22.2 (POGP 2015a).

Although rare, osteoporosis can occur during pregnancy, most commonly affecting the vertebrae, ribs, pubis (Barton 2004a) and hips, although it is not limited to these joints. The aetiology is unclear. Symptoms such as backache and groin pain may make it difficult to differentiate it from other musculoskeletal dysfunctions. It should be considered, particularly if women are subject to other risk factors, such as long-term use of corticosteroids, thyroid problems, malabsorption disorders (e.g. coeliac disease), smoking, poor diet or low body weight (Carne 2008).

Posture and moving and handling

Because every pregnant woman is affected by hormonal changes and, to varying degrees, postural adaptations to accommodate the developing fetus, all are at risk of the various musculoskeletal dysfunctions discussed. Consequently, every pregnant woman should be offered appropriate advice to minimize the chance of such problems developing. Although such advice might not be as specific as that shown in Table 22.2, it could include advice on posture in standing (Fig. 22.3a), sitting (Fig. 22.3b) and lying (Fig. 22.3c); movement on and off a bed (Fig. 22.3d); and lifting (Fig. 22.3e) (ACPWH 2013b).

Midwives can assist women in understanding the importance of posture and clarifying good back care. This includes getting up from the examination couch, which, if the woman sits up from a lying position, imitates performing a sit-up and puts great strain on the abdominals and the back. Encouraging the woman to move to a side-lying position and then swing her legs down while pushing herself up with her arms (Fig. 22.3d), and suggesting that she does this at home when getting in and out of bed, can be of great help.

Referral to physiotherapy

If there is a women's health physiotherapy service available locally, the midwife, obstetrician or general practitioner should be able to request assessment and treatment. In some places, pregnant women may be able to self-refer. When and to whom to refer may also depend on local protocol, the confidence and experience of the midwife concerned and the physiotherapy service available (see later section on women's health physiotherapy). For example, some physiotherapists might offer advice or

Table 22.2 General advice for women experiencing pregnancy-related pelvic girdle pain

Advice	Strategies
Remain active within the limits of pain.	Avoid activities that she knows make the pain worse.
Accept offers of help and involve partner, family and friends in daily chores.	Ask for other help if needed.
Rest is important.	Rest more frequently, or sit down for activities that normally involve standing (e.g. ironing).
Avoid standing on one leg.	Dress while sitting down.
Consider alternative sleeping position.	Lie on her side with pillows between legs for comfort. Turn 'under' when turning in bed, or turn over with knees together and squeeze buttocks.
Explore alternative ways to climb stairs.	Go upstairs one leg at a time with the most pain-free leg first and the other leg joining it on the step.
Plan the day.	Bring everything needed downstairs in the morning and set up changing stations both up and downstairs. Have drinks on hand (e.g. thermos flasks). A rucksack may be helpful to carry things around the house, especially if crutches have to be used.
Avoid activities that involve asymmetrical positions of the pelvis.	Avoid sitting cross-legged. Avoid reaching, pushing or pulling to one side. Avoid bending and twisting to lift or carrying anything on one hip (e.g. toddlers).
Consider alternative positions for sexual intercourse.	Try lying on the side or kneeling on all fours.
Organize hospital appointments for the same day if possible.	Combine appointments for antenatal care and physiotherapy.

POGP 2015a, reproduced with permission

exercise groups for pregnant women, whereas others may only accept referrals for women with a specific musculoskeletal dysfunction that has not responded to advice from the midwife or doctor.

Reflective activity 22.3

Are there women's health physiotherapists working in your area? What services do they offer? How can you access them? Record this information for future reference. Could you spend some time with them to discuss your respective work?

RELAXATION

The use of relaxation in pregnancy and labour goes back to the mid-20th century, if not before. Grantly Dick-Read

referred to relaxation as 'a condition in which the muscle tone throughout the body is reduced to a minimum' (Dick-Read 1954), whereas physiotherapist Helen Heardman preferred 'reduction to a minimum of mental and muscular energy conducive with life' (Heardman 1959). It has been suggested that relaxation and breathing awareness during labour may help address the *pain–anxiety–tension cycle*, act as a distraction technique, increase tolerance of pain and offer a coping strategy (Schott and Priest 2002). Although an earlier paper on complementary and alternative therapies for labour pain, including breathing (respiratory autogenic training), hypnosis and massage (Huntley et al 2004), found no proof of efficacy, a more recent review of studies into the use of relaxation therapies in labour concluded that relaxation and yoga may have a role in the reduction of pain, can increase satisfaction with pain relief and reduce the rate of assisted vaginal delivery (Smith et al 2011). Self-hypnosis has also been studied, and although results look promising, reviewers concluded that further

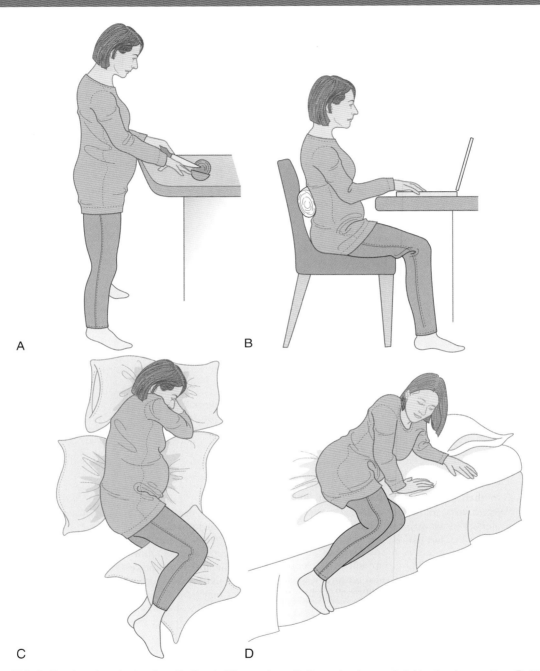

Figure 22.3 **A,** Good posture in standing. **B,** Good sitting posture. **C,** Example of a comfortable sleeping position. **D,** How to get on and off the bed.

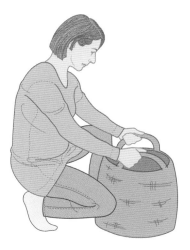

E

Figure 22.3, cont'd **E,** Good lifting technique. (Reproduced with permission from Information for Pregnant Women, FIT for Pregnancy, Association of Chartered Physiotherapists in Women's Health (ACPWH), 2013b.)

research is required to confirm its usefulness in clinical practice (Madden et al 2012).

In addition to its potential role in labour, relaxation may be considered a useful 'life skill' for dealing with stress caused by changes in lifestyle (Fordyce 2004) and managing situations such as caring for a crying baby or rebellious toddler (Schott and Priest 2002).

Health professionals teaching relaxation should ideally understand and believe in what they are teaching, and they should have practised the techniques before introducing them into their practice (Schott and Priest 2002). There are many different techniques, including the Mitchell Method of Physiological Relaxation (POGP 2014a). The Mitchell Method is based on the physiological concept of reciprocal relaxation – that is, if one group of muscles is tightened, then the opposite group will relax. People who are stressed or tense adopt a typical posture (e.g. fists clenched, shoulders hunched). The Mitchell technique addresses tension in different parts of the body with a set of instructions for each area:

- Move away from the position of stress.
- Stop.
- Be aware and feel the new position (POGP 2014a).

Physiological relaxation can be practised in any suitable, comfortable position, using the instructions in Box 22.1. Eventually, the participant should be able to memorize the instructions in bold and use the technique whenever required, and for a range of life situations that might cause stress.

POSTNATAL EXERCISE AND ADVICE

Postnatal exercises target the abdominal and pelvic floor muscles as the groups most affected by pregnancy and birth, and they are designed to aid a return to previous fitness levels (ACPWH 2013c). Transversus abdominis and pelvic floor muscle exercises may be taught as they were during pregnancy (see previous discussion), and women should be reminded that these exercises can be practised in a variety of positions and thus can be undertaken whenever and wherever they are remembered.

Whereas previous generations of new mothers might rest at home or in hospital for a period of days or even weeks before expecting to return to 'normal' activities, current expectations are for a much speedier recovery (Barton 2004b). It is therefore pertinent to encourage appropriate, safe exercises as soon as possible to help return the soft tissues to their prepregnancy condition and minimize the risk of musculoskeletal problems. Current guidance (ACPWH 2013c) gives no specific time at which to start, just suggesting as soon as possible, but a woman's choice may be influenced by any pre-existing or de novo musculoskeletal dysfunction, labour or delivery. In a study of 1193 women, Thompson et al (2002) found that primiparous women and those who had undergone an assisted vaginal delivery reported more perineal pain than others, whereas those who had undergone caesarean section reported a higher incidence of exhaustion and bowel problems.

In the absence of evidence that early appropriate exercise is detrimental to women postnatally, midwives can encourage it. Women who are not, for any reason, active in the hours or early days postdelivery may be encouraged to bend their feet and ankles up and down briskly for 30 seconds every hour to aid circulation (ACPWH 2013c). There is no evidence to support the benefit of routine postoperative chest physiotherapy to avoid respiratory complications (Silva et al 2013), but this may be indicated in high-risk cases (e.g. a pre-existing pulmonary condition or if relevant symptoms arise).

It is suggested (Barton 2004b) that the pumping action of pelvic floor exercises assists venous and lymphatic drainage, removing traumatic exudate and thus reducing symptoms. In addition, it is recommended that pelvic

---

Box 22.1 Physiological relaxation

Pull your shoulders towards your feet away from your ears, making the neck longer. Stop. Feel that your shoulders are lower down and that now there is a larger space between them and your ears.

Elbows out and open. Keep your arms supported, then push them slightly away from your sides, opening out the elbow joints. Stop. Feel the positions of your arms and elbows, and the pressure of your arms on their support, through the sensations of your skin.

Fingers and thumbs long and supported. Open out your fingers and thumbs, keeping your wrists resting on their support. Stop. Feel your fingers and thumbs fall back onto their support. Do not let your hands touch each other or they will register this instead of their own position.

Turn your hips outwards. Feel your thighs and lower legs roll outwards. Stop. Feel that your legs have rolled outwards.

Move your knees gently until comfortable. Stop. Feel the comfort in your knees.

Push your feet away from your face. Bend at the ankles downwards, gently pointing your toes. Stop. Feel that your feet are softer at the ankle joints because all the lower leg muscles are now relaxed.

Press your body into the support using the floor, bed or back of the chair – not the seat. Stop. Feel the pressure of your body on the support.

Press your head into the pillow or chair. Feel the movement in your neck as you do this. Stop. Feel the weight of your head in the hollow you have made.

Take a deep breath – feel your tummy swell out as you breathe in, **then breathe out** easily.

Repeat twice.

Drag your jaw down – do not open your mouth, just unclench your teeth inside your mouth and gently pull your jaw down. Stop. Feel the space between your upper and lower teeth, that the skin is smooth, with your lips still gently touching each other.

Bring your tongue down and let it lie in the middle of your mouth if it is stuck against the roof of your mouth. Stop. Feel the tip of your tongue touching your lower teeth.

Close your eyes if not already closed. Let your eyes close down over your eyes; do not screw them shut. Stop. Be aware of the darkness with your eyes at rest.

Smoothe the skin over your forehead from your eyebrows into your hair, continuing the movement over the top of your head and down the back of your neck – widen the space between your eyebrows and hairline, making it wrinkle free. Stop. Feel the smoothing of the skin of your forehead and your hair moving back as the large muscle of your skull slackens and relaxes.

POGP 2014a, reproduced with permission

---

floor muscle training is an appropriate treatment for persistent postnatal urinary incontinence (Boyle et al 2012).

If a woman has experienced a stillbirth or neonatal death, exercise and a return to normal physical activity may be a low personal priority. However, written advice, which can be consulted when the time is right, is a useful resource (POGP 2014b).

Women are advised to avoid strong trunk curling exercises until they have good transversus abdominis control, especially if a significant *divarication* or *diastasis* – over three fingers' width – persists (Brook et al 2013). Women can be advised that they should not undertake abdominal exercises during which they can see their abdomen dome or bulge (ACPWH 2013c).

Divarication can be assessed by asking the woman to lie flat on her back (one or no pillows), with her knees bent and feet flat on the bed. The fingers of one hand are placed widthways on her abdomen, just above or below the umbilicus. As the woman is asked to lift her head and shoulders and reach down towards her feet, it is possible to feel the recti abdominis muscle bellies pressing against the fingers, and you can then gauge the gap in finger widths (Barton 2004b).

Reflective activity 22.5

Check the recti abdominis on a friend, family member or colleague who has had children. Compare to a nulliparous woman. Are you confident in what you are doing and feeling? Could you ask a more experienced midwife or women's health physiotherapist for guidance?

In the absence of medical or surgical complications, rapid resumption of physical activities soon after delivery has not been found to result in adverse effects, but advice is that exercise routines should be gradually reintroduced (ACOG 2015), and they should not include high-impact activity too soon (RCOG 2006; ACPWH 2013c). Advice from a midwife or physiotherapist can include brisk walking, or swimming when there has been no vaginal bleeding or discharge for 7 consecutive days (ACPWH 2013c). Exercise following childbirth has, along with other interventions, been shown to improve postnatal well-being (Norman et al 2010) and help women lose weight (Amorim Adegboye and Linne 2013).

Some maternity units will have no or limited inpatient postnatal physiotherapy input. In the latter case, physiotherapists may restrict their service to women with postnatal complications, such as ongoing or delivery-related musculoskeletal dysfunctions, third or fourth degree tears, postnatal urinary retention, urinary or faecal incontinence, or rectus abdominis divarication or diastasis. Although guidance on postnatal care (NICE 2006) suggests that backache should be managed as in the general population, European guidelines on the management of pelvic girdle pain (Vleeming et al 2008) recommend specific stabilizing exercises postnatally.

WOMEN'S HEALTH PHYSIOTHERAPY

Physiotherapists in the UK have a long history of advising and treating women during pregnancy and the postnatal period (see chapter website resources). The POGP promotes high standards of physiotherapy practice within those specialties, provides means by which physiotherapists can improve their skills and acts in their professional interest. Furthermore it fosters the role of physiotherapy within the specialties, promotes health education and encourages research and interprofessional collaboration (POGP 2015b).

The role of women's health physiotherapists in the UK is diverse, usually including the care of women antenatally and postnatally, and sometimes involvement in parent education sessions. Clinicians may be specialists in the treatment of pregnancy-related musculoskeletal dysfunctions (POGP 2015b). Many treat incontinence (both female and male) and other pelvic floor muscle dysfunctions, and they may care for women undergoing gynaecological surgery. In addition, other areas of practice might include neonatal paediatrics, osteoporosis, menopause, breast care, and lymphoedema management (Brook 2007).

The Department of Health (DH) and National Health Service (NHS) have recognized the role of physiotherapists in the multiprofessional team offering antenatal care (DH 2004, NHS 2015). Physiotherapists are the experts in musculoskeletal assessment (Barton 2004a), and current evidence-based guidance on the management of pregnancy-related pelvic girdle pain (Vleeming et al 2008) recommends exercises in pregnancy; an individualized treatment programme focusing on specific stabilizing exercises as part of a multifactorial treatment for the condition postnatally; individualized physical therapy; manipulation or joint mobilization as a possible test for symptomatic relief; acupuncture; and possibly the trial of a pelvic belt for symptomatic relief. Most, if not all, of these are within the scope of practice of many physiotherapists working within women's health and are not commonly practised by other professionals working within maternity services.

Unfortunately, there appears to be little or no consistency in the provision of women's health physiotherapy around the UK (Brook 2007). This is a disadvantage to other professionals, such as midwives, who may or may not have access to such specialist services. It is reported (Brook 2007) that a unit handling 6000 deliveries a year might have anything between the equivalent of one and four full-time physiotherapists offering a range of women's health services. The last 20 years has seen a large increase in their role within continence services, with a decrease in obstetric work, possibly related to a lack of appropriate research in the specialty (Mantle 2004).

CONCLUSION

Midwives should be the lead professionals for all healthy women with straightforward pregnancies and act as key coordinators for women with more complex needs (Midwifery 2020). Because continuity of care is recommended (NICE 2008), it is ideal if midwives are knowledgeable and competent to offer advice on posture and exercise in pregnancy, the management of musculoskeletal dysfunctions and the return to normal activities postnatally. They must also know what additional services are available locally, including those offered by women's health physiotherapists. This period is an ideal time to provide advice on posture, exercise and moving and handling that women can go on to use during early parenthood and beyond.

Key Points	

- A clear understanding of the normal and altered anatomy and physiology enables the midwife to identify deviations from normal, and consult and refer appropriately.
- Appropriate exercise and the development of relaxation techniques during pregnancy and the postnatal period can have short-term and long-term health benefits for the woman.
- The midwife should provide individualized advice and information regarding exercise and posture.

References

American College of Obstetricians and Gynecologists (ACOG): *Physical activity and exercise during pregnancy and the postpartum period. ACOG Committee Opinion No 650*, Washington, ACOG, 2015.

Amorim Adegboye AR, Linne YM: Diet or exercise, or both, for weight reduction in women after childbirth, *Cochrane Database Syst Rev* (7):CD005627, 2013.

Association of Chartered Physiotherapists in Women's Health (ACPWH): *Fit and safe to exercise in the childbearing year. Advice for physiotherapists and other health professionals* (website). pogp.csp .org.uk/publications/fit-safe -physiotherapists-exercise-child bearing-year. 2013a.

Association of Chartered Physiotherapists in Women's Health (ACPWH): *Fit for pregnancy. Keep fit and cope with the physical demands of pregnancy – exercises and advice to help you* (website). pogp.csp.org.uk/ publications/fit-pregnancy. 2013b.

Association of Chartered Physiotherapists in Women's Health (ACPWH): *Fit for the future: essential exercises and advice after childbirth* (website). pogp.csp.org.uk/ publications/fit-future. 2013c.

Barton S: Relieving the discomforts of pregnancy. In Mantle J, Haslam J, Barton S, editors: *Physiotherapy in obstetrics and gynaecology*, 2nd edn, London, Butterworth-Heinemann, pp 141–164, 2004a.

Barton S: The postnatal period. In Mantle J, Haslam J, Barton S, editors: *Physiotherapy in obstetrics and gynaecology*, 2nd edn, London, Butterworth-Heinemann, pp 205–247, 2004b.

Bø K: Pelvic floor muscle training for stress urinary incontinence. In Bø K, Berghmans B, Mørkved S, et al, editors: *Evidence-based physical therapy for the pelvic floor*, 2nd edn, Edinburgh, Churchill Livingstone, pp 162–178, 2015.

Bø K, Fleten C, Nystad W: Effect of antenatal pelvic floor muscle training on labor and birth, *Obstet Gynecol* 113(6):1279–1284, 2009.

Bø K, Mørkved S: Pelvic floor and exercise science. Motor learning. In Bø K, Berghmans B, Mørkved S, et al, editors: *Evidence-based physical therapy for the pelvic floor*, 2nd edn, Edinburgh, Churchill Livingstone, pp 111–117, 2015.

Boyle R, Hay-Smith EJC, Cody JD, et al: Pelvic floor muscle training for prevention and treatment of urinary and faecal incontinence in antenatal and postnatal women, *Cochrane Database Syst Rev* (10):CD007471, 2012.

Brook G: Women's health physiotherapy service, *Natl Assoc Prim Care Rev* (summer edition):163–165, 2007.

Brook G, Brooks T, Coldron Y, et al: Physiotherapy in women's health. In Porter S, editor: *Tidy's physiotherapy*, 15th edn, Edinburgh, Churchill Livingstone, pp 605–635, 2013.

Bump R, Hurt WG, Fantl JA, et al: Assessment of Kegel pelvic muscle exercise performance after brief verbal instruction, *Am J Obstet Gynecol* 165(2):322–329, 1991.

Carne K: Osteoporosis. In Porter S, editor: *Tidy's physiotherapy*, 14th edn, Edinburgh, Churchill Livingstone, pp 182–198, 2008.

Chartered Society of Physiotherapy and Royal College of Midwives (CSP & RCM): *Personal training for your pelvic floor* (website). www.csp.org.uk/ publications/personal-training-your-pelvic-floor. 2013.

Coldron Y: *Characteristics of abdominal and paraspinal muscles in postnatal women.* Unpublished PhD thesis, St. George's, University of London, ISNI 0000 0001 3560 0100 uk.bl. ethos.429385, 2006.

Coldron Y, Stokes MJ, Cook K: Postpartum characteristics of rectus abdominis on ultrasound imaging, *Man Ther* 13(2):112–121, 2008.

Dabbas N, Adams K, Pearson K, et al: Frequency of abdominal wall hernias: is classical teaching out of date?, *J R Soc Med* 2:5, 2011.

Department of Health (DH): *National service framework for children and maternity services.* Standard 11, London, Department of Health, 2004.

Dick-Read G: *Childbirth without Fear: the principles and practice of natural childbirth*, London, William Heinemann, 1954.

Fordyce J: The antenatal period. In Mantle J, Haslam J, Barton S, editors: *Physiotherapy in obstetrics and gynaecology*, 2nd edn, London, Butterworth-Heinemann, pp 93–139, 2004.

Han S, Middleton P, Crowther CA: Exercise for pregnant women for preventing gestational diabetes mellitus, *Cochrane Database Syst Rev* (7):CD009021, 2012.

Heardman H: *Physiotherapy in obstetrics and gynaecology*, Edinburgh, Livingstone, 1959.

Huntley AL, Thompson Coon J, Ernst E: Complementary and alternative medicine for labor pain: a systematic review, *Am J Obstet Gynecol* 191(1):36–44, 2004.

Madden K, Middleton P, Cyna AM, et al: Hypnosis for pain management during labour and childbirth, *Cochrane Database Syst Rev* (11):CD009356, 2012.

Mantle J: Editorial, *J Assoc Chart Physiother Womens Health* 94(3): 2004.

Midwifery 2020: *Midwifery 2020: delivering expectations* (website). www.dhsspsni.gov.uk/midwifery _2020_report.pdf. 2010.

Miller JM, Sampselle C, Ashton-Miller J, et al: Clarification and confirmation of the Knack maneuver: the effect of volitional pelvic floor muscle contraction to preempt expected stress urinary incontinence, *Int Urogynecol J Pelvic Floor Dysfunct* 19(6):773–782, 2008.

Mørkved S, Bø K: Effect of pelvic floor muscle training during pregnancy and after childbirth on prevention and treatment of urinary incontinence: a systematic review, *Br J Sports Med* 48:299–310, 2014.

National Health Service: *Antenatal support: meet the team* (website). www.nhs.uk/conditions/pregnancy-and-baby/Pages/antenatal-team -midwife-obstetrician-pregnant .aspx#close. 2015.

National Institute for Health and Clinical Excellence (NICE): *Postnatal care. routine postnatal care for women and their babies* (website). www.nice.org.uk/guidance/cg37. 2006.

National Institute for Health and Clinical Excellence (NICE): *Antenatal care for uncomplicated pregnancies [CG62]* (website). www.nice.org.uk. 2008.

National Institute for Health and Clinical Excellence (NICE): *Weight management before, during and after pregnancy. P427 Public Health Guidance*, London, NICE, 2010.

National Institute for Health and Care Excellence (NICE): *Urinary incontinence: The management of urinary incontinence in women. CG171 NICE Clinical Guideline*, London, NICE, 2013.

National Institute for Health and Care Excellence (NICE): *Diabetes in pregnancy: management of diabetes and its complications from preconception to the postnatal period. NG3 NICE Guideline*, London, NICE, 2015.

Norman E, Sherburn M, Osborne RH, et al: An exercise and education program improves well-being of new mothers: a randomized controlled trial, *Phys Ther* 90(3):348–355, 2010.

Oteng-Ntim E, Varma R, Croker H, et al: Lifestyle interventions for overweight and obese pregnant women to improve pregnancy outcome: systematic review and meta-analysis, *BMC Med* 10:47, 2012.

Palastanga N, Field D, Soames R: *Anatomy and human movement*, 5th edn, Oxford, Butterworth-Heinemann, 2006.

Pelvic Obstetric and Gynaecological Physiotherapy (POGP): *The Mitchell method of physiological relaxation* (website). http://pogp.csp.org .uk/publications/mitchell-method -simple-relaxation. 2014a.

Pelvic Obstetric and Gynaecological Physiotherapy (POGP): *Exercise and advice after the loss of your baby* (website). http://pogp.csp.org .uk/publications/exercise-advice -after-loss-your-baby. 2014b.

Pelvic Obstetric and Gynaecological Physiotherapy (POGP): *Pregnancy-related pelvic girdle pain: guidance for health professionals* (website). http://pogp.csp.org.uk/publications/ pregnancy-related-pelvic-girdle-pain -pgp-health-professionals. 2015a.

Pelvic Obstetric and Gynaecological Physiotherapy (POGP): *About POGP* (website). http://pogp.csp.org.uk/ about-pogp. 2015b.

Royal College of Obstetricians and Gynaecologists (RCOG): *Statement No. 4. Exercise in pregnancy*, London, RCOG, 2006.

Salvesen KÅ, Mørkved S: Randomised controlled trial of pelvic floor muscle training during pregnancy, *Br Med J* 329(7462):378–380, 2004.

Schott J, Priest J: *Leading antenatal classes. A practical guide*, 2nd edn, Oxford, Books for Midwives, 2002.

Silva YR, Li SK, Rickard MJFX: Does the addition of deep breathing exercises to physiotherapy-directed early mobilisation alter patient outcomes following high-risk open upper abdominal surgery? Cluster randomised controlled trial, *Physiotherapy* 99(3):187–193, 2013.

Smith CA, Levett KM, Collins CT, et al: Relaxation techniques for pain management in labour, *Cochrane Database Syst Rev* CD009514, 2011.

Solans-Domènech M, Sánchez E, Espuña-Pons M, on behalf of the Pelvic Floor Research Group (Grup de Recerca del Sòl Pelvià; GRESP): Urinary and anal incontinence during pregnancy and postpartum: incidence, severity, and risk factors, *Obstet Gynecol* 115(3):618–628, 2010.

Stafne SN, Salvesen KÅ, Romundstad PR, et al: Regular exercise during pregnancy to prevent gestational diabetes: a randomized controlled trial, *Obstet Gynecol* 119(1):29–36, 2012.

Thangaratinam S, Rogozińska E, Jolly K, et al: Effects of interventions in pregnancy on maternal weight and obstetric outcomes: meta-analysis of randomized evidence, *Br Med J* 344:e2088, 2012.

Thompson JF, Roberts CL, Currie M, et al: Prevalence and persistence of health problems after childbirth: association with parity and method of birth, *Birth* 29(2):83–94, 2002.

Vleeming A, Albert H, Östgaard HC, et al: European guidelines for the diagnosis and treatment of pelvic girdle pain, *Eur Spine J* 17(6):794–819, 2008.

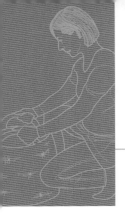

Chapter 23

Vulnerable women

Claire Homeyard and Anna Gaudion

Learning Outcomes ?

After reading this chapter, you will be able to:

- understand the importance of the woman–midwife relationship and what midwives can do to support vulnerable women
- realize how the wider determinants of health may affect pregnant women and their babies
- appreciate the effects of being a pregnant teenager
- be aware of the effects of drug and alcohol misuse in pregnancy, signs of domestic abuse and the types of questions to ask
- realize the importance of signposting women to appropriate agencies and services for further information and advice.

INTRODUCTION

In *Maternity Matters* (Department of Health (DH) 2007a) the then Labour government made explicit a commitment to tackle inequalities in access and uptake of maternity services for 'vulnerable groups'. This was followed in 2010 by the coalition government's document *Equity and Excellence* (DH 2010a). Although less implicit, it does state that all sections of society should be given the right support to enable them to have improved life chances.

A number of enquiries and reports (Marmot 2010; Manktelow et al 2015; Knight et al 2014) have highlighted that addressing the complex needs of women who are broadly described in policy terms as 'vulnerable' remains paramount. Deprivation, non-white ethnicity and maternal age

under 20 years old are associated with an increased risk of infant mortality (Marmot 2010; DH 2010b). Babies born to mothers where there is paucity of income have a 5% higher risk of dying than those whose mother is more affluent. The babies of black, black British or Asian British have a 50% increased chance of dying than mothers of white ethnicity. Maternal mortality rates are highest in areas of deprivation and in some ethnic groups, primarily Asian and black African (Knight et al 2014; Manktelow et al 2015).

Being financially disadvantaged and not being able to articulate needs because of lack of awareness of opportunity or confidence, disability, language or discrimination means that midwives, in particular, have a primary role in assessing need and making appropriate care happen. The Nursing and Midwifery Council (NMC) code states that midwives are required to 'act as an advocate for the vulnerable' (NMC 2015: 5).

This chapter provides an overview of the particular needs of vulnerable women and some introductory pointers to raise awareness and ensure that the most vulnerable women and those with chaotic lifestyles receive appropriate maternity care.

DOMESTIC VIOLENCE AND ABUSE

Domestic violence and abuse can be defined as follows:

'any incident or pattern of incidents of controlling, coercive, threatening behaviour, violence or abuse [psychological, physical, sexual, financial or emotional] between those aged 16 or over who are, or have been, intimate partners or family members regardless of gender or sexuality'.

(Taket 2013: 1)

It also includes a number of issues more prevalent in minority ethnic groups, such as forced marriage, female genital mutilation (FGM) (see Ch. 53) and 'honour' crimes. Pregnancy represents an ideal opportunity for routine enquiry because women are more likely to present to maternity services than any other health service over the course of their lives (Bowen et al 2005).

Key facts

- Around 30% of cases of abuse against women start or worsen in pregnancy (DH 2013).
- Approximately 50% of female homicide victims are killed by a partner or ex-partner (Ministry of Justice 2014).
- Disabled women are twice as likely to experience domestic violence and abuse than non-disabled women (DH 2013).
- Of maternal deaths, 14% occurred in women who had told a health professional they were in an abusive relationship (Lewis 2007).
- Approximately 75% of domestic abuse in relationships is witnessed by children (Royal College of Psychiatrists (RCPsych) 2012).
- The cost of domestic abuse to the UK taxpayer is £3.9 billion per year (British Medical Association (BMA) 2014).

Domestic abuse is underreported, mostly because of fear of reprisal, stigma and a continued relationship with the perpetrator; therefore, any statistical data needs to be interpreted with caution.

Domestic abuse is a major public health issue because it can put babies and their mothers at risk of injury or even death (Shah and Shah 2010; Lewis and Centre for Maternal and Child Enquires (CMACE) 2011; National Institute for Health and Care Excellence (NICE) 2014). Harm may also be indirect, through a woman's inability to access antenatal care (NICE 2010, 2012). Domestic abuse has long-term consequences for a woman's mental health, with increased likelihood of the victim suffering from anxiety, depression and psychosomatic symptoms (BMA 2014).

A number of professional and governmental bodies, including the Royal College of Midwives (RCM 2006), the British Medical Association (BMA 2014), the Royal College of Obstetricians and Gynaecologists (RCOG 2015) and the Royal College of Psychiatrists (RCPsych 2012), advocate that pregnant women should be seen alone and asked about domestic abuse by trained staff. This should form part of the needs, risk and choice assessment at the booking visit or at another time if the woman is not alone (Lewis and CMACE 2011; NICE 2014). It is recommended that the topic should be framed as follows:

- 'As violence in the home is so common, we now ask all women about it routinely'

- Followed by direct questions such as:
  - 'Are you afraid at home?'
  - 'Are you in a relationship with someone who hurts or threatens you?'
  - 'As an adult have you ever been emotionally or physically hurt by your partner or someone important to you?' (DH 2005; DH 2013)

The process of routine enquiry for domestic abuse has been shown to be acceptable to women (Baird et al 2011), and repeat enquiry may help to increase disclosure (Taylor et al 2011; Bacchus et al 2004); lower rates have been reported at booking (Keeling and Mason 2011). By asking all women and explaining it is a routine question, it helps to destigmatize domestic abuse and it also gives 'permission' for the woman to disclose at this time or at a later date (Homeyard and Gaudion 2009).

All women, regardless of disclosure, should be provided with information and contact helplines for support and advice in the booking information and their handheld notes (Knight et al 2015). Where a partner or other person is present, the question should be asked at a later date or an excuse found for the midwife to talk to the woman alone. In situations where a woman does not speak English, the question should be asked through an interpreter and not a family friend or relative. Where possible, the interpreter should be female and have received some instruction on domestic abuse.

A midwife's role is to let the woman know that she can disclose if and when she is ready. The midwife should refer the woman and not act as a caseworker for the woman.

It is important that a woman reaches her own decision about what to do. It may be that she takes one of the following actions:

- Calls a helpline
- Contacts the police
- Gets legal advice
- Seeks emergency accommodation
- Returns temporarily to her abusive partner after making a safety plan

Midwives need to be vigilant and sensitive to possible indicators of domestic abuse, including the following:

- Late booking or poor engagement with antenatal care
- Repeated presentation to services
- Depression, anxiety and self-harm
- Injuries of different ages, especially to the neck, breasts, head, abdomen and genital areas
- Pelvic pain, frequent urinary tract infections, vaginal infections and sexually transmitted diseases
- Partner always present during appointments and dominates the questions

Box 23.1 Home Office guidance

The Home Office guidance (Taket 2013) recommends the following mnemonic to aid the overall approach:

R   Routine enquiry

A   Ask direct questions

D   Document findings safely

A   Assess women's safety

R   Resources – give women information and respect their choices

- Poor obstetric history (e.g. repeated miscarriages) (DH 2005)

Documentation of the issues or concerns is imperative, but this should not be in the handheld notes. Confidentiality is important, but, where there is multiprofessional working, information may need to be shared; and there are limits to confidentiality. The issues of domestic violence, mental ill-health and substance misuse ('toxic trio'), are indicators of increased risk of harm to children (DH 2013). If there are reasons to suspect children are at risk, safeguarding and protection take precedence (NICE 2014). This needs to be explained to the woman. (See Box 23.1.)

Reflective activity 23.1

What ethical dilemmas can arise for the midwife when a pregnant woman with two other young children refuses to discuss the domestic abuse she is experiencing?

SUBSTANCE MISUSE (ALCOHOL AND/OR DRUGS)

The risks of physical, psychological and social harm for women who have significant problems related to substance misuse during pregnancy are well documented (DH 2007b). It is also potentially harmful for the baby. Although the risks associated with smoking during pregnancy are also recognized, they are not covered in this chapter (see Ch. 19). There are a number of illicit substances used by women in pregnancy, including cocaine, heroin, cannabis and benzodiazepines. Poly-substance misuse, for example, opiates and alcohol, is not uncommon (Lewis 2007).

Substance misuse is often compounded by other factors, such as poverty, social exclusion and homelessness (Neale 2002). Pregnant drug-using women are therefore at increased risk of poorer general health and other health-related problems, including bloodborne viruses, such as hepatitis B and C. Maternity care should be coordinated by a named midwife or doctor with specialized knowledge

of, and experience in, the care of women who misuse substances (NICE 2010; Knight et al 2015). The wider multiprofessional team, including substance misuse agencies, social care and the neonatal team, should also be involved. Substance misuse during pregnancy increases the risk of poor pregnancy and newborn outcomes (DH 2007b), including the following:

- Placental abruption (RCOG 2011)
- Stillbirth and neonatal death (Sherwood et al 2009)
- Preterm delivery and intra-uterine growth retardation (Greenough et al 2005; DrugScope 2011)
- Low birthweight and sudden infant death syndrome (Hepburn 2005)
- Neonatal abstinence syndrome (Jansson and Velez 2012; DrugScope 2011)
- Physical and neurological damage
- Fetal alcohol spectrum disorder (FASD) (BMA 2007)

Midwives should be alert to the fact that substance misuse may be associated with past or current experiences of abuse and with psychiatric or psychological problems. These women require access to assertive outreach care from mental health and specialist addiction services (Knight et al 2015).

Antenatal care

Substance misuse makes a significant contribution to maternal mortality, with 11% of all pregnant women who died between 2003 and 2005 having alcohol or drug problems (Lewis 2007). Women often book late and are poor clinic attenders. This may be the result of a number of issues, including chaotic lifestyles, poor service accessibility, fear of being judged and avoidance of social services (Lewis 2007). The use of reminder systems such as text messaging is recommended (NICE 2010). The booking history should include sensitive routine enquiry about all substance use; this includes alcohol, tobacco and pre-scribed or non-prescribed and legal and illegal drugs. For some women, pregnancy may act as a positive incentive to change substance-using behaviour.

Women should be encouraged to attend a third-sector agency that provides substance misuse services, or a specialist colocated maternity service where available (NICE 2010). A multiprofessional assessment of the extent of the woman's substance use should be arranged, including type of drugs, level, frequency, pattern and method of administration, and consider any potential risks to her unborn child from current or previous drug use.

Intrapartum care

Routine care during labour should be provided, with careful observation of mother and fetus for signs of withdrawal. Commonly seen symptoms in the mother include restlessness, tremors, sweating, abdominal pain, cramps, anxiety and vomiting. In addition, the fetus is at increased risk of hypoxia and fetal distress because the effects of drug misuse can cause placental insufficiency (DH 2007b).

Postnatal care

All mothers and babies should be transferred to the postnatal ward unless there is a medical reason for admission to the neonatal intensive care unit (NICU). Breast-feeding should be promoted where possible, with HIV being the only medical contraindication in the UK (Balain and Johnson 2014). Neonatal abstinence syndrome (withdrawal symptoms) occurs in 80% of neonates exposed to opiates in utero (Balain and Johnson 2014). Commonly seen symptoms include sneezing, poor feeding, irritability, high-pitched cry and tremors (DrugScope 2011).

Close follow-up and multiagency support to keep women in treatment programmes is essential; this is particularly significant if the baby is removed from the mother. Relapse can be a problem; the Confidential Enquiry into Maternal and Child Health (CEMACH) report highlighted that a majority of women who died with known substance misuse problems did so after 42 days postnatally (Lewis 2007). Midwives should be alert to the increased risk of postnatal depression in women who misuse substances (Ross and Dennis 2009), and provision of contraceptive advice and services should be available (Advisory Council on the Misuse of Drugs (ACMD) 2011).

Safeguarding children

It is estimated that there are between 250,000 and 350,000 children of problem drug users in the UK, representing 2% to 3% of children under the age of 16 in England and Wales and 4% to 6% in Scotland (ACMD 2011). Midwives and substance misuse services need to be aware of the laws and issues that relate to child protection. If the woman does not already have social work involvement, consent to liaise with the local service to enable appropriate assessment of her circumstances should be undertaken during pregnancy. If the woman declines referral, staff should consider any risk of significant harm to her fetus. This may override the need for the woman's consent to referral. The absence of information sharing between professional groups following serious case reviews of abuse or neglect has been highlighted as a recurring problem (National Society for the Prevention of Cruelty to Children (NSPCC) 2014). If midwives have concerns or need support and guidance, they should contact their designated named safeguarding lead or the social work children and family team manager for advice.

PREGNANT TEENAGERS

It is recognized that becoming a teenage mother can have negative consequences on a woman's physical and mental health and limits social and educational opportunities, which may affect future economic well-being (Public Health England (PHE) et al 2015). Children born to teenagers are more likely to have poorer health and social outcomes in later life compared with babies of older mothers (Swann et al 2003), and daughters are more likely to become teenage mothers themselves (Berrington et al 2005).

Teenage pregnancy involves the following effects (PHE et al 2015):

Effects on child health

- 30% higher risk of stillbirth
- 45% higher risk of infant death
- Higher risk of premature birth (20% for first and 90% for second baby)
- 15% higher risk of low birthweight (see Ch. 45)
- 30% less likely to be breastfed
- Smoke, alcohol or drug exposure during pregnancy

Effects on mental and emotional health

- Higher rate of postnatal depression
- More likely to experience mental health issues
- Negative effects on relationships
- More likely to experience physical, sexual or domestic abuse
- More likely to experience relationship breakdown

Effects on economic well-being

- Educational difficulties, which can have a negative effect on job prospects
- More likely to be from a deprived background, suffer from poor nutrition, live in poor housing and be involved in crime
- Repeat unplanned pregnancy

A number of key areas have been identified to improve outcomes (NICE 2010):

- Accessible antenatal care (e.g. held in children's centres)
- Antenatal education in peer groups
- Accessible information (e.g. www.nhs.uk/start4life/signups/new)
- A named midwife to coordinate and provide most of the care
- 'Joined-up working' and effective referral pathways – through involvement with a number of services, including health, Family Nurse Partnership (FNP), youth support, education and social care
- Involve and signpost young fathers (e.g. www.dad.info)
- Promotion of contraception to prevent second unplanned pregnancies

PARENTS WITH LEARNING DISABILITIES/INTELLECTUAL DISABILITY

In 2001, the Department of Health defined a person with a learning disability as presenting with the following:

- A significant reduced ability to understand new or complex information and/or to learn new skills
- A reduced ability to cope independently, which started in childhood, with a lasting effect on development

Valuing People (DH, 2001) set out a landscape for understanding people with learning disabilities that moves away from the stance of 'can't do' to 'can do with support'. The document starts with the proviso that people with learning disabilities are 'people first', rather than learning-disabled people. The report endorsed the right for these individuals to marry and start a family (DH 2001).

People with learning disabilities can have complex health and social needs compounded by isolation, poverty and prejudice. They experience greater inequalities in health and more unmet health needs than are present in the general population (Gibbs et al 2008; Mencap 2004, 2007 and 2012; Michaels 2008).

A systematic review looking at the existing empirical evidence on antenatal care provision for women with intellectual disabilities found a dearth of available studies (Homeyard et al 2016). However, the literature highlighted that pregnant women with learning disabilities faced a number of issues, such as the following:

- Lack of 'accessible' written information
- Limited choice
- Disempowering practices by professionals

The Disability Act of 2005 and the Mental Capacity Act of 2005 lay out a structure for the delivery of equal treatment for people with a learning disability. In 2007, both the Royal College of Midwives (RCM 2007) and the Royal College of Nursing (RCN 2007) produced guidance on caring for these women. The main areas are as follows:

- Individualized care according to need
- Working flexibly
- Making adaptations to facilitate women-centred care (Homeyard et al 2014)
- Multiple professionals working across health, social care and the third sector

Pregnant women with mild learning disabilities are most at risk of being 'invisible' to maternity services. If these women fail to engage with antenatal care at an early stage of pregnancy, they may miss out on important screening tests and available healthcare and information (Homeyard et al 2016). Because of the increased risk of adverse pregnancy outcomes (McConnell et al 2008), 'targeted' support during pregnancy has been recommended to help improve the health of both mother and baby (Mitra et al 2015).

BLACK, MINORITY AND ETHNIC WOMEN

Population movements worldwide have resulted in changes to the profile of women using National Health Service (NHS) maternity services. The number of people from black and minority ethnic (BME) communities in Great Britain is increasing. In 2013, 1 in 8 residents of the UK was born abroad, and 1 in 13 people had a non-British nationality (Office for National Statistics (ONS) 2014). There is a strong association between ethnicity, deprivation and poor outcomes in maternity care (Marmot 2010; Manktelow 2015; Wolfe et al 2014):

'One quarter of all deaths under the age of one would potentially be avoided if all births had the same level of risk as those women with the lowest level of deprivation'.

(Marmot 2010: 6)

Incoming communities – primarily from Romania and Bulgaria within Europe and those seeking asylum primarily from Eritrea, Pakistan and Syria – have also increased demand on maternity services (Darzi 2007 and 2008; ONS 2014 and 2015). These groups share the following common characteristics:

- Lack of awareness of the available UK maternity services
- Poor access and engagement

- Language and literacy difficulties
- Poor general health
- Encounters with prejudice
- Poverty

Migrants are not a homogenous group and can be divided into the following categories:

- Asylum seekers and refugees
- 'Refused' asylum seekers
- 'Illegal' immigrants
- Individuals who enter the UK with visa clearance (for reasons such as tourism, marriage, study, employment or visiting family)

Recently arrived asylum seekers and women with no recourse to public funds are likely to be more vulnerable than people who have come for employment (Taylor and Newall 2008).

Asylum seekers and refugees

Background and definitions

The 1951 Refugee Convention (United Nations High Commissioner for Refugees (UNHCR) 1951) defines a refugee as follows:

any person who … owing to a well-founded fear of being persecuted for reasons of race, religion, nationality, membership of a particular social group or political opinion, is outside the country of his (or her) nationality and is unable or, owing to such fear, is unwilling to avail himself (or herself) of the protection of that country.

An asylum seeker is defined as follows:

a person who has left their country of origin and has applied for refugee status in another country and is waiting for the decision.

(UNHCR 1951)

The term *'failed' asylum seeker* is used to describe people who have had their asylum claims refused, who have lost their appeals and who have reached the end of the process.

Pregnant women who have been displaced from their country of origin may have a number of key issues in common:

- Severe loss through the death, often traumatic and witnessed, of loved ones
- Physical assault, sexual harassment, rape
- Poor general health
- Depression
- Loneliness
- Domestic abuse

- Stress of overwhelming domestic responsibilities (Burnett and Peel 2001)

Although there are some examples of good practice and support for women who are pregnant or new mothers who are seeking asylum (e.g. Leeds, City of Sanctuary Maternity Stream, http://maternity.cityofsanctuary.org/about), many asylum seekers find it difficult to access care (Gaudion and Allotey 2008; Harris et al 2006; Shorthall et al 2014 and 2008; Qureshi and Ramaswami 2011). Access to services is made more difficult because of transience of residence, relative poverty and uncertainty within a complicated asylum process (see the chapter website resources for the video "Florence: The Experience of Becoming a Mother in Exile").

Evidence from the 2007 CEMACH report demonstrates that the care provided for women who are seeking asylum in the UK does not always provide for their needs; for example, black African women, including asylum seekers and newly arrived refugees, have a mortality rate nearly six times higher than that of their white counterparts (Lewis 2007). The report highlights that this may reflect not only cultural factors implied in ethnicity but also social circumstance. Significantly, the report recognized that for this group of women there may be additional risk factors, including poor overall health status and underlying and possible unrecognized medical conditions, such as cardiac disease.

Teenagers who are seeking asylum are particularly vulnerable because of their situation – living in poverty with uncertainty and because of a lack of familial support and a lack of experience inherent in their youth (Gaudion and Allotey 2008).

Access to maternity services

Accessing of services by women who are not well integrated into a community is challenging simply because of the principle 'you do not know what you do not know' (Gaudion et al 2007a; Homeyard and Gaudion 2008). There is little information in the public domain about how to access services (Gaudion et al 2007b; see Fig. 23.1 and chapter website resources). Current and changing entitlement to NHS maternity care is another potential barrier to accessing antenatal care (Shorthall et al 2014). The guidelines for Entitlement to Health Care state that maternity care is classed as immediately necessary care. This means that all antenatal, birth and postnatal care should be provided irrespective of ability to pay (DH 2015; Birthrights 2013).

Language and communication

Caring for women whose main language is not English may lead to women receiving suboptimal care for the following reasons:

- The woman may not be able to talk about intimate issues or discuss her past history adequately

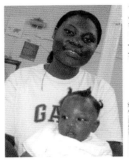

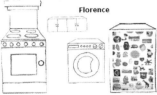

"It's easier to find out about getting a new kitchen.................. for the issue that is likely to involve many women, most women, there is nothing. What you need is advertisments telling you what to do and where to go and then of course people would "

Florence

Figure 23.1 Florence. (The Hackney Women's Wheel: Visual Diary Gaudion, Godfrey, Homeyard and Cutts page 6. Reproduced by permission of The Polyanna Project.)

- The correct information may not be conveyed when a person acting in the role of an interpreter does not have the level of language proficiency needed
- The person translating may be a perpetrator of domestic abuse

It is important to remember that women may have a basic working knowledge of the English language that enables them to go shopping or catch a bus, but this does not mean that they will have the vocabulary to fully understand issues around antenatal screening or understand the relevance of their past medical and obstetric history to their current pregnancy. The Nursing and Midwifery Council Code specifies that 'reasonable steps to meet people's language and communication needs' should be taken (NMC 2015: 7).

The Polyanna Project Maternity Wheel (Fig. 23.2) is a good example of a tool that can be used to initiate conversation. It also gives 'permission' for women to seek support for needs arising from circumstances that may be stigmatized, such as domestic abuse and mental health (NICE 2010). The numbers and web addresses can be used to inform and signpost women to relevant services.

A needs assessment conducted at Brunel University on asylum seekers in maternity services reported the following findings:

- Interpreting services often were not available
- Women did not understand the antenatal screening choices
- Women were unaware of domestic abuse services
- Women were frightened and ill prepared for the birth of their babies because they were unable to communicate their concerns
- Women often misinterpreted the body language of health professionals, leaving women frightened that something must be wrong (Gaudion and Allotey 2008)

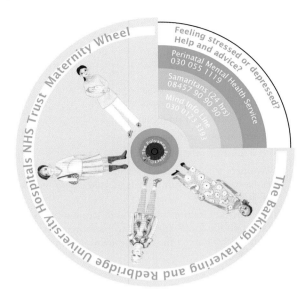

Figure 23.2 The Maternity Wheel. (Artist Heidi Cutts, The Polyanna Project. All Rights Reserved 2010©.)

Gypsy, Roma and Traveller women

In the 2011 census, 57,680 Travellers and Gypsies registered themselves in England and Wales (ONS 2014). This is likely to be a conservative figure, with government estimates being much higher at 300,000 (Cemlyn et al 2009). These populations are among the most marginalized and comprise a number of different ethnic groups. As a group, they die earlier (average life expectancy is age 60), have worse health and are less likely to receive the care they need (Cemlyn et al 2009). Poor access to care and limited information in an accessible format compounded by enforced movement affects uptake and engagement with health services (Jenkins 2004; RCN 2015). Outcomes for mothers and babies are poorer for this sector of society compared with people with fixed residency (Aspinall 2014; Parry et al 2004).

Travellers and Gypsy women may have difficulty accessing maternity services for a number of reasons:

- They may not be registered with a general practitioner and therefore unable to access care through this route
- Although many Traveller and Gypsy women live in houses, many also live in caravans or trailers. Either through choice or because they are evicted from land, they move around the country, often visiting relatives and friends. This means that continuity with a midwife or even a service is disrupted
- They may have poor literacy skills and therefore not understand information about booking times and procedures that are sent to them
- They may have encountered hostility and discriminatory attitudes within the health service previously
- Traveller sites are often in marginalized parts of town not well served by public transport, therefore making attendance more difficult (Parry et al 2004; Greenfields 2009)

Within the Traveller and Gypsy community, women marry young, and having children is an important part of their cultural identity. *Mochadi*, a term used to describe cultural issues of cleanliness and modesty, are important. The functions of cleanliness include all activities, from washing and food preparation to relationships. Washing of the hands is particularly important, especially before handling food and in the morning after getting dressed.

'Women's issues', including pregnancy, are not discussed when men are present. Although women should be offered the option of their husbands accompanying them at the birth, it should be recognized that this is not the norm for them. Childbirth is 'understood' as polluting and therefore best away from the home and in a hospital. This is a way of limiting the effects of the contamination of the process (Okley 1983). Privacy and modesty also affect uptake of breastfeeding; women do not like to 'expose' their breasts in public or even on-site where their husbands or other men might see them. Some Traveller and Gypsy women may prefer not to be cared for by a male health professional.

Improving service provision for Gypsy, Roma and Traveller women needs to include designing a flexible service near or on the site and a system so that women can directly access a midwife so that when they move, the midwife can ring ahead and arrange ongoing care.

POVERTY AND DESTITUTION

Research has shown that as poverty increases, there is a corresponding increase in infant deaths (Manktelow 2015).

In the UK there are a number of factors that can make a woman destitute, including the following:

- Ill health or pregnancy, especially for economic, illegal or irregular migrants
- Domestic abuse for migrants in cases where the woman's visa is spousal and she has no recourse to public funds
- Becoming 18 or 21 for former unaccompanied asylum-seeking children
- Women whose asylum claim has been rejected (Taylor and Newall 2008)

Women who have no recourse to public funds are particularly vulnerable, not just in terms of healthcare but the whole remit of social provision for themselves and their children. Basic provision of accommodation, food and toiletries, known as Section 4 support, may be possible for 'failed' asylum seekers before being returned to their country of origin (UK Visa and Immigration 2015). Other options include voluntary return and support from local authorities under Section 21 of the National Assistance Act 1948, Section 17 of the Children Act 1989 or Section 117 of the Mental Health Act 1995 (Taylor and Newall 2008).

CONCLUSION

Meeting the challenges of maternity service provision for women who are, because of age, ethnicity, disability, immigration status or social situation, more vulnerable, is not easy. None of the groups discussed in this chapter are homogenous; every woman is an individual and may fall into more than one of the categories. Each individual woman presents from a different culture, ethnicity, religion, identity, family structure and educational background; each has unique life experiences that inform her interpretation and uptake of maternity services. Their needs are correspondingly diverse.

The central and most important issue is communication; no midwife or other health professional should work in a silo, and information sharing is crucial. It is not necessarily about specialist services but treating women as individuals and being able to signpost to services that are specialized to maximize outcomes for mother and baby. Good practice in maternity care can help build the necessary early links with women and families and ensure that agencies are in place so that they all work together to provide a coherent and responsive service. With complex cases, it is important to consult with senior midwives or managers who can offer advice and support.

Key Points ⚷

- All midwives must be sensitive to the issues of vulnerable populations and carefully discern situations where pregnant women require multiprofessional services.

- Information sharing and communication in a language and format that women can understand is essential to promote safe and effective care.

- Women and their babies in vulnerable groups are more likely to suffer morbidity and mortality.

- All pregnant women should have a needs, risk and choice assessment by 10 weeks of pregnancy (NICE 2008).

- Midwives need to be vigilant and sensitive to the individual needs of vulnerable women.

- There is a strong association between ethnicity, deprivation, disability and poor outcomes in maternity care.

- Women who have no recourse to public funds are particularly vulnerable.

References

Advisory Council on the Misuse of Drugs: *ACMD inquiry: 'Hidden harm' report on children of drug users* (website). www.gov.uk/government/publications/amcd-inquiry-hidden-harm-report-on-children-of-drug-users. 2011.

Aspinall PJ: *Hidden needs. Identifying key vulnerable groups in data collection: vulnerable migrants, Gypsies and Travellers, homeless people and sex workers* (website). www.gov.uk/government/uploads/system/uploads/attachment_data/file/287805/vulnerable_groups_data_collections.pdf. 2014.

Bacchus L, Mezey G, Bewley S, et al: Prevalence of domestic violence when midwives routinely enquire in pregnancy, *BJOG* 111(5):441–445, 2004.

Baird K, Salmon D, White P: *A five-year follow up study of the Bristol Pregnancy Domestic Violence Programme and introduction of routine antenatal enquiry. Final report for Avon Primary Care Research Collaborative*, Bristol, University of the West of England, 2011.

Balain M, Johnson K: Neonatal abstinence syndrome: the role of breastfeeding, *Infant* 10(1):9–13, 2014.

Berrington A, Diamond I, Ingham R, et al: *Consequences of teenage motherhood: pathways which minimise the long-term negative impacts of teenage childbearing*, Southampton, University of Southampton, 2005.

Birthrights: *Foreign nationals and maternity care* (website). www.birthrights.org.uk/library/factsheets/Foreign-Nationals-and-Maternity-Care.pdf. 2013.

Bowen E, Heron J, Waylen A, et al: Domestic violence risk during and after pregnancy: findings from a British longitudinal study, *BJOG* 112(8):1083–1089, 2005.

British Medical Association (BMA): *Foetal alcohol spectrum disorders: a guide for healthcare professionals*, London, BMA, 2007.

British Medical Association (BMA): *Domestic abuse: a publication from the BMA Professional Policy Division and the Board of Science*, London, BMA, 2014.

Burnett A, Peel M: Health needs of asylum-seekers and refugees, *Br Med J* 322(7285):544–547, 2001.

Cemlyn S, Greenfields M, Burnett S, et al: *Inequalities experienced by Gypsy and Traveller Communities. Research Report No. 12*, Equality and Human Rights Commission, University of Bristol, Buckinghamshire New University, Friends, Families and Travellers, 2009.

Darzi A: *NHS next stage review, interim report. Our NHS, our future*, London, Department of Health, 2007.

Darzi A: *A framework for action. Healthcare for London*, London, NHS, 2008.

Department of Health: *Valuing people: a new strategy for learning disability for the 21st century* (website). www.gov.uk/government/uploads/system/uploads/attachment_data/file/250877/5086.pdf. 2001.

Department of Health (DH): *Responding to domestic abuse: a handbook for health professionals* (website). www.domesticviolencelondon.nhs.uk/uploads/downloads/DH_4126619.pdf. 2005.

Department of Health (DH): *Maternity matters: choice, access and continuity of care in a safe service* (website). http://webarchive.national archives.gov.uk/20130107105354/http:/www.dh.gov.uk/prod_consum_dh/groups/dh_digitalassets/@dh/@en/documents/digitalasset/dh_074199.pdf. 2007a.

Department of Health (DH): *Drug misuse and dependence: UK guidelines on clinical management*, London, DH, 2007b.

Department of Health (DH): *Equity and excellence: liberating the NHS* (website). www.gov.uk/government/uploads/system/uploads/attachment_data/file/213823/dh_117794.pdf. 2010a.

Department of Health (DH): *Tackling health inequalities in infant and maternal health outcomes: report of the infant mortality national support team* (website). www.gov.uk/government/uploads/system/uploads/attachment_data/file/215869/dh_122844.pdf. 2010b.

Department of Health (DH): *Guidance for health professionals on domestic violence* (website). www.gov.uk/government/uploads/system/uploads/attachment_data/file/211018/9576-TSO-Health_Visiting_Domestic_Violence_A3_Posters_WEB.pdf. 2013.

Department of Health (DH): *Guidance on implementing the overseas visitor hospital charging regulation 2015* (website). www.gov.uk/government/uploads/system/uploads/attachment_data/file/418634/Implementing_overseas_charging_regulations_2015.pdf. 2015.

DrugScope: *Caring for a baby with drug withdrawal symptoms* (website). www.drugscope.org.uk/Resources/Drugscope/Documents/PDF/Publications/Appendix%209_Caring%20for%20a%20baby%20with%20NAS.pdf. 2011.

Gaudion A, Allotey P: *Maternity care for refugees and asylum seekers in Hillingdon. A needs assessment*, Uxbridge, Centre for Public Health Research, Brunel University, 2008.

Gaudion A, Godfrey C, Homeyard C, et al: *The Hackney women's wheel report*, London, The Polyanna Project, 2007a.

Gaudion A, Godfrey C, Homeyard C, et al: *The Hackney women's wheel visual diary*, London, The Polyanna Project, 2007b.

Gibbs S, Brown M, Muir W: The experience of adults with intellectual disabilities and their carers in general hospitals: a focus group study, *J Intellect Disabil Res* 52(12):1061–1077, 2008.

Greenfields M: *Falling by the wayside* (website). www.diabetes.org.uk/Documents/Professionals/Referenced%20Gypsies%20and%20Travellers%20feature%20-%20Update%20Winter%2009.pdf. 2009.

Greenough A, et al: Effects of substance misuse during pregnancy, *J R Soc Promot Health* 125(5):212–213, 2005.

Harris M, Humphries K, Nabb J: Delivering care for women seeking refuge, *RCM Midwives J* 9(5):190–192, 2006.

Hepburn M: Social problems in pregnancy, *Anaesth Intensive Care Med* 6(4):125–126, 2005.

Homeyard C, Gaudion A: Safety in maternity services: women's perspectives, *Pract Midwife* 11(7):20–23, 2008.

Homeyard C, Gaudion A: Domestic abuse: are you 'asking the question'? *Pract Midwife* 12(10):36–39, 2009.

Homeyard C, Godfrey C, Gaudion A: Aiming for equal access to maternity care for all, *Pract Midwife* 17(1):13–16, 2014.

Homeyard C, Montgomery E, Chinn D, et al: Current evidence on antenatal care provision for women with intellectual disabilities: a systematic review, *Midwifery* 32:45–57, 2016.

Jansson LM, Velez M: Neonatal abstinence syndrome, *Curr Opin Pediatr* 24:252–258, 2012.

Jenkins M: *No Travellers! A report of Gypsy and Traveller women's experience of maternity care*, London, The Maternity Alliance, 2004.

Keeling J, Mason T: Postnatal disclosure of domestic violence: comparison with disclosure in the first trimester of pregnancy, *J Clin Nurs* 20(1–2):103–110, 2011.

Knight M, Kenyon S, Brocklehurst P, et al, editors: *Saving lives, improving mother's care. Lessons learnt to inform future maternity care from the UK and Ireland Confidential Enquiries into Maternal Deaths and Morbidity 2009–2012*. MBRRACE (website). www.npeu.ox.ac.uk/downloads/files/mbrrace-uk/reports/Saving%20Lives%20Improving%20Mothers%20Care%20report%202014%20Full.pdf. 2014.

Knight M, Tuffnell D, Kenyon S, et al, editors: *Saving lives, improving mothers' care – surveillance of maternal deaths in the UK 2011-13 and lessons learned to inform maternity care from the UK and Ireland Confidential Enquiries into Maternal Deaths and Morbidity 2009–13*, Oxford, National Perinatal Epidemiology Unit, University of Oxford, 2015.

Lewis G: *The Confidential Enquiry into Maternal and Child Health. Saving mothers' lives: reviewing maternal deaths to make motherhood safer 2003–2005: the seventh report on Confidential Enquiries into Maternal Deaths in the United Kingdom*, London, CEMACH, 2007.

Lewis G, Centre for Maternal and Child Enquires (CMACE): Saving mothers' lives: reviewing maternal deaths to make motherhood safer: 2006-2008. The eighth report on Confidential Enquires into Maternal Deaths in the United Kingdom, *BJOG* 118(Suppl 1):1–203, 2011.

Manktelow BN, Smith LK, Evans TA, et al: *Perinatal mortality surveillance report UK. Death for births from January to December* (website). www.npeu.ox.ac.uk/downloads/files/mbrrace-uk/reports/MBRRACE-UK%20Perinatal%20Surveillance%20Report%202013.pdf. 2013. 2015.

Marmot M: *Fair society, healthy lives*. The Marmot Review (website). www.instituteofhealthequity.org/projects/fair-society-healthy-lives-the-marmot-review. 2010.

McConnell D, Mayes R, Llewellyn G: Women with intellectual disability at risk of adverse pregnancy and birth outcomes, *J Intellect Disabil Res* 52:529–535, 2008.

Mencap: *Treat me right: better healthcare for people with a learning disability* (website). http://cddh.monash.org/assets/treat-me-right.pdf. 2004.

Mencap: *Death by indifference: following up the Treat Me Right campaign* (website). www.mencap.org.uk/sites/default/files/documents/2008-03/DBIreport.pdf. 2007.

Mencap: *Death by indifference, 74 and counting, a progress report five years on* (website). www.mencap.org.uk/sites/default/files/documents/Death%20by%20Indifference%20-%2074%20Deaths%20and%20counting.pdf. 2012.

Michaels J: *Healthcare for all: report of the independent inquiry into access for healthcare for people with learning disabilities*, London, Crown, 2008.

Ministry of Justice: *Statistics on women and the criminal justice system 2013* (website). www.gov.uk/government/uploads/system/uploads/attachment_data/file/380090/women-cjs-2013.pdf. 2014.

Mitra M, Parish SL, Clements KM, et al: Pregnancy outcomes among women with intellectual and developmental disabilities, *Am J Prev Med* 48:300–308, 2015.

National Institute for Health and Care Excellence (NICE): *Antenatal care* (website). www.nice.org.uk/guidance/cg62/chapter/1-Guidance#provision-and-organisation-of-care. 2008.

National Institute for Health and Care Excellence (NICE): *Pregnancy and complex social factors. Clinical guideline 110*, London, NICE, 2010.

National Institute for Health and Care Excellence (NICE): *QS 22, antenatal care* (website). http://publications .nice.org.uk/antenatal-care-qs22. 2012.

National Institute for Health and Care Excellence (NICE): *Domestic violence and abuse: how health services, social care and the organisations they work with can respond effectively. Public health guideline 50*, London, NICE, 2014.

National Society for the Prevention of Cruelty to Children (NSPCC): *Case reviews published in 2014* (website). www.nspcc.org.uk/ preventing-abuse/child-protection -system/case-reviews/2014/. 2014.

Neale J: *Drug users in society*, Basingstoke, Palgrave, 2002.

Nursing and Midwifery Council (NMC): *The Code* (website). www.nmc.org.uk/globalassets/ sitedocuments/nmc-publications/ revised-new-nmc-code.pdf. 2015.

Office for National Statistics (ONS): *What does the 2011 census tell us about the characteristics of Gypsy or Irish Travellers in England and Wales?* (website). www.ons.gov.uk/ons/rel/ census/2011-census-analysis/what -does-the-2011-census-tell-us-about -the-characteristics-of-gypsy-or-irish -travellers-in-england-and-wales-/ index.html. 2014.

Office for National Statistics (ONS): *Migration statistics quarterly report* (website). www.ons.gov.uk/ons/rel/ migration1/migration-statistics -quarterly-report/index.html. 2015.

Okley J: *The Traveller-Gypsies*, Cambridge, Cambridge University Press, 1983.

Parry G, Van Cleemput P, Peters J, et al: *Health status of Gypsies and Travellers in England*, Sheffield, University of Sheffield, 2004.

Public Health England (PHE), Department of Health (DH), Royal College of Midwives (RCM): *Getting maternity services right for pregnant teenagers and young fathers. A practical guide for midwives, doctors, maternity support workers and receptionists* (website). www.rcm.org .uk/sites/default/files/Getting%20 maternity%20services%20right%20 for%20pregnant%20teenagers%20

and%20young%20fathers%20 pdf.pdf. 2015.

Qureshi F, Ramaswami R: *How we plug the NHS's registration gap*. The Guardian (website). www .theguardian.com/healthcare -network/2011/sep/29/help-plug-nhs -registration-gaps-project-london. 2011.

Ross LE, Dennis C-L: The prevalence of postpartum depression among women with substance use, an abuse history or chronic illness: a systematic review, *J Womens Health* 18:475–486, 2009.

Royal College of Midwives (RCM): *Domestic abuse: pregnancy, birth and the puerperium. Guidance paper number 5*, London, RCM, 2006.

Royal College of Midwives (RCM): *Maternity care for disabled women. Guidance*, London, RCM, 2007a.

Royal College of Nursing (RCN): *Pregnancy and disability, RCN guidance for midwives and nurses*, London, RCN, 2007b.

Royal College of Nursing (RCN): *Gypsy and Traveller communities* (website). www.rcn.org.uk/ development/practice/social _inclusion/gypsy_and_traveller _communities. 2015.

Royal College of Obstetricians and Gynaecologists (RCOG): *Green-top guideline No. 63: antepartum haemorrhage* (website). www.rcog .org.uk/globalassets/documents/ guidelines/gtg63_05122011aph.pdf. 2011.

Royal College of Obstetricians and Gynaecologists (RCOG): *Working together to stop domestic violence against women* (website). www.rcog .org.uk/en/news/rcog-release -working-together-to-stop-domestic -violence-against-women/. 2015.

Royal College of Psychiatrists (RCPsych): *Domestic violence – its effects on children: the impact on children and adolescents: information for parents, carers and anyone who works with young people*, London, Royal College of Psychiatrists, 2012.

Shah PS, Shah J: Maternal exposure to domestic violence and pregnancy and birth outcomes: a systematic review and meta-analyses, *J Womens Health* 19:2017–2029, 2010.

Sherwood RA, Keating J, Kavvadia V, et al: Substance misuse in early pregnancy and relationship to fetal outcome, *Eur J Pediatr* 158:488–492, 2009.

Shorthall C, McMorran J, Taylor K, et al: *Experiences of pregnant migrant women receiving ante/peri and postnatal care in the UK: a Doctors of the World Report on the experiences of attendees at their London drop in clinic* (website). http://b.3cdn .net/droftheworld/5a507ef4b 2316bbb07_5nm6bkfx7.pdf. 2014.

Swann C, Bowe K, McCormick G, et al: *Teenage pregnancy and parenthood: a review of reviews. Evidence briefing*, London, Health Development Agency, 2003.

Taket A: *Tackling domestic violence: the role of health professionals*, 2nd edn, London, Home Office, 2013.

Taylor B, Newall N: *Maternity, mortality and migration: the impact of new communities*, Birmingham, Heart of Birmingham Teaching NHS Primary Care Trust, 2008.

Taylor J, Bradbury-Jones C, Duncan F, et al: *Health professionals' beliefs about domestic violence and the impact these have on their responses to disclosure: a critical incident technique study. Scottish Government Health Directorates Chief Scientist Office* (website). cso.scot.nhs.uk/ Publications/ExecSumms/2012/ NeedsTaylor.pdf. 2011.

UK Visa and Immigration: *Asylum support Section 4 policy and process, 2015*. www.gov.uk/government/ uploads/system/uploads/attachment _data/file/438472/asylum_support _section_4_policy_and_process _public_v5.pdf. 2015.

United Nations High Commissioner for Refugees (UNHCR): *The facts: asylum in the UK* (website). www.unhcr.org.uk/ about-us/the-uk-and-asylum.html. 1951.

Wolfe I, Macfarlane A, Donkin A, et al: *Why children die: deaths in infants, children and young people in the UK, Part A* (website). www.instituteo fhealthequity.org/projects/why -children-die-death-in-infants -children-and-young-people-in -the-uk-part-a. 2014.

354

Resources and additional reading

Cambridge J: *Language barriers: my interpretation*, Midwives Magazine 2 (website). www.rcm.org.uk/news -views-and-analysis/analysis/ language-barriers-my-interpretation. 2012.

Eboh WO, Pitchforth E, Van Teijlingen E: *Lost words: research via translation*, Midwives Magazine (website). www.rcm.org.uk/news-views-and -analysis/analysis/lost-words -research-via-translation. 2008.

National Institute for Health and Care Excellence (NICE): *Pregnancy and complex social factors* (website). www.nice.org.uk/guidance/cg110/ chapter/guidance. 2010.

Newall D, Philimore J: *Delivering in the age of super-diversity*. Midwives magazine. https://www.rcm.org .uk/news-views-and-analysis/ analysis/delivering-in-the-age-of -super-diversity. 2012.

Nursing and Midwifery Council: *NMC code for nurses and midwives* (website). http://www.nmc.org.uk/ globalassets/sitedocuments/ nmc-publications/revised-new-nmc -code.pdf. 2015.

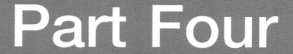

Part Four

The anatomy and physiology of fertility, embryology and fetal development

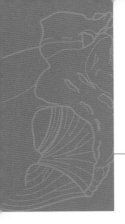

Chapter 24

Anatomy of male and female reproduction

Dr Barbara Burden and Vivien Perry

Learning Outcomes ?

After reading this chapter, you will be able to:

- describe the structures of the male reproductive system and their significance for fertility and conception
- understand the anatomical structures of the female reproductive system and their significance to midwifery practice
- identify the anatomical structures of the pelvis, its corresponding joints and ligaments and their significance for midwifery practice
- consider the dimensions, angles and axes of the pelvis and how these may influence labour and birth outcomes
- explain how the uterus changes during pregnancy, how it functions during labour, birth and the third stage of labour, and the normal processes of involution in the postpartum period.

INTRODUCTION

An understanding of the anatomy of human reproduction enables the translation of abstract concepts of anatomy to normal physiology, function and processes of conception, pregnancy, labour, birth, postpartum and related disorders. This chapter provides a reference point for application to midwifery practice, increasing understanding of the physiological aspects of the birthing process. This brings together theory and practice, enabling knowledge and understanding to be applied in the midwife's practice and health promotion. Greater understanding of the structure of the human body increases knowledge of how it functions and why it sometimes deviates from the norm.

The chapter, with its supportive literature, links with other chapters, demonstrating how anatomy and physiology may be applied to midwifery practice.

THE PELVIS

The human pelvis supports the upper body and transmits its weight to the lower limbs, enabling movement in an upright posture. In the female, the pelvis serves as a protective bony ring encircling the reproductive organs, bladder and rectum. In pregnancy, physiological processes effect subtle changes in the composition, shape, plane of inclination and internal dimensions of the true pelvis (Reitter et al 2014). These changes enable the female skeleton to support the gravid uterus and are essential to the mechanisms involved in the process of childbirth.

The pelvis consists of four pelvic bones (see Fig. 24.1):

- Two innominate
- One sacrum
- One coccyx

The innominate bones are each divided into three regions:

- Ilium
- Ischium
- Pubis

Joints and ligaments of the pelvis

The joints of the pelvis connect the innominate bones at the pubis anteriorly and to the sacrum posteriorly, and the sacrum to the coccyx (see Fig. 24.2). These joints are cartilaginous in type, consisting of plates of fibrocartilage. The pelvis also provides attachment points for ligaments,

Sacral foramina

Four pairs of foramina (or holes) are present in the sacrum, through which the four sacral nerves pass.

Ala

An ala projects laterally on each side of the sacral promontory and the superior surface of the first sacral vertebra. The alae extend to articulate with the ilium on both sides.

The anterior surfaces of the alae form part of the landmarks of the pelvic brim.

Acetabulum

A round cup-shaped socket on the external surface of the innominate bone with which the head of the femur articulates to form the hip joint. Two-fifths of the acetabulum is formed by the ilium, two-fifths by the ischium and one-fifth by the pubis.

Malformation, disease or injury of the hip joint can result in a reduction in abduction of the legs. This may result in hip and back pain in pregnancy, inability to abduct the hips during vaginal examination and delivery, and inability to adopt certain positions in labour, such as the lithotomy or squatting position.

Symphysis pubis

A cartilaginous joint between the anterior portions of the two pubic bones. There is increased mobility and size in this cartilage during the last months of pregnancy.

Ischial tuberosity

The thickened portion of the body of the ischium providing attachment points for the sacrotuberous ligament. This is the section of the pelvis that takes the full weight of the body when sitting. Women with painful perineums can be advised to sit with their knees apart and the pelvis tilted, allowing the tuberosities to take the weight of the body, so the mother is sitting on a triangular-shaped base, relieving pressure in the perineum.

The distance between the tuberosities is estimated to be 10 cm. A reduction in this dimension may indicate a reduced pelvic outlet. Although this dimension is difficult to measure, a midwife may assess the distance by placing a closed fist on the perineum between the tuberosities. The knuckles of the fist should fit comfortably between the tuberosities in a normal gynaecoid pelvis.

Sacral promontory

The prominent upper margin of the first sacral vertebra.

The measurement between the sacral promontory and the anterior surface of the pubis is the anteroposterior diameter of the pelvic brim. A reduction in this diameter can influence the descent and engagement of the presenting part of the fetus into the pelvis.

Lumbar vertebra (5th)

Articulates with the first sacral vertebra. The position of the lumbar vertebrae influences the angle of pelvic inclination.

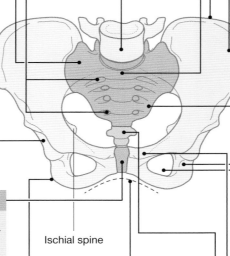

Ischial spine

Pubic arch

The arch created by the inferior rami of the pubes. The angle of the pubic arch is significant to the dimensions of the pelvic outlet. The optimal angle should be 90°, which is a feature of the gynaecoid pelvis.

Reduction in the pelvic outlet may result in obstructed labour, prolonged labour, persistent occipitoposterior positions and excessive fetal skull moulding.

Coccyx

A small triangular-shaped bone that articulates with the lower end of the sacrum. It is composed of four fused rudimentary vertebrae and provides attachment points for ligaments, muscle fibres of the anal sphincter and the ischiococcygeus muscle of the pelvic floor.

During the birth of the baby, the coccyx moves backwards to enlarge the pelvic outlet.

Ilium

Forms the upper expanded part of the innominate bone. It gives rise to the female shape of the hips.

Anterior superior iliac spine

A prominent anterior protrusion of the ilium that can be palpated through the lateral abdominal wall. The distance between the left and right anterior superior iliac spines does not necessarily indicate the capacity of the true pelvis.

Iliac crest

The curved upper border of the ilium. Women refer to this part of the pelvis as their hips.

Sacrum

Lies between the ilia, forming the rear of the pelvis. It consists of five fused vertebrae forming a wedge shape perforated by four sets of foramina through which the sacral nerves pass.

In a gynaecoid pelvis the sacrum's anterior surface is concave and a feature of the rounded cavity, allowing room for the fetal head to descend. It also plays a part in directing the baby through the pelvis around the curve of Carus (see Fig. 24.3).

Ischium

A thickened L-shaped bone that connects to the ilium posteriorly and to the pubis anteriorly. The medial surface has attachment points for the ischiococcygeus muscle of the pelvic floor.

Obturator foramen

A triangular hole created by the borders of the ischium and the pubis. It is covered by the obturator membrane, through which pass the obturator nerve and blood vessels leading to the thigh.

Pubis

Forms the anterior portion of the pelvis and has two arms called rami. The inferior ramus attaches to the ischium, and the superior ramus to the ilium at the iliopectineal eminence. It forms one-fifth of the acetabulum. The inferior ramus forms the boundary for the obturator foramen and the pubic arch, under which the baby must pass during birth.

A

Figure 24.1 The female pelvis. **A,** Anterior view of pelvis.

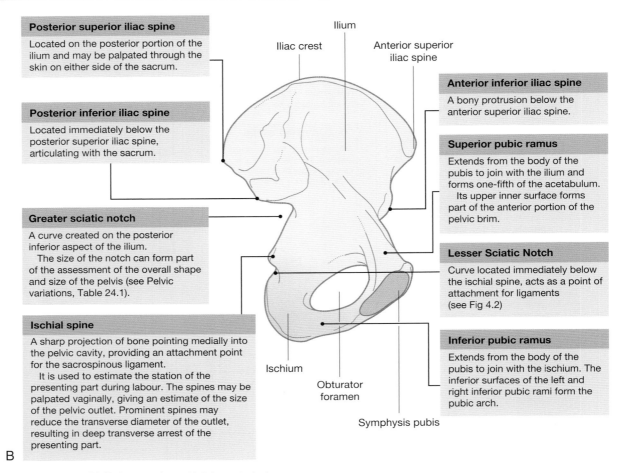

Posterior superior iliac spine

Located on the posterior portion of the ilium and may be palpated through the skin on either side of the sacrum.

Posterior inferior iliac spine

Located immediately below the posterior superior iliac spine, articulating with the sacrum.

Greater sciatic notch

A curve created on the posterior inferior aspect of the ilium.
    The size of the notch can form part of the assessment of the overall shape and size of the pelvis (see Pelvic variations, Table 24.1).

Ischial spine

A sharp projection of bone pointing medially into the pelvic cavity, providing an attachment point for the sacrospinous ligament.
    It is used to estimate the station of the presenting part during labour. The spines may be palpated vaginally, giving an estimate of the size of the pelvic outlet. Prominent spines may reduce the transverse diameter of the outlet, resulting in deep transverse arrest of the presenting part.

Anterior inferior iliac spine

A bony protrusion below the anterior superior iliac spine.

Superior pubic ramus

Extends from the body of the pubis to join with the ilium and forms one-fifth of the acetabulum.
    Its upper inner surface forms part of the anterior portion of the pelvic brim.

Lesser Sciatic Notch

Curve located immediately below the ischial spine, acts as a point of attachment for ligaments (see Fig 4.2)

Inferior pubic ramus

Extends from the body of the pubis to join with the ischium. The inferior surfaces of the left and right inferior pubic rami form the pubic arch.

Iliac crest — Ilium — Anterior superior iliac spine

Ischium — Obturator foramen — Symphysis pubis

B

Figure 24.1, cont'd **B,** Inner surface of left innominate bone.

which are bands of tissue connecting two structures. In normal circumstances, ligaments do not possess the ability to stretch, and therefore prevent excessive movements within the joints, enhancing stability.

In pregnancy, the hormones *relaxin, progesterone* and *oestrogen* affect the joints and ligaments, enabling some movement of the joints to facilitate birth. Pelvic pain sometimes occurs during pregnancy, birth or postpartum and is thought to be linked to overstretching of ligaments in the pelvis and lower spine (Rost et al 2004).

The true pelvis

The true pelvis, through which a baby negotiates passage during labour and birth, is the most significant part of the pelvis. The true pelvis incorporates the portions of the pelvis that are below the oblique plane of the pelvic brim. The portion of the pelvis that is above the pelvic brim is known as the *false pelvis*, this portion has no impact on childbirth. The *true pelvis* is divided into three regions, known as the brim, cavity and outlet (see Fig. 24.3). As the presenting part descends into the pelvis, the baby negotiates each aspect of the true pelvis simultaneously. For example, in a cephalic presentation, as the baby's head crowns, the presenting part negotiates the outlet, most of the baby's head is in the cavity and the shoulders are at the brim.

It is important to appreciate that the pelvis is three-dimensional. The pelvic measurements of the brim, cavity and outlet are viewed through a cross-section, whereas measurements incorporated in the pelvic conjugates are viewed through a sagittal section. These two measurements inform a *pelvic assessment*.

Sacroiliac ligaments

Pass in front of and behind each sacroiliac joint.

Joints and ligaments relax in pregnancy, enabling slight movement of the pelvis. Overstretching results in pelvic pain in pregnancy.

Sacrospinous ligaments

Pass from the sides of the sacrum and coccyx to the ischial spines, extending across the greater sciatic notches.

Maintain the position of the sacrum and coccyx. Maintain the interplay between the joints and ligaments of the pelvis, increasing its stability.

Form part of the boundary of the pelvic cavity.

Sacrotuberous ligaments

Extend from the sides of the sacrum and coccyx to the ischial tuberosities, crossing the greater and lesser sciatic notches.

Maintain the position of the sacrum and coccyx. Maintain the interplay between the joints and ligaments of the pelvis, increasing its stability.

Form part of the boundary of the pelvic outlet.

Sacroiliac joints

Slightly movable synovial joints at the point where the ilium joins the first two sacral vertebrae.

Mobility of these joints may increase the diameter of the pelvic brim.

Symphysis pubis

A cartilaginous joint between the anterior portions of the two pubic bones.

There is increased mobility and size in this cartilage during the last months of pregnancy. It is the site of symphysiotomy, a rarely performed surgical procedure to increase the diameters of the pelvis in obstructed labour.

Lumbosacral joint

Sited between the 5th lumbar vertebra and the sacrum.

The backward inclination of the sacrum results in stress at this joint during pregnancy, caused by weight gain as a result of the growing fetus and reproductive organs.

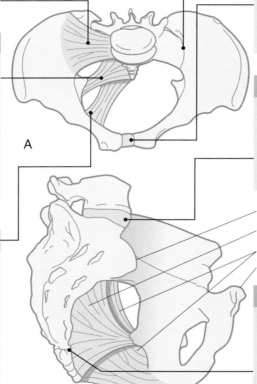

Sacroiliac joint

Sacrospinous ligaments

Sacrotuberous ligaments

Symphysis pubis

Sacrococcygeal joint

Cartilaginous joint between the sacrum and the coccyx enabling a backward movement of the coccyx in labour.

Displacement of the joint causes stretching of the surrounding ligaments with subsequent pain, particularly on sitting.

Figure 24.2 The ligaments and joints of the pelvis. **A,** Superior view. **B,** Sagittal section.

Pelvic measurements

When determining pelvic measurements (Fig. 24.4), the *pelvic brim* is the inlet to the true pelvis and is almost circular, except posteriorly, where the sacral promontory juts into the brim (see Fig. 24.5).

The landmarks of the pelvic brim describe the interplay between the fetus and the pelvis as the presenting part descends, and they are a fundamental part of the assessment of descent and engagement of the presenting part. It is not the components of the brim that are important; it is the part that the brim plays as a whole in the assessment of progress during pregnancy and labour. This is the first

test that the fetus has to pass as it descends through the pelvis. The midwife assesses engagement of the presenting part during abdominal and vaginal examinations (see Chs 35–37).

The *pelvic cavity* extends from the brim to the outlet of the pelvis. In the anteroposterior view the cavity is wedge shaped: shallow at the front and deep at the back. Viewed from above in a gynaecoid pelvis, it is *circular* in shape and designed to facilitate the descent and rotation of the presenting part. The boundaries of the cavity are as follows:

- Curve of the sacrum
- Sacroiliac joints

- Sacrospinous ligaments
- Ischia
- Superior pubic ramus
- Inferior pubic ramus
- Bodies of the pubes
- Symphysis pubis

The *pelvic outlet* is *diamond shaped* and partly bound by ligaments. It can be described in two ways:

- By anatomical structure
- By obstetric dimension – that is, the space available through which the baby must pass during birth (see Fig. 24.6)

The anatomical boundaries for the outlet of the pelvis are as follows:

- Tip of the coccyx
- Sacrotuberous ligaments
- Ischial tuberosities
- Pubic arch

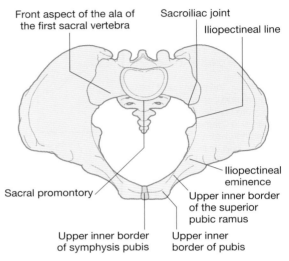

Figure 24.5 Superior view of the pelvis to show the landmarks of the pelvic brim.

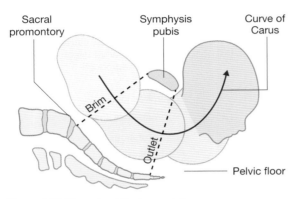

Figure 24.3 The axis of the true pelvis.

		Anteroposterior	Right and left oblique	Transverse
Brim		From upper inner border of the symphysis pubis to sacral promontory **11 cm**	From the sacroiliac joint to the iliopectineal eminence **12 cm**	Between widest points on the iliopectineal lines **13 cm**
Cavity		From inner border of the symphysis pubis to the curve of the sacrum **12 cm**	Right and left from the sacroiliac joint, fanning out to measure a point between the upper and lower pubic rami **12 cm**	From right inner surface of the ischium to left inner surface of the ischium **12 cm**
Outlet		From lower border of the symphysis pubis to sacrococcygeal joint **13 cm**	From the sacrospinous ligament to the obturator foramen **12 cm**	Transverse from the right to the left ischial spines **11 cm**

Other measurements: Sacrocotyloid diameter from sacral promontory to iliopectineal eminence – 9 cm

Figure 24.4 Pelvic measurements.

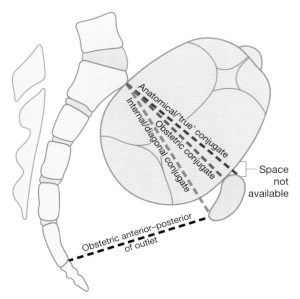

Figure 24.6 The relationship of the pelvic conjugates and the fetal negotiation of the conjugates.

The obstetric outlet is bounded by the following structures:

- Inner border of the base of the sacrum (as a result of the coccyx being deflected outwards during childbirth, thus enlarging the outlet)
- Sacrospinous ligaments
- Ischial spines
- Lower inner border of the symphysis pubis

The bones of the pelvic outlet are also points of attachment for the muscles of the pelvic floor and perineum (see Ch. 40). The muscles of the pelvic floor and perineum play a vital role in facilitating the rotation of the presenting part, so that it can negotiate the true pelvis.

Pelvic conjugates

A conjugate is a measurement taken from one point in the pelvis to another. In midwifery there are the anatomical, obstetric and internal (diagonal) conjugates (see Fig. 24.6).

Anatomical conjugate

- Measured from upper outer border of symphysis pubis, measuring across the pubic bone
- Adds approximately 1.25 cm to all measurements
- Includes space **not available** to the fetus as it enters the pelvic brim

Obstetric conjugate

- Measured from sacral promontory to upper inner border of symphysis pubis
- The fetus negotiates this smaller dimension

Internal or diagonal conjugate

- Estimated at vaginal examination as part of a pelvic assessment
- Measured from posterior inferior surface of the symphysis pubis to the sacral promontory
- Measurement varies in individual women
- Unusual to identify the sacral promontory on vaginal examination (conjugate measures between 12 and 13 cm, longer than the length of most practitioners' fingers)
- If detected, it indicates that the diameters of the pelvis are reduced, and referral for obstetric consultation should be sought

Angles and planes

Angles and planes are mathematical concepts applied to the pelvis. When standing, the pelvis slopes into a position where the pubis is lower than the sacral promontory – described as an angle of 55° to the horizontal or to the floor. This slope continues through the cavity, reducing its angle to 15° at the outlet. The fetal head must negotiate the curve created by the changing angles within the pelvis as it enters the pelvic brim in a downward and backward direction. It emerges from the outlet in a downward and forward direction as the presenting part reaches the pelvic floor. The curve created in the pelvis is known as the curve of Carus (see Figs 24.7 and 24.8).

The term *plane* describes the relationship between the pelvis and a flat surface, such as the floor, highlighting the tilt of the pelvis in a normal female skeleton. Hypothetical angles are then created in relation to the degree of tilt of a particular individual (see Figs 24.7 and 24.8), which provide a representation of the angles in relation to the planes of the pelvis. Figure 24.8 shows the axis (curve of Carus), an imaginary line through which a fetus rotates as it passes through the pelvis.

In an abnormal pelvis, the plane of the pelvis may be significantly altered, affecting the axis of the birth canal and consequently the direction of the fetus through the pelvis. The midwife needs to consider the axis of the birth canal when women adopt alternative positions for childbirth during labour and delivery (Reitter et al 2014).

1. *Sacral angle.* The angle between the plane of the brim and the anterior surface of the first sacral vertebra. The usual measurement is 90°. Measurements of less than 90° suggest a cavity smaller than the brim; more than 90°, larger than the brim.

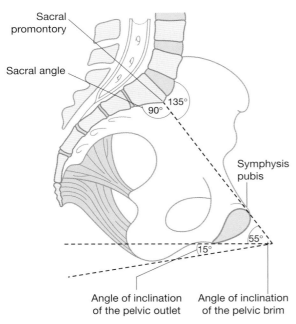

Figure 24.7 The pelvis, showing the degrees of inclination: inclination of the pelvic brim to the horizontal, 55°; inclination of pelvic outlet to the horizontal, 15°; angle of pelvic inclination, 135°; inclination of the sacrum, 90°.

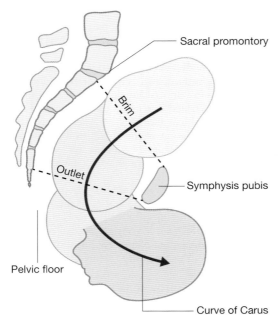

Figure 24.8 The axis of the birth canal in upright position.

2. *Angle of inclination of the pelvic brim.* The angle that the plane achieves with the horizontal when a woman is standing is approximately 55°. If greater than 55°, there may be delay in engagement of the presenting part in the pelvis.

3. *Angle of inclination of the pelvic outlet.* This is the 15° angle the upper inner border of the obstetric outlet makes with the horizontal when the woman is in a standing position.

The *subpubic angle* is between the two inferior pubic rami forming the pubic arch (see Fig. 24.1). In a gynaecoid pelvis, this should be approximately 90°, enabling two finger widths to sit in the apex of the pubic arch during vaginal pelvic assessment.

Pelvic variations

Although there are four recognized pelvic categories (Caldwell et al 1940; see Table 24.1), variations within these categories can occur. Current research by Kuliukas et al (2015) found no clustering of pelvic shapes into these four categories, thus challenging previous classifications. Some women may have mixed features, such as a gynaecoid posterior pelvis and android forepelvis. The most important factor is the true pelvic space available for the fetus to descend and emerge from the pelvis. The pelvic size and shape vary between populations and cannot be used as an indicator of risk in relation to childbirth alone; other factors such as the position and size of the fetus and processes of labour need to be taken into consideration.

Other factors that may influence the size and shape of the pelvis include the following:

- Injury and disease (Phillips et al 2000)
- Dietary deficiencies – in young women these can have a direct influence on the growth and shape of the pelvis (Velickovic et al 2013)

Other pelvic types identified

Any injury or disease of pelvic bones may significantly affect the dimensions of the pelvis, affecting the outcome of labour and birth. Table 24.2 outlines the classification and characteristics of unusual pelves, each of which may have a mixture of characteristics, with the shape depending on the degree and timing of damage. It is important that the midwife assesses women at risk of pelvic dysfunction as early as possible in the antenatal period.

Pelvic assessment

Pelvic assessment enables estimation of whether the fetus will successfully pass through the pelvis during labour and delivery, by assessing the pelvic size and outlet. Although this can be undertaken at any time before or during

Table 24.1 Pelvic categories

Characteristics	Gynaecoid/female type	Justo minor pelvis	Android/male type	Anthropoid	Platypelloid
Shape of brim	Round	Round – but small	Triangular – 'heart shaped'	Oval (widest in the anteroposterior diameter)	Bean shaped – flattened
Depth of pelvis	Shallow – straight walls	Shallow	Deep – convergent walls	Deep – straight	Shallow – divergent walls
Subpubic arch	85–90°	90°	60–75° (narrow)	More than 90°	More than 90°
Sciatic notch	Wide	Wide – but small	Narrow	Wide	Narrow
Ischial spines	Not prominent, blunt	Not prominent	Prominent and narrow interspinous diameter	Not prominent but may have narrowed interspinous diameter	Blunted, usually widely separated – not prominent
Sacrum	Deep and curved	Straight – flattened	Straight – flattened and long	Long and narrow – may be slightly curved	Broad, flat and concave
Transverse diameter of outlet	10 cm	Usually less than 10 cm. May be android characteristics present – may reduce outlet	Less than 10 cm	More than 10 cm	More than 10 cm
Implications for midwifery	Most favourable design for positive outcomes of childbirth	Miniature gynaecoid pelvis; outcomes depend on relationship between degree of size of pelvis and size of fetus	Fetal head may attempt to engage in the occipitoposterior position. Deep transverse arrest may result (see Ch. 64 discussion of excessive moulding and caput of fetal skull)	Women with this pelvis are said to be tall and 'well-built'. Pelvis is large and should accommodate the fetus as it descends during labour. Diameters may result in persistent occipitoposterior position leading to a 'face-to-pubes' delivery	Fetal head engages in the transverse diameter. This shape of pelvis may require the fetal head to negotiate the brim using a movement called asynclitism (see Fig. 24.9 and chapter website resources). This movement occurs where the baby's head tilts in one direction and then the other to enable the biparietal diameter of the fetal skull to engage in the pelvic brim and for descent to occur. Deep transverse arrest may result because the fetal head may be unable to rotate in the pelvic cavity
Estimated incidence	50%		20%	25%	Less than 5%

Table 24.2 Classified unusual pelves

Characteristics	Rachitic pelvis	Asymmetrical pelvis (Naegele's type)	Robert's pelvis	Osteomalacic pelvis	Spondylolisthetic pelvis
Shape of brim	Bean shaped Reduced anteroposterior diameter	Asymmetrical – may be absence of one sacral ala	Inlet narrow and significantly contracted	Usually grossly altered	
Depth of pelvis	Flattened	May be normal		Convergent walls	
Ischial spines		One may be prominent	Likely to be reduced interspinous diameter		
Sacrum	Lower end swings back to increase size of cavity May be bent at the middle				
Transverse diameter of outlet	Increased in size	May be altered	May be altered	Reduced bituberous diameter is less than 8 cm	May be altered – usually drastically contracted
Causes	May result following childhood rickets The soft bones are distorted by body weight. Can be caused by inadequate diet and vitamin D deficiency	Deficient development of one side of the pelvis often with bony fusion of the sacroiliac joint on the affected side. Sometimes known as Naegele's pelvis May be caused by congenital dislocation of one hip, poliomyelitis or an accident	Deficient development on both sides of pelvis with fusion of the sacroiliac joints Rare form of extreme pelvic contraction	A severe pelvis deformity occurring in adults as a result of vitamin D deficiency Distortion is different from that of childhood rickets because the condition occurs while walking and standing. Upward pressure on the legs and pelvis forces the sides of the pelvis inwards, and the weight of the body on the spine forces the sacral promontory forwards	The fifth lumbar vertebra slips forward over the sacrum. The sacral promontory is pushed backwards, and the tip of the sacrum is pushed forwards
Implications for midwifery	May lead to obstructed labour Fetal head may be deflexed, and it usually enters the pelvis with the sagittal suture in transverse Head – asynclitism (see Fig. 24.9)	May result in a reduced incidence of vaginal delivery	May result in a reduced incidence of vaginal delivery	In parts of the world where osteomalacia is endemic, a woman may develop the condition between pregnancies, resulting in a normal vaginal delivery followed by a complicated labour or delivery	Results in an extreme contraction of the true conjugate

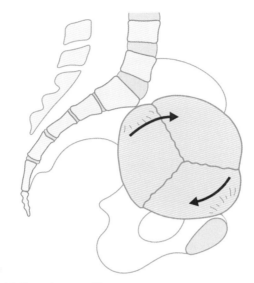

A

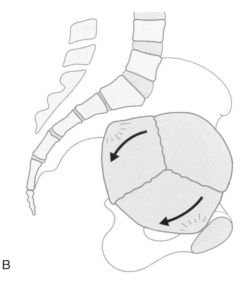

B

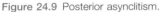

Figure 24.9 Posterior asynclitism.

pregnancy, the relationship of the pelvis to the fetal skull can only be assessed from 37 weeks gestation (antenatally or during labour). Routine pelvic assessment in the antenatal period is not recommended because of its poor predictive value (NICE 2008). Pelvic assessment is no determinant of outcome but contributes to the overall assessment of pelvic adequacy.

The assessment must include the following aspects:

- Abdominal examination – assessing engagement and descent of the presenting part
- Vaginal examination – determining the size and shape of the pelvis by assessing the following:
  - Prominence of sacral promontory (usually cannot be palpated on vaginal examination)
  - Prominence of ischial spines and, if identified, the distance between them
  - Angle of pubic arch (usually accommodates two finger widths at the apex of the arch)
  - Prominence of ischial tuberosities (usually accommodates four knuckle widths when measured externally at the level of the perineum)

It may also include the following aspects:

- X-ray examination (Harper et al 2013; Sibony et al 2006)
- Ultrasound scans
- Computed tomography and magnetic resonance imaging (Huerta-Enochian et al 2006; Chen et al 2008)

Other factors must also be considered to enable a complete assessment to be made of the overall capacity of the woman's true pelvis:

- Assessment of normality of her gait
- Height
- Shoe size less than 4
- Previous successful vaginal delivery
- Non-engagement of fetal head at 38 weeks (primigravida)
- History of rickets
- Previous pelvic injury
- Previous trial of labour or prolonged labour
- Malpresentation, such as a breech
- Extent of caput or moulding of the fetal skull during labour

FEMALE REPRODUCTIVE ANATOMY

The primary function of the female reproductive system is production and transmission of ova and provision of a nurturing environment for the fertilized ovum and developing fetus. It has the ability to accommodate the developing fetus and expel the baby and placenta at birth, returning to its near prepregnant state during the puerperium. The study of the female reproductive system is fundamental to the midwife's understanding of gynaecology, pregnancy, birth and the impact birth has on the female reproductive anatomy. The structures identified with the female reproductive system include internal and external genitalia and the pelvic organs and structures (Table 24.3), particularly the bladder, urethra and rectum. In addition, uterine muscular support, blood supply, nerve supply and lymphatics are identified. This knowledge needs to be studied in conjunction with the pelvic floor muscle structure (see Ch. 40).

Fetal development

During the first 6 weeks following fertilization, male and female gonads undergo identical forms of development. In female fetuses the ovaries descend a short distance from their position below the kidneys to sit in the pelvic cavity closely alongside the fallopian tubes. Their primary function of ovum production commences under the influence of female hormones during puberty (see Chs 25 and 31).

External genitalia

Knowledge of the anatomy of the female external genitalia (Fig. 24.10 and Box 24.1) provides a foundation for application to midwifery practice during the process of labour and birth in relation to women who require catheterization and management and care of labial and perineal tears, episiotomy, tears to the urethral meatus or clitoris, fistulae and female genital mutilation.

Any of the following structures may be damaged during the birthing process and must be assessed following birth:

- Labia majora
- Labia minora
- Clitoris
- Vestibule
- Urethral meatus
- Vaginal orifice
- Bartholin's glands

Table 24.3 Anatomical relations to the vagina

View	Section of the vagina	Associated structures
Anteriorly	Upper half Lower half	Bladder Urethra
Posteriorly	Upper third Middle third Lower third	Pouch of Douglas Rectum Perineal body
Superiorly	Centrally Above lateral	Cervix Fornices Ureters and uterine arteries
Inferiorly	Vaginal orifices and vestibule	
Laterally	Upper Middle Lower	Parametrium Pubococcygeus muscles Perineal muscle Bulbocavernosus muscles

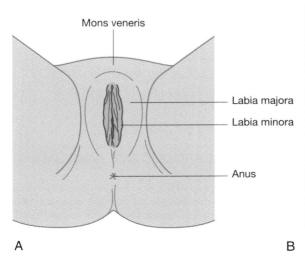

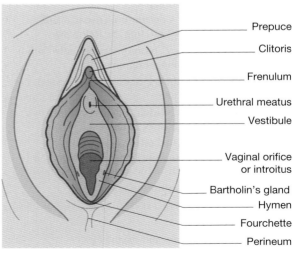

Figure 24.10 Female external genitalia. (See Box 24.1 for further information.)

Box 24.1 Female external genitalia

Mons veneris
Pad of fat over the pubic bone, covered by skin and, after puberty, hair.

Labia majora
One of two thick folds of fatty tissue (labia majora) covered with skin, extending from the mons to the perineum. The inner surface contains sebaceous glands.

Labia minora
One of two small, smooth folds of skin (labia minora) between the labia majora, containing sweat and sebaceous glands. Anteriorly, the labia minora encircle the clitoris, forming the prepuce and a smaller, lower fold called the frenulum. They meet posteriorly to form the fourchette.

Clitoris
Highly sensitive erectile tissue about 2.5 cm long. Consists of two erectile bodies called the corpora cavernosa and a glans clitoris of spongy erectile tissue.

Vestibule
Extends from clitoris to the fourchette and contains urethral and vaginal orifices. Contains the vestibular glands known as Skene's and Bartholin's glands.

Urethral meatus
Situated between the clitoris anteriorly and vaginal orifice posteriorly and is the external opening of the urethra, connecting superiorly to the bladder.

Vaginal orifice or introitus
Located posteriorly to the urethral meatus, opening into the vagina above, with the ability to stretch to accommodate the emerging baby at birth.

Hymen
A thin membrane partially occluding the vaginal introitus – easily ruptured with the use of internal tampons, physical exercise and intercourse. Further rupture occurs during vaginal delivery, resulting in the remaining tissue forming tags – carunculae myrtiformes.

Bartholin's glands
The ducts of the glands emerge on either side of the vaginal orifice on the inner surface of the labia minora. They secrete mucus to lubricate the vulva, and production increases during sexual arousal. They should not be palpable during vaginal examination unless obstructed or infected.

Fourchette
Created as the labia minora join posteriorly to the vaginal orifice, and used as a landmark for correct alignment during perineal suturing.

Perineum
Extends from the fourchette to the anal margin, covering the pelvic floor muscles.

Prepuce
A loose fold of skin covering the clitoris.

Frenulum
A small ligament maintaining the position of the clitoris.

Blood supply is via the pudendal arteries, and drainage is through corresponding veins. The external genitalia are vascular structures that facilitate healing, but they bleed heavily when traumatized.

Nerve supply is from branches of the pudendal nerve.

Lymphatic drainage occurs via the inguinal glands.

Internal genitalia

Knowledge of female internal reproductive anatomy (Fig. 24.11) enables understanding of the following:

• Pregnancy, birth and postpartum processes, including growth and development of the uterus in pregnancy

• Uterine function in labour, birth and delivery of the placenta

• Function of the muscle structures of the uterus in haemostasis and postpartum haemorrhage

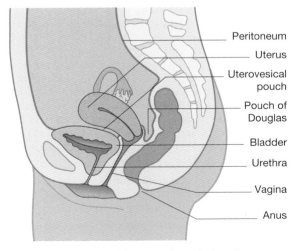

Figure 24.11 Female pelvic organs in sagittal section.

- Involution of the uterus and return of the anatomical structures to the prepregnant state
- Influence of breastfeeding on involution
- Genital tract infection
- Gynaecological conditions, such as:
  - Infection (Bartholin's abscess, postpartum infection)
  - Infertility and fertility
  - Fibroids, ectopic pregnancy, uterine prolapse, carcinoma, ovarian cysts and cervical screening

Vagina

The vagina is a fibromuscular tube directed upward and backward approximately parallel to the pelvic brim. It is important to note the angle of the vagina when conducting vaginal examinations and teaching women the correct insertion of pessaries, tampons and contraceptive diaphragms.

The vagina extends from the vulva to the cervix; the anterior wall is approximately 7.5 cm long and the posterior wall 10 cm. The walls of the vagina lie in apposition until it widens at the upper portion, where the cervix projects into the vagina at right angles, forming four recesses (*fornices*). The anterior fornix is shallow and the lateral fornices are deeper. The posterior fornix is deepest, facilitating pooling of semen during intercourse, increasing the opportunities for sperm to swim through the cervix.

There are no glands in the vagina; moisture is provided by secretions from the cervical glands and transudation of serous fluid from blood vessels. Vaginal secretions are acidic (pH 4.5); providing an unfavourable environment for spermatozoa, counteracted by the alkaline reaction of semen and cervical mucus. The vagina contains lactic acid produced by the action of lactobacilli (*Döderlein's bacilli*) on glycogen in the squamous cells of the vaginal lining, causing vaginal acidity. *Lactobacilli* normally inhabit the vagina without pathology. The lactic acid produced helps destroy pathogenic bacteria that may enter the vagina. In prepubescent girls and postmenopausal women, the vagina acidity is around pH 7, creating a favourable environment for the growth of vaginal infections, such as *Candida albicans*.

Structure The walls of the vagina have four layers:

- Interior layer of squamous epithelium arranged in transverse folds called *rugae*, enabling vaginal expansion and stretching during childbirth
- Vascular layer of elastic connective tissue
- Involuntary muscle layer with outer longitudinal fibres and inner circular fibres

- Outer layer of connective tissue – part of the pelvic fascia containing blood vessels, lymphatics and nerves

Following childbirth, the vaginal walls must be examined for damage and an assessment made to establish a plan of care.

Function The vagina is able to distend to facilitate the passage of the penis during intercourse and the baby during childbirth.

Blood supply is via the middle haemorrhoidal arteries, arising from a branch of the internal iliac arteries; drainage is through corresponding veins.

Nerve supply is via sympathetic and parasympathetic nerves from the plexus of Lee–Frankenhäuser (situated in the floor of the pouch of Douglas in the region of the uterosacral ligaments) originating from branches of the 2nd, 3rd and 4th sacral nerves.

Lymphatic drainage The lower third of the vagina drains into the inguinal glands and the upper two-thirds into the internal iliac glands.

Uterus

The uterus is a muscular, vascular, pelvic organ, often described as shaped like an upturned pear. It is situated with the bladder anteriorly and the rectum posteriorly, and normally it is in a position of anteversion (leaning forward towards the bladder) and anteflexion (curved forward on itself).

The uterus is divided into the body and the cervix. The narrow end of the uterus is inserted into the vagina and the upper body communicates with the fallopian tubes at the upper lateral surfaces (Fig. 24.12 and Box 24.2).

Structure

Endometrium is the lining of the uterus that constantly changes throughout the woman's reproductive lifecycle. It has the ability to shed during the menstrual cycle and be maintained and thickened during pregnancy.

The endometrium is composed of the following:

- Vascular connective tissue, called *stroma*, containing tubular glands. This vascular tissue is further divided into the functional and basal layer (the basal layer lies next to the myometrium). The functional layer is shed during menstruation and is regenerated from the basal layer.
- A surface layer of ciliated columnar epithelium covering the stroma
- Where the stroma dips to the level of the myometrium, it is covered with nonciliated cells.

Myometrium consists of plain muscle fibres and constitutes seven-eighths of the thickness of the uterine wall. In the non-pregnant state, the muscle layers are not clearly defined (see Fig. 24.13).

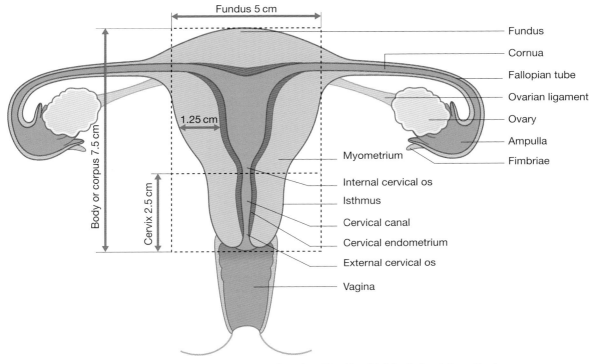

Figure 24.12 The non-pregnant uterus, fallopian tubes and ovaries. (See Box 24.2 for further information.)

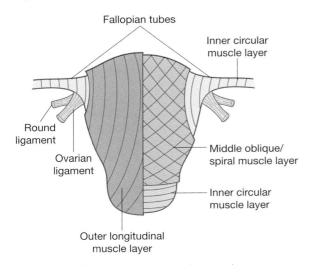

Figure 24.13 The three layers of uterine muscle.

In pregnancy, they become thicker and more defined as the following three layers of muscle:

1. *Inner circular:*
   - Sited mainly in the cornua and around the cervix
   - Assists cervical dilatation during labour

2. *Middle oblique or spiral:*
   - Thickest in the upper body of the uterus, where the placenta is normally situated
   - Have the ability to contract powerfully to act as natural ligatures to blood vessels following placental separation during the third stage of labour

3. *Outer longitudinal:*
   - Extend from the cervix anteriorly over the uterus to the cervix posteriorly
   - Have the ability to shorten in labour as the uterus contracts and retracts – facilitating descent and expulsion of the fetus, placenta and membranes

Perimetrium is a layer of peritoneum draped over the uterus and fallopian tubes, continuous with the peritoneum covering the bladder, extending to the lateral walls of the pelvis as the broad ligament (see Fig. 24.11). Folds in the peritoneum form in the following areas:

- Between the bladder and the uterus – known as the uterovesical pouch
- Between the uterus and the rectum – the *pouch of Douglas* (a recognized site for infection if the membrane is breached during surgery or trauma)

371

Box 24.2 The non-pregnant uterus, fallopian tubes and ovaries

Body or corpus

The upper two-thirds of the uterus. The cavity of the body is triangular in shape. The structure is made up of the fundus, cornua (singular cornu) and the isthmus.

Cervix

The lowest third of the uterus – cylindrical in shape with its lower half projecting into the vagina at right angles.

Internal cervical os

At the top of the cervical canal, its walls are in close apposition in the newly parous woman. It dilates and thins, becoming part of the lower uterine segment during the first stage of labour.

External cervical os

Situated at the bottom of the cervical canal, its walls are in close apposition in the prepregnant state, remaining partially dilated in parous women.

Examination of the external os forms part of the assessment of progress during labour.

Cervical endometrium or arbor vitae

The cervical endometrium is arranged in deep folds to facilitate the passage of spermatozoa through the cervical canal. The upper two-thirds is made up of columnar epithelium containing compound racemose glands secreting alkaline mucus. The cervical mucus is thin at the time of ovulation to facilitate spermatozoa. At other times it is thick in consistency, acting as a plug that assists in the prevention of infection in the uterus. The lower third is composed of stratified squamous epithelium continuous with that of the vagina.

Fundus

The upper, rounded part of the body of the uterus above the insertion of the two fallopian tubes. It may be palpated:

Antenatally:

- to assess fetal growth (weeks of gestation)
- to determine fetal lie and presentation

In labour:

- to assess uterine contractions
- to establish descent of the fetus
- to assess contractility of the uterus following expulsion of the placenta and membranes as an assessment of potential homeostasis

Postnatally:

- to determine involution

Fallopian tubes

Two tubes extending laterally from the uterus and opening into the peritoneal cavity. Each tube is approximately 10 cm long and 1 cm in diameter varying along its length. Hairs on the inner surface guide the ova towards the uterine cavity.

Scarring or obstruction caused by infection or trauma may lead to ectopic pregnancy and infertility. Tubes may be surgically ligated for sterilization purposes.

Cornu

Formed at the junction of the uterine body and fallopian tube.

Ovarian ligament

Suspends the ovary in a position close to the fimbriae of the fallopian tube to increase the probability of the ovum entering the fallopian tube.

Ovary

The female gonad that produces predetermined cells destined to become ova. Ovaries are endocrine organs producing oestrogen and progesterone and small amounts of the male hormone, androgen.

Fimbriae

Finger-like projections on the end of the fallopian tube that help to waft the ovum from the ovary to the fallopian tube.

Ampulla

Dilated distal portion of the fallopian tube where fertilization of the ovum usually occurs.

Isthmus

The junction between the body of the uterus and the cervix. During pregnancy there is growth and development of this junction, creating the lower uterine segment.

Cervical canal

This is a potential tube connecting the external os and the internal os. A plug of mucus (the operculum) forms here during pregnancy and is expelled when cervical activity and dilatation commence.

Functions of the uterus

- Provision of an environment conducive to the implantation of a fertilized ovum
- Nurture of the developing fetus
- Growth and expansion to accommodate the growing fetus and placenta
- Contraction, retraction and expulsion of the fetus, placenta and membranes during birth and maintenance of haemostasis following birth
- Return by involution to the nearly prepregnant state

Uterine ligaments maintain the normal anteverted, anteflexed position of the uterus. Damage to these ligaments

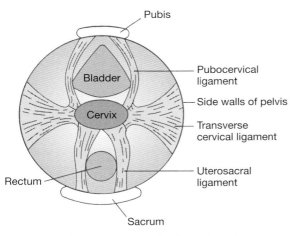

Figure 24.14 Superior view of uterine ligaments and supports.

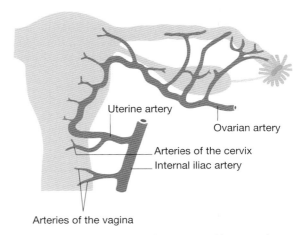

Figure 24.15 Blood supply to the uterus and its appendages.

may occur as a direct result of childbirth, especially prolonged labour; chronic constipation and straining; poor lifting techniques; poor posture; and obesity. The effect may not be seen until later in life at the menopause, where declining levels of oestrogen cause muscle and ligament atrophy and loss of function. The result of this may be uterine prolapse and associated stress incontinence and defecation difficulties (Whapples 2014).

The uterine ligaments (Fig. 24.14) are as follows:

- *Transverse cervical ligaments* (2): extend from the cervix laterally to the side walls of the pelvis (overstretching may cause uterine prolapse).
- *Uterosacral ligaments* (2): pass back from the cervix to the sacrum, encircling the rectum, and maintain the position of anteversion.
- *Pubocervical ligaments* (2): pass forwards from the cervix to the pubic bones, offering limited support to the uterus.
- *Round ligaments* (2): arise at the cornua of the uterus, descending through the broad ligament and the inguinal canals to the labia majora. They help to maintain the uterus in a position of anteversion.
- *Broad ligament:* a double fold of peritoneum extending from the lateral borders of the uterus to the side walls of the pelvis.

Blood supply The blood supply to the uterus is via uterine and ovarian arteries; drainage is by corresponding veins (Figs 24.15 and 24.16). This provides a rich supply of blood vessels to facilitate growth of the uterus and placenta during pregnancy and supports the growth and development of the fetus. Blood vessels to the uterus are twisted in the non-pregnant state and have the ability to uncoil as the uterus expands during pregnancy.

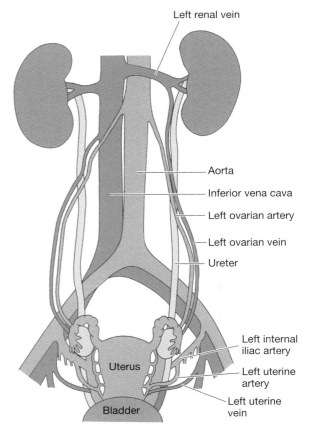

Figure 24.16 Blood supply to the uterus. Note where the ovarian vein terminates.

373

Breaches of this system can occur during pregnancy and labour and through trauma to the genital tract. This may cause severe haemorrhage, increasing the incidence of mortality and morbidity for both mother and baby (Knight et al 2014).

Uterine arteries and veins The uterine artery arises from a branch of the internal iliac artery and enters the uterus at the level of the internal cervical os, turning at right angles following a spiral course along the lateral border of the uterus, joining with the ovarian artery, with a branch to the cervix and vagina. Branches from the uterine arteries penetrate the myometrium and endometrium, enabling the regeneration and thickening of the endometrium throughout the menstrual cycle (see Ch. 25). Uterine veins follow the arteries and drain into the corresponding internal iliac veins.

Ovarian arteries and veins The ovarian arteries arise from the descending aorta and cross the urethra and internal iliac arteries before passing over the pelvic brim to enter the broad ligament just below the ovary. Branches of the ovarian artery supply the fallopian tubes and connect with the uterine artery. The right ovarian vein connects with the inferior vena cava and the left ovarian vein connects with the left renal vein.

Nerve supply The nerve supply is both sympathetic and parasympathetic. The sympathetic nervous system to the pelvis is a continuation of the aortic plexus (sometimes called the presacral nerve), and it lies in front of the fifth lumbar vertebra and the sacral promontory. It passes downwards, joining branches of the lumbar sympathetic chain lying on the floor of the pouch of Douglas. The parasympathetic nervous supply emerges from the sacral foramina to join the Lee–Frankenhäuser plexus. The nerves then pass to the uterus and other pelvic viscera (Waugh and Grant 2013).

Lymphatic drainage The lymphatic vessels and nodes draining lymph away from the pelvic organs accompany the main arteries and veins, with nodes sited along the iliac vessels and the aorta. Drainage from the upper portion of the uterus is to the lumbar and hypogastric nodes, and from the lower portion to the hypogastric nodes.

Cervix

In women who have never been pregnant the cervix can be palpated as a firm structure similar in consistency to the tip of the nose, and the cervical os is closed. In a multigravid woman who is not pregnant, the cervical os may remain partially dilated.

During pregnancy the cervix may appear to be blue because of the abundant blood supply, and towards the end of pregnancy it becomes softer as it 'ripens' in preparation for labour.

Squamocolumnar junction is where the upper columnar epithelium of the cervical canal meets the lower stratified squamous epithelium of the outer cervix. Carcinoma of the cervix is most likely to occur at this junction.

MALE REPRODUCTIVE ANATOMY

The function of the male reproductive system is the production of spermatozoa and their transfer to the female during sexual intercourse for the creation of new human life. It could be argued that once successful fertilization of the ovum has occurred, the need for knowledge of the male reproductive system is of little importance to the midwife. However, there are a number of issues that could be considered, such as sexual intercourse in pregnancy, transmission of sexually transmitted diseases (see Ch. 55), understanding of some of the causes of infertility (see Ch. 28) and examination of the male neonate (Ch. 42).

The function of the testes is the production of spermatozoa and testosterone. In the fetus the testes are sited in the abdominal cavity, gradually descending as the fetus develops, moving through the inguinal canals until they descend into the scrotum. Being sited outside of the abdominal cavity ensures that the testes are kept at a lower temperature than the body (2–3 degrees), the optimal temperature for the development of spermatozoa. The epididymis, a convoluted and coiled tube, provides the conduit for spermatozoa travel from the testes to the vas deferens and the ampulla. The vas deferens contains a muscle layer that has the potential to contract during sexually activity, pushing spermatozoa into the urethra during ejaculation.

The male reproductive system also includes a number of accessory glands; the seminal vesicles, the prostate and the bulbo-urethral glands. These three components support the development of semen, ensuring it contains the necessary nutrients and chemicals necessary for spermatozoa survival. Semen is slightly alkaline, helping to counteract the acidity of the vagina and aid motility. There is normally 2 to 6 mL of semen per ejaculation, consisting of 50 to 150 million spermatozoa. The penis consists of three areas of erectile tissue, in which there are vascular spaces, connective tissue and involuntary muscle (see Fig. 24.17). During sexual arousal the vascular spaces fill with blood to erect the penis in preparation for ejaculation.

Fetal development

In the fetus the male testes are located in the abdomen just below the kidneys, similar to the female. The gonads form distinct structures under genetic and hormonal influences (Johnson 2013). In the seventh or eighth month of

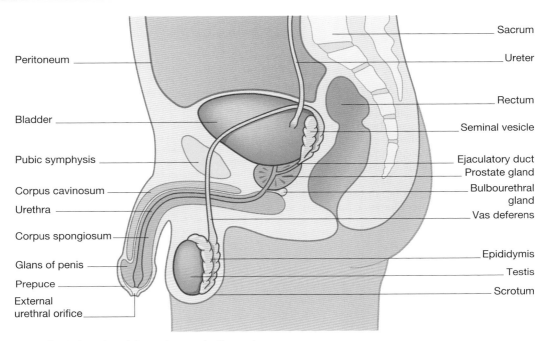

Figure 24.17 Sagittal section of the male reproductive system.

pregnancy, male testes descend with the spermatic cord through the right and left inguinal canals and at birth should be located in the scrotum of the term infant (Ellis and Mahadevan 2013) (see Ch. 42).

For more information on the male reproductive system, see the chapter website resources.

MIDWIFERY IMPLICATIONS

Knowledge of anatomy of human reproduction can help identify women who might require different care, treatment and advice, enabling the midwife to plan the most appropriate care during pregnancy, labour and puerperium, and also identify problems that may occur in the fetus and neonate. Early contact with women can identify those who may require further investigations or referral to the obstetrician for specialist care.

At the first antenatal visit ('booking'), the woman's medical and family history must be explored, identifying potential problems that may have been caused by nutritional issues, such as rickets, osteomalacia or anorexia nervosa (Dimitri and Bishop 2007; Linna et al 2014). The midwife can identify whether the pelvis may have changed from its original shape through trauma, surgery or osteoporosis (Leggon et al 2002; Phillips et al 2000; Riehi 2014) and identify normal changes in gait and in posture, pelvic arthropathy, pelvic pain and symphysis pubis diastasis (Champion 2015).

During labour, the midwife uses her understanding of pelvic anatomy to assess pelvic shape and size, using the woman's history, clinical examination, abdominal palpation and vaginal examination to provide information to help formulate a dynamic and appropriate plan of care for labour and birth. At this point, the midwife may be able to reduce the rate of prolonged labour, or identify dystocia early, and thus have a significant effect on reducing morbidity.

During the postnatal period, the midwife assesses uterine involution and return to its prepregnant state. Any deviations from normal must be swiftly identified and appropriately referred. This includes problems caused by birth trauma, stress incontinence, contraceptive methods, sexually transmitted diseases (Ch. 55) and sexual function and dysfunction. During neonatal examination (Ch. 42) the midwife establishes the normality of neonate genitalia and educates the mother accordingly.

CONCLUSION

Knowledge of human reproduction provides the foundation on which to place everyday practice. This understanding of how human reproductive anatomy is constructed and functions enables a midwife to apply the concepts to both the normal physiological process of childbirth and the concepts of obstetrics. It enables midwifery practitioners to utilize a common language to discuss midwifery and obstetric practice issues with other healthcare professionals. This supports and enhances the midwife's role as a health promoter and practitioner, interpreting complex health issues and relating them accurately and in appropriate terminology to women and their families.

Key Points

- A sound comprehension of the reproductive system provides a basis for an understanding of physiological and pathological conditions related to midwifery practice.
- Detailed anatomical information can be related to how the pelvis affects the normal and abnormal mechanisms of labour.
- Knowledge of anatomy provides a foundation for understanding how pregnancy affects the health of the pelvis and how pathological conditions and extrinsic factors affect the pelvis during parturition.
- Knowledge of anatomy of human reproduction can be applied to the study of obstetrics, gynaecological and urogenital health and pathology to enable practitioners to offer care, treatment and advice.
- An understanding of pelvic anatomy enables a midwife to assess pelvic shape and size, providing information to help formulate a plan of care for labour and birth.

References

Caldwell W, Moloy H, D'Espop A: The more recent conceptions of pelvic architecture, *Am J Obstet Gynecol* 40(4):558–565, 1940.

Champion P: Mind the gap: diastasis of the rectus abdominis muscles in pregnant and postnatal women, *Pract Midwife* 18(5):16–21, 2015.

Chen M, Coackley F, Kaimal A, et al: Guidelines for computed tomography and magnetic resonance imaging use during pregnancy and lactation, *Obstet Gynecol* 112(2):333–340, 2008.

Dimitri P, Bishop N: Rickets: new insights into a re-emerging problem, *Curr Opin Orthop* 18(5):486–493, 2007.

Ellis H, Mahadevan V: *Clinical anatomy: applied anatomy for students and junior doctors*, London, Wiley-Blackwell, 2013.

Harper LM, Odibo AO, Stamilo DM, et al: Radiographic measures of the mid pelvis to predict caesarean delivery, *Am J Obstet Gynecol* 208(460):e1–e6, 2013.

Huerta-Enochian GS, Katz VL, Fox LK, et al: Magnetic resonance-based serial pelvimetry: do maternal pelvic dimensions change during pregnancy? *Am J Obstet Gynecol* 194(6):1689–1694, 2006.

Johnson MH: *Essential reproduction*, 7th edn, Oxford, Wiley-Blackwell, 2013.

Knight M, Kenyon S, Brocklehurst P, et al, editors: *Saving lives, improving mothers' care: lessons learned to inform future maternity care from the UK and Ireland Confidential Enquiries into Maternal Deaths and Morbidity 2009–2012*, Oxford, MBRRACE-UK National Perinatal Epidemiology Unit, 2014.

Kuliukas A, Kuliukas L, Franklin D, et al: Female pelvic shape: distinct types or nebulous cloud, *Br J Midwifery* 23(7):490–496, 2015.

Leggon R, Wood G, Indeck M: Pelvic fractures in pregnancy: factors influencing maternal and fetal outcomes, *J Trauma* 53(4):796–804, 2002.

Linna M, Raevuori A, Haukka J, et al: Pregnancy, obstetric, and perinatal health outcomes in eating disorders, *Am J Obstet Gynecol* 211(4):392e1–392e8, 2014.

National Institute for Health and Care Excellence (NICE): *Antenatal care. Guideline 62*, London, NICE, 2008 (modified 2014).

Phillips A, Ostlere S, Smith R: Pregnancy-associated osteoporosis: does the skeleton recover? *Osteoporos Int* 11(5):449–454, 2000.

Reitter A, Daviss B, Bisits A, et al: Does pregnancy and/or shifting position create more room in a woman's pelvis? *Am J Obstet Gynecol* (6):2014.

Riehi J: Caesarean section rates following pelvic fracture: a systematic review, *Injury* 45(10):16–21, 2014.

Rost C, Jacqueline J, Kaiser A, et al: Pelvic pain during pregnancy: a descriptive study of signs and symptoms of 870 patients in primary care, *Spine* 29(22):2567–2572, 2004.

Sibony O, Alran S, Oury J: Vaginal birth after cesarean section: X-ray pelvimetry at term is informative, *J Perinat Med* 34(3):212–215, 2006.

Velickovic K, Makovey J, Abraham S: Vitamin D, bone mineral density and body mass index in eating disorder patients, *Eat Behav* 14(2):124–127, 2013.

Waugh A, Grant A: *Ross and Wilson anatomy and physiology in health and illness*, 12th edn, London, 2013, Churchill Livingstone.

Whapples E: Do women who have encountered vaginal childbirth experience long term incontinence or perineal pain? *Br J Midwifery* 22(10):706–715, 2014.

Resources and additional reading

Please refer to the chapter website resources.

Allotey J: *Function of the pelvis,* Manchester University UK Centre for the History of Nursing (website). www.nursing.manchester.ac.uk/ukchnm/publications/thesesand dissertations/allotey/.

Abstract from a dissertation focusing on the history of the pelvis.

Coad J: *Anatomy and physiology for midwives,* 3rd edn, London, 2011, Elsevier.

Useful midwifery-focused textbook.

Midwives Information and Resource Service (MIDIRS): www.midirs.org.

UK-based midwifery-focused information resource. This has a number of excellent resources for students and qualified midwives, including a paper on the female pelvis.

Verralls S: *Anatomy and physiology applied to obstetrics,* 3rd edn, London, Elsevier, 1993.

This is a simple, straightforward introduction to midwifery anatomy and physiology.

Waugh A, Grant A: *Ross and Wilson anatomy and physiology colouring and workbook,* 4th edn, London, Churchill Livingstone, 2014.

An interesting book for learning anatomy and physiology in a practical way. Includes a variety of activities to assist learning and provides a series of revision exercises.

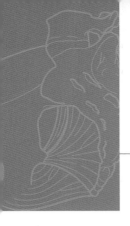

Chapter 25

Female reproductive physiology: timed interactions between hypothalamus, anterior pituitary and ovaries

Learning Outcomes ?

After reading this chapter, you will be able to:

- appreciate the essential role of gonadotrophin-releasing hormone (GnRH) neurons in the hypothalamus in regulating cyclical ovarian activity

- identify interactions between reciprocally connected neural networks in regulating pulsatile and surge release of GnRH across the ovarian cycle and their sensitivity to nutritional status

- understand the stimulatory effects of GnRH on the synthesis and pulsatile release of the gonadotrophins, and negative and positive feedback loops, generated by cyclical changes in ovarian steroid hormones in the anterior pituitary and the brain

- recognize the distinct phases of the ovarian cycle, formation and development of follicles and bidirectional communication between oocytes and surrounding somatic cells before and after ovulation

INTRODUCTION

Detailed information of menstrual and ovarian cycles, from puberty onwards, conveys a wealth of knowledge about women's nutritional status, emotional well-being and long-term health. This chapter begins with an overview of the hypothalamic–pituitary–gonadal (HPG) axis in females, identifying the unique features of gonadotrophin-releasing hormone (GnRH) neurons and the complex array of signals that impinge on this scattered population of GnRH cell bodies in the anterior hypothalamus and the cellular and molecular interactions that regulate the intermittent pulsatile and surge patterns of

release from nerve terminals in the median eminence (ME) during different phases of the infertile cycle. From here, the chapter explains the relationship between pulsatile GnRH release and the synthesis and pulsatile release of gonadotrophins, follicular-stimulating hormone (FSH), and luteinizing hormone (LH) in the anterior pituitary and describes how changing concentrations of ovarian steroid and peptide hormones exert negative and positive feedback on gonadotrophins and on the integrated neuronal networks that interact directly and indirectly with GnRH neurons. This leads to an account of events within the ovaries before, during and after ovulation, to reveal the timed interactions between ovarian follicles, maturation and ovulation of a selected follicle and formation and regression of the corpus luteum.

HYPOTHALAMIC CONTROL OF REPRODUCTION

GnRH is the final common mediator of an array of internal and external stimulatory and inhibitory regulators of fertility conveyed throughout the central nervous system (CNS). These neurons form a relatively small population scattered mainly in the medial preoptic, anterior hypothalamus and arcuate nucleus, and they send previously uncharacterized projections to a discrete area of the median eminence. The loose distribution of GnRH neurons is thought to reflect their remarkable migration during early life, from the site of origin in the olfactory placode of the developing nose, across the nasal septum, through the olfactory bulbs and into the rostral hypothalamus (Forni and Wray 2015). Following maturation of these neurons at puberty, their tightly regulated nerve terminals release GnRH in a variable pulsatile manner, into the fenestrated capillaries of the portal vasculature, where it is rapidly degraded as it travels directly to the cells of the anterior pituitary (Prevot et al 2010). Because GnRH is released in a pulsatile manner and has a half-life in blood of only 2 to 4 minutes, its receptors on the surface of pituitary gonadotrophs are stimulated intermittently. This pattern of GnRH stimulation is essential to maintain the responsiveness of gonadotrophs, which induces prolonged synthesis and pulsatile release of LH and FSH that in turn promotes gonadal development, cyclical ovarian activity and steroid hormone production (McCartney and Marshall 2014: 8–10).

From puberty to menopause, a coordinated and timely surge activation of GnRH neurons just before ovulation interrupts negative feedback regulation, with a positive feedback response to sustained elevation of oestradiol that also gives rise to elevated progesterone synthesis within the hypothalamus at the end of the follicular phase (Stephens et al 2015). During this switch, the basal, or tonic, mode of hourly pulses become more frequent, and then it shifts to a continuous elevation of GnRH concentrations in the pituitary portal blood, lasting many hours (Zhang et al 2015; Campbell and Suter 2010; Johnson 2013: 158–159). These cyclical alterations in GnRH release have been fully characterized for some time, but many questions remain about the central interactions that generate them and how these interacting neurons are sensitive to metabolic cues that vary according to nutritional status (Skorupskaite et al 2014). These brain regulators of GnRH activity effectively monitor fertility according to energy stores and markers of metabolic health (Pinilla et al 2012).

The complexity of signalling to the hypothalamic–pituitary structures that control reproduction is very striking. Successful fertility absolutely depends on GnRH responsiveness to an array of information, particularly about ovarian hormone levels, energy balance and physical and emotional stress (Pinilla et al 2012; Skorupskaite et al 2014). The neurohormonal systems that mediate dynamic alterations in these physical and emotional states must be integrated with the HPG axis to generate the appropriate patterns of GnRH release. Synchronized GnRH bursts emanate from the integral activities of a hypothalamic network, encompassing GnRH neurons, other neuropeptides and neurotransmitters that modulate its pulsatile secretion and activate the surge pattern of release in conjunction with the cycle of negative and positive stimulation by ovarian steroid and peptide hormones (Micevych and Sinchak 2011; Stephens et al 2015).

Novel aspects of GnRH neurons

To understand the complex array of interacting excitatory and inhibitory transsynaptic and glial inputs on GnRH neurons, it is necessary to begin with their functional morphology. Information processing by neurons usually occurs in discrete compartments. Dendrites receive and integrate synaptic inputs to the cell body, whereas axons initiate and conduct spikes from the cell body to distal neuronal targets. GnRH neurons do not conform to this stereotype. They are generally bipolar, with two remarkably long, relatively unbranched processes studded with dendritic spines, which are sites of excitatory synaptic input. All GnRH neurons, including those adjacent to ME, project at least one of these processes directly into the ME. At this point, the processes branch extensively and form terminals that are regulated mainly by steroid-sensitive, highly polarized glial cells. Dynamic rearrangements of these glial cells organize GnRH terminals to form reversible neurovascular junctions with the pericapillary space of the pituitary portal system, resulting in variable patterns of GnRH release (Prevot et al 2010) (see Figs 25.1, 25.2, and 25.3).

Studies on the electrical properties of GnRH projection structures demonstrate that they combine in variable degrees the functional capacities of both axon and dendrite. Sections of these 'dendrons' closest to the cell body possess a high capacity to propagate action potentials from other axon terminals, thereby mediating signal integration by controlling action potential initiation and electrical bursting (Piet et al 2015). Sections further away from the cell body receive synaptic inputs along their entire projection and propagate action potentials to the synaptic terminals in the ME. Imaging studies have shown that the great majority of GnRH neurons form multiple, close appositions with dendrons of other GnRH neurons (Campbell and Suter 2010; Piet et al 2015). These observations provide evidence that the scattered population of GnRH neurons that project to the ME are not isolated from one another but highly interconnected, through dendro-dendritic bundling and associated shared synaptic inputs. Although questions remain about the relative significance of dendrons in generating the variable pulsatile release of GnRH from the ME, they seem to provide an intrinsic mechanism to synchronize GnRH output from this scattered population of neurons (Chen and Sneyd 2014). The importance of these findings is that pituitary and therefore ovarian responsiveness to GnRH depends on the amplitude and frequency of GnRH pulses (Johnson 2013).

Neuronal orchestration of GnRH pulsatility

The essential role of GnRH in reproduction was discovered more than 40 years ago. However, it is only recently that researchers have begun to identify the interacting afferent neuronal groups and pathways that mediate the hormonal signals from ovarian follicles, nutrient signals and environmental cues that synchronize GnRH and therefore LH pulsatility with changes in body weight, temperature, and libido across the ovarian cycle (see Fig. 25.4). Two very distinct modes of GnRH release occur during the ovarian

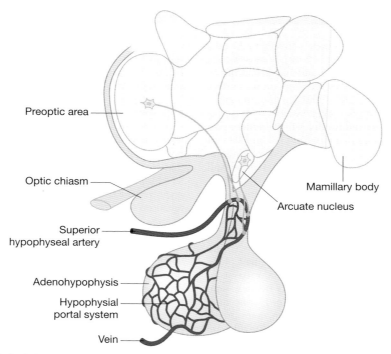

Figure 25.1 Anatomical relationships between hypothalamic GnRH neurons and their target population in the anterior pituitary gland. (Reprinted from Strauss JF, Barbieri RL, editors: Yen & Jaffe's reproductive endocrinology, 7th edn, Philadelphia, 2014, Elsevier, Saunders, 3-26, with permission from Elsevier.)

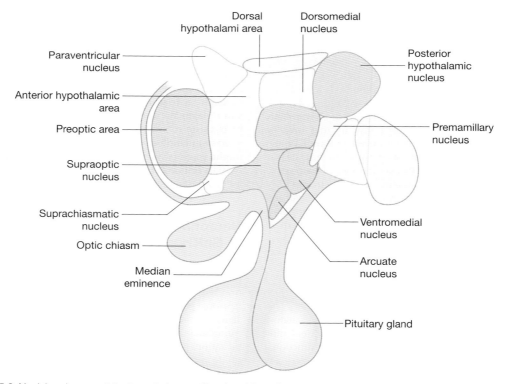

Figure 25.2 Nuclei and areas of the hypothalamus. (Reprinted from Strauss JF, Barbieri RL, editors: Yen & Jaffe's reproductive endocrinology, 7th edn, Philadelphia, 2014, Elsevier, Saunders, 3-26, with permission from Elsevier.)

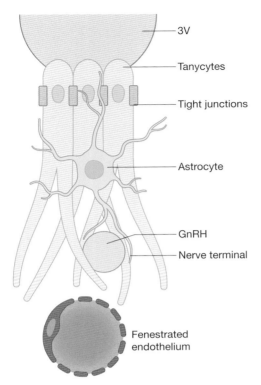

3V

Tanycytes

Tight junctions

Astrocyte

GnRH

Nerve terminal

Fenestrated
endothelium

Figure 25.3 Schematic representations of glial cells, tanycytes, astrocytes and neuroendocrine terminals in the median eminence (ME), the brain structure that forms the floor of the third ventricle. (Prevot V et al: Gonadotrophin-releasing hormone nerve terminals, tanycytes and neurohaemal junction remodelling in the adult median eminence: functional consequences for reproduction and dynamic role of vascular endothelial cells, Journal of Neuroendocrinology 22(7):639–649, 2010.)

distinct electrical properties that have a direct capacity to drive different patterns of GnRH neuronal excitation. The majority of GnRH neurons express kisspeptin receptors (kiss1r), and kiss1 induces an intense electrical activation of GnRH cells primarily through transient and sustained ionic currents (Piet et al 2015). Kiss1 neurons in the preoptic area directly innervate GnRH cell bodies and their specialized projections, and they exert their most potent stimulatory actions through high-frequency electrical currents that modulate ion channels in GnRH neurons (Piet et al 2015). Preoptic kiss1 neurons express a subthreshold persistent sodium current that dramatically alters their firing activity. They have a very low activation threshold, fire spontaneously, display a variety of firing patterns, burst-fire repetitively after a hyperpolarizing stimulus and sustain long periods of activation (Piet et al 2015). In addition, they express oestrogen receptor α, the key receptor isoform involved in the surge mechanism of GNRH/LH release, and exposure to preovulatory concentrations of oestradiol increases kiss1 mRNA expression and augments persistent sodium currents, which dramatically up-regulates their excitability (Zhang et al 2015). At present, the extent to which preoptic kiss1 neurons directly innervate GnRH nerve terminals in the ME remains to be identified (Piet et al 2015).

GnRH hourly pulsatile release

In contrast to those in the preoptic area, kiss1 neurons in the ARC are mostly quiescent or fire at low frequencies and have a much lower threshold of spontaneous electrical activation. Chronic exposure to low levels of oestradiol suppresses their kiss1 mRNA and protein levels and reduces their cell body size and dendritic spine density (Cholanian et al 2015). Consequently, during the follicular and luteal phases of the cycle, oestradiol decreases synthesis and release of kiss1 and reduces dendritic sites of excitatory synaptic input to effect an overall reduction in the capacity of ARC kiss1 neurons to stimulate GnRH and therefore LH neurons, thereby bringing about the hourly pattern of tonic pulsatile release that characterizes negative feedback regulation.

The anatomical pathways through which ARC kiss1 neurons directly innervate GnRH neurons have not been fully identified, but there is some evidence that they project to the preoptic area and provide direct innervations to GnRH neurons (Piet et al 2015). Extensive interconnected cell bodies and proximal dendrites with local branches also terminate within the ARC, and many more project to a number of other hypothalamic nuclei (Pinilla et al 2012). Numerous axonal terminals project to the ependymal layer of the third ventricle, whereas others project to GnRH terminals in the external zone of the ME. This anatomical arrangement of ARC kiss1 and GnRH neurons may provide a key mechanism for integrating the

cycle: the preovulatory GnRH surge that drives the LH surge required for ovulation and the basal or tonic GnRH release that occurs episodically, approximately every 60 to 90 minutes throughout follicular and luteal phases of the cycle. Current evidence suggests that the surge mode is driven by kisspeptin (kiss1) neurons in the preoptic area in conjunction with high concentrations of ovarian steroids, whereas the hourly clock mode is driven by another population of kiss1 neurons in the arcuate nucleus (ARC) in conjunction with low concentrations of ovarian steroids (Prevot et al 2010; Cholanian et al 2015; Zhang et al 2015).

GnRH surge release

Current evidence suggests that these two main populations of kiss1 neurons are vital presynaptic neurons, with

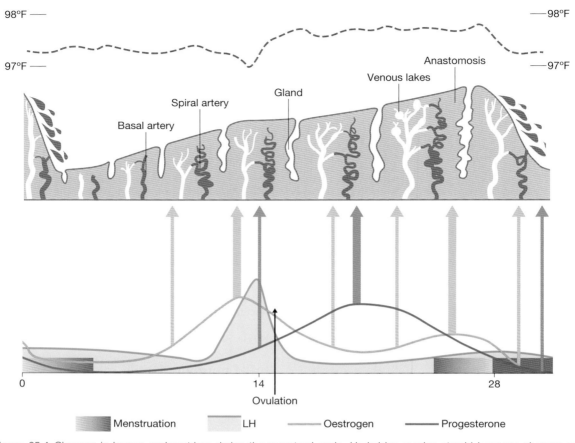

Figure 25.4 Changes in human endometrium during the menstrual cycle. Underlying ovarian steroid hormone changes are indicated below and basal temperature is indicated above. Thickness of arrows indicates strength of action. (Reproduced with permission from Johnson MH: Essential reproduction, 7th edn, Oxford, 2013, Blackwell Scientific.)

HPG axis with cyclical changes in temperature, body weight and metabolism during the follicular and luteal phases of the ovarian cycle (Mittelman-Smith et al 2012; Cholanian et al 2015).

A significant feature of kiss1 neurons in the ARC is that they also contain neurokinin B (NKB) and either dynorphin (DYN) or proenkephalin, among other neurotransmitters. They coexpress oestrogen receptor α, NKB receptor NK3 and the DYN receptor KOR (Skrapits et al 2015). This indicates that the kisspeptin/NKB/Dyn (KNDy) neurons form a network that is coupled through auto synaptic processes. Stimulation of the NKB neurons increases the action potential firing activity of KNDy neurons, which is modulated by chronic exposure to low concentrations of ovarian steroids. In contrast, DYN reduces spontaneous KNDy neuronal activity, which is also modulated by chronic exposure to ovarian steroids. KNDy neuronal exposure to dynorphin reduces subsequent responsiveness

to NKB stimulation in the presence of low concentrations of ovarian steroids (Cholanian et al 2015).

These data suggest that DYN-mediated inhibition of NKB-induced activity requires ovarian steroid feedback. This implies that KNDy neurons in the ARC comprise an oscillatory feedback loop interconnected through collaterals that synchronize the frequency of their pulsatile activity. Together, these observations support the hypotheses that coordinated activation of NKB and DYN receptors respectively can generate a pattern of alternating stimulatory–inhibitory signals on KNDy neurons that are modulated by ovarian steroids (Piet et al 2015).

KNDy neurons innervate GnRH neurons in the preoptic area and send axon collaterals to the ependymal layer of the third ventricle, where specialized cells interact with GnRH terminals and fenestrated capillaries of the pituitary portal circulation in the ME (Prevot et al 2010). In addition, they densely innervate GnRH fibres in the ME, and pulses of kisspeptin in the ME occur in temporal association with GnRH pulses (Piet et al 2015). These findings are consistent with the hypothesis that KNDy neurons in the ARC drive pulsatile GnRH and LH secretion and suggest that NKB and DYN expressed in those neurons are involved in the process of generating the rhythmic discharge of Kiss1.

THE OVARIAN CYCLE

From puberty to menopause, ovarian activity is characterized by cyclic development of several follicles and selection and maturation of the dominant follicle in preparation for the extrusion of a viable oocyte at ovulation (see Fig. 25.5). This pattern of ovulation requires cyclical release of steroid and peptide hormones that imposes a corresponding cyclicity on most organ systems, notably haemodynamics, metabolism, temperature, emotional responsiveness, libido and sexual desirability (Bobst and Lobmaier 2012; Brennan et al 2009; Chapman et al 1998; Chidambaram et al 2002; Haselton et al 2007; Lobmaier et al 2015; Salonia et al 2005; Tarin et al 2002; Mittelman-Smith et al 2012). Some of these are useful for timing ovulation, but none is as reliable as *menstruation,* the monthly shedding of bloody endometrial tissue at the end of the luteal phase triggered by cyclic decidualization of the endometrium in response to endocrine cues. Hence, the term *menstrual cycle* is invariably used as an indirect measure of the *ovarian cycle.*

The ovarian cycle has three distinct phases:

1. The *follicular* phase prepares the reproductive system to receive spermatozoa and fertilize the oocyte.

2. The *ovulatory* phase extrudes a fertilizable oocyte into the fallopian tubes.

3. The *luteal* phase prepares the reproductive system to receive and nurture the conceptus.

Phases 1 and 3 proceed over approximately 14 days, whereas the second takes about 15 minutes (Lousse and Donnez 2008).

Acquisition and maintenance of female reproductive capacity requires the extrusion of a viable oocyte at ovulation. When oocyte growth begins, somatic cells of the follicle are recruited, namely, granulosa cells (GCs) that function as the 'nurse' cells and thecal cells (TCs) that supply the GCs with the oestrogenic precursor androstenedione (Johnson 2013: 140–141). Together, these three distinct cell types form interdependent paracrine–endocrine units that make up the fundamental reproductive element of the ovary.

Fertility depends on the production of one *dominant follicle* per cycle, with the capacity to *ovulate* a fertilizable oocyte (see Fig. 25.6). From puberty to menopause, a few primary follicles are recruited every day into a pool of growing follicles, producing a continuous trickle of developing follicles. Of the 15 to 20 follicles recruited, one

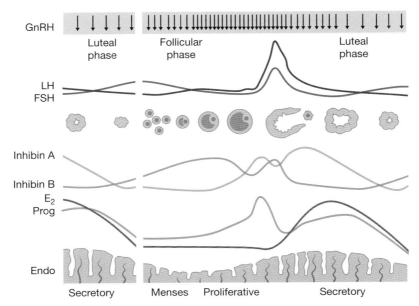

Figure 25.5 Neurohormonal, follicular and endometrial dynamics of the ovarian and menstrual cycles, with changing frequency of GnRH pulsatility in relation to low and high concentrations of LH/FSH and ovarian steroid and peptide hormones. (Reprinted from Strauss JF, Barbieri RL, editors: Yen & Jaffe's reproductive endocrinology, 7th edn, Philadelphia, 2014, Elsevier, Saunders, 3-26, with permission from Elsevier.)

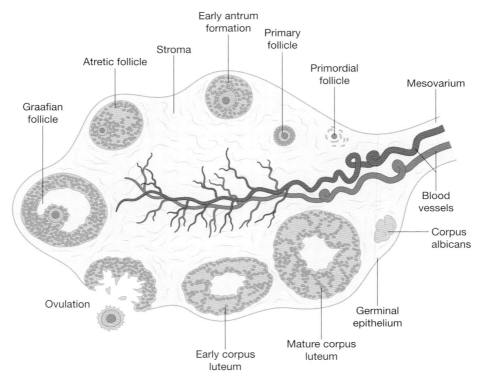

Figure 25.6 The follicular cycle of the human ovary. (Reprinted from Strauss JF, Barbieri RL, editors: Yen & Jaffe's Reproductive Endocrinology, 7th edn, Philadelphia, 2014, Elsevier, Saunders, 3-26, with permission from Elsevier.)

selected follicle demonstrates increased cell proliferation and differentiation, expansion of thecal vascularity, rapid accumulation of antral fluid and rising capacity for synthesis and secretion of steroid and peptide hormones (Geva and Jaffe 2000; Gougeon 1996; Seifer et al 2002; Tamura et al 2009; Saller et al 2010).

At midcycle, the *dominant follicle* becomes visible to the naked eye, as a large bulge under the surface epithelium of the ovary. By this stage, the fully grown oocyte has amassed lipid stores and mRNA, which is used to generate protein stores and to form organelles, including large numbers of mitochondria. These are an essential source of adenosine triphosphate (ATP) for the rise in oxidative metabolism that accompanies the energy-consuming processes of maturation and the acquisition of developmental competence, which entails a profound reorganization of the nucleus and cytoplasm in preparation for fertilization and blastocyst formation (Canipari 2000; Downs 2015; Gilchrist et al 2008; Van Blerkom 2009).

Dynamics of follicular activity

During the ovarian cycle, both ovaries recruit at least two successive waves of around 10 healthy follicles that have

reached 2 to 5 mm in diameter. As illustrated in Fig. 25.7, recruited follicles leave the dynamic pool of primary and slowly growing follicles and contain increasing amounts of steroid hormones and gonadotrophin receptors that operate in conjunction with growth factors and neurotrophic peptides (Edson et al 2009). Growing follicles also contain increasing levels of melatonin and melatonin receptors that influence steroid hormone synthesis and stimulate production of growth factors and receptors involved in cell metabolism. Melatonin also operates in a variety of ways to reduce oxidative stress, which is critical for oocyte development (Tamura et al 2009; Tamura et al 2012). These and other factors regulate the exponential growth phase in conjunction with pituitary gonadotrophins; preceding waves of growing cohorts begin to regress and undergo *atresia* or cell death (Baerwald et al 2003; Hirshfield 1991; Seifer et al 2002).

Sequences of events in the cohort of growing follicles

From the onset of the exponential growth phase, cell proliferation, fluid formation and vascularization proceed at varying speeds in the *antral follicles* recruited for

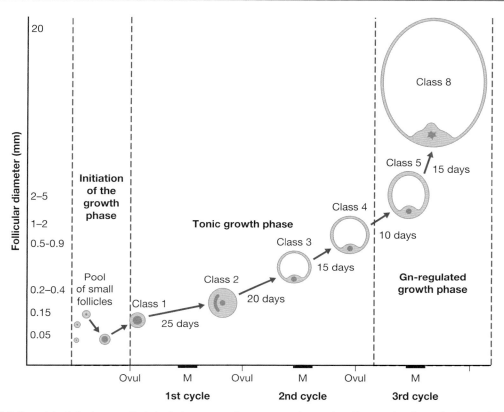

Figure 25.7 Complete follicular growth trajectories across three successive cycles. Progression through stages 1–4 relies to some extent on pituitary gonadotrophins, whereas stages 5–8 occur during the follicular phase following the third menses from initiation of the growth phase. Exponential growth, selection and dominance are regulated by rising levels of FSH and by varying sensitivity to FSH within the selected cohort. Key: M, menses; Ovul, ovulation; Gn, gonadotrophin. (This article was published in Blackburn ST (2013) Maternal, Fetal, & Neonatal Physiology: A Clinical Perspective, 3rd edn. Saunders Philadelphia, Copyright Elsevier, 2013.)

ovulation. The fastest-growing follicle is characterized by rapid cell proliferation, differentiation and vascularization; upregulation of functional FSH and LH receptors; greater uptake of gonadotrophs than the remaining follicles in the cohort; and an increased sensitivity to FSH (Gougeon 1996; Seifer et al 2002; Zackrisson et al 2000).

By day 9 of the *follicular phase,* the vascularity of the theca compartment in the selected follicle is double that in other follicles of the developing cohort, leading to increased delivery of LH to theca and FSH to mural granulosa cells (Geva and Jaffe 2000). Selected follicles also inhibit proliferation of GCs and release of oestrogens and progesterone in small follicles (Son et al 2011). This selectively inhibits GC mitosis in midsized but not large antral follicles. These interactions enhance trophic support for development of the selected follicle, whereas the remainder undergo atresia (Edson et al 2009; Saller et al 2010).

Oocyte growth

During the initial growth phase, the oocyte secretes glycoproteins that condense around it to form a translucent acellular layer called the *zona pellucid,* which creates a connecting zone between the oocyte and growing layers of GCs. Intercellular communication between GCs and between oocytes and GCs occur through gap junctions because no blood vessels penetrate beyond the *membrane propria* of the internal layer of the TCs. This bi-directional network transports ions, metabolites and low-molecular-weight substrates from the cumulus granulosa cells (CGs) to the oocyte for incorporation into larger molecules, while a large number of regulatory factors from the oocyte modulate hormonal conditions and the growth-stimulating capacity of GCs (Fig. 25.7). Throughout the growth phase of the oocyte, progression of *meiosis* is arrested at the diplotene or germinal vesicle stage of prophase by the release of inhibitory regulators from the surrounding somatic cells (Downs 2015).

Follicular fluid – the microenvironment of the cumulus–oocyte complex

The cumulus–oocyte complex (COC) is suspended in follicular fluid (FF). This fluid contains energy substrates, such as glucose, triglycerides and fatty acids, and hormones, such as insulin, leptin and melatonin, that directly regulate the growth, maturation and developmental competence of the preovulatory oocyte (Tamura et al 2009). The nutrient composition of FF varies during successive phases of follicular development and is profoundly influenced by the woman's diet and metabolism (Dunning et al 2014).

FF is composed of exudates from plasma through the follicular epithelium and secreted products of the follicle, especially GCs. This suggests that there is a 'blood–follicle barrier' for serum proteins above 300 kDa (Dunning et al 2014). At the same time, large molecules produced by the oocyte or GCs cannot cross the membrana granulosa or follicular basal lamina, thereby establishing a potential osmotic gradient, which may be responsible for recruiting fluid to the centre of the follicle (Rodgers and Irving-Rodgers 2010).

The composition of FF differs considerably from plasma: PO_2 is significantly lower and declines as the follicular diameter increases, whereas concentrations of the powerful antioxidant and free-radical scavenger melatonin are almost threefold higher than plasma concentrations (Tamura et al 2012). Glucose and lipid concentrations are lower than plasma concentrations, and concentrations of growth factors, growth inhibitory factors, angiogenic factors, anticoagulation factors and steroid and peptide hormones are very different (Antczak et al 1997; Downs 2015; Hirshfield 1991; Koga et al 2000). The presence of steroid-binding proteins allows very high concentrations of oestrogens, to match the increased capacity for steroid hormone synthesis, particularly in theca interna and mural granulosa compartments; rising levels of leptin in response to ovulatory levels of gonadotrophins and the presence of meiotic and luteinization inhibitory factor(s) indicate that FF participates in modulating oocyte maturation, progesterone secretion and onset of the final phase of cell differentiation that transforms the dominant follicle into the *corpus luteum* immediately following ovulation (Cioffi et al 1997; Dunning et al 2014; Gougeon 1996; Hinrichs et al 1991; Zackrisson et al 2000).

Recent studies have identified the significance of plasma glucose and dietary intake of saturated and polyunsaturated fatty acids for a variety of indicators of oocyte maturation and follicular development. Specifically, higher plasma glucose and total saturated fatty acids and lower concentrations of total polyunsaturated fatty acids are strongly associated with oocytes that display markers of impaired developmental capacity (Wong et al 2015). Oocyte maturation is the phase of development in which the fully grown oocyte reinitiates meiotic maturation, completes one meiotic division with extrusion of a polar body and then arrests at MII until fertilization. A prominent function of cumulus cells (CSs) during this critical phase is to channel metabolites and nutrients to the oocyte to help stimulate germinal vesicle breakdown and direct development to MII. These energy-consuming processes require precise coordination of numerous metabolic pathways and oocyte paracrine signals that direct certain aspects of CS metabolism (Dunning et al 2014; see Fig. 25.8).

The growing ratio of fluid to tissue mass in the preovulatory follicle seems to participate in temperature regulation between the dominant follicle and the surrounding stroma, resulting in a preovulatory follicle temperature 2.3 °C cooler than that of the surrounding stroma (Grinsted et al 1995). Because basal body temperature is lower during this phase of the cycle, follicle temperature is further reduced to provide a cooler internal environment for the preovulatory follicle, analogous to that provided for male germ cells in the cool scrotal sac (Bujan et al 2000). Together these regulatory mechanisms create conditions for the development of a mature oocyte with the developmental competence for fertilization, embryo formation, fetal growth and maturation.

Follicular hormonal preparation for ovulation and creation of the corpus luteum

As the dominant follicle increases in size (Fig. 25.9), rising synthesis of oestrogens and progesterone leads to a parallel rise in circulating concentrations that interact with kiss1 neurons in the preoptic area of the hypothalamus (Zhang et al 2015). The LH/FSH surge is temporally associated with attainment of peak secretion of oestrogens following a rapid rise in progesterone 12 hours earlier (Micevych and Sinchak 2008; Stouffer 2003).

Following the LH/FSH surge, fibroblasts within the *theca externa* lay down connective tissue, and *theca interna* and mural granulosa cells (GCs) begin to differentiate from a predominantly oestrogen-secreting tissue into a highly vascularized corpus luteum with progesterone as its major steroid hormone, along with a rapid rise in progesterone and melatonin receptors (Stouffer 2003; Tamura et al 2009). Before ovulation, mural GC and theca interna cells differentiate predominantly into progesterone-secreting theca-lutein and granulosa-lutein cells that remain in the ovary following ovulation and rapidly expand to form the highly vascularized corpus luteum (Niswender et al 2000; Stouffer 2003).

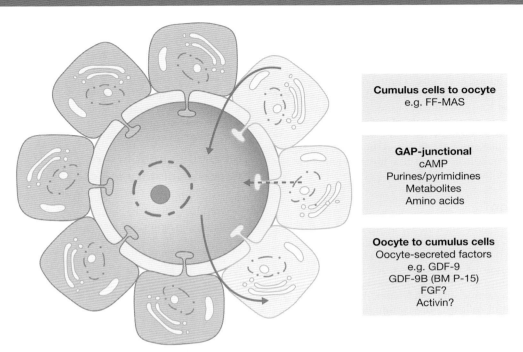

Cumulus cells to oocyte
e.g. FF-MAS

GAP-junctional
cAMP
Purines/pyrimidines
Metabolites
Amino acids

Oocyte to cumulus cells
Oocyte-secreted factors
e.g. GDF-9
GDF-9B (BM P-15)
FGF?
Activin?

Figure 25.8 Bi-directional oocyte–cumulus cell communication: paracrine (bold arrow) and gap-junctional (dashed arrow) communication between oocyte and cumulus cells. Factors transmitted include follicular-fluid meiosis-activating sterol (FF-MAS), growth differentiation factor-9 (GDF-9), fibroblast growth factor (FGF) and activin. (Sutton ML, Gilchrist RB, Thompson JG: Effects of in-vivo and in-vitro environments on the metabolism of the cumulus-oocyte complex and its influence on oocyte developmental capacity, Human Reproduction Update, 2003.9(1): p.35–48, by permission of Oxford University Press.)

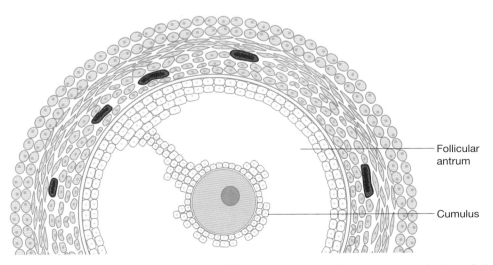

Follicular antrum

Cumulus

Figure 25.9 Expanded antral follicle with a fully developed follicular antrum leaving the oocyte surrounded by a distinct layer of granulosa cells. (Reproduced with permission from Johnson MH: Essential Reproduction, 7th edn, Oxford, 2013, Blackwell Scientific.)

During the critical preovulatory period, the oocyte also secretes molecules that enhance oestrogens and inhibit progesterone secretion by *cumulus granulosa cells* that also express oxytocin receptors (Behrens et al 1995; Gilchrist et al 2008; Sutton et al 2003). Central oxytocin appears to stimulate gonadotrophs (Evans et al 2003; Gonzalez-Iglesias et al 2015). Within the ovaries, oxytocin modulates progesterone secretion while stimulating progesterone receptors on granulosa cells, and a variety of regulatory molecules, including growth factors, integrins, prostaglandins and intracellular messengers, involved in the process of ovulation (Saller et al 2010).

Ovulation

The LH/FSH surge dramatically increases blood flow and vascular permeability in thecal capillary networks that descend to the basal lamina. The rapid increase in size and vascularization of the follicle is accompanied by local release of prostaglandin PGE_2 and vasodilatory substances such as histamine and bradykinin. PGE_2 initiates the breakdown of collagen fibres within the thecal compartment, and other molecules cause an inflammatory reaction from within. FSH and progesterone also initiate proteolytic enzyme activity that loosens, distends and finally erodes the follicle wall at its weakest point (Edson et al 2009).

Luteinization

The preovulatory LH surge also triggers luteinization or terminal differentiation of theca and granulosa cells within a few hours of ovulation (Stocco et al 2007). Both cells synthesize progesterone as the primary steroid hormone, which acts locally to sustain luteal cell function and stimulate its own secretion (Stocco et al 2007). Androgens and oestradiol are also synthesized to a lesser extent (Niswender et al 2000).

Within 12 hours of the LH/FSH surge, the fully grown oocyte is reactivated to briefly resume meiosis while complex maturational changes occur in the cytoplasm to support fertilization and the expansion of the surrounding CSs (Sutton-McDowall et al 2010). FSH receptors are present on the entire surface of human oocytes, suggesting that FSH directly controls oocyte maturation (Meduri et al 2002). At the same time, progesterone replaces oestrogens as the *dominant steroid hormone* synthesized by theca and mural granulosa cells. This shift is accompanied by a rise in prostaglandin output, which activates enzymes that weaken and distend the follicle wall. Between 36 and 42 hours following the surges, the apex of the follicle begins to bulge below the surface of the ovary, rupturing at its weakest point. This allows antral fluid to flow into the peritoneal cavity, carrying the expanded *oocyte–cumulus* complex into the fallopian tube (Edson et al 2009; see Fig. 25.9).

At ovulation, the dominant follicle releases the hugely expanded COC from the surface of the ovary. Immediately afterwards, the cumulus cell mass regulates acceptance of the oocyte by the fimbriae of the fallopian tube and subsequently functions as a hormonal and metabolic unit in the lumen of the uterine cavity, optimizing conditions for the enclosed oocyte and zona pellucida to undergo final maturational changes in preparation for fertilization, implantation and embryo formation (Talbot et al 2003).

The corpus luteum – reprogramming the postovulatory follicle

When the cumulus-oocyte complex (COC) leaves the ovary, residual cells of the dominant follicle undergo rapid remodeling, including cell growth, proliferation and final differentiation, accompanied by a rapid increase in blood flow and lymphatic drainage (Alexander et al 1998; Redmer and Reynolds 1996; Stocco et al 2007). These changes allow the corpus luteum to expand rapidly to become the most active and highly vascularized autocrine–paracrine–endocrine gland in the body, with a lifespan of approximately 14 days (Stocco et al 2007).

At the peak of its activity, in the midluteal phase of the cycle, the corpus luteum measures up to 2 cm in diameter and produces up to 25 mg progesterone per day, although the majority of its cells are nonluteal in origin (Niswender et al 2000; Redmer and Reynolds 1996).

The convoluted ovarian arterial branches are enmeshed by a responsive venous network surrounding the ovary, providing an effective means of adapting local blood flow to the dynamic state of the enclosed follicles across successive cycles (Alexander et al 1998).

CYCLICAL CHANGES IN REPRODUCTIVE ORGANS

Ovarian regulation of gonadotrophs before, during and after ovulation imposes a corresponding cycle on the functional layer of the endometrium and fallopian tubes; mucosal secretions of the cervix; and the structure, nerve density and secretions of vaginal tissue (Gipson et al 2001; Ting et al 2004). The functional zone of the endometrium undergoes successive phases of proliferation, secretion and regression, whereas mammary epithelial cells undergo proliferation and involution across the ovarian cycle (Barbieri 2014; Smith 2001).

The endometrial cycle

The endometrial cycle (Fig. 25.10) is divided into three phases, which normally take place over 28 to 30 days:

1. *Proliferative phase:* Follows menses and may last from 9 to 23 days. Under the influence of oestrogens and

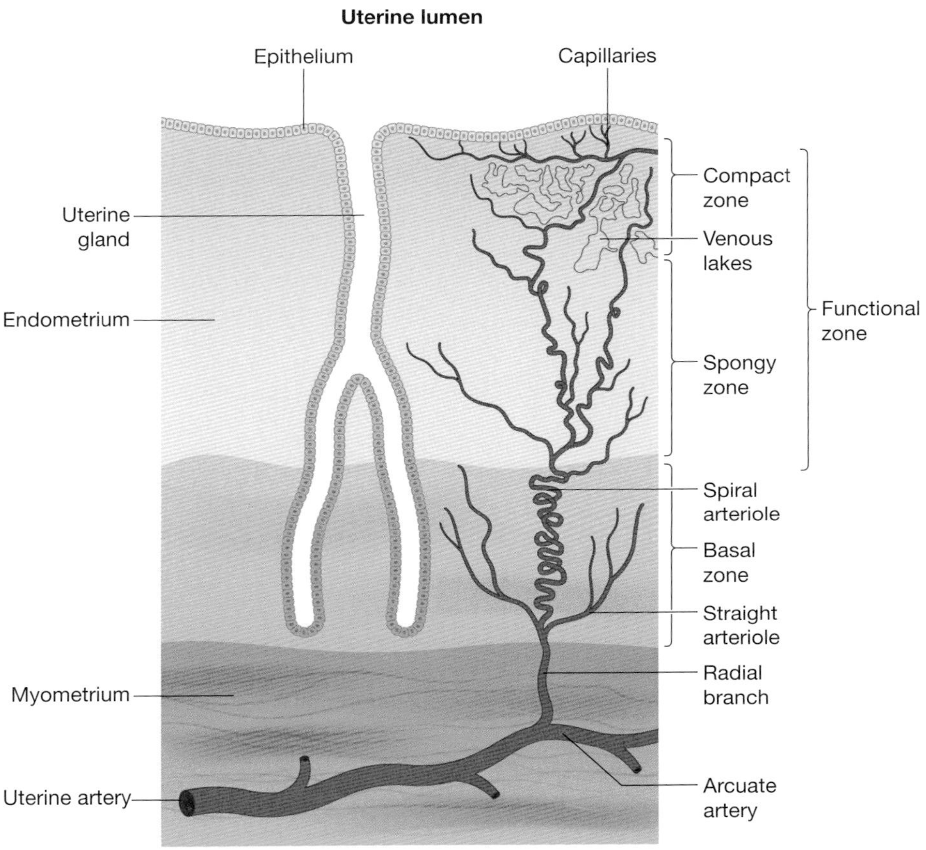

Uterine lumen

Figure 25.10 The arterial supply to the uterine endometrium. These specialized endometrial blood vessels arise within the myometrium as the arcuate arteries. Small straight arterioles supply the basal unchanging layer of the endometrium. As they leave the basal portion and enter the spongy and compact tissue that underlies the luminal epithelium, their thick smooth muscle coat formed by circular and longitudinal layers becomes progressively thinner. By the time they reach the subepithelial surface of the endometrium, they consist only of endothelial cells. (This article was published in Strauss JF, Barbieri RL, editors: Yen & Jaffe's Reproductive Endocrinology, 7th edn, Philadelphia, 2014, Elsevier, Saunders, 3-26, Copyright Elsevier, 2014.)

local growth factors, blood vessels begin to proliferate; the endometrium grows thicker and softer, and the tubular glands lengthen and become tortuous.

2. *Secretory phase:* Lasts between 8 and 17 days following ovulation. Under the influence of progesterone and oestrogens, the endometrial layer becomes even thicker; spiral arteries lengthen and become more coiled; the endometrial glands become tortuous as they expand with secretions until about 25% of the endometrium is occupied by glands.

3. *Menses:* Lasts about 4 to 6 days. Progesterone withdrawal initiates a cascade of inflammatory changes as decidualized stromal cells recruit inflammatory leucocytes, prostaglandins and matrix-degrading enzymes into the premenstrual endometrium. This intense inflammation process seems to be essential for the rapid restoration of tissue integrity that occurs following endometrial sloughing (Evans and Salamonsen 2014).

Cyclical endometrial activity

Cyclical regeneration of the functional layer of the endometrium that culminates with pre-decidualization at around 8 to 9 days after ovulation begins towards the end of menses. During the follicular phase, rising concentrations of oestrogens stimulate an intense proliferation of epithelial and stromal cells. This is followed by differentiation of glandular and stromal cells and continued growth and tubal formation of endometrial vascular cells, which is largely regulated by rising levels of progesterone, following ovulation. During the luteal phase, the functional zone is characterized by changes in cell morphology and extracellular matrix composition that transform it into a secretory paracrine/autocrine gland (Lessey and Young 2014: 202–205). Throughout the secretory phase, the endometrium clearly differentiates into three layers, with numerous gap junctions:

- A superficial compact zone containing decidualized stroma with attenuated nonsecretory glands
- A middle spongy zone consisting of distended glands with abundant secretions
- A basal zone with extensive development of protein synthesis and secretion

As illustrated in Fig. 25.10, from the midsecretory phase to the end of menstruation, the thickness of the functional layer declines from 5–8 mm to 1–3 mm as the functional layer is shed along with its connective tissue matrix, and the highly specialized arterioles are reduced to around one-third of the length reached by the onset of menses (Bakos et al 1993; Dockery et al 1990; Rogers 1996; Smith 2000). During the premenstrual phase, endometrial cells release increasing levels of proteolytic enzymes that degrade the extracellular matrix and highly potent and long-lasting vasoconstrictors called endothelins that act on the spiral arterioles (Ohbuchi et al 1995). From the second day after bleeding commences, remaining stromal cells respond to the reduced oxygen tension by synthesizing *vascular endothelial growth factor* (VEGF), which stimulates repair of the vascular bed and elongation of the remaining blood vessels, by the fifth day of the cycle (Maas et al 2001). These blood vessels have an essential role in tissue reconstruction during the proliferative phase of the cycle (Rogers 1996; Smith 2001).

The proliferative phase

By around day 5 of the endometrial cycle, cell proliferation commences when endometrial and myometrial oestrogen receptors are stimulated by increased secretion of oestrogens from the cohort of developing follicles. During this phase, oestrogens stimulate a rise in the number of ciliated cells in the luminal epithelium and expression of a variety of mitogenic factors, including VEGF, that stimulate a marked proliferation of luminal epithelial, glandular and vascular endothelial cells (Ferrara and Davis-Smith 1997). At the same time, oestrogens directly inhibit endometrial angiogenesis while vascular permeability rises and endometrial blood flow increases, to peak just before ovulation (Ma et al 2001).

Stromal fibroblasts enlarge and show signs of increased protein synthesis and association with microfibrils of collagen that become denser and thicker just before ovulation. An insoluble pericellular matrix of collagen and fibronectin forms a tight meshwork primarily around glandular and basement membranes of the luminal epithelium (Dockery et al 1990; Shiokawa et al 1996). With the surge in oestrogens that follows selection of the dominant follicle, a three- to five-fold increase occurs in endometrial thickness, and oestrogen-dependent intracellular receptors for progesterone are synthesized. During the late proliferative phase, secretory glands enlarge and become thicker and more convoluted, and proliferation in epithelial and stromal cells continues until 3 days following ovulation (Lessey and Young 2014: 202–206).

The secretory phase

Endometrial glandular cells accumulate glycogen, regulatory proteins, sugars and lipid droplets, and their secretory activity reaches a maximum around 6 days after ovulation. In anticipation of fertilization, these molecules prepare for implantation and provide essential nutritional and regulatory secretions for the conceptus (Budak et al 2006; Burton et al 2007; Cheon et al 2001). At the same time, progesterone stimulates glandular and stromal cells to release human chorionic gonadotrophin (hCG) and increased expression of two potent angiogenic factors: angiogenin in stromal cells and VEGF in stromal cells and neutrophils associated with microvessel walls (Alexander et al 1998; Gargett et al 2001; Ma et al 2001). As illustrated in Fig. 25.10, a subepithelial capillary plexus formed into a complex network of vessels by the midsecretory phase and newly regrown arterioles become increasingly more spiral as they lengthen more rapidly than the endometrium thickens (Gargett et al 2001).

Pre-decidualization

During the secretory phase, stromal cells synthesize and release a growing number of new matrix proteins together with surface expression of their receptors, including laminin, fibronectin and integrins, and the earlier cross-linking collagen fibrils are degraded. This process of matrix remodeling creates a looser and more soluble structure; from the midsecretory phase onwards, stromal cells also express a variety of regulatory peptides involved in cell replication and haemostasis. Stromal tissue undergoes further differentiation, and individual cells become larger and oedematous, which contributes to the overall thickening of the endometrium.

From the late secretory phase, further changes occur within the endometrium regulated by relaxin, progesterone, prolactin and leptin (Budak et al 2006; Gubbay et al 2002; Haig 2008). The endometrial stroma immediately surrounding the arterioles undergoes decidualization as it synthesizes a number of hormones and other molecules and is infiltrated by lymphoid cells. In the event of fertilization, these changes provide an appropriate nutritive, regulatory and immunoprotective environment for the emerging embryo until 9 to 10 weeks gestation (Alexander et al 1998; Gonzalez et al 2003; Gubbay et al 2002).

Cyclical changes in the cervix and vagina

Significant changes occur in the cervix and vagina throughout the cycle, which facilitate the passage of spermatozoa. During the follicular phase, the muscles of the cervix relax, causing the cervical os to dilate slightly (to around 3–4 mm) at the time of ovulation. The epithelial cells begin to secrete clear watery and 'stretchable' mucus midcycle.

Under the influence of rising levels of progesterone following the midcycle LH/FSH surge, the cervix becomes firmer and more tightly closed, and cervical secretions become scant, viscous and cellular, making it more difficult for spermatozoa to enter the uterus. In addition, relaxin and progesterone relax muscle layers in the isthmic portion of the tube, which assists movement of the conceptus towards the uterine cavity (Downing and Hollingsworth 1993; Johnson 2013: 184–185).

Lined with stratified squamous epithelium, the vagina is also responsive to oestrogens and progesterone. During the follicular phase, vaginal cells proliferate and begin to accumulate glycogen, which is fermented to lactic acid by the normal bacterial flora. This provides a slightly acid environment, which acts as an anti-infective agent. During sexual excitation, the acidity of vaginal fluid is partly neutralized by the increased blood flow to the pelvic region, and this alters the pH, making it more receptive for the ejaculated sperm.

The mammary cycle

The female mammary gland undergoes a surge of cell division during puberty and a cyclical pattern of proliferation and involution until approximately 35 years. During this period, hormonally induced increases in cell proliferation and *apoptosis* (programmed cell death) do not return the gland to the starting point of the previous cycle but provide for a cumulative budding of new lobules (Barbieri 2014: 236–237).

During each cycle, episodes of increased mitosis and apoptosis follow a contrasting pattern to that of the endometrium. Mammary epithelium shows decreased DNA synthesis and mitotic divisions during the first half of the cycle and maximal proliferation that peaks during the luteal phase of the cycle and is followed by a shorter period of increased apoptosis (Barbieri 2014: 236–237). A contrasting pattern of cellular activity in uterine and mammary epithelium is reflected in cyclical differences in steroid hormone receptor concentrations in the two organs of reproduction. Mammary tissue receptors for oestrogen (as in the endometrium) decline during the second half of the cycle; those for progesterone remain fairly constant throughout both phases of the cycle (Soderqvist et al 1993). During the second half of the cycle, secretory activity may also occur together with increases in breast volume because of the significant rise in extracellular levels of VEGF that stimulates angiogenesis and increases vascular permeability (Dabrosin 2003).

CONCLUSION

It is important to understand the complex mechanisms and neurohormonal pathways and interactions that synchronize ovarian, endometrial and mammary cycles, and how these are homeostatically synchronized with cyclical changes in body temperature, metabolism and emotional sensitivities. Cyclical parallels are evident in systemic and follicular homeostatic set points for glucose, insulin and lipid concentrations during the follicular and luteal phase of the ovarian cycle. The cyclical alterations in temperature and metabolism reflect the changing requirements of oocyte development and strongly indicate the elaborate connections that are made at all levels of the HPG axis to ensure optimal conditions for the cyclical release of a healthy oocyte.

Key Points

- The menstrual cycle provides reliable markers of the general health, well-being and nutritional status of women.

- During each cycle, the uterus facilitates reception, maturation and transport of spermatozoa from the vagina to the fallopian tube, and the inner layers of the uterus prepare to receive and directly nourish the blastocyst.

- The ovarian, menstrual and mammary cycles are driven by precisely timed patterns of negative and positive feedback between ovarian steroids and peptide hormones, gonadotrophins in the anterior pituitary and the interplay between ovarian steroids and the network of neurons that directly interact with GnRH neurons in the hypothalamus.

References

Alexander H, Zimmermann G, Wolkersdorfer GW, et al: Utero-ovarian interaction in the regulation of reproductive function, *Hum Reprod Update* 4(5):550–559, 1998.

Antczak M, Van Blerkom J, Clark A: A novel mechanism of vascular endothelial growth factor, leptin and transforming growth factor-B2 sequestration in a subpopulation of human ovarian follicles, *Hum Reprod* 12(10):2226–2234, 1997.

Baerwald AR, Adams GP, Pierson RA: Characterization of ovarian follicular wave dynamics in women, *Biol Reprod* 69:1023–1031, 2003.

Bakos O, Lundkvist O, Bergh T: Transvaginal sonographic evaluation of endometrial growth and texture in spontaneous ovulatory cycles – a descriptive study, *Hum Reprod* 142:142–157, 1993.

Barbieri RL: The breast. In Strauss J, Barbieri RL, editors: *Yen & Jaffe's reproductive endocrinology*, Philadelphia, PA, Elsevier, Saunders, pp 236–237, 2014.

Behrens O, Mascheko H, Kupsch E, et al: Oxytocin receptors in human ovaries during the menstrual cycle. In Ivell R, Russell J, editors: *Oxytocin*, New York, Plenum Press, pp 485–486, 1995.

Bobst C, Lobmaier JS: Men's preference for the ovulating female is triggered by subtle face shape differences, *Horm Behav* 62:413–417, 2012.

Brennan IM, Feltrin KL, Nivasinee SN, et al: Effects of the phases of the menstrual cycle on gastric emptying, glycemia, plasma GLP-1 and insulin, and energy intake in healthy lean women, *Am J Physiol Gastrointest Liver Physiol* 297:G602–G610, 2009.

Budak E, Sanchez MF, Bellver J, et al: Interactions of the hormones leptin, ghrelin, adiponectin, resistin, and PYY3-36 with the reproductive system, *Fertil Steril* 85(6):1563–1581, 2006.

Bujan L, Daudlin M, Charlet J-P, et al: Increase in scrotal temperature in car drivers, *Hum Reprod* 15(6):1355–1357, 2000.

Burton GJ, Jauniaux E, Charnock-Jones DS: Human early placental development: potential roles of the endometrial glands, *Placenta* 28(Suppl A):S64–S69, 2007.

Campbell RE, Suter KJ: Redefining the gonadotrophin-releasing hormone neurone dendrite, *J Neuroendocrinol* 22(7):650–658, 2010.

Canipari R: Oocyte–granulosa cell interactions, *Hum Reprod Update* 6(3):279–289, 2000.

Chapman AB, Abraham WT, Zamudio S, et al: Temporal relationships between hormonal and hemodynamic changes in early pregnancy, *Kidney Int* 54:2056–2063, 1998.

Chen X, Sneyd JA: Computational model of the dendron of the GnRH neuron, *Bull Math Biol* 2014.

Cheon KW, Lee H-S, Parhar IS, et al: Expression of the second isoform of gonadotrophin releasing hormone (GnRH-II) in human endometrium throughout the menstrual cycle, *Mol Hum Reprod* 7(5):447–452, 2001.

Chidambaram M, Duncan JA, Lai VS, et al: Variation in the renin angiotensin system throughout the normal menstrual cycle, *J Am Soc Nephrol* 13:446–452, 2002.

Cholanian M, Krajewski-Hall SJ, McMullen NT, et al: Chronic oestradiol reduces the dendritic spine density of KNDy (kisspeptin/neurokinin B/dynorphin) neurones in the arcuate nucleus of ovariectomised Tac2-enhanced green fluorescent protein transgenic mice, *J Neuroendocrinol* 27:253–263, 2015.

Cioffi JA, Van Blerkom J, Antczak M, et al: The expression of leptin and its receptors in pre-ovulatory human follicles, *Mol Hum Reprod* 3(6):467–472, 1997.

Dabrosin C: Variability of vascular endothelial growth factor in normal human breast tissue in vivo during the menstrual cycle, *J Clin Endocrinol Metab* 88(6):2695–2698, 2003.

Dockery P, Warren MA, Li TC, et al: A morphometric study of the human endometrial stroma during the peri-implantation period, *Hum Reprod* 5(5):494–498, 1990.

Downing SJ, Hollingsworth M: Action of relaxin on uterine contractions – a review, *J Reprod Fertil* 99:275–282, 1993.

Downs SM: Nutrient pathways regulating the nuclear maturation of mammalian oocytes, *Reprod Fertil Dev* 27:572–582, 2015.

Dunning KR, Russell DL, Robker RL: Lipids and oocyte developmental competence: the role of fatty acids and beta-oxidation, *Reproduction* 148:R15–R27, 2014.

Edson MA, Nagaraja AK, Matzuk MM: The mammalian ovary from genesis to revelation, *Endocr Rev* 30:624–712, 2009.

Evans J, Salamonsen LA: Decidualized human endometrial stromal cells are sensors of hormone withdrawal in the menstrual inflammatory cascade, *Biol Reprod* 90(1):1–12, 2014.

Evans JJ, Reid RA, Wakeman SA, et al: Evidence that oxytocin is a physiological component of LH regulation in non-pregnant women, *Hum Reprod* 18(7):1428–1431, 2003.

Ferrara N, Davis-Smith T: The biology of vascular endothelial growth factor, *Endocr Rev* 18:4–25, 1997.

Forni PE, Wray S: GnRH, anosmia and hypogonadotropic hypogonadism – Where are we?, *Front Neuroendocrinol* 36:165–177, 2015.

Gargett CE, Lederman F, Heryonto B, et al: Focal vascular endothelial growth factor correlates with angiogenesis in human endometrium. Role of intravascular neutrophils, *Hum Reprod* 16(6):1065–1075, 2001.

Geva E, Jaffe RB: Role of vascular endothelial growth factor in ovarian physiology and pathology, *Fertil Steril* 74(3):429–438, 2000.

Gilchrist RB, Lane M, Thompson JG: Oocyte-secreted factors: regulators of cumulus cell function and oocyte quality, *Hum Reprod Update* 14(2):159–177, 2008.

Gipson IK, Moccia R, Spurr-Michaud S, et al: The amount of MUC5B in cervical mucus peaks at midcycle, *J Clin Endocrinol Metab* 86(2):594–600, 2001.

Gonzalez RR, Leary K, Petrozza JC, et al: Leptin regulation of interleukin-1 system in human endometrial cells, *Mol Hum Reprod* 9(3):151–158, 2003.

Gonzalez-Iglesias AE, Fletcher PA, Arias-Cristancho JA, et al: Direct stimulatory effects of oxytocin in female rat gonadotrophs and somatotrophs in vitro: comparison with lactotrophs, *Endocrinology* 156:600–612, 2015.

Gougeon A: Regulation of ovarian follicular development in primates: facts and hypotheses, *Endocr Rev* 17(2):121–155, 1996.

Grinsted J, Kjer JJ, Blendstrup K, et al: Is low temperature of the follicular fluid prior to ovulation necessary for normal oocyte development, *Fertil Steril* 43:34–39, 1995.

Gubbay O, Critchley HOD, Bowen JM, et al: Prolactin induces ERK phosphorylation in epithelial and CD56+ natural killer cells of the human endometrium, *J Clin Endocrinol Metab* 87(5):2329–2335, 2002.

Haig D: Placental growth hormone-related proteins and prolactin-related proteins, *Placenta* 29(Suppl A):S36–S41, 2008.

Haselton MG, Mortezaie M, Pillsworth EG, et al: Ovulatory shifts in human female ornamentation near ovulation, women dress to impress, *Horm Behav* 51:40–45, 2007.

Hinrichs K, Rand WM, Palmer E: Effect of aspiration of preovulatory follicle on luteinization, corpus luteum function, and peripheral gonadotrophin concentrations in the mare, *Biol Reprod* 44:292–298, 1991.

Hirshfield AN: Development of follicles in the mammalian ovary, *Int Rev Cytol* 124:43–101, 1991.

Johnson MH: *Essential reproduction*, 7th edn, Oxford, Blackwell Scientific. 2013.

Koga K, Osuga Y, Tsutsumi O, et al: Evidence for the presence of angiogenin in human follicular fluid and the up-regulation of its production by human chorionic gonadotrophin and hypoxia, *J Clin Endocrinol Metab* 85(9):3352–3355, 2000.

Lessey BA, Young SL: The structure, function, and evaluation of the female reproductive tract. In Strauss J, Barbieri RL, editors: *Yen & Jaffe's reproductive endocrinology*, 7th edn, Philadelphia, Elsevier, Saunders, 2014.

Lobmaier JS, Probst F, Perrett DI, et al: Menstrual cycle phase affects discrimination of infant cuteness, *Horm Behav* 70:1–6, 2015.

Lousse J-C, Donnez J: Laparoscopic observation of spontaneous ovulation, *Fertil Steril* 9(3):833–834, 2008.

Ma W, Tan J, Matsumoto H, et al: Adult tissue angiogenesis: evidence for negative regulation by estrogen in the uterus, *Mol Endocrinol* 15(11):1983–1992, 2001.

Maas JW, Groothuis PG, Dunselman GA, et al: Endometrial angiogenesis throughout the human menstrual cycle, *Hum Reprod* 16(8):1557–1561, 2001.

McCartney CR, Marshall JC: Neuroendocrinology of Reproduction. In Strauss JF, Barbieri RL, editors: *Yen & Jaffe's reproductive endocrinology*, 7th edn, Philadelphia, Elsevier, Saunders, pp 3–26, 2014.

Meduri G, Charnaux N, Driancourt M-A, et al: Follicle-stimulating hormone receptors in oocytes?, *J Clin Endocrinol Metab* 87(5):2266–2276, 2002.

Micevych P, Sinchak K: Minireview: Synthesis and function of hypothalamic neuroprogesterone in reproduction, *Endocrinology* 149(6):2739–2742, 2008.

Micevych P, Sinchak K: The neurosteroid progesterone underlies estrogen positive feedback of the LH surge, *Front Endocrinol (Lausanne)* 2(90):1–10, 2011.

Mittelman-Smith MA, Williams H, Krajewski-Hall SJ, et al: Arcuate kisspeptin/neurokinin B/dynorphin (KNDy) neurons mediate the estrogen suppression of gonadotropin secretion and body weight, *Endocrinology* 153:2800–2812, 2012.

Niswender GD, Juengel JL, Silva PJ, et al: Mechanisms controlling the function and life span of the corpus luteum, *Physiol Rev* 80(1):1–29, 2000.

Ohbuchi H, Nagai K, Amaguchi M, et al: Endothelin-1 and big endothelin-1 increase in human endometrium during menstruation, *Am J Obstet Gynecol* 173(5):1483–1490, 1995.

Piet R, de Croft S, Liu X, et al: Electrical properties of kisspeptin neurons and their regulation of GnRH neurons, *Front Neuroendocrinol* 35:15–27, 2015.

Pinilla L, Aguilar E, Dieguez C, et al: Kisspeptins and reproduction: Physiological roles and regulatory mechanisms, *Physiol Rev* 92:1235–1316, 2012.

Prevot V, Bellefontaine N, Baroncini M, et al: Gonadotrophin-releasing hormone nerve terminals, tanycytes and neurohaemal junction remodelling in the adult median eminence: functional consequences for reproduction and dynamic role of vascular endothelial cells, *J Neuroendocrinol* 22(7):639–649, 2010.

Redmer DA, Reynolds LP: Angiogenesis in the ovary, *Rev Reprod* 1:182–192, 1996.

Rodgers RJ, Irving-Rodgers HF: Formation of the ovarian follicular antrum and follicular fluid, *Biol Reprod* 82:1021–1029, 2010.

Rogers PA: Structure and function of endometrial blood vessels, *Hum Reprod Update* 2(1):57–62, 1996.

Saller S, Kunz L, Dissen GA, et al: Oxytocin receptors in the primate ovary: molecular identity and link to apoptosis in human granulosa cells, *Hum Reprod* 25(4):969–976, 2010.

Salonia A, Nappi RE, Pontillo M, et al: Menstrual cycle-related changes in plasma oxytocin are relevant to normal sexual function in healthy women, *Horm Behav* 47:164–169, 2005.

Seifer DB, Feng B, Shelden RM, et al: Brain-derived neurotrophic factor: a novel human ovarian follicular protein, *J Clin Endocrinol Metab* 87(2):655–659, 2002.

Shiokawa S, Yoshimura Y, Nagamatsu S, et al: Expression of B1 integrins in human endometrial stromal and decidual cells, *J Clin Endocrinol Metab* 81(4):1533–1540, 1996.

Skorupskaite K, George JT, Anderson RA: The kisspeptin-GnRH pathway in human reproductive health and disease, *Hum Reprod Update* 20(4):485–500, 2014.

Skrapits K, Borsay BÁ, Herczeg L, et al: Neuropeptide co-expression in hypothalamic kisspeptin neurons of laboratory animals and the human, *Front Neurosci* 9, 2015.

Smith SK: Angiogenesis and implantation, *Hum Reprod* 15(Suppl 6):59–66, 2000.

Smith SK: Angiogenesis and reproduction, *Br J Obstet Gynaecol* 108(8):777–783, 2001.

Soderqvist G, von Schoultz B, Tani E, et al: Estrogen and progesterone receptor content in the breast epithelial cells from healthy women during the menstrual cycle, *Am J Obstet Gynecol* 168(3):874–879, 1993.

Son WY, Das M, Shalom-Paz E, et al: Mechanisms of follicle selection and development, *Minerva Ginecol* 63(2):89–102, 2011.

Stephens SBZ, Tolson KP, Rouse ML, et al: Absent progesterone signaling in kisspeptin neurons disrupts the LH surge and impairs fertility in female mice, *Endocrinology* 156(9):3091–3097, 2015.

Stocco C, Telleria C, Gibori G: The molecular control of corpus luteum formation, function, and regulation, *Endocr Rev* 28(1):117–149, 2007.

Stouffer RL: Progesterone as a mediator of gonadotrophin action in the corpus luteum: beyond steroidogenesis, *Hum Reprod Update* 9(2):99–117, 2003.

Sutton ML, Gilchrist RB, Thompson JG: Effects of in-vivo and in-vitro environments on the metabolism of the cumulus-oocyte complex and its influence on oocyte developmental capacity, *Hum Reprod Update* 9(1):35–48, 2003.

Sutton-McDowall ML, Gilchrist RB, Thompson JG: The pivotal role of glucose metabolism in determining oocyte developmental competence, *Reproduction* 139:685–695, 2010.

Talbot P, Shur BD, Myles DG: Cell adhesion and fertilization: steps in oocyte transport, sperm–zona pellucida interactions, and sperm–egg fusion, *Biol Reprod* 68:1–9, 2003.

Tamura H, Nakamura Y, Korkmaz A, et al: Melatonin and the ovary: physiological and pathophysiological implications, *Fertil Steril* 92:328–343, 2009.

Tamura H, Takasaki A, Taketani T, et al: The role of melatonin as an antioxidant in the follicle, *J Ovarian Res* 5:5, 2012.

Tarin JJ, Gomez-Piquer V: Do women have a hidden heat period?, *Hum Reprod* 17(9):2243–2248, 2002.

Ting AY, Blacklock AD, Smith PG: Estrogen regulates vaginal sensory and autonomic nerve density in the rat, *Biol Reprod* 71:1397–1404, 2004.

Van Blerkom J: Mitochondria in early mammalian development, *Semin Cell Dev Biol* 20:354–364, 2009.

Wong SL, Wu LL, Robker RL, et al: Hyperglycaemia and lipid differentially impair mouse oocyte developmental competence, *Reprod Fertil Dev* 27:583–592, 2015.

Zackrisson U, Mikuni M, Peterson M, et al: Evidence of the involvement of blood flow regulated mechanisms in the ovulatory process of the rat, *Hum Reprod* 15(2):264–272, 2000.

Zhang C, Bosch MA, Qiu J, et al: 17βEstradiol increases persistent Na+ current and excitability of AVPV/PeN kiss1 neurons in female mice, *Mol Endocrinol* 29:518–527, 2015.

Chapter 26

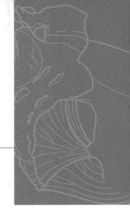

Genetics

Simon Hettle and Jean Rankin

INTRODUCTION

Genetics is the study of inheritance and variation in both individuals and populations and has its origins in curiosity about reproduction and inheritance, including inquisitiveness about both normal and abnormal development – for example, why do certain diseases 'run in families', whereas others do not?

Virtually all pregnant women will want to know if their baby is within the spectrum of that which is regarded as 'normal', and advances in genetics can both help to answer this question and have other great practical benefits in the field of human reproduction – for example, the probability that a child will suffer from a particular genetic disease can be calculated, allowing parents to make informed choices in planning their families; it may be possible, in a few cases, to replace or supplement defective genes so that the diseases they cause can be cured (*gene therapy*); and research into the possible therapeutic use of stem cells is progressing rapidly. Hence it is important that practitioners in this area are aware of both fundamental principles and relevant applications of genetics. There are many ethical questions associated with genetics, and it is also important that these are fully addressed (see Ch. 8).

GENES, CHROMOSOMES AND DNA

A gene is typically defined as a unit of inheritance. Genes are found on chromosomes, which are long, thread-like structures in the nucleus of the cell; each chromosome is made up of one DNA (deoxyribonucleic acid) molecule with many different proteins associated with it. Many genes are arranged throughout its length in a fixed manner, one after the other (Fig. 26.1).

DNA is the major single component of each chromosome and it acts as an information store: all the information necessary for the structure, function, reproduction and development of an organism is stored in a stable and coded form.

The DNA molecule is a long, thin molecule and consists of two strands wound around each other to form a double helix (Fig. 26.2); it is like a ladder in which the two uprights, while still remaining joined together by the rungs, are twisted round each other to form two interweaving spirals. In the DNA molecule, the 'uprights' are made of alternating sugar residues and phosphate groups ('sugar–phosphate backbones') and the 'rungs' are composed of organic bases, each rung consisting of two bases. There are four different bases: two purine bases – *adenine (A)* and *guanine (G)*; and two pyrimidine bases – *cytosine (C)* and *thymine (T)*. Each 'rung' is made up of a pair of bases, one purine and one pyrimidine, and the pairing arrangements in these 'rungs' are very specific:

- Adenine *always* pairs with thymine.
- Guanine *always* pairs with cytosine.

The information stored in DNA needs to be decoded and used to make cellular and organismal components

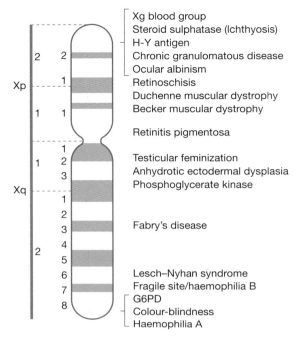

Figure 26.1 Diagrammatic representation of the human X chromosome showing some of the inherited characteristics carried.

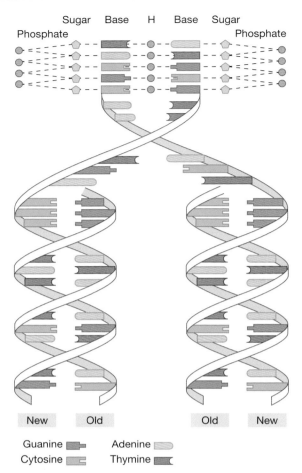

Figure 26.2 Diagram of a DNA double helix, including the process of replication.

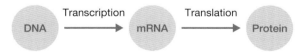

Figure 26.3 Processes involved in the expression of a gene.

(a process known as *gene expression*); most commonly, the stored information in DNA is used to direct the production of proteins. There are thousands of different proteins in the body (e.g. collagen in tendons, haemoglobin in red blood cells), each with its own specific role to play in the body. Any protein is made up of amino acids joined together in a chain. Each protein has its own specific amino acid sequence, which determines its structure and thus its function.

The encoding of information on a DNA molecule is achieved by specifying the precise order (sequence) of the bases along the molecule's length. Information is stored in the form of three-base units (*codons*). Each codon specifies a particular amino acid in a protein. Hence the sequence of bases in a DNA molecule directly determines the sequence of amino acids in a protein and thus the function of that protein. (Another definition of a gene is the part of a DNA molecule containing the series of codons necessary to encode a particular protein.)

The information stored in DNA is decoded using two processes: *transcription* and *translation*. In transcription (which takes place in the nucleus), part of the DNA molecule is used as a template to produce a molecule of messenger RNA (mRNA), and this mRNA then undergoes translation (on the ribosomes in the cytoplasm of the cell)

to produce the protein specified ultimately by the DNA (Fig. 26.3).

Ribonucleic acid (RNA) is the other kind of nucleic acid found in the cell. Unlike DNA, it is single-stranded and contains the pyrimidine base uracil (U) instead of thymine. There are three different forms of RNA in the cell, and all of these are involved in the decoding of information from DNA. These are: mRNA, rRNA (ribosomal RNA – a major component of the ribosome) and tRNA (transfer RNA – crucial in translation as an 'adaptor' molecule between mRNA and protein).

THE HUMAN GENOME

The entire genetic complement of a cell or organism is referred to as its genome. Within a typical human cell, DNA is found in the nucleus and also in the mitochondria (subcellular structures involved in energy production). In the nucleus of all nucleated human cells (apart from the gametes – sex cells – ova and spermatozoa), there are 46 chromosomes; thus, the human genome comprises 46 chromosomes. These chromosomes are arranged in 23 (homologous) pairs, and within each of these pairs, one member is derived from the father, the other from the mother. One of these pairs is the sex chromosomes: in the female, this pair consists of two X chromosomes; in the male, it consists of one X and one Y chromosome. The remaining pairs are collectively known as autosomes, and the chromosomes in this group are numbered by length, with No. 1 being the longest and No. 22 the shortest (see Fig. 26.7).

Each chromosome carries a specific and particular set of genes, and thus each individual carries two copies of any one gene, one copy derived from each parent. Any gene has different forms (or *alleles*). Commonly, a gene has two different alleles. Different alleles produce differences in the appearance (or *phenotype*) of the individual. For example, the form of the chin is controlled by a single gene that has two alleles – one allele causes the chin to be smooth, the other allele causes it to have a midline cleft.

With respect to a gene with two alleles, therefore, an individual can have two copies of one allele, two copies of the other allele (arrangements known as *homozygous*) or one copy of each *(heterozygous)*. (Thus, for the hypothetical gene A with two alleles – A and a – the combinations AA, aa and Aa are possible.) Clearly, an individual who is homozygous for one allele would have the phenotype associated with that particular allele, but what of heterozygous individuals? In this case, typically, the phenotype associated with one allele is observed in the phenotype, whereas that associated with the other allele is absent; thus, one allele *(dominant)* is said to be dominant over the other *(recessive)*.

One outcome from the Human Genome Project is that it is now known that the human nuclear genome contains a total of some 19,000 genes (Ezkurdia et al 2014).

CELL DIVISION

There are two different types of cell division:

- Mitosis, which leads to the production of two daughter cells identical in chromosome number to the parent cell (46 in humans; Fig. 26.4)
- Meiosis, which leads to the production of four daughter cells, with each containing only half the number of chromosomes of the parent cell (23 in humans; Fig. 26.5)

Mitosis occurs extensively during prenatal development to increase cell numbers, in the adult in tissues where cells are routinely lost (such as skin) and in some of the repair processes that occur following tissue damage. Meiosis only occurs during the production of gametes in the gonads. The reduction in chromosome number is essential if sexual reproduction is to take place without doubling the amount of genetic material in each generation. Note that some rearrangement of genetic material can occur during meiosis; this is an important part of the genetic variation that is an essential feature of sexual reproduction (Fig. 26.6).

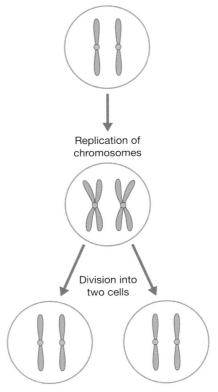

Replication of chromosomes

Division into two cells

Figure 26.4 Mitosis.

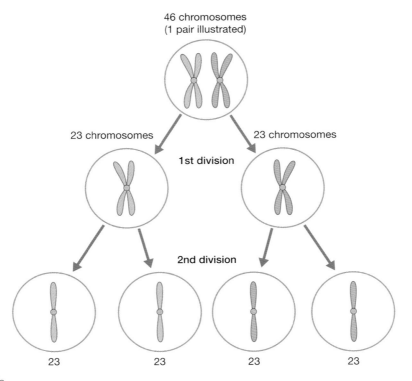

46 chromosomes
(1 pair illustrated)

23 chromosomes   23 chromosomes

1st division

2nd division

23   23   23   23

Figure 26.5 Meiosis.

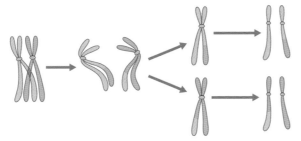

Figure 26.6 Crossover of genetic material in meiosis.

Copying (replication) of DNA occurs during both mitosis and meiosis, and it is very important that this occurs accurately, so that errors are not introduced into the DNA, with possible consequent changes in the structure and function of encoded proteins. One very important way in which this is ensured is by the 'semi-conservative' mechanism of DNA replication: a parental DNA molecule separates into its two component strands, and each of these is then used as a template for the assembly of a new strand. The strict rules of base pairing (A always pairing with T, G with C) ensure that each new double-stranded molecule is an exact copy of the parent molecule (Hartl 2011; see Fig. 26.2).

CHROMOSOMAL ANALYSIS AND ANOMALIES

The study of chromosomes is called cytogenetics. Chromosomes can be isolated from accessible adult tissues (such as lymphocytes from the blood) or from amniotic fluid or chorionic villi when information about the embryo/fetus is required. The process of examining the chromosomes is referred to as *karyotyping*, and it can provide very valuable information about the genome of the cell (Fig. 26.7a and b).

If there is an abnormal number of chromosomes present after fertilization (often as a result of abnormal events during meiosis) or if there is some alteration in structure, the pregnancy may result in miscarriage or an abnormal fetus. Generally, very major abnormalities (for example, involving whole or large pieces of chromosomes) are likely to have very serious effects. It has been shown that the majority of severe chromosomal abnormalities are not compatible with normal development. Embryos with such defects die at an early stage of development – for example, approximately 15% of pregnancies terminate in spontaneous abortion, with about 50% of these being chromosomally abnormal (Lockwood 2000).

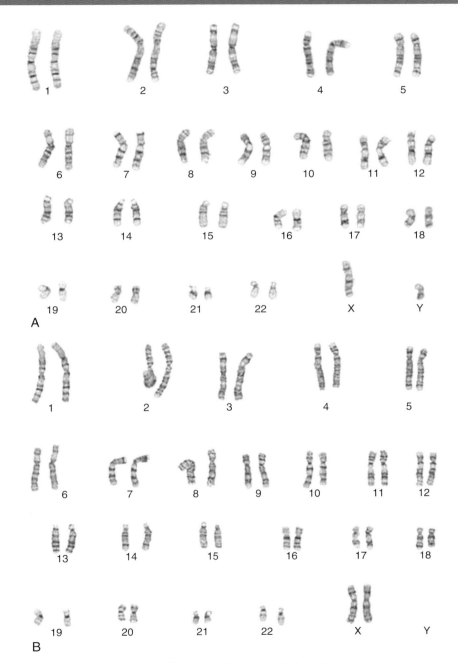

Figure 26.7 **A,** A normal human male karyotype. **B,** A normal human female karyotype.

Types of chromosome abnormalities

Several different types of chromosomal abnormalities are known:

- The presence of three chromosomes of one type is called *trisomy.*
- The presence of only one member of a pair is called *monosomy.*
- A structural change arising from the loss of a chromosome fragment is known as a *deletion.*
- A *translocation* occurs when a chromosome fragment breaks off and is added to another chromosome.
- A *reciprocal translocation* occurs if two chromosomes exchange fragments with each other.

The commonest chromosomal birth anomaly is Down syndrome, where there are 47 chromosomes instead of 46 (termed *trisomy 21* – three copies of chromosome 21; Fig. 26.8a). The incidence is 1.5/1000 live births, and this figure rises with maternal age (Cummings 2006; Hartl 2011). There are only two other examples of trisomies that are consistent with life – trisomy 13 and trisomy 18 – and even in these cases, the defects are many and severe, and affected individuals typically survive for only a short time after birth (Fig. 26.8b and c).

Other common chromosomal anomalies occur among the sex chromosomes; for example, 1.3% of implanted conceptions may carry one X chromosome without a Y or second X (monosomy X, Turner syndrome – the only viable human monosomy; Fig. 26.9). Very few of these fetuses survive – about 0.4 per 1000 live-born girls. More common at birth are other anomalies such as XXX (0.65/1000 girls), XYY, and XXY or XXXY (1.5/1000 boys) – Klinefelter syndrome (Cummings 2006; Hartl 2011; Fig. 26.10). These sex chromosome anomalies, however, generally produce fewer ill effects than the autosomal anomalies, although these effects can still be serious for the affected individual.

Reflective activity 26.2   ><

Arrange to visit a cytogenetics laboratory to observe karyotyping; ask about the processes and what information should be given to parents.

MODES OF INHERITANCE

Genetic characteristics (including genetically determined diseases) can be inherited in one of four principal ways:

- Autosomal dominant inheritance
- Autosomal recessive inheritance
- X-linked dominant inheritance
- X-linked recessive inheritance

Note that the usual patterns of dominance and recessiveness do not apply in the cases of genes carried on the sex chromosomes (see the following discussion).

Common types of genetic disease include the following:

- Enzyme deficiency states ('inborn errors of metabolism'): typically recessive in terms of inheritance, because many metabolic processes can proceed at an adequate rate with reduced levels of enzymes
- Defects in structural proteins (such as in connective tissue): typically dominant in terms of inheritance; reduced levels of these proteins and/or the presence of abnormal protein molecules will often cause pathological effects.

Autosomal characteristics/diseases

Most human genetic diseases are a result of mutations in autosomal genes, simply because there is much more genetic material in total in the 22 pairs of autosomes than in the single pair of sex chromosomes.

A homozygous person can only transmit one type of allele to any child he or she has, whereas a heterozygous person ('carrier') can transmit either of his or her two alleles to a child. Which allele a heterozygous parent transmits in any particular case is a random event, so there is a 1 in 2 (50%) chance of the child inheriting either allele. Thus, the following situations can arise:

- If both parents are homozygous for the same allele (dominant or recessive), then all their children will also inevitably be homozygous for that allele (Fig. 26.11).
- If one parent is homozygous for one allele and the other parent homozygous for the other allele, then all their children will inevitably be heterozygous (Fig. 26.12).
- If both parents are heterozygous, then there is a 1 in 4 (25%) chance of them producing a homozygous recessive child, a 1 in 4 (25%) chance of them producing a homozygous dominant child, and a 2 in 4 (50%) chance of them producing a heterozygous child. Note that in terms of phenotypes, the chance of producing a child of the dominant phenotype is 3 in 4 (75%) and of producing a child of the recessive phenotype is 1 in 4 (25%) (Fig. 26.13).

Thus, although both autosomal dominant and recessive characteristics/diseases occur in both males and females, dominant characteristics tend to be present in each generation, whereas recessive ones are not. This difference arises because a recessive characteristic can only be seen in the

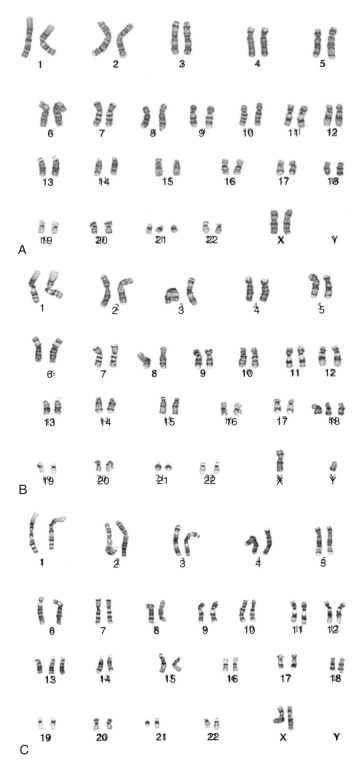

Figure 26.8 **A,** Karyotype of a female patient with Down syndrome (trisomy 21). **B,** Karyotype of a male patient with Edward syndrome (trisomy 18). **C,** Karyotype of a female patient with Patau syndrome (trisomy 13).

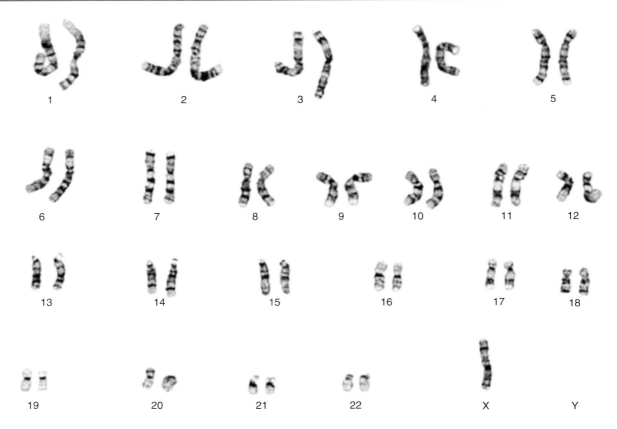

Figure 26.9 Karyotype of a patient with Turner syndrome (monosomy X).

children of a heterozygous parent and either an affected parent or another heterozygous parent. If the particular recessive allele is rare, the probability of this happening is low. In practice, it is often found that parents of an individual affected by a rare recessive characteristic are related to each other (such as first cousins); thus, so-called 'consanguineous unions' are more likely to bring together two heterozygous parents.

If two parents are themselves unaffected and have a child with a recessive characteristic/disorder, it indicates that both of them must be heterozygous. There may then be concern about whether any subsequent child they may have will also be affected. In such a case, it is important to appreciate that the risk of any one particular child suffering from the recessive condition is always 1 in 4 or 25% (Fig. 26.13).

Complications arise with diseases in which the disease process is either very variable in its severity (e.g. myotonic dystrophy) or does not become apparent until later in life (such as Huntington's disease). In the first case, it is possible

for people to have and transmit the disease without suffering any serious ill effects themselves (although subtle signs of such diseases can often be detected); in the second case, many sufferers have had their families before they realize they carry a mutant allele. In either case, parents may unknowingly pass on mutant alleles to their children and thus have several affected children.

Examples of recessively inherited autosomal conditions include phenylketonuria, galactosaemia and cystic fibrosis; examples of dominantly inherited autosomal conditions include achondroplasia, Marfan syndrome and Huntington's disease.

Sex-linked characteristics/diseases

Sex-linked conditions are those for which the relevant genes are carried on the sex chromosomes. They are more complex in their inheritance patterns than are autosomal characteristics because of the genetic difference between males and females.

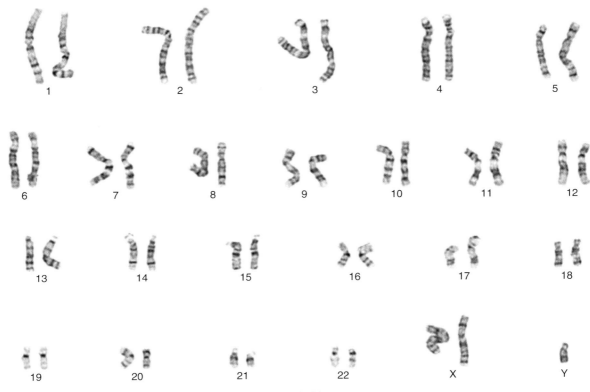

Figure 26.10 Karyotype of a patient with Klinefelter syndrome (XXY).

	Paternal alleles	
Maternal alleles	A	A
A	AA	AA
A	AA	AA

Figure 26.11 Inheritance pattern – two homozygous parents, each carrying the same allele.

	Paternal alleles	
Maternal alleles	A	a
A	AA	aA
a	Aa	aa

Figure 26.13 Inheritance pattern – two heterozygous parents.

	Paternal alleles	
Maternal alleles	A	A
a	Aa	Aa
a	Aa	Aa

Figure 26.12 Inheritance pattern – two homozygous parents, each carrying a different allele.

thus very few Y-linked characteristics. As a result of this, Y-linked characteristics are seldom considered, and the terms 'X-linked' and 'sex-linked' are often used interchangeably.

Only one of the two X chromosomes is active in any cell in a woman's body; the other is inactive (a 'Barr body'). Which X is inactive in any one cell is random and differs throughout the cells of the woman's body.

A very important consequence of the difference in sex chromosome complement between men and women is that men will always exhibit a characteristic resulting from the allele that they carry on their X chromosome because they do not have a second X chromosome. With respect to women, the situation for X-linked characteristics is very similar to that for autosomally determined characteristics: any one woman can be homozygous dominant, homozygous

Obviously, there are genes on both the X and Y chromosomes, and hence both X-linked and Y-linked characteristics are known. Note that the genes carried on the two sex chromosomes are quite different. There are very few genes on the Y chromosome (which is very small), and there are recessive or heterozygous for any gene on the X chromosome. Thus, a woman will only exhibit a recessive X-linked characteristic if she is homozygous recessive. This means that such a woman must be the child of a father who exhibits that characteristic and either a 'carrier' mother or a mother who also exhibits that characteristic, and because these combinations of parents are very rare, such women, too, are very rare.

Both X-linked dominant and recessive characteristics/diseases are known, and their patterns of inheritance can be summarized as follows:

- In X-linked recessive inheritance, there is never male-to-male transmission of the characteristic (because a father must pass on his Y chromosome if the child is to be male) (Fig. 26.14a). Also, as explained earlier, it is most usual to see only males affected by the condition. Thus, this type of disease is most typically carried by women of normal phenotype and affects mostly their sons. A woman who carries such a disease will transmit it (on average) to 1 in 2 of her children – thus, half her sons will be affected and half her daughters will be carriers (Fig. 26.14b). A man who has such a condition will pass on the disease allele whenever he passes on his X chromosome; all his daughters therefore must be carriers (assuming the mother is homozygous for the normal allele), whereas his sons cannot be affected (Fig. 26.14c).

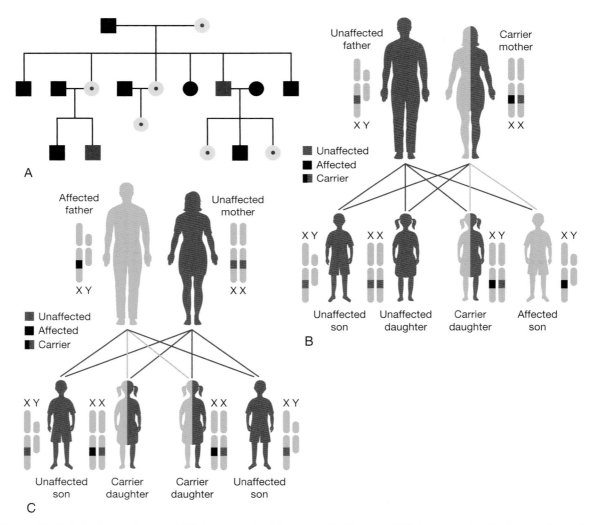

Figure 26.14 A, Pedigree diagram of X-linked recessive inheritance. **B,** Diagram of X-linked recessive inheritance with carrier mother. **C,** Diagram of X-linked recessive inheritance with affected father.

- In X-linked dominant inheritance, because the mutant allele is carried on the X chromosome, an affected male cannot pass it on to his sons, but he must pass it on to all of his daughters, whereas an affected female will pass the mutant allele on to half her sons and half her daughters. Thus, if a father is affected with the disease, only his daughters will be affected (Fig. 26.15a); if a mother is affected, then half of all her children (sons and daughters equally) will be affected (Fig. 26.15b).

Among the best-known examples of X-linked recessive diseases are Duchenne muscular dystrophy, red/green colour-blindness, and the haemophilias. There are only a few X-linked dominant diseases, one example being hypophosphataemic (vitamin D-resistant) rickets.

It is important to note that, in any generation, new mutations can arise during meiosis, and, clearly, the inheritance patterns just described will then not be applicable.

Polygenic and multifactorial characteristics

Many inherited characteristics/diseases are influenced by several genes rather than just one or two. Such characteristics are said to be polygenic (meaning 'many genes'), and the details of their inheritance patterns are often difficult to define precisely because of the interplay between the different alleles of the various genes involved (Cummings 2006).

Polygenic inheritance should not be confused with situations where several genetic disorders can cause the same effect, for example, blindness. There are many different inherited conditions that cause blindness, but most of them are simple autosomal recessive or X-linked conditions with only one mechanism operating.

If environmental factors, such as diet, and genetic ones are both important in determining the precise nature of a physical characteristic or disease process, the characteristic/disorder is said to be *multifactorial* in origin – examples of such disorders include neural tube defects and many cases of cleft lip and/or palate. Most characteristics (for example, height) and diseases (such as atherosclerosis – a very common and serious disease of larger arteries) are, in fact, multifactorial in origin, often involving several genes and several environmental factors. It can prove very difficult to determine the precise risk status of any one individual for any particular condition in such cases because of the large number of different contributory factors involved and the great range of ways in which these can vary.

ORIGIN OF GENETIC DISEASES

In considering inherited disease, the problem arises as to why such conditions exist. New mutational events occur

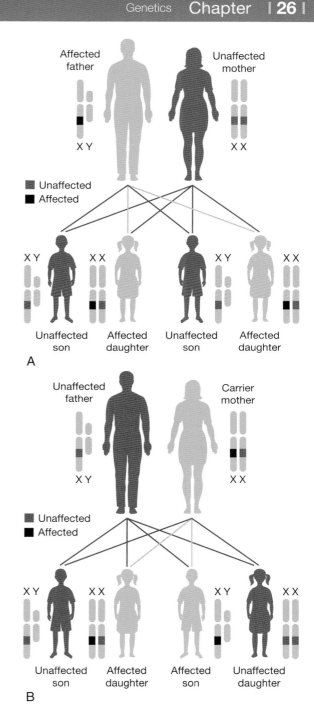

Figure 26.15 **A,** Diagram of X-linked dominant inheritance with affected father. **B,** Diagram of X-linked dominant inheritance with affected mother.

quite frequently – for example, because of errors in DNA replication during cell division or exposure to mutagenic environmental agents, such as various forms of ionizing radiation (e.g. X-rays, ultraviolet light) or mutagenic chemicals (e.g. complex organic molecules in tobacco smoke).

Single new mutations can produce a dominant auto-somal disease or a sex-linked disorder. Recessive disorders, however, cannot be explained so simply because both parents must carry the same mutation for the condition to occur. Rare recessive diseases may be explained by the lack of natural selection against a mutation that causes the heterozygous individual no ill effects, thus allowing the mutation to remain until, eventually, two people carrying the same mutation meet and produce a child who then suffers from the particular disease. There are, however, a number of relatively common recessive autosomal dis-eases (for example, sickle-cell anaemia, cystic fibrosis) for which explanations of their high frequency of occurrence must be found. In general terms, such high frequencies are thought to be explained by the existence of some selective advantage that is peculiar to the 'carrier' (heterozygous individual). In some cases, the precise nature of this advantage has been determined. For example, in the case of sickle-cell anaemia (in which the mutation occurs in the gene for one of the components of the gas transport protein haemoglobin), whereas those people who suffer from this disease (homozygous mutants) often die prema-turely, those who carry one normal allele and one mutant ('sickle-cell') allele show an increased resistance to malaria compared with people carrying two copies of the normal allele. Thus, in malarial areas, because the heterozygous person enjoys a selective survival advantage, the mutant allele is selected for and achieves a high frequency (Hartl 2011). In other cases, the precise nature of the advantage remains to be elucidated – it could be that carriers have some advantage in sexual competition, or that gametes carrying such alleles are somehow preferred, but evidence to support these hypotheses has yet to be produced.

Cummings (2006), Hartl (2011) and Klug et al (2015) provide excellent, more detailed coverage of all the mate-rial discussed thus far. Also, see the chapter website resources for further reference to diagrams, animations and other supporting material.

ASSESSMENT OF EMBRYO AND FETUS

The ability to usefully assess the genetic makeup of the embryo and fetus has improved with further understand-ing of genetic influences on disease. Parental and social expectations of the normal/perfect baby appear greater than ever before. Those involved in providing related care

need to be vigilant to the current developments emerging in this field to appropriately provide up to date informa-tion to women and their partners.

In recent years, the process of prenatal screening and diagnosing genetic disorders has advanced significantly with the advantage of assessing fetal normality earlier in pregnancy. The terms screening and diagnosis need to be differentiated. Screening, defined by the National Screen-ing Committee of the United Kingdom (National Screen-ing Committee of the United Kingdom (NSC) 2013), is 'a process of identifying apparently healthy people who may be at an increased risk of a disease or condition, they can then be offered information, further tests and appropriate treatment to reduce their risk and/or any complications arising from the disease or condition'. In contrast, the term *diagnosis* refers to the definitive confirmation of normality or abnormality as it relates to the situation, condition or disease. Prenatal screening tests are routinely available for pregnant women in line with national standards and screening programmes (National Institute for Health and Clinical Excellence (NICE 2008); National Health Service (NHS) 2013). Although screening tests often reveal the probability or degree of risk associated with the baby having a problem, many of the cases require further spe-cific diagnostic tests to confirm a more definitive diagnosis of fetal abnormality.

GENETIC COUNSELLING/ADVICE

Women and their partners in a higher-risk category are faced with some challenging decisions early in pregnancy or before conception. These individuals will often need opportunities to seek accurate, relevant, up to date infor-mation and also time to consider the options available. This is often provided through genetic counselling involv-ing trained specialists and counsellors. The midwife can also input to this process in a facilitative and sup-portive role.

The role of genetic counselling is to facilitate effective decision making, enabling deliberation on the internal and external factors that individuals need to consider to make the right choice for them and their situation. Exam-ples of internal factors may include personal values and beliefs, previous experiences and expectations of the present pregnancy or subsequent pregnancies; external factors may relate to cultural values, religious beliefs, family and friend influences, economics, education and social circumstances. It cannot be assumed when partners are involved that both parties will hold similar views and beliefs about the expectations for their baby.

Preconception counselling may be conducted in cases of a known or suspected family history of genetic disorders or a previous pregnancy affected by a genetic disorder (such as cystic fibrosis (CF)). This service allows informed decisions to be made regarding family planning. This preconception approach cannot provide absolute certainty that any baby will be disease-free. First, many diseases such as CF can be caused by a large number of different mutations, and it is both technically demanding and very resource intensive to screen for all of these. Second, even if the parents' somatic DNA is shown to be free of mutations, there is always the possibility that a new mutation could arise during gamete formation in one or both parents. However, even with this caveat, the application of molecular genetic research has proven to be of great benefit to families with a history of genetic disease.

In the majority of cases, midwives will become involved in care when meeting women during pregnancy. To facilitate the woman and partner in making informed choices, midwives should provide them with adequate explanations of the processes, risks, benefits, accuracy of the screening tests (including information on false positives/ negatives), outcomes and alternatives for any assessments offered. Other important information should include how far advanced the pregnancy will be before diagnostic tests can be completed and how long it may take for test results to become available (Chapple 2006).

Reflective activity 26.3

Arrange to attend the ultrasound department to observe a prenatal diagnostic test for a potential fetal abnormality (e.g. amniocentesis). Consider both the information requested by women and their partners when discussing the diagnostic tests and results and the information given to them by the obstetrician or midwife.

In what ways will this experience influence how you might provide information to women and partners in similar circumstances?

The key to supporting women and their partners throughout this process relies on acknowledging and respecting their values and beliefs and using communication and interpersonal skills with sensitivity. The midwife can facilitate the woman/couple making an autonomous decision by building a trusting relationship and knowing the woman and partner's expectations and fears.

Effective counselling of women and their partners facilitates them to make the right decisions for them, which includes accepting the consequences. All circumstances need to be handled with sensitivity because some individuals may not have previously considered the possibility of fetal abnormality. Unfortunately, one of the difficulties with effective decision making in pregnancy is the lack of time available to make significant decisions as gestation continues – especially for women who book late in pregnancy.

For a variety of reasons, such as limited family histories and variations observed in severity of a disease process, it can sometimes be difficult to provide clear guidelines as to inheritance, significance of outcomes and the effect(s) on individuals in any one particular counselling situation. With this in mind, any information offered needs to clarify the gaps in knowledge and the advances made in the related field.

Once risk factors have been established, information should be provided on the potential impact on the fetus and baby, including options for treatment, if any, and the nature and course of any possible resultant illnesses. Although advances in medicine have considerably altered the outlook for many conditions (e.g. persons with cystic fibrosis now have a greatly improved life and health expectancy), it is obviously important that advice is realistic, both highlighting the advances made and stressing the drawbacks currently experienced. Often, referral to specialist support groups may be useful at this time.

Equally, it is essential to discuss the impact of tests on the woman with any significant other people in her life because influences might be consequential to the responsibility and acceptance of any decisions made.

Once counselled, women (and their partners) will have decisions to make. The choices open to them may include the following:

- Not becoming pregnant and opting for fostering or adoption
- Utilizing the facilities available for infertility treatments – that is, opting for artificial insemination by donor
- Continuing with the pregnancy and 'hoping for the best'
- Undergoing prenatal diagnostic tests, with the option to:
  - Continue with the pregnancy regardless of outcome
  - Terminate the pregnancy if a positive diagnosis is made
- Utilizing other available alternatives where possible (e.g. stem cell and gene therapy)

The choices available are often complex, and consequently it is crucial that accurate knowledge is available to facilitate the best personal decisions. Case Scenarios 26.1 and 26.2 on the chapter website illustrate situations that may arise.

SCREENING FOR RISK INDICATORS

The primary aim of screening for risk indicators/markers is to provide accurate information to facilitate fully informed decisions about proceeding with diagnostic tests to confirm or exclude a genetic disorder. There are various indicators, and the utility of these in individual cases may depend on available information, previous history, the duration of gestation and parental expectations of normality. Midwives have a major role in prenatal screening programmes, which are now an integral aspect of pregnancy.

History taking

History taking has a key role in planning care for the pregnant woman (and partner). It provides detailed information and an opportunity for relationship building between the woman and the midwife, which, although always important, may be particularly relevant for further decision making. An accurate, detailed personal, family, medical and obstetric history is essential in identifying risk factors that expose the pregnancy to genetic disorders, which should ideally include relevant details of the biological father of the fetus. Sensitivity to the fact that such information is not always available is important, especially where there is no contact with the father, the woman or partner was adopted or where infertility treatment has been used to achieve the pregnancy.

Consideration of racial and/or geographical origins may also be appropriate (such as with Tay–Sachs disease in Ashkenazi Jews, or haemoglobinopathies in women of Mediterranean, African or Asiatic origin). Situations such as consanguinity (relationship by blood and descent from a common ancestor) should also be examined.

Following the history taking, the midwife and woman/partner should consider the need for further screening or testing as appropriate. Before any decisions, it is essential that the woman is aware that further screening or testing may ultimately lead to a decision about keeping or terminating the pregnancy. For some women, this may be unthinkable, and they should be clearly aware of this scenario, whereas for others, having this choice would be essential. Some women may choose to continue with screening anyway, with the view that they would like to know details and prepare for the birth accordingly.

Ultrasound scanning

In the UK, national standards recommend that all pregnant women should be routinely offered two ultrasound scans (USSs) during pregnancy (NSC 2013). The first USS should ideally be carried out at 10 weeks and before 14 weeks gestation. A second USS for detailed structural assessment of fetal abnormalities is offered between 18 and 20 weeks gestation (NICE 2008). For more details about USS, see Ch. 33. In the UK, routine USS in early pregnancy has been used for detection of clinically unsuspected fetal malformations (Whitworth et al 2010). The

early scan may predict a risk of chromosomal abnormality by measuring the amount of fluid behind the neck of the fetus, specifically the nuchal fold thickness. It is measured in millimetres, computer recorded in conjunction with maternal age and used to determine a predictive risk rate. Diagnostic USS may be carried out in a variety of specific circumstances during pregnancy, such as when the fetus is perceived to be at particularly high risk of malformation (NHS 2013).

Biochemical/maternal serum screening

- Alpha-fetoprotein (AFP) serum screening should ideally be carried out around 13 to 14 weeks gestation (see Ch. 33). AFPs are fetal proteins present in maternal serum and amniotic fluid. A raised level of AFPs may indicate intra-uterine death, multiple pregnancies or, most commonly, an open neural tube defect. A lower-than-expected reading may imply a chromosomal abnormality, for example, Down syndrome.
- Enzyme levels can be assayed to detect inborn errors of metabolism. Alpha-fetoprotein and acetylcholinesterase levels can be measured to help identify and distinguish between neural tube defects, anencephaly and ventral wall defects such as gastroschisis and omphalocele that may have been suspected during anomaly scanning. Hormone levels can be assessed to diagnose adrenogenital syndrome.

Biochemical screening tests can utilize combination tests to determine risk factors. They can incorporate serum AFPs, unconjugated oestriol and human chorionic gonadotrophin (hCG), measured with maternal age and weight in relation to gestational age.

Integrated (combined) testing

National guidelines recommend that all women should be offered a combination of tests in the first trimester to determine the risk of the fetus having Down syndrome (NICE 2008). The availability of these tests is improving, but they may not yet be available through all NHS services. The tests comprise nuchal translucency ultrasound scan plus blood tests to measure levels of beta-human chorionic gonadotrophin (β-hCG) and pregnancy-associated plasma protein-A (PAPP-A). These tests should be performed between 11 and 13 weeks and are the most efficient method of detecting Down syndrome (90% compared with 65% with second-trimester serum screening). When necessary, the tests may be repeated between 15 and 20 weeks. The benefit of the 'combined test' is that it would reduce the number of women proceeding to invasive tests. Screening by combining maternal age, nuchal scan and blood biochemistry (for maternal serum free β-hCG and

PAPP-A) gives a pickup rate of over 90% (NICE 2008). Through counselling, women and their partners need to be clear that screening tests alone do not confirm normality of the fetus.

DIAGNOSTIC TESTS

Diagnostic tests are carried out to give definitive results for abnormalities and genetic conditions when required. The procedures usually carry risk factors, and it is important that women/partners are fully informed of these and the potential outcomes before making a decision to proceed with the test. Risks include compromising the ongoing pregnancy, pregnancy loss, getting false-positive or false-negative results and having to face the dilemma of deciding whether to proceed with the pregnancy or choose termination. These choices may be more difficult for some women than for others, depending on their expectations, beliefs and needs for their pregnancy and multiple psychosocial influences.

The purpose of testing is to assess the status of the genome of an individual embryo/fetus. Each individual's genome is unique (with the exception of that of identical twins). To be able to recognize individual sequences of DNA, techniques have been developed to provide methods of analysis for the DNA of an individual. These techniques use genetic probes (which are labelled fragments of DNA) to determine whether a particular DNA sequence is present or absent. Embryonic/fetal genome analysis is only one application of this technology; others include forensic science and paternity disputes.

DNA can be isolated easily from any human cell that is alive and has a nucleus, including buccal cells and skin fibroblasts. The DNA probe is a copy of a relevant sequence that is identifiable and can be used as a 'probe' to hybridize a corresponding copy of the sample.

Preimplantation genetic diagnosis (PGD)

Preimplantation genetic diagnosis (PGD) enables people with an inheritable condition in their family to avoid passing it on to their children. Preimplantation genetic screening (PGS) (also known as aneuploidy/embryo screening) involves checking genes and/or chromosomes of embryos created through in vitro fertilization (IVF) or intracytoplasmic sperm injection (ICSI) for particular genetic disorders, to establish the sex of the embryos (where the disorder is sex linked) and other common abnormalities. Chromosomal abnormalities are a major cause of the failure of embryos to implant and miscarriages, and they can cause conditions such as Down syndrome. PGS remains an experimental intervention and comprises procedures that do not look for a specific disease but are used to identify embryos at risk.

The two major technologies (PGS) used for single-gene cell analysis involve the polymerase chain reaction (PCR – a technique to increase the amount of DNA available for analysis) and fluorescence in-situ hybridization (FISH – the use of fluorescently labelled DNA probes for the detection of single-gene defects). It is not feasible to screen for all possible genetic defects, and each embryo is screened only for those particular genetic defects likely to occur. Following the tests, healthy embryos are implanted into the mother's uterus using techniques developed for infertility treatments. The woman and partner need to carefully consider this technique before conception because it involves extrauterine assessment of the embryo itself. It can confirm with certainty that the embryo is free of the genetic defects (as diagnosed by the particular identification/screening procedure). However, many women fail to achieve a pregnancy after the transfer of good-quality embryos. A systematic review of literature has found insufficient data to determine whether PGS is an effective intervention in IVF/ICSI for improving live-birth rates (Twisk et al 2006).

Comparative genomic hybridization

A small number of clinics are now using a procedure called comparative genomic hybridization (CGH) that allows centres to test for abnormalities in all 23 chromosomes. These abnormalities may or may not be of biological significance, but their presence will lower the chance of finding suitable embryos for transfer.

These types of interventions are fraught with ethical issues, especially from those who believe in the sanctity of human life, including concerns about the numbers of embryos that may perish or become damaged during the process. Currently, PGD appears to be only used for severe/life-threatening disorders, and ongoing work is strictly regulated through the Human Fertilisation and Embryology Authority (HFEA), an independent body overseeing the use of gametes and embryos in fertility and research (see www.hfea.gov.uk).

Chorionic villus sampling

Chorionic villus sampling (CVS) is performed to obtain a biopsy of chorionic tissue from the developing embryo (see Ch. 33). The procedure involves placing a fine catheter/forceps by the transcervical or transabdominal route in conjunction with USS. DNA/cytogenetic analysis for chromosomal studies and some biochemical studies can be performed on the tissue biopsy. CVS should not be carried out before 11 weeks gestation as a precaution to prevent damage to the fetus.

Amniocentesis

Amniocentesis is performed to obtain a sample of amniotic fluid, which contains cells shed from the surface of the fetus and membranes (see Ch. 33). It can be performed at various stages of gestation but is traditionally undertaken between 16 and 18 weeks gestation when maternal age, history or screening indicates a high risk of abnormality. The cells are usually first cultured to determine the fetal karyotype and for detailed DNA analyses (including fetal sexing). The biochemical constituents of the fluid may be tested for nonspecific indicators of abnormality (e.g. AFPs), for the accumulation of specific metabolites in suspected inborn errors of metabolism, or, in later pregnancy, for fetal assessment. The main limitation of the test at this relatively advanced gestational age is the time taken to culture the cells, with results not being available until around 20 weeks gestation (see Ch. 33).

In a systematic review of 14 randomized controlled trials, Alfirevic et al (2003) compared the safety and accuracy of transcervical and transabdominal CVS with early and second-trimester amniocentesis. They concluded that second-trimester amniocentesis is safer than transcervical CVS and early amniocentesis, with transabdominal CVS being preferred when an early diagnosis is required. There appeared to be increased risks of spontaneous miscarriage, pregnancy loss and neonatal talipes associated with earlier amniocentesis compared with CVS. Regarding second-trimester amniocentesis, there was a nonsignificant increase in pregnancy loss of 1% compared with a control group (3% versus 2%), with a significant increase noted in spontaneous miscarriages (2.1% versus 1.3%). Results may occasionally be ambiguous, and there is also a small risk of cells failing to grow or contamination by maternal cells.

Fetoscopy

In fetoscopy, the fetus is observed through a fine fibreoptic telescope, during which samples of tissue may be removed under direct vision for analysis. It may be used to diagnose skin disease, such as epidermolysis bullosa lethalis, by skin biopsy. The technique may be used to perform therapeutic interventions, such as blood transfusion in rhesus incompatibility.

Cordocentesis

Cordocentesis is used to obtain a sample of fetal blood to screen for chromosomal abnormalities, haemophilia and haemoglobinopathies (see Ch. 33). It is carried out using USS to guide a fine needle to the base of the umbilical cord, where a sample of fetal blood is extracted for analysis and/or karyotyping.

All screening and diagnostic tests carry some risks, psychological and/or physical; consequently, the decision to proceed or not needs to be carefully measured. The role of the midwife is to ensure that women and their partners are given the opportunity to make fully informed autonomous decisions.

APPLICATIONS OF GENETICS

The development of molecular genetic techniques in the medical field has already yielded many benefits – for example, production of human insulin by genetically modified bacteria to treat diabetes mellitus (Cummings 2006). It is important to note that there are potential problems associated with genetic modification, and such activities are thus closely regulated by statutory bodies (e.g. Scientific Advisory Committee on Genetic Modification; Health and Safety Executive 2016). Of particular relevance to midwifery is the fact that the manipulation of human gametes is generally internationally prohibited. This is to avoid deliberately and directly changing the overall genetic constitution (the 'gene pool') of the human species, the consequences of such changes being both unpredictable and irreversible. A recent, and highly notable, exception to this occurred in the UK in 2015, where legislation to allow the mitochondrial DNA of an embryo to be manipulated to avoid diseases associated with mutations in this DNA was passed (Wellcome Trust 2015). Generally, the only human cells permitted to be genetically modified are the somatic cells (that is, all cells other than the gametes), and modifications to these cells are tightly regulated.

One of the most obvious applications of genetics in midwifery practice is genetic screening of parents and/or embryos as previously discussed. Recent research in genetics is available from which developments that decrease the morbidity and mortality currently associated with diseases may arise. In applying this research to clinical situations, the emphasis is on both prevention and cure.

Another obvious potential application of molecular genetic research in medicine is to replace or repair missing or defective alleles with normal ones – *gene therapy*. This process involves the insertion of genetic material directly into cells to alter the functioning of those cells (e.g. to allow them to produce the normal, functional version of a protein). Success has been achieved in the treatment of some diseases, such as adenosine deaminase deficiency (Klug et al 2015). However, there have been serious adverse consequences, including one fatality, during gene therapy treatment (Klug et al 2015). Despite technical and safety-related problems regarding gene therapy, this is still an active and potentially promising area of research.

Another possibility is the range of therapeutic options potentially available based on the use of stem cells

– *cell-based regenerative therapies* (National Institutes of Health 2015), which involves not only complex scientific issues but also complex ethical issues. The use of stem cells opens up a wide range of novel therapeutic options, but much work remains to be done, with respect to both the scientific and ethical issues, before these are safely and reliably available in the clinical situation.

Media reports about advances in genetic technologies and their applications are frequent, unsettling and often dramatic. Consequently, parents/prospective parents may have unrealistic expectations in this area, beyond the current limits of these technologies. The innovative approaches may well prove to be of great benefit in due course, but until both relevant complex scientific and/or ethical issues are resolved, they remain potential therapeutic options only. It is therefore important to be aware of what these technologies both can and cannot achieve when dealing with parents/prospective parents.

Finally, there are resource implications to be considered in relation to these technologies, all of which are resource intensive. Even when technology is available, consideration needs to take account of other services and limited allocation of healthcare resources. In this context, it may be possible to argue that the potential financial benefits of having children born free from genetic disease outweigh the cost of providing effective life care for a child/adult suffering from the condition. Nonetheless, this will inevitably have to be balanced with the needs of the general population in resource allocation.

CONCLUSION

The possibilities for the future are potentially profound, and the midwife will need to be aware of the range of new diagnostic and imaging technologies, emerging screening tests and innovative interventions because parents frequently request information following media coverage. For the midwife, this will also include understanding the basis of genetics and the reality of current success in genetic engineering, including the risk:benefit ratios. This area of screening and diagnostic testing is fraught with ethical dilemmas and can involve complex emotional, social and health issues for women during pregnancy. The midwife needs to provide up to date and accurate information to women and their partners in a sensitive way to facilitate and support them to make decisions regarding the best course of action for them.

Key Points

- A good understanding of cell division, chromosomes and diagnostic testing is important when talking to parents whose baby has an abnormality or to potential parents with a family history of genetic disease.

- Midwives require a sound knowledge of genetics and modes of inheritance to identify women and babies who might be at risk and to select the appropriate screening method and recognize when referral is necessary.

- Genetic engineering may have only a limited impact on the role of the midwife at present, but knowledge of the processes and possibilities in this field will become increasingly important in terms of effective communication with women and parents.

References

Alfirevic Z, Sundberg K, Brigham S: Amniocentesis and chorionic villus sampling for prenatal diagnosis, *Cochrane Database Syst Rev* (3):CD003252, 2003. (Reprinted 2007.)

Chapple J: Simplifying antenatal screening: what midwives need to know, *Br J Midwifery* 14(4):193–196, 2006.

Cummings MR: *Human heredity – principles and issues*, 7th edn, Pacific Grove (CA), Thomson/Brooks-Cole, 2006.

Ezkurdia I, Juan D, Rodriguez JM, et al: Multiple evidence strands suggest that there may be as few as 19000 human protein-coding genes, *Hum Mol Genet* 23:5866–5878, 2014.

Hartl DL: *Essential genetics: a genomics perspective*, 5th edn, Burlington (MA), Jones & Bartlett, 2011.

Health and Safety Executive: *Scientific Advisory Committee on Genetic Modification* (website). www.hse.gov.uk. 2016.

Klug WS, Cummings MR, Spencer CA, et al: *Concepts of genetics*, 11th edn,

Upper Saddle River (NJ), Pearson Benjamin Cummings, 2015.

Lockwood CJ: Prediction of pregnancy loss, *Lancet* 355(9212):1292–1293, 2000.

National Institutes of Health: *Stem cell information* (website). www.stemcells.nih.gov/. 2015.

National Health Service (NHS): *Fetal Anomaly Screening Programme (FASP) and population screening* (website). www.gov.uk/guidance/fetalanomalyscreeingprogrammeoverview/. 2013.

National Institute for health and Clinical Excellence (NICE): *Antenatal care – routine care for the healthy pregnant woman. Clinical Guideline 62*, London, NICE, 2008.

National Screening Committee of the United Kingdom (NSC): *NHS Fetal Anomaly Screening Programme. Consent standards and guidance.* Developed by the National Health Service Fetal Anomaly Screening Programme (NHS FASP) Consent Standards Review Group (website). www.screening.nhs.uk. 2013.

Twisk M, Mastenbroek S, van Wely M, et al: Preimplantation genetic screening for abnormal number of chromosomes (aneuploidies) in in vitro fertilization or intracystoplasmic sperm injection, *Cochrane Database Syst Rev* (1):CD005291, 2006.

Wellcome Trust: *Preventing mitochondrial DNA disease* (website). www .wellcome.ac.uk/About-us/ Policy/Spotlight-issues/ Mitochondrial-diseases/index.htm#/. 2015.

Whitworth M, Bricker L, Neilson JP, et al: Ultrasound for fetal assessment in early pregnancy, *Cochrane Database Syst Rev* (4):CD007058, 2010.

Chapter 27

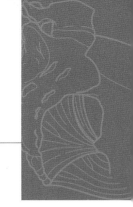

Fertility and its control

Jenny Hall (based on original work by Rosemary Towse)

Learning Outcomes ?

After reading this chapter, you will be able to:

- understand the importance of individual history taking from the woman before offering information and advice
- recognize the influence of the psychological effects of childbearing upon the reactions of the woman and her partner in resuming sexual intercourse and the use of fertility control methods
- understand the physiological principles of each method of fertility control
- evaluate the differing methods of fertility control available to women and their partners, including their advantages and disadvantages and the importance of accurate advice concerning timing of resumption of their use
- discuss the agencies and sources available where a woman and her partner can seek further information and advice

The term *contraception* means 'to prevent conception' and is usually used for a barrier or medicinal method. However, prevention of pregnancy may include methods such as sexual withdrawal or termination of a pregnancy. The control of fertility also does not just involve contraceptive techniques but is also a political issue, with governments worldwide regulating availability and access. The health of women and their families is linked to being able to control their fertility, and therefore midwives and other health professionals have an important contribution to make toward the reproductive and sexual health of women.

Worldwide, 1 in 5 pregnancies ends in abortion. In England and Wales in 2014 the abortion rate was 15.9 per 1000 women aged 15 to 44, the lowest rate for 16 years.

Rates varied from 2.5 for those under 16 years to 28 for 22-year-olds (Department of Health (DH) 2015). Although Britain still has one of the highest rates of teenage pregnancies in Europe, overall there was a one-third reduction over 2004–2014 (Office for National Statistics (ONS) 2014). Recent UK government strategy aims to continue the reduction of conception in younger women by ensuring there is appropriate education and accessibility to contraception (DH 2013: 37).

Although many couples experiencing an unplanned pregnancy will adjust well, for some it may be traumatic. Prevention of pregnancy may be improved by provision of appropriate access to information about contraception and the services available. This chapter covers details of the current methods of fertility control and the midwife's contribution to the contraceptive and sexual healthcare of the mother.

Fertility control advisory services and contraceptives are provided free under the UK National Health Service. Couples or individuals requiring sexual health advice and supplies may go either to their general practitioner (GP) or to a community contraceptive clinic. In some areas there is also a domiciliary service for select clients who, for some reason, are unable to attend the clinics. A variety of clinics may include 'drop-in' services for young people in addition to more specialized specific areas such as psychosexual counselling. Midwives should be aware of the services available locally so that they can advise women and their partners appropriately.

RESUMING SEXUAL RELATIONSHIPS FOLLOWING CHILDBEARING

Women and their partners vary in their approach to resuming physical and sexual contact following childbirth.

413

For some there will have been no change in sexual contact, whereas others will not resume for many months. Adjustment to life with a baby will bring physical and emotional challenges. The type of birth experienced has an effect on timing of resumption, with those who have had interventions such as an assisted vaginal birth, episiotomy or caesarean section less likely to resume until after 6 weeks postpartum (McDonald and Brown 2013). This may be a result of increasing levels of dyspareunia associated with some of these interventions (McDonald et al 2015). Women may have concerns around their body image that will have an effect on their responses, along with the inevitable fatigue accompanying having a new baby (Olsson et al 2005; Hipp et al 2012). Cultural and religious beliefs may also have an impact on parents' choice around resuming intimate activity.

For the father the effects of witnessing a birth can be a highly emotional experience that may be traumatic (Johansson et al 2012). However, there is evidence that partners adapt their sexual behaviour according to the needs of the mother (Olsson et al 2010; MacAdam et al 2011). There is limited research around the effect of birth on same-sex partner sexuality, although a recent study identified that women co-partners are less likely to resume penetrative sex early and more likely to gain support for being a new parent outside their relationship (Van Anders et al 2013). Partners may feel rejected when the baby is establishing a relationship with the mother, and mothers experiencing postnatal depression may find that their satisfaction with the relationship with their partners is reduced. This, in turn, may increase a partner's feelings of guilt and frustration. A midwife's role will include understanding the individual history of the couple, providing opportunity for new parents to discuss their concerns and, where necessary, offering referral to specialist counsellors.

METHODS OF FERTILITY CONTROL

The ideal method

The ideal choice should be an effective, acceptable, simple, painless method or procedure that does not rely on the user's memory (Box 27.1).

Box 27.1 The ideal method

- 100% safe and free from side effects
- 100% effective
- 100% reversible
- Easy to use
- Independent of sexual intercourse
- Used by or obviously visible to the woman
- Independent of the medical profession
- Protective against sexually transmitted diseases
- Acceptable to both partners, all cultures and religions
- Cheap and easy to distribute

Female contraception

Physiological methods

Other terms for physiological methods (Fig. 27.1) include *natural family planning*, *the Billings method* and *fertility awareness*. For some people, particularly in certain religious faiths, this is the only acceptable method of contraception. It involves the woman particularly having knowledge and awareness of how her body functions during her menstrual cycle so that she recognizes the timing of her 'safe period'. This refers to the time during the menstrual cycle when conception is less likely to take place. It is known that ovulation occurs approximately 14 days before the onset of the next menstrual period and that fertilization is possible up to 5 days before and 2 days afterwards. Allowing an extra day either end, intercourse should be avoided for these 10 or 11 days during the cycle.

Theoretically, this is very easy; however, in practice, to determine the exact time of ovulation takes time and patience. It will also depend on the regularity of the woman's menstrual cycle. If the method instructions are followed well, the method is thought to be 99% effective. It is more effective if more than one method of fertility awareness is used, such as measuring temperature changes. Following childbirth, the physiological return of ovulation is different for each woman and difficult to assess, making this method very unreliable in the first few months after childbirth. Various methods have been developed to allow the 'safe period' to be worked out.

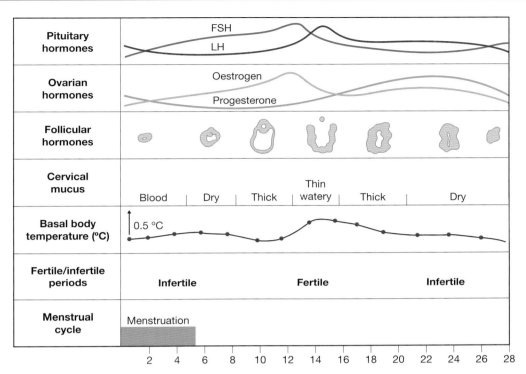

Figure 27.1 Physiological changes within the reproductive system during the menstrual cycle.

The standard days method

The standard days method (SDM) is based on abstinence from unprotected sexual intercourse at the 'fertile time' on days 8 to 19 of every cycle, assuming the woman has a regular cycle of 26 to 32 days.

The 2 day method

The 2 day method is based on recognition and presence of changes in cervical secretions seen by the woman over her monthly cycle. Fertility is assumed when any secretions are present and also the following day.

Both the SDM and the 2 day method have the advantage of being simpler than the traditional calendar, temperature, and Billings methods. They can be used in combination with measuring the woman's basal body temperature. A slightly raised temperature for 3 days may suggest that the fertile time has ended. A researched method becoming popular across Europe is the Sensiplan method, which includes a combination of the methods cited (Frank-Herrmann et al 2007). The suggested success rate is 99.6% for women who have undergone the training programme. However, any woman wanting to use any of these methods following birth must be advised to seek expert help to determine their suitability and ensure correct explanation

of the techniques even if having been familiar with the methods before.

Lactational amenorrhoea method

The lactational amenorrhoea method (LAM) method is thought to be around 99.5% effective for the fully breast-feeding mother in the first 6 months postpartum (National Institute for Health and Clinical Excellence (NICE) 2012a), providing the following criteria are met:

- The mother must be fully breastfeeding, day and night, with no feed supplements; or
- The mother is nearly fully breastfeeding with occasional other liquids; and
- The baby is under 6 months postpartum; and
- The mother should be totally amenorrhoeic. Bleeding in the first 6 weeks postpartum is not included.
- If any of the criteria change, the mother is potentially fertile.

Personal fertility monitors

Personal monitors combine the features of a microlabora-tory and a microcomputer and are designed to enable calculation of the potentially fertile and unfertile parts of the cycle. The device measures levels of luteinizing hormone (LH) and oestrogen breakdown products (E-3-G), by testing the urine with a dipstick that inserts into the machines. The devices then calculate the likely date of ovulation well in advance, and, allowing for sperm survival time, the woman is then shown high or peak days when conception could occur. To provide the machine with sufficient information for these calculations, a number of tests over the woman's cycles are required, which means that other methods to prevent pregnancy should be used. They are only recommended if the cycles are within 23 to 35 days in length.

The monitors may be of limited value immediately following childbirth because they require the woman to have two successive cycles of 23 to 35 days, which makes this method inappropriate for use by breastfeeding mothers. With perfect use, the success rate as a contraceptive tool is around 94% but may be higher (Bouchard and Genuis 2011). In addition, the monitors are also marketed to aid planning a pregnancy, although their effectiveness is underresearched.

Fertility computer 'apps'

With the increasing accessibility of personalized mobile technology, there are a number of 'apps' available for a woman to follow her menstrual cycle. These include some that provide advice on fertility control and around 'safe periods' or 'high risk' of pregnancy. Although these do help to raise awareness of personal fertility, there is minimal evidence of their accuracy in relation to aiding prevention of pregnancy. They should be used with caution, especially in women who have just given birth.

Barrier methods

Occlusive caps

Occlusive caps cover the cervix and mechanically obstruct the entrance of spermatozoa. They are made in a variety of sizes and must be fitted individually. In the UK they are free through general practice or sexual health clinics. Caps are checked for fit at regular intervals, especially after childbirth or weight loss or gain. With correct and conscientious use, the rate of pregnancy can be as low as 6 per 100 woman years, but a more typical rate within the first year of use would be 16 per 100 women (NICE 2012b). Cervical caps are less effective as a contraceptive in multiparous women.

The diaphragm or Dutch cap

The diaphragm or Dutch cap is one of the oldest methods of female contraception and has changed very little in design. A postnatal mother who wishes to use a diaphragm should not be fitted until 6 to 8 weeks postnatally, to allow the uterus and cervix to return to a non-pregnant size and the vaginal muscles to regain their tone. The shallow

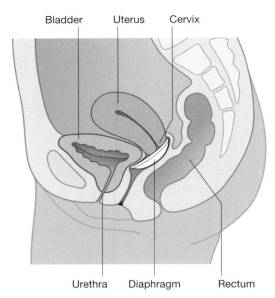

Figure 27.2 Sagittal section of the pelvis showing a diaphragm in position.

rubber or silicone diaphragm has a circular spring around the perimeter, allowing it to be compressed and inserted into the vagina rather like a tampon, with the diaphragm lying between the posterior fornix of the vagina posteriorly and the suprapubic ridge anteriorly (Fig. 27.2). The diaphragms come in graduated sizes and must be fitted individually.

A woman who has used a diaphragm before may require a larger size after childbirth, and this may need adjustment as the vaginal muscle tone improves. A diaphragm that is too large protrudes and causes discomfort, or may produce extra pressure, giving rise to urethritis-type discomfort; however, if too small, it will move around and will not provide protection. A well-fitting diaphragm is unobtrusive and will not be noticed during intercourse. It should remain in situ for 6 hours after intercourse in case ejaculate remains in the vagina and is then removed at a convenient time. Failure rates vary from 6% to 16%, depending on the care and consistency of use, when used with spermicide cream (NICE 2012b).

Other caps

Other types of cap are available that are smaller than the diaphragms and are only marketed now in the UK made from silicone. They rely on suction to remain in place over the cervix along with support from the vaginal wall. The use of spermicide is recommended, and the cap should remain in situ for at least 6 hours after intercourse and be removed before 30 hours (NICE 2012b).

Female condoms

Female condoms are thin plastic tube-shaped condoms consisting of a loose-fitting polyurethane sheath with a flexible ring at either end. The condom is inserted so that it lines the vagina. A soft but firm plastic ring at the entrance covers the genitalia and needs to be steadied in position during intercourse. This condom provides protection both from pregnancy and sexually transmitted diseases, for example, HIV, and may offer protection against cervical cancer (NICE 2012b). It is suggested the rate of pregnancy using this method is 5 in 100 if used perfectly or up to 21 in 100 if the technique is poor (NICE 2012b). Like caps, these condoms can be fitted before sexual intercourse. The female condom contains a spermicide-free lubricant. Because they are made from polyurethane, avoidance of oil-based products is not necessary.

Hormonal contraception

Oral contraception

Millions of women take oral contraceptives worldwide, and oral contraception is the most commonly used form of contraception, especially among young people. The oral contraceptive pill contains either a combination of oestrogen and progestogen (the combined pill, or COC) or progestogen on its own (the progestogen-only pill, or POP). The main controversies concern the risk of venous thromboembolism (VTE) in pill takers. The background risk for VTE in women not taking hormones is 2 per 10,000 in 1 year (Faculty of Sexual and Reproductive Healthcare (FRSH) 2014a), compared with 107 per 100,000 during pregnancy (Royal College of Obstetricians and Gynaecologists (RCOG) 2015). In women taking the COC, the risk varies from 5 to 12 per 10,000, depending on the type of pill (FRSH 2014a). Midwives should always advise any women taking the pill to seek professional advice if they have any concerns before stopping.

Combined pill

The combined pill (COC) acts by suppressing the production of luteinizing hormone (LH) and follicle-stimulating hormone (FSH) from the anterior pituitary gland and thus inhibiting ovulation. It also alters the consistency of the cervical mucus, making it impenetrable to sperm; reduces the motility of the uterine tubes so that the sperm have difficulty in passing along the tube; and causes a change in the endometrium, making it unsuitable for implantation. The latter three back-up mechanisms result from the action of progesterone.

The timing of administration of the combined pill is important to prevent ovulation from occurring. For complete efficiency, the course should begin on the first day of the menstrual period and continue for 21 days. This is followed by 7 days without tablets (or, in some cases, 'dummy' pills), during which time withdrawal bleeding occurs. The rate of conception, when taken correctly, is around 0.3 per 1000 women per year (NICE 2012c). If the woman is taking antibiotics or develops diarrhoea and vomiting, the COC will no longer provide reliable contraception. Other precautions such as condoms should be used during this time and for a further 7 days afterwards.

There are a number of contraindications to COC; women with a personal or family history of medical problems such as hypertension, migraine or venous thromboembolism should seek advice. Although there are some increased risks of use in women aged over 40, women should be assessed on their individual need because age alone does not preclude the use of COC (FRSH 2010a).

After childbirth, the mother who is not breastfeeding may start the combined pill 21 days postpartum. The regimen of 21 days of pills followed by 7 pill-free days is followed. If started on day 21, it is effective immediately. The oestrogen content of the pill is inclined to reduce lactation by suppressing prolactin and is also passed to the baby, albeit in small quantities, in the breastmilk, so the COC pill is not recommended for breastfeeding mothers (NICE 2012c).

Progestogen-only pill

The progestogen-only pill (POP) is an effective method of contraception postpartum and is ideal for breastfeeding women. The progestogen does not affect lactation, and any small quantity passing through the milk is not a problem for babies. The woman commences the POP at 21 days after delivery and takes the tablets continuously from packet to packet without a break (NICE 2015). Women should be advised that progestogen may cause erratic bleeding patterns, but this usually settles after a few months, and the periods may gradually disappear. Breastfeeding women are unlikely to see any bleeding until breastfeeding is stopped.

Progestogen acts by causing cervical mucus to form a natural plug in the cervix, which prevents the sperm entering the uterus and also reduces the motility of the fallopian tubes. In some cases, the progestogen also causes suppression of ovulation (FSRH 2009a).

The reported pregnancy rate with correct use of the POP is 1 per 300 woman years, with rates of 8 out of 100 with typical use. The traditional POP has to be taken within 3 hours of the same time each day, making this an unsuitable method if the woman has a bad memory or an erratic lifestyle. The desogestrel-only pill has a 12-hour leeway for missed pills, similar to the COC. In addition to the normal mode of action, it may prevent ovulation and in many cases cause amenorrhoea, making it a highly effective pill.

Combined transdermal patch

The combined transdermal patch (CTP) is the equivalent of the combined pill, containing oestrogen and progestogen.

The patch is applied to a clean, dry area of skin such as on the abdomen or upper arm. Each patch lasts for 7 days, after which it is replaced, for a total of 3 weeks, followed by a patch-free week. With perfect use, around 0.3 per 100 will become pregnant in the first year, or 8 per 100 with less perfect use (NICE 2012c). The patch is resistant to normal bathing, but some women find detachment of the patch to be a problem. There have been mixed results from studies in relation to the risk of VTE and the CTP. The current view is that the risk of VTE is similar with each combined hormonal product (FRSH 2014a).

Combined vaginal ring

Similar to the CTP, the combined vaginal ring (CVR) contains oestrogen and progestogen; it is placed in the vagina for 3 weeks and then removed for 1 week. During this latter time, a withdrawal bleed will occur, and at the end of the 7 days, a new ring is inserted. It has a failure rate of 1 to 2 per 100 woman years.

Long-acting reversible contraception

The term *long-acting reversible contraception* (LARC) refers to four specific contraceptive methods: intra-uterine contraceptive devices, the intra-uterine system, progesterone injections and implants. These methods are highly effective and do not affect fertility long term. In addition, they are useful for those who have compliance problems with other methods. NICE (2005) recommends that these methods should be discussed with all women who ask for information about contraception.

Intra-uterine contraceptives and intra-uterine systems

Intra-uterine contraceptives (IUCs) have been used all over the world since Biblical times. Currently IUCs are small plastic devices with copper or copper and silver stems that are placed in the uterine cavity by means of a special introducer. The mode of action of IUCs is complex and multifactorial. They act as a sterile foreign body in the uterine cavity, and the resultant physiological action is potentiated by the addition of copper. The copper is thought to have a toxic effect on sperm and ova, preventing fertilization and reducing blastocyst formation (FSRH 2015a). It is rare to find viable sperm in the uterine cavity, making it very unlikely that IUCs ever act as an abortive agent. However, if fertilization has taken place, implantation in the uterus is unlikely to occur because of the considerable change in the endometrium (FRSH 2015a). It is also thought that the device causes some reduction in tubular contraction, thereby reducing the speed of the ovum along the fallopian tube, and there is some evidence of infrequent ovulation while the device is in situ. There may also be an increased production of prostaglandins in the uterus, which increases uterine activity and causes the expulsion of a fertilized ovum. A secondary action of inhibiting implantation is relevant when used as part of emergency contraception. There is no evidence that copper IUCs increase the risk of ectopic pregnancies; however, IUC failure may increase the risk (Searle 2014).

The introduction of an IUC following birth is generally delayed until after 4 weeks postpartum (FRSH 2015a; Searle 2014), when involution of the uterus is likely to be complete. If it is inserted earlier, it may not remain in the optimum position and is more likely to be expelled. However, some trials are indicating IUCs may be successfully inserted immediately after birth, though more research is required (Lopez et al 2015). There do not appear to be any concerns regarding use of IUCs and caesarean section or breastfeeding (Goldstuck and Steyn 2013). In some cases, an IUC is inserted at the time of termination of pregnancy, if requested by the woman.

A number of types of IUC are now available (Fig. 27.3). The GyneFIX, unlike the others, is frameless, consisting of six copper bands threaded onto a length of suture material. One end is provided with a knot, which is inserted into the fundus and acts as an anchor.

An increase in the length and heaviness of menstruation with an IUC may make this an unsuitable method for women who already have menorrhagia. Women with dysmenorrhoea may find the pain is worsened by the introduction of a device for a few months following, but this should settle. Screening for sexually transmitted infection should be carried out before fitting, and women

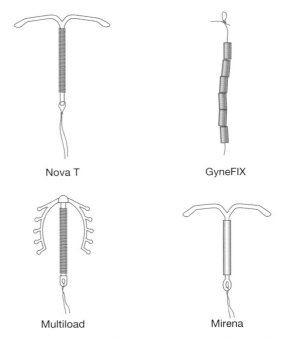

Figure 27.3 Examples of intra-uterine contraceptive devices.

with recurrent infection in the reproductive tract may be advised to use another method (FSRH 2015a).

The devices remain in situ for 5 to 10 years, depending on type, and require only minimal supervision following insertion. They have an excellent record in preventing pregnancy, with a rate of less than 20 in 1000 over 5 years (NICE 2005). If pregnancy does occur when the device is in situ, removal is advised as soon as possible because there is an increased risk of mid-trimester abortion.

Levonorgestrel-releasing intra-uterine system

The levonorgestrel-releasing intra-uterine system (IUS) is a device in which the stem also contains a reservoir of progesterone that is slowly released onto the endometrium. The effects are mostly local, so that ovulation frequently continues to occur. The thickness of the endometrium reduces after 1 month, so that, after an initial few weeks of erratic bleeding episodes, the blood loss diminishes, and amenorrhoea is common (Searle 2014). The progesterone also causes a mucus plug to form in the cervix, which safeguards the uterus from infection and impedes sperm penetration. Following pregnancy, it may be inserted from 4 weeks postpartum. It is advised that alternative contraceptive protection is used for 7 days following insertion unless it has been in the first 7 days of her menstrual cycle or if the woman is breastfeeding and fully following the LAM criteria (FSRH 2015a). Rates of pregnancy over 5 years are less than 1% (Searle 2014). It lasts for 5 years, and, following removal, fertility returns rapidly to normal.

Injectable contraceptives

Injectable contraceptives consist of a progestogen given as a deep intramuscular injection. In the UK the current formulae are Depo medroxyprogesterone acetate (DMPA) and norethisterone enantate (NET-EN). Other combined injectables are being used and researched in other countries but are not licensed in the UK. The primary action is to prevent ovulation, although there are also changes in cervical mucus and prevention of sperm penetration (FRSH 2015b). Changes to the endometrium occur, which may lead to irregular bleeding or amenorrhoea. The latter is less likely with NET-EN. There is no evidence that injectable contraceptives have any detrimental long-term effect on fertility; however, by nature of their mode of action, a return to fertility may be delayed. The average time from the last injection to conception is 1 year (FRSH 2015b). The method has a failure rate of fewer than 4 in 1000 over 2 years, with DMPA having a lower rate than NET-EN.

The injection can be given up to day 5 of the woman's cycle without need of additional protection (NICE 2005). DMPA (150 mg in 1 mL IM) is most commonly used and is repeated at 12-week intervals. NET-EN is given at 8-week intervals. There is a similar product that may be given subcutaneously instead (104 mg in 0.64 mL). It is ideal for those with a poor memory and is often used by women who are unable to take the COC. The injection may be used for those under 18 if there are no other alternatives; however, there are some concerns about the effect on bone mass density (FSRH 2015b). NET-EN (200 mg in 1 mL IM) is less commonly used and is only licensed for women after rubella immunization or when partners have had a vasectomy until there is confirmation of the success of the operation (FSRH 2015b). There is some evidence that use of injections reduces the pain of endometriosis, but there is an association with cervical cancer with use after 5 years (FRSH 2015b). Use after 2 years should be reviewed on an individual basis (NICE 2005).

DMPA can usually be commenced at any time after 21 days postpartum. Some women may experience increased or erratic bleeding patterns with the injection (FSRH 2009b). It does not affect lactation.

Progestogen-only implants

The current progestogen-only implant available in the UK is Nexplanon. It consists of a single rod of etonogestrel (ENG) on a slow-release carrier that also includes barium sulphate to enable detection by X-ray (FSRH 2014b). It is the size of a hair grip and is inserted superficially under the skin of the upper arm using a minor surgical technique and local anaesthetic. The mode of action is by inhibiting ovulation, preventing thickening of the endometrium and increasing the viscosity of the cervical mucus. This regimen has a failure rate of less than 1 out of 1000 women conceiving in the first year of use (FRSH 2014b). For around 50% of women the implant can cause irregular bleeding (NICE 2015), although this often reduces with time, with about 21% becoming amenorrhoeic (FSRH 2014b). The implant can be inserted from day 21 postpartum. The implant lasts for 3 years before needing to be replaced. When removed, fertility returns rapidly.

EMERGENCY CONTRACEPTION

There are various reasons why women may need emergency contraception. These may include unprotected sexual intercourse (no contraception used, failed coitus interruptus, rape), failure of a barrier method (split condoms, dislodged caps), missed pills or injection or expulsion of an IUC. Although some parts of the menstrual cycle may be regarded as low risk for conception, if the woman has irregular periods or is unsure of her dates, no time can be regarded as safe. In practice, therefore, most women who present with such situations will be offered emergency contraception. There are currently three options available in the UK.

Emergency contraception (oral)

The most widely used form is an oral progestogen preparation, which contains levonorgestrel (LNG) (a synthetic derivative of progesterone). This is taken as soon as possible after unprotected sexual intercourse (UPSI) and always within 72 hours. The efficacy of LNG is 97% to 99%, with higher failure the closer to ovulation UPSI takes place (Everett 2014). The pills will only affect the reported episode of UPSI and cannot protect the rest of the cycle. An alternative is oral ulipristal acetate (UPA), which inhibits or prevents ovulation and is a selective progesterone receptor modulator. This is licensed to be used within 120 hours (5 days) of UPSI. LNG is safe for breastfeeding mothers, but it is advised that breastfeeding should be avoided for 36 hours after taking UPA (FRSH 2012).

Oral emergency contraception can be obtained free from contraception clinics, sexual health clinics, GPs, NHS walk-in centres, some pharmacies or accident and emergency departments.

Emergency IUC contraception

A copper intra-uterine contraceptive device may be fitted within 120 hours of UPSI or within 5 days of the probable day of ovulation in that cycle to provide emergency contraception (NICE 2015). Its main mode of action is for the copper to be toxic on the ovum and sperm, preventing fertilization. Although less often used, it is a highly effective method of emergency contraception, with a failure rate of less than 1% (FSRH 2012).

FEMALE STERILIZATION

Tubal ligation or the application of potentially removable clips to the uterine tubes in women and ligation of the vas deferens in men (discussed later) are considered permanent methods of sterilization.

Before these procedures are carried out, it is essential that the couple is carefully counselled, with consideration being given to the psychosocial aspects of the decision and the physical factors involve in the procedure. Most couples accept sterilization without regret, but unless all eventualities have been carefully thought through, later events may lead to regret (Everett 2014). It is suggested that between 0.9% and 26% of women who are sterilized request reversal at a later date (FSRH 2014c), although the success rate is low. The advent of reliable contraceptive methods such as the IUS, which is as reliable as sterilization and yet is removable, is an option for couples who are not totally sure about future plans.

Female sterilization, unless performed at the same time as a caesarean section, is seldom carried out earlier than 6 to 8 weeks after birth, and by that time any problems affecting the baby that could influence the couple's decision are usually evident. The overall failure rate for female sterilization is 1 in 200; however, with the use of a clip, after 10 years it is 1 in 333 to 500 (NICE 2012d), and failure may occur several years after the procedure.

MALE CONTRACEPTION

Coitus interruptus (withdrawal method)

The withdrawal method is used by a large number of couples at some stage in their relationship and is widely used in accordance with some religious beliefs. It is estimated to be the choice of around 2.9% of contraceptive users worldwide (Freundl 2010). It relies on the man withdrawing his penis from the vagina before ejaculation takes place and thus requires control. This may be acceptable to some couples but may affect enjoyment and cause considerable frustration and stress in others. It may also be used alongside other natural methods.

Because of the risk of leakage of seminal fluid before withdrawal, coitus interruptus is not considered a very effective method. It is suggested there is a pregnancy rate of between 4 in 100 to 27 in 100 per year (Freundl 2010). If no other alternative is acceptable, the use of a spermicide pessary or foam would reduce the risk of conception by helping to destroy any sperm released into the vagina before withdrawal.

Condom or sheath

The condom or sheath is probably the most widely used contraception in the first few months after childbirth. It is stated to be between 85% and 98% effective (NICE 2012b). As a barrier method, it not only provides protection against conception but also is effective in preventing the transmission of sexually transmitted diseases, including HIV (Everett 2014). For this reason, many couples use this in addition to other methods, and the regular use of condoms should be encouraged as part of the promotion of safer sex. Condoms, however, cannot protect against local infestations such as scabies and lice. There is evidence that regular condom use may protect against human papillomavirus (HPV) infection, which has a link with cervical neoplasm (Winer et al 2006). However, there should be awareness that this study was related to young women in the early stages of their sexual relationships, and the effect of prevention may not be present for those who have had multiple partners.

In the UK, condoms may be obtained free from contraception or sexual health clinics, some general practice surgeries and young person's clinics or purchased at chemists or other retail outlets, with a wide variety of sizes, textures and flavours being available. Condoms lubricated with spermicide are also available but are not recommended because these are thought to increase the risk of HIV transmission (NICE 2012b). Most condoms are made from latex. Occasionally, men and women report sensitivity to the latex, and condoms made from deproteinized latex, polyurethane, or synthetic polyisoprene may be used.

The midwife should never assume that either partner knows how to use condoms correctly and safely, and if necessary the midwife should be prepared to explain the correct method for using a condom. The golden rules for safe use of condoms include the following:

- Only use condoms with the BSI or CE kite mark.
- Never use after the use-by date.
- Never use if the inner packaging around the condom is damaged.
- Condoms should only be used once.
- Take care with fingernails or rings that might snag the condom.
- Never use with oil-based products because these weaken the latex rubber and may cause it to break (these include baby or bath oil, cold cream, suntan oil, Vaseline, lipstick, aromatherapy oils and massage lotions).
- Vaginal and topical preparations such as Nystatin or other antifungal creams and pessaries and some oestrogen creams may have the same effect as oil-based products.

Following use, in the event of damage or spilling of seminal fluid, unless another contraceptive is already being used, the woman should seek advice from her GP, pharmacist or sexual health clinic regarding the need for emergency contraception.

Future developments

Male hormonal contraception is presently under research. Current trials are mainly using progestogens that inhibit production of follicle-stimulating hormone (FSH) and luteinizing hormone (LH), thus reducing sperm production, with testosterone replacement needed to prevent side effects (Chao et al 2014). Other trials are using androgens, combined with other drugs that induce sperm suppression (Chao et al 2014). The aim is to prevent sperm production while having no effect on ejaculation. Further studies are investigating prevention of sperm maturation, reduction of sperm motility or prevention of fusion of the sperm with the ovum (Chao et al 2014). Apart from the effectiveness of new types of male contraception, there are issues of acceptability to men and whether women would rely on their male partner for contraception of this type (Glasier et al 2000).

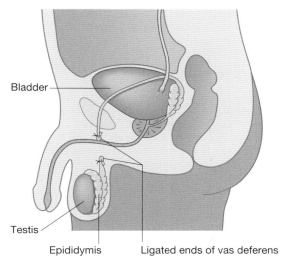

Figure 27.4 Ligation of the vas deferens.

Bladder

Testis

Epididymis   Ligated ends of vas deferens

Vasectomy

Male sterilization involves ligation of both deferent ducts (vas deferens; Fig. 27.4). It is an easier and safer procedure than tubal ligation and can be done as an outpatient procedure under local anaesthetic. Ligation of the deferent ducts prevents the sperm from reaching the seminal vesicle and ejaculatory duct. Because spermatozoa may survive in the ducts for some time, the couple should continue to take contraceptive precautions until two sperm-free specimens of seminal fluid have been produced. This will take a minimum of 3 months. Again, skilled counselling is essential before a final decision is made. The man should understand that sexual desire and activity are not affected by the operation. Despite concerns about an increased risk of testicular cancer after vasectomy, evidence is thought to be causal (FSRH 2014c). The failure rate is 1 in 2000 after clearance (FSRH 2014c).

THE ROLE OF THE MIDWIFE IN THE PROVISION OF CONTRACEPTIVE ADVICE

Many women conceive their first child unintentionally, and although this may result in a wanted child, it is not always possible to adapt well to unplanned parenthood.

Contraception advice is a specialist area, and midwives, while knowing the principles involved, also need to be aware of their limitations and when to refer the woman to a contraception or sexual health clinic. During discussions, the midwife may also detect cues that could highlight the need for specialist referral, help and advice, for example, in cases of medical disorders or where there are signs of psychosexual problems.

Factors to be considered

Discussion of fertility control with a woman and her partner needs to include consideration of a variety of issues that may influence their choice (Box 27.2). By discussing these factors, the midwife will be able to give more accurate advice to the couple about choices available and the best places to obtain contraception or gain further information. The midwife should not assume that the parents have a reliable knowledge of fertility control, and confirming their knowledge before offering advice will quickly indicate if there are misunderstandings to be

---

Box 27.2 Factors that need to be considered when choosing contraception

- Age
- General health
- Smoking
- Obesity
- Lifestyle/employment
- Experiences of family and friends
- General views on contraception
- Cultural or religious constraints
- Previous methods used which failed
- Partner's views
- Obstetric history (e.g. parity or hypertension)
- Level of intelligence/memory
- Ability or willingness to go to a family planning clinic
- Long-term plans for future pregnancies
- Stability of the relationship
- Level of efficacy demanded by the couple from their contraceptive
- Couple's feelings about each type of contraceptive
- What is available
- Any disability that could affect either partner's ability to use a particular method
- Method of infant feeding
- History of menstrual problems (e.g. premenstrual syndrome)
- Views about menstruation
- Characteristics of menstrual periods (i.e. normally 'heavy' or 'light')
- Drugs being taken
- Risk from sexually transmitted diseases

---

addressed. The midwife should appreciate that no prior contraception may have been used. It is important that the parents do not assume they continue with the prepregnancy contraception method without advice.

Reflective activity 27.3

Consider situations you have experienced where some of these factors were significant for the parents in deciding on their choice of contraception.

Timing to start contraception

The return of ovulation following birth varies individually, but evidence suggests that in non-breastfeeding women the earliest possible ovulation occurs around day 28 postpartum, with menstruation potentially returning at week 6 (FSRH 2009b). It is therefore advisable to commence protection before this time. Women who breastfeed their babies on demand are likely to suppress ovulation for a long time (see LAM method described previously). Exactly how long will depend on the suckling of the baby at frequent intervals, including regular night feedings. Babies who vary in their feeding requirements and occasionally sleep through the night will not stimulate enough prolactin to provide control of ovulation. The return of menstruation, when it occurs, indicates retrospective return of ovulation 14 days before. It is therefore important that the woman understands that printed information on packets of hormonal contraceptives does not relate to postpartum situations and that such contraception needs to be commenced independently of menstruation.

When oral contraception is started on day 21 postpartum, it provides full protection from the first day. If commenced later, other precautions such as condoms should be used for the first 7 days. For any sexual intercourse after day 21, some form of contraception should be used. Following a termination or spontaneous abortion, contraception can be started with immediate effect.

SPECIAL GROUPS

Adolescent women

The needs of young people remain one of the biggest challenges for contraceptive services. Despite the current age of consent of sex being 16 years in the UK, about 1 in 3 young people are estimated to have had intercourse by this age (FSRH 2010b). The reasons behind young people having unprotected sexual intercourse are multifactorial and related to personal knowledge and attitudes toward risk taking, contraception and motherhood, along with social and familial influences (Baxter et al 2011; FSRH 2010b). Many young people assume that approaching their GP or attending a contraception clinic will automatically involve information being passed to their parents, and some youngsters will risk a pregnancy rather than seek contraceptive advice. There is often a difference in attitude between girls and boys regarding sexual activity and contraception, with girls more likely to seek help than boys.

For young persons under 16 years of age, no contraception can be given, even condoms, unless they are shown to be Fraser competent. Following the *Gillick* ruling in 1985, the present legal situation is that individuals younger than 16 years old can independently seek medical advice and receive treatment provided they can show that they are competent to do so (see Ch. 9). In contraceptive terms, provided that the prescriber is assured that the young person understands the potential risks and benefits of the treatment/advice being given and believes that the person is likely to have sexual intercourse without contraception, the prescriber is not breaking the law by providing contraception if it is believed that it is in the person's best interest (FSRH 2010b). The value of parental support is always emphasized, and the youngsters are encouraged to talk to their parents about the consultation. All consultations are confidential, regardless of age.

Older women

With an increasing number of women having babies in their forties, contraception for this age group is an important issue. With increasing age, fertility is reduced, dependent on the quality and number of oocytes (FSRH 2010a). This suggests that some of the methods unsuitable for the highly fertile woman may be acceptable in the older woman. However, age alone is not a reason for the choice of contraception (FRSH 2010a). Decisions should be made in relation to the individual health and social needs of the woman. The COC pill can be continued until menopause in the older woman provided that she is not overweight, does not smoke and does not suffer from cardiovascular disease or migraine (FSRH 2010a). However, women over 35 should be advised that the risks of its use outweigh the benefits, and alternatives should be discussed (FSRH 2010a). Progesterone-only contraceptives tend to be recommended more, and IUSs may be particularly useful because they prevent menorrhagia, which is common in older women, and provide protection from endometrial hyperplasia and carcinoma (FSRH 2010a). Barrier methods are also popular, and many women request sterilization.

Medical disorders

Any woman with a long-standing or newly acquired medical disorder needs expert advice in relation to contraception. Some drugs can interfere with the effectiveness of hormonal methods, and some conditions require specialist knowledge. Women with conditions that make childbearing particularly hazardous may request sterilization or at least a highly effective method. Guidance for provision of contraception with medical conditions is provided within the UK Medical Eligibility Criteria for contraceptive use (FSRH 2009c). Midwives should refer parents to appropriate specialist advice and ensure that the woman knows where to seek help before deciding on any particular method of contraception.

Key Points

- Resuming sexual relationships following childbirth can be difficult for some couples.
- Various contraceptive methods are available, including physiological, barrier, hormonal and intra-uterine types.
- Methods vary in their suitability for the individual; therefore, the role of the midwife is to provide information to enable the woman and her partner to make an informed choice.
- The midwife must appreciate the individuality of each woman and her partner, considering age, family spacing and culture, religion and health backgrounds.

References

Baxter S, Blank L, Guillaume L, et al: Views regarding the use of contraception amongst young people in the UK: a systematic review and thematic synthesis, *Eur J Contracept Reprod Health Care* 16(3):149–160, 2011.

Bouchard TP, Genuis SJ: Personal fertility monitors for contraception, *Can Med Assoc J* 183(1):73–76, 2011.

Chao J, Page ST, Anderson RA: Male contraception, *Best Pract Res Clin Obstet Gynaecol* 28(6):845–857, 2014.

Department of Health (DH): *A framework for sexual health improvement in England*, London, 2013, DH.

Department of Health (DH): *Statistical bulletin. Abortion statistics, England and Wales: 2014*, London, DH, 2015.

Everett S: *Handbook of contraception and reproductive and sexual health*, 3rd edn, London, Routledge, 2014.

Faculty of Sexual and Reproductive Healthcare (FSRH): *Progestogen-only pills* (website). www.fsrh.org/pdfs/CEUGuidanceProgestogenOnlyPill09.pdf. 2009a.

Faculty of Sexual and Reproductive Healthcare (FSRH): *Postnatal sexual and reproductive health* (website). www.fsrh.org/pdfs/Ceuguidancepostnatal09.pdf. 2009b.

Faculty of Sexual and Reproductive Healthcare (FSRH): *UK medical eligibility criteria for contraceptive use* (website). www.fsrh.org/pdfs/UKMEC2009.pdf. 2009c.

Faculty of Sexual and Reproductive Healthcare (FSRH): *Contraception for women aged over 40 years* (website). www.fsrh.org/pdfs/ContraceptionOver40July10.pdf. 2010a.

Faculty of Sexual and Reproductive Healthcare (FSRH): *Contraceptive choices or young people* (website). www.fsrh.org/pdfs/ceuGuidanceYoungPeople2010.pdf. 2010b.

Faculty of Sexual and Reproductive Healthcare (FSRH): *Emergency contraception* (website). www.fsrh.org/pdfs/CEUguidanceEmergencyContraception11.pdf. 2012.

Faculty of Sexual and Reproductive Healthcare (FSRH): *Venous thromboembolism (VTE) and hormonal contraception* (website).

www.fsrh.org/pdfs/FSRHStatementVTEandHormonalContraception.pdf. 2014a.

Faculty of Sexual and Reproductive Healthcare (FSRH): *Progestogen-only implants* (website). www.fsrh.org/pdfs/CEUGuidanceProgestogenOnlyImplants.pdf. 2014b.

Faculty of Sexual and Reproductive Healthcare (FSRH): *Male and female sterilisation* (website). www.fsrh.org/pdfs/MaleFemaleSterilisationSummary.pdf. 2014c.

Faculty of Sexual and Reproductive Healthcare (FSRH): *Intrauterine contraception* (website). www.fsrh.org/pdfs/CEUGuidanceIntrauterineContraception.pdf. 2015a.

Faculty of Sexual and Reproductive Healthcare (FSRH): *Progestogen-only injectable contraception* (website). www.fsrh.org/pdfs/CEUGuidanceProgestogenOnlyInjectables.pdf. 2015b.

Frank-Herrmann P, Heil J, Gnoth C, et al: The effectiveness of a fertility awareness based method to avoid pregnancy in relation to a couple's sexual behaviour during the fertile time: a prospective longitudinal study, *Hum Reprod* 22(5):1310–1319, 2007.

Freundl G: Efficacy of natural family planning methods, *Eur J Contracept Reprod Health Care* 15(5):380–381, 2010.

Glasier AF, Anakwe R, Everington D, et al: Would women trust their partners to use a male pill?, *Hum Reprod* 15(3):646–649, 2000.

Goldstuck ND, Steyn PS: Intrauterine contraception after cesarean section and during lactation: a systematic review, *Int J Womens Health* 5:811–818, 2013.

Hipp LE, Kane Low L, van Anders SM: Exploring women's postpartum sexuality: social, psychological, relational, and birth-related contextual factors, *J Sex Med* 9(9):2330–2341, 2012.

Johansson M, Rubertsson C, Rådestad I, et al: Childbirth – an emotionally demanding experience for fathers, *Sex Reprod Healthc* 3(1):11–20, 2012.

Lopez LM, Bernholc A, Hubacher D, et al: Immediate postpartum insertion of intrauterine device for

contraception, *Cochrane Database Syst Rev* 26(6):CD003036, 2015.

MacAdam R, Huuva E, Bertero C: Fathers experiences after having a child: sexuality becomes tailored according to circumstances, *Midwifery* 27(5):e149–e155, 2011.

McDonald EA, Brown SJ: Does method of birth make a difference to when women resume sex after childbirth, *Br J Obstet Gynaecol* 120:823–830, 2013.

McDonald EA, Gartland D, Small R, et al: Dyspareunia and childbirth: a prospective cohort study, *Br J Obstet Gynaecol* 122(5):672–679, 2015.

National Institute for Health and Clinical Excellence (NICE): *Long-acting reversible contraception (update)* (website). www.nice.org.uk/guidance/cg30. 2005.

National Institute for Health and Clinical Excellence (NICE): *CKS: Contraception – natural family planning* (website). http://cks.nice.org.uk/contraception-natural-family-planning#!topicsummary. 2012a.

National Institute for Health and Clinical Excellence (NICE): *Contraception – barrier methods and spermicides* (website). http://cks.nice.org.uk/contraception-barrier-methods-and-spermicides#!scenariorecommendation:8. 2012b.

National Institute for Health and Clinical Excellence (NICE): *Contraception – combined hormonal methods* (website). http://cks.nice.org.uk/contraception-combined-hormonal-methods#!scenariorecommendation:22. 2012c.

National Institute for Health and Clinical Excellence (NICE): *Contraception – sterilization*. http://cks.nice.org.uk/contraception-sterilization#!topicsummary. 2012d.

National Institute for Health and Clinical Excellence (NICE): *Contraception – progestogen-only methods* (website). http://cks.nice.org.uk/contraception-progestogen-only-methods#!topicsummary. 2015.

Office for National Statistics (ONS): *International comparisons of teenage births* (website). www.ons.gov.uk/ons/rel/vsob1/births-by-area-of-

usual-residence-of-mother—england
-and-wales/2012/sty-international-
comparisons-of-teenage-pregnancy.
html. 2014.

Olsson A, Lundqvist M, Faxelid E, et al:
Women's thoughts about sexual life
after childbirth: focus group
discussions with women after
childbirth, *Scand J Caring Sci*
19(4):381–387, 2005.

Olsson A, Robertson E, Björklund A,
et al: Fatherhood in focus, sexual
activity can wait: new fathers'

experience about sexual life after
childbirth, *Scand J Caring Sci*
24(4):716–725, 2010.

Royal College of Obstetricians and
Gynaecologists (RCOG): *Reducing
the risk of venous thromboembolism
during pregnancy and the puerperium:
Green Top Guideline* (website).
www.rcog.org.uk/globalassets/
documents/guidelines/gtg-37a.pdf.
2015.

Searle ES: The intrauterine device
and the intrauterine system, *Best

Pract Res Clin Obstet Gynaecol*
28(6):807–824, 2014.

Van Anders SM, Hipp LE, Kane Low L:
Exploring co-parent experiences of
sexuality in the first 3 months after
birth, *J Sex Med* 10(8):1988–1999,
2013.

Winer RL, Hughes JP, Feng Q, et al:
Condom use and the risk of genital
human papillomavirus infection in
young women, *N Engl J Med*
354(25):2645–2654, 2006.

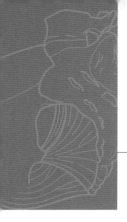

Chapter 28

Infertility and assisted conception

Debbie Barber

Learning Outcomes ?

After reading this chapter, you will be able to:

- understand the causes of female and male infertility
- be aware of the range of investigations and treatment options, including drug regimens and side effects of treatments
- apply understanding of biological functions of fertilization and embryology
- explore the social, physical and emotional impact of infertility and its impact on pregnancy and childbirth
- examine the legal, ethical, socioeconomic and psychological implications both for health professionals and for individuals with fertility issues
- use this knowledge to provide sensitive and individualized care to women and their families

INTRODUCTION

Midwives will frequently care for couples that have received assistance in achieving their pregnancy. It is important to understand the processes they have to go through to become pregnant, which can contribute to the attitudes and anxieties demonstrated by individuals and create greater challenges for the midwifery team. Most couples will have received their fertility treatment in the private sector, and occasionally the transition into normal National Health Service (NHS) care may itself be stressful. This chapter provides a background on the issues related to infertility and the factors contributing to the patients'

approach to their pregnancy. It is useful for midwives to establish links with their local fertility services to provide support and information on patients to ease the transition into their care. Improved networking between fertility nurses and midwives would complement care provided in both areas. Awareness of the range of treatment options and the side effects from treatment provides insight into both the physical and emotional condition of couples requiring midwifery care.

Multiple births are a key issue of concern in both areas of practice, and it is essential that couples understand the risks and the care required when pregnant. Singleton pregnancies with the prevention of twin and triplet pregnancies are the ultimate goal of all fertility clinics, requiring appropriate management and monitoring of treatment. Many nurses and midwives have specialized in fertility, providing care and extending their role to perform ultrasound scanning, intra-uterine insemination, embryo transfer and implications counselling (Barber 2002). Where possible, it is important for midwives and nurses to normalize pregnancies for couples, enabling them to enjoy their much-desired pregnancy.

Technological advances within the field of reproduction have increased public awareness of infertility and demand for related services. Approximately 1 in 6 couples will experience problems conceiving a child (Hull et al 1985; Templeton et al 1990) and will seek assistance to achieve a pregnancy. Since the birth of the world's first 'test-tube baby' over 30 years ago, over 1 million babies have been born in the UK from in vitro fertilization (IVF). Research has highlighted the stigma, psychological morbidity and long-term implications caused by the experience of infertility on couples (Kerr et al 1999), and these factors affect successful and unsuccessful couples. Over 95% of service provision exists within the private sector, thus providing a financial hurdle that couples must overcome before commencing their treatment.

HUMAN FERTILISATION AND EMBRYOLOGY AUTHORITY

The Human Fertilisation and Embryology Authority (HFEA) was created by the 1990 act to license and monitor clinics performing various fertility treatments (including IVF, donated egg/sperm/embryo procedures and research on embryos). All licensed clinics must have a delegated 'person responsible' who ensures that the conditions of the licence are carried out. Several forms of treatment are not controlled by the HFEA but may still potentially create similar problems to licensed treatments, including funding, ovarian hyperstimulation and multiple births. The HFEA carries out annual inspections to enable clinics to renew their licences, which include reviewing the welfare of any potential child, clinical and laboratory standards, protocols for practice in all areas and the safety of patients and their families.

In addition to providing its Code of Practice and information to staff and patients, the HFEA maintains a formal register of information regarding specific donors, donor treatments and children born from these treatments (HFEA 2009). (For more information, see the chapter website resources.)

Reflective activity 28.1

How does regulation affect the delivery and management of care of couples undergoing infertility treatments?

CAUSES OF INFERTILITY

The causes of infertility are presented in Table 28.1.

Anovulation

Anovulation may be diagnosed by the family doctor/general practitioner (GP) and may be corrected by drug therapy to initiate ovulation with an antioestrogen, such as *clomifene* – a common treatment for polycystic ovary syndrome (PCOS). Anovulation must be investigated because it may be caused by pathology, such as hyperprolactinaemia, which could be corrected, and prevent the woman from undergoing fertility treatments.

Elevated levels of prolactin inhibit the normal hormonal feedback loop that initiates ovulation. If serum prolactin is elevated to 1000 mU/L, the test should be repeated. This could be caused by stress or by a prolactin-secreting pituitary adenoma or macroadenomas diagnosed with magnetic resonance imaging (MRI). Treatment includes *bromocriptine* or *cabergoline*, which reduce the

Table 28.1 Main causes of infertility

	Incidence
Anovulation	26%
Endometriosis	3%
Tubal damage	13%
Unexplained	30%
Male factor	30%

Source: Snick et al 1997

Box 28.1 Primary and secondary amenorrhoea

Primary
Congenital abnormalities
Hyperprolactinaemia
Hypogonadotrophic hypogonadism
Hypopituitarism
Polycystic ovary syndrome
Premature ovarian failure
Secondary
Exercise related
Hyperprolactinaemia
Hypogonadotrophic hypogonadism
Hypopituitarism
Polycystic ovary syndrome
Premature ovarian failure

Source: Balen and Jacobs 2014

elevated levels of prolactin and restore normal endocrine activity and facilitate ovulation.

Anovulation can be divided into primary and secondary amenorrhoea – these are primarily caused by pituitary tumours, pituitary ablation, Kallmann syndrome and cancer treatments (see Box 28.1).

Polycystic ovary syndrome

Polycystic ovary syndrome (PCOS) is frequently detected in women undergoing investigations for anovulation (Kousta et al 1999). It is characterized by cystic ovaries with more than 10 cysts, 2 to 8 mm in diameter, distributed around and through an echodense, thickened stroma (Fig. 28.1).

Endocrine features include a raised serum level of luteinizing hormone (LH) and/or testosterone, causing

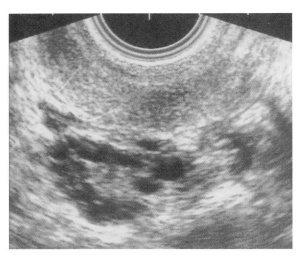

Figure 28.1 Ultrasound scan illustrating a polycystic ovary.

Box 28.2 Signs and symptoms of polycystic ovary syndrome

Obesity
Menstrual disturbance
    Amenorrhoea
    Oligomenorrhoea
Hyperandrogenism
    Acne
    Hirsutism
    Alopecia
Acanthosis nigricans
Endocrine disturbances
    Insulin
    Testosterone
    Androstenedione
    Sex-hormone-binding globulin (SHBG)
    LH
    Prolactin

---

symptoms of acne, hirsutism (hyperandrogenism), oligomenorrhoea and obesity (Box 28.2). The hypersecretion of LH is associated with menstrual irregularity and infertility. Obesity leads to hypersecretion of insulin, stimulating ovarian secretion of androgens, with increased risk of the development of type 2 diabetes (Kousta et al 2000). Anovulation is also associated with endometrial hyperplasia as a result of increased oestrogen production unopposed by progesterone (Balen and Jacobs 2014). Women with a body mass index (BMI) greater than 28 kg/m^2 and less than 20 kg/m^2 will have decreased fertility. There is an associated deficiency in gonadotrophin production with excessive weight loss as a result of diminished production of gonadotrophin-releasing hormone (GnRH).

Ovarian failure

Ovarian failure can happen at any age. If before puberty, it is commonly associated with a chromosomal abnormality, such as Turner syndrome (45X; see Ch. 26), or sterility resulting from radiotherapy or chemotherapy for childhood malignancy. Ovarian failure linked with raised gonadotrophins and cessation of periods before the age of 40 is associated with autoimmune failure, infection, previous surgery and cancer treatments. There is also a suggested link with familial forms of fragile X (Balen and Jacobs 2014).

Endometriosis

Endometriosis is a condition in which endometrial tissue is located outside the uterus, around the pelvis. This may be noted at laparoscopy as blue/black pigmentation (old lesions), red vasculated lesions (active lesions) and white nonpigmented papules (just activating) (Gould 2003). Retrograde menstruation is thought to be the most common cause of endometriosis, but altered immune function is also thought to be associated with the condition. It causes pelvic pain, dyspareunia, dysmenorrhoea and infertility. Pelvic adhesions, especially around the ovaries and tubes, with cystic lesions on the ovaries, called *endometriomas*, are common. Symptoms are linked with the menstrual cycle, age and hormonal therapy; treatments include drugs that interfere with the cycle. One group is the *GnRH agonists*, which cause *pituitary desensitization*, inducing amenorrhoea; another group is inhibitors of gonadotrophin secretion, such as *danazol*, which also have androgenic effects that cause unpleasant side effects, including hot flushes, acne, oily skin, hirsutism, reduced libido, weight gain, nausea and headaches. Both groups of drug temporarily stop menses and reduce levels of antiendometrial autoantibodies (Balen and Jacobs 2014).

Tubal factors

Tubal damage is commonly associated with pelvic inflammatory disease (PID), ectopic pregnancy, sterilization and adhesions. Increases in sexually transmitted diseases increase the risk of PID and tubal damage. Chlamydia is the most frequently reported infection and is often asymptomatic, which increases the risk of cross-contamination and failure to treat (Byrd 1993). Adhesions commonly result following pelvic infection and subsequently create further problems, including distortion and/or blockage of the fallopian tubes; development of hydrosalpinx; impaired tubal motility and movement of the oocyte; and ovarian adhesion against the pelvic sidewall, which may interfere with the movement of the oocyte into the fimbria of the fallopian tube (Dechaud and Hedon 2000), increasing the risk of ectopic pregnancy (see Ch. 53 and chapter website resources).

Unexplained infertility

Unexplained infertility is the inability to conceive after 1 year without any identified causative factors. Approximately 40% to 65% of couples in this category will conceive spontaneously within 3 years (Balen and Jacobs 2014). Age has a direct effect on the duration of time to try to conceive naturally before commencing fertility treatment.

Treatment options consist of improving fertility initially for the woman with drugs to enhance ovulation. Also it is possible to improve sperm function by inseminating prepared sperm into the uterus (intra-uterine insemination (IUI)).

Male infertility

Male factor infertility contributes to 30% of couples seeking treatment. A decline in semen quality over the last few decades has been suggested, although the evidence remains inconclusive, with little scientific knowledge of the aetiology (Shakkebaek and Keiding 1994). A full and comprehensive history of each case is an essential element in the assessment of male fertility and should include the following (Thornton 2000):

- Assessment of previous fertility
- Frequency of intercourse
- Coital difficulties
- Past history of sexually transmitted disease
- History of mumps orchitis
- History of cryptorchidism
- History of scrotal, inguinal, prostatic or bladder neck surgery
- Testicular injury
- Testicular cancer – exposure to gonadotoxic agents (e.g. chemotherapy/radiotherapy)
- Vasectomy

Causes of infertility include the following:

- Undescended testes – most common congenital abnormality, also linked with abnormal spermatogenesis
- Hypogonadotrophic hypogonadism – associated with low levels of follicle-stimulating hormone (FSH) and testosterone and is sometimes linked with Kallmann syndrome
- Cystic fibrosis – gene mutations are strongly related to congenital bilateral absence of the vas deferens

(CBAVD), a defect associated with the bilateral regression of the mesonephric duct
- Testicular failure (increased FSH levels)
- Cryptorchidism – sevenfold increased risk of testicular cancer (Thornton 2000)
- Retrograde ejaculation – congenital or following surgery to either prostate or bladder neck
- Antisperm antibodies – anything that disrupts the normal blood–testes barrier can result in the formation of antisperm antibodies, including the following:
  - Vasectomy and vasectomy reversal
  - Testicular torsion
  - Testicular biopsy
  - Varicocele
  - Inflammatory reactions in the genital tract
  - Infections (orchitis, prostatitis)
  - Congenital absence of the vas deferens (seen in the majority of cystic fibrosis patients)

Tests should include the following:

- Sperm count and analysis (see Table 28.2)
- Endocrine assessment – serum measurements of the following:
  - FSH
  - LH
  - Testosterone
  - Prolactin
- Karyotyping
- Thyroid function screening
- Genetic analysis and cystic fibrosis screening in cases of azoospermia and oligozoospermia (less than 5×10^6/mL):
  - Chromosomal microdeletions – may lead to suboptimal spermatogenesis
  - Chromosomal abnormalities responsible for suboptimal semen parameters, including Klinefelter syndrome (XXY; see Ch. 26)
  - Down syndrome – may cause hypogonadism in males, resulting in azoospermia or subfertility

Various solutions to these problems are available, and micromanipulation techniques, such as intracytoplasmic sperm injection (ICSI), have helped to overcome many male infertility problems (see chapter website resources). Previously, steroids were administered to decrease the male immune response and thus improve chances of fertilization, but now they are rarely used. Environmental factors such as pesticides, alcohol, cigarettes and drug abuse can reduce male fertility, and a decrease in consumption of recreational toxins may sometimes improve semen parameters.

Table 28.2 World Health Organization (WHO) criteria for a normal sperm count

Volume	2 mL or more
pH	7.2 or more
Count	≥20 × 10⁶/mL (Azoospermia is diagnosed when no sperm is found in the ejaculate; oligospermia is diagnosed when the concentration of sperm is vastly reduced.)
Motility	50% or more with forward progression, or 25% or more with rapid progression (within 60 minutes of ejaculation) (abnormal = asthenozoospermia)
Morphology	The 1999 edition of the WHO manual does not define normal ranges for morphology but notes that data from in vitro fertilization (IVF) programmes suggests that as sperm morphology falls below 15% normal forms (teratozoospermia), the fertilization rate decreases.
MAR test (antisperm antibodies)	<50% of motile sperm with adherent particles
Immunobead test (antisperm antibodies)	<50% of motile sperm with adherent beads

Source: WHO 2010

Female infertility – treatment and management

Ovulation induction

There are two types of drug regimens for ovulation induction – the most basic of fertility treatments:

- *Clomifene citrate* – an antioestrogen used to treat PCOS. Dosage is from 50 mg up to 100 mg to induce ovulation. It is taken from day 2 to day 6 of the cycle and should only be prescribed for up to six cycles where the woman has ovulated (Royal College of Obstetricians and Gynaecologists (RCOG) 2014). The drug can cause cervical mucus thickening, headaches and visual disturbances.

- *Gonadotrophin,* commonly subcutaneous *FSH,* to stimulate ovulation. Close monitoring is essential for these women because they are at risk of high-order multiple pregnancy and ovarian hyperstimulation syndrome (OHSS).

OHSS occurs if too many follicles are stimulated during a treatment cycle of ovulation induction (OI), intra-uterine insemination (IUI), or in vitro fertilization (IVF). Because many follicles are stimulated, especially in the case of PCO and PCOS, this causes abdominal ascites, pleural and pericardial effusions, discomfort, nausea, vomiting, difficulty breathing, electrolyte imbalance leading to dehydration and an increased risk of deep vein thrombosis. Ultrasound examination reveals enlargement of the ovaries to a diameter greater than 5 cm (Fig. 28.2).

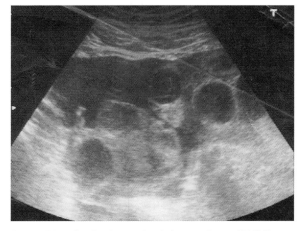

Figure 28.2 Ovarian hyperstimulation syndrome (OHSS).

Donor insemination

Donor insemination (DI) is appropriate for couples with azoospermia, paternal genetic abnormalities or those unable to afford IVF and ICSI, with national success rates of 9.6% per cycle (Thornton 2000). DI is carried out during the woman's own natural cycle or with superovulation. Monitoring with transvaginal ultrasound is undertaken to identify one leading follicle before ovulation and insemination. When more than two leading follicles are stimulated with superovulation, the cycle should be cancelled because of the risk of multiple pregnancy.

Intra-uterine insemination

Intra-uterine insemination (IUI) involves monitored superovulation and insemination of prepared sperm 35 hours after administration of human chorionic gonadotrophin (hCG) to initiate ovulation. The semen may be prepared for insemination using one of a variety of techniques, including sperm *swim-up* and *gradient-density* procedures (see chapter website resources). This treatment is appropriate for slightly suboptimal sperm parameters, unexplained infertility with normal semen parameters and factors such as female age. It does not provide information on potential problems associated with fertilization and has lower success rates than IVF.

Gamete intrafallopian tube transfer

Gamete intrafallopian tube transfer (GIFT) has generally been superseded by IVF, although it is still offered by some clinics. GIFT involves superovulation, following which the oocytes are removed via laparoscopy and a prepared sperm sample is deposited into the fallopian tube to facilitate fertilization. Consequently, this is not suitable for women with tubal damage, and it yields no information on the possible fertilization problems.

In vitro fertilization

Louise Brown was born in 1978 following pioneering work by Steptoe and Edwards, and since that time in vitro fertilization (IVF) has enabled many thousands of couples to achieve a much-desired child. The technique combines superovulation, transvaginal ultrasound-guided oocyte retrieval, insemination of oocyte with sperm in the laboratory, fertilization and replacement of embryos.

Debate surrounds the number of embryos to be replaced in the uterus, but many clinics in the UK routinely replace two embryos, achieving similar pregnancy rates to three-embryo replacements.

Current IVF treatments use daily injections of drugs (gonadotrophins) to induce the development of multiple follicles in the ovaries. The oocytes mature within these follicles, are collected and are fertilized in the laboratory.

Immature eggs from unstimulated ovaries can also be collected, matured in the laboratory for 24–48 hours and, once mature, fertilized before embryo transfer. Hence, oocyte maturation happens in the laboratory rather than the body.

Drug management

Several options are available for drug treatment of infertility (see Table 28.3). Superovulation is achieved with the administration of *FSH* injections – a purified preparation delivered subcutaneously via autoinjector (dosage from

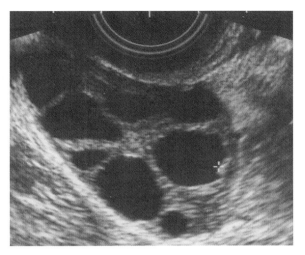

Figure 28.3 Ultrasound scan of a stimulated ovary.

50–350 IU), which recruits a cohort of follicles and promotes development and maturation (Fig. 28.3). To ensure maturation of the follicles and oocytes, administration of *hCG* is required 37 hours before oocyte retrieval.

To establish appropriate management of superovulation and avoid premature ovulation as a result of the LH surge, many units incorporate *GnRH agonists* or antagonists to prevent ovulation (administered either subcutaneously or nasally). These bind to GnRH receptors on the pituitary gonadotrophins and desensitize the pituitary. The antagonists lead to immediate suppression and are used for a much shorter time; they initiate a flare response that causes a withdrawal bleed in the woman.

Oocyte collection

Oocyte collection is undertaken as an outpatient procedure using transvaginal ultrasound (Fig. 28.4). Intravenous sedation reduces levels of pain and anxiety, and the partner can accompany the women throughout the procedure. Follicles are aspirated using gentle suction via a preset vacuum pump into small tubes, which are identified by the embryologist. A microscope is required to identify the cumulus/oocyte mass. Follicles are frequently reinflated with culture medium to encourage recovery of oocytes. Retrieved oocytes are placed in the incubator with appropriate labelling of the dishes and compartment in the incubator and are double witnessed to ensure correct safety procedures.

Sperm preparation

Sperm samples may be collected either before oocyte retrieval or following the procedure, but they should be

431

Table 28.3 Drug treatments for infertility

	Short Protocol	Long Protocol	GnRH Antagonists
Flexibility	Less flexible	Flexible regimen – can be scheduled during working week	Shorter treatment with fewer injections for the woman Currently less favoured drug choice for treatment
Success rates	Lower pregnancy rates	Better pregnancy rates	GnRH prevents LH surge.
Timing for commencement	First half of the cycle designed to use stored FSH	Luteal phase	Within the first half of the cycle
GnRH agonist	Commenced on day 2 Exogenous FSH on day 3	(Inhaled or injected) from day 21 of cycle Pituitary suppression is achieved within 14 days	 Several days of FSH administration precede GnRH
Monitoring	Transvaginal ultrasound to measure the size of the follicles (should be approximately 18 mm) before administration of hCG and then oocyte retrieval Generally lower doses of gonadotrophins are used and the time period is more patient-friendly	Hormone levels are checked for desensitization Once the woman is downregulated, daily injections of FSH to initiate superovulation are commenced. Once there are three follicles of approximately 18 mm, hCG is administrated 35 hours before oocyte retrieval	Once a woman has a leading follicle of approximately 14 mm, the drug is injected daily along with the gonadotrophin

FSH, follicle-stimulating hormone; GnRH, gonadotrophin-releasing hormone; hCG, human chorionic gonadotrophin

prepared within 30 minutes of production. Sperm preparation follows the same procedure as described in the IUI treatment. Semen samples may be frozen and subsequently defrosted for preparation before insemination. After insemination, the spermatozoa and oocytes (Fig. 28.5) are cultured overnight, then, approximately 16 to 18 hours later, are assessed for signs of fertilization and the number and grade of polar bodies extruded from the oocyte. These criteria can also aid in the detection of abnormal fertilization. The appearance of two pronuclei – one each from the sperm and oocyte – signifies normal fertilization. Occasionally, more than two pronuclei are detected, indicating abnormal fertilization, and these embryos should not be transferred.

Fertilization

Fertilization commences when the sperm binds to the zona pellucida of the oocyte (for more information, see Ch. 29 and the chapter website resources).

Embryo grading

Embryos are closely monitored for quality and potential ability to implant and create a pregnancy. Embryo grading is based on visual morphological criteria; it cannot rule out the possibility of a genetic abnormality within the embryo and therefore does not guarantee the selection of a viable embryo for replacement. Preimplantation genetic diagnosis

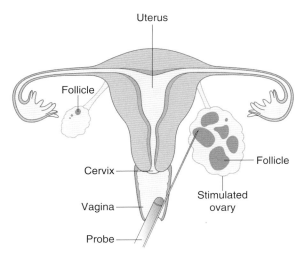

Figure 28.4 Oocyte recovery. (Courtesy of Janet Currie, Sister, Oxford Fertility Unit, Level 4, Women's Centre, Headington, Oxford.)

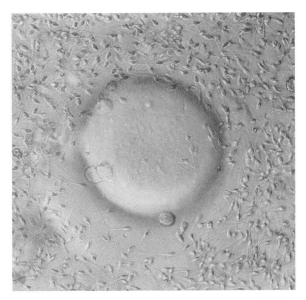

Figure 28.5 Egg and sperm. (Courtesy of Dr Susan Pickering, Senior Lecturer, Division of Women's Health, Kings College, London.)

(PGD) is the only way to identify a potential genetic anomaly, including chromosomal, X-linked, autosomal recessive and dominant and mitochondrial abnormalities (ESHRE PGD Consortium Steering Committee 2000).

For more information on embryo grading, see the chapter website resources.

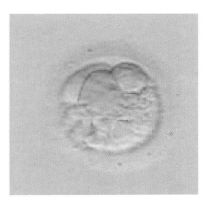

Figure 28.6 Fragmentation. (Courtesy of Dr Susan Pickering, Senior Lecturer, Division of Women's Health, Kings College, London.)

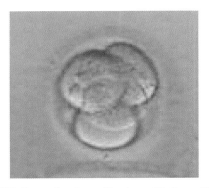

Figure 28.7 Four-cell embryo. (Courtesy of Dr Susan Pickering, Senior Lecturer, Division of Women's Health, Kings College, London.)

Fragmentation

The causes of fragmentation within the embryo (Fig. 28.6) are unknown and have been linked with poor culture conditions and blastomere loss through apoptosis, possibly from chromosomal abnormalities. Whatever the underlying pathology, fragmentation is clearly associated with decreased implantation (Scott 2002). The process of fragmentation has been identified as early as the two-cell stage and continues to develop throughout cleavage.

Embryo transfer

Embryo transfer takes place approximately 48 hours after oocyte recovery. The embryo normally contains several blastomeres at this stage, ranging from two to six in number (Fig. 28.7). Embryos may be cultured for 5 days until they have reached blastocyst stage before returning them into the uterus, but there is no evidence to prove that blastocyst replacement provides better pregnancy rates than do the day-2 transfers.

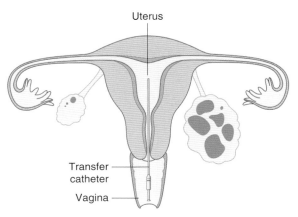

Figure 28.8 Embryo transfer. (Courtesy of Janet Currie, Sister, Oxford Fertility Unit, Level 4, Women's Centre, Headington, Oxford.)

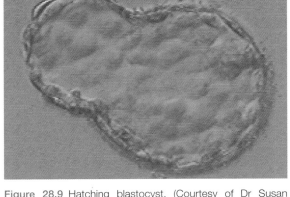

Figure 28.9 Hatching blastocyst. (Courtesy of Dr Susan Pickering, Senior Lecturer, Division of Women's Health, Kings College, London.)

A speculum is inserted into the vagina, and the cervix is wiped with a dry swab to remove excess mucus. The embryos are placed into a fine plastic catheter and passed, sometimes by ultrasound guidance, through the cervix into the endometrium (Fig. 28.8).

If the cervix is convoluted or a tight internal os is encountered, the malleable outer sheath of the catheter is adapted to pass through the obstruction. After embryo replacement, the woman is placed on luteal support to prevent a fall in progesterone levels, which could directly affect the function of the endometrium at this crucial time during potential implantation. Commonly, progesterone pessaries are administered twice daily until the pregnancy test is performed 14 days after embryo transfer. After IVF treatment, the ovaries contain multiple corpora lutea, which remain enlarged for the subsequent few weeks; these may contribute to symptoms of bloating and discomfort, and the woman should be advised of the symptoms.

Blastocyst transfer is another treatment option for couples undergoing IVF treatment. During normal physiological fertilization the sperm fertilizes the oocyte in the fallopian tube, which moves down the tract until it reaches the endometrium around day 5 following fertilization. Blastocyst development has been difficult to achieve in vitro because of inadequate culture media. As technology has developed, improved sequential media have resulted in higher rates of blastocyst development. Embryos are usually replaced on day 2 or 3, which does not correlate with implantation in vivo. Because some embryos will not reach blastocyst stage but look completely normal at the day 2 to 3 stage, it has been suggested that blastocyst transfer enables the embryologist to assess the quality of the embryo for longer and in greater detail, allowing a better choice of embryos with increased implantation

potential (Fig. 28.9). New technology associated with blastocyst transfer has improved success rates, and centres are beginning to replace single blastocysts to maintain good pregnancy rates and decrease the multiple-pregnancy rate. Blastocysts can be frozen to ensure patients can maximize their potential chance of success from a fresh cycle. *Vitrification* – a new technique of ultra-rapid freezing – allows the embryo to be chilled to liquid nitrogen temperatures ($-196\,°C$) in a fraction of a second (Mukaida et al 2006).

In vitro maturation

Women who have polycystic ovaries are most at risk of developing OHSS when undergoing fertility treatment, and *in vitro maturation (IVM)*, which does not require fertility drugs, has been licensed in the UK. Without the superovulation of the ovaries, there is no risk of the syndrome developing. This technique is established internationally, and in 2007 the first babies (twins) were born in the UK.

IVM is appropriate in women with infertility requiring assisted conception, and the success rate is known to be significantly related to the number of immature oocytes retrieved and can be predicted by the antral follicle count (AFC). IVM may be particularly beneficial to women who have an AFC of more than 20. Women with PCOS or with ultrasonographic evidence of polycystic ovaries who are ovulating may be particularly amenable to IVM (Child et al 2001).

Standard IVF involves a lengthy process of pituitary downregulation with GnRH analogues followed by stimulation by gonadotrophins. This process is time consuming, the drugs involved are known to have side effects and the typical cost of drug treatment per cycle is currently around £600–1200. The only drug used in a cycle of IVM is a single injection of *hCG* 35 hours before oocyte collection. IVM has been demonstrated to be an effective treatment for infertile women with polycystic ovaries, although IVF is currently the gold standard treatment for infertility. Approximately 25% to 50% of women attending IVF clinics have PCO or PCOS (Jurema and Nogueira 2006).

There are many women presenting for fertility treatment for whom both treatments may be appropriate. It is essential they have reliable information on which to base their choice of treatment. No randomized controlled trials currently exist that compare IVF and IVM, although there has been a case-control study comparing these methods (see Table 28.4).

There were no cases of OHSS in the IVM group. Severe OHSS occurs in around 1 in a 100 standard IVF cycles and usually requires admission to hospital for a few days.

Severe OHSS is even more common in women who have polycystic ovaries on ultrasound scan or who have PCOS.

Advantages of IVM treatment compared with IVF

Studies from Scandinavian IVM programmes, in which only one or two embryos are transferred, report pregnancy rates in the region of 15% to 25% per cycle, though this is higher (≈30%) for women less than 36 years of age. Approximately 400 babies have been born worldwide from IVM treatment. Recent studies examining the health of these children have been reassuring, showing no increase in rates of abnormality. However, it must be recognized that the number of babies born is still relatively limited (Jurema and Nogueira 2006).

Factors affecting success in IVM treatment

One of the main factors affecting the success rate of IVF treatment, and possibly IVM, is the age of the woman.

The more eggs collected, the more embryos are produced, and the greater the choice of embryos for transfer. The total number of resting follicles measured during a routine ultrasound scan is known as the antral follicle count (AFC; see chapter website resources) and has been shown to be an important predictor of success with IVM. On average, immature eggs are retrieved from half of the antral follicles present. However, as with IVF, there is always the risk that no eggs will be retrieved even when follicles are present or that those that are will not mature, fertilize or produce transfer embryos.

Cryopreservation

The cryostorage of semen, an essential service provided by most assisted conception units, is offered to patients in the following circumstances:

- Undergoing IVF treatment
- Been diagnosed with malignant disease (before chemotherapy and radiotherapy)
- Before potentially damaging pelvic surgery
- Before vasectomy procedure
- Poor-quality semen after vasectomy reversal
- A declining sperm count
- Production difficulties
- Geographical separation of the couple at the time of oocyte retrieval
- When a clean, tested sample is required

The freezing/thaw procedure, however, will damage the cells and may reduce prefreeze motility.

Embryo freezing can be performed provided that enough suitable spare embryos are available post-embryo transfer. Embryos may be frozen at the pronuclear or the

Table 28.4 Comparison of in vitro fertilization (IVF) and in vitro maturation (IVM)

	IVM	IVF
Use as treatment option	New	Well established
Fertilization rate*	77%	78%
Cleavage rate*	95%	94%
Risk of ovarian hyperstimulation syndrome (OHSS)	Reduced	High risk
OHSS rate*	0%	12.1%
Treatment cycles	Shorter	
Treatment	Human chorionic gonadotrophin (hCG) injection only	Daily injections required to stimulate ovaries
Oocytes	Fewer collected and fertilized	
Implantation, clinical pregnancy and live birth rates	Reduced rate – not significant	
Pregnancy rate	Difficult to predict at present	Good success rate

*Data from a case-control study

cleavage stage (two to eight cells) and must be of good quality (grades 1, 2 and 3 or A, B and C), with less than 20% cytoplasmic fragmentation (Dale and Elder 1997) for the best chance of survival following the freeze/thaw procedure. It has been suggested that uneven blastomeres and large amounts of fragmentation could inhibit survival potential.

Cryopreservation of oocytes provides a treatment option for women before cancer treatment that may cause temporary or permanent sterility. Unfortunately, success rates from the use of frozen eggs is very low, and only one baby has been successfully born from this technique in the UK.

Egg donation

In the UK, egg donation is maintained altruistically, primarily by anonymous donors, although occasionally donation from a family member or friend may be offered. This treatment can be used by women following the onset of premature menopause, genetic abnormality or multiple failed IVF attempts.

Because of the national shortage of donated eggs, the National Gamete Donation Trust was established to promote altruistic donation. Many fertility units have long waiting lists for donors and have introduced alternative options, such as egg sharing. This treatment provides reduced-cost IVF treatment to couples willing to donate half of their eggs to another recipient couple. This creates ethical debate, and the HFEA has produced guidelines for good practice and further review of the appropriateness of the treatment for couples (HFEA 2009). Any couple donating eggs must undergo thorough counselling, detailed history taking and investigations, including karyotyping; blood grouping; screening for infections such as hepatitis A, B and C, HIV and syphilis; and cystic fibrosis screening. To donate eggs, the donor undergoes a full IVF cycle, which is time consuming and risky. Those with pre-existing disease and familial cancers are normally dissuaded from donation. Contraindications would include any uncertainty from partners.

Some patients travel overseas to obtain donated eggs, creating further problems for UK professionals because other countries do not have regulatory bodies, such as the HFEA, so there are no restrictions on the number of embryos that can be replaced. This has led to an increase in multiple births in the UK, which has serious consequences for all involved (HFEA 2015). Issues related to treatment abroad include different legislation on management and provision of services. One key issue relates to the anonymity of the donors, which has been removed in the UK. Because most countries in the world do not have the rigorous legislation provided the HFEA, the majority of both international egg and sperm donors remain anonymous. Children born from overseas gamete donation will not be able to trace their biological parents, and

this has been a major concern of the HFEA, which manages the donor register in the UK. Another key difference is the emphasis given to counselling and the psychological preparation for egg and sperm donation in the UK. This service is not consistent throughout the world and can leave prospective parents unprepared and vulnerable while undergoing treatment and once they have achieved their goals for having children (HFEA 2015).

Surrogacy

Surrogacy involves a couple commissioning a woman to act as a host for their own genetic embryo and is a solution for women without a uterus or for whom a pregnancy may be contraindicated. It is illegal in the UK to pay a surrogate, but surrogates may have their expenses paid. In English law, the woman who gives birth to the baby is the legal mother of the child, irrespective of the genetic origin of the child. The genetic parents therefore have to apply to adopt the child from the birth mother, and this may be problematic should she change her mind about giving up her baby.

OUTCOME FROM IVF TREATMENTS

Outcome studies have closely monitored the births and development of children conceived from the techniques. Factors contributing to adverse outcome associated with assisted reproductive technology (ART) include maternal age, medical indications for infertility, paternal age and multiple pregnancies. The ICSI procedure has raised several issues because the process can potentially use sperm carrying genetic abnormalities, structural defects introduced by mechanical or biochemical damage when introducing foreign material into the oocyte and bypassing the natural selection process of fertilization (Kurinczuk 2003). Genetic screening is offered to couples with poor sperm parameters requiring ICSI (see chapter website resources).

Multiple births create further problems with morbidity and mortality of children conceived from ART (Koivurova et al 2002). Women who have IVF are 20 times more likely to have a multiple pregnancy. Approximately 24% of all IVF births are multiple, which means that 40% of IVF babies are twins or triplets (One at a Time 2009). Twins and triplets have increased risks of cerebral palsy, as follows:

- Twins – 13.2 per 1000 confinements – 8 times higher than singletons
- Triplets – 75.9 per 1000 – 47 times higher than singletons (Petterson et al 1993)

Petterson et al (1993) suggested that 1 in 10 pregnant women with twins and 1 in 5 pregnant women with triplets,

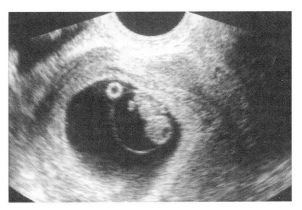

Figure 28.10 Eight-week pregnancy.

whatever the mode of conception, who reach 20 weeks gestation will experience at least one of the following: a child with cerebral palsy, an infant death or stillbirth.

One of the treatment options now offered to couples to alleviate the situation is *multifetal pregnancy reduction* – frequently performed in the United States. Data suggests that surviving twins from the procedure have an eightfold increase of cerebral palsy and an eightfold increased risk of periventricular leukomalacia (Geva et al 1998). The preferred option in the UK is to replace fewer embryos (either two or one) to reduce the incidence of multiple births (Hazekamp et al 2000) (see Fig. 28.10).

The health of the mother may also be affected. Of mothers pregnant with twins, 20% experience hypertension, 30% will develop pre-eclampsia, and they have a 12% risk of developing gestational diabetes, and this increases the likelihood of longer periods of hospitalization during pregnancy together with a negative impact on the family (see Ch. 57).

STRESS AND INFERTILITY

Infertility may have a great impact on an individual's physical and psychological well-being (Hammarberg 2003; Kerr et al 1999; Pfeffer and Woollett 1983). The process of IVF is invasive and time consuming, and it involves intimate procedures, including vaginal ultrasound scanning, transvaginal ultrasound oocyte recovery, embryo transfer, administering injections and producing a sperm sample. Couples frequently feel stigmatized and embarrassed by their infertility, and couples can experience a growing sense of isolation, creating stress and anxiety in their daily lives. Success rates are low, so many couples experience multiple episodes of grief and loss, leading to depression. Emotions described by couples include loss of

self-esteem, mourning, threat, guilt, marital problems and also health problems (Guerra et al 1998).

The costs incurred by IVF treatment are a major stress factor for couples undergoing treatment. The government has initiated a review of fertility treatments by the National Institute of Health and Care Excellence (NICE 2013) that will establish national standards for fertility treatment and end the 'postcode lottery' that currently exists. According to the latest draft, three attempts with fresh embryos and three attempts with frozen provide the best chance of achieving a pregnancy. One in six couples experience problems with fertility in Britain, and between 2010 and 2011 there were 61,726 IVF cycles; 80% of cycles take place in private practice.

Reflective activity 28.2

How would you, as a midwife, help a couple normalize their pregnancy and childbirth experience after fertility treatment?

Counselling is an integral part of the process of fertility treatment, whatever stage a couple may be undergoing, and this is provided throughout the programme independently by licensed units. Mothers who conceive by IVF have higher anxiety levels related to the survival and normality of the unborn babies, damage caused by childbirth and separation from babies after birth compared with matched controls (McMahon et al 1997). Midwife support during pregnancy is crucial to these couples, who may feel more vulnerable than parents who have conceived naturally. It is important for couples to normalize the pregnancy after the intensity of the fertility treatment, and this may be challenging for the team caring for the couples in primary, secondary and tertiary care.

CONCLUSION

Understanding the causes of infertility and the treatment processes is important so the midwife can perceive the degree of stress and the financial burden of assisted conception. Couples who experience difficulty with conception have to deal with the stress, frustration and stigma associated with being infertile. Many undergo treatments that have a low level of success and are not available from the NHS. The whole experience may damage them and their relationships and many will not achieve a long-desired pregnancy. It is important for midwives to understand the processes that couples have undergone to achieve their pregnancy. Many studies have explored the relationship between stress and negative psychosocial factors that affect fertility (Hammarberg et al 2008; Boivin 2003). It is important that individuals are informed and supported before, during and after any fertility treatments, whether basic ovulation induction programmes or highly technical IVF treatments. Published literature has identified that there are potentially increased psychological and emotional needs of successful IVF parents, which influences the support sought from midwives when these parents have transitioned from fertility treatment to antenatal through to postnatal care (Mounce 2009).

Key Points   m—O

- The midwife needs to be aware of the causes of infertility in men and women and all treatment options, including drug regimens and potential side effects.

- Infertility and its treatment can have major long-lasting social, physical and emotional effects on the women and family and their adaptation to pregnancy and childbirth.

- Infertility and its management are carefully regulated in the UK, and the midwife needs to understand current regulations and legislation.

References

Balen A, Jacobs H: *Infertility in practice*, New York, Churchill Livingstone, 2014.

Barber D: The extended role of the fertility nurse – practical realities, *Hum Fertil* 5(1):13–16, 2002.

Boivin J: A review of psychosocial interventions in infertility, *Soc Sci Med* 57:2325–2341, 2003.

Byrd C: Chlamydia trachomatis genital infections, *W V Med J* 89(8):331–333, 1993.

Child T, Adul-Juli A, Huleki B, et al: In vitro maturation of oocytes from unstimulated ovaries, normal ovaries, polycystic ovaries and women with polycystic ovarian syndrome, *Fertil Steril* 76:936–942, 2001.

Dale B, Elder K: *In vitro fertilisation*, Cambridge, Cambridge University Press, 1997.

Dechaud H, Hedon B: What effect does hydrosalpinx have on assisted reproduction? The role of salpingectomy remains controversial, *Hum Reprod* 15(2):234–235, 2000.

ESHRE PGD Consortium Steering Committee: ESHRE Preimplantation Genetic Diagnosis (PGD) Consortium: data collection II (May 2000), *Hum Reprod* 15(12):2673–2683, 2000.

Geva E, Lerner-Geva L, Stavorosky Z, et al: Multifetal pregnancy reduction: a possible risk factor for periventricular leukomalacia in premature newborns, *Fertil Steril* 69(5):845–850, 1998.

Gould D: Women's health – endometriosis, *Nurs Stand* 17(27):47–53, 2003.

Guerra D, Llobera A, Veiga A, et al: Psychiatric morbidity in couples attending a fertility service, *Hum Reprod* 13(6):1733–1736, 1998.

Hammarberg K: Stress in assisted reproductive technology: implications for nursing practice, *Hum Fertil* 6(1):30–33, 2003.

Hammarberg K, Fisher J, Wynter K: Psychological and social aspects of pregnancy, childbirth and early parenting after assisted conception: a systematic review, *Hum Reprod Update* 14(5):395–414, 2008.

Hazekamp J, Bergh C, Wennerholm U, et al: Avoiding multiple pregnancies in ART, *Hum Reprod* 15(6):1217–1219, 2000.

Hull M, Glazener C, Kelly N, et al: Population study of causes, treatment and outcome of infertility, *Br Med J* 291(6510):1693–1697, 1985.

Human Fertilisation and Embryology Authority (HFEA): *Code of practice and guidelines* (website). http://guide .hfea.gov.uk/guide/. 2009.

Human Fertilisation and Embryology Authority (HFEA): *Considering fertility treatment abroad: issues and risks* (website). www.hfea.gov.uk/ fertility-clinics-treatment-abroad .html. 2015.

Jurema M, Nogueira D: In vitro maturation of human oocytes for assisted reproduction, *Fertil Steril* 86(5):1277–1289, 2006.

Kerr J, Brown C, Balen A: The experience of couples who have infertility treatment in the United Kingdom; results of a survey performed in 1997, *Hum Reprod* 14(4):934–938, 1999.

Koivurova S, Hartikainen A, Gissler M, et al: Neonatal outcome and congenital malformations in children born after in-vitro fertilization, *Hum Reprod* 17(5):1391–1398, 2002.

Kousta E, Cela E, Lawrence N, et al: The prevalence of polycystic ovaries in women with a history of gestational diabetes mellitus, *Clin Endocrinol (Oxf)* 53(4):501–507, 2000.

Kousta E, White D, Cela E, et al: The prevalence of polycystic ovaries in women with infertility, *Hum Reprod* 14(11):2720–2723, 1999.

Kurinczuk J: From theory to reality – just what are the data telling us about ICSI offspring health and future fertility and should we be concerned, *Hum Reprod* 18(5):925–931, 2003.

McMahon C, Ungerer J, Beaurepaire J, et al: Anxiety during pregnancy and fetal attachment after in-vitro fertilization, *Hum Reprod* 12(1):176–182, 1997.

Mounce G: Assisted reproduction: what do midwives need to know?, *Midwives Magazine* February/March: 2009.

Mukaida T, Oka T, Goto K, et al: Artificial shrinkage of blastocoels using either a micro needle or a laser pulse prior to the cooling steps of vitrification improves survival rate and pregnancy outcome of vitrified human blastocysts, *Hum Reprod* 21(12):3246–3252, 2006.

National Institute for Health and Care Excellence (NICE): *Assessment and treatment for people with fertility problems*, London, NICE, 2013.

One at a Time (website). www .oneatatime.org.uk/126.htm. 2009.

Petterson B, Nelson K, Watson L, et al: Twins, triplets, and cerebral palsy in births in Western Australia in the 1980's, *Br Med J* 307(6914):1239–1243, 1993.

Pfeffer N, Woollet A: *The experience of infertility*, London, Virago, 1983.

Royal College of Obstetricians and Gynaecologists (RCOG): *Long-term consequences of polycystic ovary syndrome. Guideline No. 33*, London, RCOG, 2014.

Scott L: Embryological strategies for overcoming recurrent assisted reproductive technology treatment failure, *Hum Fertil* 5(4):206–214, 2002.

Shakkebaek K, Keiding N: Changes in semen in the testis, *Br Med J* 309(6965):1316–1317, 1994.

Snick H, Snick T, Evers J, et al: The spontaneous pregnancy prognosis in untreated subfertile couples: the Walcheren primary care study, *Hum Reprod* 12(7):1582–1588, 1997.

Templeton A, Fraser C, Thompson B: The epidemiology of infertility in Aberdeen, *Br Med J* 301(6744):148–152, 1990.

Thornton S: *Infertility in men. Update Postgraduate Centre Series – Infertility*, Amsterdam, Excerpta Medica, 2000.

World Health Organization (WHO): *WHO laboratory manual for the examination and processing of human semen* (5th edn) (website). www.who.int. 2010.

Resources and additional reading

Balen A: Management of infertility, *Br Med J* 335:608, 2007.

Brian K: *The complete guide to IVF*, London, Piatkus, 2009.

Expert Group on Multiple Births After IVF: *One child at a time: reducing multiple births after IVF report*. Human Fertilisation and Embryology Authority (website). www.hfea.gov.uk/docs/ MBSET_report.pdf. 2006.

Van Voorhis BJ: In vitro fertilisation, *N Engl J Med* 356:379–386, 2007.

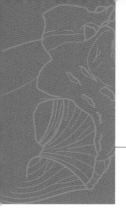

Chapter 29

Fertilization, embryo formation and feto-placental development

Mary McNabb

Learning Outcomes ?

After reading this chapter, you will be able to:

- understand the transport of spermatozoa and the cumulus–oocyte complex within the reproductive tract, and sperm–oocyte interactions during the process of fertilization

- recognize the formative influences on spermatozoa, oocyte and conceptus, of being immersed in the fluid medium of the reproductive tract

- identify the sequence of cell cleavage after fertilization and the interactive signals between blastocyst, endometrium and ovary that regulate attachment and implantation

- appreciate the characteristic features of the endometrium during the brief period of 'receptivity' required for successful attachment, implantation and placental formation

- understand the interactive signals between mother and conceptus that begin before implantation, and the synchronized functional patterns of communication between maternal-placental-fetal neurohormonal systems during fetal growth and development

INTRODUCTION

The hypothalamic-pituitary-gonadal (HPG) axis imposes cyclical variations on female physiology, metabolism and behaviour, to meet the needs of the oocyte selected for ovulation and coordinate cyclical changes in the reproductive tract, and postovulatory follicle, in readiness for fertilization, and the initiation of an interactive dialogue between mother and conceptus before implantation.

After the luteinizing hormones/human chorionic gonadatrophin/follicle-stimulating hormone (LH/hCG/FSH) surge, hormonal signals from the corpus luteum induce extensive adaptations in the maternal renal, cardiovascular, respiratory, metabolic, uterine and mammary systems. When fertilization occurs, these accelerate in response to signals from the conceptus and endometrium. Before and after implantation, paracrine 'cross-talk' between the conceptus, and the endometrium prepares for attachment and implantation; differentiation and elaboration of the trophoblast and subsequent formation of the embryo in a low oxygen environment (Colicchia et al 2014; Evans et al 2015; Fritz et al 2014; Johnson 2013: 207–212; Downs 2008; Leese et al 2008). At the same time, signals are relayed from the conceptus and postovulatory follicle that alter maternal brain sensitivities, modulate the immune response and neuroendocrine regulation of the ovarian, thyroid and adrenal axes (Cole 2010; Lei et al 1993; Lukacs et al 1995).

Taken together, these signals extend the functional lifespan of the corpus luteum; block the development of new ovarian follicles; induce adaptations in maternal thyroid, immune and stress systems; and alter maternal activity, sleep–wake cycles, food preferences and metabolism, to accommodate the fertile cycle (Lei and Rao 1994, Lancel et al 1996). In healthy, well-nourished women, these adaptations meet the distinct requirements of the conceptus and embryo during the first trimester and prepare for very different conditions needed to sustain feto-placental and neonatal development.

This chapter begins with the microenvironment of the reproductive tract where sperms, oocyte and conceptus undergo critical transformations during the first 7 days after ovulation and coitus (Downs 2008). This leads to the processes involved in fertilization that initiate a programme of cell cleavage and result in the formation of a blastocyst, containing two distinct cell types. The chapter follows unfolding events with the first paracrine-neuroendocrine signal from the blastocyst to the endometrium, ovary and maternal brain just before implantation (Cole 2010; Evans et al 2015; Lei and Rao 1994; Lukacs et al 1995). This leads to the interactive processes of attachment and implantation of extraembryonic tissues within the decidua, the elaboration and migration of these trophoblast cells into the uterine vasculature and the formation of other extraembryonic tissues. These make up the *gestational sac* within which embryo formation takes place over the next 6 to 8 weeks of pregnancy (Burton et al 2010; Burton et al 2009; Burton et al 2007; Downs 2008; Johnson 2013: 228–230).

From the events that occur during embryo formation, the chapter moves to the feto-placental phase of pregnancy, with the development of the definitive placenta, feto-placental circulation, and functional dynamics of amniotic fluid, the neuroendocrine regulation of thyroid function and the adreno-placental unit, and the development and maturation of the lungs (DiPietro et al 2004; Ivanov et al 2009; Van Leeuwena et al 2009; Butler and Bronner 2015). During this period maternal-fetal neurohormonal systems function interdependently to synchronize homeostatic functions and circadian rhythms, leading to increased coupling of maternal and fetal psycho-physiological interactions in preparation for labour, birth and attachment (de Groot et al 2003; DiPietro et al 2008; Seron-Ferre et al 2012).

The fallopian tubes

The fallopian tubes provide a critical medium for sperms and oocyte after ovulation. The inner linings and secretions facilitate bidirectional transport of oocyte and spermatozoa, and create favourable conditions for oocyte and sperm maturation, sperm storage, capacitation and fertilization, which initiate successive cleavage of the newly fertilized egg and assist transport of the conceptus towards the designated implantation site in the uterus (Leese et al 2001; Shafik et al 2005) (See Fig. 29.1).

Anatomically part of the uterus, inner layers of the fallopian tubes are continuous with those in the cavity. They are composed of an internal mucosa of ciliated and secretory epithelium, which are sensitive to changes in pituitary gonadotrophins and ovarian steroids, across the cycle (Casan et al 2000; Lei et al 1993). Intermediate layers of smooth muscle contain blood, lymph vessels and steroid-sensitive adrenergic neurons, which regulate fluid formation and coordinate tubular motility for the journey of the conceptus to the uterus (Dickens and Leese 1994; Habayeb et al 2008; Wang et al 2004 and 2006).

Around ovulation, smooth muscles display characteristic movements that bring the *infundibulum*, or distal portion of the tube, into apposition with the ovary that contains the dominant follicle, by a change in orientation of muscles surrounding the ovarian fimbriae (Zervomanolakis et al 2009). One fimbria – slightly longer than the rest – reaches out to the tubal pole of the ovary and involutes, in synchrony with ovulation, to pick up the cumulus-oocyte complex (COC) from the peritoneal cavity and release it into the enlarged trumpet-shaped *infundibulum*, lined with a very dense layer of ciliated secretory epithelium. After fertilization, the conceptus enters the *isthmus*, which has thick mucosal folds and the greatest concentration of

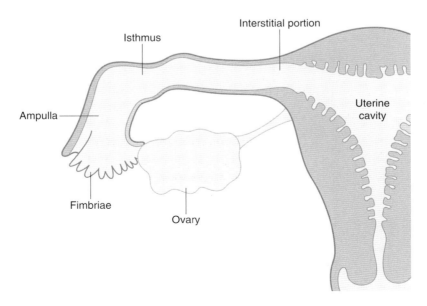

Figure 29.1 Female reproductive tract. (Carlson BM: Human embryology and developmental biology, St. Louis, 1994, Mosby.)

muscle fibres. The diameter increases from 1 to 2 mm at the uterotubal junction, to more than 1 cm at its distal end, with a lumen ranging from 1 to 100 mm (Pauperstein and Eddy 1979: 302).

The *interstitial portion* (see Fig. 29.1) is continuous with the uterine cavity and is characterized by a marked increase in ciliated cells and alterations in the shape of secretory cells. Muscles at the uterotubal junction are formed from four bundles. These hormonally sensitive interlacing spiral fibres allow strong constriction and relaxation of the interstitial portion of the tube. This regulates sperm transport and storage before fertilization and movement of the conceptus towards the uterine cavity when fertilization has been successfully completed (Evans 2002; Kaji and Kudo 2004; Talbot et al 2003; Wildt et al 1998).

Cyclical changes in the epithelial lining

Across the ovarian cycle, the tubular mucosa undergoes cyclical alterations similar to the endometrial lining of the uterus. In the first half of the cycle, secretory and ciliated cells become larger under the influence of oestrogens. Around ovulation, ciliated cells become broader and lower while secretory cells become more distended with fluid.

After ovulation, microscopic holes appear in secretory cell membranes, which coalesce to release secretions accumulated during the first half of the cycle (Hunter 2005).

Higher rates of ciliary movements within the tube on the same side as the dominant follicle are regulated by increased blood flow, higher temperature and higher concentrations of ovarian steroids, compared with the opposite tube (Zervomanolakis et al 2009). Around ovulation, beating of the dense concentration of cilia in the fimbriated portion is closely synchronized, propelling the COC into the ampulla. During this period, cilia in the ampulla also beat in the direction of the isthmus, suggesting that they further propel the COC towards the site of fertilization, taking the newly fertilized egg and surrounding cells from the ampulla and aiding subsequent movements of the conceptus towards the endometrium (Hunter 2005) (see Fig. 29.2).

Cumulus-oocyte-complex

After ovulation, the *cumulus cell mass* remains metabolically coupled to the oocyte through gap junctions. These somatic cells supply the distinct needs of the enclosed oocyte by secreting antioxidants and growth factors and

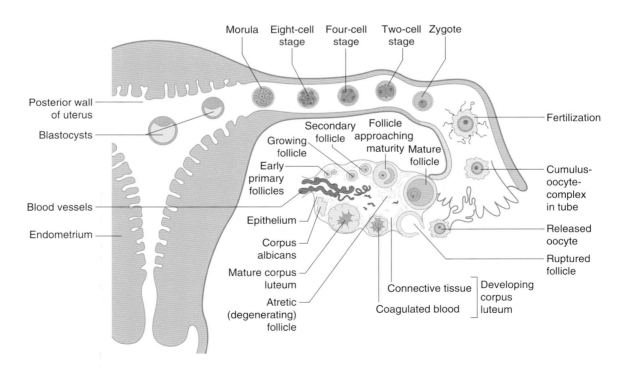

Figure **29.2** The cumulus–oocyte complex and the corpus luteum following ovulation. (This article was published in Tucker Blackburn S: Maternal, fetal and neonatal physiology, 4th edn, Maryland Heights, Elsevier, 2012. Kindle version, Copyright Elsevier, 2014.)

by selective uptake of luminal fluid to provide appropriate amino acids and form pyruvate from glucose. This is essential to limit excess glucose metabolism in the oocyte because of its negative effects on maturation and on cell cleavage after fertilization (Leese et al 2008a). At early cleavage stages, adenosine triphosphate (ATP) production is largely maintained by the oxidation of pyruvate, lactate and amino acids, reflecting a metabolically quiet state that seems to limit the formation of reactive oxygen species (ROS) and the damage they may cause to cellular and molecular processes (Lapointe et al 2005; Leese et al 2008; Leese et al 2008a; Leese 2012). Cumulus cells also activate sperm capitation by mechanisms that include binding with glycoproteins in the luminal fluid in preparation for successful fertilization (Gardner and Leese 1990; Leese et al 2001).

Transport of oocyte and conceptus within the tube is facilitated by:

- presence of cumulus cells around the oocyte and conceptus
- sweeping movements of cilia towards the uterine cavity
- presence of 'pacemaker cells' that induce smooth muscle contractions (Shafik et al 2005)
- oestrogen-induced acceleration of cumulus-oocyte movement within the tube
- LH- and progesterone-induced relaxation of the isthmic–ampullary junction, where fertilization takes place (Johnson 2013: 190–191)
- relaxation of circular muscles of the isthmus by coupling of adrenergic and endocannabinoid signaling to regulate transport through the isthmus–uterine junction (Wang et al 2004).

Sperms within the genital tract

Spermatozoa enter the genital tract in approximately 3 to 4 mL of seminal fluid. This assists in transport; buffers the acidity of vaginal secretions; provides paternal antigens and cytokines that drive events leading to immune tolerance; and supplies growth factors and nutrients that assist in the development of the conceptus (Lenicov et al 2012; Schjenken and Robertson 2014). Over 99% of spermatozoa are immediately lost by leakage from the vagina. Those remaining spend variable times in the cervix, showing differential states of motility and rates of transport through the uterus that may increase the chances of fertilization. The reservoir of spermatozoa in the cervix are actively transported in successive waves of peristalsis to a second sperm reservoir site in the isthmus and finally to the fertilization site at the isthmic–ampullary junction (Bahat et al 2003; Kunz et al 1998; Wildt et al 1998; Zervomanolakis et al 2009).

Cyclical changes in the vaginal canal around ovulation provide a protected environment for ejaculated sperm. This is mirrored by cyclical changes in cervical and vaginal tissues, including relaxation and widening of the cervix, and an increased quantity of cervical mucus, which demonstrates a characteristic 'stretchiness' that facilitates movement of seminal fluid (Drobnis and Overstreet 1992).

Microenvironment of the tubal – uterine lumen

Sperms and oocyte make reverse journeys through the genital tract. Sperms, oocyte and conceptus are composed of avascularized cells that undergo maturational changes and a highly regulated series of cleavage divisions in a fluid medium that differs considerably from plasma (Leese et al 2008; Leese et al 2008a). These cells demonstrate optimal functioning in a relatively cool environment, akin to that in the scrotum and ovarian follicle. The sperm storage site in the isthmus is cooler than the fertilization site in the ampulla. This gradient increases just after ovulation and is thought to maintain sperms in a quiescent state during storage and to guide them from quiescence to hyperactivity in the warmer ampulla. The temperature decline after ovulation also means that both sperms and oocyte are exposed to a cooler environment before the final phase of transport that culminates in fertilization (Leese et al 2008).

In healthy, well-nourished mothers, the composition of tubal and uterine fluids seems to be precisely tailored to meet the changing needs of sperms, oocyte and conceptus from ovulation to implantation. Compared with plasma, this fluid contains elevated levels of bicarbonate and potassium ions, and increased enzymatic defenses against excessive production of reactive oxygen species (ROS). Elevated potassium ions promote sperm quiescence and the development of the oocyte and conceptus by decreasing oxygen consumption and glycolysis, while elevated bicarbonate ions assist the dispersal of coronal cells around the conceptus after fertilization (Leese et al 2008a).

Concentrations of nutrients are different from plasma and vary with cyclical alterations in steroid hormones. A sixfold decline occurs in glucose from the follicular phase to the time of ovulation, and this is coupled with a simultaneous rise in lactate, which serves to limit glucose consumption (Leese et al 2001; Leese et al 2008a). Most amino acids are present in significantly higher concentrations than in plasma, which highlights the wide array of physiological activities they carry out during successive rounds of cell cleavage (Leese et al 2001; Leese 2002). These include protein synthesis, blastocyst formation and hatching, osmoregulation and pH control (Fleming et al 2004; Leese et al 2008).

Maternal nutrition and fluids within the genital tract

The nutritional composition of the fluid medium within the genital tract is directly influenced by maternal nutritional status around conception. In animal and human studies, a low protein diet changes gene expression in the blastocyst, resulting in altered proliferation and implantation of extraembryonic tissues, and persistent, systemic epigenetic changes within the inner cell mass (Eckert et al 2012; Dominguez-Salas et al 2015; Fleming et al 2015). Low protein intake and deficiencies in specific micronutrients around conception induce compensatory development pathways that alter fetal growth, leading to chronic diseases in later life (Leese 2012; Watkins et al 2015).

In studies on women with access to sufficient food, the profile of amino acids in uterine fluid supports healthy formation of the blastocyst, with a low turnover of amino acids. This minimizes mitochondrial (mt) activity and ROS formation and protects mtDNA, which is very unstable and has limited capacity for repair from degradation (Bendich 2010). Significantly, this amino acid profile occurs in women who eat a healthy diet but not among those who eat mainly processed foods and red meat (Bentov 2014; Kermack et al 2015). Together, this evidence indicates that before implantation, the blastocyst has the capacity to detect and respond to maternal nutritional status, from the nutritional profile of uterine fluids, and this information determines the subsequent pattern of implantation and placental formation and programmes fetal growth and development (Fleming et al 2015).

Reflective activity 29.1

Consider recent evidence on the effects of diet around conception. How would you explain the long-term significance of dietary intake to a woman who plans to or has just conceived?

TOWARDS FERTILIZATION – SPERM CAPACITATION

During their active transport through the genital tract, spermatozoa undergo a final series of maturational changes before a small number are ready for fertilization. The first of these is *capacitation*, caused by interactions between spermatozoa and glandular secretions of the cervix, uterus and fallopian tube during their journey to the site of fertilization. Capacitation occurs when most glycoprotein molecules added during ejaculation are removed from the cell membrane. Capitation seems to induce hyperactive motility, providing increased thrusting

power and alterations in cell surface properties, enabling entry to the zona pellucida surrounding the oocyte cell membrane (Drobnis and Overstreet 1992). Sperms also acquire:

- *thermotactic responsiveness* – enabling navigation from the cooler storage site in the *isthmus* to the warmer fertilization site at the isthmic–ampullary junction
- *short-lived chemotactic receptors* – activated in sperms reaching the isthmic storage site and precisely guide them towards the oocyte in the isthmic–ampullary junction (Bahat et al 2003).

Fusion of oocyte and spermatozoon

The final set of morphological transformations in spermatozoa is stimulated by binding to the zona pellucida. During this critical process, the acrosome swells and its membranes fuse with the overlying plasma membrane (see Fig. 29.3).

Initially, attachment is very loose, involving a number of spermatozoa. Firmer binding follows, as an oocyte-binding protein on the sperm head region is recognized by sperm receptors on the zona pellucida. The inner plasma membrane at the apical end of the spermatozoa fuses with the outer membrane of the acrosome and forms a series of membrane-bound vesicles. Proteolytic enzymes released by the *acrosome reaction* digest sections of the zona pellucida surrounding the sperm head. Subsequent movement through the zona occurs very rapidly, creating immediate access to the oocyte membrane. Only spermatozoa that have undergone this *acrosomal exocytosis* can fuse with the oocyte. Usually, the spermatozoon that makes first contact with the oocyte proceeds to fertilization. In the process of fusion, the plasma membrane of the sperm head is enveloped by microvilli on the oocyte surface (Johnson 2013: 191–194; Tosti and Boni 2004).

The *cortical reaction* occurs immediately after the fusion of the oocyte and spermatozoon. This is a series of ionic changes in the oocyte cytoplasm and cortical granules formed after ovulation, then bind to the oocyte membrane, thus releasing their content into the space between the surface of the oocyte and the surrounding zona pellucida. The vesicles contain enzymes that modify the structure of the plasma membrane, blocking the entry of further spermatozoa.

From zygote to …

The *zygote* is the newly formed cell that contains maternal and paternal chromosomes and measures about 0.15 mm in diameter (FitzGerald and FitzGerald 1994: 12). Within 2 to 3 hours of fertilization, the zygote proceeds with the final phase of meiosis that was halted immediately after fertilization, transmitting one set of chromosomes to the

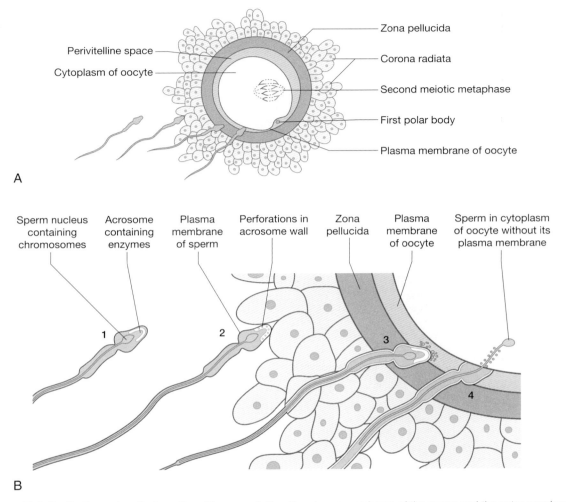

Figure 29.3 Fertilization and cortical reaction. After capacitation, the plasma membrane of the sperm and the outer membrane of the acrosome fuse and the membranes break down, releasing enzymes that allow the sperm to penetrate the corona radiata. Sperm digest their way through the zona pellucida via enzymes associated with the inner acrosomal membrane. Sperm are engulfed by the oocyte plasma membrane. Cortical granules are released when the sperm cell contacts the membrane. These granules cause other sperm in contact with the membrane to detach. (This article was published in Moore KL, Persaud TVN: The developing human, Philadelphia, Saunders, Copyright Elsevier, 2008.)

next generation. The remaining set is discarded to a second *polar body* on the periphery, which later undergoes apoptosis, along with the first one formed at ovulation (Fig. 29.3). Female chromosomes then divide mitotically, yielding one haploid set within the main body of the cytoplasm.

The cytoplasmic content of the sperm cell membrane combines with that of the oocyte and, over the next 2 to 3 hours, the sperm nuclear membrane gradually breaks down. Between 4 and 7 hours after cell fusion, two sets of haploid chromosomes are formed into male and female pronuclei,

as each becomes surrounded by distinct membranes, in opposite poles of the cell. During this period, chromosomes begin to synthesize DNA in preparation for the first mitotic division. As chromosomal content increases, the pronuclear membranes break down, bringing together two sets of male and female chromosomes. These events form the diploid complement of a new individual, and the cell immediately proceeds with a first mitotic division, passing its genetic material to two daughter cells and forming the two-cell conceptus (Downs 2008) (see Fig. 29.4).

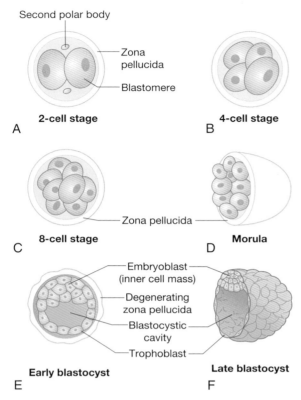

Figure 29.4 Various stages of cleavage and formation of the blastocyst. (This article was published in Moore KL, Persaud TVN: The developing human, Philadelphia, Saunders, Copyright Elsevier, 2008.)

... morula

Successive rounds of cleavages occur at approximately 12-hour intervals until 8 to 16 increasingly smaller cells are formed within the zona pellucida and remaining fragments of the cumulus cell mass. When cell cleavage has produced 8 to 16 cells, the conceptus changes its morphology and undergoes compaction to become a *morula* (resembling a mulberry; Fig. 29.4). This process establishes contiguity between adjacent cell membranes. Tight junctional complexes form between outer cell membranes and create a barrier to intercellular diffusion between inner and outer cells. At the same time, outer cells change from being radially symmetrical to being highly polarized (Edwards 2000; Downs 2008).

Glucose is consumed in increasing quantities and the *morula* utilizes a large number of growth factors for replication (Leppens-Luisier et al 2001; Leese et al 2008), including epidermal growth factor (EGF), insulin-like growth factors (IGFs) and hypoxia-inducible factors (HIFs) (Leese

1995). Acquiring the capacity to use glucose and convert it into lactate seems to occur in preparation for the hypoxic conditions that are encountered at implantation. All blastomeres show intense staining for gonadotrophin-releasing hormone (GnRH) and hCG (Casan et al 1999; Kikkawa et al 2002; Evans et al 2015). During this phase of cell cleavage, the *morula* remains within the zona pellucida. This smooth outer covering provides an overall structure that prevents premature adhesion of the blastomeres to the wall of the fallopian tube and provides an immunological barrier between maternal tissue and the genetically distinct cells of the morula (Johnson 2013: 208).

... to blastocyst

Over 24 hours, the *morula* continues cell cleavage to 16 to 32 cells. Between these two points, outer more metabolically active cells commit to trophoblast lineage, while the inner cell mass (ICM) retains the capacity for pluripotency and exhibits a quieter metabolism. Expression of critical genes for blastocyst formation commences in the 16-cell *morula* (Armant 2005; Leese et al 2008a). Outer cells begin to pump fluid internally to form a fluid-filled cavity called the *blastocoele*. Nudged to one side by this fluid, the ICM expresses gap junctions, allowing transfer of ions and small molecules from one cell to the next (Downs 2008). Meanwhile, the outer layer underlying the zona pellucida differentiates into flattened *trophectoderm* cells that combine with the zona to protect the ICM from destruction by maternal immune cells and signals the endometrium to initiate adhesion (Schultz 1998).

The fertilized egg has now become a *blastocyst* (Fig. 29.4). The trophectoderm expresses mRNA for the transcription factor, leptin, and both outer and inner cells express mRNA, protein and receptors for GnRH and the cannabinoid receptor (CB_1) (Battista et al 2008; Casan et al 1999; Edwards 2000). Composed of 34 to 64 cells, the blastocyst is programmed to prepare for the elaboration of extraembryonic tissues, beginning as a free-living organism immersed in uterine fluids that are actively accumulated by the trophoblasts (Burton et al 2002; Johnson 2013: 208). Over the next 3 days, *paracrine cross-talk* between the blastocyst and endometrium coordinates blastocyst activation with differentiation of the endometrium to a receptive state, from 7 to 9 days after ovulation (Fitzgerald et al 2008; Simon et al 1997).

ADAPTATIONS IN THE MATERNAL BRAIN, OVARY AND UTERUS

The formation of the *morula* marks the release of the first endocrine-autocrine signal from the conceptus – the glycosylated glycoprotein hCG – that elicits a wide variety of maternal adaptations to the fertile cycle and is detectable in the maternal circulation 7 days after fertilization, around the time of implantation (Cole 2012; Evans et al 2015). Recent work has shown that this signal conveys multiple messages throughout pregnancy because hCG is not a single entity, but five independent variant molecules, each with an identical amino acid sequence but with distinct arrangements and additions of other molecules that confer a wide variety of biological functions. Three of these have key regulatory functions during the fertile cycle (Cole 2010 and 2012).

A sulphated variant of hCG is produced at very low concentrations by pituitary gonadotrophs across the ovarian cycle (Cole 2012). This variant has 50 times the biological activity of LH per mole of hormone released in blood, because its metabolic clearance rate is slower (Cole 2012). Sulphated hCG matches the potency of LH in stimulating progesterone production by the corpus luteum during the luteal phase of the cycle (Cole 2012).

For the first 2 weeks after implantation, the most dominant form of hCG in maternal plasma is hyperglycosylated hCG (hCG-H), an autocrine factor initially released from trophoblasts that stimulates cell replication and differentiation of cytotrophoblast cells and remodeling of the decidua and spiral arteries during the first trimester (Evans et al 2015; Cole 2010). After this, hCG-H continues to increase up to 10 to 11 weeks gestation but comprises a smaller proportion of measured total hCG, and then declines dramatically to 1% of total hCG for the rest of the pregnancy (Evans et al 2015; Cole 2010).

The third variant is the hormone, hCG, produced by villous syncytiotrophoblast cells, that has a distinctively slow metabolic clearance rate, with a circulating half-life of 36 hours (Cole 2012). In contrast to the pattern of hCG-H secretion, hCG reaches peak levels of more than 100,000 mIU/mL around 9 to 10 weeks gestation, before falling rapidly to levels under 50,000 mIU/mL from around 18 to 20 weeks, which are maintained until the end of pregnancy (Chard et al 1995; Kosaka et al 2002). The exact mechanisms regulating this dynamic pattern of hCG secretion throughout pregnancy are not fully understood. Placental GnRH, leptin and epidermal growth factor seem to regulate secretion for the first 8 weeks of pregnancy (Islami et al 2003; Colicchia et al 2014). Thereafter, hCG secretion and uterine and placental expression of LH/hCG receptors seem to be maintained by an autoregulatory mechanism (Kikkawa et al 2002). As pregnancy progresses, the fetal kidneys and pituitary synthesize and release hCG, while rising levels of fetal adrenal steroids during the second trimester seem to have an inhibitory effect (Tsakiri et al 2002).

Throughout pregnancy, hCG performs an array of regulatory functions that include:

- stimulating progesterone production by the corpus luteum, for the first 3 weeks after implantation and inhibiting luteolysis (Myers et al 2007)

- operating on hCG/LH receptors in the maternal brain, to inhibit expression of GnRH; stimulate thyroid hormone production; increase the duration of sleep and rest and modulate food preferences and intake by stimulating a heighted sense of smell (Lei et al 1993; Lei and Rao 1994; Colicchia et al 2014)

- stimulating angiogenesis in uterine blood vessels and growth, differentiation of the placenta and a wide range of fetal organ systems (Cole 2010 and 2012)

- stimulating syncytiotrophoblast uptake of iodine (Colicchia et al 2014)

- preventing immune-rejection of the feto-placental unit by maternal tissues

- promoting uterine growth in line with the feto-placental unit and inducing myometrial quiescence until the end of pregnancy (Ticconi et al 2007; Cole 2012)

- stimulating placental formation of oestrogen towards the end of pregnancy, under the influence of fetal cortisol (Wang et al 2014).

In relation to the first trimester, the autocrine factor hCG-H regulates trophoblast infiltration of the decidua and inner third of the myometrium to create supportive conditions for embryo formation, notably low-oxygen tension, with nutrients supplied from glandular secretions (Burton et al 2001 and 2009). At the same time, the hormone hCG induces a complementary state of maternal quietness, by inducing an overwhelming desire for sleep and rest, and greater aversion to the smell and taste of food (Lukacs et al 1995; Handschuh et al 2007). Within the hypothalamus, hCG also inhibits the HPG axis to prevent the growth of new ovarian follicles, stimulates the thyroid axis to supply the needs of the embryo during neurogenesis and stimulates steroid hormone production from the corpus luteum to sustain uterine and systemic adaptations to the fertile cycle.

THE CORPUS LUTEUM OF PREGNANCY

During the fertile cycle, the functional lifespan of the corpus luteum extends from 14 to around 280 days. Over the first 6 weeks of pregnancy, it doubles in volume, as a result of hypertrophy of the luteinized granulosa and theca cells and accumulation of connective tissue and endothelial cells (Strauss and Williams 2014: 185). In fertile cycles, oestrogens and progesterone concentrations are significantly higher from days 6 and 7 after the midcycle LH/hCG/FSH surge (Stewart et al 1993). The trophic hormones for enhanced steroidogenesis from the early luteal phase seem to come from a number of hormones released from the endometrium. From 3 days' postfertilization, the secretory endometrium has the capacity to produce GnRH, hCG, FSH and progesterone (Cheon et al 2001). These findings suggest that the close connections between uterine and ovarian arteriovenous systems deliver hCG and other regulatory factors from the endometrium to the corpus luteum from the early luteal phase of fertile cycles.

In the ovary, hCG binds to LH receptors and stimulates increased synthesis of progesterone, oestrogens and relaxin. Recent evidence suggests that hCG also stimulates luteal expression of 11β-hydroxysteroid dehydrogenase, resulting in increased intraluteal generation of cortisol that prevents luteolysis during pregnancy (Myers et al 2007). Progesterone also promotes survival of the corpus luteum by autocrine stimulation of luteal cells. The marked rise in progesterone release from the corpus luteum after implantation has also been attributed to autostimulation and prostaglandins produced by the trophoblast (Baird et al 2003; Stouffer 2003).

Ovarian relaxin

After the LH/hCG/FSH surges, large luteal cells (LLCs) and small luteal cells (SLCs) develop the capacity to secrete peptide and steroid hormones in equal amounts. *Relaxin*, a peptide hormone of the insulin-like growth factor family, is a major hormone of the corpus luteum of pregnancy. Beginning during the luteal phase, under the stimulatory influence of LH/hCG, *relaxin* secretion peaks at 10 weeks gestation, decreases by around 20% and is present in maternal plasma, at stable concentrations, for the remainder of pregnancy (Bell et al 1987). **Relaxin:**

- induces endometrial stromal differentiation during the luteal phase and stimulates decidual prolactin, initiating and maintaining endometrial decidualization (Jabbour and Critchley 2001)

- operates with hCG and progesterone to activate transcription of glycodelin A, a major glycoprotein from the endometrial glands with nutritive and immunomodulatory functions (Burton et al 2002 and 2007; Glock et al 1995; Telgmann and Gellersen 1998; Tseng et al 1999)

- regulates changes in maternal thirst and osmoregulation

  Central and peripheral relaxin:

- induces renal and systemic vasodilatation, pituitary growth hormone (GH) secretion, plasma volume expansion and increased adipose tissue sensitivity to insulin during the first half of pregnancy (Chapman et al 1997; Davison et al 1990; Kristiansson and Wang 2001; Vokes et al 1988).

PREPARATION FOR IMPLANTATION

In readiness for implantation, endometrial glands accumulate glycogen, proteins, a variety of growth factors, sugars and lipid droplets, and secretory activity peaks at around 6 days after ovulation. Some secretions supply the conceptus with essential nutritional and regulatory molecules until around 9 weeks gestation (Burton et al 2002 and 2007). Ovarian progesterone stimulates increased expression of two potent angiogenic factors: *angiogenin* in stromal cells and *vascular endothelial growth factor* (VEGF) in stromal cells and neutrophils associated with microvessel walls (Gargett et al 2001; Ma et al 2001). By the mid-secretory phase, a subepithelial capillary plexus has formed into a complex network of vessels and newly regrown arterioles become increasingly spiral, as they lengthen more rapidly than the endometrium thickens (Gargett et al 2001; Starkey 1993). During the secretory phase, stromal cells release a growing number of new matrix proteins, together with the surface expression of their receptors, including laminin, fibronectin, collagen and integrins, while the earlier cross-linking collagen fibrils are degraded. This process of matrix remodeling creates a thicker, looser and more soluble structure for trophoblast infiltration.

BLASTOCYST–ENDOMETRIAL COMMUNICATION

When fertilization occurs, the designated attachment site undergoes extensive synchronized changes, transforming it from a usual state of active rejection of blastocyst attachment to a brief state of receptivity, forming a *'window of implantation'* commencing 7 days after ovulation (Fitzgerald et al 2008; Hustin 1992; Hustin and Franchimont 1992; Lessey 2000). Some changes are regulated by paracrine cross-talk with the free-floating blastocyst, while others are activated by attachment.

As the blastocyst hatches from the zona pellucida, around 6 days after fertilization, trophoblast cells surrounding the ICM make initial contact with the endometrium, by close apposition of trophoblast plasma membranes with the apical membranes of surface epithelial cells, followed by rapid proliferation and formation of junctional complexes with the surface epithelium. Apical membranes of epithelial cells display a variety of progesterone- and oestrogen-induced changes that facilitate cell recognition and interaction with the trophectoderm. These include a progressive shortening of the microvilli, creating a flatter surface, reduced thickness of the normally dense coating of glycoproteins, and inhibition of gap junctions, facilitating adhesion (Fride 2008; Hustin and Franchimont 1992; Lessey 2000).

Adhesion and attachment

Around the designated site of implantation, the luminal epithelium expresses calcitonin and the blastocyst-dependent, heparin-binding epidermal growth factor (HB-EGF). As the zona pellucida is shed, direct communication between cell adhesion molecules and their receptors on trophoblast and surface epithelium begins the dynamically balanced processes of attachment, implantation and trophoblast replication (Fitzgerald et al 2008).

IMPLANTATION – ENDOMETRIAL RESPONSE

The surface epithelium, uterine glands and decidua show distinct responses to implantation. As the tiny blastocyst lodges in the crypt of the endometrial folds and localized oedema moulds, a chamber around the trophoblast surface and epithelial cells above the newly created site multiply rapidly to form a complete cover for the embedded blastocyst, enveloped in a growing mantle of differentiating trophoblast cells, by approximately 9 days after fertilization (Armant 2005). More extensive hormone-induced changes occur within the underlying decidua, producing a range of matrix proteins to form a loose, lattice-type network, allowing free passage of water, ions and large molecules to the trophoblast cells.

Like epithelial glands, decidual cells synthesize and release specific glycoproteins. One of these has been identified as a growth factor-binding protein that may participate in regulating the pace and extent of trophoblast implantation (Hustin and Franchimont 1992). Decidual cells that release relaxin have also been found to contain prolactin, which is regulated by a number of factors from adjoining cells in the decidua, placenta and membranes. Activities of decidual prolactin include regulation of glandular secretions, expression of adhesion and proteolytic molecules and modulation of specific aspects of the immune response (Gubbay et al 2002; Jabbour and Critchley 2001).

FORMATION OF THE CYTOTROPHOBLAST SHELL AND GESTATIONAL SAC

Once the *blastocyst* has embedded in the decidua, rapidly proliferating trophoblast cells follow three distinct pathways, dividing into weakly proliferating *villous cytotrophoblasts* (vCTBs) that subsequently fuse to form a syncytium of terminally differentiated *multinucleated syncytiotrophoblasts* (STs) while the stem cell population of vCTBs forms a monolayer directly beneath the STs to renew them.

During the first trimester, STs actively take up secretions from the surrounding endometrial glands and contribute to gaseous and waste exchange (Ellery et al 2009). Throughout pregnancy, they are the major source of hormones, receptors, growth factors and regulatory enzymes (Burton et al 2007; Ferretti et al 2007; Habayeb et al 2008; Islami et al 2003; Jauniaux and Gulbis 2000; Tarrade et al 2001). These include human placental growth hormone (hPGH), prolactin, atrial natriuretic peptide (ANP), leptin, oestrogens, progesterone and a growing list of regulatory glycoproteins, including hCG-H, GnRH, corticotropin-releasing hormone (CRH) and thyrotropin-releasing hormone (TRH) (Cootauco et al 2008; Colicchia et al 2014; Evans et al 2015; Ferretti et al 2007; Pasqualini 2005).

While the cytotrophoblast shell acts as an effective barrier to maternal concentrations of oxygen, the expanding syncytiotrophoblastic mantle erodes the epithelium of surrounding endometrial glands, releasing their secretions into the extracellular matrix (Burton et al 2007). Glandular secretions enter channels forming around the cytotrophoblast shell. This activity is evident from 17 days post-conception and only begins to decline when embryo formation is complete, towards the end of the first trimester (Burton et al 2007; Jauniaux and Gulbis 2000).

HISTIOTROPHIC NUTRITION

During the first 8 to 10 weeks of pregnancy, the secretory pattern of epithelial glandular cells extends that of the *luteal phase*, with continued glycogen secretion and a rapid rise in a number of glycoproteins (Burton et al 2001 and 2007; Muller-Schottle et al 1999). These include glycodelin A, relaxin, hCG, α-tocopherol transfer protein – a powerful antioxidant and MUC-1 – a large progesterone-dependent glycoprotein (Burton et al 2002 and 2007; Jauniaux et al 2004). Synthesis of glycodelin A parallels the profile of hCG in the maternal circulation during the first trimester. This glycoprotein regulates endometrial receptivity, has potent immunosuppressive activity and is phagocytosed by the ST for recycling in anabolic pathways within the extraembryonic compartment. MUC-1 is also taken up by the syncytiotrophoblast membrane and provides a rich and energy-free source of amino acids for its synthetic requirements (Burton et al 2002; Seppala et al 2002; Tseng et al 1999). The transfer pathway for these molecules is histiotrophic (extracellular) rather than haemotrophic (vascular), which characterizes the fetal phase of gestation (Burton et al 2002) (see Fig. 29.5).

CONDITIONS FOR EMBRYOGENESIS AND EARLY PLACENTAL FORMATION

Current evidence suggests that the optimal environment for embryonic and early placental formation includes a reduced

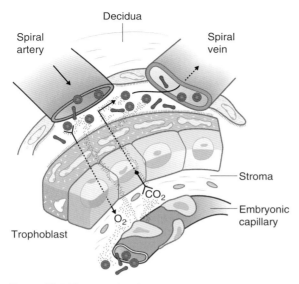

Figure 29.5 Diagram showing uteroplacental circulation and the trophoblast barrier. (Jones CJP: The life and death of the embryonic yolk sac. In Jauniaux E, Barnea ER, Edwards RG, editors: Embryonic medicine and therapy, Oxford, Oxford University Press,1997. By permission of Oxford University Press.)

oxygen tension of between 2.5% and 5% (Burton et al 2009; Fritz et al 2014). Embryonic haemoglobin, which lasts for the first 8 weeks of gestation, combines with oxygen at very low tension found in interstitial fluids. Until the middle of the second month of gestation, all embryonic erythrocytes are nucleated; hence blood viscosity remains very high and the mean radius of the emerging villous vascular system is very low (Jauniaux et al 2003). The conceptus, therefore, derives external nutritional support histiotrophically, from secretory products of the decidua and uterine glands. These secretory products are initially phagocytosed by the trophectoderm of the blastocyst, then by vCTBs and the endoderm of the yolk sac (Burton et al 2001 and 2002).

Developments within the endometrium fully complement this activity (see online Fig. 29.1). From the luteal phase of the cycle, glandular cells secrete rapidly, increasing amounts of glycoproteins, promoting cell growth and organ differentiation. The underlying decidua undergoes considerable biochemical and structural adaptations, forming an array of matrix proteins and differentiated secretory cells that provide:

- growth-promoting factors for the emerging embryo
- immunoprotection for trophoblast infiltration
- regulatory hormones, including prolactin, relaxin, renin, retinol-binding protein and prostaglandins (Burton et al 2002; Hustin and Franchimont 1992; King et al 2001; Starkey 1993).

FORMATION OF EXTRAEMBRYONIC FLUID COMPARTMENTS AND DIFFERENTIATION OF THE ICM

As implantation of the blastocyst proceeds during the first 2 weeks after ovulation, the extraembryonic mesoderm, lining the cytotrophoblast shell, progressively increases and contains isolated spaces by 12 days after fertilization. At the same time, the ICM first subdivides into a bilaminar disk of primary *endoderm* and *ectoderm* cell groups, both of which contribute to embryonic and extraembryonic tissues, then the *mesoderm* invaginates from the *ectoderm* to create a trilaminar disk (see Fig. 29.6). This marks the beginning of embryo formation (see chapter website resources).

During the second week of life, regulatory cells within the ectoderm establish a defining organizational structure called the *primitive streak*, which establishes polarity of the body axis and, consequently, initial positioning of the emerging embryo in relation to the extraembryonic compartments, while the endoderm group form a major part of the yolk sac, which performs the functions of a mature placenta during the first trimester (Downs 2008; Jones 1997).

Over the next few days, a wave of new endodermal cells migrates from the primary endoderm to line the blastocyst cavity and form the *primary yolk sac* or *exocoelomic cavity* during the fourth week of gestation. The complex fluid is derived from an ultrafiltration of maternal serum through villous stromal channels and from the secondary yolk sac, which forms at the beginning of the fourth week of gestation. Containing high concentrations of amino acids, regulatory proteins, vitamins and hormones, this fluid acts as a reservoir of molecules before their use by the yolk sac during the first 8 to 10 weeks of pregnancy (Jauniaux and Gulbis 2000; Jauniaux et al 1994).

Once the primary yolk sac forms, a thick acellular material called the extraembryonic mesoderm is secreted between the exocoelomic membrane and the cytotrophoblast. Over the next couple of days, this tissue divides to form a second chorionic cavity, between the primary yolk sac and the cytotrophoblast. An inner layer of cytotrophoblast cells delaminate to form amniogenic cells. Some differentiate into amnioblasts and organize into a specialized, semipermeable membrane composed of a single layer of cuboidal epithelial cells on a loose connective tissue matrix (Jauniaux and Gulbis 2000). Formation of the primordial amniotic cavity seems to arise by cavitation of the primary ectoderm, which opens and then reforms to create a complete membrane around the amniotic cavity, containing the emerging embryo.

Fluid formed within the amniotic cavity is largely secreted by the emerging embryo, containing much lower concentrations of all molecules and trace elements than fluid in the exocoelomic cavity (Jauniaux and Gulbis

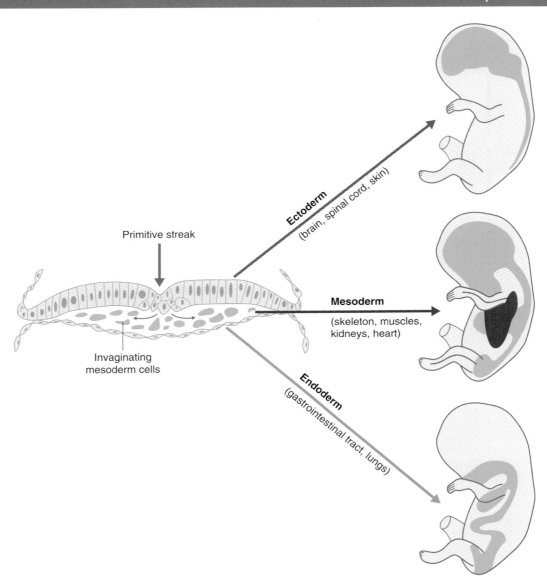

Figure 29.6 The trilaminar disc illustrating endoderm, ectoderm and mesoderm. (Dunstan GR, editor: The human embryo, Exeter, University of Exeter Press, 1990.)

2000). This indicates that the amniotic membrane separating the two compartments is not permeable to large molecules and is most glandular, and trophoblast proteins are likely absorbed by the embryo through the secondary yolk sac (Jauniaux and Gulbis 2000; Jauniaux et al 1993 and 1994). As illustrated in Fig. 29.7, during the first 8 weeks of embryonic formation, the amniotic cavity is dwarfed by the larger and highly dynamic exocoelomic cavity, containing the free-floating yolk sac, which directly nourishes and regulates the emerging embryo until around 10 weeks gestation (Jauniaux and Gulbis 1997; Jones 1997).

THE SECONDARY YOLK SAC

Around 12 days after fertilization, the primary yolk sac breaks up into a number of smaller vesicles, while the

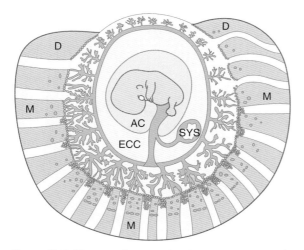

Figure 29.7 Diagram of a gestational sac at 8 to 9 weeks gestation, showing the myometrium (M), decidua (D), placenta (P) and exocoelomic cavity (EEC), the largest space inside the gestational sac from 5–9 weeks gestation. Arrows indicate uteroplacental blood circulation beginning in the periphery of the placenta. (Burton GJ, Kaufmann P, Huppertz B: Anatomy and genesis of the placenta. In Neill JD, editor: Knobil and Neill's physiology of reproduction, Amsterdam, Elsevier, 2006.)

endoderm beneath the embryonic disk grows out to form the *secondary yolk sac*. The secondary yolk sac grows rapidly, becoming larger than the amniotic cavity by the fifth week of gestation (Jones 1997). With successive folding of the emerging embryo during the dynamic process of gastrulation, between 3 and 6 weeks gestation, the neck of the secondary yolk sac is constricted to form the yolk stalk, which connects the definitive yolk sac to the primitive gut.

Until it begins to degenerate at around 9 weeks gestation, the secondary yolk sac consists of three distinct layers:

- an outer layer of *extraembryonic mesoderm* that completely lines the chorionic or exocoelomic cavity: this has a well-developed microvillous brush border and numerous pinocytotic vesicles within the cytoplasm that enhance its capacity for absorption of molecules from the surrounding exocoelomic fluid.

- a middle layer of *splanchnic mesoderm*, which contains blood islands: this contains free collagen fibrils and sinusoidal blood vessels, induced by the innermost endodermal layer of the yolk sac. Central cells of the blood islands fuse to form primitive vascular channels within the mesodermal connecting stalk, extending towards the emerging embryo where they make connections with the endothelial tubes associated with the tubular heart and major vessels (Jauniaux et al 2003; Jones 1997).

- an *endodermal layer*, which faces the yolk sac lumen (Jauniaux and Moscoso 1992; Jones 1997), is made up of large columnar cells with glycogen deposits and a well-developed capacity for protein biosynthesis. These cells are interspersed with large microvillous-lined channels that open out into the cavity of the yolk sac and seem to be involved in secretion of waste products. Many proteins and enzymes involved in energy metabolism and digestion are synthesized by the endodermal layer, including alpha-fetoprotein, antitrypsin, albumin and transferrin, before the embryonic liver takes over at around 9 to 10 weeks gestation (Jones 1997).

Blood cells and capillaries develop within the centre of the chorionic villi. At approximately 19 days, the two sets of vessels establish contact, creating the beginnings of a vascular connection between the embryonic compartment and the early placenta (Carlson 1994: 72). Blood cell formation in the secondary yolk sac continues until haematopoiesis begins in hepatic and spleen cells at around 8 weeks gestation (Jauniaux and Moscoso 1992).

THE DECIDUOCHORIAL PLACENTA

During formation of anchoring villi, proliferating extravillous cytotrophoblasts (evCTBs) extend from the syncytium, forming columns of cells that enter decidual blood vessels. As this process continues, the intervillous space begins to open, exposing the migratory extravillous trophoblast cells to a physiological increase in oxygen tension from 9 weeks gestation. This environment alters the expression of specific transcription factors, which trigger the expression of an invasive population of migratory evCTBs (Caniggia et al 2000). In addition, evCTBs express receptors for hPGH that have been found to increase the invasive potential of evCTBs in culture (Lacroix et al 2005). Further differentiation of the extravillous cells to a more invasive phenotype allows them to enter and remodel the spiral arteries and to create the low-resistance vascular system that is essential for fetal growth (Burton et al 2009; Caniggia and Winter 2002; Caniggia et al 2000; Hustin 1992).

During the first 12 weeks, extravillous trophoblast migration into the spiral arteries occurs primarily within the decidual segments (see Fig. 29.8). First the distal tips of these blood vessels are plugged with evCTBs that extend from the trophoblastic shell or the proliferating tips of the emerging villi. Sheets of these endovascular trophoblasts migrate along the capillary walls, against maternal blood flow, and accumulate within the lumen of the spiral arteries. During the subsequent process of vascular infiltration, cells strip away sections of the endothelium and burrow beneath this layer to replace elastic tissue and smooth muscle with cytotrophoblast cells that appear to surround

First trimester   **Second trimester**

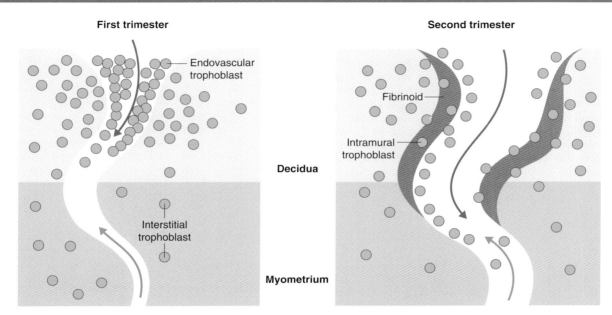

Figure 29.8 Diagram illustrating endovascular trophoblast migration into decidual segments of spiral arteries during the first trimester (left) and interstitial migration into the myometrial segments from 12 to 14 weeks. Red arrow: direction of maternal blood flow; black arrow: direction of endovascular trophoblast migration. (Pijnenborg R, Vercruysse L, Hanssens M: The uterine spiral arteries in human pregnancy: facts and controversies, Placenta 2006. 27: 939–958.)

themselves with large quantities of fibrinoid material (Burton et al 2009 and 2010). Later, surface endothelial cells grow over the new underlying tissues. Throughout, the convoluted walls of the spiral arteries are converted into tubes of fibrinoid material with no elastic tissue or smooth muscle fibres. This results in terminal coils of the spiral arteries reaching 2 to 3 mm in diameter and underlying segments undergo a generalized, nonuniform dilation as pregnancy advances and lose the capacity to respond to the vasomotor influences of continued autonomic innervation (Burton et al 2009; Hustin et al 1988; Pijnenborg et al 2006).

During the first 10 weeks of pregnancy, ultrasound studies suggest that decidual blood vessels do not reach the intervillous space. While small amounts of plasma percolate through the plugs from these low-pressure vessels, chorionic villous sampling has rarely demonstrated the presence of maternal blood. As illustrated in Fig. 29.5, current evidence suggests that during the first 9 to 10 weeks, the intervillous space is not immediately connected with the maternal circulation and is not yet bathed by maternal blood (Hustin and Schaaps 1987). As illustrated in Fig. 29.9, estimates of uterine blood flow also support this evidence. In non-pregnant women, uterine blood flow is approximately 45 mL/min, rising by around 10 mL/min during the first trimester. In contrast, much larger increases occur during the second and third trimesters, to reach over 750 mL/min by the end of pregnancy (Burton et al 2009; de Swiet 1991: 51).

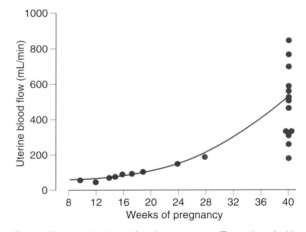

Figure 29.9 Uterine blood flow in pregnancy. (Reproduced with permission from Chamberlain G, and Broughton Pipkin F: Clinical physiology in obstetrics, Oxford, Blackwell Scientific, 1998.)

FROM EMBRYO TO FETUS

From 12 weeks onwards, trophoblast infiltration extends into myometrial segments of many spiral arteries (Burton et al 2009; Pijnenborg et al 2006). Evidence suggests that this infiltration largely occurs through the endometrial stroma to enter the vessel walls from the outside (Burton et al 2009). As in decidual segments, this activity replaces muscular and elastic tissue with fibrinoid material that converts them into widened, funnel-like tubes with no capacity to respond to the vasomotor influences of autonomic innervations that progressively decline under the influence of rising levels of oestrogen (Brauer and Smith 2015). At the same time, the trophoblast shell becomes thinner and more irregular as fetal growth enlarges its internal volume (Jauniaux et al 2003). An increasing number of extravillous cells become distinct from the shell surface and these gradually open up low-pressure flow of maternal blood within the intervillous space. Experimental evidence suggests that the velocity of blood flow from the spiral arterioles to the intervillous space is similar to an actively flowing brook entering a reed-filled marsh (Burton et al 2009; Ramsey et al 1976) (see Fig. 29.10).

This direct communication between maternal blood and placental villi coincides with the onset of rapid growth of the fetus and placenta. During this phase, the roughly formed organ systems undergo progressive differentiation and rapid growth, which requires large increases in uteroplacental size and blood volume (Mark et al 2006). Structural alterations to all segments of uterine blood vessels create conditions for the emergence of an expanding low-pressure system that optimizes gas and nutritional exchange across the placental interface (Burton et al 2009).

Growth of the amniotic compartment

Between 7 and 12 weeks gestation, production of amniotic fluid increases from 3 to 30 mL (Jauniaux and Gulbis 2000). This causes the amnion to swell until it takes over the chorionic space, bringing amnion and chorion in contact for the first time and enclosing the embryo, except for the umbilical area, within a single cavity. As the sac subsequently grows into the endometrial cavity, this portion of the chorion is gradually compressed against the decidua capsularis – the area of decidual lining surrounding the site of implantation. With continued growth, blood supply is reduced, and these villi slowly degenerate, although trophoblast cells between them remain viable for the remainder of the pregnancy. This portion of the chorion (*chorion laeve*) forms an interface between the amnion and areas of decidua not occupied by the definitive placenta (see Fig. 29.11).

The *chorion laeve* has the following features:

- Diverse layers of metabolically active tissue (despite the absence of a direct blood supply)

- Composed of a layer of fibroblast cells that are contiguous with the amnion, a reticular layer, a type of basement membrane and 2 to 10 layers of trophoblast cells closely applied to the decidua capsularis

- Produces a number of enzymes that degrade locally synthesized molecules, including prostaglandins,

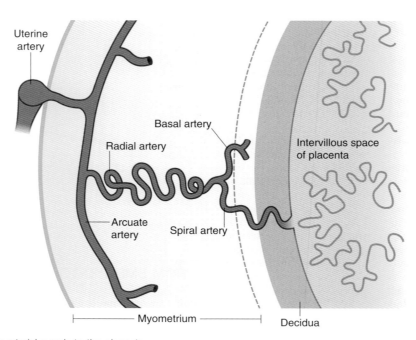

Figure 29.10 The arterial supply to the placenta.

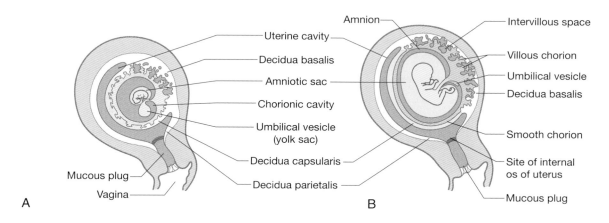

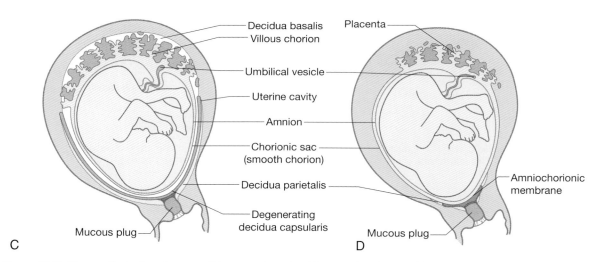

Figure 29.11 Diagram illustrating changes within compartments of the gestational sac and the changing relations of membranes to the decidua from 12 to 22 weeks gestation. (This article was published in Moore KL, Persaud TVN: The developing human, Philadelphia, Saunders, Copyright Elsevier, 2008.)

oxytocin, platelet-activating factor and brain natriuretic peptide (BNP), that inhibits oxytocin-induced contractility (Carvajal et al 2009). In this way, the chorion protects the myometrium from direct exposure to contractile forces during pregnancy (Erwich and Keirse 1992).

THE DEFINITIVE PLACENTA

As villi of the chorion laeve disappear, those attached to the decidua basalis rapidly develop to form the *mature*

placenta. The cytotrophoblast shell extends laterally and penetrates deeper into maternal tissue between the anchoring villi, and increasingly complex branching villi extend in the intervillous space. Each stem villus forms the centre of the villous tree. Fetal arterioles carrying poorly oxygenated blood enter the villi and break up into an extensive arteriocapillary–venous network. The 60 to 70 branching villi that make up the mature placenta provide a large surface area for gaseous and metabolic exchange between fetal blood within the villi and maternal blood circulating slowly around the external surface from the intervillous space (Sheppard and Bonnar 1989; see Fig. 29.12).

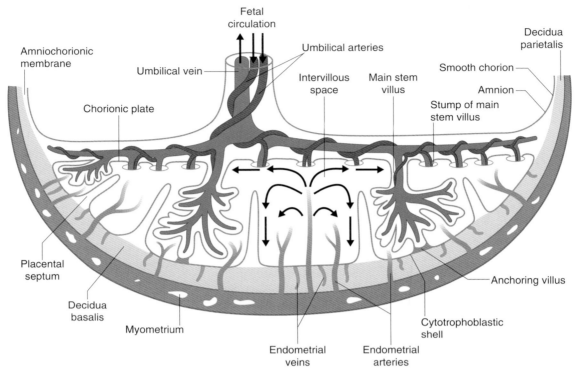

Figure 29.12 Schematic drawing of a transverse section through a full-term placenta showing the feto-placental and maternal–placental circulation. (This article was published in Moore KL, Persaud TVN: The developing human, Philadelphia, Saunders, Copyright Elsevier, 2008.)

Fetal oxygen requirements

While intraplacental and fetal concentrations of oxygen increase significantly from the end of the first trimester, a Po_2 gradient of 13.3 mm Hg persists between placenta and decidua at 16 weeks gestation and Po_2, O_2 saturation and O_2 content gradients are present between fetal blood and placenta and between placental and underlying maternal tissues (Jauniaux et al 2003). Low fetal blood Po_2 and O_2 saturation have also been found in the third trimester (Jauniaux et al 2001). The highest oxygen content is in the umbilical vein, which is 30 to 35 mm Hg and 80% to 90% saturated. By the time blood reaches the left atrium, O_2 content has fallen to 26 to 28 mm Hg, and lower concentrations supply the lungs and lower body (Tucker Blackburn 2013: 280). With homeostatic functions performed by maternal and placental systems, the fetus is therefore fully adapted to being immersed in water with significantly lower oxygen concentrations than those required by maternal and placental tissues.

Fetal regulation of amniotic fluid volume

Until about 20 weeks, the dynamics of amniotic fluid volume are thought to involve a significant transmembrane pathway from maternal blood via the placenta and movement of fluid and other molecules across the fetal skin, offering no impediment to the flow of fluid into the amniotic sac. From 17 to 25 weeks gestation, this pattern of flow diminishes, as the fetal skin begins to keratinize. During the second half of pregnancy, the fetal kidneys, lungs, gastrointestinal system and circulation make a growing contribution to the volume and circulation of amniotic fluid.

Volume increases from approximately 350 to 450 mL at 20 weeks, to 700 to 1000 mL at 36 to 39 weeks, and then begins to decline (Moore and Persaud 2008: 128). Estimates of daily volumes near term suggest that fetal urine contributes 500 mL, lung fluid 300 to 400 mL and 400 mL is removed by fetal swallowing (Moore and Persaud 2008: 130). The fluid passes into the fetal circulation and waste products cross the placental membrane and enter maternal blood in the intervillous space. Through these pathways, the water content of amniotic fluid is changed approximately every 3 hours (Moore and Persaud 2008: 128–130).

Mechanisms regulating amniotic fluid volume are poorly understood. During the second half of pregnancy, amniotic fluid is hypo-osmolar compared with maternal and fetal plasma. This osmotic gradient would be expected to drive water from the amniotic cavity into the maternal and fetal circulations via the umbilical cord, placenta and membranes. However, the precise volumes that move through these pathways remain to be confirmed (Brace 1995; Tucker Blackburn 2014/2012: 96–97).

Functions of amniotic fluid

This dynamic volume of fluid provides:

- essential space for symmetrical, external growth and movements of the fetus, aiding muscular development of upper and lower limbs and sensory stimulation
- essential space for fetal lung development
- equalization of pressure, exerted by uterine contractions, preventing compression of the umbilical vessels between the fetus and the uterine wall during fetal movements and contractions
- modulation of excessive overriding of the bones of the skull, protecting underlying cerebral membranes

and blood vessels, as the head is moulded during descent and rotation in the pelvic cavity.

LUNG FORMATION

Around 24 days after conception, a pouch-like laryngotracheal diverticulum arises as a small ventral protrusion from an area of the foregut, close to that which becomes the stomach (Tucker Blackburn 2012/14: 309–320). Once formed, the foregut elongates, separating the emerging stomach from the section that gives rise to the lungs. From an initial protrusion, the lungs take shape through a series of bifurcations, beginning with the emergence of right and left lobular buds corresponding in number to those in the mature organ.

Between 5 and 26 weeks gestation, these branch a further 16 times, to generate the respiratory trees. All bronchial airways are formed by 16 weeks and further growth proceeds by elongation and widening of existing airways. Towards the end of this phase, each terminal bronchiole divides into two or more respiratory bronchioles, while surrounding meso-dermal tissues become highly vascularized.

From 26 weeks onwards, respiratory bronchioles continually subdivide to produce approximately 20 to 70 million primitive alveoli that are vascularized by a dense network of capillaries (Moore and Persaud 2008: 202–207) (see Figs 29.13 and 29.14).

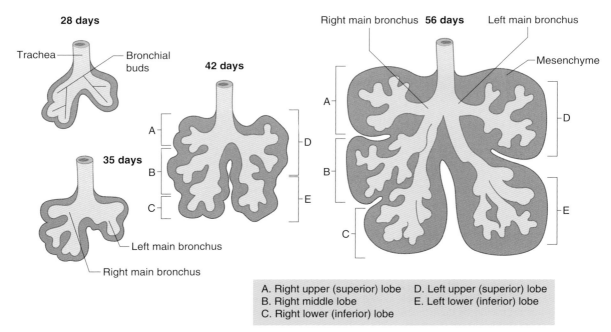

A. Right upper (superior) lobe
B. Right middle lobe
C. Right lower (inferior) lobe
D. Left upper (superior) lobe
E. Left lower (inferior) lobe

Figure 29.13 Successive stages in development of the bronchial buds, bronchi and lungs. (This article was published in Moore KL, Persaud TVN: The developing human, Philadelphia, Saunders, Copyright Elsevier, 2008.)

457

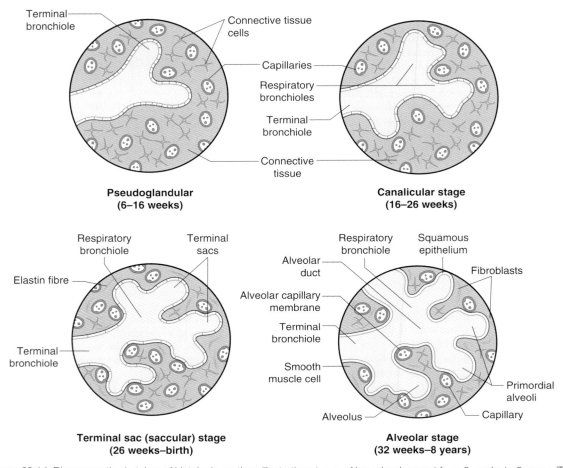

Figure 29.14 Diagrammatic sketches of histologic sections illustrating stages of lung development from 6 weeks to 8 years. (This article was published in Moore KL, Persaud TVN: The developing human, Philadelphia, Saunders, Copyright Elsevier, 2008.)

During fetal life, these potential air spaces are filled with liquid, actively secreted by the pulmonary epithelium from the surrounding circulation. Experiments have found that the volume of liquid increases from 4 to 6 mL/kg body weight at mid-gestation, to more than 20 mL/kg body weight near term. This liquid expansion of potential air space maintains a small, distending pressure in the lumen that approximates functional residual capacity of the aerated lung in the newborn. Lung fluid also assists in the formation of surfactant-producing epithelial cells that can be identified from approximately 24 weeks gestation.

There are a successive series of development, from changes within the lining of the bronchioles, to prepare the lungs for extrauterine breathing and gaseous exchange. **From 17 weeks**, the cuboidal epithelial cells provide energy and act as precursors for the development of

surfactant. Surfactant is crucial in reducing surface tension of the terminal sacs and stabilizing the membrane, which prevents lung collapsing after the onset of respiration. Intermittent breathing movements occur from approximately 11 weeks gestation and, from 24 weeks, the pattern of this activity is integrated with circadian rhythms in heart rate, temperature, body movements and sleep that seem to be mediated by maternal melatonin, which freely crosses the placenta (Tamura et al 2008). These episodic breathing movements in utero stimulate the development of lung tissue and respiratory muscles and some experimental evidence suggests that they may increase cardiac output and blood flow to vital organs, including the heart, brain and placenta. Rhythmic breathing movements are regulated by brainstem adrenergic respiratory neural networks and adrenaline from the adrenal medulla.

Hormonal regulation of lung development and maturation

Differentiation of type II pneumocytes and production of surfactant are closely associated with increasing levels of different hormones within the fetal circulation, particularly cortisol, oestrogens, adrenaline, hPL, prolactin, triiodothyronine (T_3) and placental CRH (see website for further information).

FETO-PLACENTAL CIRCULATION

The fetus relies on the placenta for respiration, nutrition and excretion, and fetal blood circulates throughout the placenta to realize these requirements (see Fig. 29.15). Fetal circulation differs from adult circulation in that blood is oxygenated in the placenta and not in the lungs. This system requires:

- larger and more numerous red cells (6 to 7 million/mm^3)
- higher haemoglobin content (20.7 g/dL) to pick up the maximum amount of oxygen
- a modified form of haemoglobin (HbF), which is active in the slightly more acid blood
- additional fetal structures:
  - ductus arteriosus
  - ductus venosus
  - foramen ovale
  - two hypogastric arteries

The intra-uterine circulation takes shape during early embryonic formation: umbilical veins bring oxygenated blood to the primitive heart from the *chorion frondosum*; *vitelline veins* return blood from the yolk sac; and *cardinal veins* return blood from the rest of the body. Blood enters the heart via the sinus venous and flows through a single atrium and ventricle. When the ventricle contracts, blood is pumped through the *bulbus cordis*, passes into the dorsal aorta and eventually returns to deliver waste products to the chorion (Moore and Persaud 2008: 292).

During fetal life, the vascular system becomes more extensive as it parallels the increasing size and complexity of individual organs and tissues. Oxygenated blood returns from a greatly enlarged placenta, via the umbilical vein. Approximately 50% of this blood enters a hepatic microcirculation and later joins the inferior vena cava via the hepatic veins. The remaining blood passes directly to the inferior vena cava, through a shunt called the *ductus venosus*. Blood flow through this vascular bypass is thought to be regulated by a physiological sphincter that responds to changing volume in the umbilical vein, which helps protect the fetus from erratic fluctuations in blood pressure (Walker 1993).

In addition to well-oxygenated blood from the placenta, the inferior vena cava receives less-oxygenated blood from the abdomen, pelvis and lower limbs, representing more than 66% of total venous return. Before entering the heart, the inferior vena cava bifurcates into two channels: the foramen ovale links it to the left atrium and a small inlet links it to the right atrium. In the left atrium, the foramen ovale ends in a one-way valve that only permits blood flow from right to left. Flow patterns in the right atrium allow 50% of oxygenated blood returning from the placenta to be shunted to the left atrium. This right-to-left flow through the foramen ovale is maintained by the larger quantity and greater speed of blood flow from the inferior vena cava on the right, compared with that entering the left atrium via the pulmonary veins from the lungs. During fetal life, lung tissue *extracts* oxygen from the low circulating blood volume entering from the right ventricle and returns poorly oxygenated blood to the left atrium. Low venous return from the lungs is actively maintained by the exposure of pulmonary vessels to blood PO_2, which keeps them in a state of hypoxic vasoconstriction (Walker 1993).

A small volume of well-oxygenated blood from the inferior vena cava enters the right atrium. This is mixed with poorly oxygenated blood returning from the head via the superior vena cava, which mainly enters the right ventricle through the tricuspid valve. From the right ventricle, only 10% of blood enters the lungs via pulmonary arteries. The remaining 90% is diverted into the descending aorta via a muscular artery called the *ductus arteriosus*, which connects the main pulmonary artery to the aorta. Throughout fetal life, patency and therefore relaxation of this muscular artery is actively maintained by the low fetal PO_2, high circulating levels of PGE_2 and local release of PGI_2 (Amash et al 2009). As a result of this shunt, most blood leaving the right ventricle perfuses the lower body and the placenta (Moore and Persaud 2008: 325; Walker 1993).

In the left atrium, the pulmonary component combines with a much larger volume of more highly oxygenated blood from the inferior vena cava. From the left atrium, blood passes into the left ventricle. A small amount of this blood supplies the heart, two-thirds leaves via the ascending aorta to perfuse the upper part of the body with highly oxygenated blood, while the remaining one-third flows through the aortic isthmus to the descending aorta, and then to the lower body and placenta (Walker 1993). Two hypogastric arteries convey deoxygenated blood to the placenta.

Shunting of blood on the venous side by the foramen ovale and on the arterial side by the ductus arteriosus are structural devices that enable the blood to bypass the lungs and be directed to the placenta. This large volume of poorly oxygenated blood returning to the placenta flows much more rapidly than the more highly oxygenated blood supplying the upper body. The rate of flow tends to

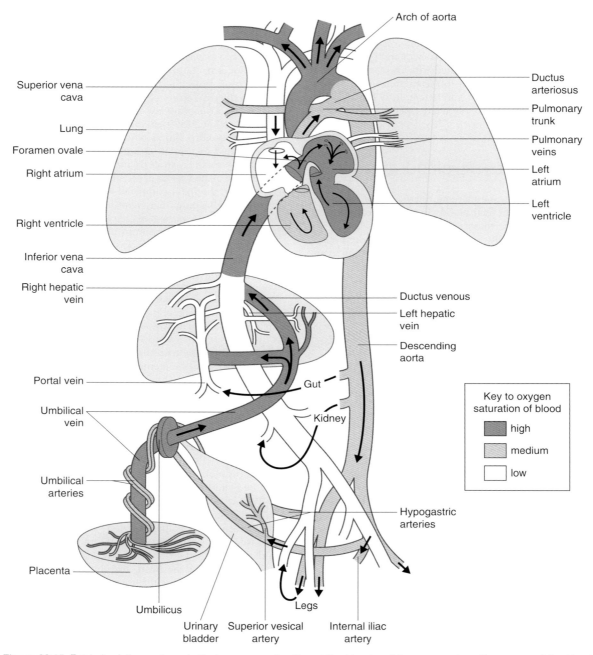

Arch of aorta

Superior vena cava

Lung

Foramen ovale

Right atrium

Right ventricle

Inferior vena cava

Right hepatic vein

Portal vein

Umbilical vein

Umbilical arteries

Placenta

Ductus arteriosus

Pulmonary trunk

Pulmonary veins

Left atrium

Left ventricle

Ductus venous

Left hepatic vein

Descending aorta

Gut

Kidney

Hypogastric arteries

Key to oxygen saturation of blood

high
medium
low

Umbilicus

Urinary bladder

Superior vesical artery

Legs

Internal iliac artery

Figure 29.15 Fetal circulation: colours indicate oxygen saturation of the blood and the arrows show the course of the blood from the placenta to the heart. (This article was published in Moore KL, Persaud TVN: The developing human, Philadelphia, Saunders, Copyright Elsevier, 2008.)

be most rapid in the descending aorta. From this vessel, blood is directly pumped into the umbilical arteries and returns for gaseous exchange in the placenta (Walker 1993; Fig. 29.15).

During intra-uterine life, the fetal–placental circulation operates as a single unit, providing a low-resistance, high-capacity reservoir in the vascular bed of the placenta, maintained by the absence of valves in the umbilical veins. From animal experiments, total fetal–placental blood volume is estimated at 100 to 120 mL/kg body weight, with 80 to 90 mL/kg representing fetal blood volume at any given time, while the remainder is contained within the umbilical–placental circulation. This additional capacity helps protect the fetal circulation from fluctuations in blood pressure and blood flow distribution at a time when autoregulation of regional blood flow is not fully developed.

MATERNAL–FETO-PLACENTAL NEUROHORMONAL INTERACTIONS

Adrenal and thyroid hormones are essential for the regulation of intra-uterine homoeostasis, and for the timely differentiation and maturation of fetal organs. These hormones play complex roles during fetal life and are believed to underlie the cellular communication that coordinates maternal-fetal interactions.

Central role of adrenal cortex and placenta

Steroidogenic enzymes are present in the emerging adrenal cortex from 6 to 7 weeks gestation. Synthesis of the main hormones, dehydroepiandrosterone (DHEA), its sulphate, DHEA-S, and pregnenolone sulphate begins from 6 weeks gestation, while cortisol synthesis occurs between 7 and 12 weeks gestation (Goto et al 2006; Kempna and Fluck 2008; Tsakiri et al 2002).

From 8 to 10 weeks onwards, DHEA-S and pregnenolone sulphate are increasingly utilized by the placenta as essential substrates for formation of oestrogens and progesterone (Pasqualini 2005). Transfer of maternal glucocorticoids to the fetus is regulated by a placental glucocortical 'barrier'. Regulatory mechanisms are essential to stimulate placental and fetal growth, and protect rapidly growing fetal organs from excess glucocorticoid exposure (Wyrwoll et al 2009). This also enables the preparation of intra-uterine tissues and fetal organs for the transition from pregnancy to labour.

Development of the adrenal cortex

The significance of the adrenal glands is indicated by their spectacular growth and secretory capacity during intra-uterine life. Cells forming the cortex appear at 3 to 4 weeks gestation and enlarge rapidly to equal the size of the kidneys by the end of the first trimester. By 6 to 8 weeks gestation, the cortex forms these distinct zones:

- a large inner fetal zone
- an outer definitive zone that forms a thin subcapsular rim
- an indistinct transitional area between the two (Goto et al 2006; Tsakiri et al 2002)

During the second trimester, the adrenals enlarge in direct proportion to the increase in total body weight. At this time, their relative weight is 35 times the adult value. In the third trimester, gland weights continue to increase but at a slower rate than the rest of the body. At term, the fetal adrenals are similar in size to those in the adult (Pearson Murphy and Branchaud 1994; Seron-Ferre and Jaffe 1981).

Adrenal growth seems to be largely regulated by hCG, ACTH, oestradiol, prolactin, melatonin and growth factors derived from within the glands, along with those from other fetal organs, including the placenta, liver and kidneys (Freemark et al 1997; Tsakiri et al 2002). Until the latter part of pregnancy, the active steroid-producing fetal zone is predominantly involved in synthesizing DHEA-S for the placenta (Pepe and Albrecht 1990). During the last 3 months of pregnancy, maternal melatonin stimulates adrenal weight gain and synthesis of DHEA-S, while at the same time negatively regulates the process of maturation by inhibiting ACTH- and CRH-induced production of cortisol.

Adrenal medulla

In contrast to the cortex, the chromaffin cells are formed from adjacent sympathetic ganglia that are derived from the neural crest. Unlike the cortex, this part of the gland does not become a discrete structure during fetal life. During this period, small islands of chromaffin cells are scattered throughout the cortex and larger and much more active islets form independently of the medulla, along the outside of the aorta (Mesiano and Jaffe 1997). Immature chromaffin cells have been observed from approximately 8 weeks and significant concentrations of noradrenaline have been found from 15 weeks gestation. No degeneration has been found to occur in these cells until the postnatal period (Phillippe 1983).

Within the adrenal gland, small groups of cells that contain measurable amounts of noradrenaline have been observed at 9 weeks, but their content remains low until the third trimester. While noradrenaline remains predominant in the fetal response to stress, the rising capacity for cortisol production near term produces a sharp increase in the capacity of chromaffin cells to produce adrenaline. The proportion of adrenaline increases progressively from approximately 28 weeks to term, when it constitutes around 50% of total catecholamine content of the gland. As measured in amniotic fluid, catecholamine metabolites increase between the second and third trimester and plasma catecholamine concentrations rise progressively during the course of labour. These changes mediate a range of cardiovascular, metabolic and respiratory responses to labour and birth (Lagercrantz and Marcus 1992; Lagercrantz and Slotkin 1986; Phillippe 1983).

CONCLUSION

Maternal adaptations to support implantation and formation of the distinct biological environments for embryo formation and feto-placental development begin during the luteal phase of the cycle. The presence of the conceptus is recognized through intracellular and hormonal signals that accelerate adaptations in central and peripheral maternal organ systems. Intra-uterine conditions for embryo formation during the first trimester are very different from those that emerge to support the feto-placental system. Knowledge of these transformations enables women to understand the dramatic changes in their bodily experiences from early to late pregnancy.

Key Points

- Fertilization and blastocyst activation takes place in a fluid medium that is determined by maternal nutritional status
- Successful fertilization, implantation and placental formation depend on cyclical changes in steroid hormones across the ovarian cycle
- Intense activity occurs within the uterus after fertilization, as extraembryonic tissues proliferate ahead of embryo formation in a low-oxygen environment
- At the end of feto-placental development, maturational changes have taken place in organs, such as the lungs and liver, while the HPA axis is briefly activated to regulate the onset of labour

References

Amash A, Holcberg G, Sheiner E, et al: Lipopolysaccharide differently affects prostaglandin E_2 levels in fetal and maternal compartments of perfused human term placenta, *Prostaglandins Other Lipid Mediat* 88:18–22, 2009.

Armant DR: Blastocysts don't go it alone. Extrinsic signals fine-tune the intrinsic development program of trophoblast cells, *Dev Biol* 280:260–280, 2005.

Bahat A, Tur-Kaspa I, Gakamsky A, et al: Thermotaxis of mammalian sperm cells: a potential navigation mechanism in the female genital tract, *Nat Med* 9(2):149–151, 2003.

Baird DD, Weinberg CR, McConnaughey DR, et al: Rescue of the corpus luteum in human pregnancy, *Biol Reprod* 68:448–456, 2003.

Battista N, Pasquariello N, Di Tomaso M, et al: Interplay between endocannabinoids, steroids and cytokines in the control of human reproduction, *J Neuroendocrinol* 20(Suppl 1):82–89, 2008.

Bell RJ, Eddie LW, Lester AR, et al: Relaxin in human pregnancy serum measured with a homologous radioimmunoassay, *Obstet Gynecol* 69:585–589, 1987.

Bendich AJ: Mitochondrial DNA, chloroplast DNA and the origins of development in eukaryotic organisms, *Biol Direct* 5:42, 2010.

Bentov Y: 'A Western diet side story': the effects of transitioning to a Western-type diet on fertility, *Endocrinology* 155(7):2341–2342, 2014.

Brace RA: Current topic: progress toward understanding the regulation of amniotic fluid volume: water and solute fluxes in and through the fetal membranes, *Placenta* 16:1–18, 1995.

Brauer MM, Smith PG: Estrogen and female reproductive tract innervations: cellular and molecular mechanisms of autonomic neuroplasticity, *Auton Neurosci* 187:1–15, 2015.

Burton GJ, Hempstock J, Jauniaux E: Nutrition, genetics and placental development, *Placenta* 22(Suppl A):S70–S76, 2001.

Burton GJ, Watson AL, Hempstock J, et al: Uterine glands provide histotrophic nutrition for the human fetus during the first trimester of pregnancy, *J Clin Endocrinol Metab* 87(6):2954–2959, 2002.

Burton GJ, Kaufmann P, Huppertz B: Anatomy and genesis of the placenta. In Neill JD, editor: *Knobil and Neill's physiology of reproduction*, Amsterdam, Elsevier, 2006.

Burton GJ, Jauniaux E, Charnock-Jones DS: Human early placental development: potential roles of the endometrial glands, *Placenta* 28(Suppl A):S64–S69, 2007.

Burton GJ, Woods AW, Jauniaux E, et al: Rheological and physiological consequences of conversion of the maternal spiral arteries for uteroplacental blood flow during human pregnancy, *Placenta* 30:473–482, 2009.

Burton GJ, Jauniaux E, Charnock-Jones DS: The influence of the intrauterine environment on human placental development, *Int J Dev Biol* 54:303–311, 2010.

Butler SJ, Bronner ME: From classical to current: analyzing peripheral nervous system and spinal cord lineage and fate, *Dev Biol* 398:135–146, 2015.

Caniggia I, Winter JL: Hypoxia inducible factor-1: oxygen regulation of trophoblast differentiation in normal and pre-eclamptic pregnancies – a review, *Placenta* 23(Suppl A):S47–S57, 2002.

Caniggia I, Mostachfi H, Winter J, et al: Hypoxia-inducible factor-1 mediates the biological effects of oxygen on human trophoblast differentiation through TGFβ3, *J Clin Invest* 105(5):577–587, 2000.

Carlson BM: *Human embryology and developmental biology*, St. Louis, Mosby, 1994.

Carvajal JA, Delpiano AM, Cuello MA, et al: Brain natriuretic peptide (BNP) produced by human chorioamnion may mediate pregnancy myometrial quiescence, *Reprod Sci* 16(1):32–42, 2009.

Casan EM, Raga F, Polan ML: GnRH mRNA and protein expression in human preimplantation embryos, *Mol Hum Reprod* 5(3):234–239, 1999.

Casan EM, Raga F, Bonilla-Musoles F, et al: Human oviductal gonadotrophin-releasing hormone: possible implication in fertilization, early embryonic development, and implantation, *J Clin Endocrinol Metab* 85(4):1377–1381, 2000.

Chamberlain G, Broughton Pipkin F: *Clinical physiology in obstetrics*, Oxford, 1998, Blackwell Scientific.

Chapman AB, Zamudio S, Woodmansee W, et al: Systemic and renal hemodynamic changes in the luteal phase of the menstrual cycle mimic early pregnancy, *Am J Physiol* 273(42):F777–F782, 1997.

Chard T, Iles R, Wathen N: Why is there a peak of human chorionic gonadotrophin (HCG) in early pregnancy?, *Hum Reprod* 10(7):1837–1840, 1995.

Cheon KW, Lee H-S, Parah IS, et al: Expression of the second isoform of gonadotrophin-releasing hormone (GnRH)-II in human endometrium throughout the menstrual cycle, *Mol Hum Reprod* 7(5):447–452, 2001.

Cole LA: Biological functions of hCG and hCG-related molecules, *Reprod Biol Endocrinol* 8:102, 2010.

Cole LA: hCG, five independent molecules, *Clin Chim Acta* 413:48–65, 2012.

Cootauco AC, Murphy JD, Maleski J, et al: Atrial natriuretic peptide production and natriuretic peptide receptors in the human uterus and their effects on myometrial relaxation, *Am J Obstet Gynecol* 199(429):e1–e6, 2008.

Colicchia M, Campagnolo L, Baldini E, et al: Molecular basis of thyrotropin and thyroid hormone action during implantation and early development, *Hum Reprod Update* 20(6):884–904, 2014.

Davison JM, Shiells EA, Phillips PR, et al: Influence of hormonal and volume factors on altered osmoregulation of normal human pregnancy, *Am J Physiol* 258(27):F900–F907, 1990.

de Groot RHM, Adamc JJ, Hornstrab G: Selective attention deficits during human pregnancy, *Neurosci Lett* 340:21–24, 2003.

De Swiet M: The cardiovascular system. In Hytten F, Chamberlain G, editors: *Clinical physiology in obstetrics*, Oxford, Blackwell Scientific, 1991.

Dickens CJ, Leese HJ: The regulation of rabbit oviduct fluid formation, *J Reprod Fertil* 100:577–581, 1994.

DiPietro JA, Irizarry RA, Costigan KA, et al: The psychophysiology of the maternal–fetal relationship, *Psychophysiology* 41:510–520, 2004.

DiPietro JA, Costigan KA, Nelson P, et al: Fetal responses to induced maternal relaxation during pregnancy, *Biol Psychol* 77(1):11–19, 2008.

Dominguez-Salas P, Moore SE, Baker MS, et al: Maternal nutrition at conception modulates DNA methylation of human metastable epialleles, *Nat Commun* 5:3746, 2015.

Downs KM: Embryological origins of the human individual, *DNA Cell Biol* 27(1):3–7, 2008.

Drobnis EZ, Overstreet JW: Natural history of mammalian spermatozoa in the female reproductive tract, *Oxf Rev Reprod Biol* 14:1–45, 1992.

Dunstan GR, editor: *The human embryo*, Exeter, University of Exeter Press, 1990.

Eckert JJ, Porter R, Watkins AJ, et al: Metabolic induction and early responses of mouse blastocyst developmental programming following maternal low protein diet affecting life-long health, *PLoS One* 7(12):e52791, 2012.

Edwards RG: The role of embryonic polarities in preimplantation growth and implantation of mammalian embryos, *Hum Reprod* 15(Suppl 6):1–8, 2000.

Ellery PM, Cindrova-Davies T, Jauniaux E, et al: Evidence for transcriptional activity in the syncytiotrophoblast of the human placenta, *Placenta* 30:329–334, 2009.

Erwich JJHM, Keirse MJMC: Placental localisation of 15-hydroxyprostaglandin dehydrogenase in early and term pregnancy, *Placenta* 13:223–229, 1992.

Evans JP: The molecular basis of sperm–oocyte membrane interactions during mammalian fertilization, *Hum Reprod Update* 8(4):297–311, 2002.

Evans J, Salamonsen LA, Menkhorst E, et al: Dynamic changes in hyperglycosylated human chorionic gonadotrophin throughout the first trimester of pregnancy and its role in early placentation, *Hum Reprod* 30(5):1029–1038, 2015.

Ferretti C, Bruni L, Dangles-Marie V, et al: Molecular circuits shared by placental and cancer cells, and their implications in the proliferative, invasive and migratory capacities of trophoblasts, *Hum Reprod Update* 13(2):121–141, 2007.

FitzGerald MJT, FitzGerald M: *Human embryology*, London, Baillière Tindall, 1994.

Fitzgerald JS, Poehlmann TG, Schleussner E, et al: Trophoblast invasion: the role of intracellular cytokine signaling via signal transducer and activator of transcription 3 (STAT3), *Hum Reprod Update* 14(4):335–344, 2008.

Fleming TP, Kwong WY, Porter R, et al: The embryo and its future, *Biol Reprod* 71:1046–1054, 2004.

Fleming TP, Watkins AJ, Sun C, et al: Do little embryos make big decisions? How maternal dietary protein restriction can permanently change an embryo's potential, affecting adult health, *Reprod Fertil Dev* 27:684–692, 2015.

Freemark M, Driscoll P, Maaskant R, et al: Ontogenesis of prolactin receptors in the human fetus in early gestation, *J Clin Invest* 99(5):1107–1117, 1997.

Fride E: Multiple roles for the endocannabinoid system during the early stages of life: pre- and postnatal development, *J Neuroendocrinol* 20(s1):75–81, 2008.

Fritz R, Jain C, Armant DR: Cell signaling in trophoblast-uterine communication, *Int J Dev Biol* 58:261–271, 2014.

Gardner DK, Leese HJ: Concentrations of nutrients in mouse oviduct fluid and their effects on embryo development and metabolism *in vitro*, *J Reprod Fertil* 88:361–368, 1990.

Gargett CE, Lederman F, Heryonto B, et al: Focal vascular endothelial growth factor correlates with angiogenesis in human endometrium. Role of intravascular neutrophils, *Hum Reprod* 16(6):1065–1075, 2001.

Glock JL, Nakajima ST, Stewart DR, et al: The relationship of corpus luteum volume to relaxin, estradiol, progesterone and human chorionic gonadotrophin levels in early normal pregnancy, *Early Pregnancy* 1:206–211, 1995.

Goto M, Hanley KP, Marcos J, et al: In humans, early cortisol biosynthesis provides a mechanism to safeguard female sexual development, *J Clin Invest* 116(4):953–960, 2006.

Gubbay O, Critchley HO, Bowen JM, et al: Prolactin induces ERK phosphorylation in epithelial and CD56+ natural killer cells of the human endometrium, *J Clin Endocrinol Metab* 87(5):2329–2335, 2002.

Habayeb OMH, Taylor AH, Bell SC, et al: Expression of endocannabinoid system in human first trimester placenta and its role in trophoblast proliferation, *Endocrinology* 149(10):5052–5060, 2008.

Handschuh K, Guibourdenche J, Tsatsaris V, et al: Human chorionic gonadotrophin expression in human trophoblasts from early placenta: comparative study between villous and extravillous trophoblastic cells, *Placenta* 28:175–184, 2007.

Hunter RHF: The fallopian tubes in domestic mammals: how vital is their physiological activity?, *Reprod Nutr Dev* 45:281–290, 2005.

Hustin J: The maternotrophoblast interface: uteroplacental blood flow. In Barnea ER, Hustin J, Jauniaux E, editors: *The first twelve weeks of gestation*, Berlin, Springer-Verlag, 1992.

Hustin J, Franchimont P: The endometrium and implantation. In Barnea ER, Hustin J, Jauniaux E, editors: *The first twelve weeks of gestation*, Berlin, Springer-Verlag, 1992.

Hustin J, Schaaps J-P: Echocardiographic and anatomic studies of the maternotrophoblast border during the first trimester of pregnancy, *Am J Obstet Gynecol* 157(1):162–168, 1987.

Hustin J, Schaaps J-P, Lambotte R: Anatomical studies of the utero-placental vascularization in the first trimester of pregnancy, *Trophoblast Res* 3:49–60, 1988.

Islami D, Bischof P, Chardonnens D: Modulation of placental vascular endothelial growth factor by leptin and hCG, *Mol Hum Reprod* 9(7):395–398, 2003.

Ivanov PCh, Ma QDY, Bartsch RP: Maternal-fetal heartbeat phase synchronization, *Proc Natl Acad Sci USA* 106(33):13641–13642, 2009.

Jabbour HN, Critchley HOD: Potential roles of decidual prolactin in early pregnancy, *Reproduction* 121:197–205, 2001.

Jauniaux E, Gulbis B: Embryonic physiology. In Jauniaux E, Barnea ER, Edwards RG, editors: *Embryonic medicine and therapy*, Oxford, Oxford University Press, 1997.

Jauniaux E, Gulbis B: In vivo investigation of placental transfer early in human pregnancy, *Eur J Obstet Gynecol Reprod Biol* 92:45–49, 2000.

Jauniaux E, Moscoso JG: Morphology and significance of the human yolk sac. In Barnea ER, Hustin J, Jauniaux E, editors: *The first twelve weeks of gestation*, Berlin, Springer-Verlag, 1992.

Jauniaux E, Gulbis B, Jurkovic D, et al: Protein and steroid levels in embryonic cavities in early human pregnancy, *Hum Reprod* 8(5):782–787, 1993.

Jauniaux E, Gulbis B, Jurkovic D, et al: Relationship between protein concentrations in embryological fluids and maternal serum and yolk sac size during human early pregnancy, *Hum Reprod* 9(1):161–166, 1994.

Jauniaux E, Wilson A, Burton G: Evaluation of respiratory gases and acid-base gradients in human fetal fluids and uteroplacental tissue between 7 and 16 weeks' gestation, *Am J Obstet Gynecol* 184(5):998–1003, 2001.

Jauniaux E, Gulbis B, Burton GJ: The human first trimester gestational sac limits rather than facilitates oxygen transfer to the fetus – a review, *Placenta* 24(Suppl A):S86–S93, 2003.

Jauniaux E, Cindrova-Davies T, Johns J, et al: Distribution and transfer pathways of antioxidant molecules inside the first trimester human gestational sac, *J Clin Endocrinol Metab* 89(3):1452–1458, 2004.

Johnson MH: *Essential reproduction*, 7th edn, Oxford, Blackwell Scientific, 2013.

Jones CJP: The life and death of the embryonic yolk sac. In Jauniaux E, Barnea ER, Edwards RG, editors: *Embryonic medicine and therapy*, Oxford, Oxford University Press, 1997.

Kaji K, Kudo A: The mechanism of sperm-oocyte fusion in mammals, *Reproduction* 127:423–429, 2004.

Kempna P, Fluck CE: Adrenal gland development and defects, *Best Pract Res Clin Endocrinol Metab* 22(1):77–93, 2008.

Kermack AJ, Finn-Sell S, Cheong Ying C, et al: Amino acid composition of human uterine fluid: association with age, lifestyle and gynaecological, pathology, *Hum Reprod* 30(4):917–924, 2015.

Kikkawa F, Kajiyama H, Watanabe Y, et al: Possible involvement of placental peptidases that degrade gonadotrophin-releasing hormone (GnRH) in the dynamic pattern of placental hCG secretion via GnRH degradation, *Placenta* 23:483–489, 2002.

King AE, Critchley HO, Kelly RW: The NF-kappa B pathway in human endometrium and first trimester decidua, *Mol Hum Reprod* 7:175–183, 2001.

Kosaka K, Fujiwara H, Tatsumi K, et al: Human chorionic gonadotrophin (HCG) activates monocytes to produce interleukin-8 via a different pathway from luteinizing hormone/HCG receptor system, *J Clin Endocrinol Metab* 87(11):5199–5208, 2002.

Kristiansson P, Wang JX: Reproductive hormones and blood pressure during pregnancy, *Hum Reprod* 16(1):13–17, 2001.

Kunz G, Noe M, Herbertz M, et al: Uterine peristalsis during the follicular phase of the menstrual cycle: effects of oestrogen, antioestrogen and oxytocin, *Hum Reprod Update* 4(5):647–654, 1998.

Lacroix M-C, Guibourdenche J, Fournier T, et al: Stimulation of human trophoblast invasion by placental growth hormone, *Endocrinology* 146(5):2434–2444, 2005.

Lagercrantz H, Marcus C: Sympathoadrenal mechanisms during development. In Polin RA, Fox WW, editors: *Fetal and neonatal physiology*, Philadelphia, Saunders, 1992.

Lagercrantz H, Slotkin TA: The 'stress' of being born, *Sci Am* 254:92–102, 1986.

Lancel M, Faulhaber J, Holsboer F, et al: Progesterone induces changes in sleep comparable to those of agonistic GABAA receptor modulators, *Am J Physiol* 271(34):E763–E772, 1996.

Lapointe J, Kimmins S, McLaren LA, et al: Estrogen selectively up-regulates the phospholipid hydroperoxide glutathione peroxidase in the oviducts, *Endocrinology* 146(6):2583–2592, 2005.

Leese HJ: Metabolism of the preimplantation embryo: 40 years on, *Reproduction* 143:417–427, 2012.

Leese HJ, Baumann C, Brison G, et al: Metabolism of the viable mammalian embryo: quietness revisited, *Mol Hum Reprod* 14(12):667–672, 2008.

Leese HJ, Hugentobler SA, Gray SM, et al: Female reproductive tract fluids: composition, mechanism of formation and potential role in the developmental origins of health and disease, *Reprod Fertil Dev* 20:1–8, 2008a.

Leese HJ: Quiet please, do not disturb: a hypothesis of embryo metabolism and viability, *Bioessays* 24(9):845–849, 2002.

Leese HJ, Tay JI, Reischi J, et al: Formation of fallopian tubal fluid: role of a neglected epithelium, *Reproduction* 121:339–346, 2001.

Leese HJ: Metabolic control during preimplantation mammalian development, *Hum Reprod* 1(1):63–72, 1995.

Lei ZM, Rao CV, Kornyei JL, et al: Novel expression of human chorionic gonadotrophin/luteinizing hormone receptor gene in brain, *Endocrinology* 132(5):2262–2270, 1993.

Lei ZM, Rao CV: Novel presence of luteinizing hormone/human chorionic gonadotrophin (hCG) receptors and the down-regulating action of hCG on gonadotrophin-releasing hormone gene expression in immortalized hypothalamic gt1-7 neurons, *Mol Endocrinol* 8:1111–1121, 1994.

Leppens-Luisier G, Urner F, Sakkas D: Facilitated glucose transporters play a crucial role throughout mouse preimplantation embryo development, *Hum Reprod* 16(6):1229–1236, 2001.

Lessey BA: The role of the endometrium during embryo implantation, *Hum Reprod* 15(Suppl 6):39–50, 2000.

Lukacs H, Hiatt ES, Lei ZM, et al: Peripheral and intracerebroventricular administration of human chorionic gonadotrophin alters several hippocampus-associated behaviors in cycling female rats, *Horm Behav* 29:42–58, 1995.

Ma W, Tan J, Matsumoto H, et al: Adult tissue angiogenesis: evidence for negative regulation by estrogen in the uterus, *Mol Endocrinol* 15(11):1983–1992, 2001.

Mark PJ, Smith JT, Waddell BJ: Placental and fetal growth retardation following partial progesterone withdrawal in rat pregnancy, *Placenta* 27:208–214, 2006.

Mesiano S, Jaffe RB: Development and functional biology of the primate fetal adrenal cortex, *Endocr Rev* 18(3):378–403, 1997.

Moore KL, Persaud TVN: *The developing human*, Philadelphia, Saunders, 2008.

Muller-Schottle F, Classen-Linke I, Alfer J, et al: Expression of uteroglobin in the human endometrium, *Mol Hum Reprod* 5(12):1155–1161, 1999.

Myers M, Lamont MC, van den Driesche S, et al: Role of luteal glucocorticoid metabolism during maternal recognition of pregnancy in women, *Endocrinology* 148:5769–5779, 2007.

Pauperstein CJ, Eddy CA: Morphology of the fallopian tube. In Beller FK, Schumacher, editors: *The biology of the fluids of the female genital tract*, Elsevier Science Ltd, 1979.

Pasqualini JR: Enzymes involved in the formation and transformation of steroid hormones in the fetal and placental compartments, *J Steroid Biochem Mol Biol* 97:401–415, 2005.

Pearson Murphy BE, Branchaud CL: The fetal adrenal. In Tulchinsky D, Little BA, editors: *Maternal–fetal endocrinology*, Philadelphia, Saunders, 1994.

Pepe GJ, Albrecht ED: Regulation of the primate fetal adrenal cortex, *Endocr Rev* 11(1):151–176, 1990.

Phillippe M: Fetal catecholamines, *Am J Obstet Gynecol* 146(7):840–855, 1983.

Pijnenborg R, Vercruysse L, Hanssens M: The uterine spiral arteries in human pregnancy: facts and controversies, *Placenta* 27:939–958, 2006.

Ramsey EM, Houston ML, Harris JW: Interaction of the trophoblast and maternal tissues in three closely related primate species, *Am J Obstet Gynecol* 124(6):647–652, 1976.

Remes Lenicov F, Rodriguez Rodrigues C, Sabatté J, et al: Semen promotes the differentiation of tolerogenic dendritic cells, *J Immunol* 189:4777–4786, 2012.

Schjenken JE, Robertson SA: Seminal fluid and immune adaptation for pregnancy – comparative biology in mammalian species, *Reprod Domest Anim* 49(Suppl 3):27–36, 2014.

Schultz RM: Blastocyst. In Knobil E, Neill JD, editors: *Encyclopedia of reproduction*, vol 1, San Diego, Academic Press, 1998.

Seppala M, Taylor RN, Koistinen H, et al: Glycodelin: a major lipocalin protein of the reproductive axis with diverse actions in cell recognition and differentiation, *Endocr Rev* 23(4):401–430, 2002.

Seron-Ferre M, Mendez N, Abarzua-Catalan L, et al: Circadian rhythms in the fetus, *Mol Cell Endocrinol* 349:68–75, 2012.

Seron-Ferre M, Jaffe RB: The fetal adrenal gland, *Annu Rev Physiol* 43:141–162, 1981.

Shafik A, Shafik AA, El Sibai O, et al: Specialized pacemaking cells in the human fallopian tube, *Mol Hum Reprod* 11(7):503–505, 2005.

Sheppard BI, Bonnar J: The maternal blood supply to the placenta, *Prog Obstet Gynecol* 7:27–30, 1989.

Simon C, Gimeno J, Mercader A, et al: Embryonic regulation of β_3, α_4 and α_1 in human endometrial cells in vitro, *J Clin Endocrinol Metab* 82(8):2607–2616, 1997.

Starkey PM: The decidua and factors controlling placentation. In Redman CWG, Sargent IL, Starkey PM, editors: *The human placenta*, Oxford, Blackwell Scientific, 1993.

Stewart DR, Overstreet JW, Nakajima T, et al: Enhanced ovarian steroid secretion before implantation in early human pregnancy, *J Clin Endocrinol Metab* 76(6):1470–1476, 1993.

Stouffer RL: Progesterone as a mediator of gonadotrophin action in the corpus luteum: beyond steroidogenesis, *Hum Reprod Update* 9(2):99–107, 2003.

Strauss JF, Williams CJ: The ovarian life cycle. In Strauss JF, Barbieri RL, editors: *Yen & Jaffe's reproductive endocrinology*, 7th edn, Philadelphia, Elsevier, Saunders, 2014.

Talbot PD, Shur BD, Myles DG: Cell adhesion and fertilization: steps in oocyte transport, sperm-zona pellucida interactions, and sperm-egg fusion, *Biol Reprod* 68:1–9, 2003.

Tamura H, Nakamura Y, Terron MP, et al: Melatonin and pregnancy in the human, *Reprod Toxicol* 25:291–303, 2008.

Tarrade A, Kuen RL, Malassine A, et al: Characterization of human villous and extravillous trophoblasts isolated from first trimester placenta, *Lab Invest* 81(9):1199–1211, 2001.

Telgmann R, Gellersen B: Marker genes of decidualisation: activation of the decidual prolactin gene, *Hum Reprod Update* 4:472–479, 1998.

Ticconi C, Zicari A, Belmonte A, et al: Pregnancy-promoting actions of HCG in human myometrium, and fetal membranes, *Placenta* 28(Suppl A):S137–S143, 2007.

Tosti E, Boni R: Electrical events during gamete maturation and fertilization in animals and humans, *Hum Reprod Update* 10(1):53–65, 2004.

Tsakiri SP, Chrousos GP, Margioris AN: Molecular development of the hypothalamic-pituitary-adrenal (HPA) axis. In Eugster EA, Pescovitz OH, editors: *Developmental endocrinology*, Totowa, Humana Press, 2002.

Tseng L, Zhu HH, Mazella J, et al: Relaxin stimulates glycodelin mRNA and protein concentrations in human endometrial glandular epithelial cells, *Mol Hum Reprod* 5(4):372–375, 1999.

Tucker Blackburn S: *Maternal, fetal & neonatal physiology*, 4th edn, Maryland Heights, Elsevier. Kindle version 2014, 2012.

Van Leeuwen P, Geue D, Thiel M, et al: Influence of paced maternal breathing on fetal-maternal heart rate coordination, *Proc Natl Acad Sci USA* 106(33):13661–13666, 2009.

Vokes TJ, Weiss NM, Schreiber J, et al: Osmoregulation of thirst and vasopressin during normal menstrual cycle, *Am J Physiol* 254(23):R641–R647, 1988.

Walker AM: Circulatory transitions at birth and the control of neonatal circulation. In Hanson MA, Spencer JAD, Rodeck CH, editors: *Fetus and neonate: physiology and clinical applications, vol 1, The circulation*, Cambridge, Cambridge University Press, 1993.

Wang H, Guo Y, Wang D, et al: Aberrant cannabinoid signaling impairs oviduct transport of embryos, *Nat Med* 10(10):1074–1080, 2004.

Wang H, Xie H, Guo Y, et al: Fatty acid amide hydrolase deficiency limits early pregnancy events, *J Clin Invest* 116(8):2122–2131, 2006.

Wang WS, Liu C, Li WJ, et al: Involvement of CRH and hCG in the induction of aromatase by cortisol in human placental syncytiotrophoblasts, *Placenta* 35:30–36, 2014.

Watkins AJ, Lucas ES, Marfy-Smith S, et al: Maternal nutrition modifies trophoblast giant cell phenotype and fetal growth in mice, *Reproduction* 149:563–575, 2015.

Wildt L, Kissler S, Licht P, et al: Sperm transport in the human female genital tract and its modulation by oxytocin as assessed by hysterosalpingoscintigraphy, hysterotonography, electrohysterography and Doppler sonography, *Hum Reprod Update* 4(5):655–666, 1998.

Wyrwoll CS, Seckl JR, Holmes MC: Altered placental function of 11β-hydroxysteroid dehydrogenase 2 knockout mice, *Endocrinology* 150(3):1287–1293, 2009.

Zervomanolakis I, Ott HW, Seeber BE, et al: Uterine mechanisms of ipsilateral directed transport: evidence for a contribution of the utero-ovarian countercurrent system, *Eur J Obstet Gynecol Reprod Biol* 144S:S45–S49, 2009.

Resources and additional reading

Please refer to the chapter website resources.

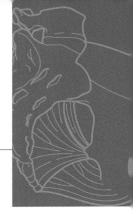

Chapter **30**

The fetal skull

Dr Barbara Burden and Amanda Willetts

Learning Outcomes ?

After reading this chapter, you will be able to:

- describe the process of fetal development of the structures of the skull
- be familiar with the components of the fetal skull and their significance
- assess the structures, circumference and diameters of the fetal skull and their importance in clinical practice
- identify internal structures within the fetal skull and possible complications that can occur during the birthing process
- describe the structures of the fetal skull and evaluate how this knowledge enables midwives to assess progress during labour and care through the neonatal period

INTRODUCTION

It is essential for a midwife to understand the parameters and characteristics of the fetal skull because of its significance during the mechanism of labour. Two key functions of the fetal skull are the protection of the brain, which is subjected to pressure as it descends through the birth canal during labour, and an ability to change shape, adapting to the process of labour in response to uterine contractions and the size and shape of the pelvis. By assessing the landmarks of the fetal skull, such as sutures and fontanelles, a midwife is able to diagnose the position and attitude of the fetal head in the pelvis, effectively assess progress of labour and determine the most likely mechanism of labour and mode of delivery.

DEVELOPMENT OF THE FETAL SKULL

As the fetus develops in utero, the *mesenchyme layer* surrounding the brain starts to ossify, forming the various bones of the fetal skull (see Ch. 29). This process is called *intramembranous ossification* and begins between 4 to 8 weeks gestation. The initial development of the skull occurs from this intramembranous structure, derived from neural crest cells and mesoderm. The intramembranous structure is divided into two major components, the *neurocranium*, which forms the protective case of the skull, and the *viscerocranium*, forming the bones of the face.

The neurocranium can be subdivided into the *chondrocranium* and the *dermatocranium*. The chondrocranium (cartilaginous part) is formed by the fusion of cartilages and, after ossification, becomes the occipital, temporal, sphenoid and ethmoid bones. The dermatocranium (membranous part) is thought to arise from the external dermal scales, developed to protect the brain. This lies under the superficial layers of the skin, covering and protecting the dorsal section of the brain, giving rise to the parietal and frontal bones.

The earliest visible signs of development can be seen on ultrasonography at about 4 to 6 weeks gestation with calcification of the membranes and the development of the occiput. This becomes easier to determine from approximately 8 weeks, when intramembranous ossification is more prominent. At 12 weeks, the outline of the individual bones become evident (Moore, Persaud and Torchia 2015; Sadler 2015; see Fig. 30.1).

Ossification of the bones continues throughout pregnancy with individual bones ossifying from their centre. At term, the bones of the skull are thin and pliable, enabling some movement of bones to take place during labour. The two frontal bones have usually united by term.

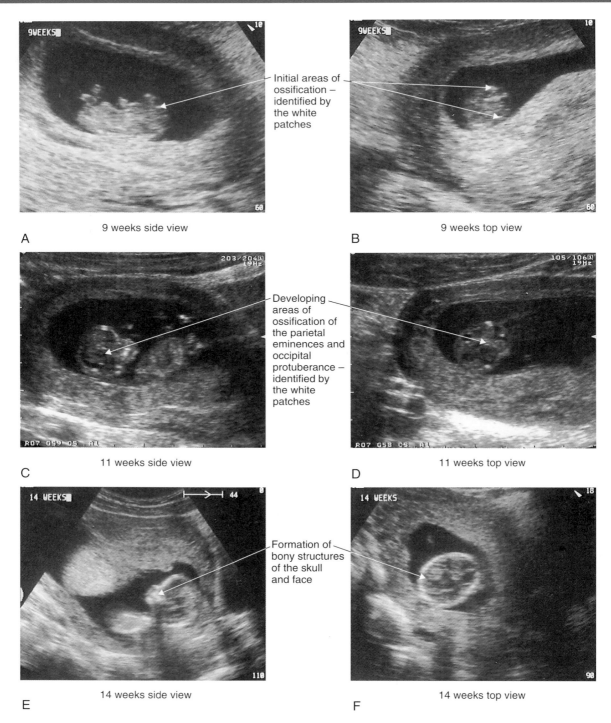

Initial areas of ossification – identified by the white patches

A   9 weeks side view

B   9 weeks top view

Developing areas of ossification of the parietal eminences and occipital protuberance – identified by the white patches

C   11 weeks side view

D   11 weeks top view

Formation of bony structures of the skull and face

E   14 weeks side view

F   14 weeks top view

Figure 30.1 Ultrasound images illustrating development and ossification of the fetal skull at 9, 11 and 14 weeks gestation. (Reproduced by kind permission of the Ultrasound Department at the Luton and Dunstable Hospital NHS Trust.)

THE EXTERNAL STRUCTURES OF THE NEWBORN SKULL

After birth, the midwife examines the external structures of the newborn head to identify any unusual characteristics or abnormalities in the skull structure (see Fig. 30.2). A baseline measurement of the newborn skull is sometimes taken during this procedure and documented within the child's neonatal records.

Layers of the external structures of the skull

The external structures of the skull are those from the skin through to the lining of the skull bones and are reflected in the acronym SCALP:

- Skin
- Connective tissue – a type of fascia that contains blood vessels and hair follicles. This may become oedematous during labour, resulting in a caput succedaneum
- Aponeurosis – a fibrous sheet of tissue connected to bone
- Loose connective tissue – a loose layer enabling movement of the scalp
- Periosteum – a double layer of connective tissue covering and nourishing the bone, which is attached to the edges of bone

THE SKULL

The fetal skull is a complex structure composed of 29 irregular flat bones with 22 of these paired symmetrically: 8 bones form the cranium, 14 the face and 7 the base (see Fig. 30.3). Knowledge of the fetal skull in the antenatal period enables a midwife to assess the size of the fetal head in relation to the size of the pelvis and assess engagement of the fetal skull in the pelvis (Barbera et al 2009). This also helps inform clinicians of analysis of ultrasonography parameters before and during labour (Tutschek, Torkildsen and Eggebø 2013).

Sutures

The sutures of the fetal skull are soft, fibrous tissues linking some bones of the skull. They enable moulding of the head to take place during labour and expansion of the brain as it develops during childhood.

The sutures of the skull are:

- frontal (metopic) suture (See Fig. 30.4)
- sagittal suture
- lambdoid (lambdoidal) suture
- coronal suture

Fontanelles

A fontanelle is a membranous, non-ossified area of the skull where three or more sutures meet (Fig. 30.4).

The significant fontanelles of the skull are:

- anterior fontanelle or bregma
- posterior fontanelle
- anterolateral or temporal fontanelles
- posterolateral or mastoid fontanelles

Sinuses

A sinus is a naturally occurring cavity in the body. Sinuses enable blood to circulate throughout the skull and into the brain membranes. The sinuses associated with the frontal, ethmoidal, sphenoidal and maxillary bones change shape during puberty and are thought to be associated with voice tone.

The bones and regions of the skull

The skull is divided into three main regions:

- the vault
- the base
- the face

The vault of the skull comprises:

- two frontal bones
- two parietal bones
- two temporal bones
- one occipital bone

Measurements of the fetal skull

The presentation and position of the fetal head in relation to the pelvic brim influence the degree of flexion or extension of the head and determine the precise realignment of the skull bones during labour and delivery. To assess the skull size in relation to various diameters of the maternal pelvis, diameters of the fetal skull have been measured to correspond with common postures adopted by the fetal head as it enters the pelvic brim (Figs 30.5 and 30.6). Each of these diameters and degree of flexion and extension of the fetal head has a direct effect on the progress and possible outcome of labour. By understanding this, the midwife can suitably inform the mother so that decisions can be made on positions in labour, pain relief and subsequent care of the baby at birth. It is important to remember, though, that these measurements are only an estimate and vary considerably, depending on the baby's size and weight.

Text continued on p. 474

Scalp

This is the thick, soft tissue covering the pericranium. It comprises skin, hair follicles, blood vessels, connective tissue and muscle fibres.

The scalp may have puncture marks or lacerations from fetal scalp electrodes if these are used intrapartum.

The tissues of the scalp may swell during labour owing to pressure of the maternal cervix on the presenting part of the head.

Circumference – suboccipitobregmatic

Measured from the base of the head where it joins the neck, around to the centre of the anterior fontanelle and back to the neck (33 cm).

This circumference is the measurement when the fetal head is well flexed in the lower uterine segment, aiding easy entrance to the pelvic brim.

Position of anterior fontanelle under the scalp

Felt as a diamond-shaped 'cavity' under the scalp.

The fontanelle in the healthy infant is soft and spongy to touch.

A sunken fontanelle is indicative of dehydration in the newborn.

A swollen fontanelle may be indicative of raised intracranial pressure in the newborn.

Brow

Also called the sinciput, it is the area covering the frontal bone.

Vertex

This area is bordered by the anterior fontanelle, the posterior fontanelle and laterally by the parietal eminences.

This is the most common presenting part of the fetus during labour and shows that the head is well flexed.

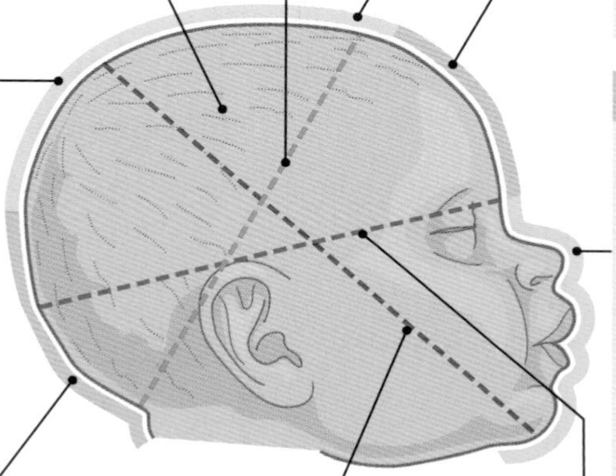

Face

The face of the newborn baby is smaller in relation to the head than that of an adult.

It extends from the supraorbital ridges to the chin.

It cannot mould during labour.

It may sustain severe swelling or bruising in labour when the face is the presenting part.

Occiput

This is the area over the occipital bone. The occiput is the denominator of the vertex used to assess and record the fetal presentation and position during the antenatal period and in labour. In a well-flexed cephalic presentation, the occiput will meet the pelvic floor and produce the internal rotation of the head necessary for extension of the head under the subpubic arch of the pelvis.

Circumference – mentovertical

Measured from the point of the chin to the highest point of the vertex and back to the chin (39 cm).

This circumference presents in a brow presentation.

Circumference – occipitofrontal

Measured from the glabella (bridge of the nose) to the occipital protuberance and back to the bridge of the nose (35 cm).

This is the measurement of the skull of the newborn baby recorded at birth.

This measurement is also the presenting circumference of a deflexed head during prolonged labour associated with premature rupture of membranes.

Figure 30.2 External structures and circumferences of the newborn skull.

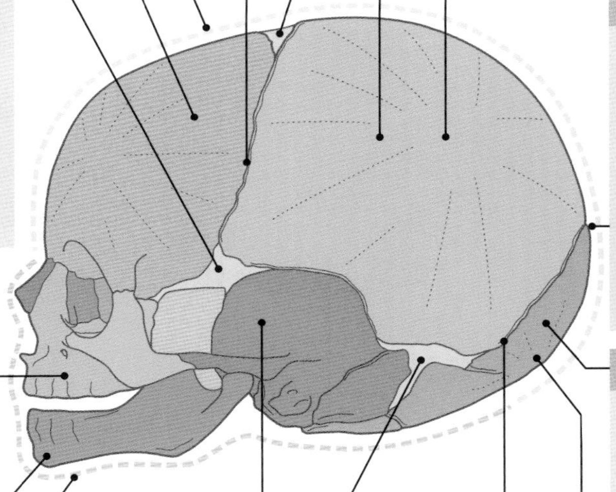

Vault

Extends from the orbital ridges to the nape of the neck.

This is the section of the fetal skull possessing the ability to compress during labour, facilitating the presentation of the smallest presenting part.

Coronal suture (2)

Passes from the anterolateral (temporal) fontanelle to the anterior fontanelle on both sides of the skull between the frontal and parietal bones.

Anterior fontanelle (bregma)

A diamond-shaped structure connecting four sutures. Usually 2–2.5 cm across and 2.5–3 cm long. Can be detected on vaginal examination when the head is deflexed as in an occipitoposterior position. Does not close for 16–18 months following birth.

Parietal bones (2)

These are the largest bones in the skull. The two bones are united at the top of the skull by the sagittal suture.

Parietal eminence

This is the point of origin of ossification in the parietal bone.

Frontal bones (2)

These bones are usually already fused together in the newborn baby at term.

Anterolateral fontanelle

This is situated between the temporal, frontal and parietal bones.

It has no significance in midwifery practice, but it is thought to enable expansion of the skull to facilitate growth of the brain during childhood.

Posterior fontanelle (lambda)

The fontanelle is triangular in shape and connects the lambdoidal sutures and the sagittal suture.

It is a key landmark used during vaginal examination to assess the fetal position and denominator in relation to parts of the maternal pelvis and is usually felt when the head is well flexed.

Maxilla

Upper jaw

Occipital bone

This is a triangular-shaped bone at the back of the skull, the boundary of which defines the area called the occiput.

Mandible

Jaw bone

Temporal bones (2)

Occipital protuberance

The point from which ossification commences in the fetus, forming the occipital bone.

Base

The bones of the base of the skull are united with the bones of the face. The bones of the base and face are unable to compress and therefore do not possess the ability to mould during labour.

Mastoid fontanelle

Fontanelle between the temporal, parietal and occipital bones.

Supports growth of the skull after birth.

Lambdoidal suture

Passes from the mastoid fontanelle to the posterior fontanelle on either side of the skull, connecting the posterior elements of the parietal bones with the occipital bone.

It has the ability to enable the occipital bone to move under the parietal bones during labour, helping to reduce the presenting diameter of the skull.

Figure 30.3 Characteristics of the fetal skull.

471

Lambdoidal suture

Passes from the mastoid fontanelle to the posterior fontanelle on either side of the skull, connecting the posterior elements of the parietal bones with the occipital bone.

It enables the occipital bone to move under the parietal bones during labour, helping to reduce the presenting diameter of the skull.

Occipital bone

Is connected to the parietal bones by the lambdoidal suture.

Posterior fontanelle (lambda)

The fontanelle is triangular in shape and connects the lambdoidal sutures and the sagittal suture.

It is a key landmark used during vaginal examination to assess the fetal position in relation to parts of the maternal pelvis and is usually palpated when the head is well flexed.

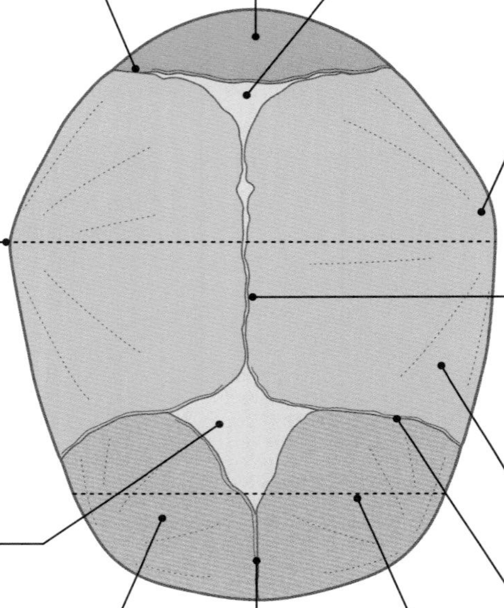

Parietal eminence

This is the point of origin of ossification in the parietal bone.

Biparietal diameter – 9.5 cm

This is the measurement of the distance between the two parietal eminences on the parietal bones.

Crowning of the baby's head occurs once this diameter is delivered vaginally.

Sagittal suture

This suture connects the anterior and posterior fontanelles and unites the two parietal bones at the top of the skull.

Parietal bone

The parietal bones are the largest bones in the skull. The two bones are united at the top of the skull by the sagittal suture.

Anterior fontanelle

A diamond-shaped structure connecting four sutures. Usually 2–2.5 cm across and 2.5–3 cm long.

Coronal suture

Passes from the temporal fontanelle to the anterior fontanelle on both sides of the skull, linking the frontal bones to the parietal bones.

Frontal bone

Consists of two bones, which are fused together in the full-term infant.

Frontal suture

This suture unites the frontal bones and is central to the brow. It is fused by adulthood.

Bitemporal diameter – 8 cm

This is the measurement along the coronal suture from its widest part at the temples.

Figure 30.4 The bones, sutures and fontanelles of the fetal skull.

Suboccipitofrontal – 10 cm

Measured from the junction of the head with the neck just below the occipital protuberance to the centre of the frontal suture.

This diameter presents when the fetal head is almost completely flexed and engages in the pelvis in a vertex presentation.

May result in normal moulding of the skull and possible caput succedaneum.

Submentobregmatic – 9.5 cm

Measured from the junction of the chin with the neck to the centre of the anterior fontanelle.

This diameter engages when the head is fully extended in a face presentation.

Mentovertical – 13.5 cm

Measured from the point of the chin to the central point of the top of the head at the vertex.

This diameter presents in a brow presentation where the head is midway between flexion and extension.

Suboccipitobregmatic – 9.5 cm

Measured from the junction of the head with the neck just below the occipital protuberance to the centre of the anterior fontanelle.

This diameter presents when the fetal head is flexed and engages in the pelvis in a vertex presentation.

This is the optimum diameter and shape for dilatation of the cervix in labour.

May result in normal moulding of the skull and possible caput succedaneum.

Occipitofrontal – 11.5 cm

Measured from the glabella (bridge of the nose) to the occipital protuberance.

This diameter presents in an occipitoposterior or occipitolateral position when there is insufficient flexion of the head. The outcome at birth may be a face-to-pubes delivery of the head following a persistent occipitoposterior position.

Submentovertical – 11 cm

Measured from the junction of the chin with the neck to the highest point on the vertex.

This diameter presents in a face presentation when the head is not fully extended.

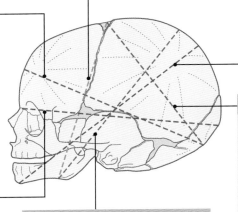

Figure 30.5 Diameters of the fetal skull.

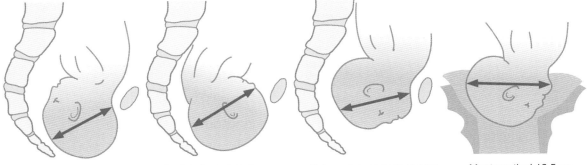

Suboccipitobregmatic 9.5 cm
vertex presentation

Occipitofrontal 11.5 cm
persistent occipitoposterior position

Submentobregmatic 9.5 cm
face presentation

Mentovertical 13.5 cm
brow presentation

Figure 30.6 Diameters of the fetal head in relation to the maternal pelvis.

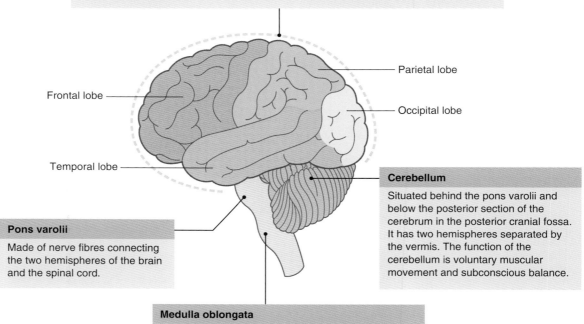

Cerebrum

Occupies the anterior and middle cranial fossae and is the largest part of the brain. It is divided by a cleft called the longitudinal cerebral fissure, giving the impression of two halves of the brain. These are called the right and left hemispheres. The superficial part of the cerebrum is composed of grey matter (nerve cell bodies), forming the cerebral cortex and the deep layers of white matter (nerve fibres).

Parietal lobe

Frontal lobe

Occipital lobe

Temporal lobe

Cerebellum

Situated behind the pons varolii and below the posterior section of the cerebrum in the posterior cranial fossa. It has two hemispheres separated by the vermis. The function of the cerebellum is voluntary muscular movement and subconscious balance.

Pons varolii

Made of nerve fibres connecting the two hemispheres of the brain and the spinal cord.

Medulla oblongata

A pyramid-shaped structure extending from the pons varolii above to the spinal cord below. Associated with elements of autonomic reflex activity such as cardiac and respiratory actions and reflexes such as vomiting, coughing, sneezing and swallowing.

Figure 30.7 External structures of the brain.

Reflective activity 30.1

When you examine a baby next, pay particular attention to the skull bones, sutures and fontanelles, which can easily be felt under the scalp. Note the degree of tension of the anterior fontanelle to assess the well-being of the newborn. Familiarize yourself with the importance of these structures within midwifery practice.

INTERNAL STRUCTURES OF THE FETAL SKULL

The anatomy of the brain

The internal structures of the fetal skull, although protected by the cranium, are at risk because of the skull's ability to change shape during labour and birth. Altering the shape of the skull can result in overstretching of the internal structures and trauma to tissues or blood vessels. (See Figs 30.7, 30.8 and 30.9.)

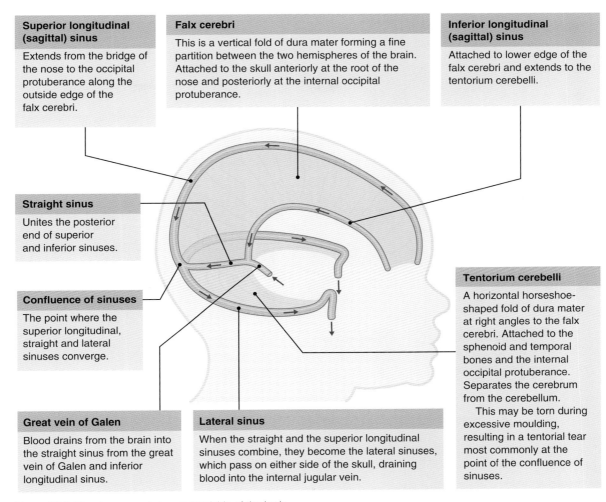

Superior longitudinal (sagittal) sinus

Extends from the bridge of the nose to the occipital protuberance along the outside edge of the falx cerebri.

Falx cerebri

This is a vertical fold of dura mater forming a fine partition between the two hemispheres of the brain. Attached to the skull anteriorly at the root of the nose and posteriorly at the internal occipital protuberance.

Inferior longitudinal (sagittal) sinus

Attached to lower edge of the falx cerebri and extends to the tentorium cerebelli.

Straight sinus

Unites the posterior end of superior and inferior sinuses.

Confluence of sinuses

The point where the superior longitudinal, straight and lateral sinuses converge.

Tentorium cerebelli

A horizontal horseshoe-shaped fold of dura mater at right angles to the falx cerebri. Attached to the sphenoid and temporal bones and the internal occipital protuberance. Separates the cerebrum from the cerebellum.

This may be torn during excessive moulding, resulting in a tentorial tear most commonly at the point of the confluence of sinuses.

Great vein of Galen

Blood drains from the brain into the straight sinus from the great vein of Galen and inferior longitudinal sinus.

Lateral sinus

When the straight and the superior longitudinal sinuses combine, they become the lateral sinuses, which pass on either side of the skull, draining blood into the internal jugular vein.

Figure 30.8 The sinuses and dura mater folds of the brain.

Regions of the cerebrum

The regions of the cerebrum are divided according to the bones under which they lie:

- parietal lobe
- temporal lobe
- frontal lobe
- occipital lobe

Meninges of the brain

The three membranous coverings of the brain are called:

- dura mater
- arachnoid mater
- pia mater (see Fig. 30.9)

MOULDING OF THE FETAL SKULL DURING LABOUR

The fetal skull has a unique ability to flex during birth, while adapting to prolonged compression, to enhance its passage through the birth canal. This adaptation process is termed *moulding*, a process during which bones of the skull override each other as a result of pressure from labour force and the pelvic girdle (Pu et al 2011; see Fig. 30.10).

Moulding can increase or reduce the diameters of the skull by up to 1.5 cm. In the normal moulding process, the frontal bones move under the anterior aspects of the parietal bones, with the occiput moving under the parietal bones at the rear. This enables the skull to change *shape* but not *volume*. Where one diameter is decreased, another will be increased to accommodate the volume (see Table 30.1

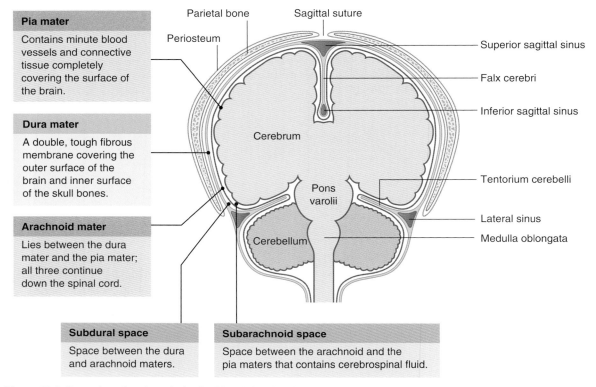

Pia mater

Contains minute blood vessels and connective tissue completely covering the surface of the brain.

Dura mater

A double, tough fibrous membrane covering the outer surface of the brain and inner surface of the skull bones.

Arachnoid mater

Lies between the dura mater and the pia mater; all three continue down the spinal cord.

Parietal bone

Periosteum

Sagittal suture

Superior sagittal sinus

Falx cerebri

Inferior sagittal sinus

Cerebrum

Tentorium cerebelli

Pons varolii

Lateral sinus

Cerebellum

Medulla oblongata

Subdural space

Space between the dura and arachnoid maters.

Subarachnoid space

Space between the arachnoid and the pia maters that contains cerebrospinal fluid.

Figure 30.9 Coronal section through the fetal head showing the internal structures of the brain.

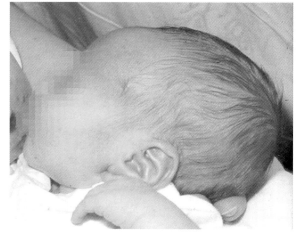

Figure 30.10 Normal moulding.

Table 30.1 Variations in the diameters of the fetal skull because of compression and moulding

Presentation	Effect on diameter
Vertex presentation with good flexion	Suboccipitobregmatic decreased Biparietal decreased Mentovertical increased
Persistent occipitoposterior position of the vertex (POP)	Occipitofrontal decreased Biparietal decreased Submentobregmatic increased
Face presentation	Submentobregmatic decreased Biparietal decreased Occipitofrontal increased
Brow presentation	Mentovertical decreased Biparietal probably decreased Suboccipitobregmatic increased

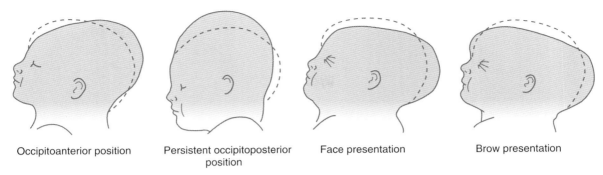

Occipitoanterior position

Persistent occipitoposterior position

Face presentation

Brow presentation

Figure 30.11 Moulding of the head.

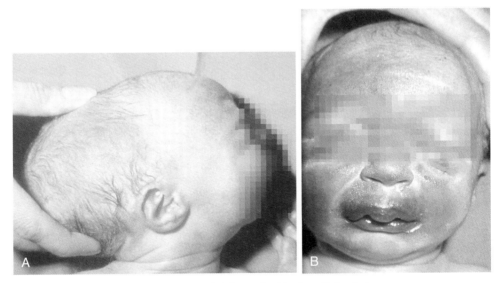

Figure 30.12 Moulding following face presentation and delivery: **A**, side view. **B**, front view.

and Figs 30.11 and 30.12). Where there is extreme or rapid moulding or abnormal compression of the fetal skull, a tear in the cerebral falx (*falx cerebri*) or cerebellar tentorium (*tentorium cerebelli*) can occur (see Fig. 30.9).

The midwife must record the degree of moulding present at birth. During the neonatal examination, the midwife reassesses moulding to ensure it is decreasing, and this may include taking measurements of the occipitofrontal circumference. Posterior moulding reduces within a few hours of birth, whereas anterior moulding is visible longer, decreasing over the first 48 hours of life.

INJURIES TO THE FETAL SKULL AND SURROUNDING TISSUES

Caput succedaneum

A caput succedaneum is an oedematous swelling within the superficial connective tissue layer of the scalp (see Figs 30.13 and 30.14). The swelling results from the pressure exerted on the fetal head by the cervix during labour. Oedema collects in the unsupported section of the fetal

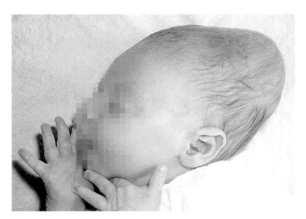

Figure 30.13 A neonate with caput succedaneum.

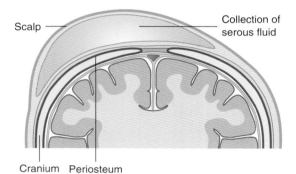

Scalp

Collection of
serous fluid

Cranium   Periosteum

Figure 30.14 Caput succedaneum.

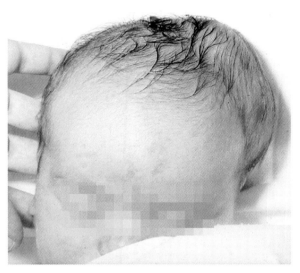

Figure 30.15 A neonate with cephalhaematoma.

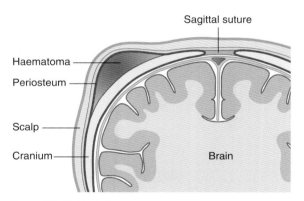

Sagittal suture

Haematoma

Periosteum

Scalp

Cranium

Brain

Figure 30.16 Cephalhaematoma.

head, which protrudes through the opening developed by the dilating cervix.

This results in an extraperiosteal collection of fluid (outside of the periosteum). The size of this swelling depends on the stage of cervical dilatation and, at full dilatation, it may cover an extensive section of the presenting part. Not all babies develop caput, as factors such as duration of labour, strength of contractions and descent of the presenting part all influence its development.

Characteristics of caput succedaneum

- Present at birth
- Moulding of the skull is present
- Usually a soft swelling that pits on pressure
- May cross suture lines
- Tends to decrease in size after delivery
- No treatment is required as it generally disappears within 24 to 48 hours as the fluid is reabsorbed

Cephalhaematoma

A cephalhaematoma is bleeding between the periosteum and the bone of the fetal skull (Figs 30.15 and 30.16). It is caused by friction of the skull against the pelvis or forceps during labour, and is associated with *asynclitism* of the fetal skull (the sideways rocking mechanism of the fetal head as it descends), or trauma after a vacuum extraction (see Chs 24 and 59). Injury to the fetal skull results in the periosteum separating from the underlying bone with subsequent bleeding between the bone and periosteum layers. The resulting swelling is confined to the area of the affected skull bone by the periosteum layer. A cephalhaematoma can be present in more than one bone but occurs most commonly in the parietal bones. The affected area is initially soft, but, as osmosis occurs, fluid is removed and the area becomes firm.

Characteristics of cephalhaematoma

- Appears 12 to 72 hours after delivery.
- Tends to enlarge after delivery.
- Is circumscribed and does not pit on pressure.
- May be bilateral.
- Can persist for weeks and, in rare cases, months.
- May contribute to jaundice.

Treatment for this condition is rare, as most cephalhaematomas disperse naturally. The neonate is usually unperturbed by the injury, but some may be slightly irritable and require gentle handling. As with any blood loss, the baby must be monitored for signs of anaemia and jaundice as lysis of blood occurs, and vitamin K is administered to increase prothrombin levels and assist with clotting.

It is important to consider that, in some babies, there may be both caput and cephalhaematoma present.

Lacerations

Lacerations to the scalp or face can result from fetal scalp electrodes, fetal blood monitoring or instrumental delivery. They usually require little or no treatment and heal quickly, but the midwife needs to identify these, document their situation and monitor for healing and well-being. The aim of neonatal care in this instance involves prevention and detection of infection and promotion of wound healing.

Chignon

A chignon may result after application of a vacuum extraction cup to the fetal scalp during delivery (Fig. 30.17). The vacuum cup is applied to the scalp and suction applied, drawing the scalp into the cup. Any slight movement of the scalp layers results in the area under the cup becoming oedematous and bruised.

The result is an oedematous structure the same size and shape as the vacuum cup. This condition usually disappears within a week following delivery. In rare cases, vacuum extraction has been associated with *subaponeurotic haemorrhage*, when bleeding occurs below the epicranial aponeurosis (see the following discussion).

Subaponeurotic haemorrhage/subgaleal haemorrhage

A subaponeurotic haemorrhage (sometimes referred to as a subgaleal haemorrhage) is a rare, but serious condition in which rupture of the emissary veins (the connection from the extracranial to intercranial venous systems) leads to bleeding into the space between the periosteum and the epicranial aponeurosis (see Fig. 30.18). This causes the epicranial aponeurosis to be pulled away from the membranous lining of the skull bones (the periosteum), and thus can allow a large space for bleeding to be significant (50%–75% of the baby's blood volume). It is often associated with instrumental delivery, especially that of vacuum

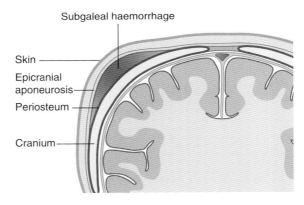
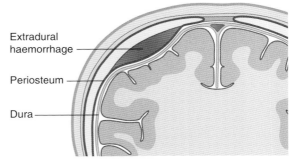

Figure 30.18 Subaponeurotic hemorrhage/subgaleal haemorrhage.

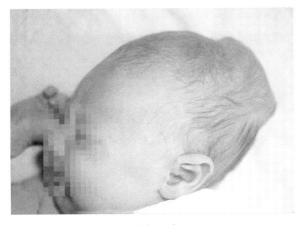

Figure 30.17 A ventouse 'chignon'.

extraction. Bleeding in this instance may be extensive, and so admission to a neonatal unit for observation and treatment is necessary.

The subaponeurotic haemorrhage can be felt as a mass that can cross suture lines, with or without the presence of pitting oedema to the head and ears. This can further be seen as swelling to the surrounding tissues, such as the eyelids and ear lobes (The Royal Australian and New Zealand College of Obstetricians and Gynaecologists 2015).

The risks to the baby after birth are *hypovolaemic shock*, related *anaemia* and *death* (Chadwick et al 1996). Treatment should consist of early recognition and diagnosis, resuscitation and urgent referral to a specialist neonatal team.

INTERNAL INJURIES

Tentorial tear

The tentorium cerebelli is a fold of dura mater within which are present the venous sinuses, which contains blood being removed from the brain (see Fig. 30.8). On rare occasions, the fetal head can be compromised by a difficult delivery or excessive or abnormal moulding, resulting in tearing of the membranes, followed by cerebral bleeding or haemorrhage (Fig. 30.19). This damage is often labelled as a *tentorial tear*.

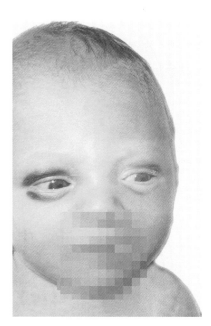

Figure 30.19 External signs of cerebral bleeding.

The baby presents with signs of cerebral irritation and raised intracranial pressure, including a tense, expanded anterior fontanelle, asphyxia (bradycardia and apnoea), and convulsions. In these instances, the midwife must seek urgent medical assistance and arrange transfer to a neonatal intensive care unit for observation (see Ch. 49).

Reflective activity 30.2

Revise the internal structures of the fetal skull.

Visit your local neonatal intensive care unit to discuss the current treatment and care required by a baby with a tentorial tear or subdural bleed.

Make notes on the advice given, including signs and symptoms to enable you to detect this condition and current patterns of care available for this baby.

THE RELEVANCE OF THE FETAL SKULL TO PARENTS

It is important midwives share their knowledge with parents to expand understanding of the needs of their baby. This commences in the antenatal period when the midwife discusses the nutritional needs of the fetus during development and growth, and explains the link between the mother's pelvis and the fetal skull during labour.

Immediately after delivery, during examination of the neonate, the midwife can point out to parents the key features of the skull and their significance, including the fontanelles and sutures, and the presence of any deviations from normal, for example, a chignon or caput.

During the postnatal period, it is important that the midwife discusses checking the anterior fontanelle as a measure of the neonate's well-being. Box 30.1 provides a useful checklist for the midwife to use in educating mothers and others in the care of the baby.

Reflective activity 30.3

Use the diagrams of the fetal skull in Fig. 30.20 to revise the information outlined within this chapter. Photocopy the diagrams and revise the structures until you are confident that you know all of the components of the fetal skull and their application to midwifery practice.

CONCLUSION

Knowledge of the anatomy of the brain and fetal skull enables practitioners to understand the role they play during labour and birth, helping them to assess, prevent,

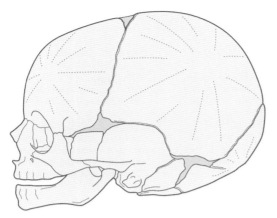
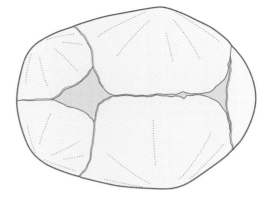

Figure 30.20 Diagrams of the fetal skull.

- Handle the head of the newborn carefully to avoid injury.
- Do not shake the baby, as damage can occur to the internal structures of the skull.
- Support the baby's head for 3 months until the baby has developed some control over movement.
- The top of the head of the baby should be washed carefully because of the soft anterior fontanelle.
- Babies need to maintain a neutral thermal environment after birth. As most body heat is lost through the head, in cooler environments, their head should be covered.
- Observe the anterior fontanelle for signs of dehydration in the newborn (indented), but remember to allow time for the baby to absorb a feed once fed. The anterior fontanelle (see Fig. 30.2) is diamond shaped and feels soft and spongy to touch in a normal and healthy baby.
- Presence of a raised or bulging anterior fontanelle could indicate raised intracranial pressure and review by a clinician is recommended.
- Injuries to the baby's head should be reported immediately to a doctor so assessment can take place.
- A caput succedaneum usually disappears within 48 hours.
- A cephalhaematoma is absorbed within 1 to 4 weeks.

predict and diagnose potential and actual morbidity, while understanding the process of natural changes within the skull that help facilitate the birth of a baby.

After birth, the midwife uses skills of observation and diagnosis to ensure the baby's health and well-being. Knowledge of the structures outlined in this chapter enable the midwife to provide health promotion information and advice to parents, on both the process and outcome of birth, and the subsequent care their new baby requires.

Key Points

- It is important for midwives to be conversant with the structure and development of the fetal brain and skull.
- The fetal skull effects upon labour, influencing its duration, pain relief required and outcome.
- Labour effects upon the fetal skull by influencing the amount and type of moulding and internal injuries that occur during birth.
- The midwife must anticipate and assess injuries relating to the fetal skull, including the presence of caput succedaneum, cephalhaematoma, subaponeurotic/subgaleal haemorrhage, chignon and scalp electrode injury. Assessment must include consideration of injuries relating to internal structures of the skull, such as tentorial tears.
- Midwives use their knowledge to inform practice and assist families in developing knowledge and confidence in caring for their baby.

References

Barbera A, Imani F, Becker T, et al: Anatomic relationship between the pubic symphysis and ischial spines and its clinical significance in the assessment of fetal head engagement and station during labor, *Ultrasound Obstet Gynecol* 33(3):320–325, 2009.

Chadwick LM, Pemberton PJ, Kurinczuk JJ: Neonatal subgaleal haematoma: associated risk factors, complications and outcome, *J Paediatr Child Health* 32(3):228–232, 1996.

Moore K, Persaud T, Torchia G: *Before we are born: essentials of embryology and birth defects*, 9th edn, London, WB Saunders, 2015.

Pu F, et al: Effect of different labor forces on fetal skull molding, *Med Eng Phys* 33(5):620–625, 2011.

Royal Australian and New Zealand College of Obstetricians and Gynaecologists (RANZOG): Prevention, detection, and management of subgaleal haemorrhage in the newborn, RANZOG, 2015.

Sadler T: *Langman's medical embryology*, 13th edn, London, Wolters Kluwer Health, 2015.

Tutschek B, Torkildsen EA, Eggebø TM: Comparison between ultrasound parameters and clinical examination to assess fetal head station in labor, *Ultrasound Obstet Gynecol* 41(4):425–429, 2013.

Resources and additional reading

Please refer to the chapter website resources.

Kapit W, Elson LM: *The anatomy coloring book*, 4th edn, Pearson, 2013.

Detailed text, which invites user to learn through reviewing and colouring diagrams.

Websites:

The Open University Antenatal Care Module: 6. *Anatomy of the female pelvis and fetal skull study session 6 anatomy of the female pelvis and fetal skull*.

http://www.open.edu/openlearnworks/mod/oucontent/view.php?id=36&printable=1.

Royal College of Obstetricians and Gynaecologists (RCOG) 'StratOG' - elearning resource https://stratog.rcog.org.uk/tutorial/pelvic-anatomy/the-fetal-skull-5109.

Fetal skull revision quiz.

Stanford Childrens Health 2016 Anatomy of the Newborn Skull http://www.stanfordchildrens.org/en/topic/default?id=anatomy-of-the-newborn-skull-90-P01840.

Presentation of fetal skull and access to further information.

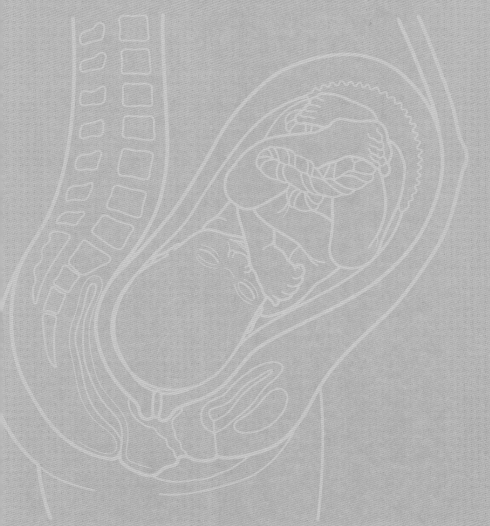

Part Five

Pregnancy

Chapter 31

Maternal neurohormonal and systemic adaptations to feto-placental development

Mary McNabb

Learning Outcomes ❓

After reading this chapter, you will be able to:

- recognize the effects of prolonged maternal brain exposure to steroid and peptide hormones from early pregnancy
- identify the factors that regulate the dramatic changes in maternal cardiovascular, respiratory and fluid regulatory systems before and during pregnancy, and the significance of these adaptations for fetal growth and development
- understand the hormonal regulation of uterine and mammary adaptations, and the significance of these changes for fetal and neonatal development
- recognize the altered regulation of maternal neurohormonal systems during different phases of pregnancy and the role of placental hormones in the homeostatic regulation of intra-uterine conditions for fetal growth and maturation
- appreciate the changes in maternal autonomic nervous system during different phases of pregnancy in relation to the developing capacity for synchronized, psychophysical interactions between mother and fetus

INTRODUCTION

This chapter will outline the time course and regulation of adaptive responses of maternal renal, cardiovascular and haemodynamic systems to pregnancy. This will be followed by the adaptations that occur in the uterus and mammary gland. The chapter will conclude with the adaptations in maternal hypothalamic–pituitary regulation of gonadotrophs, prolactin and growth hormone and the adaptive responses of the hypothalamic–pituitary–adrenal (HPA) axis from early and late pregnancy (Brunton et al 2008; Brunton and Russell 2010; Douglas 2010).

While embryo formation is taking place in a low-oxygen environment within the uterus, the first hormonal signal from the conceptus has already entered the maternal brain, to induce a complementary state of quietness and increased maternal desire for sleep during the first trimester (Lukacs et al 1995). Within the brain, human chorionic gonadotrophin (hCG) also increases the activity of the thyroid gland, which participates in regulating implantation and placental formation, and provides iodine for neural cell formation in the embryo (Colicchia et al 2014). Outside the brain, hCG stimulates increased production of progesterone and relaxin from the corpus luteum, to regulate maternal uterine, renal, circulatory, haemodynamic and respiratory adaptations in preparation for the luteal–placental shift towards the end of the first trimester (Conrad and Baker 2013).

Suppression of gonadotrophin-releasing hormone (GnRH) stimulation of pituitary gonadotrophs by hCG is accompanied by a gradual rise in the production of prolactin from the anterior pituitary gland. This is sustained throughout pregnancy by the combined influences of oestrogens and progesterone and the rise in brain opioid peptides during the third trimester (Brunton and Russell 2008; Grattan et al 2008). Within the brain, prolactin reduces maternal stress responsiveness from early pregnancy onwards, and this plays a key role in reducing fetal exposure to the adverse programming effects of glucocorticoids (Grattan and Kokay 2008). From early pregnancy, prolactin also stimulates neurogenesis in the olfactory system, resulting in improved odour recognition of the infant after birth (Grattan et al 2008; Douglas 2010 and 2011). Throughout pregnancy and lactation, prolactin also has a central inhibitory effect on the release of GnRH and luteinising hormone (LH), while simultaneously increasing maternal appetite and gastrointestinal absorption, to meet the increased energy demands of fetal growth and lactation (Douglas 2011; Grachev et al 2015).

The maternal brain is also influenced by the rapid rise in progesterone. In addition to its inhibitory effect on

GnRH release, progesterone reduces maternal anxiety from early pregnancy onwards and operates on respiratory centres to stimulate ventilation (Marcouiller et al 2014; Zuluaga et al 2005). In addition, progesterone stimulates maternal appetite and reduces responsiveness of the stress axis by increasing the level of brain opioid peptides that directly reduce the reactivity of the hypothalamic-pituitary adrenal (HPA) axis to a wide variety of physical, cognitive and psychological stressors (Brunton and Russell 2010). The progesterone-induced rise in brain opioid peptides also facilitates their restraining influence on the electrical activity of oxytocin neurons in the hypothalamus and on oxytocin nerve terminals in the posterior pituitary gland (Brunton and Russell 2008).

Outside the brain, progesterone and prolactin induce alterations in the immune system that create an active immunological tolerance of fetal–placenta antigens. Once these antigens are detected, the maternal immune system responds with a wide range of protective immune-regulatory mechanisms, which positively influence the fetal immune and central nervous systems, with lasting consequences for health in later life (Marques et al 2015). Besides functioning as an anti-inflammatory and immune-steroid, progesterone also plays an essential role in the decidualization of the endometrium and actively maintains myometrial quiescence until the end of pregnancy (Mesiano 2014: 255–256).

Detailed information on the pattern of steroid and peptide hormone production and the time course of maternal vascular adaptations provide useful indicators of maternal well-being and feto-placental development at different phases of pregnancy. For example, women who feel sleepy during the early weeks of pregnancy and calmer and less anxious by the end of the first trimester are expressing the central effects of hCG, progesterone and prolactin in early pregnancy (Brunton and Russell 2008; Douglas 2011). Plasma concentrations of progesterone and relaxin in early pregnancy are also associated with lower mean systolic blood pressure in the second and third trimester, and a positive correlation exists between the extent of plasma volume expansion and fetal growth, reduced risk of pregnancy complications and preterm labour (Khraibi et al 2003; Kristiansson and Wang 2001; Steer 2000).

PULMONARY AND CARDIOVASCULAR ADAPTATIONS

Regulation of fluid balance, cardiovascular volume and blood pressure varies across the follicular and luteal phase of the ovarian cycle (Chapman et al 1997). This includes some degree of hyperventilation and changing alveolar and arterial tensions of carbon dioxide (CO_2) levels that are influenced by oestrogens and progesterone (Duvekot

and Peeters 1998). A slight degree of hyperventilation develops during the luteal phase, and alveolar and arterial tensions of carbon dioxide (CO_2) are significantly lower than before ovulation (Chapman et al 1997). This occurs through the combined neuronal actions of oestrogens and progesterone within the respiratory centre in the medulla. Rising levels of oestrogens during the luteal phase stimulate synthesis of progesterone receptors in superficial medullary chemoreceptors, while the simultaneous increase in progesterone reduces their activation threshold and increases their sensitivity to P_{CO_2} (Duvekot and Peeters 1998; Marcouiller et al 2014). After conception, hyperventilation increases and the magnitude of decline in P_{CO_2} correlates with arterial concentrations of progesterone (Chapman et al 1998; Jensen et al 2005).

During the luteal phase of the cycle, mean arterial pressure (MAP) declines significantly, leading to a reflexive rise in cardiac output, while blood volume remains fairly constant (Chapman et al 1997; Williams et al 2001). In most studies, systolic blood pressure is slightly raised compared with the follicular phase, while diastolic pressure is 5% lower. After conception, the greatest change in blood pressure occurs around 6 to 8 weeks gestation (Mahendru et al 2012 and 2014). In early pregnancy, 80% to 90% of the total pregnancy-related fall in MAP and systemic vascular resistance (SVR) has already taken place (Duvekot and Peeters 1998). After 8 weeks, MAP continues to fall, reaching its lowest level by 24 weeks (Robson et al 1989; Mahendru et al 2014). The pregnancy-related decline in MAP seems to be largely mediated by the fall in diastolic pressure that begins during the luteal phase of the cycle (Duvekot and Peeters 1998). Systolic blood pressure declines in early pregnancy and remains constant until 20 weeks, rising significantly in some studies during the second half of pregnancy, while diastolic pressure reaches its lowest point at 24 weeks, and rises significantly for the remainder of pregnancy (Mabie et al 1994; Mahendru et al 2014; Volman et al 2007) (see Fig. 31.1).

Current research on maternal vascular adaptations suggests that the circulatory system is profoundly dilated during pregnancy and the process begins during the luteal phase of the cycle. Using serial blood pressure to measure the time course of cardiovascular changes, therefore, requires a baseline value during the follicular phase of the cycle against which to identify the significant fall in both diastolic and systolic blood pressure that happens as early as 6 weeks gestation (Mahendru et al 2012 and 2014) (see Fig. 31.2).

ADAPTATIONS IN FLUID REGULATION

Osmotic thresholds for thirst and vasopressin secretion decline during the luteal phase, leading to a comparable

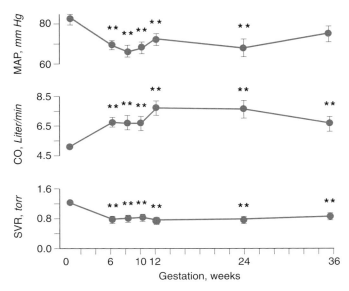

Figure 31.1 Systemic haemodynamic changes before and during pregnancy. Mean arterial pressure (MAP) decreases and cardiac output (CO) increases significantly by 6 weeks gestation in association with a decline in systemic vascular resistance (SVR). (This article was published in Chapman AB, Abraham WT, Zamudio S, et al: Temporal relationships between hormonal and hemodynamic changes in early pregnancy, Kidney Int 54: 2056-2063, Copyright Elsevier, 1998.)

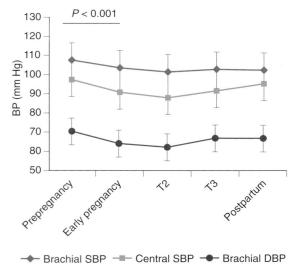

Figure 31.2 Changes in brachial, central systolic and diastolic blood pressure from preconception to postpartum period. T2 = second trimester and T3 = third trimester. Significant changes in BP in very early pregnancy. (Mahendrua AA, Everetta TR, Wilkinsonb IB, Leesa CC, McEniery CM: A longitudinal study of maternal cardiovascular function from preconception to the postpartum period, J Hypertens, 32:849–856, 2014.)

reduction in plasma osmolality through a fall in plasma sodium and its associated *anions*, primarily chloride and bicarbonate (Chapman et al 1997; Vokes et al 1988). When conception occurs, plasma osmolality continues to decline to 8 to 10 mOsmol/kg below midfollicular values by 10 weeks gestation, and this new set-point for thirst and vasopressin secretion is maintained throughout pregnancy and labour (Chapman et al 1998; Davison et al 1981). These changes are stimulated by a primary renal and systemic vasodilation, which creates a fall in total vascular resistance (see Fig. 31.3).

In the absence of any increase in plasma volume, the postovulatory fall in renal and systemic vascular resistance initiates a decline in ventricular afterload. This activates a reflex rise in cardiac output, followed by a significant expansion in plasma volume by 6 weeks gestation, increasing rapidly to around 45% to 50% of non-pregnant values by 36 weeks (Chapman et al 1998). The fall in SVR from the luteal phase stimulates renal sodium and water retention by activating fluid-retaining components of the renin–angiotensin–aldosterone system (RAAS), while blunting the vasoconstrictive effects (Chapman et al 1997; Chidambaram et al 2002; Conrad and Davison 2014; Sealey et al 1987).

When conception occurs, *plasma renin* activity, *aldosterone* and *atrial natriuretic peptide* (ANP) increase significantly by 6 weeks gestation (Chapman et al 1997 and 1998;

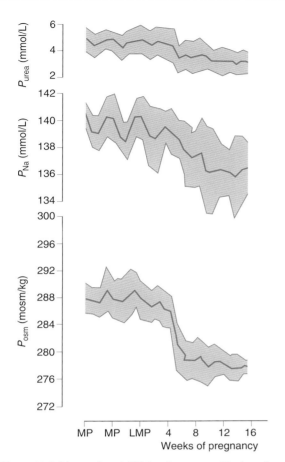

Figure 31.3 Mean values (±SD) for plasma urea (P$_{urea}$), sodium (P$_{Na}$) and osmolality (P$_{osm}$) measured at weekly intervals during the infertile cycle and following conception to 16 weeks gestation. (Baylis C, Davison J. The urinary system. In Chamberlain G, Broughton Pipkin F, editors: Clinical physiology in obstetrics, Oxford, Blackwell Science, 263–307, 1998.)

Sealey et al 1985). Despite higher basal activity of the RAAS during pregnancy, the early fall in plasma sodium sets a lower response threshold, and renal reactions to natriuretic stimuli-like ANP and vascular responses to vasoconstrictor components, notably vasopressin and angiotensin II, are significantly blunted, as occurs during the luteal phase.

These responses are largely mediated by rising levels of hCG, oestrogens, progesterone and relaxin (Fig. 31.4). Oestrogens stimulate hepatic synthesis of angiotensinogen (renin substrate) and promote formation of angiotensin-(1–7) (ANG-[1–7]) over angiotensin II (ANG II). ANG-(1–7) opposes the pressor effects of ANG II by

releasing nitric oxide, bradykinin and prostacyclin (Valdes et al 2001; Zhang et al 2001). Rising levels of hCG and relaxin in early pregnancy simultaneously attenuate the pressor effects of ANG II, while progesterone counteracts its vasoconstrictive actions by decreasing mean arterial pressure (Conrad 2010). Progesterone also stimulates aldosterone synthesis, promoting water retention, while the natriuretic actions of progesterone are inactivated in the kidneys (Hermsteiner et al 2002; Quinkler et al 2001; Szmuilowicz et al 2006). Together, these modifications of the RAAS sustain volume expansion without an attendant increase in blood pressure (Duvekot and Peeters 1998; Nakamura et al 1988; Sudhir et al 1995).

RENAL HAEMODYNAMIC ADAPTATIONS

Although the kidneys constitute less than 0.5% of total body weight, in resting non-pregnant adults, blood flow is equal to 25% of cardiac output, reflecting their key role in regulating fluid and electrolyte balance (Stanton and Koeppen 1993). From the midluteal phase of the cycle, significant changes occur in renal haemodynamics, as vascular resistance declines, while plasma flow and glomerular filtration rate increase significantly, by 6 weeks gestation, compared with values obtained during the midfollicular phase of the cycle. Minimal renal vascular resistance occurs at 8 weeks gestation, and this coincides with a peak rise in plasma flow of around 70%, which remains at slightly lower values for the remainder of pregnancy (Baylis and Davison 1998; Chapman et al 1998; Conrad and Davison 2014) (Fig. 31.5).

These findings suggest that the relaxin and progesterone released by the corpus luteum before and after conception stimulate a primary fall in renal and systemic vascular resistance. This initiates a chain of events that begin with a reflexive rise in cardiac output and renal sodium and water retention, despite the increase in glomerular filtration rate, leading to an expansion in plasma volume before any increase occurs in basal metabolic rate (Spaanderman et al 2000; Conrad and Davison 2014). A primary reduction in vascular resistance of non-reproductive organs, particularly in the kidneys, seems to be initiated before conception in preparation for the dramatic increase in uteroplacental blood flow during the second and third trimesters (Conrad and Davison 2014).

Considerable evidence suggests that the luteal decline in vascular resistance and plasma osmolality, and the subsequent rise in plasma volume and total body water are positive indicators of maternal adaptations to pregnancy and long-term health because of their strong association with increased fetal growth, reduced perinatal mortality and risk of cardiovascular disease in later life

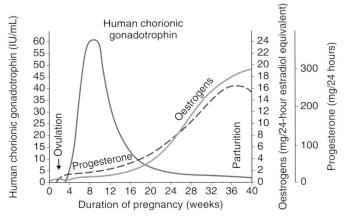

Figure 31.4 Patterns of excretion of human chorionic gonadotrophin, progesterone and oestrogens during pregnancy. (Blackburn ST: Maternal fetal and neonatal physiology: a clinical perspective, 4th edn, Philadelphia, Saunders, 2013.)

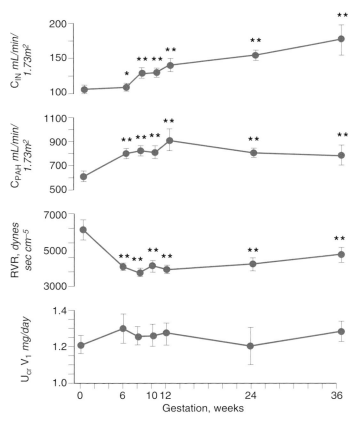

Figure 31.5 Renal haemodynamic changes before and during pregnancy. Changes in glomerular filtration rate, effective renal plasma flow and renal vascular resistance from mid-follicular phase until 36 weeks gestation. (This article was published in Chapman AB, Abraham WT, Zamudio S, et al: Temporal relationships between hormonal and hemodynamic changes in early pregnancy. Kidney Int 54:2056–2063, Copyright Elsevier, 1998.)

(Duvekot et al 1995; Longnecker et al 2014; Mahendru et al 2014; Steer et al 1995; Steer 2000).

HORMONAL REGULATION OF MATERNAL CARDIOVASCULAR ADAPTATIONS

Current findings suggest that the renal and systemic fall in vascular resistance and the reflexive rise in cardiac output and increase in global arterial compliance are stimulated by the postovulatory increase in *relaxin, oestrogens* and *progesterone* from the corpus luteum. This is followed by a significant rise in *adrenomedullin*, a long-lasting vaso-relaxant, from a variety of tissues by 8 weeks gestation, and possibly *calcitonin gene-related peptide*, another potent vasodilator that rises in the maternal circulation in early pregnancy (Conrad 2010, Conrad and Davison 2014; Di Iorio et al 1999; Hermsteiner et al 2002; Nakamura et al 1988; Novak et al 2001; Sudhir et al 1995). From around 18 weeks gestation, angiogenic factors, particularly *vascular endothelial growth factor* (VEGF) and *placental growth factor* (PGF), appear to sustain these vasodilatory mechanisms by synergistic interactions with relaxin-signaling pathways within the vascular system (Conrad 2010, McGuane et al 2011). This continues until the third trimester when PGF levels decline, as placental vascular growth seems to be progressively modulated by a rise in antiangiogenic factors (Levine et al 2004).

FROM CORPUS LUTEUM TO PLACENTA

In pregnancy, relaxin is detectable in the peripheral circulation 6 days after the midcycle LH/hCG/FSH surge. By 11 days, concentrations are significantly higher in fertile than in non-fertile cycles and concentrations increase rapidly up to 20 weeks gestation (Johnson et al 1991; Stewart et al 1993). Limited human studies have demonstrated that higher plasma concentrations of relaxin and progesterone in early pregnancy are associated with lower mean systolic blood pressure in late pregnancy (Kristiansson and Wang 2001). Recent evidence suggests that although oestrogens have a stimulatory effect on cardiac output, and oestrogens and progesterone stimulate systemic and uterine vasodilation, neither seems to influence renal blood vessels, which show a marked degree of dilation after ovulation and are known to be responsive to relaxin (Chapman et al 1997; Conrad and Davison 2014; Nakamura et al 1988; Sudhir et al 1995) (Fig. 31.6).

Relaxin has a unique spectrum of effects on the vascular system that encompass both rapid and sustained vasodilation of the arterial system in selected organ systems, particularly the renal circulation. Short-term relaxin administration stimulates a rapid dilation of selected small arteries and is mediated by interactions between relaxin receptors and a number of endothelial factors, including nitric oxide synthase (McGuane et al 2011 and 2011a). Prolonged relaxin administration decreases systemic and renal vascular resistance, and increases renal plasma flow, cardiac output and global arterial compliance. These effects depend on a cascade of interactions between relaxin receptors and an array of angiogenic growth factors and regulatory enzymes that actively inhibit vasoconstriction by altering the molecular composition of the small and medium arteries, and blunting the response to a number of vasoconstrictors, including angiotensin, vasopressin and catecholamines (Conrad and Davison 2014; McGuane 2011).

Within the vascular system, relaxin stimulates increased expression of at least two angiogenic factors, VEGF and the closely related PGF. After ovulation, there is a sustained rise in VEGF from granulosa cells, which plays a key role in the formation of the vascular network in the corpus luteum (Strauss and Williams 2014: 182). After implantation, VEGF is involved in forming and restructuring uteroplacental blood vessels. Circulating levels of free VEGF rise from early pregnancy, peak at around 20 weeks, then gradually decline towards term (Ren et al 2014). Circulating levels of free PGF rise from around 17 weeks gestation, peak around 30 to 32 weeks and also decline towards terms (Saffer et al 2013). Both of these angiogenic factors function as intermediaries in the sustained relaxin vasodilatory pathway (McGuane et al 2011).

CARDIOVASCULAR ADAPTATIONS

The maternal cardiovascular system undergoes an extensive expansion in response to pregnancy. The first event is decreased vascular resistance of non-reproductive organs, leading to a profound fall in SVR, which reaches its lowest point at the end of the first trimester (Poppas et al 1997). By reducing cardiac afterload, this primary adaptation stimulates an overall rise of approximately 40% to 50% in cardiac output (Duvekot et al 1995; Volman et al 2007). Most longitudinal studies suggest that cardiac output rises significantly during the first trimester, and peaks at 20 to 32 weeks, with no significant changes thereafter, or continues to show further small rises until term (Chapman et al 1997; Desai et al 2004; Duvekot and Peeters 1998; Mabie et al 1994; Mahendru et al 2014; Volman et al 2007). Measures of the pattern and relative contribution of heart rate (HR) and stroke volume (SV) to increased cardiac output suggest that HR rises progressively throughout pregnancy, while in some studies, SV increases significantly by 8 weeks and rises further to reach maximum

489

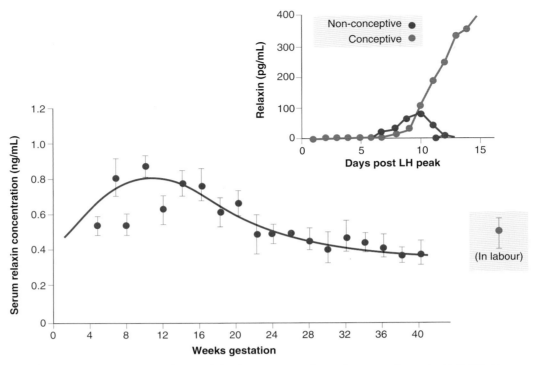

Figure 31.6 Serum relaxin concentrations from ovulation in a nonconceptive and a conceptive cycle. (Jaffe RB: Neuroendocrine metabolic regulation of pregnancy. In: Yen SSC, Jaffe RB, editors: Reproductive endocrinology, Philadelphia, Saunders, 775, 2009.)

values between 20 and 37 weeks, declining slightly over the remainder of the pregnancy (Desai et al 2004; Mahendru et al 2014; Robson et al 1989; Volman et al 2007).

Stroke volume increases significantly by 8 weeks, peaks at 16 to 22 weeks and plateaus or shows further small increases during the third trimester (Volman et al 2007). This represents a rise of 21% to 22% over prepregnancy values. In different studies, HR has been found to increase significantly above prepregnancy values by 5 and 16 weeks gestation. Data on the remainder of pregnancy suggests that the increase peaks at 31 to 36 weeks and shows little significant change a thereafter. Current evidence indicates that HR may increase by between 11% and 17% over prepregnancy values (Capeless and Clapp 1989; Duvekot et al 1993; Robson et al 1989; Volman et al 2007).

Peripheral arterial vasodilatation

Cardiac output rises in early pregnancy in response to a fall in systemic vascular resistance that reduces afterload in the myocardial fibres during left ventricular ejection. Decreases in both MAP and total peripheral resistance are evident at 8 weeks gestation, reaching their lowest point

by the middle of pregnancy, before returning to similar or slightly above prepregnancy values at term (Desai et al 2004). The decline in peripheral vascular resistance is brought about by early reduced vasomotor tone; remodeling of resistance-sized arteries; relaxation of systemic, renal and pulmonary vascular tone and development of new vascular beds in the placenta during the second trimester (Conrad and Novak 2004; Kelly et al 2004; McGuane et al 2011).

The initial fall in peripheral vascular resistance is induced during the luteal phase by rising levels of relaxin, oestrogens and progesterone. Progesterone has been shown to reduce vascular muscle tone (Magness and Rosenfeld 1989; Omar et al 1995). When fertilization occurs, the further decline creates a state of relative hypovolaemia, causing a reflexive increase in stroke volume and heart rate (Clapp et al 1988; Davison and Noble 1981; Duvekot et al 1993).

The compensatory rise in cardiac output produces a rise in vascular filling state characterized by a rise in left atrial diameter, a rise in glomerular filtration rate and little change in plasma renin, between 5 and 8 weeks gestation (Duvekot et al 1995). Studies have demonstrated that the fall in vascular resistance precedes the rise in circulating blood volume during pregnancy.

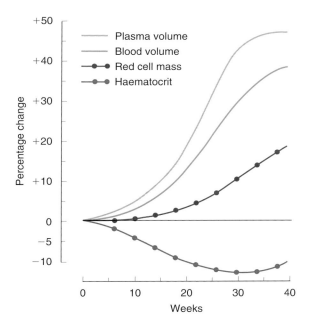

Figure 31.7 Changes in plasma volume, blood volume, red cell mass and haematocrit during normal pregnancy, expressed as a percentage of prepregnancy levels. (Rosso P: Nutrition and metabolism in pregnancy, New York, 1990, Oxford University Press. By permission of Oxford University Press.)

This suggests that systemic vasodilatation is a primary adaptation to pregnancy that initiates a rise in cardiac output and maintains overall tissue perfusion and blood pressure before significant increases in circulating blood volume occur (Capeless and Clapp 1989; Phippard et al 1986) (see Fig. 31.7).

Blood volume

The increase in blood volume is composed of a maximum rise of 45% to 50% in plasma volume and a 20% rise in red cell volume above non-pregnant values. The time course of the increase in plasma volume differs from the rise in red cell mass. Plasma volume begins to rise in the first trimester, increases more rapidly in the second and only slightly during the remainder of the pregnancy, and is reversed after birth. In contrast, expansion in red cell mass begins in the second trimester and achieves highest increases in the third. Because of the different pace at which these changes proceed, haemoglobin concentration and haematocrit decline progressively until about 30 weeks gestation. From then onwards, this trend is reversed, because increases in red cell volume outstrip plasma volume expansion during the third trimester (Steer et al 1995; Steer 2000).

ADAPTATIONS IN THE VASCULAR RENIN–ANGIOTENSIN–ALDOSTERONE SYSTEM

Current evidence suggests that plasma volume expansion is primarily stimulated by the decline in total peripheral vascular resistance, which activates multiple changes in different components of the maternal vascular renin–angiotensin–aldosterone system (August et al 1995; Irani and Xia 2008; Joyner et al 2007; Skinner 1993).

Angiotensinogen or renin substrate increases very early in pregnancy and closely mirrors levels of oestrogens in individual women (Skinner 1993). During pregnancy, placental oestrogens are largely converted in a series of enzymatic transformations from dehydroepiandrosterone (DHEA-S) and related androgens in the fetal zone of the adrenal glands and fetal liver (Pasqualini 2005). When these androgens reach the placenta and membranes, they undergo enzymatic conversion to a form that serves as a substrate for the synthesis of oestrogens (Ticconi et al 2006). Rising concentrations of oestrogens in the maternal circulation and the simultaneous fall in MAP stimulates renal production of renin, and oestrogens provide the main stimulus for hepatic production of angiotensinogen, which acts as a substrate for renin (Romen et al 1991).

Renin, angiotensins and angiotensin-converting enzymes

Renin is a proteolytic enzyme synthesized and released mainly by specialized smooth muscle cells of afferent arterioles entering the glomeruli of the kidney, in response to low blood pressure, low circulating levels of sodium chloride, a rise in effective renal plasma flow and rising levels of oestrogens (Irani and Xia 2008; Romen et al 1991; Valdes et al 2001). In pregnancy, plasma renin remains fairly stable between 5 and 10 weeks and measures of active renin show a modest rise after 20 weeks gestation (Duvekot et al 1995; Skinner 1993). On reaching the bloodstream, renin cleaves off part of angiotensinogen, triggering an enzymatic cascade that initially forms a biologically inactive peptide called *angiotensin I* (ANG I). In pregnancy, the next phase involves an oestrogen-induced down-regulation of angiotensin-converting enzyme (ACE), which circulates in plasma and is found in most tissues; however, particularly high activities of the enzyme have been found in the lungs (Valdes et al 2001). This glycoprotein cleaves off part of ANG I to form the biologically active peptide, ANG II. Within the kidneys, ANG II stimulates increased fluid reabsorption in the proximal tubular cells by enhancing reabsorption of bicarbonate. Within the adrenals, ANG II stimulates cells in the outer zone of the cortex to secrete aldosterone. In the non-pregnant state, ANG II also acts on peripheral arterioles as a potent vasoconstrictor (Skinner 1993).

During pregnancy, the vasodilatory peptide ANG-(1–7) is formed from ANG II, by angiotensin-converting enzyme 2 (ACE2), and from the biologically inactive peptide, ANG I, in the vasculature (Heitsch et al 2001). Current evidence shows a progressive rise in urinary excretion of ANG-(1–7) from 6 weeks gestation (Brosnihan et al 2003; Valdes et al 2001). Although plasma levels of ANG II are double than those in the non-pregnant state by the second week of pregnancy, its pressor effects are attenuated by hCG, ANG-(1–7) and relaxin (Conrad and Davison 2014; Heitsch et al 2001; Krane and Hamrahian 2007; Skinner 1993; Weiner et al 1994). Oestrogens also inhibit adrenal receptors for ANG II, reducing its stimulatory effect on aldosterone (Wu et al 2003).

Aldosterone, progesterone and deoxycorticosterone

Aldosterone reduces sodium excretion primarily by acting on distal portions of the renal tubules, where it stimulates reabsorption of sodium ions. Plasma levels increase significantly by 12 weeks gestation and reach a plateau at 30 weeks that is three to five times higher than non-pregnant values. During the first half of pregnancy, effective renal plasma flow increases by 70% to 80%, and then declines slightly in the third trimester but remains 50% to 60%

above non-pregnant values, which is greater than occurs in any other physiological state. The resulting increase in glomerular filtration rate increases the sodium load from 20,000 to 30,000 mmol/day (Skinner 1993). In pregnancy, aldosterone plays a key role in stimulating sodium retention (Quinkler et al 2001).

In the non-pregnant state, progesterone acts to enhance the excretion of sodium by decreasing its reabsorption in the proximal tubules and by blocking the increased reabsorption of sodium by aldosterone in the distal tubules. Although progesterone concentrations exceed those of aldosterone at least 50-fold during pregnancy, the renal activity of aldosterone is preserved by the enzymatic conversion of progesterone to a number of different metabolites (Quinkler et al 2001). Current findings suggest that progesterone is effectively converted to various metabolites in the kidneys, which reduces its binding to mineralocorticoid receptors, thereby attenuating its capacity to competitively inhibit aldosterone (Quinkler et al 2001). Some of the increase in progesterone is also converted to *deoxycorticosterone* (DOC), which acts on the distal tubules to promote the reabsorption of sodium. Rising levels of DOC occur by approximately 8 weeks gestation and increase 10- to 15-fold, to a peak of approximately 100 mg/dL at term, which is higher than aldosterone. However, the salt-retaining properties of this hormone are 30 to 50 times less potent than aldosterone (Nolten and Rueckert 1981; Skinner 1993) (Fig. 31.8).

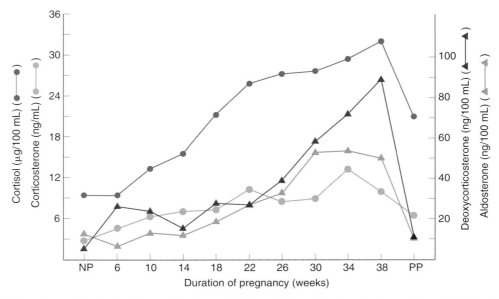

Figure 31.8 Mean adrenocorticosteroid levels in 11 women throughout pregnancy and postpartum (PP) compared to levels in non-pregnant (NP) women. (Reproduced from Wintour EM, Coghlan JP, Oddie CJ, et al: A sequential study of adrenocorticosteroid level in human pregnancy, Clin Exp Pharmacol Physiol 5(4):399–403, 1978.)

Atrial natriuretic peptide

Atrial natriuretic peptide (ANP) is a diuretic, natriuretic and vasodilator hormone, produced in the atrial chambers of the heart. Outside of pregnancy, secretion is primarily stimulated by stretching of the atrial wall that accompanies volume expansion or increases in blood pressure. ANP acts in a variety of ways to decrease fluid intake, promote salt and water excretion, and counter all components of the RAAS (Cootauco et al 2008; Duvekot and Peeters 1998; Kaufman 1995). Within the kidneys, ANP directly inhibits renin production and tubular reabsorption of sodium, and inhibits production of aldosterone in the adrenals. In vitro studies have also shown that ANP produces marked relaxation of vascular smooth muscle and antagonizes the vasoconstrictive effects of ANG II (Cootauco et al 2008; Steegers 1991).

Conflicting evidence currently exists on the pattern of ANP secretion during normal pregnancy and the extent to which its actions are blunted. Plasma levels have been reported to decline from 20 weeks gestation, reaching its lowest levels at 36 weeks and returning to non-pregnant values by 12 weeks postpartum (Thomsen et al 1993). Other studies have reported a modest rise with advancing gestation, declining at term or at placental separation and then falling significantly by 72 hours postpartum (Lowe et al 1992; Yoshimura et al 1994).

All experimental evidence indicates that atrial, renal and adrenal responsiveness to ANP is blunted during pregnancy. Oestrogens and progesterone reduce ANP receptors in the zona glomerulosa, thereby inhibiting its aldosterone-suppressant effects, while the kidneys display a blunted response to the diuretic effects of both ANP and nitric oxide (Knight et al 2006; Vaillancourt et al 1997). At the same time, the relaxin-induced rise in nitric oxide blunts the activity of atrial volume receptors, which attenuates the reduction in renal tubular sodium reabsorption, thus facilitating the expansion in extracellular fluid volume (Tam and Kaufman 2002 and 2010). These regulatory mechanisms persist until late pregnancy when ANP responsiveness to intravenous volume expansion is enhanced (Lowe et al 1992). Experimental evidence suggests that activation of the cardiac oxytocin system induces a rapid rise in ANP, which may stimulate the rapid diuresis that takes place postpartum (Mukaddam-Daher et al 2002; Yosimura et al 1994).

Erythropoiesis

During pregnancy, erythropoiesis rises from the second trimester, peaks during the third and returns to non-pregnant levels by 5 weeks postpartum (Choi and Pai 2001). The increase in red cell mass is stimulated by *erythropoietin*. This glycoprotein hormone is synthesized in ground tissue, in the kidneys and, to a lesser extent, in the liver. Levels of serum immunoreactive erythropoietin remain at non-pregnant values during the first trimester, begin to rise during the second and reach maximum levels during the third trimester (Beguin et al 1990). Within the bone marrow, erythropoietin acts on erythrocyte colony-forming cells. These give rise to increasing numbers of mature erythrocytes within 2 days of increased levels of erythropoietin within the circulation.

At present, the precise mechanisms involved in stimulating erythropoietin during pregnancy remain unclear. The evidence suggests that components of the maternal plasma renin–angiotensin system may be involved. Angiotensinogen and erythropoietin share a number of similarities. Both compete for specific binding to erythropoietin receptors on human bone marrow cells, and bone marrow cells show binding of angiotensinogen that is inhibited by erythropoietin. These findings suggest that angiotensinogen is a precursor for erythropoietin. Both components are increased in the maternal circulation during pregnancy, but the timing and possible interactions between angiotensinogen and erythropoietin remain to be identified. A number of pregnancy hormones have stimulatory and inhibitory influences on the actions of erythropoietin. Progesterone partly prevents the inhibitory influence of oestrogen on stem cell utilization of erythropoietin, while placental lactogen and prolactin enhance the stimulatory action of erythropoietin on red cell production. At present, the relative significance of these hormonal influences remains unclear (Tucker Blackburn 2013: 217).

VENTILATION

Extensive anatomical and functional changes occur in the respiratory system. These accommodate both the progressive increase in gas exchange required by rising blood volume and the growing space occupied by the uterus. From early pregnancy onwards, the overall shape of the chest alters by flaring of the lower ribs that seems to occur independently of any mechanical pressure from the growing uterus. This progressively increases the subcostal angle from 68 degrees in early pregnancy to 103 degrees at term, and increases the transverse diameter of the chest by approximately 2 cm. Because of flaring of the lower ribs, the diaphragm rises by a maximum of 4 cm, and its contribution to respiratory effort increases and shows no evidence of being impeded by the uterus. Studies on diaphragmatic movements during respiration – either sitting or lying down – have found them to be larger than in the non-pregnant state. This implies that breathing during pregnancy is more diaphragmatic than costal (de Swiet 1991a; Romen et al 1991) (Fig. 31.9).

The main functional change within the lungs is the gradual increase in the amount of air that is inspired or

493

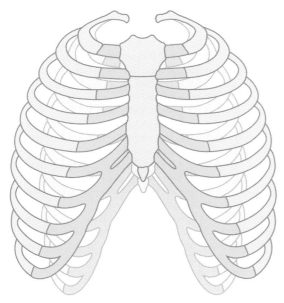

Figure 31.9 The ribcage in pregnancy (**coloured**) and the non-pregnancy state (**grey**) showing the increased subcostal angle, the increased transverse diameter and the raised diaphragm in pregnancy. (Reproduced with permission from de Swiet M: The respiratory system. In Hytten F, Chamberlain G, editors: Clinical physiology in obstetrics, Oxford, Blackwell Scientific, 83–100, 1991a.)

expired with a normal breath. This functional capacity (tidal volume) increases from 500 mL in the non-pregnant state to approximately 700 mL at term. As a result of this change, women breathe more deeply during pregnancy than in the non-pregnant state (Fig. 31.10).

Because the maximum amount of air that can be expired forcibly after maximum inspiration only increases by 100 to 200 mL, the increase in tidal volume is produced at the expense of the expiratory reserve volume. This means that a smaller amount of air remains in the lungs at the end of quiet expiration. As less residual air is mixed with the next inspiration of fresh air, this results in lower levels of P_{CO_2} that bring about a reciprocal rise in P_{O_2}. P_{CO_2} declines from approximately 39 mm Hg in the non-pregnant state to 31 mm Hg during pregnancy, while P_{O_2} increases from 93.4 to 101.8 mm Hg, over the same period (de Swiet 1991a).

Oxygen consumption

The progressive increases in cardiac output and pulmonary ventilation are proportionately greater than those occurring in maternal and fetal oxygen consumption during pregnancy. Oxygen consumption shows a linear increase with body weight as pregnancy advances, increasing to 38 mL/min (15%) above average values in the non-pregnant state (de Swiet 1991a). It is composed of the overall increase in tissue mass, higher metabolic rate of fetal and placental tissue, along with that of some maternal organs, particularly the heart, lungs and kidneys (Fig. 31.11).

The increase in oxygen consumption is facilitated by a 40% to 50% increase in ventilation and by an 18% increase in the oxygen-carrying capacity of the blood. Because of this relative oversupply of oxygen, higher concentrations are returned to the heart from the venous circulation, making the arteriovenous oxygen difference significantly smaller than in the non-pregnant state. The extent of the arteriovenous oxygen difference is smallest in early pregnancy and does not reach average non-pregnant values until term (de Swiet 1991a).

The increase in ventilation during pregnancy reduces alveolar and plasma concentrations of carbon dioxide. Studies have demonstrated that arterial partial pressure of carbon dioxide (P_{CO_2}) is about 30 mm Hg in late pregnancy, compared with 39 mm Hg during the follicular phase of the cycle. Because fetal P_{CO_2} remains at approximately 41 mm Hg, the lower levels in the maternal circulation encourage the diffusion of CO_2 from the fetal blood across the placental membranes.

Reflective activity 31.1

Consider the time course of circulatory and haemodynamic adaptations from the luteal phase until the end of pregnancy. How would you measure these changes to accurately assess maternal cardiovascular and haemodynamic adaptations to pregnancy?

ADAPTATIONS IN THE MAMMARY GLANDS/BREAST

See Ch. 44 and chapter website resources.

ADAPTATIONS IN THE REPRODUCTIVE TRACT

During pregnancy, the uterus is transformed from a small pelvic organ, with a cavity of around 10 mL and weighing approximately 50 g. By 36 weeks, uterine weight has increased to an estimated 1100 g, representing almost a 20-fold increase in mass, and its average volume is 5 litres. At this point, the uterus comes in contact with the anterior abdominal wall and extends as far as the xiphisternum. The uterus is a central recipient of the increases in circulating blood volume from the second trimester. In the follicular phase of the cycle, uterine blood flow is approximately 45 mL/min (Burton et al 2009). This

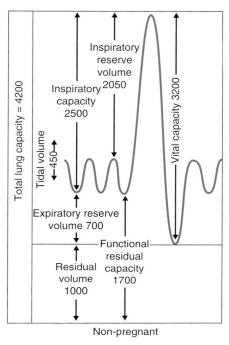
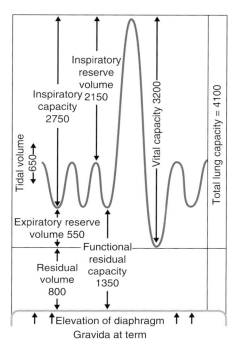

Figure 31.10 Lung volume changes in pregnancy. (This article is published in Tucker Blackburn S: Maternal, fetal and neonatal physiology, St. Louis, Saunders, Copyright Elsevier, 2013.)

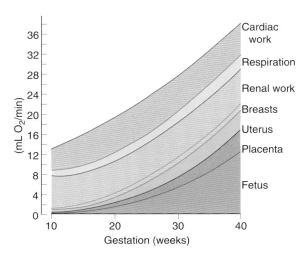

Figure 31.11 Partition of the increased oxygen consumption in pregnancy among the organs concerned. (Reproduced with permission from de Swiet M: The respiratory system. In Hytten F, Chamberlain G, editors: Clinical physiology in obstetrics, Oxford, Blackwell Scientific, 83–100, 1991a.)

changes very little during early pregnancy but rises sharply from about 20 weeks, to reach approximately 750 mL/min at term, when it receives nearly 20% of total cardiac output (Burton et al 2009; Steer 1991).

Uterine growth is characterized by a highly regulated process of myometrial cell differentiation:

- proliferation and reduced apoptosis in early pregnancy
- hypertrophy of existing cells and increased matrix elaboration during the remainder of pregnancy (Shynlova et al 2009)

Growth is stimulated by hCG, relaxin, progesterone, growth factors, oestrogens and oxytocin, and by progressive distension exerted by the fetus, placenta and amniotic fluid, particularly during the third trimester. These factors promote synthesis of structural and contractile proteins (Shynlova et al 2009; Ticconi et al 2006). During the first few months of pregnancy, growth is accompanied by increasing thickness of the myometrium in the corpus and the fundus. As the organ increases in length from around 12 weeks, the isthmus is gradually formed as an area with reduced density of muscle fibres (Steer 1991). Until the end of pregnancy, uterine growth keeps pace with fetal and

495

placental growth and the increased volume of amniotic fluid. Towards term, uterine growth is slower than that of the fetus, which results in increased mechanical stretch (Arrowsmith and Wray 2014; Kawamata et al 2007).

Myometrial changes

Bundles of smooth muscle fibres within the uterus are arranged in three or four layers embedded in a matrix of connective tissue and ground substance. The former acts as intramuscular tendons, while the latter transmits contractile forces from individual cells along the muscle bundle during labour (Tucker Blackburn 2013: 116–118). Two outer layers contain longitudinal and circular fibres that are partly continuous with the supporting ligaments. The middle layers that hold the vascular supply have a criss-cross pattern of fibres that run in all directions. Finally, the inner layer is composed of longitudinal fibres and covers the decidua (Steer 1991).

The smooth muscle forming the myometrium does not have the precise transverse alignment of thick and thin filaments that characterizes the organization of skeletal fibres. Filaments of smooth muscle are situated in random bundles throughout the cells, and myosin filaments are arranged alongside actin in uninterrupted unidirectional order. In addition to these main contractile filaments, smooth muscle also contains intermediate filaments. These are attached to all areas of cell membrane, which allows them to form networks across the cell. As a result of this organization, contractions can generate force in any direction and also produce a much greater degree of shortening than in skeletal muscle. For most of the pregnancy, this action remains local, as few intracellular connections are formed and quiescence is actively maintained by hormonal mechanisms that regulate the process of differentiation, until the last few weeks of pregnancy (Mendelson 2009; Shynlova et al 2009).

Neurohormonal regulation

Current evidence suggests that smooth muscle cells, such as the myometrium, have a very distinct phenotype compared with cardiac and skeletal muscle (Shynlova et al 2009). Myometrial cells display remarkable cellular plasticity during and after pregnancy, and are uniquely regulated by hCG, relaxin, oestrogens, progesterone, placental CRH, prostacyclin, nocturnal melatonin and oxytocin (Grazzini et al 1998; Olcese 2012; Sharkey and Olcese 2007; Shynlova et al 2009; Smith 2007).

From the luteal phase of the cycle, oestrogens modify the properties of the myometrium to reduce its capacity to support sympathetic and sensory innervations and, during pregnancy, this neurodegeneration also affects cholinergic neurons (Brauer and Smith 2015). Although prolonged exposure to rising levels of oestrogens during pregnancy seems to be the main regulator of this process, local elevation of progesterone after implantation has also been directly associated with nerve degeneration and progressive mechanical stretch, and placental growth and attachment may also be involved (Brauer and Smith 2015; Fuchs 1995) (Fig. 31.12).

Prolonged exposure to oestrogens also reduces vaginal sympathetic, cholinergic and nociceptive innervations (Ting et al 2004). Therefore, at term, high levels of oestrogens can facilitate increased vaginal stretching without activating afferent nociceptive pathways (Brauer and Smith 2015; Ting et al 2004).

Taken together, these findings suggest that placental steroids temporarily disable neuronal regulation of the myometrium and simultaneously facilitate increased hormonal control. The dominance of progesterone, hCG and relaxin during the first and second trimester actively maintains myometrial quiescence, while the increasing dominance of oestrogens and nocturnal increases in oxytocin/oxytocin receptors and melatonin during the third trimester stimulate a circadian pattern of myometrial activity during the third trimester (Olcese 2012). Recent experiments suggest that the uterus is responsive to circadian cues because it expresses circadian clock genes both before and during pregnancy (Akiyama et al 2010).

Until late pregnancy, hCG increases the number and size of myometrial cells, inhibits formation of gap junctions and actively maintains myometrial quiescence (Ticconi et al 2006). Progesterone also stimulates uterine growth and myometrial quiescence, while oestrogens induce synthesis of structural and contractile proteins and enzymes that supply energy for the process of contraction (Shynlova et al 2009). Oestrogens also influence molecules within the plasma membrane that control permeability for ions like sodium, potassium, calcium and chloride. These ion fluxes determine the resting potential and electrical excitability of myometrial cells (Arrowsmith and Wray 2014; Fuchs and Fuchs 1984; Kawamata et al 2007; Pepe and Albrecht 1995).

Besides having a direct effect on the structure of myometrial cells, oestrogens also regulate the formation of oxytocin receptors, which promote uterine contractions, in conjunction with highly regulated influxes of $Ca2+$ (Kawamata et al 2007). During pregnancy, myometrial and decidual receptors for oxytocin also increase from 27.6 fmol/mg DNA in the non-pregnant state, to 171.6 fmol/mg DNA at mid-gestation and to 1391 fmol/mg DNA at term (Fuchs 1995).

Cervical changes

The cervix forms a continuous anatomical connection between the anterior surface of the vagina and the lower uterine segment. In nulliparous women, the wall of the

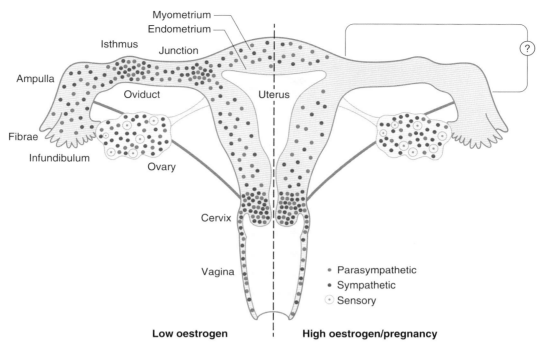

Figure 31.12 Schematic diagram of major reproductive tract structures showing a "consensus" depiction of associated innervation. The low oestrogen state is depicted on the left. Axon distribution under high oestrogen conditions at term pregnancy are shown on the right. (Brauer MM, Smith PG: Estrogen and female reproductive tract innervation: cellular and molecular mechanisms of autonomic neuroplasticity, Auton Neurosci 187:1–17, 2015.)

cervix is largely composed of dense fibrous connective tissue, formed by thick, cross-linked collagen fibrils that are invested in a ground substance, composed of elastin and core proteins attached to large numbers of unbranched polysaccharide chains. These form an interconnecting lattice that actively binds to collagen fibrils in a way that positions them to provide maximal mechanical strength. The smaller muscle content is organized in bundles lying in longitudinal, spiral and circular orientation throughout cervical tissue (Rudel and Pajntar 1999).

Few structural changes occur in the cervix until the latter part of pregnancy. There is an overall increase in size accompanied by a rise in total collagen content, some hypertrophy of external muscle fibres and a progressive rise in vascularity. As pregnancy advances, some biopsy studies have reported a gradual reduction in collagen density, a rise in polysaccharide chains and a possible redistribution of core proteins in favour of those that are highly absorbent. In addition to the increased vascularity, these findings may explain the increasing water content and slightly softer consistency of the cervix during pregnancy (Hughesdon 1952; Jeffrey 1991; Uldbjerg et al 1983). More recent studies using magnetic resonance imaging of the cervix and surrounding structures, from the

second to the third trimester, have shown that the cervix becomes shorter, as the upper aspect is pulled into the lower segment, which is stretched by growth and descent of the fetal head (House et al 2009).

MATERNAL NEUROENDOCRINE ADAPTATIONS TO THE FERTILE CYCLE: SYNCHRONIZED INTERACTIONS AND INTERDEPENDENT DEVELOPMENT OF MOTHER AND FETUS

This section covers maternal neurohormonal adaptations to fertility that begin with suppression of the hypothalamic–pituitary–gonadal (HPG) axis after conception, and altering the secretory capacity of gonadotrophs and lactotrophs within the anterior pituitary gland. These changes facilitate a rise in maternal prolactin release that operates in the brain and periphery to induce a range of alterations in metabolism, immune function, mammary adaptations, stress responsiveness and expansion of olfactory brain

497

regions in preparation for maternity. The section continues with the switch from maternal, to placental growth hormone within the maternal circulation and its effects on metabolism, particularly during the latter half of pregnancy. The section concludes with neurohormonal interactions between mother, placenta and fetus that facilitate increased basal activity of the maternal HPA axis required to sustain the cardio-respiratory and metabolic adaptations, and the gradual activation of the fetal HPA axis during the last trimester. During this period, the fetus is protected from the detrimental effects of exposure to maternal levels of cortisol by placental endocrine/paracrine regulation of an enzyme that converts biologically active cortisol to inactive cortisone. At the same time, circadian cues from the mother, contrasting changes in maternal and fetal autonomic systems and development of the fetal auditory system synchronize maternal-fetal behavioural states that seem to alter maternal emotional responses and enhance maternal closeness with her unborn infant in preparation for attachment after birth. See chapter website resources.

CONCLUSION

Maternal cardiovascular, respiratory and haemodynamic adaptations to pregnancy begin during the luteal phase of the cycle. After fertilization, the first hormonal signal from the conceptus enters the maternal brain to induce behavioural changes that are conducive to the needs of the emerging embryo for a state of quiet metabolic activity. Meanwhile, the maternal circulatory system is profoundly dilated, creating a large increase in plasma volume in anticipation of the rapid growth phase of the fetus and

placenta during the second half of pregnancy. From the second trimester, placental hormones become increasingly important regulators of maternal vascular and uterine adaptations, while maternal neuroendocrine adaptations critically depend on the development and maturation of the feto-placental unit. During the second half of pregnancy, the maternal brain is exposed to the rising levels of placental steroid and peptide hormones that stimulate an enhanced emotional sensitivity and increased desire for interpersonal trust. Over the same period, synchronized interactions occur between mother and fetus that coordinate autonomic and neuroendocrine activities and circadian rhythms that are essential for regulating fetal maturation and the circadian timing of birth.

Key Points

- Maternal brain and systemic systems undergo progressive alterations from the luteal phase of the cycle that anticipate the needs of the embryo, fetus and neonate.

- These adaptations are driven by hormonal signals from the hypothalamic-pituitary axis, the conceptus and the feto-placental unit.

- Adaptations in maternal neuroendocrine and autonomic nervous systems take shape through interdependent, synchronized interactions between mother-embryo and feto-placental systems.

- These adaptations heighten maternal brain sensitivity to the needs of the fetus and neonate.

References

Akiyama S, Ohta H, Watanabe S, et al: The uterus sustains stable biological clock during pregnancy, *Tohoku J Exp Med* 221:287–298, 2010.

Arrowsmith S, Wray S: Oxytocin: its mechanism of action and receptor signalling in the myometrium, *J Neuroendocrinol* 26:356–369, 2014.

August P, Mueller FB, Sealey JE, et al: Role of renin-angiotensin system in blood pressure regulation in pregnancy, *Lancet* 345:896–897, 1995.

Baylis C, Davison J: The urinary system. In Chamberlain G, Broughton Pipkin F, editors: *Clinical physiology*

in obstetrics, Oxford, Blackwell Science, 1998.

Beguin Y, Lipscei G, Oris R, et al: Serum immunoreactive erythropoietin during pregnancy and in the early postpartum, *Br J Haematol* 76:545–549, 1990.

Brauer MM, Smith PG: Estrogen and female reproductive tract innervation: cellular and molecular mechanisms of autonomic neuroplasticity, *Auton Neurosci* 187:1–17, 2015.

Brosnihan KB, Neves LAA, Joyner J-N, et al: Enhanced renal immunocytochemical expression of ANG-(1-7) and ACE2 during

pregnancy, *Hypertension* 42(2): 749–753, 2003.

Brunton PJ, Russell JA: The expectant brain: adapting for motherhood, *Nat Rev Neurosci* 9:11–25, 2008.

Brunton PJ, Russell JA, Douglas AJ: Adaptive responses of the maternal-hypothalamic-pituitary-adrenal axis during pregnancy and lactation, *J Neuroendocrinol* 20:764–776, 2008.

Brunton PJ, Russell JA: Endocrine induced changes in brain function during pregnancy, *Brain Res* 1364:198–215, 2010.

Burton GJ, Woods AW, Jauniaux E, et al: Rheological and physiological consequences of conversion of the maternal spiral arteries for uteroplacental blood flow during human pregnancy, *Placenta* 30:473–482, 2009.

Capeless EL, Clapp JF: Cardiovascular changes in early pregnancy, *Am J Obstet Gynecol* 161(6):1449–1452, 1989.

Chapman AB, Zamudio S, Woodmansee W, et al: Systemic and renal haemodynamic changes in the luteal phase of the menstrual cycle mimic early pregnancy, *Am J Physiol* 273(42):F777–F782, 1997.

Chapman AB, Abraham WT, Zamudio S, et al: Temporal relationships between hormonal and hemodynamic changes in early pregnancy, *Kidney Int* 54:2056–2063, 1998.

Chidambaram M, Duncan JA, Lai VS: Variation in the renin angiotensin system throughout the normal menstrual cycle, *J Am Soc Nephrol* 13:446–452, 2002.

Choi JW, Pai SH: Change in erythropoiesis with gestational age during pregnancy, *Ann Hematol* 80:26–31, 2001.

Clapp JF, Seaward BL, Sleamaker RH, et al: Maternal physiologic adaptations to early pregnancy, *Am J Obstet Gynecol* 159(6):1456–1460, 1988.

Colicchia M, Campagnolo L, Baldini E, et al: Molecular basis of thyrotropin and thyroid hormone action during implantation and early development, *Hum Reprod Update* 20(6):884–904, 2014.

Conrad KP, Novak J: Emerging role of relaxin in renal and cardiovascular function, *Am J Physiol* 287:R250–R261, 2004.

Conrad KP: Unveiling the vasodilatory actions and mechanisms of relaxin, Is this in the text?, *Hypertension* 56:2–9, 2010.

Conrad KP, Baker VL: Corpus luteal contribution to maternal pregnancy physiology and outcomes in assisted reproductive technologies, *Am J Physiol* 304:R69–R72, 2013.

Conrad KP, Davison JM: The renal circulation in normal pregnancy and preeclampsia: is there a place for relaxin?, *Am J Physiol* 306:F1121–F1135, 2014.

Cootauco AC, Murphy JD, Maleski J, et al: Atrial natriuretic peptide production and natriuretic peptide receptors in the human uterus and

their effects on myometrial relaxation, *Am J Obstet Gynecol* 199:429.e1–429.e6, 2008.

Davison JM, Noble MCB: Serial changes in 24 hour creatinine clearance during normal menstrual cycles and the first trimester of pregnancy, *Br J Obstet Gynaecol* 88:10–17, 1981.

Davison JM, Vallotton MB, Lindheimer MD: Plasma osmolality and urinary concentration and dilution during and after pregnancy: evidence that lateral recumbency inhibits maximal urinary concentrating ability, *Br J Obstet Gynaecol* 88:427–479, 1981.

Desai DK, Modley J, Naidoo DP: Echocardiographic assessment of cardiovascular hemodynamics in normal pregnancy, *Obstet Gynecol* 104:20–29, 2004.

de Swiet M: The respiratory system. In Hytten F, Chamberlain G, editors: *Clinical physiology in obstetrics*, Oxford, Blackwell Scientific, 1991a.

Di Iorio R, Marinoni E, Letizia C, et al: Adrenomedullin production is increased in normal human pregnancy, *Eur J Endocrinol* 140:201–206, 1999.

Douglas AJ: Baby on board: do responses to stress in the maternal brain mediate adverse pregnancy outcome?, *Front Neuroendocrinol* 31(3):359–376, 2010.

Douglas AJ: Mother-offspring dialogue in early pregnancy: impact of adverse environment on pregnancy maintenance and neurobiology, *Prog Neuropsychopharmacol Biol Psychiatry* 35:1167–1177, 2011.

Duvekot JJ, Peeters LLH: Very early changes in cardiovascular physiology. In Chamberlain G, Broughton Pipkin F, editors: *Clinical physiology in obstetrics*, Oxford, Blackwell Science, 1998.

Duvekot JJ, Cheriex EC, Pieters FAA: Early pregnancy changes in hemodynamics and volume homeostasis are consecutive adjustments triggered by a primary fall in systemic vascular tone, *Am J Obstet Gynecol* 169(6):1382–1392, 1993.

Duvekot JJ, Cheriex EC, Pieters FAA, et al: Maternal volume homeostasis in early pregnancy in relation to fetal growth restriction, *Obstet Gynecol* 85(3):361–367, 1995.

Fuchs A-F, Fuchs F: Endocrinology of human parturition: a review, *Br J Obstet Gynaecol* 91:948–967, 1984.

Fuchs A-F: Plasma membrane receptors regulating myometrial contractility and their hormonal modulation, *Semin Perinatol* 19(1):15–30, 1995.

Grachev P, Li XF, Goffin V, et al: Hypothalamic prolactin regulation of luteinizing hormone secretion in the female rat, *Endocrinology* 156(8):2880–2892, 2015.

Grattan DR, Steyn FJ, Kokay IC, et al: Pregnancy-induced adaptation in the neuroendocrine control of prolactin secretion, *J Neuroendocrinol* 20:407–507, 2008.

Grattan DR, Kokay IC: Prolactin: a pleiotropic neuroendocrine hormone, *J Neuroendocrinol* 20:752–763, 2008.

Grazzini E, Guillon G, Mouillac B, et al: Inhibition of oxytocin receptor function by direct binding of progesterone, *Nature* 392:509–512, 1998.

Heitsch H, Brovkovych S, Malinski T, et al: Angiotensin-(1-7) stimulated nitric oxide and superoxide release from endothelial cells, *Hypertension* 37:72–76, 2001.

Hermsteiner M, Zoltan DR, Kunzel W: Human chorionic gonadotrophin attenuates the vascular response to angiotensin II, *Eur J Obstet Gynecol Reprod Biol* 102:148–154, 2002.

House M, Bhadelia RA, Myers K, et al: Magnetic resonance imaging of three-dimensional cervical anatomy in the second and third trimester, *Eur J Obstet Gynecol Reprod Biol* 144S:S65–S69, 2009.

Hughesdon PE: The fibromuscular structure of the cervix and its changes during pregnancy and labour, *J Obstet Gynaecol Br Emp* 59:763–776, 1952.

Irani RA, Xia Y: The functional role of the renin-angiotensin system in pregnancy and preeclampsia, *Placenta* 29:763–771, 2008.

Jeffrey JJ: Collagen and collagenase: pregnancy and parturition, *Semin Perinatol* 15(2):118–126, 1991.

Jensen D, Wolfe LA, Slatkovska L, et al: Effects of human pregnancy on the ventilatory chemoreflex response to carbon dioxide, *Am J Physiol* 288:R1369–R1375, 2005.

Johnson MR, Okokon E, Collins WP, et al: The effect of human chorionic gonadotrophin and pregnancy on the circulating level of relaxin, *J Clin Endocrinol Metab* 72(5):1042–1047, 1991.

Joyner J, Neves LAA, Granger JP, et al: Temporal-spatial expression of ANG-(1-7) and angiotensin-converting enzyme 2 in the kidney of normal and hypertensive rats, *Am J Physiol* 293:R169–R177, 2007.

Kawamata M, Tonomura Y, Kimura T: Oxytocin-induced phasic and tonic contractions are modulated by the contractile machinery rather than the quantity of oxytocin receptor, *Am J Physiol* 292:E992–E999, 2007.

Kaufman S: Control of intravascular volume during pregnancy, *Clin Exp Pharmacol Physiol* 22:157–163, 1995.

Kelly BA, Bond BC, Poston L: Aortic adaptation to pregnancy: elevated expression of matrix metalloproteinases-2 and -3 in rat gestation, *Mol Hum Reprod* 10(5):331–337, 2004.

Khraibi AA, Yu T, Tang D: Role of nitric oxide in the natriuretic and diuretic responses in pregnant rats, *Am J Physiol* 285:F938–F944, 2003.

Knight S, Snellen H, Humphreys M, et al: Increased renal phosphodiesterase-5 activity mediates the blunted natriuretic response to ANP in the pregnant rat, *Am J Physiol* 292:F655–F659, 2006.

Krane NK, Hamrahian M: Pregnancy: kidney diseases and hypertension, *Am J Kidney Dis* 49(2):336–345, 2007.

Kristiansson P, Wang JX: Reproductive hormones and blood pressure during pregnancy, *Hum Reprod* 16(1):13–17, 2001.

Levine RJ, Maynard SE, Qian C, et al: Circulating angiogenic factors and the risk of preeclampsia, *N Engl J Med* 350(7):672–683, 2004.

Longnecker MP: Maternal glomerular filtration rate in pregnancy and fetal size, *PLoS One* 9(7):e101897, 2014.

Lowe SA, Macdonald GJ, Brown MA: Atrial natriuretic peptide in pregnancy: response to oral sodium supplementation, *Clin Exp Pharmacol Physiol* 19:607–612, 1992.

Lukacs H, Hiatt ES, Lei ZM, et al: Peripheral and intracerebroventricular administration of human chorionic gonadotrophin alters several hippocampus-associated behaviors in cycling female rats, *Horm Behav* 29:42–58, 1995.

Mabie W, DiSessa TG, Crocker LG, et al: A longitudinal study of cardiac output in normal human pregnancy, *Am J Obstet Gynecol* 170(3):849–856, 1994.

Magness RR, Rosenfeld CR: Local and systemic estradiol-17 beta: effects on uterine and systemic vasodilation, *Am J Physiol* 256:E536–E542, 1989.

Mahendru AA, Everett TR, Wilkinson IB, et al: Maternal cardiovascular changes from prepregnancy to very early pregnancy, *J Hypertens* 30:2168–2172, 2012.

Mahendrua AA, Everetta TR, Wilkinsonb IB, et al: A longitudinal study of maternal cardiovascular function from preconception to the postpartum period, *J Hypertens* 32:849–856, 2014.

Marcouiller F, Boukari R, Laouafa S, et al: The nuclear progesterone receptor reduces post-sigh apneas during sleep and increases the ventilatory response to hypercapnia in adult female mice, *PLoS One* 9(6):e100421, 2014.

Marques AH, Bjørke-Monsen A-L, Teixeira AL, et al: Maternal stress, nutrition and physical activity: impact on immune function, CNS development and psychopathology, *Brain Res* 1617:28–46, 2015.

McGuane JT, Debrah JE, Sautina L, et al: Relaxin induces rapid dilation of rodent small renal and human subcutaneous arteries via PI3 kinase and nitric oxide, *Endocrinology* 152:2786–2796, 2011a.

McGuane JT, Danielson LA, Debrah JE, et al: Angiogenic growth factors are new and essential players in the sustained relaxin vasodilatory pathway in rodents and humans, *Hypertension* 57:1151–1160, 2011.

Mendelson CR: Minireview: fetal-maternal hormonal signalling in pregnancy and labor, *Mol Endocrinol* 23:947–954, 2009.

Mesiano S: The endocrinology of human pregnancy and fetal-placental neuroroendocrine development. In Strauss JF, Barbieri RL, editors: *Yen & Jaffe's reproductive endocrinology*, 7th edn, Philadelphia, Elsevier, 2014.

Mukaddam-Daher S, Jankowski M, Wang D, et al: Regulation of cardiac oxytocin system and natriuretic peptide during rat gestation and postpartum, *J Endocrinol* 175:211–216, 2002.

Nakamura T, Matsui K, Ito M, et al: Effect of pregnancy and hormone treatments on pressor responses to angiotensin II in conscious rats, *Am J Obstet Gynecol* 159(5):989–995, 1988.

Nolten WE, Rueckert PA: Elevated free cortisol index in pregnancy: possible regulatory mechanisms, *Am J Obstet Gynecol* 139(4):492–498, 1981.

Novak J, Danielson LA, Kerchner LJ, et al: Relaxin is essential for renal vasodilation during pregnancy in conscious rats, *J Clin Invest* 107(11):1469–1475, 2001.

Olcese J: Circadian aspects of mammalian parturition: a review, *Mol Cell Endocrinol* 349(1):62–67, 2012.

Omar HA, Ramirez R, Gibson M: Properties of a progesterone-induced relaxation in human placental arteries and veins, *J Clin Endocrinol Metab* 80(2):370–373, 1995.

Pasqualini JR: Enzymes involved in the formation and transformation of steroid hormones in the fetal and placental compartments, *J Steroid Biochem Mol Biol* 97:401–415, 2005.

Pepe GJ, Albrecht ED: Actions of placental and fetal adrenal steroid hormones in primate pregnancy, *Endocr Rev* 16(5):608–648, 1995.

Phippard AF, Horvath JS, Glynn EM: Circulatory adaptations to pregnancy – serial studies of haemodynamics, blood volume, renin and aldosterone in the baboon, *J Hypertens* 4:773–779, 1986.

Poppas A, Shroff SG, Korcarz CE, et al: Serial assessment of cardiovascular system in normal pregnancy: role of arterial compliance and pulsatile arterial load, *Circulation* 95:2407–2415, 1997.

Quinkler M, Johanssen S, Bumke-Vogt C, et al: Enzyme-mediated protection of the mineralocorticoid receptor against progesterone in the human kidney, *Mol Cell Endocrinol* 171:21–24, 2001.

Ren Y, Wang H, Qin H, et al: Vascular endothelial growth factor expression in peripheral blood of patients with pregnancy induced hypertension syndrome and its clinical significance, *Pak J Med Sci* 30(3):634–637, 2014.

Robson SC, Hunter S, Boys RJ, et al: Serial study of factors influencing changes in cardiac output during human pregnancy, *Am J Physiol* 256:H1060–H1065, 1989.

Romen Y, Masaki DI, Mittelmark RA: Physiological and endocrine adjustments to pregnancy. In Mittelmark RA, Wiswell RA, editors: *Exercise in pregnancy*, Baltimore, Williams and Wilkins, 1991.

Rosso P: *Nutrition and metabolism in pregnancy*, New York, Oxford University Press, 1990.

Rudel D, Pajntar M: Contractions of the cervix in the latent phase of labour, *Contemp Rev Obstet Gynaecol* December:271–279, 1999.

Saffer C, Olson G, Boggess KA, et al: Determination of placental growth factor (PlGF) levels in healthy pregnant women without signs or symptoms of preeclampsia, *Pregnancy Hypertens* 3:124–132, 2013.

Sealey JE, Atlas SA, Glorioso N, et al: Cyclical secretion of prorenin during the menstrual cycle: synchronization with luteinizing hormone and progesterone, *Proc Natl Acad Sci USA* 82:8705–8709, 1985.

Sealey JE, Cholst I, Glorioso N, et al: Sequential changes in plasma luteinizing hormone and plasma prorenin during the menstrual cycle, *J Clin Endocrinol Metab* 65(1):1–5, 1987.

Shynlova O, Tsui P, Jaffer S, et al: Integration of endocrine and mechanical signals in the regulation of myometrial functions during pregnancy and labour, *Eur J Obstet Gynecol Reprod Biol* 1445:S2–S10, 2009.

Sharkey J, Olceses J: Transcriptional inhibition of oxytocin receptor expression in human myometrial cells by melatonin involves protein kinase c signaling, *J Clin Endocrinol Metab* 92(10):4015–4019, 2007.

Skinner SL: The renin system in fertility and normal human pregnancy. In Robertson JIS, Nicholls MG, editors: *The renin–angiotensin system*, vol 1, London, Gower Medical, pp 50.1–50.16, 1993.

Smith R: Parturition, *N Engl J Med* 356:271–283, 2007.

Spaanderman MEA, Meertens M, Van Bussell M, et al: Cardiac output increases independently of basal metabolic rate in early pregnancy, *Am J Physiol* 278:H1585–H1588, 2000.

Stanton BA, Koeppen BM: The kidney. In Berne RM, Levy MN, editors: *Physiology*, St. Louis, Mosby Year Book, 1993.

Steegers EAP: Atrial natriuretic peptide during human pregnancy and puerperium, *Fetal Med Rev* 3:185–196, 1991.

Steer PJ: The genital system. In Hytten F, Chamberlain G, editors: *Clinical physiology in obstetrics*, Oxford, Blackwell Scientific, 1991.

Steer PJ: Maternal hemoglobin concentration and birth weight, *Am J Clin Nutr* 71(5):1285S–1287S, 2000.

Steer P, Ash Alam M, Wadsworth J, et al: Relation between maternal haemoglobin concentration and birth weight in different ethnic groups, *Br Med J* 310:489–491, 1995.

Stewart DR, Overstreet JW, Nakajima ST, et al: Enhanced ovarian steroid secretion before implantation in early human pregnancy, *J Clin Endocrinol Metab* 76(6):1470–1476, 1993.

Strauss JF, Williams CJ: The ovarian life cycle. In Strauss JF, Barbieri RL, editors: *Yen & Jaffe's reproductive endocrinology*, 7th edn, Philadelphia, Elsevier, 2014.

Sudhir K, Chou TM, Mullen WL, et al: Mechanisms of oestrogen induced vasodilation: in vivo studies in canine coronary conductance and resistance arteries, *J Am Coll Cardiol* 26:807–814, 1995.

Szmuilowicz ED, Adler GK, Williams JS, et al: Relationship between aldosterone and progesterone in the human menstrual cycle, *J Clin Endocrinol Metab* 91(10):3981–3987, 2006.

Tam S, Kaufman S: NOS inhibition restores renal responses to atrial distension during pregnancy, *Am J Physiol* 282:R1364–R1367, 2002.

Thomsen JK, Fogh-Andersen N, Jaszczak P, et al: Atrial natriuretic peptide (ANP) decrease during normal pregnancy as related to hemodynamic changes and volume regulation, *Acta Obstet Gynecol Scand* 72:103–110, 1993.

Ticconi C, Belmonte A, Piccione E, et al: Feto-placental communication system with the myometrium in pregnancy and parturition: the role of hormones, neurohormones, inflammatory mediators, and locally active factors, *J Matern Fetal Neonatal Med* 19(3):125–133, 2006.

Ting AY, Blacklock AD, Smith PG: Estrogen regulates vaginal sensory and autonomic nerve density in the rat, *Biol Reprod* 71:1397–1404, 2004.

Tucker Blackburn S: *Maternal, fetal & neonatal physiology*, St. Louis, Saunders Elsevier, 2013.

Uldbjerg N, Ulmsten U, Ekman G: The ripening of the human uterine cervix in terms of connective tissue biochemistry, *Clin Obstet Gynaecol* 26(1):14–26, 1983.

Vaillancourt P, Omer S, Palfree R, et al: Downregulation of adrenal atrial natriuretic peptide receptor mRNAs and proteins by pregnancy in the rat, *J Endocrinol* 155:523–530, 1997.

Valdes G, Germain AM, Corthorn J, et al: Urinary vasodilator and vasoconstrictor angiotensins during menstrual cycle, pregnancy, and lactation, *Endocrine* 16(2):117–122, 2001.

Vokes TJ, Weiss NM, Schrieiber J, et al: Osmoregulation of thirst and vasopressin during normal menstrual cycle, *Am J Physiol* 254(23):R641–R647, 1988.

Volman MNM, Rep A, Kadzinska I, et al: Haemodynamic changes in the second half of pregnancy: a longitudinal, noninvasive study with thoracic electrical bioimpedance, *Br J Obstet Gynaecol* 114(5):576–581, 2007.

Weiner CP, Lizasoain I, Baylis SA, et al: Induction of calcium dependent nitric oxide synthases by sex hormones, *Proc Natl Acad Sci USA* 91:5212–5216, 1994.

Williams MR, Westerman RA, Kingwell BA: Variations in endothelial function and arterial compliance during the menstrual cycle, *J Clin Endocrinol Metab* 86(11):5389–5395, 2001.

Wintour EM, Coghlan JP, Oddie CJ, et al: A sequential study of adrenocorticosteroid level in human pregnancy, *Clin Exp Pharmacol Physiol* 5(4):399–403, 1978.

Wu Z, Zheng W, Sandberg K: Estrogen regulates adrenal angiotensin type 1 receptors by modulating adrenal angiotensin levels, *Endocrinology* 144(4):1350–1356, 2003.

Yoshimura T, Yoshimura M, Yasue H, et al: Plasma concentration of atrial

501

natriuretic peptide and brain natriuretic peptide during normal human pregnancy and the postpartum period, *J Endocrinol* 140:393–397, 1994.

Zhang Y, Stewart KG, Davidge ST: Endogenous estrogen mediates vascular reactivity and distensibility in pregnant rat mesenteric arteries, *Am J Physiol* 280:H956–H961, 2001.

Zuluaga MJ, Agrati D, Pereira M, et al: Experimental anxiety in the black and white model in cycling, pregnant and lactating rats, *Physiol Behav* 84:279–286, 2005.

Resources and additional reading

Please refer to the chapter website resources.

Chapter 32

Confirming pregnancy and care of the pregnant woman

Kuldip K. Bharj and Lesley Daniels

Learning Outcomes

After reading this chapter, you will be able to:

- discuss the role of the midwife in the provision of personalized care during pregnancy giving due consideration to women's physiological, educational, psychological and socioeconomic needs and recognize the importance of culture, ethnicity, age, disability and sexual orientation in the provision of responsive care
- describe the physical and biochemical assessments that may enable the diagnosis and confirmation of pregnancy
- discuss opportunities for women to make early contact with the maternity service and discuss the purpose of the initial visit, identifying the importance of taking a comprehensive antenatal history, and consider the relevance of the information obtained in determining future care and the options for place of birth
- examine the physiological changes during pregnancy that might lead to disturbance and discomfort within the various body systems and discuss their implications and the ways in which these may be alleviated or minimized

- describe the physical examination, including the abdominal examination, undertaken during initial and subsequent antenatal visits, and discuss the relevance of the information obtained in planning prospective care
- discuss the psychological needs of women during pregnancy and explore the role of the midwife in supporting women during their transition into pregnancy, childbirth and early parenting
- recognize the importance of health education and promotion during the antenatal period to maintain and/or improve the woman and her baby's health
- describe the signs and symptoms of pelvic girdle pain and discuss its possible physical and psychological effects and its management during the antenatal, intranatal and postnatal period
- appreciate the importance of effective communication with women and their families during the antenatal period to provide sensitive and responsive care and to develop positive relationships with them

---

INTRODUCTION

This chapter focuses on the care and services available to women during the antenatal period from the point at which a woman believes she may be pregnant to the onset of labour. During this period, pregnant women experience tremendous anatomical, physiological and psychological changes to assist them to adapt, prepare for birthing and transition to parenting. Care during pregnancy is one of the essential preventative health services. During this period, midwives are key professionals who work in

partnership with women and doctors, where appropriate, to assess women's individual needs and to plan and implement the most appropriate care to women and their families.

CONFIRMATION OF PREGNANCY

Many women of childbearing age who are sexually active may suspect that they are pregnant, especially if their menstrual period is delayed and/or other symptoms of pregnancy, such as nausea or vomiting, are experienced. Often, women say that they 'just feel different'. Women may choose to confirm their pregnancy either by using a home pregnancy test or by seeking diagnosis through their midwife or general practitioner (GP). Confirmation of pregnancy is established by a detailed history and a clinical examination based on the symptoms and signs of pregnancy, resulting from the physiological alteration in the body's systems and organs. These include amenorrhoea, breast changes and tenderness, nausea and vomiting, increased frequency of micturition, enlargement of the uterus and skin changes. These symptoms and signs become obvious to the woman as her pregnancy advances, but, as some of these symptoms and signs may be found in other conditions not associated with pregnancy, it is important that the midwife is aware of these conditions, as she may need to refer the woman for further investigations or specialist advice.

Reflective activity 32.1

When you next undertake a first 'history taking' interview, discuss with the woman and, if appropriate, her partner the following:

- What made her suspect that she was pregnant?
- How did she confirm the pregnancy? Did she use a home pregnancy test?
- How many weeks pregnant was she when the pregnancy was confirmed?
- How, and at what gestation, did she make contact with her midwife and/or GP?

Signs and symptoms of pregnancy may be considered as presumptive, probable and positive, as illustrated in Table 32.1.

First 4 weeks

Amenorrhoea: If a woman misses her period (amenorrhoea), this may be suggestive that she is pregnant. After implantation of the fertilized ovum, the endometrium undergoes decidual change and normally menstruation does not occur throughout pregnancy, although some women can be pregnant and still have a small amount of bleeding during the first few months of their pregnancy at the time their period is normally due.

Amenorrhoea almost invariably accompanies pregnancy and, in a sexually active woman who has previously menstruated regularly, can be considered to be caused by pregnancy unless this is disproved. However, the possibility of secondary amenorrhoea should be considered. There may be other reasons that cause amenorrhoea, for example, illness, stress, shock, anorexia or strenuous exercise.

Breast changes: Discomfort, tenderness or tingling and a feeling of fullness of the breasts may be noticed as early

as the third or fourth week of pregnancy, as the blood supply to the breasts increases; however, not every woman will experience or notice such changes.

Nausea and vomiting: These are common symptoms experienced by women in early pregnancy, affecting approximately 80% to 90% of pregnant women, albeit at varying levels (Badell et al 2006; Ebrahimi et al 2010; Naumann et al 2012). Although nausea, retching and vomiting are experienced by most pregnant women, nausea affects 50% to 80% women and about 50% experiencing vomiting and retching (Miller 2002; Woolhouse 2006); vomiting on its own is rare (Badell et al 2006). Nausea, vomiting and retching is most common in the first trimester, and only a small percentage experience it in the morning, but many suffer from it throughout the day.

Vomiting is also a feature of a variety of other conditions, such as gastroenteritis, urinary tract infection and hydatidiform mole, and these should be excluded.

Around 8 weeks

Nausea and vomiting: These usually persist in those women who are affected.

Frequency of micturition: This is due to increased vascularity of the bladder and lasts until about the 16th week of pregnancy when the gravid uterus rises out of the pelvic girdle.

Breast changes: The breasts enlarge and the superficial veins on both the chest and breasts dilate. The enlarged breasts may be painful.

Around 12 weeks

Nausea and vomiting: These may decrease, and, for some women, cease altogether. The mean duration of nausea is about 34.6 days and, in about 50% of women, it lasts until 14 weeks gestation (Lacroix et al 2000).

Enlarged uterus: The enlarged uterus is just palpable above the symphysis pubis at about 12 weeks. Other reasons for an enlarged uterus include tumours such as ovarian cysts or fibroids. Ascites may be mistaken for a pregnant uterus.

Skin changes: Profound physiological endocrine, immunological, metabolic and vascular alterations in pregnancy contribute to a variety of skin changes (Tunzi et al 2007). Areas of hyperpigmentation, which are more prominent in darkly pigmented skin, include the nipples and areolae; the linea nigra (the line of pigmentation from the symphysis pubis to the umbilicus); and chloasma, also referred to as the 'mask of pregnancy' (Bolanca et al 2008) (see chapter website resources). The nipples become more prominent and Montgomery's tubercles are visible on the areola.

Table 32.1 Signs and symptoms of pregnancy

Time – weeks gestation	Presumptive signs	Probable signs	Positive signs	Differential diagnosis
4+	Amenorrhoea			Emotional disturbance Illness such as tuberculosis or thyrotoxicosis Hormonal imbalance
4 onwards			Presence of human chorionic gonadotrophin (hCG) in blood and urine	Hydatidiform mole
4–14	Nausea and vomiting			Gastroenteritis Urinary tract infection Hydatidiform mole
3–4+	Breast changes			
5–6			Visualization of gestational sac and pulsation of fetal heart on ultrasound	
6–10		Hegar's sign – softening of the vagina and cervix		
First 12	Frequency of micturition			Urinary tract infection
6–12	Skin changes			
8 onwards		Goodell's sign – softening of the cervix and vagina – accompanied by increased leukorrhoeal discharge Osiander's sign – pulsation of the uterine arteries through the lateral fornices Chadwick's sign – lilac discoloration of the vaginal mucous membrane Changes in the uterus – size increases and the shape changes		Pelvic congestion
10			Fetal heart sounds audible with Sonicaid	

Continued

505

Table 32.1 Signs and symptoms of pregnancy—cont'd

Time – weeks gestation	Presumptive signs	Probable signs	Positive signs	Differential diagnosis
14–16			Fetal skeleton visible on radiological examination, although unlikely to be used because of the risks of irradiation	
16 onwards	Quickening – first fetal movements felt by the woman			Intestinal movement possibly because of wind
16		Colostrum may be expressed from the breasts Uterine souffle Abdominal enlargement		Increased blood flow to uterus in, for example, ovarian tumours
16–28	Internal ballottement			
From 20	Braxton Hicks contractions			
From 22		Fetal parts felt by examiner		
24		Fetal heart audible with Pinard's stethoscope		

Around 16 weeks

Colostrum: The breasts may begin to secrete colostrum, which persists throughout pregnancy and for the first few days after delivery until milk is produced. A secondary areola may appear in darkly pigmented skin.

Quickening: The first fetal movements may be felt by primigravid women at 19+ weeks and by multiparous women at 17+ weeks. The time scale over which fetal movements are felt first by the woman varies (Kraus and Hendricks 1964) and ranges from 15 to 22 weeks in primigravid and from 14 to 22 weeks in multiparous women (O'Dowd and O'Dowd 1985). Quickening, often described as 'flutters', or a feeling of 'bubbles coming to the surface' rather than recognizable movements, is an unreliable indicator of gestational age, as sometimes these feelings can be attributed to flatulence.

Around 20 weeks

For 70% to 90% of women, nausea and vomiting have usually diminished by 22 weeks gestation (Lacroix et al 2000; Badell et al 2006; Ebrahimi et al 2010). The secondary areola, if not already present, may appear. The fundus of the uterus is normally palpated just below the umbilicus.

Around 24 weeks

The fundus can be felt just above the umbilicus, and the fetal parts and movements may be felt on abdominal palpation. The fetal heart sounds may be heard with a fetal stethoscope, and at 24 weeks the fetus is considered to be capable of an independent existence.

From 28 to 40 weeks

The fundus continues to rise until 36 weeks, when it reaches the xiphisternum and remains at that level until the fetal head engages. Braxton Hicks contractions, painless irregular uterine contractions, may be palpated from about 16 weeks and these persist until the end of pregnancy.

Engagement of the fetal head occurs from approximately 36 weeks gestation, the fundus descends slightly, causing, together with the increased flexion of the fetus, a relief of pressure that is experienced by the woman in the form of 'lightening'. This may not occur in multigravidae, as the head often does not engage until labour is established. This lightening allows the woman to breathe with more comfort; however, the descent of the head may cause pressure on the bladder, resulting in increased frequency of micturition.

Signs of pregnancy found by vaginal examination

It is now uncommon to undertake a vaginal examination in early pregnancy; however, if performed, the following signs of pregnancy may be observed:

- *Goodell's sign.* This is a softening and increasing vascularity of the cervix and vagina and is accompanied by increased leukorrhoeal discharge (Blackburn 2007).
- *Hegar's sign.* The softening and increased compressibility of the lower uterine segment makes it possible, on bimanual examination, for the fingers in the anterior fornix and those on the abdomen almost to meet (Blackburn 2007).
- *Osiander's sign.* The increased pulsation of the uterine arteries through the lateral fornices can be detected.
- *Chadwick's sign*, also referred to as 'Jacquemier sign', is a purplish discoloration of the vaginal and cervical mucous membrane resulting from increased vascularity of those tissues (Blackburn 2007).
- *Enlargement of the uterus* is noted and compared with the period of gestation.

Positive signs of pregnancy

Although there are many physical changes experienced by the woman that might suggest pregnancy, there are a number of positive signs that will confirm pregnancy:

1. *Fetal heart sounds:* may be detected from 10 weeks gestation using Sonicaid ultrasonic equipment and from 24 weeks gestation can be heard with the Pinard fetal stethoscope.
2. *Fetal movements:* felt by the examiner.
3. *Palpation of fetal parts:* felt by the examiner.
4. *Fetal skeleton:* is visible on radiological assessment at 14 to 16 weeks, although x-rays are now rarely used because of the risks of damage to the developing fetus through irradiation.

5. *Gestational sac:* may be visualized by ultrasonography at about 5 weeks and the fetal heart may be seen pulsating at 6 weeks using abdominal ultrasound. Vaginal ultrasound scanning may detect these signs a week earlier (Chudleigh and Pearce 1994). A viable intra-uterine pregnancy is confirmed when fetal heart pulsations can be seen in the gestational sac in the uterus.

Laboratory diagnosis of pregnancy

Chorionic tissue, which later forms the placenta, starts producing the hormone *human chorionic gonadotrophin* (hCG), which is excreted in the urine. This hormone is usually detected in the urine from the time of the first missed period. Immunological tests depend on the detection of hCG in the urine. Pregnancy tests fall into three categories with varying sensitivities to hCG:

- *Direct latex agglutination tests* (Fig. 32.1), where a small amount of latex particle reagent is placed on a dark glass slide; the latex particles are coated with antibodies that will bind to hCG. The reagent is milky in appearance, but when urine with hCG is added, the antibodies bind to the hCG, causing the particles to agglutinate. The liquid changes to a granular consistency, indicating a positive test result. Where no hCG is present, agglutination does not occur and the liquid remains milky (Wheeler 1999).
- *Monoclonal antibody tests/indirect agglutination tests.* Latex particles or red blood cells are coated with hCG. When the antibody solution is added, the particles or cells agglutinate. When urine containing hCG is added, the hormone binds to the antibodies, preventing them from attaching to the hCG on the cells, and no agglutination occurs (Wheeler 1999).

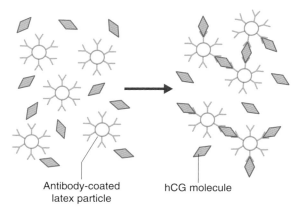

Antibody-coated latex particle   hCG molecule

Figure 32.1 The principle of direct latex agglutination tests. (From Wheeler 1999.)

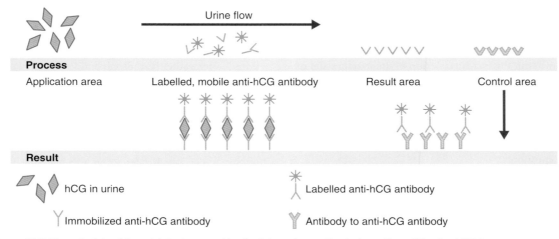

Figure 32.2 The principle of the wick test as used in dipstick and cassette devices. (From Wheeler 1999.)

- *The wick or cassette method* (Fig. 32.2). This may be a simple dipstick test with an absorbent wick on a cardboard or plastic backing, or a more sophisticated wick enclosed in a case to give a cassette-type test as with home pregnancy tests; it may also contain a control window. The absorbent wick is passed through the urine stream or dipped into the urine, or drops of urine are placed upon the sample window. Antibodies labelled with a coloured dye and placed between the application area and the result area bind to the hCG. As the urine is absorbed, it travels along the wick to the result area – this appears as a coloured band. The excess urine moves further along the wick to the control panel, where it is bound to another antibody and a further coloured band is displayed. When hCG is present and the test is performed correctly, the result window and the control window will show coloured bands. If hCG is not present, no band will be visible in the result window, only in the control window. If the control window is blank, the test has not been performed correctly and should be repeated.

Up to 40 types of laboratory test kits are available in the UK (Wheeler 1999). These have a wide range of different sensitivities, from 20 to 1000 IU/L of hCG.

Home pregnancy tests (over-the-counter pregnancy tests) have a more consistent range of sensitivity, from 25 to 50 IU/L, take from 1 minute to obtain a result, appear easy to use and manufacturers claim a 99% accuracy rate. However, the sensitivity and specificity of tests is variable and the diagnostic efficiency of home pregnancy tests is affected by the characteristics of the users (Bastian et al 1998; Cole et al 2009); therefore, it is possible to have either a false-positive, although this is rare, or a false-negative test. A false-positive result could result if

pregnancy loss happens soon after the test. False-negative results are more likely to arise from testing before the recommended number of days from the last menstrual period, or from a failure to read or follow the instructions. Therefore, a negative result in a woman who does not menstruate within a week may be repeated, although other symptoms and signs may be suggestive of the diagnosis. The advantages of using home pregnancy tests are that a woman can confirm pregnancy in the privacy of her home and be the first to have the information. It provides a quick result at an early point in the pregnancy and after confirmation of pregnancy, women are encouraged to contact their midwife or doctor to commence their antenatal care.

Pseudocyesis

This is a phantom or false pregnancy and may occur in women with an intense desire to become pregnant. Amenorrhoea will be present. The woman will complain of all the subjective symptoms of pregnancy, usually in a bizarre order; the abdomen may be distended and the breasts may secrete a cloudy liquid (American Psychiatric Association 2013). However, she is not pregnant. The signs on which a certain diagnosis of pregnancy can be made – namely, palpation of the fetus or hearing the fetal heart – are not present. Referral to a psychologist or psychiatrist may be required (Tarín et al 2013).

ANTENATAL CARE

Over the past two centuries, antenatal services have seen major developments in terms of their provision and delivery and are widely acknowledged to have contributed to the positive maternal and neonatal outcomes. Contemporary antenatal services have quality at their heart, with safety, women's experience and satisfaction and effectiveness of care as their central tenets. All women seek a healthy outcome to their pregnancy; they want high-quality, personalized care that is coupled with greater information and education to enable them to make informed choices about the place and nature of their care so that they can access services in a timely fashion (Renfrew et al 2014). Women want to be cared for by healthcare professionals who are compassionate, friendly and communicate with them in a respectful manner with whom they can work together and decide the type and nature of care they want and need.

The UK maternity services aim to provide a world-class service to women and their families, with the overall vision for the services to be flexible and personalized. Services should be designed to fit around the individual needs of the woman, baby and family circumstances, with due consideration being given to factors that may render some women and their families to become vulnerable and disadvantaged. Pregnancy is a normal physiological process for the majority of women. Women and their families need support to have as normal a pregnancy and birth as possible, with medical intervention being offered only if it is of benefit. However, in some circumstances, both midwifery and obstetric care are indicated and care should be based on providing good clinical and psychological outcomes for the woman and her baby (Department of Health (DH) and Department for Education and Skills (DfES) 2004; DH 2007; National Institute for Health and Clinical Excellence (NICE) 2008).

Aims of antenatal care

The purpose of antenatal care is to improve and maintain maternal and fetal health by monitoring the progress of pregnancy to confirm normality and detect any deviation early so that corrective care can be provided. The aims of antenatal care are to:

- facilitate the development of partnership between the woman and the professionals involved in her care
- exchange information about all aspects of care with the woman and her family, enabling them to make informed decisions about pregnancy, birth and parenting
- increase the woman's understanding of public health issues to maintain and promote her health, and make positive lifestyle choices during childbirth and onwards
- regularly monitor maternal and fetal health in pregnancy to confirm normality and to detect early any complications of pregnancy and refer women to

appropriate healthcare professionals from the multidisciplinary team

- prepare the woman and her family for the physical, psychological and emotional adaptation to pregnancy and for safe birth, and, where possible, drawing up a birth plan to facilitate a fulfilling experience for them
- afford opportunities for the woman and her family to increase their knowledge of aspects essential for childbirth and for early parenthood
- provide evidence-based information for the woman and her family, supporting them to make informed choices about methods of infant feeding
- prepare for the period after birth, including family planning advice

Care during pregnancy

Pregnant women are encouraged to seek professional healthcare as early as possible in pregnancy, typically within the first 10 weeks of pregnancy (NICE 2012), so that they can obtain and use evidence-based information to plan their pregnancy and to benefit from antenatal screening and health promotion activities. With early information about the available models of antenatal care, women, in partnership with healthcare professionals, can make decisions about the most appropriate pathway of their care best suited to their personal, social and obstetric circumstances.

Where women seek care at a later stage in pregnancy, they will have reduced access to antenatal care. It is likely that the woman will have reduced options in terms of antenatal screening tests, and some investigations, for example, serum screening for Down syndrome (see Ch. 33), are accurate only if carried out at specific times, in this case between 15 and 18 weeks. Early detection of these conditions enables further investigations, such as ultrasound scan or amniocentesis, to be carried out at the optimum time.

Early access to antenatal care enables healthcare professionals to obtain baseline measures, facilitating accurate monitoring of the effect of physiological changes on vital systems and organs of the body and early detection of any complications. For example, the recording of the blood pressure in the first trimester of pregnancy provides a baseline against which the physiological changes in the blood pressure can be assessed. In some cases, complications may have already arisen by the time the woman seeks antenatal care. If such complications are not managed in a timely manner, they can adversely affect maternal and fetal outcomes (Centre for Maternal and Child Enquiries (CMACE) 2011; Knight et al 2015).

The woman should be able to choose whether her first contact in pregnancy is with a midwife or her GP. However, antenatal services vary; in many parts of the UK, for many women, the first point of contact for maternity services is the GP, although increasingly women contact midwives as their first contact with maternity (Redshaw et al 2014).

To achieve the principles of antenatal care, pregnant women require evidence-based information. Evidence suggests that women desire accurate and timely information about pregnancy and childbirth so that they can develop their knowledge and understanding of pregnancy, childbirth and related issues, enabling them to make informed decisions about the care they want and prefer (Bharj 2007; Kirkham and Stapleton 2001; Mander 2001). Women need information, which is based on current evidence that is clearly understood and in a format they can easily access. When offering information, healthcare professionals must take into account the requirements of women who have physical and sensory learning disabilities and women whose competence in speaking and reading English is low, exploring appropriate ways of exchanging meaningful information.

Midwives are key healthcare professionals who work with women to support them to make informed choices regarding preferred arrangements for antenatal care, place of birth and postnatal care. In addition to being knowledgeable, midwives should be friendly, kind, compassionate, caring, approachable, nonjudgemental, respectful, have time for women and be good communicators, providing support and companionship (Nicholls and Webb 2006; Bharj and Chesney 2010; Freedman et al 2014). These attributes are essential for the development of the woman–midwife relationship. Many worldwide studies highlight that all women perceive the woman–midwife relationship to be central to their pregnancy, childbirth and postnatal experiences (Anderson 2000; Davies 2000; Kirkham 2010; Edwards 2005; Bharj 2007; Lundgren and Berg 2007). Midwives, therefore, play an essential role in the life of women during their most significant period and have the power to either augment or mar women's experiences of pregnancy and childbirth.

Reflective activity 32.2

Reflect on the discussions you have had or have observed with women during the initial visit. Do you think that you provided sufficient information for the woman to make informed decisions about patterns of antenatal care, home birth and who she would wish to see during the antenatal period?

Outline of present pattern of maternity services in the UK

There are a wide range of models of care available across the UK because of its geographical and demographic variations and new models of care are continuing to develop.

Some examples are care in the community through Children's Centre, GP Surgery, Independent midwifery or the woman's home, or a hospital setting or a mixture of hospital and the community setting. The organization of maternity services varies throughout the UK, with care being planned and delivered through clinical commissioning groups (CCG) in England (NHSCC 2013). The maternity and obstetric units are often formed as a part of the larger general hospitals, and the maternity and midwifery services are normally provided through such units and are integrated within the community and hospital. Midwifery units are designed and staffed according to the birth rates; therefore, the sizes of the units are variable dependent on the birth rates. Some National Health Service (NHS) hospitals provide tertiary maternity and neonatal services for part of the regions. Generally, midwifery staff are employed by an acute maternity unit and may work either in the community or in the hospital, or, in some models of care, in both.

Birth settings

Women are offered choices in the place of birth and the four main settings are: 'consultant-led obstetric units' (CLU), 'midwifery-led units' (MLU), either alongside (AMLU) or free standing/standalone (FMU) and 'home' (Hall 2003) (for choices of place of birth, see Ch. 34). CLUs are usually attached to the district or regional units and deliver care both for women who have complex healthcare needs and for those with no complications of pregnancy, labour and birth. CLUs are staffed by midwives and obstetricians. Women may be referred to an obstetrician who becomes the lead professional for the duration of their childbirth continuum or receive their care from a midwife. Women with complex healthcare needs will be referred to an obstetrician and may access all their care in the antenatal, intranatal and postnatal period within these settings.

Some women with less complex healthcare needs may access some of their care in the hospital setting and some in the community setting. A full range of obstetric facilities (such as anaesthesia, surgery, blood transfusion and neonatal intensive care) are readily available in CLUs.

MLUs, sometimes known as 'low-risk maternity units' (Hall 2003), are often located close to, but separate from, CLUs. These units normally aim to provide care to women with uncomplicated pregnancies; the women, however, have to meet the criteria for the unit throughout pregnancy, labour and birth. MLUs are staffed predominantly by midwives, although they may be jointly run by midwives and GPs. If a deviation from normal is detected during pregnancy, labour or birth, the woman will be referred to an obstetrician, or, if appropriate, a GP, and may have to transfer place of care to the CLU. Normally, women access the majority of their antenatal care in the community setting with minimal care in the hospital setting.

Women may choose to have their babies at home instead of a hospital setting (see Ch. 34). Each of the midwifery units in the UK has its own arrangements for providing a home birth service and its own guidelines and attitudes towards these. The provision of this service depends on local resources, local practices and policies, and the beliefs, skills and commitment of individual practitioners providing the service. Women who choose to have a home birth are normally given care in the community by the lead professional who may be either a midwife or GP. In circumstances where the maternity needs of the woman cannot be managed in the home setting, then she and/or her baby is transferred to the nearest CLU.

The purpose of the FMUs is to offer a 'home-like' environment within an institutional setting. The philosophy and the kind of care offered by an FMU are very similar to those of the MLUs, and the main difference is that the FMU is geographically situated away from the CLU. Typically, women who access care at these settings are less likely to require interventions and assimilate with the guidelines and protocols of these units. Should an intervention be required for a woman, a decision will need to be made about transferring to the CLU.

To meet the maternity needs of the local populations, two things have happened concomitantly in some areas of England. The move to centralize maternity services has seen a number of mergers and, at the same time, there have appeared a small number of new community units or birth centres to provide a limited service for women who would otherwise have to travel long distances to have their babies in large obstetric units (for example, see Kirkham 2003). However, in light of recent evidence (Hatem et al 2008; Sandall et al 2015), highlighting clinical outcomes are not adversely affected for women who have uncomplicated pregnancies and who birth in MLUs, maternity services are exploring other models of care.

Team midwifery

Maternity services for women in the NHS are normally provided by a multiprofessional team composed of community midwives, GPs, and hospital-based midwives or doctors in the antenatal period and usually by hospital-based midwives or doctors in the intrapartum period (unless they have a home birth) and by midwives and the GPs in the postnatal period. However, many maternity units are maximizing a multiprofessional approach to service provision and delivery and are collaborating with other relevant healthcare professionals to develop a multiagency, integrated care pathway, involving shared care, for example, with the drug and alcohol treatment services. This collaborative approach to care has improved the experience and outcome for women and babies.

A variety of approaches to *team midwifery* have emerged since the 1990s, after the publications of the Winterton Report (1992) and the Changing Childbirth Report (DH 1993); they strive to provide choice and continuity, and these can include team midwifery normally based in the community, *one-to-one midwifery practice* care for women (Green et al 1998; Page et al 2000), that is, a complete episode of care from the booking interview to transfer to the health visitor after birth, including intrapartum care. Other approaches include *caseload midwifery*, or, as it is sometimes referred to, *midwifery group practice*. This comprises a small number of midwives organized into a team who are responsible for the delivery of a full range of maternity care. The midwives in the team are each responsible for approximately 30 to 40 women in a year.

In addition, groups of self-employed midwives are being commissioned to provide some maternity services. For example, *Neighbourhood Midwives* provide private maternity services alongside commissioned NHS care. Although many parts of the UK have some sort of team arrangement for providing maternity services, these teams may vary from two or three midwives to over 30. The teams are responsible for providing care in the hospital setting, community settings or both. There are four possible options of care:

- a team of community midwives, with support from the GP, deliver antenatal and postnatal care in the community setting and also provide care during labour and birth at home
- most of the antenatal and postnatal care is provided in the community with some hospital visits in the antenatal period, particularly for routine scans, antenatal screening, obstetric and any medical care; intrapartum care is in the hospital setting by team midwives, and then early transfer home
- antenatal care is shared by the hospital and community and is determined by the health needs of the woman; intranatal care is given in the hospital by hospital midwives, and then postnatal care in the community setting by community midwives
- antenatal and intrapartum care are offered in the hospital setting, together with specialized services, and then postnatal care is determined by the woman's health needs.

The type of care offered is dependent on the health needs of the woman and local practices and protocols. Where women do not have any perceived complications in the antenatal and intrapartum period, they may choose to have all their care in the community setting or a mixture of both community and hospital. However, those women who have or develop complications in pregnancy or the intrapartum period access services in the hospital setting.

Increasingly, there are developments where the NHS is collaborating with the local authority to offer maternity services from children's centres. In addition to this, some midwives are seconded to specialist outreach services, particularly *Sure Start* (integrated health, education and welfare support services for children under 4 and their families) and smoking cessation services.

In many areas, antenatal day assessment units have been developed to provide outpatient care. In circumstances where complications arise, such as moderate pregnancy-induced hypertension, the pregnant women can be referred to the antenatal assessment unit, where her and her baby's health may be assessed and monitored. Referral to such units can be made by the women themselves, by midwives or by other healthcare professionals.

To meet the needs of pregnant women, the last two decades have seen development of many different models of care. With this, there has been a decline of other models such as the 'domiciliary in and out scheme (DOMINO scheme)'. Within this model, antenatal care is delivered by a community midwife as it would be for a home birth. The community midwife provides care at home during labour, and continues care when the woman is transferred into hospital for birth. After birth, the woman and her baby, when healthy, are transferred home with postnatal care provided by the community midwife.

Independent midwifery services

Independent midwives (IM) are currently in the minority, approximately 180 in the UK, delivering a high standard of maternity care around to 3000 women and their babies every year (Gardner 2014). The midwives are self-employed and offer maternity services to individual women. Their education and governance is the same as that of any other practising midwife within the UK and within the same regulatory body. The Health Care and Association Professionals (Indemnity Arrangements) Order 2013, which came into force on 25 October 2013, required all healthcare professionals, including midwives, to have Professional Indemnity Insurance (PII) in place as a condition of their registration. This legislation had a major consequence for independent midwives. Unlike midwives working in NHS organizations and other public organizations who are covered by their employers' insurance schemes, IMs who are self-employed have no vicarious liability or indemnity. To secure their personal PII was unaffordable, Independent Midwives UK (a membership organization for independent midwives in the UK), supported by women and their families, midwives and other birth organizations, successfully developed their own PII.

The other main differences are that IMs set up their protocols for practice, using evidence-based practice, and usually offer a home birth service, meeting women's individual requirements; usually practise in small groups of two or three or in some cases single-handed. Some midwives have honorary contracts with their local hospitals and offer a DOMINO service, though where midwives are unable to secure contracts, when a woman booked with them requires medical services, the independent midwife can only accompany her to hospital as a friend or doula.

Place of birth

During pregnancy, women need unbiased information to consider where they wish to give birth. This is discussed in more detail in Chapter 34. The most common place of birth continues to remain the hospital setting, and the rate of home births has not changed significantly over the past few decades, despite calls for increasing women's choice in the place of birth. Although the rate of home birth remains low, there are marked geographical variations, and this appears to depend on midwives and doctors supporting the idea of healthy women having their babies at home. Where this was the case, the numbers of women having home births increased.

Pattern of care

Historically, irrespective of their personal needs, individual risk status or parity, all pregnant women were encouraged to routinely attend an antenatal clinic every 4 weeks up to 28 weeks gestation, then 2-weekly up to 36 weeks, and then weekly thereafter. Evidence in the 1980s suggested that healthy women were at no greater risk of maternal or perinatal mortality if they attended fewer antenatal visits than the historical pattern of care (Hall et al 1985) and, in 1982, the Royal College of Obstetricians and Gynaecologists (RCOG) recommended that maternity care providers should reduce the number of antenatal visits for women who do not have any complications of pregnancy from the historical pattern of 14 to 16 visits for all women to 5 to 7 visits for multiparous women and 8 or 9 visits for primigravid women (RCOG 1982). Maternity services were slow to implement this recommendation; however, more recently, the NICE guidance (2008) recommended that for nulliparous women with uncomplicated pregnancies, 10 antenatal appointments 'should be adequate', and that for parous women with uncomplicated pregnancies, seven antenatal appointments 'should be adequate'. Although this reduction in the frequency of antenatal appointments does not result in adverse clinical maternal and neonatal outcomes (Sikorski et al 1996; Villar et al 2001), there is a possibility of poorer psychological outcomes and dissatisfaction with frequency of visits, such as concerns about fetal well-being, and they had increased negative attitudes towards their babies, both in pregnancy and in the postnatal period (Sikorski et al 1996; Hildingsson et al 2005). It is essential, however, that the number of antenatal visits should be tailored to meet women's individualized health needs instead of attending antenatal appointments in a ritualistic pattern.

Throughout the childbearing period, all women should be provided with the opportunity to discuss issues and to ask questions (NICE 2008). To enable women to make informed choices about their care, midwives need to work in partnership with women and their families to develop and maintain relationships based on effective communication skills, empathy and trust. To communicate effectively and discuss matters fully with women, antenatal appointments need to be structured in such a way as to ensure the woman has sufficient time to make informed decisions (NICE 2008), and midwives need to develop the knowledge required to ensure they are able to offer up-to-date, consistent, evidence-based information and clear explanations, using terminology that women and their families are able to understand. Adjustments may need to be made to ensure that women with additional communication needs are able to access information in a format they are able to understand. This may include using interpreters, online resources or DVDs and leaflets and books to support discussions.

THE FIRST ANTENATAL VISIT

The first antenatal visit and taking of the woman's history may occur in the woman's home, a health centre or GP surgery, or at the first visit to the hospital antenatal clinic. If a combined approach is taken, this will reduce the visits that the woman may have to make.

Women may feel apprehensive at their first visit, especially if they have not previously met the midwives or medical staff. Good communication skills and a non-judgemental attitude are important to enable women to feel at ease in discussing very intimate personal details. A warm, friendly greeting and a pleasant, comfortable environment can also help put women at their ease. Although many women may be rather apprehensive at the first visit, teenagers, women who are less proficient in speaking English and those who are unhappy about their pregnancy may feel especially vulnerable. Interpreters are required for women who have limited fluency in speaking and understanding English and, where possible, such women should be given information in formats that enable them to access and understand the information easily – for example, written information in their own language, audiovisual tapes or in Braille. In many areas, a care pathway approach is being adopted, for example, specialist midwives and specialist teams deliver care to teenage women to ensure that women's individual needs are met.

Whatever the background of the woman, or her reactions to her pregnancy, building a positive relationship with her is one of the midwife's most important aims during this first antenatal visit. This provides a foundation upon which the trust between a midwife and a woman will be built during the rest of the pregnancy. The woman needs open communication with a midwife who is well informed and committed to supporting her as an individual, encouraging the development of mutual respect, trust and partnership. There is growing evidence of women's views of the maternity services that consistently highlights the importance of the quality of the women's relationship with their midwife and the importance of this relationship in their satisfaction levels (Kirkham 2010).

The importance at the beginning of the interview is for the woman to establish confidence in the midwife, and so the purpose and process of the interview and issues such as confidentiality must be addressed initially. The woman needs to understand the midwife's professional responsibilities, in terms of information which may be shared and which may need to be discussed with other members of the team. Similarly, the midwife needs to ensure that a woman's request that information is kept confidential is respected.

History taking

When the history is taken at home or in a community clinic, the woman is likely to be more at ease. If the interview takes place in the hospital, the midwife should prepare the interview room to be as pleasant and nonclinical as possible to facilitate communication and the development of a relationship of mutual trust. The midwife must also provide privacy and sufficient time for the interview, and make this clear to the woman.

During early pregnancy, the woman may be experiencing nausea and fatigue and will appreciate not having to travel to attend a busy clinic among strangers. Any problems can usually be discussed in private and the midwife can give information and offer advice as appropriate. When other members of the family are present during this initial assessment, this gives the midwife the opportunity to meet them, but she should also be sensitive that there may be information that the woman considers private or confidential and would prefer not to discuss in their presence. Some time alone spent between the midwife and woman is essential and this should be facilitated.

The interview should be a two-way process of interaction between the woman and midwife. It involves assessment of the woman's social, psychological, emotional and physical condition and obtaining information about the present and previous pregnancies, and the medical and family history. Care can then be planned in conjunction with the woman to meet her specific needs and wishes.

An antenatal booking interview should comprise more than merely recording an obstetric history; it should be about communicating information and promoting a relationship between the woman and the midwife (Methven 1982a and 1982b). Factors conducive to a more relaxed atmosphere and which promote communication should be considered, for example, the environment of the setting where the history is going to be taken, arrangements of the furniture in the room, body language and interpersonal skills. A few minutes spent by the midwife in introducing herself and talking informally enables the woman to settle down and relax before personal issues are discussed. A skilled midwife can elicit most of the information required from the woman in a pleasant conversational manner without the woman realizing that she is being closely questioned. Open questions, rather than closed questions, should be employed because these encourage free responses and promote two-way interaction between the woman and midwife. During the interview, the midwife should be sensitive to the woman's attitude to her pregnancy and, if possible, to that of her partner. Unusually adverse attitudes and body language should be noted and counselling and support given as required.

Personal details

The woman's full name, address, telephone number, age, date of birth, ethnicity, religion and occupation (and that of her partner) are accurately recorded. Information regarding the woman's status with a partner/husband/wife is elicited to determine whether the woman is in a stable relationship or if the woman is alone and may need additional support from the midwife and other agencies.

The woman's ethnicity is ascertained because some medical and obstetric conditions are more likely to occur in certain ethnic groups and appropriate diagnostic tests are required. However, asking about ethnicity is complex (Dyson 2005) and midwives need to develop competence in accomplishing this sensitively. The religion of the woman is recorded because of the special requirements and rituals that may be practised and affect the mother and her baby. Occupation gives an indication of socioeconomic status. Women in socioeconomic groups IV and V (see chapter website resources) may experience social and economic inequalities. These wider determinants of health, coupled with poverty, are most likely to adversely affect their or their fetus's/baby's health and clinical outcomes. The midwife needs to work with other agencies to provide the woman and her family with appropriate support to promote and improve her health.

Present pregnancy

The date of the first day of the last menstrual period (LMP) is ascertained, care being taken to check that this was the last *normal* menstrual period. Some women have a slight blood loss when the fertilized ovum embeds into the decidual lining of the uterus and many mistake this for the last period. Pregnancy has been assumed to last 280 days, and to overcome the irregularity of the calendar, a working rule of thumb was devised by Naegele. By counting forwards 9 months and adding 7 days from the first

day of the last normal menstrual period, it is possible to arrive at an estimated date of delivery (EDD); alternatively, count back 3 months and add 7 days. This method of calculating the EDD is known as *Naegele's rule*. However, as February is a short month and the remaining months have 30 or 31 days, 280 to 283 days may be added to the date of the LMP. It is unclear whether the length of pregnancy is affected by social, ethnic or obstetric factors (Rosser 2000). It is important to explain that it is quite normal for the actual day of delivery to be up to 2 weeks before or after the EDD.

Details of the woman's menstrual history should be sought: the age at which menstruation began, the duration of the periods and the number of days in the cycle. Conception occurs shortly after ovulation. With a regular cycle of about 28 days, the standard calculation is reasonably accurate to within a few days, provided that the woman knows the date of her last normal menstrual period.

In a 35-day cycle, ovulation would normally occur 21 days after the period; in a 21-day cycle, only 7 days after. Adjustments may be made, therefore, when the woman has a regular long or short cycle. If the cycle is long (for example, 33 days), the days in excess of 28 are added when calculating the EDD (Table 32.2). With a regular short cycle, such as 23 days, the number of days less than 28 is subtracted from the EDD.

The calculation is difficult if the woman does not know the date of her last menstrual period, cycles are irregular or a normal cycle has not resumed since taking the oral contraceptive pill or after a previous birth. If the woman has a good idea of when conception occurred, the EDD can be calculated by adding 38 weeks to this date, or subtracting 7 days from 9 months.

Women should be asked to note the date when fetal movements are felt first. Primigravidae normally become aware of fetal movements between 18 and 20 weeks, whereas multigravidae recognize the sensation a little earlier, between 16 and 18 weeks. This may be used to confirm the expected date of delivery, although with the widespread use of ultrasound in the UK, the gestational age is usually established during an ultrasound examination (see Ch. 33). A dating ultrasound offered to a woman

Table 32.2 Calculation of the EDD

Cycle 28 days	Cycle 33 days	Cycle 23 days
LMP: 12 Aug 2016	LMP: 12 Aug 2016	LMP: 12 Aug 2016
+7 days + 9 months	+7 days +5 days +9 months	+7 days −5 days +9 months
EDD: 19 May 2017	EDD: 24 May 2017	EDD: 14 May 2017

between 10 and 13 weeks of pregnancy normally measures the crown–rump length (CRL), and, for pregnancies beyond 14 weeks, the fetal gestational age is determined by the measurement of the head circumference or biparietal diameter (BPD) (NICE 2008).

Although the use of ultrasound to estimate gestational age is very useful, some women may find it distressing if there are discrepancies between the date estimated by Naegele's rule and that given after an ultrasound examination, especially those who are certain of the date of conception or who have a regular cycle and are certain of the date of the first day of their last menstrual period. In most cases, it would be inappropriate to alter the expected date of delivery without the mother's agreement, especially when there is less than 10 to 14 days discrepancy with the previously given date.

Other pregnancy symptoms such as breast changes, nausea and vomiting and increased frequency of micturition are noted. Nausea and vomiting may range from occasional slight nausea to frequent, severe vomiting with ketosis, when immediate medical treatment is necessary (Ch. 52). Any history of bleeding per vaginam since the last normal menstrual period is recorded, and the woman is requested to seek medical attention immediately should further bleeding occur (see Ch. 53).

In the first trimester of pregnancy, a woman is quite likely to feel tired, perhaps nauseated and generally rather off-colour. A caring, approachable midwife who provides support, encourages the woman to express any worries and ask questions and gives clear information can be a great help to the woman at this time.

Previous pregnancies

It is necessary to ask about all previous pregnancies, including miscarriages or terminations of pregnancy. If the woman has had a miscarriage, she is asked at what stage in pregnancy it occurred, whether she knows of any possible cause, if she was transferred to hospital and, if so, whether she needed either an operation to remove retained products of conception or a blood transfusion or both.

Similar questions are asked about terminations of pregnancy, including the reason for termination and how it was performed. Some women may not wish this information to be recorded in handheld notes and their autonomy should be respected; however, the information should be recorded within hospital notes, and the reasons for this discussed with the woman.

Details of all pregnancies, labours and puerperia are essential:

- Was the pregnancy uncomplicated or complicated – for example, did the woman experience vomiting, hypertension or haemorrhage?
- Was the birth of baby at term and were there any complications?
- What was the length of the labour?
- Was the baby born in hospital or at home?
- Was the birth of the baby with or without assistance – for example, was the birth assisted with a forceps, ventouse extraction or caesarean section? If so, why was the intervention required?
- Did she have a normal, healthy baby and was the baby well at birth? And now?
- If the baby died, she is asked if she knows why, and what happened. This information is important to record, as the reasons for the baby's death may indicate risks to the current pregnancy.
- The birthweight of any previous baby is important because this gives some indication of the capacity of the woman's pelvis.
- Was the woman unwell after her baby's birth, or were there any problems such as haemorrhage or any other complications?
- She is asked if she breastfed her previous baby, if this was an enjoyable experience and for how long she was able to breastfeed. Her previous experience may influence how she intends to feed her expected baby. If she fed artificially, the reasons for this are explored. The midwife will ensure that the woman is fully informed of the health benefits of breastfeeding, to both herself and her baby, to enable her to make an informed choice of feeding method and she is asked how lactation was suppressed.

All pregnancies are dealt with in chronological order. If the history reveals any obstetric or pediatric complications and previous notes are not accessible, the information should be sought from the hospital where care was delivered.

This is a useful part of the interview, as this may be the first opportunity that the woman has had for reviewing and reflecting on her previous childbirth experiences, and this provides a forum for clarifying management of problems both previously and in the future.

Medical and surgical history

This includes enquiry about any illness, operation or accident, which could complicate pregnancy. It is important to enquire about any cardiac diseases, including rheumatic fever, prosthetic heart valves, hypertension (with or without proteinuria) and any haematological conditions such as haemophilia, thrombocytopenia or haemoglobinopathies and thromboembolic occurrences. Severe respiratory problems requiring hospital admission, such as asthma or cystic fibrosis, and endocrine disorders, such as pre-existing diabetes, thyroid disease and renal and liver disease, are noted. Neurological conditions, such as epilepsy, and any autoimmune disease or previous or current malignancy are significant. Also diseases of the gastrointestinal tract, for example, Crohn's or ulcerative colitis, are recorded. A woman should be given an opportunity to discuss whether there are any other conditions she may have. If a woman has any of the mentioned conditions, then information is needed about the treatment she has had or is having. Many of the pre-existing diseases may complicate the pregnancy, and pregnancy may aggravate the condition. Some women have complex health and social care needs, so the medical history must be taken accurately, as she might require referral to specialists or care during her pregnancy and might need to be managed by a multidisciplinary team or a specific care pathway to achieve the best outcome for the woman and her fetus.

A history of mental illness, especially postnatal depression or psychosis, is of significance because such conditions may recur in a subsequent pregnancy. The woman is asked about previous infectious diseases and bloodborn viruses, such as tuberculosis, HIV and hepatitis B or C. Although immunization programmes are well established in the UK, some women may not be immune to rubella, especially those born elsewhere and need to be advised to avoid contact with the disease in pregnancy because rubella virus, if contracted in pregnancy, can cross the placenta and cause fetal abnormality.

All women should be asked about female genital mutilation (FGM). If a woman has had FGM, explanation should be given to the woman that since April 2015, it is mandatory to submit this information to the Health and Social Care Information Centre (HSCIC) FGM Enhanced Dataset. If the pregnant woman with FGM is under 18 years of age, then it is a legal requirement to report this to the police (RCOG 2015a).

Operations on the uterus or the pelvic floor are significant. After a caesarean section or myomectomy, there may be a weakened uterine scar, especially if the wound was infected, and there is a slight risk that it could rupture during a subsequent pregnancy or labour. Women of childbearing age sometimes have to undergo extensive pelvic floor repair operations. If a woman has had a successful operation for the relief of stress incontinence, both the woman and the obstetrician will be concerned about the mode of delivery; sometimes, another vaginal delivery is considered inadvisable and a caesarean section is planned.

Relevant accidents include those involving the spine and pelvis, particularly if a fracture has occurred and deformity resulted. Deformity of the spine or pelvis after poliomyelitis or congenital dislocation of the hip would cause similar concern because in all these instances, the bony pelvis may be asymmetrical and, accordingly, have a smaller capacity. Enquiry may be made about back pain or pelvic girdle pain, and appropriate support and advice given and referral made, if appropriate.

Details of any blood transfusions are important, including the reason and any adverse reactions.

Drugs and medications

It is important to ask the woman whether she is taking any drugs because many drugs that are quite safe for the woman may have a teratogenic effect on the fetus. The woman should be informed about the risk of taking over-the-counter drugs without medical advice (NICE 2008).

Drug dependency in women of childbearing age is an increasing problem, and it is important that the midwife ascertains whether the woman has previously taken or is currently taking prescribed drugs and/or drugs for 'social or recreational' use. The misused substances are likely to have a detrimental effect on the health of the woman and her fetus/baby; however, this is dependent on the type, dose and route of the drug being used. Women with drug dependency are at an increased risk of developing medical and obstetric problems than are women who do not misuse drugs, and their babies are at an increased risk of neonatal complications (Hepburn 1993).

Women who misuse drugs may have a multitude of social, emotional, financial and sexual health problems that necessitate multiagency involvement to try to minimize harm to themselves, their children and families. It is essential that the approach and attitude of the midwife is caring, nonjudgemental and constructively helpful when discussing health needs and the support that can be offered to the woman; otherwise, the woman may reject the help that the health and other specialist services can offer.

Smoking in pregnancy

Smoking during pregnancy is a most significant contributing factor for poor health, poor clinical outcomes and health inequalities, increasing, for example, the risk of miscarriage, placental abruption, placenta praevia, preterm birth, stillbirth, perinatal death, sudden unexpected death in infancy and congenital abnormalities, such as development of a cleft lip and cleft palate in babies. Therefore, reducing smoking in pregnant women is an area of priority for all. Midwives are ideally placed to give health promotion advice to the woman and her partner on the detrimental effects of smoking on the woman, fetus and newborn baby. The initial interview and antenatal visits are ideal times to discuss whether the woman smokes, the implications of this and whether she would like to give up smoking (NICE 2008 and 2012).

Women should be encouraged to either stop or reduce smoking during pregnancy. See Box 32.1 for Antenatal Quality Standard, statement 5 (NICE 2012). Women should be provided with unbiased and evidence-based information, aiming to encourage them to stop smoking, rather than cause fear or stress. Discussion with the women's partner and enlisting their support in reducing smoking may also be beneficial. Women should be offered details of how to access local NHS Stop Smoking Services

Box 32.1 Antenatal care quality standard: quality statements

The NICE quality standard for antenatal care sets out how a high-quality antenatal care service should be organized so that the best care can be offered to people using NHS services in England.

Statement Number	Quality Statement
1	Pregnant women are supported to access antenatal care, ideally by 10 weeks, 0 days.
2	Pregnant women are cared for by a named midwife throughout their pregnancy.
3	Pregnant women have a complete record of the minimum set of antenatal test results in their handheld maternity notes.
4	Pregnant women with a body mass index of 30 kg/m^2 or more at the booking appointment are offered personalized advice from an appropriately trained person on healthy eating and physical activity.
5	Pregnant women who smoke are referred to an evidence-based stop smoking service at the booking appointment.
6	Pregnant women are offered testing for gestational diabetes if they are identified as at risk of gestational diabetes at the booking appointment.
7	Risk assessment – pre-eclampsia.
8	Pregnant women at intermediate risk of venous thromboembolism at the booking appointment have specialist advice provided about their care.
9	Pregnant women at high risk of venous thromboembolism at the booking appointment are referred to a specialist service.
10	Pregnant women are offered fetal anomaly screening in accordance with current UK National Screening Committee programmes.
11	Pregnant women with an uncomplicated singleton breech presentation at 36 weeks or later (until labour begins) are offered external cephalic version.
12	Nulliparous pregnant women are offered a vaginal examination for membrane sweeping at their 40- and 41-week antenatal appointments, and parous pregnant women are offered this at their 41-week appointment.

Source: NICE 2012

and the NHS pregnancy smoking helpline. Psychosocial interventions for smoking cessation in pregnancy, such as providing information on the effects of smoking, effects of inhalation of passive smoking, advantages of stopping and strategies to stop, particularly combined with individual counselling, are effective in smoking cessation in pregnancy and contribute to improvement in maternal and neonatal clinical outcomes (Lumley et al 2000; Chamberlain et al 2013).

The National Institute for Health and Clinical Excellence (NICE) has published guidance on public health intervention aimed at stopping smoking in pregnancy and after childbirth that would further assist midwives and other healthcare professionals to access and utilize recommendations for good practice (NICE 2008 PH10).

Alcohol consumption during pregnancy

Alcohol has detrimental effects on the fetus. Women who consume high levels of alcohol before and during pregnancy and those who are alcohol dependent are more likely to have babies with varying forms of congenital abnormalities, often described as *fetal alcohol syndrome* (RCOG 2006).

The midwife should use the opportunity to take a history of alcohol use, assess the risk of alcohol dependence or risk to the fetus from alcohol consumption, and advise and refer appropriately. There is no conclusive evidence regarding what is a safe amount of alcohol to drink during pregnancy and the advice given to the expectant mother should be based upon the current recommendation of NICE (2008). The NICE guidance recommends that women should be advised to avoid alcohol during pregnancy where possible. If they do choose to drink, they should not drink more than 1 to 2 UK units per week (1 unit equals half a pint of ordinary-strength lager or beer or one shot (25 mL) of spirit; one small (125 mL) glass of wine is equal to 1.5 UK units). However, evidence suggests that getting drunk or binge drinking (that is, more than 5 standard drinks or 7.5 UK units on a single occasion) may be harmful to the baby (NICE 2008). It also appears that alcohol consumption in the first trimester of pregnancy is more likely to adversely affect neonatal outcomes (Nykjaer et al 2014). This suggests that the most consistent and safest advice for women is alcohol abstinence.

Diet and supplements in pregnancy

It is important to ask about the woman's diet and nutritional intake. Advice should be tailored to her individual circumstances, taking into account her cultural, faith and socioeconomic background (see Ch. 17). General advice to all women should include the need for a well-balanced diet that contains proteins (beans, pulses, lentils, meat and fish), dairy products (milk, cheese, yoghurt), fruit and vegetables, carbohydrates (bread, pasta, rice and potatoes) and fibre (wholegrain flour, wholegrain bread and fruit and vegetables) (NICE 2008).

Pregnant women should be advised to avoid foods that may place their fetus at risk of *Listeria monocytogenes* infection, for example, unpasteurized milk, unpasteurized soft cheeses and mould-ripened cheeses. Uncooked or undercooked ready meals and pâtés, including vegetarian options (which may be a source of *Listeria*, *Escherichia coli* and *Toxoplasma*) should also be avoided; raw eggs and products containing raw eggs, such as mayonnaise, should be avoided because of the risk of salmonella infection. Vegetable and salad foods should be washed before eating, and food should be stored at the correct temperature in the refrigerator and on the appropriate shelves to reduce the risk of infections such as listeriosis, *E. coli* and toxoplasmosis. Women should be advised to wash their hands before any food preparation.

Women should be advised to take folic acid and vitamin D supplements. Folic acid (400 microgrammes) should be taken in the preconception period and up to 12 weeks gestation. Vitamin D (10 microgrammes daily) should be taken throughout pregnancy. Women should be informed about the importance of vitamin D for their health and their fetus's health and encouraged to eat foods such as oily fish, eggs, nuts, meat and foods fortified with vitamin D. As high intakes (more than 10 times the recommended daily allowance) of retinol – the animal form of vitamin A – may be associated with congenital abnormality, the NICE (2008) recommendation is that foods containing vitamin A, such as liver and liver products, should be avoided.

Iron supplements should only be taken when medically advised.

Family history

The woman's family medical history is important. Familial diseases, such as hypertension and diabetes, are sometimes discovered during routine antenatal examinations, and it is useful to know the woman's medical background. It is essential to know if any near relative has pulmonary tuberculosis because the newborn child is very vulnerable to the infection and must be protected. Arrangements are made for the child to receive Bacillus Calmette–Guérin (BCG) vaccination before leaving hospital and being segregated from the infected person.

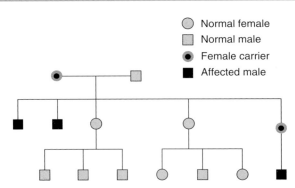

Figure 32.3 A medical pedigree showing three generations with X-linked haemophilia.

As there is a familial tendency to produce twins, especially dizygotic twins, it is important to ask whether there are twins in the family and, if so, whether they are monozygotic (identical) or dizygotic (non-identical) (Ch. 57).

The woman should be asked whether there is any history of congenital abnormality in the family (Fig. 32.3), as she and her partner may need referral for genetic counselling (see Ch. 26). A number of diagnostic techniques are available for the diagnosis of congenital conditions in pregnancy, and these may be discussed with the couple.

The midwife also carefully observes and enquires about the woman's reaction to her pregnancy, whether she is happy about it and coping with the initial minor disorders, or appears anxious, tense and unhappy. Guiding the conversation in a skillful, relaxed, unhurried manner and active listening, with interpretation of both verbal and nonverbal communications, helps elicit the woman's feelings and concerns. Appropriate support and help can then be offered.

It might appear that history taking is a lengthy procedure; however, in most cases it can be completed within about an hour, as the majority of clients are healthy young women who have never been seriously ill. However, the initial interview is also a time when the midwife informs the woman of aspects of screening and the rest of the pregnancy and this can take considerable time in addition to the history taking. This personal history provides a basis on which it is possible to assess the woman's physical, psychological and emotional health and well-being and, to some extent, anticipate the outcome of her pregnancy. An important aspect of this time spent taking the history is that the midwife and woman can meet and develop the relationship, which has such a fundamental influence on the woman's subsequent experience of pregnancy and childbirth.

On completion, the midwife can make a holistic assessment of the woman that influences the discussion around her particular needs and wishes. The midwife gives clear, accurate information about the variety of services available to enable the woman to make informed choices. Only then can a care plan for pregnancy and childbirth be discussed, tailored and agreed to the woman's individual needs. The woman should be given appropriate literature for her reference after her visit, such as *The Pregnancy Book* (DH/Public Health Agency 2015). A future appointment may be made with the midwife, and arrangements are made for any antenatal diagnostic tests to be undertaken.

Domestic abuse

Domestic abuse during pregnancy is of major concern; it affects the physical and mental health and safety of the woman and her fetus. (This is discussed in Ch. 23, but a brief overview is given here as part of the antenatal care routine.) Pregnancy may trigger or exacerbate abuse, and this may result in injury, obstetric complications such as miscarriage, placental abruption, antepartum haemorrhage, preterm labour, intra-uterine growth restriction and stillbirth and maternal death (Janssen et al 2003; Shah and Shah 2010; Jahanfar et al 2014).

All women should be routinely asked about domestic abuse. Although midwives may find it difficult to recognize domestic abuse (Mauri et al 2015), they may be the first point of contact for possible help for a woman who is abused, and the opportunity to initiate questions that may lead to disclosure of abuse can arise at the booking interview or during subsequent antenatal care. Suspicion may arise where the woman is always accompanied by her partner, especially where he constantly answers questions and undermines her. In addition to having an understanding of domestic abuse, including the symptoms and signs of abuse, the midwife needs to be skilled in asking difficult questions (see Ch. 23). All women should be afforded an opportunity to disclose domestic abuse in a safe environment (NICE 2008). Women who experience domestic abuse should be offered information about the choices available to them and the resources to support them. Documentation of abuse should be made with the woman's consent but not in handheld records. Medical evidence of abuse may be needed should the case proceed to court. If the woman does not wish her disclosure to be recorded, her autonomy should be respected.

Antenatal screening

At the first visit, women should be offered evidence-based information in relation to screening for fetal anomalies and assistance to make an informed choice about having or not having a scan (NICE 2008) (see Chs 26 and 33).

For further information see Antenatal Screening Time Line http://cpd.screening.nhs.uk/timeline.

SUBSEQUENT ANTENATAL APPOINTMENTS

When the woman and midwife meet for an antenatal appointment, the midwife should greet the woman in a friendly manner, introduce herself, review with the woman the purpose of the appointment, and elicit from the woman any concerns or questions she may have regarding the well-being of herself or her fetus or any other issues.

Antenatal appointments offer women opportunities to discuss and ask questions about their maternity care. They also provide the midwife with an opportunity to offer women information about pregnancy, health promotion and preparation for parenthood. Issues that should be discussed during the antenatal period include infant feeding, management of breastfeeding, care of the baby, vitamin K prophylaxis and newborn screening tests and information about changes that the woman may experience during the postnatal period, including 'baby blues' and postnatal depression (NICE 2008).

Details of all discussions between the woman and the maternity care provider, including information discussed, advice offered and plans of care developed, should be agreed and then recorded in the woman's handheld records, using terminology that the woman is able to understand.

Antenatal appointments may take place in a range of settings, such as the woman's home, a GP surgery, hospital or children's centre. Although easy access to the setting for women is essential, the midwife must carefully consider the environment in which the antenatal appointment will take place and ensure that women have the opportunity to discuss issues they regard as sensitive in a confidential manner.

Infant feeding

An important area of discussion relates to the woman's intended method of feeding (see Ch. 44). The woman should be asked about whether in previous pregnancies she commenced breastfeeding and for how long she fed her baby. It is useful to explore whether she had any difficulty previously and/or whether she is aware of the health benefits of breastfeeding for herself and her baby.

The difficulties that women have in breastfeeding can be overcome, and the rate and duration of breastfeeding increased, if the woman has access to evidence-based information and care (see Ch. 44). During the antenatal period, women should have the opportunity to have a meaningful conversation about feeding their baby with a midwife (United Nations Children's Fund 2012), for example, detailed discussion about how successful breastfeeding can be initiated and maintained. This can include information on analgesia in labour, offering the baby skin-to-skin contact and an early opportunity to suckle after delivery, correct 'latching' and positioning, the value of breastmilk, baby-led feeding (both day and night), rooming in and the management of common breastfeeding problems. Midwives need to be aware, when discussing infant feeding, that 'How do you intend to feed your baby – breast or bottle?' is a loaded question and the two choices should never be offered as if they are equal. Many women are unaware of the risks associated with artificial feeding and need appropriate and accurate information on which to make an informed choice. Women who choose to artificially feed their baby will need information to enable safe feeding. For women who have decided to breastfeed, the values of breastfeeding should be reinforced, with positive encouragement of how they can succeed. For women who express a preference for artificial feeding, the reasons for their choice should be explored and information offered to support them to make an informed choice.

Assessments in pregnancy

Maternal weight

Many women are concerned about their weight during pregnancy. To identify which women may be at increased risk of complications as a result of underweight or obesity, women's body mass index (BMI) is calculated during the first antenatal appointment (see Box 32.2). Women who are underweight (weight less than 18.5 kg/m^2) before the start of pregnancy and do not gain adequate weight during pregnancy may lack the reserves to support optimal growth and development of the embryo/fetus. This could adverse affect neonatal outcomes.

Although maternal obesity is increasing becoming a major cause of maternal mortality and morbidity (Knight et al 2014), weight loss is not encouraged during the antenatal period. It is essential, however, that healthy nutrition and weight management are discussed with pregnant women. Referral to a dietician may be appropriate. Traditionally, women were weighed during each antenatal appointment; however, it is now recommended that repeated maternal weighing, as part of routine antenatal care, should not be undertaken (NICE 2008), although some women may express a preference to be weighed to monitor their weight.

Blood pressure and urinalysis

At each antenatal visit, the woman's blood pressure must be measured and a sample of her urine tested for protein (NICE 2008). These tests are performed to screen for hypertensive disorders and pre-eclampsia (see Ch. 54). The midwife needs to ensure that the results of these screening tests are accurate, as clinical decision making and subsequent care will be informed by the results.

Box 32.2 Calculation of body mass index (BMI)

$$BMI = \frac{\text{Weight in kilograms}}{(\text{Height in metres})^2}$$

Example 1 Weight 57 kg (9 stone); height 1.68 m (5' 6"):

$$BMI = \frac{57}{1.68^2} = 20.3$$

Example 2 Weight 64 kg (10 stone); height 1.57 m (5' 2"):

$$BMI = \frac{64}{1.57^2} = 25.6$$

Example 3 Weight 76 kg (12 stone); height 1.57 m (5' 2")

$$BMI = \frac{76}{1.57^2} = 30.7$$

BMI score	Category
<18.5	Underweight
18.5–24.9	Normal
25.029.9	Overweight
30.0–34.9	Moderately obese
35.0–39.9	Obese
≥40	Severely obese

Source: Adapted from World Health Organisation (WHO)

Accuracy of the results may be affected by poor technique, or the use of inaccurate or inappropriate equipment.

During antenatal appointments, it is usual to measure blood pressure when the woman is sitting upright with her back supported for comfort (see Ch. 54). The woman should rest for 5 minutes before the measurement being taken, and the midwife should instruct the woman not to talk or eat during the measurement, as this may result in an inaccurate higher measurement being recorded (McAlister and Straus 2001). Tight clothing on the arm should be removed, the measurement should not be taken over clothing; the upper arm supported at heart level and the sphygmomanometer cuff placed at heart level. This is because measurements made with the arm lower than heart level can be 11 to 12 mm Hg higher than those made with the arm supported and the cuff at heart level (Dougherty and Lister 2008). Conversely, if the arm is raised above the heart level, the measurement may be falsely low (Beevers et al 2001). Selection of the appropriate-sized cuff for the individual woman is important to obtain an accurate reading; the cuff should cover 80% of the circumference of the woman's upper arm (British Hypertensive Society 2015).

Urine testing for protein can be performed by quickly dipping a reagent strip into a sample of fresh urine. The reagent strips are impregnated with chemicals that react with abnormal substances in the urine and change colour. It is important to inform women that the urine sample should be fresh, as urine that has been stored deteriorates quickly, and this can affect the final result (Higgins 2008). To ensure reliable results, it is essential that the reagent strips are stored and used according to the manufacturer's instructions. The reagent strips usually need to be stored in a dry, dark place, so it is important to make certain that the lid is always replaced between antenatal consultations during a clinic.

During pregnancy, it is common for women to report an increase in the amount of vaginal discharge they experience. This discharge may contaminate the urine sample and protein be detected in the urine. If abnormal substances are detected in the urine, culture and sensitivity testing under laboratory conditions may be indicated. For example, if a reagent stick test indicated the presence of nitrites or leucocyte esterase in the urine, culture and sensitivity testing would identify the organism and specify the most appropriate treatment (Dougherty and Lister 2008).

Blood testing

Anaemia

During pregnancy, maternal iron requirements increase because of the requirements of the fetus and placenta and an increase in maternal red cell mass (NICE 2008). Maternal plasma volume increases by up to 50% and the red cell mass increases by up to 20%, resulting in a drop in the haemoglobin concentration in the blood, which resembles iron deficiency anaemia. In addition to testing for anaemia in early pregnancy, all women should be offered testing for anaemia at 28 weeks gestation (NICE 2008). If anaemia is detected, treatment should be considered, as treatment at this point should allow sufficient time for correction of anaemia before term. Haemoglobin levels outside the normal UK range (10.5 g per 100 mL at 28 weeks) should be investigated (NICE 2008). Irrespective of their Rhesus D status, it is recommended that all women are screened for atypical red cell antibodies at 28 weeks gestation (NICE 2008) (for further details, see Ch. 33). If the woman is Rhesus negative, routine anti-D prophylaxis is recommended.

All women should be provided with information on sickle cell and thalassemia screening and carrier status before the 10th week of pregnancy and be offered screening for these conditions. Completion of the Family Origin Questionnaire and prevalence in the local population will indicate the appropriate screening options (NICE 2008).

Abdominal examination

During the antenatal period, abdominal examination is carried out to determine the symphysis fundal height and, from 36 weeks gestation, to determine the presentation and lie of the fetus. To perform an abdominal examination, the midwife needs to be able to observe, palpate and auscultate the woman's abdomen. Some women may find the nature of this examination intimate and embarrassing. Attention to privacy and the woman's comfort should reassure the woman. Sensitive communication skills are required to enable the midwife to explain the purpose and procedure of the examination, and, as the midwife performs the examination, she should ensure that the woman understands the findings by explaining them using appropriate language and terminology.

Before commencing the abdominal examination, the woman should be asked to empty her bladder if she has not done so recently. This is to ensure that the examination does not cause the woman undue discomfort and that a full bladder does not distort either the measurement of symphysis–fundal height or the palpation.

The woman should then lie as flat as she finds comfortable in the supine position. One or two pillows may be required for comfort, and she may wish to slightly flex her legs. Some women experience a condition called supine hypotensive syndrome when lying flat on their back, which results from compression of the inferior vena cava and the abdominal aorta by the gravid uterus. Signs that a woman may be suffering from supine hypotensive syndrome include dizziness, pallor, tachycardia, sweating, nausea and hypotension. These unpleasant signs should resolve when the woman is assisted to turn onto her side and blood flow is no longer obstructed. To reduce the risk of this syndrome, the midwife should consider using a wedge, or pillows, under the woman's right side to alter the centre of gravity and reduce compression of the inferior vena cava and abdominal aorta. Only the woman's abdomen needs to be exposed, and sheets, or a blanket, can be used to cover legs if required. The midwife should wash and dry her hands before commencing the abdominal examination.

During the antenatal period, an abdominal examination consists of the following parts:

- observation
- palpation and measurement of the symphysis–fundal height
- auscultation of the fetal heart

Observation

The approximate size and shape of the uterus should be observed. The size of the uterus should correspond to the estimated period of gestation calculated by the dating scan or, if this is not available, the date of the last known menstrual period. When making this assessment, take into account the height of the woman.

If the uterus appears to be larger than that indicated by the period of gestation, the main possibilities include:

- large-for-gestational-age fetus
- multiple pregnancies
- polyhydramnios
- uterine fibroids
- hydatidiform mole (Sasaki 2003)

If the uterus appears to be smaller than that indicated by the period of gestation, the most likely causes are:

- small-for-gestational-age fetus
- oligohydramnios
- fetal death

The gravid uterus is usually a longitudinal ovoid in shape. Sometimes, during late pregnancy, the shape of the uterus may be described as 'unusual'. This may be because of the fetus lying in either an oblique or transverse position.

While observing the size and shape of the uterus, the midwife may note abdominal scars, *striae gravidarum* (also called stretch marks), or a line of dark pigmentation called the *linea nigra*, which extends from the umbilicus to the pubis. If not already noted in the maternity records, the reason for abdominal scars should be ascertained and this recorded in the maternity records. Striae gravidarum may be seen as red marks, if they are new, or silver-coloured marks, if they date from a previous pregnancy or weight gain. Fetal movements may also be observed.

Palpation

Palpation of the abdomen should be carried out gently and smoothly using both hands, warmed. Although it is the pads of the fingers that are used to palpate the fetal parts, it is essential that nails are short to avoid causing the woman discomfort. Undue pressure may cause the woman pain and tightening of the abdominal muscles and stimulate uterine contractions, all of which will make the palpation more difficult. During the palpation, the midwife should position herself so that she is able to observe the woman's face for signs of discomfort, such as grimacing. If signs of discomfort are observed, the midwife should ascertain the reason for the discomfort, reassure the woman and amend her technique.

Symphysis pubis–fundal height may be estimated from 24 weeks gestation onwards by palpation, or, as recommended by NICE (2008), measured using a tape measure. If the midwife is estimating the fundal height by palpation, the ulnar border of the hand is placed at the uppermost point of the fundus of the uterus and the height compared with the size expected for the period of gestation (see Fig. 32.4).

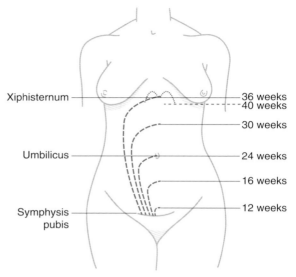

Figure 32.4 The height of the fundus at different stages of pregnancy.

While NICE currently recommends that the symphysis–fundal height is measured using a tape measure, there are some limitations to this procedure. A review of the current evidence base revealed a wide variation in accuracy and limited predictive value in the use of symphysis–fundal height measurement in detecting both small- and large-for-gestational-age babies (NICE 2008). Research has also shown that clinicians are biased in their measurement of fundal height if they have knowledge of the gestational age of the pregnancy or if they use a marked tape measure (Ross 2007).

The Perinatal Institute for Maternal and Child Health (2007) recommends using a non-elastic tape measure with the centimetre markings placed on the underside next to the woman's abdomen to reduce observer error and bias. The tape measure should be secured at the top of the fundus with one hand and, with the tape measure staying in contact with the skin; the tape measure should be run along the longitudinal axis of the uterus to the top of the symphysis pubis, without correcting to the midline of the woman's abdomen. The measurement should be recorded in the woman's antenatal maternity record and plotted on a growth chart. Customized symphysis–fundal height charts, adjusted for maternal weight, height, parity and ethnic group, are available. If the midwife suspects that the fetus is small-for-gestational age, then referral should be made for ultrasound biometric testing (RCOG 2013).

From 36 weeks gestation, the abdominal examination should include palpation to determine the position of the fetus. Assessment of fetal presentation by abdominal palpation before 36 weeks gestation should not be routinely offered to women because it is not always accurate, is of little predictive value and may cause unnecessary discomfort (NICE 2008).

The following terms are used in relation to the position of the fetus in utero:

- presentation
- denominator
- position
- attitude

- engagement
- lie

The presentation of the fetus in utero is determined by the part of the fetus lying in the lower pole of the uterus (Fig. 32.5). After 36 weeks gestation, the most common presentation is cephalic. Other possible presentations are breech, face, brow and shoulder.

The lie is the relationship of the long axis of the fetus to the long axis of the uterus (Fig. 32.6). The lie of the

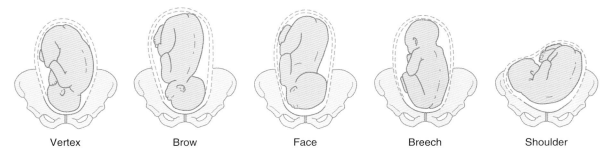

| Vertex | Brow | Face | Breech | Shoulder |

Figure 32.5 The presentation of the fetus.

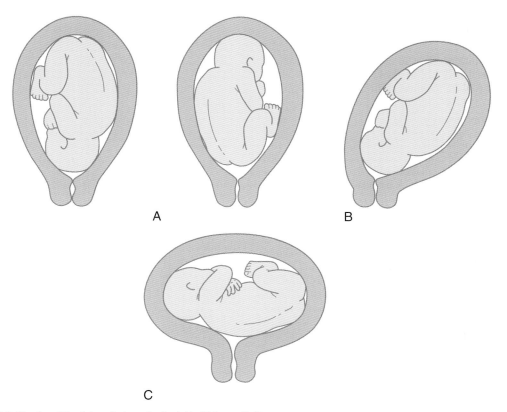

A   B

C

Figure 32.6 The lie of the fetus. **A**, Longitudinal. **B**, Oblique. **C**, Transverse.

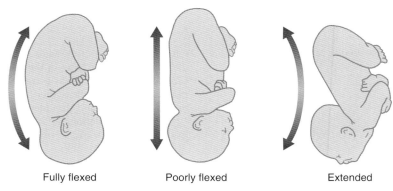

Fully flexed   Poorly flexed   Extended

Figure 32.7 The attitude of the fetus.

fetus may be longitudinal, oblique or transverse. In the later weeks of pregnancy, the lie should be longitudinal.

The denominator is a fixed point on the presenting part that is used to indicate the position:

- In a cephalic presentation, the denominator is the occiput.
- In a breech presentation, the denominator is the sacrum.
- In a face presentation, the denominator is the mentum (chin).

The position of the fetus in utero is the relationship of the denominator to the six areas of the woman's pelvis (see chapter website resources). The areas of the woman's pelvis are:

- left and right anterior
- left and right lateral
- left and right posterior

In a cephalic presentation, the denominator is the occiput, so the position of the fetus is described as:

- left or right occipitoanterior (LOA, ROA)
- left or right occipitolateral (LOL, ROL)
- left or right occipitoposterior (LOP, ROP)

Anterior positions are more common than posterior positions and help promote flexion of the fetus. In the anterior position, the fetal back is uppermost and can flex more easily against the woman's soft abdominal wall than when it lies against the woman's spinal column, as occurs in a posterior position.

The attitude is the relationship of the fetal head and limbs to its body. The attitude of the fetus may be described as being fully flexed, deflexed, partially extended or completely extended (Fig. 32.7). When fully flexed, the fetal head and spine are flexed, the arms are crossed over the chest, and the legs and thighs are flexed, forming a compact ovoid that fits the uterus comfortably.

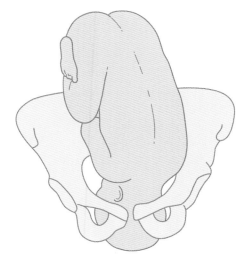

Figure 32.8 Engagement of the fetal head.

Engagement of the fetal head occurs when the transverse diameter of the fetal skull has passed through the brim of the pelvis (that is, the biparietal diameter measuring 9.5 cm) (Fig. 32.8). Engagement of the fetal head may be measured in fifths. The amount of head palpable above the brim of the pelvis is assessed and described as follows (Fig. 32.9):

5/5: Five-fifths of the fetal head are palpable above the brim of the pelvis on abdominal palpation. That is, the whole head can be palpated.

4/5: Four-fifths of the fetal head are palpable above the brim of the pelvis on abdominal palpation. One-fifth is below the pelvic brim and cannot be palpated per abdomen.

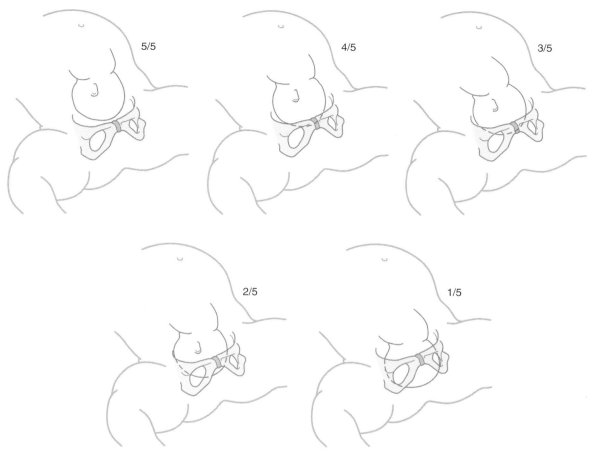

Figure 32.9 Abdominal examination to determine the descent of the fetal head in fifths.

3/5: Three-fifths of the fetal head are palpable above the brim of the pelvis on abdominal palpation. Two-fifths are below the pelvic brim and cannot be palpated per abdomen.

2/5: Two-fifths of the fetal head are palpable above the brim of the pelvis on abdominal palpation. Three-fifths are below the pelvic brim and cannot be palpated per abdomen. The widest transverse diameter of the fetal head has now passed through the brim of the pelvis and the fetal head is described as being engaged.

1/5: One-fifth of the fetal head is palpable above the brim of the pelvis on abdominal palpation. Four-fifths are below the pelvic brim and cannot be palpated per abdomen. The fetal head is sometimes described as being 'deeply engaged' in the pelvis.

To determine the presentation, position, attitude, engagement and lie of the fetus in utero by abdominal examination, the midwife will use three distinct manoeuvres:

- pelvic palpation
- fundal palpation
- lateral palpation

For palpation of the abdomen, see Fig. 32.10.

Pelvic palpation

This is the most important manoeuvre in abdominal palpation, as it is during the pelvic palpation that the presentation of the fetus is determined. Traditionally, midwives may have performed a fundal palpation, followed by a lateral palpation and then a deep pelvic palpation. However, for some women, palpation of the uterus may cause tightening of the uterine and abdominal

525

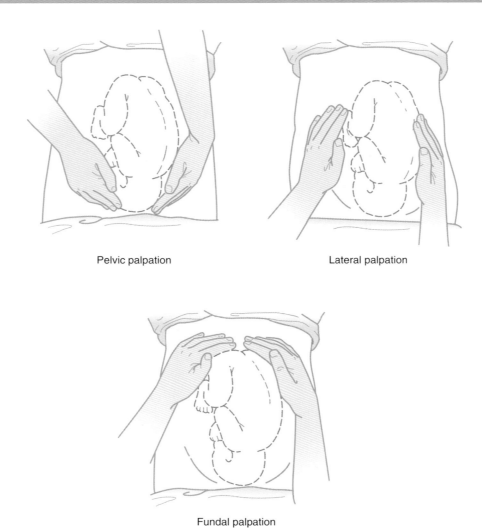

Pelvic palpation

Lateral palpation

Fundal palpation

Figure 32.10 Palpation of the abdomen.

muscles, which may make it very difficult to determine fetal presentation, so consideration should be given to performing the pelvic palpation first, when the muscles of the uterus and abdomen are relaxed. In addition to determining the presentation of the fetus, the attitude and degree of engagement of the fetal head may also be identified. To perform a deep pelvic palpation, the midwife stands alongside the woman, facing the woman's feet. The midwife then places one hand on each side of the uterus near the pelvic brim. The fingertips should then sink gently and smoothly into the pelvis to feel the presentation. The fetal head feels hard and round. If the fetal head is not engaged, it may be possible to ballotte it. This means that if the fetal head is given a gentle tap by an examining

finger, the head floats away from the finger and then is felt to return to the examining finger. If the fingertips can sink further into the pelvis, more on one side than the other, this may mean that the head is flexed and the occiput is lying on the side into which the fingers sink more deeply. Occasionally, some midwives or obstetricians may also perform pelvic palpation using a manoeuvre called 'Pawlick's grip'. The thumb and first finger of the hand are spread open and placed just above the symphysis pubis with the thumb and finger tips pointing towards the woman's face. The thumb and finger then grasp the lower part of the abdomen to determine the presentation and engagement of the presenting part. Some practitioners find this manoeuvre useful if the presenting part is above the pelvic brim; however, it is unlikely that all the information required during a pelvic palpation can be ascertained by use of Pawlick's grip alone, and deep pelvic palpation may need to be carried out in addition to Pawlick's grip. To minimize discomfort for the woman, it may be more prudent to perform deep pelvic palpation first.

Fundal palpation

Fundal palpation is carried out to determine which part of the fetus is lying in the fundus of the uterus. Still turned to face the woman, the midwife uses both hands to gently palpate the fundus. If the fetal presentation is cephalic, then the breech will be felt in the fundus. The breech feels irregular in outline, less hard than the fetal head, and fetal lower limbs may be felt near it. If the presentation of the fetus is breech, then the fetal head will be felt in the fundus. The fetal head feels smooth, round and hard. It is usually ballottable and separated from the trunk by a groove, the fetal neck. It is possible to move the fetal head more freely than the breech, which can only be moved from side to side.

Lateral palpation

Lateral palpation is carried out to determine the position of the fetal back. The midwife turns to face the woman's face. One hand is placed flat on one side of the woman's abdomen to steady it, while the other hand gently palpates down the length of the other side of the maternal abdomen. The process is then reversed, with the hand that was being used to steady the abdomen being used to palpate the length of the abdomen and the hand that was used first to palpate the abdomen being used to steady the uterus. The fetal back is felt as a continuous, smooth resistant object, whereas the fetal limbs are felt as being small, irregular objects that may move while they are being palpated. If the fetal back cannot be palpated, but fetal limbs are felt on both sides of the midline of the uterus, the fetal position is most likely to be occipitoposterior.

Auscultation

This is carried out when women visit the antenatal clinic. The early sounds are heard through ultrasound and from about 16 weeks may be heard via the electronic monitor (see Ch. 33).

Auscultation can be undertaken with the Pinard monaural fetal stethoscope or the binaural stethoscope and/or with an electronic fetal heart monitor. Ideally, the midwife should use the Pinard, and then the electronic monitor, as the means of monitoring the heartbeat are different, and the former is more likely to identify a true fetal heartbeat (Gibb and Arulkumaran 1997). Having palpated the abdomen, the midwife should know where to listen for the fetal heart sounds, which are heard at their maximum at a point over the fetal shoulder. When the fetus is lying in an occipitoanterior or occipitolateral position, the heart

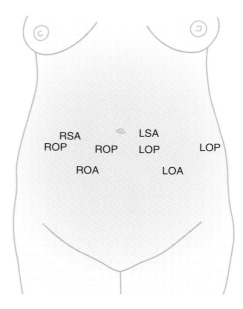

Figure 32.11 The approximate points of the fetal heart sounds in vertex and breech presentations.

sounds are heard from the front and to the right or left according to the side on which the fetal back lies (Fig. 32.11). The fetal heart sounds like the ticking of a watch under a pillow, the rate being about double that of the woman's heartbeat observed at the wrist. The woman and her partner usually enjoy listening to their baby's heartbeat too.

A uterine souffle, caused by the flowing of blood through the uterine arteries, may be heard; this is a soft, blowing sound, the rate of which corresponds to the woman's pulse.

Abdominal findings throughout pregnancy

At first, only the height of the fundus is ascertained (see Fig. 32.4).

- *Week 12* (sometimes earlier): The fundus is just palpable above the symphysis.
- *Week 16:* The fundus is halfway to the umbilicus. At this stage, a multigravida may have felt fetal movements.
- *Week 20:* The fundus reaches the lower border of the umbilicus and all women should be asked about movements. Fetal heart sounds may be audible.
- *Week 24:* The fundus reaches the upper border of the umbilicus, the fetus may just be palpable and fetal heart sounds are heard.
- *Week 28:* The fundus of the uterus is one-third of the distance from the umbilicus to the xiphisternum. The

fetus is now easily palpable, very mobile and may be found in any lie, presentation or position.

- *Week 32:* The uterus is two-thirds of the distance from the umbilicus to the xiphisternum. The fetus lies longitudinally and, usually, the head presents. If the midwife finds a breech presentation, she should refer the woman to a doctor. It may be decided to turn the fetus, though the doctor will probably want to wait to see whether it turns spontaneously.

- *Week 34:* The uterus extends nearly as far as the xiphisternum. Almost always the lie is longitudinal; usually the presentation is cephalic. If the breech presents, then external cephalic version may be attempted or left to term.

- *Week 36:* The fundus reaches the xiphisternum. The presentation should be cephalic. In a primigravida, the head may be engaged or engagement may occur a little later. If the head is engaged, the fundus will be lower, at about the level of a 34-week pregnancy, and the woman will have experienced 'lightening'.

- *Weeks 37 to 40:* The findings will all be similar except that the fetus becomes more stable and the amount of liquor diminishes slightly. The midwife must observe the woman carefully for signs of supine hypotensive syndrome during abdominal examinations, especially as pregnancy advances and the weight of the uterus increases.

Engagement of the fetal head

There is a popular myth that engagement of the head occurs at 36 weeks in a primigravida. In about 50% of primigravidae, engagement of the head occurs between 38 and 42 weeks (Weekes and Flynn 1975), and in 80% of cases labour ensues within 14 days of the head engaging. In multigravidae, because of lax uterine and abdominal muscles, engagement may not take place until labour is established. If the head is engaged, the pelvic brim is certainly of adequate size and the probability is that the cavity and outlet are also adequate.

Engagement is often referred to as *lightening*, because of the sense of lightness women feel as the pressure is lessened on the diaphragm. In some women, the fetal head may not be engaged at term. This may be because of a full bladder or rectum or an occipitoposterior position, where the presenting part tends to be deflexed. A steep angle of inclination of the pelvic brim tends to delay engagement until labour is well established. This is seen more commonly as a racial characteristic in West African and West Indian women.

If the fetal head is high, an ultrasound scan may be performed to exclude placenta praevia. It is difficult to determine cephalopelvic disproportion before labour because of the factors involved in labour itself.

After this examination, the findings are recorded and the woman is informed of these.

Helping women to manage and cope with pregnancy changes

Most women experience physical changes during pregnancy which, although they are not life threatening, may be a source of anxiety and discomfort. These changes are sometimes referred to as 'minor disorders of pregnancy'. However, for many women, the effect of these changes is certainly not minor; they have to manage and cope with the 'minor disorders' in addition to their ongoing responsibilities for family, home and employment at a time when they may also be experiencing pregnancy-related fatigue and discomfort. It is important that the midwife treats the woman with sensitivity, compassion and respect when these changes are being discussed, offering evidence-based information and advice to support the woman at this time (NMC 2015).

Reflective activity 32.3

Ask a pregnant woman what it felt like when her abdomen was palpated.

When you are present at an antenatal examination, observe the verbal and nonverbal communication that occurs between the mother and the midwife, and consider the points that were particularly good and those that may be improved.

PHYSIOLOGICAL CHANGES IN PREGNANCY

The gastrointestinal tract

Periodontal disease

Many women experience periodontal disease during pregnancy, resulting in local (gingival) and systemic inflammatory and immune responses (Boggess et al 2003; Mukherjee and Almas 2010). Periodontal disease has been associated with preterm birth, pre-eclampsia, second trimester miscarriage and small-for-gestational-age infants (Boggess et al 2003; Moore et al 2004), although the precise links between periodontal disease and an adverse pregnancy outcome are yet unknown.

Gingivitis occurs as food debris and calcified dental plaque collect in the minute spaces between the teeth and the gum, causing irritation and inflammation. Bleeding of the gums may occur during eating, brushing or if the gums are probed. Some women may also report an increase in tooth mobility. All women should be encouraged to attend the dentist (care is free for pregnant women and for a year after the birth of the baby in the UK). Women who experience bleeding gums should be advised to use a soft toothbrush to brush their teeth.

Nausea and vomiting

Nausea and vomiting are the most common gastrointestinal symptoms experienced in early pregnancy, with up to 85% of women experiencing nausea and 50% of women actually vomiting (Jewell and Young 2010) (see Ch. 52). While the aetiology is unclear, rising levels of human chorionic gonadotrophin during pregnancy have been implicated. Jewell and Young (2010) suggested that nausea is less common in women who experience miscarriage and more common in multiple pregnancies and molar pregnancies.

Nausea and vomiting during pregnancy are often referred to as 'morning sickness', yet many women report experiencing symptoms throughout the day or in the evening rather than only in the morning. Women may become concerned about the effect of nausea and vomiting on their pregnancy. The midwife should reassure women that there are no harmful effects upon the fetus as a result of nausea and vomiting, while acknowledging the detrimental effect the condition can have upon the woman's day-to-day activities (NICE 2008).

A number of non-pharmacological and pharmacological treatments for the relief of nausea in pregnancy have been suggested, including ginger, P6 acupressure and antihistamines (NICE 2008) (see Ch. 18). Rest and regular small amounts of carbohydrate are thought to be helpful (Jewell and Young 2010).

A small number of women may develop a condition called *hyperemesis gravidarum*, where excessive vomiting during early pregnancy alters fluid and electrolyte balance (see Ch. 52). Women with hyperemesis gravidarum generally feel very unwell. They may have signs of dehydration, including a dry mouth and mucous membranes, and dipstick urine testing may show the presence of ketones in the urine. Admission to a hospital is usually required to correct the fluid and electrolyte imbalance via intravenous fluid therapy.

Heartburn

Heartburn is a frequent complaint during pregnancy, reported by up to 72% of women during the third trimester of pregnancy (Marrero et al 1992). Heartburn is described as a burning sensation, or discomfort, felt behind the sternum or throat. It may be accompanied by regurgitation of the acidic stomach contents into the throat or mouth, causing a bitter taste. Regurgitation may be caused by the effects of progesterone relaxing the lower oesophageal sphincter, resulting in gastrooesophageal reflux. Although heartburn is not associated with adverse outcomes of pregnancy, it is important to distinguish between the pain caused by heartburn and epigastric pain associated with pre-eclampsia (NICE 2008). Measuring the woman's blood pressure and testing her urine for protein enables the midwife to exclude pre-eclampsia.

Treatment of heartburn is aimed at providing relief of symptoms. An upright position, especially after meals, and sleeping in a propped-up position may resolve the symptoms of heartburn. Additionally, eating small, frequent meals and reducing the quantity of high-fat foods and gastric irritants, such as caffeine and caffeine derivatives, may prove effective. Antacids may also be considered for the relief of heartburn where lifestyle and dietary modification has not been effective at relieving symptoms.

Constipation

Constipation may occur as a result of rising progesterone levels in pregnancy, causing a reduction in gastric motility and hence increased gastric transit time. Constipation is associated with poor dietary fibre intake and may cause abdominal discomfort and pain during defecation. Constipation has also been found to be a predisposing factor for haemorrhoids (Quijano and Abalos 2005).

As a preventative measure, and for women who experience constipation, information regarding the benefits of increasing the amount of fibre and fluid within the diet should be offered. Some women may not understand which foods are high in fibre and the midwife may need to discuss how the woman's diet can be modified to include more fibre-rich foods and fluids. Many women drink carbonated drinks or drinks containing caffeine, and rather than increasing their intake of these fluids, midwives should encourage them to drink additional water or caffeine-free drinks.

If constipation is not resolved by these simple measures, women may choose to take a fibre supplement (NICE 2008).

Haemorrhoids

Haemorrhoids are swollen veins at, or near, the anus. The aetiology of haemorrhoids is unclear, but predisposing factors include a history of constipation, a low-fibre, low-fluid diet and bowel disease associated with an increase in intra-abdominal pressure or diarrhoea (Quijano and Abalos 2005). Haemorrhoids are normally asymptomatic, but during pregnancy they may become symptomatic as a result of altered tone and position of the pelvic floor and sphincter muscles. Some women report that haemorrhoids cause them to experience a burning sensation or itching around the anus. Intermittent bleeding of the anus and leakage of mucus, faeces or flatus have also been reported (Quijano and Abalos 2005). The symptoms of haemorrhoids are usually transient and in most cases mild, but they can cause some woman discomfort or pain. Treatment of haemorrhoids during pregnancy is aimed at relieving symptoms, especially pain control, and any corrective treatment is usually deferred until after the birth of the baby (Quijano and Abalos 2005). Women should be offered information about increasing the amount of fibre and fluid, particularly water, within their diet, as this has been shown to be an effective treatment for symptomatic haemorrhoids and bleeding (Alonso-Coello et al 2005). A fibre supplement may be considered and local ointments containing an anaesthetic are widely used, although there is currently no evidence regarding their effectiveness or safety in pregnancy (NICE 2008).

The circulatory system

Varicose veins

Varicose veins occur when a valve within the vein weakens and allows a backflow of blood, putting more pressure on the other valves and causing blood to pool and stagnate. The vein then becomes distended and swollen near to the surface of the skin. The veins of the leg are the most commonly affected, but veins in the vulva (vulval varicosities) and anus (haemorrhoids) can also be affected. During pregnancy, the veins are placed under increased pressure as a result of an increase in circulating blood volume and the effect of progesterone relaxing the muscular wall of the blood vessels. Varicose veins are thought to affect up to 40% of pregnant women (Rabhi et al 2000) with multiparous women having a greater risk of developing varicose veins than primiparous women (Beebe-Dimmer et al 2005). Symptoms of varicose veins and oedema include heavy, achy legs, which the woman may feel are unsightly, and pain, night cramps, tingling or numbness. The skin around the varicose vein may feel itchy. Some women report a burning sensation or throbbing. Carr (2006) suggests that for up to 80% of the women who develop problems with varicose veins during pregnancy, these symptoms appear during the first trimester of pregnancy. Treatment for varicose veins may be surgical removal, pharmacological treatments, where liquid sclerosing drugs are injected into the affected veins to make them shrink, or non-pharmacological treatments, such as compression bandages, rest, leg elevation, exercise, immersion in water and reflexology. During pregnancy, treatment focuses upon relief of symptoms, with surgical and pharmacological treatments being deferred until after the birth. The most common treatments for the relief of symptoms of varicose veins and oedema during pregnancy are compression stockings, elevation of the feet, water immersion and reflexology; however, there is insufficient available evidence to make reliable recommendations for clinical practice (Smyth et al 2015). For the majority of women, the varicose veins resolve on their own within the first 3 or 4 months after the baby's birth.

The vaginal tract

Vaginal discharge

Leucorrhoea describes the change in the amount and type of vaginal discharge that many women experience during pregnancy; this often increases, and is usually white, non-offensive and non-irritant. However, if the change is associated with an itch, soreness, offensive smell, or pain when passing urine, the underlying cause should be determined (NICE 2008). It is essential that when discussing these issues with women, the midwife asks appropriate questions, in a sensitive manner, to determine which investigations and treatment may be required.

The most common causes of vaginal discharge during pregnancy are *bacterial vaginosis, vaginal trichomoniasis* and *vaginal candidiasis* (commonly called *thrush*). Bacterial vaginosis is a common condition caused by an overgrowth of bacteria within the vagina and characterized by a white–grey vaginal discharge, which may smell fish-like. The discharge does not usually cause soreness or itching of the vagina or vulva.

Trichomoniasis is one of the most commonly sexually transmitted infections and is characterized by a green–yellow frothy vaginal discharge and pain on urination. The discharge may have an unpleasant or fish-like smell (see Ch. 55).

Vaginal candidiasis is caused by the yeast *Candida albicans* and is characterized by a white vaginal discharge, which may smell of yeast. The discharge may be thicker than the woman's usual discharge, but in some women, it is more watery.

Investigation of the cause of vaginal discharge includes taking vaginal and cervical swabs. If the test result is positive, referral to a medical practitioner will be required. This may be the woman's own GP or a sexual health clinic.

The recommended treatment of vaginal candidiasis during pregnancy is a 1-week course of a topical imidazole cream and/or vaginal pessaries (NICE 2008). As yet, the safety of oral treatments for vaginal candidiasis in pregnancy has not been ascertained, and so they should not be offered to pregnant women (NICE 2008). The midwife should offer the woman information about self-help measures that may reduce the discomfort associated with vaginal candidiasis, including avoiding perfumed soaps, bubble baths and vaginal deodorants, which may further irritate the sore skin of the vulva and vagina, and keeping the perianal area as cool as possible by wearing loose clothing and cotton underwear. Cold compresses or ice cubes wrapped in a cloth and placed against the vulva may reduce soreness and itching. (For further information on sexually transmitted diseases, see Ch. 55.)

The skin in pregnancy

Hyperpigmentation of the skin during pregnancy is very common, occurring in up to 90% of pregnant women. Hyperpigmentation results in a darkening of areas that are already pigmented, like the areola, nipples, vulva and perianal region. Some women also note hyperpigmentation of the skin in the inner thigh region and axilla. It is usually more noticeable in women with dark complexions. The cause of hyperpigmentation is unclear, but it is thought to be related to an increase in serum oestrogen, serum progesterone and melanocyte-stimulating hormone.

Connective tissue changes

Approximately 90% of pregnant women experience striae gravidarum, commonly called 'stretch marks', by the end of the second trimester of pregnancy, as a result of abdominal distension, maternal weight gain, genetic predisposition and the hormonal changes that occur in pregnancy (Muallem and Rubeiz 2006). Striae gravidarum appear as red–purple linear streaks over the abdomen, thighs, arms, breasts and buttocks, and gradually fade into pale, skin-coloured, or silver streaks; itching may accompany the striae gravidarum. A number of preventative measures, including the application of creams and oils, have been suggested as beneficial in preventing the development of striae gravidarum; however, there is lack of high quality evidence to suggest their effectiveness (Brennan et al 2012).

The musculoskeletal system in pregnancy

Backache

Back and pelvic pain are common in pregnancy, with the 20% to 90% of women reporting back pain at some point during their pregnancy (Sabino et al 2008; Han 2010). It is thought that loosening of the ligaments in the pelvic area under the influence of relaxin and progesterone and altered maternal posture are the main causes of back and pelvic pain during pregnancy.

Posture is altered as pregnancy advances because the curvature of the lower spine becomes exaggerated to balance the increasing anterior weight of the gravid uterus. Many women report that back and pelvic pain are worse during the evening and in the last trimester of pregnancy, disturbing sleep and interfering with ordinary daily activities, such as walking, sitting and working. Pennick and Liddle (2013) confirmed that pregnant-specific exercise programmes, physiotherapy and acupuncture appeared to reduce back or pelvic pain, while some women reported pain relief by using pillows to support their stomachs when lying down. Back strain may be reduced by women turning onto their sides when sitting up and as they swing their legs down when they get up off a couch or bed, rather than attempting to raise themselves from their back without using their arms for support.

Pregnancy-related pelvic girdle pain

Pregnancy-related pelvic girdle pain (PPGP) affects approximately one in five pregnant women (Association of Chartered Physiotherapists in Women's Health 2007), although the actual incidence of PPGP is unclear because symptoms of PPGP are dismissed by many women and their maternity carers, as being the 'aches and pains' of pregnancy. Women experience pain in the joints of the pelvis; the symphysis pubis joint at the front of the pelvis and the sacroiliac joints at the back of the pelvis.

The exact cause of this pain is not understood, but there is little evidence to support the common belief that it is caused by loosening of the ligaments in the pelvic area under the influence of relaxin and progesterone, especially if it develops into pelvic girdle pain although it is associated with pelvic girdle instability (Vleeming et al 2008). It is thought that the pain is caused by abnormal stretching of the pelvic joints during pregnancy (Wellock 2002).

For non-pregnant women, the average gap between the pelvic bones at the pubic joint is 4 to 5 mm. During pregnancy, this gap may widen by 2 to 3 mm (Leadbetter et al 2004). Studies have shown that many women experience significant pain without great separation of the bones and the degree of pain is unrelated to the degree of separation (Leadbetter et al 2004). Stability of the pubic joint is essential for efficient weight-bearing and mobility, and instability may cause pain in the symphysis pubis.

The onset of symptoms of PPGP may occur gradually or acutely during the second or third trimester of pregnancy, or during labour or birth. The pelvic pain is of varying intensity, mild ache to severe pain, anywhere between the posterior iliac crest and the gluteal fold, particularly in the vicinity of the sacroiliac joints, either at the front or back (Leadbetter et al 2004). Women experience pain during walking or while performing activities that require them to part, or lift, their legs, such as climbing stairs, getting dressed or turning over in bed (Leadbetter et al 2004, Wellock and Crichton 2007). Women with pelvic girdle pain may be observed walking with a 'waddling' gait, although some women report hearing or feeling a clicking, snapping or grinding within the symphysis pubis (Leadbetter et al 2004). Moderate to severe pain affects women's quality of life, profoundly limiting all aspects of their daily activities, such as caring for their homes, families and themselves. Women may not be able to care for their children and may experience social isolation (Crichton and Wellock 2008).

In some rare cases, the gap between the pelvic bones widens by more than 10 mm, causing a partial or complete rupture of the symphysis pubis. This condition is called diastasis symphysis pubis (DSP) and may occur as a result of traumatic separation of the symphysis during a spontaneous or operative delivery or as a result of accidental injury to the pelvis during pregnancy (Leadbetter et al 2004). Although pelvic girdle pain may be diagnosed by taking a history of the symptoms experienced by the woman, DSP is diagnosed by x-ray.

During the antenatal period, the aim of management of the condition is to reduce activities that exacerbate pain. Most cases are managed conservatively, and so it is important that women understand the aetiology of the condition and what lifestyle changes they may need to make. These changes may include reducing nonessential activities and accepting help regarding childcare and household chores. Self-help measures, such as placing pillows between the knees, may make it more comfortable for women when they are side-lying in bed.

Conservative management of PPGP involves exercise, advice on posture and mobility, physiotherapy and acupuncture; however, there is limited evidence of the effectiveness of these interventions (Pennick and Liddle 2013). Women who experience severe pain and where mobility is significantly impaired, elbow crutches or a wheelchair may be required. Some women find that a trochanteric, or pelvic, support belt relieves pain, but the belts do not correct pelvic asymmetry, and the woman may still require analgesia. Women may be seek further support from a charitable organization. 'The Pelvic Partnership', which aims to raise awareness of the condition (see http://www.pelvicpartnership.org.uk/), offers literature on Pelvic girdle pain and pregnancy (RCOG 2015b) to assist women to gain further information to manage their condition.

During labour, women with pelvic girdle pain may find it difficult to move into different positions, and the midwife may need to be an advocate for the woman, facilitating her to move in ways that do not exacerbate her symptoms. This may include either a lateral or a supported 'all fours' position for vaginal examinations and birth. The lateral position may be preferable for fetal blood sampling, assisted deliveries or suturing of the perineum if required. Immersion in water may be beneficial for some women, as water relieves weight bearing and allows for ease of position change, but entering and exiting a birth pool may cause pain and, in some cases, delay treatment. An individual assessment of the woman's mobility will be required before her entering the water.

If the woman chooses either epidural or spinal anaesthesia for labour and birth, the woman and midwife need to be aware of the possibility of the symptoms of pelvic girdle pain being masked and excessive mobilization of the joint, causing increased pain during the postpartum period. Before receiving either epidural or spinal anaesthesia, the range of hip abduction should be measured and recorded in the woman's notes. The midwife needs to ensure that this range is not exceeded while the anaesthesia is effective.

During the postnatal period, women with pelvic girdle pain may require assistance with personal hygiene and care of their baby. This may include assisting the woman to the toilet and providing aids within the shower, such as handrails and chairs. Assistance with bathing and changing the baby may be needed and help in handing the baby to the mother rather than the mother having to get up to attend to the baby's needs. Consideration needs to be given to the position the woman adopts to feed her baby;

a lateral position may be more comfortable for women who wish to breastfeed their babies. During this period, the midwife should make an assessment of the woman's risk of being predisposed to a deep vein thrombosis. Antiembolic stockings may be worn and thromboprophylaxis prescribed if appropriate. Women with moderate to severe symptoms may need referral to an obstetric physiotherapist during the postnatal period, and if the symptoms fail to resolve, referral to an orthopaedic surgeon may need to be considered. Very rarely, pelvic suturing may be required.

Leg cramp

The cause of leg cramps during pregnancy is unclear. It has been suggested that leg cramps may occur as a result of either circulatory changes during pregnancy or changes in calcium and magnesium levels during pregnancy. Although leg cramps do not cause any lasting damage, they can be very painful. The pain is caused by a build up in lactic and pyruvic acid, which leads to an involuntary contraction of the calf muscle. Leg cramps are often experienced during the night, so women may suddenly wake in pain; this can be extremely distressing.

During an episode of leg cramps, women may find that getting out of bed, walking around, stretching and massaging the affected muscle helps. Calcium, sodium and magnesium supplementation are sometimes used; however, their effectiveness is not conclusive (Zhou et al 2015). Sodium supplements may decrease the episodes of cramps; however, their effect is slight. Calcium appears to have no effect, and there is some evidence that in some women, magnesium supplementation stopped them from having leg cramps altogether and for others, the frequency of attacks was reduced although this was not consistent (Zhou et al 2015).

Carpal tunnel syndrome

Carpal tunnel syndrome occurs as a result of oedema in the carpal tunnel; this compresses the median nerve, causing paraesthesia, swelling and pain in the hand or hands and impairs sensory and motor function of the hand (NICE 2008). Interventions to reduce the symptoms of carpal tunnel syndrome include wrist splints and analgesia. Referral to the physiotherapist should be considered.

CONTINUOUS ASSESSMENT OF MATERNAL AND FETAL WELL-BEING

Women's physical and mental health is assessed throughout pregnancy to ensure that their health is maintained and, where possible, improved. Any signs of complications are identified early and appropriate referral pathways are followed. Midwife should also observe woman's mental health status. During pregnancy, women experience emotional and psychological changes, and many feel anxious and worried. They are also vulnerable to developing mental health illnesses, particularly if they have any pre-existing mental illnesses. Midwives should enquire about women's emotional well-being at each routine antenatal contact (Quality standard 4, NICE 2016).

Fetal well-being is assessed at each subsequent antenatal visit. Fetal growth is assessed by palpation of the uterus, to check that it is compatible with the gestational age. The pattern of fetal movements is checked and, although perception of fetal movements is variable, most women are aware of fetal movements, particularly during the second half of pregnancy. Fetal heart rate should be regular and variable between the range of 110 to 160 beats per minute. In the majority of the pregnancies, these are adequate to determine fetal status, but on occasions where fetal well-being is of concern, then detailed monitoring is necessary.

CONCLUSION

As this chapter has demonstrated, the antenatal period is a time of tremendous psychological and physical adjustment for the pregnant woman and her family. The midwife can work in partnership with the woman to increase the woman's understanding of these changes and to help her prepare for the birth and parenthood by offering evidence-based information and individualized plans of care and support, taking into account women's diverse, and sometimes complex, backgrounds. Many women experience physiological changes in pregnancy that may lead to disturbance and discomfort within various body systems. The midwife is ideally placed to offer women information and support to enable them to cope with these changes and the

challenges they might present to them in their day-to-day life. Initial and subsequent antenatal care should be provided within an environment of respect and partnership, and the midwife should aim to make every woman feel valued and every antenatal visit positive and informative.

Key Points

- The midwife should be aware of the main pregnancy tests available to women and the accuracy of these.
- The initial antenatal-history-taking visit is an important opportunity to assess the physical, psychological, educational and social needs of the woman and, accordingly, the plan of care.
- The antenatal period is a time of physical, psychological and social adjustment for the woman and her family, through which the midwife can guide and assist both.
- The significance of the woman's social, family, medical and obstetric histories should be carefully assessed to identify any potential problems and highlight her individual needs throughout the antenatal period in preparation for childbirth.
- The physiological changes that are shaped by pregnancy may have effects that are uncomfortable or of concern to the woman. An important part of the midwife's role lies in assessing these changes, ensuring the woman understands why they are occurring and suggesting strategies for increasing the comfort and well-being of the woman and her growing fetus.
- The midwife should be conversant with the physiology of pregnancy, be able to identify when pregnancy deviates from the norm and be able to refer to the appropriate practitioner.
- The antenatal period offers an ideal opportunity for the midwife in terms of health promotion and wider public health, from advising on smoking cessation to diet and exercise.

References

Alonso-Coello P, Guyatt G, Heels-Ansdell D, et al: Laxatives for the treatment of haemorrhoids, *Cochrane Database Syst Rev* (4):CD004649, 2005.

American Psychiatric Association: *Diagnostic and statistical manual of mental disorders (DSM-5)*, 5th edn, Arlington, VA, American Psychiatric Association 2013.

Anderson T: Feeling safe enough to let go: the relationship between a

woman and her midwife during the second stage of labour. In Kirkham M, editor: *The midwife-mother relationship*, London, Macmillan, 2000.

Association of Chartered Physiotherapists in Women's Health: Pregnancy related pelvic girdle pain. *Guidance for mothers to be and new mothers* (website). www.acpwh.org.uk/docs/ACPWH-PGP_Pat.pdf. 2007.

Bastian L, Nanda K, Hasselblad V, et al: Diagnostic efficiency of home pregnancy test kits, *Arch Fam Med* 7(5):465–469, 1998.

Badell ML, Ramin SM, Smith JA: Treatment options for nausea and vomiting during pregnancy, *Pharmacotherapy* 26(9):1273–1287, 2006.

Beebe-Dimmer JL, Pfeifer JR, Engle JS, et al: The epidemiology of chronic venous insufficiency and varicose veins, *Ann Epidemiol* 15(3):175–184, 2005.

Beevers G, Lip GYH, O'Brien E: Blood pressure measurement (Part 1). sphygomanometry: factors common to all techniques, *Br Med J* 322(7292):981–985, 2001.

Bharj KK: *Pakistani Muslim women birthing in northern England: exploration of experiences and context*, Unpublished thesis, Sheffield, Sheffield Hallam University, 2007.

Bharj KK, Chesney M: Pakistani Muslim women and midwives relationship: what are the essential attributes? Chapter 9. In Kirkham M, editor: *The midwife-mother relationship*, 2nd edn, Basingstoke, Palgrave Macmillan, 2010.

Blackburn ST: *Maternal, fetal and neonatal physiology*, Philadelphia, WB Saunders, 2007.

Boggess KA, Lieff S, Murtha AP, et al: Maternal periodontal disease is associated with an increased risk for pre-eclampsia, *Obstet Gynecol* 10(2):227–231, 2003.

Bolanca I, Bolanca Z, Kuna K, et al: Grubisić G: Chloasma—the mask of pregnancy, *Coll Antropol* 32(Suppl 2):139–141, 2008.

Brennan M, Young G, Devane D: Topical preparations for preventing stretch marks in pregnancy, *Cochrane Database Syst Rev* (11):CD000066, 2012.

British Hypertensive Society: *Blood pressure measurement* (website). www.bhsoc.org/files/9013/4390/7747/BP_Measurement_Poster_-_Manual.pdf. 2015.

Carr S: Current management of varicose veins, *Clin Obstet Gynecol* 49(2):414–426, 2006.

Centre for Maternal and Child Enquiries (CMACE): Saving mothers' lives, reviewing maternal deaths to make motherhood safer: 2006–2008, the eighth report on confidential enquiries into maternal deaths in United Kingdom, *Br J Obstet Gynaecol* 118(Suppl 1):1–203, 2011.

Chamberlain C, O'Mara-Eves A, Oliver S, et al: Psychosocial interventions for supporting women to stop smoking in pregnancy, *Cochrane Database Syst Rev* (10):CD001055, 2013.

Chudleigh P, Pearce M: *Obstetric ultrasound*, 2nd edn, Edinburgh, Churchill Livingstone, 1994.

Cole LA, Ladner DG: Background hCG in non-pregnant individuals: need for more sensitive point of care and over the counter pregnancy tests, *Clin Biochem* 42:168–175, 2009.

Crichton MA, Wellock VK: Pain, disability and symphysis pubis dysfunction: women talking, *Evidence Based Midwifery* 6(1):9–17, 2008.

Davies J: Being with women who are economically without. In Kirkham M, editor: *The midwife-mother relationship*, London, Macmillan, 2000.

Department of Health (DH): *Changing childbirth: report of the expert maternity group (Cumberlege report)*, London, HMSO, 1993.

Department of Health (DH): *Maternity matters: choice, access and continuity of care in a safe service*, London, The Stationery Office, 2007.

Department of Health (DH), Department for Education and Skills (DfES): *National service framework for children, young people and maternity services*, London, HMSO, 2004.

Department of Health (DH), reproduced by Public Health Agency: *The pregnancy book*, 2015 (website). www.publichealth.hscni.net/publications/pregnancy-book-0. 2015.

Dougherty L, Lister S: *The Royal Marsden Hospital manual of clinical nursing procedures*, Chichester, Wiley-Blackwell, 2008.

Dyson S: *Ethnicity and screening for sickle cell/thalassaemia*, Oxford, Elsevier, 2005.

Ebrahimi N, Maltepe C, Einarson A: Optimal management of nausea and vomiting of pregnancy, *Int J Womens Health* 2:241–248, 2010.

Edwards N: *Birthing autonomy: women's experiences of planning home births*, London, Routledge, 2005.

Freedman LP, Kruk ME: Disrespect and abuse of women in childbirth: challenging the global quality and accountability agendas, *Lancet* 384:e42–e43, 2014.

Gardner S: Save independent midwives!, *Br J Midwifery* 22(4):232, 2014.

Gibb DME, Arulkumaran S: *Fetal monitoring in practice*, 2nd edn, London, Butterworth Heinemann, 1997.

Green JM, Curtis P, Price H, et al: *Continuing to care, the organisation of maternity services in the UK: a structured review of evidence*, Hale, Books for Midwives, 1998.

Hall J: Free-standing maternity units in England. In Kirkham M, editor: *Birth centres, a social model for maternity services*, London, Books for Midwives, 2003.

Hall M, MacIntyre S, Porter M: *Antenatal care assessed: a case study of an innovation in Aberdeen*, Aberdeen, Aberdeen University Press, 1985.

Han IH: Pregnancy and spinal problems, *Curr Opin Obstet Gynecol* 22(6):477–481, 2010.

Hatem M, Sandall J, Devane D, et al: Midwife-led versus other models of care for childbearing women, *Cochrane Database Syst Rev* (4):CD004667, 2008.

Hepburn M: Drug use in pregnancy, *Br J Hosp Med* 49(1):51–55, 1993.

Higgins D: Patient assessment (Part 6) – urinalysis, *Nurs Times* 104(12):24–25, 2008.

Hildingsson I, Rådestad I, Waldenström U: Number of antenatal visits and women's opinion, *Acta Obstet Gynecol Scand* 84(3):248–254, 2005.

Jahanfar S, Howard LM, Medley N: Interventions for preventing or reducing domestic violence against pregnant women, *Cochrane Database Syst Rev* (11):CD009414, 2014.

Janssen PA, Holt VL, Sugg NK, et al: Intimate partner violence and adverse pregnancy outcomes: a population based study, *Am J Obstet Gynecol* 188(5):1341–1347, 2003.

Jewell D, Young G: Interventions for nausea and vomiting in early pregnancy, *Cochrane Database Syst Rev* (9):CD000145, 2010.

Kirkham M, editor: *The midwife-mother relationship*, 2nd edn, Basingstoke, Palgrave Macmillan, 2010.

Kirkham M, editor: *Birth centres, a social model for maternity services*, London, Books for Midwives, 2003.

Kirkham M, Stapleton H, editors: *Informed choice in maternity care: an evaluation of evidence-based leaflets*. NHS Centre for Reviews and Dissemination (Report 20), York, University of York, 2001.

Knight M, Tuffnell D, Kenyon S, et al, editors: *on behalf of MBRRACE-UK: saving lives, improving mothers' care – surveillance of maternal deaths in the UK 2011–13 and lessons learned to inform maternity care from the UK and Ireland confidential enquiries into* maternal deaths and morbidity 2009–13, Oxford, National Perinatal Epidemiology Unit, University of Oxford, 2015.

Knight M, Kenyon S, Brocklehurst P, et al, editors: *on behalf of MBRRACE-UK: saving lives, improving mothers' care – lessons learned to inform future maternity care from the UK and Ireland confidential enquiries into maternal deaths and morbidity 2009–12*, Oxford, National Perinatal Epidemiology Unit, University of Oxford, 2014.

Kraus GW, Hendricks CH: Significance of the quickening date in determining duration of pregnancy, *Obstet Gynecol* 24(2):178–182, 1964.

Lacroix R, Eason E, Melzack R: Nausea and vomiting during pregnancy: a prospective study of its frequency, intensity, and patterns of change, *Am J Obstet Gynecol* 182(4):931–937, 2000.

Leadbetter RE, Mawer D, Lindow SW: Symphysis pubis dysfunction: a review of the literature, *J Matern Fetal Neonatal Med* 16(6):349–354, 2004.

Lumley J, Oliver S, Waters E: Interventions for promoting smoking cessation during pregnancy, *Cochrane Database Syst Rev* (2):CD001055, 2000.

Lundgren I, Berg M: Central concepts in the midwife-woman relationship, *Scand J Caring Sci* 18(2):368–375, 2007.

Mander R: *Supportive care and midwifery*, Oxford, Blackwell Science, 2001.

Marrero JM, Goggin PM, Caestecker JS: Determinants of pregnancy heartburn, *Br J Obstet Gynaecol* 99(9):731–734, 1992.

Mauri EM, Nespoli A, Persico G, et al: Domestic violence during pregnancy: midwives' experiences, *Midwifery* 31:498–504, 2015.

McAlister FA, Straus SE: Evidence based treatment for hypertension, *Br Med J* 322(7291):908–911, 2001.

Methven RC: The antenatal booking interview: recording an obstetric history or relating with a mother-to-be? *Research and the Midwife Conference Proceedings*, Glasgow 63–76, 1982a.

Methven RC: The antenatal booking interview: recording an obstetric history or relating with a mother-to-be? *Research and the Midwife*

Conference Proceedings, Glasgow 77–86, 1982b.

Miller F: Nausea and vomiting in pregnancy: the problem of perception—is it really a disease?, *Am J Obstet Gynecol* 186(5 Suppl):S182–S183, 2002.

Moore S, Ide M, Coward PY, et al: Periodontal disease and adverse pregnancy outcome, *Br Dent J* 197(5):251–258, 2004.

Muallem MM, Rubeiz NG: Physiological and biological skin changes in pregnancy, *Clin Dermatol* 24(2):80–83, 2006.

Mukherjee PM, Almas K: Orthodontic considerations for gingival health during pregnancy, a review, *Int J Dent Hyg* 8(1):3–9, 2010.

National Health Service Clinical Commissioning (NHSCC): (website). www.nhscc.org/ccgs/. 2013.

National Institute for Health and Clinical Excellence (NICE): *NICE clinical guideline 62. Antenatal care: routine care for the healthy pregnant woman*, London, NICE, 2008.

National Institute for Health and Clinical Excellence (NICE): *Public health guidance (PH10), draft scope on 'how to stop smoking in pregnancy and following childbirth'* (website). http://pathways.nice.org.uk/path ways/smoking#path=view%3A/path ways/smoking/smoking-cessation-in -maternity-services.xml&content =view-node%3Anodes-prescribers -of-quit-smoking-drugs. 2008.

National Institute for Health and Care Excellence (NICE): *Quality standard for antenatal care*, London, QS22, 2012.

National Institute for Health and Clinical Excellence (NICE): Antenatal and postnatal mental health, *Quality standard* 115:2016.

Naumann CR, Zelig C, Napolitano PG, et al: Nausea, vomiting, and heartburn in pregnancy: a prospective look at risk, treatment, and outcome, *J Matern Fetal Neonatal Med* 25(8):1488–1493, 2012.

Nicholls L, Webb C: What makes a good midwife? An integrative review of methodologically-diverse research, *J Adv Nurs* 56(4):414–429, 2006.

Nursing and Midwifery Council (NMC): *The code: professional standards of practice and behaviour for nurses and midwives*, London, NMC, 2015.

Nykjaer C, Alwan NA, Greenwood DC, et al: Maternal alcohol intake prior to and during pregnancy and risk of adverse birth outcomes: evidence from a British cohort, *J Epidemiol Community Health* 68(6):542–549, 2014.

O'Dowd M, O'Dowd T: Quickening – a re-evaluation, *Br Med J* 92(10):1037–1039, 1985.

Page AL, Cooke P, Percival P: Providing one-to-one practice and enjoying it. In Page L, editor: *The new midwifery: science and sensitivity in practice*, London, Churchill Livingstone, 2000.

Pelvic Partnership (website). www .pelvicpartnership.org.uk/index2 .html. 2008.

Pennick V, Liddle SD: Interventions for preventing and treating pelvic and back pain in pregnancy, *Cochrane Database Syst Rev* (8):CD001139, 2013.

Perinatal Institute for Maternal and Child Health: *Fetal growth fundal height measurements* (website). www.pi.nhs.uk/growth/fhm.htm. 2007.

Quijano CE, Abalos E: Conservative management of symptomatic and/ or complicated haemorrhoids in pregnancy and the puerperium, *Cochrane Database Syst Rev* (3):CD004077, 2005.

Rabhi Y, Charras-Arthapignet C, Gris JC, et al: Lower limb vein enlargement and spontaneous blood flow echogenicity are normal sonographic findings during pregnancy, *J Clin Ultrasound* 28(8):407–413, 2000.

Redshaw M, Henderson J: *Safely delivered: a national survey of women's experience of maternity care*, Oxford, National Perinatal Epidemiology Unit, 2014.

Renfrew MJ, McFadden A, Bastos MH, et al: Midwifery and quality care: findings from a new evidence-informed framework for maternal and newborn care, *Lancet* 384:1129–1145, 2014.

Ross MG: Clinical bias in fundal height measurement, *Obstet Gynecol* 110(4):892–899, 2007.

Rosser J: Calculating the EDD – which is more accurate, scan or LMP?, *Pract Midwife* 3(3):28–29, 2000.

Royal College of Obstetricians and Gynaecologists (RCOG): *Report from the RCOG working party on antenatal* and intrapartum care, London, RCOG, 1982.

Royal College of Obstetricians and Gynaecologists (RCOG): Alcohol consumption and the outcomes of pregnancy. RCOG Statement No 5, London, RCOG, 2006.

Royal College of Obstetricians and Gynaecologists (RCOG): The investigation and management of the small-for-gestational-age fetus, Greentop Guideline 31 (2nd edn), February 2013 (website). https://www.rcog.org.uk/en/guidelines-research-services/guidelines/gtg31. 2013 (Minor revisions – January 2014).

Royal College of Obstetricians and Gynaecologists (RCOG): Greentop Guideline 53. Female genital mutilation and its management (2nd edn), RCOG. (website). www.rcog.org.uk/globalassets/documents/guidelines/gtg-53-fgm.pdf. 2015a.

Royal College of Obstetricians and Gynaecologists (RCOG): Pelvic girdle pain and pregnancy, RCOG. (website). www.rcog.org.uk/globalassets/documents/patients/patient-information-leaflets/pregnancy/pi-pelvic-girdle-pain-and-pregnancy.pdf. 2015b.

Sabino J, Grauer JN: Pregnancy and low back pain, Curr Opin Obstet Gynecol 1(2):137–141, 2008.

Sandall J, Soltani H, Gates S, et al: Midwife-led continuity models versus other models of care for childbearing women, Cochrane

Database Syst Rev (9):CD004667, 2015.

Sikorski J, Wilson J, Clement S, et al: A randomised controlled trial comparing two schedules of antenatal visits: the antenatal care project, Br Med J 312(7030):546, 1996.

Sasaki S: Clinical presentation and management of molar pregnancy, Best Pract Res Clin Obstet Gynaecol 17(6):885–892, 2003.

Shah PS, Shah J: Maternal exposure to domestic violence and pregnancy and birth outcomes: a systematic review and meta-analyses, J Womens Health 19(11):2017–2031, 2010.

Smyth RMD, Aflaifel N, Bamigboye AA: Interventions for varicose veins and leg oedema in pregnancy, Cochrane Database Syst Rev (10):CD001066, 2015.

Tarín JJ, Hermenegildo C, García-Pérez MA, et al: Endocrinology and physiology of pseudocyesis, Reprod Biol Endocrinol 11:39, 2013.

Tunzi M, Gray GR: Common skin conditions during pregnancy, Am Fam Physician 75(2):211–218, 2007.

United Nations Children's Fund: The UNICEF Baby Friendly Initiative standards (website). www.unicef.org.uk/Documents/Baby_Friendly/Guidance/Baby_Friendly_guidance_2012.pdf. Updated 2012.

Villar J, Carroli G, Khan-Neelofur D, et al: Patterns of routine antenatal care for low-risk pregnancy,

Cochrane Database Syst Rev (4):CD000934, 2001.

Vleeming A, Albert HB, Östgaard HC, et al: European guidelines for the diagnosis and treatment of pelvic girdle pain, Eur Spine J 17(6):794–819, 2008.

Weekes ARL, Flynn MJ: Engagement of the fetal head in primigravidae and its relationship to the duration of gestation and time of onset of labour, Br J Obstet Gynaecol 82(1):7–11, 1975.

Wellock VK: The ever-widening gap: symphysis pubis dysfunction, Br J Midwifery 10(6):348–353, 2002.

Wellock VK, Crichton MA: Understanding pregnant women's experiences of symphysis pubis dysfunction: the effect of the pain, Evidence Based Midwifery 5(2):40–46, 2007.

Wheeler M: Home and laboratory testing pregnancy testing kits, Prof Nurse 14(8):571–576, 1999.

Winterton N: 1992 House of Commons Health Committee, Second Report, Maternity Services (Vol 1), HMSO, 1992.

Woolhouse M: Complementary medicine for pregnancy complications, Aust Fam Physician 35(9):695, 2006.

Zhou K, West HM, Zhang J, et al: Interventions for leg cramps in pregnancy, Cochrane Database Syst Rev (8):CD010655, 2015.

Resources and additional reading

http://cks.nice.org.uk/antenatal-care-uncomplicated-pregnancy#!scenario.

http://www.nhs.uk/Conditions/pregnancy-and-baby/pages/pregnancy-and-baby-care.aspx.

http://bestpractice.bmj.com/best-practice/monograph/493.html.

See UNICEF guidelines on 'How to prepare infant formula and sterilize feeding equipment to minimize the risks to your baby'. (website). www.unicef.org.uk/Documents/Baby_Friendly/Leaflets/guide_to_bottle_feeding.pdf.

Your booking appointment is your first official antenatal appointment. It provides your midwife with valuable background information about you. http://www.babycentre.co.uk/a551015/your-booking-appointment#ixzz3zF6FM64h.

Chapter 33

Antenatal investigations

Maureen Boyle

Learning Outcomes ?

After reading this chapter, you will be able to:

- discuss the range of routine and specialized tests available to the woman and her family during the antenatal period
- be aware of the research and evidence around screening and diagnostic tests, and the means by which the midwife and mother can access this information
- be conversant with the necessity and strategies for information sharing between the woman and midwife to ensure informed choice by the woman

INTRODUCTION

The field of antenatal investigations has grown greatly in the past several years. Screening tests are currently being offered and women are required to make decisions that would have previously been unthinkable. Although National Institute for Health and Care Excellence (NICE) (2014) guidelines for antenatal care recommend a schedule of antenatal tests, there is still a wide variation in what tests are considered 'routine' in various parts of the UK. The increase in the use of information technology has meant that women and their partners often have accessed much specialized information themselves, and this may shape their questions.

Midwives need to have a better-than-ever knowledge of what tests are being offered so that they can ensure women are making their choices based on up to date and comprehensive information. Midwives also need to be effective counsellors, as it is acknowledged that the skills and attitudes of midwives influence the uptake of screening tests (van den Berg et al 2007; McNeill et al 2014). The midwife should also appreciate that the complete clinical antenatal examination is one of the most effective and efficient screening and diagnostic tools, if undertaken systematically and skillfully.

SCREENING AND DIAGNOSIS

Although the meanings of screening and diagnosis are very different, they are often confused, and the midwife must ensure that the woman fully understands the difference.

Screening can be defined as determining the risk or likelihood of a condition, whereas a *diagnostic test* will give a definite answer. Sometimes, action will be taken after the results of a screening test. For example, a low haemoglobin (Hb) result in pregnancy may be assumed to be caused by pregnancy-induced anaemia, and iron tablets will probably be given without further investigation, although in a few rare cases, the anaemia may be caused by uncommon conditions, such as chronic renal infection, which would need further investigations to obtain a diagnosis. However, it would not be cost-effective to do an infinite range of investigations for every woman who presented with a positive screening test where the usual cause can be easily treated.

Some screening tests will produce results that mean an invasive test will be necessary to obtain a diagnosis. This needs to be made clear to the woman by the midwife providing counselling – for example, a woman may not want to undertake a Down syndrome test if she would not undergo amniocentesis in the case of a 'high risk' result. Some tests, such as an ultrasound, can be both screening and diagnostic (see Table 33.1). For instance, a scan can diagnose a missing limb or neural tube defect, but it can also discover anomalies (for example, 'soft markers'), which would need further investigations to determine a diagnosis.

Table 33.1 Common procedures used for fetal assessment

Test		Time
Nuchal translucency (screening)	Chromosomal abnormality	10-14 weeks
Chorionic villus sampling (diagnostic)	Chromosomal abnormality Genetic disease Metabolic disorders Haemoglobinopathies Infection	>10 weeks
Amniocentesis (diagnostic)	Chromosomal abnormality Genetic disease Metabolic disorders Haemoglobinopathies Infection	10-14 weeks (early) 15-18 weeks
Ultrasound (screening and diagnostic)	Assess fetus (dates/growth/viability/number) Diagnosis of some abnormalities (e.g. structural) Screening for abnormalities (e.g. soft markers) Assessment of placental site Liquor volume measurement	All gestations
Cordocentesis (diagnostic)	Obtain fetal blood sample	2nd/3rd trimester
Doppler (screening)	Assess fetal/placental/uterine blood flow	2nd/3rd trimester

It is not enough to just explain the test, the midwife should discuss the implications of both positive and negative results that need to be explored before a woman can be said to be making an informed choice. Literature such as 'Screening tests for you and your baby' (Public Health England 2014a) may prove a valuable resource, but it is not a substitute for specific discussion with a midwife. As tests become more varied and complex and midwives' time more limited, ensuring properly informed choice is becoming a greater challenge for midwives.

BLOOD TESTS

Blood is taken from a woman during pregnancy to detect conditions that may influence her well-being and that of the developing fetus.

Blood tests for assessment of maternal well-being

ABO and Rhesus blood grouping

Blood is typed as A, B, AB or O, depending on specific agglutinogens on the erythrocytes. The Rhesus factor identifies the blood group as negative or positive, depending on whether the Rhesus factor antigen is present.

Because of the risk of anaemia, haemorrhage and shock in pregnancy and during birth, and the possible need to provide transfusion, it is important that the blood group is identified early in the pregnancy.

Antibodies

Maternal blood is examined for the presence of antibodies, particularly Rhesus antibodies if the woman is Rhesus negative. If the fetus is Rhesus positive, antibodies can be stimulated by the occurrence of a fetomaternal haemorrhage, when 'leaks' occur and some fetal Rhesus-positive cells pass into the maternal circulation. This can happen as pregnancy progresses, during procedures such as amniocentesis, chorionic villus sampling (CVS) or external cephalic version (ECV), in situations such as an antepartum haemorrhage, or at delivery. The Rhesus negative woman may respond by producing antibodies, which may then cross the placenta in the current or subsequent pregnancies, to the fetal circulation and cause haemolysis in a Rhesus-positive fetus. The administration of anti-D immunoglobulin is effective in preventing the production of these antibodies (Qureshi et al 2014). Recent guidance from NICE (2014) suggests that routine antenatal anti-D prophylaxis should be offered to all non-sensitized, Rhesus-negative women. It is crucial that careful discussion takes place regarding this prophylaxis, as the woman must appreciate that she is being given a blood product. If the woman knows that the father of the child is Rhesus negative also, prophylaxis will be unnecessary, and partner testing may be considered (NICE 2014).

ABO incompatibility and less common antibodies, such as anti-c ('little c') and anti-K (Kell), can also affect the fetus or newborn. Antibody screening is usually undertaken initially at booking and then repeated later in the pregnancy.

Full blood count

Full blood counts are taken routinely at booking and intervals during pregnancy, primarily to detect a pathological fall in haemoglobin (Hb), which may indicate iron deficiency anaemia. No woman should reach term with a potentially dangerous anaemia because this exposes her to the risk of an amount of blood loss at delivery that she is unable to tolerate. It must be remembered, however, that other rare conditions may be discovered 'accidentally'; for example, a low white cell count may lead to a diagnosis of leukaemia. It is important, therefore, that no abnormal result ever be disregarded and that the woman understands each test.

Haemoglobin

Because of physiological changes in pregnancy, haemoglobin (Hb) levels will normally reduce, with the lowest reading expected at about 34 weeks. The World Health Organisation (WHO 2011) cites 11 g/dL (110 g/L) as the lowest acceptable reading, although other authorities quote figures down to 10 g/dL (100 g/L). A result of 10.5 g/dL (105 g/L) would be considered normal at 28 weeks. A low Hb reading needs further investigation to establish the cause, so that appropriate treatment can be commenced.

Serum ferritin levels and total iron-binding capacity (TIBC) may be assessed and causes of insidious blood loss, such as from chronic renal infection or parasitic infestation, may be investigated.

Measurement of serum ferritin at booking may predict those who will develop anaemia during pregnancy and, therefore, treatment could be commenced before the Hb becomes low (Letsky 2002; Ribot et al 2014).

Mean corpuscular volume

The earliest effect of iron deficiency is a reduced mean corpuscular volume (MCV). MCV is also reduced with alpha- and beta-thalassaemia minor. A raised MCV is associated with folate deficiency (high alcohol intake can reduce absorption of folic acid) or B_{12} deficiency.

Platelets

Platelets usually stay within the normal range for non-pregnant women, although levels may fall during pregnancy within this range. An abnormal fall could indicate various medical conditions and would need further investigation.

White cell count

The total number of white cells rises in pregnancy, mainly because of the increase of neutrophils. However, an abnormal rise could indicate an infection, and this cause needs additional exploration.

Haemoglobinopathies

Haemoglobinopathies are a diverse group of inherited single-gene disorders involving abnormal haemoglobin patterns, which constitute two major conditions: *thalassaemia (minor or major)* and *sickle cell* disorders: *sickle cell trait (SCT or HbAS); sickle cell haemoglobin C disease (HbSC); and sickle cell disease/anaemia (HbSS).*

Both sickle cell disease and thalassaemia are recessive conditions; therefore, only those inheriting an affected gene from each parent will have the disease. If a woman is found to be carrying either the *HbS* gene or the thalassaemia trait (thalassaemia minor), it is necessary to test the baby's father before a prediction about the baby's condition can be made. If both parents carry the gene, antenatal diagnosis can be made by chorionic villus sampling (CVS), amniocentesis or, more rarely, cordocentesis.

Currently, in high-prevalence areas, booking bloods for all women are automatically screened by hospital laboratories. In areas considered low prevalence, the Family Origin Questionnaire (Public Health England (PHE) 2014b) should be used by midwives to identify which women to test.

Maternal infection screening

Rubella

This common viral infection is a significant condition in pregnancy because of the teratogenic effect on the developing fetus caused by transplacental transmission of the virus. Detection of rubella antibodies is carried out by serological testing to identify immunity (IgG antibodies) or infection (IgM antibodies).

The majority of women in the UK are immune as a result of routine vaccination against rubella at 11 to 14 years of age, although those not growing up in the UK may not have been vaccinated. Since 1988, vaccination is now part of the measles, mumps and rubella (MMR) vaccine, usually administered before 15 months to male and female infants. Previously, all pregnant women were tested for rubella immunity at antenatal booking; however, currently the advice is for women to ensure they are fully immunized before becoming pregnant, and routine antenatal screening is not recommended (PHE 2016).

If a woman is not immune and comes into contact with rubella, she may develop the disease. Rubella can cause the loss of the pregnancy or the birth of a rubella-infected baby with various physical and mental anomalies.

The fetus is most vulnerable up until 16 weeks, but the infection can cross the placenta at any gestation. To avoid the danger of rubella in future pregnancies, the non-immune woman can be offered vaccination in the puerperium, initially by the midwife and the second dose usually by the general practitioner (GP). She will need to ensure effective contraception for a minimum of 1 month after receiving the vaccinations.

Hepatitis

Hepatitis means inflammation of the liver. There are several different viruses that affect the liver (A, B, C, D, E and G), but B and C are the types with the most direct relevance to midwives at present.

Hepatitis B (HBV)

Hepatitis B is an infectious bloodborne viral disease. It can cause a range of symptoms from very mild to life threatening. About 10% of adults infected become chronic carriers, and this may then progress to serious and fatal liver disease. Transmission is by contact with body fluids or vertically to the fetus. However, although there is a high chance of perinatal transmission, interventions after birth can greatly reduce the risk of the baby becoming a chronic carrier, and, therefore, identification of the mother's HBV status during pregnancy is important. All pregnant women should be screened for HBV infection (NICE 2014) and, if a positive result is identified, procedures detailed in 'Hepatitis B Antenatal Screening and Newborn Immunisation Programme: best practice guidance' (Department of Health (DH) 2011) should be commenced.

Because of its high level of infectivity, all healthcare workers (especially midwives) who have contact with body fluids should be vaccinated against HBV.

Hepatitis C (HCV)

Although HCV is very similar to hepatitis B, many more people infected with it will become chronic carriers and develop liver damage. There is no vaccine against HCV. At present, universal antenatal screening for HCV is not undertaken, but previous research has demonstrated a 0.8% prevalence rate in inner London, and in this study the majority of the infected women had no identified risk factors (Ward et al 2000). Similar findings were obtained in more recent research in Ireland (Lambert et al 2013).

Human immunodeficiency virus infection

NICE (2014) guidelines state that human immunodeficiency virus (HIV) testing should be recommended to all women as part of routine antenatal screening, as there are now clearly identified strategies that can reduce transmission to the fetus and maintain/improve the woman's health. As with all tests, informed consent is necessary, and the midwife must ensure her knowledge base in this very fast-changing area is up to date in order that she can offer explanations and answer questions. This is a condition where new research is frequently being published and, therefore, all maternity units should have an identified resource person to whom the more complex enquiries can be referred.

Toxoplasmosis

Toxoplasmosis is a parasitic infection caused by the protozoon *Toxoplasma gondii*, which may cause congenital infection in the fetus. It can be transmitted from domestic cat faeces, soil, raw meat and unpasteurized milk. Pregnant women are also advised to avoid contact with sheep during lambing.

The test, which examines the immunity status of the woman by looking at IgG and IgM antibodies, should be performed in a toxoplasmosis reference laboratory, as diagnosis is not straightforward. NICE (2014) does not recommend routine testing.

Listeriosis

Listeriosis can cause upper respiratory disease, septicaemia and encephalic disease. In pregnancy it can result in preterm labour, stillbirth or meningitis (in the woman or fetus/baby). It is caused by a common bacterium usually transmitted via contaminated food, and advice is given to pregnant women to specifically avoid soft cheeses and pâtés, and to ensure 'cook-chill' meals are well heated through. Pregnant women are advised to avoid contact with sheep during lambing. Diagnosis is made by culture of blood or cerebrospinal fluid.

Cytomegalovirus

Cytomegalovirus (CMV) is a herpes virus that can be passed on by many routes, including sexual activities. CMV can lie latent in maternal tissues and become reactivated during pregnancy. The presence of CMV antibodies in the blood is indicative of infection, and virus-specific IgM antibody is present in acute infections. It is the most common cause of intra-uterine infection, and the fetus can be assessed by amniotic fluid studies (Yinon et al 2010).

Serology

Serological tests, both non-treponemal and treponemal, can be undertaken in the antenatal period, and most women in the UK are routinely screened for syphilis at booking, as there is evidence that this is still an appropriate test (UK National Screening Committee (UK NSC) 2013) (see Ch. 55).

It is possible to get false-positive results with conditions such as malaria, tuberculosis and glandular fever, and those infected with pinta and yaws may test positive. Those who abuse narcotics can also test as a false positive.

Blood glucose screening

Gestational diabetes is defined as carbohydrate intolerance, resulting in hyperglycaemia with onset or first recognition during pregnancy. NICE (2015) recommends that women at risk are screened in pregnancy, usually by means of a 75 g oral glucose tolerance test at 24 to 28 weeks, as identifying women with gestational diabetes can lead to improved pregnancy outcomes, and potentially benefitting the woman who is at increased risk of developing type 2 diabetes. Note that type 2 diabetes actually may be already established but undiagnosed, and midwives must stress to the woman the importance of attending the postnatal appointment that will be arranged for her, to confirm her diabetic status.

ANTENATAL MATERNAL BLOOD TESTS TO ASSESS THE FETUS

Maternal serum screening for Down syndrome (MSSDS)

In the late 1980s, workers at St Bartholomew's Hospital, London, developed a method of screening all women for the risk factor of Down syndrome (chromosome anomaly trisomy 21) in a current pregnancy by means of a maternal blood test (Loncar et al 1995). Since then, the test has been refined, expanded and a nuchal translucency (NT) ultrasound assessment added. Combined with the woman's age (it has long been recognized that the incidence of Down syndrome increases with the age of the woman), these calculations result in an individual risk estimation.

Currently, there are several variations of the test and local National Health Service (NHS) Trust policies will determine the specific tests offered. NICE (2014) recommends the combined test between 11 weeks and 13 weeks 6 days, with the triple or quadruple test, if booking later, at 15 to 20 weeks.

- *Triple or quadruple test:* alpha-fetoprotein (AFP), unconjugated oestriol, beta-hCG and – if quadruple – inhibin-A, undertaken in the second trimester.
- *Integrated test:* pregnancy-associated plasma protein A (PAPP-A) and NT in the first trimester, plus the quadruple test in the second trimester, and the results integrated to provide one result.
- *Combined test:* NT plus beta-hCG and PAPP-A, done in the first trimester.
- *Serum integrated test:* serum only (PAPP-A in the first trimester and the quadruple test in the second trimester).

It is important the woman realizes that the outcome is only a risk assessment and if her result is considered a 'screen positive', she will probably be offered an amniocentesis for a diagnosis. It is also possible that a 'screen negative' may well occur despite an affected fetus, and this also needs to be made clear.

An increased level of AFP has been previously used on its own as a screening test for neural tube defects (spina bifida and anencephaly), to be followed by amniocentesis to detect diagnostic levels in the amniotic fluid. Most neural tube defects are now diagnosed by ultrasound examination.

Not all pregnancies are suitable for routine MSSDS screening. Levels can be influenced by a multiple pregnancy, intra-uterine bleeding, obesity or the woman having insulin-dependent diabetes. The midwife must ensure she includes all relevant information on the laboratory form, such as the woman's weight, her ethnic origin and her smoking status (NHS Antenatal and Newborn Screening 2014).

Non-invasive prenatal testing (NIPT)

It has recently become possible to test cell-free fetal DNA from the plasma of pregnant women to provide information about the potential risks for fetal aneuploidy (Robinson et al 2015), chromosomes 21, 18, 13 and sex chromosomes being most commonly assessed. This technique is still being developed, but it has already been introduced in some parts of the world (Williams et al 2015).

ASSESSMENT OF FETAL WELL-BEING

Fetal heart rate

In assessing the fetal heart rate as an indication of fetal well-being, it is usual practice to assess baseline rate, variability and alteration in heart rate in reaction to stress or movement.

The fetal heart rate varies through the antenatal period, ranging between 110 and 160 beats per minute (bpm), with an average baseline of:

- 155 bpm at 20 weeks
- 144 bpm at 30 weeks
- 140 bpm at term

During this time, variations around 20 bpm above and below these baselines are considered within normal limits and signify changes in fetal oxygenation. Tachycardia is more common in the preterm fetus, but may also indicate reaction to maternal medication, maternal pyrexia or tachycardia, acute blood loss, fetal anaemia, fetal infection or conditions, such as Wolff–Parkinson–White disease. Tachycardia may be seen in fetal hypoxia but not usually without other indications.

Bradycardia (heart rate under 110 bpm) is most likely to be caused by hypoxia, fetal heart block or vagal nerve stimulation.

Fetal movements

Monitoring fetal movements as a test of fetal well-being was introduced by Sadovsky in the 1970s (Sadovsky et al 1983), and this led to extensive use of the Cardiff 'Count to ten kick chart'. This required the woman to count 10 movements over a 12-hour period, with instructions to contact her midwife or GP, should the 10 movements not be achieved. Despite many perceived problems (for example, non-compliance, increased anxiety), some still consider fetal movements to be an effective means of assessing well-being and reduced fetal activity as one of the most accurate means of identifying the fetus at risk of intra-uterine death (Heazell and Froen 2008); however, NICE does not recommend routine fetal movement counting, as there is no clear research evidence of benefit at present (Mangesi et al 2012).

Maternity services have a variety of approaches, but whatever system is in place, it is important to encourage the woman to become familiar with her own baby's pattern of movement and for her to be aware of what actions she should take should there be a significant change in the movements.

Reflective activity 33.1   ><

Explore the policies regarding fetal movement assessment in your Trust and, if possible, compare these with policies from other hospitals.

ULTRASOUND

In the UK, ultrasound scanning (Fig. 33.1) is a routine part of antenatal care for women and is integral to many of the specialized investigations. Ultrasound imaging is a non-invasive (when done with an abdominal transducer) screening and diagnostic technique using sound waves with a frequency well above the range of human hearing. Although at present the usual method of ultrasound scanning is abdominal, vaginal ultrasound, using a special probe, is becoming more common in early pregnancy or for specialized assessment.

Ultrasound scans can be performed for a variety of reasons, from the earliest gestation up to and including when in labour, and postnatally to detect complications in the mother (for example, retained products) or to assess the baby. However, antenatal ultrasound is most common, and it is important to remember that a scan for any reason during this period may result in findings apart from the purpose for which it was being done – for instance, a scan to assess the placental site may result in the discovery of a fetal abnormality. A woman undergoing ultrasound scanning should be aware of a scan's capabilities, that a raised body mass index (BMI) can make ultrasound difficult and therefore less accurate, and that the finding of no abnormalities by ultrasound is not a guarantee that no problems will develop.

Increased technology has made 3D (still) and 4D (moving 3D) scans available; however, at present the NHS usually only uses these images in Fetal Medicine Units to diagnose and assess abnormalities as necessary.

Reflective activity 33.2   ><

With the woman's and ultrasonographer's permission, sit in on some ultrasound scans at various gestations in pregnancy so you can become familiar with the findings of the ultrasonographer and with the questions women may ask.

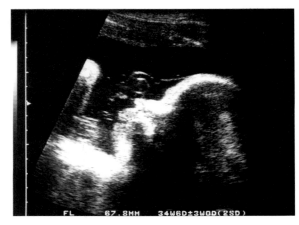

Figure 33.1 Ultrasound scan.

Indications for first trimester ultrasound

Booking/early/dating scans

Historically, first trimester scans were only routinely offered to women ensure their last menstrual period, and an estimated delivery date (EDD) was able to be calculated from fetal measurements taken during scanning. However, at present, NICE guidelines (2014) suggest all women should be offered an ultrasound between 10 and 13+6 weeks, not only to determine gestational age and identify multiple pregnancies, but also as part of screening for anomalies.

Parameters that may be used to determine gestational age are *crown–rump* length, *biparietal diameter, femur length* and *head circumference.* Measurements will be recorded to act as a baseline from which fetal growth can be monitored later in pregnancy.

The gestational sac is sometimes assessed early in the first trimester to confirm an intra-uterine pregnancy, to calculate the gestational age before the fetus is visible, or to diagnose an anembryonic pregnancy (no embryonic tissue).

Diagnosis of pregnancy

The embryonic sac may be identified as early as 5 weeks gestation using a transabdominal probe, and at 4 weeks with a transvaginal probe. Fetal heart movements can be visualized at 6 to 7 weeks gestation, and lack of fetal heart movement is a reliable method of diagnosing fetal death after this time. Actual movements of the fetus can be observed from 8 to 9 weeks. Doppler ultrasound equipment, which produces amplified sound waves (that is, Sonicaid/Doptone), may be used to hear the fetal heart after about 12 weeks gestation, but failure to hear the fetal heart should not be assumed to indicate fetal death. Fetal viability should be checked by an ultrasound scan.

Ectopic pregnancy

This may be detected by ultrasound scan, the transvaginal route being more accurate than the abdominal route. Diagnosis is not always easy, but identification of high-risk groups, clinical examination and biochemical tests usually assist the diagnosis.

Miscarriage/missed abortion/vaginal bleeding

If a woman reports no longer 'feeling pregnant', or there are no signs of expected growth, an ultrasound scan may show the fetal sac failing to grow and a visible fetal pole but no fetal heartbeat. One advantage of routine early scans is identification of missed miscarriages, potentially avoiding traumatic bleeding and possible emergency admission for these women.

Vaginal bleeding is not uncommon in early pregnancy and often the cause is never determined. Ultrasound is extremely valuable in assessing fetal viability when bleeding occurs to determine what action, if any, should be taken.

Hydatidiform mole

Ultrasound scan confirms the diagnosis after clinical signs such as painless vaginal bleeding, a large-for-dates uterus, hyperemesis gravidarum and absence of fetal heart sounds by 14 weeks gestation using Doppler ultrasound occur.

Multiple pregnancies

Multiple pregnancies can be identified by ultrasound from 4 weeks transvaginally and 5 weeks abdominally. Initially, it is suspected when more than one fetal sac is seen, the presence of two (or more) viable fetuses confirms the diagnosis.

Many twin pregnancies result in a singleton birth. Because of the increased number of first trimester ultrasound scans, the 'vanishing twin' syndrome has been described, where twins are seen on an early scan but one is then lost – this is sometimes associated with vaginal bleeding but often is not. The figures for this are uncertain and range between 20% and 50% of twin pregnancies (see Ch. 57).

Nuchal translucency scan

Nuchal translucency (NT) is the measurement of the fluid level at the back of the fetal neck. It is usually performed between 11 and 14 weeks gestation as part of the combined screening test for chromosomal abnormalities. A raised result may also indicate a cardiac anomaly. Later in the gestation, the nuchal translucency cannot be assessed, and if this scan is undertaken, it is called a nuchal fold scan and increased thickness will have the same implications as an increased NT.

Indications for second trimester ultrasound

In the UK since the 1980s, women have been offered routine ultrasound assessment between 18 and 20 weeks gestation, often called the 'anomaly', 'mid-pregnancy', '20-week' or 'mid-trimester' scan. By this time, most fetal organs are formed and many abnormalities can be seen. However, it must be stressed that not all structures and their functions can be assessed; some may need later scans and many abnormalities may not be able to be assessed by ultrasound at all. In spite of this, women frequently see this routine scan as a signal that 'everything is alright' and a guarantee of a problem-free pregnancy and baby, which can be a very misleading assumption. The quality of the assessment is dependent on accessing a good image, and some circumstances (such as position of the fetus or maternal obesity) may compromise this.

Estimation of fetal age

If an earlier scan has not been performed, the accuracy of the gestational age by dates can be confirmed by fetal measurements. For accuracy, the measurements to assess gestational age should be undertaken in the first or early second trimester, as prediction of gestational age by ultrasound scan cannot be accurately made after 24 weeks, because of the wide spread of normal measurements. Measurements will be recorded, to act as a baseline in case fetal growth needs to be monitored later in pregnancy.

Placental location

During every ultrasound examination, identification of the placenta is made, but it is routinely done during the second trimester scan. If the placental site is low in the mid-trimester scan, a repeat scan is usually offered in the third trimester, and the woman is advised as to what to do in the case of bleeding before this. Only a minority of placentae will fail to become fundal by 32 weeks, but if the placenta remains partially or wholly in the lower uterine segment, it is a placenta praevia and appropriate care must be instigated.

Identification of fetal anomalies

Although fetal anomalies can be detected during any ultrasound scan, the mid-trimester scan is used routinely for this examination.

Fetal anatomy is assessed and many conditions, mainly structural, can be diagnosed (although some may need referral to a specialist centre for a definitive diagnosis). In addition, the ultrasonographer can also note any 'soft markers' – for example, extra digits, choroid plexus cysts or talipes. These can be benign anomalies that either disappear (for example, most choroid plexus cysts) or can be easily treated after birth. However, they can also be a manifestation of more serious underlying conditions, such as a chromosomal abnormality. An amniocentesis may be offered to exclude this. The use of soft markers is a controversial subject and can be a cause of great anxiety for many (Loughna 2006; Roshanai et al 2015).

Cervical incompetence

In some cases, serial ultrasound may be used from about 14 weeks to assess the condition of the cervical canal and detect shortening.

Indications for third trimester ultrasound

Assessment of fetal growth

Fetal growth is assessed clinically at every antenatal visit. If the midwife or doctor feels growth is suboptimal, a referral for ultrasound assessment is usually made to confirm the clinical findings (NICE 2014).

To assess fetal growth by ultrasound, the age of the fetus must be accurately established before 24 weeks gestation. Fetal growth may be monitored by serial ultrasound measurements of various parameters every 2 to 4 weeks. Measurements of head and abdominal circumference are commonly used to estimate the growth in small-for-gestational-age fetuses (both asymmetrical and symmetrical) and large-for-gestational-age fetuses. In a fetus with symmetrical intra-uterine growth restriction (IUGR), the normal growth shows deviation below the 5th (or 10th) centile. In the asymmetrical condition, the abdominal circumference growth is slow and may stop, and eventually the head circumference growth also slows. IUGR can be diagnosed by plotting serial scans along centile lines, previously defined as the normal growth pattern for that population. Many Trusts are now using customized antenatal charts rather than standard ones (Perinatal Institute 2016) (see Ch. 45). If IUGR occurs, a fall-off of growth can be seen. Growth acceleration (large abdominal circumference) above the 90th centile may be because of maternal diabetes mellitus, especially if associated with polyhydramnios and a large placenta.

Estimation of fetal weight

Estimation of fetal weight can be made by using measurements obtained during ultrasound assessment. For the preterm fetus, and especially very preterm and multiples, ultrasound estimation of weight is the method of choice. This may provide vital information when consideration is being given to expediting a premature delivery.

However, at term it has been shown that parous women can often estimate the weight of the fetus as accurately as professionals using palpation (Diase and Monga 2002). Clinical assessment can also be as accurate as ultrasound (Banerjee et al 2008) in estimating fetal weight around term; however, research studying this has specified using experienced professionals to do the assessments. It may be that a generation of practitioners, who are becoming increasingly dependent on ultrasound in their practice, may not be able to replicate this research in the future. Since there will always be situations where ultrasound cannot be accessed, it is a reminder for all midwives to maintain their clinical skills of palpation and weight estimation.

Reflective activity 33.3

When carrying out an antenatal check in late pregnancy or when caring for a woman in labour, try to estimate the fetal weight during your routine abdominal examination and palpations. Check after the birth to assess your skill.

Malpresentations/malpositions

Late in the third trimester, an ultrasound scan can be used to confirm clinical findings regarding the presentation and position of the fetus (or each fetus in the case of a multiple pregnancy). This information can be used to help decision making if there is a question over the mode of delivery.

Ultrasound will also be used to guide the clinician if external cephalic version (ECV) is undertaken to turn a breech presentation.

Additional fetal assessment

Doppler ultrasound

As well as being used to monitor the fetal heart (for example, Sonicaid), this technique is also used to measure blood flow in the fetal and uterine/placental vessels from a waveform recording on a monitor screen. The blood flow pattern will change as an adaptation to poor placental function, so it is thought that alterations in the fetal umbilical blood flow may occur in early fetal compromise. Women may be referred for Doppler assessment in the second and third trimester because of oligohydramnios, differing growth in multiple pregnancies, IUGR (or a history of IUGR in a previous pregnancy) or maternal conditions (such as hypertensive disorders of pregnancy). It may also form part of post-date fetal assessment.

Amniotic fluid measurement

As a routine clinical assessment during palpation in the second and third trimester, amniotic fluid quantity may be estimated to be reduced (oligohydramnios) or increased (polyhydramnios). Both these conditions, if suspected, need to be referred for ultrasound evaluation. Oligohydramnios may be associated with various fetal abnormalities or with fetal compromise. Polyhydramnios may also be present with a fetal abnormality (for example, oesophageal atresia) or be associated with maternal disease (such as diabetes mellitus) and a large fetus. All these conditions will need expert assessment, especially in determining timing and mode of delivery and planning aftercare. Amniotic fluid volume will also be evaluated as part of the assessment of fetal well-being for a woman with a medical condition (for example, pre-eclampsia) or as part of a post-term assessment.

INVASIVE TESTS

Chorionic villus sampling

Chorionic villus sampling (CVS) can be undertaken at any gestation but is used primarily as a first trimester test. Under continuous ultrasound visualization of the placenta, chorionic villi are obtained, usually by syringe, and these can be analysed for fetal chromosomal abnormalities. A provisional result is usually available within a few days. Depending on the position of the placenta, the procedure can be done either transabdominally or via the cervix.

The advantage of an early diagnostic test for chromosomal abnormality is that the woman would probably have the option of a first trimester termination, if that was her decision. Disadvantages include a rate of pregnancy loss usually quoted at more than amniocentesis; however, it has been suggested that rates of loss are reducing substantially (Akolekar et al 2015).

Difficulty in analysing the miscarriage rate is, however, complicated by the higher rate of spontaneous miscarriage in the first trimester. There is also a risk of results failure and studies have indicated a link between CVS and limb abnormality, probably restricted to procedures undertaken before 10 weeks gestation (Royal College of Obstetricians and Gynaecologists (RCOG) 2005).

After the procedure, Rhesus-negative women will usually be given anti-D immunoglobulin to prevent possible isoimmunization.

Amniocentesis

Amniotic fluid can be used to test for fetal conditions such as chromosomal abnormalities, genetic diseases or some fetal infections.

In the UK, amniocentesis is usually performed at about 15 to 18 weeks gestation using ultrasound to visualize the uterus and its contents. A fine needle is passed through the abdominal wall into the uterus and about 20 mL of amniotic fluid is extracted. The fetal cells in the amniotic fluid must be cultured and the time taken for their growth (about 2–3 weeks) accounts for the wait for a diagnosis, which women find difficult. Where there are the resources to use DNA analysis on the amniotic fluid, a much quicker result is possible. Some amniocentesis will fail to give a result when the fetal cells do not grow, and the woman must be aware of this small risk (about 1:500) and other disadvantages before she can make an informed choice to have an amniocentesis.

After the procedure, the fetal heart is auscultated or visualized on an ultrasound, and the woman should be allowed to hear/see this. She will usually be advised to rest for that day and avoid strenuous activity for a few days. Rhesus-negative women will receive anti-D immunoglobulin to prevent possible Rhesus isoimmunization.

The risk of pregnancy loss after amniocentesis is about 0.5% to 1%, but this can vary according to operator and centre. There is also a risk of infection after any invasive procedure.

Some tests on amniotic fluid, such as diagnosis of neural tube defects (which is now done by ultrasound) or assessing the lecithin:sphingomyelin ratio for fetal pulmonary maturity, are now no longer considered a reason for an invasive test.

Cordocentesis

This is an invasive investigation performed under ultrasound imaging, whereby a sample of fetal blood is obtained from the umbilical cord or intrahepatic vein, usually in the second or third trimester of pregnancy. The site of sampling is selected on considerations of accessibility, quality of visualization, gestational age and safety. The investigation was developed from a number of earlier interventions, including fetoscopy, for the purpose of antenatal diagnosis.

Cordocentesis carries a risk of pregnancy loss and also a risk of maternal infection and haemorrhage.

CONCLUSION

The suggestion of even a minor defect or anomaly in the fetus can cause extreme anxiety for parents, especially as even if all further tests show no abnormality no professional can guarantee a 'perfect' baby.

There is some evidence that the anxiety engendered on identification of a potential problem does not go away even after a reassuring diagnosis (Lawrence 1999; Yarcheski et al 2011) and also that maternal anxiety during pregnancy may affect the physiological development of the fetus (Teixeira et al 1999; Ding et al 2014).

However, the concept of antenatal screening is popular with most women, and the ability to identify many abnormal fetuses leads to women having a choice of terminating the pregnancy. There are also many healthy children – and their mothers are alive today because of the provision of the tests described in this chapter.

The midwife's role is to ensure that the woman receives accurate, evidence-based and up to date information in language she can understand to make an informed decision. Where possible, the midwife should provide written information to support any discussions, and should also be aware of other sources of information or support that may be helpful, such as through the Internet and through voluntary groups. Whatever range of tests the woman and her family choose to access, for whatever reasons, the midwife should continue to provide support and respect throughout her care.

Key Points

- Investigations offered to women in the antenatal period are increasing in number and complexity.

- Midwives need to keep up to date in the changing field of antenatal investigations, and have access to contemporary sources of information.

- Antenatal tests, and their potential consequences, need to be fully understood by the woman before they are undertaken. Written information should support any verbal discussion where possible.

- The well-being of the woman and fetus/baby, and the successful outcome of a pregnancy, can be dependent on antenatal investigations.

References

Akolekar R, Beta J, Picciarelli G, et al: Procedure-related risk of miscarriage following amniocentesis and chorionic villus sampling: a systematic review and meta-analysis, *Ultrasound Obstet Gynecol* 45(1):16–26, 2015.

Banerjee K, Mittal S, Kumar S: Clinical vs. ultrasound evaluation of fetal weight, *Int J Gynaecol Obstet* 86(1):41–43, 2008.

Department of Health (DH): *Hepatitis B antenatal screening and newborn immunisation programme: best practice guidance, 2011.* (website). www.dh.gov.uk/publications. 2011.

Diase K, Monga M: Maternal estimates of neonatal birth weight in diabetic patients, *South Med J* 95(1):92–94, 2002.

Ding XX, Wu YL, Xu SJ, et al: Maternal anxiety during pregnancy and adverse birth outcomes: a systematic review and meta-analysis of prospective cohort studies, *J Affect Disord* 159(2):103–110, 2014.

Heazell A, Froen J: Methods of fetal movement counting and the detection of fetal compromise,

J Obstet Gynaecol 28(2):147–154, 2008.

Lambert J, Jackson V, Coulter-Smith S, et al: Universal antenatal screening for hepatitis C, *Ir Med J* 106(5):136–138, 2013.

Lawrence S: Counselling for Down syndrome screening, *Br J Midwifery* 7(6):368–370, 1999.

Letsky E: *Blood volume, haematinics, anaemia* (Ch. 2). In de Swiet M, editor: *Medical disorders in obstetric practice*, 4th edn, Oxford, Blackwell, 2002.

Loncar J, Barnabei J, Larsen J: Advent of maternal serum markers for Down syndrome screening, *Obstet Gynecol Surv* 50(4):316–320, 1995.

Loughna P: Soft markers for congenital anomaly, *Curr Obstet Gynaecol* 16(2):107–110, 2006.

Mangesi L, Hofmeyr GJ, Smith V: Fetal movement counting for assessment of fetal well-being, *Cochrane Database Syst Rev* 2012.

McNeill J, Alderdice F, Rowe R, et al: Down's syndrome screening in Northern Ireland: women's reasons for accepting or declining serum

testing, *Int J Evid Based Healthc* 7(3):76–83, 2014.

National Institute for Clinical Excellence (NICE): *Antenatal care: routine care for the healthy pregnant woman, NICE clinical guideline 62, London, 2008, modified 2014.*

National Institute for Clinical Excellence (NICE): *Diabetes in Pregnancy. NICE clinical guideline NG3: 2015.*

National Health Service (NHS): *Antenatal and Newborn Screening Timeline.* (website). www.screening.nhs.uk. 2014.

Perinatal Institute: *Customised fetal growth charts.* (website). www.perinatal.org.uk. 2016.

Public Health England (PHE): *Rubella susceptibility screening in pregnancy to end in England PHE press release 27th January 2016.* (website). https://www.gov.uk/government/news/rubella-susceptibility-screening-in-pregnancy-to-end-in-england. 2016.

Public Health England: *Screening tests for you and your baby.* (website). www.gov.uk. 2014a.

Public Health England: *Family origin questionnaire: sickle cell and thalassaemia screening.* (website). www.gov.uk. 2014b.

Qureshi H, et al: BCSH guideline for the use of anti-D immunoglobulin for the prevention of haemolytic disease of the fetus and newborn, *Transfus Med* 24(1):8–20, 2014.

Ribot B, Aranda N, Viteri F, et al: Depleted iron stores without anaemia early in pregnancy carries increased risk of lower birthweight even when supplemented daily with moderate iron, *Hum Reprod* 27(5):1260–1266, 2014.

Robinson C, van den Boom D, Bombard AT: Noninvasive prenatal detection of aneuploidy, *Clin Obstet Gynecol* 57(1):210–225, 2015.

Roshanai AH, Ingvoldstad C, Lindgren P: Fetal ultrasound examination and assessment of genetic soft markers in Sweden: are ethical principles respected?, *Acta Obstet Gynecol Scand* 94(2):141–147, 2015.

Royal College of Obstetricians & Gynaecologists (RCOG): Amniocentesis and chorionic villus sampling, Guideline No. 8, London, 2005.

Sadovsky E, Ohel G, Havazeleth H, et al: The definition and the significance of decreased fetal movements, *Acta Obstet Gynecol Scand* 62(5):409–413, 1983.

Teixeira J, Fisk N, Glover V: Association between maternal anxiety in pregnancy and increased uterine artery resistance index: cohort based study, *Br Med J* 318(7177):153–157, 1999.

UK National Screening Committee (UK NSC): *Screening for syphilis in pregnancy: external review against programme appraisal criteria for the UK national screening committee.* (website). www.screening.nhs.uk/syphilis. 2013.

Van den Berg M, Timmermans D, Kleinveld J, et al: Are counsellors' attitudes influencing pregnant women's attitudes and decisions on prenatal screening?, *Prenat Diagn* 27(6):518–524, 2007.

Ward C, Tudor-Williams F, Cotzias T, et al: Prevalence of hepatitis C among pregnant women attending an inner London obstetrics department: uptake and acceptability of named antenatal testing, *Gut* 47(2):277–280, 2000.

Williams J, Rad S, Beauchamp S, et al: Utilization of noninvasive prenatal testing: impact on referrals for diagnostic testing, *Am J Obstet Gynecol* 213(1):102–104, 2015.

World health Organization (WHO): *Haemoglobin concentration for diagnosis of anaemia and assessment of severity WHO 2011.* (website). www.who.int/vmnis/indicators/haemoglobin.pdf. 2011.

Yarcheski A, Mahon NE, Yarcheski TJ, et al: A meta-analytic study of predictors of maternal-fetal attachment, *Int J Nurs Stud* 46(5):708–715, 2011.

Yinon Y, Farine D, Yudin M: Screening, diagnosis and management of cytomegalovirus infection in pregnancy, *Obstet Gynecol Surv* 65(11):736–743, 2010.

Resources and additional reading

The NHS Screening programme has online learning resources for continuing professional development: https://cpdscreening.phe.org.uk/elearning.

More information on Population Screening Programmes and the NHS fetal anomaly screening programme (FASP) can be found at https://www.gov.uk/topic/population-screening-programmes/fetal-anomaly.

Chapter 34

Choice, childbearing and maternity care: the choice agenda and place of birth

Sheena Byrom OBE and Anna Byrom

INTRODUCTION

Choice is a complex concept that has long been promoted as a cornerstone of effective maternity care provision. Midwifery philosophy advocates choice as the power or opportunity to actively choose among alternatives, marking a shift away from medical notions of informed consent, a term that implies more passive compliance with care (Spoel 2004). Translated into midwifery practice, the choice agenda requires midwives to support women and families to make fully informed decisions throughout their childbearing and childrearing journeys. However, the process of making informed decisions is challenging, affected by a range of subjective, contextual factors. Enabling effective, informed decision making requires more than providing full information about the choices available. Consideration of how, when, where and who provides the information is also relevant. In this chapter, concepts of choice and decision making are considered, including a review of the choice agenda throughout maternity services, focusing specifically on choice related to place of birth.

CHOICE RHETORIC AND MATERNITY CARE

Choice for childbearing women became a key focus for policy makers in the UK in 1993 with the publication of *Changing Childbirth* (Department of Health (DH) 1993). This landmark report advocated *choice, continuity and control* and became the new rhetoric of maternity services. Before that, the voices of mothers-to-be were at best unspoken or unheard and at worst, suppressed. Pressure groups such as the National Childbirth Trust (NCT) and the Association of Improvements in Maternity Services (AIMS) became important catalysts for change, along with more recent organizations such as Birthrights and Birth-ChoiceUK (see also Ch. 2).

In England, *Maternity Matters: Choice Access and Continuity of Care* (DH 2007) remains as the government's focal policy document, which explicitly stipulates four national choice guarantees (see Table 34.1). These guarantees aimed to ensure women and their families were given the opportunity to make informed choices throughout the maternity care pathway (see Fig. 34.1). Even though there continues to be a policy commitment to supporting childbearing women and families to choose how to access maternity services, the type of antenatal care they receive, where to have their baby and options for postnatal care, this is still far from reality for all throughout maternity services.

Table 34.1 *Maternity Matters*: four national choice guarantees

National choice guarantees:	
Choice of how to access maternity care	When they first learn that they are pregnant, women and their partners will be able to go straight to a midwife if they wish or to their general practitioner. Self-referral into the local midwifery service is a choice that will speed up and enable earlier access to maternity services.
Choice of type of antenatal care	Depending on their circumstances, women and their partners will be able to choose between midwifery care or care provided by a team of maternity health professionals, including midwives and obstetricians. For some women, team care will be the safest option.
Choice of place of birth	Depending on their circumstances, women and their partners will be able to choose where they wish to give birth. In making their decision, women will need to understand that their choice of place of birth will affect the choice of pain relief available to them. **Options for place of birth are:** • birth supported by a midwife at home • birth supported by a midwife in a local midwifery facility (e.g. birth centre) • birth supported by a maternity team in a hospital
Choice of postnatal care	After going home, women and their partners will have a choice of how and where to access postnatal care. This will be provided either at home or in a community setting, such as a Sure Start Children's Centre.

Source: DH 2007: 12–13

Choice constrained

Research and audit findings continue to identify how women remain unaware of the choices available to them throughout childbearing, birth and beyond (Garcia et al 1998; Kirkham and Stapleton 2001; Hundley et al 2001; Lavender and Chapple 2005; Madi and Crow 2003; Dodwell and Gibson 2009; Redshaw and Heikkila 2010; National Federation of Women's Institutes (NFWI) 2013). Denial of choice can cause significant biopsychosocial harm for women and their families (Cook and Loomis 2012) because decisions about childbearing and birth involve social, economic and political, rather than merely medical, issues (Wolfson 1986). Choice for women in all aspects of their childbirth journey remains a 'postcode lottery'; controlled by organizational culture, leadership, financial constraints and clinical guidelines.

Women's autonomy for decision making is frequently restricted by lack of caregiver time, available knowledge and personal bias (Kirkham 2004). The experience and personal beliefs of maternity care workers can influence what and how information is shared with women (Levy 2004). Although women report feeling overwhelmed with the amount of information imparted to them during pregnancy (Nolan 2009), many will continue to be influenced by messages communicated via television, the

Internet, social media and the use of smartphone apps (Byrom and Byrom 2014). The choices women make during pregnancy and childbirth are most frequently shaped by cultural norms, passed on through friends, family and the media (American Sociological Association (ASA) 2015).

In the UK, hospital birth is the norm, reinforced by the processes of socialization, cultural imagery around labour and birth and the language of safety and risk; therefore, choices are set within this context. In the context of choice and place of birth, Knightly (2007) comments that people are overloaded with information, especially from the media. In a sophisticated media age characterized by the swiftness of 'sound bites', it is difficult to get messages across based on 'evidence'. The increasing evidence and government support of the suitability of birth at home or in midwife-led units needs to be matched with the messages conveyed in the media. The overriding notion that hospital birth is safe is supported by portrayals in popular culture of home birth as risky and fraught with danger. As such, concepts of choice need to be viewed against a backdrop of consumerism, information-giving, risk, litigation and maternity services resources.

Although choice can appear constrained for individuals, there is a continued focus on increasing the choices for women across maternity services, to promote providers

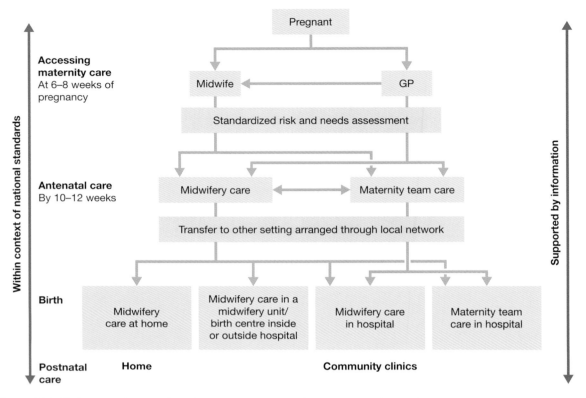

Figure 34.1 Choice commitments along the maternity pathway. (Department of Health Maternity matters: choice, access and continuity of care in a safe service. London, 2007, DH.)

within the current marketplace of healthcare service structures. Midwives aim to give women choices, and women are encouraged to make them. However, as outlined previously, making choices is not straightforward, particularly around the choice of place of birth. Choices are relative and are not solely made by what is on offer in any specific place or at any particular time; choices are influenced by the values and beliefs of women, midwives and doctors (Edwards 2005). An offer of choice must be matched with having the capacity to provide that choice. This applies to the choice of a hospital birth with availability of epidural anaesthesia or water birth, a freestanding birth centre or birth at home.

Birth place – challenging choices

In the UK, the move from home to hospital for place of birth was the result of a policy mandate (Ministry of Health 1970; see also Ch. 2). The decision was made without the evidence that it would improve safety, and members of the public, namely childbearing women, were

not consulted (Beech 2011). Since the 1960s, home birth has declined in the UK, as demonstrated in Figure 34.2 (Office for National Statistics (ONS) 2016).

However, policy recommendations in England (DH 2007) and organizational reconfigurations of maternity services in the country have resulted in an increase in alongside maternity units (AMUs), whereas the number of freestanding maternity units (FMUs) has remained static (see Fig. 34.3) (Dodwell/BirthChoiceUK 2015).

A midwifery-led unit (MLU) or birth centre is a maternity unit designed to provide a homely and tranquil environment. MLUs are run by experienced midwives and offer a social model of care in which birth is viewed primarily as a physiological event. Midwifery-led units are situated either 'alongside' a labour ward or delivery suite in an obstetric unit (hospital) or 'freestanding' in a community setting, usually some distance from an obstetric unit.

The Birthplace in England Research Programme (National Perinatal Epidemiology Unit (NPEU) 2011) provided robust evidence about care in midwifery units

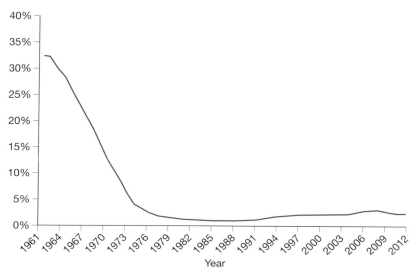

Figure 34.2 Home birth rates for England and Wales, 1961–2012. (Office for National Statistics (ONS) (2016). Birth characteristics in England and Wales: 2015. ONS, London.)

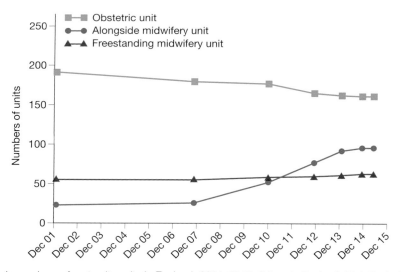

Figure 34.3 Change in numbers of maternity units in England, 2001–2015. (Miranda Dodwell, BirthChoiceUK, 2015.)

and planned home births and how the safety and quality compares with planned care in an obstetric unit. The findings on clinical outcomes are from a large prospective cohort study (Hollowell 2011). The main focus of the study was the care of *healthy women with uncomplicated pregnancies,* and it concluded that giving birth in a midwifery unit (birth centre) achieves optimal clinical outcomes for mother and baby and reduces healthcare costs (Hollowell 2011; Schroeder et al 2011; National Institute for Health and Care Excellence (NICE) 2014).

The *Birthplace* study demonstrated that planned care in a midwifery unit results in lower rates of regional analgesia, caesarean section, instrumental birth and episiotomy; reduced need for blood transfusion and higher-level medical care and an overall decrease in maternal morbidity (Hollowell 2011). Importantly, there were positive outcomes for babies too. For babies, planned midwifery unit care provided similar rates of healthy and adverse outcomes as traditional labour ward care, and initiation of breastfeeding was higher (Hollowell 2011).

> **Box 34.1** Questions women should ask about where to have their babies
>
> Questions you might like to ask about where to have your baby:
> - What are the different places where I can choose to have my baby?
> - What are the advantages and disadvantages of these different places?
> - Where can I find more information or support for my choice about where I have my baby?
> - Can I change my mind about where to have my baby?
> - How likely am I to have a midwife I know looking after me during labour?
> - What different types of pain relief are available in the different places?
> - Can my birth companion(s) stay with me after the birth?
> - What types of serious medical problems can affect babies, and how common are they?
>
> Source: NICE 2014

The NICE (2014) reiterated the *Birthplace* findings and, using other research evidence, formulated key recommendations on place of birth for women who are healthy and unlikely to experience complications. The guidance provides information for the public to help with decision making by recommending specific points to consider (see Box 34.1).

Based on the *Birthplace* study findings (NPEU 2011) and NICE (2014) recommendations, several Web-based and interactive tools have been developed to assist women in making the right decisions regarding their care (Coxon 2014; NICE 2014; Which? 2015).

WHERE DO WOMEN GIVE BIRTH?

On a global level, political agendas, accessibility of universal health services, private medical practice and the availability of midwives are all factors that influence a woman's ability to choose where and how to give birth (Sandall 2015). In low-income countries, access to appropriate maternity care is hindered by lack of finances, lack of transport services and the actual availability of maternity services (Renfrew et al 2014). In addition, women's cultural beliefs around birth, particularly in relation to safety, mean that they may make choices deemed 'risky' to maternity care workers (Dahlen 2014).

This pattern is replicated throughout Europe, with choice in place of birth available to women varying greatly. Some countries such as the Netherlands offer access to home birth and midwife-led units; in other countries, home birth is illegal, with restrictions placed on midwives to provide the service (Schiller 2016). In eastern European countries most babies are born in hospital. Although the case of *Ternovsky* v. *Hungary* (European Court of Human Rights (ECHR) 2011) established the human rights of a woman to choose the circumstances in which she gives birth, this is far from what happens in reality. In Bulgaria, for example, it is illegal for health professionals to attend women for a home birth, and midwifery-led units do not exist.

Choices for women living in the UK vary from country to country, depending on availability and accessibility of options. The home birth rate in Scotland is lower than in England, and even within the country the rate fluctuates, potentially because of the availability of midwife-led units. A survey carried out in 2013 (Cheyne et al 2015) revealed that 24% of women were not offered any choice of where to give birth, and only 25% were offered the choice of a home birth. In Northern Ireland the choice is even more limited in that only three midwife-led units exist. In 2014 over 1000 women were surveyed, and 44.6% of women were not offered any choice in place of birth, and only 15.5% of women were offered a home birth (McCann et al 2015).

Despite the plethora of evidence and guidance, most women in England still give birth in obstetric units (Birth-ChoiceUK 2014) (see Fig. 34.4), and reform is slow.

There is potential for many more women in the UK to be referred for care in an MLU (Newburn et al 2015). There were 698,512 live births in England and Wales during 2013 (Office for National Statistics (ONS) 2014), and estimates suggest that 45% of women giving birth in National Health Service (NHS) settings are at low risk of complications (Sandall et al 2014). On this basis, approximately 314,330 women were therefore eligible for MLU care, but only 89,000 in England received intrapartum care away from an obstetric unit. As a result, many thousands of 'low-risk' women and babies in England and Wales (225,330) are receiving care in settings with more medicalized approach, exposing them to unnecessary routine intervention.

Why is this happening?

From the information noted earlier, it is known that birth outside an obstetric unit depends on availability – not all maternity services offer MLU care, and some have a restricted or nonexistent home birth service. Women view hospital birth as the safest place to give birth based on cultural norms, and those who choose to have their baby in a hospital the first time usually do so again with subsequent pregnancies (Coxon 2015). However, even when

Where women gave birth in England, 2012
Total number of women = 686,500

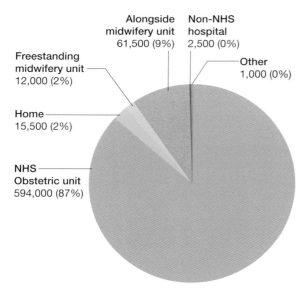

Alongside midwifery unit
61,500 (9%)

Non-NHS hospital
2,500 (0%)

Freestanding midwifery unit
12,000 (2%)

Other
1,000 (0%)

Home
15,500 (2%)

NHS Obstetric unit
594,000 (87%)

Figure 34.4 Where women gave birth in England, 2012. ©BirthChoiceUK 2014, (Miranda Dodwell 2014, pers. comm. 18 February). Data sources: Office for National Statistics (2013) and Comptroller and Audit General (2013).

services provide the full range of choice for place of birth, uptake of out-of-hospital birth is variable (McLachlan et al 2015) and dependent on staffing models and how information is articulated. Sometimes choices are influenced by clinical guidelines and the caregiver's interpretation of a guideline (see Case Study 34.1). How caregivers communicate choice also influences place of birth decisions.

Reflective activity 34.1

Take a look at Case Study 34.1. Think about how you might use the NICE recommendations to help Fatima make her decision about where to have her baby.

Communicating choice

The work of midwives involves sharing information and knowledge with childbearing women and being their advocate when required. The language maternity workers use when articulating choice is as crucial as the content (Furber and Thomson 2010). Both the language and content used can be influenced by caregiver bias (Levy 2004), shortage of time (Kirkham 2004) and the actual or perceived inability of the caregiver to provide full details

CASE STUDY 34.1

Fatima is worried. She is 32 weeks pregnant with her second baby. Fatima was distressed when she discovered that she was expecting another baby because she still had not recovered from the trauma of her first experience.

Through connecting with other mothers via social media, Fatima heard some women talking about midwifery units (birth centres), and those who had given birth there seemed to have positive feelings about them. Fatima asked her midwife if there was a birth centre nearby that she could use this time. The midwife explained that the nearest midwifery unit was 15 miles away, but suggested that Fatima that would not be allowed to give birth in a birth centre anyway because her first baby had been born by caesarean section.

Fatima felt disappointed, and she expressed this to the online community of mothers. Several responses on the forum were reassuring, but others made her feel even more confused. It seemed some mothers who had had a previous caesarean section were supported in their choice to have their next baby at home or in an MLU. Fatima was encouraged to contact a supervisor of midwives at the hospital where she was receiving care, and she did so after finding a telephone number in her handheld's records.

A meeting was arranged, and Fatima felt much better because her fears were listened to. An appointment was made with Fatima's obstetrician, and an action plan that accommodated Fatima's requests was made and recorded in her records.

of an intervention or to engage in a conversation that may ensue.

It has been argued that although some women prefer to relinquish any autonomy on offer and to be directed by the those caring for them, health professionals need more education on facilitating decision making (Lokugamage and Bourne 2015). Interventions such as ultrasound scanning, blood tests during pregnancy and immunizations are viewed as the norm, and not a choice, potentially leaving women feeling alienated should they choose to opt out. When a woman makes a decision not to have an intervention or follow a proposed care pathway, it is often documented that she has 'refused' it. This in itself portrays a compulsory status. Use of the word *decline* in these situations deflects any power status back to the mother, and it influences the focus and meaning of choice by giving a sense that the procedure was 'on offer' rather than a given.

Additional work by Glasser, a psychologist (2013), can be useful in rethinking habits in ways of thinking and acting that might have been adopted by the midwife/ maternity care worker and that may stifle choices being

Table 34.2 Choice theory – seven caring habits versus seven deadly habits

Seven caring habits	Seven deadly habits
1. Supporting	1. Criticizing
2. Encouraging	2. Blaming
3. Listening	3. Complaining
4. Accepting	4. Nagging
5. Trusting	5. Threatening
6. Respecting	6. Punishing
7. Negotiating differences	7. Bribing or rewarding to control

Source: Glasser 2013: 10–11

provided to women and their families and also might affect practitioners themselves (see Table 34.2). The contrast between *caring* and *deadly* habits is stark, and it is useful to consider how the woman might experience these habits and how this might influence her whole experience and perspective of the maternity service.

How parents interpret evidence provided depends on their perception of how 'risky' they think the proposed intervention or pathway of care is (Dahlen 2014) and what and how their midwife or doctor presents an option as a 'risk' (Coxon 2012). Consider women who are healthy and not expecting any complications who are deciding where to have their babies. They are given the evidence from the *Birthplace* study (NPEU 2011) and NICE (2014) to help them decide. For some women, even if the recommendations for out-of-hospital birth are clearly advantageous, they will not feel safe. Alternatively, for others, being at home to give birth feels less 'risky', even if there has been the suggestion to give birth in an obstetric unit because of an identified clinical risk.

Articulating evidence or clinical guidance based on population studies is not easy. 'What if it happens to me?' or 'What would you do?' are questions frequently asked by women searching for the right decision for themselves and their babies. The discussion that ensues will be hugely influenced by the midwife's knowledge base and her own personal and professional philosophy. Scamell (2014) explored aspects of communication between a midwife and a pregnant woman when discussing choices for place of birth, finding that that the language used by midwives was disempowering and limiting. Indeed, an exploration of women's views of how choice was articulated revealed that the communication style of midwives played a significant part in the women's childbirth experience (Hallam et al 2016).

In their study of women's choices, expectations and experiences of childbirth, Malcrida and Boulton (2014) found that women attempted to gain control by obtaining

information to have as natural a birth as possible, but they were also influenced by medical knowledge and yielded to medical interventions. Women then blamed themselves (Malcrida and Boulton 2014) for a dissatisfying experience when their choices did not go as planned or criticized the antenatal education programme they engaged with (Geddes 2013). Women are frequently seen as irresponsible and blamed for the choices they make (Dahlen 2010). This is heightened by the risk agenda that has grown in maternity services in response to litigation, service improvements and quality surveillance measures.

Reflective activity 34.2

Think about the way *you* communicate choice regarding place of birth to childbearing women and their families. How do you begin the conversation? What information do you share? What information and evidence have you accessed to inform your discussion. What factors influence the information sharing and/or conversation?

Managing risk or facilitating safety?

Choice in maternity care is synonymous with the 'risk agenda'. At each contact with maternity services, women are expected to navigate their childbearing journey via messages of risks and benefits. Paradoxically, as new technologies are developed and medical interventions in childbirth expand, the discourse of 'risk' increases (Symon 2006). When considering the choices presented, navigating conversations around risk and safety is not easy for women using maternity services. The complexity behind the individual decisions they make is constrained by cultural, historical and social factors, in addition to tensions within medical systems relating to responsibility and control (Coxon et al 2014; Malcrida and Boulton 2014).

In addition, if midwives themselves view childbirth through a 'risk' lens, it negatively influences their perception of birth outside the hospital (Mead and Kornbrot 2004). According to some, the risk discourse has framed childbirth as a dangerous journey (Lupton 1999; Walsh 2006). Childbearing and birth, along with many life events, have been increasingly medicalized, catalyzed when birth moved from the home to the hospital. The 'medical model' continues to present birth as safe retrospectively, with the concept of 'safe' being the delivery of a live mother and baby. Other outcomes such as iatrogenic damage and the experience of childbirth are frequently discounted. Schiller (2015) and Hill (2015) highlight the fact that a live baby is not 'all that matters', as is often suggested when women feel traumatized following childbirth.

The media report risk in a way that focuses on severity or potential harm, rather than on probability (Symon 2006; Coxon 2012; Rogers et al 2012). They look for a headline to attract readers, and television programmes such as *One Born Every Minute* do little to instil confidence in women's ability to give birth, with highly edited shots of childbirth scenes giving a sense of drama and chaos (Hill 2015). These influence societal attitudes and women's perceptions of how childbirth is, and they potentially add to the general sense of fear. The word *risk* has negative connotations, a more positive alternative being *chance* (Symon 2006). Women describe feeling concerned and fearful of the forthcoming birth of their baby when labelled 'high risk' during pregnancy (Williams and MacKey 1999).

For all childbearing women, safety is paramount for themselves and their babies. Although it is widely accepted that the recognition of potential risks and avoidance of harm is a good thing in healthcare, Dahlen describes the focus on risk in maternity services as a contributor to the fear in childbirth and highlights the difference between managing risk and facilitating safety (Dahlen 2014). If maternity care is centred on risk avoidance, with an absence of acknowledgement of social and spiritual perspectives, anxiety replaces joy, and safety may be compromised (Dahlen 2014). As mentioned previously, a woman may feel safer in her own surroundings at home, even though 'risks' of complications have been explained. When these important aspects of safety are ignored, women report feeling threatened and make choices that potentially increase risk – for example, *freebirthing* (Dahlen 2014). When midwives articulate and facilitate choice, they should consider Dahlen's (2012a) proposal to 'dance in the grey zone' between normality and risk. This can be achieved by being alert and responsive while facilitating the joy of childbirth (Dahlen 2012a). Building partnerships with women shares responsibility and builds trust, and it results in positive outcomes for mothers and babies (Dahlen 2014). Replacing care focused on systems and processes with relationship-based care and using the concept of 'safety' instead of 'risk' could make maternity care safer for women, healthcare workers and organizations (Dahlen 2014). Dahlen and Gutteridge (2015: 100) suggest that it is time to bring joy back into maternity care and to begin by seeing 'women as being full of capacity not full of catastrophe'.

Human rights and birth choice

In her chapter on human rights and childbirth, lawyer Elizabeth Prochaska suggests that by focusing on dignity as a guiding principle, maternity care providers can maximize the potential for delivering respectful, compassionate care that values the individuality of each woman and her choices (Prochaska 2015). When women are expected to comply with rigid clinical guidelines, protocols or power structures within health services, their care becomes depersonalized.

Even if armed with the best information, women will not always be in a position to make choices or be 'allowed' to follow their preferences. Conveyer-belt care, where the ultimate goal is to produce a live baby without the risk of litigation, leads to defensive practice (Symon 2000).

Maternity care workers must always consider the human rights of the mother, and that she is not merely a container or 'vessel' to carry her baby (Prochaska 2015; Hill 2015; Schiller 2015).

A woman's experience of childbirth is an important outcome of labour and birth (Hill 2015; McLachlan et al 2015). There is compelling evidence that continuity models of midwifery care are associated with higher satisfaction levels (McLachlan et al 2015) and improved outcomes for women and their babies (Sandall et al 2013), including those experiencing social disadvantage (Rayment-Jones et al 2015). When this is not available, some women choose to employ an independent midwife to ensure continuity, and others would rather give birth unattended (freebirth) rather than fight for the type of birth experience they want (Dahlen 2012b). Other women (or partners) choose a doula to help them negotiate the childbirth journey, for many reasons. Doulas are birth companions employed to provide emotional and practical support to women and families from pregnancy, during birth, and through to the postnatal period, and they should complement the midwife–mother relationship (McMahon 2015).

Facilitating choice: what can the midwife do?

Continuity of midwifery care by one or two midwives maximizes the potential for individualized decision making. However, all maternity services should provide evidence-based written information to help childbearing women make the best decision for themselves and their babies, and some organizations are using technology to support the process, such as smartphone applications. Although these are helpful, verbal discussions between all involved in the woman's maternity journey are essential. Indeed, the 2015 *Montgomery* v. *Lanarkshire* ruling of the United Kingdom Supreme Court states clearly that health professionals must impart information in a way that is understandable, to enable appropriate consent.

To support midwives and doctors to facilitate information sharing in a user-friendly way, NICE (2012a and b) has developed a guide to providing generic patient information on how best to frame risks and benefits. This guidance directs practitioners to use pictograms and animations to help with understanding the evidence.

Midwives can also direct women to other reliable resources, such as the *Baby Buddy* smartphone application (app) (Best Beginnings 2015). This app is free of charge and is endorsed by the Royal College of Midwives. It provides information about the benefits and risks of many interventions and pathways during childbirth and the early years, in a way that is easily accessed and attractive to service users, especially younger mothers. The NHS (2015) also provides information via the World Wide Web.

In relation to choice in place of birth, NICE (2014) has developed a detailed resource for midwives with helpful information charts. It is important that midwives know about reliable sources of information to signpost women and families to help them to decide where to give birth. Which? (2015) provides a useful interactive Web-based tool, and Coxon (2014) has developed an attractive and easy-to-use evidence-based "Birth Place Decisions" document that can be downloaded from the Internet.

Other resources that the midwife can use are included in Boxes 34.2–34.4, and these will assist in day-to-day practice.

Box 34.2 Recommendation 1.5.24: patient experience in adult NHS services

Use the following principles when discussing risks and benefits with a patient:

- Personalize risks and benefits as far as possible.
- Use absolute risk rather than relative risk (e.g. 'the risk of the event increases from 1 in 1000 to 2 in 1000', rather than 'the risk of the event doubles').
- Use natural frequency (e.g. 10 in 100) rather than a percentage (e.g. 10%).
- Be consistent in the use of data (e.g. use the same denominator when comparing risk: 7 in 100 for one risk and 20 in 100 for another, rather than 1 in 14 and 1 in 5).

- Present a risk over a defined period of time (months or years) if appropriate (e.g. 'if 100 people are treated for 1 year, 10 will experience a given side effect').
- Include both positive and negative framing (e.g. 'treatment will be successful for 97 out of 100 patients and unsuccessful for 3 out of 100 patients').
  - Be aware that different people interpret terms such as *rare, unusual* and *common* in different ways, and use numerical data if available.
- Think about using a mixture of numerical and pictorial formats (e.g. numerical rates and pictograms)

Source: NICE 2012a and b

Box 34.3 CHOICE mnemonic

CHOICE top tips for maternity care workers:

Culture – Think about the culture in your maternity service; is it supportive and empowering, or is it fearful and restricting? If it is the latter, discuss with your supervisor of midwives, and put your concerns in writing. Always consider each woman's cultural background – 'safety' is much more than managing risk.

Human rights – Maternity care must be based on compassion and respect; it must promote and protect each woman's human rights and her right to make fully informed and autonomous decisions about her body and her baby. Control, whether to keep it or pass it on for a while, is a human right.

Opinion – Should only be offered if requested, and should be delivered with caution. Should not be biased or scaremongering. Use non-threatening language; try to use words that focus on 'wellness' rather than 'risk'.

Individual – See each woman this way, and use population data as a 'guide' not as a definitive rule. Each woman

has her own back story and reasons for choosing a particular path of care. Perceptions of 'risk' are individual too; what may be acceptable to one woman may be an enormous concern to another.

Courage – Remember why you came to do the work you do, and hold woman-centred principles at the heart of everything you do. Try to influence others by example, and remember that not speaking up is another form of colluding. Look after yourself! It is not easy to be courageous. Seek positive support to help you.

Evidence – Accessing and understanding reliable research findings is not always straightforward, and even the best research does not always help. Do you know how to critique research papers? Do you understand the importance of articulating evidence? How are your clinical guidelines developed and used in your service? How can you influence? Print off the fabulous *aide-memoire* from NICE (see Box 34.2) and keep it in your pocket – use when discussing choices with women.

© Sheena Byrom 2015

Box 34.4 Practice points – choices

- Reflect on your beliefs and knowledge, and consider how they may influence the way you provide information to facilitate decision making.
- Observe conversations between professionals and women using the service. How is choice communicated? What language is used? How are childbearing women included in the discussion? Do they have time to ask questions, and if so, what questions do they ask?
- Familiarize yourself with and use Kirstie Coxon's (2014) resource, the Which? (2015) toolkit and the NICE intrapartum guideline (2014) resource for midwives.

- Use the NICE (2012a and b) guidance on patient information (Box 34.2) aide-memoire to help you to articulate evidence in a nonbiased way.
- Use the CHOICE mnemonic (Box 34.3) to help you to focus on the important aspects of choice in childbirth.
- Check out websites such as Understanding Uncertainty to help you to understand the different ways of framing risks and benefits (http://understandinguncertainty.org).

CONCLUSION

Midwives have a responsibility to develop confidence and skills in having women- and family-centred conversations about the choices available throughout maternity services – evidence-informed conversations that respect the rights of women and families to make truly informed choices about the care they receive. Using tools that have been developed (see NICE (2012a and b) recommendations in Box 34.4, the CHOICE mnemonic in Box 34.3 and the NICE (2014) *Choosing Place of Birth: Resource for Midwives*) to guide approaches to choice facilitation can help. Improving continuity of care and investing in models of midwifery that enhance it are vital in future maternity services. However, more effort is also required to drive a cultural shift to address fear within maternity services, childbearing women and society more generally. This can only be achieved by engaging with the media, becoming involved in politics and working closely with childbearing families. Additionally, developing services that offer an appropriate range of choices for place of birth and models of midwifery care is essential if services are to meet the needs of all childbearing women and families.

Key Points

- The concept of 'choice' around place of birth is complex; women are influenced by a wide range of social, medical, historical and cultural factors.
- Information giving by midwives is influenced by personal perspectives, clinical guidance, organizational cultures and dominant obstetric ideologies around birth.
- Clinical guidelines provide guidance for women and their caregivers, and they should not be mistaken with policies and protocols.
- Hospital birth for healthy women not expecting complications increases the risk of unnecessary medical intervention.
- Whether birth takes place at home or in hospital, the experience should be positive and empowering for both mother and midwife.

References

American Sociological Association (ASA): TV's subliminal influence on women's perception of pregnancy and birth, *Science Daily* (website). www.sciencedaily.com/releases/2015/08/150822154852.htm. 2015.

Beech B: Challenging the medicalisation of birth, *AIMS Journal* 23(2). (website).

http://aims.org.uk/Journal/Vol23No2/challengingmedicalisation.htm. 2011.

Best Beginnings: *Baby buddy app* (website). www.bestbeginnings.org.uk/babybuddy. 2015.

BirthChoiceUK: *Home birth rates for England and Wales 1961 to 2012* (website). www.birthchoiceuk.com/Professionals/BirthChoiceUKFrame

.htm?http://www.birthchoiceuk.com/Professionals/MainIndex.htm. 2014.

Byrom S, Byrom A: Social media: connecting women and midwives globally, *MIDIRS Midwifery Digest* 24(2):141–149, 2014.

Cheyne H, Critchley A, Elders A, et al: *Having a baby in Scotland 2015: listening to mothers.* The Scottish

Government (website). www.gov.scot/Resource/0049/00490953.pdf. 2015.

Comptroller and Audit General: *Maternity services in England, session 2013–14, HC 794*, London, National Audit Office. Available at: https://www.nao.org.uk/wp-content/uploads/2013/11/10259-001-Maternity-Services-Book-1.pdf. 2013.

Cook K, Loomis C: The impact of choice and control on women's childbirth experiences, *J Perinat Educ* 21(3):158–168, 2012.

Coxon K: Making evidence about risks and benefits available to parents, *Perspective – NCT's journal on preparing parents for birth and early parenthood* 16 (website). http://ow.ly/Qpj9Q. 2012.

Coxon K: *Birth place decisions: information for women and partners on planning where to give birth* (website). www.nhs.uk/Conditions/pregnancy-and-baby/Documents/Birth_place_decision_support_Generic_2_.pdf. 2014.

Coxon K: How does place of birth influence planned birth setting in subsequent pregnancies?, *Midwives* 18:35–36, 2015.

Coxon K, Sandall J, Fulop NJ: To what extent are women free to choose where to give birth? How discourses of risk, blame and responsibility influence birth place decisions, *Health Risk Soc* 16(1):51–67, 2014.

Dahlen H: Undone by fear? Deluded by trust?, *Midwifery* 26:156–162, 2010.

Dahlen H: *Dancing in the grey zone between normality and risk (conference paper)*. Paper presented at the Normal Labour and Birth: 7th International Research Conference, 2012a.

Dahlen H: *Home births: it's time to broaden the focus of the debate* (website). www.hannahdahlen.com.au/articles/home-births-it's-time-to-broaden-the-focus-of-the-debate/. 2012b.

Dahlen H: Managing risk, or facilitating safety?, *Int J Childbirth* 4(2):2014.

Dahlen H, Gutteridge K: Stop the fear and embrace birth. In Byrom S, Downe S, editors: *The roar behind the silence: why kindness, compassion and respect matter in maternity care*, London, Pinter and Martin, 2015.

Department of Health (DH): *Changing childbirth: the report of the Expert Maternity Group (the Cumberlege Report)*, London, HMSO, 1993.

Department of Health (DH): *Maternity matters: choice, access and continuity of care in a safe service*, London, DH, 2007.

Dodwell M, BirthChoiceUK: *Personal communication: Change in numbers of maternity units in England, 2001–2015*, with permission from Rod Gibson Associates Ltd, 2015.

Dodwell M, Gibson R: *An investigation into choice of place of birth*, London, NCT, 2009.

Edwards NP: *Birthing autonomy: women's experiences of planning home birth*, Abingdon, Routledge, 2005.

European Court of Human Rights (ECHR): *Case of Ternovsky v. Hungary Strasbourg* (website). http://hudoc.echr.coe.int/eng?i=001-102254#{"itemid":["001-102254"]}. 2011.

Furber CM, Thomson AM: The power of language: a secondary analysis of a qualitative study exploring English midwives' support of mother's baby-feeding practice, *Midwifery* 26(2):232–240, 2010.

Garcia J, Redshaw M, Fitzsimons B, et al: *First class delivery: Audit Commission Report on the maternity services. Part 1*. National Perinatal Epidemiology Unit, Oxford, 1998.

Geddes L: *Does the NCT tell women the truth about birth?* (website). www.lindageddes.com/123/does-the-nct-tell-women-the-truth-about-birth_2013. 2013.

Glasser W: *Take charge of your life: how to get what you need with choice-theory psychology*, Bloomington, iUniverse, 2013.

Hallam JL, Howard CD, Locke A, et al: Communicating choice: an exploration of mothers' experiences of birth, *J Reprod Infant Psychol* 45(3):300–307, 2016.

Hill M: *A healthy baby is not ALL that matters* (website). www.positivebirthmovement.org/pbm-blog/a-healthy-baby-is-not-all-that-matters_2015. 2015.

Hollowell J: *Birthplace programme overview: background, component studies and summary of findings. Birthplace in England research programme. Final report part 1*, NIHR Health Services Delivery and Organisation Programme, London, National Institute for Health Research, 2011.

Hundley V, Ryan M, Graham W: Assessing women's preferences for intrapartum care, *Birth* 28:254–263, 2001.

Kirkham M: *Informed choice in maternity care*, London, McMillan, 2004.

Kirkham M, Stapleton H, editors: *Informed choice in maternity care: An evaluation of evidence based leaflets*, York, NHS Centre for Reviews and Dissemination, 2001.

Knightly R: Delivering choice: where to birth, *Br J Midwifery* 15(8):475–478, 2007.

Lavender T, Chapple J: How women choose to give birth, *Pract Midwife* 8(7):10–15, 2005.

Levy V: How midwives used protective steering to protect informed choice in pregnancy. In Kirkham M, editor: *Informed choice in maternity care*, London, McMillan, 2004.

Lokugamage A, Bourne T: They don't know what they don't know. In Byrom S, Downe S, editors: *The roar behind the silence: why kindness compassion and respect matter in maternity care*, London, Pinter and Martin, 2015.

Lupton D: Risk and the ontology of pregnant embodiment. In Lupton D, editor: *Risk and sociocultural theory*, Cambridge, Cambridge University Press, 1999.

Madi BC, Crow R: A qualitative study of information about available options for childbirth venue and pregnant women's preference for a place of delivery, *Midwifery* 19(4):328–336, 2003.

Malcrida C, Boulton T: The best laid plans? Women's choices, expectations and experiences in childbirth, *Health (London)* 18(1):41–59, 2014.

McCann P, Boulter D, Devine B: *Stakeholder engagement. Community Maternity Services Project. Report of the findings from online surveys of women, midwives, general practitioners and obstetricians, June–September 2014*, Belfast, Community Maternity Services, 2015.

McLachlan HL, Forster DA, Davey M-A, et al: The effect of primary midwife-led care on women's experience of childbirth: results from the COSMOS randomised controlled trial, *Br J Obstet Gynaecol* 2015.

McMahon M: *Why doulas matter*, London, Pinter and Martin, 2015.

Mead MMP, Kornbrot DE: The influence of maternity units' intrapartum intervention rates and midwives' risk perception for women suitable for midwifery-led care, *Midwifery* 20(1):61–71, 2004.

Ministry of Health: *Domiciliary midwifery and maternity bed needs: the Report of the Standing Maternity and Midwifery Advisory Committee (Sub-committee Chairman J. Peel)*, London, HMSO, 1970.

Montgomery v. Lanarkshire, United Kingdom Supreme Court (UKSC): *Summary Judgement 11*. http://bit .ly/1gb5Zyl. 2015.

National Clinical Guideline Centre: *Patient experience in adult NHS services: improving the experience of care for people using adult NHS services*. Clinical Guidelines CG138. London, National Clinical Guideline Centre at the Royal College of Physicians, 2012a.

National Federation of Women's Institutes (NFWI): *Support overdue: women's experiences of maternity services* (website). www.thewi.org .uk/__data/assets/pdf_file/0006/ 49857/support-overdue-final-15 -may-2013.pdf. 2013.

National Health Service (NHS): *NHS choices: your health your choice. Pregnancy and baby.* (website). www .nhs.uk/conditions/pregnancy-and -baby/pages/birth-plan.aspx#close. 2015.

National Institute for Health and Care Excellence (NICE): *Patient experience in adult NHS services: improving the experience of care for people using adult NHS services* (website). www .nice.org.uk/guidance/cg138. 2012b.

National Institute for Health and Care Excellence (NICE): *Intrapartum care: care of healthy women and their babies during childbirth* (website). www .nice.org.uk/guidance/cg190_2014. 2014.

National Perinatal Epidemiology Unit (NPEU): *The Birthplace cohort study: key findings*. Birthplace in England Research Programme (website). www.npeu.ox.ac.uk/birthplace/ results. 2011.

Newburn M, Byrom S, Rocca-Ihenacho L, et al: *Evidence of clinical effectiveness. Midwifery Unit Network – policy research briefing 2* (website). www.mid wiferyunitnetwork.com. 2015.

Nolan M: Information giving and education in pregnancy: a review of qualitative studies, *J Perinat Educ* 18(4):21–30, 2009.

Office for National Statistics: *Characteristics of birth 2, England and Wales, 2012*, References tables – Table 8: Maternities: place of birth and whether area of occurrence is the same as area of usual residence, or other than area of usual residence. London, 2013, ONS. Available at: http://www.ons.gov.uk/ ons/rel/vsob1/characteristics-of- birth-2--england-and-wales/2012/ rft-characteristics-of-birth-2.xls. 2012.

Office for National Statistics (ONS): *Births in England and Wales by characteristics of birth 2, 2013* (website). www.ons.gov.uk/ons/ rel/vsob1/characteristics-of-birth -2--england-and-wales/2013/sb -characteristics-of-birth-2.html. 2014.

Office for National Statistics (ONS): *Birth characteristics in England and Wales*, London, 2015, ONS, p 2016.

Prochaska E: Dignity in maternity: the power of human rights to improve care for childbearing women. In Byrom S, Downe S, editors: *The roar behind the silence: why kindness compassion and respect matter in maternity care*, London, Pinter and Martin, 2015.

Rayment-Jones H, Murrells T, Sandall J: An investigation of the relationship between the caseload model of midwifery for socially disadvantaged women and childbirth outcomes using routine data - a retrospective study, *Midwifery* 31(4):409–417, 2015.

Redshaw M, Heikkila K: *Delivered with care: a national survey of women's experience of maternity care in England*, Oxford, NPEU, 2010.

Renfrew MJ, Homer C, Downe S, et al: Midwifery: an executive summary for the *Lancet's Series* (website). www.thelancet.com/pb/assets/raw/ lancet/stories/series/midwifery/ midwifery_exec_summ.pdf. 2014.

Rogers C, Yearley C, Littlehales C: The Birthplace study: turning the tide of childbirth, *Br J Midwifery* 20(1):28– 33, 2012.

Sandall J: *Place of birth in Europe, birth in Europe in the 21st century*, Entre Nous, The European Magazine for Sexual and Reproductive Health *81*, WHO Europe (website). www.euro.who.int/entrenous. 2015.

Sandall J, et al: Midwife led models of midwifery care for childbearing women and other models of care for childbearing women, *Cochrane Database Syst Rev* (8):CD004667, 2013.

Sandall J, Murrells T, Dodwell M, et al: The efficient use of the maternity workforce and the implications for safety and quality in maternity care: a population-based, cross-sectional study, *Health Serv and Del Res* 2(38):2014.

Scamell M: 'She can't come here!' Ethics and the case of birth centre admission policy in the UK, *J Med Ethics* 40(12):813–816, 2014.

Schiller R: *All that matters: women's rights in childbirth*. Guardian Shorts (website). http://guardianshorts .com. 2015.

Schiller R: *Dubska ECHR judgment: disappointing but not the last word, birthrights*. http://www.birthrights. org.uk/category/legal-cases/. 2016.

Schroeder L, Petrou S, Patel N, et al: *Birthplace cost-effectiveness analysis of planned place of birth: individual level analysis. Birthplace in England research programme. Final report part 5, NIHR Service Delivery and Organisation Programme*, London, National Institute for Health Research, 2011.

Spoel P: *The meaning and ethics of informed choice in Canadian midwifery*. Laurentian University, Canada (website). www.persons.org .uk/mso/hid/hid3/spoel%20paper .pdf. 2004.

Symon A: Litigation and defensive clinical practice: quantifying the problem, *Midwifery* 16(1):8–14, 2000.

Symon A: *Risk and choice in maternity: an international perspective*, London, Elsevier, 2006.

Walsh D: Risk and normality in maternity care: revisioning risk for normal childbirth. In Symon A, editor: *Risk and choice in maternity care*, London, Elsevier, 2006.

Which?: *Birth choice: find the right place for you to give birth* (website). www .which.co.uk/birth-choice/. 2015.

Williams S, MacKey M: Women's experience of preterm labour: a feminist critique, *Health Care Women Int* 20:29–48, 1999.

Wolfson C: Midwives and home birth: social, medical and legal perspectives, *Hastings Law J* 909:57, 1986.

Resources and additional reading

Byrom S, Downe S: *The roar behind the silence: why kindness, compassion and respect matter in maternity care*, London, Pinter and Martin, 2015.

This book is focussed on kindness and compassion, and it includes chapters from leading midwives and researchers in maternity care.

McCourt C, Rance S, Rayment J, et al: *Birthplace qualitative organisational case studies: how maternity care systems may affect the provision of care in different birth settings. Birthplace in England Research Programme. Final report part 6. NIHR Service Delivery and Organisation Programme*, London, National Institute for Health Research, 2011.

This website includes orginal and continuing information and resources from the Birthplace in England Research Programme.

National Institute for Health and Care Excellence (NICE): *Intrapartum care: care of healthy women and their babies during childbirth* (website). www.nice.org.uk/guidance/cg190_2014. 2014.

Offers a full range of information, evidence and tools to assist in providing choice to women and families.

Rogers J, Barber T, Marsh S, et al: *Birth Place Choices (BPC) project* (website). www.uhs.nhs.uk/Media/SUHT Internet/Services/ObsMidwifery Gynae/BirthPlaceChoice/Birth ChoiceProjectFinalReport.pdf. 2006.

Report from a 2005 project supported by the Department of Health.

Schiller R: *All that matters*, The Guardian Short book, 2015.

This book examines women's rights in childbirth, setting birth in context amid the struggle for reproductive rights across the world.

Symon A: *Risk and choice in maternity: an international perspective*, London, Elsevier, 2006.

This book explores the changing reality of risk management in maternity care and highlights some of the difficulties encountered in offering or exercising choice.

Wilks J: *Choices in pregnancy and childbirth*, London, Singing Dragon, 2015.

Interesting book that provides evidence and research to underpin a positive pregnancy and birth experience.

Useful websites:

AIMS: http://www.aims.org.uk.

Association of Radical Midwives: http://www.midwifery.org.uk.

Choices in Childbirth: https://choicesin childbirth.org.

Midwives for Choice http://midwives forchoice.ie.

The Positive Birth Movement http://www.positivebirthmovement.org.

Tell Me a Good Birth Story: http://tellmeagoodbirthstory.com.

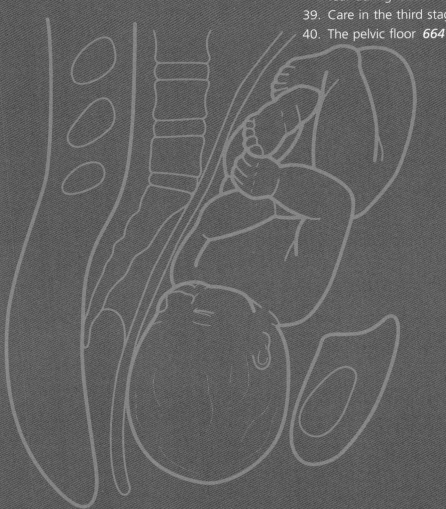

Part Six

Labour and birth

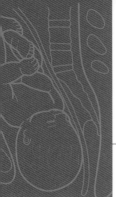

Chapter 35

Physiological changes from late pregnancy until the onset of lactation: from nesting to suckling-lactation and parent-infant attachment

Mary McNabb

Learning Outcomes ?

After reading this chapter, you will be able to:

- identify synchronized brain transformations in mothers and fathers during pregnancy and after birth
- understand maternal–feto-placental neurohormonal interactions that coordinate maturation of fetal organ systems with maternal uterine and brain alterations in preparation for labour, birth and lactation
- recognize key hormonal interactions that regulate the shift from uterine quiescence to nocturnal myometrial activation
- understand why mothers need a safe place with a trusted companion for labour and birth
- identify the significance of undisturbed maternal–infant and paternal–infant attachment following birth

INTRODUCTION

By nature, humans are highly sociable. From early life, the number and quality of intimate social connections play a critical role in promoting physical and mental well-being (Holt-Lunstad et al 2010). Humans typically have one or more long-lasing sexual partners during the reproductive life span and belong to complex social networks that incorporate siblings, parents, extended family, friends, community groups and pets. From an evolutionary perspective, loving relationships and successful participation and cooperation in a variety of social networks across generations seems to make a substantial contribution to the development of cognitive abilities, empathy, emotionality, language and creativity (Neumann 2009; Carter 2014).

Across the life span, relationships that have the greatest significance for long-term health and well-being are those between sexual partners, mother and child. There is extensive research on the enduring effects of loving couple interactions on physical and emotional health, and a large body of evidence shows that infants totally depend on intimate attachment to their mothers following birth to maintain mutual homeostatic regulation of essential physiological functions and brain and neuroendocrine developments that began during uterine life (Hofer 2006; Light et al 2005; Van Leeuwen et al 2009; Van Puyvelde et al 2015; Zheng et al 2014). The quality and duration of maternal care experienced during this critical period of development shape adult social behaviour, through altered patterns of gene expression following birth (Champagne 2008; Feldman et al 2010). In female infants, the quality of maternal sensory interactions regulates the level of central oestrogen receptors that is maintained into adult life, and these determine the level of expression of brain oxytocin receptors that mediate their own capacity for mothering (Champagne 2008).

In keeping with this high level of sociality, humans typically provide biparental care and protection for their infants and young children, with help from extended family members. Recent experimental studies have begun to reveal that couples experience synchronized neurohormonal changes during and after pregnancy, and extensive transformations occur in neural networks and central hormonal receptor concentrations of mothers and fathers as a result of their contact with each other and their infant- and child-care experiences (Abraham et al 2014; Conde and Figueiredo 2014; Gettler et al 2011; Gordon et al 2010a and 2010b; Leuner et al 2010). Current research findings have revealed a high degree of overlap in the brain transformations and neurohormonal changes that mediate the emergence and development of maternal and paternal behaviours (Perea-Rodriguez et al 2015). Human and animal studies on the impact of paternal care, on long-term health and development of offspring, have shown extensive sex-specific effects of early paternal involvement on cognitive, emotional, social and parenting capacities during the adult lives of the offspring (Bales and Saltzman 2016; Tabak et al 2015).

The chapter explores the neurohormonal basis of maternal emotional and cognitive changes that become increasingly apparent during the latter half of pregnancy. The hormonal and intracellular regulation of myometrial quiescence; synchronization of maternal–fetal cardiorespiratory systems and regulation of fetal circadian rhythms by maternal melatonin are examined. The chapter continues with hormonal regulation of the circadian onset of increasingly synchronized uterine contractions from around 24 to 30 weeks gestation and the rise in maternal pain threshold from late pregnancy until 24 hours following birth (Germain et al 1993; Gintzler and Liu 2001; Smith et al 2015). The significance of maternal sleep during late pregnancy; fetal maturational changes in preparation for labour and the role of the fetal-adreno-placental system and fetal lung maturation in regulating the shift from pregnancy to labour (Mendelson 2009; Smith 2007); and the changes in central and peripheral oxytocin systems in preparation for labour, birth, maternal–infant interactions and lactation are described.

After identifying maternal and feto-placental regulators of the shift from pregnancy to labour, the chapter elaborates the dynamic process of uterine activation, progressive transformations in the cervix and fetal membranes and the intracellular processes involved. The environmental influences and patterns of care that optimize the circadian rhythm of labour; pulsatile release of maternal oxytocin; fetal neurohormonal responses to the physiological stress of labour; spontaneous birth of the baby and the process of placental separation, the onset of tonic uterine contractions and hemostasis will be brought together, concluding with the physiological shift from intra-uterine to extrauterine dependence and the neurohormonal basis of maternal behaviour and maternal–infant attachment.

MATERNAL AUTONOMIC AND NEUROENDOCRINE ADAPTATIONS

The first half of pregnancy and lactation are characterized by a low ratio of sympathetic to parasympathetic activity, reflecting greater vagal activation during embryo formation, early feto-placental development and maternal–infant attachment. From early pregnancy onward, the hypothalamic–pituitary–adrenal (HPA) axis also becomes increasingly hyporesponsive to a variety of physical and emotional stressors (Bosch et al 2004; Brunton et al 2005; Douglas 2011; Groer et al 2002; Kammerer et al 2002; Levy et al 2004;

Terenzi and Ingram 2005). During late pregnancy and lactation, brain alterations in neuropeptide and steroid interactions serve to heighten emotional sensitivities and enhance women's capacity to form trusting relationships and intimate social bonds (Kinsley et al 1999; Kim et al 2010; Kosfelt et al 2005; Leng et al 2008; Neumann 2009; Pearson et al 2009; Uvnas Moberg 2013). In late pregnancy, anxiety behaviours in response to stressful stimuli are attenuated by central oxytocin and prolactin, whereas aggressive defensive behaviours and reduced fearfulness in response to perceived threats to the fetus and neonate increase from late pregnancy to advanced labour and peak during lactation (Kinsley 2008; Neumann 2009). Several neurotransmitters and neuropeptides are implicated in regulating maternal aggression, including local release of oxytocin within selected areas of the hypothalamus during and after birth (Brunton and Russell 2008; Neumann 2009; Russell and Brunton 2009).

In late pregnancy, responsiveness of the HPA axis is increasingly attenuated, whereas sympathetic activation gradually increases and peaks during active labour and birth (Di Pietro et al 2012). Over the last 6 weeks of pregnancy, women experience significant emotional and cognitive changes associated with 'nesting' and other signs of the emergence of maternal responsiveness and affiliation, and women often experience periods of heightened apprehension relating to fetal and neonatal well-being (Brunton and Russell 2008; Douglas 2011; Douglas et al 2005; Grattan 2002; Kask et al 2008; Neumann 2009; Russell and Brunton 2006).

Prolactin – maternal stress and anxiety

In humans, levels of prolactin and human placental lactogen (hPL) rise throughout pregnancy. During advanced labour, prolactin levels decline rapidly but rise again soon after birth (see chapter website resources). Following placental separation, hPL disappears from the maternal circulation, but suckling stimulates ongoing prolactin secretion that peaks within the first 3 months of lactation (Diaz et al 1989; Grattan 2002). In the brain, prolactin initiates key elements in the repertoire of behaviours involved in nest-building during late pregnancy and nurturing, protecting and nourishing the infant during lactation (Lucas et al 1998): reduction of maternal fearfulness and anxiety and reduced stress responsiveness during pregnancy and lactation (see chapter website resources).

Regulation of myometrial quiescence

Various factors regulate uterine quiescence until the end of pregnancy, particularly *progesterone, human chorionic gonadotrophin (hCG), corticotropin-releasing hormone (CRH), relaxin, nitric oxide* and *melatonin*. These hormonal influences interact with alterations in myocytes from early pregnancy and depress the formation of *gap junctions*

563

between individual cells that ensure low frequency of cell-to-cell communication (Garfield et al 1995; Shynlova et al 2009). Towards the end of pregnancy, localized myometrial contractions occur spontaneously in response to uterine distension, when uterine growth declines relative to the fetus (Shynlova et al 2009). This increases uterine wall stretch, facilitating a prelabour rise in myometrial oxytocin receptors, and melatonin receptor expression declines relative to non-pregnant values, attenuating its suppressive effects on myometrial oxytocin receptors. At the same time, a shift occurs in the ratio of placental oestrogens of maternal and fetal origin, particularly during the hours of darkness (Hedriana et al 2001; McGregor et al 1997; Smith et al 2009). This activates oestrogen receptors, which stimulates the increased expression of gap-junction and contractile proteins between myocytes (Fetalvero et al 2008; Smith et al 2015; Terzidou et al 2005).

Myometrial quiescence – placental steroids

Plasma concentrations of oestrogens and progesterone increase progressively throughout pregnancy and labour, but target tissue responsiveness is controlled by changes in expression and activation of their nuclear and non-nuclear receptor subtypes and by pregnancy-induced expression of progesterone metabolites, which maintain uterine quiescence by binding directly to membrane-bound receptors and inhibiting signalling pathways (Condon et al 2003; Dong et al 2009; Mesiano et al 2002; Mesiano and Welsh 2007; Sheehan et al 2005; Smith et al 2009). The capacity of steroid and peptide hormones to maintain uterine quiescence is also enhanced by functional inactivation of autonomic innervation in the myometrium and by increased receptors for peptides and neurotransmitters that promote relaxation and inhibit the contractile effects of oxytocin (Brauer and Smith 2015; Casey et al 1997; Dong et al 2003; Ferguson et al 1998; Grammatopoulos et al 1996; Price and Lopes Bernal 2001).

Changing balance of placental steroid hormone receptors

Circulating levels of oestrogens and progesterone increase throughout pregnancy, but myometrial excitability in response to oestrogens is inactivated by subtle interactions between their receptor subtypes and by antioestrogenic effects of the low ratio of oestriol to oestradiol that persists until the end of pregnancy, when changes occur in progesterone receptor subtypes that weaken its capacity to inhibit the formation of gap junctions between myocytes (see chapter website resources).

Myometrial quiescence – placenta and fetal membranes

During pregnancy, spontaneous oxytocin and prostaglandin-induced myometrial contractions are inhibited by the placenta and chorio-amniotic membranes surrounding the uterus. The placenta produces *atrial natriuretic peptide* (ANP), and the chorion and amnion produce *brain natriuretic peptide* (BNP). Both peptides inhibit oxytocin-induced contractions (Carvajal et al 2006 and 2009; Cootauco et al 2008). These are ideally positioned to protect the fetus from oxytocin and other inflammatory mediators, with the capacity to stimulate myometrial contractility (Keelan et al 2003) (see chapter website resources).

Amnion, chorion and decidua also express enzymes to synthesize and metabolize oestrogens, progesterone (PR), and oxytocin (Blanks et al 2003). Current evidence suggests that the dominance of PR-B is maintained in these tissues until the end of pregnancy, when enzymatic changes stimulate concurrent *increases* in the potent oestrogen oestradiol and more inactive forms of progesterone and reduced interaction between all forms of PR and coregulatory transcription factors (Blanks et al 2003; Dong et al 2009). The feto-placental membranes and maternal decidual tissues therefore establish endocrine–paracrine networks regulating the length of gestation and the onset and progress of labour (Chibbar et al 1995; Cootauco et al 2008; Henderson and Wilson 2001; Ticconi et al 2006).

Circadian rhythms and maternal–fetal synchronization

Maternal circadian cues play a key role in the physiological development of the embryo, fetus and infant. During intra-uterine life, circadian signals are directly relayed from the uterus. These, together with other peripheral organ systems such as the heart, lungs and kidneys, express clock genes that are coordinated by the central clock in the suprachiasmatic nucleus (SCN) in the anterior hypothalamus. Axons of SCN cells project to adjacent hypothalamic neurons, where they synchronize overt circadian rhythms, such as body temperature, sleeping/waking, feeding and release of adrenocorticotropic hormone and cortisol from the pituitary–adrenal connection. Additionally, via a more complex neural route involving central and peripheral sympathetic neurons, the SCN regulates nocturnal production and release of melatonin from the pineal gland (Reiter et al 2014).

Experimental findings on rats have shown that uterine and decidual tissues provide circadian rhythms to the embryo and fetus (Akiyama et al 2010). The human fetus displays 24-hour rhythms in temperature and oxygen consumption by 32 to 33 weeks gestation (Bauer et al 2009). Evidence from studies conducted in humans and non-human primates has also revealed entrained 24-hour rhythms in fetal heart rate and respiratory movements during the latter half of pregnancy (Seron-Ferre et al 2007).

Recent studies on maternal–fetal cardiorespiratory activity from 34 weeks gestation have identified fetal–maternal heart rate synchronization under conditions of spontaneous and controlled maternal breathing. At night, mean hourly fetal heart rate decreases in synchrony with mean maternal heart rate, and synchronization at the beat-to-beat time scale has also been demonstrated, particularly during higher-paced maternal breathing. The underlying mechanisms remain to be discovered, but the authors hypothesize that maternal–fetal cardiac coupling may be mediated by fetal auditory responses to maternal heartbeat, and this synchronization has been shown to continue for the first 2 months following birth (Van Leeuwen et al 2009; Van Puyvelde et al 2015). These findings demonstrate the existence of a dynamic interconnectedness of maternal–fetal/maternal–neonatal integrated physiological systems during fetal and neonatal development.

Circadian rhythms in the myometrium

From mid-pregnancy onward, nocturnal increases in maternal melatonin from the pineal gland are stimulated by an unidentified placental hormone (Tamura et al 2008). Current evidence suggests that oxytocin, oestriol, and melatonin are involved in the emergence of circadian rhythms in myometrial contractility during the third trimester, which orchestrate the gradual transition from pregnancy to labour and the circadian timing of birth. During the third trimester melatonin levels rise significantly during the rest phase of the light–dark cycle. Although uterine melatonin receptor concentrations do not rise until the onset of labour, acute inhibition of endogenous melatonin levels by exposure to light reversibly suppresses nocturnal uterine contractions in late pregnancy (Olcese et al 2013; Olcese and Beesley 2014). Experimental findings suggest that melatonin operates in a number of ways to prepare the myometrium for labour by regulating nocturnal oxytocin release, increasing gap junction formation and synergistically enhancing oxytocin induced contractility while also modulating the increase in myometrial receptors for oxytocin (Sharkey et al 2009; Sharkey and Olcese 2007).

Over the same period, melatonin readily crosses the placenta. Within the fetal compartment melatonin stimulates adrenal growth, modulates cortisol release and together with circadian information from the uterus and decidua, generates a circadian rhythm in the activity of the fetal zone of the adrenal gland and other fetal organ systems (Torres-Farfan et al 2003, 2006 and 2011). This indicates that the fetal adrenal gland becomes a strong peripheral clock that is regulated by maternal melatonin.

The emergence of circadian rhythms in the fetal adrenal gland leads to a nocturnal surge in placental oestriol that mirrors myometrial activity. The dominance of oestradiol during the hours of darkness stimulates oxytocin release, which, along with melatonin, increases myometrial sensitivity to oxytocin (McGregor et al 1997; Murphy Goodwin 1999).

Gestational analgesia

A significant rise in maternal pain threshold occurs between late pregnancy and 24 hours following birth (Gintzler and Liu 2001; Whipple et al 1990). Findings from animal and human studies indicate that maternal pain threshold rises gradually from 30 weeks gestation, accelerates during the last 3 to 4 weeks of pregnancy, rises further during labour and then falls precipitously within 24 hours of birth (Draisci et al 2012; Gintzler and Liu 2001; Ohel et al 2007). Evidence indicates that placental steroids augment pelvic afferent tone. These nerves entering the spinal cord from the cervix and uterus activate multiple analgesic synergies between spinal κ/δ opioid systems, non-opioid peptides and spinal noradrenergic pathways descending from the brainstem (Liu and Gintzler 2003). The opioid effects are further enhanced by a steroid-induced downregulation of spinal opioid-modulating peptides, vasoactive intestinal peptide (VIP) and substance P (Gintzler and Liu 2001). Following the onset of labour, utero-cervical stimulation exerts presynaptic inhibition of primary sensory neurons transmitting painful stimuli that seem to be mediated primarily by noradrenergic and serotoninergic pathways within the spinal cord (Komisaruk and Sansone 2003).

Other findings have shown that melatonin has sedative, hypnotic and analgesic effects that seem to be primarily involved in inhibiting spinal nociception (Ambriz-Tututi et al 2009; Reiter et al 2014). Thus, the placental-induced rise in nocturnal melatonin from late pregnancy until birth may operate in addition to the placental steroid activated rise in spinal nociception that extends from late pregnancy until around 24 hours following birth (Gintzler and Liu 2001). Together these multiple modulatory systems induce a progressive rise in maternal pain threshold from late pregnancy until 12 to 24 hours following birth (see chapter website resources).

Maternal sleep and melatonin

During late pregnancy, women seem to have a greater need for nocturnal sleep. Current evidence suggests that women who do not have 7 to 8 hours of undisturbed nocturnal sleep during the third trimester have a lower pain threshold in early labour and are more likely to require medical interventions because of inefficient uterine activity (Beebe et al 2007; Lee and Gay 2004). Animal experiments have demonstrated an adverse effect of prolonged exposure to light on the fetal SCN resulting in altered circadian rhythms following birth and long-term alterations in glucose metabolism (Ferreira et al 2012). These findings highlight the potential dangers of exposure to constant light, unusual light–dark cycles or night-shift work for women, *especially* during the second half of pregnancy (Reiter et al 2014). Risk factors include night work and light pollution in urban areas. In this increasingly urbanized world, it is becoming increasingly difficult to avoid light exposure at night that is sufficient to alter the function of the biological clock and reduce circulating melatonin levels (Reiter et al 2014).

Studies in healthy non-pregnant adults have also found that work-related sleep restriction, or sleep restriction for one or more days, increases sensitivity to experimentally evoked pain and leads to the development of new onset spontaneous pains (Haack et al 2012; Schestatsky et al 2013). Nocturnal release of maternal melatonin during the latter half of pregnancy seems to be enhanced by creating 'night-like' conditions before bedtime. Research on non-pregnant adults shows that room lighting has a profoundly suppressive effect on the nocturnal release of melatonin and shortens the duration of melatonin release (Gooley et al 2011).

FETAL PREPARATIONS FOR LABOUR

The progressive nocturnal rhythm in uterine activity during the last trimester gradually shifts the fetus towards the lower pole of the uterus, and the presenting part descends into the pelvis. This helps the fetus to increase flexion and descent and to follow the curve of Carus. Activation of the fetal HPA axis during the third trimester produces physiological increases in cortisol, which interacts with other hormones to induce maturational changes in the thyroid axis, lungs, and liver, pancreas, and gut and thermogenic proteins in brown adipose tissue (Freemark 1999; Garbrecht et al 2006; Liggins 1994). In the brain, catecholaminergic neurons have a key role in cortical differentiation and maturation of respiratory neural networks in the brainstem (Fujii et al 2006). Cortisol and adrenaline also stimulate a gradual increase in blood pressure in preparation for pulmonary expansion and cessation of the feto-placental circulation soon after birth (see chapter website resources).

During the last couple of days before the onset of labour, fetal breathing activity is reduced, and production of lung fluid occurs at a gradually decreasing rate (Bland 2001). Fetal breathing may be depressed by endogenous opioids and rising concentrations of prostaglandin E_2 (PGE_2), whereas the decline in lung liquid volume is associated with increased production of cortisol and catecholamines from late pregnancy to birth (Jain and Duddell 2006;

Lagercrantz and Herlenius 2002). It is suggested that the fetal brain is protected from reduced oxygen and glucose supplies around the time of birth by an increase in central oxytocin, beginning just before the onset of labour and peaking around 2 hours before birth (Brown and Grattan 2007). The fetal brain is exposed to elevated levels of oxytocin, which triggers a transient but significant switch of the gamma-amino butyric acid (γ-aminobutyric acid) (GABA) neurotransmitter, from excitatory to inhibitory. This reduces brain requirements for nutrients and oxygen during transition to air-breathing and suckling (Khazipov et al 2008; Tyzio et al 2006). Current evidence suggests that the oxytocin in the fetal brain is derived from both mother and fetus (Khazipov et al 2008).

THE FETAL ADRENO-PLACENTAL 'CLOCK'

The duration of pregnancy is strongly associated with the rising profile of placental CRH in the maternal circulation (Smith 2007; Tyson et al 2009). CRH levels rise exponentially in maternal and fetal circulatory systems during the last 12 weeks of pregnancy, peak during labour, and fall precipitously following birth (Chan et al 1993; Goland et al 1986). In individual women, the exponential increase tends to mirror the duration of pregnancy: women who give birth prematurely have higher mid-pregnancy levels of CRH than those who give birth at term (McLean et al 1995; Smith 2007). The bioavailability of CRH is regulated by a circulating binding protein, which declines at the end of pregnancy, further increasing maternal and fetal tissue exposure to CRH (Grammatopoulos 2008) (Fig. 35.1).

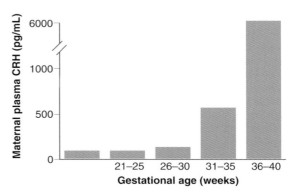

Figure 35.1 Mean plasma corticotropin-releasing hormone (CRH) concentrations in eight women followed sequentially during the second half of pregnancy. (This article was published in Goland RS, Jozak RN, Conwell I: Placental corticotropin-releasing hormone and the hypercortisolism of pregnancy, Am J Obstet Gynecol 171(4):1287–1291, Copyright Elsevier, 1994.)

During pregnancy and labour, placental CRH targets a number of maternal, placental and fetal organ systems. In the fetal compartment, CRH receptors have been identified in the pituitary gland, adrenal cortex, lungs, placenta and membranes (Grammatopoulos 2007 and 2008). In the adrenals, placental CRH directly stimulates the fetal zone to produce DHEA-S and the definitive zone to produce cortisol, in a dose-dependent manner (Jaffe 2001; Rehman et al 2007). The rapid rise in CRH during late pregnancy enhances fetal production of DHEA-S, and this leads to a more rapid rise in placental formation of oestriol over oestradiol, which is largely derived from the maternal adrenal DHEA-S (Smith et al 2009 and 2015). The maternal pituitary–adrenal axis is also a target organ for CRH and the myometrium is both a source and target for CRH and a related family of urocortin peptides (Goland et al 1994; Grammatopoulos 2007; Markovic et al 2007; Smith 2007) (see chapter website resources).

Myometrial actions of placental CRH

During pregnancy, human myometrial cells express a large number of CRH and CRH-related urocortin peptides and their major receptor subtypes CRH-R1 and CRH-R2 (see chapter website resources).

As term approaches, oxytocin and inflammatory cytokines also stimulate expression of many variants of the CRH-R1 receptor with reduced signalling capacities, and the expression of CRH-R1 variants with reduced signalling capacity is increased in the lower uterine segment with the onset of labour (Grammatopoulos and Hillhouse 1999; Hillhouse and Grammatopoulos 2001; Markovic et al 2007).

In contrast to CRH-R1, activation of CRH-R2 stimulates signalling pathways that enhance myometrial contractility. Recent experiments on gene profiles in different regions of the uterus have identified expression of fundal genes for CRH-R2 that increase significantly during labour (Grammatopoulos 2008; Stevens and Challis 1998). These findings indicate that dynamic changes in the balance of myometrial CRH-R1 receptor subtypes at term stimulate concomitant physiological changes in the fundus and lower uterine segment from late pregnancy to birth. Whereas muscles in the upper segment generate coordinated forceful contractions, those in the lower segment have reduced stimulatory influences, and this contrast facilitates increased contractility of the fundus, elongation of the lower segment over the presenting part, and progressive cervical dilation as labour advances (Bukowski et al 2006).

CRH activity in placenta and membranes

The placenta and membranes also express two major CRH receptor subtypes: *CRH-R1* and *CRH-R2*. In the placenta, the CRH-R1 subtype seems to increase expression of *type 2 cyclo-oxygenase* (COX-2), which stimulates biosynthesis of prostaglandin precursors and decreases expression of *prostaglandin dehydrogenase* (PGDH) – the key enzyme produced by the placenta and membranes that metabolizes active primary prostaglandins to an inactive form and inhibits production of progesterone (Amash et al 2009; Gao et al 2008; Grammatopoulos 2008) (see chapter website resources).

NEUROENDOCRINE AND CENTRAL OXYTOCIN SYSTEMS FROM LATE PREGNANCY

In pregnancy, magnocellular oxytocin neurons in the supraoptic nucleus (SON) and paraventricular nucleus (PVN) are restrained from premature activation to prevent preterm labour and preserve accumulating oxytocin stores in the neurohypophysis in preparation for labour, birth and the onset of lactation (Higuchi and Okere 2002; Russell and Brunton 2006 and 2009; Russell et al 2003). The secretory response of magnocellular neurons to various physiological stimuli are progressively restrained at several levels by opioid systems, which are largely stimulated by allopregnanolone – a neurosteroid metabolite of progesterone (Brunton and Russell 2008; Higuchi and Okere 2002; Russell and Brunton 2009). In late pregnancy, brainstem and forebrain neuronal projections to the SON and PVN are activated in preparation for labour, birth, the induction of maternal behaviours and lactation (de Kock et al 2003; Douglas et al 2002; Ortiz-Miranda et al 2005; Russell et al 2003) (see chapter website resources).

Central oxytocin

Two distinct and independently regulated oxytocin systems exist within the brain that are highly activated during the peripartum period. Parvocellular neurons act as neurotransmitters within PVN neurons that project to the forebrain, limbic system and autonomic centres in the brainstem and spinal cord (Neumann 2009; Russell and Brunton 2009). Oxytocin is also released in much larger quantities from soma and dendrites of magnocellular neurons within the SON, PVN and other associated nuclei throughout labour and lactation (Leng et al 2008; Russell et al 2003) (see chapter website resources).

Central oxytocin receptors

In experimental studies dramatic changes have been identified in the expression of oxytocin receptor mRNA over the peripartum period in key areas relating to neural regulation of uterine contractions during labour, control of maternal heart rate, pain perception and the initiation and intensity of maternal behaviours and lactation (Ingram and Wakerley 1993; Ingram et al 1995; Insel 1990; Leng et al 2008; Levy et al 2004; Meddle et al 2007; Terenzi and Ingram 2005; Wilson and Ingram 2003). In the bed nucleus of the stria terminalis (BNST) and the ventrolateral septum, responsiveness to oxytocin increases from late pregnancy to early lactation, and receptor concentrations in the BNST increase by 40% between day 15 of pregnancy and the first 6 days postpartum (Insel 1990). Relative to the non-pregnant state, oxytocin receptors are elevated in the medial preoptic area and the ventrolateral septum in late pregnancy; peak concentrations have been measured in the SON and brainstem regions during labour and birth; and those in the ventromedial nucleus and the amygdala increase during labour and lactation (Bealer et al 2006; Meddle et al 2007; Terenzi and Ingram 2005).

Because the PVN is the main source of oxytocin neurons that project within the brain and spinal cord, locally released oxytocin stimulates receptors on parvocellular neurons, simultaneously activating all terminal regions during and after birth (Kendrick 2000). Each of these initiate specific components of maternal behaviour, including social recognition through olfactory memory, modulation of anxiety and facilitation of aggression in response to perceived dangers to the offspring during late pregnancy and lactation, and enhanced spatial memory immediately following birth (Bale et al 2001; Bosch et al 2004; Insel 1997; Kinsley et al 1999; Kinsley 2008; Levy et al 2004; Lipschitz et al 2003; Neumann 2009; Terenzi and Ingram 2005; Tomizawa et al 2003).

Uterine oxytocin receptors

During pregnancy, myometrial receptors for oxytocin (OTR) increase from 27.6 fmol/mg DNA in the non-pregnant state to 171.6 fmol/mg DNA at mid-gestation and 1391 fmol/mg DNA at term (Fuchs et al 1984). Maximum receptor concentrations have been found in early labour at term, 3583 fmol/mg DNA – significantly higher than before labour begins (Fuchs et al 1982). Concentrations of decidual receptors are relatively low in mid-pregnancy and reach maximal values following the onset of labour. Within the fetal membranes, increased OTR binding has been found between late pregnancy and labour, with highest increases in the amnion (Takemura et al 1994).

Myometrial receptor concentrations are highest in the fundus and corpus, significantly lower in the lower segment, and lowest in the cervix, whereas decidual receptors are highest in sections surrounding the corpus and lowest around the lower segment (Blanks et al 2003; Arrowsmith and Wray 2014). During early labour, myometrial receptor concentrations are uniformly high in the upper segment and progressively lower in the isthmus and cervix, whereas those in the decidua are highest in the corpus, followed by the fundus and the isthmus (Fuchs et al 1984; Fuchs and Fuchs 1991; Hirst et al 1993) (see chapter website resources).

Gap junctions have a critical role in coordinating cellular responsiveness to oxytocin. At term, higher concentrations of myometrial gap junctions occur in the fundus compared with the lower segment, and the difference becomes increasingly pronounced during labour. This creates increasing *fundal dominance* during the course of labour and regulates progressive conductance of electrical activity, from fundus to cervix, to propagate multicellular synchronization of myometrial responsiveness to neuroendocrine, pulsatile and intra-uterine oxytocin systems (Blanks et al 2003; Fuchs et al 1991; Kimura et al 1996; Russell et al 2003; Shmygol et al 2006).

During spontaneous labour, myometrial and decidual OTR concentrations decline significantly in advanced labour, particularly in the lower segment (Fuchs et al 1984). Although findings in the lower segment are unreliable because of progressive incorporation of the cervix into the lower segment, available evidence suggests that oxytocin receptor mRNA significantly declines in the lower segment with increasing duration of labour. In spontaneous labour, the decline occurs gradually over 12 to 16 hours, but in oxytocin-induced and oxytocin-augmented labour, it is much steeper, especially when the infusion is constant rather than pulsatile (Robinson et al 2003; Willcourt et al 1994) (see chapter website resources).

NOCTURNAL MYOMETRIAL ACTIVATION AND CERVICAL RIPENING

The uterus has a well-defined 24-hour rhythm of contractility and electrical and endocrine activation (Schlabritz-Loutsevitch et al 2003). In human pregnancy, increased contractile activity has been observed between 8:30 pm to 2 am from 24 weeks gestation (Fuchs et al 1992; Germain et al 1993; Moore et al 1994; Sharkey et al 2009). Current research suggests the emergence of a nocturnal surge in rhythmic myometrial contractions is a key indication of uterine activation in preparation for the shift from pregnancy to labour. Nocturnal surges in oestriol, melatonin and oxytocin occur from around 35 to 36 weeks gestation, and these coincide with the 24-hour rhythm of spontaneous birth (Fuchs et al 1992; McGregor et al 1997; Schlabritz-Loutsevitch et al 2003; Tamura et al 2008).

The nocturnal surge in oestriol, which originates from fetal adrenal DHEA-S and interactions between fetal cortisol, CRH and hCG occur from 35 weeks gestation; nocturnal plasma melatonin rises from 36 weeks gestation; and nocturnal peaks in plasma concentrations of oxytocin occur from 37 to 39 weeks gestation (Fuchs et al 1991 and 1992; Germain et al 1993; Moore et al 1994; Murphy Goodwin 1999; Schlabritz-Loutsevitch et al 2003; Tamura et al 2008; Wang et al 2014). Oestrogens and melatonin increase gap junctions and oxytocin receptors, and melatonin also synergizes with oxytocin, increasing oxytocin-induced contractility in a dose-dependent manner (Sharkey et al 2009; Smith et al 2015).

From approximately 36 weeks onward, structural alterations become more apparent in cervical stroma and mucosal tissues, which alters its dimensions in relation to the lower uterine segment (House et al 2009). Within cervical connective tissue, alterations occur in the composition and concentration of the gel-like material called ground substance (*proteoglycans*) in which connective tissue cells and fibres are embedded. At the same time, an increase occurs in enzymes that degrade collagen. The concentration of ground substance relative to collagen is thought to reach a maximum during cervical softening before the onset of labour. This overall increase is characterized by the emergence of a higher proportion of molecules with a weaker affinity for collagen fibrils (see chapter website resources).

Cervical and uterine muscles

During late pregnancy and the latent phase of labour, myometrial components of the cervix contract in characteristic short, high-frequency pressure increases, which are independent of the rest of the uterus, until the onset of established labour (Rudel and Pajntar 1999). These contractions may stimulate local connective tissue changes associated with cervical ripening (Olah et al 1993; Pajntar 1994). In primiparous women, softening of cervical tissue proceeds alongside effacement and is thought to occur in response to increased formation of gap junctions between adjacent cells in the myometrium of the uterine cavity. *Gap junctions* are composed of symmetrical portions of plasma membrane from adjacent cells. These form intercellular channels for passage of ions and small molecules, facilitating rapid intracellular transmission of electrical impulses and chemical signals between cells. Gap junctions emerge in late pregnancy and undergo further increases in size and number during early labour. Formation and permeability of gap junctions are stimulated by oestrogens, prostaglandins and melatonin, and inhibited by progesterone, hCG and relaxin (Ambrus and Rao 1994; Burghardt et al 1993; Chow and Lye 1994; Sharkey et al 2009; Smith et al 2015). Before labour begins, myometrial expression of gap junctions is much higher in the fundus than in the lower segment, and this difference accelerates during labour (Sparey et al 1999).

By facilitating the propagation of action potentials from cell to cell, gap junctions synchronize myometrial activity. Tension is transmitted from the myometrium by the outer layer of muscle that extends along the periphery of the supravaginal portion of the cervix (Pajntar 1994; Smith et al 2015). This facilitates stretching of the lower uterine segment, which elongates as pressure is exerted by the fetus during descent into the pelvis. These combined forces seem

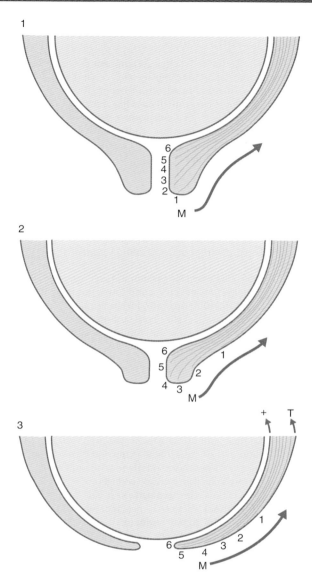

Figure 35.2 Diagram representing a hypothesis concerning differential movement of tissue planes at the time of cervical effacement and dilatation. M, direction of movement of collagen bundles; T, +, differential tension across the myometrium. (Reproduced with permission from Gee H: Uterine activity and cervical resistance determining cervical change in labour. MD thesis, University of Liverpool, UK, 1981 (fig 14.5).)

to produce a differential rate of tissue uptake in the cervix and the adjacent lower segment of the uterus. Maximum uptake occurs at the lower peripheral end of the cervix, producing a gradual upward movement of soft cervical tissue that eventually merges with the lower segment (Gee and Olah 1993; Havelock et al 2005) (Fig. 35.2).

Uterocervical changes and inflammation

Local pro-inflammatory changes accompany the remodeling and stretching of uterine muscle and cervical connective tissue during the latter part of pregnancy. The progressive release of inflammatory mediators like *nuclear factor kappa B (NF-κB)*, *cytokines* and *interleukins* seems to gradually overwhelm the selective suppression of inflammatory and immune responses established from the beginning of pregnancy by *progesterone, prolactin* and *cortisol* (Gubbay et al 2002; Johnson et al 2008; Rosen et al 1998; Shynlova et al 2009; Vaisanen-Tommiska et al 2003). Remodeling of the cervical connective tissue and stretching of the lower uterine segment and fetal membranes overlying the cervix produce local alterations in the relative activity of mediators of inflammatory and anti-inflammatory reactions (Allport et al 2001; Moore et al 2006; Vaisanen-Tommiska et al 2003).

These include increased concentrations of a key cytokine, *interleukin (IL)-8*, in the cervix and lower uterine segment with cervical ripening; higher concentrations of enzymes that synthesize prostacyclin, PGE_2 and $PGF_{2\alpha}$ in the lower segment compared with the fundus both before and during labour; raised cervical production of cytokines and nitric oxide (NO) at term and during labour; increased expression of NF-κB and *decreased* expression of glucocorticoid receptors in cervical tissue from late pregnancy to birth; and downregulation of *placental cortisol receptors* (Allport et al 2001; Johnson et al 2008; Keelan et al 2003; Sparey et al 1999). The COX-2 enzymes that stimulate prostaglandin synthesis are activated in cervical tissue by *NO* and *NF-κB*. The higher concentrations of these enzymes in the lower compared with the upper segment before labour may also increase collagenolytic activity of cervical tissue, thus contributing to cervical ripening. With the onset of labour, these enzymes increase further in the lower but not the upper segment, which suggests that prostaglandins may actively promote relaxation of the lower uterine segment throughout the course of labour (Myatt and Lye 2004; Sparey et al 1999).

Remodeling gestational tissues

Fetal membranes consist of amnion and chorion layers connected by an *extracellular matrix (ECM)* of collagen fibres that provides the main tensile strength of the membranes. Current findings suggest that membranes undergo a regulated process of tissue remodeling similar to that in the cervix from late pregnancy to birth (Moore et al 2006). In the cervix and membranes, remodeling and maturation processes involve changes in collagen fibres.

The amnion lies in direct contact with amniotic fluid, which contains elevated concentrations of pro- and anti-inflammatory cytokines from early pregnancy (Keelan et al 2003). During the third trimester, surfactant proteins

and phospholipids also enter amniotic fluid in increasing quantities and these have macrophage-activating properties that stimulate NF-κB activity, which regulates expression of *MMP enzymes*. Cytokines stimulate the prostaglandin H synthase 2 enzyme, which stimulates synthesis of prostaglandins, and concentrations of $PGF_{2\alpha}$ increase significantly in the amnion from around 38 weeks gestation (Keelan et al 2003; Lee et al 2008; Smith 2007). NO has been found to stimulate release of PGE_2 in amnion-like cells and fetal membranes, and recent evidence suggests that oxytocin is involved in stimulating the release of NO and pro-inflammatory cytokines from fetal membranes during labour (Ticconi et al 2004).

The amnion is separated from the myometrium by the chorion and decidua. Research findings suggest that the chorion, decidua and placenta produce anti-inflammatory cytokines, and the placenta and chorion also produce the enzyme *prostaglandin dehydrogenase* (PGDH), which is a potent in activator of prostaglandins (Amash et al 2009; Keelan et al 2003). Late in pregnancy, chorionic PGDH activity declines, whereas the expression of the inducible isoform of the *prostaglandin-generating enzyme COX-2* increases significantly in the adjacent amnion (Ticconi et al 2006). Many anti-inflammatory cytokines are produced in the decidua, which decrease local prostaglandin production, and their levels remain elevated following the onset of labour, whereas those in the placenta seem to decline during the course of labour (Keelan et al 2003) (see chapter website resources).

FROM LATE PREGNANCY TO BIRTH

The transition from nocturnal myometrial contractions to the onset of labour extends from around 30 weeks gestation, particularly in primigravid women. During this period, cervical tissues become less resistant, interrelated anatomical changes occur in the cervix and lower uterine segment, and the myometrium is activated nocturnally by episodes of rhythmic contractions (House et al 2009). Under the influence of the rapid rise in CRH, placental synthesis of oestriol accelerates towards the end of pregnancy (Smith et al 2009; Wang et al 2014). From late pregnancy to birth, progesterone dominance declines within uterine tissues, and related forces that promote myometrial quiescence and inhibit multicellular interactions are progressively modulated, in a region-specific manner, within the myometrium and surrounding intrauterine tissues (Bukowski et al 2006; Henderson and Wilson 2001; Mesiano and Welsh 2007; Sparey et al 1999).

From around 32 weeks, the onset of increased nocturnal release of oxytocin coincides with the decrease in the plasma oestrogen/progesterone ratio and the rise in oxytocin receptor density in the uterus. Under these conditions, a small rise in the pulsatile release of oxytocin seems to stimulate episodes of uterine contractions during the hours of darkness (Fuchs et al 1991; Germain et al 1993; Moore et al 1994). Expression of oestrogen-, melatonin- and prostacyclin-induced gap-junction proteins in the myometrium also increases from around 37 weeks, particularly in the fundus, and these provide low-resistance pathways between smooth muscle cells that increase the coordination of contractile activity throughout the uterus (Chow and Lye 1994; Fetalvero et al 2008; Sharkey et al 2009) (see chapter website resources).

These dynamic changes progressively generate functionally distinct sections of the uterus from late pregnancy to birth. Towards the end of pregnancy, the recurring episodes of nocturnal contractions become stronger and more frequent, until the functionally differentiated myometrium expresses its intrinsic capacity to propagate progressively stronger contractions from the fundus to the cervix during labour and birth (Bukowski et al 2006; Sparey et al 1999; Ticconi et al 2006).

MATERNAL–FETAL READINESS FOR LABOUR

In women, the transition from nocturnal rhythms in uterine contractions to latent labour is highly variable and is influenced by a host of additional factors, including maternal cognitive activity, fetal position and emotional readiness for labour (Wuitchik et al 1989). Throughout the last 4 weeks of pregnancy, physiological adaptations seem to be enhanced when women relax in the evenings to enhance the duration of sleep (Lee and Gay 2004). Using favoured ways of relaxing in late pregnancy, particularly during the early hours of darkness, facilitates the nocturnal rise in oxytocin and melatonin, which mediate the physiological increase in myometrial activity (Fuchs et al 1992; Sharkey et al 2009). This phase of preparatory changes in uterine smooth muscle and cervical tissue accelerates at term and indicates the combined preparation of maternal and fetal organ systems for labour and birth (Majzoub and Karalis 1999).

Reduced cognitive stimulation, relaxation and sleep are key elements of preparation because of the positive association between low cognitive activation and expressions of maternal love; between sleep duration in late pregnancy and shorter duration of labour; and between chronic anxiety, heightened levels of fear, pain perception and labour complications (Bartels and Zeki 2004; Haddad et al 1985; Lee and Gay 2004; Saisto et al 2001). Research evidence also indicates that low cognitive anxiety enables women to experience less discomfort during early labour, suggesting that the absence of fear modulates maternal pain perception (Wuitchik et al 1989).

When nocturnal uterine activation continues to accelerate beyond the hours of darkness, mothers need to be with their trusted companions and provided with a quiet, warm, "night-like" environment and minimal cognitive stimulation communication (Hodnett et al 2008). These conditions are conducive to the release of central oxytocin and melatonin and induce a timeless hypnotic state that deepens as labour progresses (Wierrani et al 1997). Maintaining a calm, secure, low-lit environment also prevents a stress-induced rise in *catecholamines,* which have been shown to inhibit oxytocin and attenuate uterine contractions (Levinson and Shnider 1979).

Neuroendocrine oxytocin

The release of oxytocin from the neurohypophysis during labour occurs in response to neuronal feedback to the brainstem from the uterus, cervix and vagina. During late pregnancy and labour, innervation is low in the body of the uterus and significantly higher in the cervix and adjacent parts of the pelvic cavity. Stretching and distension of these areas activates sensory afferent nerve pathways that transmit signals via the spinal cord and brainstem to oxytocin neurons in the hypothalamus. These respond with discrete bursts of accelerated discharge that transport the stored hormone along axons of hypothalamic neurons, and each of these give rises to numerous varicosities or large vesicles in the neurohypophysis. From here, oxytocin is released in intermittent pulses into the general circulation (Rossoni et al 2008) (Fig. 35.3).

Throughout labour and birth, increasing vaginocervical stimulation produced by downward pressure of the fetus transmits nerve impulses via the vagal and pelvic nerves, through spinal and brainstem pathways, to the hypothalamus (Russell et al 2003). These recurring episodes of sensory stimulation trigger characteristic bursts of magnocellular oxytocin neurons, resulting in minute-to-minute variation in plasma oxytocin levels during spontaneous labour (Fuchs et al 1991). As illustrated in Fig. 35.4, pulse frequency increases significantly during labour, but pulse amplitude remains low until the active phase, when it rises sharply, particularly during the final moments around birth. After birth, this pattern of oxytocin release accelerates in response to sensory contact and suckling, and it peaks during the middle of lactation (Fuchs et al 1991; Johnston and Amico 1986; Rossoni et al 2008) (see chapter website resources).

Oxytocin receptors are regulated by *oxytocinase,* an enzyme that rapidly degrades oxytocin. Placental oxytocinase is released into the maternal circulation during pregnancy and reaches its highest levels just before the onset of labour (Ito et al 2001; Nomura et al 2005). This enzyme prevents receptor desensitization during prolonged oxytocin release, as happens during labour and lactation. Oxytocinase may also suppress the pain of uterine contractions before and after birth by rapidly

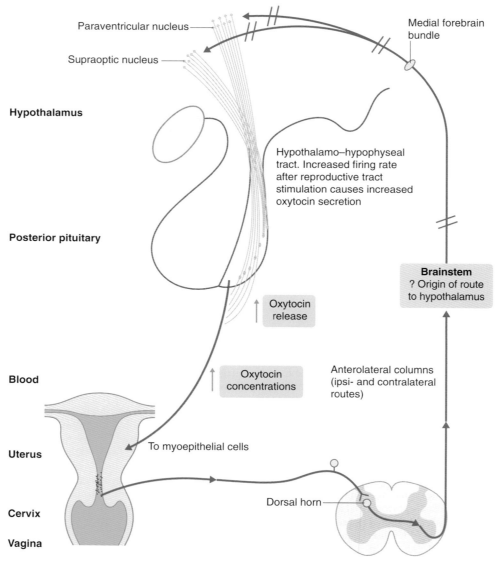

Figure 35.3 The neuroendocrine reflex underlying oxytocin synthesis and secretion. Stretching of the cervix and lower segment (black line) activates the reflex, leading to oxytocin release (red line). (Reproduced with permission from Johnson MH: Essential reproduction, Oxford, Blackwell Science, 2013.)

inactivating oxytocin following its release (see chapter website resources). Because of the increase in oxytocinase before the onset of labour, receptor concentrations remain elevated for approximately 20 hours of labour, after which they begin to decline (Ito et al 2001).

Established labour

Once cervical effacement has been completed and dilation of the external os is under way, sensory touch techniques during contractions seem to induce pain relief, relaxation and slow breathing patterns, in a quiet private "night-like" environment that enables women to sleep between contractions. When couples have established *a trusted relationship with the midwife*, labour usually progress quickly and women experience very little pain during contractions, especially when the process of labour follows a circadian rhythm.

During established labour, the supported upright position helps fetal descent with contractions, and it helps

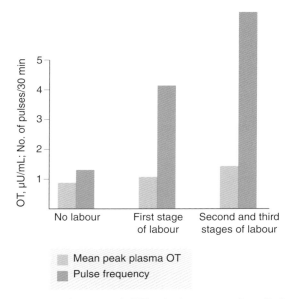

Figure 35.4 Mean oxytocin (OT) pulse frequency and amplitude determined in women at term, not in labour ($n = 11$), during the first stage of labour ($n = 13$) and combined second and third stages ($n = 8$). n = number in each group. (Fuchs A-R, Romero R, Keefe D, et al: Oxytocin secretion and human parturition: pulse frequency and duration increase during spontaneous labour. Am J Obstet Gynecol 165(5):1515–1523, 1991.)

women to use hip rotation to relieve discomfort (Ben Regaya et al 2010). A related study has found that a kneeling squat position significantly increases the bony transverse and antero-posterior dimension in the midpelvic plane and the pelvic outlet (Reitter et al 2014). Together these findings suggest that supported upright position is optimal during established labour, whereas a kneeling squat position has specific benefits during established labour, particularly during the expulsive phase.

Towards the expulsive phase

Just before the fetal head reaches the pelvic floor, the frequency of contractions may slow down, particularly in primigravid women. When uterine and fetal dynamics are not completely synchronized, this presents as a slowing down of the labour process and may require experimenting with different maternal positions to allow the fetus to fully descend into the pelvic outlet and complete anterior rotation (Reuwer et al 2009). A slow pace of descent allows the simultaneous surge in fetal adrenaline and vasopressin to complete the removal of lung liquid, dilate pulmonary blood vessels and stimulate production of surfactant, all of which enhance cardiorespiratory adaptations immediately following birth (Bland 2001; Wellmann et al 2010; Burkhardt et al 2012).

In biological terms, the expulsive phase is reached when the fetal head exerts pressure on the pelvic floor and the cervix becomes incorporated into the lower uterine segment, which becomes progressively thinner as expulsive contractions induce a progressive vagino-cervical stretch that activates positive afferent nerve pathways to oxytocin neurons in the supraoptic and paraventricular nuclei in the hypothalamus to set up positive afferent nerve pathways to the hypothalamus (Antonijevic et al 1995; Sansone et al 2002). This reflexive mechanism stimulates increased central release of oxytocin, and with increasing flexion and anterior rotation of the fetal head, pressure from the vertex against the gutter-shaped pelvic floor muscles stimulates their stretch receptors that activate both neuroendocrine and neurotransmitter oxytocin systems (Sansone et al 2002).

During the expulsive phase, vagino-cervical stretch activates magnocellular and parvocellular neurons. The former release oxytocin in characteristic pulses into the systemic circulation, whereas the latter release oxytocin into the spinal cord. The spinal projection stimulates sympathetic neurons that project to radial muscles of the iris, producing a characteristic dilation of the pupils, and brainstem sympathetic neurons stimulate a rise in blood pressure that maintains blood flow to the active uterus during the expulsive phase of labour (Ingram et al 1995; Komisaruk and Sansone 2003). The reflexive mechanism induced by vagino-cervical stretch also activates presynaptic inhibition of primary sensory neurons that convey painful stimuli within the spinal cord, which may account for the further increase in pain threshold that occurs in women during labour (Komisaruk and Sansone 2003; Ohel et al 2007) (Fig. 35.5).

Any unresolved maternal anxieties or perceived threats or dangers to the fetus may stimulate catecholamines, particularly adrenaline, which inhibits the pulsatile release of oxytocin, leading to a decline or cessation of uterine contractions, excessive blood loss following birth and delay in the onset of suckling and lactation (Chen et al 1998; Levinson and Shnider 1979; Odent 1992). Current evidence suggests that a private, warm, low-lit environment with a trusted companion enhances the release of central and neuroendocrine oxytocin and melatonin, minimizing the rise in maternal cortisol and catecholamines activated by heightened fear and anxiety that may occur just before expulsive contractions begin (Chen et al 1998; Levinson and Shnider 1979; Wuitchik et al 1989).

The expulsive phase is accompanied by a physiological increase in maternal catecholamine levels, particularly noradrenaline. This increases cardiac output and pulmonary circulation, providing the physical energy that usually coincides with the final moments of labour (Odent 1987). Many women find that they focus on rhythmic breathing during the expulsive phase and this 'hypnotic-like' state enables them to follow their bodies' expulsive efforts. This

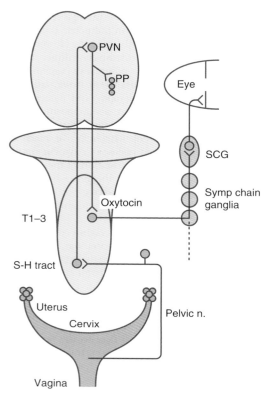

Figure 35.5 Schematic view of the pathway mediating the reflexive release of oxytocin in response to vaginocervical stimulation and the pathway mediating the pupil dilation response to vaginocervical stimulation. PVN, Paraventricular nucleus. PP, Posterior pituitary. SGC, Superior cervical ganglion. S-H tract, Spinohypothalamic tract. T1-3, Thoracic spinal cord level 1-3. (Reproduced with permission from Komisaruk BR, Sansone G: Neural pathways mediate vaginal function: the vagus nerves and spinal cord oxytocin, Scand J Psychol 44:241–250, 2003.)

encourages the woman to move the rest of the fetal body down the birth canal, without undue stress on herself or her baby.

Reflective activity 35.1

How would you use this knowledge to promote spontaneous labour in a primigravid woman who thinks she may be in labour at 09.00 am?

Spontaneous maternal breathing

To maintain uterine blood flow and adequate oxygenation to the fetus during the expulsive phase, maternal hyperventilation and breath-holding need to be avoided. Over prolonged periods, breath-holding (*Valsalva manoeuvre*) increases intrathoracic pressure, which reduces venous return to the heart. Consequently, cardiac output falls and blood pressure drops, leading to a reduction in uteroplacental perfusion (Blackburn 2013: 132). In a recent randomized study comparing Valsalva and spontaneous pushing, the expulsive phase of labour was shorter and umbilical arterial pH, PO_2 and Apgar scores were higher in the *spontaneous* pushing group (Yildirim and Beji 2008).

Fetal neurohormonal responses to labour and birth

Labour and birth induce increased secretion of *adrenomedullin, catecholamines, vasopressin cortisol* and *thyroid-stimulating hormone (TSH)*. Adrenomedullin is a potent vasodilator of the pulmonary circulation that facilitates a rapid increase in pulmonary blood flow at birth (Boldt et al 1998). Free cortisol levels double in association with labour, rising further in the 1–2 hours following birth. As well as stimulating maturational changes in key organ systems, cortisol induces increased deiodination of *thyroxine (T₄)* to produce *triiodothyronine (T₃)*. This works in conjunction with the dramatic surge in TSH at birth, stimulating striking increases in T_3 during the first 24 hours of neonatal life, which is particularly important for regulating thermogenesis (Nathanielsz et al 2003).

In the fetus, catecholamine levels rise throughout labour, reaching 20 times adult resting values immediately following birth. The intermittent squeezing of the fetal head during human labour triggers a rapid surge in catecholamine release (see chapter website resources).

Cardiovascular responses

Contractions induce transient reductions in uteroplacental perfusion altering the feto-placental circulation pattern. Ultrasonic studies suggest that at the beginning of a uterine contraction, maternal venous outflow is halted, and the content of the uterine veins is expressed into the maternal circulation. Simultaneously, arterial inflow that coincides with the onset of contractions is retained within the intervillous space. During contractions, this blood forms an increased pool that creates marked distension and vascular engorgement in the intervillous space. Transient reduction in uteroplacental perfusion during contractions may be partly compensated by the increased volume of maternal blood made available for gaseous exchange. To ensure the perfusion of the placenta, maternal blood pressure and cardiac output also rise in response to contractions. During the phase of uterine relaxation following each contraction, an increased blood flow has been observed, which may also compensate for decreased oxygen delivery during the preceding contraction (Bleker et al 1975; Robson et al 1987).

The circulation of a healthy fetus in spontaneous labour is not thought to be compromised by contractions. The umbilical circulation does not seem to be altered by changes in intra-uterine pressure or by short-term changes in fetal–placental or maternal–placental blood flow that accompany contractions. Fetal cardiac output rises in response to increased intra-uterine pressure during contractions, allowing fetal blood pressure to maintain a relatively constant pressure difference between the inside and outside of its vascular system. Concurrently, raised levels of fetal adrenaline specifically act to facilitate increases in heart rate and blood pressure, both of which serve to increase the rate of feto-placental blood flow between contractions (see chapter website resources).

The effect of fetal head pressure and the resulting catecholamines activates the maturing parasympathetic system and inhibits cardiac pacemakers, resulting in decreased cardiac output, slowing of the heart rate and reduced blood pressure. Slowing of the heart rate during contractions reduces the oxygen requirements of cardiac muscle. Parasympathetic influences on heart rate can be counteracted by adrenaline but not by noradrenaline. In the fetus at term, sufficient levels of adrenaline may be released to produce variable increases or decreases in heart rate in response to uterine contractions (see chapter website resources).

Birth, placental separation and cardiorespiratory adaptations

As the fetus leaves the uterine cavity, the surface area of the contracting uterus declines rapidly to produce a uterine diameter of around 10 cm. This reduction encompasses the site of placental attachment to the decidual lining, leading to compression of placental tissue and uteroplacental blood vessels, including approximately 100 spiral arteries that have supplied the placenta at a rate of 500 to 800 mL/min throughout the course of labour (Letsky 1998). Tonic myometrial compression of these blood vessels is greatly facilitated by placental-induced adaptations in the constituents of decidual and myometrial segments of the spiral arteries (Kawamata et al 2007). During the first and second trimesters, structural transformations of the vessel walls replace elastic lamina and smooth muscle layers with a matrix containing fibrin (Matijevic et al 1996).

When the mother is free to reach down and take the baby into her arms at birth, she brings herself into an upright position. This prevents compression of uterine blood flow returning to the right atrium via the inferior vena cava and allows gravity to assist the process of placental ejection, and the sight, smell, sounds and sensations of sensory contact between mother and infant stimulate a significant increase in central and peripheral release of oxytocin, as opioid restraint on maternal oxytocin neurons is removed immediately after birth. Basal levels of oxytocin rise significantly, and sensory stimulation and suckling

increase pulse frequency and amplitude of oxytocin release, compared with labour and birth (Matthiesen et al 2001).

The enhanced release of oxytocin into the peripheral circulation following birth of the infant stimulates tonic contraction and retraction of the myometrium, which squeezes the spongy placental tissue and forces blood in the collapsing intervillous spaces back into the veins of the decidua (Kawamata et al 2007; Shynlova et al 2009). Spontaneous flow of blood through the intact umbilical cord further reduces placental size by transferring approximately 120 mL of blood into the neonatal circulation (Dunn 1985).

As illustrated in Fig. 35.6, the intact cord continues to supply oxygenated blood to the infant as placental separation is progressing. This allows volume adjustments for new capillary beds that are opened by the dramatic fall in pulmonary vascular resistance as lung capillaries dilate with the onset of ventilation, which begins pulmonary gas exchange following birth (Boldt et al 1998; Dunn 1985;

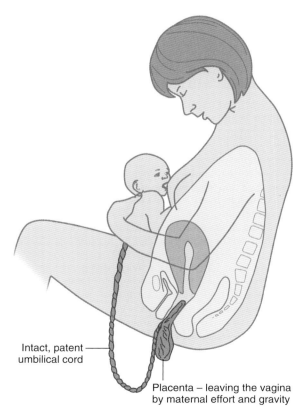

Intact, patent umbilical cord

Placenta – leaving the vagina by maternal effort and gravity

Figure 35.6 Maternal–infant sensory contact, placental separation and the transition from placental to mammary nutrition. (Inch S: Birthrights, London, Merlin Press, 1989.)

Hooper et al 2015; Kluckow and Hooper 2015). Before birth, the majority of right ventricular output flows from the main pulmonary artery to the descending aorta via the *ductus arteriosus* (DA). Because pulmonary venous return is low, left ventricular preload depends on umbilical venous return via the *ductus venosus* (DV), inferior vena cava and *foramen ovale* (FO) to the left atrium. During birth, the airways are cleared of fluid, and lung aeration soon after birth triggers a large decrease in pulmonary vascular resistance (PVR), which results in a sharp increase in pulmonary blood flow (PBF). These two events initiate the switch from umbilical to pulmonary venous return that maintains cardiac output throughout the transition process, thereby avoiding large fluctuations in blood pressure and blood supply to vital organs immediately following birth. As ventilation becomes established, pulmonary venous return replaces umbilical venous return as the major source of preload for the left ventricle. At the same time, the labour- and birth-induced increases in vasopressin, adrenomedullin and catecholamines combine to stimulate pulmonary blood flow, dilate bronchioles and pulmonary blood vessels, promote fluid retention, stimulate metabolism, enhance alertness and promote attachment. Therefore, the time required by individual infants to effect the successful transition from placental to pulmonary gas exchange provides the physiological basis for timing cord clamping (Hooper et al 2015).

Haemostasis and fibrinolysis

With sustained myometrial contraction, the congested decidual veins are severed and sealed by the shearing forces of the crisscrossed network of muscle fibres surrounding them. As illustrated in Fig. 35.7, the placenta is simultaneously torn from the uterine wall, at the line of the decidua basalis, and falls into the uterine cavity, peeling off the membranes as it descends towards the cervix and falls into the vagina (Benirschke 1992). Placental separation leaves behind a surface wound of 300 cm^2 containing approximately 100 severed arteries in which maternal blood coagulates rapidly because of a major increase in the concentration of several coagulation factors and decreased fibrinolytic activity, which characterizes pregnancy, labour and the first couple of hours following birth (Letsky 1998). Pregnancy is also accompanied by marked increases in *clotting factors VII, VIII, X and XII* and by a significant rise in vascular and placental *plasminogen activator inhibitors (PAIs)* leading to a marked increase in plasma fibrinogen by the third trimester (Dalaker 1986; Letsky 1998).

Before and after birth, these systemic haemostatic changes are accompanied by a local activation of *clotting factors V and VIII* and increased levels of *fibrinogen*, which results in a pronounced shortening of whole blood clotting time that is more pronounced in uterine than peripheral blood. Because of their combined effects, torn blood

vessels are sealed, and the site of placental separation is rapidly covered by a fibrin mesh that represents 5% to 15% of total circulating fibrinogen (Letsky 1998). Prostaglandin metabolites are simultaneously released into the general circulation from the torn surface tissues of the decidua basalis at the site of separation, where they stimulate *sustained* uterine contractions (Noort et al 1989).

When women do not experience prolonged stress-induced catecholamine release or severe vaginal or perineal lacerations during labour and birth, immediate blood loss from the vagina constitutes a small proportion of the increase in plasma and red cell volume that occurs during pregnancy. Most of the pregnancy-induced increase in blood volume is lost over a longer time period, through diuresis during the first 48 hours and lochia discharge from the placental site over the first 2 months postpartum (Hytten 1995: 119–122). Although visual estimates of blood loss within the first hour following birth are highly inaccurate, the significance of estimated blood loss at birth needs to be judged in relation to the expansion in blood volume during pregnancy (Bloomfield and Gordon 1990; Gyte 1992).

FROM UTERO-PLACENTA CIRCULATION TO MAMMARY SECRETIONS

Until birth, the fetus is essentially a parenterally nourished organism receiving a fairly constant supply of simple nutrients from the maternal circulation across the feto-placental barrier. During this period of enhanced anabolic metabolism, the maternal circulation supplies the placenta with glucose, amino acids and relatively smaller amounts of essential and nonessential fatty acids for selective uptake and transfer to the fetus (Hay 1995; Herrera 2000). Soon after birth, placental transfer of nutrients and gaseous exchange between maternal and fetal circulatory systems ends along with placental hormonal interactions with the fetal adrenal gland (Ben-Davis et al 2007) (see chapter website resources).

The expression of innate mother–infant interactions, particularly during the early weeks after birth, is critical for the infant's long-term general health and emotional well-being (Moriceau and Sullivan 2006; Neumann 2009; Stern 1997). Close body contact between mother and infant regulates homeostatic mechanisms, promotes a physiological increase in glucocorticoid and mineralocorticoid brain receptors, and prevents a rise in the infant's stress axis, which is highly sensitive to periods of separation, particularly during the first 3 days after birth (Bystrova et al 2003; Christensson et al 1995; Hofer 1994 and 2006; Hammock and Levitt 2013; Sarrieau et al 1988).

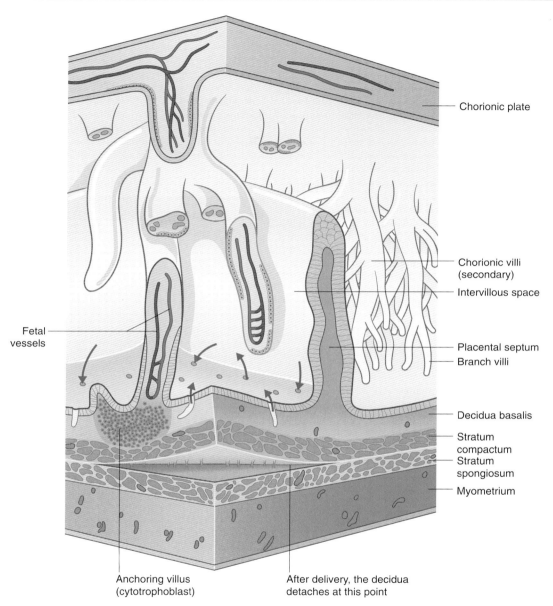

Figure 35.7 Diagrammatic representation of placental, decidual and myometrial tissue near term, illustrating the line of placental separation. Arrows indicate blood flow from uteroplacental arteries to the intervillous space and back to the uteroplacental veins. (This article was published in Blackburn ST: 2013. Maternal, fetal and neonatal physiology, ed 4. St. Louis, Saunders Elsevier, Copyright Elsevier, 2013.)

Initiation of maternal behaviour and attachment

Following spontaneous vaginal birth, mother and baby are highly motivated to remain in intimate sensory contact to initiate attachment, suckling and lactation. This includes an oxytocin-induced synaptic reorganization of the hippocampus, which improves maternal spatial memory, enabling the mother to develop a 'laser-like' focus for everything relating to the needs of her infant (Kinsley 2008; Monks et al 2003; Pedersen and Boccia 2002; Tomizawa et al 2003) (see chapter website resources).

Women's stated preference for intimate 'social affection' over participating in large social groups is mediated by suckling-induced activation of the *mesocorticolimbic dopamine system*, which is regulated by oxytocin (see chapter website resources). The pleasurable effects of intimate contact between mother and infant set up the desire for further maternal stimulation and infant suckling, which reinforces and strengthens the maternal–infant bond, partly by increasing central oxytocin receptors and release of oxytocin into the central nervous system (see chapter website resources).

CONCLUSION

Reproduction is a transformative process for mothers, fathers and babies. Extensive brain changes occur in mothers and fathers during pregnancy and following birth. Synchronized interactions occur between mother and fetus during the latter half of pregnancy, and mothers provide the fetus with circadian cues that are an essential part of maturational development. Circadian rhythms also characterize uterine activation and the shift from pregnancy to labour and birth. A complex interplay occurs between maternal–feto-placental systems that is finely regulated by neurohormonal systems. These coordinate maternal brain changes with fetal preparation for labour, birth and dependent development following birth. When midwives understand these dynamic interactions, they can learn to become attuned to the unfolding processes, support normal physiological processes and gain parental trust well before the onset of labour.

Key Points

- The shift from pregnancy to labour commences during the last trimester.

- Circadian rhythms of uterine activation, labour and birth are controlled by maternal and feto-placental neuro-endocrine-paracrine systems.

- A detailed understanding of these systems provides current evidence for practices to complement the dynamic changes in mother and fetus from late pregnancy until the onset of suckling-lactation.

- Current evidence suggests that regular sleep in late pregnancy and trusted companionship in a quiet, private environment for labour and birth facilitates a circadian pattern of uterine activation leading to spontaneous labour and birth.

- The establishment of ventilation following birth regulates cardiopulmonary adaptations that bring about the shift from fetal to neonatal circulation.

References

Abraham E, Hendler T, Shapira-Lichter I, et al: Father's brain is sensitive to childcare experiences, *Proc Natl Acad Sci USA* 111(27):9792–9797, 2014.

Akiyama S, Ohta H, Watanabe S, et al: The uterus sustains stable biological clock during pregnancy, *Tohoku J Exp Med* 221:287–298, 2010.

Allport VC, Pieber D, Slater DM, et al: Human labour is associated with nuclear factor-κB activity which mediates cyclo-oxygenase-2 expression and is involved with the 'functional progesterone withdrawal', *Mol Hum Reprod* 7(6):581–586, 2001.

Amash A, Holcberg G, Sheiner E, et al: Lipopolysaccharide differently affects prostaglandin E_2 levels in fetal and maternal compartments of perfused human term placenta, *Prostaglandins Other Lipid Mediat* 88:18–22, 2009.

Ambriz-Tututi M, Rocha-González H, Cruz SL, et al: Melatonin: a hormone that modulates pain, *Life Sci* 84:489–498, 2009.

Ambrus G, Rao CV: Novel regulation of pregnant human myometrial smooth muscle cell gap junctions by human chorionic gonadotrophin, *Endocrinology* 135(6):2772–2779, 1994.

Antonijevic IA, Leng G, Luckman SM, et al: Induction of uterine activity with oxytocin in late pregnant rats replicates the expression of c-fos in neuroendocrine and brain stem neurons as seen during parturition, *Endocrinology* 136(1):154–163, 1995.

Arrowsmith S, Wray S: Oxytocin: its mechanism of action and receptor signalling in the myometrium, *J Neuroendocrinol* 26:356–369, 2014.

Bale TL, Davis AM, Auger AP, et al: CNS region specific oxytocin receptor expression: importance in regulation of anxiety and sex behaviour, *J Neurosci* 21(7):2546–2552, 2001.

Bales KL, Saltzman W: Fathering in rodents: neurobiological substrates and consequences for offspring, *Horm Behav* 77:249–259, 2016.

Bartels A, Zeki S: The neural correlates of maternal and romantic love, *Neuroimage* 21:1155–1166, 2004.

Bauer J, Janecke A, Gerss J, et al: Circadian variation in oxygen consumption in preterm infants, *J Perinat Med* 37:413–417, 2009.

Bealer SL, Lipschitz DL, Ramoz G, et al: Oxytocin receptor binding in the hypothalamus during gestation in rats, *Am J Physiol Regul Integr Comp Physiol* 291:R53–R58, 2006.

Beebe KR, Lee KA: Sleep disturbances in late pregnancy and early labour, *J Perinat Neonatal Nurs* 23(2):103–108, 2007.

Ben Regaya L, Fatnassi R, Khlifi A, et al: Role of deambulation during labour: a prospective randomized study, *J Gynecol Obstet Biol Reprod (Paris)* 39(8):656–662, 2010.

Ben-Davis S, Zuckerman-Levin N, Epelman M, et al: Parturition itself is the basis for fetal adrenal involution, *J Clin Endocrinol Metab* 92(1):93–97, 2007.

Benirschke K: Placental separation at birth. In Polin RA, Fox WW, editors: *Fetal and neonatal physiology*, Philadelphia, Saunders, pp 95–96, 1992.

Blackburn ST: *Maternal, fetal and neonatal physiology*, 4th edn, St. Louis, Saunders Elsevier, 2013.

Bland RD: Loss of liquid from the lung lumen in labour: more than a simple 'squeeze', *Am J Physiol Lung Cell Mol Physiol* 280(4):L602–L605, 2001.

Blanks AM, Vatish M, Allen MJ, et al: Paracrine oxytocin and estradiol demonstrate a spatial increase in human intrauterine tissues with labour, *J Clin Endocrinol Metab* 88(7):3392–3400, 2003.

Bleker OP, Kloosterman GJ, Mieras DJ, et al: Intervillous space during uterine contractions in human subjects: an ultrasonic study, *Am J Obstet Gynecol* 123(7):697–699, 1975.

Bloomfield TH, Gordon H: Reaction to blood loss at delivery, *J Obstet Gynaecol* 10(Suppl 2):S13–S16, 1990.

Boldt T, Luuhleainen P, Tyhrquist F, et al: Birth stress increases adrenomedullin in the newborn, *Acta Paediatr* 87(1):93–94, 1998.

Bosch OJ, Kromer SA, Brunton PJ, et al: Release of oxytocin in the hypothalamic paraventricular nucleus, but not central amygdala or lateral septum in lactating residents and virgin intruders during maternal defense, *Neuroscience* 124:439–448, 2004.

Brauer MM, Smith PG: Estrogen and female reproductive tract innervation: cellular and molecular mechanisms of autonomic neuroplasticity, *Auton Neurosci* 187:1–17, 2015.

Brown CH, Grattan DR: Does maternal oxytocin protect the fetal brain?, *Trends Endocrinol Metab* 18(6):225–226, 2007.

Brunton PA, Russell JA: The expectant brain: adapting for motherhood, *Nat Rev Neurosci* 9:11–25, 2008.

Brunton PJ, Meddle SL, Ma S, et al: Endogenous opioids and attenuated hypothalamic-pituitary-adrenal axis responses to immune challenge in pregnant rats, *J Neurosci* 25(21):5117–5126, 2005.

Bukowski R, Hankins GDV, Saade GR, et al: Labour-associated gene expression in the human uterine fundus, lower segment and cervix, *PLoS Med* 3(6):918–928, 2006.

Burghardt RC, Barhoumi R, Dookwah H: Endocrine regulation of myometrial gap junctions and their role in parturition, *Semin Reprod Endocrinol* 11(3):250–260, 1993.

Burkhardt T, Schwarbe S, Morgenthaler NG: Copeptin: a marker for stress reaction in fetuses with intrauterine growth retardation, *Am J Obstet Gynecol* 2012.

Bystrova K, Widstrom A-M, Mattheisen A-S, et al: Skin-to-skin contact may reduce negative consequences of 'the stress of being born': a study on temperature in newborn infants, subjected to different ward routines in St Petersburg, *Acta Paediatr* 92(3):320–326, 2003.

Carter CS: Oxytocin pathways and the evolution of human behavior, *Annu Rev Psychol* 65:17–39, 2014.

Carvajal JA, Delpiano AM, Cuello MA, et al: Brain natriuretic peptide (BNP) produced by human chorioamnion may mediate pregnancy myometrial quiescence, *Reprod Sci* 16(1):32–42, 2009.

Carvajal JA, Vidal RJ, Cuello MA, et al: Mechanisms of paracrine regulation by fetal membranes of human uterine quiescence, *J Soc Gynecol Investig* 13(5):343–349, 2006.

Casey ML, Smith J, Alsabrook G, et al: Activation of adenylyl cyclase in human myometrial smooth muscle cells by neuropeptides, *J Clin Endocrinol Metab* 82(9):3087–3092, 1997.

Champagne FA: Epigenetic mechanisms and the transgenerational effects of maternal care, *Front Neuroendocrinol* 29:386–397, 2008.

Chan E-C, Smith R, Lewin T, et al: Plasma corticotrophin-releasing hormone, β-endorphin and cortisol inter-relationships during human pregnancy, *Acta Endocrinol* 128:339–344, 1993.

Chen DC, Nommsen-Rivers L, Dewey KG, et al: Stress during labour and delivery and early lactation performance, *Am J Clin Nutr* 68(2):335–344, 1998.

Chibbar R, Wong S, Miller FD, et al: Estrogen stimulates oxytocin gene expression in human chorio-decidua, *J Clin Endocrinol Metab* 80(2):567–572, 1995.

Chow L, Lye SJ: Expression of the gap junction protein connexin-43 is increased in the human myometrium toward term and with the onset of labour, *Am J Obstet Gynecol* 170(3):788–795, 1994.

Christensson K, Cabrera T, Christensson E, et al: Separation distress call in the human neonate in the absence of maternal body contact, *Acta Paediatr* 84(5):468–473, 1995.

Conde A, Figueiredo B: 24-h urinary free cortisol from mid-pregnancy to 3-months postpartum: gender and parity differences and effects, *Psychoneuroendocrinology* 50:264–273, 2014.

Condon JC, Jeyasuria P, Faust JM, et al: A decline in the levels of progesterone receptor coactivators in the pregnant uterus at term may antagonize progesterone receptor function and contribute to the initiation of parturition, *Proc Natl Acad Sci USA* 100(16):9518–9523, 2003.

Cootauco AC, Murphy JD, Maleski J, et al: Atrial natriuretic peptide production and natriuretic peptide receptors in the human uterus and their effects on myometrial relaxation, *Am J Obstet Gynecol* 199:429.e1–429.e6, 2008.

Dalaker K: Clotting factor VII during pregnancy, delivery and puerperium, *Br J Obstet Gynaecol* 93:17–21, 1986.

de Kock CPJ, Wierda KDB, Bosman LWJM, et al: Somatodendritic secretion in oxytocin neurons is upregulated during the female reproductive cycle, *J Neurosci* 23(7):2726–2734, 2003.

Di Pietro JA, Mendelson T, Williams EL, et al: Physiological blunting during pregnancy extends to induced relaxation, *Biol Psychol* 89:14–20, 2012.

Diaz S, Seron-Ferre M, Cardenas H, et al: Circadian variation of basal plasma prolactin, prolactin response to suckling, and length of amenorrhoea in nursing women, *J Clin Endocrinol Metab* 68(5):946–955, 1989.

Dong X, Yu C, Shynlova O, et al: p54nrb is a transcriptional corepressor of the progesterone receptor that modulates transcription of labor-associated gene, connexin 43(Gja1), *Mol Endocrinol* 23(8):1147–1160, 2009.

Dong Y-L, Wimalawansa SJ, Yallampalli C: Effects of steroid hormones on calcitonin gene-related peptide receptors in cultural human myometrium, *Am J Obstet Gynecol* 188(2):466–472, 2003.

Douglas AJ: Mother-offspring dialogue in early pregnancy: impact of adverse environment on pregnancy maintenance and neurobiology, *Prog Neuropsychopharmacol Biol Psychiatry* 35:1167–1177, 2011.

Douglas AJ, Bicknell RJ, Leng G, et al: β-Endorphin cells in the arcuate nucleus: projections to the supraoptic nucleus and changes in expression during pregnancy and parturition, *J Neuroendocrinol* 14:768–777, 2002.

Douglas AJ, Meddle SL, Toschi N, et al: Reduced activity of the noradrenergic system in the paraventricular nucleus at the end of pregnancy: implications for stress hyporesponsiveness, *J Neuroendocrinol* 17:40–48, 2005.

Draisci G, Catarci S, Vollono C, et al: Pregnancy-induced analgesia: a combined psychological and neurophysiological study, *Eur J Pain* 16:1389–1397, 2012.

Dunn P: The third stage and fetal adaptation. In Clinch J, Matthews T, editors: *Perinatal medicine*, Lancaster, MIT Press, pp 47–54, 1985.

Feldman R, Gordon I, Zagory-Sharon O: The cross-generation transmission of oxytocin in humans, *Horm Behav* 58:669–676, 2010.

Ferguson JE, Seaner RM, Bruns DE, et al: Expression and specific immunolocalization of the human parathyroid hormone/parathyroid hormone-related protein receptor in the uteroplacental unit, *Am J Obstet Gynecol* 179(2):321–329, 1998.

Ferreira DS, Amaral FG, Mesquita CC, et al: Maternal melatonin programs the daily pattern of energy metabolism in adult offspring, *PLoS One* 7(6):e38795, 2012.

Fetalvero KM, Zhang P, Shyu M, et al: Prostacyclin primes pregnant human myometrium for an enhanced contractile response at parturition, *J Clin Invest* 118(12):3966–3979, 2008.

Freemark M: The fetal adrenal and the maturation of the growth hormone and prolactin axes, *Endocrinology* 140(5):1963–1965, 1999.

Fuchs A-R, Behrens O, Liu H-C: Correlation of nocturnal increase in plasma oxytocin with a decrease in plasma estradiol/progesterone ratio in late pregnancy, *Am J Obstet Gynecol* 167(6):1559–1563, 1992.

Fuchs A-R, Fuchs F: Physiology of parturition. In Gabbe SG, editor: *Obstetrics, normal and problem pregnancies*, New York, Churchill Livingstone, pp 147–174, 1991.

Fuchs A-R, Fuchs F, Husslein P, et al: Oxytocin receptors and human parturition: a dual role for oxytocin in the initiation of labour, *Science* 215:1396–1398, 1982.

Fuchs A-R, Fuchs F, Husslein P, et al: Oxytocin receptors in the human uterus during pregnancy and parturition, *Am J Obstet Gynecol* 150(6):734–741, 1984.

Fuchs A-R, Romero R, Keefe D, et al: Oxytocin secretion and human parturition: pulse frequency and duration increase during spontaneous labour, *Am J Obstet Gynecol* 165(5):1515–1523, 1991.

Fujii M, Umezawa K, Arta A: Adrenaline contributes to prenatal respiratory maturation in rat medulla-spinal cord preparation, *Brain Res* 1090:45–50, 2006.

Gao L, Liu C, Xu C, et al: Differential regulation of prostaglandin production mediated by corticotrophin-releasing hormone receptor type 1 and 2 in cultured placental trophoblasts, *Endocrinology* 149(6):2866–2876, 2008.

Garbrecht MR, Klein JM, Schmidt TJ, et al: Glucocorticoid metabolism in the human fetal lung: implications for lung development and the pulmonary surfactant system, *Biol Neonate* 89:109–119, 2006.

Garfield RE, Ali M, Yallampalli C, et al: Role of gap junctions and nitric oxide in control of myometrial contractility, *Semin Perinatol* 19(1):41–51, 1995.

Gee H: *Uterine activity and cervical resistance determining cervical change in labour*, MD thesis, Liverpool, University of Liverpool, 1981.

Gee H, Olah KS: Failure to progress in labour. In Studd J, editor: *Progress in obstetrics and gynaecology*, vol 10, Edinburgh, Churchill Livingstone, pp 159–181, 1993.

Germain AM, Valenzuela GJ, Ivankovic M, et al: Relationship of circadian rhythms of uterine activity with term and preterm delivery, *Am J Obstet Gynecol* 168(4):1271–1277, 1993.

Gettler LT, McDade TW, Feranil AB, et al: Longitudinal evidence that fatherhood decreases testosterone in human males, *Proc Natl Acad Sci USA* 108(39):16194–16199, 2011.

Gintzler AR, Liu N-J: The maternal spinal cord: biochemical and physiological correlates of steroid-activated antinociceptive processes, *Prog Brain Res* 133:83–97, 2001.

Goland RS, Jozak RN, Conwell I: Placental corticotrophin-releasing hormone and the hypercortisolism of pregnancy, *Am J Obstet Gynecol* 171(4):1287–1291, 1994.

Goland RS, Wardlaw SL, Stark RI, et al: High levels of corticotrophin-releasing hormone immunoreactivity in maternal and fetal plasma during pregnancy, *J Clin Endocrinol Metab* 63(5):1199–1203, 1986.

Gooley JJ, Chamberlain K, Smith KA, et al: Exposure to room light before bedtime suppresses melatonin onset and shortens melatonin duration in humans, *J Clin Endocrinol Metab* 96:E463–E472, 2011.

Gordon I, Zagoory-Sharon O, Leckman JF, et al: Prolactin, oxytocin and the development of paternal behavior across the first six months of fatherhood, *Horm Behav* 58:513–518, 2010a.

Gordon I, Zagoory-Sharon O, Leckman JF, et al: Oxytocin and the development of parenting, in humans, *Biol Psychiatry* 68:377–382, 2010b.

Grammatopoulos DK: The role of CRH receptors and their agonists in myometrial contractility and quiescence during pregnancy and labour, *Front Biosci* 12:561–571, 2007.

Grammatopoulos D: Placental corticotrophin-releasing hormone and its receptors in human pregnancy and labour: still a scientific enigma, *J Neuroendocrinol* 20:432–438, 2008.

Grammatopoulos D, Stirrat GM, Williams SA, et al: The biological activity of the corticotrophin-releasing hormone receptor–adenylate cyclase complex in human myometrium is reduced at the end of pregnancy, *J Clin Endocrinol Metab* 81(2):745–751, 1996.

Grammatopoulos DK, Hillhouse EW: Activation of protein kinase C by oxytocin inhibits the biological activity of the human myometrial corticotrophin-releasing hormone receptor at term, *Endocrinology* 140(2):585–594, 1999.

Grattan DR: Behavioural significance of prolactin signaling in the central nervous system during pregnancy and lactation, *Reproduction* 123:497–506, 2002.

Groer MW, Davis MW, Hemphell J: Postpartum stress: current concepts and the possible protective role of breastfeeding, *J Obstet Gynecol Neonatal Nurs* 31(4):411–417, 2002.

Gubbay O, Critchley HO, Bowen JM, et al: Prolactin induces ERK phosphorylation in epithelial and CD56⁺ natural killer cells of the human endometrium, *J Clin Endocrinol Metab* 87(5):2329–2335, 2002.

Gyte G: The significance of blood loss at delivery, *MIDIRS Midwifery Digest* 2(1):88–92, 1992.

Haack M, Scott-Sutherland J, Santangelo G, et al: Pain sensitivity and modulation in primary insomnia, *Eur J Pain* 16:522–533, 2012.

Haddad PF, Morris NF, Spielberge CD: Anxiety in pregnancy and its relation to use of oxytocin and analgesia in labour, *J Obstet Gynaecol* 6:77–81, 1985.

Hammock EAD, Levitt P: Oxytocin receptor ligand binding in embryonic tissue and postnatal brain development of C57BL/6J mouse, *Front Behav Neurosci* 7:195, 2013.

Havelock JC, Keller P, Muleba N, et al: Human myometrial gene expression before and during parturition, *Biol Reprod* 72:707–719, 2005.

Hay WW: Metabolic interrelationships of placenta and fetus, *Placenta* 16(1):19–30, 1995.

Hedriana HL, Munro CJ, Eby-Wilkens EM, et al: Changes in rates of salivary oestiol increases before parturition at term, *Am J Obstet Gynecol* 184(2):123–130, 2001.

Henderson D, Wilson T: Reduced binding of progesterone receptor to its nuclear response element after human labour onset, *Am J Obstet Gynecol* 185(3):579–585, 2001.

Herrera E: Metabolic adaptations in pregnancy and their implications for the availability of substrates to the fetus, *Eur J Clin Nutr* 54(Suppl 1):S47–S51, 2000.

Higuchi T, Okere CO: Role of supraoptic nucleus in regulation of parturition and milk ejection revisited, *Microsc Res Tech* 56:113–121, 2002.

Hillhouse EW, Grammatopoulos DK: Control of intracellular signaling by corticotrophin-releasing hormone in human myometrium, *Front Horm Res* 27:66–74, 2001.

Hirst JJ, Chibbar R, Mitchell BF: Role of oxytocin in the regulation of uterine activity during pregnancy and in the initiation of labour, *Semin Reprod Endocrinol* 11(3):219–233, 1993.

Hodnett ED, Gates S, Hofmeyr GJ, et al: Continuous support for women during childbirth (Cochrane Review). In *The Cochrane Library*, Issue 1, Chichester, John Wiley, 2008.

Hofer MA: Early relationships as regulators of infant physiology and behaviour, *Acta Paediatr* 397:9–18, 1994.

Hofer MA: Psychobiological roots of early attachment, *Curr Dir Psychol Sci* 15(2):84–88, 2006.

Holt-Lunstad J, Smith TB, Layton JB: Social relationships and mortality risk: a meta-analytic review, *PLoS Med* 7(7):e1000316, 2010.

Hooper SB, Polglase GR, te Pas AB: A physiological approach to the timing of umbilical cord clamping at birth, *Arch Dis Child Fetal Neonatal Ed* 100:F355–F360, 2015.

House M, Bhadelia RA, Myers K, et al: Magnetic resonance imaging of three-dimensional cervical anatomy in the second and third trimester, *Eur J Obstet Gynecol Reprod Biol* 144S:S65–S69, 2009.

Hytten F: *The clinical physiology of the puerperium*, London, Farrand Press, 1995.

Inch S: *Birthrights*, London, Merlin Press, 1989.

Ingram CD, Adams TST, Jiang QB, et al: Limbic regions mediating central actions of oxytocin on milk-ejection reflex in the rat, *J Neuroendocrinol* 7(1):1–13, 1995.

Ingram CD, Wakerley JB: Post-partum increase in oxytocin-induced excitation of neurons in the bed nuclei of the stria terminalis in vitro, *Brain Res* 602:325–330, 1993.

Insel TR: Regional changes in brain oxytocin receptors post-partum: time course and relationship to maternal behaviour, *J Neuroendocrinol* 2(4): 539–545, 1990.

Insel TR: A neurobiological basis of social attachment, *Am J Psychiatry* 154(6):726–735, 1997.

Ito T, Nomura S, Okada M, et al: Transcriptional regulation of human placental leucine aminopeptidase/ oxytocinase gene, *Mol Hum Reprod* 7(9):887–894, 2001.

Jaffe RB: Role of the human fetal adrenal gland in the initiation of parturition, *Front Horm Res* 27:75–85, 2001.

Jain L, Dudell GG: Respiratory transition in infants delivered by cesarean section, *Semin Perinatol* 30:296–304, 2006.

Johnson MH: *Essential reproduction*, 7th edn, Oxford, 2013, Blackwell Scientific.

Johnson RF, Rennie N, Murphy V, et al: Expression of glucocorticoid receptor messenger ribonucleic acid transcripts in the human placenta at term, *J Clin Endocrinol Metab* 93(12):4887–4893, 2008.

Johnston JM, Amico JA: A prospective longitudinal study of the release of oxytocin and prolactin in response to infant suckling in long term lactation, *J Clin Endocrinol Metab* 62(4):653–657, 1986.

Kammerer M, Adams D, von Castelberg B, et al: Pregnant women become insensitive to cold stress, *BMC Pregnancy Childbirth* 2:8, 2002.

Kask K, Backstrom T, Gulinello M, et al: Lower level of prepulse inhibition of startle response in pregnant women compared to postpartum women, *Psychoneuroendocrinology* 33:100–107, 2008.

Kawamata M, Tonomura Y, Kimura T, et al: Oxytocin-induced phasic and tonic contractions are modulated by contractile machinery rather than the quantity of oxytocin receptor, *Am J Physiol Endocrinol Metab* 292:E992–E999, 2007.

Keelan JA, Blumenstein M, Helliwell RJA, et al: Cytokines, prostaglandins and parturition – a review, *Placenta* 17(Suppl A):S33–S46, 2003.

Kendrick KM: Oxytocin, motherhood and bonding, *Exp Physiol* 85S:111S–124S, 2000.

Khazipov R, Tyzio R, Ben-Air Y: Effects of oxytocin on GABA signalling in the fetal brain during delivery, *Prog Brain Res* 170:243–257, 2008.

Kim P, Mayes LC, Wang X, et al: The plasticity of human maternal brain: longitudinal changes in brain anatomy during the early postpartum period, *Behav Neurosci* 124(5):695–700, 2010.

Kimura T, Takemura M, Nomura S, et al: Expression of oxytocin receptor in human pregnant myometrium, *Endocrinology* 137(2):780–785, 1996.

Kinsley CH: The neuroplastic maternal brain, *Horm Behav* 54:1–4, 2008.

Kinsley CH, Madonia L, Gifford GW, et al: Motherhood improves learning and memory, *Nature* 402:137–138, 1999.

Kluckow M, Hooper SB: Using physiology to guide cord clamping, *Semin Fetal Neonatal Med* 20:225–231, 2015.

Komisaruk BR, Sansone G: Neural pathways mediate vaginal function: the vagus nerves and spinal cord oxytocin, *Scand J Psychol* 44:241–250, 2003.

Kosfelf M, Heinrichs M, Zak PJ, et al: Oxytocin increases trust in humans, *Nature* 435:673–676, 2005.

Lagercrantz H, Herlenius E: Neurotransmitters and neuromodulators. In Lagercrantz H, Hanson M, Evrard P, et al, editors: *The newborn brain*, Cambridge, Cambridge University Press, pp 139–165, 2002.

Lee KA, Gay CL: Sleep in late pregnancy predicts length and type of delivery, *Am J Obstet Gynecol* 191:2041–2046, 2004.

Lee SE, Romero R, Park I-S, et al: Amniotic fluid prostaglandin concentrations increase before the onset of spontaneous labour, *J Matern Fetal Med* 21(2):89–94, 2008.

Leng G, Meddle SL, Douglas AL: Oxytocin and the maternal brain, *Curr Opin Pharmacol* 8:731–734, 2008.

Letsky EA: The haematological system. In Chamberlain G, Broughton Pipkin F, editors: *Clinical physiology in obstetrics*, Oxford, Blackwell Science, pp 1–110, 1998.

Leuner B, Glasper ER, Gould E: Parenting and plasticity, *Trends Neurosci* 33(10):465–473, 2010.

Levinson G, Shnider SM: Catecholamines: the effects of maternal fear and its treatment on uterine function and circulation, *Birth Fam J* 6(3):167–174, 1979.

Levy F, Keller K, Poindron P: Olfactory regulation of maternal behavior in mammals, *Horm Behav* 46:284–302, 2004.

Liggins GC: The role of cortisol in preparing the fetus for birth, *Reprod Fertil Dev* 6:141–150, 1994.

Light KC, Grewen KM, Amnico JA: More frequent partner hugs and higher oxytocin levels are linked to lower blood pressure and heart rate in premenopausal women, *Biol Psychol* 69:5–21, 2005.

Lipschitz DL, Crowley WR, Bealer SL: Central blockade of oxytocin receptors during late gestation disrupts systemic release of oxytocin during suckling in rats, *J Neuroendocrinol* 15:743–748, 2003.

Liu N-J, Gintzler AR: Facilitative interactions between vasoactive intestinal polypeptide and receptor type-selective opioids; implications for sensory afferent regulation of spinal opioid action, *Brain Res* 959:103–110, 2003.

Lucas BK, Ormandy CJ, Binart N, et al: Null mutation of the prolactin receptor gene produces a defect in maternal behaviour, *Endocrinology* 139(10):4102–4107, 1998.

Majzoub JA, Karalis KP: Placental corticotrophin-releasing hormone: function and regulation,

Am J Obstet Gynecol 180(1):S242–S246, 1999.

Markovic D, Vatish M, Giu M, et al: The onset of labour alters corticotrophin-releasing hormone type 1 receptor variant expression in human myometrium: putative role of interleukin-1β, *Endocrinology* 148(7):3205–3213, 2007.

Matijevic R, Meekins JW, McFaden IR, et al: Physiological changes of spiral arteries and blood flow in the placental bed during early pregnancy, *Contemp Rev Obstet Gynaecol* 8:127–131, 1996.

Matthiesen A-S, Ransjo-Arvidson A-BR, Nissen E, et al: Postpartum maternal oxytocin release by newborns: effects of infant hand massage and suckling, *Birth* 28(1):13–19, 2001.

McGregor J, Barrett J, Hastings C: Diurinal variation of salivary estriol in pregnancy, *Am J Obstet Gynecol* S56, 1997.

McLean M, Bistits A, Davies J, et al: A placental clock controlling the length of human pregnancy, *Nat Med* 1(5):460–463, 1995.

Meddle SL, Bishop VR, Gkoumassi E, et al: Dynamic changes in oxytocin receptor expression and activation at parturition in the rat brain, *Endocrinology* 148(10):5095–5104, 2007.

Mendelson CR: Minireview: fetal-maternal hormonal signaling in pregnancy and labor, *Mol Endocrinol* 23(7):947–954, 2009.

Mesiano S, Chan E-C, Fitter JT, et al: Progesterone withdrawal and estrogen activation in human parturition are coordinated by progesterone receptor A expression in the myometrium, *J Clin Endocrinol Metab* 87(6):2924–2930, 2002.

Mesiano S, Welsh TN: Steroid hormone control of myometrial contractility and parturition, *Semin Cell Dev Biol* 18:321–331, 2007.

Monks DA, Lonstein JS, Breedlove SM: Got milk? Oxytocin triggers hippocampal plasticity, *Nat Neurosci* 6(4):327–328, 2003.

Moore TR, Iams JD, Creasy RK, et al: Diurnal and gestational patterns of uterine activity in normal human pregnancy, *Obstet Gynecol* 83(4):517–523, 1994.

Moore RM, Mansour JM, Redline RW, et al: The physiology of fetal membrane rupture: insights gained from the determination of physical properties, *Placenta* 27:1037–1051, 2006.

Moriceau S, Sullivan RM: Maternal presence serves as a switch between learning fear and attraction in infancy, *Nat Neurosci* 9(8):1004–1006, 2006.

Murphy Goodwin T: A role for estradiol in human labour, term and preterm, *Am J Obstet Gynecol* 180(1):S208–S213, 1999.

Myatt L, Lye SJ: Expression, localization and function of prostaglandin receptors in myometrium, *Prostaglandins Leukot Essent Fatty Acids* 70:1337–1348, 2004.

Nathanielsz PW, Berghorn KA, Derks JB, et al: Life before birth: effects of cortisol on future cardiovascular and metabolic function, *Acta Paediatr* 92:766–772, 2003.

Neumann ID: The advantage of living social: brain neuropeptides mediate the beneficial consequences of sex and motherhood, *Front Neuroendocrinol* 30:483–496, 2009.

Nomura S, Ito T, Yamamoto E, et al: Gene regulation and physiological function of placenta leucine aminopeptidase/oxytocinase during pregnancy, *Biochim Biophys Acta* 1751:19–25, 2005.

Noort WA, van Bulck B, Vereecken A, et al: Changes in plasma levels of $PGF_{2\alpha}$ and PGI_2 metabolites at and after delivery at term, *Prostaglandins* 37(1):3–12, 1989.

Odent M: The fetus ejection reflex, *Birth* 14(2):104–108, 1987.

Odent M: The nature of birth and breastfeeding, *Bergin, Garvey, Westport*, 1992.

Ohel I, Walfisch A, Shitenberg D, et al: A rise in pain threshold during labour: a prospective clinical trial, *Pain* 132:S104–S108, 2007.

Olah KS, Gee H, Brown JS: Cervical contractions: the response of the cervix to oxytocic stimulation in the latent phase of labour, *Br J Obstet Gynaecol* 100:635–640, 1993.

Olcese J, Beesley S: Clinical significance of melatonin receptors in the human myometrium, *Fertil Steril* 102(2):329–335, 2014.

Olcese J, Lozier S, Paradise C: Melatonin and the circadian timing of human parturition, *Reprod Sci* 20(2):168–174, 2013.

Ortiz-Miranda S, Dayanithi G, Custer E, et al: Micro-opioid receptor preferentially inhibits oxytocin release from neurohypophysial terminals by blocking R-type Ca2+ channels, *J Neuroendocrinol* 17:583–590, 2005.

Pajntar M: The smooth muscles of the cervix in labour, *Eur J Obstet Gynecol Reprod Biol* 55(1):9–12, 1994.

Pearson RM, Lightman SL, Evans J: Emotional sensitivity for motherhood: late pregnancy is associated with enhanced accuracy to encode emotional faces, *Horm Behav* 56:s57–s63, 2009.

Pedersen CT, Boccia ML: Oxytocin links mothering received, mothering bestowed and adult stress responses, *Stress* 5(4):259–367, 2002.

Perea-Rodriguez JP, Takahashi EY, Amador TM, et al: Effects of reproductive experience on central expression of progesterone, oestrogen α, oxytocin and vasopressin receptor mRNA in male California mice (*Peromyscus californicus*), *J Neuroendocrinol* 27:245–252, 2015.

Price SA, Lopez Bernal A: Uterine quiescence: the role of cyclic AMP, *Exp Physiol* 86(2):265–272, 2001.

Rehman K, Sirianni R, Parker R, et al: The regulation of adrenocorticotrophic hormone receptor by corticotrophin-releasing hormone in human fetal adrenal definitive/transitional zone cells, *Reprod Sci* 14(6):578–587, 2007.

Reiter RJ, Dun Xian T, Korkmaz A, et al: Melatonin and stable circadian rhythms optimize maternal, placental and fetal physiology, *Hum Reprod Update* 20(2):293–307, 2014.

Reitter A, Daviss B-A, Bisits A: Does pregnancy and/or shifting positions create more room in a woman's pelvis?, *Am J Obstet Gynecol* 211(6):662.e1–662e9, 2014.

Reuwer P, Bruinse H, Franx A: *Proactive support of labor: the challenge of normal childbirth*, Cambridge, Cambridge University Press, 2009.

Robinson C, Schumann R, Zhang P, et al: Oxytocin-induced desensitization of the oxytocin receptor, *Am J Obstet Gynecol* 188(2):497–502, 2003.

Robson SC, Dunlop W, Boys RJ, et al: Cardiac output during labour, *Br Med J* 295(6607):1169–1172, 1987.

Rosen T, Krikun G, Ma Y, et al: Chronic antagonism of nuclear factor-κB activity in cytotrophoblasts by dexamethasone: a potential mechanism for anti-inflammatory action of glucocorticoids in human placenta, *J Clin Endocrinol Metab* 83(10):3647–3652, 1998.

Rossoni E, Feng J, Tirozzi B, et al: Emergent synchronous bursting of oxytocin neuronal network, *PLoS Comput Biol* 4(7):e1000123, 2008.

Rudel D, Pajntar M: Contractions of the cervix in the latent phase of labour, *Contemp Rev Obstet Gynaecol* 11(4):271–279, 1999.

Russell JA, Brunton PJ: Neuroactive steroids attenuate oxytocin stress responses in late pregnancy, *Neuroscience* 138:879–889, 2006.

Russell JA, Brunton PJ: Oxytocin (peripheral/central actions and their regulation). In Bloom F, Squire LF, Spitzer N, editors: *Encyclopedia of neuroscience*, Amsterdam, Elsevier, pp 337–347, 2009.

Russell JA, Leng G, Douglas AJ: The magnocellular oxytocin system, the fount of maternity: adaptations in pregnancy, *Front Neuroendocrinol* 249(1):27–61, 2003.

Saisto T, Kaaja R, Ylikorkala O, et al: Reduced pain tolerance during and after pregnancy in women suffering from fear of labour, *Pain* 93:123–127, 2001.

Sansone GR, Gerdes CA, Steinman JL, et al: Vaginocervical stimulation releases oxytocin within the spinal cord in rats, *Neuroendocrinology* 75:306–315, 2002.

Sarrieau A, Sharma S, Meaney MJ: Postnatal development and environmental regulation of hippocampal glucocorticoid and mineralocorticoid receptors, *Brain Res* 471:158–162, 1988.

Schestatsky P, Dall-Agnol L, Gheller L, et al: Pain–autonomic interaction after work-induced sleep restriction, *Eur J Neurol* 20:638–646, 2013.

Schlabritz-Loutsevitch N, Middendorf HR, Muller D, et al: The human myometrium as a target for melatonin, *J Clin Endocrinol Metab* 88(2):908–913, 2003.

Seron-Ferre M, Valenzuela GJ, Torres-Farfan C: Circadian clocks during embryonic and fetal development, *Birth Defects Res C Embryo Today* 81:204–214, 2007.

Sharkey J, Olcese J: Transcriptional inhibition of oxytocin receptor expression in human myometrial cells by melatonin involves protein kinase c signaling, *J Clin Endocrinol Metab* 92(10):4015–4019, 2007.

Sharkey JT, Puttaramu R, Word A, et al: Melatonin synergizes with oxytocin to enhance contractility of human myometrial smooth muscle cells, *J Clin Endocrinol Metab* 94(2):421–427, 2009.

Sheehan PM, Rice GE, Moses EK, et al: 5β-reductase decrease in association with human parturition at term, *Mol Hum Reprod* 11(7):495–501, 2005.

Shmygol A, Gullam J, Blanks A, et al: Multiple mechanisms involved in oxytocin-induced modulation of myometrial contractility, *Acta Pharmacol Sin* 27(7):827–832, 2006.

Shynlova O, Tsui P, Jaffer S, et al: Integration of endocrine and mechanical signals in the regulation of myometrial functions during pregnancy and labour, *Eur J Obstet Gynecol Reprod Biol* 144(Suppl 1):S2–S10, 2009.

Smith R: Parturition, *N Engl J Med* 356:271–283, 2007.

Smith R, Imtiaz M, Banney D, et al: Why the heart is like an orchestra and the uterus is like a soccer crowd, *Am J Obstet Gynecol* 181–185, 2015.

Smith R, Smith J, Shen X, et al: Patterns of plasma corticotrophin-releasing hormone, progesterone, estradiol, and estriol change and the onset of human labor, *J Clin Endocrinol Metab* 94:2066–2074, 2009.

Sparey C, Robson SC, Bailey J, et al: The differential expression of myometrial connexin-43, cycloxygenase-1 and -2, and Gs alpha proteins in the upper and lower segments of the human uterus during pregnancy and labour, *J Clin Endocrinol Metab* 84(5):1705–1710, 1999.

Stern JM: Offspring-induced nurturance: animal–human parallels, *Dev Psychobiol* 31:19–37, 1997.

Stevens MY, Challis JRG: Corticotrophin-releasing hormone receptor subtype 1 is significantly up-regulated at the time of labour in the human myometrium, *J Clin Endocrinol Metab* 83(11):4107–4115, 1998.

Tabak BA, Meyer ML, Castle E, et al: Vasopressin, but not oxytocin, increases empathic concern among individuals who received higher levels of paternal warmth: a randomized controlled trial, *Psychoneuroendocrinology* 51:253–261, 2015.

Takemura M, Kimura T, Nomura S, et al: Expression and localization of human oxytocin receptor mRNA and its protein in chorion and decidua during parturition, *J Clin Invest* 93:2319–2323, 1994.

Tamura H, Nakamura Y, Terron MP, et al: Melatonin and pregnancy in the human, *Reprod Toxicol* 25:291–303, 2008.

Terenzi MH, Ingram CD: Oxytocin induced excitation of neurones in the rat central and medial amygdaloid nuclei, *Neuroscience* 132:345–354, 2005.

Terzidou V, Soporanna SR, Kim LU, et al: Mechanical stretch up-regulates the human oxytocin receptor in primary human uterine myocytes, *J Clin Endocrinol Metab* 90(1):237–246, 2005.

Ticconi C, Belmonte A, Piccione E, et al: Feto-placental communication system with the myometrium in pregnancy and parturition: the role of hormones, neurohormones, inflammatory mediators, and locally active factors, *J Matern Fetal Neonatal Med* 19(3):125–133, 2006.

Ticconi C, Zicari A, Realacci M, et al: Oxytocin modulates nitric oxide generation by human fetal membranes at term pregnancy, *Am J Reprod Immunol* 52:185–191, 2004.

Tomizawa K, Iga N, Lu Y-F, et al: Oxytocin improves long-lasting spatial memory during motherhood through MAP kinase cascade, *Nat Neurosci* 6(4):384–390, 2003.

Torres-Farfan C, Mendez N, Abarzua-Catalan L, et al: A circadian clock entrained melatonin is ticking in the rat fetal adrenal, *Endocrinology* 152(5):1891–1900, 2011.

Torres-Farfan C, Richter HG, Germain AM, et al: Maternal melatonin selectively inhibits cortisol production in the primate fetal adrenal gland, *J Physiol (Lond)* 554(3):841–856, 2003.

Torres-Farfan C, Valenzuela FJ, Germain AM, et al: Maternal melatonin stimulates growth and prevents maturation of the capuchin monkey fetal adrenal gland, *J Pineal Res* 41:58–66, 2006.

Tyson EK, Smith R, Read M: Evidence that corticotrophin-releasing hormone modulates myometrial contractility during human pregnancy, *Endocrinology* 150(12):5617–5625, 2009.

Tyzio R, Cossart R, Khalilov I, et al: Maternal oxytocin triggers a transient inhibitory switch in GABA signalling in the fetal brain during delivery, *Science* 314:1788–1792, 2006.

Uvnas Moberg K: *The hormone of closeness: the role of oxytocin in relationships*, London, Pinter and Martin, 2013.

Vaisanen-Tommiska M, Nuutila M, Aittomaki K, et al: Nitric oxide metabolites in cervical fluid during pregnancy: further evidence for the role of cervical nitric oxide in cervical ripening, *Am J Obstet Gynecol* 188(5):779–785, 2003.

Van Leeuwen P, Geue D, Thiel M, et al: Influence of paced maternal breathing on fetal-maternal heart rate coordination, *Proc Natl Acad Sci USA* 106(33):13661–13666, 2009.

Van Puyvelde M, Lotts G, Meys J, et al: Whose clock makes yours tick? How maternal cardiorespiratory physiology influences newborns' heart rate variability, *Biol Psychol* 108:132–141, 2015.

Wang WS, Liu C, Li WJ, et al: Involvement of CRH and hCG in the induction of aromatase by cortisol in human placental syncytiotrophoblasts, *Placenta* 35:30–36, 2014.

Wellmann S, Benzing J, Kappa G, et al: High Copeptin concentrations in umbilical cord blood after vaginal delivery and birth acidosis, *J Clin Endocrinol Metab* 95(11):5091–5096, 2010.

Whipple B, Josimovich JB, Komisaruk BR: Sensory thresholds during the antepartum, intrapartum, and postpartum periods, *Int J Nurs Stud* 27(3):213–221, 1990.

Wierrani F, Grin W, Hlawka B, et al: Elevated serum melatonin levels during human late pregnancy and labour, *Am J Obstet Gynecol* 17(5):449–451, 1997.

Willcourt RJ, Pager D, Wendel J, et al: Induction of labour with pulsatile oxytocin by computer-controlled pump, *Am J Obstet Gynecol* 170(2):603–608, 1994.

Wilson BC, Ingram CD: Convergent effects of oxytocin and an opioid agonist in the bed nuclei of the stria terminalis of the peripartum rat, *Brain Res* 991:267–270, 2003.

Wuitchik M, Bakal D, Lipshitz J: The clinical significance of pain and cognitive activity in latent labour, *Obstet Gynecol* 73(1):35–42, 1989.

Yildirim G, Beji NK: Effects of pushing techniques in birth on mother and fetus: a randomized study, *Birth* 35:25–30, 2008.

Zheng J-J, Li S-J, Zhang X-D, et al: Oxytocin mediates early experience-dependent cross-modal plasticity in the sensory cortices, *Nat Neurosci* 17(3):391–399, 2014.

Resources and additional reading

Please refer to the chapter website resources.

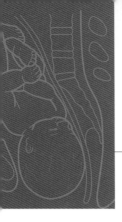

Chapter 36

Care in the first stage of labour

Dr Denis Walsh

Learning Outcomes ?

After reading this chapter, you will be able to:

- understand the importance of the context of childbirth
- recognize the onset of labour and appreciate the normal physiology of labour
- provide evidence-based care appropriate to the needs of the woman and her baby
- understand principles such as woman-centred care
- have insight into the key roles of environment and relationships with carers
- have an awareness of the holistic elements of labour care

INTRODUCTION

Labour and birth are an amazing integration of powerful physiological and psychological forces that bring a new human life into the world. It is difficult not to devalue labour and birth when it is analysed, dissected and examined to make it understood, because it works best as a coherent whole. There are key physical, emotional and social dimensions to the process of labour, in that the arrival of a baby heralds the birth or extension of a family. Throughout history, labour and birth had special meaning for every culture and their occurrence is often marked by spiritual and cultural symbols (Kitzinger 2000). In the UK today, such rituals have been marginalized by the medical environment in which most parturition takes place, with about 87% of births occurring in consultant units, 2% at home (National Audit Office (NAO) 2013) and 11% either in alongside midwifery units or in free-standing midwifery units (NAO 2013). For the midwife, a holistic understanding of labour and birth requires an awareness of the physiological/psychological changes and ability to see these remarkable events as having transformative potential for women and families, and having social and even political ramifications. This perspective has, as a starting point, a profound respect for and trust in women's innate ability to birth without technology or medical intervention. The chapter attempts to describe the changes, the events and the care from these personal, social and political dimensions.

Two birth stories (Case Studies 36.1 and 36.2) reveal the complexity of labour and birth.

CASE STUDY 36.1 EMILY'S BIRTH STORY

Emily was a 'no-nonsense' sort of person. She approached the birth of her first baby in a straightforward way. 'I'll know what to do at the time', she kept telling me. 'You just tag along and I'll ask if I need anything'. She called me out one Sunday morning and when I arrived told me her labour had started, and although she did not want me to do anything, she asked me to stay for a few hours. Later, she said I could go because she had hours to go yet. She called me again early the next morning and said it was time for the baby to come. I drove over to her house, and 2 hours later her son was born into the birthing pool, and there were tears all round. Emily was in tune with her body. She understood it and how the birth process would go for her far better than I did.

CASE STUDY 36.2 JUDY'S BIRTH STORY

Judy just avoided induction of labour because she was 10 days past her due date when her waters broke. The contractions arrived 8 hours later and were huge from the start. Despite fantastic support from Ben, her partner, she felt out of control with the labour's intensity. Her cervix was 7 cm dilated when she requested a vaginal examination 2 hours later. After an hour, her contractions became even more intense, and I suspected she was approaching the pushing phase. Then suddenly, everything stopped. She dozed on and off for 4 hours, when suddenly she was bearing down and the baby was born within two contractions. Judy felt traumatized by her rollercoaster ride, which she felt swept along by.

The midwife's description of these births shows how the experience of labour can vary for different women. The time spans were different – the first in excess of 24 hours and the second had a 'rest phase' of 4 hours before the birth. The women adapted to their experience in contrasting ways – one confident and controlled, the other feeling swamped by the power of her labour. In neither case is the midwife's role described, but different strategies of support would have been required to care appropriately for each woman.

Other aspects are key to assisting our understanding of these births. Both babies were born at home. Both women had people in attendance that they knew and had chosen to be there. Neither woman had any drugs, or common birth interventions. They did it 'naturally'. Their births were not typical of 21st-century childbirth experience in the UK. More typically, childbirth occurs in hospital with carers who have not been previously met, using routine interventions such as continuous electronic fetal monitoring. One in three births results in an instrumental vaginal birth or a caesarean section (NAO 2013). It could be argued that normal labour and birth is under threat, with only about 47% of women in England having a drug-free normal birth (NAO 2013).

Being in hospital requires conforming to an environment where the woman inevitably becomes a 'patient' and carers assume the status of experts. Labour is expected to conform to clinical guidelines designed for the 'average', triggering a range of interventions if deviation occurs from this 'average'. This chapter explores normal labour and birth from the perspective of non-intervention, viewing the birth environment as crucial to physiological processes. Having a baby on a labour ward may be viewed as a 'care intervention', likely to upset a delicate balance of physical, psychological and social processes that need to work in harmony for birth to be humane and life-enhancing. But it must also be said that the midwife can do much to neutralize the environmental effects and biomedical ethos of a labour ward by her support of physiological processes and her relationship with the woman.

THE CONTINUUM OF LABOUR

Labour has been traditionally divided into stages but this demarcation has its origins in a preoccupation with the time duration of each stage and its historical link to complications for the mother and baby. When learning about labour, practitioners are introduced to notions of time at the outset, which is consistent with a biomedical understanding of parturition that anticipates pathology in an effort to treat it as early as possible.

An alternative approach is beginning to gain exposure through the writings of midwives such as Downe and McCourt (2008) and Dixon et al (2013), where labour is a continuum from onset to completion, characterized by particular physiological and psychological behaviours at various points on that continuum. Some of these behaviours are anatomical changes, for example, changes in the cervix; some are physiological, such as release of body hormones; and some psychological, such as an alertness and focusing just before birth.

Individual behaviours and responses vary, and the importance of knowing and intuitively connecting with women is a key challenge for the midwife and allows care to be appropriate and tailored to individual need.

Although the demarcations of the stages of labour in the traditional biomedical model are intended to aid clarity in understanding physiology and care for the professional caregiver, they may also effectively silence the woman and discredit her version of events. For the woman, labour is a continuing physiological, psychological and emotional experience, the culmination and main focal point of the reproductive process, where artificial compartmentalization may be neither relevant nor important (Dixon et al 2013). The significance of labour, a biologically and socially creative life event, is reflected in the minutiae of detail women can recall about their particular labour(s). Events that are relatively common and usual from a midwife's perspective acquire much meaning and importance in the eyes of the woman and her family. To maximize the potential for a satisfactory outcome of labour, it is therefore essential that women's stories and details of events are listened to and valued.

Reflective activity 36.1 ＞＜

Ask your mother or close female relative about your birth and note the phrases she uses to describe it, the memories that have stayed with her and the overall impression of the experiences that she communicates to you. If you are not able to do this, ask another woman whom you know well to talk about her birth experience.

If the midwife anticipates a normal outcome to labour and birth, and trusts the woman's physiology will function optimally, this can positively influence the woman's own attitude. Women with an optimistic demeanour towards childbirth have better experiences and outcomes than those beset by anxiety and fear of what could go wrong

(Green et al 1998). This is particularly relevant in an era where media exposure of hospital birth is contributing towards an epidemic of fear in first time mothers (Morris and McInerney 2010). Midwives, therefore, can play a key role in empowering women as they approach childbirth within contemporary culture.

CHARACTERISTICS OF LABOUR

Normal labour naturally follows a sequential pattern that usually involves painful regular uterine contractions stimulating progressive effacement and dilatation of the cervix with descent of the fetus through the pelvis, culminating in the spontaneous vaginal birth of the baby, followed by the expulsion of the placenta and membranes. This traditional and orthodox biomedical definition of normal labour divides labour into three stages:

- *First stage:* from the onset of regular uterine contractions, accompanied by effacement and dilatation of the cervix, to full dilatation of the cervix.
- *Second stage:* from full dilatation of the cervix and the onset of expulsive, bearing-down contractions to the birth of the baby.
- *Third stage:* from the birth of the baby to the complete expulsion of the placenta and membranes.

The social model is more holistic and has contrasting values to the biomedical model (see Table 36.1).

The alternative values of the social model mean that the strenuous work of labour is acknowledged as fundamental. Gould (2000) acknowledged this along with the crucial role of movement. This highlights the courage and perseverance demonstrated by women as they 'work' during labour and the importance of an environment where movement will be facilitated.

PHYSIOLOGY OF LABOUR

Several physiological factors integrate as labour develops (Box 36.1), and these will be examined in turn.

Cervical effacement and dilatation

Cervical effacement and dilatation occur as a result of contraction and retraction of the uterine muscle.

Effacement (taking up) of the cervix may start in the latter 2 or 3 weeks of pregnancy and occurs as a result of changes in the solubility of collagen present in cervical tissue. This is influenced by alterations in hormone activity, particularly oestrogen, progesterone, relaxin, prolactin and prostaglandins (Blackburn 2013; see also Ch. 35).

Table 36.1 Biomedical and social models

Biomedical model	Versus	Social model
Body as machine		Whole person
Reductionism – powers, passages, passenger		Integrate – physiology, psychosocial, spiritual
Control and subjugate		Respect and empower
Expertise/objective		Relational/subjective
Environment peripheral		Environment central
Anticipate pathology		Anticipate normality
Technology as master		Technology as servant
Homogenization		Celebrate difference
Evidence		Intuition
Safety		Self-actualization

Source: Walsh and Newburn 2002

Box 36.1 Summary of the physiological changes in the first stage of labour

- Completion of effacement of the cervix and dilatation of the os uteri caused by uterine activity:
  - Contraction and retraction of uterine muscles
  - Fundal dominance
  - Active upper uterine segment, passive lower segment
  - Formation of the retraction ring
  - Polarity of the uterus
  - Intensity or amplitude of contractions
  - Resting tone
- Formation of the bag of forewaters and the hindwaters
- Rupture of the membranes
- Show

Braxton Hicks contractions, which become stronger in the final weeks of pregnancy, may also enhance the process. Effacement is completed in labour as the cervix becomes shorter and dilates slightly, becoming funnel shaped as the internal os opens to form part of the lower uterine segment (see Fig. 36.1).

Progressive dilatation of the cervix (see Fig. 36.2) is a definitive sign of labour.

When the cervix is dilated sufficiently to allow the fetal head to pass through, full dilatation has been achieved. Although this is usually 10 cm, it may be more or less depending on the size of the fetal head.

In primigravidas, effacement of the cervix usually precedes dilatation; however, in multigravidas, effacement and dilatation of the cervix normally occur simultaneously (see Fig. 36.2).

Uterine contractions

Uterine contractions are responsible for achieving progressive effacement and dilatation of the cervix and for the descent and expulsion of the fetus in labour. Contractions of the uterus in labour have the following characteristics:

- They are involuntary.
- They are intermittent and regular.
- In almost all labours, they are painful.

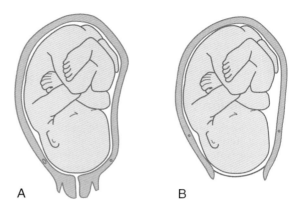

Figure 36.1 The uterus. **A,** Cervix before effacement. **B,** Effacement and dilatation of the cervix and the stretched lower uterine segment.

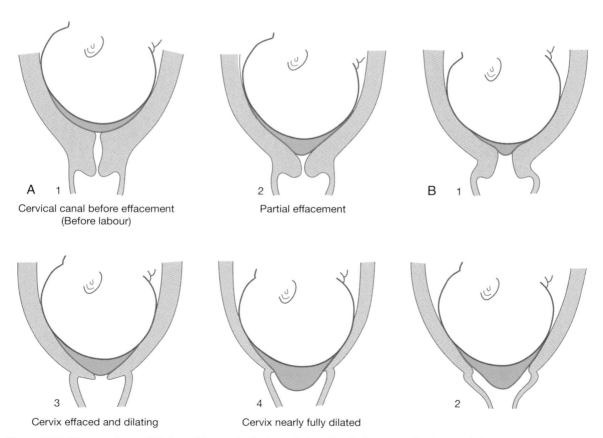

A 1 Cervical canal before effacement (Before labour)

2 Partial effacement

B 1

3 Cervix effaced and dilating

4 Cervix nearly fully dilated

2

Figure 36.2 Effacement and dilatation of the cervix. **A,** In a primigravida. **B,** Occurring simultaneously in a multigravida.

The pain may be in part a result of ischaemia developing in the muscle fibres during contractions. The backache that may accompany cervical dilatation is caused by stimulation of sensory fibres that pass via the sympathetic nerves to the sacral plexus.

Coordination of contractions

Contractions start from the cornua of the uterus, passing in waves, inwards and downwards. In normal uterine action, the intensity is greatest in the upper uterine segment and lessens as the contraction passes down the uterus. This is called fundal dominance. The upper segment of the uterus contracts and retracts powerfully, whereas the lower segment contracts only slightly and dilates. Between contractions the uterus relaxes.

The coordinated uterine activity characteristic of normal labour occurs as a result of near-simultaneous contraction of all myometrial cells. During pregnancy, increasing numbers of gap junctions form between the cells of the myometrium (see Ch. 35 also). These low-resistance communication channels enhance electrical conduction velocity and facilitate the coordination of myometrial contraction (Blackburn 2013).

Retraction

Retraction is a state of permanent shortening of the muscle fibres and occurs with each contraction (see Fig. 36.3).

The muscle fibres gradually become shorter and thicker, especially in the upper uterine segment. This exerts a pull on the less-active lower uterine segment, the maximum pull being directed towards the weakest point, the cervix, and the os uteri. Hence the cervix is gradually 'taken up', or effaced, and the upward pull then dilates the os uteri.

As the space within the upper uterine segment diminishes with the contraction and retraction of the muscle fibres, the fetus is forced down into the lower segment and the presenting part exerts pressure on the os uteri. This aids

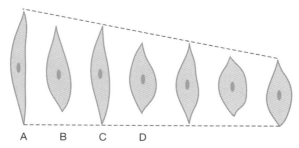

Figure 36.3 Retraction of the uterine muscle fibres. **A,** Relaxed. **B,** Contracted. **C,** Relaxed but retracted. **D,** Contracted but shorter and thicker than those in B.

dilatation, and also causes a reflex release of oxytocin from the posterior pituitary gland, promoting further uterine action. A ridge gradually forms between the thick, retracted muscle fibres of the upper uterine segment and the thin, distended lower segment. This is called a *retraction ring* – a normal physiological occurrence in every labour.

Polarity

The rhythmical coordination (*polarity*) between the upper and lower segments is balanced and harmonious in normal labour. Whereas the upper segment contracts powerfully and retracts, the lower segment contracts only slightly and dilates.

Intensity or amplitude

Contractions cause a rise in intra-uterine pressure – the *intensity* or *amplitude* of contractions – which can be measured by placing a fine catheter into the uterus and attaching it to a pressure-recording apparatus. Each contraction rises rapidly to a peak and then slowly declines to the resting tone. In early labour the contractions are weak, with an amplitude of about 20 mmHg, last 20 to 30 seconds and occur without any particular pattern. As labour progresses, the contractions become stronger, longer and more frequent. At the end of the first stage they are strong, with an amplitude of 60 mmHg, last 45 to 60 seconds and occur every 2 to 3 minutes.

Resting tone

The uterus is never completely relaxed, and between contractions a measured resting tone is usually 4 to 10 mmHg. During contractions the blood flow to the placenta is curtailed; thus, oxygen and carbon dioxide exchange in the intervillous spaces is impeded. The period of relaxation between contractions when the uterus has a low resting tone is therefore vital for adequate fetal oxygenation.

Formation of the forewaters and hindwaters

As the lower uterine segment stretches and cervical effacement commences, some chorion becomes detached from the decidua and both membranes form a small bag containing amniotic fluid, which protrudes into the cervix. When the fetal head descends onto the cervix, it separates the small bag of amniotic fluid in front, the forewaters, from the remainder, the hindwaters (see Fig. 36.4).

The forewaters aid effacement of the cervix and early dilatation of the os uteri, and the hindwaters help to equalize the pressure in the uterus during uterine contractions, providing some protection to the fetus and placenta.

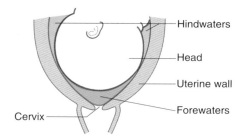

Figure 36.4 Formation of hindwaters and forewaters.

Labels on figure: Hindwaters, Head, Uterine wall, Forewaters, Cervix

Rupture of the membranes

The membranes are thought to rupture as a result of increased production of prostaglandin E2 in the amnion in labour (McCoshen et al 1990) and the force of the uterine contractions, causing an increase in the fluid pressure inside the forewaters and a lessening of the support as the cervix dilates. In normal labour the membranes usually rupture during the second stage of labour.

Show

The 'show' is the *operculum* from the cervical canal passed per vaginam in labour, displaced when effacement of the cervix and dilatation of the os uteri occur. It is usually mucoid and may be slightly streaked with blood as a result of some separation of the chorion from the decidua around the cervix.

Hormones of labour

In the previous chapter, the role of labour and birth hormones was explained. Principally these involve oxytocin, beta endorphins, catecholamines, cortisol and prolactin. All of these hormones interconnect with each other and are highly sensitive to environmental effects and caring behaviours. Mammals and therefore humans have evolved over thousands of years to marry feeling safe during labour and birth with optimum physiological and hormonal interactions (Buckley 2015). There is increasing awareness of the relationship between oxytocin, endorphin release and the level of catecholamines and cortisol (see Ch. 35). Anxiety and fear stimulate the release of adrenaline (epinephrine), noradrenaline (norepinephrine) and cortisol, and inhibit oxytocin; hence the importance of birth environment and birth relationships in promoting calm and confidence in birthing women. Dixon et al (2013) capture this 'dance of labour' in paralleling hormonal effects with physiological changes and their accompanying emotional responses in women during labour (see Fig. 36.5). This understanding of labour and birth brings a much needed holistic dimension, foregrounding what has been missing in the past – women's lived experience of these events.

CARE DURING THE FIRST STAGE OF LABOUR

The aims of midwifery care in labour are to achieve a safe labour and birth for mother and baby, and a pleasurable, fulfilling experience of childbirth for the mother and her partner.

Now that deaths in childbirth for women and babies in the Western world are rare, women's experience of childbirth has taken on greater significance and has become a major focus for the professionals assisting childbirth. Most early research on labour and birth did not explore women's experiences and was based around professionals' priorities and their interests. Recent studies have determined women's views on various aspects of care (Lally et al 2008; Redshaw et al 2007; Rudman et al 2007) and these can be summarized under the following themes:

- Information that is full, accurate, evidence-based and individualized
- Choice
- Control
- Continuity

These themes need to underpin the philosophy of care and its application, helping to define woman-centred care, as described and endorsed in maternity care policy at government level (Department of Health (DH) 2007a and 2007b).

To provide woman-centred care, the midwife should do the following:

1. Assess the needs and expectations of each individual woman regarding labour and birth.
2. Plan care with each woman in labour, tailored to meet her specific needs and expectations.
3. Put the care plan into practice.
4. Evaluate the care given to measure its effectiveness.

Partnership in care

The relationship between the woman and her midwife is ideally a partnership (Pairman 2000) that should begin in pregnancy, and it has been described as 'skilled companionship' or the 'professional friend' in its intimacy and reciprocity (Pembroke and Pembroke 2008). The partnership ethos requires a social rather than biomedical model of maternity care, endorsing the involvement of the woman and her partner in decision making from the very

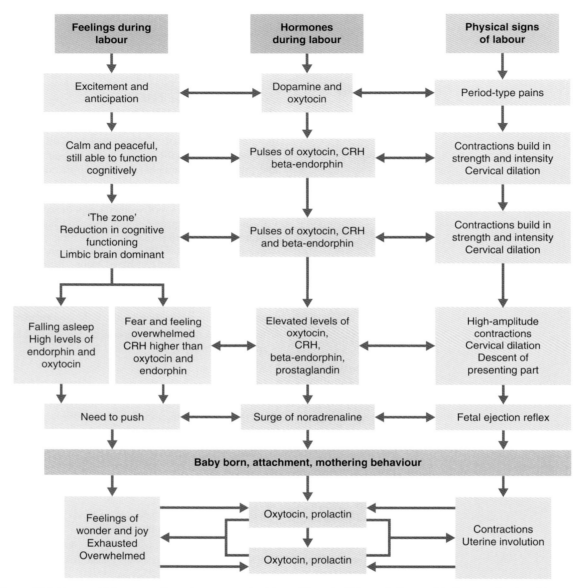

Figure 36.5 Dance of labour: emotions, hormones, physiology. (Dixon L, Skinner J, Foureur M: The emotional and hormonal pathways of labour and birth: integrating mind, body and behaviour, New Zealand College of Midwives Journal 48:15, 2013.)

start of pregnancy, and requiring the woman to be able to voice her needs and wishes freely. The midwife should strive to build a relationship of mutual trust and create an environment in which expectations, wishes, fears and anxieties can be readily discussed. This requires good communication, which results from a two-way interaction between equals.

Emotional and psychological care

The midwife needs to have a good understanding of a woman's feelings in labour. Attitudes and reactions to childbirth vary considerably and are influenced by differing social, cultural and religious factors. For a multigravida, previous experience of birth will also be important.

Many women anticipate labour with mixed feelings of fear and excitement. Some may eagerly anticipate the birth, confident in their ability to cope, seeing birth as an emotionally fulfilling and enriching experience involving all immediate family members. They may have attended teaching sessions for natural or active childbirth and have a particular plan of action for their labour, often called a *birth plan*. Others may be excited at the prospect of actually seeing their babies, yet fearful of labour and anxious about their ability to cope with pain and 'perform' well. Some expect labour to be painful and unpleasant, controlled by obstetricians and midwives, and to be achieved with as little pain and active participation as possible.

The woman may be apprehensive about entering an unknown, and perhaps threatening, hospital environment and concerned about relinquishing her personal autonomy and identity. Alternatively, expectations of labour may be unrealistic, and may be unfulfilled, leading to feelings of disappointment, failure or loss. Multigravidas are often anxious about children they have left at home. The midwife can do much to alleviate these worries.

Birth partners may also have particular concerns that they feel unable to share. Reservations may be influenced by the role society attributes to gender – a man being expected to be strong and able to cope; or may be caused by fear of the unknown and concern for someone who is loved. Same-sex partners may feel anxious about the reception they or their partners may receive. With a partnership and individual approach to care, particularly if established during the antenatal period, the midwife has a valuable opportunity to encourage the couple to voice their particular needs and anxieties, and explore and agree ways of dealing with them. Whatever the needs of the individual couple, they are influenced by the desire to do what is best for their baby and, if they are confident that the midwife will respect and comply with their wishes in normal circumstances, they will usually readily agree to modify expectations should labour complications arise.

Throughout labour there should be a free flow of information between the woman, her partner and the midwife. Being fully informed and involved in decision making helps the woman to retain a sense of autonomy and control (Healthcare Commission 2008). The midwife should be aware that not all individuals may feel sufficiently secure or freely able to express fears or anxieties during labour. Circumstances such as an unwanted pregnancy, fear or previously poor relationships with professional caregivers may engender feelings of unhappiness, hostility and resentment. The midwife needs to be particularly sensitive to nonverbal indicators of such feelings and give the necessary help and support needed by the woman. Above all, though, the midwife should be compassionate, empathic and nonjudgemental. Extensive research has shown that caring behaviours directly stimulate the affiliative, soothing regulatory centre in the mammalian brain

(Gilbert 2010) and facilitating labour physiology by augmenting oxytocin release (Moberg 2011)

The role of the birth supporter

Evidence from a number of studies indicates the positive effect of continuous support in labour (Hodnett et al 2008 and 2013). Although it is usual in the UK for a couple to support each other in labour, some women may choose to have a relative, friend or doula as labour companions. Whoever has been chosen, the midwife should explore with supporters their experiences of childbirth, their role expectations during labour and their ability to undertake the supporter role. It has been suggested that if chosen supporters have had negative childbirth experiences, these need to be addressed by the midwife if they are not to hinder the supporting relationship with the woman.

The midwife involves the birth supporter as part of the team, with a defined role, which can include massaging back, abdomen or legs, helping with breathing awareness and relaxation, and offering drinks and other means of sustenance. Such activities, during a highly anxious time, can be very valuable in helping the partner to feel usefully occupied and involved in the birthing event.

The midwife must be sensitive to the possible need for personal space and privacy and should judge when, and if, it is appropriate to leave the woman and partner alone. This is usually more acceptable in early labour but less so when labour is strong and well advanced, when to be left alone might be frightening. If the midwife must leave for a short period, she must ensure that the couple can summon help if necessary. The midwife must also be sensitive to the emotional needs of the partner and other members of staff and recognize that, particularly during a long labour, a short break may be beneficial in helping to replenish energy levels.

Advocacy

For some women, fear of the unknown, being cared for in hospital by unfamiliar people, experiencing greater pain than expected or the effect of analgesic drugs can cause feelings of vulnerability, loss of personal identity and powerlessness. This may be magnified for women for whom English is not their first language. Vulnerable individuals can lose the ability to adequately express their needs, wishes, values and choices and adopt a passive recipient role. The midwife may need to act as advocate, to ensure that personal needs are met (Walsh 2007a). This includes informing, supporting and protecting women, acting as intermediary between them and obstetric and other professional colleagues and facilitating informed choice. To achieve this, the midwife must be professionally confident, have a clear awareness of the woman's needs and be able to communicate these to other colleagues to ensure effective collaboration. Developing and trusting intuition is central to this activity. The midwife's rapport and connectedness with the woman for whom she is caring mean that appropriate decision making and a facilitatory birth environment is more likely (Walsh 2007b). Using these skills, the midwife is more able to empower the woman and her partner so that both feel sufficiently informed and confident to participate in decision making during this important life experience.

THE BIRTH ENVIRONMENT

Practitioners of normal birth and women themselves know how significant the birth environment is for the experience and outcomes of birth, including the birth setting, the relational components of care and congruence of values about birth.

Home

Home birth has long generated an intense debate, and birth at home has become a rallying point for midwives and women who endorse childbirth's essential normality against those who can only view its normality retrospectively. Tew (1998) first challenged the dominant 1970s/1980s view that the safest environment for birth was hospital. She exposed the fundamental flaw of assigning a single cause (hospitalization of birth) to a discrete effect (lowering perinatal mortality rates) without consideration of alternative explanations. This spurious logic had led to a nationwide movement of birth to hospitals over 20 years before an alternative explanation gained credibility – that the fall was attributable to the dramatic improvement in the general health of women in the post-war period coupled with an even more dramatic rise in living standards (Campbell and McFarlane 1994; Tew 1998).

It is now acknowledged that current evidence does not provide justification for requiring that all women give birth in hospital (Olsen and Clausen 2012) and that women should be offered an explicit choice when they become pregnant of where they want to have their babies (DH 2007a). Within the UK, the Birthplace study found that nulliparous women's babies were at a slightly elevated risk of a poor perinatal outcome compared with birthing in a midwifery unit or an obstetric unit (Brocklehurst et al 2011). However, other comprehensive literature reviews of home birth research, which included 26 studies from many parts of the developed world, concluded that 'studies demonstrate remarkably consistency in the generally favourable results of maternal and neonatal outcomes, both over time and among diverse population groups' (Fullerton and Young 2007: 323). The outcomes were also favourable when viewed in comparison to various reference groups (midwifery unit births, planned hospital births).

Randomized controlled trials (RCTs) have demonstrated clear benefit in a number of associated elements of the home birth 'package of care', including continuity of care during labour and birth (Hodnett et al 2008 and 2013) and midwife-led care (Hatem et al 2008), both of which are probably universal aspects of home birth provision.

Though official UK government policy up to the present is to offer women a choice about place of birth, the UK home birth rate remains just above 2%, compared with 25% in the early 1960s (NAO 2013). There are anecdotal stories of women either being discouraged from choosing the home birth option or being told that staff shortages may affect the availability of midwives.

One practical measure to reduce the bias to hospital birth may be to keep the option for home birth open until labour begins. Requiring a firm decision in early pregnancy regarding home birth may be problematic for the following reasons:

- Some women may develop complications during pregnancy that require hospital care.
- Some women have access to midwifery support at home in early labour and may prefer to stay there rather than face an uncomfortable journey to hospital.

Midwifery units

There are two types of midwifery unit: freestanding and alongside. The Birthplace study recommended that these terms (freestanding and alongside) be adopted to replace the numerous alternative names such as *birth centres, midwifery-led units, community midwifery units* and so forth. Maternity services across the UK are merging, driven by the growth of neonatal tertiary referral centres and by rationalizing of management and clinical structures of individual hospitals that are no longer seen as cost-effective if they remain separate. These pressures are leading to stakeholders choosing to combine birth facilities on one site with neonatal services or retain present infrastructures and open midwifery-led units or birthing units (DH 2007b). The benefit of midwifery units for women and midwives has been comprehensively established by the Birthplace study, which found that caesarean section and epidural rates among other common birth interventions were significantly lowered when women at low obstetric risk accessed them (Brocklehurst et al 2011). In addition, costs per woman were reduced and markers of physiological birth like physiological third stage increased. As a consequence, the National Institute for Health and Care Excellence (NICE) Intrapartum Guidelines, updated in 2014 and 2016, now encourage low-risk women to birth in midwifery units (NICE 2014 and 2016).

A systematic review of alongside midwifery units (Hodnett et al 2012) has consistently shown a reduction in labour and birth interventions and increased satisfaction for women.

All of this evidence is resulting in increased numbers and size of midwifery units across England, though currently they only provide for around 12% of all births (NAO 2013), a figure that could be expanded to around 30%.

Qualitative literature on home birth and freestanding midwifery units highlights two other aspects of care: how temporality is enacted and how smallness of scale affects the ethos and ambience of care. The regulatory effect of 'clock time' is less evident both at home and in midwifery units. Labour rhythms rather than labour progress tend to be emphasized by staff and there is usually greater flexibility with the application of the labour record, the partogram (Fig. 36.6). Part of the reason for this lies in the absence of an organizational imperative to 'get women through the system' (Walsh 2006a). Small numbers of women birthing mean less stress on organizational processes and a more relaxed ambience in the setting. This appears to suit women and staff well, suggesting attunement to labour physiology, inherently manifesting as biological rhythms based on hormonal pulses of activity, rather than regular clock time rhythms (Adam 1995). This increases the perception of clinical freedom, satisfaction and feeling of belonging for midwives (Walsh 2006b).

Significant research undertaken into different organizational models of midwifery care including teams, caseloads and midwifery group practices has been premised on the principle that women benefit from establishing an ongoing relationship with their carers rather than being cared for by strangers within a fragmented model. Common sense may suggest that journeying through such significant rites of passage in the experience of childbirth is best done in the company of known carers. Even without the studies, it could be argued that indigenous birth practices have much to inform maternity care in the West. For thousands of years, traditional birth attendants working with local women have harnessed the power of known birth companions in facilitating birth for the uninitiated woman. Western-style birth lost this crucial dimension when birth was hospitalized and supported by professionals who were usually unknown to labouring women. After the advent of doulas in US hospitals in the late 1970s, recognition was given to this fundamental aspect of labour care.

Doula studies examined the value of being supported throughout the entire labour and this aspect of care has now been extensively researched. A systematic review of 22 RCTs (Hodnett et al 2013) concluded that continuous support during labour had the following advantages:

- Women were more likely to have shorter labours.
- Women were less likely to have a baby with a low Apgar score.
- Reduced caesarean sections, pharmacological analgesia, assisted vaginal birth, low Apgar scores, and labour length
- Resulted in women experiencing more positive births
- Could provide the most effective support from those not employed by the institution
- Will be less effective in a highly medicalized environment

A review of eight studies of labour support provided by five different categories of persons concluded that care by known, untrained laywomen, starting in early labour, was most effective (Rosen 2004). A study echoing childbirth physiology found that oxytocin was released in women exposed to stress and this triggered 'tending' and 'befriending' behaviours rather than the classical (male) response of 'fight and flight'. In a further mirroring of the hormonal cascade of labour, endogenous opiates, also released during the experience of stress, augment these effects (Taylor et al 2000).

The number of carers a woman has during her period of continuous support may also be relevant to outcome, as caesarean section rates appear to increase in direct line with increasing number of carers. Keeping the number of changes of labour support persons to a minimum has been recommended (Gagnon et al 2007).

Midwives have argued for decades to provide continuous support in labour so that they can genuinely be 'with woman'. It is likely that this organizational aspect alone would increase normal birth rates substantially. Yet achieving this goal remains an objective rather than an imperative for most maternity services.

Continuity has been the subject of research and debate in midwifery for two decades. Examination of wider health literature reveals that continuity has been of interest for many other areas, summarized by Haggerty et al (2003) as being centred on the following:

- Informational continuity (patient story available to all relevant agencies)
- Management continuity (consistent, coherent care)
- Relational continuity (known carers)

All three contribute to a better patient experience and, arguably, better care. Midwifery care has focused more

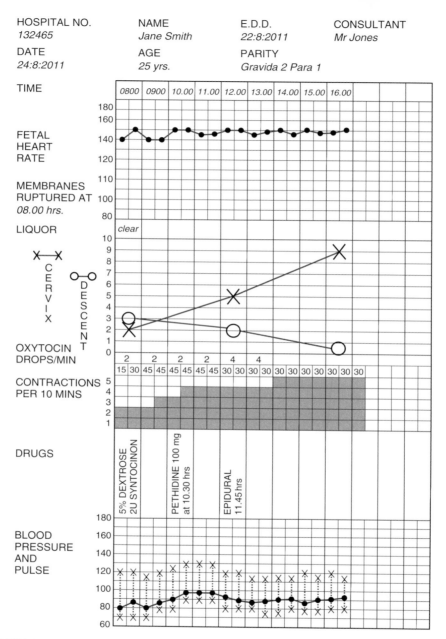

Figure 36.6 A partogram.

on relational continuity, possibly believing that the other two will follow, although this may not be the case. A case can be made for this focus because of the unique features of the midwife/woman relationship: its biologically determined longevity, its journey through a major rites of passage experience, and the intimate nature of its focus.

There are many organizational variants of continuity of care in midwifery services, including named midwife, teams, caseloads and group practices. Research has suggested the following:

• Teams should number no more than six because as numbers increase, 'a known midwife' becomes 'someone met once or twice' to eventually 'someone spoken of by a colleague' and continuity becomes meaningless (Flint 1993).

- Continuity needs differ depending on phases of care. Keeping the number of carers to a minimum may be more important for labour and the postnatal period than antenatally (Green et al 1998).
- Continuity between phases, especially having a known midwife for labour, is highly valued by women (Walsh and Devane 2012) and reduces labour interventions (Tracey et al 2013; Hartz et al 2012).

In relation to clinical outcomes and satisfaction with care, team and continuity variants generally reduce interventions, including epidural, induction of labour, episiotomy and neonatal resuscitation rates and improve satisfaction.

Midwifery-led care

All of the previously discussed models and settings of care demonstrate the value added of trained midwives leading the provision of care. The importance of midwifery-led care has been established by Sandall et al's (2013) systematic review, which showed a lowering of intervention rates in labour and birth and a reduction in preterm birth and fetal and neonatal death. Walsh and Devane's (2012) meta-synthesis of midwifery-led care found that the probable mechanism by which benefits are realized has to do with the greater autonomy for midwives and greater agency for women that this model provides.

ONSET OF LABOUR

Physiological changes occurring in late pregnancy are described in Chapter 35 and lead to signs heralding the onset of labour. Some women will follow a particular physiological pattern, but allowance should be made for individual variations, which may be associated with differences in pain perception and response, parity, and expectations of labour. These factors must be considered by the midwife in assisting the woman to recognize when she is in labour.

Uterine contractions

Women become aware of the painless, irregular, Braxton Hicks contractions of pregnancy, which increase as pregnancy advances. In labour these become regular and painful. Initially the woman may experience minimal discomfort and complain of sacral and/or lower abdominal pain, not necessarily immediately associated with labour. Such discomfort may later be noted to coincide with tightening or tension of the abdomen, occurring at regular intervals of 20 to 30 minutes and lasting 20 to 30 seconds. These uterine contractions can be felt by the midwife on abdominal palpation. As labour progresses, contractions become longer, stronger and more frequent, resulting in progressive effacement and dilatation of the cervix.

Show

Show, the mucoid, often blood-stained, discharge is passed per vagina, representing the passage of the operculum, which previously occupied the cervical canal. This is indicative of a degree of cervical activity – that is, softening and stretching of tissues, causing separation of the membranes from the decidua around the opening of the internal os. The show is often the first sign that labour is imminent or has started.

Rupture of the membranes

Rupture of the membranes can occur before labour or at any time during labour (see Ch. 35). Although significant, it is not a true sign of labour unless accompanied by dilatation of the cervix. An estimated 6% to 19% of women at term will experience spontaneous rupture of the membranes before labour starts (Tan and Hannah 2002), and in 85% of women the membranes rupture spontaneously at a cervical dilatation of 9 cm or more (Schwarcz et al 1979). The amount of amniotic fluid lost when the membranes rupture depends largely on how effectively the fetal presentation assists in the formation of the forewaters. In the presence of a normal amount of amniotic fluid, if the head is not engaged in the pelvis and the presenting part is not well applied to the os uteri, rupture of the membranes is easily recognized by a significant loss of fluid. If the presenting part is engaged and well applied, rupture of the forewaters may result in minimal fluid loss. This is usually followed by further seepage of amniotic fluid, which may be mistaken for urinary incontinence (not uncommon in late pregnancy). Usually the woman's history or evidence of amniotic fluid confirms the rupture of the membranes.

Contact with the midwife

Changing patterns of care reflect recent research highlighting the importance of consistent advice and continuity of care for this early phase of labour (Walsh 2007a). The woman should therefore be advised to contact the midwife when regular contractions are recognized, the membranes rupture or if she is concerned for any reason.

Clear and written instructions, given well in advance of the expected date of birth, including relevant telephone numbers of the community or team midwives and their location, are necessary and useful for anxious partners/birth supporters.

If the woman does not know the midwife, the midwife must be aware of the sensitivity of the first meeting and the importance of the initial interaction with the woman, which forms the basis for their future relationship. Women experience a variety of conflicting emotions and it is important that at the initial meeting, the midwife makes a rapid assessment of the woman and context to prioritize her care.

Information should be calmly and sensitively sought, allowing sufficient time for the woman to express her feelings and identify needs. In particular, a woman's story of how labour started should be validated, not dismissed as not fitting with what the textbooks say (Gross et al 2003). The midwife can achieve a relaxed, confident and reassuring approach while acquiring the necessary information and enabling the woman's verbal contribution to be valued, fostering the desired supportive partnership in care.

Before examining the woman, the midwife should review the woman's notes and ensure that all required information is present. The birth plan should indicate the special needs and wishes of the woman and her partner and can assist in providing continuity of care and may provide reassurance to the woman that her particular needs and wishes are recorded for staff caring for her to see. Such plans may also be instrumental in enabling the woman to retain control of labour events and can provide the midwife with a valuable opportunity for health education in relation to birth.

OBSERVATIONS

General examination

The midwife assesses the woman's appearance and demeanour, looking for features of general health and well-being. Observations of temperature, pulse, blood pressure and urinalysis are undertaken, providing a baseline for the labour. Recommendations regarding the frequency of recording the vital signs in labour are based on tradition rather than evidence. Commonly, in early labour the temperature and blood pressure are recorded every 4 hours and the pulse hourly (NICE 2014 and 2016).

Abdominal examination

A detailed abdominal examination is carried out, between contractions, to determine the lie, presentation, position and level of engagement of the presenting part. This includes a process of assessing visually, palpation and finally auscultation. This must be a gentle process, avoiding pain or discomfort and involving the couple as much as possible. The lie should be longitudinal. It is also important to determine the presentation and whether the presenting part is engaged, or will engage, in the pelvis. Auscultation of the fetal heart completes the abdominal examination; it should be strong and regular with a rate of between 110 and 160 beats per minute.

Vaginal examination

This procedure is one of the options to help confirm the onset of labour. However, it is invasive and often very uncomfortable for the woman and also poses a potential infection risk. Women may request it in seeking reassurance about the status of labour.

Records

When labour is established, all observations, examinations and any drug treatment are recorded on the partogram, enabling observations to be detailed on one sheet (see Fig. 36.6). The midwife's record constitutes a legal document, and throughout labour, accurate, concise and comprehensive records must be maintained in accordance with the midwives' rules and record-keeping guidance (NMC 2012 and 2015). Notations must be made at the time of the event, or as near as possible, and authenticated with the midwife's full, legible signature and status.

Contemporaneous records also facilitate continuity of care in the event that care has to be transferred to another member of the team.

GENERAL MIDWIFERY CARE IN LABOUR

Assessment of progress

Labour progression has been the focus of extensive research over the past 40 years, although such research generally suffers from contextual narrowness, having been exclusively carried out in large maternity hospitals. This limits the ability to premise writing on conventional evidence sources and undermines attempts to explain the rich variety of personal anecdote around individual women's labours. Research into out-of-hospital birth settings is urgently needed to explore and explain labour patterns.

Origins of the progress paradigm

Friedman's seminal work in measuring and recording cervical dilatation over time with a cohort of women in the mid-1950s influenced understanding of average lengths of labour for primigravid and multigravid women. The resulting sigmoid-shaped Friedman curve, representing early, middle and later phases of the first stage of labour, was incorporated into obstetric and midwifery textbooks for 50 years (Friedman 1954) (Fig. 36.7).

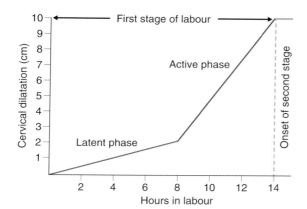

Figure 36.7 A cervicograph.

In the early 1970s, while working in remote area of Rhodesia, concerned about the disastrous consequences of obstructed labours, Philpott and Castle (1972) added the partogram to labour records and amplified the cervicograph to give guidance regarding slow labours, with three action lines used in the active phase of the first stage of labour:

1. *Alert line* at 1-cm/hour rate – signalling the need for close monitoring.
2. *Transfer line* – 2 hours behind the alert line – need for transfer physically to a major hospital.
3. *Action line* – 2 hours behind the transfer line – rupture membranes and administer Syntocinon.

Studd (1973) measured cohorts of women admitted to UK hospitals at differing stages of labour, plotting cervical dilatation over time, raising the possibility that British women might labour at different rates than African or North American women.

Organizational factors

This clinical imperative that long labours could indicate pathology may not have gained credence without the changes in organizational structures in how maternity care was delivered, in particular the centralizing movement of the second half of the 20th century. With more women giving birth in larger hospitals, organizational pressure increased towards processing women through labour wards and postnatal wards. Martin (1987) railed against assembly-line childbirth in the 1980s, and Perkin's (2004) comprehensive and considered critique of US maternity care policy, likening the Henry Ford car assembly line to the organization of maternity hospital activity, highlighted the explicit adoption of an essentially business/industrial model by maternity hospitals.

A study of childbirth at a freestanding midwifery unit (FMU) in the UK (Walsh 2006a) highlighted temporal differences as being the most striking factor differentiating the FMU from maternity hospitals. Women's labours were not on a time line and there was no pressure to 'free up' rooms for new occupants. The corollary of hospitals with time restrictions on labour length is that more women can labour and birth within their space. It comes as little surprise to find that the hospitals still practising active management of labour are among the largest in Europe, with over 8000 births per year (Murphy-Lawless 1998). Midwives' anecdotes and ethnographic research point to the pressures that exist in big units to 'get through the work' (Hunt and Symonds 1995).

A backlash against the clinical imperative of labour progress began to appear in the late 1990s when Albers's research (1999) concluded that nulliparous women's labours were longer than suggested by Friedman. In a low-risk population of women cared for by midwives in nine different centres in the United States, some active phases of labour were twice the length of Friedman's cohort (17.5 hours vs. 8.5 hours for nulliparas, and 13.8 hours vs. 7 hours for multiparas) without any consequent morbidity. A later study found an average length of labour similar to that of Friedman but with a wider range of 'normal' (Cesario 2004). Primiparous women remained in the first stage for up to 26 hours, and multiparous women for 23 hours, without adverse effects. A recent RCT showed that if prescriptive action lines that limit labour length are used with primigravid women, then over 50% will require intervention, with the authors calling for a review of labour length orthodoxies (Lavender et al 2006).

One study examined patterns of cervical dilatation in 1329 nulliparous women, finding slower dilatation rates in the active phase, especially before 7 cm, where the slowest group were all below Friedman's 1-cm/hour threshold. Conclusions suggested that current diagnostic criteria for protracted or arrested labour may be too stringent, citing important contextual differences in current practice to Friedman's day (Zhang et al 2002). Improvement in the general health of the current generation of women compared with 50 years ago probably makes them less vulnerable to the effects of long labours.

These papers suggest more physiological variation between women than previously thought. Midwives have always known that many women do not fit the average of a 1-cm/hour dilatation rate and, more fundamentally, may not physiologically mimic the parameters of the 'average' cervix. The cervix may be fully dilated at 9 or 11 cm. Given the infinite variety in women's physical appearance and psychosocial characteristics, it seems reasonable to expect subtle differences in their birth physiology.

Better understanding of the hormones regulating labour contributes to this more complex picture of physiological variation. Odent (2001) and Buckley (2004) illustrated that the 'hormonal cocktail' influencing these processes is appropriately called the 'dance of labour', the hormones' delicate interactions mediated by environmental and relational factors resembling the rhythm, beauty and harmony of skilled dancers.

Rhythms in early labour

The division of the first stage of labour into latent and active is clinician-based and not necessarily resonant with the lived experience of labour, especially for women with a long latent phase. Early labour is an area that continues to generate complaints from labouring women who often feel they are being prevented from accessing labour wards (Eri et al 2015). Much of the problem stems from inadequate and inflexible norms of understanding around the transition from latent phase to active phase in the first stage of labour. Traditionally, the latent phase of labour has been understood to be of varying length, culminating in a transition to the active phase at around 4-cm dilatation of the cervix (NICE 2014). However, more recent research by Zhang et al (2010) has questioned this threshold. His extensive studies in the United States demonstrated that cervical dilatation in many women does not accelerate significantly until 6 cm dilated (see Fig. 36.8). His research has resulted in the American College of Obstetrics and Gynaecology changing its guidance so that active phase of the first stage of labour is now 6-cm dilatation. As yet, guidance from NICE remains unchanged at 4-cm dilatation. Gross et al (2003) increased understanding of the phenomenon of early labour by revealing how eclectically it presents in different women and how they vary in their self-diagnosis: 60% of woman experienced contractions as the starting point of their labours and the remainder described a variety of other symptoms. Gross suggests the direction of questioning be changed from eliciting the pattern of contractions to simply enquiring 'How did you recognize the start of labour?'

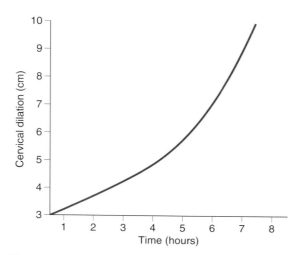

Figure 36.8 Zhang curve. Zhang et al 2002.

The midwifery diagnosis of labour in hospital is not simply a unilateral clinical judgement but a complex blend of balancing the totality of the woman's situation with institutional constraints including workloads, guidelines, continuity concerns, justifying decisions to senior staff and risk management (Burvill 2002; Cheyne et al 2006). This can be contrasted with care at a home birth or in an FSBC, where the organizational and clinical parameters are secondary to women's lived experience and care is driven by the latter (Walsh 2006a).

Twenty-five years ago, Flint (1986) counselled that early labour was best experienced at home with access to a midwife, and this remains the ideal for low-risk women. Maternity services have realized that the worst place may be on a labour ward, because, as research shows, this can result in more labour interventions (Hemminki and Simukka 1986; Rahnama et al 2006).

Recent studies demonstrate the value of triage facilities or early labour assessment centres if home assessment in early labour is not an option, as this results in fewer labour interventions (Lauzon and Hodnett 2004). The value of attending an FSBC (Jackson et al 2003) and seeing a midwife rather than an obstetrician (Turnbull et al 1996) have been suggested. Individualising care, and ongoing informational and relational continuity are all important elements of best practice for the latent phase of labour.

Rhythms in mid labour

Midwives' understanding of the active phase of the first stage of labour has been the main focus of partogram recordings over the past 50 years. Having discussed the relaxation in timelines around this issue in recent years, the decoupling of the phenomenon of labour slowing or stopping, from the presumption that this represents pathology, can be explored. A retrospective examination of thousands of records of home birth women discovered that some had periods when the cervix stopped dilating temporarily in active labour (Davis et al 2002). This was not interpreted as pathology by birth attendants, and after variable periods of time, cervical progression began again. Apart from strong anecdotal evidence that some women experience a latent period in advanced labour, this was the first to record data on labour 'plateaus' (see Fig. 36.9).

Since then, Zhang et al (2010) have argued that a step-like partogram (see Fig. 36.10) more accurately reflects the quiescent and acceleratory phases of labour and this alternative partogram is being researched in Sweden and Australia.

Gaskin's (2003) description of 'pasmo' indicated that physiological delays were known about in the 19th century. Accepting the individuality of the labour experience for different women, the subtlety of hormonal interactions and the mediating effects of environment and companions, it is entirely feasible that labour could be understood as a 'unique normality', varying from woman to woman (Downe and McCourt 2008). Midwifery skill lies in facilitating this individual expression.

Recent research into the use of differing action lines (2 hours and 4 hours behind the 1 cm/hour line) in the active phase of labour indicates that allowing for a slower rate of cervical dilatation does not result in more caesarean sections and, importantly, women are just as satisfied with longer labours (Lavender et al 2006). A cervical dilatation rate of 0.5 cm/hour in nulliparous women is now recommended (Enkin et al 2000).

Vaginal examinations

The ubiquity of vaginal examination as a practice in labour, inextricably linked to the progress paradigm, means that the vaginal examination remains the most common procedure on labour wards. Appraisal of this common childbirth intervention is required to examine

whether widespread use is justifiable. In recent years, a number of critical review papers have challenged the ubiquity, purpose and impact of regular vaginal examinations in labour (Keely 2015; Dahlen et al 2013). Earlier, Devane's (1996) systematic literature review failed to identify a research basis for this procedure, which reveals the power of the labour progress paradigm, effectively driving adoption of the procedure on the basis of custom and practice. The literature around sexual abuse (Robohm and Buttenheim 1996) and post-traumatic stress disorder (Menage 1996) indicates that women who have these experiences find vaginal examinations very problematic. A study by Bergstrom et al (1992), based on videotaped vaginal examinations in US labour wards, revealed the ritual that has evolved around the practice to legitimize such an intrusion into a person's private space, showing the surgical construction of a practice undertaken by strangers that would be totally unacceptable in any other circumstance except in an intimate sexual context between consenting adults. The adoption of a passive patient role and the marked power differential between the patient and the clinician were other taken-for-granted behaviours. In a UK-based study, similar conclusions were postulated (Stewart 2005).

Two important questions need asking before any vaginal examination is carried out (Warren 1999):

- Why do I need to know this information now?

- Is there any other way I can obtain it?

Finally, when examination is clinically justifiable, can the findings be accepted with confidence? The poor inter-observer reliability of the procedure (Clement 1994), illustrated by 'guesstimate' rather than 'estimate' scenarios of some clinical practice, may be assisted by practitioners

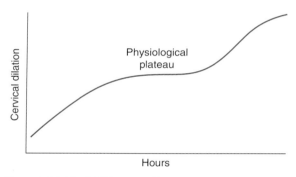

Figure 36.9 The MANA curve. (Davis et al 2002.)

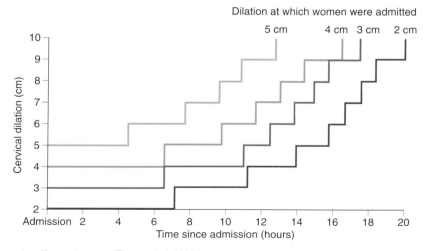

Figure 36.10 Zhang step-like partogram. (Zhang et al 2010.)

ensuring that they undertake the examination systematically, and seek a 'second opinion' should the findings be unclear.

It is imperative that midwives approach vaginal examinations guided by negotiated and explicit consent, clear clinical justification and with sensitivity for the discomfort, embarrassment and pain that may be caused.

Indications for vaginal examination

1. To confirm the onset of labour and establish a baseline for further progress
2. To aid in assessing labour progress through determining the dilatation and condition of the cervix. (It is good practice to precede this with an abdominal examination to determine the fetal lie, presentation and position, the engagement or otherwise of the presentation and to auscultate the fetal heart.)
3. To diagnose the presentation when this is in doubt
4. To rupture the membranes when necessary

Method

The woman is made comfortable in a semirecumbent or lateral position with legs separated and as relaxed as possible. She can be encouraged to practice relaxation exercises. Appropriate cleansing is carried out, then the examining fingers (index and forefinger) are generously lubricated and gently inserted into the vagina.

During the examination, the midwife should note any abnormalities or deviations from normal, such as vulval varicosities, lesions (such as warts or blisters), vaginal discharge/loss, oedema and any previous scarring. She should also note the tone of the vaginal muscles and pelvic floor, and other characteristics, such as vaginal dryness or excess heat, which might indicate pyrexia.

Cervix

The cervix is assessed for consistency, effacement and dilatation (as discussed previously and in Ch. 35).

Consistency: The cervix is usually soft and pliable to the examining fingers. It may feel thick and is often described as having a consistency comparable to that of the lips.

Effacement and dilatation: The cervical canal, which usually projects into the vagina, becomes shorter, until no protrusion can be felt. This shortening, often referred to as the 'taking up' of the cervix, results from the dilatation of the internal cervical os and the gradual opening out of the cervical canal.

During and following effacement, the cervical consistency alters and it becomes progressively thinner. Complete effacement may be present in primigravidae before the onset of labour and before dilatation. In the multiparous woman, although a degree of effacement may be present before labour, completion of the process occurs simultaneously with cervical dilatation as labour advances.

A soft, stretchy cervix, closely in contact with the presenting part, indicates potential for normal cervical dilatation. A tight, unyielding cervix or one loosely in contact with the presenting part is less favourable and may be associated with long labour.

Membranes

In early labour the membranes can be difficult to feel as they are usually closely applied to the head. During a contraction the increase in pressure may cause the bag of forewaters to become tense and bulge through the os uteri. The membranes may be inadvertently ruptured if pressure is applied at this time. If the head is poorly applied to the cervix, the bag of forewaters may bulge unduly early in the first stage, and early rupture of membranes is likely to occur. This tends to occur with an occipitoposterior position.

Presentation

The presentation is normally the smooth, round, hard vault of the head. Sutures and fontanelles can be felt with increasing ease as the os uteri dilates, thereby enabling confirmation of the presentation and determination of the position and attitude of the head. The degree of moulding of the fetal head can also be assessed. As labour continues, particularly if the membranes are ruptured, subsequent formation of a caput succedaneum may make recognition of sutures and fontanelles difficult and sometimes impossible. Rarely, a prolapsed cord may be felt as a soft loop lying in front of or alongside the fetal head. If the fetus is still alive, the cord will be felt to pulsate.

Position

This can be determined by identification of the fontanelles and the sutures (Figs 36.11 and 36.12). An occipitoanterior position is identified by feeling the posterior fontanelle towards the anterior part of the pelvis. In an occipitoposterior position, the anterior fontanelle will be felt anteriorly. The fontanelles are identified by the number of sutures that meet (see Ch. 30). See Table 36.2 and the chapter website resources.

Occasionally, the sagittal suture is found in the transverse diameter of the pelvis between the ischial tuberosities. It is then necessary to identify one or both fontanelles to determine the position. It may also be possible to feel an ear under the symphysis pubis, and this may give an indication of the position of the fetus. Before birth, when the fetal head has rotated on the pelvic floor, the sagittal suture should be in the anteroposterior diameter of the pelvis.

A summary of how to assess the position of the fetus is given in Table 36.2.

Table 36.2 Assessing the position of the fetus

Position of sagittal suture	Position of fontanelle	Position of fetus
Right oblique	Posterior fontanelle anteriorly to the left	LOA
	Anterior fontanelle anteriorly to the left	ROP
Left oblique	Posterior fontanelle anteriorly to the right	ROA
	Anterior fontanelle anteriorly to the right	LOP
Transverse diameter of the pelvis	Posterior fontanelle to the left	LOL
	Posterior fontanelle to the right	ROL
Anteroposterior diameter of the pelvis	Posterior fontanelle felt anteriorly	OA
	Anterior fontanelle felt anteriorly	OP

LOA, left occipitoanterior; LOL, left occipitolateral; LOP, left occipitoposterior; OA, occipitoanterior; OP, occipitoposterior; ROA, right occipitoanterior; ROP, right occipitoposterior; ROL, right occipitolateral.

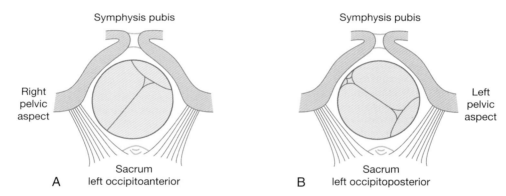

Symphysis pubis — Symphysis pubis

Right pelvic aspect — Left pelvic aspect

Sacrum — Sacrum

A left occipitoanterior — B left occipitoposterior

Figure 36.11 Identifying the position of the fetus. **A,** Left occipitoanterior: the sagittal suture is in the right oblique diameter of the pelvis. **B,** Left occipitoposterior: the sagittal suture is in the left oblique diameter of the pelvis. (Simkin P, Ancheta R: The labor progress handbook, Oxford, 2000, Blackwell Science.)

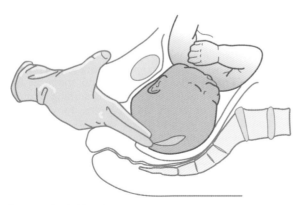

Figure 36.12 Identifying the sagittal suture and fontanelles during vaginal examination. (Simkin P, Ancheta R: The labor progress handbook, Oxford, 2000, Blackwell Science.)

Flexion and station

The fetal head may or may not be flexed at the onset of labour. In the presence of efficient uterine action and as a result of fetal axis pressure, the fetal head usually flexes, further facilitating a well-fitting presenting part. Unless the pelvis is particularly roomy or the fetal head small, deflexion of the head, and palpation of the posterior and anterior fontanelles, may be indicative of malposition of the fetal head, poor cervical stimulation and prolongation of labour.

The station or level of the presenting part refers to the relationship of the presenting part to the ischial spines. The maternal ischial spines are palpable as slight protuberances covered by tissue on either side of the bony pelvis. Descent in relation to the maternal ischial spines should be progressive and is expressed in centimetres, as indicated in Fig. 36.13.

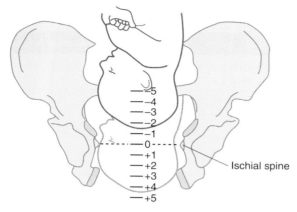

Figure 36.13 Stations of the head in relation to the pelvis. Descent in relation to the maternal ischial spines is expressed in centimetres. (Simkin P, Ancheta R: The labor progress handbook, Oxford, 2000, Blackwell Science.)

The examination is completed by applying a vulval pad, changing any soiled linen and making the woman comfortable. The fetal heart is then auscultated. All findings are recorded and the midwife analyses the findings to establish a total picture on which to make an accurate assessment of the progress of labour and to forecast how the labour is likely to advance. The midwife is able to relate to the woman and her partner the progress to date, and review with them the original birth plan for any adjustments that the woman and the midwife feel are necessary.

Alternative skills for 'sussing out' labour

There is a dearth of any research examining alternatives to vaginal examinations for labour care, given the rich anecdotes that surround this area. Midwives have always taken into account the character of contractions, a woman's response to them and the findings from abdominal palpation. Stuart (2000) is possibly unique in relying on abdominal palpation instead of vaginal examination to ascertain progress, and most midwives weigh the results of vaginal examination above contractions and behaviour. It is the practices that are substitutional for vaginal examinations that are the most interesting. Hobbs (1998) advocated the 'purple line' method – observing a line that runs from the distal margin of the anus up between the buttocks, said to indicate full dilatation when it reaches the natal cleft. Shepherd et al (2010) reported in their longitudinal study that 76% of women developed the line. In a comprehensive manual of care during normal birth, Frye (2004) identified monitoring temperature change in the lower leg. As labour progresses, so a coldness on touch

is noted to move from the ankle up the leg to the knee. Another marker may be the forehead of a woman. Possibly originating from traditional birth attendant practices in Peru, this involves feeling for the appearance of a ridge running from between the eyes up to the hairline as labour progresses.

Other wisdom comes from intuitive perceptions that many midwives may recognize but find hard to articulate and even harder to write down, as illustrated by the story to be found on the chapter website.

The transitional phase between the first and second stages has been studied by Baker and Kenner (1993), who noted the common vocalizations that mark it. These are just a few examples of anecdotes that abound in this area. It is an area ripe for observational research and for articles mapping the richness of midwives' experience.

Finally, there is the domain of emotional nuance reading, which may have a huge impact on how labour unfolds (Kennedy et al 2004). One such episode occurred in the midwifery units study by Walsh (2006b), when a teenage girl arrived in early labour, very distressed. The midwife asked her mother and sister to leave the room and gently enquired as to how she was. She burst into tears, and over the next 2 hours the midwife held her in an embrace on a mattress on the floor as the girl sobbed and sobbed. Then she said she was ready and went on to have a normal, rather peaceful birth. In other settings, the girl may have been offered an epidural, but this was emotional rather than pain distress. The skill of the midwife was in her intuitive emotional nuance reading of that and how to bring comfort and support.

'Being with', not 'doing to', labouring women

The quest to dismantle assembly-line birth, removing women from the intrapartum timeline and rehabilitating belief in 'unique normality' of labour for individual women, challenges a radical rethink of the focus and orientation to normal labour care. Hints of a different way of midwives situating themselves with women are in the writings of midwives and they speak in paradox and metaphor. Leap (2000) tells of 'the less we do, the more we give', and Kennedy et al (2004) of 'doing nothing' in their insightful study of expert US midwives. Fahy (1998) conceptualizes the work of the midwife as 'being with' women, not 'doing to' them, and Anderson (2004) quips that good labour care requires the midwife 'to drink tea intelligently'. These writers are alluding not to a temporally regulated activity marked by task completions but to a disposition towards compassionate companionship with women that is a 'masterly inactivity' (Royal College of Midwives (RCM) 2010). As a midwifery unit midwife offered during an interview: 'It's about being comfortable when there is nothing to do'.

Loss per vagina and rupture of the membranes

The time at which the membranes rupture should be recorded, together with the appearance of the liquor. A minor amount of blood-stained loss is consistent with a show or detachment of the membranes occurring with increasing cervical dilatation. Copious mucoid blood-stained loss may herald full cervical dilatation. A greenish colour is indicative of meconium staining, sometimes associated with fetal distress. Frank bleeding per vagina is abnormal; if this occurs, the midwife must consult with the obstetrician, who will ascertain the source – whether maternal or fetal – and determine the appropriate action. Measurement of loss and monitoring of the woman's condition is vital.

Bladder care

The woman is encouraged to empty her bladder every 2 hours. A full bladder is uncomfortable and may delay the progress of labour by inhibiting descent of the fetal head if it is above the ischial spines. This will reflexively inhibit efficient uterine contractions and cervical dilatation. Pressure on the distended bladder by the fetal head may give rise to oedema and bruising, leading to possible difficulties in micturition in the early days of the puerperium.

Mobility and ambulation

Twenty-five RCTs were included in a systematic review, which concluded that ambulation reduced caesareans, epidurals and the length of labour (1 hr 22 min) and contributed to fewer neonatal unit (NNU) admissions (Lawrence et al 2013).

MacLennan et al's (1994) meta-analysis of their own trial with five others also found a reduction in the need for analgesia and noted that 46% of women in their study who declined entry to the trial did so because they did not want to lose the choice of ambulation. One of the largest trials (Bloom et al 1998) found that 99% of ambulant women would choose this mobility again. No other differences were noted compared with the recumbent group.

Movement appears to be a central characteristic of normal labour (Gould 2000). In an overview of trials of ambulation, Smith et al (1991) found that when given the choice, women changed position an average of seven to eight times in the course of their labours.

Upright posture

Positive effects of gravity and lessened risk of aortocaval compression (and therefore improved fetal acid–base outcomes) were described by Bonica (1967) and Humphrey et al (1973). Mendez-Bauer et al (1975) demonstrated stronger, efficient uterine contractions. In upright postures the flexion and abduction of the hips, combined with the freedom for the coccyx to articulate backwards, provide greater room at the pelvic outlet, both in the anterior/posterior and transverse dimensions (Michel et al 2002).

Gupta et al's (2012) review of position in the second stage of labour support these earlier findings. They concluded that upright posture for second stage and birth resulted in a significant reduction in assisted vaginal birth, fewer episiotomies, fewer fetal heart abnormalities and a nonsignificant reduction in the length of second stage, although an increase in second degree tears and blood loss.

Flint (1986) discussed the idea of midwives 'fitting around women', emphasizing that nearly all common procedures, such as fetal monitoring and vaginal examinations, could be done without asking the woman to get on the bed. Props, such as beanbags and birth balls, can be used to facilitate positional and postural changes. Certainly, the mass trend towards lying down for childbirth, at least in Western cultures, was never tested empirically and occurred largely to assist the birth practitioners to carry out technical interventions, such as forceps deliveries and administration of anaesthetics (Donnison 1988) (see Ch. 2). This will continue to be tacitly endorsed by midwives as long as the 'bed birth myth' of childbirth remains. Many midwifery units have removed beds entirely from the birth room and replaced them with thick floor mattresses. This simple, cosmetic alteration would be deeply symbolic and may have a significant impact on birth positions. Figure 36.14 illustrates a variety of positions for the first stage of labour.

Reflective activity 36.3

Review the records of the births you have attended, and consider the positions women adopted. Begin to include this component of the birth in your records, and evaluate the effect on the woman and on you.

Moving and handling

Moving and handling concerns, and worries about back injuries, may preclude some midwives from assisting women who opt for an upright birth posture. If this is a real issue for practitioners, it may also have implications for assisting at recumbent births as well because these sometimes require awkward twisting and bending. Midwives are now usually trained in 'good back care' with mandatory moving and handling sessions run by hospitals. The application of these principles should not interfere with assisting women to birth in upright postures, as these postures probably also protect women's joints and backs more than conventional bed birth.

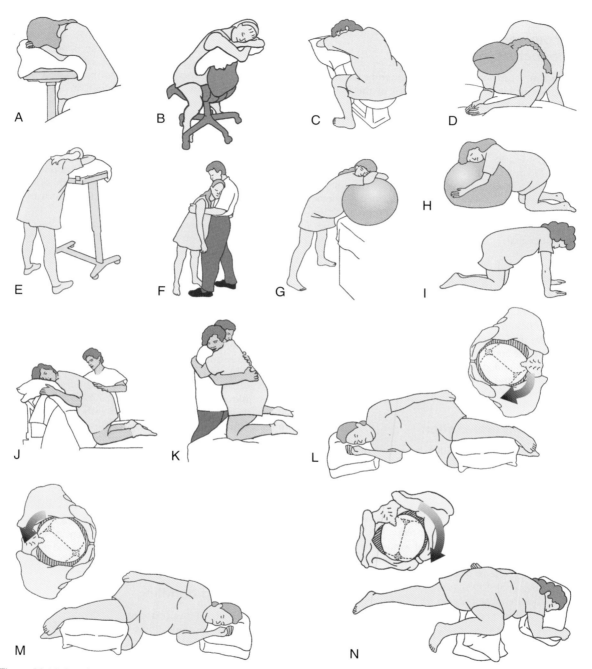

Figure 36.14 A variety of positions for the first stage of labour. **A,** Sitting, leaning on a tray table. **B,** Straddling a chair. **C,** Straddling toilet, facing backwards. **D,** Standing, leaning on bed. **E,** Standing, leaning on a tray table. **F,** Standing, leaning forward on partner. **G,** Standing, leaning on ball. **H,** Kneeling with a ball. **I,** On hands and knees. **J,** Kneeling over bed back. **K,** Kneeling, partner support. **L,** Pure side-lying on the 'correct' side, with fetal back 'toward the bed'. Gravity pulls fetal head and trunk towards ROL. **M,** Pure side-lying on the 'wrong' (left) side for an ROP fetus. Fetal back is 'toward the ceiling'. Gravity pulls fetal occiput and trunk towards direct OP. **N,** Semi-prone on the 'correct side' – with fetal back 'toward the ceiling'. If the fetus is ROP, the semi-prone woman lies on her left side. Gravity pulls fetal occiput and trunk towards ROL, then ROA. OP, occipitoposterior; ROA, right occipitoanterior; ROP, right occipitoposterior; ROL, right occipitolateral. (Reproduced with permission from Simkin P, Ancheta R: The labor progress handbook, Oxford, 2000, Blackwell Science.)

Home birth practitioners are familiar with birth taking place in living rooms and bedrooms, and with the restlessness of labour, during which women move freely within the privacy of their chosen birthing space, and may choose the bed only as a prop. It is probably time to expunge the term 'confinement' from the vocabulary of childbirth once and for all, and ensure that the environment 'belongs' to the woman and her partner.

Prevention of infection

In labour, both mother and fetus are vulnerable to infection, particularly following membrane rupture. The possibility is increased when the immune response is undermined by suboptimal health – for example, anaemia, malnourishment, chronic illness – or when the woman is exhausted by a long and arduous labour. The hospital environment itself may increase the woman's risk of infection as she is exposed to a variety of unfamiliar organisms and possible sources of infection.

The midwife must ensure, as far as possible, a safe environment for the woman and prevent infection and cross-infection. Such measures include good standards of hygiene and care, correct handwashing of the carers before and after attending the woman, frequent changing of vulval pads, and meticulous aseptic techniques when undertaking vaginal examination and other invasive procedures such as catheterization.

General measures, such as limiting the flow of traffic within the birthing area, scrupulous cleansing of communal equipment (for example, beds, baths, toilets and trolleys) and increasing staff awareness of the potential for, and prevention of, infection, must all be observed. A formal mechanism for infection control within hospitals must include maternity departments. One survey of surveillance of hospital-based obstetric and gynaecological infection showed a significant reduction in the incidence of infection when regular feedback to staff was implemented (Evaldon et al 1992).

NUTRITION IN LABOUR

Controlling women's behaviours and choices in labour has traditionally included restrictions on what they can eat and drink. This was driven by concerns about aspirating stomach contents (*Mendelson's syndrome*) should general anaesthesia be required in an emergency. However, as regional anaesthesia has become common and anaesthetic techniques have improved, the incidence of aspiration has plummeted (Chang et al 2003). Apart from the medical risks, controlling what women eat and drink in normal labour is paternalistic and, arguably, an infringement of human rights. At home and in midwifery unit births, the sensible approach of self-regulation has operated for decades. Women eat and drink when they feel hungry and thirsty, more commonly in early labour. Some women experience nausea as labour progresses and therefore forsake food, although they do usually continue to drink small amounts.

Odent (1998) and Anderson (1998) suggested that the smooth muscle structure of the uterus works much more efficiently than skeletal muscle, making comparatively small energy demands and utilizing fatty acids and ketones readily as an energy source. It is suggested that because the woman in physiological labour becomes withdrawn from higher cerebral activity, and as skeletal muscles are at rest, energy requirements are less than normal.

Tranmer et al (2005) tested the hypothesis that unrestricted eating and drinking during labour might reduce the incidence of labour dystocia. Though no effect was shown, it did highlight that when women self-regulate, many do choose to eat and drink, usually small amounts and often in the early stages of labour.

Ssengabadda (2014) has undertaken a recent extensive literature review in this area and concluded that self-regulated eating and drinking was beneficial to labouring women.

Imposed fasting in labour for all women should be challenged in the light of evidence discussed previously. Restrictions may lead to dehydration and ketosis, resulting in unnecessary intervention (Johnson et al 1989).

Many maternity units require the administration of an acid inhibitor like *ranitidine* (see Ch. 10) to increase the pH of the stomach contents. However, this is only appropriate in women of high-risk status who might be more at risk of emergency procedures and should not be applied to women in normal labour.

ASSESSING THE FETAL CONDITION

The midwife needs to understand the mechanisms that control fetal heart response to interpret the fetal response to labour. The cardioregulatory centre of the brain, situated in the medulla oblongata, is influenced by many factors. Baroreceptors situated in the arch of the aorta and carotid sinus sense alterations in blood pressure and transmit information to the cardioregulatory centre. Chemoreceptors situated in the carotid sinus and arch of the aorta will respond to changes in oxygen and carbon dioxide tensions. The cardioregulatory centre is controlled by the autonomic nervous system and, in response to varying physiological factors, either the sympathetic or parasympathetic nervous system will be stimulated. The sympathetic nervous system, via the sinoatrial node, causes an increase in heart rate, whereas the parasympathetic nervous system causes a rate reduction. The continuous interaction of these two systems results in minor fluctuations in the heart rate that are recognized as variability. Development of the sympathetic nervous system occurs early in fetal life, whereas the parasympathetic nervous response does not become pronounced until later in pregnancy. This accounts for the higher baseline rate of the fetal heart during early pregnancy and the lower rate at term.

Monitoring the fetal heart

The activity of the fetal heart may be assessed intermittently using the Pinard fetal stethoscope or a hand held Doppler device. This provides the midwife with sample information regarding the rate and rhythm of the fetal heart. At commencement of intermittent auscultation, it is important to distinguish the maternal pulse from the fetal heart, as the former can mimic a fetal heart and, therefore, can be falsely reassuring to the midwife. An understanding of the workings of the Doppler is useful, and reinforces the value of the use of the Pinard stethoscope at regular intervals even if the Doppler is used (Gibb and Arulkumaran 2007).

Intermittent auscultation of the fetal heart is usually undertaken every 15 minutes during the first stage of labour, though this is based on custom and practice, not research. In the second stage of labour, this increases to every 5 minutes. NICE (2014 and 2016) recommends intermittent auscultation and abandonment of the 'admission trace' for women in normal labour.

Healthy fetal heart patterns

The normal fetal heart has a baseline rate of between 110 and 160 beats per minute (bpm). The baseline rate refers to the heart rate present between periods of acceleration and deceleration. Baseline variability refers to the variation in heart rate of 5 to 15 bpm, occurring over a time base of 10 to 20 seconds. Figure 36.15 demonstrates normal baseline variability. The presence of good variability is an important sign of fetal well-being (NICE 2007).

Acceleration patterns of the fetal heart of 15 bpm from the baseline, as shown in Fig. 36.16, are often associated with fetal activity and stimulation and are thought to be useful indicators of absence of fetal acidemia in labour (Spencer 1993). They are not considered to be clinically significant if of short duration – that is, less than 15 seconds. When two are present within a 20-minute period, the trace is described as 'reactive' (Gibb 1988). This is considered to be a positive sign of fetal health, indicating good reflex responsiveness of the fetal circulation.

Electronic fetal monitoring

In normal labour, continuous electronic fetal monitoring (EFM) is not required because it results in more birth interventions without a demonstrable improvement in fetal outcome (Alfirevic et al 2013). Inter- and intra-observer reliability is poor with EFM, and maternity units should regularly update all labour ward staff in the interpretation of traces as recommended by the Confidential Enquiry into Maternal and Child Health (CEMACH) (Edwards 2004). The International Federation of Gynaecology and Obstetrics (FIGO) has recently produced guidelines on intrapartum fetal monitoring that are evidence-based and therefore recommended (FIGO 2015).

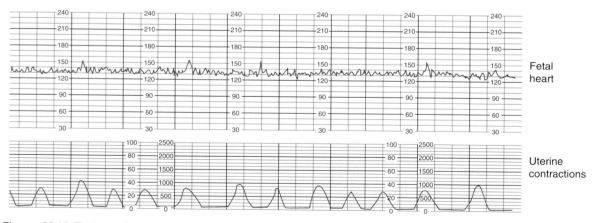

Figure 36.15 Electrocardiogram (ECG) trace showing baseline variability in fetal heart rate. (Courtesy of Sonicaid, Abingdon, Oxon.)

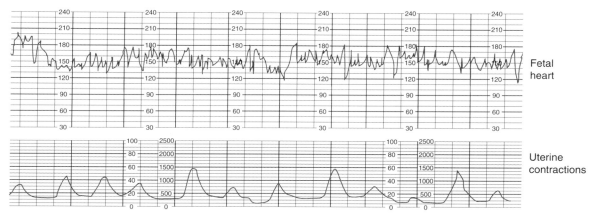

Fetal heart

Uterine contractions

Figure 36.16 Fetal heart rate accelerations. (Courtesy of Sonicaid, Abingdon, Oxon.)

CONCLUSION

Care during the first stage of labour is as much about trusting the birth process and intuitively connecting with labouring women as it is about monitoring and understanding the physiology. A social model of birth emphasizes the relational aspects of this experience and the key role of the birth environment. When these are understood and appropriately applied, physiology will be maximized, and complications will occur in only a small minority of women. However, against the backdrop of increasing medicalization of childbirth, midwives may feel caught between the social and biomedical models and will need the support of each other if they are to facilitate empowering birth experiences for women in their care.

Key Points

- Labour is an intense, individual event, in which the midwife can play a pivotal role in supporting normality and enabling and facilitating birth to be a positive and empowering experience.

- The midwife should be knowledgeable about the psychological, physiological and social aspects of labour to work in partnership with the woman and plan care appropriately.

- The midwife must be conversant with contemporary research and evidence and committed to sharing this knowledge with the woman and her partner.

- Continuity of care and carer provides a valued model of care and improves the outcomes of labour – where possible, this should be worked towards. Effective use of notes and records, including partograms, is a crucial part of this.

- One-to-one care during the active phase of the first stage of labour should be utilized as a means of monitoring maternal and fetal well-being and as an educational opportunity for the woman and birth partner.

- The growth in midwifery units, both freestanding and alongside, provides an opportunity to develop women-centred care and increase midwifery autonomy.

References

Adam B: *Timewatch: the social analysis of time*, Cambridge, Polity Press, 1995.

Albers L: The duration of labour in healthy women, *J Perinatol* 19(2):114–119, 1999.

Alfirevic Z, Devane D, Gyte G: Continuous cardiotocography (CTG) as a form of electronic fetal monitoring (EFM) for fetal assessment during labour, *Cochrane Database Syst Rev* (3):CD006066, 2013.

Anderson T: Is ketosis in labour pathological? *Pract Midwife* 1(9):22–26, 1998.

Anderson T: *The impact of the age of risk for antenatal education.* NCT conference, Coventry, March 13, 2004.

Baker A, Kenner A: Communication of pain: vocalisation as an indicator of the stage of labour, *Aust N Z J Obstet Gynaecol* 33(4):384–385, 1993.

Bergstrom L, Roberts J, Skillman L, et al: 'You'll feel me touching you, sweetie'. Vaginal examinations during the second stage of labour, *Birth* 19(1):10–18, 1992.

Blackburn ST: *Maternal, fetal and neonatal physiology*, 4th edn, Philadelphia, 2013, WB Saunders.

Bloom S, McIntyre D, Beimer M: Lack of effect of walking on labour and delivery, *N Engl J Med* 339(2):76–79, 1998.

Bonica J: *Principles and practice of obstetric analgesia and anaesthesia*, Philadelphia, F.A. Davis, 1967.

Brocklehurst P, Hardy P, Hollowell J, et al: Perinatal and maternal outcomes by planned place of birth for healthy women with low risk pregnancies: the Birthplace in England national prospective cohort study, *Br Med J* 343(7840):d7400, 2011.

Buckley S: Undisturbed birth – nature's hormonal blueprint for safety, ease and ecstasy, *MIDIRS* 14(2):203–209, 2004.

Buckley SJ: *Hormonal physiology of childbearing: evidence and implications for women, babies, and maternity care*, New York, Childbirth Connection, 2015.

Burvill S: Midwifery diagnosis of labour onset, *Br J Midwifery* 10(10):600–605, 2002.

Campbell R, McFarlane A: *Where to be born: the debate and the evidence*, 2nd edn, Oxford, National Perinatal Epidemiology Unit, 1994.

Cesario S: Reevaluation of Friedman's labor curve: a pilot study, *J Obstet Gynecol Neonatal Nurs* 33(6):713–722, 2004.

Chang J, Elam-Evans L, Berg C, et al: Pregnancy-related mortality surveillance – United States, 1991–1999, *MMWR Surveill Summ* 52(2):1–8, 2003.

Cheyne H, Dowding D, Hundley V: Making the diagnosis of labour: midwives' diagnostic judgement and management decisions, *J Adv Nurs* 53(6):625–635, 2006.

Clement S: Unwanted vaginal examinations, *Br J Midwifery* 2(8):368–370, 1994.

Dahlen H, Downe S, Duff M, et al: Vaginal examination during normal labor: routine examination or routine intervention? *Int J Childbirth* 3(3):142–152, 2013.

Davis B, Johnson K, Gaskin I: The MANA curve – describing plateaus in labour using the MANA database, Abstract No. 30, 26th Triennial Congress ICM, Vienna, 2002.

Department of Health (DH): *Making it better for mother and baby: clinical case for change*, London, DH, 2007a.

Department of Health (DH): *Maternity matters: choice, access and continuity of care in a safe service*, London, DH, 2007b.

Devane D: Sexuality and midwifery, *Br J Midwifery* 4(8):413–420, 1996.

Dixon L, Skinner J, Foureur M: The emotional and hormonal pathways of labour and birth: integrating mind, body and behaviour, *NZCOM Journal* 48:15, 2013.

Donnison J: *Midwives and medical men: a history of the struggle for the control of childbirth*, London, Historical Publications, 1988.

Downe S, McCourt C: From being to becoming: reconstructing childbirth knowledge. In Downe S, editor: *Normal birth: evidence and debate*, London, Elsevier Science, 2008.

Edwards G: *Adverse outcomes in maternity care*, Cheshire, Books for Midwives, 2004.

Enkin M, Kierse M, Neilson J, et al: *A guide to effective care in pregnancy and childbirth*, Oxford, Oxford University Press, 2000.

Eri TS, Bondas T, Gross M, et al: A balancing act in an unknown territory: a metasynthesis of first-time mothers' experiences in early labour, *Midwifery* 31(3):e58–e67, 2015.

Evaldon GR, Frederici H, Jullig C, et al: Hospital-associated infections in obstetrics and gynaecology. Effects of surveillance, *Acta Obstet Gynecol Scand* 71(1):54–58, 1992.

Fahy K: Being a midwife or doing midwifery, *Aust Coll Midwives Inc J* 11(2):11–16, 1998.

Flint C: *Sensitive midwifery*, London, Heinemann, 1986.

Flint C: *Midwifery teams and caseloads*, London, Butterworth Heinemann, 1993.

Friedman E: The graphic analysis of labour, *Am J Obstet Gynecol* 68:1568–1575, 1954.

Frye A: *Holistic midwifery. Volume 2: Care of the mother and baby from onset of labour through the first hours after birth*, Portland, Labry's Press, 2004.

Fullerton J, Young S: Outcomes of planned home birth: an integrative review, *J Midwifery Womens Health* 52(4):323–333, 2007.

Gagnon A, Meier K, Waghorn K: Continuity of nursing care and its link to caesarean birth rate, *Birth* 34(1):26–31, 2007.

Gaskin IM: Going backwards: the concept of 'pasmo', *Pract Midwife* 6(8):34–36, 2003.

Gibb D: *A practical guide to labour management*, London, Blackwell Scientific, 1988.

Gibb DMF, Arulkumaran S: *Fetal monitoring in practice*, 3rd edn, London, Butterworth-Heinemann, 2007.

Gilbert P: *The compassionate mind: a new approach to life's challenges*, Oakland, New Harbinger Publications, 2010.

Gould D: Normal labour: a concept analysis, *J Adv Nurs* 31(2):418–427, 2000.

Green J, Coupland B, Kitzinger J: *Great expectations: a prospective study of women's expectations and experiences* of childbirth, Cambridge, Child Care and Development Group, 1998.

Gross M, Haunschild T, Stoexen T, et al: Women's recognition of the spontaneous onset of labour, Birth 30(4):267–271, 2003.

Gupta JK, Hofmeyr GJ, Shehmar M: Position in the second stage of labour for women without epidural anaesthesia, Cochrane Database Syst Rev (5):CD002006, 2012.

Haggerty J, Reid R, Freeman G, et al: Continuity of care: a multidisciplinary review, Br Med J 327(7425):1219–1221, 2003.

Hartz DL, Foureur M, Tracey S: Australian caseload midwifery: the exception or the rule, Women Birth 25(1):39–46, 2012.

Hatem M, Sandall J, Devane D, et al: Midwife-led versus other models of care for childbearing women, Cochrane Database Syst Rev (4): CD004667, 2008.

Healthcare Commission: Towards better births: a review of maternity services in England, London, Commission for Healthcare Audit and Inspection, 2008.

Hemminki E, Simukka R: The timing of hospital admission and progress of labour, Eur J Obstet Gynecol Reprod Biol 22:85–94, 1986.

Hobbs L: Assessing cervical dilatation without VEs, Pract Midwife 1(11):34–35, 1998.

Hodnett ED, Downe S, Walsh D: Alternative versus conventional institutional settings for birth, Cochrane Database Syst Rev (8):CD000012, 2012.

Hodnett ED, Gates S, Hofmeyr GJ, et al: Continuous support for women during childbirth, Cochrane Database Syst Rev (2):2008.

Hodnett ED, Gates S, Hofmeyr GJ, et al: Continuous support for women during childbirth, Cochrane Database Syst Rev (7):CD003766, 2013.

Humphrey M, Hounslow D, Morgan S: The influence of maternal posture at birth on the fetus, J Obstet Gynaecol Br Commonw 80(12):1075–1080, 1973.

Hunt S, Symonds A: The social meaning of midwifery, Basingstoke, Macmillan, 1995.

International Federation of Gynecology and Obstetrics (FIGO): FIGO intrapartum fetal monitoring guidelines

(website). www.figo.org/news/available-view-figo-intrapartum-fetal-monitoring-guidelines-0015088. 2015.

Jackson D, Lang J, Ecker J, et al: Impact of collaborative management and early admission in labor on method of delivery, J Obstet Gynecol Neonatal Nurs 32(2):147–157, 2003.

Johnson C, Kierse MJNC, Enkin M, et al: Nutrition and hydration in labour. In Chalmers I, Enkin M, Kierse MJNC, editors: Effective care in pregnancy and childbirth, vol 2, Oxford, Oxford University Press, 1989.

Keely S: The role and impact of vaginal examinations in contemporary practice, MIDIRS 25(1):60–66, 2015.

Kennedy H, Shannon M, Chuahorm U, et al: The landscape of caring for women: a narrative study of midwifery practice, J Midwifery Womens Health 49(1):14–23, 2004.

Kitzinger S: Rediscovering birth, London, Simon & Schuster, 2000.

Lally J, Murtagh M, Macphail S, et al: More in hope than expectation: women's experience and expectations of pain relief in labour: a review, BMC Med 6:7, 2008.

Lauzon L, Hodnett ED: Labour assessment programs to delay admission to labour wards, Cochrane Database Syst Rev (1):CD000936, 2004.

Lavender T, Alfirevic Z, Walkinshaw S: Effect of different partogram action lines on birth outcomes, Obstet Gynecol 108(2):295–302, 2006.

Lawrence A, Lewis L, Hofmeyr GJ, et al: Maternal positions and mobility during first stage labour, Cochrane Database Syst Rev (8):2013.

Leap N: The less we do, the more we give. In Kirkham M, editor: The midwife-mother relationship, London, Macmillan, pp 1–18, 2000.

MacLennan A, Crowther C, Derham R: Does the option to ambulate during spontaneous labour confer any advantage or disadvantage? J Matern Fetal Med 3(1):43–48, 1994.

Martin E: The woman in the body: a cultural analysis of reproduction, Milton Keynes, Open University Press, 1987.

McCoshen JA, Hoffman DR, Kredentser JV, et al: The role of fetal membranes in regulating production, transport, and

metabolism of prostaglandin E2 during labor, Am J Obstet Gynecol 163(5 Pt 1):1632–1640, 1990.

Menage J: Post-traumatic stress disorder following obstetric/gynaecological procedures, Br J Midwifery 4(10):532–533, 1996.

Mendez-Bauer C, Arroyo J, Garcia-Ramos C: Effects of standing position on spontaneous uterine contractility and other aspects of labour, J Perinat Med 3(2):89–100, 1975.

Michel SC, Rake A, Treiber K: MR obstetric pelvimetry: effect of birthing position on pelvic bony dimensions, AJR Am J Roentgenol 179(4):1063–1067, 2002.

Moberg K: The oxytocin factor, 2nd edn, London, Pinter & Martin Ltd, 2011.

Morris T, McInerney K: Media representations of pregnancy and childbirth: an analysis of reality television programs in the United States, Birth 37(2):134–140, 2010.

Murphy-Lawless J: Reading birth and death: a history of obstetric thinking, Cork, Cork University Press, 1998.

National Audit Office (NAO): Maternity services in England, London, NAO, 2013.

National Institute for Health and Care Excellence (NICE): Intrapartum care: care of healthy women and their babies during childbirth, CG190, London, NICE, 2007; 2014 and 2016.

Nursing and Midwifery Council (NMC): Midwives rules and standards, London, NMC, 2012.

Nursing and Midwifery Council (NMC): The Code: professional standards of practice and behaviour for nurses and midwives, London, NMC, 2015.

Odent M: Labouring women are not marathon runners, Pract Midwife 1(9):16–18, 1998.

Odent M: New reasons and new ways to study birth physiology, Int J Gynaecol Obstet 75:S39–S45, 2001.

Olsen O, Clausen JA: Planned hospital birth versus planned home birth, Cochrane Database Syst Rev (9):CD000352, 2012.

Pairman S: Women-centred midwifery: partnerships or professional friendships? In Kirkham M, editor: The midwife–mother relationship, London, Macmillan, 2000.

Pembroke NF, Pembroke JJ: The spirituality of presence in midwifery care, Midwifery 24(3):321–327, 2008.

Perkins B: *The medical delivery business: health reform, childbirth and the economic order*, London, Rutgers University Press, 2004.

Philpott R, Castle W: Cervicographs in the management of labour on primigravidae 1. The alert line for detecting abnormal labour, *J Obstet Gynaecol Br Commonw* 79:592–598, 1972.

Rahnama P, Ziaei S, Faghihzadeh S: Impact of early admission in labour on method of delivery, *Int J Gynaecol Obstet* 92(3):217–220, 2006.

Redshaw M, Rowe R, Hockley C, et al: *Recorded delivery: a national survey of women's experience of maternity care 2006*, Oxford, NPE, 2007.

Robohm J, Buttenheim M: The gynaecological care experience of adult survivors of childhood sexual abuse: a preliminary investigation, *Women Health* 24(3):59–75, 1996.

Rosen P: Supporting women in labour: analysis of different types of caregivers, *J Midwifery Womens Health* 49:24–31, 2004.

Royal College of Midwives (RCM): *Campaign for normal birth* (website). http://www.rcmnormalbirth.org.uk/stories/on-the-crest-of-a-wave/masterly-inactivity/. 2010.

Rudman A, El-Khouri B, Waldenstrom U: Women's satisfaction with intrapartum care – a pattern approach, *J Adv Nurs* 59(5):474–487, 2007.

Sandall J, Soltani H, Gates S, et al: Midwife-led continuity models versus other models of care for childbearing women, *Cochrane Database Syst Rev* (8):2013.

Schwarcz R, Diaz AG, Fescina R, et al: Latin American collaborative study

on maternal posture in labour, *Birth Fam J* 6(1):1979.

Shepherd A, Cheyne H, Kennedy S: The purple line as a measure of labour progress: a longitudinal study, *BMC Pregnancy Childbirth* 10(1):54, 2010.

Simkin P, Ancheta R: *The labor progress handbook*, Oxford, Blackwell Science, 2000.

Smith M, Acheson L, Byrd J, et al: A critical review of labour and birth care, *J Fam Pract* 35:107–115, 1991.

Spencer JA: Clinical overview of cardiotocography [Review], *Br J Obstet Gynaecol* 100(Suppl 9):4–7, 1993.

Ssengabadda P: Effects of eating and drinking in labour on maternal and perinatal outcomes in low-risk women, *MIDIRS* 24(4):467–475, 2014.

Stewart M: 'I'm just going to wash you down': sanitizing the vaginal examination, *J Adv Nurs* 51(6):587–594, 2005.

Stuart C: Invasive actions in labour: where have all the 'old tricks' gone? *Pract Midwife* 3(8):30–33, 2000.

Studd J: Partograms and nomograms of cervical dilatation in management of primigravid labour, *Br Med J* 4(5890):451–455, 1973.

Tan BP, Hannah ME: Oxytocin for prelabour rupture of membranes at or near term (Cochrane Review) (Substantive update: 28 August 1996), *The Cochrane Library*, Issue 3, Oxford, Update Software, 2002.

Taylor S, Klein L, Lewis B, et al: Biobehavioural responses to stress in females, *Psychol Rev* 107(3):411–429, 2000.

Tew M: *Safer childbirth? A critical history of maternity care*, London, Free Association Books, 1998.

Tranmer J, Hodnett E, Hannah M, et al: The effect of unrestricted oral carbohydrate intake on labor progress, *J Obstet Gynecol Neonatal Nurs* 34(3):319–328, 2005.

Turnbull D, Holmes S, Cheyne H, et al: Randomised controlled trial of efficacy of midwifery-managed care, *Lancet* 348(9022):213–218, 1996.

Walsh D: Subverting assembly-line birth: childbirth in a free-standing birth centre, *Soc Sci Med* 62(6):1330–1340, 2006a.

Walsh D: Birth centres, community and social capital, *MIDIRS* 16(1):7–15, 2006b.

Walsh D: *Evidence-based care for normal labour & birth: a guide for midwives*, London, Routledge, 2007a.

Walsh D: *Improving maternity service. Small is beautiful: lessons for maternity services from a birth centre*, Oxford, Radcliffe Publishing, 2007b.

Walsh D, Newburn M: Towards a social model of childbirth. Part 1, *Br J Midwifery* 10(8):476–481, 2002.

Walsh D, Devane D: A metasynthesis of midwife-led care, *Qual Health Res* 22(7):897–910, 2012.

Warren C: Invaders of privacy, *Midwifery Matters* 81:8–9, 1999.

Zhang J, Landy H, Branch W: Contemporary patterns of spontaneous labor with normal neonatal outcomes, *Obstet Gynecol* 116(6):1281–1287, 2010.

Zhang J, Troendle J, Yancey M: Reassessing the labour curve, *Am J Obstet Gynecol* 187(4):824–828, 2002.

Resources and additional reading

Useful websites:

Please refer to the chapter website resources for more information.

Royal College of Midwives (RCM): *The Royal College of Midwives' survey of positions used in labour and birth* (website). www.rcm.org.uk/sites/default/files/Birth%20position%20Report%20FINAL%20Aug2011_0.pdf. 2010.

Walsh D: *Evidence and skills for normal labour and birth: a guide for midwives,* London, Routledge, 2011.

Which: www.which.co.uk/birth-choice/find-and-compare?gclid=CMP1tpbkh8gCFc-6GwodTHMLQg.

Follow this link to see a template for a birth plan and to explore the excellent site for place of birth choices hosted by Which.

The Cochrane Collaboration resources, for example:

Hodnett ED, et al: *Review on continuous care during labour.* http://onlinelibrary.wiley.com/doi/10.1002/14651858.CD003766.pub5/full. 2013.

MBRRACE-UK—Mothers and babies: reducing risk through audits and confidential enquiries across the UK: www.npeu.ox.ac.uk/mbrrace-uk.

Royal College of Midwives (RCM)—Electronic learning module on active birth: www.rcm.org.uk.

Free for RCM members.

Evidence Based Midwifery Network—Evidence-based midwifery guidelines for midwifery-led care in normal labour: www.rcm.org.uk/clinical-practice-and-guidance/evidence-based-guidelines.

Useful resource for different aspects of care.

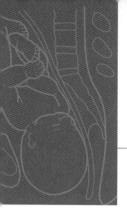

Chapter 37

Care in the second stage of labour

Soo Downe

Learning Outcomes ?

After reading this chapter, you will be able to:

- understand maternal behaviours associated with transition and the expulsive stage of labour
- understand the basic physiology of transition and the second stage
- understand some of the techniques that are currently used in childbirth
- recognize that many midwifery practices in the area of physiological birth are based on empirical but not formal evidence
- understand the importance of clear, comprehensive, accurate record keeping

INTRODUCTION

The anatomical second stage of labour has been traditionally defined as the period from full dilatation of the os uteri to the birth of the baby. However, women do not experience labour and birth by its anatomical divisions or by the dilatation of the cervix (Gross et al 2006), and labours do not usually progress at a uniform rate.

The distinctive physiological changes that occur just before or around the time the cervical os is fully dilated are traditionally defined as 'transition'. There is a paucity of formal evidence about the nature of transition, although some observational studies have been undertaken (Crawford 1983; Roberts and Hanson 2007). During or following this phase, the woman begins to feel a variable urge to bear down. Anecdotal evidence indicates that it is not uncommon for midwives to offer women pharmacological pain relief if the urge to bear down occurs when vaginal examination indicates that the anatomical second stage is

still some way off. If she then progresses more quickly than expected, such pain relief may inhibit the natural urge to bear down actively. It is thus essential that midwives know how to recognize the transitional phase of labour, and how to support women effectively at this time.

SIGNS OF PROGRESS

Transition

Transition occurs at variable times between the late first stage and early second stage of labour. It is recognizable by a change in the behaviour of the woman and, sometimes, by a change in the nature of the contractions she is experiencing. Any or all of the following may be noted:

- Loss of control; panic
- Belief that she cannot carry on
- Fearfulness (sometimes of dying)
- Disorientation
- Nausea
- Uncontrollable shivering
- Demands for pain relief
- A need to shout and scream
- A slowing of contractions
- A heavy 'show' – a loss per vaginam, which is usually a mixture of blood and mucus
- A period when the woman dozes, and goes 'inside herself' (the so-called 'rest and be thankful' phase)
- A variable urge to bear down or to push

If a vaginal examination is undertaken, the woman's cervical os will typically be found to be between 7 and 9 cm dilated, although smaller dilations have been reported (Borrelli et al 2013; Downe et al 2008; Roberts et al 1987).

Reflective activity 37.1

Next time you are with a woman in transition and/or the expulsive phase of labour, ask yourself the following questions.

- Does she want/need pain relief? Could reassurance, support, and faith in her capacity to birth the baby be just as effective?
- Will firm direction be helpful for her, or will it lead her to panic?
- If her contractions are decreasing in length and strength, is this a result of underlying pathology, or is it only part of a physiological transition? Does she need to rest for a short time? Is she hungry?
- Is she well hydrated?
- Does she want to be touched or not?
- Is the early pushing urge being felt because of fetal malposition, or is the head just descending very rapidly? Should she push spontaneously if you are not sure the cervical os is fully dilated?
- Is she enabled to adopt any position she wants? What would you do if she throws her arms back and brings her hips forward when she begins pushing?
- Is it difficult not to say 'hold your breath and push'? If so, why do you think this is?

If the answers conflict with local guidelines or with the usual actions midwives are expected to take locally, consider how these guidelines or informal expectations can be examined by you and your colleagues, with a view to revision.

Expulsive phase

Initially, the strength and consistency of the pushing urge tends to vary in intensity, becoming more consistent over time. The woman usually makes a characteristic grunting noise at the height of the contraction. She may feel that her bowels are emptying, which may be very embarrassing for her. The perineum bulges and is stretched thin as it is distended by the descending fetus. The anus initially pouts and then dilates with contractions. The vagina begins to gape, and finally the presenting part is visible. If she is upright and mobile at this point, the woman may lean forward with her arms placed higher than her head, brace herself against a wall or something solid and move towards a squatting position by bending her legs and abducting her thighs, which results physiologically in widening the pelvic capacity, and straightening the *curve of Carus*, to optimize the fetal passage through the birth canal. Women who are semirecumbent may throw their arms backwards and try to hold on to something behind them, possibly as an instinctive response to the same need. Other women will spontaneously adopt an all-fours position.

Some midwives have noted the appearance of a rounded area at the level of the lower back when the woman is in an upright or all fours position: the *rhombus of Michaelis* (Sutton and Scott 1996). Sutton and Scott note that it is caused by the pressure of the fetal head which lifts the sacrum and the coccyx out of the way. Others have noted anecdotally that women who have an epidural in situ may experience discomfort under the ribs at around about the time of full cervical dilatation. This may be a function of fetal realignment as the fetal head descends, causing a sensation of pressure above the level of the epidural block. In upright forward positions, a 'purple line' may be visible, which shows promise when used as a sign that the expulsive phase might be imminent (Kordi et al 2014; Shepherd et al 2010). This is a purplish line that develops from the anal margin and that can be seen to move up the anal cleft as labour progresses, possibly as a result of the pressure of the fetal head on blood vessels in the sacral region, causing distension that can be visible on the skin.

The efficacy of all these observations in predicting the transition to the expulsive phase of labour for individual women remains to be researched.

It is not always necessary to carry out a vaginal examination to confirm the onset of the anatomical second stage of labour, especially if the woman's behaviour indicates that expulsive contractions have begun (Downe et al 2013; National Institute for Health and Care Excellence (NICE) 2014: 29). However, where there is some uncertainty about this, or where the woman requests an examination, this can be done in conjunction with an abdominal examination and palpation, to confirm the station and position of the presenting part, and full dilatation of the os uteri. If no cervix is felt, there is positive confirmation of the onset of the anatomical second stage of labour. However, this might not signal the onset of spontaneous maternal pushing because, in some cases, the fetus still needs to rotate and descend to be in an optimum position to trigger active expulsive contractions. For this reason, the time between diagnosis of full dilatation of the cervix and active pushing is termed the *passive second stage of labour*. There is little established evidence on the optimal limits to this phase, and, in general, it should be led by the woman's sensations and the well-being of her and of her fetus. If she has regional analgesia in situ, local guidelines usually recommend a passive second stage of an hour or more, to allow for descent and rotation of the fetal head, given that there is usually less pelvic floor resistance under these circumstances, so rotation tends to take longer.

Once organized bearing down commences, the *active second stage of labour* is deemed to have commenced.

PHYSIOLOGY OF THE ACTIVE SECOND STAGE OF LABOUR

Contractions

On average, at this stage, studies have indicated that contractions have amplitude of 60 to 80 mmHg, occur every 2 to 3 minutes and last for 60 to 70 seconds, although other patterns of second-stage contractions can be effective. Marked retraction of the uterus further aids the descent of the fetus through the birth canal. There is no appreciable fall in the height of the fundus, however, because the fetal back tends to uncurl from its flexed attitude and the lower uterine segment stretches. The force of the uterine contractions and secondary powers is transmitted down the fetal spine to its head. This is *fetal axis pressure* and helps the descent of the fetus through the birth canal.

Secondary powers

The expulsion of the fetus is further aided by the voluntary muscles of the diaphragm and abdominal wall. In general (although there are distinct variations between individuals), the presenting part descends to approximately 1 cm above the level of the ischial spines, pressure from the fetal presentation stimulates nerve receptors in the pelvic floor and the woman experiences the desire to bear down. This is termed the 'Ferguson reflex' (Ferguson 1941). This sensation may occur before the end of the anatomical first stage of labour or at or after cervical full dilatation. The voluntary muscles of the chest and abdominal wall act reflexively in concert with the uterine contractions to overcome the resistance of the vagina, pelvic floor muscles and external parts. During this process, the diaphragm is lowered and the abdominal muscles contract.

The pelvic floor

The advancing fetus gradually stretches the vagina and displaces the pelvic floor. Anteriorly, the pelvic floor is pushed up and the bladder is drawn up into the abdomen, where it is less likely to be damaged. Posteriorly, the pelvic floor is pushed down in front of the presenting part. The rectum is compressed; thus, any faecal contents will be expelled. The perineal body becomes elongated and paper-thin as it is flattened by the advancing fetus.

MECHANISM OF LABOUR

As labour progresses, the fetus is moved through the birth canal and induced to make various twists and turns as a result of the forces that occur, causing it to respond to the contours and planes of the maternal pelvis. These movements are called, collectively, the *mechanism of labour*. An understanding of this mechanism enables assessment of progress in labour and recognition of when physiological support may be required or if a call for assistance should be made.

There is a mechanism for every fetal presentation and position. The widest diameter of the brim of the pelvis is transverse, whereas the widest diameter of the outlet is anteroposterior. To make the best use of available space, the widest presenting diameter of the fetal head usually enters the pelvis in the transverse diameter. As it descends, the fetal head and then the shoulders rotate to emerge in the anteroposterior diameter. The mechanism for the most common presentation is as follows, although it should be noted that the specific physiology of individual women and fetal dyads can alter this mechanism.

The lie is longitudinal, the presentation is cephalic and the presenting part is the area of the vertex. The attitude is one of flexion and therefore the denominator is the occiput. The engaging diameter is the suboccipitobregmatic (on average, approximately 9.5 cm). The position may be either right or left occipitoanterior.

Descent

Descent is the process whereby the fetal head moves into the pelvis (Fig. 37.1). Engagement occurs when the widest

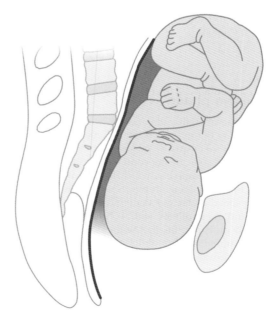

Figure 37.1 Descent of a fetus with a well-flexed head presenting. The sagittal suture is in the transverse diameter of the pelvis. (Mother in upright position.)

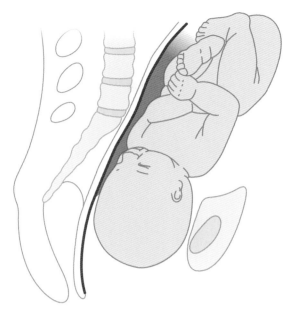

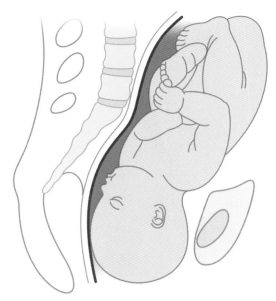

Figure 37.2 Internal rotation occurs. The sagittal suture is in the oblique diameter of the pelvis. (Mother in upright position.)

Figure 37.3 Internal rotation complete – the head is descended to the vulval outlet. The sagittal suture is now in the anteroposterior diameter of the pelvis. As the head deflexes slightly with descent, the sacrum and coccyx are displaced posteriorly. (Mother in upright position.)

diameter of the presenting part enters the pelvis. This is more likely to occur before the onset of labour in nulliparous rather than multiparous women.

Flexion

At the beginning of labour the fetal head is usually in an attitude of natural flexion. As labour progresses, the head meets the resistance of the pelvic floor muscles, and flexion increases. Fetal axis pressure is then transmitted through the occiput, which is pushed down lower as a consequence. The forehead is pushed upwards by the resistance of the soft parts, and so complete flexion is obtained.

Internal rotation

When the occiput meets the resistance of the pelvic floor, it rotates forward approximately 45 degrees (Fig. 37.2). The slope of the pelvic floor aids this internal rotation forwards, allowing the head to emerge in the longest diameter of the pelvic outlet, that is, the anteroposterior diameter (Fig. 37.3). The occiput then escapes under the pubic arch and the head is crowned.

Crowning of the head

The head is *crowned* when it has emerged under the pubic arch and no longer recedes between contractions. The

widest transverse diameter of the head (the biparietal diameter) is born (Fig. 37.4).

Extension

Once the head is crowned, extension takes place to allow the bregma, forehead, face and chin to pass over the perineum.

Restitution

When the head is born, it rights itself with the shoulders (Fig. 37.5). During the movement of internal rotation, the head is slightly twisted because the shoulders do not rotate at that time. The baby's neck is untwisted by restitution.

Internal rotation of the shoulders

The shoulders undergo an internal rotation similar to that of the head and then lie in the anteroposterior diameter of the outlet. The head, being free outside the birth canal, moves approximately 45 degrees at the same time, so internal rotation of the shoulders is accompanied by external rotation of the head. Rotation follows the direction of restitution; thus, the occiput turns to the same side

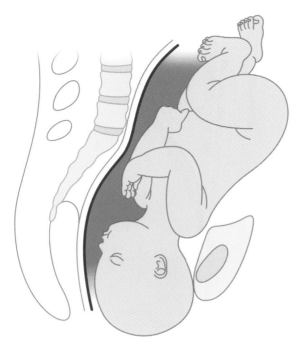

Figure 37.4 The head is crowned. The sacrum and coccyx regain their normal position. (Mother in upright position.)

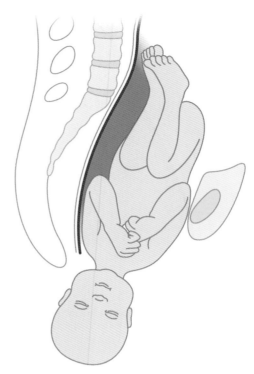

Figure 37.6 Internal rotation of the shoulders leads to external rotation of the head. (Mother in upright position.)

of the maternal pelvis as it was at the beginning of labour (Fig. 37.6).

Lateral flexion of the shoulders

The curve of the birth canal (the *curve of Carus*) causes the trunk of the baby to flex sideways as it is born. If the mother is semirecumbent, the angles of inclination of the birth canal mean that uterine pressure is exerted on the fetal shoulder anterior to her, and so the anterior shoulder is born under the pubic arch first, then the posterior shoulder passes over the perineum, causing the trunk of the baby to flex anteriorly, towards the mother's abdomen. If the mother is in a forward-leaning position (upright or on all fours) the angle of inclination of the birth canal and the forces of gravity usually cause the posterior shoulder to emerge first, with the anterior shoulder and trunk then following, again in lateral flexion towards the mother's abdomen.

After the birth

Once the baby is born, there is a marked retraction of the uterus, which starts the process of placental separation. This is completed in the third stage of labour.

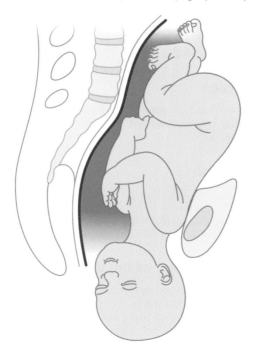

Figure 37.5 The head restitutes to the oblique, in line with the position of the shoulders. (Mother in upright position.)

DURATION OF THE SECOND STAGE OF LABOUR

The midwife should be aware of the rapidity with which the second stage can progress, especially for multiparous women, in whom it can sometimes last only a few minutes. For this reason, and because this is a time when a woman needs intense support and reassurance, she, and her birth companion(s), should not be left without a midwife in continuous attendance after the late first stage has commenced.

The NICE guidelines recommend the offer of abdominal examination and palpation and vaginal examination to assess progress after around an hour of active pushing for nulliparous women, and after about half an hour for multigravida women, if there are no clear signs of progress at this point (NICE 2014: 65). The guidelines also note that birth will usually take place within about 3 hours of the start of the active second stage for nulliparous women and within about 2 hours for a multiparous woman. Both rotation and/or descent of the presenting part are indicators of progress. If there is no fetal rotation or descent within this time span, this could be grounds for discussion with the woman and senior staff to decide if interventions are needed to ensure progress (NICE 2014: 65). These are, however, guidelines. In the presence of effective uterine activity, where there is progressive descent of the presenting part, and the condition of the woman and fetus does not give rise for concern, time alone does not provide sufficient grounds for curtailment of the second stage. Studies in this area demonstrate increased intervention and morbidity over time, but it is not clear if this is a result of actual or anticipated pathology (Altman and Lydon-Rochelle 2006). Positive, respectful communication between the woman and her birth companion(s), the midwife, senior colleagues and obstetric staff are all essential in maximizing good decision making in this area.

Many midwives take note of the pattern of progress in previous labours if the woman is multigravida; or that of labour in the sisters and mother of the labouring woman. This way of individualizing assessment of labour progress has not yet been tested in formal research studies.

Factors that may slow the progress of the active second stage but that can be corrected by time or by technique include a *malpositioned or deflexed fetus* (see the chapter website for Case Study 37.1) and use of pain relief (particularly *pethidine* or *epidural analgesia*). Corrective techniques for the former include the use of optimal fetal positioning (Sutton and Scott 1996). The effect of pethidine will ameliorate with time. NICE guidelines recommend that women with regional analgesia should be enabled to move around and adopt upright positions where possible (using telemetry if possible for continuous electronic fetal monitoring); that analgesia should be continued through the second stage and until after perineal repair where this is necessary; that pushing be delayed for at least 1 hour to allow for descent and rotation of the fetal head, if all other parameters are normal; and that the second stage should ideally be completed within 4 hours in these circumstances (NICE 2014: 37).

POSITIONS IN THE SECOND STAGE OF LABOUR

If supported to respond instinctively to labour, most women will move around spontaneously and adopt different positions during their labour and birth as they adapt to the position of the baby and the progress of the labour. Based on the latest Cochrane review in this area (Gupta et al 2012), current NICE intrapartum guidelines recommend that women avoid the use of supine positions in labour (NICE 2014: 54).

A woman who does adopt a semirecumbent position for whatever reason should be well supported by pillows and perhaps a wedge to prevent her from sliding down into the dorsal position. Should this happen, the heavy gravid uterus is likely to compress the vena cava, causing subsequent hypotension, reduced placental perfusion and fetal hypoxia (Humphrey et al 1974; Johnstone et al 1987).

Whatever position the woman chooses, the midwife should be able to adapt the principles of care in labour and management of birth appropriately.

Reflective activity 37.2

Consider how you could make the environment where you work a space where women feel they can mobilize freely and spontaneously depending on their instincts as the second stage progresses. How should the labour and birth space be laid out? What kind of support techniques will you use? How can you use the current resources in the labour and birth environment to maximum effect? What kind of conversations will you have with the woman/partner so that the birth partner is confident in helping the woman, and so that the woman can trust her instincts enough to adopt a range of positions spontaneously as her birth progresses? How will you fulfil monitoring and recording requirements for women who adopt the full range of possible birth positions?

MIDWIFERY CARE

During this period of maximum exertion, the woman should be praised for her efforts, and both she and her partner should be kept fully informed of progress made.

Information should be given between contractions, when the woman can relax and attend to what is being said. The midwife can help to promote confidence and allay anxiety by adopting a quiet, calm manner, and through tone of voice, tactile gestures and other nonverbal means of communication. Privacy is essential. It may help to have a 'do not disturb' sign on the door. Casual conversation between staff over the woman is never acceptable, and it is particularly disrespectful at this time.

Hygiene and comfort measures

The extreme exertion of the woman during the second stage of labour is likely to make her feel hot and sticky. She may appreciate having her face and hands sponged frequently. However, some women find this distracting because it breaks their concentration: it is very much a matter of personal choice. The woman may find drinks of iced water welcome and refreshing. If oral fluids are contraindicated, mouthwashes should be offered.

If leg cramps are experienced, these may be relieved by massage and by extending the leg and dorsiflexing the foot—that is, keeping the heel on the ground or bed, and pushing the toes towards the leg to stretch the calf muscle—as long as this is not uncomfortable.

A full bladder may delay progressive descent of the fetus, and the bladder may also be damaged by pressure as the fetus advances. Occasionally, if the fetal head has descended deeply into the pelvis and has caused upward displacement of the maternal urinary bladder, the woman may be unable to pass urine and the midwife may also find the passage of a catheter difficult. For this reason it is advisable to encourage regular micturition throughout labour, especially once the midwife recognizes that the expulsive stage of labour is imminent.

Support during transition

This phase of labour can be difficult for the woman and for those attending and supporting her. The midwife needs to be a calm and reassuring presence and must assess each woman carefully because individuals react in extremely diverse ways at this time. It is important that the midwife responds to the transitional phase appropriately in each individual case. The aim is to enable the woman to regain her capacity to cope and to trust in her own ability to birth her baby, so that she can take a positive approach to the active second stage of labour. The midwife should also pay attention to the woman's other birth companions, to ensure that they are reassured that this is a normal part of labour and an indication that the birth of the baby is not far away. Requests for epidural analgesia at this time from women who had previously said they did not want this form of pain relief should be considered in the light of the woman's behavioural cues. If she is showing signs of transition, the best approach might be to ask her if she wants close support through a few contractions, until she has a strong urge to push. If this is acceptable to the woman, the midwife needs to provide her with very active 'presencing', or being empathically there for her, and fully engaged with her, rather than simply being in the room (Fleming 1998) as she faces the next few contractions. The skills needed in this situation include emotional support, reassurance and encouragement and, for some women, therapeutic physical touch through massage and counterpressure, paying close attention to the woman's responses to see what is helpful and what is not.

Support during the expulsive phase of labour

Early bearing-down efforts

Traditionally, midwives in the UK have discouraged women from bearing down until the cervical os is known to be completely dilated, particularly in the case of the primigravid woman. This has usually been advised on the assumption that active pushing before full cervical dilatation may cause oedema of the os uteri, which will impede or prevent the vaginal birth of the baby (Downe et al 2008). However, a few small-scale observational studies and surveys (Bergstrom et al 1997; Borrelli et al 2013; Downe et al 2008; Petersen and Besuner 1997; Roberts et al 1987) have noted that the urge to push before full dilation of the cervix is not uncommon. This has led to suggestions that, where the fetal head is well positioned, and the cervix is more than 8 cm dilated, spontaneous pushing may be physiological (Roberts and Hanson 2007). Indeed, there is some evidence that preventing women from responding to the urge to push is very distressing for them, and that they remember this as one of the most distressing aspects of their birth (Bergstrom et al 1997). However, given the small size and localized context of these studies to date, best practice in this area remains uncertain.

If it is in the interests of a specific woman/fetus/baby to minimize the bearing-down urge, methods of doing this include the offer of Entonox, or coaching in controlled breathing techniques, to give women some distraction from the sensations; adoption of the left lateral position, which reduces the effect of gravity; or, at the extreme, the administration of opiod or epidural pain relief. The impact of these techniques on labour progress in this situation has not been subject to formal research.

See the chapter website for Case Study 37.2.

Delayed bearing-down efforts and the passive second stage of labour

The passive second stage probably occurs because although the cervix is fully dilated, the fetal head has not yet descended to compress the tissues of the pelvic floor and therefore to stimulate muscular contractions, as in the 'Ferguson reflex' (Ferguson 1941). The role of the midwife in this situation is to ensure that the woman is well hydrated and to ensure that maternal and fetal well-being are maintained. Assuming all is well, as noted previously, a watch-and-wait policy can be adopted until the woman begins to experience the bearing-down sensation.

Pushing technique

Organized sustained pushing with contractions, involving breath-holding (closed glottis pushing, known as the Valsalva manoeuvre), is still practised by some midwives in the belief that it reduces the duration of the second stage of labour and therefore the period of highest risk to the fetus. This practice has been challenged intermittently since the late 1950s (Beynon 1957; Bloom et al 2006). The most recent authoritative statement on the subject (NICE 2014: 66) concludes that *the woman should be informed that in the second stage she should be guided by her own urge to push.* The guidance goes on to recommend: *If pushing is ineffective or if requested by the woman, strategies to assist birth can be used, such as support, change of position, emptying of the bladder and encouragement.*

The observation that women in the semirecumbent position tend to push their pelvis forward and arch themselves backwards during the second stage of labour throws into question the common practice in many consultant maternity units of encouraging women who use the semirecumbent position to abduct their legs by bending them and pushing them towards their hips, and to lean forwards as they push. This practice, and the alternatives, require more examination. There is, as yet, no good evidence on the optimum advice on how to help women with bearing down when they have minimal sensation as a result of regional analgesia. However, in the absence of maternal sensation, some degree of direction from the midwife is probably necessary.

Perineal practices

A number of practices are used by midwives in the second stage of labour in an effort to minimize trauma to the perineum. These include the use of hot or cold compresses; perineal massage as the fetal head advances; and guarding with a gentle, or, in some cases, firm pressure, to maintain fetal flexion, and to support the perineal tissues as they stretch. NICE guidelines do not recommend perineal massage (NICE 2014: 67) or any other specific techniques to prevent perineal damage, although the current Cochrane review in this area does find evidence to support the use of warm compresses (Aasheim et al 2011). It is not clear whether the techniques used in the study would benefit women using upright positions in labour.

There is controversy currently about the 'hands off the perineum' policy that resulted from the HooP trial (McCandlish et al 1998). However, NICE guidance continues to be that either hands-on or poised approaches are equally acceptable, based on the best available evidence (NICE 2014: 66).

Assessing the need for episiotomy

An episiotomy is a surgical incision of the perineum to enlarge the vulval orifice. The midwife should be aware that pelvic floor and perineal trauma may have long-term implications for the woman and her partner and should not be performed as a routine practice, even where women have had previous third and fourth degree perineal tears (Carroli and Belizan 2004; Hartmann et al 2005; NICE 2014: 66–67). The possibility of perineal trauma should be discussed with the woman before the labour. Her informed choices for this element of labour should be recorded. If an episiotomy becomes necessary, she should be informed, and the midwife must only proceed with her consent (see Ch. 40 for more details).

OTHER MIDWIFERY TECHNIQUES

Optimal fetal positioning

In recent years, the technique of optimal fetal positioning has become increasingly popular (Sutton and Scott 1996). Techniques are proposed for shifting a baby that is malpositioned or asynclitic in labour, including raising one hip or rotating the hips, to change the angles of inclination of the pelvis (Hanson 2009). These observations and techniques have empirical credibility, but they remain to be tested formally for their efficacy.

Water birth

Therapeutic use of water in childbirth has grown in popularity. Some women may wish to spend most of their labour and birth in the water pool, others choose to spend short periods and some women may wish to leave the water for the actual birth of the baby and birth of the placenta.

Systematic review evidence indicates that there are some clinical benefits to labouring in water, including pain relief (Cluett and Burns 2009). The benefits and risks of the actual birth of the baby in water are less well researched (NICE 2014: 26, 35–36,68; Royal College of Midwives (RCM) 2012).

The essential issues to consider are as follows; some of these are also relevant to the use of water in the first stage of labour.

Temperature of the water

Too high a temperature will be uncomfortable for the woman and may cause fetal tachycardia: a maximum temperature of 37.5°C is recommended (NICE 2014: 35). Temperatures that are comfortable for the woman are recommended (RCM 2012).

Infection of mother or baby

Infection risk appears to be very low and can be minimized by using disposable bath linings, where possible, and by thorough cleaning and drying of the bath after use in accordance with current methods of prevention of cross-infection.

Water embolism

In theory, water embolism may occur when maternal placental bed sinuses are torn in the third stage of labour. Water may then enter the circulation. Although there have been no recorded cases of water embolism, some (but not all) local guidelines recommend that the third stage of labour should be conducted out of the water, and that any oxytocic preparation, if used, should be given when the woman has left the water. However, in other sites, the third stage is conducted while the woman is still in the pool. This is an area that is significantly underresearched at present, and so best practice is not established.

Perineal trauma

The possibility of perineal trauma must be borne in mind, although the counterpressure of the water on the perineum tends to slow down the birth somewhat. If necessary, the midwife can provide verbal support to the woman to allow the head and shoulders to emerge slowly.

Cord snapping

There have been occasional case reports of cord snapping during water births (RCM 2012). Although this is a very rare occurrence, it is good practice to keep two cord clamps nearby when the baby is being born, so that they can be applied rapidly if this event occurs.

Monitoring maternal and fetal health

The fetal heart can be auscultated using an underwater ultrasonic monitor, wireless electronic fetal monitoring or Pinard's stethoscope. If pain relief is required, inhalational analgesia (Entonox) is suitable. The woman must not be left unattended while using inhalational analgesia during a water birth. If narcotic analgesia is required, the woman should be asked to leave the water because the drowsiness induced by the drugs compromises safety.

The baby

The baby should be brought to the surface immediately after birth by the woman, birth partner or midwife. The umbilical cord should not be clamped and cut while the baby is still under water because the sudden reduction in placental-fetal blood flow may initiate respiration, and thus water inhalation.

PREPARATION FOR THE BIRTH

This is a time of great anticipation, and it is now that the value of the midwife–woman relationship that has been developed, the strength of the mother and the skills of the midwife are demonstrated. If the midwife has established a good relationship with the woman and her partner, has enabled the woman to work through her labour with confidence and has kept the woman and her supporting companions informed of progress and what to expect in the second stage, then the woman and her companions can approach the actual birth with confidence. The atmosphere in the birth room should be calm and unhurried, so that the woman can emerge from the experience with positive memories and intact self-respect. Privacy for the mother must be ensured because it is embarrassing and stressful for her if people repeatedly enter her room.

The midwife should prepare for birth as soon as she suspects that the second stage is imminent. This is especially the case for multigravida women, who can progress very quickly, but some primigravid woman also have very short pushing phases of labour. It is essential to include the women's vocalizations and behaviour in the judgement of progress, and not to rely simply on the findings of a vaginal examination, or on stereotypes of 'typical' patterns of progress.

The room should be clean and warm for the birth of the baby. A warm cot is prepared and resuscitation equipment is checked.

THE ACTIVITIES OF THE MIDWIFE DURING THE BIRTH

The actual methods of supporting women during birth can be learned only by experience. However, the principles remain the same and can be applied to whatever position the woman adopts for birth. She must be kept informed at all times, and her wishes must be respected.

A clean area is prepared, including a clean gown or apron and gloves for the midwife. To minimize the risk of contamination from blood or liquor splashes, and of infection with diseases such as HIV, the midwife can also wear unobtrusive eye protection, such as plain spectacles. Any other person likely to come into contact with blood or other body fluids should be similarly protected.

Local anaesthetic and syringe are made available for perineal infiltration before an episiotomy, should it be necessary. If the mother has consented to active management of the third stage of labour, a suitable oxytocic drug is checked and drawn up in readiness for use. NICE guidelines recommend 10 IU of oxytocin alone, rather than combined oxytocin and syntometrine (NICE 2014: 72);

discussion should have taken place previously regarding active and expectant management (see Ch. 39).

If the woman is recumbent, the vulva can be washed with warm solution, the birth area draped with clean or sterile towels, and a clean pad placed over the anus to minimize faecal contamination. There is no evidence that infection rates are increased if plain water is used, and the practice of draping has not been evaluated in terms of infection rates (Keane and Thornton 1998). If a woman is in an upright position, a clean area should be prepared on the surface beneath her.

If the woman does not have an epidural in situ, and if the labour has progressed normally to this point, her spontaneous pushing efforts will usually be effective. The midwife will need to provide support and encouragement. If a 'hands off the perineum' ('hands poised') approach is used, and the woman is semirecumbent, it is important to ensure that rapid progress does not threaten the integrity of the perineum. If the fetal head is advancing very fast, one hand can be cupped over the perineum to provide gentle counterpressure to the descending head, and/or flexion maintained by placing the palm of the other hand lightly on the emerging head with fingers pointing to the sinciput. However, the head must not be held back by excessive pressure because this risks overstretching and tearing of the deeper structures of the pelvic floor. When women are in more upright positions, the 'hands poised' approach is the norm, but similar attention should be paid, and the woman should be guided verbally if there is very rapid descent of the presenting part.

Until the head crowns, it will recede between contractions. The head crowns when the widest transverse diameter, the biparietal diameter, distends the vulva, and then no longer recedes. After crowning, as the head extends from its position of flexion, and sweeps the perineum to be born, the woman is usually asked to breathe steadily in and out to prevent the birth taking place too quickly. Inhalational analgesia can help at this point. Until recently, it has been standard practice to check for cord around the neck of the emerging baby, before the birth of the shoulders, and to clamp and cut a nuchal cord if it is tight. However, given the evidence on the benefits of keeping the cord intact (see following discussion) and a lack of evidence that nuchal cord compromises the vast majority of babies (Kong et al 2015), there is a shift away from this practice. A technique called the 'somersault manoeuvre' (Schorn and Blanco 1991) is widely practised in the United States (see Fig. 37.7) and has been adopted by some midwives in the UK. There is, however, no evidence that unlooping the cord as opposed to leaving it in situ improves fetal oxygenation, and some midwives report that they will not check for the cord unless the birth seems to be impeded. In this case and, rarely, if the cord is so tightly round the neck or shoulders as to prevent the birth of the baby, two pairs of artery forceps must be applied 2 to 5 cm apart, and the cord cut between them and unwound. However, this procedure should only be performed when absolutely necessary, because once the cord is severed, the baby is no longer oxygenated, and the loss of placental blood flow may further compromise the baby if there is any subsequent delay with the shoulders. Even if this doesn't happen, allowing the cord to pulsate after birth is now usual practice, to optimize the transfer of blood from the placental circulation to the baby, and cutting the cord prevents this from occurring (see following discussion).

At this stage, some mothers like to be helped into a position to see the baby's head, possibly with the aid of a mirror, and watch, or perhaps assist with, the birth of the trunk.

Following *restitution* and *external rotation* of the head, the shoulders will normally be in the anteroposterior diameter of the pelvis, although some babies are born with the shoulders in the oblique. If the mother has consented to active management of the third stage of labour, an oxytocic is given by the second attending midwife, as the anterior shoulder is born, or immediately following the birth.

The baby will usually be born spontaneously, but if the mother is in the semirecumbent position, and if the midwife is sure that internal rotation of the shoulders has occurred, the birth can be assisted by placing one hand each side of the baby's head. With the next contraction, gentle downward traction may be applied to the baby's head. The anterior shoulder will then emerge below the symphysis pubis. The baby is then lifted up to allow the posterior shoulder to sweep the perineum, and the baby's trunk is carried towards the woman's abdomen, being born by lateral flexion. The baby can then be placed on the woman's abdomen, or in her arms, where she can immediately see and touch it. The time of birth is noted. Skin-to-skin contact at this time is important for improved breastfeeding outcomes and reduced neonatal distress/ crying (Moore et al 2012; NICE 2014: 78).

If the mother is in an upright forward-leaning position, the midwife usually only needs to be in a position to receive the baby to ensure that it is brought safely to the ground or into its woman's arms.

For most babies, nasopharyngeal suctioning is unnecessary once they are born; however, in the presence of meconium or of excessive mucus, it may be required.

It is now widely accepted that there are benefits to delaying umbilical cord clamping for at least 1 minute and up to 5 minutes, or until the cord has stopped pulsating (McDonald et al 2013; NICE 2014: 72). Whenever the cord is cut, before division, the cord is first clamped with two artery forceps, cut between the forceps with blunt-ended scissors and then sealed close to the umbilicus, usually with a plastic clamp. It is important to ensure that the baby is thoroughly and gently dried and covered warmly to prevent excessive heat loss while maintaining the skin-to-skin contact with its mother.

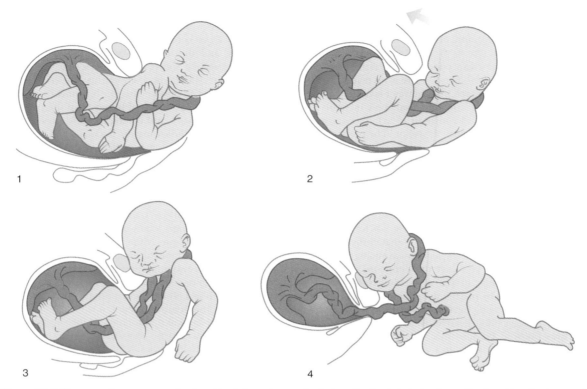

Figure 37.7 Somersault manoeuvre: the head is delivered normally, but as the body is being born, the head is raised towards the symphysis pubis and the body is moved away from the perineum. This allows for minimum tension on the cord; the midwife can more easily unwrap it and allow the infant to reperfuse. (From Mercer J, Skovgaard R, Peareara-Eaves J, Bowman T: Nuchal cord management and nurse-midwifery practice, *J Midwifery Womens Health*, September/October 2005. Reproduced with permission of Elsevier.)

This is an ecstatic moment for the parents, and the midwife is privileged to share their joy in the birth of their baby.

OBSERVATIONS AND RECORDINGS

Transition and the second stage of labour are very demanding for both woman and fetus. It is a time when the capacity of the woman to birth her baby is most tested. It is also a time when the possibility of fetal hypoxia in a previously compromised baby increases as the alteration in uterine activity reduces placental-fetal oxygenation (Katz et al 1987). It is therefore important to continually assess the well-being of mother and fetus.

Recordings should include any discussions with the woman and any decisions she has taken about the way the labour is conducted. The decisions and actions of the midwife must also be recorded. The woman's general condition and state of mind are noted. Her pulse is taken regularly to rule out rare acute problems, such as intra-uterine infection or a concealed intrapartum haemorrhage, and to ensure that the fetal rather than maternal heart rate is being auscultated. Blood pressure should be checked hourly, and temperature every 4 hours, if the second stage lasts that long (NICE 2014: 64). NICE guidelines also recommend that the woman is offered abdominal examination and palpation and vaginal examination hourly in the active second stage, and that the fetal heart is auscultated for a minute every 5 minutes. The frequency, strength and duration of uterine contractions are observed, in addition to the relaxation of the uterus between contractions. Any sustained loss of uterine activity will result in delayed progress. The midwife will need to reassess the situation to establish the likely cause, and either remedy the situation or seek assistance if necessary.

Continuous electronic fetal heart monitoring does not provide benefits for the healthy woman and fetus in labour (Alfirevic et al 2013; NICE 2014: 39), but if it is in progress as a result of complications in mother and/or fetus, the cardiotocograph trace should be analysed and assessed for normality after every contraction.

The amniotic fluid is observed for meconium staining. Current NICE guidelines (NICE 2014: 32) recommend continuous electronic fetal monitoring (and transfer for women who are out of hospital) for women with significant meconium-stained liquor, which is defined as either dark green or black amniotic fluid that is thick or tenacious, or any meconium-stained amniotic fluid containing lumps of meconium. For women with light meconium staining, NICE only recommends continuous electronic fetal monitoring (and transfer) when there are other indications of complications in mother or baby (NICE 2014: 39–40).

All observations, including the timing of the various stages and phases of the labour, must be recorded in locally approved labour records. Independent midwives are advised to agree their records in collaboration with their local supervisor of midwives. All actions taken by the midwife must be noted. Each entry must be dated, timed, and signed legibly. Entries made by students must always be countersigned by the attending midwife.

FUTURE RESEARCH IN THIS AREA

As noted earlier, there are research gaps in terms of maternal behavioural cues and of physiological symptoms of progress throughout the second stage of labour, and these all need to be researched. The normal physiology of transition requires particular attention. This includes the relative value of vaginal examination in the assessment of labour progress, when set against both maternal cues and symptoms, and other means that have been proposed, such as second stage ultrasound assessment of cervical dilation and fetal position/descent. There is little evidence about the mechanisms of labour in upright or all-fours positions, or on how the family histories of women might help to predict which labour and birth patterns are physiological for this particular mother/baby dyad and which are not. Techniques for helping women to push when they have an epidural in situ need more research, as does the use of optimal fetal positioning. The question of the best approach to supporting the perineum in a range of positions and circumstances is currently under debate, both for births in and out of the water. Third stage management in water is very underresearched at present.

In addition to these concerns, over the last few years there has been an increased awareness of the consequences of events in labour, particularly in terms of the microbiome (Maynard et al 2012; Jašarević et al 2015) and epigenome (Dahlen et al 2013) and potential associated interactions between events in labour and later autoimmune disease for the neonate (Sevelsted et al 2015). Concern about disrespect and abuse in childbirth is on the rise and has precipitated a range of research studies that are currently in progress around the world (Bohren et al 2015; Bowser and Hill 2010). These areas are likely to stimulate an expanded research agenda with relevance to second stage labour over the next few years.

CONCLUSION

For many years it has been assumed that the second stage of labour can be strictly delimited and predicted. Increasing attention to women's actual experiences has led to more formal recognition of the fluidity of the phases of labour and to an acknowledgement of the nature of transition. Whatever the eventual findings of future research in this area, transition and the expulsive stage of labour remain times of intense hard work, profound psychological impression, and great exhilaration, joy and happiness for the mother, her partner and possibly her baby. The empathetic and skilled midwife is an essential companion on the journey to motherhood that is represented by this stage of labour.

Key Points

- Transition and second stage can be physically and emotionally intense, and maternal behaviour is usually a good indication of progress during this time.

- It is essential for midwives to understand the physiology and mechanisms of this phase of labour and to be able to apply this knowledge in different situations.

- A skilled midwife can offer unobtrusive support and care while ensuring the well-being of the mother and baby.

- Clear, comprehensive and contemporaneous record keeping is essential.

- Empirical evidence indicates that traditional and new midwifery skills can be beneficial, but there are many gaps in the research evidence in this area and in understanding the nature of normal and optimal birth.

- Such studies as there have been in this area generally indicate that the second stage of labour can usually be left to progress according to the pattern and activities of the individual woman when mother and baby are healthy and well supported.

References

Aasheim V, Nilsen ABV, Lukasse M, et al: Perineal techniques during the second stage of labour for reducing perineal trauma, *Cochrane Database Syst Rev* (12):CD006672, 2011.

Alfirevic Z, Devane D, Gyte GML: Continuous cardiotocography (CTG) as a form of electronic fetal monitoring (EFM) for fetal assessment during labour, *Cochrane Database Syst Rev* (5):CD006066, 2013.

Altman MR, Lydon-Rochelle MT: Prolonged second stage of labor and risk of adverse maternal and perinatal outcomes: a systematic review, *Birth* 33(4):315–322, 2006.

Bergstrom L, Seidel J, Skillman-Hull L, et al: 'I gotta push. Please let me push!' Social interactions during the change from first to second stage labor, *Birth* 24(3):173–180, 1997.

Beynon CL: The normal second stage of labour: a plea for reform of its conduct, *J Obstet Gynaecol Br Emp* 64(6):815–820, 1957.

Bloom SL, Casey BM, Schaffer JI, et al: A randomized trial of coached versus uncoached maternal pushing during the second stage of labor, *Am J Obstet Gynecol* 194(1):10–13, 2006.

Bohren MA, Vogel JP, Hunter EC, et al: The mistreatment of women during childbirth in health facilities globally: a mixed-methods systematic review, *PLoS Med* 12(6):2015.

Borrelli SE, Locatelli A, Nespoli A: Early pushing urge in labour and midwifery practice: a prospective observational study at an Italian maternity hospital, *Midwifery* 8:871–975, 2013.

Bowser D, Hill K: *Exploring evidence for disrespect and abuse in facility-based childbirth. Report of a Landscape Analysis*, Washington, DC, USAID Traction Project, 2010.

Carroli G, Belizan J: *Episiotomy for vaginal birth (Cochrane Review), The Cochrane Library*, Issue 1, Chichester, John Wiley, 2004.

Cluett ER, Burns E: Immersion in water in labour and birth, *Cochrane Database Syst Rev* (2):CD000111, 2009.

Crawford JS: The stages and phases of labour: an outworn nomenclature that invites hazard, *Lancet* 2(8344):271–272, 1983.

Dahlen HG, Kennedy HP, Anderson CM, et al: The EPIIC hypothesis: intrapartum effects on the neonatal epigenome and consequent health outcomes, *Med Hypotheses* 280(5):656–662, 2013.

Downe S, Trent Midwifery Research Group, Young C, et al: Multiple midwifery discourses: the case of the early pushing urge. In Downe S, editor: *Normal birth: evidence and debate*, Oxford, Elsevier, 2008.

Downe S, Gyte GM, Dahlen HG, et al: Routine vaginal examinations for assessing progress of labour to improve outcomes for women and babies at term, *Cochrane Database Syst Rev* (7):CD010088, 2013.

Ferguson JK: A study of the motility of the intact uterus of the rabbit at term, *Surg Gynecol Obstet* 73:359–366, 1941.

Fleming VE: Women-with-midwives-with-women: a model of interdependence, *Midwifery* 14(3):137–143, 1998.

Gross MM, Hecker H, Matterne A, et al: Does the way that women experience the onset of labour influence the duration of labour?, *Br J Obstet Gynaecol* 113(3):289–294, 2006.

Gupta JK, Hofmeyr GJ, Shehmar M: Position in the second stage of labour for women without epidural anaesthesia, *Cochrane Database Syst Rev* (5):CD002006, 2012.

Hanson L: Second-stage labor care: challenges in spontaneous bearing down, *J Perinat Neonatal Nurs* 23(1):31–39, 2009.

Hartmann K, Viswanathan M, Palmieri R, et al: Outcomes of routine episiotomy: a systematic review, *J Am Med Assoc* 293(17):2141–2148, 2005.

Humphrey MD, Chang A, Wood EC, et al: A decrease in fetal pH during the second stage of labour when conducted in the dorsal position, *J Obstet Gynaecol Br Commonw* 81(8):600–602, 1974.

Jašarević E, Howerton CL, Howard CD, et al: Alterations in the Vaginal microbiome by maternal stress are associated with metabolic reprogramming of the offspring gut and brain, *Endocrinology* 156(9):3265–3276, 2015.

Johnstone FD, Aboelmagd MS, Harouny AK: Maternal posture in second stage and fetal acid-base status, *Br J Obstet Gynaecol* 94(8):753–757, 1987.

Katz M, Lunenfeld E, Meizner I, et al: The effect of the duration of the second stage of labour on the acid-base state of the fetus, *Br J Obstet Gynaecol* 94(5):425–430, 1987.

Keane HE, Thornton JG: A trial of cetrimide/chlorhexidine or tap water for perineal cleaning, *Br J Midwifery* 6(1):34–37, 1998.

Kong CW, Chan LW, To WW: Neonatal outcome and mode of delivery in the presence of nuchal cord loops: implications on patient counselling and the mode of delivery, *Arch Gynecol Obstet* 292(2):283–289, 2015.

Kordi M, Irani M, Tara F, et al: The diagnostic accuracy of purple line in prediction of labor progress in Omolbanin Hospital, Iran, *Iran Red Crescent Med J* 16(11):e16183, 2014.

Maynard CL, Elson CO, Hatton RD, et al: Reciprocal interactions of the intestinal microbiota and immune system, *Nature* 489(7415):231–241, 2012.

McCandlish R, Bowler U, van Asten H, et al: A randomised controlled trial of care of the perineum during second stage of normal labour, *Br J Obstet Gynaecol* 105(12):1262–1272, 1998.

McDonald SJ, Middleton P, Dowswell T, et al: Effect of timing of umbilical cord clamping of term infants on maternal and neonatal outcomes, *Cochrane Database Syst Rev* (7):CD004074, 2013.

Moore ER, Anderson GC, Bergman N, et al: Early skin-to-skin contact for mothers and their healthy newborn infants, *Cochrane Database Syst Rev* (5):CD003519, 2012.

National Institute for Health and Care Excellence (NICE): Intrapartum care: care of healthy women and their babies during childbirth (website). www.nice.org.uk/guidance/cg190/resources/guidance-intrapartum-care-care

-of-healthy-women-and-their-babies
-during-childbirth-pdf. 2014.

Petersen L, Besuner P: Pushing
techniques during labor: issues and
controversies, *J Obstet Gynecol
Neonatal Nurs* 26(6):719–726, 1997.

Roberts J, Hanson L: Best practices
in second stage labor care: maternal
bearing down and positioning,
J Midwifery Women's Health
52(3):238–245, 2007.

Roberts JE, Goldstein SA, Gruener JS,
et al: A descriptive analysis of
involuntary bearing down efforts

during the expulsive phase of
labour, *J Obstet Gynecol Neonatal
Nurs* 16(1):48–55, 1987.

Royal College of Midwives (RCM):
Evidence based guidelines for
midwifery-led care in labour;
immersion in water for labour and
birth (website). www.rcm.org.uk/sites/
default/files/Immersion%20in%20
Water%20%20for%20Labour%20
and%20Birth_0.pdf. 2012.

Schorn MN, Blanco JD: Management of
the nuchal cord, *J Nurse Midwifery*
36(2):131–132, 1991.

Sevelsted A, Stokholm J, Bønnelykke K:
Cesarean section and chronic
immune disorders, *Pediatrics*
135(1):e92–e98, 2015.

Shepherd A, Cheyne H, Kennedy S,
et al: The purple line as a measure
of labour progress: a longitudinal
study, *BMC Pregnancy Childbirth*
16(10):54, 2010.

Sutton J, Scott P: *Understanding and
teaching optimal fetal positioning*, 2nd
edn, Tauranga (NZ), Birth Concepts,
1996.

Resources and additional reading

Byrom S, Downe S: *The roar behind the
silence; why kindness and compassion
matter in maternity care*, London,
2015, Pinter and Martin.

Kennedy HP: A model of exemplary
midwifery practice: results of a
Delphi study, *J Midwifery Womens
Health* 45(1):4–19, 2000.

Kennedy HP, Shannon MT: Keeping
birth normal: research findings on

midwifery care during childbirth,
J Obstet Gynecol Neonatal Nurs
33(5):554–660, 2004.

Renfrew MJ, McFadden A, Bastos MH,
et al: Midwifery and quality care:
findings from a new evidence-
informed maternity care framework,
The Lancet 384(9948):1129–1145,
2014.

Simkin P, Ancheta R: *The labor progress
handbook: early interventions to
prevent and treat dystocia*, Chichester,
John Wiley and Sons, 2011.

Walsh D, Downe S, editors: *Essential
midwifery practice: intrapartum care*,
Chichester, Wiley-Blackwell, 2010.

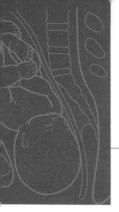

Chapter 38

Supporting choices in reducing pain and fear during labour

Cecelia M Bartholomew

Learning Outcomes ?

After reading this chapter, you will be able to:

- understand the physiological aspect of pain processes in labour and its effect on the woman
- appreciate the impact of fear and other psychological interactions on the pain processes and how they affect the woman's perception of pain and her experience of childbirth
- be aware of the effect of culture and the environment on the birth process
- understand the nature of support in labour and its relationship to the woman's coping mechanisms
- be familiar with a range of approaches available to support the woman to take control of her childbirth experience, which will enable her to be involved in the management of her pain during labour

INTRODUCTION

The 9 months of pregnancy brings with them a whirlwind of emotions that culminates in birth, an event that women look forward to, but often fear, because the process is accompanied by unwanted aches and pains. Many women become anxious about their ability to cope with pain, and this may affect their perceptions of control during labour and their overall satisfaction with their birth experience. The challenges for the midwife lie in enabling each woman to understand the various factors that influence her own interpretation and experience of the uncomfortable sensations that accompany birth. The midwife's role is to assist the woman to be prepared, alleviate her fears, facilitate the optimum choices for pain relief to match the woman's

individual needs and ensure the best outcome for both mother and the newborn.

AN EXPLORATION OF PAIN IN LABOUR

Pain is a complex, subjective phenomenon influenced by psychological, physiological and sociocultural factors. Although pain is universally experienced and acknowledged, it is not completely understood (Lowe 2002). Pain is usually associated with injury and tissue damage and tends to be a warning to rest and protect the area. In childbirth, however, it has a different meaning because it is part of a naturally occurring and generally welcomed life event. Increasing pain at the end of a normal pregnancy is often the first sign that labour has commenced (McDonald 2006), with psychological implications for the woman and those around her as they recognize the need to prepare for the baby's arrival.

The pain in labour can be described as having both a visceral and somatic component (Wong 2013). Visceral pain relates to the deeper organs, such as the uterus, whereas somatic pain sensations is from the skin and muscles, such as in the perineum. During the first stage of labour, as the uterus contracts, the arteries supplying the myometrium are squeezed, and the cervix begins to efface and dilate (Lowe 2002) (see Chs 35–37). The pain is cramp-like and visceral in origin, occurring as a result of mechanoreceptors being stimulated, with a consequential reduction of oxygen to the uterine and cervical tissues resulting in ischaemia (Novikova and Cluver 2012). The contractions, which cause pushing and pulling on pelvic structures (Lowe 2002), also induce discomfort. The pain in labour may be felt in the abdominal wall, lumbosacral region, the gluteal regions and commonly in the thighs as the pain is referred to these areas (Novikova and Cluver 2012; Wong 2013).

In the second stage of labour the visceral pain continues but is accompanied by somatic sensations resulting from the distension of the pelvic floor, perineum and vagina (Lowe 2002). This pain is thus more severe than in the first stage, and as the sensations combine, the woman also experiences rectal pressure and discomfort with the descent and expulsion of the fetus (Novikova and Cluver 2012).

Uterine, cervical and perineal nerve supply

The autonomic nervous system serves the uterus and the cervix (see Ch. 35), with the body of the uterus being supplied by the sympathetic fibres emanating from the tenth, eleventh and twelfth thoracic vertebrae (T10, T11, T12) and the first lumbar vertebra (L1); the cervix is supplied by the parasympathetic fibres from the 2nd, 3rd and 4th sacral vertebrae (S2, S3, S4) (see Fig. 38.1). In the second stage of labour, pain in the perineum is transmitted via the pudendal nerve and branches, derived from the 2nd and 3rd sacral nerve roots meeting the branched

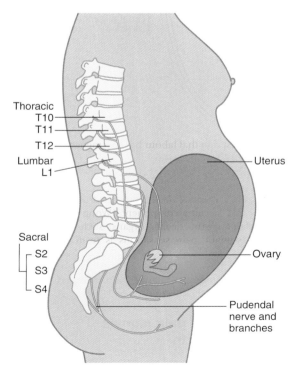

Thoracic
T10
T11
T12
Lumbar
L1

Uterus

Sacral
S2
S3
S4

Ovary

Pudendal nerve and branches

Figure 38.1 Pain pathways. (This article was published in Yerby M, editor: Pain in childbearing, London, 2000, Baillière Tindall, Copyright Elsevier.)

network from the uterus at the uterovaginal plexus, also called the *Lee–Frankenhäuser plexus*.

Nociceptors

The nerve receptors that are activated by noxious stimuli, causing pain, are called *nociceptors*. There are two main types of nociceptors: the fast, thinly *myelinated alpha-delta (Aδ) nerve fibres*, and the slower, smaller, *unmyelinated C nerve fibres*. They are physiologically specialized peripheral sensory neurons (Bridgestock and Rae 2013) activated by thermal, mechanical and/or chemical changes in tissues (Tracy et al 2015). In the first stage of labour, stimulation of the C fibres dominates (Wong 2013). These fibres are found in the deep viscera, such as the uterus, and give rise to the deep prolonged pain of labour when stimulated by muscular contractions and chemical substances (McDonald 2006; McGann 2007). In the second stage, the sharp pain from the vagina and perineum occur as a result of stimulation of the Aδ fibres. Notably, running laterally to the two types of fibres are alpha-beta (Aβ) nerve fibres, which respond to non-painful stimuli such as vibration and light touch, that inhibit sensations (Steeds 2013). Stimulation of the large Aβ nerve fibres in the skin modulates the transmitted signals of pain in labour and may be the effective source of non-pharmacological forms of pain relief such as transcutaneous electrical nerve stimulation (TENS), hydrotherapy and massage (Mander 2011).

Transduction, transmission and interpretation of pain signals in labour

In labour, chemicals are produced as a result of ischaemia when myometrial blood vessels are occluded during contractions and because of trauma to cervical tissues as the cervix dilates. The ensuing inflammatory response summons a mixture of chemicals, including *histamine, serotonin, bradykinins* and *prostaglandins*. Transduction occurs as these inflammatory mediators douse the nociceptors; the nerve fibres become sensitized and activated (Steeds 2013) to stimulate an action potential in the nerve. *Substance P*, a neuropeptide, is also released from the afferent nerves as part of the 'signalling process' of pain on its way to the dorsal horn of the spinal cord; it could be termed a potentiator of pain sensation.

Pain signals transmitted as action potentials from the afferent neurons enter the spinal cord through the posterior (dorsal) root into the grey matter in an area of the spine called the dorsal horn, where the primary afferent neurons synapse with second-order neurons (Steeds 2013; Bridgestock and Rae 2013) (Fig. 38.2a). The dorsal horn is divided into 10 layers called laminae, where various types of stimuli, including the noxious messages, are decoded. The C fibres terminate in lamina II, which is also known as the substantia gelatinosa, whereas the Aδ fibres terminate in laminae I and V (Steeds 2013) (Fig. 38.2b).

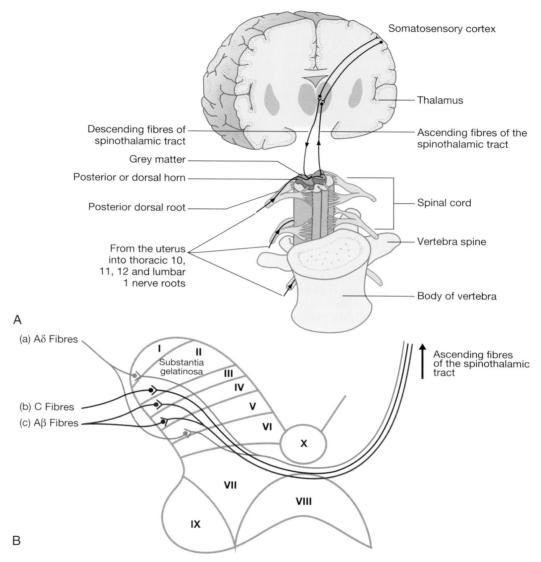

Somatosensory cortex

Thalamus

Descending fibres of spinothalamic tract

Ascending fibres of the spinothalamic tract

Grey matter

Posterior or dorsal horn

Posterior dorsal root

Spinal cord

From the uterus into thoracic 10, 11, 12 and lumbar 1 nerve roots

Vertebra spine

Body of vertebra

A

(a) Aδ Fibres

I
II
Substantia gelatinosa
III
IV

Ascending fibres of the spinothalamic tract

(b) C Fibres

(c) Aβ Fibres

V

VI

X

VII

VIII

IX

B

Figure 38.2 **A,** Brain and spinal cord connections. (This article was published in Yerby M, editor: Pain in childbearing, London, 2000, Baillière Tindall, Copyright Elsevier.) **B,** Layers of the dorsal horn where the Aδ, Aβ and C efferent nerve fibres synapse.

The pain signals subsequently cross the spinal cord to the opposite side before ascending up the spinothalamic tract to the thalamus then on to the higher centres of the cerebral cortex, where they are perceived and interpreted (McCool et al 2004). Simultaneously, there are descending tracts from the brain, with returning signals to the spinal cord. These nerve fibres in the descending tracts release endorphins at the spinal level that inhibit some of the noxious messages ascending to the brain (Mander 2011). The naturally occurring endorphins act like

exogenous opioids modulating pain messages (McGann 2007; Millan 2002).

Modulation of pain signals during childbirth

If the midwife has a good understanding of the hormonal interplay that has an impact on the pain signals that reach the brain, this will help with the selection of an appropriate strategy to change the woman's perception and experience of her pain. Melzack and Wall (1965) described mechanisms for modulating pain at spinal cord level. At the dorsal horn in the substantia gelatinosa of the spinal cord, pain stimuli may be blocked by a 'gating' mechanism. When the 'gate' is open, pain sensations reach the higher centres. When the 'gate' is closed, pain is blocked and does not become part of the conscious; therefore, pain is reduced. The theory has been examined and has been shown to be not completely accurate (Mendell 2014); however, it has helped with the development and understanding of various methods to relieve pain by interrupting pain signals reaching the higher brain centre.

Endorphins

One mechanism of pain modulation involves opioid-like substances that are released as a result of a process initialized by a noxious stimulus. One of these naturally occurring hormonal groups is *endorphins*, the neuropeptides, which are produced by the hypothalamus and pituitary gland and released by the descending nerve fibres at the spinal cord level. With greater understanding of endorphins and their opiate-like properties, it was noted that they work by suppressing the release and effect of the neurotransmitter *Substance P*. They do so by binding to opioid receptors, thus hindering the relay of pain messages to the brain, affecting the perception of pain as the individual becomes cognizant of the feeling of discomfort.

In a physiological labour, positive perception of stress raises *beta-endorphin* levels in the blood, which in turn affects how the woman experiences pain. Beta-endorphins are the hormones involved in the feelings generated in relationships and are also released through social, emotional and physical interventions (Kirkham and Jowitt 2012; Sanders 2015; Buckley 2015), which can produce a sense of euphoria and pleasure. This has implications for some of the non-pharmacological methods of pain relief, which are discussed further on in this chapter.

Reflective activity 38.1

With your current knowledge and understanding, consider a time when you have experienced acute pain.
  Try to recall what you did immediately as the pain occurred. Did you touch/stroke the area? Did you want to move around or sit/lie quietly? You should now be able to relate this to the phenomenon of modulation of pain signals.

FEAR AND OTHER PSYCHOLOGICAL ELEMENTS RELATED TO PAIN

Although it may be easy to acknowledge the physical and sensory dimensions of pain, the experience in labour has a psychological component, which midwives and other maternity healthcare professionals must appreciate to address the subjective nature of the phenomenon for each woman. As such, the perceived intensity of labour pains and resulting responses involve more than the sensory input from the stimulation of nociceptors in the uterus and perineum. There is an affective dimension that relates to unpleasant feelings and discomfort (Price 2000), wherein the experienced strength of the pain is influenced by cognitive factors such as vigilance, beliefs, emotional state, alertness, expectations and level of attention (Legrain et al 2009; Atlas and Wager 2012) and heightened by feelings of fear and anxiety, which may accompany the woman's experience of labour. In turn, fear in childbirth promotes the activation of the catecholamine response, contributing to uterine dystocia and a protracted labour (Rouhe et al 2009; Hodnett et al 2013; Collins 2015).

As labour progresses, signs of the effect of pain on the woman become evident. Pain causes an increased release of stress hormones called *catecholamine* (e.g. *epinephrine*) that results in vasoconstriction, leading to a rise in heart rate, cardiac output and blood pressure and possibly causing hyperventilation. This combination decreases cerebral and uterine blood flow, which may affect the contractility of the uterus (McDonald 2006), causing uncoordinated uterine activity (McDonald and Noback 2003) and resulting in a lengthened labour. Hyperventilation tends to alter oxygen balance, which may modify the acid–base status of the blood, causing maternal alkalosis, and may in turn cause fetal hypoxia (Lowe 2002). By supporting the woman, the midwife can enable a level of containment of catecholamines concentration so that uterine activity may be efficient and effective, expediting the labour and shortening the accompanying discomfort of labour pains.

Although fear may be considered negative, anxiety related to pain may have a protective role by facilitating appropriate behaviours (Carleton and Asmundson 2009) that are necessary for the woman to prepare for the impending birth. However, individuals with high levels of anxiety sensitivity tend to become fearful of the symptoms of pain and doubtful of their ability to cope, demonstrating states of hypervigilance (Thompson et al 2008; Whitburn et al 2014). This exhibition of fear may relate to the pain that is currently present but also to perceptions and concerns of what *could* occur (Carleton and Asmundson 2009). Most individuals would normally choose to avoid what they consider to be potentially pain-inducing situations as a result of their fears (Hirsh et al 2008), but labour cannot be avoided. As such, this fearful state may result in what Hirsh et al (2008) described as pain catastrophizing.

Although a minor level of catastrophic thinking and hypervigilance may be necessary for the woman to cope with the labour pain and birth, over a prolonged period it can increase the degree of suffering and hamper her ability to take control of her thoughts, preventing her from focusing her mind on the beneficial aspects of her pain (Whitburn et al 2014). This may then lead to a predisposition to underestimate her personal coping ability while exaggerating the threat of the anticipated pain (Hirsh et al 2008; Veringa et al 2011). Catastrophizing has been shown to be positively associated with avoidance behaviour (Flink et al 2009), even to the point of ignoring or rejecting information and guidance that are provided on how to deal with fear and pain (Klomp et al 2014).

Fundamentally, what the midwife should understand is that perceptions of pain will vary among women even when the stimuli are similar; they will react to their labour pains in different ways (Morley 2008). Maternity caregivers will therefore need to be cognizant of the woman's expectations when dealing with her individualized pain and provide clear and precise communication that is repeated and explained where necessary, making every effort to provide consistent information and guidance (Klomp et al 2014).

CULTURAL ASPECT OF PAIN

The definition, understanding and manifestation of pain will be influenced by the cultural experiences of the woman, her family and her caregivers. Culture therefore affects attitudes toward pain in childbirth as a result of coping strategies and mechanisms (Callister et al 2003; Klomp et al 2012). Although some individuals may accept intervention when in pain, others may demonstrate a more stoic approach and avoid help because of their socialization towards behaviour in such circumstances (Peacock and Patel 2008; Gibson 2014).

Over the years, qualitative studies have shown that women from different backgrounds perceive and deal with the pain associated with childbirth in different ways. In their critical review of such research, Van De Gucht and Lewis (2015) highlighted that women's perception of how to deal with the pain in labour was significantly influenced by sociocultural ideals, supporting studies such as that undertaken by Johnson et al (2004), who showed that the Dutch women had a fundamental belief that birth was a normal phenomenon accompanied by pain, which, although difficult, should not be feared, but used effectively. Finnström and Söderhamn (2006) observed that for the Somalian women in their study, it was not acceptable to cry or wail when in pain; instead they thought that it was necessary to stay in control, tolerate the pain and involve a friend or a family member to help them cope with the event. In Jordan, Abushaikha and Sheil (2006) observed that the women were expected to labour silently, ensuring they were not overheard while utilizing spiritual methods to cope. They were required to demonstrate

patience and endurance towards the pain as a show of strong faith. A more recent finding from New Zealand (Doering et al 2014) highlighted that Japanese women demonstrated a sense of resistance to pharmacological pain relief because of the spiritual meaning of birth.

Midwives' own cultural experiences and meaning of pain will also affect their interpretation and attention to women in labour, as a study by Cheung (2002) that compared Chinese women with Scottish women indicated. One midwifery manager commented that a loud vocalization as a coping strategy was occasionally misconstrued by health workers, who were more likely to interpret this as a sign of inability to cope and offer the women analgesia or anaesthetics, whereas those who remained quiet were often unnoticed (Cheung 2002). This misconception and oversight represents a need for cultural sensitivity and competence when caring for women in childbirth (Brathwaite and Williams 2004). Awareness of the cultural meanings of childbirth pain and how different women cope and are likely to behave will assist in the provision of culturally competent care (Callister et al 2003). Nonetheless, it should not be ignored that cultural assumptions made by midwives may lead to stereotyping and prevent individualized and appropriate care.

Reflective activity 38.2 ><

How would you establish what a woman's cultural response to pain is? What would you do to prevent yourself from making an assumption about this?

Midwives must also develop their ability to interpret and understand the verbal communication of pain, and body language, to address the needs of individuals from culturally diverse groups (Finnström and Söderhamn 2006). In Sweden, Bergh et al (2013) showed that midwifery students attributed different quantitative meanings to the pain descriptors used by women, indicating how imperative it is that midwives become familiar with the value of different words that women use to describe their pain because their interpretation may affect the assessment of the woman's discomfort.

The birthing environment

Beliefs and trends on birthing environment have changed significantly over the last 50 years. Jones et al (2012) and Crafter (2000) both highlighted that the physical and cultural setting of the place of birth have a significant impact on the woman's experience of pain in labour and birth. In the 1970s, the Peel Report (DHSS 1970) recommended hospitalization for all births. With the provision of pharmacological methods to relieve pain for all women, the opportunity may have contributed to an increase in the medicalization of labour in women of low risk over the years. Admission to the hospital milieu means women that are expected to adapt to the unfamiliar environment as they endeavour to cope with their labour. Midwives need to be aware that in such unfamiliar surroundings, women may have raised levels of anxiety and subsequently be prevented from identifying and adopting their own coping mechanisms during labour. These hospital settings and routines can sometimes have a negative impact on the normal birthing process for women (Olsen and Calusen 2012; Zielinski et al 2015), with many women accepting this as a normal part of the experience of birth.

A Cochrane systematic review (Hodnett et al 2012) highlighted that the levels of satisfaction were increased in women in an alternative setting such as a midwifery-led unit during the experience of labour and birth without analgesia. Another more recent review of the literature noted that women who birthed in their own homes had a sense of control of their environment, which they described as empowering (Zielinski et al 2015). The National Collaborating Centre for Women's and Children's Health (NCC-WCH) recommended that low-risk multiparous and nulliparous women who choose to give birth at home as a way of reducing interventions and managing their labour pain should be supported to do so (NCC-WCH 2014). However, if the woman chooses to or needs to birth away from her home, such as in a midwifery-led unit, the environment within the rooms should be set to promote a relaxed atmosphere that encourages belief in her ability to cope and manage her labour with her midwife. Therefore, furnishings, music and artwork can be used to promote a relaxing, home-like environment.

Antenatal education and preparation for birth

Dick-Read (1944) and Lamaze (1958) both proposed that labour was not inherently painful. Dick-Read (1944), who appears to be the original authority in this area, endorsed the view that pain was influenced by women's socioculturally conditioned fear and expectation of birth. They both suggested that labour pains could be controlled by psychoprophylactic techniques, such as muscle relaxation and breathing exercises. Dick-Read (1944) also postulated that providing information and encouraging women to communicate are useful aspects in preparing women for pain in childbirth. Herein lies the potential value of antenatal education and preparation in reducing the fear and anxiety associated with childbirth.

The previously described concepts and techniques have been incorporated into antenatal classes, used as a basis of empowering the woman to identify and develop confidence in her own body's resources to enhance the childbirth experience (Gagnon and Sandall 2007; Leap

et al 2010). As a result, this increases women's ability to cope while lowering the levels of the affective aspect of pain and encourages less use of pharmacological pain relief in labour (Spiby et al 2003).

However, the literature regarding the effectiveness of childbirth education highlights the difficulties in evaluating its full value because of inconsistencies in the content or method of delivery (Gagnon and Sandall 2007; Ferguson et al 2013). Although there should be some core content, on balance, antenatal classes need to support women to make well-informed choices to manage their pain and fear in labour. Antenatal course leaders should explore women's subjectivity around pain in labour (Schott 2003) and help them to explore how their own values, expectations and preferences can influence their choices (Lally et al 2014). Women should also be presented with a realistic but positive approach to the pain they will experience (Schott 2003). Brief but accurate information on the relevant physiology will assist in their understanding of normality, which underpins the sensations experienced and how they change over the duration of labour.

During antenatal classes women can be helped to explore and articulate the range of coping strategies they have used in previous experiences of pain; those positive methods can then be enhanced to replace negative strategies (Escott et al 2009). Nolan (2000) and Lally et al (2014) implied that women find it difficult to make choices about the management of their pain in labour because they are ignorant of the body's resources for coping with pain and find it difficult to imagine what the pain would be like. However, if they are encouraged during the classes to recall and develop their own preexisting methods of managing and tolerating pain, it may be easier for them to develop a greater sense of self-efficacy to deal with their pains once labour commences (Escott et al 2009).

Continuous support in labour

Each woman needs to feel supported during labour. This support may be informational, practical or emotional (Hodnett et al 2013), all being essential elements in the art of midwifery (Berg and Terstad 2006). Support in labour affects the sympathetic element of the autonomic nervous system, by breaking the *fear–tension–pain cycle* observed by Dick-Read (Mander 2000) and giving women a sense of security and reassurance in their ability to cope with the pain (Van der Gucht and Lewis 2015). A correlation study in the United States by Abushaikha and Sheil (2006) examined the relationship between the feeling of stress and continuous professional support in labour, concluding that women who felt supported for the duration of their labour reported less stress compared with those who felt they had received less support.

From an international perspective, the main sources of support for women in labour depends on the society and culture to which they belong and varies in the different countries. In Western societies it tends to be the midwife and the woman's partner who provide help at this emotional time. However, in some countries, support may also come from untrained laywomen, female relatives, nurses, monitrices (midwives who are self-employed birth attendants) and doulas (Rosen 2004).

Doulas are experienced individuals who provide non-medical support for women in childbirth to enable them to achieve a rewarding birth experience (Koumouitzes-Dovia and Carr 2006). Now professionally trained in some cases, they may also be referred to as a labour/birth companion or a labour support specialist/assistant (Hodnett et al 2013; Steel et al 2015). They work alongside the midwife during the labour to help the woman and her partner through the discomforts and rewards of birthing her baby.

McGrath and Kennell (2008), in a randomized controlled trial, reported that women who were supported by a doula required less analgesia compared with those in the control group. Doulas provide care that is continuous and address psychological factors resulting from the physical processes of childbirth (Paterno et al 2012). In the UK, doulas may be used as supportive friends for vulnerable women who may not have access to such assistance from their families.

Koumouitzes-Dovia and Carr (2006) examined women's perceptions of their doulas and found that the women felt that doulas were a source of reassurance and encouragement who also provided support for their husbands. A doula can act as a mediator between the partner and the midwife to provide stability that makes the woman calm and secure (Berg and Terstad 2006). In a review of 22 trials involving 15,288 women, Hodnett et al (2013) demonstrated that women who had continuous support in the intrapartum period were more likely to have shorter labours and less likely to have analgesia. The benefit of this support was greater when the provider was not a member of the hospital staff. Thus, the companionship that can be provided by lay individuals and certified doulas can present women with an opportunity to use non-pharmacological/non-medical resources to enable them to cope with the pain in labour.

COMPLEMENTARY AND ALTERNATIVE THERAPIES

Complementary and alternative therapies (see Ch. 18) involve practices that are not always categorized as conventional medicine (Smith et al 2006). The NCC-WCH (2014) recommended that women who want to use acupuncture, acupressure, hypnosis, breathing and relaxation techniques to cope with pain should not be discouraged from engaging in these practices; however, it does not encourage standard provision of such services. There is some evidence that they may work to relieve perception of pain and improve satisfaction with the whole experience of childbirth (Jones et al 2012). However, although there is support for these and other forms of coping strategies such as music and massage (McNabb et al 2006), more research is required in this area (Smith et al 2006; NCC-WCH 2014).

There is increasing interest in the use of hypnosis, biofeedback, sterile water for injections and aromatherapy as alternative methods women can utilize to cope with pain in labour. In the Cochrane Collaborations systematic review on pain management in labour (Jones et al 2012), it was suggested that most of these non-pharmacological methods are safe for both mother and baby, but there is insufficient high-quality evidence to support their efficacy in relieving pain in childbirth. One example is the use of injected water papules, which has been shown in a few systematic reviews to help with back pain in labour (Huntley et al 2004; Hutton et al 2009); however, because of variation in research methods and results, it is not currently recommended for use in midwifery practice (NCC-WCH 2014; NICE 2014).

Hydrotherapy

It is well known that a warm bath or shower is useful for relaxation and is a simple and cost-effective means of reducing muscular aches and pains. Hydrotherapy continues to be used worldwide to provide comfort for women in labour, and it includes the use of the shower, bath and birthing pool. According to the Royal College of Midwives (RCM), the practice encourages a woman-centred approach to care, in line with the aim to normalize birth and promote maternal choices in labour (Harding et al 2012). Women who choose to use water as a pain-relieving strategy in labour and who qualify to do so should be given the opportunity to utilize this method (NCC-WCH 2014). There is evidence to suggest that immersion in warm water during the first stage of labour decreases reports of pain and the use of analgesia, without any adverse effects on the duration of labour or neonatal outcome (Cluett and Burns 2012; Othman et al 2012). Therapeutic showering in labour is also a form of hydrotherapy (Stark et al 2011) in which women can feel a sense of control, deciding how and when they use this method to relieve their pain. Although research and guidelines on therapeutic showering in labour are lacking, this method of pain relief is also being considered a preference for women during childbirth (Madden et al 2013; Vargens et al 2013).

The mechanism that underpins hydrotherapy in labour is unclear, but it is thought that warm water decreases the perception of pain by stimulating the larger Aδ nerve fibres blocking impulses from the smaller C fibres (Teschendorf and Evans 2000) in accordance with the gate-control theory of pain modulation. In addition to inducing muscle relaxation and reducing anxiety, immersion or showering in warm water may also decrease the release of catecholamines and encourage the release of endorphins (Labor and Maguire 2008). Labouring in birthing pools also enables free movement and change of positions to facilitate progress (Cluett and Burns 2012), making it possible for the woman to be an active participant in her experience of birth (da Silva et al 2009). Women in a study by Maude and Foureur (2007) who chose to use hydrotherapy to cope reported that they felt protected, supported and comforted while using the water.

It has been postulated that the environment in which the pool/bath is situated and the interaction with the caregivers also have a significant part to play on the effectiveness of this method (Cluett and Burns 2012). The ambience created by the environment of the water pool is important; for example, women may feel less relaxed labouring in a bath in a hospital setting compared with one that is situated in a specially designed birthing unit or located in the woman's own home.

Maternal safety is paramount while the woman uses a birthing pool, particularly if she requires additional analgesia, such as Entonox, because she may relax and may become drowsy while in the water. The midwife needs to be vigilant and must not leave the woman unattended in a birthing pool. The temperature of the woman and the water need to be monitored hourly; the water temperature

should be maintained below 37.5°C (NCC-WCH 2014). These measures will ensure that the woman is kept safe and does not become hyperthermic, which may have adverse effects on the fetus. Whether at home, at the birthing centre or in the hospital, the bath or pool needs to be clean and should be maintained in accordance with hospital and manufacturer guidelines to maintain hygiene (NCC-WCH 2014).

Transcutaneous electrical nerve stimulation

TENS is the application of pulsed electrical current through surface electrodes placed on the skin, parallel to each other and on each side of the spine, overlying the areas on the skin (dermatomes), which are supplied by the nerves responsible for labour pain. These areas are thoracic 10 (T10) to lumbar 1 (L1) and spinal 2 to spinal 4 (S2–S4) (El-Wahab and Robinson 2014) (see Fig. 38.3).

TENS produces small electrical sensations, which can be described as tingling and prickling. The effect of the sensation is thought to assist in the interruption of pain impulses at the spinal level. The way it works can be partially explained by Melzack and Wall's (1965) gate-control theory of pain. The large and faster Aβ fibres are stimulated by the electrical pulses, transferring the message from the stimulation of nerve endings in skin more quickly than that of pain impulses (Johnson 2014), interrupting the nociceptic messages travelling along the smaller Aδ and C nociceptor fibres from the uterus, vagina and the perineum. In addition, Aδ fibres are stimulated at spinal and

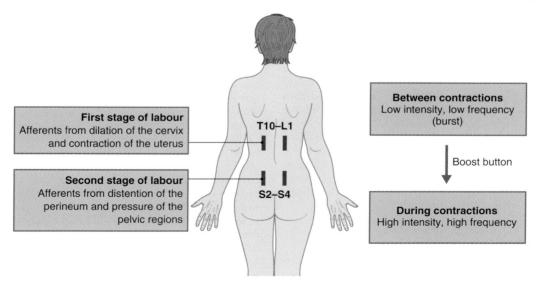

Figure 38.3 TENS electrode positioning for use during labour. (Johnson MI: Transcutaneous electrical nerve stimulation (TENS): research to support clinical practice. Oxford, 2014, Oxford University Press, by permission of the publisher, Oxford University Press.)

supraspinal levels, causing a release of endogenous opiates such as endorphins that bind to opioid receptors in the brain to produce further analgesic effect (van der Spank et al 2000; El-Wahab and Robinson 2014).

However, NCC-WCH (2014) has recommended that TENS should not be used in established labour. This is in light of reviews by Dowswell et al (2011) and Bedwell et al (2011), who found that there was limited evidence that it was useful to reduce pain in established labour. This could be partially explained by the fact that it takes about 40 minutes for the maximum endorphin level to be established (Rodriguez 2005). If women choose TENS to help them cope in labour, for it to be maximally effective, they should be advised to apply it in the early phases of labour to enable the endorphins to build up naturally as their labour progresses (Price 2000).

The advantages of TENS include the fact that it is a non-invasive form of pain relief and may be used with no systematic effects on the woman or the fetus. Because it is self-regulated, it can give the woman a feeling of control and responsibility for managing her pain relief (de Ferrer 2006; Bedwell et al 2011). When correctly positioned, the electrodes supply a residual voltage, which can be boosted by the woman as the contraction commences and maintained for the duration of the pain. This experience can provide the woman with autonomy and help her achieve greater emotional satisfaction from her experience of childbirth. Although more robust studies are required on this form of pain relief, in light of the absence of adverse side effects, it seems logical to support its use in those women who choose it for their labours (Bedwell et al 2011).

PHARMACOLOGICAL PAIN RELIEF

Midwives need to be able to give advice and explain the side effects of pharmacological pain relief. This means midwives must keep up to date with current medications and their side effects, following unit policies at all times (Nursing and Midwifery Council (NMC) 2010). An understanding of pharmacokinetics, including the changing drug absorption, metabolism, distribution and excretion in both the woman and that of her fetus/baby, is important in providing information and advice to the woman regarding choices of pain relief (see Ch. 10 and chapter website resources).

Nitrous oxide (Entonox)

Nitrous oxide, known as 'laughing gas', has been widely used since the 1930s in the UK to alleviate women's experience of pain in childbirth. It has no distinctive taste or smell and is used during labour in a mixture of 50% nitrous oxide and 50% oxygen, mainly under the trade

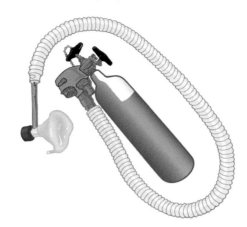

Figure 38.4 Portable Entonox apparatus.

name Entonox, which is supplied by the British Oxygen Company (BOC) as small portable cylinders (Fig. 38.4) or piped directly to the birthing suite.

Entonox is self-administered via a mouthpiece or face mask through a one-way demand valve. Inhalation causes the valve to open, and it closes when the woman stops. This ensures that there is not a continuous supply of gases when it is not intended, which can lead to unconsciousness. The effects of Entonox are quite rapid, commencing 20 seconds after breathing in, with a maximum effect at 60 seconds. To obtain effective relief from pain at the height of the contraction, inhalation should commence immediately as the contraction begins (Rosen 2002), with breathing at the normal rate. Taking into consideration the manufacturer's guidelines, the midwife will need to ensure that the woman is given clear instructions on how to use the apparatus, preferably in the antenatal period.

The way that it works is unclear, but it has been hypothesized that Entonox stimulates the release of an endogenous opioid in the brain that modulates pain stimuli through the descending spinal cord nerve pathways (Maze and Fujinaga 2000; Rosen 2002; Klomp et al 2012; Collins 2015). Although some women who have used it found it of limited benefit in relieving their pain, they often report that they were less concerned about the discomfort of their contractions (Bishop 2007). This is because it has an analgesic and anxiolytic effect on the woman (Collins 2015).

Some of the advantages include its rapid onset and reversal of its effect when discontinued (Rosen 2002; Bishop 2007). Although it may not totally relieve pain for some women, it may give them a sense of control over the management of their labour pain. The anxiolytic effect is advantageous because it lessens the anxiety and fear in labour that some women may have. For example, it may be useful for young mothers, women with histories of traumatic births and women who are concerned with birthing in unfamiliar surroundings (Collins 2015).

Rosen's (2002) systematic review of randomized controlled trials regarding the efficacy and safety of Entonox suggested that it is generally safe for both mother and fetus. However, some women may be uncomfortable with the feeling of euphoria or dysphoria that accompanies its use (Bishop 2007). Women should also be warned about this and other common side effects, such as dry mouth or even vomiting (NCC-WCH 2014), so that they can make an informed decision about its use. It seems that, very rarely, the gas may cause unconsciousness if the woman is hypoxic or if continuously inhaled, for example, when someone is assisting in holding the apparatus. Consequently, the woman must be able to hold the breathing apparatus herself while using this method. Respiratory depression may occur in the mother when it is combined with opioids (Yeo et al 2007), so where an opioid has been administered, the midwife must also include careful respiratory observation for any signs of changes in breathing patterns or hypoxia.

When Entonox is used by the woman there is complete absorption through the placenta (Yeo et al 2007). Thus, there is some equilibrium between the maternal and the fetal blood levels of the gases. At the same time, it is rapidly cleared from the fetal system when the mother stops inhaling, with little effect on Apgar scores, neurological and adaptive capacity scores or acid–base balance (Reynolds 2010).

Midwives should be cognizant that prolonged use of Entonox for more than 24 hours can cause inactivation of vitamin B_{12} (BOC 2015). Therefore, before administering this form of pain relief, the woman should have been assessed antenatally for vitamin B_{12} deficiency or impaired oxygen intake (Collins 2015).

If cylinders of Entonox are being used, storage should also be considered because the two gases separate at cold temperatures, with oxygen rising and nitrous oxide settling at the bottom. According to the BOC, to ensure that the gas is suitable for use, the cylinders should be maintained at a temperature above $10\,^{\circ}C$ for at least 24 hours before it being used (BOC 2011). Without warming to the correct temperature, the woman will get little analgesia at the start, and risk inhaling a concentrated hypoxic mixture of nitrous oxide (Howie and Robinson 2013). It is important, therefore, to follow the manufacturer's essential safety information to enable safe administration of gases to the woman. It is particularly significant for midwives who attend home births and keep cylinders in their cars for transportation to and from the woman's home.

Parenteral opioids

Opioid analgesia is one of the most widely utilized forms of pharmacological pain relief in labour. This group of medication includes *morphine, diamorphine, pethidine* (*meperidine* in the United States) and *meptazinol, fentanyl* and *remifentanil*. Approximately 95% of obstetric units in the UK use bolus doses of intramuscular pethidine or diamorphine for women in labour (Howie and Robinson 2013). Increasingly, obstetric units are providing women with the option of self-administration via an individually controlled pump to deliver the opioids (Saravanakumar et al 2007), enabling the woman to take a more active part in managing her pain relief.

The use of opioids continues despite limited evidence of their impact on pain in childbirth (NCC-WCH 2014). The mode of action is similar in all opioids; what differs is the variation in effect. There continues to be concerns about the unwanted results on the woman with regard to nausea, vomiting and sedation (El Wahab and Robinson 2014). For example, as a result of the sedative effect of opioids, it is recommended that the woman should not use the bath or birthing pool within 2 hours of administration or if she feels drowsy (NICE 2014), limiting her access to this additional form of pain relief and method of relaxation in labour.

Jones et al (2012) also relate concerns about the consequence opioids may have on the woman's ability to make decisions about her care. Together with undesired effects such as hyperventilation, urine retention and slowing down of gastric emptying, her ability to mobilize during labour may be reduced, thereby lengthening her labour. In the newborn, opioids may also cause respiratory depression and drowsiness that may last for a few days and as a result may negatively affect sucking and breastfeeding (Reynolds 2010; NICE 2014). Current UK national guidelines recommend that an antiemetic is administered with intravenous and intramuscular opioids (NICE 2014).

Naloxone is an opioid antagonist that is available for use in the UK. It blocks the receptors to which the opiate binds, impairing their actions and reversing the depressive effect on respiration. When a newborn demonstrates severe respiratory distress as a result of opiate effect, the drug can be used to reverse this side effect. However, *Naloxone* is not a first-line emergency drug but can be used after restoration of a normal heart rate and colour achieved by positive-pressure ventilation (Moe-Byrne et al 2013). It should not be given routinely because there are no studies to recommend its use in this way (Guinsburg and Wyckoff 2006), and it is contraindicated if the mother is narcotic dependent (Moe-Byrne et al 2013).

Pethidine

Pethidine is a synthetic opioid and has been widely used in midwifery for women in the labour since the 1950s. It is the most used intramuscular opioid in UK consultant-led units (Tuckey et al 2008; Howie and Robinson, 2013), although Wee (2007) suggested that the intramuscular route is not ideal because of variation in absorption rate. The doses range from 50 to 150 mg, with no more than 400 mg in 24 hours. Another method of administration is through a bolus intravenous dose or through a pump that is controlled by the woman; the amount administered is dependent on the woman's weight, degree of pain, stage of labour and the rate of progress.

Pethidine acts in 20 to 40 minutes, with 2 to 3 hours of clinical effect (Howie and Robinson 2013). It works by binding to receptor proteins that diffuse through cell membranes to exert its effect within the central nervous system. It acts on efferent nerve pathways descending from the brain at the dorsal horn, thus playing a role in the 'gating' of pain at the spinal column level (Rang et al 2015). Pethidine is metabolized by the liver to *norpethidine* and *pethidinic acid* and further conjugated with glucuronic acid before excretion in urine (Howie and Robinson 2013).

Notably, one of the main concerns about the use of pethidine is the effect on the fetus. The high lipid solubility of the drug, and its metabolite norpethidine, allows rapid transfer across the placenta, which is route and the dose dependent. There is evidence of the drug being found in cord blood within 2 minutes of intravenous administration and 30 minutes following intramuscular administration (Briggs et al 2012), with the mean cord blood concentration ranging between 75% to 90% of the maternal venous level (Howie and Robinson 2013).

If the birth of the baby follows within 2 to 5 hours of administration, there may well be respiratory depression in the neonate; furthermore, although this is the peak time range for neonatal effect, it may also occur if delivery occurs before 2 hours (Hunt 2002). The half-life of the drugs in the fetus is lengthened because of immature metabolic and excretory pathways, which means that the adverse effects on the fetus may be exhibited up to 72 hours after delivery (El-Wahab and Robinson 2014). Babies affected tend to be less alert, quicker to cry when disturbed and more difficult to settle. It is therefore crucial to monitor the newborn during this time.

Diamorphine

Diamorphine is a synthetic form of morphine that in itself has no analgesic properties until administration, when it undergoes a process of hydrolysis in the plasma and is converted to morphine (Rawal et al 2007; Howie and Robinson 2013). During labour it is usually given intramuscularly or subcutaneously in a dose of 5 to 10 mg, which varies according to the weight of the woman, with an effect that lasts up to 4 hours. Although it is used far less than pethidine, some obstetric-led units do offer women the drug as one of the options for pain relief. Compared with pethidine, diamorphine has been shown to have the same sedative result but less side effects, such as vomiting, and better neonatal Apgar scores at 1 minute and no difference

at 5 minutes (Ullman et al 2010). Pain scores for labour are reduced far more than when pethidine is used (El Wahab and Robinson 2014). Despite these findings, pethidine's popularity within units continues, possibly because of its availability, its relatively low cost and the fact that it has been approved for use by midwives since the 1950s by the midwifery governing body – the Central Midwives Board, whose role has been now taken over by the NMC (Reynolds 2010). In light of current evidence, it may be time for midwives to challenge its continued use in favour of diamorphine and call for the change in practice.

When providing care for a woman requesting opiates, the midwife needs to be aware of the length of time it takes for the particular opioid to become effective and how long the effect lasts after administration. Care can be tailored appropriately and the woman made aware of such factors to assist her decisions about choosing this option for pain relief. The midwife needs to observe the woman for any of the side effects and be able to take the appropriate action.

Epidural anaesthesia

Epidural anaesthesia involves an invasive procedure that requires specialized intervention by an anaesthetist. It incorporates the administration of anaesthetic agents into the epidural space, accessed between the 2nd and 3rd lumbar vertebrae. It is completed using an aseptic technique. Following cleansing of the skin and application of local anaesthetic, a Tuohy needle is carefully inserted into the potential space, which is identified when there is loss of resistance (Hawkins 2010). This is made easier by increasing the flexion of the spine because the tough ligamentum flavum has to be overcome before the insertion of the needle into the 1 to 7 mm thick potential epidural space between the dura mater and arachnoid mater (Figs 38.5 and 38.6).

The Tuohy needle contains a large bore with centimetre marking and a bevelled end to aid insertion and positioning of a fine catheter, which is threaded through once the correct position is achieved. The catheter is left in situ to allow access, initial administration and topping up of the analgesia. Throughout the procedure, the midwife should support the woman and her partner both physically and psychologically. Following induction of the anaesthesia, the analgesia is usually managed by the midwife. However, if the facility is available, it can be controlled by the woman using a pump and monitored by the midwife. The anaesthetic agent is given in bolus doses, and the current recommendation is a low concentration of local anaesthetic and opioid solution such as 0.0625% to 0.1% bupivacaine or equivalent, with 1.0 to 2.0 µg/mL fentanyl (NCC-WCH 2014).

The epidural space is the section of the vertebral canal that is not occupied by the dura and its contents,

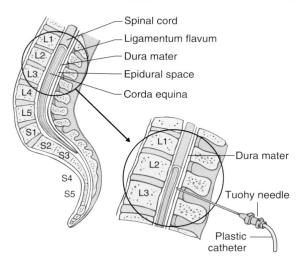

Figure 38.5 Epidural induction: insertion of the Tuohy needle. (This article was published in Yerby M, editor: Pain in childbearing, London, 2000, Baillière Tindall, Copyright Elsevier.)

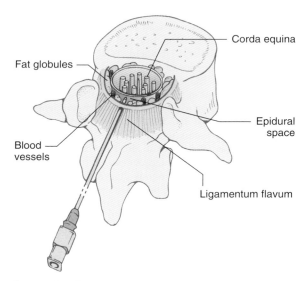

Figure 38.6 Epidural induction: Tuohy needle positioned in the epidural space. (This article was published in Yerby M, editor: Pain in childbearing, London, 2000, Baillière Tindall, Copyright Elsevier.)

extending from the foramen magnum of the skull to the sacral hiatus (Ellis 2009). The epidural space contains blood vessels, nerve roots and fat (Westbrook 2012). The fat enables the injected local anaesthetic to easily diffuse throughout the epidural space (Ellis 2009). At the level of the first lumbar vertebra, the spinal cord becomes a collection of nerve fibres termed the *cauda equina*. The injection of the bupivacaine and fentanyl into the epidural

space bathes the nerves of the cauda equina, blocking the autonomic nerve pathways that supply the uterus, thus changing action potentials in the nerves and preventing pain. The epidural analgesia acts on the sympathetic nervous system by altering adrenaline and noradrenaline levels in the blood (May and Leighton 2007).

The effect on the autonomic nervous system produces vasodilatation in the peripheral circulation, causing the extremities to feel warm, so this is a test that can be used to observe if the epidural is taking effect. Pooling of the circulation in the periphery also occurs and may cause hypotension because there is a loss of peripheral resistance in the lower limbs.

The woman's blood pressure must be monitored regularly after the first dose and following every 'top up'. In the UK, the national guidelines recommend that the blood pressure should be monitored every 5 minutes for 15 minutes, at the point the anaesthetic agent is administered when the epidural is inserted and with subsequent top-ups of 10 mL or more (NICE 2014). Any sign of hypotension is usually managed by increasing intravenous fluids and repositioning the woman. If there is no sign of recovery, the anaesthetist must be informed immediately to administer a bolus dose of a vasopressor, such as ephedrine. The sensory level and motor block should be assessed hourly (El Wahab and Robinson 2014) to monitor for potential complications. The assessment of the height of the sensory block can be conducted through a dermatome assessment using an approved cold spray or ice to compare the sensation on the skin between a nonaffected area, such as the arm, with the level of the height of the block on the abdomen. The desired effect of an epidural in normal labour is a sensory block extending from T10–L1 (Aitkenhead and Moppett 2013). The height of the block is usually kept at T8–T10 and should be assessed on the right and left side for comparison of the effect of the epidural (see Fig. 38.7). The motor block can be assessed with a tool such as the Bromage Scale (Bromage 1978; Lacassie et al 2007; Aitkenhead and Moppett 2013) (see Table 38.1).

It is also important to appreciate that because the epidural causes a lack of feeling, the woman will not be able to move as normal. It is therefore critical that the midwife monitor the woman's pressure areas (elbows, knees, heels and sacrum) and institute a regime of regular movement to change the woman's position, taking care avoid any dragging of the skin on the bedsheets (Bailey 2010; Prior 2002). There have been instances of *decubitus ulcers* (also known as pressure ulcers or bedsores) reported (Hughes 2001; Alfirevic et al 2004), and for a young woman this injury can cause weeks, if not months, of pain and suffering and often requires specialist treatment.

The development of decubitus ulcers following epidural analgesia should be considered unacceptable in good midwifery practice, and it poses a risk of clinical negligence claims.

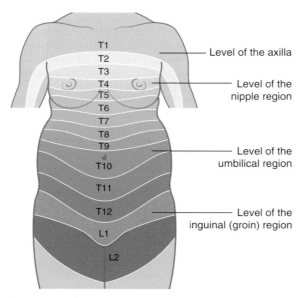

T1
T2 — Level of the axilla
T3
T4 — Level of the
T5   nipple region
T6
T7
T8
T9 — Level of the
T10   umbilical region
T11
T12 — Level of the
L1   inguinal (groin) region
L2

Figure 38.7 Sensory dermatomes on the pregnant woman with key landmarks to help indicate the desired levels of the effect of the epidural.

Table 38.1 Method of scoring the effect of an epidural on motor block

Observation	Degree of block	Score
The woman is able to freely raise her legs, bend her knees and rotate her ankles.	There is no motor block.	0
The woman is only able to bend her knees but can freely rotate her ankles.	There is partial motor block.	1
The woman is not able to bend her knees but can rotate her ankles.	There is almost a complete motor block.	2
The woman is unable to move her legs or rotate her ankles.	There is a complete motor block.	3

Source: Adapted from Bromage 1978: 144

The effect of an epidural on the fetus is indirect as a result of maternal physiological and biochemical changes (Reynolds 2010). For example, with hypotension, the placental bed is unable to compensate for lowered delivery of blood to the uterus, so bradycardia in the fetus may be

an issue (O'Connor 2007). On a whole, the effects of epidurals on the baby are more consistently beneficial compared with systemic analgesia, not only with regard to the Apgar score but also to the fetal acid–base status, and on breastfeeding (Reynolds 2010). It is recommended that there should be continuous fetal monitoring for at least 30 minutes with the induction of the epidural, then following each top-up bolus dose of 10 mL or more of the anaesthetic agent (NCC-WCH 2014).

An epidural is a very effective form of pain relief. The midwife can immediately observe a change in a woman's demeanour following its introduction. However, there are occasions when the epidural injections are unsuccessful, with unwanted consequences of the procedure. The anaesthetist should be informed immediately of such incidences. One such side effect is urine retention. The midwife will need to observe for signs of this happening during labour and in the postnatal period. As pain sensation is lost, normal bladder function may be affected (Ching-Chung et al 2002), but women tend to have fewer problems with micturition when low-dose epidurals are used (Wilson et al 2009). Other side effects include pyrexia and pruritus (NCC-WCH 2014), but the main concern in such instances is that the symptoms may lead to unnecessary investigations when the cause is unclear and independent of any infection (McGrady and Litchfield 2004).

Another consequence of the epidural is that the pelvic floor muscles become relaxed, and this may have an effect on fetal head rotation (Odibo 2007), so the woman may not feel the sensation to push; both of which may lengthen the second stage. If the fetal condition is satisfactory, delayed pushing seems to decrease the need for instrumental deliveries (Roberts et al 2005) and does not appear to increase the number of caesarean sections. As such, NCC-WCH (2014) recommends delaying pushing for 1 hour after diagnosis of the second stage, with delivery of the baby before the completion of 4 hours.

Other undesirable risks the midwife needs to be aware of, but that must be sensitively communicated by the anaesthetist as part of the preadministration counselling, are respiratory arrests and accidental dural puncture.

Respiratory arrest may be caused by the accidental induction of a high nerve block or the injection of bupivacaine into a vein. The first sign will be a tingling tongue with a rapid deterioration; therefore, the midwife needs to be prepared for immediate resuscitation.

Accidental dural puncture occurs in 0.5% to 2% of persons receiving regional anaesthetics, with 70% to 80% of these developing a postural headache. The headaches are caused by a lowering of pressure of circulating cerebrospinal fluid, causing a stretching of brain tissue, in turn causing pain. A dural puncture is treated with an autologous blood patch of 10 to 20 mL of the woman's own blood injected near the site of the epidural to seal the dura. Rest is important following the procedure, which is done to rectify the condition and prevent more spinal fluid leakage from increasing headaches until the dura is healed. Smaller-gauge needles are used for spinal anaesthetic and could prevent a dural tap (Sprigge and Harper 2008)

A Cochrane review (Anim-Somuah et al 2011) concluded that epidurals created more instrumental deliveries, but there was no statistical evidence to suggest that epidurals caused long-term backache or increased the incidence of caesarean section. It is known that ligaments are altered by the hormones of pregnancy, which permits some movement, increasing pelvic size to facilitate birth. Consequently, backache is a common complaint in pregnancy and following birth and may not be specifically caused by the epidural.

As shown, there are benefits and associated risks with this form of analgesia, which must be fully discussed and understood by the woman so that she may make an informed decision about choosing it as an option to manage pain during her birth. The midwife's role is to support her during and after the procedure while maintaining safety for the woman and the fetus throughout the labour.

helps to decrease anxiety, it does not always lessen women's pain. It also must be remembered that many women do not attend antenatal classes, and this might mean that the midwife must provide information during labour. Support has been shown to be valuable, whether by partner, midwife or doula, and is most effective when provided continuously by a known midwife. Women with continuous support seem to require less pain relief, but when a labour becomes long and pain increases, women tend to require systemic pain relief. Research should continue to investigate women's needs and the continued use of systemic analgesia that is safe in labour for both mother and fetus. Midwives are duty bound to continue to develop their skills in supporting women's choices in labour, whether with or without pain relief.

Reflective activity 38.3

Having explored the pharmacological and alternative methods midwives can use to modulate pain, write down other actions the midwife can take to relieve the woman's fear and anxiety that may present during labour. Think about how *you* would describe to the woman the different choices that she has for pain management during labour.

CONCLUSION

Pain is a multifaceted phenomenon of pregnancy, without which women would not know they were in labour. Fear and other psychological factors affect women's perceptions of pain in labour, and although antenatal education

---

Key Points

- An understanding of what pain is and how it may be experienced is influenced by women's expectations, previous experience and the effect of childbirth education on their experiences and the fear–pain–anxiety triangle.

- The midwife must take account of the physiological aspects of pain, its transmission, pain substances and the gate-control theory of pain control.

- The cultural and social aspects of pain will influence the environment and coping mechanisms of women in labour and how support may be provided by families and friends.

- There is a wide range of pain-management strategies, from the use of distractive techniques or TENS to pharmacological methods of pain relief, including Entonox, opioids and epidural analgesia.

- It is critical that midwives ensure that whatever pain management strategy is chosen by the woman, risks of complications or problems are fully explained, and the midwife monitors the maternal and fetal well-being throughout.

References

Abushaikha L, Sheil E: Labor stress and nursing support: how do they relate? *J Int Womens Stud* 7(4):198–208, 2006.

Aitkenhead AR, Moppett I, Thompson J: *Smith and Aitkenhead's textbook of anaesthesia*, London, Elsevier Health Sciences, 2013.

Alfirevic A, Argalious M, Tetzlaff JE: Pressure sore as a complication of labor epidural, *Anesth Analg* 98:1783–1784, 2004.

Anim-Somuah M, Smyth RMD, Jones L: Epidural versus non-epidural or no analgesia in labour, *Cochrane Database Syst Rev* 12:2011.

Atlas LY, Wager TD: How expectations shape pain, *Neurosci Lett* 520(2):140–148, 2012.

Bailey J: How to… prevent pressure sores. Evidence based care and practice, *RCM Midwives J* (website). www.rcm.org.uk/system/files/5.%20Midwives%20Sept%202010.pdf. 2010.

Bedwell C, Dowswell T, Neilson JP, et al: The use of transcutaneous electrical nerve stimulation (TENS) for pain relief in labour: a review of the evidence, *Midwifery* 27(5):e141–e148, 2011.

Bergh IH, Ek K, Mårtensson LB: Midwifery students attribute different quantitative meanings to 'hurt', 'ache' and 'pain': a cross-sectional survey, *Women Birth* 26(2):143–146, 2013.

Berg M, Terstad A: Swedish women's experiences of doula support during childbirth, *Midwifery* 22(4):330–338, 2006.

Bishop JT: Administration of nitrous oxide in labor: expanding the options for women, *J Midwifery Womens Health* 52(3):308–309, 2007.

Brathwaite AC, Williams CC: Childbirth experiences of professional Chinese Canadian women, *J Obstet Gynecol Neonatal Nurs* 33(6):748–755, 2004.

Bridgestock C, Rae CP: Anatomy, physiology and pharmacology of pain, *Anaesth Intensive Care* 14(11):480–483, 2013.

Briggs GG, Freeman RK, Yaffe SJ: *Drugs in pregnancy and lactation: a reference guide to fetal and neonatal risk*, Philadelphia, Lippincott Williams and Wilkins, 2012.

British Oxygen Company (BOC): *Entonox essential safety information* (website). www.boconline.co.uk/internet.lg.lg.gbr/en/images/entonox410_43539.pdf. 2011.

British Oxygen Company (BOC): *Entonox the essential guide* (website). www.bochealthcare.co.uk/internet.lh.lh.gbr/en/images/entonox_essential_guide_hlc401955_Sep10409_64836.pdf. 2015.

Bromage PR: *Epidural analgesia*, Philadelphia, Saunders, 1978.

Buckley SJ: Executive summary of hormonal physiology of childbearing: evidence and implications for women, babies, and maternity care, *J Perinat Educ* 24(3):145–153, 2015.

Callister LC, Khalaf I, Semenic S, et al: The pain of childbirth: perceptions of culturally diverse women, *Pain Manag Nurs* 4(4):145–154, 2003.

Carleton RN, Asmundson GJ: The multidimensionality of fear of pain: construct independence for the Fear of Pain Questionnaire-Short Form and the Pain Anxiety Symptoms Scale-20, *J Pain* 10(1):29–37, 2009.

Cheung NF: The cultural and social meanings of childbearing for Chinese and Scottish women in Scotland, *Midwifery* 18(4):279–295, 2002.

Ching-Chung L, Shuenn-Dhy C, Ling-Hong T, et al: Postpartum urinary retention: assessment of contributing factors and long-term clinical impact, *Aust N Z J Obstet Gynaecol* 42(4):367–370, 2002.

Cluett ER, Burns E: Immersion in water in labour and birth, *Cochrane Database Syst Rev* (2):CD000111, 2012.

Collins M: A case report on the anxiolytic properties of nitrous oxide during labor, *J Obstet Gynecol Neonatal Nurs* 44(1):87–92, 2015.

Crafter H: Psychology of pain in labour. In Yerby M, editor: *Pain in childbearing*, London, Baillière Tindall, 2000.

da Silva FMB, de Oliveira SMJV, Nobre MRC: A randomised controlled trial evaluating the effect of immersion bath on labour pain, *Midwifery* 25(3):286–294, 2009.

de Ferrer G: TENS: non-invasive pain relief for the early stages of labour, *Br J Midwifery* 14(8):480–482, 2006.

Department of Health and Social Security (DHSS): *Domiciliary and maternity bed needs. Report of the Sub-committee of the Standing Midwifery and Maternity Advisory Committee (Peel Report)* 197, London, HMSO, 1970.

Dick-Read G: *Childbirth without fear*, New York, Harper Row, 1944.

Doering K, Patterson J, Griffiths CR: Japanese women's experiences of pharmacological pain relief in New Zealand, *Women Birth* 27(2):121–125, 2014.

Dowswell T, Bedwell C, Lavender T, et al: Transcutaneous electrical nerve stimulation (TENS) for pain management in labour, *Cochrane Database Syst Rev* (2):CD007214, 2011.

Ellis H: The anatomy of the epidural space, *Anaesthesia and Intensive Care Medicine* 10(11):533–535, 2009.

El-Wahab N, Robinson N: Analgesia and anaesthesia in labour, *Obstet Gynaecol Reprod Med* 24(4):97–102, 2014.

Escott D, Slade P, Spiby H: Preparation for pain management during childbirth: the psychological aspects of coping strategy development in antenatal education, *Clin Psychol Rev* 29(7):617–622, 2009.

Ferguson S, Davis D, Browne J: Does antenatal education affect labour and birth? A structured review of the literature, *Women Birth* 26(1):e5–e8, 2013.

Finnström B, Söderhamn O: Conceptions of pain among Somali women, *J Adv Nurs* 54(4):418–442, 2006.

Flink IK, Mroczek MZ, Sullivan MJL, et al: Pain in childbirth and postpartum recovery: the role of catastrophizing, *Eur J Pain* 13(3):312–316, 2009.

Gagnon AJ, Sandall J: Individual or group antenatal education for childbirth or parenthood, or both, *Cochrane Database Syst Rev* (3):CD002869, 2007.

Gibson E: Women's expectations and experiences with labour pain in medical and midwifery models of birth in the United States, *Women Birth* 27(3):185–189, 2014.

Guinsburg R, Wyckoff MH: Naloxone during neonatal resuscitation: acknowledging the unknown, *Clin Perinatol* 33(1):121–132, 2006.

Harding C, Munro J, Jokinen M: *Evidence based guidelines for midwifery-led care in labour: immersion in water for labour and birth*, London, RCM, 2012.

Hawkins JL: Epidural analgesia and anesthesia. In Duke J, editor: *Anesthesia secrets*, Philadelphia, Mosby/Elsevier, pp 458–465, 2010.

Hirsh AT, George SZ, Bialosky JE, et al: Fear of pain, pain catastrophizing, and acute pain perception: relative prediction and timing of assessment, *J Pain* 9(9):806–812, 2008.

Hodnett ED, Downe S, Walsh D: Alternative versus conventional institutional settings for birth, *Cochrane Database Syst Rev* (8):CD000012, 2012.

Hodnett ED, Gates S, Hofmeyr GJ, et al: Continuous support for women during childbirth, *Cochrane Database Syst Rev* (7):CD003766, 2013.

Howie LA, Robinson C: Non-neuraxial analgesia in labour, *Anaesth Intensive Care* 14(7):272–275, 2013.

Hughes C: Obstetric care. Is there risk of pressure damage after epidural anaesthesia? *J Tissue Viability* 11(2):56–58, 2001.

Hunt S: Pethidine: love it or hate it? *MIDIRS Midwifery Digest* 12(3):363–365, 2002.

Huntley AL, Coon JT, Ernst E: Complementary and alternative medicine for labor pain: a systematic review, *Am J Obstet Gynecol* 191(1):36–44, 2004.

Hutton EK, Kasperink M, Rutten M, et al: Sterile water injection for labour pain: a systematic review and meta-analysis of randomised controlled trials, *Br J Obstet Gynaecol* 116:158–166, 2009.

Johnson MI: *Transcutaneous electrical nerve stimulation (TENS): research to support clinical practice*, Oxford, Oxford University Press, 2014.

Johnson TR, Clark Callister L, Freeborn DS, et al: Dutch women's perception of childbirth in the Netherlands, *MCN Am J Matern Child Nurs* 32(3):170–177, 2004.

Jones L, Othman M, Dowswell T, et al: Pain management for women in labour: an overview of systematic reviews, *Cochrane Database Syst Rev* (3):CD009234, 2012.

Kirkham M, Jowitt M: Optimising endorphins, *Pract Midwife* 15(10):33–35, 2012.

Klomp T, Manniën J, de Jonge A, et al: What do midwives need to know about approaches of women towards labour pain management? A qualitative interview study into expectations of management of labour pain for pregnant women receiving midwife-led care in the Netherlands, *Midwifery* 30(4):432–438, 2014.

Klomp T, van Poppel M, Jones L, et al: Inhaled analgesia for pain management in labour, *Cochrane Database Syst Rev* (9):CD009351, 2012.

Koumouitzes-Dovia J, Carr CA: Women's perceptions of their doula support, *J Perinat Educ* 15(4):34–40, 2006.

Labor S, Maguire S: The pain of labour, *Rev Pain* 2(2):15–19, 2008.

Lacassie HJ, Habib AS, Lacassie HP, et al: Motor blocking minimum local anesthetic concentrations of bupivacaine, levobupivacaine, and ropivacaine in labor, *Reg Anesth Pain Med* 32(4):323–329, 2007.

Lally JE, Thomson RG, MacPhail S, et al: Pain relief in labour: a qualitative study to determine how to support women to make decisions about pain relief in labour, *BMC Pregnancy Childbirth* 14(1):6, 2014.

Lamaze F: *Painless childbirth* (LR Celestine Translation), London, Burke, 1958.

Leap N, Sandall J, Buckland S, et al: Journey to confidence: women's experiences of pain in labour and relational continuity of care, *J Midwifery Womens Health* 55(3):234–242, 2010.

Legrain V, Van Damme S, Eccleston C, et al: Neurocognitive model of attention to pain: behavioral and neuroimaging evidence, *Pain* 144(3):230–232, 2009.

Lowe NK: The nature of labor pain, *Am J Obstet Gynecol* 186(5 Suppl Nature):S16–S24, 2002.

Madden KL, Turnbull D, Cyna AM, et al: Pain relief for childbirth: the preferences of pregnant women, midwives and obstetricians, *Women Birth* 26(1):33–40, 2013.

Mander R: Does social support affect pain in labour? *Br J Midwifery* 8(11):667–672, 2000.

Mander R: *Pain in childbearing and its control: key issues for midwives and women*, 2nd edn, Oxford, Wiley and Blackwell, 2011.

Maude RM, Foureur MJ: It's beyond water: stories of women's experience of using water for labour and birth, *Women Birth* 20(1):17–24, 2007.

May A, Leighton R: *Epidurals for childbirth: a guide for all delivery suite staff*, 2nd edn, London, Cambridge University Press, 2007.

Maze M, Fujinaga M: Recent advances in understanding the actions and toxicity of nitrous oxide, *Anaesthesia* 55(4):311–314, 2000.

McCool WF, Smith T, Aberg C: Pain in women's health: a multi-faceted approach toward understanding, *J Midwifery Womens Health* 49(6):473–481, 2004.

McDonald JS: Obstetric pain. In McMahon SB, Koltzenburg M, editors: *Wall and Melzack's textbook of pain*, 5th edn, Edinburgh, Elsevier, 2006.

McDonald JS, Noback CP: Obstetric pain. In Melzack R, Wall PD, editors: *Handbook of pain management*, Edinburgh, Churchill Livingstone, pp 147–161, 2003.

McGann K: The anatomy and physiology of pain. In *Fundamental aspects of pain assessment and management*, Gateshead, Quay Books, 2007.

McGrady E, Litchfield K: Epidural analgesia in labour, *Continuing Education in Anaesthesia, Critical Care and Pain* 4(4):114–117, 2004.

McGrath SK, Kennell JH: A randomized controlled trial of continuous labor support for middle-class couples: effect on cesarean delivery rates, *Birth* 35(2):92–97, 2008.

McNabb MT, Kimber L, Haines A: Does regular massage from late pregnancy to birth decrease maternal pain perception during labour and birth? A feasibility study to investigate a programme of massage, controlled breathing and visualisation, from 36 weeks of pregnancy until birth, *Complement Ther Clin Pract* 12(3):222–231, 2006.

Melzack R, Wall PD: Pain mechanisms: a new theory, *Science* 150:971–979, 1965.

Mendell LM: Constructing and deconstructing the gate theory of pain, *Pain* 155(2):210–216, 2014.

Millan MJ: Descending control of pain, *Prog Neurobiol* 66(6):355–474, 2002.

Moe-Byrne T, Brown JVE, McGuire W: Naloxone for opiate-exposed newborn infants, *Cochrane Database Syst Rev* (2):CD003483, 2013.

Morley S: Psychology of pain, *Br J Anaesth* 101(1):25–31, 2008.

National Collaborating Centre for Women's and Children's Health (NCC-WCH): *Intrapartum care: care of healthy women and their babies during childbirth*, London, NCC-WCH, 2014.

National Institute for Health and Care Excellence (NICE): *Intrapartum care; care of healthy women and their babies during childbirth*, London, NICE, 2014.

Nolan M: The influence of antenatal classes on pain relief in labour, *Pract Midwife* 3(6):26–31, 2000.

Novikova N, Cluver C: Local anaesthetic nerve block for pain management in labour, *Cochrane Database Syst Rev* (4):CD009200, 2012.

Nursing and Midwifery Council (NMC): *Standards for medicine management*, London, NMC, 2010.

O'Connor PJ: Complication of obstetric regional anaesthesia. In Finucane BT, editor: *Complications of regional anaesthesia*, 2nd edn, New York, Springer, pp 242–262, 2007.

Odibo L: Does epidural analgesia affect the second stage of labour? *Br J Midwifery* 15(7):429–435, 2007.

Olsen O, Clausen JA: Planned hospital birth versus planned home birth, *Cochrane Database Syst Rev* (9):CD000352, 2012.

Othman M, Jones L, Neilson JP: Non-opioid drugs for pain management in labour, *Cochrane Database Syst Rev* (7):CD009223, 2012.

Paterno MT, van Zandt SE, Murphy J, et al: Evaluation of a student-nurse doula program: an analysis of doula interventions and their impact on labor analgesia and cesarean birth, *J Midwifery Womens Health* 57:28–34, 2012.

Peacock S, Patel S: Cultural influences on pain, *Rev Pain* 1(2):6–9, [DATR], 2008.

Price S: Pain relief: a practical guide to obstetrics TENS machines, *Br J Midwifery* 8(9):550–552, 2008. 2000.

Prior J: The pressure is on: midwives and decubitus ulcers, *RCM Midwives J* 5(5):196–200, 2002.

Rang HP, Ritter JM, Flower RJ: *Rang and Dale's pharmacology*, 8th edn, London, Elsevier/Churchill Livingstone, 2015.

Rawal N, Tomlinson AJ, Gibson GJ, et al: Umbilical cord plasma concentrations of free morphine following single-dose diamorphine analgesia and their relationship to dose-delivery time interval, Apgar scores and neonatal respiration, *Eur J Obstet Gynecol Reprod Biol* 133(1):30–33, 2007.

Reynolds F: The effects of maternal labour analgesia on the fetus, *Best Pract Res Clin Obstet Gynaecol* 24(3):289–302, 2010.

Roberts CL, Torvaldsen S, Cameron CA, et al: Delayed versus early pushing in women with epidural analgesia, a systematic review and meta-analysis, *MIDIRS Midwifery Digest* 15(2):212–218, 2005.

Rodriguez MA: Transcutaneous electrical nerve stimulation during birth, *Br J Midwifery* 13(8):522–526, 2005.

Rosen M: Nitrous oxide for relief of labor pain: a systematic review, *Am J Obstet Gynecol* 186(5 Suppl Nature):S110–S126, 2002.

Rosen P: Supporting women in labor: analysis of different types of caregivers, *J Midwifery Womens Health* 49(1):24–31, 2004.

Rouhe H, Salmela-Aro K, Halmesmäki E, et al: Fear of childbirth according to parity, gestational age, and obstetric history, *Br J Obstet Gynaecol* 116(1):67–73, 2009.

Sanders R: Functional discomfort and a shift in midwifery paradigm, *Women Birth* 28:e87–e91, 2015.

Saravanakumar K, Garstang JS, Hasan K: Intravenous patient-controlled analgesia for labour: a survey of UK practice, *Int J Obstet Anesth* 16(3):221–225, 2007.

Schott J: Antenatal education changes and future developments, *Br J Midwifery* 11(10):S15–S17, 2003.

Smith CA, Collins CT, Cyna AM, et al: Complementary and alternative therapies for pain management in labour, *Cochrane Database Syst Rev* (4):CD003521, 2006.

Spiby H, Slade P, Escott D, et al: Coping strategies in labor: an investigation

of women's experiences, *Birth* 30(3):189–194, 2003.

Sprigge JS, Harper SJ: Accidental dural puncture and post dural puncture headache in obstetric anaesthesia: presentation and management: a 23-year survey in a district general hospital, *MIDIRS Midwifery Digest* 18(3):391–396, 2008.

Stark MA, Craig J, Miller MG: Designing an intervention: therapeutic showering in labor, *Appl Nurs Res* 24(4):73–77, 2011.

Steeds CE: The anatomy and physiology of pain, *Surgery (Oxford)* 31(2):49–53, 2013.

Steel A, Frawley J, Adams J, et al: Trained or professional doulas in the support and care of pregnant and birthing women: a critical integrative review, *Health Soc Care Community* 23(3):225–241, 2015.

Teschendorf ME, Evans CP: Hydrotherapy during labor: an example of developing a practice policy, *MCN Am J Matern Child Nurs* 25(4):198–203, 2000.

Thompson T, Keogh E, French CC, et al: Anxiety sensitivity and pain: generalisability across noxious stimuli, *Pain* 134(1):187–196, 2008.

Tracy LM, Georgiou-Karistianis N, Gibson SJ, et al: Oxytocin and the modulation of pain experience: implications for chronic pain management, *Neurosci Biobehav Rev* 55:53–67, 2015.

Tuckey JP, Prout RE, Wee MYK: Prescribing intramuscular opioids for labour analgesia in consultant-led maternity units: a survey of UK practice, *Int J Obstet Anesth* 17:3e8, 2008.

Ullman R, Smith LA, Burns E, et al: Parenteral opioids for maternal pain management in labour, *Cochrane Database Syst Rev* (9):CD007396, 2010.

Van der Gucht N, Lewis K: Women's experiences of coping with pain during childbirth: a critical review of qualitative research, *Midwifery* 31(3):349–358, 2015.

Van der Spank JT, Cambier DC, De Paepe HMC, et al: Pain relief in labour by transcutaneous electrical nerve stimulation (TENS), *Arch Gynecol Obstet* 264(3):131–136, 2000.

Vargens OM, Silva AC, Progianti JM: Non-invasive nursing technologies for pain relief during childbirth – the Brazilian nurse midwives' view, *Midwifery* 29(11):e99–e106, 2013.

Veringa I, Buitendijk S, de Miranda E, et al: Pain cognitions as predictors of the request for pain relief during the first stage of labor: a prospective study, *J Psychosom Obstet Gynecol* 32(3):119–125, 2011.

Wee M: Analgesia in labour: inhalational and parenteral, *Anaesth Intensive Care* 8(7):276–278, 2007.

Westbrook JL: Anatomy of the epidural space, *Anaesth Intensive Care* 13(11):551–554, 2012.

Whitburn LY, Jones LE, Davey MA, et al: Women' s experiences of labour pain and the role of the mind: an exploratory study, *Midwifery* 30(9):1029–1035, 2014.

Wilson MJA, MacArthur C, Shennan A: Urinary catheterization in labour with high-dose vs mobile analgesia: a randomized controlled trial, *Br J Anaesth* 102(1):97–103, 2009.

Wong C: Current management of labour pain. In Chin ML, Fillingim RB, Ness TJ, editors: *Pain in women*, New York, Oxford University Press, 2013.

Yeo ST, Holdcroft A, Yentis SM, et al: Analgesia with sevoflurane during labour: II. Sevoflurane compared with Entonox for labour analgesia, *Br J Anaesth* 98(1):110–115, 2007.

Zielinski R, Ackerson K, Low LK: Planned home birth: benefits, risks, and opportunities, *Int J Womens Health* 7:361–377, 2015.

Resources and additional reading

Arendt KW, Tessmer-Tuck JA: Nonpharmacologic labor analgesia, *Clin Perinatol* 40(3):351–371, 2013.

Craig KD, Versloot J, Goubert L, et al: Perceiving pain in others: automatic and controlled mechanisms, *J Pain* 11(2):101–108, 2010.

Gibson E: Women's expectations and experiences with labour pain in medical and midwifery models of birth in the United States, *Women Birth* 27(3):185–189, 2014.

Lindholm A, Hildingsson I: Women's preferences and received pain relief in childbirth – a prospective longitudinal study in a northern region of Sweden, *Sex Reprod Healthc* 6(2):74–81, 2015.

Petersen A, Penz SM, Gross MM: Women's perception of the onset of labour and epidural analgesia: a prospective study, *Midwifery* 29(4):284–293, 2013.

Steel A, Adams J, Frawley J, et al: The characteristics of women who birth at home, in a birth centre or in a hospital labour ward: a study of a nationally-representative sample of 1835 pregnant women, *Sex Reprod Healthc* 6(3):132–137, 2015.

Active Birth Centre: http://activebirth centre.com

This is the official UK website for the Active Birth Centre born from the Active Birth movement founded by Janet Balaskas in the 1980s. The website provides links to the services offered by the centre, such as courses for healthcare professionals, preparation for childbirth classes for women and their partners and a range of complementary services related to childbirth.

Lamaze International: www.lamazeinternational.org

Lamaze is a well-known international organization situated in the United States. The website provides information on useful resources and training with regard to conducting classes on preparation for childbirth.

Expectancy: www.expectancy.co.uk

This UK-based organization provides training for midwives in complementary therapies. The website provides useful information on various therapies for labour, where to find a UK trained professional and guidance on a range of resources for midwives.

The Journal of Pain: www.jpain.org

This website links to the journal and enables access (based on subscription) to up to date information on all aspects of issues related to pain in general, including childbirth, with emphasis on clinical and basic research, patient care, education and health policy.

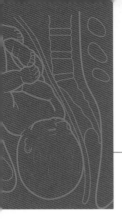

Chapter 39

Care in the third stage of labour

Tina Harris

Learning Outcomes ?

After reading this chapter, you will be able to:
- describe the physiology of the third stage of labour
- differentiate between expectant and active management
- identify variations in management of the third stage of labour and their potential benefits and limitations
- explore the debate between expectant and active management and the implications for midwifery practice
- identify how to examine the term placenta and membranes

INTRODUCTION

The period from the birth of the baby to the expulsion of the placenta and membranes is known as the third stage of labour (Begley et al 2015). It is a time of great importance, when mother and child meet face to face for the first time and when the actions of those present can have a long-term effect on developing family relationships and successful breastfeeding. It is also a time when the placenta and membranes will separate from the uterine wall, descend into the lower uterine segment and be expelled. The skill and expertise of the midwife is needed to support this special time between mother, baby and family while monitoring successful completion of the childbirth process.

Traditionally, this period of childbirth has been regarded as 'hazardous' because of the risk of excessive bleeding. Haemorrhage is a major cause of maternal death in the world (World Health Organisation (WHO) 2012 and 2014); however, within the UK, a very small number of women die as a result of excessive bleeding (Knight et al

2014). This low rate of haemorrhage has been attributed to active management during the third stage of labour. Active management includes the administration of an oxytocic drug, clamping and cutting of the cord, and the speedy delivery of the placenta, usually by controlled cord traction (Begley et al 2015).

Despite a lack of high-quality research evidence (Begley et al 2015), active management of the third stage of labour continues to be recommended in guidelines for all women (International Confederation of Midwives-International Federation of Gynecology and Obstetrics (ICM-FIGO) 2006, National Institute for Health and Care Excellence (NICE) 2014; WHO 2012). However, active management is not without risk. While it is suggested that giving a uterotonic reduces bleeding and the risk of severe haemorrhage, the benefit of early cord clamping and controlled cord traction in terms of blood loss is less clear (Begley et al 2015). A more targeted approach for active management has therefore been suggested, rather than its indiscriminate use for all women (Harris 2001; Soltani 2008), with further investigation of the risk and benefits of the individual components of active management.

An alternative to active management is *expectant management*, sometimes called 'physiological' management. With this approach there is no intervention in the normal physiological processes, with the woman birthing the placenta and membranes herself; the midwife's role being one of 'watchful waiting'.

The role of the midwife during the third stage of labour is:

- to offer women a choice of care relevant to their individual needs
- to support and monitor the normal physiological, sociological and psychological processes at work
- to detect those women who deviate from the norm and offer appropriate care, which may include active management of the third stage

In achieving this, midwives need to have an understanding of the physiology of the third stage, be aware of the latest research evidence and be able to develop partnerships with women to achieve successful delivery of the placenta and membranes with the appropriate, rather than indiscriminate, use of intervention.

It is suggested that often women are not given information about the third stage and do not choose how it will be managed (Harris 2005; Selfe and Walsh 2015). Some midwives struggle in offering women this choice for a variety of reasons.

- NICE guidance recommends prophylactic active management for all women (NICE 2014).
- Active management remains the most common form of management of the third stage of labour for women giving birth in the UK (Farrar et al 2010).
- Some midwives may have either little or no experience in managing the third stage of labour expectantly and lack confidence in this form of care (Harris 2005; Godfrey 2010).

If women are to have a real choice, then consideration needs to be given to educating and supporting midwives in clinical practice and in developing a reflective analytical approach to discussions between midwives and women about the third stage. The discussion of third stage management should ideally take place during the antenatal period and include the benefits and limitations of both active and expectant management. The midwife needs to pay careful attention to offering women clear information, which should be as value-free as possible, while being responsive to the woman's individual circumstances. After the discussion, the woman's choice should be recorded clearly in her notes.

Reflective activity 39.1

Read the paper by Judith Mercer on rethinking placental transfusion and cord-clamping issues (2012). Reflect upon the evidence in the paper and consider how you can incorporate delayed cord clamping into your everyday practice. What are the challenges to implementing a change in cord-clamping practice among midwives and how might these be managed?

Reflect on how the paper may influence your own practice.

Reflective activity 39.2

Take a few minutes to reflect upon your experience of discussing third stage management with a woman. Consider what factors influenced the approach you adopted, the content of the discussion and the woman's decision. How may your personal feelings influence a woman's choice of management during the third stage?

PHYSIOLOGY OF THE THIRD STAGE

The third stage of labour is not really a stage at all. It is an extension of what has happened before (that is, the process of giving birth) and what will happen afterwards (the control of bleeding and the return of the uterus to its non-pregnant state). During labour, the uterine muscles contract and retract under the influence of naturally produced oxytocin. These muscles continue to contract and retract during the third stage to expel the placenta and membranes. The control of bleeding is brought about by the same physiological processes.

Separation of the placenta usually begins with the contraction that delivers the baby's trunk and is completed with the next one or two contractions. As the body of the baby is delivered, there is a marked reduction in the size of the uterus. The myometrium in the upper uterine segment increases in thickness as the lower uterine segment musculature thins, facilitating detachment and expulsion of the placenta. An uncoordinated approach between the two segments has been associated with a longer third stage and an increased risk of bleeding (Patwardhan et al 2015).

Initially, placental separation was thought to be brought about by the bursting of decidual sinuses under pressure and the subsequent forming of a retroplacental blood clot, which tore the septa of the spongiosa layer of the decidua basalis, detaching the placenta from the uterine wall (Brandt 1933). However, ultrasound studies suggest separation is caused by the active placental site uterine wall thickening and reducing in size, causing the placenta to 'shear off'. Krapp et al (2000 and 2003) describe three phases to the third stage of labour (see Fig. 39.1). These three phases have now been widely accepted as describing the process of placental detachment and expulsion.

- *Latent phase:* period of time from delivery of the infant until the beginning of placental separation. During this phase, the placenta-free uterine wall thickens under the influence of intermittent contraction and retraction of muscle fibres, with minimal thickening of the uterine wall over the placenta (101 ± 87 seconds).
- *Detachment phase:* period of placental separation and detachment from the uterine wall, brought about by gradual thickening of the uterine wall over the site of placental attachment. The myometrium adjacent to the lower edge of the placenta contracts, thickens and reduces its surface area overall, which leads to a shearing off of the placenta in that area. This wave of placental wall thickening and placental separation continues upwards and outwards until the whole placenta is detached (56 ± 45 seconds). Separation of the placenta from the uterine wall is normally achieved within 3 minutes.

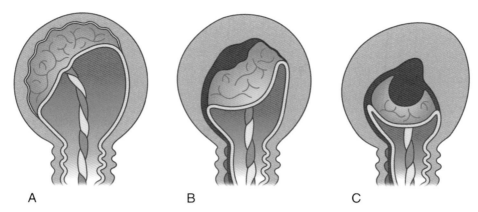

Figure 39.1 Phases in the third stage of labour. **A,** *Latent phase*: characterized by a thick placenta-free wall and thin placental site wall. **B,** *Detachment phase*: characterized by a gradual thickening of the uterine wall over the site of placental attachment. This process can be monophasic (a constant shearing-off movement) or multiphasic (which is characterized by pauses between phases of active detachment). **C,** *Expulsion phase*: the uterine wall is uniformly thickened and drives the placenta into the lower segment for expulsion.

- *Expulsion phase:* period from complete separation of the placenta to vaginal expulsion. The upper uterine segment contracts strongly, forcing the placenta to fold in on itself and descend into the lower segment and from there to the vagina. Gravity, and sometimes maternal effort brought about by stimulation of the pelvic floor, leads to expulsion of the placenta and membranes (77 ± 63 seconds).

The mean length of the third stage is calculated to be approximately 6 minutes (365 ± 270 seconds) (see Fig. 39.2). Herman et al (2002) and, more recently, Altay et al (2007) have identified that with a placenta attached at the fundus, detachment is normally bipolar and is linked to a shorter third stage duration. An anterior placental location influences onset, progress of labour and postpartum outcome (Di et al 2015) and prolongs the third stage of labour (Torricelli et al 2015).

Cord clamping

If the umbilical cord remains intact during the third stage, blood can pass to and from the infant until cord pulsation has ceased. The amount of blood gained or lost by the baby will depend on its position (loss or gain), and whether cord milking (gain) or a uterotonic drug (gain) is administered (Mercer and Erickson-Owens 2012). There is the potential for continued delivery of oxygenated blood to the newborn via the cord (Mercer and Erickson-Owens 2012; Hutchon 2006), of particular importance in those babies born prematurely or asphyxiated (Ghavam et al 2014). There is a recommendation to initiate resuscitation at the bedside to avoid cord clamping (Mercer and Erickson-Owens 2014).

Deferred cord clamping (DCC) also leads to a net gain of 80 mL (Yao and Lind 1974) or up to 30% of the baby's total blood volume (Mercer and Erickson-Owens 2012 and 2014). This gain has been associated with benefits for the infant with no additional risk to the woman (Hutton and Hassan 2007; McDonald et al 2013) (see Box 39.1). The consensus therefore is to delay/defer cord clamping in third stage management unless there is a clear indication to do otherwise (Duley et al 2015). Early cord clamping (ECC) has also been associated with fetomaternal transfusion; this is of particular importance in women who are rhesus negative (Lapido 1972).

With DCC now being recommended in third stage management, a tension is created when a woman chooses to donate her baby's cord blood, as ECC is needed to ensure a high volume collection (Brown 2013). As DCC is associated with benefits for mother and baby, women need to consider these when deciding about cord blood donation. In the future, strategies such as combining smaller cord blood donations from multiple donors may allow women to continue to gift their baby's cord blood with DCC.

Reflective activity 39.3   ><

Read Brown's (2013) *Contradictions of Value: Between Use and Exchange in Cord Blood Bioeconomy*. Do you consider cord blood to be clinical waste? What are your own thoughts and feelings about cord blood donation? What do you think are the ethical dilemmas around cord blood donation? How can midwives support women's informed choice to donate cord blood?

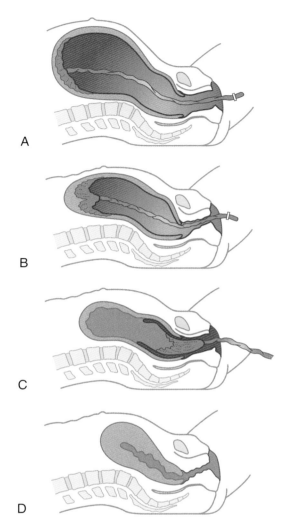

Figure 39.2 The mechanism of placental separation. **A,** The placenta before the child is born. **B,** The placenta partially separated immediately after the birth of the child. **C,** The placenta completely separated. **D,** The placenta expelled and the uterus strongly contracted and retracted.

It is suggested that with ECC, the resulting extra fetal blood retained in the placenta prevents it from being so tightly compressed by the uterus. As a result, contraction and retraction of the uterus may be less effective, and maternal blood loss increased, leading to a greater retro-placental blood clot being formed. Botha (1968) does not consider the formation of a retroplacental blood clot a physiological process. Rather, it occurs as a result of this intervention. To reduce the size of the placenta, shorten the third stage and reduce blood loss after ECC, Asicioglu et al (2015) have suggested adopting placental cord drainage (PCD). This involves releasing the clamp from the cut end of the severed cord closest to the placenta. However, while this study showed a reduction in the mean estimated blood loss and duration of the third stage with PCD, the intervention group also received cord traction; the control group did not, which may have influenced results. Soltani et al (2011) advise caution in the interpretation of available PCD trials because of the lack of high-quality research. As such, using PCD in practice remains open to debate.

During the process of separation, descent and expulsion of the placenta, a number of clinical signs may be seen.

- A small amount of blood oozes from the placental bed and tracks down between the membranes,

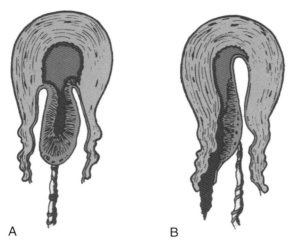

A B

Figure 39.3 Expulsion of the placenta: **A,** Schultze method. **B,** Matthews Duncan method.

appearing as a gush of blood from vagina (sign of separation).

- Abdominally, the uterus rises up to sit on top of the descended placenta, which can resemble a full bladder as it lies in the lower uterine segment (sign of descent).
- Lengthening of the cord (sign of descent)
- Presentation of the placenta at the vulva

During the expulsive phase, the placenta may appear at the vagina in one of two ways (see Fig. 39.3).

Schultze

The placenta appears fetal surface first, like an inverted umbrella with the membranes trailing behind. Any blood lost during the third stage will collect on the maternal surface of the placenta and be encased by the membranes. Over 80% of placentae are delivered in this way (Akiyama et al 1981).

Matthews Duncan

Less commonly, the placenta slips from the vagina sideways and the maternal surface appears at the vulva first. Midwives often use the term 'dirty Duncan' for this type of presentation because more bleeding is seen vaginally – blood escapes immediately from the placental site because it is not encased in the membranes. This is often associated with slower separation of the placenta and ragged membranes.

Detachment of the membranes begins in the first stage of labour, when separation occurs around the internal cervical os. In the third stage, complete separation takes place assisted by the weight of the descending placenta, peeling them from the uterine wall.

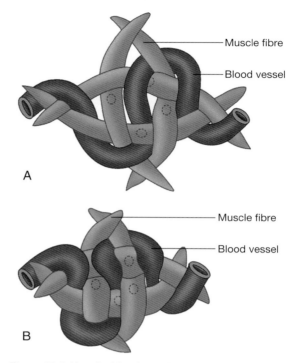

Figure 39.4 How the blood vessels run between the interlacing muscle fibres of the uterus. **A,** Muscle fibres relaxed and blood vessels not compressed. **B,** Muscle fibres contracted, blood vessels compressed and bleeding arrested.

Control of bleeding

After placental expulsion, several mechanisms come into play to control bleeding from maternal sinuses at the site of placental attachment.

1. The empty uterus fully contracts and the uterine walls come into apposition.
2. The myometrium continues to contract and retract intermittently. The interlacing muscle fibres become living ligatures, constricting the torn blood vessels and sealing them (see Fig. 39.4). The absence of these oblique muscle fibres in the lower uterine segment is attributed to the increased blood loss seen with placenta praevia.
3. The process of blood clotting at the site of placental attachment is initiated and the area quickly becomes covered with a fibrin mesh, using up to 10% of a woman's circulating fibrinogen.
4. Breastfeeding, the baby nuzzling at the breast and skin-to-skin contact increases the release of oxytocin from the posterior pituitary, enhancing uterine contractility.

- Previous postpartum haemorrhage
- Anaemia
- Clotting disorders
- Pregnancy-induced hypertension
- Chronic hypertension
- Overdistended uterus, as in polyhydramnios, multiple pregnancies and fibroids
- Grand multiparity
- Induction/augmentation of labour
- Poor uterine action during labour and delivery
- Long first or second stage of labour
- Dehydration during labour
- Instrumental delivery
- Oxytocic drugs
- Full bladder at onset of the third stage of labour
- How the third stage of labour is managed
- The psychological environment of birth

Any factor that interferes with the normal physiological processes can influence the outcome of the third stage of labour (see Box 39.2). This includes a variety of complications of pregnancy and childbirth and the actions of individual midwives. Oxytocic drugs given before and during the third stage of labour also influence events. A woman's ability to avoid complications will also be based on her general health and by avoiding predisposing factors, such as dehydration, anaemia, ketosis, exhaustion and hypotonic uterine action.

MANAGEMENT OF THE THIRD STAGE OF LABOUR

Commonly, midwives describe two ways of managing the third stage: **active management** and **expectant management**. However, difficulties remain in defining what these terms mean, as midwives practice both methods in a variety of different ways (Harris 2005; Schorne et al 2015), leading to mixed approaches. The most commonly described form of each management will be outlined here with discussion about where variation may take place.

The woman and her midwife will have discussed options for the third stage during the antenatal period and again during labour and made a decision over which management she would like.

Expectant management

Expectant management is one of 'watchful anticipation' and draws upon the normal physiological processes to bring about expulsion of the placenta and membranes through contraction of the uterus, stimulated by an increase in oxytocin release at the time of the birth of the baby. The woman is active during this process and the midwife's role is a passive one, involving close observation and encouragement.

The effectiveness of this physiological process can be influenced by inhibition of oxytocin release, as can happen when excess adrenaline is produced by anxiety (Buckley 2004). Therefore, a woman requires positive psychological support from a midwife for physiological processes to be effective (Saxton et al 2014 and 2015; Fahy et al 2010; Hastie et al 2009). This includes encouraging a woman to be aware and respond to what her body is telling her to do (Hodnett et al 2013; Sandall et al 2013).

Drug administration during labour can also inhibit oxytocin release and, therefore, expectant management is usually not recommended for women at high risk, when a woman has induction/augmentation of labour with oxytocics, and where epidural anaesthesia or narcotic analgesia has been given (Buckley 2004; Fry 2007).

Principles of expectant management

In accordance with the principles of non-intervention in expectant management, no uterotonic drug is administered and the cord is not clamped and cut.

The time of birth is recorded, which indicates the start of the third stage of labour.

Whichever position in which a woman chooses to give birth, the newborn infant will be placed either on the bed/floor covering between the woman's legs or on the woman's abdomen, depending on her choice. As the cord is not clamped, there is a free flow of blood from baby to and from the placenta until cord pulsation has ceased. Usually, no matter the position in which a woman gives birth, she will choose to sit once the baby is born. This allows her the opportunity to touch, hold and examine her baby. Early skin-to-skin contact is advantageous in stimulating oxytocin release (Marin Gabriel et al 2010), maintaining the infant's temperature, promoting successful breastfeeding and supporting development of mother–infant attachment (Moore et al 2012). The midwife then leaves the woman and her family to experience the powerful first meeting with their new baby, undisturbed while remaining in the room to observe and monitor physical well-being, including vaginal blood loss and maternal pulse. If the woman is prevented from holding her baby by a short cord, the woman may choose to have the cord clamped and cut once it has stopped pulsating. The midwife notes the time when the cord is clamped for recording later (O'Brien 2015).

Detection of separation and descent of the placenta

As the uterus begins to contract again, the woman will usually indicate this and may have an urge to bear down. The midwife may also notice abdominal changes; the fundus rises up and becomes more globular. The separated placenta may be seen as a bulge, similar to a full bladder, just above the symphysis pubis, with the well-contracted uterus sitting above it. A gush of blood per vagina may occur, which tends to be larger than that observed in active management when a uterotonic has been given. The cord also lengthens. There is no necessity to palpate the abdomen, unless there is cause for concern or the midwife suspects there may be some delay. If it is needed, gentle palpation of the fundus will ascertain uterine tone without disturbing the physiological process. The midwife must avoid 'fundal fiddling', which can lead to increased bleeding. Encouraging the woman to adopt an upright position at this time will lead to rapid expulsion of the placenta and membranes. Care needs to be taken when assisting the woman to move into an upright position, as she will have the baby in her arms. Standing, squatting and sometimes using a toilet, bucket or bedpan can be used.

Delivery of the placenta and membranes

The placenta is delivered by maternal effort. Normally, the woman in an upright position will feel the placenta as it descends to the pelvic floor, which triggers an urge to push, or the placenta will just fall out under the influence of gravity.

The midwife's role is to let the woman know what is happening, to encourage her to adopt an upright position once she feels a contraction, and respond to urges to push or bear down if she wants to. A flat hand placed across the lower abdomen may assist the woman to birth the placenta, as the counter pressure compensates for poor muscle tone. The placenta and membranes are then delivered either onto the bed/floor or into a bedpan/bucket. If the membranes trail behind, they can be eased out of the vagina by turning the placenta to make a rope of the membranes, by applying gentle traction on the membranes with the fingers (usually in an up-and-down motion), or

by asking the woman to cough. Once the placenta is completely expelled, the time is noted to calculate the length of the third stage for recording later. The midwife then palpates the abdomen to ensure the uterus is well contracted and observes for signs of excessive blood loss. The cord can then be clamped and cut and cord blood taken as necessary. The placenta and membranes are then checked in front of the parents.

It is suggested by midwives that the third stage normally takes between 5 and 15 minutes but can take up to an hour (Harris 2005). While some authors suggest the length of the third stage is longer with expectant management than active management (Prendiville et al 1988; Rogers et al 1998), other authors looking specifically at ultrasound images suggest there is no difference (Herman et al 1993; Krapp et al 2000). If physiologically the length of the third stage is similar for both active and expectant management, perhaps time differences may be attributed to the actions of either the midwife or the woman. It has been noted that the use of an upright posture after separation appears to reduce blood loss and the length of the third stage in expectant management (Rogers et al 1998).

If there is delay in placental delivery, a number of actions can be taken. Odent (1998) suggests gently pressing upwards on the abdominal wall just above the pubic bone (with the woman lying on her back). If the cord does not move, then placental separation can be confirmed. Emptying the bladder, changing the woman's position and encouraging the woman to walk a short way may assist in placental delivery. Encouraging a woman to blow into an empty bottle has also been described (Fry 2007). In a small study exploring midwives' expertise in expectant management, Begley et al (2012) identified that midwives alluded to using the cord to easy out a placenta sitting in the vagina, although such an approach is not normally recommended in practice guidelines. According to NICE guidance (2014), an expectant management is prolonged if not completed by 60 minutes.

Principles of active management

Active management is an intervention in the normal physiological processes and involves the prophylactic administration of a uterotonic at the end of the second stage of labour, cord clamping and controlled cord traction (CCT) to bring about delivery of the placenta and membranes. The woman for the most part is a passive participant in this process.

History of active management

Active intervention in the third stage of labour became popular after the isolation of ergometrine (Dudley and Moir 1935) and the development of synthetic oxytocin (Syntocinon) (du Vigneaud and Tippett 1954). Initially, ergometrine was used as a treatment for postpartum haemorrhage (PPH), and it was then given after the third stage to prevent PPH. Syntometrine (a mixture of Syntocinon and ergometrine) was marketed in the 1960s (Embrey et al 1963) as a uterotonic drug, administered at the birth of the baby's anterior shoulder and followed by early clamping and cutting of the umbilical cord and CCT. This approach became known as active management and its popularity quickly spread. It has been so successful that it has become normal practice throughout the UK, irrespective of the degree of risk.

Uterotonic drugs

Uterotonic drugs (drugs that make the uterus contract) are used during the third stage in three ways as a:

- *prophylaxis:* to prevent PPH irrespective of the risk status of the woman
- *planned treatment:* when a risk of PPH has been identified, for example, when a woman has a low haemoglobin level or a history of previous PPH
- *treatment in an emergency:* when uncontrolled bleeding occurs as a result of uterine atony

Active versus expectant management

While the benefits of oxytocic drugs in treating atonic PPH are recognized, their routine use in preventing the problem has been the subject of much debate and various clinical trials. The most recent systematic review of three studies comparing active versus expectant management in low risk women (Begley et al 2015) concluded that there was an overall reduction in mean maternal blood loss of less than 100 mL in women having an active third stage of labour over expectant management (mean weighted difference −78.80 mL), with no statistical difference in severe PPH (1000 mL or more). The review also highlighted that active management showed an average increase in diastolic blood pressure over 90 mmHg, administration of analgesia after birth up until discharge from the delivery suite, after pains and the return of a woman to hospital because of bleeding. It has been suggested for some time that Syntocinon replace Syntometrine as the drug of choice in active management, as some of the complications previously mentioned have been associated with the ergometrine component of Syntometrine (McDonald et al 1993; NICE 2007 and 2014; Begley 2015).

Critics of research studies comparing active and expectant management highlight a number of factors that may have influenced the findings reported.

Lack of skill in expectant management among midwives. Three of four studies were conducted in hospitals where active management was the norm (Gyte 1994). In one study, where authors indicated that expectant management was more common, statistics were not available as to the rate of expectant management before the trial began (Rogers et al 1998). In an observation study in New Zealand, in birth environments where expectant management is the norm, no reduction in blood loss was seen with active management (New Zealand College of Midwives (NZCM) 2009). It is proposed that these findings suggest a link between normal blood loss and expectant management, where midwives are skilled in the technique and women have had a normal physiological first and second stage of labour (Begley et al 2015). This may add weight to the growing evidence that, for low-risk women, an expectant management approach may not significantly increase blood loss after birth, making it a realistic option.

Difficulty in defining what constitutes excessive blood loss. It is recognized that blood loss estimation is inaccurate, with over and under estimation common among clinicians (Razvi et al 1996; Razvi et al 2008). In addition, as the reduced loss associated with active management has become the norm, midwives may interpret the slightly higher blood loss rate in expectant management as abnormal. While oxytocics may appear to reduce blood loss at delivery in the short term, when the action wears off after transfer from the delivery suite, the blood will be lost then (Kashanian et al 2010; Wickham 1999). Wickham (1999) observed that after active management, women often experienced a heavy blood loss when going to the bathroom for the first time, and Kashanian et al (2010) confirmed this, noting statistically significant higher blood loss in the 'fourth stage of labour' (see p. 657) in women having active management. This hypothesis has been further strengthened by the most recent Cochrane review, comparing active and expectant management, which found an increased rate of women returning to hospital with bleeding after active management (Begley et al 2015) This may suggest that the use of uterotonics during the third stage merely delays blood loss until a time when it is less likely to be noticed. It is possible that women are supposed to lose blood at this time, as they no longer require such a high circulating blood volume to supply the placental bed, and the haemodilution of pregnancy may support a woman's ability to cope with this. It has been suggested that blood loss less than 750 mL is not severe in normal healthy women (Begley et al 2015), although further research is needed to look at what constitutes normal blood loss after childbirth and the implications of actively reducing it.

Variation in practice. When comparing research protocols of published trials, no consensus can be reached on a definition of what constitutes active and expectant management, which implies there is variation in practice (Begley 1990; Prendiville et al 1988; Rogers et al 1998; Thilaganathan et al 1993). Gyte (1994) suggests that a 'piecemeal' approach, a combination of active and expectant management techniques, was used by a significant number of midwives within the Bristol trial. Inter- and intra-third-stage-practice variation among midwives has subsequently been reported (Harris 2005; Rogers et al (2012), as has variation in third stage policies (Winter et al 2007), intra- and inter-country variation in third stage care (Festin et al 2003; Stanton et al 2008) and variation in management between maternity care providers (Tan et al 2008; Schorne et al 2015). Variation in active management has also increased with the introduction of DCC, delayed or omitted administration of a uterotonic and evidence suggesting that CCT can be omitted without increased risk of PPH (Downey and Bewley 2010; Hutton et al 2013; Baker 2014; Hofmeyr et al 2015). This highlights the difficulty in evaluating the results of comparative studies where variation in practice could have occurred and suggests the need for further research to explore the risks and benefits of individual components of active management as it evolves. At present, evidence suggests that it is the uterotonic element of active management that reduces blood loss, but there is no consensus on when it should be given and whether it is necessary in low-risk women who have had a physiological labour and birth (Begley et al 2015).

Logue (1990) looked at PPH rates among doctors and midwives and found considerable variation, with some individuals having consistently much higher rates of PPH than others. She suggests that when managing the third stage, 'more conservative and patient operators show the lowest PPH rates, compared with the more impatient and heavy-handed who show the highest rates' (Logue 1990: S11). This implies that the action or inaction of practitioners may have a direct effect on the outcome of the third stage and requires further exploration. This is supported in the literature by reference to the potential dangers of 'fundal fiddling' and inappropriate cord traction leading to uterine inversion (Pena-Mari and Comunian-Carrasco 2007; McDonald 2009; WHO 2012).

Current options

Currently, the following uterotonic drugs are available to manage the third stage of labour:

Syntocinon. This is a synthetically produced form of oxytocin, given either intravenously (5 IU) or intramuscularly (5–10 IU). It can be given with delivery of the anterior shoulder or shortly after the birth. Intramuscular (IM) Syntocinon acts within 2 to 3 minutes of administration. A dose of 10 IU of Syntocinon administered IM is considered the oxytocic drug of choice for active management (NICE 2014; WHO 2012). Although some authors have suggested that

Syntometrine remains the most effective uterotonic in reducing blood loss (McDonald et al 2004), it causes nausea, vomiting and hypertension, making Syntocinon, which has fewer side effects, an appropriate alternative. Any product containing Syntocinon needs to be stored at 2 to 8°C, as it deteriorates at high temperatures (emc. medicines.org.uk; EMC 2016).

Intramuscular Syntometrine 1 mL. This is usually given with the birth of the anterior shoulder or shortly after. Syntometrine contains ergometrine 500 μg and oxytocin 5 units in 1 mL. The oxytocin fraction induces strong, rhythmic contraction of the muscle fibres of the upper segment of the uterus within 2 to 3 minutes of administration. Its effect lasts for approximately 5 to 15 minutes (Baskett 1999). This rapid-acting, short-duration component is designed to initiate strong uterine action, which is sustained by the action of the ergometrine fraction that will induce a strong, non-physiological spasm of uterine muscle within 6 to 8 minutes (Sorbe 1978). The effect of ergometrine is maintained for approximately 60 to 90 minutes (Baskett 1999). Because of the spasm-inducing properties of ergometrine, there is a theoretical risk of retained placenta and, therefore, the midwife should aim to deliver the placenta before ergometrine takes effect. Syntometrine becomes inactive at high temperatures and therefore needs careful storage.

Intramuscular ergometrine 500 μg. This will cause a strong, sustained uterine contraction. If intramuscular ergometrine is administered *instead of* Syntometrine, it is given a little earlier, at the crowning of the head, as it takes longer to act, at 6 to 8 minutes. The World Health Organization (WHO 2012) does not support its use for routine management in the third stage, owing to its effect on blood pressure and the potential risk of shoulder dystocia. The conclusion of a review of ergot alkaloids in the third stage suggests that although these drugs are effective, other drugs such as oxytocin and prostaglandins may be preferable (Liabsuetrakul et al 2007).

Intravenous ergometrine 250 to 500 μg. This takes effect approximately 45 seconds after administration; it is usually given by a doctor but may be given by a midwife in an emergency situation, usually to control postpartum bleeding.

Prostaglandins

There is currently some interest in exploring the use of a prostaglandin E1 analogue (misoprostol) for management of the third stage. Misoprostol (in doses of 400–600 mg) can be given orally or rectally, needs no equipment to administer and does not become inactive at high temperatures. This makes it an ideal therapy for countries in the developing world where refrigeration and health services are limited. However, it is associated with shivering and transient pyrexia. In a systematic review of prostaglandins for preventing PPH (Tuncalp et al 2012), findings suggested that neither intramuscular prostaglandins nor oral misoprostol were as effective at preventing PPH as injectable uterotonics.

Nipple stimulation

A simple alternative to parenteral oxytocics for the third stage of labour is nipple stimulation, which according to Irons et al (1994) tends to reduce the length of the third stage and the amount of blood loss. However, in the outcome of a recent systematic review (Abedi et al 2016) it was highlighted that there is currently insufficient evidence to evaluate the effect of nipple stimulation for reducing PPH and larger high-quality trials are needed.

Principles of active management

Currently, active management is recommended for all women, although those at low risk who request expectant management should be supported in their choice (NICE 2014). The package of care recommended includes routine use of a uterotonic drug (10 IU Syntocinon), administered before clamping and cutting the cord, DCC from 1 to 5 minutes and CCT after signs of placental separation (NICE 2014).

Positioning the baby after birth

Where the infant is placed at birth will depend on the position that the woman chooses for birth. As discussed previously, there are significant benefits for both mother and child of early skin-to-skin contact. There is also a need to provide a safe, warm and draught-free environment.

When to give the uterotonic

It has been recommended that during active management, a uterotonic drug is administered either at the birth of the baby's anterior shoulder or shortly after the birth of the baby (if a midwife is alone), and before the cord is clamped and cut (NICE 2014).

When to cut the cord

Traditionally, midwives were advised to clamp and cut the umbilical cord as soon as possible after the birth of the baby to prevent an excess of placental blood being forced into the infant's circulation under the influence of the administered oxytocic, preventing hypervolaemia and hyperbilirubinaemia in the neonate. Early clamping lowers postnatal levels of plasma bilirubin, with a lower incidence of neonatal jaundice that requires phototherapy (McDonald 2013; Rabe et al 2012). However, evidence now suggests there is a benefit to delaying cord clamping for up to 5 minutes and that any subsequent polycythaemia in the neonate appears to be benign (Hutton and Hassan 2007).

Detection of separation and descent of the placenta

In active management, it is normally the midwife who detects the first uterine contraction after the baby's birth by means of placing a hand gently on the woman's abdomen and waiting for the uterus to rise up and contract beneath it. Midwives are often warned at this time of the dangers of 'fundal fiddling', which may lead to partial separation of the placenta, with the potential for excessive bleeding to occur. Although CCT, as described by Spencer (1962), should commence as soon as the uterus contracts, Levy and Moore (1985) suggest waiting until signs of separation are present. This latter study found no significant difference in the incidence of PPH or the length of the third stage between those who started CCT as soon as the uterus contracted and those who waited for signs of separation. However, the rate of PPH appeared to be significantly higher when the midwife unsuccessfully used CCT without waiting for these signs. Current best practice is to observe signs of placental separation before commencing CCT.

Signs of separation and descent

As the uterus contracts and the placenta separates, the fundus rises up and becomes more globular. The separated placenta may be seen as a bulge, similar to a full bladder, just above the symphysis pubis, with the well-contracted uterus sitting above it. Combined with the abdominal findings, the midwife may notice that there is a gush of blood per vagina and that more of the cord becomes visible as the placenta descends. The blood seen tends to be less than that observed in expectant management. The woman may experience pain at this time and also feel the urge to bear down as the placenta enters the vagina.

Delivery of the placenta and membranes

The placenta is delivered by cord traction with the woman in a sitting/semirecumbent position. The midwife either wraps her fingers around the cord or uses a clamp to apply downward sustained traction until the placenta appears at the vulva. When the placenta becomes visible, traction is applied upwards (following the curve of Carus) to extract the placenta from the vagina (Spencer 1962). The placenta is delivered into the midwife's hands or into a bowl placed close to the introitus.

While applying cord traction, some midwives place a hand above the symphysis pubis and push the uterus upwards (known as 'guarding of the uterus') (see Fig. 39.5). This is said to prevent uterine inversion; however, there is currently no evidence available to support this practice. Some midwives use this hand to apply counter pressure when performing cord traction, and others suggest it provides valuable information on descent, as the placenta can be felt beneath the hand, moving down into the vagina (Harris 2005).

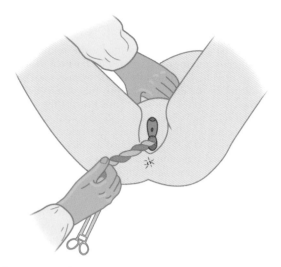

Figure 39.5 Controlled cord traction whilst guarding the uterus.

In some units, women are encouraged to deliver the placenta by maternal effort (see p. 658). In unskilled hands cord traction, as a part of active management, is not recommended (WHO 2012).

After placental delivery, the time is noted to calculate the length of the third stage for recording in the notes. The midwife palpates the abdomen to ensure the uterus is well contracted and notes vaginal blood loss.

Reflective activity 39.5 ›‹

It has been suggested that midwives consider deferring cord clamping when a newborn baby requires resuscitation (Mercer and Erickson-Owens 2014). Read the paper by Mercer and Erickson-Owens and consider how practical it would be to adopt this in practice and the rationale for doing so.

Reflective activity 39.6 ›‹

Consider the form of words you would choose when discussing active and expectant management of labour. What are the key points you would make, and which research and evidence would you use to explain the woman's choices?

Examination of the placenta and membranes

The placenta and membranes are carefully and systematically examined as soon after delivery as possible so

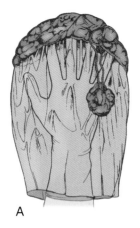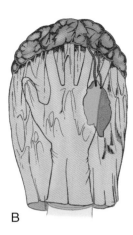

Figure 39.6 **A,** Succenturiate lobe. **B,** The torn membrane – the missing lobe is in the uterus.

that, if incomplete, action can be taken immediately. The examination is to determine completeness and to detect any abnormalities, which may suggest problems in the neonate (see Box 39.3).

Initially, the placenta is held up by the cord to view the membranes; a discrete hole, which the baby passed through, may be seen. Sometimes membranes are ragged and every attempt should be made to piece them together to ensure completeness.

The placenta is placed on a flat surface and thoroughly examined in a good light. The amnion is stripped from the chorion up to the umbilical cord to confirm that both membranes are present. The maternal surface is wiped clear of blood clots and carefully examined to ensure all the cotyledons are present. Any areas of infarction (firm whitish patches) are noted and the placental edge examined for blood vessels running into the membranes. These vessels may track back to the placenta (an erratic vessel) or go to an accessory lobe in the membranes (a succenturiate lobe). If a vessel ends at a hole in the membranes (see Fig. 39.6), a succenturiate lobe may have been left behind in the uterus and the woman will need referral to an obstetrician.

The cord is examined, noting its insertion and length (though this is no longer routinely measured) and the number of umbilical vessels. Usually the cord insertion is central and the length is approximately 50 cm. Occasionally, only one umbilical artery is present; this is associated with congenital anomalies, especially renal agenesis (absence of kidneys). The paediatrician would need to be informed and a detailed examination of the newborn requested.

The placenta is usually weighed; weight at term is normally about one-sixth of the baby's birthweight. ECC increases the placental weight, as it contains a greater residual blood volume.

Box 39.3 The normal placenta and membranes at term

Placenta
- Shape: flat and round or oval
- Diameter: 18–20 cm
- Thickness: 2.5 cm at centre, becoming thinner at the edges
- Weight: 1/6th of baby's birthweight (Haeussner et al 2013)
- Two surfaces (see Fig. 39.7)
  - Maternal
    - Attached to the uterine decidua
    - Deep red in colour
    - Divided by grooves or sulci into approximately 15–20 irregular lobes
    - Lobes (called cotyledons) contain masses of chorionic villi
    - Observations
      - A thin greyish layer can be seen (part of the basal decidua)
      - The placenta may feel gritty due to calcium deposits
  - Fetal
    - Lies adjacent to the fetus
    - Pearly white appearance
    - Covered in amnion
    - Cord normally inserted centrally
    - Blood vessels are seen radiating out to the edges, like the roots of a tree
    - Branches of these blood vessels penetrate the substance of the placenta
    - Each cotyledon has its own supply of fetal blood
    - In the centre of each cotyledon there is a main branch of the umbilical artery and vein

Membranes
- Two membranes
  - Chorion
    - Outer membrane
    - Continuous with the edge of the placenta
    - Derived from trophoblast
    - Opaque, friable and roughened by pieces of decidua adherent to it
    - This membrane lines the uterine cavity
  - Amnion
    - Inner membrane
    - Can be stripped back to insertion of the cord
    - Derived from inner cell mass
    - Smooth, transparent and stronger than the chorion
    - Secretes amniotic fluid/liquor amnii which, at term, measures 1000–1500 mL

Umbilical cord (funis)
- Connects the placenta to the fetus
- Approximately 50 cm long and 2 cm thick
- Structure
  - The cord contains three blood vessels
    - One large umbilical vein carrying oxygenated blood to the fetus
    - Two umbilical arteries winding around the vein carrying deoxygenated blood from the fetus back to the placenta
  - A jelly like substance (Wharton's jelly) cushions the blood vessels, reducing the risk of compression in utero
  - Amnion covers the cord and provides additional support and protection
  - The cord also has a spiral twist: this torsion gives some protection from pressure
- The function of the cord ceases as pulmonary respiration is established shortly after birth
- Lacking a blood supply, the cord becomes dead tissue and quickly atrophies, as do the internal structures continuous with it
- It can provide access for bacteria to enter the body; therefore, care needs to be taken to keep it dry until the cord stump separates (see chs. 42 and 48)

Finally, any blood loss collected is measured and added to the estimated amount of loss that has soaked into linen and pads. Particular care is needed in estimating losses in excess of 300 mL, when amounts are often underestimated (Levy and Moore 1985), with the level of error increasing with the amount lost.

The findings are recorded in the mother's notes. Immediate referral to a doctor is made if it is thought that a piece of placental tissue has been retained.

CARE AFTER BIRTH (THE FOURTH STAGE)

A midwife should remain with the woman for the first hour after birth.

After the delivery of the placenta and membranes, the midwife palpates the woman's abdomen to ensure the uterus is well contracted, assesses vaginal blood loss and

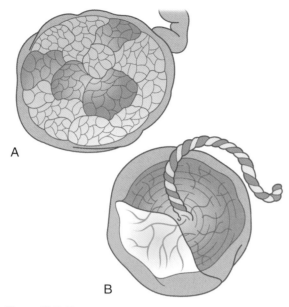

Figure 39.7 The placenta. **A,** The maternal surface, showing the cotyledons. **B,** The fetal surface.

examines the woman for any soft tissue damage that may require repair. The midwife makes the mother comfortable. This is an ideal time for the midwife to share the couple's delight in their baby and encourage any questions and affords the midwife an excellent opportunity for health education to facilitate parent–baby attachment. Most women will enjoy early contact with their baby and there is evidence that this early and unhurried contact significantly affects maternal emotional well-being when measured 6 weeks postnatally (Ball 1994). The father/partner, too, usually wishes to share this time with his family and should be encouraged to do so. This must be given priority over many routine procedures (Sheridan 2010). Sensitivity is required in caring for women who appear to show little interest in their baby at birth.

Women who plan to breastfeed should be encouraged to do so soon after birth, usually within the first hour. At this time, the baby usually displays a strong urge to suck, and a successful feed benefits both mother and baby. Early feeding is associated with ongoing breastfeeding success and the release of endogenous oxytocin, which stimulates uterine contractions and helps maintain haemostasis (see Ch. 44).

Ongoing care includes regular examination of the woman's abdomen to ensure the uterus remains contracted and observation of the lochia. The woman is encouraged to pass urine, as a full bladder predisposes to a relaxed uterus and heavy blood loss. If this occurs, the bladder is emptied, and then the midwife can massage the fundus of the uterus to stimulate a contraction. Assessing and recording blood loss during the first hour after the third stage could add to knowledge of the risks and benefits of third stage management approaches (Williams 2014).

Observation of the infant will include colour, respirations and general activity. The umbilical cord is checked to ensure the cord clamp is firmly in place and that there is no bleeding. Care is taken to ensure that the baby does not become chilled; body temperature can be maintained by skin-to-skin contact or warm wrapping and cuddling by the parents. It is good practice that the midwife remains with the woman and baby for at least 1 hour after delivery, whether at home or in hospital.

RECORDS

A complete and accurate account of labour must be recorded and must be sufficiently comprehensive to enable other carers to have a clear picture of events, thus facilitating communication and avoiding discontinuity of care (Nursing and Midwifery Council (NMC) 2015).

Statute requires that a birth notification form be completed. This is normally completed by the midwife shortly after the baby's birth.

Abnormalities of the placenta

Succenturiate lobe

A succenturiate lobe (see Fig. 39.8) is a small portion or lobe of placenta that is separated from the main body. This is formed from some of the villi of the chorionic membrane that have continued to develop instead of becoming atrophied. It is attached to the main placenta by blood vessels that pass through the membrane. A succenturiate lobe may be retained in the uterus after the placenta has been expelled and can cause PPH and sepsis. When there is a small hole in the fetal membranes with placental vessels running towards it, a retained succenturiate lobe may be suspected, and the woman should be referred to an obstetrician for assessment.

Circumvallate placenta

In this type of placenta, the chorion is not attached to the edge of the placenta, but to the fetal surface at some distance from the edge (see Fig. 39.9). A thickened ring of membrane is seen on the fetal surface.

Bipartite placenta

This is a placenta divided into two main lobes (see Fig. 39.10).

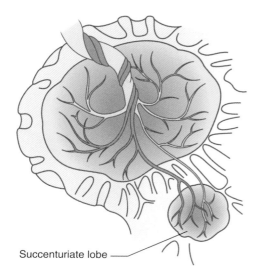

Succenturiate lobe

Figure 39.8 Placenta with succenturiate lobe.

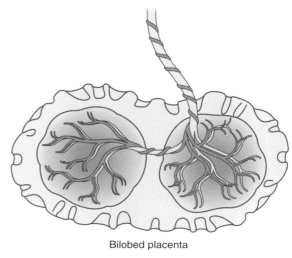

Bilobed placenta

Figure 39.10 Bipartite placenta.

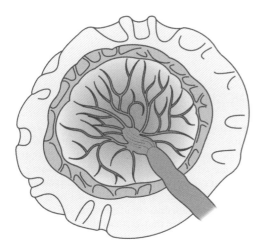

Figure 39.9 Circumvallate placenta.

Placenta accreta

This is a placenta that becomes abnormally adherent to the uterine muscle over the whole or part of its surface. It is very rare with an incidence of 1.7 per 10,000 maternities in the UK (Fitzpatrick et al 2012).

Infarcts

Red or white patches are sometimes seen on the maternal surface of the placenta. These are caused by localized death of placental tissue because of interference with the blood supply.

Infarcts are red at an early stage of their development; they later become white and appear as patches of white fibrous tissue. They may be seen occasionally in any placenta, but they are often associated with pre-eclampsia.

Calcification

On the maternal surface of the placenta, small greyish-white patches are often to be seen, particularly on the post-mature placenta, owing to calcium deposits. They convey a gritty sensation to the fingers and are not significant.

Abnormalities of the umbilical cord

The cord may be too short (which may cause delay during labour) or too long, when there is a risk of cord prolapse. Occasionally, it is very thick or very thin; in either case, great care is required in tying the cord and subsequently watching for haemorrhage. Rarely, a piece of fetal intestine may protrude into the cord, which may be diagnosed on ultrasound antenatally. After birth, the abnormality will be suspected if the cord is swollen close to the umbilicus, the size of the swelling depending on the amount of intestine that has protruded (see Ch. 49). Knots are caused by movements of the fetus before birth, by the fetus slipping through a loop of the cord. False knots may be caused by the blood vessels being longer than the actual cord, and so doubling back on themselves in the Wharton's jelly, or to irregularities and the formation of nodes (see Fig. 39.11).

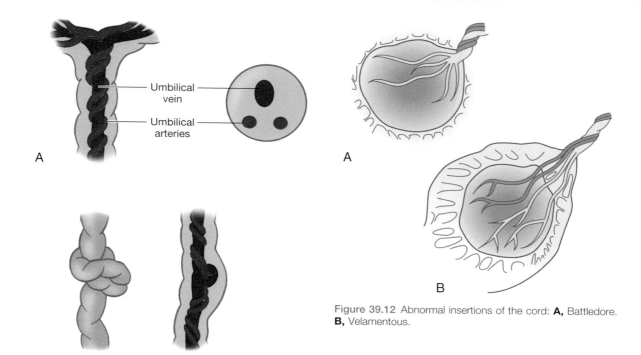

Figure 39.11 A, The umbilical cord in side view and cross-section, showing the one umbilical vein with the two umbilical arteries twisting spirally around it. The vein and arteries lie in Wharton's jelly; the cord is enclosed within the amnion. **B,** True and false knots.

Figure 39.12 Abnormal insertions of the cord: **A,** Battledore. **B,** Velamentous.

Abnormalities of insertion

The cord may be attached to one side of the placenta (an eccentric insertion) or to the margin of the placenta (a battledore insertion), or the vessels of the cord may break up and run into the membrane before reaching the placenta (a velamentous insertion) (see Fig. 39.12). This is particularly dangerous if the unprotected blood vessels should lie near the internal cervical os. This very rare condition is called vasa praevia (vessels in advance of the fetus). Should a blood vessel so situated be compressed when the membranes rupture, the fetus will suffer hypoxia. If a vessel should rupture during artificial rupture of membranes (ARM), blood will be lost from fetal vessels in the membrane. Such fetal haemorrhage is dangerous and may lead to stillbirth or the necessity for a neonatal blood transfusion. Ebbing et al (2015) have found that anomalous cord insertion, marginal and especially velamentous, is associated with increased risk of complications in the third stage, such as the need for manual removal, curettage and postpartum haemorrhage.

CONCLUSION

The third stage of labour is an important period for mother and baby, when the significance of their first meeting cannot be overestimated. The midwife supports this special time while monitoring successful delivery of the placenta and membranes. If midwives are to offer women a choice of third stage management, midwifery skills in both active and expectant management are required with a body of knowledge that enables the detection of those women who deviate from the norm, in whom active management may be the most appropriate form of care. In this way, women at low risk may be spared unnecessary intervention in the normal process of giving birth. In addition, midwives need to remain aware of the changing evidence base in relation to the benefits of active management over expectant management, including what element, if any, of active management reduces blood loss, and which combination of elements are necessary to provide the greatest benefit for all women, but particularly those at increased risk of bleeding. In addition, midwives need to be aware that DCC is beneficial to both mother and baby and should be part of routine management of the third stage. Finally, midwives need to be aware of the changing evidence base around the necessity for CCT in active management.

References

Abedi D, Jahanfar S, Namvar F: Nipple stimulation or breastfeeding for preventing post partum hemorrhage in the third stage of labour: protocol for systematic review, *Cochrane Database Syst Rev* 2016.

Akiyama H, Kohzu H, Matsuoka M: An approach to detection of placental separation and expulsion with new clinical signs: a study based on haemodynamic method and ultrasonography, *Am J Obstet Gynecol* 140(5):505–511, 1981.

Altay MM, Ilhan AK, Haberal A: Length of the third stage of labor at term pregnancies is shorter if placenta is located at fundus: prospective study, *J Obstet Gynaecol Res* 33(5):641–644, 2007.

Asicioglu O, Unal C, Asicioglu BB, et al: Gulova S: Influence of placental cord drainage in management of the third stage of labor: a multicenter randomized controlled trial, *Am J Perinatol* 32(4):343–350, 2015.

Baker K: How to…conduct active management of the third stage of labour, *Midwives* 16(6):34–35, 2014.

Ball JA: *Reactions to motherhood,* Hale, Books for Midwives, pp 113–115, 1994.

Baskett TF: *Essential management of obstetric emergencies,* 3rd edn, Bristol, Clinical Press, 1999.

Begley CM, Guilliland K, Dixon L, et al: Irish and New Zealand midwives' expertise in expectant management of the third stage of labour: the MEET study, *Midwifery* 28:733–739, 2012.

Begley C: A comparison of 'active' and 'physiological' management of the third stage of labour, *Midwifery* 6(1):3–17, 1990.

Begley C, Gyte GML, Devane D, et al: Active versus expectant management for women in the third stage of labour, *Cochrane Databse Syst Rev* (3):CD007412, 2015.

Botha MA: The management of the umbilical cord in labour, *S Afr J Obstet Gynaecol* 16(2):30–33, 1968.

Brandt M: The mechanism and management of the third stage of labour, *Am J Obstet Gynecol* 23:662–667, 1933.

Brown N: Contradictions of value: between use and exchange in cord blood bioeconomy, *Sociol Health Illn* 35(1):97–112, 2013.

Buckley SJ: Undisturbed birth – nature's hormone blueprint for safety, easy and ecstasy, *MIDIRS Midwifery Digest* 14(23):203–209, 2004.

Di M, Severi FM, Petraglia F: Anterior placental location influences onset and progress of labor and postpartum outcome, *Placenta* 35(4):463–466, 2015.

Downey C, Bewley S: Childbirth practitioners' attitudes to third stage management, *Br J Midwifery* 18(9):576–582, 2010.

Dudley HW, Moir JC: The substance responsible for the traditional clinical effect of ergot, *Br Med J* 1:520–523, 1935.

Duley LMM, Drive JO, Soe A, et al: *Clamping of the umbilical cord and placental transfusion. RCOG Scientific Impact Paper No. 14.* RCOG: London (website). https://www.rcog.org.uk/globalassets/documents/guidelines/scientific-impact-papers/sip-14.pdf. 2015.

Ebbing C, Kiserud T, Johnsen SlL, et al: Third stage of labor risks in velamentous and marginal cord insertion: a population-based study, *Acta Obstet Gynecol Scand* 94(8):878–883, 2015.

Embrey MB, Barber DTC, Scudamore JH: The use of 'Syntometrine' in prevention of post-partum haemorrhage, *Br Med J* 1(5342):1387–1389, 1963.

EMC (Electronic Medicines Compendium): *Syntocinon 10 IU/ml Concentrate for solution for infusion. Summary of product characteristics.* London, Datapharm Communications Ltd. Accessed at https://www.medicines.org.uk/emc/medicine/30336. 2016.

Fahy K, Hastie C, Bisits A, et al: Holistic physiological care compared with active management of the third stage of labour for women at low risk of postpartum haemorrhage: a cohort study, *Women Birth* 23(4):146–152, 2010.

Farrar D, Tuffnell D, Airey R, et al: Care during the third stage of labour: a postal survey of UK midwives and obstetricians, *BMC Pregnancy Childbirth* 10:23, 2010.

Festin MP, Lumbiganon P, Tolosa JE, et al: International survey on variations in practice of the management of the third stage of labour, *Bull World Health Organ* 81(4):286–291, 2003.

Fitzpatrick KE, Seller S, Kurinczuk JJ, et al: Incidence and risk factors for placenta accrete/increta/percreta in the UK: a national case-control study, *PLoS One* 7(12):e52893, 2012.

Fry J: Physiological third stage of labour: support it or lose it, *Br J Midwifery* 15(11):693–695, 2007.

Ghavam S, Dushyant B, Mercer J, et al: Effects of placental transfusion in extremely low birthweight infants: meta-analysis of long and short term outcomes, *Transfusion* 54(4):1192–1198, 2014.

Godfrey E: Off the record: third stage of labour, *Midwives* 13(4):7, 2010.

Gyte G: Evaluation of the meta analyses on the effects, on both mother and baby, of the various components of 'active' management of the third stage of labour, *Midwifery* 10(4):183–199, 1994.

Haeussner E, Schmitz C, von Koch F, et al: Birth weight correlates with size but not shape of the normal human placenta, *Placenta* 34(7):574–582, 2013.

Harris T: Changing the focus for the third stage of labour, *Br J Midwifery* 9(1):7–12, 2001.

Harris T: Midwifery practice in the third stage of *labour*, PhD thesis, Leicester, De Montfort University, 2005.

Hastie C, Fahy KM: Optimising psychophysiology in the third stage of labour: theory applied to practice, *Women Birth* 22(3):89–96, 2009.

Herman A, Zimerman A, Arieli S, et al: Down-up sequential separation of the placenta, *Ultrasound Obstet Gynecol* 19(3):278–281, 2002.

Herman A, Weinraub Z, Bukovsky I, et al: Dynamic ultrasound imaging of the third stage of labour: new perspectives into third stage mechanisms, *Am J Obstet Gynecol* 168(5):1496–1499, 1993.

Hofmeyr GJ, Mshweshwe NT, Gulmezoglu AM: Controlled cord traction for the third stage of labour, *Cochrane Database Syst Rev* (1):CD008020, 2015.

Hodnett ED, Gates S, Hofmeyr GJ, et al: Continuous support for women during childbirth, *Cochrane Database Syst Rev* (7):2013.

Hutchon DJR: Delayed cord clamping may be beneficial in rich settings, *Br Med J* 333(7577):1073, 2006.

Hutton EK, Stoll K, Taha N: An observational study of umbilical cord clamping practices of maternity care providers in a tertiary care center, *Birth* 40(1):39–45, 2013.

Hutton EK, Hassan ES: Late vs early clamping of the umbilical cord in full-term neonates, *J Am Med Assoc* 297(11):1241–1252, 2007.

ICM and FIGO: *Joint statement: Management of the third stage of labour to prevent postpartum haemorrhage* (website). www.pphprevention.org/files/ICM_FIGO_Joint_Statement.pdf. 2006.

Irons DW, Sriskandabalan P, Bullough CH: A simple alternative to parenteral oxytocics for the third stage of labour, *Int J Gynecol Obstet* 46(1):15–18, 1994.

Kashanian M, Fekrat M, Masoomi Z, et al: Comparison of active and expectant management on the duration of the third stage of labour and the amount of blood loss during the third and fourth stages of labour: a randomised controlled trial, *Midwifery* 26(2):241–245, 2010.

Knight M, Kenyon S, Brocklehurst P, et al: *Saving lives: improving mothers' care. Lessons learnt to inform future maternity care from the UK and Ireland Confidential Enquiries into Maternal Deaths and Morbidity 2009-2012*, Oxford, NPEU, 2014.

Krapp M, Baschat AA, Hankeln M, et al: Gray scale and color Doppler sonography in the third stage of labour for early detection of failed placental separation, *Ultrasound Obstet Gynecol* 15(2):138–142, 2000.

Krapp M, Katalinic A, Smrcek J, et al: Study of the third stage of labor by color Doppler sonography, *Arch Gynecol Obstet* 267(4):202–204, 2003.

Lapido OA: Management of third stage of labour with particular reference to reduction of feto-maternal transfusion, *Br Med J* 1(5802):721–723, 1972.

Levy V, Moore J: The midwife's management of the third stage of labour, *Nurs Times* 81(39):47–50, 1985.

Liabsuetrakul T, Choobun T, Peeyananjarassri K, et al: Prophylactic use of ergot alkaloids in the third stage of labour, *Cochrane Database Syst Rev* (2):CD005456, 2007.

Logue M: Management of the third stage of labour: a midwife's view, *J Obstet Gynaecol* 10(Suppl 2):10–12, 1990.

Marin Gabriel MA, Llana Martin I, Lopez Escobar A, et al: Randomised controlled trial of early skin-to-skin contact: effects on the mother and the newborn, *Acta Paediatr* 99(11):1630–1634, 2010.

McDonald S: Physiology and management of the third stage of labour. In Fraser D, Cooper M, editors: *Myles textbook for midwives*, Edinburgh, Churchill Livingstone, 2009.

McDonald SJ, Middleton P, Dowswell T, et al: Effect of timing of umbilical cord clamping of term infants on maternal and neonatal outcomes, *Cochrane Databse Syst Rev* (7):CD004074, 2013.

McDonald SJ, Abbott JM, Higgins SP: Prophylactic ergometrine-oxytocin versus oxytocin for delivery of the placenta, *Cochrane Database Syst Rev* (1):CD000201, 2004.

McDonald SJ, Prendiville WJ, Blair E: Randomised controlled trial of oxytocin alone versus oxytocin and ergometrine in active management of labour, *Br Med J* 307(6913):1167–1171, 1993.

Mercer JS, Erickson-Owens DA: Rethinking placental transfusion and cord clamping issues, *J Perinat Neonatal Nurs* 26(3):202–217, 2012.

Mercer JS, Erickson-Owens DA: Is it time to rethink cord management when resuscitation is needed?, *J Midwifery Womens Health* 59(6):635–644, 2014.

Moore ER, Anderson GC, Bergman N, et al: Early skin-to-skin contact for mothers and their healthy newborn infants, *Cochrane Database Syst Rev* (15):(5):2012.

National Institute for Health and Care Excellence (NICE): *Intrapartum care: care of healthy women and their babies during childbirth*, London, London, Royal College of Obstetricians and Gynaecologists (RCOG) Press, 2007.

National Institute for Health and Care Excellence (NICE): *Intrapartum care: care of healthy women and their babies during childbirth*, NICE guideline CG190 (website). www.nice.org.uk/guidance/cg190/resources/guidance-intrapartum-care-care-of-healthy-women-and-their-babies-during

-childbirth-pdf. London, Royal College of Obstetricians and Gynaecologists (RCOG) Press, 2014.

New Zealand College of Midwives (NZCM): Third stage management practices of midwife lead maternity carers: an analysis of The New Zealand College of midwives database information 2004–2008, Christchurch, The New Zealand College of Midwives, 2009.

Nursing and Midwifery Council (NMC): *The code*, London, NMC, 2015.

O'Brien P: Delayed cord clamping: the new norm, *Br J Midwifery* 23(5):312, 2015.

Odent M: Don't manage the third stage of labour, *Pract Midwife* 1(9):31–33, 1998.

Patwardhan M, Herandez-Andrade E, Ahn H, et al: Dynamic changes in the myometrium during the third stage of labor, evaluating using two-dimensional ultrasound in women with normal and abnormal third stage of labor and in women with obstetric complications, *Gynecol Obstet Invest* 80(1):26–37, 2015.

Pena-Mari GE, Comunian-Carrasco G: Fundal pressure versus controlled cord traction as part of the active management of the third stage of labour, *Cochrane Database Syst Rev* (4):CD005462, 2007.

Prendiville WJ, Harding JE, Elbourne DR, et al: The Bristol third stage trial: active versus physiological management of the third stage of labour, *Br Med J* 297(6659):1295–1300, 1988.

Rabe H, Diaz-Rossello JL, Duley L, et al: Effect of timing on umbilical cord clamping and other strategies to influence placental transfusion at preterm birth on maternal and infant outcomes, *Cochrane Database Syst Rev* (8):2012.

Razvi K, Chua S, Arulkumaran S, et al: A comparison between visual estimation and laboratory determination of blood loss during the third stage of labour, *Aust N Z J Obstet Gynaecol* 36(2):152–154, 1996.

Razvi K, Chua S, Arulkumaran S, et al: A comparison between visual estimation and laboratory determination of blood loss during the third stage of labour, *Aust N Z J Obstet Gynaecol* 36(2):152–154, 2008.

Rogers C, Harman J, Selo-Ojeme D: The management of the third stage of labour – a national survey of current practice, *Br J Midwifery* 20(12):850–857, 2012.

Rogers J, Wood J, McCandlish R, et al: Active versus expectant management of the third stage of labour: the Hinchingbrooke randomised controlled trial, *Lancet* 351(9104):693–699, 1998.

Sandall J, Soltani H, Gates S, et al: Midwife-led continuity models versus other models of care for childbearing women, *Cochrane Database Syst Rev* (8):2013.

Saxton A, Fahy K, Hastie C: Effects of skin-to-skin contact and breastfeeding at birth on the incidence of PPH: a physiologically based theory, *Women Birth* 27(4):250–253, 2014.

Saxton A, Fahy K, Rolfe M, et al: *Does skin-to-skin contact and breastfeeding affect the rate of primary postpartum haemorrhage: results of a cohort study. Midwifery.* (website). http://dx.doi.org/10.1016/j.midw.2015.07.008. 2015.

Schorne MN, Minnick A, Donaghey B: An exploration of how midwives and physicians manage the third stage of labor in the United States, *J Midwifery Womens Health* 60(2):187–198, 2015.

Selfe K, Walsh D: The third stage of labour: are low-risk women really offered an informed choice?, *MIDIRS Midwifery Digest* 25(1):66–71, 2015.

Sheridan V: Organisational culture and routine midwifery practice on labour ward: implications for mother-baby contact, *Evidence Based Midwifery* 8(3):76–84, 2010.

Soltani H: Global implications of evidence 'biased' practice: management of the third stage of labour, *Midwifery* 24(2):138–142, 2008.

Soltani H, Poulose TA, Hutchon DR: Placental cord drainage after spontaneous vaginal delivery as part of the management of the third stage of labour, *Cochrane Database Syst Rev* (9):CD004665, 2011.

Sorbe B: Active pharmacologic management of the third stage of labor, *Obstet Gynecol* 52(6):694–697, 1978.

Spencer PM: Controlled cord traction in management of the third stage of labour, *Br Med J* 1(5294):1728–1732, 1962.

Stanton C, Armbruster D, Knight R, et al: How do physicians and midwives manage the third stage of labour?, *Birth* 35(3):220–229, 2008.

Tan WM, Klein MC, Saxell L, et al: How do physicians and midwives manage the third stage of labour?, *Birth* 35(3):220–229, 2008.

Thilaganathan BCA, Cutner A, Latimer J, et al: Management of the third stage of labour in women at low risk of postpartum haemorrhage, *Eur J Obstet Gynaecol Reprod Biol* 48(1):19–22, 1993.

Torricelli M, Vannuccini S, Moncini I, et al: Anterior placental location influences onset and progress of labor and postpartum outcome, *Placenta* 36(4):463, 2015.

Tuncalp O, Hofmeyr GJ, Hulmezoglu AM: Postaglandins for preventing postpartum haemorrhage, *Cochrane Database Syst Rev* (8):CD000494. 2012.

du Vigneaud V, Ressler C, Tippett S: The sequence of amino acids in oxytocin with a proposal for the structure of oxytocin, *J Biol Chem* 205:949, 1954.

Wickham S: Further thoughts on the third stage, *Pract Midwife* 2(10):14–15, 1999.

Williams C: Should midwives measure blood loss in the fourth stage of labour?, *Br J Midwifery* 22(6):394–398, 2014.

Winter C, Macfarlane A, Deneux-Tharaux C, et al: Variation in policies for management of the third stage of labour and the immediate management of postpartum haemorrhage in Europe, *Br J Obstet Gynaecol* 114(7):845–854, 2007.

World Health Organization (WHO): *WHO recommendations for the prevention of postpartum haemorrhage*, Geneva, WHO (website). http://apps.who.int/iris/bitstream/10665/75411/1/9789241548502_eng.pdf. 2012.

World Health Organization (WHO): *Maternal mortality fact sheet No 348.* (website). www.who.int/mediacentre/factsheets/fs348/en/. 2014.

Yao AC, Lind J: Placental transfusion, *Am J Dis Child* 127(1):128–141, 1974.

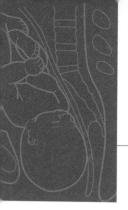

Chapter 40

The pelvic floor

Dr Angie Wilson

Learning Outcomes ?

After reading this chapter, you will be able to:

- develop comprehensive knowledge and understanding of the anatomical structures and function of the pelvic floor in relation to episiotomy, perineal injury, repair and wound healing
- integrate best evidence into clinical practice
- identify factors associated with short- and long-term perineal morbidity
- be familiar with national and employing authorities' guidelines and policies in relation to perineal care and management
- apply statutory, professional and legal principles associated with inadequate or incorrect repair of the perineum

INTRODUCTION AND BACKGROUND

Perineal trauma and subsequent management of the perineum at birth has changed significantly throughout the decades. This change has been in part influenced by the attending accoucheur, changing the role of the midwife and trends in perineal management and repair (Kettle 2005). Midwives are now working with an increasingly well-informed client group, and this is particularly evident as seen in the steady rise in the number of women seeking help and advice in midwifery-run perineal care clinics because of prolonged perineal morbidity or fear of severe perineal trauma occurring in a subsequent birth (Bosan-quet 2010; Dugdale et al 2005; Fitzpatrick et al 2002; Thakar et al 2007; Wilson 2014). In recent years, there has been an identifiable trend towards women requesting an elective caesarean section to avoid pain, severe pelvic floor dysfunction and long-term sexual difficulties (Dahlen

2015; Nerum et al 2006; Sekhon 2010). The midwife plays a pivotal role in normalizing childbirth, working in partnership with women (Nursing and Midwifery Council (NMC) 2015a) and providing high-quality evidence-based care. Part of that role is applying evidence-based knowledge and information for women, and promoting strategies that can minimize perineal trauma during childbirth and the puerperium. This chapter aims to enable the midwife to consider critically, the care and management of the perineum during childbirth to minimize the risk of perineal trauma and its subsequent morbidity.

THE PELVIC FLOOR

The curved shape of the gynaecoid pelvis and funnel-shaped pelvic floor encourages fetal descent into the pelvic cavity. During the mechanism of labour, the fetus adopts a series of rotational movements, which is assisted by the resistance of the pelvic floor (Stein 2009) see Ch. 37 for the mechanism of labour.

Situation and structure

The perineum is situated between the buttocks laterally, the vagina superiorly and anus posteriorly. The pelvic floor, collectively, is all the muscles, nerves, fascia and ligaments that connect the whole and act as a hammock to support the pelvic organs. The pelvic floor is a vital part of the body's core, centre of gravity and power and movement within the skeletal frame. A strong and healthy pelvic floor, therefore, is essential to the positive outcome of childbirth and the woman's health and well-being.

The pelvic floor corresponds to the diamond shape of the pelvic outlet. It resembles a funnel or hammock because of its attachment at various levels of the pelvic outlet. The boundaries of the pelvic outlet on which the muscles and soft tissues are attached are the pubic arch anteriorly, ischial tuberosities, ischiopubic rami and sacrotuberous ligaments laterally and coccyx posteriorly. The pelvic floor is higher posteriorly because of the curve of Carus. In the female, the urethra, vagina and anus pass through this structure. The pelvic floor is subdivided into two triangular parts. An imaginary line can be drawn between the ischial tuberosities, dividing the anterior urogenital and posterior anal triangles. The anterior triangle contains the external urogenital organs and urogenital diaphragm. The posterior triangle contains the anal sphincter complex (Kettle 2005; Tortora et al 2009). At rest, the pelvic floor supports the pelvic organs. When contracted, muscles close the urethra, anus and vagina. With increased intra-abdominal pressure, the pelvic floor muscles contract further to raise the pelvic organs and maintain the support mechanism of the pelvic floor.

The pelvic floor consists of the following six layers, which extend from the uppermost pelvic peritoneum, to the skin of the vulva and external genitalia, perineum and buttocks:

- Pelvic peritoneum
- Endopelvic fascia
- Deep muscles
- Superficial muscles
- Subcutaneous fat
- Skin

Pelvic peritoneum

This is a covering of smooth, thin translucent membrane, which covers the uterus and fallopian tubes. Anteriorly, it forms the uterovesicle pouch, covering the bladder. Posteriorly, it forms the pouch of Douglas.

Endopelvic fascia

Endopelvic fascia is composed of connective tissue, collagen fibres and elastin and is one continuous unit. These compact the space between the pelvic organs and sidewalls of the pelvic cavity (Tortora et al 2009). The function of this connective tissue is to stabilize and provide support to pelvic organs. They become thickened when extra support is needed, forming pelvic ligaments:

- *Transverse cervical ligaments, known as Mackenrodt's, or Cardinal* – attached to the upper vagina, lateral margins of supravaginal cervix and lateral walls of the pelvis
- *Uterosacral ligaments* – attached to the upper vagina fornices, supravaginal cervix and uterus to sacroiliac joint
- *Round ligaments*– attached below the cornua of the uterus and inserted within the labia majus and mons pubis. This ligament maintains the uterus in an anteverted (tilted forwards) and anteflexed (bent back on itself) position

- *Pubocervical ligaments* – attached bilaterally to the inner pubic rami, attached posteriorly to bladder, upper vagina and supravaginal cervix
- *Broad ligaments* – these are folds of peritoneum, which act as ligaments that extend laterally between the uterus and side walls of the pelvis

These ligaments play an important role together with pelvic floor muscles in maintaining support to the uterus. Overstretching may result in pelvic organ prolapse (Smith 2004).

Pelvic floor muscles

Tables 40.1 and 40.2 describe the superficial and deep levator ani muscle layers of the pelvic floor, respectively. Each muscle has its own distinct function, which combined as a whole provides the main strength and function of the pelvic floor. Figure 40.1 illustrates the superficial and deep muscles.

The main functions of the pelvic floor are to:

- Support the bladder, vagina, uterus and rectum, maintaining optimal mechanical orientation of the urethra and angle of the anorectum for continence
- Assist in the process of childbirth and rotation of the presenting part through the mechanism of labour
- Maintain intra-abdominal pressure when laughing, coughing, sneezing, vomiting or lifting heavy objects
- Assist in the process on micturition and defecation
- Aid the mechanism of sexual function and appreciation

Properties of perineal muscle structure

Skeletal, striated muscle fibres function under conscious voluntary control and are strengthened on stimulation. Good muscular control prevents the prolapse of pelvic organs. There are two distinct types of muscle fibres, characterized by two speeds of activity. These are type 1 (slow twitch) fibres and type 2 (fast twitch) fibres (Best et al 1965). See chapter website resources.

The functional characteristics of pelvic floor muscle

- Excitable – twitch muscle fibres contract when stimulated, receive and respond to neurotransmitting chemicals, such as during labour and sexual activity
- Contractile – muscles are able to forcibly stretch when adequately stimulated
- Extensible – during the second stage of labour, the pubococcygeus undergoes the greatest stretch up to 3.26 its original length (Baessler et al 2008; Lien et al 2004)
- Elastic – muscle fibres are able to recoil, resuming their resting length after stretching

The protein collagen provides muscles, tendons and ligaments with their firmness and strength. Elastin and keratin work in conjunction with collagen to provide elasticity;

Table 40.1 Superficial muscles of the pelvic floor

	Description	Origin	Insertion	Innervation	Function
Ischiocavernosus	Bilateral muscles	Arise from the ischial tuberosities, pass upwards and along the pubic arch	Inserted into corpora cavernosa of the clitoris. Some fibres interwoven to unite with membraneous urethral sphincter	Branches of pudendal nerve – 2nd, 3rd and 4th sacral nerve	Assists in maintaining clitoral erection
Bulbospongiosus/ Bulbocavernosus	Encircle the vagina and urethral orifice The Bartholin's glands are situated anteriorly to this muscle and vestibular bulbs beneath	Extend from the central tendon of the perineal body	Inserted anteriorly into the dorsal root of the corpora cavernosa clitoris of the clitoris. Unite with fibres of transverse perinei and borders of anal sphincter	Branches of pudendal nerve 2nd, 3rd and 4th sacral nerve	Initiates erection of clitoris, vaginal contractions and orgasm during sexual activity
Superficial transverse perinei	Traverses the ischial tuberosities to central tendon in perineal body	Arise from ischial tuberosities	Interlocks with bulbospongiosus, border of external sphincter perineal body forming central perineal body	Branches of pudendal nerve 2nd, 3rd and 4th sacral nerve	Provides strength and support to the perineal body
Deep transverse perinei	Traverses the ischial tuberosities	Arise from ischial tuberosities and deep rami	Interlocks with bulbospongiosus, at a deeper level border of external sphincter perineal body forming central perineal body	Branches of pudendal nerve 2nd, 3rd and 4th sacral nerve	Provides collectively, the total strength of the perineal body
Membranous urethral sphincter muscle	Not a true sphincter	Arises from one pubic bone	Encircles urethra and inserts at opposite pubic bone	Posterior labial nerves and dorsal nerve of clitoris	Closes urethra and controls end micturition

External anal sphincter (EAS)

Superficial EAS	Oval shaped circle of muscle surrounding the anus and subdivided into: a. subcutaneous b. superficial c. deep Sultan et al (2007:5-6)	Fuses with bulbocavernosus, transverse perinei anteriorly	Attached to anal coccygeal ligament and tip of coccyx	Inferior rectal branch of pudendal nerve	Keeps anal canal and anus closed Maintains voluntary control of faeces and flatus Contributes to 30% unconscious resting tone
Deep EAS	Circular striated voluntary muscle interwoven with puborectalis posteriorly	Inseparable from puborectalis	Attached to anal coccygeal ligament and tip of coccyx	Inferior rectal branch of pudendal nerve	Keeps anal canal and anus closed Maintains voluntary control of faeces and flatus Contributes to 30% unconscious resting tone

Internal anal sphincter (IAS)

	3-4 cm long and 2-3 mm thick with rounded edge (Sultan et al 2007:6)	Thickened continuation of circular smooth muscle of bowel, 6-8 mm above anal margin at junction of superficial and subcutaneous portion of EAS		Sympathetic lumbar 5 nerve and parasympathetic sacral nerves 2 to 4	Keeps anal canal and anus closed Maintains tonic contraction, preventing involuntary passage of faeces and flatus (vital during sleep) Contributes to 50%-85% resting tone

Table 40.2 Deep muscles of the pelvic floor

LEVATOR ANI	Description	Origin	Insertion	Innervation	Function
Pubococcygeus A broad muscular sheet of paired muscles of variable thickness	Combination of fast and slow twitch muscles	Arise from the inner pubic rami, posterior to bladder, urethra, upper vagina and anal canal	Central tendon of perineal body and anococcygeal body and coccyx	Branches of 3rd and 4th sacrospinous nerves	Provides a strong sling to support the pelvic organs and resists an increase in intra-abdominal pressure when coughing, sneezing and laughing Constricts the anus and contracts during orgasm (Stein 2009:4)
Puborectalis	Pale in colour and fast twitch muscle fibres	Wraps around the ano-rectal junction and forms a sling located beneath the pubococcygeus	Posterior fibres connect with external anal sphincter	Branches of 3rd and 4th sacrospinous nerves	Maintains anterior angle of rectum. Fast twitch muscles control contraction of urethral and anal orifice to maintain continence and are activated during sexual activity
Iliococcygeus	Thin layer of muscle, darker in colour relating to slow twitch muscles (Stein 2009:8) These fill the space from one side wall to the other	Arise from the inner border of white line of fascia on the inner aspects of the iliac bones and ischial spines	Inserted at the midline and inserted posteriorly into anal-coccygeal raphe and coccyx	Branches of 3rd and 4th sacrospinous nerves	Maintains endurance of supportive function through slow twitch muscle activity, which are slow to tire Remains toned when at rest
Ischiococcygeus (coccygeus muscles)	Triangular sheets of muscle and fibrous tissue	Arise from the ischial spine	Pass down to upper coccyx and lower sacral border	Branches of 3rd and 4th sacrospinous nerves	Stabilizes sacroiliac and sacrococcygeal joints

*Obturator internus and piriformis – conduit for pudendal nerve which controls perineal function. (Sourced from: Carola et al 1992, Tortora et al 2009, Verralls 1980.)

however, effectiveness reduces with age (Halperin et al 2010). Collagen can be enhanced through the intake of vitamin C-rich foods (Tortora et al 2009). Women can be encouraged to undertake perineal massage after 34 weeks gestation to boost the production of collagen.

Ischiorectal fossa

The ischiorectal fossa is a deep, fatty wedge-shaped area between the gluteus maximus, anal sphincter, transverse perinei and bulbospongiosus muscles.

Perineal body

The perineal body is a pyramid-shaped mass of fibro-muscular tissue that is also referred to as the central tendon. It intersects the levator ani; pubococcygeus deep and superficial transverse perinei; bulbospongiosus and external anal sphincter muscles. It is the central point separating the urogenital and anal triangles between the vagina and anus and ischial tuberosities laterally, with the rectovaginal septum at the apex. The perineal body provides total strength to the pelvic floor. The triangle measures approximately 3.5 cm in length on each side. The perineal body may be damaged during labour through stretching, tearing or an episiotomy (Hamilton-Fairley 2009). Blood is supplied via the pudendal arteries and venous return is via the corresponding veins. Lymphatic drainage enters the inguinal and external iliac glands. Nerve supply is via the perineal branch of the pudendal nerve.

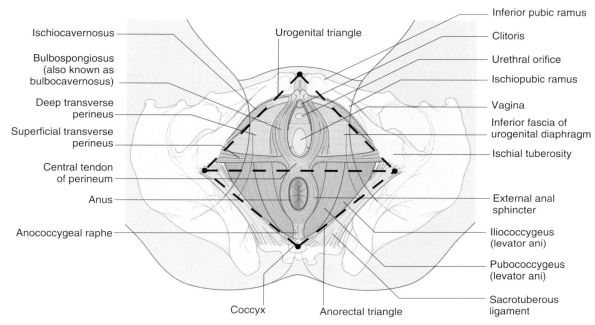

Figure 40.1 Superficial and deep muscles identifying urogenital and anogenital triangles.

Labels (clockwise):

- Ischiocavernosus
- Bulbospongiosus (also known as bulbocavernosus)
- Deep transverse perineus
- Superficial transverse perineus
- Central tendon of perineum
- Anus
- Anococcygeal raphe
- Coccyx
- Urogenital triangle
- Anorectal triangle
- Inferior pubic ramus
- Clitoris
- Urethral orifice
- Ischiopubic ramus
- Vagina
- Inferior fascia of urogenital diaphragm
- Ischial tuberosity
- External anal sphincter
- Iliococcygeus (levator ani)
- Pubococcygeus (levator ani)
- Sacrotuberous ligament

Blood, lymph and nerve supply

Branches of the internal iliac arteries supply blood to the muscles of the pelvic floor and venous return is via corresponding veins. Lymph drains into the internal iliac glands. Innervation is via the pudendal nerve and 3rd and 4th nerves of the sacral plexus.

Fat

Excessive fat may impose extra stress and pressure on the pelvic floor.

Skin

Elasticity of perineal skin is influenced by the amount of collagen in underlying connective tissue. The extent of striae gravidarum noted during pregnancy is a useful, non-invasive measure to determine the woman's elastic skin index and how well the perineum will stretch during labour (Halperin et al 2010; Magdi 1949).

CONSIDERATIONS FOR MIDWIFERY PRACTICE

Changes during pregnancy

- *relaxin*, together with an increased blood supply, modifies connective tissue and collagen, providing greater elasticity and stretching of the muscles, and ligaments of the pelvic floor to facilitate the birth of the baby during vaginal delivery (Baessler et al 2008)
- *progesterone* diminishes smooth-muscle tone and support to the ureters, bladder and urethra
- increased body mass index (BMI) has been shown to correlate with increased intraabdominal pressure, which may predispose to stress urinary incontinence during pregnancy and in later life (Morkved 2007)

Changes during labour and delivery

- during fetal descent into the pelvis, the pelvic floor muscles become displaced, pushing the bladder upwards towards the symphysis pubis. Changes occur despite mode of delivery
- the presenting part meets the resistance of the U-shaped pelvic floor and rotates towards the symphysis pubis during the mechanism of labour
- flexion of the fetal head is affected by poor uterine contractibility and perineal muscle tone, which can result in malposition
- the fetal head causes normal stretching and distension to pelvic floor muscles and connective tissue, adding pressure on the pudendal nerve
- the bulbocavernosus, pubococcygeus and puborectalis muscles are distended and thinned posteriorly to

minimize perineal trauma. These muscles can stretch up to 3.26 times the muscles' original lengths (Lien et al 2004)

Changes during the puerperium

- after delivery, the pelvic floor resumes its original supporting function because of its contractibility and elasticity
- recovery and future integrity of the pelvic floor is dependent on the length of labour and the degree of damage and tissue repair during the months after delivery (Lavin et al 1996)

A prolonged labour with repeated and excessive stretching to the pelvic floor and pudendal nerve can result in loss of tone, elasticity and nerve damage (Sultan et al 1994a). This presents the highest risk for stretch-related injury and subsequent problems associated with urinary incontinence postpartum and pelvic organ prolapse in later life (Haadem et al 1991).

Understanding the mechanism of labour and the capacity of the pelvic floor to stretch during the second stage of labour is an important consideration for the midwife. Close observation of the slowly distending perineum and emerging fetal head will enable the midwife to develop confidence and competence in their ability to assist the woman in birthing their baby with minimal intervention and trauma.

PERINEAL TRAUMA

Definition

Obstetric perineal trauma is any damage to the genitalia during childbirth. It occurs spontaneously or intentionally by a surgical incision (episiotomy) (Kettle 2004). Trauma includes bruising, grazing, tearing, stretching or indirectly by denervation injury (Pregazzi et al 2002).

Approximately 350,000 (85%) women in the UK annually will sustain some degree of perineal trauma. Of these women, 65% to 75% women will require perineal repair after birth (Ismail et al 2013; Kettle et al 2002; Morris et al 2013; Willer et al 2014). Lack of recognition, accurate assessment and repair after delivery can result in long-term physical and psychological morbidity, such as pain, stress urinary or anal incontinence, dyspareunia or some degree of sexual difficulties (Andrews et al 2005a; Bick et al 2012; Moore et al 2013; Pergialiotis et al 2014; Reid et al 2014; Williams et al 2007). These disabilities can have a significant effect on women's breastfeeding success and attachment to the new baby, sexual relations with their partner and the adaptation to family life in the early puerperium and long term (Andrews et al 2005a; Kettle et al 2002; MacArthur et al 2001; Sultan et al 1994a).

Types of trauma

Trauma can occur spontaneously during vaginal birth or after an episiotomy. Trauma can be divided into anterior or posterior perineal trauma. Anterior trauma is defined as injury to the labia, anterior vaginal wall, urethra or clitoris. Maternal morbidity is minimal in these areas of trauma. Posterior trauma includes injury to the posterior vaginal wall, perineal muscles and/or anal sphincter complex (Spendlove 2005). Severe perineal trauma (SPT) during vaginal birth can occur naturally or as a result of obstetric intervention. This type of trauma is defined as a third or fourth degree tear, also referred to as obstetric anal sphincter injuries (OASIS) (Andrews et al 2006a). The incidence varies internationally and ranges between 0.5% to 17.3% of vaginal births, depending on level of obstetric intervention (Organisation for Economic Cooperation and Development (OECD) 2013). These injuries are associated with increased maternal morbidity (Dahlen 2015: 697; Priddis et al 2013).

Classification of trauma

Spontaneous trauma has been classified as follows:

- **First degree tear** – injury to anterior or posterior vaginal epithelium, perineal skin or vaginal mucosa
- **Second degree tear** – injury to superficial perineal muscles: bulbocavernosus and transverse perinei; perineal body. Deeper trauma involves the pubococcygeus and puborectalis muscles
- **Third degree tear** – injury to the perineum, involving the anal sphincter muscles, subdivided into:
  - 3a – less than 50% of external anal sphincter thickness torn
  - 3b – more than 50% of external anal sphincter torn
  - 3c – internal anal sphincter torn
- **Fourth degree tear** – injury to the perineum, involving the anal sphincter muscles (external and internal anal sphincter) and anal epithelium

Classifications of third and fourth degree tears. (National Institute for Health and Care Excellence (NICE) Intrapartum Care 2014, Royal College of Obstetricians and Gynaecologists (RCOG) 2015a, Sultan et al 2007:14.) See Fig. 40.2.

All practitioners caring for women with perineal trauma need to be familiar with the trauma classifications mentioned so that an accurate assessment of the type of trauma is identified and managed appropriately after a vaginal delivery.

Labial tears or lacerations

Labial tears are classified as a superficial graze or as deep tears. They can occur unilaterally or bilaterally.

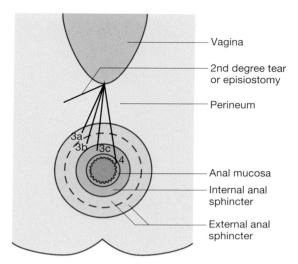

Figure 40.2 Position of a second, third and fourth degree tear/episiotomy.

Vagina

2nd degree tear or episiostomy

Perineum

Anal mucosa

Internal anal sphincter

External anal sphincter

Clitoral and periurethral tears

Clitoral and periurethral tears are rare but extremely painful and are more likely to be associated with a wider presenting diameter of the fetal head at birth with a malposition, such as persistent occipitoposterior position.

Cervical tears

Cervical tears may be caused during the second stage of labour when the woman forcibly pushes before the cervix is completely dilated, during a forceps or ventouse delivery before the cervix is fully dilated, because of multiple births or internal manoeuvres for shoulder dystocia. Severe bleeding is likely and may lead to a postpartum haemorrhage (PPH).

Prevalence of perineal trauma

Obstetric perineal trauma has been reported by the UK Government Statistical Service for the Department of Health (GSSDH) as the most common complication of childbirth occurring in 48% of vaginal deliveries (Gillard et al 2010). The *Hospital Episodes Maternity Statistics 2013–2014* (Health and Social Care Centre 2015) identified that the main complication in delivery episodes was because of 'perineal lacerations', occurring in 56% women. During this period, 74% women experienced significant perineal trauma. It is difficult, however, to establish the true incidence of perineal trauma internationally because of the wide variance in reported obstetric and midwifery practice and the multivariable factors, which contribute to trauma. For example, the rate and angle of the episiotomy and the type of instrumental delivery that influences reported

outcomes between studies. Careful and critical analysis is also required when evaluating perineal outcomes between primiparous and multiparous women, births at home and midwifery-led units and hospital settings. An absence of international trauma classification reported in some studies makes comparability difficult. Midwives' and obstetricians' philosophies and experience will influence perineal management and care specifically during labour and further internationally. In countries where there is predominantly obstetric led care, such as in South America and the Middle and Far East, episiotomy rates may exceed 70% regardless of parity, which increases SPT rates (da Silva et al 2012). In obstetric units where there is liberal use of episiotomy, the rate of women requiring repair can be as high as 85% to 90% in Eastern Europe (Hospital Episodes Statistics (HES 2012)). Performance of midline or medio-lateral episiotomy, assisted by an instrumental delivery, increases perineal trauma rates with variations between and within countries. An estimated 4 million (50%) childbearing women in the US receive an episiotomy, and an additional 28% require perineal repair for spontaneous lacerations (Renfrew et al 1998). In contrast, in Australia, as few as 13.4% women receive an episiotomy and 28% women have an intact perineum (Dahlen 2015: 694). The rate of SPT after an instrumental delivery (both forceps and vacuum) shows high variations across countries. Reported rates vary from under 2% in Poland, Israel, Italy, Slovenia and Portugal to 3.5% in Finland and 7.1% in the UK, Switzerland and New Zealand, 7.3% and 11.1% in the US. Rates higher than 17% have been reported in Canada and Denmark. Rates of SPT without instrumental delivery internationally are considerably less but still show equally wide variations between the two indicators, from less than 0.1% in Poland, 0.7% in Finland, 1.5% in the US, 2.2% to 5% in Australia and UK, respectively, and 3.1% to 3.7% in Canada, Denmark, Sweden and Switzerland, respectively (OECD 2013). Individual management strategies need to be clearly identified, reporting logistic regression analysis among women in study variables to understand why some countries report higher rates than others. In Brazil, 98.4% of multiparous women are reported to have 'mild' perineal trauma, sustaining first and second degree tears (combined classifications) and 1.6% sustaining SPT. Among primiparous women, 95.8% are reported to have first and second degree tears, with 4.2% sustaining SPT (Oliveira et al 2014).

Trauma rates vary internationally, with in-home birth or freestanding units compared with hospital care. Smith et al (2013) reported intact perineum rates of 9.6% (125 out of a group of 1302 nulliparous women) and 31% (453 out of 1452 multiparous women), with higher incidences in the home setting or freestanding midwifery-led units in southeast England. In addition, there was a lower incidence of OASIS and fewer second degree tears sutured in the community, compared with the hospital setting.

Similar findings were reported by Lindgren et al (2008) in Sweden, whereby the risk of sustaining perineal trauma, including a sphincter tear, was lower in the planned home birth group. Taking a low risk population into account, it is important that perineal trauma rates are drawn from primiparous and multiparous women in both the hospital and community settings and evaluated and reported separately.

Standardized classifications and guidelines of perineal trauma (RCOG 2007 and 2015) and levels of competency in midwives and obstetricians may contribute to variations in perineal trauma rates, although labial and clitoral tears/grazes are not classified currently. Underreporting in clinical practice, because of the risk of litigation, may be reflected in study statistics or may be associated with nonreferral to international classifications of perineal trauma in clinical trials. Misdiagnosis or misinterpretation of classifications of trauma may lead to inconsistency and reliability of coding and reporting in clinical practice.

Changes in perineal management that embrace high standards of evidence-based practice, alongside highly competent midwives and obstetricians, has provided a useful indicator of the quality of obstetric and midwifery care reported in European countries in relation to SPT (Hals et al 2010; OECD 2013).

Short- and long-term effects of perineal trauma

Pain and infection continues to be the major cause of short- and long-term morbidity for women (Bick et al 2012; Glazener et al 1995; MacArthur et al 2004). Stress urinary or anal incontinence, which is largely underreported, can result from relaxed pelvic floor muscles, denervation or more severe trauma (East et al 2009; Leeman et al 2009). Dyspareunia and sexual difficulties are not uncommon, with up to 53% women having difficulties at 8 weeks postdelivery, and 49% still having problems at 12 to 18 months (Buhling et al 2006; Glazener 1997; Sayasneh et al 2010; Williams et al 2007; Wu et al 2007).

Risk factors associated with perineal trauma

Predisposing risk factors need to be viewed independently and in conjunction with the woman's obstetric history. Interventions in labour and delivery will compound existing predisposing risk factors. The aim is to minimize these in the first instance.

Maternal risk factors include

- Nulliparity (up to 4%)
- Maternal age, very young and older women
- Tissue type – elastin index or abnormal collagen synthesis
- Asian ethnicity – pelvic floor anatomy, e.g. short perineum

Associated risk factors:

- Induction of labour and oxytocin augmentation
- Precipitate labour
- Prolonged second stage of labour greater than 1 hour
- Malposition – persistent occipito-posterior or transverse position
- Birthweight over 4000 kg and male gender
- Epidural analgesia
- Instrumental delivery, forceps specifically
- Episiotomy, leading to extension
- Midline or medio-lateral episiotomies, with postdelivery angles of less than 30 and greater than 60 degrees linked to OASIS
- Directed pushing (Valsalva manoeuvre) during second stage of labour
- Previous OASIS
- Shoulder dystocia, associated with episiotomy and internal manoeuvres
- Accoucheur
- Poor nutritional status
- Smoking – affecting wound healing through poor vasoconstriction and tissue ischemia
- Female genital mutilation (Type 11 or 111)

RCOG (2015a; Dahlen 2007a: 699; Thakar and Sultan 2005). For full references see website.

MIDWIVES' DUTIES AND RESPONSIBILITIES

All midwives have a duty of care and responsibility to ensure all women receive evidence-based information and advice in their pregnancy about how they can minimize perineal trauma at their birth. Women who have experienced severe or problematic perineal trauma previously should be identified early in pregnancy and offered an appointment to visit the specialist perineal care midwife or consultant obstetrician for perineal assessment and an individualized care pathway and perineal care plan. A patient information leaflet provided by the RCOG (2015b) – 'Information for You' – is clearly set out for women who have experienced a third or fourth degree tear. This can be helpful to support the discussion and provide information so that the woman can make a fully informed choice regarding elective caesarean section or vaginal delivery. It is also important that women who have *female genital mutilation* (FGM) and who may require de-infibulation are identified early in their pregnancy for optimum maternal and neonatal outcomes (Royal College of Midwives

(RCM) et al 2013) (see Ch. 56). It is now mandatory that all women who have a history of FGM and those being treated are identified and have their details recorded for the purposes of FGM prevalence data set statistics in England (Department of Health (DH) 2015).

An audit of women's level of satisfaction of a one-to-one consultation at a perineal care clinic, including mode of delivery and severity of perineal trauma, identified that women found the discussion an empowering experience. They disclosed that partnerships were enhanced with their midwife in labour. Fewer women requested caesarean section, and there was a reduction in the incidence of SPT as classified by the RCOG (2007) (Wilson 2014).

Interventions that may prevent or minimize perineal trauma

The following interventions have shown to enhance maternal comfort or reduce the incidence of perineal trauma at birth and during the puerperium.

- Perineal massage at 34 weeks gestation (Beckmann et al 2013). (See chapter website resources for details)
- Mobilization during labour and adopting an upright, lateral position during delivery reduces incidence of epidural anaesthesia and instrumental deliveries (Baker 2010; Meyvis et al 2012; Pearson 2012; RCM 2010; Shorten et al 2002)
- Spontaneous pushing during the second stage of labour (Albers et al 2005; Laine et al 2012; Prins et al 2011; Sampselle et al 2010)
- Warm compresses to the perineum during the second stage of labour, resulting in significantly reduced risk of third and fourth degree tears (Aasheim and Nilson 2012; Albers et al 2005; Dahlen et al 2007; RCOG 2015a). (See chapter website resources for further details)
- 'Hands on' perineal support and protection at crowning (Hals et al 2010; Laine et al 2012; RCOG 2015a)
- Continuous support, and working in partnership with midwife using good communication and compassionate care (Dahlen 2015)
- Birth at home or in a birth centre
- 'Breathing' the head out between contractions (Albers et al 2005).
- Restricted episiotomy and preference for vacuum extraction, if required (Dahlen 2015)
- Assessment of perineal trauma at delivery including bidigital anal sphincter assessment (Andrews et al 2006; NICE 2014; Stevenson 2010; Sultan et al 2007)

- Repair of all second degree perineal trauma (Kettle et al 2002 and Kettle 2004; NICE 2014). See key practice points Fig. 40.3

Interventions that require further research or remain controversial:

- Pelvic floor muscle training (PFMT) and pelvic floor exercises (PFEs) (Boyle et al 2012)
- Water emersion for delivery (Cortes et al 2011: 27; Harper 2000)
- Restricted mediolateral episiotomy when performed, at wider angle of 60 degrees (Freeman et al 2014; Kalis et al 2011; Stedenfeldt et al 2012)
- 'Hands on' or 'hands poised' (Aasheim and Nilson 2012: 4; Laine et al 2012; McCandlish et al 1998). (See chapter website resources for further details)
- *Elastolabo* (Reggiardo et al 2012)

The National Institute of Health and Care Excellence Intrapartum Care Pathway (NICE 2014: 5) recommends:

'Either the "hands on" (guarding the perineum and flexing the baby's head) or the "hands poised" (with hands off the perineum and baby's head but in readiness) technique can be used to facilitate spontaneous birth'.

However, the RCOG (2015a) advocates manual perineal protection/'hands on' technique to reduce the incidence of OASIS (Hals et al 2010; Laine et al 2012). This includes:

- Using the left hand to slow down the delivery of the head
- Using the right hand protecting the perineum
- The woman not pushing when the head is crowning
- Clear rationale for episiotomy in risk groups and performance of correct angle

No sound evidence available

- Perineal stretching devices – Epi-no (Kovacs et al 2004; Ruckharberle et al 2009)
- Perineal ice packs in the second stage of labour (Dahlen 2007b)

See chapter website resources for video – 'Hands on or poised'

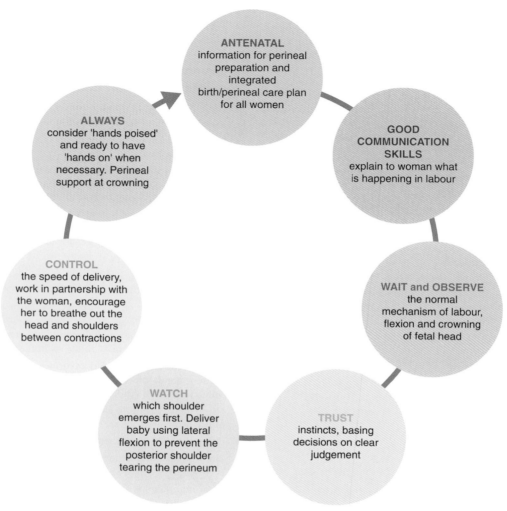

ANTENATAL information for perineal preparation and integrated birth/perineal care plan for all women

GOOD COMMUNICATION SKILLS explain to woman what is happening in labour

WAIT and OBSERVE the normal mechanism of labour, flexion and crowning of fetal head

TRUST instincts, basing decisions on clear judgement

WATCH which shoulder emerges first. Deliver baby using lateral flexion to prevent the posterior shoulder tearing the perineum

CONTROL the speed of delivery, work in partnership with the woman, encourage her to breathe out the head and shoulders between contractions

ALWAYS consider 'hands poised' and ready to have 'hands on' when necessary. Perineal support at crowning

Figure 40.3 Key practice points.

EPISIOTOMY (SURGICAL INCISION)

An episiotomy is a 'surgical incision through the perineum and perineal body during the last part of the second stage of labour, beginning in the perineal midline but directed laterally at an angle of at least 60 degrees in the direction of the ischial tuberosity' (Kalis 2011: 223). It is undertaken to enlarge the diameter of the vulval outlet to facilitate a vaginal delivery (Kalis et al 2011; NICE 2014). (See Fig. 40.2.)

There are three types of incision:

Right mediolateral:

- The incision line commences from the vaginal fourchette in the midline, which avoids cutting into the Bartholin's gland.

- Directed from the midline, and laterally at an angle of at least 45 to 60 degrees in the direction of the right ischial tuberosity.

Midline (median, medial):

- The incision commences at the vaginal fourchette and directed along the midline through the central tendon of the perineal body.

Anterior de-infibulation for women with female genital mutilation:

- An anterior incision for Type 111 FGM. Performed during the late second stage of labour. The practitioner's forefinger is inserted into the introitus and directed towards the pubis (see Fig. 40.4).

- An incision is made anteriorly, along the line of the finger to free scar tissue and fused labia towards the urinary meatus. A mediolateral episiotomy may also be required. See Figure 40.5 for how to perform a right medio-lateral episiotomy.

Midline incisions are no longer performed in the UK because of the high incidence of anal sphincter injuries

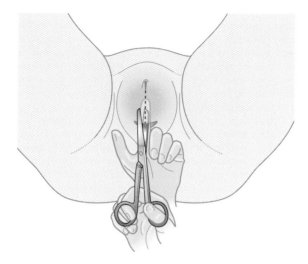

Figure 40.4 Anterior incision for Type 111 FGM.

(ASI) (Kalis et al 2011 and 2012; Stedenfeldt et al 2012; Tincello et al 2003). Mediolateral episiotomy is now the UK standard because of the reduced incidence of OASIS when directed 45 to 60 degrees away from the perineal midline (Andrews et al 2005a; NICE 2014; Revicky et al 2010; Silf et al 2015). A 60 degree episiotomy from the centre of the introitus results in a postdelivery and suture angle of 45 degrees (Kalis et al 2011). Eogan et al (2006) have demonstrated in their small case control study of 100 women that there was a 50% relative reduction in the risk of a woman sustaining a third degree tear for every 6 degrees away from the perineal midline that an episiotomy was performed. Clinical updates for doctors, midwives and student midwives is essential to familiarize them with the recommended incision angle of 60 degrees.

Structures involved in an episiotomy

An episiotomy is equivalent to a second degree tear. Structures include the perineal skin, bulbospongiosus, transverse perinei and pubococcygeus. The puborectalis is involved if a deep incision is made. The difference between a second degree tear and episiotomy is in the pathway of the trauma. An episiotomy cuts through muscle fibres, nerves and other structures. A tear works around these structures, following a natural pathway, which is why this

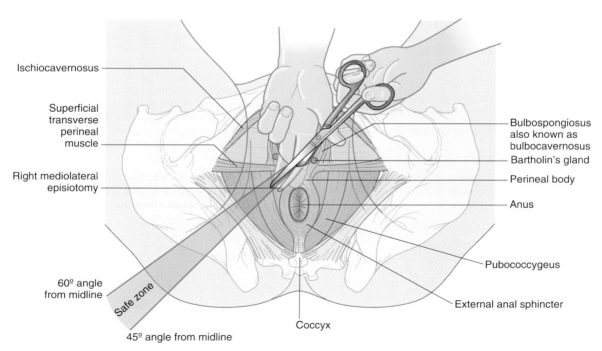

Figure 40.5 A diagrammatic representation of a right mediolateral episiotomy directed at a 60 degree angle, identifying the muscles involved when the incision is made.

type of trauma may be less painful than an episiotomy (Dahlen 2015: 702).

Episiotomy rate

Episiotomy rates vary considerably on an international and national level because of individual practice, experience and continuing controversial views related to the benefits and risks of the procedure. Rates vary between countries from 14% in England, 13.4% in Australia, 50% in the United States, 91% in Thailand and 99% in Eastern Europe (HES 2011), with Finland demonstrating the lowest figures of 5% (Dahlen 2015; Raisanen et al 2010; Trinh et al 2015). Higher episiotomy rates have been associated with anal sphincter tears (Kalis et al 2011; Raisanen et al 2010; Renfrew et al 1998). The recommended rate of episiotomy advocated is 10% (World Health Organisation (WHO) 1996).

Indications

Restricted use of episiotomy is recommended because of the risks of the procedure and limited benefits of its liberal use (Lappen et al 2010; Melo et al 2014; Sleep et al 1984). Episiotomy should be restricted to:

- situations when there is a nonreassuring fetal heart rate with early or late decelerations
- facilitate instrumental delivery (specifically forceps)
- malpresentation or malposition of fetal head because of wider diameters or lack of moulding with face presentation
- vaginal breech with forceps for the after-coming head
- a rigid, thick and inelastic perineum that will not stretch, causing delay in the second stage of labour
- assist with shoulder dystocia for internal manoeuvres, if necessary
- those affected by FGM (Type 111)
- excessive vaginal and perineal scar tissue after reconstructive vaginal surgery
- maternal request
- prolonged second stage of labour (Robinson et al 2000)
- 'button holing' of the perineum

(NICE 2014, RCOG 2012)

Contraindications

- inflammatory bowel disease
- perineal malformation
- coagulation disorders
- the woman's refusal to have the procedure performed

When to make the incision

The rationale and decision for performing an episiotomy must be based on strong clinical evidence and good clinical judgement (NMC Code 2015). Informed consent from the woman must be sought at all times (NMC 2015). Effective analgesia must be provided before the procedure, except in an emergency when there is acute fetal compromise (NICE 2014). Straight or curved blunt-ended Mayo episiotomy scissors are used to protect the fetal head at the time of incision. The incision should only be made when the presenting part is distending the perineum; failure to do this will fail to accelerate the delivery and lead to excessive blood loss.

Preparation includes the delivery trolley being laid according to local protocol. Correct safety precautions and avoiding needlestick injury are essential. Use of personal protective equipment (PPE), including sterile gloves, need to be carried out in accordance with the local Standard Infection Control to protect the practitioner from HIV and hepatitis infection. *Lidocaine* for perineal infiltration before episiotomy is used in accordance with Patient Group Directives under Standards for Medicine Management (NMC 2010). See Table 40.3 for instructions for perineal infiltration and right-mediolateral episiotomy. The woman's comfort and dignity must be maintained throughout the procedure.

Risks associated with episiotomy

Episiotomy and instrumental delivery (forceps) is associated with an increased incidence of OASIS because of the spontaneous extension of the incision (Dahlen et al 2015; Mullally et al 2011). Dyspareunia and sexual dysfunction is increased in women after an episiotomy (Rathfisch et al 2010) compared with women with spontaneous lacerations (Carroli and Mignini 2009; Sleep et al 1984; Raisanen et al 2010). Rates of HIV transmission to the neonate may be increased as a result of increased blood loss (Siegfried et al 2011).

Complications

- Injury to the Bartholin's gland and possible cyst formation
- Extension of the episiotomy to a third or fourth degree tear
- Complex repair
- Excessive blood loss and potential PPH associated with instrumental delivery
- Wound infection and dehiscence
- Haematoma formation at time of repair
- Increased need for analgesia on day 10
- Decreased vaginal lubrication, postpartum dyspareunia and sexual difficulties

Table 40.3 Procedure for perineal infiltration and right mediolateral episiotomy

Action	Rationale
1. Explain the rationale and procedure to the woman and her partner. *Only undertake the procedure when the presenting part is distending the perineum, to thin out perineal muscles	1. To reassure the woman and confirm consent To prevent excessive blood loss and deep perineal damage
2. Place the woman in a comfortable position with her legs open	2. To ensure that the whole perineal area is accessible
3. Cleanse the perineal area using the agreed aseptic technique	3. To minimize infection
Infiltration before episiotomy 4. Place the less dominant index and middle fingers into the vagina between the presenting part and perineum. Insert the needle fully into the perineal tissue, starting at the centre of the fourchette and directing it midway between the ischial tuberosity and anus in a 'fan' shape. Aim to infiltrate between 20 and 90 degrees	4. To protect the baby from accidental damage To provide maximum analgesia for incision
5. Draw back the plunger of the syringe before injecting 5–10 mL of local anaesthetic, 1% *lidocaine,* slowly into the tissue as the needle is withdrawn Wait 1–2 minutes before incision, if time permits	5. To check that the *lidocaine* is not accidentally injected into a blood vessel and to provide effective anaesthesia to facilitate a pain-free incision
6. Insert the middle and index fingers into the vagina and gently pull the perineum away from the presenting fetal part	6. To protect the presenting fetal part from accidental damage
7. Perform the incision when the presenting part has distended the perineum	7. To minimize pain and blood loss
8. Insert the open scissors between the two fingers and make the incision in one single cut, ideally at the height of a contraction to minimize discomfort	8. To ensure a straight cut, minimize severe perineal damage and facilitate optimum anatomical realignment
9. Perform the incision – it should extend at least 3–4 cm into the perineum. The incision should start midline from the centre of the fourchette and then extend outwards in a mediolateral direction at a 60 degree angle towards the right ischial tuberosity, avoiding the anal sphincter(s). Withdraw the scissors carefully	9. To increase the vulval outlet, facilitate delivery and minimize the risk of anal sphincter injury
10. Control delivery of the presenting part and shoulders	10. To prevent sudden expulsion of the presenting part and extension of the episiotomy incision
11. Apply pressure to the episiotomy incision between contractions if there is a delay in delivering the baby	11. To control bleeding from the wound
12. Thoroughly inspect the vagina and perineum, including a rectal examination, after completion of the third stage of labour	12. To identify the extent of trauma before repair
13. Record episiotomy in woman's case notes together with clear rationale	13. Complies with Midwives Code (2015) of good practice and safeguards against litigation

Adapted from Kettle (2011)

- Necrotizing fasciitis is a rare but potential fatal consequence of episiotomy
- Excessive perineal scar tissue

(Mullally et al 2011).

The 'unkindest cut'

Women's negative experience of episiotomy has left them with feelings of revulsion, fear and anger. The incision has been described as the 'unkindest cut of all' (Kitzinger et al 1981 and 1986), and remains one of the most commonly performed surgical procedures globally (Silf et al 2015). The resultant scar and experience can have a major effect on the woman's body image and self-worth, affecting their psychological and physical well-being (Way 1996), including their sexuality. (See Ch. 13.)

Reported benefits of episiotomy have included the prevention of severe lacerations, pelvic floor relaxation and fetal injury (Woolley 1995). Episiotomy may afford protection to nulliparous women from anal sphincter injury and prevent faecal incontinence because of the inelasticity of their perineal muscles (Poen et al 1997). Bertozzi et al (2011) reports lower scores for dyspareunia, stress and urge urinary incontinence and better personal and sexual relationships, sleep energy and emotions at twelve months for both primiparous and multiparous women after episiotomy. A systematic Cochrane review of episiotomy (Carroli and Mignini 2009) has since identified that a restricted policy prevents less SPT such as OASIS, results in less suturing by 30% and fewer healing complications at 7 days' postpartum, reducing associated risks and morbidity by 12% to 31%. Episiotomy has also been associated with delayed wound healing and increased pain in the first 10 postnatal days (Klein et al 1994; Williams et al 2007). Secondary benefits with a restricted policy include increased bonding and restoration of a normal sex life (Wu et al 2013). However, clinicians should explain to women that the evidence for the protective effect of episiotomy remains conflicting (RCOG 2015a).

A restricted policy of episiotomy was introduced in the UK in 1986 as a result of two major studies undertaken by Sleep et al (1984) and the Argentine Episiotomy Trial Collaborative Group (1993). The outcomes revealed that there were no statistical differences in maternal or neonatal outcomes between groups of women when a restricted or liberal policy was implemented in labour. As a result, WHO (1996) stated that the systematic use of episiotomy was unjustified. A Randomized Controlled Trial (RCT) is currently being proposed by Melo et al (2014) to investigate selective episiotomy versus no episiotomy, and these results will be of interest to review. The judicious use of episiotomy among practitioners will inevitably make a substantial difference to future episiotomy rates with improved perineal morbidity. With the reduction in the rate of episiotomies performed by midwives and doctors, student midwives need to observe this procedure being undertaken, attend in-service training and practise the procedure using a bespoke training model, such as the Keele and Staffs Episiotomy Repair Trainer (Limbs and Things, UK 2015). Despite the integration of episiotomy practise with perineal repair workshops, Silf et al (2015) report wide variations in both midwives' and doctors' predictions and performance of a right mediolateral episiotomy performed at a 60 degree angle. Results were collected from an audit of practice and multiprofessional workshops held at a national midwifery conference in the UK. Similar findings are reported by Wong et al (2014), whereby the predicted degree of incision was performed 8 degrees closer to the midline. Results demonstrated that, despite training, the angle of incision is very subjective to the individual practitioner. The introduction of the *Episcissors-60*, an instrument with a fixed marker guide of an angle of 60 degrees, enables the practitioner to cut an accurate angle when the fetal head has distended the perineum, ensuring a postdelivery angle of 43 degrees (Freeman et al 2014). This tool is currently being piloted in a local National Health Service (NHS) Trust (personal communication) and would replace 'eyeballing' the current angle of incision (see website for history of episiotomy).

Reflective activity 40.2 ><

From observation in clinical practice, reflect on the rationale provided by the midwife or doctor for undertaking an episiotomy. Was it justified? What was the angle of incision? What was the classification of perineal trauma?

THE PRINCIPLES OF PERINEAL REPAIR

Initiation into episiotomy and perineal repair have been integrated into midwifery programmes since 1983 (NMC 2009) and formally reiterated in the European Union Directives 80/154/EEC and 80/155/EEC (Wallace 2001). Episiotomy and perineal repair falls within the scope of midwifery practice (International Confederation of Midwives (ICM) 2013).

The principles of repair are to achieve haemostasis and anatomical integrity, restoring the perineal muscles to their prepregnancy function by primary intention healing. The true incidence of the type of perineal trauma sustained is often difficult to estimate because of incomplete or inaccurate assessment and classification of the trauma, lack of anatomical knowledge, confidence, expertise or training of both midwives and doctors (Andrews et al 2006b; Bick et al 2012; Morris et al 2013).

Perineal pain is the most frequently reported complication after repair, and its severity may be associated with the gravity of the trauma (MacArthur et al 2004). Levels of pain also vary, depending on whether the tear is repaired or left to heal naturally. The competence of the practitioner, choice of technique and materials chosen to undertake the repair can also influence pain levels and will therefore make a substantial difference to the woman's comfort after the repair (Kettle et al 2002).

Methods and materials for repair

It was traditional for the majority of midwives to repair perineal trauma, adopting a locking stitch to the vaginal wall and an interrupted technique to the muscle layer and perineal skin. Midwives' choice of this method of repair has largely stemmed from their initial instruction, experience, ease of removal if stitches are too tight, and not feeling confident using a continuous technique (Wilson 2009). The current recommendations advocate a continuous technique of perineal repair using a rapidly absorbable suture material, such as *Vicryl Rapide* (RCOG 2007; NICE 2014). Comparing continuous versus an interrupted repair technique with standard or rapidly absorbed suture material shows that significantly fewer women reported pain at 10 days with the continuous technique. However, there was no difference in superficial dyspareunia reported at 3 months using either technique, using standard or rapidly absorbed suture material. However, the need for suture removal was significantly less with the continuous technique using the rapidly absorbed suture material (Kettle et al 2002). Similar findings were reported by Fleming (1990), Gemynthe et al (1996) and Olah (1994).

Two-stage technique leaving perineal skin unsutured

A two-stage repair technique, leaving the perineal skin unsutured, has been compared with the traditional repair in three layers in the Ipswich Childbirth Study (Gordon et al 1998). Findings demonstrated there was no difference in perineal pain at 24 or 48 hours and 10 days, no difference in the number of wound dehiscence and fewer women reporting tight stitches in the two-stage technique. At 3 months' postpartum, fewer women reported pain and were able to resume pain-free intercourse using the two-stage technique. In a follow-up study 1 year later, fewer women reported the perineum as feeling different from before the delivery (Grant et al 2001). Similar findings were reported by Oboro et al (2003) in a multicentre evaluation in Nigeria. However, the rate of clinically assessed gaping of the perineum was higher in the two-layer technique at 48 hours.

'To suture or not to suture' second degree perineal tears?

There is still debate among some midwives and women as to whether to suture or leave a tear to heal naturally. A small RCT undertaken by Lundquist et al (2000) found that minor perineal lacerations – those not bleeding and not extending 2×2 cm – healed as well as lacerations repaired. A further small RCT undertaken by Fleming et al (2003), comparing suturing versus nonsuturing of first and second degree tears indicated that there was no significant difference between the types of management in terms of perineal pain or depression. However, women in the nonsutured group experienced slower wound healing at 6 weeks. High levels of morbidity, such as increased urinary frequency at 10 days and an increased rate of self-referral for perineal problems and higher postnatal Edinburgh depression scores at 12 months, were found in the nonsutured group. There was no difference in reported pain (Metcalfe et al 2006). It is important, therefore, to consider other outcomes in addition to levels of pain. Small qualitative studies, reporting women's experiences, have identified that perineal repair can be a negative experience for some women recalling these as barbaric and horrific (Clement et al 1999; Head 1993; Salmon 1999). Midwives have a responsibility and are accountable to the women in their care to act as their advocate, providing unbiased information based on the best available evidence to assist them in their choice and decision of perineal management (NMC 2015a). See chapter website resources for further discussion.

Tissue adhesive

Four studies have shown favourable outcomes for closing the perineal skin with tissue adhesive compared with using subcuticular stitches (Bowen et al 2002; Feigenberg et al 2014; Mota et al 2009; Rogerson et al 2000). However, these trials are small and the methodological design is variable. Adopting a two-stage repair may alleviate some of the problems related to skin sensitivity.

Rationale for perineal repair

- To control bleeding
- Close 'dead' space
- Minimize the risk of infection
- Assist perineal healing by primary intention
- Achieve correct anatomical alignment
- Achieve an aesthetically pleasing result
- Minimize postpartum sexual difficulties

Recommendations for clinical practice

- Repair to first degree trauma to improve healing unless skin edges are well opposed and not bleeding
- Repair to second degree tear – muscles should be sutured to improve healing
- If the skin edges are opposed after suturing of the muscle in second degree trauma, the skin layer may be left to heal naturally

(RCOG 2007, NICE 2014).

SYSTEMATIC ASSESSMENT OF PERINEAL TRAUMA

A systematic visual and digital assessment of perineal trauma should be undertaken, including a bi-digital rectal examination for all women after a vaginal delivery, irrespective if they have an intact perineum, to avoid missing overt and occult (sphincter damage not identified at delivery) anal sphincter injuries (OASIS) (Bick et al 2012; Sultan et al 2007). See Boxes 40.1 and 40.2. Failure to undertake a rectal examination after a vaginal delivery is considered a breach of duty and represents substandard care (Symon 2008). See Box 40.3.

Where there is any doubt, a senior midwife or obstetrician should be sought to double assess. Re-examination of trauma has shown to identify 40% of missed or incorrectly classified sphincter injuries (Groom et al 2002) or doubled, with midwives missing 87% and doctors 28%, respectively (Andrews et al 2006a; Sultan et al 1995b; Sultan et al 2007).

Procedure

Perineal repair must be undertaken under aseptic conditions with a good light source. Placing a woman's legs in lithotomy using poles is not necessary, as this may over extend her legs and cause excessive stretching of the perineum and possible wound breakdown. Restraining the woman's legs may also invoke negative feelings of previous sexual abuse or FGM (Walton 1994). A working epidural should be tested for adequate analgesia and topped up if necessary. Infiltration of the perineum using lidocaine 0.5% or 1% 10 to 20 mL needs to be administered 2 to 3 minutes before repair. Adequate analgesia during repair is essential, as the procedure can be associated with considerable pain (Sanders et al 2002). The midwife must prepare and check the suture trolley, undertake a needle and swab count before and after the procedure in accordance with employing authority practice guidelines, which includes checking the expiry date of the suture material and local anaesthetic. Cleansing the vulva and perineum with tap water has been shown to be as effective as chlorhexidine antiseptic (Keane and Thornton 1998). The repair should be undertaken within 30 minutes of the birth or as soon as possible to minimize pain, excessive blood loss and infection (Odibo 1997). The woman's comfort and dignity must be maintained at all times. The procedure and rationale for perineal repair is shown in Table 40.4 and the method for performing the repair is shown in Fig. 40.6.

An accurate description and diagram of the trauma and repair must be documented in the woman's notes for future referral as appropriate.

Box 40.2 Anal sphincter assessment

Obtain verbal consent

Identify if perineal tear extends to anal margin

Visual observation – check absence of anal puckering around the anterior section of the anus between 9 and 3 o'clock. This is suspicious of anal sphincter trauma

Perform rectal examination to exclude injury to internal and external anal sphincters and ano-rectal mucosa – in a fourth degree tear, the anal canal is opened

Insert lubricated index finger into the woman's anus and ask her to squeeze (if epidural not in situ)

Torn anal sphincter muscle may be visualized by retraction of separated ends of the muscle backwards, towards the ischio-rectal fossa – an apparent gap will be felt anteriorly (see Fig. 40.7)

Feel the muscle bulk of the sphincter palpating between thumb and finger (pill rolling), particularly when regional epidural in situ, as muscle power will be affected (Tohill and Kettle 2013)

Feel the muscle bulk of the sphincter palpating between thumb and finger (pill rolling), particularly when regional epidural in situ, as muscle power will be affected (Tohill and Kettle 2013)

Box 40.3 Mnemonic for performing a rectal examination

Verbal consent

Adequate analgesia

Good lighting

Insert index finger into anal canal, thumb into vagina using pill-rolling action to palpate anal sphincter

Not sure? Ask the woman to squeeze her buttocks, if OASIS is present, you will feel a gap anteriorly; separated ends retract

Absence of anal puckering anteriorly

Reproduced by kind permission of Karen Woodward (2015)

Box 40.1 Genital and vaginal assessment

Good lighting for accurate visual assessment

Explanation and verbal consent from woman

Offer inhalation analgesia

Position woman comfortably for clear visibility of genitalia

Inspect genitalia and vagina, labial tears and grazes

Vaginal examination to identify anterior and posterior wall lacerations, apex of the injury exploring the full extent of the trauma

Extent of blood loss, consider a cervical tear

Table 40.4 Procedure for continuous method of perineal repair

Action	Rationale
1. Explain the rationale for genital, vaginal and rectal assessment. Explain the steps of the repair procedure to the woman and her partner	1. To inform and reassure the woman about the procedure and confirm verbal consent. Ensure sensitivity and the woman's needs throughout
2. Check maternal baseline observations, uterus and PV blood loss to exclude PPH before and after repair	2. To ensure that the woman's general condition is stable before and after commencing the repair
3. Assist the woman into a comfortable and appropriate position. Lithotomy may be used if necessary (be aware of history of FGM or sexual abuse) Ensure good lighting	3. To avoid women's distress To ensure that the whole perineal area is accessible with clear visibility of all structures involved
4. Cleanse the vulva and perineal area with tap water. Drape the area with a sterile lithotomy towel	4. To minimize risk of infection
5. Count swabs, needles, suture material and instruments on trolley and record in notes	5. To confirm equipment and materials used for repair
6. Offer inhalation analgesia	6. To minimize pain on digital inspection
7. Undertake thorough and systematic visual and digital assessment of the vagina, perineum and anorectum to determine extent of perineal trauma in all women after a vaginal delivery, even with an apparent intact perineum	7. To ensure the repair is not beyond the scope of the clinicians' level of competence and to avoid missing an overt or occult anal sphincter tear Refer to more a competent practitioner, as required
8. Identify anatomical landmarks. These may include hymenal remnants and muscular tissue of superficial and deep muscles	8. To assist the practitioner to correctly align and approximate the traumatized tissue and facilitate healing. *NB:* Misalignment may cause long-term morbidity such as dyspareunia
9. Check for allergy to local anaesthesia before perineal infiltration	9. To avoid anaphylactic shock
10. Check *Lidocaine* as per Medicines Management protocol (NMC 2012) Draw back the plunger of the syringe before injecting 10–20 mL of local anaesthetic, 1% *lidocaine,* slowly into the four aspects of the trauma, from fourchette along vaginal wall and into the full length of both sides of perineal muscle to distal end, ensuring even distribution Check effectiveness of analgesia	10. To check for expiry date and that the *lidocaine* is not accidentally injected into a blood vessel To provide effective anaesthesia to facilitate a pain-free repair
11. Identify the apex of the vaginal trauma and insert the first anchoring stitch 5–10 mm above this point to secure bleeding points not visible with a surgeon's square knot for stability (see website for more information)	11. To ensure haemostasis of any bleeding vessels that may have retracted beyond the apex
12. Suture posterior vaginal trauma using a loose, continuous non-locking stitch. Continue to the hymenal remnants, taking care not to make the stitches too wide	12. To appose the edges of traumatized vaginal mucosa and muscle without causing shortening or narrowing of the vagina
13. Check depth of trauma and repair perineal muscle in one or two layers in same continuous stitch. Ensure that each stitch reaches the trough of the traumatized tissue.	13. To close dead space, achieve haemostasis and prevent paravaginal haematoma formation

Continued

Table 40.4 Procedure for continuous method of perineal repair—cont'd

Action	Rationale
14. Visualize the needle at the trough of the trauma each time it is inserted and match each stitch on either side of the wound for depth and width	14. To prevent sutures being inserted through the rectal mucosa *NB:* A recto-vaginal fistula may form if this occurs
15. Bring the needle through the tissue behind the hymenal ring, closing this and emerge in the centre of the perineal muscle, checking depth of the trauma. Continue to repair the deep and superficial muscles using a loose, continuous stitch ending at the inferior aspect of the trauma Two layers may be necessary if deep muscles are involved	15. To realign the perineal muscles, close the dead space, achieve haemostasis and minimize the risk of haematoma formation
16. Repair the skin layer by repositioning the needle and reversing the stitching direction at the inferior aspect of the trauma. Place the stitches loosely and fairly deeply under the surface of the skin and in the subcutaneous layer, approximately 5–10 mm apart	16. To align and appose skin edges and complete the perineal repair without contact to nerve endings, considering cosmetic results
17. Check tension of stitch. Do not pull the stitches too tight	17. To prevent discomfort from over tight sutures if reactionary oedema and swelling occur
18. Complete the subcutaneous repair to the hymenal ring, sweep the needle behind the fourchette and into the vagina and complete the repair using a loop or Aberdeen knot (see website for more information)	18. To secure the stitches and invert the knot in the vaginal mucosa with minimal bulk
19. Inspect the repaired perineal trauma	19. To ensure the trauma has been sutured correctly and that haemostasis has been achieved. To check that there is no excessive bleeding from a missed bleeding point or from the cervix or uterus
20. Insert two fingers gently into the vagina	20. To confirm that the introitus and vagina have not been stitched too tightly
21. Perform a bidigital rectal examination. *Diclofenac acid* (100 mg) suppositories may be inserted per rectum at this point	21. To confirm that no sutures have penetrated the rectal mucosa To provide continuing analgesia
22. Cleanse and dry the perineal area. Apply a sterile pad	22. To minimize infection
23. Check and record that all swabs, needles and instruments are correct against the ones checked in at the commencement of the procedure	23. To confirm that all equipment and materials used are complete and accounted for
24. Place the woman in the position of her choice and advise her regarding hygiene and analgesia	24. To ensure that the woman is made comfortable after the procedure and supported
25. Document and sign a detailed account of the assessment and repair using a picture to identify the extent of the trauma in the woman's records NMC (2010) Record Keeping: *guidance for nurses and midwives* and local units requirements	25. To fulfil statutory requirements and to provide an accurate account of the repair for future reference

Adapted from Kettle 2011; Tohill and Kettle 2013; NICE 2014

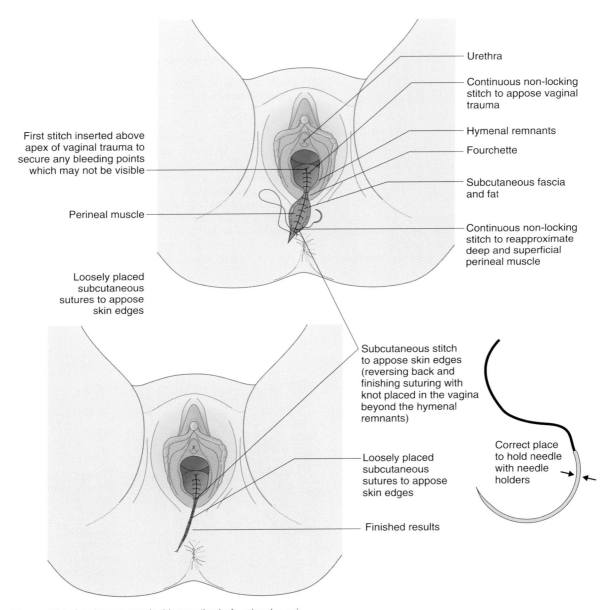

First stitch inserted above apex of vaginal trauma to secure any bleeding points which may not be visible

Perineal muscle

Loosely placed subcutaneous sutures to appose skin edges

Urethra

Continuous non-locking stitch to appose vaginal trauma

Hymenal remnants

Fourchette

Subcutaneous fascia and fat

Continuous non-locking stitch to reapproximate deep and superficial perineal muscle

Subcutaneous stitch to appose skin edges (reversing back and finishing suturing with knot placed in the vagina beyond the hymenal remnants)

Loosely placed subcutaneous sutures to appose skin edges

Finished results

Correct place to hold needle with needle holders

Figure 40.6 Continuous non-locking method of perineal repair.

Reflective activity 40.3 ✗❮

Reflect on the information and rationale you would discuss with a woman to enable her to make an informed decision about her perineal trauma management.

Advice after perineal repair

- Type of trauma and need for follow-up care as appropriate
- Wound healing process
- Methods of pain relief
- Personal hygiene and recommended hand washing technique
- Rest, diet and fluid intake to minimize constipation
- Pelvic floor exercises
- Self-referral to specialist perineal care midwife or appropriate clinician if perineal pain, dyspareunia or continence problems persist

The National Institute for Health and Care Excellence (NICE 2014): Postnatal Care – provide recommendations for perineal care. See website for postpartum perineal care, wound healing and postpartum sexual difficulties.

See Chs 41 (postnatal care), 66 (postnatal morbidity) and 13 (sexuality).

Third and fourth degree tears

Third and fourth degree tears (OASIS or SPT) are the major cause of anal incontinence in women affecting approximately 15% to 61% worldwide (Andrews et al 2013; Reid et al 2014). See Fig. 40.7. The reported rate of OASIS occurring in singleton, term, cephalic and first vaginal births in England appears to have tripled between 2000 and 2012 from 1.8% to 5.9%, with an overall incidence in the UK of 2.9% (range 0%–8%). The incidence is higher in primiparae (6.1%) compared with 1.7% in multiparae (RCOG 2015a). The incidence of SPT would appear to have increased in other developed nations, such as Australia (Dahlen et al 2015). This is a serious concern and all practitioners need to evaluate their care and give careful consideration to perineal management

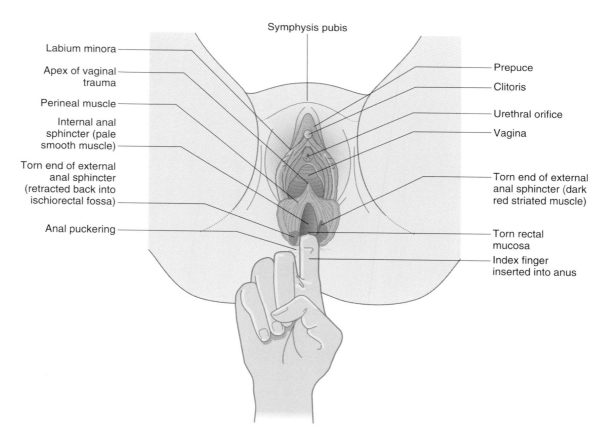

Figure 40.7 Anal sphincter injury.

and anal sphincter assessment in association with a clear protocol for the management of OASIS together with risk management strategies and audit of perineal trauma (NHS Litigation Authority 2011). Clinically detectable OASIS are reported by Andrews et al (2006a and 2006b) to occur in 0.4% to 19% of vaginal births in centres where mediolateral or midline episiotomies are practiced. The wide variation in reported incidences is likely to be caused by underreporting by women themselves as a result of embarrassment or social stigma, or better recognition and classification in midwifery practice. Midwives can make a significant difference to the woman's experience as two-thirds of all third degree tears occur during spontaneous vaginal births (Bedwell 2006). Approximately 30% of women will report faecal, flatal or urinary incontinence or sexual problems 3 months postpartum. Results after a prospective cohort study in the UK identified that of the 435 women who sustained OASIS, 96% of women were faecally continent 3 months after a primary repair. However, 34% of women reported faecal urgency, 25% complained of poor flatal control, and 30% reported pain and bleeding on defecation, while 51% of women reported urinary problems. Sexual intercourse was resumed by 57% women. However, dyspareunia was reported by 32% of women (Marsh et al 2011). The psychological effect of SPT is extensive and complex and Priddis et al (2014) has identified that the lack of sensitivity by the care provider can make a significant difference to how the woman perceives herself, her body and is able to adapt to personal, family and sexual life long term.

See chapter website resources for further information.

Labial and clitoral tears

Occurrence of labial tearing after a vaginal birth has been reported as 35.4% (McCandlish et al 1998). Fusion of labia minora may occur when both labia are torn, causing adhesions, thin bands or a 'tissue bridge' occurring as a by-product of the normal healing of the wound. This occurrence is rare but can lead to difficulties when resuming sexual activity and voiding (Arkin et al 2001; Seehusen et al 2007). No adverse outcomes have been reported, leaving single labial tears to heal naturally, although the aesthetic effects on the woman must be considered and discussed. Clitoral tears must be repaired by a competent senior obstetrician in theatre under regional anaesthesia using a rapidly absorbable suture material, such as *Vicryl Rapide* 3.0 on a small needle. Clitoral tears can be very painful. Substandard repair can result in sexual difficulties and failure to reach orgasm.

Cervical tears

These tears need to be repaired in theatre under regional or general anaesthesia.

DISCUSSION

In the UK, midwives attend 60% of normal vaginal births and are responsible for the repair of the majority of uncomplicated second degree perineal trauma (NHS Maternity Statistics in England 2013–2014 (2015). Therefore, midwives have a major responsibility, as they are often the only practitioners who will be assessing and classifying perineal trauma after a normal birth. The expertise of the midwife is therefore paramount.

In a systematic review of six studies addressing midwives' and doctors' perceived knowledge and training in the anatomy, assessment and classification of perineal trauma, the majority of doctors and/or midwives reported this area of expertise to be poor (Andrews et al 2005b; Bick et al 2012; Cornet et al 2012; Fernando et al 2002; Mutema 2007; Sultan et al 1994b). In a more recent survey of perineal management completed by midwives and doctors in Australia, 71% of midwives had received training in assessing for ASI. However, only 16% were confident in making a correct diagnosis (East et al 2015). This is a major concern and may be attributed to feelings of guilt or shame of reporting a third degree tear with a woman in the midwives' care.

Structured hands-on training has been shown to be an effective way of improving midwifery skills and knowledge in perineal anatomy and correct identification of perineal trauma (Andrews et al 2005b and 2009; Kettle et al 2002; Selo-Ojeme et al 2009; Sultan et al 1995b). A quasi-experimental study to address midwives' perceived level of confidence and competency in perineal repair in 2003, identified that although 90% of midwives claimed to undertake repair, only 27.1% perceived that they were confident to undertake the procedure. After an interventional educational programme in perineal repair across five UK NHS maternity units, significantly greater numbers of midwives were able to practice perineal repair at higher levels of competency. Frequent undertaking of the procedure, educational support and one-to-one instruction at the bedside made the strongest contribution to perceived confidence and competency in the skill. Factors inhibiting confidence and competence were limited access to in-service training or continuing professional development; limited supervision and mentoring; trend not to repair and time and staff shortages. In addition, an increased number of senior student midwives were able to participate in perineal repair confidently under the direct supervision of their midwife mentor, when they perceived that their midwife mentor was confident and competent to undertake the procedure (Wilson 2009 and 2012).

More recently, a UK-wide survey of midwifery practice (The Perineal Assessment and Repair Longitudinal Study (PEARLS)) identified that 58% of midwives did not suture all second degree tears, and only 6% of midwives used evidence-based suturing methods to repair all layers of perineal trauma. Further findings revealed that only 34% of midwives felt confident to assess trauma all the time and 50% most of the time. There was a significant association with years of practice and confidence. When asked about performing repair, only 21.6% of midwives felt confident to perform repair all of the time and 54.1% most of the time (Bick et al 2012). After this survey, the PEARLS matched–pair cluster randomized control study (Ismail et al 2013) introduced a standardized multiprofessional perineal training package across 22 UK maternity units, enrolling 3681 women who had sustained a second degree perineal tear during 2010–2012. Results were positive, demonstrating an improvement in the uptake of evidence–based midwifery practice in perineal trauma management. Training also had a significant effect on the reduced numbers of women reporting perineal wound infections and the need for suture removal. Practitioners now have access to the MaternityPEARLS perineal repair training electronic learning package through the Royal College of Midwives (*i-learn*) and the Royal College of Obstetrics and Gynaecology *StratOg* learning sites. This is the first validated perineal management e-learning package, which improves knowledge and skills, and is comparable to traditional in-service training, external study days and workshops. Electronic learning has the advantage of enabling practitioners to access education at any time and place worldwide (Mahmud et al 2013).

Professional and legal responsibilities

Midwives have a duty of care within their scope of practice. They are professionally accountable for their actions and omissions in accordance with the guidelines and policies set out by their employing authorities, the Midwives Rules and Standards (NMC 2012), the Code (NMC 2015) and the principles of good Record Keeping (NMC 2012). Every healthcare professional has a duty of candour and must be open and honest with women about the outcomes of their care and with their colleagues and organization, reporting concerns related to any aspects of care or management (NMC 2015b). Midwives need not fear the risk of litigation if their everyday practice is underpinned by current best evidence. Failure to undertake the role expected of the experience and expertise of the midwife is a breach of that duty to the woman, the NMC and profession (Griffith et al 2010). The importance of good communication, documentation, team working, continuing professional development and risk management strategies must not be underestimated in minimizing perineal morbidity and preventing medico-legal claims (see Ch. 9).

CONCLUSION

Midwives can make a significant difference to women's postpartum perineal morbidity. Empowering women to take an active role in their perineal management during pregnancy, labour and the puerperium can alleviate many of the physical and psychosocial problems identified in the literature. Because of the lower rates of episiotomy reported in the UK, midwives and students need to be proactive in seeking knowledge and experience in practising episiotomy at the recommended 60 degree angle to gain confidence in performing this skill when indicated. Recognition of risk factors, accurate and timely assessment and management of all categories of perineal trauma, specifically, anal sphincter damage, is imperative to avoid unnecessary perineal morbidity. Accessing regular multiprofessional surgical skills, perineal repair workshops and online learning, including episiotomy, has shown to increase the midwives' level of confidence and competency, enabling them to work sensitively in partnership with and acting as true advocates for the women in their care. Professional credibility, accountability and self-regulation are the cornerstones of best practice and are the duties of all midwives.

Key Points

- Access to evidence-based information in minimizing perineal trauma at birth for midwives and women can reduce the incidence of short- and long-term perineal morbidity.
- A restricted policy of episiotomy at a 60 degree angle reduces the rate of severe perineal trauma.
- 'Hands-on' perineal support at crowning may reduce trauma.
- Performing a bidigital anal sphincter (rectal) assessment after all vaginal deliveries can avoid missing a third degree tear.
- A continuous method of perineal repair using a rapidly absorbable suture material is associated with less pain in the first 10 days' postpartum.
- Vigilance is the keyword for recognizing genital tract infection and sepsis in all women.
- Pelvic floor exercises during pregnancy and the puerperium reduces stress urinary incontinence both in the short and long term.
- Provision of follow-up care for all women who have sustained problematic perineal trauma with a specialist perineal care midwife or obstetrician is important for good long-term outcomes.

References

Aasheim V, Nilsen AB: Perineal techniques during the second stage of labour for reducing perineal trauma (Review), *The Cochrane Collaboration*, The Cochrane Library, (2):2012.

Albers LL, Sedler K, Bedrick E, et al: Midwifery care measures in the second stage of labour and reduction of genital tract trauma at birth, *J Midwifery Womens Health* 50(5):365–372, 2005.

Andrews V, Shelmeridine S, Sultan AH: Anal and urinary incontinence 4 years after a vaginal delivery, *Int Urogynecol J* 24:55–60, 2013.

Andrews V, Sultan AH, Thakar R, et al: Occult anal sphincter injuries – myth or reality? *Br J Obstet Gynaecol* 113:195–200, 2006a.

Andrews V, Sultan AH, Thakar R, et al: Risk factors for obstetric anal sphincter injury: a prospective study, *Birth* 33:117–122, 2006b.

Andrews V, Thakar R, Sultan AH: Structured hands-on training in repair of obstetric anal sphincter injuries (OASIS): an audit of clinical practice, *Int Urogynecol J Pelvic Floor Dysfunct* 20:193–199, 2009.

Andrews V, Thakar R, Sultan AH, et al: Are mediolateral episiotomies actually mediolateral? *Br J Obstet Gynaecol* 112:1156–1158, 2005a.

Andrews V, Thakar R, Sultan AH, et al: Can hands-on perineal repair courses affect clinical practice? *Br J Midwifery* 13(9):562–566, 2005b.

Argentine Episiotomy Trial Collaborative Group: Routine vs selective episiotomy: a randomised controlled trial, *Lancet* 342(8886):1517, 1993.

Arkin AE, Chern-Hughes B: Case report: labial fusion postpartum and clinical management of labial lacerations, *J Midwifery Womens Health* 47(4):290–292, 2001.

Baessler K, Schussler B, Bugio K, et al: *Pelvic floor re-education – principles and practice*, 2nd edn, London, Springer-Verlag, 2008.

Baker K: Midwives should support women to mobilise during labour, *Br J Midwifery* 18(98):492–497, 2010.

Beckmann MM, Stock OM: *Antenatal perineal massage for reducing perineal trauma* (Review), The Cochrane Collaboration, Cochrane Library Issue 4, Oxford, John Wiley and Sons Ltd., 2013.

Bedwell C: Are third degree tears unavoidable? The role of the midwife, *Br J Midwifery* 14(4):212, 2006.

Bertozzi S, Londero AP, Fruscalzo A, et al: *Impact of episiotomy on pelvic floor disorders and their influence on women's wellness after the sixth month postpartum, a retrospective study.* BMC Women's Health 11, Biomed Central Ltd., 2011.

Best C, Taylor N: *The living body*, 4th edn, London, Chapman and Hall Ltd 1965.

Bick DE, Ismail KM, Macdonald S, et al: How good are we at implementing evidence to support the management of birth related perineal trauma? A UK wide survey of midwifery practice, *BMC Pregnancy Childbirth* 12:57, 2012.

Bosanquet A: A day in the life of a specialist perineal midwife, *Midwives* 58, 2010.

Bowen ML, Selinger M: Episiotomy closure comparing enbucrilate tissue adhesive with conventional sutures, *Int J Gynaecol Obstet* 78:201–205, 2002.

Boyle R, Hay-Smith EJC, Cody JD, et al: *Pelvic floor muscle training for prevention and treatment of urinary and faecal incontinence in pregnant women and women who have recently given birth.* The Cochrane Library, Issue 10, Oxford, Update Software, 2012.

Buhling K, Schmidt S, Robinson J, et al: Rate of dyspareunia after delivery in primiparae according to mode of birth, *Eur J Obstet Gynecol Reprod Biol* 124:42–46, 2006.

Carola R, Hartley J, Noback C: *Human anatomy and physiology*, 2nd edn, New York, McGraw-Hill Inc, 1992.

Carroli G, Mignini L: *Episiotomy for vaginal birth*. Cochrane Database of Systematic Reviews, Issue 1, Chichester, John Wiley and Sons, 2009.

Clement S, Reed B: To stitch or not to stitch? *Pract Midwife* 2(4):20–28, 1999.

Cornet A, Porta O, Pineiro L, et al: Management of obstetric perineal tears: do obstetric and gynaecological residents receive adequate training? Results of an anonymous survey, *Obstet Gynecol Int* 2012:316983, 2012.

Cortes E, Basra R, Keller C: Waterbirth and pelvic floor injury: a retrospective study and postal survey using ICIQ modular long form questionnaires, *Eur J Obstet Gynecol Reprod Biol* 155:27–30, 2011.

da Silva F, de Oliveira S, Bick D, et al: Risk factors for birth-related trauma: a cross-sectional study in a birth centre, *J Clin Nurs* 21:2209–2218, 2012.

Dahlen H: Perineal care and repair. In Pairman S, Pincombe J, Thorogood C, et al, editors: *Midwifery preparation for practice*, 3rd edn, Sydney, Churchill Livingstone Elsevier, 2015.

Dahlen H, Priddis H, Thornton C: Severe perineal trauma is rising, but let us not overreact, *Midwifery* 31:1–8, 2015.

Dahlen HG, Ryan M, Homer CSE, et al: An Australian prospective cohort study of risk factors for severe perineal trauma during childbirth, *Midwifery* 23(2):196–203, 2007a.

Dahlen HG, Homer CSE, Cooke M: Perineal outcomes and maternal comfort related to the application of perineal warm packs in the second stage of labour: a randomized controlled trial, *Birth* 34(4):282–290, 2007b.

Department of Health (DH): *Female Genital Mutilation Risk and Safeguarding Guidance for Professionals*, London, 2015.

Dugdale AF, Hill SR: Midwifery-led care: establishing a postnatal perineal clinic, *Br J Midwifery* 12(10):648–653, 2005.

East C, Forster D, Nagle C, et al: Women's experience perineal pain following childbirth, *J Paediatr Child Health* 45:PO38, 2009.

East CE, Lau R, Biro MA: Midwives' and doctors' perceptions of their preparation for and practice in managing the perineum in the second stage of labour: a cross-sectional survey, *Midwifery* 31(1):122–131, 2015.

Eogan M, Daly L, O'Connell PR, et al: Does the angle of episiotomy affect the incidence of anal sphincter injury? *Br J Obstet Gynaecol* 113:190–194, 2006.

Feigenberg T, Maor-Sagie E, Zivi E, et al: Using adhesive glue to repair first degree perineal tears: a prospective randomized controlled trial, *Biomed Res Int* 2014:526590, 2014.

Fernando RJ, Sultan AH, Radley S, et al: Management of obstetric anal sphincter injuries: a systematic review and national survey of practice, *BMC Health Serv Res* 2(1):9, 2002.

Fitzpatrick M, Cassidy M, O'Connell PR, et al: Experience with an obstetric perineal clinic, *Eur J Obstet Gynecol Reprod Biol* 100:199–203, 2002.

Fleming N: Can the suturing method make a difference in postpartum perinea pain? *J Nurse Midwifery* 35(1):19–25, 1990.

Fleming VEM, Hagen S, Niven C: Does perineal suturing make a difference? The SUNS trial, *Br J Obstet Gynaecol* 110:684–689, 2003.

Freeman RM, Hollands HJ, Barron LF, et al: Cutting a mediolateral episiotomy at the correct angle: evaluation of a new device, the Episcissors-60, *Med Devices (Auckl)* 7:23–28, 2014.

Gemynthe A, Langhoff-Roos J, Sahl S, et al: New VICRYL formulation: an improved method of perineal repair? *Br J Midwifery* 4(5):230–234, 1996.

Gillard S, Shamley D: Factors motivating women to commence and adhere to pelvic floor muscle exercises following a perineal tear at delivery: the influence of experience, *J Assoc Chart Physiother Womens Health* 106:5–18, 2010.

Glazener CM: Sexual function after childbirth: women's experiences, persistent morbidity and lack of professional recognition, *Br J Obstet Gynaecol* 104:330–335, 1997.

Glazener CA, Stroud P, Naji S, et al: Postnatal maternal morbidity: extent, causes, prevention and treatment, *Br J Obstet Gynaecol* 102:282–287, 1995.

Gordon B, Mackrodt C, Fern E, et al: The Ipswich childbirth study: 1. A randomised evaluation of two stage postpartum perineal repair leaving the skin unsutured, *Br J Obstet Gynaecol* 105:435–440, 1998.

Grant A, Gordon B: The Ipswich childbirth study: one year follow up

of alternative methods used in perineal repair, *Br J Obstet Gynaecol* 108:34–40, 2001.

Griffith R, Tengnak C, Patel C: *Law and professional issues in midwifery* (website). www.learningmatters.co.uk. 2010.

Groom K, Patterson-Brown S: Can we improve on the diagnosis of third degree tears? *Eur J Obstet Gynaecol Reprod Biol* 101:19–21, 2002.

Haadem K, Ling L, Ferno M, et al: Estrogen receptors in the external anal sphincter, *Am J Obstet Gynecol* 164(2):609–610, 1991.

Halperin O, Raz I, Ben-Gal L, et al: Prediction of perineal trauma during childbirth by assessment of striae gravidarum score, *J Obstet Gynecol Neonatal Nurs* 39:292–297, 2010.

Hals E, Oian P, Pirhonen T, et al: A multicentre interventional program to reduce the incidence of anal sphincter tears, *Am J Obstet Gynecol* 116:901–908, 2010.

Hamilton-Fairley D: *Obstetrics and gynaecology*, 3rd edn, Oxford, Wiley-Blackwell, 2009.

Harper B: Waterbirth basics: from newborn breathing to hospital protocols, *Midwifery Today Int Midwife* (54):9–15, 68, 2000.

Head M: Dropping stitches, *Nurs Times* 89(33):64–65, 1993.

Health and Social Care Information Centre (HSCIC): *National Health Service*. Maternity Statistics, England 2013-2014 (website). http://www.hscic.gov.uk/catalogue/PUB16725/nhs-mate-eng-2013-14-summ-repo-rep.pdf. 2015.

Hospital Episodes Statistics: NHS Maternity Statistics 2011-2012 Survey Report 2012. www.hesonline.nhs.uk. 2012.

International Confederation of Midwives: *Essential competencies for basic midwifery practice* (website). www.internationalmidwives.org/what-we-do/education-core documents/essential-competencies-basic-midwifery-practice/. 2013.

Ismail KMK, Kettle C, Macdonald SE, et al: Perineal Assessment and Repair Longitudinal Study (PEARLS): a matched-pair cluster randomised trial, *BMC Med* 11:209, 2013.

Kalis V, Laine K, de Leeuw JW, et al: Classification of episiotomy: towards a standardisation of

terminology, *Br J Obstet Gynaecol* 119:522–526, 2012.

Kalis V, Landsmanova J, Bednarova B, et al: Evaluation of the incision angle of mediolateral episiotomy at 60 degrees, *Int J Gynaecol Obstet* 112:220–224, 2011.

Keane HE, Thornton JG: A trial of chlorhexidine or tap water for perineal cleaning, *Br J Midwifery* 6(1):34, 1998.

Kettle C: *Perineal care. Clinical evidence* (website). www.clinicalevidence.com/ceweb/conditions/pac/1401/1401_background.jsp. 2004.

Kettle C: The management of perineal trauma. In Henderson C, Bick D, editors: *Perineal care: an international issue*, Quay Books, Salisbury, 2005.

Kettle C: The pelvic floor. In Macdonald S, Magill-Cuerden J, editors: Mayes' Midwifery, London, Bailliere Tindall, 2011.

Kettle C, Hill RK, Jones P, et al: Continuous versus interrupted perineal repair with standard or rapidly absorbed sutures after spontaneous vaginal birth: a randomised controlled trial, *Lancet* 359:2217–2223, 2002.

Kitzinger S, Simpkin P, editors: *Episiotomy and the second stage of labour*, 2nd edn, Seattle, Penny Press, 1986.

Kitzinger S, Walters R: *Some women's experiences of episiotomy*, London, National Childbirth Trust, 1981.

Klein M, Gauthier R, Robbins J, et al: Relationship of episiotomy to perineal trauma and morbidity, sexual dysfunction, and pelvic floor relaxation, *Am J Obstet Gynecol* 171(September):591–598, 1994.

Kovacs C, Heath P, Heather C: First Australian trial of the birth training device Epi-No: a highly significant increased chance of an intact perineum, *Aust N Z J Obstet Gynaecol* 44:347–348, 2004.

Laine K, Skjeldestad FE, Sandvik L, et al: Incidence of obstetric anal sphincter injuries after training to protect the perineum: cohort study, *BMJ Open* 2:e001649, 2012.

Lappen JR, Gosssett D: Changes in episiotomy practice: evidence-based medicine in action, *Expert Rev Obstet Gynecol* 5(3):301–309, 2010.

Lavin J, Smith AR: Pelvic floor damage, *Mod Midwife* 6(5):14–15, 1996.

Leeman L, Fullilove MIS, Borders N, et al: Postpartum perineal pain in low episiotomy settings: association with severity of genital trauma, labour care, and birth variables, *Birth* 36(4):283–288, 2009.

Lien KCMS, Mooney B, DeLancey JOL, et al: Levator ani muscle stretch induced by simulated vaginal birth, *Obstet Gynecol* 103(1):31, 2004.

Limbs and Things, UK (website). http://limbsandthings.com/global/products/keele-staffs-episiotomy-repair-trainer/.

Lindgren HE, Radestad IJ, Christensson K, et al: Outcome of planned home births compared to hospital birth in Sweden between 1992 and 2004. A population-based register study, *Acta Obstet Gynecol Scand* 87(7):751–759, 2008.

Lundquist M, Olsson A, Nissen E, et al: Is it necessary to suture all lacerations after a vaginal delivery? *Birth* 27(2):79–85, 2000.

MacArthur C, Glazener CM, Wilson PD: Obstetric practice and faecal incontinence three months after delivery, *Br J Obstet Gynaecol* 108:678–683, 2001.

MacArthur AJ, Macarthur C: Incidence, severity and determinants of perineal pain after vaginal delivery: a prospective cohort study, *Am J Obstet Gynecol* 191(4):1119–1204, 2004.

Magdi I: Obstetric injuries of the perineum, *J Obstet Gynaecol Br Emp* 687–700, 1949.

Mahmud A, Kettle C, Bick D, et al: The development and validation of an internet-based training package for the management of perineal trauma following childbirth: MaternityPEARLS, *Postgrad Med J* 89:382–389, 2013.

Marsh F, Rogerson L, Landon C, et al: Obstetric anal sphincter injury in the UK and its effects on bowel, bladder and sexual function, *Eur J Obstet Gynaecol Reprod Biol* 153:223–227, 2011.

McCandlish R, Bowler U, van Asten H, et al: A randomised controlled trial of care of the perineum during second stage of normal labour, *Br J Obstet Gynaecol* 105:1262–1272, 1998.

Melo I, Katz L, Coutinho I, et al: Selective episiotomy vs. implementation of a non episiotomy protocol: a randomised clinical trial, *Reprod Health* 11:66, 2014.

Metcalfe A, Bick D, Tohill S, et al: A prospective cohort study of repair

and non-repair of second degree perineal trauma: results and issues for future research, *RCM Evidence Based Midwifery* 4(2):60–64, 2006.

Meyvis I, Rompaey B, Goormans K, et al: Maternal positions and other variables: effects on perineal outcomes in 557 births, *Birth* 39(2):115–120, 2012.

Moore E, Morehead C: Promoting normality in the management of the perineum during the second stage of labour, *Br J Midwifery* 21(9):115–120, 2013.

Morkved S: Evidence for pelvic floor physical therapy for urinary incontinence during pregnancy and after childbirth. In Bo K, et al, editors: *Evidence-based physical therapy for the pelvic floor, bridging science and clinical practice*, Philadelphia, Elsevier, 2007.

Morris A, Berg M, Dencker A: Professional's skills in assessment of perineal tears after childbirth: a Systematic Review, *Open J Obstet Gynecol* 13(3):7–15, 2013.

Mota R, Costa F, Amaral A, et al: Skin adhesive versus subcuticular suture for perineal skin repair after episiotomy: a randomized controlled Trial, *Acta Obstet Gynecol Scand* 88(6):660–666, 2009.

Mullally A, Murphy D: Episiotomy, *Global library of women's medicine* (website). doi: 10.3843/GLOWM.10128. 2011.

Mutema EK: A tale of two cities: auditing midwifery practice and perineal trauma, *Br J Midwifery* 15(8):511–513, 2007.

National Health Service (NHS): *Litigation Authority, CNST Maternity Clinical: Risk Management Standards*. London, NHSLA, 2011.

National Institute for Health and Care Excellence (NICE): *Intrapartum Care: Care of Healthy Women and Their Babies During Childbirth*, CG190, London, NICE, 2014.

Nerum H, Halvorsen L, Sorlie T, et al: Maternal request for caesarean section due to fear of birth: can it be changed through crisis orientated counselling? *Birth* 33(3):221–228, 2006.

Nursing and Midwifery Council (NMC): *Standards for Pre-registration Midwifery Education*, London, NMC, 2009.

Nursing and Midwifery Council (NMC): *Standards for Medicines Management*, London, NMC, 2010.

Nursing and Midwifery Council (NMC): *Midwives rules and standards*, London, NMC, 2012.

Nursing and Midwifery Council (NMC): *Record Keeping: Guidance for nurses and midwives*, London, NMC, 2012.

Nursing and Midwifery Council (NMC): *The Code: Professional standards of practice and behavior or nurses and midwives*, London, NMC, 2015a.

Nursing and Midwifery Council (NMC): *Openness and Honesty when things go wrong: Professional Duty of Candour*, London, NMC, 2015b.

Oboro VO, Tabowei TO, Loto OM, et al: A multicentre evaluation of the two-layered repair of postpartum perineal trauma, *J Obstet Gynaecol* 23(1):5–8, 2003.

Odibo L: Suturing of perineal trauma: how well are we doing? An audit, *Br J Midwifery* 5(11):690–692, 1997.

Olah K: Subcuticular perineal repair using a new, continuous technique, *Br J Midwifery* 2(2):67–71, 1994.

Oliveira LS, Brito G, Quintanas M, et al: *Perineal trauma after vaginal delivery in healthy pregnant women* (website). doi: 10.1590/1516-3180.2014.1324710. 2014.

Organisation for Economic Cooperation and Development (OECD): *Health at a glance* (website). www.oecd.org/health/health-at-a-glance.htm. 2013.

Pearson S: Warwick midwives are delivering women in upright positions, *Br J Midwifery* 20(7):522–523, 2012.

Pergialiotis V, Vlachos D, Protopapas A, et al: Risk factors for severe perineal lacerations during childbirth, *Int J Gynaecol Obstet* 125:6–14, 2014.

Poen AC, Felt-Bersma RJF, Dekker GA, et al: Third degree obstetric perineal tears: risk factors and the preventive role of mediolateral episiotomy, *Br J Obstet Gynaecol* 104:563–566, 1997.

Pregazzi R, Sartore A, Bortoli P, et al: Immediate postpartum perineal examination as a predictor of puerperal pelvic floor dysfunction, *Obstet Gynecol* 99(4):581–584, 2002.

Priddis H, Dahlen HG, Schmied V, et al: Risk of occurrence, subsequent mode of birth and morbidity for women who experienced severe perineal trauma in a first birth in New South Wales between

2000-2008: a population based data linkage study, *BMC Pregnancy Childbirth* 13:89, 2013.

Priddis H, Schmied V, Dahlen H: Women's experience s following severe perineal trauma: a qualitative study, *BMC Womens Health* 14:2–11, 2014.

Prins M, Boxem J, Lucas C, et al: Effect of spontaneous pushing versus valsalva pushing in the second stage of labour on mother and fetus: a systematic review of randomised trials, *Br J Obstet Gynaecol* 118(6):662–670, 2011.

Räisänen S, Vehviläinen-Julkunen K, Heinonen S: Need for and consequences of episiotomy in a vaginal birth: a critical approach, *Midwifery* 26:348–356, 2010.

Rathfisch G, Dikencik BK, Beji NK, et al: Effects of perineal trauma on postpartum sexual function, *J Adv Nurs* 66(12):2640–2649, 2010.

Reggiardo G, Fasani R, Mignini F: Multicentre, open label study to evaluate the efficiency and tolerability of a gel (Elastolabo®) for the reduction of the incidence of perineal traumas during labour and related complications in the postpartum period, *Trends in Medicine* 12(3):143–149, 2012.

Reid A, Beggs A, Sultan AH, et al: Outcome of repair of obstetric anal sphincter injuries after three years, *Int J Gynaecol Obstet* 127:47–50, 2014.

Renfrew MJ, Hannah W, Albers L, et al: Practices that minimise trauma to the genital track in childbirth: a systematic review of the literature, *Birth* 25(3):143–160, 1998.

Revicky V, Nirmal D, Mukhopadhyay S, et al: Could a mediolateral episiotomy prevent obstetric anal sphincter injury? *Eur J Obstet Gynecol Reprod Biol* 150:142–146, 2010.

Robinson JN, Norwitx ER, Cohen AP, et al: Predictors of episiotomy use at first spontaneous vaginal delivery, *Obstet Gynecol* 96(2):214–218, 2000.

Rogerson L, Mason GC, Roberts AC: Preliminary experience with twenty perineal repairs using Indermil tissue adhesive, *Eur J Obstet Gynecol Reprod Biol* 88:139–142, 2000.

Royal College of Midwives (RCM): The *Royal College of Midwives' Survey of Positions Used in Labour and Birth*. London, RCM, 2010.

Royal College of Midwives (RCM), RCN, Royal College of Obstetricians and Gynaecologists (RCOG), Equality Now, UNITE: *Tackling FGM in the UK: Intercollegiate Recommendations for identifying, recording, and reporting*. London, Royal College of Midwives, 2013.

Royal College of Obstetricians and Gynaecologists (RCOG): *Green top guidelines, methods and materials in perineal repair (23)*, 2007.

Royal College of Obstetricians and Gynaecologists (RCOG): *Bacterial sepsis following pregnancy, green-top guideline* No. 64b, 2012.

Royal College of Obstetricians and Gynaecologists (RCOG): *The management of third- and fourth-degree perineal tears, green top guideline* No. 29, 2015a.

Royal College of Obstetricians and Gynaecologists (RCOG): *Information for you. A third- or fourth-degree tear during birth (also known as obstetric anal sphincter injury-OASI)*, 2015b.

Ruckharberle E, Jundt K, Bauerle M, et al: Prospective randomised multicentre trial with birth trainer EPI-NO® for the prevention of perineal trauma, *Aust N Z J Obstet Gynaecol* 49:478–483, 2009.

Salmon D: A feminist analysis of women's experiences of perineal trauma in the immediate post-delivery period, *Midwifery* 15(4):247–256, 1999.

Sampselle C, Hines S: Spontaneous pushing during birth: relationship to perineal outcomes, *J Nurse Midwifery* 44(1):36–39, 2010.

Sanders J, Campbell R, Peters T: Effectiveness of pain relief during perineal suturing, *Br J Obstet Gynaecol* 109:1066–1068, 2002.

Sayasneh A, Pandeva I: Postpartum sexual dysfunction: a literature review of risk factors and mode of delivery, *British Journal of Medical Practitioners* 3(2):316–321, 2010.

Seehusen DA, Earwood JS: *Postpartum labial adhesions* (website) www.jabfm.org doi: 10.3122/jabfm.2007.04.060214. 2007.

Sekhon L: Changing patient needs: issues and ethics of maternal requested caesarean section, *RCSI Medical Student* 3(1):61–64, 2010.

Selo-Ojeme D, Ojutiku D, Ikomi A: Impact of a structured, hands-on, surgical skills training programme for midwives performing perineal repair, *Int J Gynaecol Obstet* 106(3):239–241, 2009.

Shorten A, Donsante J, Shorten B: Birth position, accoucheur, and perineal outcomes: informing women about choices for vaginal birth, *Birth* 29(1):18–27, 2002.

Siegfried N, van der Merve L, Brockelhurst P, et al: Antiretrovirals for reducing the risk of mother to child transmission of HIV infections, *Cochrane Database Syst Rev* 6(7):CD003510, 2011.

Silf K, Woodhead N, Kelly J, et al: Evaluation of accuracy of mediolateral episiotomy incisions using a training model, *Midwifery* 31:197–200, 2015.

Sleep J, Grant A, Garcia J, et al: West Berkshire perineal management trial, *Br Med J (Clin Res Ed)* 289:587–590, 1984.

Smith DB: Female pelvic floor health, *J Wound Ostomy Continence Nurs* 31(3):130–137, 2004.

Smith L, Price N, Simonite V, et al: Incidence and risk factors for perineal trauma: a prospective observational study, *BMC Pregnancy Childbirth* 13:59, 2013.

Spendlove Z: To suture or not to suture? Decisions, decisions, decisions. A grounded theory study to explore the decision making-process of midwives regarding management of perineal trauma following spontaneous childbirth, *Evidence Based Midwifery* 3(1):45–50, 2005.

Stedenfeldt M, Pirhoen J, Blix E, et al: Episiotomy characteristics and risks for obstetric anal sphincter injuries: a case-control study, *Br J Obstet Gynaecol* 119:724–730, 2012.

Stein M: *Heal pelvic pain*, New York, McGraw Hill, 2009.

Stevenson L: Guideline for the systematic assessment of perineal trauma, *Br J Midwifery* 18(8):498–501, 2010.

Sultan AH, Kamm MA, Hudson CH: Pudendal nerve damage during labour: prospective study before and after childbirth, *Br it J Obstet Gynaecol* 101:22–28, 1994a.

Sultan AH, Kamm M: Third degree obstetric anal sphincter tears: risk factors and outcomes of primary repair, *Br Med J* 308:887–891, 1994b.

Sultan AH, Kamm MA, Hudson CH: Obstetric perineal trauma: an audit of training, *J Obstet Gynecol* 15:9–23, 1995b.

Sultan A, Thakar R, Fenner D: *Perineal and anal sphincter trauma*, London, Springer-Verlag Ltd, 2007.

Symon A: Third degree tears: the three-stage negligence test, *Br J Midwifery* 16(30):192–193, 2008.

Thakar R, Sultan A: Prevention of obstetric perineal trauma. In Henderson C, Bick D, editors: Replace with: *Perineal Care: an international issue*, Salisbury, Quay Books, 2005.

Thakar R, Sultan AH: Postpartum problems and role of a perineal clinic. In Sultan A, Thakar R, Fenner D, editors: *Perineal and anal sphincter trauma*, London, Springer-Verlag Ltd, 2007.

Tincello DG, Williams A, Fowler GE, et al: Differences in episiotomy technique between midwives and doctors, *Br J Obstet Gynaecol* 110:1041–1044, 2003.

Tohill S, Kettle C: How to suture correctly, *Midwives* 16(1):32, 2013.

Tortora G, Derrickson B: *Principles of anatomy and physiology* (vol 2), 12th edn, Asia, John Wiley and Sons Pte Ltd, 2009.

Trinh A, Roberts C, Ampt A: Knowledge, attitude and experience of episiotomy use amongst obstetricians and midwives in Vietnam, *BMC Pregnancy Childbirth* 15:101, 2015.

Verralls S: Anatomy and physiology applied to obstetrics, Guildford, Pitman Medical, 1980.

Wallace M: *The European Union Standards for Nursing and Midwifery: Information for Accession Countries*. Copenhagen, World Health Organisation (WHO) Regional Office for Europe, 2001.

Walton I: *Sexuality and motherhood*, Hale, Books for Midwives, 1994.

Way S: Episiotomy and body image, *Mod Midwife* 6(9):18–19, 1996.

Willer H, Aabakke AJM, Krebs L: The effect of primary delivery of the anterior compared with the posterior shoulder on perineal trauma: a study protocol for a randomised controlled trial, *Trials* 15:291, 2014.

Williams A, Herron-Marx S, Hicks C: The prevalence of enduring postnatal perineal morbidity and its relationship to perineal trauma, *Midwifery* 23:392–403, 2007.

Wilson AE: *A quasi-experimental study to evaluate an educational in perineal repair for midwives and students*, Ph.D. thesis, University of Surrey, Guildford, 2009.

Wilson AE: Effectiveness of an educational programme in perineal repair for midwives, *Midwifery* 28:236–246, 2012.

Wilson AE: *Audit of Antenatal Perineal Care Clinic: 2013-2014*. Royal Surrey County Hospital, RSCH Foundation Trust, Guildford, Surrey, 2014.

Wong KW, Ravindran K, Thomas J, et al: Mediolateral episiotomy: are trained midwives and doctors approaching it from a different angle? *Eur J Obstet Gynecol Reprod Biol* 174:46–50, 2014.

Woodward K: *Labour Ward Coordinator, Delivery Suite*, Rotherham National Health Service (NHS) Foundation Trust. Personal Communication, 2015.

Woolley RJ: Benefits and risks of episiotomy: A review of the English – language literature since 1980. Part II, *Obstet Gynaecol Surv* 50(11):821–835, 1995.

World Health Organisation (WHO): *Division of Family Health, and Safe Motherhood: Care in Normal Birth: A Practical Guide. Report of Technical Working Group*. Geneva, WHO, 1996.

Wu LC, Lie D, Malhorta R, et al: What factors influence midwives' decision to perform or avoid episiotomies? A focus group study, *Midwifery* 29:943–949, 2013.

Xu X, Wang H, Su L: Women's sexual health: improve our health, improve the world, WHO position paper. Fourth World Conference on women. Geneva, WHO, 2007.

Resources and additional reading

Please refer to chapter website resources.

Dahlen HG, Homer C, Leal N, et al: From social to surgical – historical perspectives on perineal care during labour and birth, *Women Birth* 24(3):105–111, 2010.

Frohlich J, Kettle C: Perineal care best – practice. Systematic review, *BMJ Clin Evid* 2015.

Olsson A, Robertson E, Falk K, et al: Assessing women's sexual health after childbirth: the role of the postnatal check, *Midwifery* 27:195–202, 2011.

Priddis H, Schmied V, Kettle C, et al: "A patchwork of services" – caring for women who sustain severe perineal trauma in New South Wales – from the perspective of women and midwives, *BMC Pregnancy Childbirth* 14:236, 2014.

Swain J, Dahlen HG: Putting evidence into practice: a quality activity of proactive pain relief for postpartum perineal pain, *Women Birth* 26:65–70, 2013.

Tohill S, Kettle C: How to suture correctly, *Midwives* 16(1):30–31, 2013 (website). www.rcm.org.uk/ news-views-and-analysis/analysis/ how-to-suture-correctly.

Useful websites

Perineal massage

https://www.youtube.com/ watch?v=DK2P8Ziqc6Y.

Hands on or poised – HOOP study

https://www.youtube.com/ watch?v=oaEnLD96lzg.

Episiotomy and perineal repair

https://stratog.rcog.org.uk/tutorial/ episiotomy-repair/undertaking -the-repair-5334.

DVD – episiotomy and perineal repair

http://www.perineum.net/product/ repair-of-mediolateral-episiotomy -and-diagnosis-of-acute-obstetric -perineal-trauma-dvd/44857/.

The Keele & Staffs Episiotomy Repair Trainer (Limbs and Things, UK. http://limbsandthings.com/global/ products/keele-staffs-episiotomy -repair-trainer/).

Royal College of Midwives (RCM): www.rcm.org.uk.

For:

RCM: Evidence based guidelines for midwifery-led care in labour: Care of the perineum, London, 2012, RCM.

RCM I-learn PEARLS e-learning programme.

Part Seven

Postnatal care and the care of the newborn baby

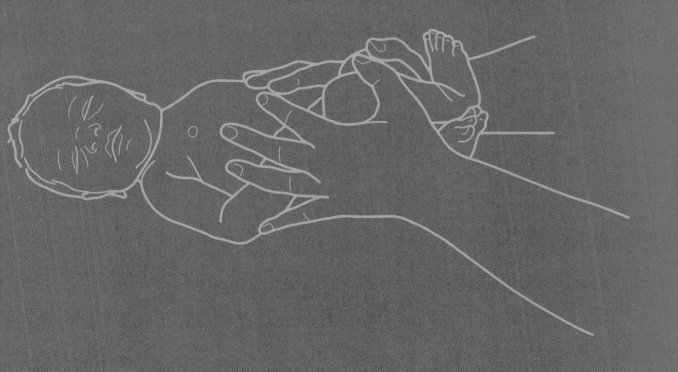

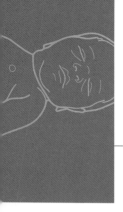

Chapter **41**

Content and organization of postnatal care

Debra Bick and Caroline Hunter

Learning Outcomes ?

After reading this chapter, you will be able to:

- understand the range of normal physical and psychological changes during the puerperium
- be knowledgeable about evidence-based advice and support to meet the needs of each woman
- be aware of the importance of providing culturally sensitive, individualized postnatal care for women during the puerperium
- understand the need for care provision to be undertaken in partnership with women and other care providers to ensure a seamless, high-quality service

INTRODUCTION

The days, weeks and months after birth are a crucial time to monitor and support a woman's physical and psychological recovery from giving birth, to ensure she is able to fully care for her infant and that she, her partner and other family members are supported in their transition to parenthood and family life. In many countries, the puerperium is usually defined as a period of around 6 to 8 weeks after the birth, although there is no evidence base to support this as an optimal duration of recovery from birth, with a number of studies conducted during the last two decades that show widespread and persistent maternal physical and psychological morbidity (MacArthur et al 2002; Woolhouse et al 2014). In recognition of this, this chapter also uses the term 'postnatal period' to suggest a longer and less-defined timespan during which the recovery from birth and transition to motherhood may take place.

Compared with the focus of care during pregnancy and labour and birth, care during the postnatal period has remained relatively 'invisible', with limited efforts made by healthcare providers to revise the content or duration of care to meet the needs of individual women. This situation may change, however, given findings from the most recent MBBRACE-UK inquiry that more women die after having a baby than during their pregnancy or labour (Knight et al 2014), and the opportunities postnatal care presents to implement interventions to improve the life and health of women and their infants, which is recognized by policy makers, including NICE (National Institute for Health and Care Excellence (NICE) 2014a) and the Chief Medical Officer for England (Davies 2015; Bick et al 2015). This chapter considers the most recent evidence to support the physiological changes women experience after birth, the content and organization of services for postnatal women, the role of the health professionals who provide postnatal care and consideration of how more effective care could be provided.

AIMS OF POSTNATAL CARE

The purported aims of postnatal care are to:

- Promote and monitor the physical well-being of mother and baby
- Promote and monitor the psychological well-being of mother and baby
- Help women, their partners and other family members to adapt to parenthood with confidence within a supportive environment
- Identify and promote opportunities for ongoing health promotion in both mother and baby

The organization of postnatal care

The organization of routine postnatal midwifery care in the UK is underpinned by a range of guidelines and standards for maternity care (NICE 2014a; NICE 2014b; Department of Health, Social Services and Public Safety Northern Ireland (DHSSPSNI) 2012; Maternity Services Action Group (MSAG) 2011). Recommendations in general underpin the need for services that are efficient, effective and responsive to the needs of local populations. With respect to postnatal care, each individual woman should have a named health-care professional coordinating her care (NICE 2014a) and, in most cases, this will be the community midwife.

Postnatal care for most women begins in a hospital, although length of in-patient postnatal stay has changed significantly over the last 20 years, decreasing from several days in the 1990s to 6 to 24 hours for women who have had a straightforward delivery in 2006 (Redshaw et al 2007; Royal College of Midwives (RCM) 2014). Evidence for the optimum length of a postnatal stay is lacking; however, many commentators suggest that the focus should be on the level of support available to individual women in the days and weeks after birth (Schmied and Bick 2014) rather than on arbitrary time limits.

Core midwifery postnatal care was traditionally delivered over a series of home visits by a community midwife, which, in reality for most women, has included contacts up to 10 to 14 days post-birth. NICE postnatal guidance made no specific recommendations for the total number of contacts but did recommend a minimum of three contacts (NICE 2014a), and, in practice, current provision is variable, with an average of three episodes of contact within a 2-week period, some of which may take place in postnatal clinics in the community. In most cases, care of the mother and baby is transferred to the health visiting services towards the end of the second postnatal week. Maternity service workers play an increasingly visible role in the provision of postnatal care, both in hospital and community settings, although there has been limited analysis or evaluation of their role. Continuity of care in the form of case-loading teams has been shown in some studies to increase women's satisfaction with postnatal provision (Sandall et al 2015), but there is significant disparity across the UK in the provision of this service. Recent research suggests that, although most women are generally positive about the postnatal care they receive (National Audit Office (NAO) 2013; Care Quality Commission (CQC) 2015; RCM 2014), fragmentation, poor communication between practitioners and underresourcing within the service is having a negative effect on the well-being of many women, with both physical and psychological requirements remaining unmet.

The content of postnatal care

NICE (2014a) guidelines identify core dimensions of care to be provided to all women during the postnatal period (see Box 41.1 – NICE guidelines for routine postnatal care). It recommends that an individualized and documented care plan is developed with the woman, ideally from around 28 weeks of pregnancy, with information about a woman's care from the antenatal, intrapartum and immediate postnatal period added to the care plan over the continuum of pregnancy and birth and before her transfer home after the birth. During all postnatal episodes of contact, whether in a hospital or at home, the care plan should be reviewed and adjusted where necessary, with discussions taking place with the woman about the timing and content of her next contact. Furthermore, women should be asked about their physical, mental and emotional well-being at each contact and encouraged to report any concerns they may have about themselves or their baby.

Although most women may only experience minor or transient health issues, the incidence and prevalence of medical complications in the postnatal period is increasing. Older maternal age, obesity, comorbidities associated with pre-existing cardiac disease, diabetes or severe mental health problems, increased rates of caesarean section and inequalities arising within growing migrant populations are all contributing to outcomes of maternal morbidity in the postnatal period (Knight et al 2014). The NICE postnatal guidelines and quality standards emphasize that care in the puerperium should be underpinned by a philosophy of respect for individual choice, while also recognizing that the postnatal period represents an opportunity to promote long-term health, well-being and, if necessary, lifestyle and health behaviour changes (NICE 2014a and b). Despite this, research suggests that postnatal care, either in a hospital or community setting, still focuses mainly on routine observations and superficial enquiry and that opportunities to make a difference to women's physical or emotional well-being are often missed (Bick et al 2015). However, it is essential that midwives and other health professionals acknowledge that women will experience physiological and psychological changes within the broader context of their social and cultural influences, including those of family, friends and the environment of care. Midwives must, therefore, approach postnatal care from a holistic perspective, which takes into account the wide variety of individual women's needs and experiences, rather than relying simply on a formulaic 'tick box' approach to care.

Physiological changes during the postnatal period

The postnatal period offers opportunities to reduce longer-term physical and mental health issues. The data around maternal morbidity and mortality highlights the importance of maintaining a high index of suspicion around

---

Box 41.1 NICE guidelines for routine postnatal care

Routine core postnatal care and information for women and their infants (adapted from NICE Clinical Guideline No. 37: Routine postnatal care of women and their babies 2014)

Within the first 24 hours after birth:

1. Measure and document BP and urine void within 6 hours after birth.
2. Encourage all women to mobilize.
3. Provide ongoing support for breastfeeding, including advice on skin-to-skin contact.
4. All women should be given information about the physiological process of recovery from birth.
5. All women should be provided with information about the signs and symptoms of deteriorating maternal or infant health and emergency contact numbers.
6. All women should have a written care plan for the postnatal period, including details of any forthcoming appointments or referrals.

Between 2 and 7 days' post-birth:

1. All women should receive the Department of Health 'Birth to Five' handbook within 3 days, and its use should be discussed with women and their families.
2. At every postnatal visit, women should be asked about the following and offered reassurance and/or referral and treatment regarding:
   - Perineal pain (offer visual assessment if the woman reports discomfort)
   - Perineal and hand hygiene
   - Wound healing (perineal or abdominal)
   - Urinary incontinence
   - Bowel function
   - Fatigue
   - Headaches
   - Back pain
   - Normal patterns of emotional changes in the postnatal period
   - Contraception, with contact details for contraceptive advice
3. Women should be offered advice and ongoing support in their infant's feeding choices, including information about local breastfeeding support groups.

4. Midwives should encourage all women to use self-care techniques, including rest and gentle exercise.
5. All women should be asked at every postnatal contact about their emotional well-being and their support networks. Women and their families/partners should be encouraged to tell their health professional about any changes in emotional state and/or behaviour that are outside of the woman's normal pattern.
6. Midwives should be aware of the signs and symptoms of domestic abuse and know where to access help and advice.
7. Anti–D immunoglobulin should be offered to every non-sensitized Rh–D–negative woman within 72 hours after the delivery of an Rh–D–positive baby.
8. Women found to be seronegative on antenatal screening for rubella should be offered an MMR (measles, mumps, rubella) vaccination after the birth and before discharge from the maternity unit, if they are in hospital.

Weeks 2 to 8

1. All women should be advised to report common health issues or any further concerns.
2. Discuss resumption of sexual activity, contraception and possible dyspareunia.
3. All women should continue to be asked about their general emotional and physical well-being.
4. At around 10 to 14 days after birth, all women should be asked about resolution of symptoms of 'baby blues'. If symptoms have not resolved, the woman's psychological well-being should continue to be monitored and, if symptoms persist, evaluated for postnatal depression.
5. Continue to observe for indications of domestic abuse.
6. At the end of the postnatal period, the coordinating healthcare professional should ensure that the woman's physical, emotional and social well-being is reviewed. Screening and medical history should also be taken into account.

---

symptoms of deteriorating health post-pregnancy (Bick et al 2015) and midwives need to be fully aware of the physiological changes that women experience during the puerperium to offer appropriate and timely advice and care. Although more research is needed into the effectiveness of specific interventions, potentially life-threatening conditions such as sepsis, hypertensive disorders or postpartum psychosis will require immediate treatment. It is, therefore, essential that midwives use this time as an opportunity to discuss signs and symptoms of health deterioration with women and encourage women and their families to report their concerns.

Involution of the uterus

The term *involution* describes the return of the gravid uterus to its original size and shape as a pelvic organ. After the birth of the baby and the expulsion of the placenta, a process of ischaemia begins, whereby the uterine muscles constrict the blood vessels to significantly reduce the volume of circulating blood. As the vagina, uterine ligaments and pelvic floor musculature begin to return to their prepregnancy state, redundant muscle, fibrous and elastic tissue require disposal. The mechanism of phagocytosis deals with elastic and fibrous tissues; however, the process is usually incomplete and some elastic tissue remains, meaning that a once-pregnant uterus will never return completely to its nulliparous state. Muscle fibres undergo a process of autolysis, or digestion by proteolytic enzymes, and waste products from this mechanism are passed into the bloodstream to be eliminated by the kidneys.

The decidual lining of the uterus is shed in the lochia, which also contains blood and serum. Around the tenth postnatal day, a new endometrium begins to grow from the basal layer. This process is usually completed in about 6 weeks, although the evidence base for this is sparse and variations have been reported within a range of 4 to 8 weeks (Marchant et al 1999). Changes in the colour of the lochia are described in three stages: *lochia rubra* (red), *lochia serosa* (pink) and *lochia alba* (white). These terms have long formed the basis of practice; however, research suggests that they do not accurately represent the wide range of experience of women in the postnatal period (Marchant et al 1999; Fletcher et al 2012).

Hormonal changes

After the delivery of the placenta, circulating levels of oestrogen and progesterone fall rapidly, along with a corresponding rise in prolactin, stimulating lactation and milk secretion. An increase in the level of oxytocin occurs when the baby suckles or skin-to-skin contact occurs, contracting the cells around the alveoli and increasing the pressure that propels milk along the ducts. This is often felt as a tingling sensation ('let-down') and/or as abdominal cramps, as a result of further uterine contractions.

The ovaries and fallopian tubes will become pelvic organs again, and negative feedback mechanisms prompted by the drop in oestrogen and progesterone will trigger the resumption of the ovarian menstrual cycle, even in the presence of exclusive breastfeeding practices. Ovulation takes place before menstruation is noted; therefore, pregnancy may occur before the first period, and women should be advised that contraception will be necessary from day 21 post-birth. Long-acting reversible contraception (LARC) has been shown to be clinically more effective than the combined oral contraceptive pill, but midwives must be aware of the need to discuss all appropriate options for individual women (NICE 2005; Bick et al 2015) (see Ch. 27).

Cardiovascular system

The volume of blood in the circulatory system decreases to prepregnancy levels and blood regains its viscosity. This is due to the diuretic effect of the removal of uterine waste products via the bloodstream. Smooth muscle tone in the vessel walls improves as progesterone falls, allowing cardiac output, stroke volume and blood pressure to return to prepregnancy levels. Midwives should note that cardiac disease was the leading single cause of maternal death in the last triennial review (Knight et al 2014). International research emphasizes the importance of multidisciplinary working in this area, although research is urgently needed on the structure and working practices of these teams, in terms of their effect on maternal and infant outcomes and use of healthcare resources (Bick et al 2014).

Respiratory system

Changes in the respiratory system are affected by the full ventilation of the basal lobes of the lungs, which are no longer compressed by the enlarged uterus. Chest wall compliance, tidal volume and respiratory rate should return to normal parameters within 1 to 3 weeks (Stables and Rankin 2010).

Musculoskeletal system

The musculoskeletal system returns gradually to its prepregnancy state over a period of approximately 3 months after birth. Ligaments of the uterus and the muscles of the pelvic floor and abdomen should return to their prepregnant state as progesterone levels fall. This process can be aided by early ambulation and undertaking postnatal exercises (Boyle et al 2012); however, approximately one-third of women experience urinary incontinence in the weeks and months after pregnancy, with a high proportion (up to 75%) of these women still reporting symptoms several years later (Gyhagen et al 2013; Brown et al 2015). Most women do not seek treatment for this condition, either because of embarrassment, because they believe incontinence to be a 'normal' part of childbearing or because they feel it is a 'minor' issue that they should be able to manage themselves (Hägglund and Wadensten 2007; O'Donnell et al 2005). This highlights the importance of midwives' raising the issue with women at an early stage in the postnatal period so that appropriate management may be undertaken.

Urinary system

Changes in the urinary tract include a marked diuresis, which lasts for 2 to 3 days after delivery. Fluid and electrolyte balance returns to normal after approximately 3 weeks. Dilatation of the urinary tract, which occurs during pregnancy because of increased progesterone and vascular volume, resolves, and the renal organs return to their prepregnancy state. Urinary retention may still occur during this period as a result of stretching of the bladder and bruising of the urethra during labour. Midwives should ensure that women are informed of the importance of emptying the bladder frequently to avoid further bladder distension and the need for catheterization (Stables and Rankin 2010).

CARE OF WOMEN'S HEALTH DURING THE POSTNATAL PERIOD

For many women, the period after giving birth may be marked by minor and transient physical discomforts, which require monitoring and/or pain relief that, in most cases, can be self-managed by the woman, with advice as needed from the midwife or general practitioner (GP). However, in view of the increasing evidence that postnatal morbidity is more widespread and persistent than previously considered (Knight et al 2014; NICE 2014a; Woolhouse et al 2012; Bhavnani and Newburn 2010), all women need to be carefully assessed during the puerperium to identify conditions that may require more urgent treatment to avoid long-term morbidity or even mortality. Women should be encouraged to report any physical signs or symptoms in the postnatal period that are impacting on their normal activity or well-being and midwives need to maintain awareness of when they need to act quickly and refer women appropriately when necessary.

Uterine involution and vaginal loss

The process of involution has traditionally been assessed by the midwife during the postnatal period by the use of a tape measure or abdominal palpation to measure the distance between the symphysis pubis and the fundus. There is little evidence of the accuracy or reliability of either method in monitoring normal involution (Cluett et al 1997), and current NICE postnatal guidance does not support routine measurement in the absence of other risk factors (NICE 2014a). Of the few studies that have been undertaken, these have suggested that the normal duration and composition of vaginal loss is much more varied than previously assumed (Fletcher et al 2012; Marchant et al 1999). Concerns about the pattern of involution or blood loss may be raised if factors such as pyrexia, abdominal pain, heavy or offensive lochia or maternal malaise are also present. Secondary postpartum haemorrhage, occurring from 24 hours after delivery and usually due to the retention of placental tissue, is among the leading causes of postnatal readmission to hospitals, but timely and accurate diagnosis can be difficult (Aiken et al 2012) (see

Ch. 67). Therefore, midwives should encourage women to report any changes in vaginal bleeding in order to accurately assess and treat any potential problems.

Perineal care

The majority of women who have had a vaginal birth will experience some level of perineal pain and will require effective pain relief and advice on perineal care. NICE postnatal guidance recommends that women who have had a vaginal birth are asked about perineal healing and whether they have any concerns about this at each postnatal contact (NICE 2014a). Visual assessment of the perineum should be offered by the midwife if the woman reports any pain or discomfort, ensuring that the whole perineal area is observed and the woman is asked about symptoms such as pain and offensive vaginal loss. It is particularly important to emphasize good perineal hygiene, such as hand washing before and after changing sanitary protection or going to the toilet, while any perineal trauma (sutured or unsutured) is healing to reduce the risk of genital tract sepsis (Royal College of Obstetricians and Gynaecologists (RCOG) 2012). While bruising and tears to the vagina and perineum will usually heal rapidly in the presence of good hygiene and general health, evidence is lacking around the 'normal' length of recovery time. It is, therefore, imperative that the midwife regard each case as individual and refer any concerns promptly. Figures for the rate of perineal wound infection vary, but studies suggest that around 1 in 10 women will develop an infection (Johnson et al 2012) and that women who undergo an instrumental delivery are at particular risk. Midwives should take risk factors into account when assessing perineal trauma and ensure that regular examination in the postnatal period is prioritized to ensure prevention and timely treatment.

Perineal pain should be managed with a combination of localized and systemic pain management. First-line management, in most cases, will be oral analgesia, most commonly paracetamol (Chou et al 2013). This may be combined in the short-term with codeine unless contraindicated, but may predispose the woman to constipation. Ibuprofen may be used in the postnatal period (and while breastfeeding), but midwives should be aware of any contraindications with the use of Non-Steroidal Anti-Inflammatory Drugs (NSAIDs). NSAIDs are contraindicated in women with a history of asthma, preeclampsia or stomach ulcers. In those women who have experienced severe perineal trauma or have had an instrumental delivery, NSAIDs may be administered via suppository. They can provide relief for up to 24 hours and result in less additional pain relief being required (Hedayati et al 2003).

Local pain relief options may be recommended in addition to analgesia. In a Cochrane Library review,

Hedayati et al found insufficient evidence to recommend the use of topical anaesthetics (e.g. creams) for the relief of perineal pain (Hedayati et al 2005). However, a recent systematic review found that the use of ice packs or cooling gel pads brought short-term pain relief to some women (East et al 2007), although they should be used with caution to minimize the possibility of 'ice burns' to the perineal skin. No demonstrable effect was found on healing outcomes of use of other cooling methods, such as sitting in cool water. There is no evidence to suggest that the use of aromatherapy oils (e.g. lavender) added to bathwater is effective in reducing perineal pain or aiding healing; however, women may find warm baths soothing.

Micturition and bowels

Various urinary symptoms may present in the perineal period, and it is important that the midwife is able to identify these to advise on appropriate management and refer if necessary. In the hospital setting, toilet facilities should be clean and privacy ensured. Urine voided within the first 6 hours of birth should be documented as an intervention to ensure that women who may be going into urinary retention are identified and that preventative measures are taken before considering if catheterization is needed (NICE 2014a). It may be 2 to 3 days before the woman has a bowel movement, especially if she has a painful perineum and/or has had inadequate dietary/fluid intake during labour. Constipation – defined as decreased frequency and regularity of defecation and alteration in the composition of stool – is identified by maternal self-reporting. Women should be asked within 3 days of birth if they have opened their bowels, and those who report experiencing discomfort should have their diet and fluid intake assessed. A gentle laxative may be recommended if dietary measures are not effective. A recent Cochrane review (Turawa et al 2014) of treatments for postpartum constipation, which included five trials of 1208 women in total, was unable to make any recommendations as to the efficacy of current interventions to treat postpartum constipation, although it suggested that a high-fibre diet and increased fluid intake could be helpful. For the treatment of haemorrhoids in the postnatal period, one systematic review suggests that topically applied anaesthetic creams may also be useful in managing pain (Vazquez 2010). Midwives should also be aware of the link between severe perineal trauma and faecal incontinence in the postpartum period. A 2010 systematic review of 31 longitudinal studies noted that third and fourth degree perineal tears were strongly associated with faecal incontinence (Bols et al 2010), while Gartland et al noted that this condition may still be prevalent up to 4 years' postpartum (Gartland et al 2015). Given the effect of this condition on lifestyle and emotional health, it is essential that midwives address this

issue with women and encourage early referral of symptoms (Lo et al 2010).

Infant feeding

Midwives need to be able to offer high-quality evidence-based support to women who wish to breastfeed, as successful breastfeeding is linked with maternal well-being and confident adaptation to motherhood (Britton et al 2007). Exclusive breastfeeding for a minimum of 6 months has also been linked to a reduction in childhood asthmas, infant gastroenteritis, Sudden Infant Death Syndrome (SIDS) and respiratory disease (Horta and Victora 2013). There is also evidence to suggest that children who have never been breastfed may exhibit poorer cognitive development and higher rates of behavioural issues than those who have (Horta and Victora 2013) and that breastfeeding may be protective against both maternal and child obesity (Woo and Martin 2015; Gibbs and Forste 2014). However, despite extensive evidence around the benefits of breastfeeding for women and their infants, 99% of UK women give up exclusive breastfeeding before the end of the recommended 6-month period (McAndrew et al 2012). Evidence shows that women under 20 of white British ethnicity who live in economically and educationally deprived environments are less likely to start or continue breastfeeding than older and more economically secure women (McAndrew et al 2012). Midwives are ideally placed to educate and empower women in the feeding choices for their infants. However, more research is needed around the most appropriate and effective ways of providing this support. Midwives should be aware of the *UNICEF Baby Friendly Initiative*, which offers advice and guidelines on how to support and encourage women to develop a successful breastfeeding relationship. Baby-led feeding should be practised, with no restriction on the duration or frequency of feeds, and advice on the benefits of skin-to-skin contact (UNICEF 2012) (see Ch. 44).

Midwives should also be able to support those women who make an informed choice not to breastfeed. Despite the low rates of breastfeeding continuation in the UK, some women report lack of support, unequal treatment and feelings of pressure to breastfeed when they choose to give formula feeds to their infants (Wirihana and Barnard 2012). It is important that women are supported in all their choices, even if these do not match the choice of the health professional.

CARE OF WOMEN'S PSYCHOLOGICAL HEALTH

Pregnancy and childbirth are major life events. In addition to physical health, changes to emotional and psychological well-being are also experienced. Depression and anxiety are the most common mental health problems during pregnancy, with around 15% to 20% of women experiencing these symptoms in the first year after childbirth and the prevalence range reflecting findings from studies that have assessed symptoms at different time periods after birth and using a range of measures of identification (NICE 2014b). Mood disorders of the puerperium are often divided into three entities in ascending order of severity: postnatal blues, postnatal depression and puerperal psychosis. However, it is important to note that there is debate as to whether these classifications represent separate clinical disorders or a single disorder ranged along a continuum of severity (Miles 2011). Midwives have a vital role to play in monitoring women for signs and symptoms of mental health issues and providing support and referral where necessary (Grier and Geraghty 2015). It should also be noted that depression should not be regarded as a 'catch-all' term for psychological disorders during pregnancy and the postnatal period. Women may also have anxiety disorders, eating disorders or self-harm issues that may have been present before birth and require ongoing treatment and support.

Postpartum 'blues'

Often known as the 'baby blues', this transient, self-limiting condition usually occurs between the third and tenth day after the birth. It is considered a normal reaction and is estimated to be experienced by around 70% to 85% of all postnatal women (Morris-Rush et al 2003). Commonly reported symptoms include tearfulness, irritability and lability of mood. Women and their family members require support during this time and reassurance that, owing to its transient nature, professional intervention is not generally indicated. However, women should be encouraged to seek further evaluation if postnatal blues symptoms persist beyond 10 to 14 days. NICE guidance recommends use of self-care techniques to minimize symptoms such as regular physical activity and sleep and good nutrition, with limited intake of alcohol (NICE 2014b).

Postnatal depression

Most cases of postnatal depression (PND) start in the first 3 months' postpartum, with a peak onset at around 4 to 6 weeks (Brealey et al 2010). Symptoms may include persistent low mood, fatigue, tearfulness, insomnia, poor appetite, feelings of uselessness and helplessness, despair or even suicidal thoughts, and women who have a previous history of antenatal depression or PND are at increased risk (Jones et al 2012). It can be a debilitating condition with long-term adverse effects on the woman, her family and the mother/baby relationship and is considered a

public health concern as a result of its association with higher rates of maternal suicide (NICE 2014b; Tabb et al 2013). However, it is important for midwives to recognize that women may experience significant barriers to seeking help for PND, among them fear of failure or of being labelled an 'unfit mother' (McLoughlin 2013). Midwifery care should be delivered in an empathetic and empowering way to allow women to feel confident in voicing their concerns without being stigmatized (Grier and Geraghty 2015; McCarthy and McMahon 2008). Women should be encouraged to access support from their GP and health visitor and may find that peer-support groups, such as breastfeeding cafés, or postnatal groups can help ameliorate a sense of isolation (Miles 2011).

Puerperal psychosis

This condition affects approximately 1 to 2 in every 1000 new mothers and is more common in those who have a previous history of psychiatric disorders or a family history of psychosis. The recurrence rate is between 25% and 57% (Essali et al 2012). Onset is within the first month postbirth and may be as early as 48 hours after delivery. Symptoms appear rapidly and may include aural and visual hallucinations, delusions, paranoia and significantly altered behaviour (Bergink and Kushner 2014). Midwives must be aware of the risk factors and signs of puerperal psychosis and make immediate emergency referrals for any women in whom the condition is suspected. Admission to a mother and baby psychiatric unit is usually the most appropriate treatment, and most women will recover within a few months, although relapse is possible in a subsequent pregnancy (Austin et al 2008). However, recent reports have highlighted the uneven provision of acute perinatal mental health services across the UK. Continued underfunding has led to a significant reduction in the number of available beds in mother and baby units, and only 27% of maternity services have a specialist mental health midwife (Mental Health Network (MHN) 2014; Gilburt 2015).

Postnatal debriefing and psychosocial support

There has been considerable debate as to the appropriateness of implementing postnatal debriefing to prevent post-traumatic stress disorder (PTSD), particularly among women who have experienced traumatic births. The definition of traumatic birth may be subjective, but risk factors include emergency caesarean section, operative delivery and concerns about infant well-being (Beck 2004; Andersen et al 2012). It is also important to note that women who had a normal vaginal birth may also experience symptoms of PTSD.

A recent Cochrane review, which included data from seven randomized controlled trials (RCTs) from the UK, Australia and Sweden, found little or no evidence to support debriefing interventions (compared with standard postnatal care) to prevent psychological trauma in women after childbirth, with most studies having poor methodological quality (Bastos et al 2015). Some evidence from general population studies suggests that interventions may in fact have an adverse effect in individuals at risk of PTSD (Bisson et al 2015). Despite the paucity of robust evidence in maternal postnatal populations, midwives need to be acutely aware and assess the social and psychological support available to individual women to ensure additional contacts are planned if required (NICE 2014b; McKenzie-McHarg et al 2015).

THE ROLE OF HEALTH PROFESSIONALS DURING THE POSTNATAL PERIOD

The midwife remains the core provider of care for the majority of women during the postnatal period. However, for postnatal care to meet the needs of an increasingly varied demographic, multidisciplinary teams of health professionals should work together to ensure equitable provision of high-quality care. Effective multidisciplinary working is essential, particularly during transfers of care from acute to primary care teams (e.g. from midwife to health visitor) to ensure safe and comprehensive care provision that meets the physical, emotional and social needs of the women, her baby and her family (NICE 2014a).

Over the last 20 years, policy changes have limited the role that GPs play in maternity care, and the current NICE guidance on routine postnatal care of healthy women and babies do not refer to GP involvement but that contacts are undertaken by the health professionals with the 'right skills and competencies' (NICE 2014a). In current practice, the GP role in postnatal care is usually limited to performing the 6 to 8 week 'discharge' check, which is not supported by an evidence base, although a King's Fund report suggested that all GP practices should be able to provide a full postnatal assessment, including a review of mental health and provision of contraception (Smith et al 2010). Of note is that the current National Health Service (NHS) England Standard General Medical Services Contract defines the duration of GP contact as only the first 14 days' postpregnancy. As there is evidence that the routine 6 to 8 week check does not meet the needs of women, recommendations have been made that the content, timing and care provider are reviewed, although

this has yet to be addressed from a research perspective (Bick et al 2015).

Maternity support workers (MSWs) are now employed in many areas of maternity care to undertake aspects of the care previously given by midwives. In the postnatal period, this can include home visits and breastfeeding support. However, there is no nationally agreed role for an MSW and some commentators have raised concerns that this may lead to a lack of clarity, which may affect the safety and accountability if MSWs are, for example, delegated inappropriate tasks (Hussain and Marshall 2011; Lindsay 2014). The midwife remains the lead professional at all times, even when care is undertaken by an MSW.

A health visitor will make contact with the woman and her baby during the postnatal period (with contacts likely to have commenced during pregnancy) and for a number of years afterwards until the child reaches school age. Postnatal contacts may commence when the midwife is still visiting the woman, and it is important that clear communication and a comprehensive handover is given when the midwife discharges the woman and baby from maternity care. The health visitor role in specialist community health nursing, aims to reduce inequalities by working with individuals, families and communities, promoting good health and preventing ill health, with an emphasis on partnership working that cuts across disciplinary, professional and organizational boundaries (Nursing and Midwifery Council (NMC) 2004). Health visitors also play a central role in recognizing deteriorations in maternal mental health by asking the depression identification questions ('Whooley questions') and administering the Edinburgh Postnatal Depression Score where appropriate (Axford et al 2015).

CONCLUSION

There are significant opportunities for postnatal care to make a demonstrable difference to the health and wellbeing of women and infants in both the short- and longterm. Through the promotion of evidence-based midwifery care and effective interdisciplinary workings, women and their families can be encouraged to make positive changes to promote their health and help safeguard future pregnancies.

However, the current model of postnatal care in the UK often falls short of this standard, providing care that is still highly fragmented, rarely individualized and often inflexible. Although examples of high-quality care do exist, in too many cases women are left with their physical and psychological needs unmet at a time of significant transition and lifestyle adjustment. All women should be offered compassionate and holistic care that suits their individual needs, but, as the health profile of birthing women changes and becomes more complex, midwives and other associated health professionals must ensure that their knowledge and skills are adequate to provide the high-quality care that these women require.

Acknowledgement

Debra Bick is supported by the National Institute for Health Research (NIHR) Collaboration for Leadership in Applied Health Research and by the Care South London at King's College Hospital NHS Foundation Trust. The views expressed are those of the author[s] and not necessarily those of the NHS, NIHR or Department of Health.

Key Points

- Postnatal care must be planned, organized and delivered in partnership with women and their families, tailored to their physical, emotional and cultural needs. For many women, the current structure of postnatal care does not always meet their requirements.
- The postnatal period offers an opportunity to promote ongoing health and well-being for mothers and their infants. However, more evidence is required as to the most effective ways of addressing the increasing rates of complex maternal health problems during this time.
- Midwives should utilize available evidence and research, such as is available in the NICE guidelines for postnatal care, to provide high-quality care.

References

Aiken C, Mehasseb M, Prentice A: Secondary postpartum haemorrhage, *Fetal Matern Med Rev* 23:1–14, 2012.

Andersen LB, Melvaer LB, Videbech P, et al: Risk factors for developing post-traumatic stress disorder following childbirth: a systematic review, *Acta Obstet Gynecol Scand* 91:1261–1272, 2012.

Austin MP, Priest SR, Sullivan EA: Antenatal psychosocial assessment for reducing perinatal mental health morbidity, *Cochrane Database Syst Rev* (4):CD005124, 2008.

Axford N, Barlow J, Coad J, et al: Rapid Review to Update Evidence for the Healthy Child Programme 0–5. *London: Public Health England* (website). https://www.gov.uk/government/uploads/system/uploads/attachment_data/file/40, 9772. 2015.

Bastos MH, Furuta M, Small R, et al: Debriefing interventions for the prevention of psychological trauma in women following childbirth, *Cochrane Database Syst Rev* (4):CD007194, 2015.

Beck CT: Birth trauma: in the eye of the beholder, *Nurs Res* 53:28–35, 2004.

Bergink V, Kushner S: Postpartum psychosis. In Galbally M, Snellen M, Lewis A, editors: *Psychopharmacology and pregnancy*, Springer Berlin Heidelberg, 2014.

Bhavnani V, Newburn M: Left to your own devices: the postnatal care experiences of 1260 first-time mothers. London, NCT, 2010.

Bick D, Beake S, Chappell L, et al: Management of pregnant and postnatal women with pre-existing diabetes or cardiac disease using multi-disciplinary team models of care: a systematic review, *BMC Pregnancy Childbirth* 14:428, 2014.

Bick D, MacArthur C, Knight M, et al: Post-pregnancy care: missed opportunities in the reproductive years. In Davies S, editor: *Annual Report of the Chief Medical Officer 2014, the Health of the 51%: Women*, London, Department of Health, 2015.

Bisson JI, Cosgrove S, Lewis C, et al: Post-traumatic stress disorder, *Br Med J* 351:h6161, 2015.

Bols EM, Hendriks EJ, Berghmans B, et al: A systematic review of etiological factors for postpartum fecal incontinence, *Acta Obstet Gynecol Scand* 89:302–314, 2010.

Boyle R, Hay-Smith EJC, Cody JD, et al: Pelvic floor muscle training for prevention and treatment of urinary and faecal incontinence in antenatal and postnatal women, *Cochrane Database Syst Rev* (10):CD007471, 2012.

Brealey SD, Hewitt C, Green JM, et al: Screening for postnatal depression– is it acceptable to women and healthcare professionals? A systematic review and meta-synthesis, *J Reprod Infant Psychol* 28:328–344, 2010.

Britton C, McCormick F, Renfrew M, et al: Support for breastfeeding mothers, *Cochrane Database Syst Rev* (1):CD001141, 2007.

Brown S, Gartland D, Perlen S, et al: Consultation about urinary and faecal incontinence in the year after childbirth: a cohort study, *Br J Obstet Gynaecol* 122:954–962, 2015.

Care Quality Commission (CQC): *Maternity Services Survey 2015*. Care Quality Commission, 2015.

Chou D, Abalos E, Gyte GM, et al: Paracetamol/acetaminophen (single administration) for perineal pain in the early postpartum period, *Cochrane Database Syst Rev* (1):CD008407, 2013.

Cluett ER, Alexander J, Pickering RM: What is the normal pattern of uterine involution? An investigation of postpartum uterine involution measured by the distance between the symphysis pubis and the uterine fundus using a paper tape measure, *Midwifery* 13:9–16, 1997.

Davies S: *Annual Report of the Chief Medical Officer 2014, The Health of the 51%: Women*. In Health DO, editor: London, 2015.

DHSSPSNI: *A Strategy for Maternity Care in Northern Ireland 2012–2018*. Belfast, 2012.

East CE, Begg L, Henshall NE, et al: Local cooling for relieving pain from perineal trauma sustained during childbirth, *Cochrane Database Syst Rev* (4):CD006304, 2007.

Essali A, Alabed S, Guul A, et al: Treatments to help prevent psychosis in women who have just given birth, *Health* 2012.

Fletcher S, Grotegut CA, James AH: Lochia patterns among normal women: a systematic review, *J Womens Health* 21:1290–1294, 2012.

Gartland D, MacArthur C, Woolhouse H, et al: Frequency, severity and risk factors for urinary and faecal incontinence at 4 years postpartum: a prospective cohort, *Br J Obstet Gynaecol* 123(7):1203–1211, 2015.

Gibbs B, Forste R: Socioeconomic status, infant feeding practices and early childhood obesity, *Pediatr Obes* 9:135–146, 2014.

Gilburt H: *Mental health under pressure*, London, 2015, The King's Fund.

Grier G, Geraghty S: Mind matters: Developing skills and knowledge in postnatal depression, *British Journal of Midwifery* 23:110–114, 2015.

Gyhagen M, Bullarbo M, Nielsen T, et al: The prevalence of urinary incontinence 20 years after childbirth: a national cohort study in singleton primiparae after vaginal or caesarean delivery, *Br J Obstet Gynaecol* 120:144–151, 2013.

Hägglund D, Wadensten B: Fear of humiliation inhibits women's care-seeking behaviour for long-term urinary incontinence, *Scand J Caring Sci* 21:305–312, 2007.

Hedayati H, Parsons J, Crowther CA: Rectal analgesia for pain from perineal trauma following childbirth, *Cochrane Database Syst Rev* (3):CD003931, 2003.

Hedayati H, Parsons J, Crowther CA: Topically applied anaesthetics for treating perineal pain after childbirth, *Cochrane Database Syst Rev* (2):CD004223, 2005.

Horta BL, Victora CG: *Long-term effects of breastfeeding – a systematic review.* 2013.

Hussain CJ, Marshall JE: The effect of the developing role of the maternity support worker on the professional accountability of the midwife, *Midwifery* 27:336–341, 2011.

Johnson A, Thakar R, Sultan AH: Obstetric perineal wound infection: is there underreporting? *Br J Nurs* 21:S28–S35, 2012.

Jones CJ, Creedy DK, Gamble JA: Australian midwives' awareness and management of antenatal and postpartum depression, *Women Birth* 25:23–28, 2012.

Knight M, Kenyon S, Brocklehurst P, et al: *Saving Lives, Improving Mothers' Care Lessons Learned to Inform Future Maternity Care from the UK and Ireland Confidential Enquiries into Maternal Deaths and Morbidity 2009–2012.* 2014.

Lindsay P: Maternity support workers and safety in maternity care in England, *Pract Midwife* 17:20–23, 2014.

Lo J, Osterweil P, Li H, et al: Quality of life in women with postpartum anal incontinence, *Obstet Gynecol* 115:809–814, 2010.

MacArthur C, Winter HR, Bick DE, et al: Effects of redesigned community postnatal care on womens' health 4 months after birth: a cluster randomised controlled trial, *Lancet* 359:378–385, 2002.

Marchant S, Alexander J, Garcia J, et al: A survey of women's experiences of vaginal loss from 24 hours to three months after childbirth (the BLiPP study), *Midwifery* 15:72–81, 1999.

Maternity Services Action Group (MSAG): *A Refreshed Framework for Maternity Care in Scotland.* Edinburgh, Scottish Government, 2011.

McAndrew F, Thompson J, Fellows L, et al: Infant feeding survey 2010, *Leeds: Health and Social Care Information Centre*, 2012.

McCarthy M, McMahon C: Acceptance and experience of treatment for postnatal depression in a community mental health setting, *Health Care Women Int* 29:618–637, 2008.

McKenzie-McHarg K, Ayers S, Ford E, et al: Post-traumatic stress disorder following childbirth: an update of current issues and recommendations for future research, *J Reprod Infant Psychol* 1–19, 2015.

McLoughlin J: Stigma associated with postnatal depression: A literature review, *British Journal of Midwifery* 21:784–791, 2013.

Mental Health Network (MHN): *A Good Start in Life: Improving Perinatal and Maternal Mental Health Provision*, London, Mental Health Network, NHS Confederation, 2014.

Miles S: Winning the battle: a review of postnatal depression, *Br J Midwifery* 19:221–227, 2011.

Morris-Rush JK, Freda MC, Bernstein PS: Screening for postpartum depression in an inner-city population, *Am J Obstet Gynecol* 188:1217–1219, 2003.

National Audit Office (NAO): *Maternity Services in England: report by the Comptroller and Auditor General.* London, National Audit Office, 2013.

National Institute for Health and Care Excellence (NICE): *Long-acting reversible contraception*, NICE, 2005.

National Institute for Health and Care Excellence (NICE) (ed.): *CG 37: Postnatal care - routine postnatal care of women and their babies*, NICE, 2014a.

National Institute for Health and Care Excellence (NICE): *CG 192 Antenatal and postnatal mental health: clinical management and service guidance*, NICE, 2014b.

Nursing and Midwifery Council (NMC): *Standards of proficiency for specialist community public health nurses*, London, Nursing and Midwifery Council, 2004.

O'Donnell M, Lose G, Sykes D, et al: Help-seeking behaviour and associated factors among women with urinary incontinence in France, Germany, Spain and the United Kingdom, *Eur Urol* 47:385–392, 2005.

Redshaw M, Rowe R, Hockley C, et al: *Recorded Delivery: A National Survey of Women's Experience of Maternity Care 2006*, National Perinatal Epidemiology Unit NPEU, 2007.

Royal College of Midwives (RCM): *Postnatal care planning. Pressure Points*, London, Royal College of Midwives, 2014.

Royal College of Obstetricians and Gynaecologists (RCOG): *Green-Top Guideline 64b: Bacterial Sepsis Following Pregnancy*, London, Royal College of Obstetricians and Gynaecologists, 2012.

Sandall J, Soltani H, Gates S, et al: Midwife-led continuity models versus other models of care for childbearing women, *Cochrane Database Syst Rev* (9):CD004667, 2015.

Schmied V, Bick D: Postnatal care – current issues and future challenges, *Midwifery* 30:571–574, 2014.

Smith A, Shakespeare J, Dixon A: *The role of GPs in maternity care – what does the future hold*, London, The King's Fund, 2010.

Stables D, Rankin J: *Physiology in childbearing: with anatomy and related biosciences*, Elsevier Health Sciences, 2010.

Tabb KM, Gavin AR, Guo Y, et al: Views and experiences of suicidal ideation during pregnancy and the postpartum: findings from interviews with maternal care clinic patients, *Women Health* 53:519–535, 2013.

Turawa EB, Musekiwa A, Rohwer AC: Interventions for treating postpartum constipation, *Cochrane Database Syst Rev* (9):CD010273, 2014.

UNICEF: *Guide to the Baby Friendly Initiative standards*. London, UNICEF, 2012.

Vazquez JC: Constipation, haemorrhoids, and heartburn in pregnancy, *Clin Evid* 2010.

Wirihana LA, Barnard A: Women's perceptions of their healthcare experience when they choose not to breastfeed, *Women Birth* 25:135–141, 2012.

Woo JG, Martin LJ: Does breastfeeding protect against childhood obesity? Moving beyond observational evidence, *Curr Obes Rep* 4:207–216, 2015.

Woolhouse H, Gartland D, Perlen S, et al: Physical health after childbirth and maternal depression in the first 12 months postpartum: results of an Australian nulliparous pregnancy cohort study, *Midwifery* 30:378–384, 2014.

Woolhouse H, McDonald E, Brown S: Women's experiences of sex and intimacy after childbirth: making the adjustment to motherhood, *J Psychosom Obstet Gynaecol* 33:185–190, 2012.

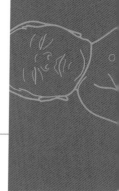

Chapter 42

Physiology, assessment and care of the newborn

Stephanie Michaelides

Learning Outcomes ?

After reading this chapter, you will be able to:

- have a clear understanding of applied anatomy and physiology and the transition from fetal to neonatal life
- identify the importance of providing evidence-based, physiologically appropriate care and management to the neonate
- commit to allocating the same time and attention to the assessment and examination of the newborn as to its mother and family
- explore a framework for undertaking an assessment of the newborn, educating the woman about her baby's needs and how they might be met

INTRODUCTION

Providing the woman with support and guidance in her adjustment to motherhood is an important aspect of the midwife's role. To achieve this, the midwife works with a range of agencies and professionals to support a seamless process from the antenatal period through early parenthood.

As well as being a screening test, the examination of the newborn provides the practitioner with important knowledge throughout the assessment, which can be used to start baseline observations and a care plan. This enables the team to support the care given so that development problems that may occur from fetal to postnatal life can be identified and treated early to reduce morbidity and mortality. The examination of the newborn also provides an opportunity to facilitate maternal/paternal–infant interaction through better understanding the baby's unique development and behaviour.

This chapter will begin with an overview, followed by the application of physiology to the assessment of the newborn. The examination of the newborn is then presented, largely in systems order. The chapter then completes with the daily care of the newborn.

The baby as an individual

Woman-centred care has been an important development in providing choice, continuity and control to women and their families. However, it is likely that the time and attention paid to the assessment and care of the baby, even on a day-to-day basis, has been a fraction of that paid to the woman. It is crucial that babies are viewed as individuals in their own right and that midwives allocate the same attention to their assessment and care. This requires in-depth knowledge of neonatal psychological and physiological development, and complex communication and educational skills.

The baby is recognized as a person (Children Act 1989) with individual needs that require the midwife to act as an advocate and act with duty of care for those needs. Rather than relying on verbal responses, the midwife communicates with the baby via sight, touch and hearing. This must be a focused activity to absorb all information provided by the baby's responses and behaviour. Upon completion of any examination, the findings must be discussed with the parents so that the baby's management and care can be planned in partnership. A documented care plan is then recorded in the baby's notes and updated as the baby's individual needs require. If consent is withheld, then further information, support of a peer or medical advice may be sought. Consent needs to be obtained by the person providing the care (i.e. if the baby deviates from normal, the decision of how to proceed must be made in partnership with a senior neonatologist) (see also Ch. 9).

If the woman wishes the baby to be given oral (or no) vitamin K preparation, the midwife has a duty (NMC 2015), to ask the neonatologist to see the mother and ensure that the decision-making outcome is recorded in the baby's notes. If invasive treatment is required, then consent needs to be obtained by the person implementing the invasive procedure, so that the parents can be given the information they need. If the parents feel that they have not been given adequate information, then consent may not be deemed valid (Department of Health (DH) 2009a).

If the parents refuse life-saving care for the baby, the midwife needs to work with the appropriate professionals (general practitioner or senior neonatologist) to enable the parents in understanding the severity of the situation. It is crucial to record what information has been given and any discussions that take place.

The midwife should clearly document the decisions and justify actions and omissions, providing a clear picture of the transitional events that occurred at birth and during the first 28 days of postnatal life.

Assessment of the newborn

This assessment is not a 'one-off' procedure, but a complex, dynamic and continuous activity throughout the antenatal period, labour, at birth and in the neonatal period. Quick recognition – and appropriate referral of the fetus/neonate with any deviations from normal – results in an enhanced quality of life for that baby and family. In order to achieve this, a formalized communication system between the baby and midwife is vital.

For a period of 9 months, the fetus has been in a safe, untouched and warm environment in which every need is catered for, free movement is allowed and psychological attachment to the mother is developed.

The long-term effects of the birth experience and transition from this safe environment are unknown, and it is imperative that birth attendants consider the baby and the environment he/she has recently left with equal empathy and care as that offered to the mother.

APPLIED PHYSIOLOGY

The midwife's knowledge of the normal fetal physiology, transitional events that occur at birth and the changes to the newborn's physiology can be applied to recognition of normal and abnormal events at birth and the difference between primary and secondary apnoea and their management. In this way, the midwife is able to provide thoughtful and reasoned practice and justify all actions.

Respiratory system

In this section, the embryological development of lungs, role of lung fluid, fetal breathing movements and development and function of surfactant will be explored (see also Ch. 46). It is important to understand the growth and development of the respiratory system from its initial development at embryonic stage through pre-birth (See chapter website resources for additional information.)

The respiratory system consists of:

- upper respiratory tract: the nasal cavity, pharynx and associated structures
- lower respiratory tract: the larynx, trachea, bronchi and lungs

At birth, the umbilical cord is clamped and cut; this allows the major circulatory changes that divert the blood to the fetal lungs rather than to the placenta for oxygenation. The transitional events that take place for the baby to take the initial breath change the lungs from passive organs filled with fluid to structures of air-absorbent cells, which play a vital role in aerobic metabolism.

In uterine life, the fetus obtains oxygen and excretes carbon dioxide via the placenta. Although the lungs are not used for gaseous exchange, *fetal breathing movements* occur from 11 weeks gestation to exercise the muscles of respiration. As the fetus grows, the strength and frequency of breathing movements increase until they are present between 40% to 80% of the time at a rate of 30 to 70 breaths per minute (Davis and Bureau 1987).

Hormones – including steroids, insulin, prolactin and thyroxine – influence lung maturity and dictate how well the baby's lung will function after birth.

Lung fluid, a silky clear fluid that may be seen draining from the baby's mouth at birth is different to surfactant. Its function appears to be mainly for cell proliferation and differentiation. At birth, the lungs must switch function from the secretion of fluid to absorption of gases and exchange of gases. The catecholamine surge, which occurs during labour, is probably the final catalyst to complete this change (Milner and Vyas 1982). Some lung fluid is swallowed and then excreted via the fetal kidneys and into the amniotic fluid. At term, 10 to 25 mL/kg of body weight of liquid remains, which is either expelled via the upper airways or absorbed via the lymphatic system of the lungs, a process commenced at the onset of labour and completed at birth (Gleason and Devaskar 2011).

If delivered by elective lower section caesarean section (ELSCS), the burst of catecholamines provided by the onset of labour will not occur. The lungs will not have been compressed to expel lung fluid. The lung fluid is not absorbed and may be present after birth; therefore, the midwife will need to observe the baby closely for signs and symptoms of *transient tachypnoea of the newborn* (TTN) (see Ch. 46).

Respiration in the neonate

Ribcage and respiratory musculature are immature and will continue to develop into adulthood (Harris 1988). The diaphragm and abdominal muscles are used for respiratory movement, and it may be difficult to see movement of the chest when counting respiratory rate (more easily measured by observing the rise and fall of the baby's abdomen).

For the first 2 to 3 months of life, the baby is an obligatory nose breather and is unable to breathe through the mouth, thus it is vital that the nose is kept clear at all times of any obstacles such as eye protection pads or when nursing the baby, where skin-to-skin contact is made.

Breathing rate is a simple guide to well-being but needs to be assessed alongside the baby's behaviour while validating normality. The respiratory rate is usually between 40 and 60 breaths per minute; however, this rate will need to be considered in relation to the baby's behaviour and activity. Newborns are periodic rather than regular breathers and premature babies more so than full-term babies (Kumar et al 2014).

They may have periods of even and uneven breathing with long gaps between breaths. A baby that has been very active or crying may have a respiratory rate above 70 to 80 per minute and during sleep, the rate may be less than 40.

Tachypnoea (rate of greater than 60) is a result of increased carbon dioxide and chemoreceptors, providing the information to the medulla; thus, an increased respiratory rate may indicate respiratory acidosis, which requires urgent referral to a senior neonatologist for immediate management to prevent the baby from developing metabolic acidosis and collapse (see Ch. 46).

Breathing movements should be *symmetrical*. Babies can generate spontaneous pressures above 70 cm H_2O and develop a spontaneous pneumothorax; therefore, symmetrical movement of the chest confirms normality.

Babies mainly use the diaphragm to aid breathing, and so the *diaphragm* should also move symmetrically, confirming *phrenic nerve* integrity. Damage to the phrenic nerve can occur after shoulder dystocia, and it is important to validate normality at an early stage to avoid later respiratory arrest.

Control of respiration: The control of the respiratory system is mainly autonomic, involving the cortex, brainstem, airways, aortic/carotid chemoreceptors and central control by the medulla. The development and maturity of the central nervous system influences control of respiration, as does temperature, drugs, hypoxia, acidosis and the sleep state of the infant. Drugs such as opiates or epidural given to the mother during labour can affect the control of the respiratory system and can cause respiratory distress within the first 12 hours of life (Kumar et al 2014).

Abnormal signs

Behaviour – the baby is not able to provide eye-to-eye contact with its carer

Muscle tone – the newborn is limp on handling

Tachypnoea at rest – due to the baby attempting to reverse respiratory acidosis

Stridor – suggests upper airway obstruction, which could be caused by oedema or abnormal growths

Expiratory grunting – where the epiglottis closes prematurely – and does not exhale all carbon dioxide, and may be caused by lower airway problems such as surfactant not functioning appropriately or meconium inhalation into the alveoli. This may be seen in a baby who is over 37 weeks gestation who is hypothermic. If not treated promptly by increasing the baby's temperature, respiratory acidosis will result, followed by metabolic acidosis and collapse.

Nasal flaring – the baby increases its ability to inhale oxygen by flaring the nostrils.

Increased respiratory effort – in the form of intercostal and subcostal recession: in response to poor efficiency of surfactant

Cyanosis in room air – a late sign, indicating that the baby has large amounts of unsaturated haemoglobin and is short of oxygen. Cyanosis is best observed by looking at the central circulation, such as in the gums and tongue, because they are more likely to show the level of central perfusion. A baby that is cyanosed needs to be close to resuscitation equipment, as reserves to sustain breathing are at a minimum.

Note: It is important to note that if there are signs of respiratory distress, the practitioner ascertains the correct oxygenation of the newborn (see the next section).

Cardiovascular system in the embryo and fetus

The first functioning system in the embryo, the cardiovascular system (CVS), is composed of the heart and blood vessels and is a closed system that continuously circulates a given blood volume. Blood can be seen circulating in the body by the end of 3 weeks.

Fetal circulation

The structure of the heart provides a circulatory process different from that needed to maintain cardiovascular function after birth. In utero, the lungs have a low systemic pressure and an increased pulmonic pressure, leading to very little blood flow to the lungs, which are nonfunctional in utero. The fetal brain requires the highest oxygen concentration and the fetal circulation is designed to provide the vital organs, such as the brain, liver and tissues, with the maximum concentration of vital materials.

Within the fetal system, oxygen content varies throughout the circulation and is lower than in the neonate or adult, with a concentration of fetal haemoglobin of 18 to 20 g/dL; fetal blood has a high affinity for oxygen to support the fetus through the hypoxia, which occurs during labour contractions. (See Chs 29 and 46.)

Changes at birth

After the birth and the taking of the first breath, the right atrial pressure is lowered and the left atrial pressure is increased slightly, causing closure of the *foramen ovale.* Aeration of the lungs opens up the pulmonary capillary bed, lowering vascular resistance and increasing the pulmonary bed blood flow. The neonate can generate a pressure of up to 70 cm H_2O during inspiration (Strang 1977). This is thought to force fluid out of the lungs to overcome the high resistance and surface tension of the alveoli and to be necessary to establish lung volumes, distributing gas through the lungs.

Oxygenation and the reduction of endogenous prostaglandins from the maternal circulation further *reduces* the vascular resistance and initiates the closure of the *ductus arteriosus.* As a result of pressure changes within the heart, the *foramen ovale* closes functionally at or soon after birth from compression of the two portions of the atrial septum. The *ductus arteriosus* is closed functionally between the fourth to seventh day, closing structurally later when fibrin is laid down – which can take several months to complete.

These physiological changes normally start when the neonate takes the first breath. The neonatal brain must be functioning adequately for the baby to continue to breathe at a sufficient rate to allow homeostasis of oxygen and carbon dioxide within the body.

The vessels which in intra-uterine life carried deoxygenated blood to the placenta, the umbilical and *hypogastric arteries* and those which conveyed oxygenated blood from the placenta to the fetus, the *umbilical vein* and the *ductus venosus*, also close and later become ligaments.

These circulatory changes take place over a period of hours or even days. Respiratory and cardiac disorders accompanied by hypoxia and acidosis may delay, or even reverse, the circulatory changes in the heart and lungs.

Changes in the blood

At birth, the baby has a high haemoglobin concentration (about 17 g/dL), mostly fetal type, HbF, which is required in utero to increase the oxygen-carrying capacity of the blood. Because oxygenated blood from the placenta is soon mixed with deoxygenated blood from the lower part of the fetus, the overall oxygen saturation of fetal blood is therefore reduced.

After birth, the high number of red blood cells is not required, so haemolysis of excess red blood cells takes place, which may result in physiological jaundice of the newborn within 72 hours of birth (see Ch. 47). The conversion from fetal to adult haemoglobin (HbA) starts in utero and is completed during the first year or two of life. By the age of 3 months, the haemoglobin has fallen to about 12 g/dL.

At birth, the prothrombin level is low because of lack of *vitamin K,* a cofactor required for the activation of several clotting proteins in the blood. A deficiency may result; for example, after ventouse birth, the baby can develop a subgaleal haemorrhage (bleeding in the potential space between the skull and galea aponeurosis). Vitamin K administration can rapidly correct such a clotting problem. By the fifth or sixth day, milk feeding is usually established, and the bacteria necessary for the synthesis of vitamin K are present in the intestine.

Skin and temperature control

After birth, the baby must adjust to a lower and labile environmental temperature. The heat-regulating mechanism in the newborn is inefficient, and the body temperature may drop unless great care is taken to avoid chilling. Heat is lost by *radiation, convection, evaporation* and *conduction.* These factors can be rectified if the baby is born into a warm environment of 26°C, dried carefully and wrapped warmly or provided with skin-to-skin contact with the mother (see Ch. 43).

The full-term newborn's skin is well developed, opaque with few veins visible, has limited pigmentation and wrinkles around joints.

The layers of the skin include the epidermis, dermis and subcutaneous layers. The epidermis is a thin, effective barrier preventing penetration and absorption of potential toxins and microorganisms and retaining water, heat and other substances (see chapter website resources).

The skin of full-term newborns is covered with a varying amount of vernix caseosa, a thick, white, creamy substance. This forms between 17 and 20 weeks gestation and by 40 weeks, is found primarily in creases such as the axilla, neck and groins, acting as protection during uterine life (Moore et al 2015). Vernix is a perfectly balanced moisturizer and any surplus should be massaged gently into the baby's skin after the birth.

Gastrointestinal system

Normal function of the gastrointestinal (GI) system should be established before artificially feeding the newborn baby. This can be achieved through reviewing the woman's history and antenatal profile. Polyhydramnios, for example, may indicate obstruction of the GI tract, specifically the oesophagus.

The midwife needs to understand glucose metabolism of the fetus and newborn to support the woman in her chosen method of infant feeding (de Rooy and Hawdon 2002) (see Ch. 44).

After birth, the maturation of the GI tract is stimulated by specific peptides, enteroglucagon and motilin. Enteroglucagon stimulates intestinal mucosa to develop, and motilin encourages gut motor activity.

Nutritive/non-nutritive sucking is the baby's main pleasure and may be satisfied by breast- or bottle-feeding alone. Babies will find solace in sucking their fingers or thumbs or suckling at the breast. Mothers need to understand why the baby is frequently demand feeding, so that they are reassured and not concerned that they have insufficient milk to satisfy their baby. It is important that the midwife explains to the woman, that during the third trimester, the fetus lays down adipose tissue to support ketogenesis, which will support the baby in the first few days of life while awaiting the initiation of feeding.

The knee-to-abdomen position increases abdominal pressure and may cause vomiting of newly ingested food; therefore, nappy changing should be avoided soon after a feed. The supporting gastric and intestinal musculature of the newborn is relatively deficient, shown by the reduced peristaltic movement and the tendency towards distension. The use of pethidine or morphine during labour may decrease peristalsis, and, in association with a weak cardiac sphincter, it will in some cases increase regurgitation for several days after birth.

Meconium, a soft, greenish-black viscid substance, which has gradually accumulated in the intestine from about the 16th week of intra-uterine life, consists of mucus, epithelial cells, swallowed amniotic fluid, fatty acids and bile pigments.

- 0 to 2 days – meconium is passed – the first stool being passed within the first 48 hours. This indicates that the lower bowel is patent, although certain conditions, such as a fistula connecting the urethra and anus, may allow an apparent passage of meconium, despite the absence of the anus.
- 2 to 4 days – as food is digested, the residue mixes with the remaining meconium and the stool changes colour to a greenish-brown *(changing stool)*, indicating that the GI tract is patent.
- 5th day onwards – the stools become yellow.
  - The breastfed baby passes:
    - soft, bright-yellow, inoffensive stools
    - may pass stools five or more times a day as lactation is establishing
    - after 3 or 4 weeks (when lactation fully established) may only pass one soft yellow stool every 2 or 3 days, as there are few waste products from breastmilk

- The artificially fed baby passes:
  - paler, more formed stools with a slightly offensive odour
  - more regular stools when feeding is established, although constipation is more likely
  - It is also important to note that babies who are artificially fed obtain vitamin k and thus will not require to be given vitamin K orally or intramuscularly.

See chapter website resources for more information.

Renal system

The fetus passes urine into the amniotic fluid during pregnancy and *oligohydramnios* (reduced amniotic fluid) may indicate renal abnormalities. At term, the kidneys are relatively immature, especially the renal cortex. Glomerular filtration rate and the ability to concentrate urine are limited. Relatively large amounts of fluid are required to excrete solids.

The baby should pass urine, which has a low specific gravity, within 24 hours of birth. Initially, urinary output is about 20 to 30 mL per day, rising to 100 to 200 mL daily by the end of the first week as fluid intake increases.

If the baby becomes dehydrated, excretion of solids such as urea and sodium chloride is impaired. Dehydration can be recognized by a sunken anterior fontanelle, dry mouth and skin inelasticity, and, most importantly, more than 10% loss of birthweight. It is important to note that a baby who is dehydrated will continue to pass the normal amount of urine; thus, a wet nappy does not validate normality.

Glucose metabolism

See chapter website resources for more information on fetal metabolism.

In utero, the fetus relies on the intravenous transfer of glucose and other nutrients via the umbilical vein for growth and development. Fetal metabolism is directed to anabolism under the influence of insulin, utilizing glycogen, fat and protein.

After birth, normoglycaemia must be maintained to protect brain function and to adapt to the intermittent delivery of milk into the gut for nutritional needs. A neonate over 37 completed weeks gestation and deemed 'normal' is able to adapt physiologically to episodes of starvation by utilizing ketone bodies. This is reflected in a postnatal fall in blood glucose concentration, which may be wrongly viewed as pathological and managed accordingly (de Rooy and Hawdon 2002). After birth, the breakdown of glucose continues under the influence of insulin, but about 8 hours after birth, the baby begins to switch to *glucagon metabolism* (Hawdon 2008).

Musculoskeletal system

The musculoskeletal system provides stability and mobility for all physical activity and includes the bones, joints and supporting and connecting tissue. This provides a means of protection for vital organs (brain, spinal cord), mineral storage (calcium, phosphorus) and production of red blood cells. In comparison with an adult or child's skeleton, the newborn's skeleton is flexible, with the bones mainly composed of cartilage, and joints are elastic, facilitating the passage through the birth canal.

Normal variations in shape, size, contour or movement may be because of position in utero or genetic factors and should be distinguished from congenital anomalies and birth trauma. Early diagnosis of disorders and early intervention often prevent long-term deformity and the need for surgery.

Central nervous system

The development of the neurological system commences 18 days' postconception (see chapter website resources). After birth, the brain continues to grow rapidly within the first year of life, follows a more gradual growth rate until the age of 10, and then there is minimal growth to adolescence. Physiological and psychological well-being are vital to the development of full neurological potential.

Babies born at term can be active participants in their environment and are capable of *social interaction*. It has been shown that they are able to mimic the expression of their carers and are able to some extent to self-regulate themselves.

At birth, the baby's autonomic system maintains homeostasis of all major organs, regulating temperature and cardiorespiratory function. The well newborn will have mature autonomic and motor systems, which can be assessed by the ability to maintain stable cardiorespiratory function. If the baby is unwell or premature, handling will stress the autonomic system, and the baby can become cyanosed and bradycardic (Rennie and Kendall 2013).

State of consciousness in the newborn is influenced by the reaction to stimuli, and understanding the baby's level of consciousness ensures sensitive care and management in assisting in the adaptation to the environment and advance through stages of consciousness. Providing this information to the mother assists her in caring for her baby, may assist feeding and utilizes the baby's energy and available resources effectively (see Box 42.1).

Babies are able to 'tune out' noxious stimuli, and this occurs through the process of habituation. The baby stores the memory of the stimulus and with repeated episodes, learns not to respond to it. Overstimulation of babies who are on 'system overload' will cause them to suffer further stress, requiring appropriate care such as limited

---

Box 42.1 States of consciousness in the newborn

Sleep states

1. *Deep sleep.* Hard to awaken; eyes closed; some jerky movements.
2. *Light sleep.* Eyes closed; moves from deep to light sleep; light sleep to drowsy state – may be sucking present.

Awake states

3. *Drowsy or semi-dozing.* Eyes open or closed; reacts to source of sensory stimuli; minimal motor activity; eyes with bright look.
4. *Quiet alert.* Focuses on stimuli source; minimal motor activity in relation to stimuli; may or may not be fussing.
5. *Active alert.* Much motor activity; increased startles or activity in relation to stimuli; may or may not be fussing.
6. *Crying.* Difficult to get a response to stimuli; will need to bring infant down to state 5 to begin response to stimuli or to feed baby.

(Brazelton and Nugent 1995)

---

handling and an environment with minimal noise and lights to support recovery.

The newborn baby has very poor motor development compared with other mammals but highly developed senses (sight, hearing, taste, smell); hence, it is important to pick up babies and talk to them, stroking them to stimulate and evoke response. Maternal–infant interaction is facilitated by eye-to-eye contact with the mother. A 12-day-old baby is able to imitate the facial and manual gestures of adults, and this may operate as a positive feedback mechanism to caregivers.

Protection against infection

In utero, the fetus is protected from infection by the intact amniotic sac and the barrier mechanism of the placenta, although certain microorganisms do cross the placenta and may infect the fetus (see Ch. 48). During the last trimester of pregnancy, there is a transplacental transfer of immunoglobulin G (IgG) from the mother to the fetus, providing protection against the infectious diseases to which the mother has antibodies. These antibodies provide baby passive immunity for about 4 to 6 months (Wilson et al 2015).

The newborn baby has no immunity to common organisms and, when exposed to them at birth for the first time, is highly susceptible to infection. Soon after birth, the baby becomes colonized by the mother's set of microorganisms, facilitated by early and frequent contact.

Clinical infection occurs when the number and virulence of the organisms overwhelm the poorly developed defense mechanisms of the baby. Breastfeeding encourages specific bacteria to multiply in the bowel, and the acid conditions that result from this may help to prevent the overgrowth of potential pathogens, providing some protection from infection.

CARE AT BIRTH

Preparation

The midwife is obliged to support the birth of any baby showing signs of life at any gestation – in all environments, including outside hospital. It is crucial that midwives are knowledgeable about the physiology of the baby born at different gestations, and how this changes their care and management needs.

Preparations should be made before the baby's birth, and these include identifying women whose babies are at increased risk or who will require specialist care after delivery. The midwife must be prepared to provide care for 'high-risk' and 'low-risk' women (see Box 42.2), although research indicates that the classification of risk factors remains a debatable area, and the focus needs to be on providing safe, quality care for all women and avoiding the label of 'high risk/low risk' (Lancet 2014; Renfrew 2015).

The development of complications during labour and birth is a major contributor to increased neonatal mortality and morbidity (Maternal and Child Health Research Consortium (MCHRC) 2001; Manktelow on behalf of MBRRACE 2015; Chou et al 2015). The midwife can identify that all is normal, detect any deviations and make appropriate referral or alter management of care accordingly.

This action plan begins antenatally to ensure that the woman is prepared and informed to self-manage her body and pregnancy so that she becomes confident and seeks appropriate support should deviations occur.

At birth, the transition to independent life involves a significant physiological shift. The midwife needs to have a good insight into changes of fetal physiology to evaluate the care each individual newborn baby requires.

The Apgar score

The Apgar score, devised by Virginia Apgar in 1953 (American College of Obstetricians and Gynecologists (ACOG) 2015; Levene et al 2008), is a universally and commonly used quantitative measure of the neonate's well-being at and around birth, although it is criticized for its simplicity and limited prognostic significance (ACOG 2015; Levene et al 2008; Sinha et al 2012; National Institute for Health and Care Excellence (NICE) 2014). Five indicators are used:

Box 42.2 Risk factors for specialist resuscitation care

High-risk pregnancy
- Rhesus isoimmunization
- Moderate to severe pre-eclampsia
- Severe IUGR
- Insulin-dependent diabetic (mother)
- Antepartum haemorrhage
- Prolonged rupture of membranes

Abnormal labour
- Fetal distress, prolapsed cord
- Deep transverse arrest
- Cephalopelvic disproportion

Abnormal delivery
- Emergency caesarean section
- Heavy meconium staining of liquor
- Prolapsed cord
- Vacuum or high rotational, medium forceps

Abnormal presentation
- Breech
- Face
- Brow
- Compound/shoulder

Abnormal gestation
- Preterm birth

Abnormal fetus
- Severe oligohydramnios or polyhydramnios
- Known congenital abnormality
- Past history of abnormality
- Multiple births

(Adapted from Sinha et al 2012)

---

heart rate, respiratory effort, colour, muscle tone and response to stimuli (see Table 42.1).

Recording the numerical score alone provides insufficient information concerning the neonatal condition. The important factor is that the neonate's physiological condition and progress is recorded verbally and in writing, until the neonate is in a good condition.

It is advisable, if more than one practitioner is present at a delivery where resuscitation is undertaken, that the baby's Apgar score is agreed between practitioners before the formal record being made. Disagreements can be discussed with the supervisor of midwives and senior neonatologist. It is important for the future management of the newborn's well-being that an accurate assessment is given (UK Resuscitation Council 2016).

Tone, heart and respiratory rate, the most important measures within this scoring system, will indicate the nature and timing of active resuscitation. An Apgar score

Table 42.1 The Apgar score

Sign	Score		
	0	1	2
Heart rate	Absent	Slow < 100	Fast > 100
Respiratory effort	Absent	Slow irregular	Good/crying
Muscle tone	Limp	Some flexion of extremities	Active
Reflex irritability	No response	Grimace	Cry, cough
Colour	Pale or blue	Body pink, extremities blue	Completely pink

of 8 to 9 indicates that the neonate is in good condition. The midwife should expect that most mature babies would obtain a score of about 9 as those over 37 weeks gestation will have a mature neurological system, restricting blood flow to the extremities to supply the brain and other major organs with extra-oxygenated blood. Therefore, the baby will have *acrocyanosis*, and this continues until after 48 hours because of poor peripheral circulation (see chapter website resources).

Maternal–infant relationship

The relationship between mother and baby begins at birth. The experience of the pregnancy may act as a positive or negative foundation for this relationship. The mother's reaction to her baby will vary greatly according to her culture, experience, expectations and environment and will be affected by her physical and emotional state. In some cultures, the mother will wish to have immediate and close contact with her baby from the moment of birth. Others will want the baby cleansed before holding. So that individual needs can be appropriately met, the midwife needs to discuss the mother's wishes, expectations and fears before the labour.

'Bonding' is a term to be used with caution, as it may imply an immediate and strong relationship at the moment of first sight. This may be very threatening and inhibiting for some mothers who will build up their relationship with their new baby in a slower and less obvious way, although the end result is as enduring and strong (see chapter website resources).

Research illustrates mothers' reactions to newborn infants. The mother's first response is to touch her baby (easier if the baby is naked) with fingertips, progressing to a protective caressing movement. The mother will often then move the baby to a position to facilitate face-to-face

eye contact. Throughout this time, she talks to the baby in a higher-pitched voice than usual (Klaus and Kennell 1976). Early research suggested the existence of a 'sensitive time' around the birth, at which the mother and baby should be encouraged to be together, and that women missing this time were at risk of neglecting or abusing their infants. However, Brazelton postulated that even should parent and child have to be separated, if the attendants ensure that the mother has photographs of her baby and is involved in the baby's management and care, cuddling or even just touching her child, the relationship can be effectively preserved and nurtured (Brazelton 1983).

The right hemisphere in the brain is thought to be the emotional sense of self, and, in the newborn, the critical growth period is from the last trimester to 2 years of age.

A mother who is well will cradle her baby, mainly using her left hand; however, a depressed mother will cradle with her right hand (Reissland et al 2007). Some research has also highlighted that stress and depression may impact the ongoing interaction between mother and baby (Reissland and Burt 2010). Working hard to form relationships with the mother and the baby is important in recognizing difficulties involving relationship issues between mother and baby. For example, the personality of the mother may not match that of her baby, and a placid mother may give birth to a baby who is anxious, active and require more attention. It is important to recognize that the relationship of mother and baby can be affected by not knowing what to do, feeling overwhelmed, losing independence, fear of inadequacy, hurting the baby and, ultimately, being a bad parent.

The psychologically healthy mother can cope with professionals, but the psychologically unhealthy mother who may be driven by fear of her baby rather than love may find professionals, such as midwives, dominant and persecutory. That mother may need the care of the professional herself and, left alone, she cannot care for her baby.

Depressed mothers may not be able to decode and respond appropriately to infant's facial expression (Arteche et al 2011).

Warmth

The baby, accustomed to a constant intra-uterine temperature of 37.8°C, is born into a much cooler atmosphere, ideally at 26°C. At birth, the baby should be dried while the assessment of the APGAR is being undertaken before making a decision to cut or keep the cord intact and provide delayed cord clamping. Drying and removing the wet towel will prevent evaporation, and then the baby can be handed to the mother to keep warm, avoiding unnecessary exposure (NICE 2014). Warm covers are placed over the baby, and later the baby should be dressed, covered appropriately and placed in a preheated cot. Within an hour of birth, the baby's axillary temperature is taken and the result validated with comparison between the palpation of arms/legs and abdomen (see Ch. 43).

Identification

Two identification labels record name, date of birth and sex are used to identify the baby. These should be shown to the mother or partner and applied to the baby's ankles or wrists in the mother's presence. Should a label become detached, a replacement must be completed and placed on the baby using the same procedure. Ideally, the labels should not be removed until the baby is in his/her own home. During daily examination, these labels are checked by the midwife for cleanliness, comfort – neither too tight nor too loose for the baby's wrist or ankle – and number (i.e. two).

Several maternity units have developed systems to ensure that babies are properly identified and secure, including recording footprints and handprints, and these should include the names of the mother and baby.

Ideally, a Resuscitaire should be situated in the delivery room because, should the baby need resuscitation, removing him/her from the parents can add significantly to the parent's distress. If the baby has to be separated from the mother, a relative must accompany the baby to enable feedback to be given to the mother, as to what events took place, and to validate that the baby returned to the mother and is, indeed, her own baby.

Vitamin K

After birth, free-circulating vitamin K is low, decreasing during the first few days of life and gradually rising after 3 to 4 days. This may result in excessive bleeding if trauma occurs, for example, during instrumental delivery.

In the UK, it has been advised that all babies should be given vitamin K (NICE 2006; Department of Health (DH) 1998), supported by research (Busfield et al 2013), and parents should be provided with information on whether or not to give vitamin K, and the route of administration, as advised in the Drugs and Therapeutics Bulletin (DTB 2016).

Vitamin K deficiency bleeding (VKDB) (formerly known as haemorrhagic disease of the newborn) is a bleeding tendency that results from a lack of ability in the newborn to utilize vitamin K (see Ch. 47).

Signs and symptoms include bleeding from:

- the GI tract
- the intracranial space
- mucosal surfaces
- circumcision site
- venipuncture site
- heel-prick sites
- the umbilical stump (delayed)

Oral use of vitamin K

Absorption from the gastrointestinal tract is erratic in the newborn, and there is the possibility of regurgitation, inhalation and loss of vitamin K. Additional evidence is required before firm recommendations can be made concerning the optimal dose and form of the vitamin K.

The blood spot (Guthrie) screening test provides a simple method for assessing VKDN. Three minutes of pressure should be applied to the site after taking the blood sample, and a note made of the time taken for the bleeding to stop. Plasters damage the baby's skin and should not be used unless absolutely necessary.

It is also important to note that the vitamin K solution contains beef products and appropriate informed consent requires recognizing that topical or intramuscular administration may be accepted by specific groups, as it is not taken orally.

EXAMINATION OF THE NEWBORN

The first question parents ask is whether or not their newborn baby is 'normal', as they examine him/her from head to toe in minute detail, equal to that of any dedicated professional. This is always an important adjunct to the midwife's assessment and, before any examination, parents' participation is welcomed and any concerns they have should be identified and discussed.

Four types of examination of the newborn are carried out:

- the initial post-birth examination
- the holistic examination from head to toe, which includes the Newborn and Infant Physical Examination (NIPE) screening process
- the NIPE screening test, which focuses on the assessment of eyes, heart, hips and testes
- daily examination for general well-being

Each examination has a slightly different purpose, but all should follow a systematic process and be undertaken with the principles set over the next pages, which will provide the midwife with the best means of assessment (see Fig. 42.1). The next sections include information provided in a systematic way, to enable the full holistic examination; however, some examinations, such as the initial post-birth examination will not include all of these components.

Initial post-birth examination

The midwife will undertake a thorough examination of the newborn soon after birth (NICE 2014). Before examining the baby, the midwife needs to recognize that the baby

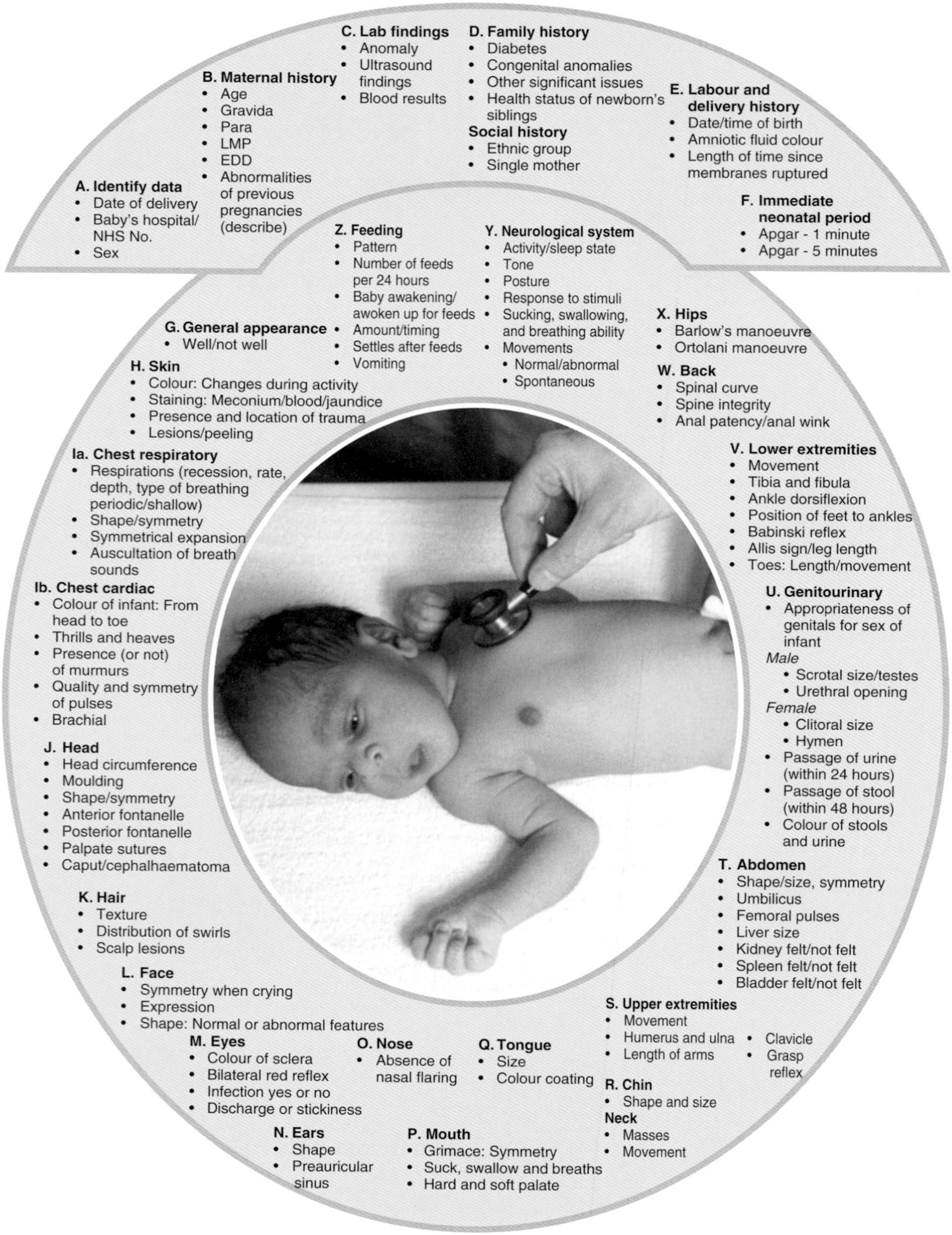

C. Lab findings
- Anomaly
- Ultrasound findings
- Blood results

D. Family history
- Diabetes
- Congenital anomalies
- Other significant issues
- Health status of newborn's siblings

Social history
- Ethnic group
- Single mother

B. Maternal history
- Age
- Gravida
- Para
- LMP
- EDD
- Abnormalities of previous pregnancies (describe)

E. Labour and delivery history
- Date/time of birth
- Amniotic fluid colour
- Length of time since membranes ruptured

A. Identify data
- Date of delivery
- Baby's hospital/ NHS No.
- Sex

F. Immediate neonatal period
- Apgar - 1 minute
- Apgar - 5 minutes

Z. Feeding
- Pattern
- Number of feeds per 24 hours
- Baby awakening/ awoken up for feeds
- Amount/timing
- Settles after feeds
- Vomiting

Y. Neurological system
- Activity/sleep state
- Tone
- Posture
- Response to stimuli
- Sucking, swallowing, and breathing ability
- Movements
  - Normal/abnormal
  - Spontaneous

G. General appearance
- Well/not well

X. Hips
- Barlow's manoeuvre
- Ortolani manoeuvre

H. Skin
- Colour: Changes during activity
- Staining: Meconium/blood/jaundice
- Presence and location of trauma
- Lesions/peeling

W. Back
- Spinal curve
- Spine integrity
- Anal patency/anal wink

Ia. Chest respiratory
- Respirations (recession, rate, depth, type of breathing periodic/shallow)
- Shape/symmetry
- Symmetrical expansion
- Auscultation of breath sounds

V. Lower extremities
- Movement
- Tibia and fibula
- Ankle dorsiflexion
- Position of feet to ankles
- Babinski reflex
- Allis sign/leg length
- Toes: Length/movement

Ib. Chest cardiac
- Colour of infant: From head to toe
- Thrills and heaves
- Presence (or not) of murmurs
- Quality and symmetry of pulses
- Brachial

U. Genitourinary
- Appropriateness of genitals for sex of infant
- *Male*
  - Scrotal size/testes
  - Urethral opening
- *Female*
  - Clitoral size
  - Hymen
- Passage of urine (within 24 hours)
- Passage of stool (within 48 hours)
- Colour of stools and urine

J. Head
- Head circumference
- Moulding
- Shape/symmetry
- Anterior fontanelle
- Posterior fontanelle
- Palpate sutures
- Caput/cephalhaematoma

T. Abdomen
- Shape/size, symmetry
- Umbilicus
- Femoral pulses
- Liver size
- Kidney felt/not felt
- Spleen felt/not felt
- Bladder felt/not felt

K. Hair
- Texture
- Distribution of swirls
- Scalp lesions

L. Face
- Symmetry when crying
- Expression
- Shape: Normal or abnormal features

S. Upper extremities
- Movement
- Humerus and ulna
- Length of arms
- Clavicle
- Grasp reflex

M. Eyes
- Colour of sclera
- Bilateral red reflex
- Infection yes or no
- Discharge or stickiness

O. Nose
- Absence of nasal flaring

Q. Tongue
- Size
- Colour coating

R. Chin
- Shape and size

Neck
- Masses
- Movement

N. Ears
- Shape
- Preauricular sinus

P. Mouth
- Grimace: Symmetry
- Suck, swallow and breaths
- Hard and soft palate

Figure 42.1 The A–Z examination of the newborn tool, detailing the different systems.

at birth has no history, except that noted in the records of maternal and family history and fetal well-being, and the midwife needs to review these records before the examination. The midwife might also need to check for any other issues that might affect the neonate.

This initial examination uses information elicited from intuitive knowledge gained from experience, the Apgar score and physiological assessment using the senses – sound, vision and touch. It provides basic information, detects any *obvious abnormalities* or deviations from normal that require referral and provides an opportunity for the midwife to support the parents in their role as carers for the new addition to their family.

Before this first examination, the baby should have at least 1 hour after birth to recover (NICE 2006) – sometimes referred to as the 'golden hour'. This allows mother and baby time to adapt to physiological changes and gives the baby time to adapt to the environment and, if breastfeeding, to feed successfully.

The NIPE screening examination and the holistic examination

These examinations are similar. Both assessments must be undertaken by an appropriately trained health professional. Some of these skills require postgraduate training at present, although increasingly, it is being integrated into pre-registration education programmes.

However, the *NIPE screening tests* focuses on four key aspects to the examination: eyes, heart, hips and testes. The *Holistic examination* – sometimes referred to as the *Neurobehavioural Physical Assessment of the Newborn* (NBPAN) – will also include these areas but will also include additional assessments. For example, the examination for NIPE (UKSC 2005) will be used to exclude cataracts and retinoblastoma, and the holistic assessment of eyes will include the exclusion of Down syndrome through the shape of the eye, jaundice through the exclusion of yellow sclera, sexually transmitted infections and trauma such as conjunctival haemorrhages.

The holistic assessment includes an examination of all systems as a whole, plus neurological behaviour and psychological development of each newborn. The main aim of the holistic examination is to validate normality through the exclusion of abnormality and, where possible, identify abnormalities and communicate any action required to the parents.

Since 1994, increasingly midwives have undertaken the holistic examination rather than their medical colleagues, providing continuity of care as recommended in *Changing Childbirth* (DH 1993), facilitating the midwife's self-audit and having the potential for improving interprofessional partnerships (Hall and Elliman 2006; Hall 1999).

Midwives have a vital role to recognize and validate normality and refer when deviation from the norm is detected. Any possible problems should be ascertained at the outset, providing stabilization and minimizing any future harm before transfer in order to ensure future well-being.

The United Kingdom National Screening Committee (UKNSC) of the Newborn and Infant Physical Examination (NIPE) (UKNSC 2008) advocates the first NIPE screening be undertaken within 72 hours of birth, allowing the postnatal transition of major organs, such as the heart, to take place before the examination. This is done before transfer to the community and the discharge to the care of a health visitor and GP. It is expected that the midwife (NICE 2006) will care for the newborn from birth to 6 to 8 weeks. It is intended that the second holistic examination is combined into a single postnatal visit at 6 weeks to validate the woman's well-being. In between those two examinations, the midwife will assess each baby, reviewing past and present individual history before deciding which criteria need assessment during physical examination and which can be validated through observation alone.

Examination of the newborn assessment tool

A clinical assessment tool (see chapter website resources) has been designed to assess the physiological and behavioural cues to assist the midwife to validate normality through the exclusion of abnormality and identify deviations from normal (Michaelides 2010).

Using a tool enables important information to be gathered through assessment and analysis of the woman's oral and recorded history. A systematic framework, beginning with examination of the heart while the baby is quiet, goes through to the most intrusive testing – the Moro reflex and measuring the head circumference – at the end. The latter is undertaken last, as the baby will find it uncomfortable and will require comforting upon completion.

The tool consists of 26 criteria (Fig. 42.1 a–z), the number of which that will be fully examined at each examination being dependent on the purpose of the examination and the experience and training of the midwife.

Preparation

Preparation is vital to ensure a smooth and effective examination process. An area, to provide privacy and a controlled environment, needs to be set aside; an examining table with an overhead heater and light source can be utilized to examine babies at a height that will prevent back strain in the practitioner. It provides a safe environment for the baby (see Fig. 42.2) and a safe storage space for the required equipment (see Box 42.3). In the home environment, the midwife can use a changing mattress or table (or similar surface area) covered with a warm sheet/towel to examine the baby.

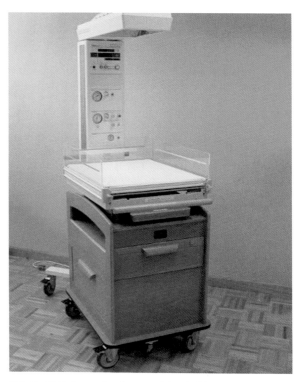

Figure 42.2 Apparatus for examining babies.

Box 42.3 Resources and equipment required to undertake the examination

- Where possible, an overhead heater/heated mattress
- Firm surface
- Sheets and blankets
- A spare nappy
- Cleaning equipment (bowl and cotton wool)
- Ophthalmoscope (cleaned and preset to the practitioner's eyesight)
- Stethoscope
- Small torch
- Tape measure
- Thermometer
- Sterilized spatula
- Mediswabs
- Gloves
- Cord-clamp remover
- Bag for used nappy, used gloves, etc.
- Non-stretchable tape measure
- Scales
- Supine stadiometer/roll-measuring mat

Communication

Before the examination, the woman/parents need to be given full information regarding the rationale for the examination (for example the 72 hours assessment) and the importance of identifying deviations from normal in order to facilitate early treatment and minimize long-term sequalae. After the examination, the midwife must give the parents feedback on the assessment as a whole and, if a deviation from normal is identified, provide information on what the concern may be and discuss future management. For women who are unable to speak English, link workers or translators are essential. The midwife must demonstrate an ability to communicate with the baby, have an understanding of his/her 'language' and to observe and note physiological and behavioural well-being.

Informed consent

The NIPE booklet, *Screening tests for you and your baby* (Public Health England (PHE) England 2015) (see chapter website resources), offered to mothers at booking, provides information about the NIPE examination and suggests that parents should ask their midwife for any further information.

Daily examination

As part of the postnatal examination, the midwife will examine the baby, including checking behaviour, the eyes, skin, umbilicus and napkin area, feeding patterns and (if in hospital) the presence of two identification labels. This examination provides an opportunity to both establish the baby's progress and well-being, and to teach the mother what to look for in monitoring her baby's well-being and to learn skills in baby care.

PHYSICAL ASSESSMENT OF THE NEWBORN

Birth

The baby enters postnatal life from a quiet, dark, warm and wet environment, with boundaries provided by the uterus, entering a whole new world. While drying the baby or, in the case of waterbirth, when the baby reaches the surface, the midwife assesses adaptation to extrauterine life by undertaking the Apgar score at 1 and 5 minutes with a brief physical assessment to exclude gross structural abnormalities. It is important to delay validating gender until the midwife has assessed this, and there is no doubt. Once given, this will be publicized immediately to family and friends and causes great distress if, after later assessment, the gender is questioned.

During the first hour of life, the baby is given to the mother or father and interaction begins. As the baby is alert in this first hour, the mother should be supported to give a first breastfeed. If artificially fed, the midwife needs to undertake a fuller assessment of the gastrointestinal system. The baby who breastfeeds will take in a small, but valuable, quantity of colostrum. A baby given formula is likely to take an amount of fluid which, if the GI tract is incomplete, such as in cleft palate or imperforate anus, may cause preventable damage. It is also important to recognize the first successful artificial feed may also exclude oesophageal fistula and, thus, a midwife must always be present when the first feed is given to recognize the baby that may become cyanosed as a result of milk entering the lungs.

Formal assessment of the newborn

Physical examination of the newborn baby should be performed systematically, examining each physiological system to ensure entirety (see Fig. 42.1), using the skills of observation, palpation and, where relevant, auscultation.

It is important to recognize that the baby will provide information on his/her health and well-being. It is through expert knowledge and experience of neonatal behavioural and physiological assessment of the newborn that the practitioner will be able to identify the infant who requires special care.

The midwife needs to explain that the assessment of well-being is a continual process and that each examination only validates normality through the exclusion of abnormality for that moment in time. With continual observation, care and professional support through education and physical assessment, there is a growing reassurance.

History

During the antenatal period, a full record is taken of the family and previous medical and obstetric histories of the woman and partner. The present pregnancy, labour and prenatal period should be reviewed to identify any risk factors that may affect the baby.

When obtaining a history from women, it is important that the communication process is open and interactive. Women should be given the reasons for certain questions and how this affects the care provided (see chapter website resources and Ch. 32).

Laboratory results need to be assessed by the midwife for their relevance to the assessment of the newborn. For example, a group O-positive mother with a baby who is jaundiced may trigger consideration of the possibility of *ABO incompatibility*.

Kell antibodies can attack the bone marrow, reduce red cell production and may result in the baby being anaemic at the time of birth. Anaemia in the newborn will render the baby hypoxic, requiring resuscitation at the time of birth and administration of fresh blood.

Sexually transmitted diseases, if not treated in the antenatal period, may affect the baby postnatally and, therefore, the baby will need to be observed for signs of infection (see Ch. 48).

Health education is important, although it is not always possible to reduce at-risk behaviour of women, and a nonjudgemental and supportive approach is required in obtaining true and accurate information to facilitate appropriate care (see chapter website resources).

Information such as the date of the first day of the last menstrual period (LMP) and the estimated date of conception (EDC) is crucial in the calculation of gestational age, an important aspect in the management of care.

When undertaken correctly, fetal surveillance (see Ch. 36) can assist the midwife to have the relevant practitioners present at birth. The type of birth may affect the management of the baby – after a protracted labour, the baby may be traumatized and may require an initial superficial examination to validate well-being, followed by a full examination when signs of recovery are apparent. Minimal handling may assist the shocked newborn to recover. The physical examination should ideally last no longer than 15 minutes, as newborn babies cannot deal with excessive handling.

Maternal concerns are an important guide in the focus of the examination, as the majority of women will spend time examining, feeling, stroking and counting their baby's fingers and toes. In the majority of cases, they themselves will recognize if their baby deviates from normal.

General appearance

A baby's age and gestation will influence his/her general appearance. Type of birth, postnatal age, and the timing of the last feed affects the baby's behaviour. A hungry baby will be difficult to examine as many of the assessments require a quiet, calm baby, able to tolerate handling for 10 to 15 minutes in order to complete the physical examination.

A baby who has had a difficult birth may be very irritable or be in a deep sleep (State 1 – see Box 42.1), and the midwife needs to use the baby's behaviour to guide the examination.

Observation

A 'hands-off' approach is used when observing the baby. The baby over 38 weeks gestation will display a flexed posture, indicating good muscle tone (Fig. 42.3). General features are noted for dysmorphia.

Gestational assessment

Previously, weight defined term and preterm babies; a baby weighing less than 2500 g was deemed to be premature. Further research (Battaglia and Lubchenco 1967)

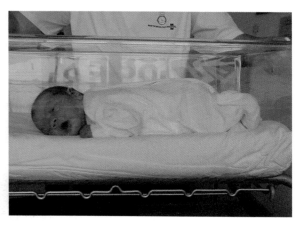

Figure 42.3 A well-flexed baby.

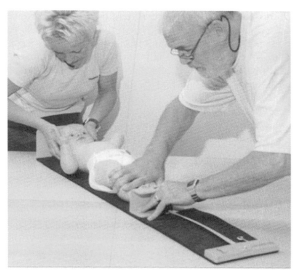

Figure 42.4 Measurement of height. (From Jokinen M: Measuring newborns: does size really matter? RCM Midwives J 5(5):186–187, 2002.)

showed that gestational age and whether the baby's growth is appropriate for that age is a greater predictor of outcome.

Assessment tools, such as the Dubowitz scoring system (Dubowitz et al 1970), are used to assess the gestational age of the newborn using a neurological scale (see Ch. 45). This assessment is used with babies deemed to be less than 38 weeks gestation. The main assessment of gestational age can be carried out using approximate estimates of fetal development, i.e. the LMP, the estimated date of delivery (EDD), ultrasound and physical characteristics (see chapter website resources).

Measurements

The UK World Health Organisation growth charts

These are based on measurements collected over time by the World Health Organisation (WHO) from healthy breastfed babies whose mothers did not smoke and were not deprived (see website). Plotting the baby's weight and head circumference enables the midwife to identify those 'at risk' and validate the normal baby to plan future care.

Weight

Scales need to be regularly maintained for accurate measurement and recording. Care should be taken to minimize the baby's heat loss while weighing by placing the baby safely in the scales and ensuring that the surroundings are warm and free from draughts.

The weight can be plotted on the centile chart, and babies who are small- or large-for-gestational age identified and a plan of action developed, agreed and recorded in the baby notes. Babies below the ninth centile have reduced glycogen stores and may be more prone to hypothermia and hypoglycaemia, so thermoregulation and feeding must be given extra attention.

The baby will lose 5% to 10% of body weight in the first week of life, then steadily gain at an average rate of 25 to 30 g per day until 6 months of age (Wilkinson 1997).

Note: A baby who has not reached his/her birthweight by day 10 needs to be reviewed to exclude signs of poor feeding, thermoregulation issue or underlying urinary tract infection.

Dehydration: This is seen in babies who have yet to establish breastfeeding; identification is vital to prevent hypoglycaemia and hypernatraemia. Signs of dehydration include loss of skin turgor, dry mucous membranes, lethargy and a sunken fontanelle; a weight loss of greater than or equal to 10% is also significant. Urine output is normally 1 to 3 mL per hour, and this will continue regardless of the presence of dehydration; thus, a wet nappy does not indicate well-being.

Length

There is debate as to whether or not babies should be measured. Now, for accurate measurement, a supine stadiometer (Wilkinson 1997) newborn length instrument or a rollamat (Fig. 42.4) may be used. Both methods require the baby to be stretched; therefore, two persons are required to undertake the measurement accurately.

Head circumference

This measurement is taken with a non-stretchable tape applied closely around the scalp, using the posterior eminence and the frontal and parietal eminences as markers. The largest estimate of three is taken. Immediately after birth, the measurement may be increased by oedema or caput; therefore, it needs to be repeated when any swelling has subsided.

Vital signs

The temperature is measured while the respiratory rate is counted. If the baby is cold (less than 36.5°C), the examination may be discontinued or the baby may be continued to be examined under a radiant heater. The midwife needs to include in her action plan, a reassessment of the temperature after 1 hour to exclude infection, completion of records and may require medical support.

The respiratory rate is usually between 40 and 60 breaths per minute, although the baby's behaviour before counting the respiratory rate needs to be taken into account. As periodic rather than regular breathers, the baby may have periods of even and very uneven breathing and long gaps between breaths. It is important to concentrate on a small area of the abdomen, and this makes counting a little easier.

Note: A baby that is otherwise well but has tachypnoea greater than 50 at rest may be exhibiting a sign of respiratory acidosis and must be referred to a senior paediatrician.

Skin

The skin protects the baby against infection, enables communication and is sensitive to touch, pressure, temperature and pain. After birth, the baby is rubbed dry – touch should be gentle to minimize discomfort to the baby.

The epidermis of the skin of a newborn is thin and delicate and, in post-mature babies, is dry and sometimes peeling (see chapter website resources).

The best environment to observe the colour of the baby is in natural daylight, as artificial light can affect the depth of colour observed. Pink is the normal colour of newborns. A red/plethoric colour which, when the baby cries, becomes dusky/purple, may be caused by an excessively high packed cell volume (PCV) and is deemed to be pathological, as it may indicate *polycythaemia* (see chapter website resources).

Pale skin or pallor is an indication of poor perfusion and anaemia. Infants of diabetic mothers tend to be pinker than average and 'post-mature' infants are paler.

Asian and dark-skinned babies may have *blue naevi* scattered around any area of the body, which may be mistaken for bruises. Parents are sometimes concerned and can be reassured that this deep pigmentation of the skin will fade in a few months.

Petechiae (tiny subcutaneous haemorrhages) – normally are a result of traumatic delivery, for example, a tight cord around the neck, and should disappear within 24 to 48 hours. If this does not happen and they appear to multiply, this might be pathological and the baby needs to be referred for diagnosis.

Jaundice may occur physiologically after 72 hours because of extra red cell breakdown in combination with an immature liver, which cannot metabolize all unconjugated bilirubin; the latter leaks under the skin and gives a jaundiced colour. The use of a transcutaneous bilirubinometer to estimate the level of jaundice on all at-risk newborns daily for 72 hours (see Ch. 47) enables estimation of jaundice.

Common variations of the skin include tiny milia on the nose (plugged sweat glands).

Erythema toxicum may be noted. These papular lesions with an erythematous base are found more on the trunk than on the extremities and fade away without treatment by 1 week of age. Occasionally their profusion is alarming.

Haemangiomata

- *Vascular naevi* are superficial capillary haemangiomata, which may occur over the upper eyelids and the nape of the neck, sometimes hidden by the hairline. These usually diminish in size and fade by 1 year of age.

- *Capillary* (*strawberry*) *haemangioma* usually presents between birth and 2 months of age. These are most common on the face, scalp, back or chest. This haemangioma enlarges before diminishing by 1 year of age and disappears by the age of 5 to 7 years.

- *Port wine stain* (*naevus flammeus*), if situated on an area of skin over a nerve pathway, such as the trigeminal area on the face, may be associated with meningeal haemangioma (Sturge–Weber syndrome). Large areas of discoloration may require later laser treatment.

The skin is observed daily for soreness, rashes and septic spots.

Dry skin

A normal skin barrier has cells that are packed tightly together. Applying olive oil for moisturizing or massaging baby skin has been used for years. However, *oleic acid*, a core component of vegetable oils, disrupts the structure of skin cells, weakening the skin barrier, so either avoiding oils completely (Lavender et al 2009) or using mineral based oils may be preferable (Cooke et al 2015).

Cardiorespiratory system

The heart and lung assessments are interlinked to reduce handling and ascertain how both function, to distinguish between heart and lung normal physiology and pathology.

Observation

Colour

The infant's colour is an important index of the function of the cardiorespiratory system.

- 'Good' colour in Caucasian infants means a reddish-pink hue all over, except for possible cyanosis of hands, feet and, occasionally, lips (*acrocyanosis*).

- Mucous membranes of dark-skinned babies are more reliable indicators of cyanosis (and degree of jaundice) than the skin.

- The baby's colour should be assessed at regular intervals during the postnatal period.

- Examinations, whenever possible, should be undertaken with the baby naked to ascertain colour symmetry from head to toe.

Chest

The general appearance of the chest is noted, observing the neck and collarbone area. The chest and abdomen are examined while observing respirations.

- Position of nipples, and presence of skin tags, accessory nipples or skin discoloration are noted.

- Chest should be rounded.

- Both sides of the chest cavity should move symmetrically, with breathing actioned by the diaphragm and abdominal muscles.

- Respiratory rate and pattern are observed for symmetrical movement of the diaphragm. (Asymmetrical movement of the diaphragm should alert the midwife to possible *phrenic nerve* damage. Although babies may have periodic breathing, episodes of true apnoea longer than 20 seconds are deemed abnormal and may indicate neurological damage or abnormality.)

- Breathing should not draw on accessory muscles; indrawing of intercostal or subcostal muscles. Signs of accessory muscle use indicate *severe respiratory distress*.

- Breathing should be quiet – audible sounds are a sign of deviation from normal and can help identify the origins of respiratory difficulty depending on the type. For example, inspiratory grunting could indicate a problem in the upper airway, i.e. oedema or mass. An expiratory grunt suggests the cause is in the lower airways and may be caused by *hypothermia, surfactant deficiency* or *meconium aspiration*.

Palpation

The chest is palpated gently, as there may be breast enlargement because of maternal hormones, and pressure can cause discomfort and pain.

- Position of the heart is checked to see whether it is on the left or right side of the chest. This is best done by auscultation (see next section) but can be confirmed occasionally by palpation.

- This is followed by validation of the absence of *heaves* and *thrills* and identification of the point of maximum impulse (see chapter website resources).

- *Capillary filling time* is measured using applied pressure on the chest or gently squeezing of the earlobe or toe and expecting the blood flow to return within 3 seconds.

- *Brachial and femoral pulses* are identified and palpated for strength, rhythm and volume.

- *Femoral pulses* are best palpated when the baby is quiet and often feel quite weak in the first day or two. It is vital to validate their presence in the assessment of cardiovascular function.

- *Dorsalis pedis* pulses may be palpated in preference to femoral pulses.

Auscultation

Normal or abnormal breath sounds may be noticed by the practitioner before the use of the paediatric stethoscope to identify heart and breath sounds (see chapter website resources). Performed after a period of observation, this can enhance the examiner's perception, knowledge of and communication with the baby. Warming the chest piece by applying friction to the stethoscope head reduces disturbance of the baby, facilitating auscultation.

Auscultation of breath sounds in the newborn is easier than in a child, as breath sounds are being established with the absence of crackles and wheezes (see Fig. 42.5).

The heart should be examined alongside other aspects such as femoral pulses. To determine whether the heart is on the right or left side, the examiner should observe precordial activity, rate, rhythm, quality of the heart sounds and the presence or absence of murmurs.

When the baby is peaceful, the rate, rhythm and presence of murmurs can be determined much more easily than when the baby is a crying or 'fussy'. The midwife could encourage the mother to pacify the baby by the use of her little finger or a dummy.

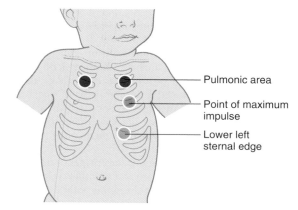

Figure 42.5 The areas of auscultation of heart and lung sounds.

— Pulmonic area
— Point of maximum impulse
— Lower left sternal edge

The heart rate normally is a sinus rhythm between 120 and 160 beats per minute, varying with gestational and chronological age and degree of activity (Begum et al 2012).

Murmurs mean less in the newborn period than at any other time. A neonate may be found to have an extremely serious heart anomaly without any murmurs (Hall and Elliman 2006). A closing *ductus arteriosus* may cause a murmur that, in retrospect, is only transient, but, at the time, is very loud, worrisome and misleading. Gallop sounds may be an ominous finding, while the presence of a split 'S2' (i.e. *lub dub dub*) may be reassuring. If new to auscultation of heart sounds, it is difficult to ascertain S1 and S2 (see chapter website resources). Simultaneous palpation of the brachial pulse and auscultation of the *lub dub* makes identification of sounds easier.

The stethoscope aids assessment of the cardiovascular system. However, the best assessment is to observe or obtain an accurate maternal/family history of cardiac problems and also the baby's behaviour. A baby who has been active, then suddenly becomes lethargic, appears to have less tone, is not interested in feeding or is tachypnoeic on effort, especially after feeds, needs urgent referral and admission by ambulance to the nearest acute neonatal unit.

Major congenital abnormalities can be *duct dependent*; therefore, most cardiac conditions will be diagnosed in the community after the transfer to the home. It is important for the parents to understand normal behaviour of the newborn and to seek advice if their baby deviates from this.

The cardiovascular assessment is not complete until the liver is palpated and deemed to be of normal size, i.e. less than 2 cm below the costal margin on palpation.

Congenital heart disease

Significant congenital heart disease (CHD) may be diagnosed at virtually any age. Some conditions are discovered in neonates; others rarely are identified during infancy. The profound haemodynamic transitions that occur at the time of birth make the clinical presentation of heart disease a challenge to practitioners to identify CHD. An understanding of the fetal circulation and transition to postnatal life can provide the clinician with the tools to anticipate and treat problems safely as they arise. For example, a baby who is suspected of having CHD and is cyanosed is **not** given oxygen, as this will encourage the ductus arteriosus to close faster.

Although they cannot be prevented, there are many treatments for the defects and any related health problems. Babies in the UK have the physical examination within 72 hours after birth. While the ductus arteriosus is patent, it is difficult to identify the murmur (see Ch. 49).

Pulse oximetry

Research in Sweden and in the UK has identified the use of pulse oximetry as a test that can provide an improved means of identifying at-risk newborns (Singh et al 2014; de-Wahl Granelli et al 2009; Knowles et al 2005). Pulse oximetry is a non-invasive diagnostic test used for detecting the percentage of haemoglobin (Hb) that is saturated with oxygen. Oxygen saturation is a measure of how much oxygen the blood is carrying as a percentage of the maximum it could carry. A normal pulse reading is 98 to 100; a reading under 95 is too low and may indicate a baby at risk of CHD.

To obtain accurate recordings, it is important to apply the probe correctly, making sure the two light sources and receiver face each other, the probe is placed on the right hand of the baby and, depending on the size of the baby, whether the thumb or wrist is used. It is important to review the makers instructions on how to apply and maintain the necessary equipment (Thangaratinam et al 2012).

Morphological examination

Accurate assessment of the morphological system is essential for identifying the baby who will need more thorough examination, medical/support services or family counselling. External assessment of dysmorphic features offers clues to the presence of internal anomalies. This examination requires a systematic approach to assessment, including observation and palpation.

The head

Because of moulding, the shape of the head after birth can be round, bullet-shaped or an elongated oval, which may concern parents. They need to be reassured that the head will assume its natural shape, given time. This needs to be noted, as the measurement of the head circumference will differ from birth to that taken 4 or 5 days later. The average full-term head circumference, occipital–frontal diameter measurement, should be approximately 33 to 38 cm avoiding the ears.

The vault of the head is held in the midline while the size, shape and symmetry are assessed. The scalp and face should be inspected for cuts, abrasions or bruises. Trauma sites, such as fetal blood sample site, should be identified and recorded, to support follow-up care and management.

The presence of caput succedaneum or cephalhaematoma (Fig. 42.6) should be noted (see Ch. 30).

The mobility and width of suture lines and the degree and direction of moulding of the skull bones is noted. Fontanelles are examined: large fontanelles may reflect a delay in ossification of bones and may be associated with hypothyroidism. In its normal state, the anterior fontanelle is flat and at the same level as the surrounding bones. A sunken fontanelle can be a symptom of *dehydration*, and a full and bulging fontanelle and wide sutures are characteristic of *hydrocephalus*.

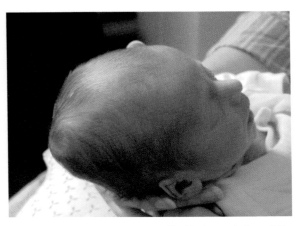

Figure 42.6 Cephalhaematoma. (By kind permission of Dr. Raoul Blumberg.)

Exclusion of *craniosynostosis* (a condition which affects males twice as often as females) needs to be undertaken by assessing all sutures to validate normality through mobility or overriding of sutures. This condition in which the sutures close too early causes pressure inside the vault and can be recognized as the baby grows older by an asymmetrical appearance, for example, closure of the lambdoid suture causes a flat occiput and if not identified can cause brain damage.

The hair

The condition and amount of hair is also noted, as this can be affected by certain metabolic disturbances (e.g. *hypothyroidism*).

The face

This is examined for normal appearance and symmetry of eyes, ears and features during crying and rest.

The eyes

Both eyes should be observed together to identify and exclude any trauma, *petechiae* and *naevi*, as any naevi over the trigeminal area may involve the trigeminal nerve and requires referral. The eyes should be observed for oedema or discharge because this may indicate infection, such as a sexually transmitted disease, and, if not identified and treated, can swiftly progress to a systemic infection.

Eyes should be observed for position, size and symmetry, as eyes that are wide apart (*hypertelorism*) may indicate a syndrome. Eyes that appear large can be associated with glaucoma (Tappero and Honeyfield 2014).

The baby should be able to provide eye-to-eye contact with its carer; however, *ptosis* (drooping) of the eye lids warrants an immediate referral, as it may be a congenital abnormality of neurological origin.

The eyes are tested for the *red reflex* by means of an ophthalmoscope. The purpose of this test is to detect abnormalities of the retina, lens and cornea. The red reflex must be deemed to be intact and complete to exclude *cataracts, brushfield spots*, which may indicate Down syndrome, or incomplete, which may indicate *retinoblastoma*. This assessment can be undertaken when the baby opens his/her eyes during the examination. Alternatively, the baby then can be taken into a darkened room after the full examination. When using the ophthalmoscope, the retina is seen as clear and red, with the amount of red pigment being dependent on race (for more information see chapter website resources).

Ophthalmia neonatorum is conjunctivitis that occurs in the newborn. Conjunctivitis is an inflammation of the conjunctiva, the surface or covering of the eye, resulting from infectious or noninfectious causes. It is identified by an inflamed conjunctiva and watery solution or pus secreted from the eye. Simple infective conjunctivitis is often caused by *Staphylococcus aureus, streptococci* or *Escherichia coli*. If infection is suspected, appropriate swabs for *Chlamydia trachomatis* and *gonorrhoea* must be taken to exclude these infections, which are associated with corneal ulceration and blindness (UKNSC 2008).

The ears

Both are examined for symmetry and normal position on the baby. An imaginary line can be drawn from the inner canthus of the eye to the posterior fontanelle, and the helix of the ear should be above the line to validate normality. The pinna of the ear should be flexible and recoil easily. Accessory auricles, skin tags and sinuses should be noted, as they may indicate further abnormalities, such as those affecting the renal system (Roth et al 2008) (see chapter website resources).

Hearing: Sensitivity to sounds should be noted. The ability to hear enables babies to communicate and learn about the world in which they live. However, one baby will sleep through the loudest music and another will be startled by someone speaking softly.

Since March 2006, all babies in the UK have been offered a hearing screen test soon after birth. The screening for a hearing defect involves two painless tests – the otoacoustic emissions test (OAE) and the automated auditory brainstem response test (AABR).

Babies are sometimes referred because of the results being affected by the baby being unsettled at the time of the test or because fluid, such as vernix or liquor, was in the ear. The test can be repeated.

The mouth

This should be checked, commencing with the rooting and sucking reflexes, examining the gums for clefts and to ensure that there are no deciduous teeth present. Epstein's pearls (small white inclusion cysts clustered about the midline at the juncture of the hard and soft palate) are a normal finding. Tongue-tie, in which the frenulum restricts the movement of the tongue, should be identified correctly utilizing evidence-based tools (Cawse-Lucas 2015).

The midwife should ensure that there are neither hard nor soft palatal clefts (Bannister 2001). The palpation and visualization of both the hard and soft palates is imperative – it is necessary to use a torch and tongue depressor. Midwives and doctors have been shown to have missed a cleft palate (Hunter and Habel 2014; Habel et al 2006).

To examine the mouth with a tongue depressor, the baby should be swaddled and the head held gently held to avoid movement during the examination. A sterilized spatula is inserted and the tongue is depressed, which enables the visualization of hard and soft palates. It is vital to inspect right back to the *uvula* to exclude minor degrees of cleft palate (Hunter and Habel 2014). Wood carries bacteria and multiple spatulas in one box can become contaminated when accessing individual spatulas, thus encouraging cross-infection to the newborn; consequently, spatulas require sterilization before use.

The mouth should be examined at regular intervals to validate normality and exclude infection, for example, *Candida albicans.*

The nose

This is examined for normal position and the presence of nares and possible unilateral *choanal atresia*, which may or may not be easily identifiable (see Ch. 49).

Suctioning of babies is no longer advisable, except in specific circumstances – for example, the presence of meconium or blood at birth. If a suction catheter is introduced into the nasal passages, the delicate epithelial lining and dissection of the mucous glands may be damaged and the baby may become snuffly. Unless the baby has a problem with breathing, time will heal the damage and breathing should be normal within several days.

The neck

This is passively examined for rotation and for anterior and lateral flexion and extension.

- Anterior flexion – the chin should touch or almost touch the chest.
- On extension, the occipital part of the head should touch or almost touch the back of the neck.

When there is asymmetrical rotation or lateral flexion or when range of motion is limited, this is recognized as abnormal. The neck should also be examined for *goitre* and thyroglossal or brachial arch sinus tracks, and the spaces hidden by creases, for evidence of septic spots or irritated skin.

Sharing information with parents

If there are concerns that the baby is dysmorphic, it is important to communicate this sensitively to the parents before referral to a senior neonatologist, as a dysmorphic baby may be a clue to the presence of other congenital anomalies (e.g. cardiac or gastrointestinal). One useful way to begin the discussion is to ask the parents whom the baby resembles. The parents may then feel they can disclose their concerns. Even if the baby does have a resemblance to other family members, it does not exclude genetic abnormalities, and the baby should be referred to a neonatologist for follow-up. The words used to describe a dysmorphic baby need to accentuate the positive; for example, words such as 'distinctive facial features' (Aase 1990) rather than 'abnormal' or 'deformed' should be expressed.

Musculoskeletal system

History

Prenatal history is vital to musculoskeletal assessment because the uterine environment affects the musculoskeletal development of the fetus. Any event or condition that changes the intra-uterine environment can alter fetal growth, movement or position. Factors such as oligohydramnios, breech presentation, abnormal growth patterns and exposure to teratogenic agents may adversely affect the development and maturation of the musculoskeletal system in utero. The skeletal system is interlinked with the neurological system; therefore, factors such as possible birth trauma need to be considered.

The birth history, such as duration of labour, signs of fetal distress and type of birth (vaginal or caesarean), has a bearing on conditions such as cerebral palsy and brachial palsy.

In multiple gestations, the birth order is worth noting because there is a higher incidence of congenital hip dysplasia in first-born children.

An accurate gestational age assessment is necessary for assessment of the infant's posture and muscle tone.

Careful scrutiny and recording of the musculoskeletal system during the first newborn physical examination is imperative, as this forms the basis for all future examinations.

Examination

A thorough and systematic physical examination of the skeletal system, including the skull, clavicles, upper limbs, legs, spine and the hips, should be done within the first 24 hours after delivery. Then, should an abnormality of the spine be noted, the senior neonatologist will undertake the hip examination, thereby limiting stress to the newborn. As with other systems, skeletal examinations are undertaken while watching the newborn or while examining other systems.

Evaluation of the musculoskeletal system includes an appraisal of:

- posture, position and gross anomalies
- discomfort from bone or joint movement

- range-of-joint motion
- muscle size, symmetry and strength
- the configuration and mobility of the back

Observation proceeds from the general to the specific and includes the ratio of extremity length to body length. General inspection includes observation for symmetry of movement and size, shape, general alignment, position and symmetry of different parts of the body.

Soft tissue and muscles should be observed for swelling, muscle wasting and symmetry. Asymmetry of length or circumference, constrictive bands or length deformities of the extremities should not be present.

Palpation, along with inspection, is used on each extremity to identify component parts (for example, the two bones – radius and ulna – in the forearm), function and normal range of motion.

Clavicles are inspected and palpated for size, contour and crepitus (grating that can be felt or heard on movement of ends of broken bone). A fractured clavicle, one of the most common birth injuries, should be suspected when there is a history of a difficult delivery, irregularity in contour, shortening, tenderness or crepitus on palpation. It can be very uncomfortable and painful. The midwife may notice this when undressing the baby.

Humerus length and contour should be noted. A fractured humerus should be suspected if there is a history of difficult delivery. A mass, due to a haematoma formation or signs of pain during palpation, may also be noted. If there is an injury, to minimize the pain and discomfort, the baby's affected arm should be placed at right angles to its body and the 'babygro' can be used to hold it in position. Alternatively, the arm can be gently bandaged against the baby's body, to reduce movement. The mother must also be given information how to dress and undress her baby and also the positions to adopt to support the baby to feed comfortably and minimize the level of pain.

Elbow, forearm and wrist are examined for size, shape and number of bones and for range-of-joint motion.

Hands should be examined for shape, size and posture, and fingers for number, shape and length. Inspection of palm creases should also be included. Although a single simian crease across the palm is usually associated with Down syndrome, it is often found in normal babies.

The fingers are usually flexed in a fist with the thumb under the fingers. The nails, usually smooth and soft and extending to the fingertips, should be examined for size and shape. The mother should be advised how to cut the nails to avoid causing infection to the nail bed, which can cause septicaemia.

Lower extremities

From observation, the position of the baby's lower limbs will give a picture of the position adopted in utero. The majority of babies will lie with the legs folded on the abdomen, appearing externally rotated and bowed with everted feet. The baby delivered in a breech presentation often has flexed, abducted hips and extended knees. This positional adaptation of the lower limbs should not be confused with congenital malformations; however, a midwife who is in doubt should seek a second opinion from a peer or a neonatologist.

The midwife should examine the baby for normal appearance and for length, shape and movement of limbs, ensuring that the baby is able to move each limb fully and that the joints are functional. The legs are palpated to ascertain the presence of the femur, tibia and fibula. Femoral length can be observed by straightening both legs together and noting the length or by testing for the *Allis sign* as follows. Keeping the feet flat on the bed and the femurs aligned, flex both of the baby's knees. With the tips of the big toes in the same horizontal plane, face the feet, bend so that the baby's knees are at eye level and note the height of both knees. It will be apparent if one knee is higher than the other. This is a *positive Allis sign* and may indicate developmental hip displacement.

Ankles and feet: Examination includes observation of resting and active movement. Passive motion of the ankle in dorsiflexion and plantar flexion varies depending on the infant's position in utero. For example, ankle and forefoot adduction, a positional deformity, can be differentiated from *congenital equinovarus* (clubfoot) malformation by passively positioning the foot in the midline and gently applying pressure to dorsiflex the foot to form a 'square window'. A clubfoot or other structurally abnormal foot and ankle will not have a full range of motion, will resist dorsiflexion and will not be able to form a square window (Bridgens and Kiely 2010).

The feet should be examined for shape, size and posture; checking that the baby is moving both feet and adopts a normal position when at rest. The toes are examined for number, position, spacing, the presence of webbing and whether the nails are a normal shape and appearance. The soles of the feet should be inspected as part of the gestational age assessment and should, therefore, each be opened fully. This part of the examination is undertaken when eliciting the *Babinski reflex* (see the next section).

Assessment of the back: Neural tube defects (NTD) are usually detected before birth as a result of *maternal alpha-fetoprotein* (AFP) measurement or ultrasound examination. Babies with NTD normally would have been born in an appropriate unit with the relevant staff, neonatologist and neonatal nurses available at birth and afterwards. However, not all women choose antenatal screening and some may not have had antenatal care; thus, spinal neural defects could still present without warning.

On completing the examination of the lower limbs, the baby is briefly lifted and held suspended with the examiner's hand under the chest so that the back is observed to view the curvature of the spine and the baby's ability to

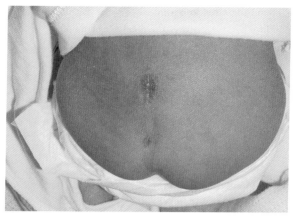

Figure 42.7 Lumbar and sacral "dimples". Ultrasound revealed tethering of the spinal cord. (By kind permission of Dr. Raoul Blumberg.)

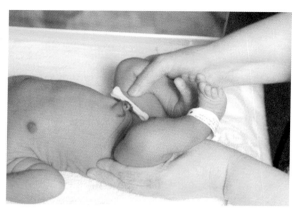

Figure 42.8 Examination of the hips.

lift the head. The spine should be straight, excluding *scoliosis, kyphosis* and *lordosis.*

The back continues to be observed with the baby lying prone. The spine is then examined from the base of the skull to the coccyx, noting any *skin disruption, tufts of hair, soft* or *cystic masses, haemangioma, pilonidal dimple cysts* or *sinus tract* (see Fig. 42.7). These deviations from normal may be signs of congenital spinal anomaly.

The position of the scapulae should also be noted while the infant is in the prone position to rule out *Sprengel's deformity,* a winged or elevated scapula.

The entire length of the spine should be gently palpated to ensure that it is complete and that there is no sign of pain.

A baby born at home found to have a *meningocele* (herniation of meninges) requires urgent referral and transport to hospital. Before and during transport, the lesion – especially if ruptured – should be covered with a sterile, non-adherent dressing. If that is not available, gently place sterile gauze soaked in normal saline and wrap in cling film. Pressure on the affected area must be avoided, the baby must be nursed in the prone position and gently transferred into hospital.

Hips: Developmental dysplasia of the hip (DDH) is the preferred term for the disease previously referred to as congenital dislocation of the hip (CDH). The new term takes into consideration that dislocation of the hip can develop after birth and although the hips can be deemed to be normal at birth, the baby can later have a positive screening for a *dislocated* or *dislocatable* hip joint.

The assessment of the baby's hips is undertaken within the first 72 hours of birth to detect conditions that may need early treatment. The UKNSC has produced standards and competencies to ensure consistency throughout the UK for improved and early detection of abnormalities to enable non-invasive treatment and avoid surgical intervention. These standards detail how the examination should be undertaken and by whom (UKNSC 2008). The assessment of the hips should be undertaken on a firm surface and one hip at a time examined by a trained professional. The left hip is more frequently affected than the right.

The neonate's pelvic girdle is not fully ossified and does not have the same characteristics as the adult pelvic girdle; the acetabula are shallower than in the adult. The acetabulum is still developing and it is quite possible for the femoral head to be able to move outside the acetabulum (*luxation* or *dislocation*) or through an abnormality within the acetabulum (*subluxation* or *partial dislocation*).

Early detection is vital to avoid surgical intervention. Left untreated, the hip joint develops abnormally and surgical reduction is required. Early diagnosis enables the use of splints, allowing the hip joint to develop normally.

It is important for parents to be informed that one assessment is not sufficient to validate the hip stability. It is important that they continually observe for signs of dislocated hip, such as difficulty in putting the nappy on the baby or any apparent difficulty in walking and inform their GP if they have any concerns.

Examination

The ideal time to undertake examination of the hip (Fig. 42.8) is within the first 72 hours. Before the examination, the practitioner needs to recognize the importance of history in identifying the babies at risk. High-risk factors for DDH include (Keay and Morgan 1982):

- family history of DDH
- abnormal rotation of the developing hip during the first trimester
- neuromuscular disease, especially in the second trimester
- abnormal mechanical forces (e.g. oligohydramnios)

- breech presentation in utero for a significant part of fetal life
- female infants (who are more susceptible to the maternal hormone *relaxin*).

Aspects of care that can prevent DDH include postnatal application of mechanical forces, associated with the baby able to fully abduct the hips, such as being allowed to lie in the prone position when awake and being carried in a sling with hips fully abducted – African babies whose mothers transport them in this way have a low incidence of DDH.

The hips should be examined at regular intervals for congenital dislocation, which may be identified by the use of one of two tests:

- *Ortolani test*, which detects a *dislocated hip reducing* during the examination
- *Barlow test*, which detects a hip *dislocating or subluxing* during the examination (Sewell et al 2009)

A distinctive 'clunk' is of significance and is usually felt rather than heard by the examiner. However, 'clicks' often felt while performing these tests are not predictive of DDH but can be confusing for an inexperienced examiner.

Ideally, examination of the hips should be the final part of the examination, as it is often disruptive and uncomfortable for the baby. The midwife can utilize methods to reduce discomfort, such as encouraging the baby to suck the mother's finger or, if bottle-feeding, using the pacifier.

Practitioners undertaking the examination of the hips must have undertaken training during which they have been both taught and observed by an expert in the examination (STEPS 2011). Practice on the '*Baby Hippy*' manikin is advised before examining a baby. An inexperienced practitioner can cause damage to the baby by failing to diagnose a false negative test because of poor practice or use of excessive force on a dislocated hip during abduction, causing damage to blood supply and ligaments.

The midwife should observe the baby and note any difficulties with abduction. For example, if the baby found the procedure of examining the femoral pulses distressing or the *Allis sign* (see chapter website resources) was positive, this may be an indication that the right or left hip may be dislocated.

Ortolani and Barlow tests

The baby should be lying relaxed on a flat, firm surface in an environment warm and free from draughts. It is vital that the practitioner examines only one hip at a time with a full focus on undertaking the manoeuvre correctly.

Ortolani test

- Stabilize one hip by bending the knee and hip, keeping the pelvis stable and firmly on the mattress (see Fig. 42.8)

- Bend the other knee and hip
- Place two fingers over the greater trochanter (outer upper leg)
- Position the thumb on the inner trochanter
- Attempt to *abduct* (away from the midline of the body) the thigh to 90 degrees by applying pressure with the two fingers on the greater trochanter.

If the hip is dislocated, it will not be possible to abduct it, and the neonate will keep the thigh at an angle less than expected. This angle is noted and recorded.

Barlow test

- Continue to stabilize one hip, keeping the pelvis stable and firmly on the mattress (Fig. 42.8)
- Bend the other knee and hip
- Place two fingers over the greater trochanter (outer upper leg)
- Position the thumb on the inner trochanter
- The thigh is lifted and *adducted* (moved towards the midline of the body)
- With pressure applied with the thumb laterally, the femur is telescoped to note any movement of the head of the femur away from the acetabulum. Normality is confirmed when no movement is noted.

These two manoeuvres are then repeated with the other hip joint. If any deviations from normal are noted, the examiner should refer the baby to a senior medical practitioner.

If undertaken by a competent practitioner, the Ortolani and Barlow manoeuvres remain the best screening method for DDH.

Additional investigations

X-rays are unhelpful in assessment, as the femoral head is cartilaginous until 6 months of age. Ultrasound examination of the hips is undertaken as part of screening for DDH; however, its effectiveness is not recognized by all.

The leaflet on developmental dysplasia of the hip, congenital *talipes equinovarus* (clubfoot) and lower limb deficiencies (STEPS 2011) should be given to parents of affected babies. This will inform them of facts relating to deviations from normal in the lower limbs and raise awareness that, although the baby's hips may be stable at the first examination, it is important to have the hips examined once again at 6 to 8 weeks to exclude the development of an abnormality.

Gastrointestinal system

Abdomen

During fetal life, the fetus relies on the placenta for food and elimination of waste products. To sustain life after birth, the newborn baby must adapt to the intermittent intake of nutrients necessary for the body's metabolic requirements of growth, replacement and energy production, followed by their digestion and utilization and the excretion of waste products. The baby is able to suck and swallow, but the digestive process and glucose metabolism take time to adapt to postnatal life.

Physical assessment of the gastrointestinal system, therefore, commences with the mouth and completes on examination of the anus. Normality needs to be confirmed before the baby being able to undertake artificial feeding, as this entails a comparatively large intake volume.

The shape of the abdomen should be rounded, soft, symmetrical and slightly protruding. A flat abdomen may signify decreased tone and may herald the presence of abdominal contents in the chest cavity through a diaphragmatic hernia or abnormalities of the abdominal musculature.

Abdominal skin in the term baby is smooth and opaque with a medium-thick texture. Post-term babies have thick, parchment-like skin with superficial or sometimes deep cracking in the creases of the skin and no vessels seen over the trunk.

Diastasis recti (separation of the rectus muscles) is a common finding in the newborn. Another midline malformation is an umbilical hernia, which reduces spontaneously within 2 years. If it is large, it will require surgical treatment.

Midline defects such as *omphalocele* or *gastroschisis* may be seen at birth (see Ch. 49). As the fetus grows during the first trimester of pregnancy, the developing intestines extend into the umbilical cord and should return to the abdomen by the 11th week of fetal development. However, if the muscles in the abdominal wall fail to close properly, the intestines may partially return to the abdominal cavity. Immediate management is to avoid fluid loss and maintain a clean environment; therefore, the baby's body is placed in a special plastic bag, tied below the arms. The umbilical cord is examined before cutting (Fig. 42.9) and applying the Hollister clamp, to exclude herniation of intestine into the cord itself and to visualize the presence of three vessels (Lissauer et al 2015). Two vessels, one artery and a vein, sometimes indicate renal anomaly (Thummala et al 1988). The cord is a bluish-white colour and gelatinous at birth. The quantity of Wharton's jelly affects the thickness of cord. Large-for-gestational-age infants have thick, gelatinous cords. Babies with congenital syphilis may also have thick cords. A thin, small cord is another indication of intrauterine growth restriction.

The cord darkens and shrivels as it dries and separates by a process of dry gangrene, usually between the fifth and seventh day. It should be dry and without drainage of any type. Discharge of any colour before or after separation is not deemed normal; for example, clear discharge indicates

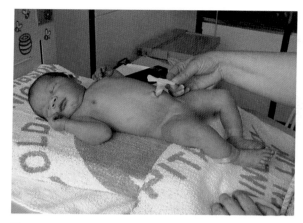

Figure 42.9 The correct length for clamping and cutting the cord.

a *patent urachus* or *omphalomesenteric duct* (Tappero and Honeyfield 2014).

The area around the cord is observed for any redness, which needs to be dealt with quickly to avoid serious septicaemia. The mother needs to understand the potential for infection from urine and faeces if the umbilical cord is placed inside the nappy, and the midwife can support the mother by showing her how to achieve this (Zupan et al 2004).

Cleaning the cord: A good handwashing technique is essential before attending to the cord to avoid a spread of the highly dangerous bacterium, *Staphylococcus aureus*. The umbilical cord is inspected daily by the midwife for signs of infection and separation. If the cord is soiled by a dirty nappy, it should be cleaned with water only and dried with cotton wool swabs (NICE 2006). In low resource countries, however, the use of antiseptics such as chlorhexidine may be used to reduce infection risk (Karumbi et al 2013; WHO 2013).

Peristaltic movement

The midwife should observe for patterns and shape of movement, observing movement from the side of the abdomen and at eye level.

Normal abdominal movements are synchronous with chest movements. After 1 hour of life, intermittent peristaltic movement is visible. Continuous peristaltic movement can imply intestinal obstruction (see Fig. 42.10).

It is important for the midwife to auscultate numerous neonatal bowel sounds to confidently validate normality.

Palpation

Before palpating the abdomen, the midwife needs to check that the baby has not been fed a large amount before the examination, as the baby will not be able to tolerate the

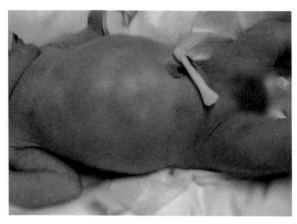

Figure 42.10 A distended abdomen with visible loops of bowel. (By kind permission of Dr. Raoul Blumberg.)

palpation. The midwife should stand at the right side of the baby and the hands must be warm and the nails short to enable palpation of the organs to take place without discomfort to the baby. The baby should be lying supine and be relaxed. Palpation should be informed by knowledge of the anatomy of the intestinal organs in the position and depth of palpation. The baby's facial expression needs to be observed for signs of discomfort or pain during the palpation, and the baby's respirations need to be synchronized with the palpation to identify an enlarged liver during respiration. Flexing the baby's knee at the hip can allow the abdominal muscles to relax and aid palpation.

Light palpation of the four quadrants assesses the texture and warmth of the skin (see chapter website resources). It also reveals tenderness and guarding. Deep palpation identifies the absence of masses.

The liver is a superficial organ and palpation needs to take that into consideration. The liver edge should not be more than 2 cm inferior to the right costal margin. Babies in heart failure, where the liver acts as a sponge for fluid, will have an enlarged liver that can be palpated more than 2 cm below the costal margin. Slight oedema can sometimes also be seen around the eyelids.

The spleen is a deep organ but, if enlarged, becomes a superficial organ; thus, firm but light pressure is applied to confirm normality. A non-palpable spleen equates to normality.

The abdominal area overlying the kidneys is also balloted, applying firm even pressure. The kidney should not be felt (Royal College of Midwives (RCM) 2015a).

Vomiting

Most babies vomit at some time and mostly this is unimportant (Orenstein 1999). However, there are circumstances when the type of vomiting is important, the main

one being green bile (Walker et al 2006). It cannot be assumed that this is meconium that was ingested at birth, and the baby should be examined by a senior neonatologist to exclude obstruction such as a *volvulus*, which can lead to occlusion of the blood supply to the intestines and cause necrosis of the intestinal tract.

Possets are small, frequent vomits, particularly common in the first few days after birth. 'Posseting' is also common when the milk flow is excessive. Most babies cope with these episodes quite well and either swallow or vomit out the regurgitated contents. The parents need to be informed how to manage these episodes. The baby should be left slightly on his/her side, while the posset is wiped away, and should not be lifted or patted on the back as both may cause overstimulation, affecting the coordination of sucking, swallowing and breathing. It is important for parents to be aware that if the baby is to vomit green-colour fluid, this is an emergency and the baby needs to be seen immediately.

If the baby has inhaled a large amount of vomit, appropriate resuscitation needs to take place (Page and Jeffery 2000). Before any resuscitation involving mask ventilation, and when the baby has had a feed, the midwife needs to be prepared to pass a nasogastric tube to empty the contents of the stomach to avoid inhalation (RCM 2015b) (see website for guidelines on how to undertake this).

The groin

When lying quietly, the baby's groin is flat, and if it is thin, visible pulsation of the femoral pulse may be noted. Any visible swelling on crying or on palpation must be referred urgently for diagnosis and management, as this might indicate inguinal hernia or undescended testis – in the male or female – querying the sex of the baby.

Genitourinary system

Male infant genitalia

Scrotum: All embryos are initially female. Under the influence of testosterone, the labia enlarge to become a scrotum, brownish in pigmentation, and should be fully rugated.

Testes: Normally, the testes of a full-term newborn are approximately 1.5 to 2 cm in length (Conner 2014). They should be palpated and have a consistency similar to that of a pea. If the scrotum appears discoloured and the testes feel solid, urgent referral is required.

The differential diagnosis for the presence of a solid scrotal mass includes *testicular torsion, scrotal haematoma* and *testicular infarction* (Diamond and Gosalbez 1998).

Hydrocele: The signs of a hydrocele include palpation of a cystic mass in the scrotal pouch. The whole scrotum appears swollen and firm – like a balloon filled with water – and it allows the passage of light from a torch (*transillumination*) (Diamond and Gosalbez 1998). Transillumination of the hydrocele excludes herniation of intestinal contents into the sac. Hydroceles are common and will disappear in time, unless they are communicating types.

Undescended testes (UDT): is a common finding and, in most cases, the aetiology is unknown. There is an increased risk of infertility and testicular cancer in men with a history of UDT. The testes are very sensitive to temperature and can sometimes be seen moving up the inguinal canal. It can take up to 3 years for UDT to descend; therefore, the baby will be followed up until descent. A timeline and pathway of care is provided by the NIPE standards (UKNSC 2008; Public Health England (PHE) 2015).

Hypospadias: Congenital abnormalities rarely appear singly; therefore, if the baby is noted to have UDT, extra vigilance is required to assess whether the urethral opening is central on the glans. In *hypospadias*, the opening is found on the undersurface and in *epispadias*, it is above the surface. Observing the baby pass urine is a good method of validating normality.

The penis shape and length are noted. *Chordee* is a lack of ventral tissue on the penis, leading to it being curved ventrally. Surgery is required to correct the condition.

Female infant genitalia

In the female newborn, the labia majora cover the labia minora and the clitoris.

Before designating a sex to an apparently female infant, the labia majora must be parted and the clitoris observed to be an appropriate size. The hymen should then be identified through appropriate examination. The hymen is a thickened and avascular structure, with a central opening, and can be easily identified during the first few days of life. The practitioner can then identify a non-perforated hymen, which may cause peritonitis when menstruation begins and, if not identified appropriately, can lead to the teenager having the reproductive organs removed and become unable to reproduce (RCM 2015a). If imperforate, the hymen appears like a tiny, smooth bald head (Tappero and Honeyfield 2014). A discharge from the vagina will indicate that the hymen is perforated. The discharge is usually creamy white at birth, occasionally being replaced after the second day by one appearing bloodstained (*pseudomenses*), as maternal hormones diminish.

Disorders of sex development (DSDs)

Disorders of sex development (DSDs) are also sometimes called intersex conditions and these are a group of rare conditions where the reproductive organs and genitals do not develop as expected.

If there is any doubt as to the sex of the baby, it is important that the concerns are discussed sensitively with the parents (Ahmed and Hughes 2002). Parents will often be very distressed and continually apply pressure to be told the sex of the baby. They will take on board any

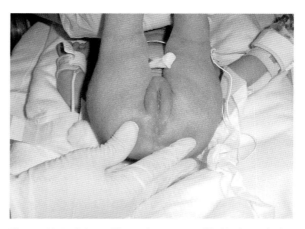

Figure 42.11 Infant with an absent anus. (By kind permission of Dr. Raoul Blumberg.)

terminology used, so it is important to avoid the terms 'he' or 'she' or 'it'. At the same time, the sex of the baby cannot be entered on the birth certificate until further investigations have been undertaken to confirm the sex. If the 'wrong' sex is registered, it is an extremely difficult and lengthy process to correct the mistake (Reiner 1999; Hiort et al 2014).

Anus and rectum

The anus and rectum should be checked for patency and position. The practice of using a clinical thermometer to ensure anal patency is now considered outmoded. The anal sphincter is assessed by gently touching the anus and eliciting the anal 'wink' – the contraction and retraction of the muscle proving the anus is patent. (See also Fig. 42.11.)

Stools: Record the number and character of all stools passed.

Constipation: occurs most commonly in babies who are artificially fed. Breastfed babies may not pass a stool for 2 or 3 days once feeding is established, but this is quite normal, providing the stools are yellow and soft.

Urinary output: This is often less than 1 mL/kg/h during the first 12 to 18 hours after birth. Most healthy term babies urinate within the first 12 hours; however, a small number of healthy infants may not urinate until 24 to 36 hours after birth. If in doubt as to whether or not a baby has passed urine, place a piece of cotton wool at the end of the penis or urethra to elicit the passage of urine. Using bags should be avoided, as the adhesive can cause skin damage. Persistent oliguria beyond 36 hours should be evaluated in an otherwise healthy infant (Moghal and Embleton 2006).

The odour and colour of the urine are also noted. Occasionally, a red stain is found on the napkin because of urates colouring the urine.

Neurological examination

Assessment of neurological function is important in assessing successful transition from extrauterine life and environmental factors in the perinatal period that may have caused a pathological response of the central and peripheral nervous systems. Early identification of deviations from normal can significantly reduce mortality and improve the quality of life for the newborn and family.

The Apgar score and its running commentary may indicate a baby who requires focus on the neurological system. The type of delivery, such as shoulder dystocia, can cause *brachial plexus damage, facial* and *Erb's palsy,* paralyzed vocal cords and damage to one or both of the phrenic nerves, all of which need to be excluded (see Ch. 64).

The examination of the neurological system is, in large part, undertaken by examining the other systems.

Physical examination

Probably the most reliable information that can be obtained quickly from a neurological evaluation is through discussing the baby's behaviour with the mother and the baby's response to handling during the preceding parts of the physical examination.

Level of consciousness: One of the most important areas of the examination is the neonate's alertness and interaction with his/her mother, his/her overall behaviour and movement preceding and during the examination.

Cry: This is the baby's main method of communication to alert carers to pain, hunger, discomfort or suffering. It is important that the carers understand the types of crying to give appropriate care. When listening to the sound of crying, the tone and its clarity should be noted; it should be without hoarseness, or a nasal tone. Equally, the type of pain and whether or not pain relief is required by the baby needs to be established. Change from an uncomfortable position, a soothing bath, massage, or sucking on a finger or breast might bring relief. It takes time and skill to interpret the different sounds, and conscious effort needs to be given to listening and observing babies to perfect this form of communication.

Head: The shape and size, fontanelle and suture size are examined as stated during the morphological examination. *Cranial bruit* may indicate an intracranial vascular malformation.

Face: Facial dysmorphism may indicate a genetic syndrome, such as *trisomy 18,* and facial features are observed during crying for facial palsy.

Eye examination: The baby should be alert and provide eye-to-eye contact and through and exclude brain tumours, such as retinoblastoma.

Skin: Cutaneous birthmarks such as *café-au-lait spots* may indicate the presence of a genetic disorder, such as *neurofibromatosis. Naevi* over nerve(s), such as the trigeminal area or spine may also be identified.

Skeletal system: The skeletal and neurological systems are interlinked and examination of the baby can indicate an abnormality; for example, a hair tuft over the spinal region may indicate a degree of spina bifida.

Tone: The strength and reflexes of limbs can indicate normal or abnormal movements, indicating neurological damage

Reflexes

It is now known that babies are aware of their in-utero environment and at birth are equipped for survival. They can hear, smell, taste, see up to a distance of 30 cm (Wilkinson 1997) and favour the colours black and white. The majority of reflexes are deemed to be primitive involving the brainstem and spinal cord.

- *Rooting reflex* – a primitive survival reflex in which a touch on the baby's cheek will cause the baby to move the mouth to the site of touch, searching for food. When the upper lip is touched, the mouth will open. These are useful reflexes for the mother to utilize when preparing the baby for feeding, whether breast-, bottle- or cup-feeding.

- *Sucking reflex* – can be tested by placing a clean, little finger into the baby's mouth or observing the baby feeding. The baby will tend to make sucking efforts, whether hungry or not. This confirms the baby's ability to coordinate breathing, sucking and swallowing – an important measure of neural integrity.

- *Grasp reflex* – can be tested by brushing the infant on the back of the hand, which will then open to grasp an offered finger. The midwife should then extend the baby's arms and lift the baby gently, observing the head and how well controlled or lax is the way in which it is held. This tests the *traction reflex.* This reflex will also need to be checked after a traumatic birth to note nerve damage that may not be obvious by observing the tone and position of the arms.

- *Moro reflex* (startle reflex) – can be observed physiologically or tested for. The baby may already have demonstrated this reflex during the examination and, therefore, a further demonstration is not required. If it has not been seen, the reflex can be tested by first ensuring the baby is calm and at rest. The midwife supports the baby's head with the left hand from the neck to the lower back and brings the baby's chin to the chest. The baby is then elevated several centimetres off the bed, with the head allowed to drop gently to the right-supporting hand. The baby will throw the arms back and then forwards, towards the chest, allowing the fists to close. The baby may also cry. The aim of this examination is to enable the baby's head to appear to fall into an empty space; it is not to fall from a height, and the head must never touch the mattress. This procedure must not be undertaken if the baby is not relaxed.

- *Asymmetrical tonic neck reflex* – the baby will extend the limbs on the side of the body, with the head turned towards.
- *Stepping or walking reflex* – the baby is supported by the practitioner, with the soles of the feet flat against the mattress. This will encourage the baby to put one foot in front of the other, straighten the spine and attempt to 'walk'.
- *Babinski reflex* – the baby's foot is supported in the left hand and pressure is applied with the index finger of the other hand on the outer part of the sole of the foot up to the small toe and across to the big toe. The normal response is for the baby to extend and fan the toes and finally to flex them. The midwife can take the opportunity to note webbing of the toes when eliciting this reflex.

The complete behavioural examination is quite dependent on infant–examiner interaction and, thus, the midwife should aim to examine the baby with gentleness and respect, communicating with the baby on both verbal and nonverbal levels.

Cranial nerves

The 12 pairs of cranial nerves are referred to by name or Roman numerals. They originate from different parts of the brain and assessment of their function confirms normality and recognizes deviations from normal (see chapter website resources).

Assessment of the autonomic nervous system

The autonomic nervous system is involved in a complex of reflex activities essential to sustain life, and these are dependent on sensory input to the brain or spinal cord. Normal autonomic function in a baby at term is well developed and can be observed through the following reflex actions:

- ability to adapt temperature to the environment
- respiratory rate and heart rate changes with physical activity
- responses of the pupils to light
- contraction of the external anal sphincter (*anal wink*) in response to touch or when air is blown over it – the muscular opening of the anus should have a firm appearance and not be distended and lax
- skin – *harlequin sign* – when the baby is lying on one side, the upper area is light and the lower area dark red

Identifying and managing pain and stress in the term newborn

Until the 1980s, it was thought that babies did not feel pain; therefore, pain relief was rarely given (see also Ch. 49).

Years ago, dummies laced with brandy and sugar were sometimes used to pacify a very distressed newborn; however, procedures that required pain relief in children or adults were undertaken on newborns without pain relief. Today, the physiology of pain pathways in babies is better understood, and it is now recognized that the baby's spinal sensory nerve cells are more excitable than those of adults. Midwives, doctors and nurses rely on patients to report their pain and its severity. The baby is unable to speak, so practitioners need to be aware of evidence of pain and obtain experience of the normal behaviour of the baby. The inability to communicate in no way negates the possibility that the baby is experiencing pain and is in need of appropriate pain relief (Lago et al 2009). Time spent observing babies is invaluable in trying to understand how to adapt the care provided to minimize stress and pain to the newborn.

The physiological response to painful stimulus in the baby is greater and lasts for a longer period of time than in the adult. Adults have a sophisticated nerve pathway that can narrowly pinpoint the area of painful stimulus. In the newborn, this pathway is still developing, which means the baby is unable to localize pain but can feel pain in response, not only to painful stimuli but also to touch over a wide area of the body (Anand and Scalzo 2000). Damaged skin, either from a heel prick or from ventouse or other instrumental birth, will be very sensitive to touch, and this sensitivity can last several weeks (see chapter website resources) (Anand 2001). Therefore, painful procedures should be kept to a minimum and comfort measures used, plus information to mothers and families about the effects of pain on their baby's behaviour (Maxwell et al 2013).

Causes of pain

The effect of certain procedures needs to be considered in relation to the amount of pain caused to the baby, including:

- long or short/precipitate labour – headache
- type of labour, e.g. occipitoposterior position
- instrumental birth – bruising/trauma from ventouse cap
- heel pricks undertaken for the Guthrie test, etc.
- removal of plasters
- insertion of intravenous needles for antibiotic therapy
- delivery of fluid to the subcutaneous tissue, after blockage of an intravenous cannula

Signs of pain

One of the best indicators is vocal expression, heard in long-lasting crying. Facial expressions – brow bulge, eye squeeze and nasolabial furrow – are also reliable indicators of pain.

Other behavioural signs of pain include pedalling movement of the legs, toes spread, legs tensed and pulled up, agitation of arms and a withdrawal reaction (Bellieni 2012).

Comfort measures – sucrose and breastfeeding

Research on pain, undertaken on the blood spot screening and venipuncture procedures, recognizes these as being very painful for the newborn **and** for the parents observing a distressed newborn. There needs to be clear justification to undertake every heel-prick procedure. From the research, it is recommend that, before term babies undergoing the heel prick procedure, the baby should:

- if breastfeeding, be held by the mother and be enabled to suckle for several minutes
- be given a dummy/finger to suck throughout the procedure (Carbajal et al 2003)
- be given 2 mL of 12% to 25% sucrose and allowed to suck for 2 minutes

One study indicated that breastfeeding alone can reduce crying; however, a number of randomized controlled trials provide unequivocal evidence that babies cry less when given a combination of nutritive or non-nutritive sucking and sucrose (Carbajal et al 2003; Shah et al 2012).

Many cultures recognize that the taste of sweetness reduces pain, as does massage, talking gently and obtaining eye contact with the baby.

Jitteriness versus seizures

Jitteriness, although not a type of seizure, is a movement disorder characterized by movements with qualities primarily of tremulousness and occasionally of clonus. It is important to distinguish jitteriness from seizures.

If the limb that is tremulous is pressed down very gently against the mattress and the tremors stop, seizure is excluded; if movement continues, it is a positive sign of seizure. The midwife must call for help and stay with the baby to observe the progress and length of seizures; this is also important to provide support if the respiratory system is involved (Silverstein and Jensen 2007).

Assessment of feeding

The final and crucial part of the assessment is to ascertain well-being by reviewing the baby's feeding. A baby who has been feeding well and is able to show that the brain is able to coordinate sucking, swallowing and breathing validates appropriate brain function.

Bad news

Before undertaking the examination of the newborn, it is important for practitioners to have had training in 'giving bad news', recognizing that what they might deem good news may not produce the same reaction in the parents. A girl rather than a boy is a disaster for some parents. The smallest of deformities, such as an extra digit, can cause major concerns for parents who wished for the 'perfect' baby. For major congenital abnormalities, it is important to know specialist centres in the area and the latest management and treatment to have some insight when the parents start asking questions about the well-being of their baby.

Consequently, it is important that the examination of the newborn is undertaken where privacy is guaranteed and the parents feel that they can ask questions and that they have the professionals' full attention. If the midwife is not able to convey bad news, the examination should be delayed until the support of a senior colleague, with training and experience, is available.

Mother–baby attachment

Parent–infant interaction is believed to play a central role in the baby's social, emotional and physiological development. The quality of the interaction between mother and baby can provide the baby with an environment for optimal development and growth. The foundation of this relationship is trust and affection. If there is failure to develop this relationship, the baby is at risk of delays in neurological developmental, child abuse, neglect and failure to thrive (Pridham et al 1999). Research has shown that educating the mother to understand her baby and his/her behaviour can have a positive effect on maternal–infant interaction (Anderson 1981).

Today in the UK, women often stay in hospital less than 24 hours for a non-complicated birth, and, therefore, teaching opportunities are limited. Antenatal classes are an ideal opportunity to provide the necessary education that serves as a valuable health-promotion tool to affect positive parenting, beginning at birth.

After the birth, mother and baby should be given a minimum of 1 hour of supported privacy together in the labour ward, and this should then be followed by keeping mother and baby together as much as possible during the early neonatal period when they are getting to know one another and mothering skills are developing. This is easily achieved if the birth takes place in the home; however, this is more difficult to achieve in the hospital setting and if there has been a complicated birth (Noyman-Veksler et al 2015).

The Maternity Services Advisory Committee (MASC 1985) were early advocates of having the baby's cot beside the mother's bed, and this has been supported more recently by UNICEF (UNICEF 2011). Restricted contact between mother and baby in the early postnatal period is associated with less affectionate maternal behaviour and maternal feelings of incompetence and lack of confidence (Thomson and Westreich 1989). Maternal–infant attachment established from birth is strengthened by the woman getting to understand her baby, and because handling can aid this process, the mother is encouraged to care for her baby soon after birth. The use of strategies such as using the shortened *Brazelton Neonatal Behavioural Assessment Scale* (see chapter website resources) can assist parents to learn more about their baby's capabilities (Nugent 2004). Unrestricted access allows the mother freedom to respond to her baby whenever the baby is awake. Although this aspect of initiating the relationship between mother and baby is important, the ability to enhance that relationship is dependent on the mother's physiological well-being (Rubertsson et al 2015).

There must be communication between mother and baby for interaction to take place. Mother and baby need to respond to each other's cues and the environment must be such as to facilitate that interaction. It is difficult for a woman who has had a difficult birthing to respond physically if she is unable to move and handle her baby. The midwife needs to provide the response to the cues given by the baby while allowing the mother to recover, and, in doing so, act as a role model, educating the woman about the different cues, such as hunger, boredom, discomfort and pain, which the baby provides. A crying baby can overwhelm the woman's psychological well-being at this vulnerable time after birth. The father or partner, too, should be involved in the baby's care and progress; otherwise, they may feel neglected and become jealous of the close relationship developing between mother and baby.

Three stages have been described in the maternal–infant attachment process.

1. The first is when the mother and baby first become acquainted and involves early physical contact.
2. The next is the care-taking relationship when the mother learns to care for – feed, change, wash and bathe – her baby.
3. The final stage, called identity, occurs when the child is incorporated into the family.

To reach this final stage, mother and baby grow to know and love each other as they interact. The baby may initiate interaction by crying. The mother responds by rocking the cot or picking the baby up and cuddling him/her. This is the expression of a mother's instinct to tend and protect her child. The baby stops crying when picked up and becomes alert and responsive. The mother should be encouraged to talk and establish eye-to-eye contact. In turn, the baby gazes at his/her mother and responds; thus, mother–baby interaction is synchronized and attachment develops.

At times, mother and baby have to be separated because of maternal illness or because the baby needs intensive or special care; most mothers are likely to overcome any adverse effects of this separation (Thomson and Westreich 1989). Some consider that the degree to which a mother perceives separation as having an adverse effect on her mothering ability may be related to the outcome (Richards 1978; Ross 1980) and also the contact between mother and baby while the baby is in hospital (Moore and Nelson 2003). Women of low socioeconomic status and/or with poor social support may be more adversely affected by restricted contact with their baby than their more affluent counterparts (Thomson and Westreich 1989). One study demonstrated this, highlighting the benefits of early and prolonged contact after birth to women and babies with low social support (Anisfeld and Lipper 1983).

Not uncommonly, some mothers are worried that they do not feel a maternal instinct or really love their baby during the early days of motherhood. They need reassurance that their feelings are quite normal and that, as they and their baby learn to know each other, love will follow.

Each society and culture has its behavioural norms about what is accepted as normal and appropriate maternal–infant interaction, and it is important to acknowledge these differences.

Newborn behaviour

For the first 6 weeks of life, the baby does not distinguish night from day and spends 24 hours sleeping, waking, crying and feeding. Newborns have a very small stomach and require regular intake of food; they will, on the whole, feed every 3 to 4 hours. What parents often find difficult is that the baby is awake at night and asleep during the day. Babies move from one sleep state to another, from quietly looking around, actively responding to sounds, to crying. Parents are sometimes concerned not to 'spoil' their babies and sometimes delay in answering their baby's cries. Before 6 months of age, the neural processes are not mature enough to enable the baby to manipulate the carer (to think 'if I cry, I will get my mother to come to see to me'). If and when the baby cries, it is for a reason such as hunger, fear, discomfort, pain or boredom. Rather than spoiling the baby, if the mother/carer answers the cries immediately, the baby will develop securely, knowing his/her needs will be answered (Bell and Ainsworth 1972).

A baby's primary needs are for food, fluid, sleep, warmth, security and love, and the method of expressing those needs is crying. This is a signal to the carer to communicate with the baby, recognize the cry and meet the need; parents and practitioners need time to understand and interpret. Parents need to be given this information to recognize their baby's needs and know what to do to help the baby calm down.

When responding to the baby's cry, the mother/carer must be 10 to 12 inches in front of the baby, establish eye contact and, at the same time, find a way to control the baby's flailing arms and legs while firmly and gently talking to the baby (Ludington-Hoe et al 2002). The baby can alternatively be held against the mother's body and talked to gently.

Another method of satisfying the baby is to provide non-nutritive sucking by giving the baby fingers or a dummy to suck or by putting the baby to the breast. Teaching the baby the difference between night and day is also helpful. That could be accomplished by placing the baby in an environment of light and normal sounds during the day and at night, making sure the environment is dark or the lights dimmed and sounds are gentle. Parents need to understand that they will not always succeed immediately in stopping the baby from crying; however, a variety of methods should be tried until successful. Scientifically, it is recognized that crying in the newborn can cause pathological changes to the cardiorespiratory system (Anderson 1988); therefore, listening to the baby crying without taking action to stop the crying is no longer acceptable practice.

Placing the cot near the bed will make access to the baby easier at night-time. The baby will develop an organized pattern of sleep by the age of 16 weeks (Matsuoka et al 1991). At 6 weeks the baby should begin to smile, and at 3 months take note of the surroundings.

Sleep versus play time

After any physical examination, the baby is dressed and given to a parent to hold. When the baby is placed in the cot, the position of the baby in the cot is informed by the 'Back to sleep' campaign to prevent sudden infant death syndrome (SIDS) (see Ch. 51). It is important to recognize that the baby is positioned on the back for sleep, but when awake, evidence recommends that the baby can be placed in the prone position for about 15 minutes a day. This can prevent conditions such as delays in motor skills, *positional plagiocephaly* (flattening of the occipital region of the head), positional *torticollis* (contracture of the sternocleidomastoid muscle) and *shoulder retraction*. None of these is life-threatening or should lead to abandoning the 'back to sleep' position (Fig. 42.12) (Chung-Park 2012).

POSTNATAL CARE

Care of the newborn is based on the philosophy of a continuum of quality care that commences with antenatal and intrapartum care. This begins with getting to know the fetus both antenatally and during the intrapartum period, and that knowledge informs the management of care given to the baby from the moment of birth to 28 days.

Preparation of the parents for early detection of deviations from normal and management of the newborn is vital wherever the birth takes place. It is expected that preparation for parenthood has taken place to reduce the psychological stress to both the baby and family.

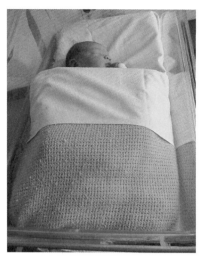

Figure 42.12 Baby in cot in the recommended position for sleep.

The UK is a multicultural society and for a partnership of care to be developed with parents, the cultural norms of the ethnic groups need to be understood. Many traditional practices need to be understood rather than feared. One of these practices, cup-feeding, utilized effectively today in neonatal units, was brought to the UK from Africa, where the survival of high-risk newborns was achieved by cup-feeding well before its introduction to the UK. The midwife needs to make links with women's ethnic groups and religious leaders to learn and understand traditional practice so that safe care can be provided to the newborn by supporting and, where necessary, sensitively changing practice.

Hygiene

Because newborn infants have little resistance to microorganisms, they are highly susceptible to infection. An apparently mild infection can rapidly become a serious condition in the newborn, so every effort must be made to protect the newborn from infection.

There are three main factors in avoiding infection:

1. Keep the baby's skin healthy and intact so bacteria have no portal of entry for invasion of tissues.

2. Limit the bacteria in the baby's surroundings.

3. Adopt a barrier-nursing technique to avoid cross-infection.

Sources of infection

The infant may be infected in a number of ways:

Attendants: The nose, throat or skin of those dealing with the baby may harbour dangerous organisms (staphylococci and streptococci). This includes not only the midwife and doctor but also the parents themselves.

Hands and clothing: Facilities for washing the hands must be available after personal toileting and in the nursery and wards. Disposable hand towels are preferable for use. The hands must be washed before and after attending each baby. Antiseptic hand cream applied to the hands after washing is valuable. Long fingernails not only hinder many examination procedures but also can cause the baby discomfort and harbour infection.

Dust: The air and dust in maternity wards and nurseries contain many bacteria, one of which, *Staphylococcus aureus*, is most liable to cause infection. The ward and nursery should be adequately ventilated. Cleaning must be thorough and should minimize dust being scattered around the room. Floors are cleaned using vacuum cleaners with filters, preventing bacteria passing out of the machine into the air. Damp dusting is advisable. Cots, trolleys and tables can be wiped over with dilute antiseptic and dried well.

Fomites: Infection may be spread by unsterilized instruments, bowls and dressings. Clothing and napkins may be the source. Before the era of pre-packed feeds and disposable bottles and teats in hospitals, inadequately sterilized bottles and teats were a source of infection. This may still be the case in some homes.

Cross-infection: Rooming-in, in which babies are nursed beside the mother's bed, is the usual practice nowadays. This aids the bonding process and reduces the risk of cross-infection. Overcrowding in wards and nurseries should be avoided. Individual equipment for bathing and changing should be provided, disposable articles being used whenever possible. Any baby suspected of infection should be isolated from other babies.

The main routine care of the baby involves changing the napkins (nappies), washing or bathing and feeding. Soiled linen and napkins should be handled, with gloved hands, as little as possible and placed in bags and closed while carried to the waste bin.

Bathing the baby

The issue of transmission of human immunodeficiency virus (HIV) through maternal vaginal secretions has encouraged the practice of the baby being given a bath soon after birth. Currently, there are no studies to support the reduction of HIV from this. Vernix is deemed to protect the skin, and may act as an antibacterial agent and promote healing from the trauma of birth. Bathing the baby removes this skin-protecting vernix. Work undertaken so far suggests the importance of the newborn's condition and temperature being stabilized in the normal range for 2 to 4 hours before the bath being given to avoid hypothermia (see Ch. 43) (WHO 2013).

Bath time offers parents a time to get to know their baby through tactile interaction.

To protect the skin pH, it is important that any cleansing agents that are used have a neutral pH and minimal dyes and perfumes, and that the baby's skin is rinsed well to reduce the risk of allergic sensitization (Cetta et al 1991; NICE 2006; Crozier and Macdonald 2010; WHO 2013).

While the baby is being bathed, care must be taken to prevent abrasions of the skin which might allow entry of bacteria. Great care must also be taken with the eyes and cord, which are both sites of potential infection.

Chafing or intertrigo, caused by friction between two skin surfaces, is usually seen in the groin or axilla and in the folds of the neck. It indicates that the baby's skin has not been adequately dried after being washed or bathed. The energetic removal of vernix caseosa may also be the cause. After a bath, a soft dabbing movement with a soft towel should dry the folds in the skin. Where chafing has occurred, drying and a very light dusting with an antiseptic powder will heal the lesion.

Dermatitis of the groin, buttocks and anus

Redness and excoriation may be produced around the groin, anus and buttocks. The development of this condition may be influenced by wetness of the skin (see chapter website resources). When the skin is exposed to urine, the pH rises and changes from acid to alkaline, enabling penetration of microorganisms into the building blocks of the stratum corneum.

Treatment and care

- Use of appropriate barrier creams containing petroleum (soft paraffin) protects skin, maintains the acid pH and aids healing
- Application of zinc oxide enables skin healing
- Exposure to air is unhelpful
- As much urine and faeces as possible should be removed and barrier cream reapplied to the affected areas
- If *Candida albicans* is suspected:
  - Inspect the baby's mouth
  - Take swabs for culture and sensitivity testing
  - Antifungal ointment or cream should be used
- Dermatitis is a very painful condition and great care is needed in its treatment
- The affected area should be washed with soft absorbent cotton wool and well dried with gentle dabbing
- Avoid use of soap or cleansing substances, as they also may cause irritation to the skin
- Maintain high standards of hygiene

Newborn screening tests

Various tests and examinations may be carried out in the early neonatal period to detect the presence of specific abnormal conditions. Early diagnosis and treatment may ameliorate the effects of many conditions. Thus, some inborn errors of metabolism may be managed with diet and/or drugs (see Chs 49 and 50 plus chapter website resources).

Blood spot screening test

The UK National Screening Committee recommend that all babies in the UK are offered screening for *phenylketonuria* (PKU), *congenital hypothyroidism* (CHT), *sickle cell disorders* (SCD), *cystic fibrosis* (CF) and *medium-chain acyl-CoA dehydrogenase deficiency* (MCADD). The test is offered to all babies in the UK at the age of 5 to 8 days.

- **Phenylketonuria** is an autosomal recessive genetic condition where babies are unable to metabolize phenylalanine (an amino acid found in proteins).
- **Congenital hypothyroidism** affects 1 in 4000 babies in the UK. Screening is done by measuring the level of thyroxine or thyroid-stimulating hormone (TSH) in the blood sample. Further investigations of thyroid function will be required, if the test result is abnormal. If the condition is confirmed, early treatment with levothyroxine (thyroxine) sodium by the age of 21 days will prevent mental handicap and promote normal growth (Kelnar et al 1995).
- **Sickle cell disorders** affect 1 in 2500 babies in the UK, and the aim of screening is to identify the babies who are affected to commence penicillin prophylaxis. This baby is at risk of infections and severe acute anaemia in the first few years of life if left untreated (Quinn 2013).
- **Deficiency of medium-chain acyl-CoA dehydrogenase** causes the accumulation of medium-chain fatty acids and impairs ketone production.
- **Cystic fibrosis (CF)** affects 1 in 2500 babies across the UK. It is an autosomal recessive inherited condition that mainly affects babies' digestion and lung function. Diagnosis enables nutrition and growth to be improved and reduces chest infection (Lim et al 2014) (see Ch. 50).
- **Medium-chain acyl-CoA dehydrogenase deficiency** (MCADD)

METABOLIC DISEASES

Bodies break down protein in foods, such as meat and fish, into amino acids. Amino acids that are not needed are usually broken down and removed from the body. However, babies with inherited metabolic diseases will not be able to break down amino acids and, thus, are at risk, which can cause the neonate to become seriously ill. Public Health England (PHE) is responsible for the NHS

Screening Programmes, and, in early 2015, has added another 4 metabolic diseases, allowing the Blood spot to now test for:

- maple syrup urine disease (MSUD)
- isovaleric acidaemia (IVA)
- glutaric aciduria type 1 (GA1)
- homocystinuria (pyridoxine unresponsive) (HCU)

These conditions can all be treated with a carefully managed diet and, in some cases, with medication. With early diagnosis, morbidity can be reduced (see also Chs 49 and 50).

Hearing tests

Recent technological advances have led to improved screening methods that can identify the majority of children with impaired hearing; therefore, it is recommended that babies should be screened before leaving hospital.

The test is non-invasive and involves the measurement of *otoacoustic emissions* (OAE), which are low-level inaudible sounds produced by the inner ear. The screening of newborns is part of the continuum of early childhood hearing tests, which screen and diagnose to improve identification of hearing impairment in young children.

The value of such a test is that children with hearing impairments can be given extra help at an early age to develop speech since the critical period for language and speech development is generally regarded as the first 2 years of life.

Vaccinations

Infants are known to be susceptible to infections in the first 2 months of life as the immune system of the newborn is immature and takes some time to develop. The UK Joint Committee for Vaccination and Immunisation (JCVI) recommends that parents give informed consent for their babies to be vaccinated against two of the most serious infections – tuberculosis (BCG) and hepatitis B – where it is necessary (DH 2009b).

Vaccination is now offered in the early postnatal period to babies whose parents have emigrated from a country with high prevalence of tuberculosis or whose family members have previously been infected.

Hepatitis B vaccine is given within the first 12 hours after birth to babies whose mothers are chronic carriers of hepatitis B virus or who have had acute hepatitis B during pregnancy.

FOLLOW-UP OF THE BABY

When the baby is deemed to be well and no longer requires midwifery care, the baby is discharged from the midwife to the health visitor, who usually visits the mother and baby at home. The health visitor discusses problems with the mother, gives advice on topics such as childcare and family planning, and encourages the mother to take her baby to the child health clinic or to her GP regularly. The baby's development will be followed closely by initiating the vaccination programme and developmental assessments. The GP is responsible for general medical care, but some babies with medical problems are also followed up by a neonatologist/paediatrician.

RECORD-KEEPING

Record-keeping is an important aspect of care given to the newborn. The examination and any care needs to be recorded along with the underpinning rationale for present and future management (NICE 2006). This commences with completing the case notes and birth notification (within the first 36 hours), which must be sent to the appropriate medical officer. Important information, such as whether or not the baby has fed or has passed urine and meconium, needs to be documented in the notes to form a baseline for further assessments.

To midwives, the hands-on care may be seen as more important than documentation, but medico-legal experts and the NMC advise that contemporaneous records must be kept (NMC 2015). Good record-keeping provides evidence of actions and omissions, protects the newborn by promoting high standards of clinical care, promotes team communication, gives an accurate account of treatment and provides the ability to detect problems at an early stage (Walton and Bedford 2007; NMC 2015).

A common core content record is available for every child and parent and, for each professional engaged in delivery, to record the progress and care given, and this record is the *UK Parent-held Child Health Record (PHCHR or 'Red Book')*.

The new WHO growth charts are included to document and support the decisions the practitioners make in regard to the care of the newborn.

After the first holistic physical examination, the practitioner should complete the PHCHR and give it to parents to commence the documentation of the forthcoming journey.

CONCLUSION

The aim of this chapter has been to introduce the reader to the physiology applied to the examination of the newborn, the range of assessments and examinations undertaken and the care given to newborn babies and their families. For more detail, the reader is referred to the website for other resources and links, providing the in-depth knowledge required to undertake the examination of the newborn.

Key Points

- The transition from fetus to neonate is a complex process, and the midwife needs to be knowledgeable about fetal and neonatal physiology to recognize that the progression has been completed.
- Care of the neonate should be based on supporting and enhancing normal transition, in early identification of deviations from normal and appropriate management and referral.
- Midwives should allocate the same time and attention to the examination and assessment of the baby, as for they would for the woman.
- Midwives need to have a clear understanding of neonatal anatomy, physiology and behaviour to help women understand the behaviours, responses and care needs of their newborn baby.
- The midwife must not undertake any elements of care without completing the necessary training and education (NMC 2012 and 2015).
- Clear, accurate and contemporaneous record-keeping is essential in ensuring continuity of care, and effective information to the parents and carers of the neonate.

References

Aase JM: *Diagnostic dysmorphology*, New York, Plenum Medical Book Company, 1990.

Ahmed SF, Hughes IA: The genetics of male undermasculinization, *Clin Endocrinol (Oxf)* 56(1):1–18, 2002.

American College of Obstetricians and Gynecologists (ACOG): The Apgar score. Committee Opinion No. 644, *Obstet Gynecol* 126:e52–e55, 2015.

Anand KJ: International evidence-based group for neonatal pain: consensus statement for the prevention and management of pain in the newborn, *Arch Pediatr Adolesc Med* 155:173–180, 2001.

Anand KJ, Scalzo FM: Can adverse neonatal experiences alter the brain development and subsequent behaviour? *Biol Neonate* 77:69–82, 2000.

Anderson CJ: Enhancing reciprocity between mother and neonate, *Nurs Res* 30:89–93, 1981.

Anderson GC: Crying, foramen ovale shunting, and cerebral volume, *J Pediatr* 113(2):411–412, 1988.

Anisfeld E, Lipper E: Early contact, social support and mother–infant bonding, *Pediatrics* 72:79–83, 1983.

Arteche A, Joormann J, Harvey A, et al: The effects of postnatal maternal depression and anxiety on the processing of infant faces, *J Affect Disord* 133(1–2):197–203, 2011.

Bannister P: Early feeding management. In Watson ACH, Sell DA, Grunwell P, editors: *Management of cleft lip and palate*, London, Whurr, 2001.

Battaglia FC, Lubchenco LO: A practical classification of newborn infants by weight and gestational age, *J Pediatr* 71(2):159–163, 1967.

Bell SM, Ainsworth MD: Infant crying patterns and maternal responsiveness, *Child Dev* 43(4):1171–1190, 1972.

Bellieni CV: Pain assessment in human fetus and infants, *AAPS J* 14(3):2012.

Begum E, Bonno M, Sasaki N, et al: Blunted heart rate circadian rhythms in small for gestational age infants during the early neonatal period, *Am J Perinatol* 29(5):369–376, 2012.

Brazelton TB: *Infants and mothers*, New York, Delacourt Press, 1983.

Brazelton TB, Nugent JK: *Neonatal behavioral assessment scale*, Cambridge, Mac Keith Press, 1995.

Bridgens J, Kiely N: Current management of clubfoot (congenital talipes equinovarus), *Br Med J* 340:c355, 2010.

Busfield A, Samuel R, McNinch A, et al: Vitamin K deficiency bleeding after NICE guidance and withdrawal of Konakion Neonatal: British Paediatric Surveillance Unit study, 2006–2008, *Arch Dis Child* 98(1):41–47, 2013.

Carbajal R, Veerapen S, Couderc S, et al: Analgesic effect of breast feeding in term neonates: randomised controlled trial, *Br Med J* 326(7379):13, 2003.

Cawse-Lucas J, Waterman S, St Anna L: Clinical inquiry: does frenotomy help infants with tongue-tie overcome breastfeeding difficulties? *J Fam Pract* 64(2):126–127, 2015.

Cetta F, Lambert GH, Ros SP: Newborn chemical exposure from over-the-counter skin care products, *Clin Pediatr (Phila)* 30(5):286–289, 1991.

Children Act, London, HMSO, 1989.

Chou D, Daelmans CB, Jolivet RR, et al: On behalf of the Every Newborn Action Plan (ENAP) and Ending Preventable Maternal Mortality (EPMM) working groups 2015 Analysis Women's, Children's, and Adolescents' Health Ending preventable maternal and newborn

mortality and stillbirths, *Br Med J* 351:h4255, 2015.

Chung-Park MS: Knowledge, opinions, and practices of infant sleep position among parents, *Mil Med* 177(2):235–239, 2012.

Conner GK: Genitourinary assessment. In Tappero EP, Honeyfield ME, editors: *Physical assessment of the newborn: a comprehensive approach to the art of physical examination*, 5th edn, Neonatal Network, NICU Ink, 2014.

Cooke A, Cork MJ, Victor S, et al: Olive oil, sunflower oil or no oil for baby dry skin or massage: a pilot, assessor-blinded, randomized controlled trial (the Oil in Baby SkincaRE [OBSeRvE] Study), *Acta Derm Venereol* (website), 2015.

Crozier K, Macdonald SE: Effective skin-care regimes for term newborn infants: a structured literature review, *Evidence Based Midwifery* 8(4):128–135, 2010.

Davis GM, Bureau MA: Pulmonary and chest wall mechanics in the control of respiration in the newborn, *Clin Perinatol* 14(3):551–579, 1987.

Department of Health (DH): *Changing Childbirth. Report of the Expert Maternity Group*, London, HMSO, 1993.

Department of Health (DH): *Vitamin K for newborn babies*, London, DH, 1998.

Department of Health (DH): *Reference Guide to Consent for Examination or Treatment*, 2nd edn, London, DH, 2009a.

Department of Health (DH): *Birth to Five*, London, DH, 2009b.

De Rooy L, Hawdon J: Nutritional factors that affect the postnatal metabolic adaptation of full-term small- and large-for-gestational-age infants, *Pediatrics* 109(3):e42, 2002.

De-Wahl Granelli A, Wennergren M, Sandberg K, et al: Impact of pulse oximetry screening on the detection of duct dependent congenital heart disease: a Swedish prospective screening study in 39 821 newborns, *Br Med J* 338:a3037, 2009.

Diamond DA, Gosalbez R: Neonatal urologic emergencies. In Walsh PC, Retik AB, Vaughan ED, et al, editors: *Campbell's urology*, 7th edn, Philadelphia, WB Saunders, 1998.

Drugs and Therapeutics Bulletin (website). www.dtb.org.uk/dtb/index.html. 2016.

Dubowitz LM, Dubowitz V, Goldberg C: Clinical assessment of gestational age in the newborn infant, *J Pediatr* 77(1):1–10, 1970.

Gleason CA, Devaskar SU: *Avery's diseases of the newborn*, 9th edn, Elsevier, 2011.

Habel A, Elhadi N, Sommerlad B, et al: Delayed detection of cleft palate: an audit of newborn examination, *Arch Dis Child* 91:238–240, 2006.

Hall D, Elliman D: *Health for all children: revised fourth edition paperback*, Health Surveillance, Oxford University Press, 2006.

Hall DMB: The role of the routine neonatal examination, *Br Med J* 318:619–620, 1999.

Hiort O, Birnbaum W, Marshall L, et al: Management of disorders of sex development, *Nat Rev Endocrinol* 10:2014.

Hunter L, Habel A: *Palate examination: identification of cleft palate in the newborn: best practice guide*, Royal College of Paediatrics and Child Health (RCPCH), 2014.

Harris TR: Physiologic principles. In Goldsmith J, Karotkin E, editors: *Assisted ventilation of the neonate*, 2nd edn, Philadelphia, WB Saunders, 1988.

Hawdon JM: Investigation and management of impaired metabolic adaptation presenting as neonatal hypoglycaemia, *Paediatr Child Healt* 18(4):161–165, 2008.

Jokinen M: Measuring newborns: does size really matter? *RCM Midwives* 5(5):186–187, 2002.

Keay AJ, Morgan DM: *Craig's care of the newly born infant*, 7th edn, Edinburgh, Churchill Livingstone, 1982.

Karumbi J, Mulaku M, Aluvaala J, et al: Topical umbilical cord care for prevention of infection and neonatal mortality, *Pediatric Infect Dis J* 32(1):78–83, 2013.

Kelnar JH, Harvey D, Simpson C: *The sick newborn baby*, London, Baillière Tindall, 1995.

Klaus MH, Kennell JH: *Maternal–infant bonding*, St. Louis, Mosby, 1976.

Knowles R, Griebsch I, Dezateux C, et al: Newborn screening for congenital heart defects: a systematic review and cost-effectiveness analysis, *Health Technol Assess* 9(44):1–152, 2005.

Kumar M, Chandra S, Ijaz Z, et al: Epidural analgesia in labour and neonatal respiratory distress: a case-control study, *Arch Dis Child Fetal Neonatal Ed* 99(2):F116–F119, 2014.

Lago P, Garetti E, Merazzi D, et al: Guidelines for procedural pain in the newborn, *Acta Paediatr* 98:932–939, 2009.

The Lancet Midwifery Series (website). www.thelancet.com/series/midwifery. 2014.

Lavender T, Bedwell C, Tsekiri-O'Brien E, et al: Qualitative study exploring women's and health professionals' views of newborn bathing practices, *Evidence Based Midwifery* 7(4):112–121, 2009.

Levene M, Tudehope D, Sinha S: *Essential Neonatal Medicine*, 4th edn, Oxford, Blackwell, 2008.

Lim MTC, Wallis C, Price JF, et al: Diagnosis of cystic fibrosis in London and South East England before and after the introduction of newborn screening, *Arch Dis Child* 99(3):197–202, 2014.

Lissauer T, Fanaroff AA, Miall L, et al: *Neonatology at a Glance*, 3rd edn, Chicester, Wiley-Blackwell, 2015.

Ludington-Hoe SM, Cong X, Hashemi F: Infant crying: nature, physiologic consequences and select interventions, *Neonatal Netw* 21(2):29–36, 2002.

Manktelow BM, Smith SL, Evans TA, Hyman-Taylor P, et al: On Behalf of the MBRRACE-UK Collaboration, *Perinatal Mortality Surveillance Report UK Perinatal Deaths for Births from January to December 2013*. Leicester, The Infant Mortality and Morbidity Group, Department of Health Sciences, University of Leicester, 2015.

Maternal and Child Health Research Consortium (MCHRC): *Confidential Enquiry into Stillbirths and Deaths in Infancy: 8th Annual Report*, London, MCHRC, 2001.

Maternity Services Advisory Committee: *Maternity care in action, Part 3: Postnatal care*, London, HMSO, 1985.

Matsuoka M, Segawa M, Higurashi M: The development of sleep and wakefulness cycle in early infancy and its relationship to feeding habits, *Tohoku J Exp Med* 165:147–154, 1991.

Maxwell LG, Malavolta CP, Fraga V: Assessment of pain in the neonate, *Clin Perinatol* 40(3):457–469, 2013.

Michaelides S: *Clinical Assessment Tool*. In *Neuro-Behavioural Physiological*

Assessment of the Newborn, London, Middlesex University, 2010.

Milner AD, Vyas H: Lung expansion at birth, *Pediatrics* 101(6):879–886, 1982.

Moghal NE, Embleton N: Management of acute renal failure in the newborn, *Semin Fetal Neonatal Med* 11(3):207–213, 2006.

Moore KL, Nelson AM: Transition to motherhood, *J Obstet Gynecol Neonatal Nurs* 32:465–477, 2003.

Moore KL, Persaud TVN, Torchia M: *The developing human: clinically oriented embryology*, 10th edn, Philadelphia, Saunders, 2015.

National Institute for Health and Clinical Excellence (NICE): *Routine Postnatal Care of Women and Their Babies*, London, NICE, 2006.

National Institute for Health and Clinical Excellence (NICE): *Intrapartum Care for Healthy Women and Babies*, London, NICE, 2014.

Noyman-Veksler G, Herishanu-Gilutz S, Kofman O, et al: Post-natal psychopathology and bonding with the infant among first-time mothers undergoing a caesarian section and vaginal delivery: sense of coherence and social support as moderators, *Psychol Health* 30(4):441–455, 2015.

Nugent JK: *A Relationship-Building Approach to Family Centred Care at Enriching Early Parent–Infant Relationships Conference*, London, Brazelton/JJP, 2004.

Nursing and Midwifery Council (NMC): *Midwives Rules and Standards*, London, NMC, 2012.

Nursing and Midwifery Council (NMC): *The Code: Professional Standards of Practice and Behaviour for Nurses and Midwives*, London, NMC, 2015.

Orenstein SR: Gastroesophageal reflux, *Pediatr Rev* 20:24–28, 1999.

Page M, Jeffery H: The role of gastro-oesophageal reflux in the aetiology of SIDS, *Early Hum Dev* 59:127–149, 2000.

Pridham K, Kosorok MR, Greer F, et al: The effects of prescribed versus ad libitum feedings and formula caloric density on premature infant dietary intake and weight gain, *Nurs Res* 48(2):86–93, 1999.

Public Health England (PHE), Newborn and infant physical examination (NIPE): *Standards and care pathways* (website). www.gov.uk/government/

publications/newborn-and-infant-physical-examination-care-pathway. 2015.

Public Health England (PHE): *Screening tests for you and your baby*. Available at: https://www.gov.uk/government/publications/screening-tests-for-you-and-your-baby-description-in-brief. 2016.

Quinn CT: Sickle cell disease in childhood: from newborn screening through transition to adult medical care, *Pediatr Clin North Am* 60(6):1363–1381, 2013.

Reiner WG: Assignment of sex in neonates with ambiguous genitalia, *Curr Opin Pediatr* 11(4):363–365, 1999.

Reissland N, Burt M: Bi-directional effects of depressed mood in the postnatal period on mother–infant non-verbal engagement with picture books, *Infant Behavior and Development* 33(4):613–618, 2010.

Reissland N, Hopkins B, Helms P, et al: Maternal stress and depression and the lateralisation of infant cradling, *J Child Psychol Psychiatry* 50:263–269, 2009.

Renfrew MJ: *Rebalancing Care, Transforming Lives, RCM Zepherina Vietch Memorial Lecture*, London, Royal College of Obstetricians and Gynaecologists (RCOG), 2015.

Rennie J, Kendall G: *A manual of neonatal intensive care*, London, CRC Press, 2013.

Richards MPM: Possible effect of early separation on later development. In Brimblecombe FSW, Richards MPM, Roberton NRC, editors: *Early separation and special care nurseries*, London, SIMP/Heinemann Medical Books, 1978.

Ross GS: Parental responses to infants in intensive care: a separation issue re-evaluation, *Clin Perinatol* 7:47–61, 1980.

Roth DA, Hildesheimer M, Bardenstein S, et al: Preauricular skin tags and ear pits are associated with permanent hearing impairment in newborns, *Pediatrics* 122:e884, 2008.

Royal College of Midwives (RCM): *2015 Examination of the Newborn: Electronic Learning Programme* (website). www.ilearn.rcm.org.uk. 2015a.

Royal College of Midwives (RCM): *Royal College of Midwives (RCM) i-learn: Electronic Learning Module: Practical Guide to Neonatal Jaundice* authored by Michaelides S

739

(website). www.ilearn.rcm.org.uk/ user/view.php?id=6939&course=104, 2015b.

Rubertsson C, Pallant JF, Sydsjö G, et al: Maternal depressive symptoms have a negative impact on prenatal attachment – findings from a Swedish community sample, *J Reprod Infant Psychol* 33(2):153–164, 2015.

Sewell MD, Rosendahl K, Eastwood DM: Developmental dysplasia of the hip, *Br Med J* 339:b4454, 2009.

Shah PS, Herbozo C, Aliwalas LL, et al: Breastfeeding or breast milk for procedural pain in neonates, *Cochrane Database Syst Rev* 12: N.PAG, 2012.

Silverstein FS, Jensen FE: Neonatal seizures, *Ann Neurol* 62(2):112–120, 2007.

Sinha S, Miall L, Jardine L: *Essentials of neonatal medicine*, 5th edn, Wiley-Blackwell, 2012.

Singh A, Rasiah SV, Ewer AK: The impact of routine predischarge pulse oximetry screening in a regional neonatal unit, *Arch Dis Child Fetal Neonatal Ed* 99(4):F297–F302, 2014.

STEPS: *Baby hip health: a guide to hip development* (website). www.steps-charity.org.uk/. 2011.

Strang LB: Pulmonary circulation at birth. In *Neonatal respiration, physiological and clinical studies*, Oxford, Blackwell Scientific, 1977.

Tappero EP, Honeyfield ME: *Physical assessment of the newborn: a comprehensive approach to the art of physical examination*, NICU Ink, 2014.

Thangaratinam S, Brown K, Zamora J, et al: Pulse oximetry screening for critical congenital heart defects in asymptomatic newborn babies: a systematic review and meta-analysis, *Lancet* 379(9835):2459–2464, 2012.

Thomson M, Westreich R: Restriction of mother–infant contact in the immediate postnatal period. In Chalmers I, Enkin M, Keirse MJNC, editors: *Effective care in pregnancy and childbirth*, Oxford, Oxford University Press, 1989.

Thummala MR, Raju TN, Langenberg P: Isolated single umbilical artery anomaly and the risk for congenital malformations: a meta analysis, *J Pediatr Surg* 33(4):580–585, 1988.

Walker GM, Neilson A, Young D, et al: Colour of bile vomiting in intestinal obstruction in the newborn: questionnaire study, *Br Med J* 332(7554):1363, 2006.

Walton S, Bedford H: Parents' use and views of the national standard Personal Child Health Record: a survey in two primary care trusts, *Child Care Health Dev* 33(6):744–748, 2007.

Wilkinson A: Infants and children. In Epstein O, de Bono DP, Perkin GD, et al, editors: *Clinical examination*, 2nd edn, St. Louis, Mosby, 1997.

Wilson CB, Nizet V, Maldonado YA, et al: *Remmington and Klein's infectious diseases of the fetus and newborn infant*, 8th edn, Philadelphia, WB Saunders, 2015.

World Health Organization (WHO): *WHO recommendations on postnatal care of the mother and newborn* (website). http://apps.who.int/iris/bitstream/10665/97603/1/9789241506649_eng.pdf. 2013.

UNICEF: *How to Implement Baby Friendly Standards – A Guide for Maternity Setting*, UNICEF UK (website). www.unicef.org.uk/Documents/Baby_Friendly/Guidance/Implementation%20Guidance/Implementation_guidance_maternity_web.pdf. 2011.

United Kingdom Resuscitation Council: *Resuscitation at birth, Newborn Life Support Provider Course Manual*, London, Resuscitation Council UK, 2016.

UK National Screening Committee (UKNSC): *Child Health Sub-Group Report on Congenital Cataract* (website). http://legacy.screening.nhs.uk/screening-recommendations.php. 2005.

UK National Screening Committee (UKNSC): *Newborn and Infant Physical Examination Programme* (website). http://legacy.screening.nhs.uk/screening-recommendations.php. 2008.

Zupan J, Garner P, Omari AAA: Topical umbilical cord care at birth, *Cochrane Database Syst Rev* (3):CD001057, 2004.

Resources and additional reading

Gleason CA, Devaskar SU: *Avery's diseases of the newborn*, 9th edn, Elsevier, 2011.
An excellent practical and clinical resource.

Royal College of Midwives (RCM): *Examination of the Newborn: Electronic Learning Programme* (website). www.ilearn.rcm.org.uk. 2015. (EON modules, London, RCM).
This electronic learning resource is available to national and international members and has a range of modules. The Examination of the Newborn is a comprehensive programme that includes theory, reflective activities, plus audio and video clips to illustrate the examination of the newborn. It also features an excellent clip, detailing a hip examination.

Royal College of Paediatrics and Child Health: The Personal Child Health Record (The Red Book) at http://www.rcpch.ac.uk/PCHR.
Information and links concerning the national standard health and development record book provided to parents/carers after birth. There is also an online version.
STEPS Charity: http://www.steps-charity.org.uk
Useful resources for parents and professionals.

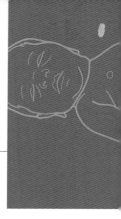

Chapter 43

Thermoregulation

Stephanie Michaelides

Learning Outcomes ?

After reading this chapter, you will be able to:

- describe the mechanisms of heat loss and identify examples of each
- define the appropriate and neutral thermal environment for the newborn infant
- identify signs and symptoms of cold stress
- describe methods of preventing and correcting hypothermia and hyperthermia
- discuss the role of the midwife in providing a safe environment for mother and baby prior to and after birth
- include information and advice regarding thermoregulation in antenatal and parenting education, and in the provision of postnatal care

INTRODUCTION

Practitioners involved in the care of the newborn need to master the art of thermoregulation to support and maintain a suitable environment for the baby's well-being, achieve safe and competent practice, and provide information and advice for parents and other relevant persons involved in the baby's care.

No newborn baby can afford the effects of cold stress. Those least able to tolerate hypothermia include the late-preterm and/or growth-restricted and ill babies. Maintenance of an optimal thermal environment, which studies have shown to influence growth and survival, is a vital part of neonatal care (Kumar et al 2009).

Globally, it is recognized that hypothermia is one of the leading causes of neonatal death, and rather than just the adaptation to a colder environment, low temperature in the newborn is often a sign of sepsis, which may ultimately cause the death from an otherwise treatable condition (Kirkup 2015; Lawn et al 2005).

This chapter focuses on the physiology and the pathophysiology of hypothermia and identification and management of maintaining a safe environment for the newborn in the maintenance of a neutral thermal environment.

PHYSIOLOGY OF THERMOREGULATION

Information from temperature receptors distributed widely in many parts of the body is transmitted to the following brain areas:

- The hypothalamus, where autonomic responses are coordinated
- The cerebral cortex, for behavioural responses

When the body temperature rises, the typical adult human autonomic response is peripheral vasodilatation and sweating to cool the skin; the behavioural response is to seek a cooler environment and remove clothing. When body temperature falls, the typical responses are peripheral vasoconstriction and shivering, seeking warmth and putting on more clothing.

Normal thermoregulatory function ensures that over a wide range of ambient temperatures, body core temperature is controlled at a relatively stable level – generally between 36.5°C and 37.5°C (Blackburn 2013). The ambient temperature range over which normal body temperature is achieved with minimal activation of metabolic and evaporative process is called the *thermoneutral zone*. For a naked adult, this zone is between approximately 27°C and 33°C.

Deviations of body temperature may take three forms:

1. Heat gain exceeds heat loss despite compensatory reactions – body temperature rises → hyperthermia.
2. Heat loss exceeds heat gain – temperature falls → hypothermia.
3. Control mechanisms break down and temperature alters according to environmental factors. If the rectal temperature rises above 40.8°C or falls lower than 35.8°C, there is increasing malfunction and risk of tissue damage and, ultimately, death.

Fetal perspective

During pregnancy, the heat generated by the mother increases by 30% to 35%, and thus the woman can be expected to have a temperature of 37.5°C during pregnancy. This is a result of the effect of progesterone on metabolism and the basal metabolic rate (BMR), leading to the mother's perception of being more comfortable in a cool environment. In the maternal system, there is an increase of 4 to 7 times the cutaneous blood flow and activity of sweat glands.

Fetal temperature is tightly linked to maternal temperature regulation and cannot be autonomously controlled by the fetus (the *heat clamp*). Fetal temperature is generally about 0.3 to 1.0°C above maternal body temperature (Liebeman et al 2000) – usually 37.6 to 37.8°C (Blackburn 2013; Polin et al 2011).

The placenta is an effective heat exchanger for the fetus, and thermoregulation is influenced by the following factors:

• Fetal and placental metabolic activity

• Thermal diffusion capacity of heat exchange within the placenta

• Rates of blood flow in the placental and intervillous spaces (Asakura 2004)

Some fetal generated heat is dissipated into the amniotic fluid via the umbilical cord (Hartman and Bung 1999; Blackburn 2013). Heat transfer is facilitated by the maternal–fetal gradient, apparent when the mother is exposed to changes in temperature, either during exercise or illness or through environmental factors such as sitting in a sauna.

Unstable uterine temperature, especially in the embryological state, can cause teratogenic abnormalities in the newborn (American College of Obstetricians and Gynaecologists (ACOG) 2015; Artal and Hopkins 2013). In these cases the gradient may be reversed or reduced, which can lead to the fetal temperature rising. Changes in fetal temperature tend to be slower than maternal changes because of the insulating effects of the amniotic fluid (Blackburn 2013).

Neonatal perspective

Thermoregulation is a critical physiological function in the neonate – closely linked to survival and health status.

Birth precipitates the baby into a harsh and cold environment that requires major physiological adaptations and changes, including thermoregulatory independence. Newborn babies are less efficient than adults in the ability to thermoregulate.

The ability to generate heat depends on age, body mass and environmental heat loss, and a large surface-area-to-mass ratio (about 3 times higher than in the adult) leads to difficulty in maintaining body temperature in a cold environment.

Babies with a low body mass are more at risk. Although full-term babies have control over peripheral vascular circulation equal to that of adults, the autonomic thermoregulatory responses are not fully developed. The healthy baby can increase basal heat production by 2.5 times in response to cold within 1 to 2 days of birth, although less so in the first 24 hours. Newborn babies are rarely able to shiver, and the increased heat comes from the *noradrenergic lipolysis* of the brown fat deposits characteristic of the neonate and activation of specially adapted mitochondria in the brown fat to produce heat.

The most dangerous time for the newborn to lose heat is during the first 10 to 20 minutes of life. If measures are not taken to halt heat loss, the baby becomes *hypothermic* (temperature <36.5°C) soon after birth. A premature or sick baby who becomes hypothermic will be at risk of developing health problems and of dying (Confidential Enquiries into Stillbirth and Deaths in Infancy (CESDI) 2003; de Almeida et al 2014), but the chances of survival are greatly increased if the temperature stays above 36°C. Birth should always take place in an environmental temperature above 25°C.

Hyperthermia (temperature >37.5°C) can occur and in extreme cases can cause death within the first 24 hours after birth. Hyperthermia increases the metabolic rate, leading to increased oxygen and glucose consumption plus water loss through evaporation. This causes hypoxia, metabolic acidosis and dehydration. A core temperature above 42°C may lead to neurological damage (World Health Organisation (WHO) 1994).

Hyperthermia can be caused by infection; it is not possible to distinguish between infection and environmental factors by measuring the body temperature or by clinical signs. Therefore, a temperature above 37.7°C in the newborn is a deviation from normal, and the baby must be urgently referred to the neonatologist for assessment, diagnosis and management.

Internal and external gradients

The external and internal gradients are interdependent. The *internal gradient* is the temperature differential between the core of the body and the skin and results in the transfer of heat from within the body to its surface. This process relies on an effective and extensive blood flow in capillaries and venous plexi influenced by tissue insulation provided by subcutaneous fat and the convective movement of heat through the blood. Heat conduction is under sympathetic control that results in changes in the skin blood flow by vasoconstriction and vasodilatation.

In the neonate, heat loss through this gradient is increased because of the thinner layer of subcutaneous fat and larger surface-to-volume ratio than in the adult (Blackburn 2013).

The *external gradient* results in heat loss from the body surface to the environment – the rate of heat loss is directly proportional to the difference between the temperature of the skin and that of the environment.

Heat transfer by the external gradient is increased in the neonate because of an increased surface area and thermal transfer coefficient. The neonate maintains temperature by means of the external gradient – that is, temperature skin changes –whereas the adult uses the internal gradient. This is especially significant for the preterm baby, for whom the control and effects of changes in the environmental temperature are more profound (Lunze and Hamer 2012).

Heat loss and gain

Babies at term are *homeotherms*, meaning they have the ability to produce heat to maintain body temperature within a comparatively narrow range. The newborn cannot regulate body temperature as well as an adult can, and when the environment becomes too cold or hot, the baby is unable to respond and maintain temperature, therefore tolerating a limited range of environmental temperatures (Gardner et al 2011). Thermal stability improves gradually as the baby increases in weight and age.

There are four main routes of heat loss (Hammarlund and Sedin 1986):

1. *Evaporation:* heat loss through evaporation of water from the skin and respiratory tract; highest immediately following delivery and bathing, and reduced by the following actions:
   - Drying baby's head after birth and following a bath
   - Placing a hat on the baby
   - Removing wet towels quickly following birth
   - Delaying bathing until the baby's temperature is stable and above 36.8 °C

2. *Convection:* heat loss to moving air or fluid around the neonate; dependent on the difference between skin and air or fluid temperature, the amount of body surface exposed to the environment and the speed of air or fluid movement. Heat loss can be prevented by the following actions:
   - Increasing the birthing room temperature
   - Keeping room temperature above 25 °C when the baby is naked

   - Reducing draughts in the birth area
   - Covering the baby with a blanket

3. *Radiation:* heat is radiated from the skin to surrounding colder solid objects, including windows or incubator walls. This is the predominant mode of heat loss after the first week of life in babies born before 28 weeks and in all other babies throughout the neonatal period. Heat loss can be prevented by the following action:
   - Keeping the baby away from windows and draughts

4. *Conduction:* heat loss through contact with cold objects, including cold mattresses, scales and radiograph plates (Blackburn 2013). Heat loss can be prevented by the following action:
   - Warming all surfaces that the baby is likely to come in contact with (Resuscitaire, scales, bedding)

(See chapter website resources for more information.)

Insensible water loss (i.e. loss through the skin, urine, faeces and respiratory tract) may lead to significant heat loss – increased in preterm and low birthweight babies (Rutter 1985) because of the large ratio of surface area to body mass, limited subcutaneous fat, immature epidermal skin layer structure and increased body water content. Risks rise in environments where insensible water loss is increased because 0.58 kcal of heat is lost with each gram of water lost through evaporation (Hammarlund and Sedin 1986).

The appropriate temperature of a baby depends upon the baby's age, gestation and weight. If left wet and naked, the newborn infant cannot cope with environmental temperatures of less than 32 °C. If a thermometer is not available in a room, the environment must be assessed through personal comfort – what appears very warm and uncomfortable for an adult dressed in thin clothes with short sleeves is likely to be appropriate for the newborn.

Neonatal heat production

The hypothalamus and the autonomic and sympathetic nervous systems are important aspects of maintaining the temperature within narrow set limits of 36.5 to 37.5 °C in the newborn (see chapter website resources). Constant body temperature is achieved by a functioning neurological system balancing heat-gain with heat-loss effector systems.

In the newborn, heat production results from metabolic processes that generate energy by oxidative metabolism of glucose, fats and proteins. The organs that generate the greatest energy are the brain, heart and liver. To maintain a constant body temperature, *heat loss* from the surface of the body must equal *heat gain*.

In the baby, although the hypothalamus will receive cold alert messages from the skin, abdomen, spinal cord and internal organs, to regulate temperature stimuli from other areas of the body, the most sensitive receptors are contained within the *trigeminal area* of the face (Hackman 2001).

The responses of the skin surface are determined by the following:

- Skin temperature
- Rate and direction of temperature change
- Size of area stimulated

Physical mechanisms include involuntary reactions, including shivering, and voluntary reactions involving muscular activity, through crying, restlessness and hyperactivity. These responses can be affected by anaesthetics, damage to the brain, muscle relaxants or sedative drugs.

The baby may generate heat by crying and become hyperactive when cold stress is severe enough to cause jitteriness, although shivering does not appear. If cold stress is not eliminated at this point, the baby may become extremely hypothermic, hypoglycaemic, hypoxic, acidotic and lethargic, and eventually death will ensue, caused by cold injury. The full-term baby can flex the body into the 'fetal' position, which provides some protection against cold stress, but the lack of muscle tone and flaccid posture of an immature or ill baby result in greater heat loss. Babies can also reduce shunting of internal heat to body surfaces by constricting peripheral vessels.

Chemical or *non-shivering thermogenesis* is the process by which the neonate generates heat through an increase in the metabolic rate and through *brown adipose tissue (BAT)* metabolism. This process can be utilized by adults and neonates – in the adult the metabolic rate can be increased by about 10 to 15%, whereas the neonate can increase the metabolic rate by up to 100% (Cannon and Nedergaard 2004).

Heat production and brown adipose tissue

A cold-stressed baby depends primarily on mechanisms that cause chemical thermogenesis. Neonatal heat production is mainly through non-shivering thermogenesis. When the baby becomes hypothermic, noradrenaline and thyroid hormones are released, inducing lipolysis in brown fat. This process can be affected by pathological events, including hypoxia, acidosis and hypoglycaemia.

BAT is believed to constitute 2% to 7% of the newborn's weight, depending on gestation and weight. Brown fat starts to be deposited in the fetus from 28 weeks gestation (Blackburn 2013). The brown adipocyte is uniquely suited to its role in newborn thermogenesis and differs from white adipose tissue because it is capable of rapid metabolism, heat production and heat transfer to the peripheral circulation.

The total amount of heat produced in the neonate is unknown, but may be up to 100% of its requirements (Blackburn 2013). The sympathetic nervous system stimulates the adrenal gland to release adrenaline, increasing the metabolism of brown fat and catecholamines and releasing the required glucose. The thyroid gland is also stimulated by the pituitary to release thyroid-stimulating hormone, also producing thyroxine (T_4) – known to enhance heat production from BAT.

BAT contains high concentrations of complex mitochondria, stored triglycerides, sympathetic nerve endings and a rich capillary network to carry heat around the body. The presence of an uncoupling protein within the mitochondria of brown fat cells supports the combustion of fatty acids to produce heat.

BAT is especially prominent in the mammalian fetus, and anatomical distribution is important to its function. The largest mass of tissue envelops the kidneys and adrenal glands; smaller masses are present around the blood vessels and muscles in the neck, and there are extensions of these deposits under the clavicles and into the axillae. Further extensions accompany the great vessels entering the thoracic inlet. The proximity of BAT to large blood vessels and vital vascular organs provides the ability for rapid transfer of heat to the circulation. The activation of BAT metabolism *only* occurs following birth. During intrauterine life, maternal prostaglandins and adenosine do not allow non-shivering thermogenesis to take place. With the clamping of the cord, this mechanism is blocked, enabling the hypothalamus to react to hypothermia (Hall 2016; Polk 1988) (see chapter website resources).

Feeding

From birth, the baby requires water, glucose and certain electrolytes. Calories are utilized for growth and energy to maintain body temperature and metabolism. The method of feeding the neonate, whether orally, by nasogastric tube or intravenously, and the frequency and volume of feeds depend on gestational age and physical condition. When gastric feeds have to be delayed for days and certainly if for more than a week, as in a case of a baby with severe respiratory distress, parenteral nutrition is required to ensure adequate calorific intake. Milk contains far more calories than dextrose given intravenously or orally (Faranoff and Fanaroff 2012).

Drugs

Medication given to pregnant women can affect thermoregulation, as in the following examples:

- *Analgesia in labour* (such as pethidine given intramuscularly or intravenously and the use of bupivacaine for epidurals) – causes maternal vasodilatation and heat loss, rendering the fetus vulnerable to heat loss after birth.

- *Tranquillizers, antidepressants* and *hypnotics* in large doses, and *general anaesthetics* and *muscle relaxants* during caesarean section – tend to affect the neonate's muscle activity, leading to flaccidity and a resulting hypothermia.
- *Babies of women addicted to drugs* are often hyperactive with a higher metabolic rate, which can upset the thermoregulatory balance – potentially leading to hyperthermia.

THE ROLE OF THE MIDWIFE

During pregnancy

Advice is provided regarding maintaining a stable temperature, especially during the first trimester of pregnancy when cell division and differentiation are occurring. There is a higher risk of congenital fetal abnormalities in women who use a sauna, especially if this is a new activity to which the mother's physiology has not adapted (ACOG 2015; Artal and Hopkins 2013; Cohen 1987; Smith et al 1988; Tikkenhan and Heinonen 1991). Care should be taken with other activities, such as hectic exercise or 'hot yoga', which significantly increase the maternal temperature.

Many women complain of heat during their pregnancy. The midwife can offer realistic and practical advice, including wearing natural fabrics, such as cotton, thin wool, silk or linen, and having cool baths/showers. The midwife should also assess the woman's health, excluding infection and/or pyrexia, taking appropriate and swift action should either be identified.

Labour and birth

Midwives' actions prior to labour and delivery determine the well-being of the newborn baby. This includes controlling the neonatal environment, ensuring that the labour and delivery room (or home) is sufficiently warm, above 25°C. Monitoring and recording this every 4 hours is important. Attention must also be paid to the warmth of the towels used for wrapping the baby and other factors that may affect the neonate's well-being, and any deviations from normal must be acted upon. A raised maternal temperature may be an indication of infection or maternal ketosis (see Ch. 36) and may have implications for mother, fetus and neonate.

Water birth

Warm water as pain relief during labour and for giving birth is increasingly being chosen by women, and it is believed that warm water can improve uterine perfusion and uterine contractions, leading to a less painful birth.

The temperature of the water must be comfortable for the woman and should be between 34 and 37°C (Royal College of Midwives and Royal College of Obstetricians and Gynaecologists (RCM and RCOG) 2006; RCM 2012a, 2012b). Therefore, water temperature must be frequently measured and recorded. When the baby is delivered in warm water, it is believed that breathing will not be initiated until the baby's head is lifted above the water. If the baby is asphyxiated or the water cold, then the baby may inhale some pool water (Gilbert and Tookey 1999).

Birth room

Whether in home or in hospital, the midwife should ensure that all professionals, the woman and her family understand the importance of the birthing room being warm (temperature at 25–28°C) and free from draughts caused by open windows, doors or fans. It is also helpful to discuss safe skin-to-skin contact for warmth after delivery with the parents (RCM 2010; 2012a).

It is good practice to record the temperature of the birthing room/theatre in maternal and neonatal notes (WHO 1997).

The midwife should prepare warmed soft towels, blankets and baby clothing (including a hat) by using the radiant heater of the Resuscitaire, radiator or warming pad. Blankets should be warm but not hot enough to cause any trauma to the neonate.

Prior to the birth, the cleaned Resuscitaire is prepared – putting the radiant heater on 'pre-warmed' mode and heating sheets and blankets. Portable/transport incubators must always be fully charged and heated, with additional warmed blankets, ready to go at short notice.

Risk factors in labour

The following aspects may lead to neonatal hypothermia or hyperthermia:

- Fetal hypoxia/distress
- Maternal distress resulting in pyrexia
- Maternal infection resulting in pyrexia or hypothermia
- Epidural anaesthesia
- Substance abuse

If the neonate is considered to be at high risk, the midwife needs to inform the paediatrician and the special care baby nursery staff before birth.

Initial newborn care

A knowledge of physiology increases understanding of the implications of the neonate being exposed to heat or cold stress and directs care needs.

The neonate's head (the largest surface area) should be dried by the midwife, or possibly birth partner, as it enters the cooler birthing environment. A full-term baby's temperature may drop by 1 to 2°C within 30 minutes of birth if heat loss is not prevented (Martin et al 2014).

As the neonate is born, he or she may, according to maternal wishes, be placed on the mother's abdomen – a source of heat and comfort to the newborn baby – and an effective method of preventing heat loss regardless of gestational age. The midwife dries the baby, discards the damp towel, then covers the baby with a fresh, dry, warm towel. To reduce heat loss, a hat may be applied while parents provide skin-to-skin contact (Hall 2016; Blackburn 2013).

Skin-to-skin contact

Recognition of the importance of close and direct contact between mother and baby immediately following birth has led to the widespread adoption of the practice of 'skin-to-skin' care, in which the infant is placed naked and almost always prone directly onto the mother's chest very shortly after birth.

Skin-to-skin care is also recognized as a potential benefit to encourage breastfeeding and to improve maternal attachment behaviour and reduce crying by infants, together with improving cardiorespiratory stability for preterm infants. It is also utilized in warming a baby when he or she becomes hypothermic. A Cochrane review notes that this practice has 'no apparent short or long term negative effects' (Moore et al 2012).

Following birth, the midwives often leave mother and baby to breastfeed alone to facilitate the maternal–infant relationship. The mother may also be encouraged to utilize skin-to-skin care if the baby is not interested in breastfeeding and also as a means of improving newborn temperature if the infant becomes hypothermic; many times the mother and baby are left alone while this care is provided.

Strategies and practices for the prevention of sudden infant death syndrome are actively promoted by health professionals during early neonatal life, and parents are explicitly warned of the dangers of placing their baby prone to sleep and informed of the importance of appropriate covering and correct positioning of the baby within the cot. Parents are also discouraged from co-sleeping if taking sedative drugs, drinking alcohol or being excessively tired (UNICEF UK Baby-Friendly Initiative and Foundation for the Study of Infant Deaths (FSID) 2008; UNICEF UK and Scottish Cot Death Trust 2011).

For the significant majority of newborn infants, it is clear that breastfeeding and skin-to-skin practices are safe and beneficial and should be recommended. There have been situations in the UK and Ireland where apparently healthy term infants have had an unexplained collapse,

and although a rare event, it is one that may lead to death or long-term neurological disability (Nakamura and Sano 2008). Therefore, in balancing the benefits of skin-to-skin care, for such recommendations to be safe for all infants, the midwife needs to ensure appropriate vigilance of babies receiving skin-to-skin care following birth within the first 24 to 48 hours (see Table 43.1). It is useful to explain to the mother and her family or visitors that the mother and baby should be watched, and if the mother becomes sleepy, then the baby should be placed on his or her back in his or her own cot.

Parental knowledge about breathing, colour and activity in the infant is important, too, because many unsuspected collapses occur in the first few days of life (Herlenius and Kuhn 2013).

Babies of less than 32 weeks gestation will have inadequate keratinization of the skin, enabling evaporation of water and heat through the skin. Some units place the baby up to the neck in a special plastic bag after being dried (Doglioni et al 2014).

This can be useful in preventing heat and fluid loss in babies born with a congenital abnormality, such as exomphalos (see Ch. 49). It is important to note that plastic bags are only used if the baby is nursed under a radiant heater.

Care given in the first hour of life is crucial to the physiological well-being of the newborn baby, and equally important is the care he or she receives to remove fear, discomfort and pain from the environment in which the infant now lives. Supporting the woman to breastfeed her baby within the first hour of birth can provide the same human contact that the baby has known for the previous 40 weeks gestation and enables the development of maternal–infant interaction (Lamb 1983; Moore et al 2012); additionally, it provides a high level of nutrients to the baby to maintain brown fat metabolism (see chapter website resources).

Bathing

The timing of the first bath depends on the hospital culture and its carers and the wishes of the parents. Bathing babies soon after birth should be avoided. Babies are cleaned by initially gently drying with a warm towel and bathed at least 24 hours to 5 days later to maintain temperature and also to minimize harm to the delicate newborn skin.

Awareness of blood as a potential risk for hepatitis B virus and HIV transmission (Hudson 1992) has led to many hospitals encouraging staff to routinely bathe babies soon after birth to reduce exposure to blood-borne pathogens for healthcare workers and family members (Varda and Behnke 2000).

Midwives owe a duty of care to the newborn and should work towards individualized care for mother and baby. Care should be driven by the needs of the neonate and the

Table 43.1 Assessment criteria prior to supporting skin-to-skin care

	Well	Not Well
Assessment of the respiratory system	Quiet breathing with respiratory rate 40/minute and no extra effort on breathing	Nasal flaring Expiratory/Inspiratory grunting, visible respiratory effort Costal/subcostal recession Respiratory rate above 50/minute
Behaviour of the newborn	Quite alert, active alert, crying	Asleep or difficult to rouse
Perfusion	Colour of skin and mucous membranes, gums and hard palate should be pink	Appears cyanosed or pale

Correct Positioning and Covering of the Baby While Receiving Skin-to-Skin to Care	
Head	Baby should be upright and turned to one side.
Face	Baby's face can easily be seen by the mother.
Neck	Neck should be erect in midline, not bent.
Mouth and nose	Mouth and nose should be uncovered and visible (note that a baby is an obligatory nose breather).
Extremities	Arms and legs should be well flexed when the baby is lying prone on his or her abdomen.
Chest	Baby is well flexed on mother's/father's chest and is chest-to-chest with mother, not over a breast.
Shoulders	Baby's shoulders are flat against the mother's or father's chest.
Clothing – head	Hair should be dry and covered with a hat.
Covers	The covers should be wrapped all the way around the baby and mother, avoiding heat loss and maintaining the position of the baby against the mother's chest.

mother, avoiding routine practice and 'care by the clock'. Premature babies may be unable to tolerate the additional oxygen and glucose demands of maintaining a temperature above 36.5°C and may become cold stressed (Lyon and Freer 2011).

Resuscitation

Home environment

The area prepared for resuscitation must be warm. A changing mat can be used, with a nest of warmed towels in which the baby is placed after being dried and the wet towel discarded. This can be achieved by the use of heat pads or hot-water bottles which must be removed before the baby is placed in the towels.

Hospital/birth centre

Resuscitaires have an overhead *radiant heater*, which can work on three different settings:

- *Pre-warm* – the setting used prior to birth to warm the mattress and towels.

- *Manual mode* – heat output is manually set between 50% and 60% (a higher output than 60% may lead the baby to become overheated).

- *Baby mode/skin probe* – the temperature is controlled by a preset setting, usually 36.5°C.

Thermoregulation is a life-or-death issue to the premature infant, and it has been recommended that 'all delivery suites and neonatal/paediatric staff should be trained in the thermal care of the infants at resuscitation' (CESDI 2003; UK Resuscitation Council 2015, 2016).

The moment the baby is placed on the Resuscitaire and under the radiant heater, the midwife needs to put the setting to either manual or *servocontrol*. When servocontrolled baby mode is used, the temperature is set to 36.8°C. A small area on the upper part of the baby's abdomen is cleaned of vernix using a *Mediswab*; the silver side of the probe is placed on the abdomen and secured with a reflective disc. This protects the probe from the infrared heat source, ensuring that it does not overheat. Overheating may result in inaccurate information going to the computerized sensor, causing radiant heat source output to be reduced and the baby to become hypothermic. The probe must be monitored regularly to ensure that it remains attached properly and keeps the baby's temperature stable.

The baby should be positioned to ensure the whole of the body is under the heat – the baby may move down the table, away from the radiant heater, during resuscitation. It is also important not to occlude the radiant heat source.

Poor radiant heater use can lead to hyperthermia and dehydration or hypothermia, which causes respiratory and metabolic acidosis, increasing the risk of morbidity and mortality.

Warm gel pads can be used to provide conductive heat gain and support thermoregulation when transferring the newborn from the labour ward to the neonatal intensive care unit (NICU).

Oxygen therapy

Oxygen is cold, and it is important that when administered facially, a flow of 1 to 2 litres only is used, with the mask firmly over the baby's face, avoiding the whole face/head becoming cold. In some units, Resuscitaires have humidifiers attached to them, which replace fluid lost and also provide warmed oxygen.

The temperature should be recorded at 30 minutes of age to facilitate taking appropriate action if heat is being lost rapidly (CESDI 2003).

Examination of the newborn

The midwife usually performs an examination of the neonate soon after birth, and this requires a warm and draught-free environment because the baby is usually exposed. The more in-depth examination requires a safe surface area and will be undertaken with the baby naked; therefore, it needs to be carried out under a radiant heater and on a firm mattress at the correct height (see Ch. 42).

A superficial examination can be performed while the baby is in the mother's or father's arms. It is vital that the baby is dried prior to being exposed naked by parents, and the environment must be at least 25°C. This keeps the baby warm through the warmth of the parent's skin and provides an opportunity for the midwife to educate the parents about what is being looked for and why. This is a time for parents to wonder at the miracle that is their baby and for the midwife to assist in this and not to rush or bustle or make it seem like an everyday episode.

Temperature assessment

Within a short time, the baby's temperature begins to adjust to the extrauterine environment.

Using the rectal route for routine temperature measurement is no longer a justifiable procedure. Historically, this was carried out to confirm the patency of the anus (now examined visually by observing whether the anus is in the midline and patent – see Ch. 42).

Temperature is normally measured via the axilla (see Fig. 43.1). If the baby becomes cold, BAT begins to metabolize, which may give rise to a normal temperature reading and/or the area of BAT concentration being warm. The baby must be assessed by touching the limb and comparing with the abdomen (see Fig. 43.2). This should identify whether the temperature in both is equal

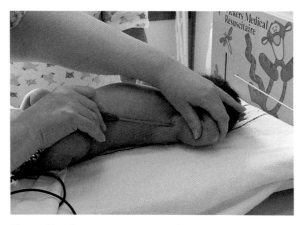

Figure 43.1 Correct measurement of temperature via the axilla.

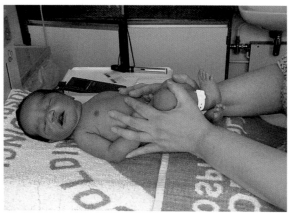

Figure 43.2 Measuring the newborn temperature of the limbs versus abdomen.

to validate the probe/thermometer reading. If the abdomen is warmer than the limbs, the practitioner may consider that the baby is hypothermic and take appropriate action to warm the baby and exclude infection (Tuitui et al 2010; Agarwal et al 2010).

Transfer

On transfer from one environment to another, there is an increased risk of temperature loss in transit. Transferring the baby from the labour ward to the postnatal ward is best done by placing the baby next to the mother, covered loosely. If transported in the cot, the baby needs to be dressed appropriately, including a hat. If the mother has not brought clothes for the baby, the neonatal unit always has clothing that can be utilized.

The best method to transport *sick and premature babies* to the neonatal unit is to place the baby in a stable environment, such as the *transport incubator*, facilitating warmth, observation and care. In the case of transporting the newborn baby from home to hospital, the baby is normally transported in the mother's arms, and although this is an appropriate position, there is a concern in regard to the event of a collision and the safety of the baby; therefore, the use of an incubator that is small and portable in the form of the *Baby Pod* can be utilized (see Fig. 43.3). This portable incubator provides safe transport and also provides a stable internal heat source.

If accompanying a woman with an in utero transfer, the midwife must be prepared for the birth and should have towels and space blankets available to minimize heat loss while in transit.

The ideal and safe environment to transfer a baby from home to hospital is by using the portable incubator to maintain a stable warm environment. If, however, one is not available, the ambulance must be sufficiently warm to allow observation of colour and respiratory effort. If the baby has no breathing problems, skin-to-skin contact can be used to support thermoregulation.

The midwife should record the temperature before and after leaving one area for another, whether in the hospital or community.

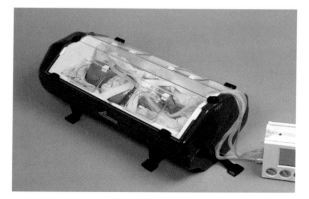

Figure 43.3 Baby Pod infant transport device. (Used with permission from Advanced Healthcare Technology (AHT).)

MONITORING AND MAINTAINING TEMPERATURE

Monitoring

Mercury devices are gradually being replaced by *infrared electronic probes* or *electronic probes* and occasionally *tympanic thermometers*. Electronic and infrared thermometers predict the temperature within 60 seconds (Leick-Rude and Bloom 1998; De Curtis et al 2008). Servocontrol is used to reduce handling and maintain an automatic response to temperature changes in the baby.

The *rectal temperature* is one of the most accurate measurements. The rectum bends sharply to the right, and the passing of the hard thermometer may potentially cause a perforation. The probe must be well lubricated with Vaseline or soft paraffin prior to insertion, and inserted no more than 3 cm into the rectum of the term baby and no more than 2 cm in the preterm (Blackburn 2013; Fleming et al 1983). Stool in the rectum can also influence the accuracy of readings.

Many clinicians continue to consider rectal temperature measurement as the gold standard because it closely approximates the neonate's core temperature, and it continues to be used in babies who are undergoing therapeutic hypothermia. However, because of the possible trauma caused by this method, it is not used in the well newborn, in whom the axilla is the site used.

Core temperature drops only when the baby's effort to produce heat has failed. A rectal/axilla temperature in the normal range does not, therefore, mean no cold stress; it may mean that the baby has activated brown fat metabolism and is producing chemical heat to maintain his or her temperature. This is achieved as the hypothalamus recognizes a temperature of less than 36.0 °C and switches on the 'central heating' in the form of non-shivering thermogenesis. The cause of the hypothermia needs to be isolated and removed prior to the baby utilizing brown fat stores and becoming cold stressed and sick.

Temperature is now measured in the axilla, which contains a large area of brown fat tissue that, when non-shivering thermogenesis takes place, releases chemical energy, causing the area to become warmer than core temperature. Therefore, the reading will be higher than the core reading in a hypothermic baby (Bliss-Holtz 1991), up to 0.49 °C from the core temperature, providing a false-positive result and making it difficult to recognize hypothermia. Following positioning of the probe (see Fig. 43.1), the arm is brought down and held firmly against the body, which encloses the probe to avoid inaccurate results being recorded. Midwives must assess the temperature of the individual baby through behavioural and physiological signs and symptoms of cold stress.

Tactile reading/human touch can validate the reading given by the axillary site. Comparing the abdominal temperature, which is representative of the core temperature, with that of the extremities can identify a cold baby (see Fig. 43.2). Warm, pink feet and abdomen indicate that the baby is in thermal comfort. Cold feet and warm trunk indicate that the baby is in cold stress. In *hypothermia*, the feet and trunk are cold to touch (WHO 1997). If the feet are red and hot, the face is flushed and the baby is restless, the baby could be overheated.

Use of the *inguinal site* may be beneficial because there is good blood flow and no brown adipose tissue to confuse readings, but research has yet to validate it as an accurate means of monitoring temperature in the newborn.

Tympanic temperature appears to be an excellent and accurate way to take the temperature of children and adults but is *less accurate* for newborn babies (Craig et al 2002).

The majority of babies maintain their temperature well, but there are times when parents become concerned about their baby and need to be taught a safe method to assess their baby's temperature to detect hypothermia or hyperthermia early. This can be done by using a thermometer or by feeling the baby's skin (touch assessment) and observing for other signs.

Another non-invasive method for taking the temperature of the baby is the *Thermospot* – a 12-mm sticky black disc that changes to a 'smiley' face when the reading is complete. Parents are asked to place this high in the axilla or over the liver area in the epigastrium. This method is not reliable if the temperature of the baby is below 35.5 °C (Morley and Blumenthal 2000).

Maintaining temperature

The mother is a great source of heat for the baby when the baby is held in her arms. The midwife should encourage the mother to hold her baby close to her body to promote warmth and also engender a greater sense of intimacy. This method of maintaining temperature was investigated in a study at the Hammersmith Hospital in 1987, earning the term *kangaroo care*, also known as *skin-to-skin care*, and is often used for very small neonates (Whitelaw et al 1988). A similar approach to care was used in a study in Colombia, in which very preterm and small-for-gestational-age babies were nursed inside their mothers' clothing between their breasts (Sleath 1985). There was a 95% survival rate

for babies of 500 to 2000 g, improved rate of breastfeeding and closer maternal–baby interaction. Similar good outcomes have been found using the same approach in London. A Cochrane review suggests this might be a useful means of stabilizing the well-being of small infants, although the review noted that more research is required (Conde-Agudelo et al 2011).

Babies requiring surgery have particular needs that must be assessed according to the reason for and type of surgery (see chapter website resources).

MINIMIZING THE RISKS OF HYPOTHERMIA

Wrapping and swaddling

Warm towels or blankets and clothing for the baby are essential; however, tight swaddling that restricts movement may have a detrimental effect on thermoregulation and respiration during sleep and is discouraged, especially for a baby left in a cot.

When placing the *very premature baby* under the radiant heater, the baby is usually placed into the plastic bag wet because this minimizes water and heat loss through evaporation (Laptook and Watkinson 2008; UK Resuscitation Council 2015 and 2016).

Hats and clothes

The use of hats for the newborn, especially for those that are small for gestational age and preterm and babies who are being resuscitated, has proven effective in reducing heat loss from the largest surface area of the baby.

The midwife should ensure that babies' clothing is of natural fabrics and not too close-fitting. It is better to use several layers of thin clothing rather than one or two thick layers. The midwife needs also to ensure that there are no loose threads that may become wrapped around the neonate's fingers or toes, as these can cause considerable trauma if not discovered quickly.

Bathing

Bathing the baby cleanses and provides an opportunity to assess and validate the baby's well-being by observing physiological behavioural patterns, and it is an excellent time for baby and family to interact (Karl 1999). This may be viewed by some midwives as a time-consuming or mundane task, better delegated to a healthcare support worker. If midwives delegate this task, they must ensure that the person providing care is able to assess the well-being of the baby prior to the bath, provide information and advice at an appropriate level to the parents and provide a report back on the baby's well-being. Throughout the bath, well-being should be assessed following the cues the baby is providing, and these should be pointed out to the mother (see Ch. 42).

Parent education

Educating parents in the care of their babies at home includes giving advice on suitable clothing for the baby in terms of material and the number of layers required to maintain both heat and ventilation. A checklist can be useful for educating parents of small babies going home, which includes practical advice on helping babies keep warm indoors and outdoors (see chapter website resources for information leaflet). This information should be translated into appropriate languages for those whose first language is not English, particularly for those who have little knowledge of newborn care in the UK climate.

Social workers can be mobilized in circumstances where financial help is needed to assist with heating bills and adequate home insulation or ventilation.

THE SICK NEONATE

Hypothermia

Hypothermia is a temperature less than 36.5°C. The baby is more at risk of becoming hypothermic during the first 12 hours following birth, although it can occur at other times during the neonatal period.

Signs and symptoms of cold stress initially include the following (Table 43.2):

- Are nonspecific
- May indicate other severe diseases
- May be confused with bacterial infection

If these signs and symptoms are not addressed the baby will develop *sclerema*, which causes a classic range of symptoms, including hardening of the skin, with an apparent redness of the face and extremities, giving a superficial impression of healthy rosiness.

As the baby utilizes oxygen to metabolize brown fat, it reaches its limit, and because there may already be hypoxia, this leads to impaired cardiac function and haemorrhage

Table 43.2 Signs of a baby with hypothermia

Thermoregulation: Signs of heat conservation and vasoconstriction	The baby will be pale and mottled, with cool extremities and warmer abdomen.
Gastrointestinal tract: Decreased peristalsis and absorption	Will have a history of: • Poor feeding • Decreased volume intake if artificially feeding • Possets • If fed by nasogastric tube (NGT), increased gastric aspirates, abdominal distension and vomiting
Neurological system: Increased physical activity to generate heat	The baby may communicate through his or her behavior: • Irritability • Crying • Increase in spontaneous activity, such as moving down or up the cot • In severe cases, lethargy, poor tone, and decrease in spontaneous activity
Respiratory system: Hypoxia and acidosis Respiratory acidosis and metabolic acidosis May have increased demand for oxygen	• Increasingly weak cry • If premature, may have episodes of bradycardia and apnoea • Increasing episodes of apnoea • In the baby above 38 weeks gestation, may show tachypnoea at rest and also signs of shallow and slow breathing as hypothermia is not rectified
Cardiovascular system: Reduced metabolic metabolism	• Decreased heart rate
Environmental factors and infection	Long-term chronic hypothermia will lead to difficulty in gaining weight; thus, a baby who has difficulty in gaining weight may be utilizing calories to maintain well-being, or this may indicate an underlying infection, such as infection of the urinary tract.

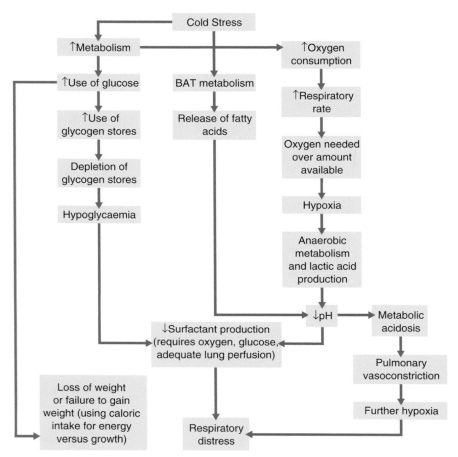

Figure 43.4 Physiological consequences of cold stress BAT, brown adipose tissue. (Blackburn ST: Maternal fetal and neonatal physiology: a clinical perspective, 4th edn, Philadelphia, Saunders, 2013.)

(especially pulmonary). Cellular function switches from *aerobic* to *anaerobic metabolism*, leading to the production of lactic acid and metabolic acidosis (Fig. 43.4). Hypoglycaemia can also cause acidosis, and because the brain does not tolerate lack of glucose, neurological damage can occur. If severe cold stress is not treated, the baby develops clotting disorders and dies (Blackburn 2013; Rennie 2012).

Management

There is no general agreement on the management of hypothermia, but prevention is the best treatment. A baby with a temperature of less than 36.5°C must be urgently referred to the paediatrician/neonatologist, and the midwife needs to enable the baby to increase his or her temperature by adding more warmed clothing, increasing the environmental temperature or placing the infant close to the mother, either dressed or naked and covered. The

baby must be observed closely to monitor his or her well-being and airway.

Mild hypothermia (temperature range 36–36.4°C)

Rewarming the *mildly hypothermic* neonate is not problematic, but debate continues about the virtues of *rapid* versus *slow* rewarming and their respective advantages and disadvantages in severe cold stress. Slow rewarming is the usual practice.

Moderate hypothermia (temperature range 32–35.9°C)

The baby is placed clothed, but not covered, under a radiant heater or in an incubator set at a temperature of 35 to 36°C. Alternatively, the baby can be warmed using a gel- or water-filled mattress set at 36.5°C, with the room temperature set at 32 to 34°C (Carmichael et al 2007).

In the home environment, if clinically stable, skin-to-skin contact with the mother in a room with a temperature of at least 25°C can be used.

Severe cold stress

The main aim in severe cold stress is to maintain a thermal environment in which the baby is not required to increase his or her basal metabolic rate. The baby is rewarmed **slowly** to avoid hypotension resulting from vasodilatation of the peripheral circulation and acidosis. Rapid rewarming may induce apnoea and cardiac failure. Because oxygen consumption is minimal with gradients of less than 1.5°C, the incubator temperature is set at 1.5°C higher than the baby's core temperature and adjusted every 15 to 30 minutes. The baby must be naked to allow the heat from the incubator or radiant warmer to warm him or her. The baby should preferably not be fed gastrically because hypothermia reduces evacuation of gastric contents and reduces peristalsis. Intravenous fluids ensure adequate fluid and glucose intake, but it is important to warm all fluids given to the baby prior to administration.

Hyperthermia

Hyperthermia is a temperature of more than 37.8°C. This is less common in newborn care. Pyrexia may result from excessive environmental temperatures, incubator overheating (or the greenhouse effect of an incubator in the sunlight), overdressing the baby, infection, dehydration or a change in central control resulting from drugs or cerebral damage.

As with cold stress, hyperthermia results in increased metabolism and oxygen consumption. It is important that the baby is cooled slowly. This means removing woollens or leaving the baby with only one blanket. Extreme measures, including leaving the baby in thin clothes or restricted bedding, must be avoided.

Reversal of heat stress

The aim in reversing hyperthermia is to reduce metabolic heat production. The baby will attempt to assume an extended position, allowing heat loss via the external gradient to the environment, and to aid this process the baby should have most of his or her clothes removed. Damp-sponging babies is not recommended. This encourages rapid heat loss, which may then lead to cold stress and shock (Kenner et al 1993).

Once the cause of the hyperthermia has been corrected, the temperature should return to normal within 1 hour. If improvement is not noted within that hour and the baby remains pyrexial and looks unwell, infection must be excluded, and brain damage needs to be investigated (Jain 2012).

Effects and signs of hyperthermia

Hyperthermia increases the metabolic rate and the evaporative water loss rate, which can cause dehydration. The baby is unable to fully utilize the mechanism of sweating to reduce heat. The exception is the baby born to a mother with substance abuse, in which case the baby may become sweaty and wet when stressed and hyperactive. In the normal term baby, the only area of the body on which sweating takes place is the head and, in times of shock, the palms of the hands.

Signs of hyperthermia are not readily apparent and include restlessness and crying. As a result of metabolic rate increases, there may be *tachypnoea* and *tachycardia*. The baby's face and extremities are red because of vasodilatation. This is a serious sign of hyperthermia and must be acted upon to reverse heat gain by isolating the cause. If this does not occur and the temperature rises above 42°C, the baby will go into shock; convulsions and coma may occur.

As with hypothermia, the main cause of hyperthermic stress in the newborn is a result of misinterpreting the environmental temperature and its effect on the baby. This can happen by leaving the baby in a closed car on a hot and sunny day, overdressing the baby on a cold day while inside or putting the baby too close to a heat source.

Reflective activity 43.1

Review your local guidelines and protocols for thermoregulation, and measure these against national guidelines and your knowledge of physiology. Consider whether these provide sufficiently up to date, practical information.

EQUIPMENT

Equipment must be used appropriately and with consideration of the thermoregulatory effect.

- *Incubators:* These should be used only for those babies who are ill, likely to become ill, or at a weight less than the 9th percentile. Modern incubators now have double walls to stop radiant heat loss. The air temperature can be controlled manually or automatically. Incubators and radiant warmers also have an automatic servocontrol skin probe attachment.

- *The transport incubator:* This is more familiar to the neonatal nurse than to the midwife, and it provides the means of transferring, monitoring and supporting the small or sick neonate. The midwife should, however, gain a basic understanding of this equipment and its use (see chapter website resources).

- *Heated mattress:* Two types of mattress are used:
  - *Gel filled:* this type has heat-conducting properties and is surrounded by a soft film that does not irritate the baby's skin.

- **Water filled:** when used in the cot, it should have holes in the base as an emergency outlet in case there is an accidental slow leak.

- See the chapter website resources for more information.

- *Phototherapy:* This can be delivered to the baby in an incubator, cot or open bassinet with a servocontrolled overhead radiant heating source. The neonate's temperature must be monitored via the axilla, and recorded every 3 to 4 hours, because the baby can become hyperthermic or hypothermic during this treatment.

- *Heat shields:* Modern incubators have reduced the need for these, but, if used, they should be checked for cracks, ease of movement and safety. Heat shields should be used when nursing a baby naked in an incubator and in other situations to prevent, or help treat, hypothermia.

- *Oxygen therapy:* When given in percentages greater than 30%, oxygen should be humidified and warmed. If given via an endotracheal tube, it should be given at body temperature. If given via a head box, it should be at the same temperature as the incubator to avoid causing *physiological confusion.*

CONCLUSION

Although a homeotherm in the true sense of the word, the neonate has higher heat and water losses than those of the adult, so a thermal environment that allows a minimal resting metabolic rate must be provided. Midwives should give special attention to the maintenance of a 'normal' temperature, particularly for the at-risk neonate. An understanding of the physiology of temperature control, calorific intake and application to practice is vital so as to provide a safe transition to extrauterine life.

The midwife is a key practitioner in preparing, supporting and educating the mother and her family in thermoregulation, its impact on the baby and deviations from normal.

Key Points   ⊓—O

- Thermoregulation is a crucial part of ensuring neonatal well-being, regardless of gestation and risk factors.
- The midwife requires a high level of knowledge and understanding of the applied physiology of thermoregulation to provide safe and effective care to the woman and her baby.
- Prevention and early identification of deviations from normal can prevent long-term morbidity and mortality.
- Hypothermia and hyperthermia may be caused by sepsis, cerebral malfunction or an inadequately stable thermal environment.
- The midwife oversees and controls the environment and ensures the provision of a neutral thermal environment, contributing to preventing hypothermia and hyperthermia.
- An important part of the midwife's role is in educating and preparing parents and other professionals regarding the thermoregulatory needs of the neonate and integrating this into a framework of care, allowing parents to learn more about their child.
- Appropriate and effective management of hypothermia and hyperthermia, and effective use of appropriate equipment and monitoring, will reduce long-term morbidity and mortality.

References

Agarwal S, Sethi V, Srivastava K, et al: Human touch to detect hypothermia in neonates in Indian slum dwellings, *Indian J Pediatr* 77:759–762, 2010.

American College of Obstetricians and Gynecologists (ACOG): Physical activity and exercise during pregnancy and the postpartum period. Committee Opinion No. 650, *Obstet Gynecol* 126:e135–e142, 2015.

Artal R, Hopkins S: Exercise, *Clin Updates Womens Health Care* 7(2):1–105, 2013.

Asakura H: Fetal and neonatal thermoregulation, *J Nippon Med Sch* 71(6):360–370, 2004.

Blackburn ST: *Maternal, fetal, & neonatal physiology: a clinical perspective,* 4th edn, Philadelphia, Elsevier, 2013.

Bliss-Holtz J: Determining cold stress in full term newborns through temperature site comparisons, *Sch Inq Nurs Pract* 5(2):113–123, 1991.

Cannon B, Nedergaard J: Brown adipose tissue: function and physiological significance, *Physiol Rev* 84:277–359, 2004.

Carmichael A, McCullough S, Kempley ST: Critical dependence of acetate thermal mattress on gel activation temperature, *Arch Dis Child Fetal Neonatal Ed* 92:44–45, 2007.

Cohen FL: Neural tube defects: epidemiology, detection and prevention, *J Obstet Gynecol Neonatal Nurs* 16(2):105–115, 1987.

Conde-Agudelo A, Belizán JM, Diaz-Rossello J: Kangaroo mother care to reduce morbidity and mortality in low birthweight infants, *Cochrane Database Syst Rev*. Cochrane Neonatal Group, Cochrane Library, Wiley Online Library, 2011.

Confidential Enquiries into Stillbirth and Deaths in Infancy (CESDI): *Project 27/28. An enquiry into quality of care and its effect on the survival of babies born at 27–28 weeks*, London, The Stationery Office, 2003.

Craig J, Lancaster G, Taylor S, et al: Infrared ear thermometry compared with rectal thermometry in children: a systematic review, *Lancet* 360(9333):603–609, 2002.

de Almeida MF, Guinsburg R, Sancho GA, et al: Brazilian Network on Neonatal Research. Hypothermia and early neonatal mortality in preterm infants, *J Pediatr* 164(2):271–275, 2014.

De Curtis M, Calzolari F, Marciano A, et al: Comparison between rectal and infrared skin temperature in the newborn, *Arch Dis Child Fetal Neonatal Ed* 93(1):F55–F57, 2008.

Doglioni N, Cavallin F, Mardegan V, et al: Total body polyethylene wraps for preventing hypothermia in preterm infants: a randomized trial, *J Pediatr* 165(2):261–266, 2014.

Fanaroff AA, Faranoff JM: *Klaus and Fanaroff's care of the high-risk neonate: expert consult*, 6th edn, Philadelphia, Elsevier, 2012.

Fleming M, Hakansson H, Svenningsen NW: A disposable temperature probe for skin measurement in the newborn nursery, *Int J Nurs Stud* 10(2):89–96, 1983.

Gardner SL, Carter BS, Enzman-Hines MI, et al: *Merenstein & Gardner's handbook of neonatal intensive care*, 7th edn, St. Louis, Mosby Elsevier, 2011.

Gilbert RE, Tookey PA: Perinatal mortality and morbidity among babies in water: national surveillance study, *Br Med J* 319(7208):483–487, 1999.

Hackman PS: Recognizing and understanding the cold-stressed term infant, *Neonatal Netw* 20(8):35–41, 2001.

Hall JE: *Guyton and Hall textbook of medical physiology*, 13th edn, Philadelphia, Elsevier Saunders, 2016.

Hammarlund K, Sedin G: Heat loss from the skin of preterm and full term newborn infants during the first weeks after birth, *Biol Neonate* 50(1):1–10, 1986.

Hartman S, Bung P: Physical training during pregnancy – physiological considerations and recommendations, *J Perinat Med* 27(3):204–215, 1999.

Herlenius E, Kuhn P: Sudden unexpected postnatal collapse of newborn infants: a review of cases, definitions, risks, and preventive measures, *Transl Stroke Res* 4:236–247, 2013.

Hudson CN: HIV infection in obstetrics and gynaecology, *Baillières Clin Obstet Gynaecol* 6(1):137–148, 1992.

Jain A: Ch. 15. In Rennie JM, editor: *Rennie & Roberton's textbook of neonatology: expert consult: online and print*, 5th edn, Edinburgh, Churchill Livingstone, 2012.

Karl D: The interactive newborn bath: using infant neurobehavior to connect parents and newborns, *MCN Am J Matern Child Nurs* 24(6):280–286, 1999.

Kenner C, Brueggemeyer A, Gunderson LP: *Comprehensive neonatal nursing: a physiologic perspective*, Philadelphia, WB Saunders, 1993.

Kirkup B: *The report of the Morecambe Bay investigation: an independent investigation into the management, delivery and outcomes of care provided by the maternity and neonatal services at the University Hospitals of Morecambe Bay NHS Foundation Trust from January 2004 to June 2013*, London, Stationery Office, 2015.

Kumar V, Shearer JC, Kumar A, et al: Neonatal hypothermia in low resource settings: a review, *J Perinatol* 29:401–412, 2009.

Lamb ME: Early mother–neonate contact and mother child relationship, *J Child Psychol Psychiatry* 24(3):487–494, 1983.

Laptook AR, Watkinson M: Temperature management in the delivery room, *Semin Fetal Neonatal Med* 13(6):383–391, 2008.

Lawn JE, Cousens S, Zupan J: 4 Million neonatal deaths: when? where? why? *Lancet* 365(9462):891–900, 2005.

Leick-Rude MK, Bloom LE: A comparison of temperature taking methods in neonates, *Neonatal Netw* 17(5):21–37, 1998.

Liebeman E, Lang J, Richardson DK, et al: Intrapartum maternal fever and neonatal outcome, *Pediatrics* 105(1):8–13, 2000.

Lunze K, Hamer DH: Thermal protection of the newborn in resource-limited environments, *J Perinatol* 32:317–324, 2012.

Lyon AJ, Freer Y: Goals and options in keeping preterm babies warm, *Arch Dis Child Fetal Neonatal Ed* 96(1):F71–F74, 2011.

Martin RJ, Fanaroff AA, Walsh MC: *Fanaroff and Martin's neonatal-perinatal medicine*, 10th edn, Philadelphia, Saunders, 2014.

McCall EM, Alderdice F, Halliday HL, et al: Interventions to prevent hypothermia at birth in preterm and/or low birthweight infants, *Cochrane Database Syst Rev* (1):CD004210, 2008.

Moore ER, Anderson GC, Bergman N, et al: Early skin-to-skin contact for mothers and their healthy newborn infants, *Cochrane Database Syst Rev* (3):CD003519, 2012.

Morley D, Blumenthal I: A neonatal hypothermia indicator, *Lancet* 355(9204):659–660, 2000.

Nakamura T, Sano Y: Two cases of infants who needed cardiopulmonary resuscitation during early skin-to-skin contact with mother, *J Obstet Gynaecol Res* 34(4 Pt 2):603–604, 2008.

Polin SH, Fox RA, Abman WW: *Fetal and neonatal physiology: expert consult – online and print*, 4th edn, Philadelphia, Saunders Elsevier, 2011.

Polk DH: Thyroid hormone effects on neonatal thermogenesis, *Clin Perinatol* 12:151–156, 1988.

Rennie JM: *Rennie & Roberton's textbook of neonatology: expert consult: online and print*, 5th edn, Edinburgh, Churchill Livingstone, 2012.

Royal College of Midwives (RCM): *Revealing the evidence behind the magic of touch*, London, RCM, 2010.

Royal College of Midwives (RCM): *Midwifery practice guidelines, 'immediate care of the newborn'* (website). https://www.rcm.org.uk/sites/default/files/Immediate%20

Care%20%20of%20the%20 Newborn.pdf. 2012a.

Royal College of Midwives (RCM): *Immersion in water for labour and birth: evidence-based guidelines for midwifery-led care in labour*, London, RCM, 2012b.

Royal College of Midwives (RCM) & Royal College of Obstetricians and Gynaecologists (RCOG): *RCOG/The Royal College of Midwives Joint Statement No. 1: Immersion in water during labour and birth*, London, RCOG, 2006.

Rutter N: The evaporimeter and emotional sweating in the neonate, *Clin Perinatol* 12:63–77, 1985.

Sleath K: Lessons from Colombia, *Nurs Mirror* 160(14):14–16, 1985.

Smith M, Upfold J, Edwards M: The dangers of heat to the newborn, *Patient Management* 3:157–165, 1988.

Tikkenhan J, Heinonen O: Maternal hyperthermia during pregnancy and cardiovascular malformations in the offspring, *Eur J Epidemiol* 7(6):628–635, 1991.

Tuitui RL, Suwal SN, Shrestha S: Hand-touch method for detection of neonatal hypothermia in Nepal, *J Trop Pediatr* 57:236–238, 2010.

UK Resuscitation Council: *Newborn life support – resuscitation at birth manual*, 3rd edn, London, UK Resuscitation Council, 2015.

UK Resuscitation Council: *Resuscitation and support of transition of babies at birth* (website). www.resus.org.uk/ resuscitation-guidelines/ resuscitation-and-support-of-transition-of-babies-at-birth/. 2016.

UNICEF UK & Scottish Cot Death Trust: *Reduce the risk of cot death leaflet* (website). www.unicef.org.uk/ Documents/Baby_Friendly/Leaflets/ Scotland_Reduce_the_Risk_of_Cot_ Death_Leaflet.pdf. 2011.

UNICEF UK Baby-Friendly Initiative with the Foundation for the Study of Infant Deaths (FSIDS): *Sharing a bed with your baby. A guide for breastfeeding mothers*, London, UNICEF UK/FSID, 2008.

Varda KE, Behnke R: The effect of timing of initial bath on newborn's temperature, *J Obstet Gynecol Neonatal Nurs* 29(1):27–32, 2000.

Whitelaw A, Heisterkamp G, Sleath K, et al: Skin to skin contact for very low birthweight infants and their mothers, *Arch Dis Child* 63:1377–1381, 1988.

World Health Organisation (WHO), Division of Reproductive Health, Maternal and Newborn Health/Safe Motherhood: Thermal protection and/or management of neonatal hypothermia and hyperthermia. Report of a technical working group. In *Essential newborn care*, Geneva, WHO, 1994.

World Health Organisation (WHO): *Thermal protection of the newborn: a practical guide*, Geneva, WHO, 1997.

Resources and additional reading

MacDonald MG, Seshia MK: *Avery's neonatology: pathophysiology and management of the newborn*, Philadelphia, Lippincott Williams and Wilkins, 2015.

A key internationally appropriate textbook presenting the pathophysiology and a range of useful resources.

Polin RA, Spitzer A: *Fetal & and neonatal secrets*, 3rd edn, St. Louis, Mosby, 2013.

An interestingly set out text, with clinical issues centred on the newborn.

Royal College of Midwives (RCM): *Electronic learning programme: examination of the newborn module* (website). www.rcm.org.uk. 2015.

This is an excellent resource (free to members) that includes examination of the newborn and thermoregulation issues for newborns.

Chapter 44

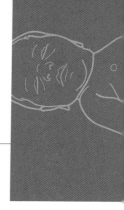

Infant feeding and relationship building

Francesca Entwistle

Learning Outcomes ?

After reading this chapter, you will be able to:

- explain the anatomy and physiology of breastfeeding and how to support a mother in pregnancy and after birth to get breastfeeding off to a good start so that she can continue to breastfeed her baby for as long as she wishes
- understand the influence of breastmilk and breastfeeding on the health and well-being outcomes for the mother and baby
- understand the importance of secure mother–infant attachment and how this can be encouraged to support close and loving relationships between mothers and babies so that all mothers are able to keep their babies close and be responsive to their cues for feeding and comfort
- explain the challenges that may arise when a mother is breastfeeding, know how to provide support with effective management options and know when and where to seek further help
- support mothers who are bottle feeding to be responsive to their baby's needs, to prepare feeds safely and to use appropriate infant formula
- describe infant feeding cultures, social and political, within the UK and how these influence women's decisions to feed their infants
- know how to practise as a midwife within the *International Code of Marketing of Breastmilk Substitutes*

INTRODUCTION

Mother–baby interactions are intuitive, and at birth the mother is physiologically programmed to communicate with, feed and care for her baby. Left alone, she will respond to her baby's needs, and the hormone *oxytocin* will be released (Cadwell 2007). Oxytocin (sometimes referred to as the love hormone) promotes very early attachment behaviours, breastfeeding and the baby's brain development (Uvnäs-Moberg and Francis 2003; Winberg 2005).

The World Health Organization (WHO 2011); UK Department of Health (DH 2009/2011); APPG (2015); Scottish government (2011); Department for Health, Social Services and Public Safety Northern Ireland (DHSSPS 2013); Welsh government (2015); and Public Health England (PHE 2015) recommend that all infants are exclusively breastfed for 6 months, and thereafter alongside other foods for 2 years and beyond (WHO 2016). Other countries also recommend this standard, including Australia (Australian Health Ministers Conference 2009); America, as cited by the American Academy of Pediatrics (AAP 2012); and New Zealand, as cited by the New Zealand Ministry of Health (NZMH 2012 and 2016).

In the UK, breastfeeding initiation rates are improving, from 62% in 1990 to 76% to 81% in 2005 (McAndrew et al 2012), but there are large social and demographic variations, and only small numbers of women continue to breastfeed exclusively. In 2010, only 17% of all mothers were still exclusively breastfeeding at 3 months, 12% at 4 months and 1% at 6 months (McAndrew et al 2012). Low breastfeeding rates lead to increased incidence of illness, which has significant implications for children, families, societies and the health services.

Many women in the UK grow up in a 'bottle-feeding' culture in which initiating and establishing breastfeeding can be challenging. Young mothers and those from lower socioeconomic groups are least likely to breastfeed and have the worst health and social outcomes for themselves and their babies. Mothers who bottle feed should be supported to keep their babies close, so they too can learn to respond to the baby's cues for feeding and comfort; in addition, they should be taught how to safely prepare and choose appropriate formula.

WHY ARE BREASTMILK AND BREASTFEEDING SO IMPORTANT?

Investing in breastfeeding and relationship building is now recognized as a positive, proactive mechanism to promote mother–infant attachment behaviours and improve mental health and well-being for the mother and the child (*Acta Paediatrica* 2015; Britton et al 2011; Ekstrom et al 2006; Groër 2005; Gutman et al 2009; Heikkilä et al 2011; Kim et al 2011; National Institute for Health and Care Excellence (NICE) 2012; Oddy et al 2009; Oddy et al 2011; Sacker et al 2006; Strathearn et al 2009; Sunderland 2007; Unite/CPHVA 2008).

Not breastfeeding increases a baby's risk of obesity, diabetes, respiratory infections, gastroenteritis, ear infections, allergic disease and sudden infant death syndrome (*Acta Paediatrica* 2015; AAP 2012; Arenz et al 2004; Bartok and Ventura 2009; Cathal and Layte 2012; Chivers et al 2010; Harder et al 2005; Horta et al 2007; Ip et al 2007; *Lancet* 2016; Quigley et al, 2007; Renfrew et al 2012b; Scott et al 2012; Shields et al 2006).

Not breastfeeding also increases a baby's risk of being admitted to hospital, and the effect on the child's IQ and other measures of development is now recognized in high-quality studies (Ajetunmobi et al 2015; Horta and Victoria 2013; Iacovou and Sevilla-Sanz 2010; Kramer et al 2008; *Lancet* 2016; Renfrew et al 2009).

Breastfeeding and skin-to-skin contact at birth and in the early days and weeks helps parents to initiate and build a close, loving and nurturing relationship with their baby (Unicef 2013). Breastfeeding provides a unique opportunity for attachment between mother and baby and can protect the child from maternal neglect (Strathearn et al 2009).

Women who do not breastfeed have an increased risk of developing breast and ovarian cancer (*Lancet* 2016; World Cancer Research Fund International/American Institute for Cancer Research (WCRF/AICR) 2009).

One in 10 babies born alive need specialist neonatal care of some sort. Breastfeeding or providing breastmilk for premature and sick babies improves their short- and long-term health and well-being outcomes, reducing both mortality and morbidity (Renfrew et al 2009; Lancet 2016).

PUBLIC HEALTH AND INFANT FEEDING

'Breastfeeding is a natural safety net against the worst effects of poverty......exclusive breastfeeding goes a long way towards cancelling out the health difference between being born into poverty or being born into affluence. It is almost as if breastfeeding takes the infant out of poverty for those few vital months in order to give the child a fairer start in life and compensate for the injustices of the world into which it was born'.

James P. Grant, Executive Director
of Unicef, 1980–1995

Commissioning services to increase and sustain breastfeeding would make an important contribution to improving public health and reducing health inequalities, and it would save significant costs to the National Health Service (NHS) (Renfrew et al 2012b; Public Health England (PHE) and Unicef 2016).

It is known that some vulnerable mothers – including young mothers and mothers from lower socioeconomic groups, who are least likely to breastfeed (McAndrew et al 2012; Scientific Advisory Committee on Nutrition (SACN) 2008) – have the worst health and social outcomes for themselves and their babies. Breastfeeding provides one solution to this long-standing problem, as an intervention to help tackle health inequality. One study found that those low-income mothers who breastfed for 6 to 12 months had the highest scores of any group on quality of parenting interactions at age 5 (Gutman et al 2009). Evidence has also demonstrated that a child from a low-income background who is breastfed is likely to have better health outcomes than a child from a more affluent background who is formula-fed (Wilson et al 1998). However, in line with previous infant feeding surveys, in 2010, low maternal age and low educational level were found to be the strongest predictors of infant feeding outcomes, other than previous feeding experience, even when other factors were taken into consideration (McAndrew et al 2012).

In the UK, NICE (2012, 2013 and 2015a), the Chief Medical Officer (CMO) (Davies 2013), Public Health England (2015), Department of Health (2014), Scottish government (2011), Public Health Wales (2013), Welsh government (2010) and Health Improvement, Northern Ireland (DHSSPS 2013) *all* recognize worrying trends in low breastfeeding rates. They highlight the importance of improving breastfeeding rates to promote child and maternal health and well-being and call for implementation of the Unicef UK Baby Friendly Initiative in all maternity and community healthcare settings as a minimum standard to support breastfeeding, as a way of reducing risk, improving services and helping families to give their babies the best start in life. The CMO also calls for monitoring and examination of the effects of the marketing of breastmilk substitutes (Davies 2013; WHO 2013b).

Midwives are in an ideal place to expand their public health role (CNO 2010) in working with women and their families to help them understand the value of breastfeeding and in supporting mothers to breastfeed. They can help to reduce inequalities and social deprivation by implementing the Healthy Child Programme (DH 2015) and working closely with health visitors and those specialist nurses providing the *Family Nurse Partnership Programme* to support women who breastfeed to continue to do so (DH 2011). The first 1001 days (24 months) of a child's life are vitally important for ensuring that the brain achieves its optimum development and the foundations of nurturing are laid down to ensure all babies achieve the best start in life (All Party Parliamentary Group (APPG) 2015).

A multidisciplinary and longitudinal approach is required, in line with governments' public health strategies, to support women during pregnancy, birth and in the postpartum period (NICE 2012).

THE BABY FRIENDLY INITIATIVE

In 1989, *Protecting, Promoting and Supporting Breastfeeding: The Special Role of Maternity Services* (WHO/Unicef 1989) was published. This was adopted as a global initiative by policymakers at a meeting in Florence, Italy, now referred to as the *Innocenti Declaration* (Henschel and Inch 1996). In June 1991, the *Baby-Friendly Hospital Initiative* (BFHI) was launched at the International Paediatric Association Conference, Ankara, providing a global focus for the intent of the Innocenti Declaration. The principles of the declaration were embodied in the 'Ten Steps to Successful Breastfeeding', designed as a set of standards that could be followed by maternity units all over the world and audited to demonstrate measurable improvements (see Box 44.1).

The Unicef UK Baby Friendly Initiative (BFI) was introduced in 1994 (Unicef UK 1998). At this time, breastfeeding initiation and prevalence rates were low, and the programme acted as a foundation to implement evidence-based care to support more women to breastfeed their infants. To achieve this, it was recognized that there was a need to update education for healthcare staff and to implement evidence-based service policy to underpin minimum standards that would support breastfeeding. The BFI programme used a focused approach to implement significant changes to healthcare practice and to lift the bar on what was required to improve care. The BFI has succeeded in gaining national recognition for the importance of breastfeeding. It has also created a new 'common knowledge' related to breastfeeding practice within the health service and among policymakers. Topics that were once hotly debated, such as skin-to-skin contact, rooming-in, teaching mothers how to breastfeed and avoiding supplementation, are now accepted as good practice. Indeed, for many student midwives, 'normal practice' is offering all women skin-to-skin contact with their babies immediately after birth, and they do not know a time when this did not happen. Although not every

---

Box 44.1 The WHO/Unicef (1989) International ten steps to successful breastfeeding

All providers of maternity services should:
1. Have a written breastfeeding policy that is routinely communicated to all healthcare staff.
2. Train all healthcare staff in the skills necessary to implement the breastfeeding policy.
3. Inform all pregnant women about the benefits and management of breastfeeding.
4. Help mothers initiate breastfeeding soon after birth.
5. Show mothers how to breastfeed and how to maintain lactation even if they are separated from their babies.
6. Give newborn infants no food or drink other than breastmilk, unless medically indicated.
7. Practise rooming in, allowing mothers and infants to remain together 24 hours a day.
8. Encourage breastfeeding on demand.
9. Give no artificial teats or dummies to breastfeeding infants.
10. Foster the establishment of breastfeeding support groups and refer mothers to them on discharge from the hospital or clinic.

Source: WHO/Unicef (1989)

---

mother in the UK receives this level of support, overall standards have improved, and most health professionals, including pre-registration midwives and health visitors, now have knowledge of what good care should be, and the skills to best to support mothers and babies.

The current body of evidence demonstrates that a multitude of interventions, including full implementation of the Ten Steps and the BFI standards, is associated with significant improvements in infant feeding practices within relevant healthcare environments (*Acta Paediatrica* 2015; Broadfoot et al 2005; Caldeira and Goncalves 2007; Cattaneo and Buzzetti 2001; Del Bono and Rabe 2012; Figueredo et al 2012; Kramer et al 2001; *Lancet* 2016). Since the BFI was introduced, UK breastfeeding initiation rates have risen from 62% to 81% (McAndrew et al 2012).

The WHO/Unicef UK Baby Friendly Hospital Initiative is a globally recognized programme that forms a key strand of the WHO Global Strategy on Infant and Young Child Feeding (WHO 2003). In the UK, the BFI is recognized as the minimum standard for care provision (NICE 2011, 2013 and 2015a). UK-wide government policy has resulted in the majority of maternity and community facilities having made some progress towards achieving Baby-Friendly accreditation and improving breastfeeding rates. In 2010, only 21% were fully Baby-Friendly accredited; this had increased to 60% of maternity services and

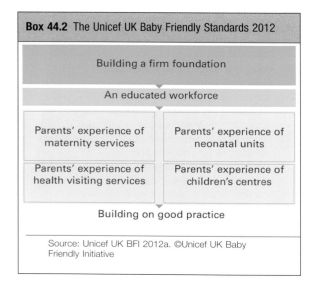

Box 44.2 The Unicef UK Baby Friendly Standards 2012

Building a firm foundation

An educated workforce

| Parents' experience of maternity services | Parents' experience of neonatal units |
| Parents' experience of health visiting services | Parents' experience of children's centres |

Building on good practice

Source: Unicef UK BFI 2012a. ©Unicef UK Baby Friendly Initiative

Box 44.3 The Unicef UK Baby Friendly Maternity Standards

1. Support pregnant women to recognize the importance of breastfeeding and early relationships for the health and well-being of their baby.
2. Support all mothers and babies to initiate a close and loving relationship and feeding soon after birth.
3. Enable mothers to get breastfeeding off to a good start.
4. Support mothers to make informed decisions regarding the introduction of food or fluids other than breastmilk.
5. Support parents to have a close and loving relationship with their baby.

Source: Unicef UK BFI 2012a. ©Unicef UK Baby Friendly Initiative

63% of health visiting services in November 2016 (Unicef UK BFI 2016a).

Over the past decade, new and emerging evidence and understanding of what works to support women to breast-feed and respond to their infants' needs has become apparent. Evidence regarding the importance of early care practices and the future well-being of the child indicates that a broader approach to the BFI could result in better outcomes for all children, including strategies that promote a greater emphasis on early brain development, emotional attachment and positive parenting interactions (Gerhardt 2004; Heikkilä et al 2011; Sacker et al 2006; Schore 2000 and 2001; Shonkoff and Phillips 2000; Zeedyk et al 2008).

In 2012, Unicef UK implemented new Baby Friendly standards in maternity, neonatal, health visiting and children's centre services to enable each mother to get breastfeeding off to a good start and build a close and loving relationship with her baby (see Box 44.2). This universal multifaceted approach aims to build a mother's confidence and ability to feed her baby based on her individual needs, preferences and desires from a biological, psychological and cultural perspective (Unicef UK BFI 2012a).

The UN Convention on the Rights of the Child

Unicef is a child rights organization, and therefore the best interests of children are at the very core of everything it does. In practice, this means that when decisions are made about children, those decisions must not be swayed by what is convenient for governments, institutions or individual adults at the expense of what is best for the

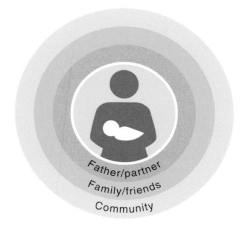

Figure 44.1 The mother and baby at the 'heart' of care.

child. Therefore, the defining principle of the BFI has been that every standard must have the best interests of babies at its very heart (Unicef UK 1992, Article 24; UN 2016) (see Box 44.3).

When thinking about child rights for babies, it is impossible to consider babies in isolation. Their rights will only be fully met if they are considered in conjunction with their main carer. The very best main carer for a new baby is the baby's mother. She is biologically programmed to love her baby, and the relationship between a mother and her baby has been described as the foundation on which all other relationships are built (Fig. 44.1). Influences of partners and close family have a huge impact and will ultimately provide much needed support to mothers. It is vitally important that this relationship is nurtured and protected. This does not mean negating the role of fathers and other partners and family members; it is more a recognition of where it is important to start if the very best for the baby is to be achieved: mother as primary care, father/partner as important second carer, other family members and friends as backup and then health professionals and other members of the community as support.

The needs of the newborn baby – food and love

Mothers and infants form a biological and social unit; a mother's breastmilk is unique, specifically designed and the ideal food for her baby – it is a living fluid, packed full of antibodies, hormones, enzymes and other factors that help the baby to grow and develop. For the mother, breastfeeding is an integral part of the reproductive process and provides important physiological health protection properties; for example, the release of oxytocin while feeding has multiple functions, including aiding milk flow, involution of the uterus following birth and, for all mothers (breastfeeding or formula feeding), helping the mother to fall in love with her baby (Gerhardt 2004; Strathearn et al 2012). Midwifery practices in the labour room and in the early days are critical in providing a nurturing environment that helps to keep oxytocin levels high and cortisol (stress hormone) levels low.

An emerging body of evidence suggests that nurturing the mother–infant relationship in the early days aids the baby's brain development. Brain growth is rapid from birth; at 1 year the baby will have developed 70% of its 'neural wiring' for the future and 90% by age 3 (Zeedyk et al 2008).

The nutritional needs of a healthy term infant can be met by exclusively breastfeeding for the first 6 months. A child's short- and long-term health is not improved by complementary feeding before this time (Dewey and Lutter 2001). By around 6 months, most infants are developmentally ready for other foods, and human milk alone will not meet the infant's nutritional needs (Dewey and Lutter 2001). Infants should therefore be offered other foods alongside breastmilk for 2 years and beyond (WHO 2013a and 2016).

PHYSIOLOGY OF THE INFANT GASTROINTESTINAL TRACT

The maturation of the neonatal gut is stimulated by initiation of feeding, milk composition, hormonal regulation and genetic encoding (Blackburn 2013). Initiation of early breastfeeding is a major stimulus for the increase of plasma concentrations of peptide hormones, for example, *enteroglucagon*, which stimulates growth of the intestinal mucosa; *gastrin*, which stimulates growth of the gastric mucosa and exocrine pancreas; and *motilin* and *neurotensin*, which stimulate gut activity. Colostrum stimulates epithelial cell turnover and maturation. *Epidermal growth factor* and *cortisol* also assist in the growth and development of

the neonatal gastrointestinal system. None of these crucial components are available in formula milk.

Breastmilk aids the passage of meconium through the gut, whereas formula milk does not. Delayed passage of meconium is associated with elevated bilirubin levels as a result of reabsorption of unconjugated bilirubin and recirculation to the liver; therefore, physiological jaundice may be problematic if feeding is delayed.

Until the baby is 9 months old, intake of formula milk stimulates a greater insulin response than intake of breastmilk (Blackburn 2013), thus initiating an unnecessary increase in the metabolism of glucose stores. Exclusive breastfeeding for the first 6 months of life, followed by the introduction of appropriate complementary foods, is a significant factor in reducing the risk of obesity and Type II diabetes (Lancet 2016; WHO 2015).

One of the most notable actions is that of *secretory IgA*, which has important antitoxic and antiallergic properties, protecting the neonatal gut from bacteria, viruses and other harmful organisms, which cannot be replicated in artificial formulae. IgA acts to 'line the gut', restricting the permeability of harmful infections and allergens. IgA is found in very high concentration in the colostrum and declines to lower levels as the baby develops and milk volumes increase (Coad and Dunstall 2011).

NORMAL NEONATAL METABOLISM

All mammalian milks contain water, fat, protein, carbohydrate, minerals and vitamins. Human breastmilk contains other important factors that are absent from infant formula, including hormones, enzymes, growth factors, essential fatty acids, immunological and nonspecific protective factors that cannot be reconstituted in other substances.

The immature neonatal exocrine pancreatic function is a major factor in the digestion of foods in the first few weeks of life. The neonate relies on alternative/additional means for digestion of proteins, carbohydrates and fats, and compensation occurs by use of enzymes in the saliva, intestine and breastmilk.

Infants have a very slow growth compared with other species; therefore, human breastmilk has low protein concentrations. High protein concentrations could present excessive solute load for the immature kidney. Protein digestion in the neonate is slow because of the limited production of gastric *pepsin*, with *pancreatic enterokinase* output less than 10% that of adults. The acidic environment of the infant's stomach helps to separate out the proteins into whey and casein; the whey is more dominant in breastmilk and more easily digested (Xiao-Ming 2008).

Neonatal carbohydrate digestion relies on amylase in breastmilk, which remains high during the first 6 weeks of lactation. Neonatal salivary amylase is only one-third of adult levels, and pancreatic amylase represents only 2.5% to 5% of adult levels.

Fat is the principal source of energy for infants, and in human milk it is very easily digested. Fat digestion has been shown to be greater in breastfed versus formula-fed preterm neonates. Although the neonate has raised gastric lipase, there is reduced pancreatic lipase for fat digestion. This is compensated for by the stimulus of suckling at the breast, stimulating secretion of lingual lipase in the neonate, which aids digestion (Blackburn 2013).

The composition of breastmilk is not always the same and varies with the stage of lactation, with the transition of colostrum to mature milk, with time of day and during the course of a breastfeed – it is uniquely tailored to assist the neonate in independent metabolism.

CONSTITUENTS OF COLOSTRUM AND BREASTMILK

Colostrum is produced from 16 weeks gestation and continues for the first 3 to 4 days postpartum, when it gradually changes to mature milk. It is a yellow-orange, thick, sticky fluid that assumes its colour from beta-carotene (Lawrence and Lawrence 2015); it has a lower calorific value than breastmilk (approximately 67 kcal/100 mL versus 75 kcal/100 mL for breastmilk).

The daily volume ranges from 2 to 29 mL per feed, and protein, fat-soluble vitamins and mineral percentages are higher than in breastmilk, with lower levels of carbohydrate and fat. It is unique in its high concentration of protective constituents – immunoglobulins, macrophages, lymphocytes, neutrophils and mononuclear cells – giving it a higher protein content. The concentration of growth factors is up to five times higher in colostrum than in mature milk.

Transitional breastmilk is produced between colostrum (from 3–4 days) and mature milk and lasts for approximately 10 days to 2 weeks postpartum (Lawrence and Lawrence 2015). During this time, protein and immunoglobulin levels decrease, whereas carbohydrate and fat levels increase. Water-soluble vitamins increase, and fat-soluble vitamins decrease.

Mature breastmilk contains approximately 90% water, with 10% proteins, carbohydrate and fats along with vitamins and minerals. The main solid constituent is the fatty acid component that provides 50% of the calorific requirements. Fat content varies at and during each feed according to the neonate's requirement.

Protein

Human milk is very low in protein, approximately 0.9%, which consists of whey and casein. In breastmilk, the *whey* is dominant and easily digested. The ratio is reported to be 9/1 to 6/4 whey/casein at different lactating periods

(Xiao-Ming 2008). Whey is an easily digested antioxidant and can act as an antihypertensive, anticancerous, antiviral, antibacterial and chelating agent (Xiao-Ming 2008). The main components are *alpha-lactalbumin, beta-lactoglobulin, serum albumin, immunoglobulins, lactoferrin* and *lysozyme.* Casein constitutes the smaller portion of the protein. In cow's milk, the protein content is reversed, with a ratio of approximately 80% casein to 20% whey (Lawrence and Lawrence 2015). Out of the 20 amino acids present, eight are essential and provide the important nitrogen content required by the neonate. Two of the most abundant amino acids are *cystine* and *taurine.* Taurine is absent from cow's milk but plays an important role in brain maturation and is thought to function as a neurotransmitter. It was originally presumed to be involved only in conjugation of bile acids. Cystine is essential for somatic growth (Wambuch and Riordan 2015).

Carbohydrates

Carbohydrates comprise mainly lactose, with small quantities of oligosaccharides, galactose and fructose. Lactose increases calcium absorption and is readily metabolized into galactose and glucose (assisted by the intestinal enzyme lactase), providing the necessary energy to feed the growing brain (Wambuch and Riordan 2015). These levels remain constant and are unaffected in malnourished women (Lawrence and Lawrence 2015).

Some oligosaccharides promote the growth of *Lactobacillus bifidus,* which increases the acidity of the neonatal gut, protecting it from pathogenic invasion (Kunz et al 1999). *L. bifidus* may inhibit the growth of harmful bacteria, and it gives breastfed babies' stools their yoghurt-like smell.

Fats

The fat content varies at different times of the day and during a feed, with higher amounts towards the end of a feed (Kunz et al 1999). Preterm fat concentrations may be 30% higher (Wambuch and Riordan 2015), although other studies did not detect any major differences in lipid composition between term and preterm breastmilk apart from more *medium- and intermediate-chain fatty acids* (Rodriguez-Palmero et al 1999). *Long-chain polyunsaturated fatty acids (LCPUFAs)* are important for normal visual and brain development and are absent from formula milk.

The majority of LCPUFAs are derived from maternal body stores rather than diet. Maternal diet may directly affect the fatty acid composition of breastmilk (Kunz et al 1999; SACN 2007). Vegetarian women are able to maintain a high milk content of *arachidonic acid* (AA) and *docosahexaenoic acid* (DHA). DHA is the LCPUFA associated with improved visual and neurological function (Makrides et al 1995; SACN 2007).

Approximately 98% of the fat components are triglycerides that are broken down to fatty acids and glycerol by the enzyme lipase, found in breastmilk itself. The remaining fats are *phospholipids* (0.7%), *cholesterol* (0.5%) and other lipolysis products. Digestion of triglycerides is initiated in the stomach, where gastric lipase commences lipolysis, and this is continued in the intestine by *pancreatic lipase*. Pancreatic lipase is, however, poorly developed at term, so the infant's own lingual and gastric lipase and another found only in breastmilk, called *bile salt stimulated lipase* (BSSL), is of particular importance to the newborn in aiding digestion of the fat. The resulting monoglycerides have potent bactericidal properties and maintain infection control in the stomach and small intestine (Rodriguez-Palmero et al 1999).

Vitamins

Water-soluble vitamins C (ascorbic acid), B_1 (thiamine), B_2 (riboflavin and niacin), B_6 (pyridoxine), folate (pteroylglutamic acid), B_{12} (cobalamin), pantothenic acid and biotin are all present in breastmilk. Niacin, B_{12} and Vitamin D can be increased by maternal intake (Rodriguez-Palmero et al 1999; SACN 2016).

Fat-soluble vitamins A (retinol), beta-carotene (carotenoids), D (cholecalciferol), E (alpha-tocopherol) and K (phylloquinone) are all present in breastmilk.

Minerals

Minerals include *sodium, potassium, chloride, calcium, magnesium, phosphorus, free phosphate* and *sulphur*. Citrate binds some minerals and is soluble in water, so it is important even though it is not a mineral. Trace elements such as *iron, zinc, copper, manganese, selenium, iodine* and *fluorine* are all present in breastmilk, although the latter two are absent from colostrum (Rodriguez-Palmero et al 1999).

The uptake of iron in breastmilk is facilitated by the high levels of lactose and vitamin C, enabling up to 70% of absorption to take place. Absorption of exogenous iron from formula milk is limited and can adversely affect the action of lactoferrin from breastmilk in the gut if the woman is mixed-feeding.

Unabsorbed iron is a contributory factor to the increased incidence of gastroenteritis in formula-fed infants (see Fig. 44.2 and Table 44.1).

'*Worldwide 830,000 deaths could be prevented if all babies were breastfed within an hour of birth*'.

Mason et al (2013)

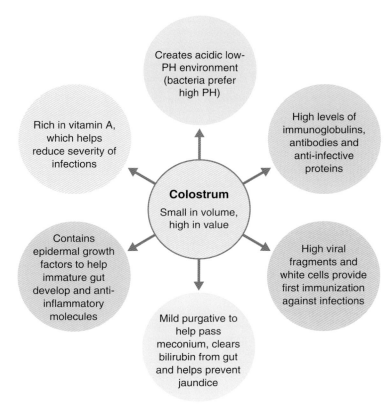

Colostrum
Small in volume, high in value

- Creates acidic low-PH environment (bacteria prefer high PH)
- High levels of immunoglobulins, antibodies and anti-infective proteins
- High viral fragments and white cells provide first immunization against infections
- Mild purgative to help pass meconium, clears bilirubin from gut and helps prevent jaundice
- Contains epidermal growth factors to help immature gut develop and anti-inflammatory molecules
- Rich in vitamin A, which helps reduce severity of infections

Figure 44.2 Why colostrum is important.

Table 44.1 How breastmilk provides protection for the baby

Substance	Action
1. Antimicrobial agents	
Lymphocytes	Kill infected cells directly or mobilize other components of the immune system (T cells)
Macrophages and neutrophils	The most common leucocytes in breastmilk; surround and destroy bacteria
Immunoglobulins Secretory IgA, IgG, IgM and IgD	Important in providing passive immunity The most important is IgA synthesized and stored in the breast. 'Paints' the baby's tract and gut, preventing the entry of pathogenic bacteria and enteroviruses. Provides resistance to a range of pathogens in gastrointestinal and respiratory tracts. Neutralizes viruses and toxins from microorganisms such as *Escherichia coli*, *Salmonella*, *Clostridium difficile*, shigellae, streptococci, staphylococci, pneumococci, poliovirus and the rotaviruses.
Lysozyme	Enhances the ability of IgA and attacks *E. coli*; acts with peroxide and ascorbate to destroy gram-positive and other bacteria in the gut and respiratory system
Lactoferrin	A protein that binds to iron; competes with bacteria for iron, thus depriving bacteria of nutrients for proliferation; enhances iron absorption in neonate's intestinal tract; kills *E. coli* bacteria
Bifidus factor – nitrogen-containing carbohydrate	Promotes growth of anaerobic lactobacilli in the neonatal gut, providing a protective acid medium
Mucin	Attaches to bacteria and viruses that enter the baby's body
Cytokines	Play a role in immune modulation and immune protection of breastmilk
B_{12}-binding protein	Deprives bacteria of vitamin B_{12}
Oligosaccharides – carbohydrates (monosaccharides)	Bacteria attach to these oligosaccharide 'binding' sites and form a compound that the baby excretes. They influence microflora, increasing the number of probiotics, which defend against pathogens in otitis media, respiratory tract infections, urinary tract infections and diarrhoea.
Fatty acids	Disrupt membranes surrounding certain viruses and destroy them
Complement (C3 and C4 components)	Has the ability to fuse bacteria bound to a specific antibody and destroy them through lysis
Fibronectin	Facilitates the uptake of bacteria by mononuclear phagocytic cells
Mucins – protein and carbohydrate molecules	Adhere to bacteria and viruses (including HIV) and prevent them from attaching to mucosal surfaces
2. Anti-inflammatory factors	
Secretory IgA, lactoferrin and lysozyme	Multipurpose anti-inflammatory role; lactoferrin inhibits the complement system and suppresses cytokine release from macrophages that have been stimulated by bacteria.
Antioxidants (alpha-tocopherol, beta-carotene cystine, ascorbic acid)	Absorbed into the circulation and have systemic anti-inflammatory effects

Table 44.1 How breastmilk provides protection for the baby—cont'd

Substance	Action
Epithelial growth factors	Enhance maturation of the neonatal gut and limit entry of pathogens
Other anti-inflammatory factors include platelet-activating factor, antiproteases (alpha-antichymotrypsin and alpha-antitrypsin) and prostaglandins.	
3. Immunomodulators	
Nucleotides, cytokines and anti-idiotypic antibodies	Appear to promote development of the neonatal immune system and help with cell repair
4. Leucocytes (white blood cells) During the first 10 days there are more white cells per mL of human milk than there are in blood.	
Approximately 90% of leucocytes in breastmilk are *neutrophils* and *macrophages.*	Eliminate bacteria and fungi by phagocytosis
80% of the *lymphocytes* are T cells.	T cells play an important role in establishing and maximizing the capabilities of the immune system.
5. Recent discoveries	
Alpha lactalbumin	When alpha lactalbumin mixes with acid (as found in breastmilk and the stomach of breastfed infants) it has the potential to attack cancer cells.
Stem cells	Remaining in the body long after breastfeeding cessation, they have the potential to serve as an internal repair system for some long-term conditions.
Lactoferrin	Currently being investigated as a treatment for autoimmune conditions such as rheumatoid arthritis, multiple sclerosis and septic shock.
The Broncho-Mammary Pathway: 'A mother will use her own immune system to protect herself from 'germs' within her immediate environment. When breastfeeding she transfers this immunity via her lymph nodes into the milk she gives to her baby, thereby protecting her baby on a continuous basis. The system is known as GALT (gastro-associated lymph tissue) and BALT (broncho-associated lymph tissue)' (Unicef UK BFI 2012a).	
For more information, go to www.analyticalarmadillo.co.uk/2010/10/ask-armadillo-whats-in-breastmilk-but.html	

Source: Ballard and Morrow 2013; Hanson 2004; Lawrence and Lawrence 2015; Minchin 2015; Wambach and Riordan 2015

The risks to the infant of not being breastfed

Breastfeeding has beneficial effects on the psychological and physical well-being of mother and baby. A review of the evidence on the effects of breastfeeding on short- and long-term infant and maternal health outcomes in developed countries found that a history of breastfeeding was associated with a reduction in the risk of acute otitis media, nonspecific gastroenteritis, severe lower respiratory tract infections, atopic dermatitis, asthma (young children), obesity, type 1 and 2 diabetes, childhood leukaemia, sudden infant death syndrome (SIDS) and necrotizing enterocolitis (Ip et al 2007) (see Table 44.1).

The action of sucking at the breast helps to initiate production of saliva that increases absorption of carbohydrate and fat. Neonatal saliva contains amylase that assists in glucose absorption and lipase that increases uptake of fatty acids (Blackburn 2013). These enzymes will be reduced if the baby is preterm and unable to suckle because tube-feeding bypasses this process, so it is important for the midwife to assist the woman to initiate suckling as soon as the reflex is present. In addition, pancreatic secretory trypsin inhibitor is a major motogenic and protective factor in human breastmilk; its presence influences gut integrity and repair (Marchbank et al 2009).

Breastmilk's immune properties have been specifically highlighted (*Acta Paediatrica* 2015; Chien and Howie 2001;

Duijts et al 2009; Hanson 2004; Ip et al 2007; Renfrew et al 2012b) (see Table 44.1). It helps to provide protection from leukaemia (Guise et al 2005; Kwan et al 2004), rotavirus infection, gastrointestinal infections (Quigley et al 2006), respiratory tract infection (Bachrach et al 2003), *Haemophilus influenzae* meningitis (Silfverdal et al 1999), urinary tract infection and otitis media (*Lancet* 2016; Lubianca et al 2006) and necrotizing enterocolitis (Henderson et al 2009; Lin et al 2008). The Millennium Cohort Study estimated that a 53% reduction of readmissions of children to the hospital with diarrhoea and lower respiratory tract infections could have been made if women exclusively breastfed for 6 months (Quigley et al 2007).

Other benefits include improved motor/personal and social development (Michaelsen et al 2009); improved IQ (Horta and Victoria 2013; Iacovou and Sevilla-Sanz 2010; Kramer et al 2008; *Lancet* 2016); protection from noninsulin-dependent diabetes mellitus (Chertok et al 2009; Robertson and Harrild 2010), eczema, asthma, and food allergies (Davidson et al 2010; Oddy 2009); and protection from cardiovascular disease in later life (Horta et al 2007; Holmes et al 2010; Leon and Ronalds 2009; Ravelli et al 2000).

Further benefits include possible protection from schizophrenia (McCreadie 1997) and postnatal depression (Kendall-Tackett 2009); juvenile rheumatoid arthritis (Mason et al 1995); inflammatory bowel disease (Mikhailov and Furner 2008); Crohn's disease and coeliac disease (Akobeng et al 2006); development of the physiological integrity of the oral cavity, ensuring alignment of teeth and fewer problems with malocclusions (*Lancet* 2016); and protection from sudden infant death (McVea et al 2000; *Lancet* 2016). The action of breastfeeding has beneficial effects on dental caries and mouth and jaw development, and it reduces the risk of childhood obesity (Arenz and Von Kries 2009; Bartok and Ventura 2009; Cathal and Layte 2012; Horta et al 2007; O'Tierney et al 2009).

Breastfeeding provides a unique opportunity for attachment between mother and baby and can protect the child from maternal neglect (Strathearn et al 2009). Breastfeeding provides one solution as an intervention to help tackle health inequality. One study found that those low-income mothers who breastfed for 6 to 12 months had the highest scores of any group on quality of parenting interactions at age 5 (Gutman et al 2009). Evidence has also demonstrated that a child from a low-income background who is breastfed is likely to have better health outcomes than a child from a more affluent background who is formula-fed (Wilson et al 1998).

Breastfeeding and the preterm baby

Breastfeeding confers all of the previously noted advantages, and because of the reduced capability of the preterm baby's immune system, it is vital for early protection against infection. Preterm infants are particularly vulnerable to necrotizing enterocolitis, so it is very important that women are supported to breastfeed fully (*Lancet* 2016; Renfrew et al 2009). Women who give birth prematurely provide perfectly balanced breastmilk for their babies – the nonprotein nitrogen content is 20% higher than in those who give birth at term, providing the necessary free amino acids essential for growth (Wambach and Riordan 2015). Preterm breastmilk contains higher concentrations of *polymeric immunoglobulin A* (pIgA), lactoferrin, lysozyme and epidermal growth factor. In addition, the numbers of *macrophages*, *neutrophils* and *lymphocytes* are higher in the colostrum (Wambach and Riordan 2015). Lingual lipases will be reduced if the baby is preterm and unable to suckle because tube-feeding bypasses this process. Long-term neurodevelopment outcomes are improved when preterm infants receive human milk (AAP 2012), and the UK Millennium Cohort Study found that not breastfeeding is associated with reduced cognitive ability, particularly in children born preterm (Quigley et al 2012).

Protective effects of breastfeeding for the mother

For mothers, breastfeeding is associated with a reduction in breast and ovarian cancers (*Lancet* 2016; WCRF/AICR 2009), improved bone density and reduction of anaemia. It can also be an effective postpartum contraceptive during 'total' breastfeeding (WHO Task Force 1999), having the added advantage of delaying menstruation and reducing anaemia.

CONTRAINDICATIONS TO BREASTFEEDING

There are very few absolute contraindications to breastfeeding.

Neonatal conditions (WHO/Unicef 2009)

Galactosemia

A galactose-free formula must be given.

Maple-syrup urine disease

A special formula that is free from leucine, isoleucine and valine is required.

Phenylketonuria

A phenylalanine-free formula must be given for a period of time, with possible breastfeeding later.

Maternal conditions

HIV

In the UK, where formula milk is available, it is recommended that mothers who are known to be HIV infected refrain from breastfeeding from birth, except where exceptional circumstances prevail; for example, a mother who is an asylum seeker may not have access to formula feed and sterilizing equipment and may need to return to her own country (Taylor et al 2011).

Worldwide, where avoidance of breastfeeding is not acceptable, feasible, affordable, sustainable or safe (AFASS), exclusive breastfeeding together with antiretroviral drugs helps to prevent HIV transmission (Horvath et al 2010; WHO 2010; WHO 2016).

Drugs – maternal medication

Certain drugs pass through breastmilk and may be harmful to the neonate, and temporary or permanent avoidance of breastfeeding may be recommended, depending on the prescription of drugs currently in use by the woman (e.g. antipsychotic, anticarcinogenic, iodides, antiepileptics). Midwives need to update their knowledge using the most recent *British National Formulary* (BNF), the Breastfeeding Network Drugs in Breastmilk web resources https://www.breastfeedingnetwork.org.uk/ or the local pharmacy drug information service within their trust/hospital service.

Substance misuse

Substances such as nicotine, alcohol, ecstasy, amphetamines and cocaine are known to have harmful effects on the baby through breastmilk. Opioids, benzodiazepines and cannabis can all cause sedation in the mother and baby. Women should be asked to abstain and cease to breastfeed while under the influence of these substances (WHO/Unicef 2009). It is important for the midwife to explain to the woman why she should abstain and what the effect on the baby might be; the midwife should record the discussion in the notes.

Conditions where a woman can continue to breastfeed but health problems may be of concern

Hepatitis B

The baby should be given a hepatitis B vaccine within the first 48 hours or as soon as possible thereafter (WHO/Unicef 2009). The woman can continue breastfeeding.

Hepatitis C

A small study of the breastmilk of seropositive women indicated a very low risk of transmitting the virus to the baby (Zimmermann et al 1995). The advice is to continue breastfeeding.

Pollutants in breastmilk

A variety of pollutants in the environment may arise in breastmilk, which should not prevent breastfeeding or its promotion because breastfeeding itself offers a degree of protection against many pollutants.

Research by environmental scientists found that because of human milk's nutritional, immunological, anticancer and detoxifying effects, women should be encouraged to continue to breastfeed even in the context of widespread pollution while also avoiding known contaminants such as alcohol and drugs and removing themselves from polluted environments where possible. In addition, they should be involved in creating healthier, safer, and cleaner environments for themselves and their children (Mead 2008).

THE MIDWIFE'S ROLE IN SUPPORTING, PROTECTING AND PROMOTING BREASTFEEDING AND HELPING A MOTHER TO BUILD A CLOSE AND LOVING RELATIONSHIP WITH HER BABY

Midwives need to be knowledgeable about the anatomy and physiology of breastfeeding and about how best they can enhance and facilitate an environment conducive to successful breastfeeding.

Understanding how breastfeeding works

Anatomy of the breast

See Fig. 44.3 for the anatomy and applied physiology of the breast (see also chapter website resources).

The breast is made up of the nipple, areola, mammary tissue, supporting connective tissue and fat, blood and lymphatic vessels and nerves.

There are approximately 20 lobes in the breast. Within the breast tissue are alveoli, small sacs with milk-secreting cells (lactocytes); the alveoli are surrounded by a basket of cells known as the myoepithelial cells, which contract to help the milk flow out of the ducts. The nipple has an average of nine openings, surrounded by the areola, where Montgomery glands secrete an oily fluid that protects the skin and has an individual smell that attracts the baby to its mother (WHO 2009).

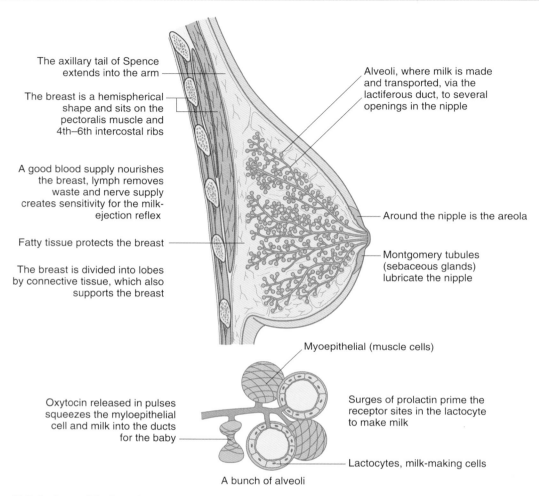

The axillary tail of Spence extends into the arm

The breast is a hemispherical shape and sits on the pectoralis muscle and 4th–6th intercostal ribs

A good blood supply nourishes the breast, lymph removes waste and nerve supply creates sensitivity for the milk-ejection reflex

Fatty tissue protects the breast

The breast is divided into lobes by connective tissue, which also supports the breast

Alveoli, where milk is made and transported, via the lactiferous duct, to several openings in the nipple

Around the nipple is the areola

Montgomery tubules (sebaceous glands) lubricate the nipple

Myoepithelial (muscle cells)

Oxytocin released in pulses squeezes the myloepithelial cell and milk into the ducts for the baby

Surges of prolactin prime the receptor sites in the lactocyte to make milk

Lactocytes, milk-making cells

A bunch of alveoli

Figure 44.3 Anatomy of the breast.

PHYSIOLOGY OF LACTATION

Puberty to pregnancy (mammogenesis)

Oestrogen and growth hormone stimulate the growth of the mammary ducts during puberty. In the second half of the menstrual cycle, progesterone stimulates development of the lactiferous ducts and alveoli. Proliferation of the epithelial tissue is a gradual process at each menstrual cycle.

First trimester: myoepithelial cells hypertrophy, and blood vessels become more prominent under the influence of oestrogen, with a 50% increase in blood flow to the breast (Blackburn 2013).

Second trimester: secretion of colostrum is facilitated.

Third trimester: progesterone and human placental lactogen ensure that alveoli mature and milk begins to be produced. Progesterone circulates in high concentrations in pregnancy and prevents milk secretion until the birth takes place (Neville 1999).

Prolactin is a single-chain peptide hormone released from the anterior pituitary gland, and serum levels increase during pregnancy. It is thought to be essential for the development and final stages of the differentiation of the alveoli and ducts in pregnancy (Blackburn 2013; Neville 1999). Prolactin-inhibiting factor, produced by the hypothalamus, maintains low prolactin levels to prevent milk secretion in pregnancy.

Oxytocin is an octapeptide hormone produced in the hypothalamus and stored and secreted in the posterior pituitary gland (Blackburn 2013). It is produced in low levels during pregnancy (possibly as a result of the action of a placental enzyme). It stimulates electrical activity and muscle contractions in the myometrium during labour and is critical in the milk-ejection reflex postpartum.

Other hormones, such as *human placental lactogen (hPL), human chorionic gonadotrophin (hCG), growth hormone* and *adrenocorticotropic hormone (ACTH)*, act synergistically with prolactin and progesterone to influence the growth of the glandular tissues of the alveoli to promote mammogenesis (Blackburn 2013). Human placental lactogen assists in mobilization of free fatty acids and inhibition of peripheral glucose utilization and stimulates mammary growth. ACTH stimulates the adrenals to secrete corticosteroids.

Initiation of lactation (lactogenesis)

Initiation of milk production involves a complex interaction of several hormones and factors. Following the birth, oestrogen and progesterone levels decline rapidly, allowing a rise in prolactin and oxytocin levels. Prolactin (the milk-releasing hormone) released from the anterior pituitary gland stimulates alveolar cells to produce milk while acting synergistically with growth hormone, insulin, cortisol and thyrotropin-releasing hormone (TRH) (Blackburn 2013).

Oxytocin stimulates contraction of the myoepithelial cells surrounding the alveoli, causing an ejection reflex, and milk is propelled down the lactiferous ducts.

The action required to stimulate both of these hormones is known as the neurohormonal reflex (or 'let-down' reflex). This stimulus is controlled by the effect of the neonate sucking at the breast, but it is also stimulated by skin-to-skin contact; warmth; massage; stroking; nipple stimulation from the baby's hands 'kneading' the breasts and the baby's legs 'kicking'; and the mother seeing, smelling, touching and hearing her baby.

Suckling stimulates prolactin release from the anterior pituitary gland, and therefore it is imperative that the midwife helps the mother to initiate skin-to-skin contact and to breastfeed as soon as possible after the birth. This helps the mother and baby to spend time together to enable instinctive behaviours and self-attachment. It is suggested that sucking movements reach a peak at 45 minutes and decline within 2 to 2.5 hours after the birth (Righard and Alade 1990; WHO/Unicef 1989), in line with a physiological reduction in adrenaline levels (Widström et al 1990). Lack of 'priming' the alveolar prolactin receptor cells may result in shutdown or reduction of milk supply. Sensory nerve endings are activated in the nipple and areola area, and this stimulates the hypothalamus via the spinal cord. As a result, oxytocin is released, prolactin-inhibiting factor is suppressed and prolactin is released.

The levels of prolactin are increased towards the end of a feed, after approximately 20 to 30 minutes following a feed and at night, thus maintaining a diurnal increase (Blackburn 2013; WHO 2009). The midwife needs to explain this to the mother so she understands that breastfeeding at night promotes and stimulates the production of prolactin; helping her to be responsive to her baby's needs day and night will help her to get breastfeeding off to a good start.

Prolactin release works on a *supply-and-demand* principle. When the baby suckles at the breast, prolactin-releasing factor is released by the hypothalamus and stimulates prolactin release from the anterior pituitary gland. When the baby stops suckling, a negative feedback *prolactin-inhibiting factor* (known as *PIF or FIL feedback inhibitor of lactation*) is released (Fig. 44.4).

Prolactin-inhibiting factor (PIF) is a protein secreted in the breastmilk itself that increases in amount as breastmilk accumulates in the breast. Its function is to exert negative feedback to block future milk production when there is ineffective milk removal from the breast. Whereas prolactin and oxytocin are released systemically, therefore influencing milk production in both breasts, PIF build-up can occur in one breast, only affecting milk production in that breast. Therefore, if a baby is ineffectively attached and unable to effectively remove milk from the breast, the build-up of PIF will ultimately result in a reduced milk supply. Milk production can be 'stepped up' again by effectively removing milk from the breast, thereby reducing the amount of circulating PIF in the breastmilk. Conversely, if the mother 'complements' with formula milk following breastfeeds, the baby's desire to feed will be reduced at subsequent feeds, which ultimately interferes with the body's ability to produce the required amount of breastmilk.

Prolactin can also be inhibited by oestrogen. Following birth, midwives may have a conversation with women about their contraceptive choices. If the mother chooses to use an oral contraception, the 'progesterone-only' pill (minipill POP) is advisable when she is breastfeeding (www.breastfeedingnetwork.org.uk). Regular suckling suppresses secretions of gonadotrophin-releasing hormone (GnRH), luteinizing hormone (LH) and follicle-stimulating hormone (FSH), which results in suppression of ovulation and menstruation. *Lactation amenorrhoea* as a method of contraception has an efficacy rate of 98% if the mother is **exclusively** breastfeeding (including at least once at night), the baby is less than 6 months old and the mother has no periods. If any of these three indicators changes (e.g. the baby starts to have other foods or drink, and/or is over 6 months old), then the mother should use another form of contraception (NICE 2016; WHO 2009).

Maintenance of lactation (lactogenesis)

Breastmilk production is a supply-and-demand mechanism and thus is individualized to the mother–infant pair.

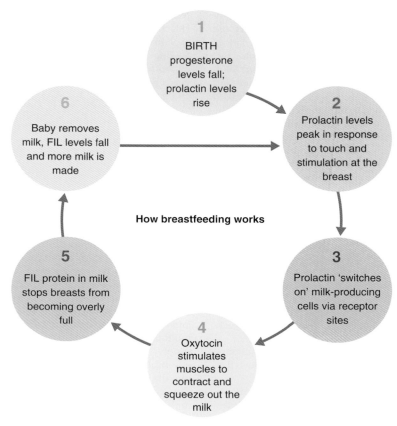

Figure 44.4 Physiology: how breastfeeding works. FIL, feedback inhibitor of lactation.

Walker (2015) defines lactogenesis I as the colostrum stage, with 100 mL of colostrum available to the infant on day 1 postpartum, approximately 7 mL per feed in the first 24 hours and 14 mL per feed in the second 24 hours (Royal College of Midwives (RCM) 2002). Lactogenesis II defines the onset of copious milk production between 32 and 96 hours postpartum, and lactogenesis III is the maintenance of milk production. This phase is reliant on an intact hypothalamic–pituitary axis regulating prolactin and oxytocin levels and maintenance of frequent sucking and removal of milk by the neonate (Blackburn 2013). Growth hormone, corticosteroids, thyroxine and insulin continue to play an important part in maintaining established lactation. Sodium and chloride levels in breastmilk fall in the first few days, followed by an increase in lactose concentrations. Lactoferrin and secretory IgA rise immediately, then fall with the increase in volume in the first few days.

Helping mothers to get breastfeeding off to a good start – antenatally

Midwives' contribution to the support and education of women in the antenatal and immediate postnatal period has an enormous effect on women's satisfaction, on breastfeeding success and on breastfeeding rates overall (NICE 2006, 2010b and 2015a). Getting breastfeeding off to a good start in the very early days through skin-to-skin contact at birth, an early feed and helping the mother learn how to be responsive to her babies needs is important. Evidence suggests that breastfeeding continuation is increased and promoted by face-to-face support delivered before and after the birth by a trained breastfeeding professional or peer counsellor (Dyson et al 2008; Renfrew et al 2007).

Discussion regarding infant feeding with the woman and her partner during the antenatal period should aim to involve them in a discussion based on their individual needs, hopes and aspirations. A meaningful conversation will help them prepare for the birth and the postnatal period in a safe environment to explore and discuss how breastfeeding might be experienced within their own family and social context (Box 44.4). Evidence suggests that parents benefit from knowing how to position and attach their baby at the breast, how to overcome common breastfeeding challenges, how to respond to and meet their newborn baby's needs and how to build a close and loving relationship with their baby (Unicef UK BFI 2012b).

Supporting infant feeding at birth

The birth environment and labour ward practices influence a mother's infant feeding choices and breastfeeding success. The 2010 Infant Feeding Survey highlights that mothers who used pethidine for pain relief in labour had the lowest breastfeeding initiation rates (77%) and were less likely to be breastfeeding at 1 and 2 weeks postdelivery (McAndrew et al 2012).

The healthy, term newborn baby can see, hear, smell, taste and also respond to touch. The baby's rooting reflex is mature. The baby moves his or her head and can bring the hand to the mouth; gravity and the use of leg and arm movement enables the baby to 'crawl' to the breast in search of food. Skin-to-skin contact will elicit pre-feeding

behaviours, and the baby will move towards the breast, locating the nipple and often self-attaching for the first feed (Cadwell 2007; Colson et al 2008; Henderson 2011). It is important that skin-to-skin contact takes place in an unhurried environment for an unlimited period immediately (or as soon as possible) after the birth (Moore et al 2012; NICE 2006). It increases the duration of breastfeeding, maternal–infant interaction, neonatal temperature and glucose levels at 90 minutes, and it reduces crying of the neonate (Moore et al 2012; NICE 2006). When undisturbed, a series of behaviours have been identified following the birth that enable the baby to self-regulate his or her feeding and sleeping (Widström et al 2011). When the infant is peaceful and in skin-to-skin contact with its mother, he or she will go through nine behavioural phases: birth cry, relaxation, awakening, activity, crawling, resting, familiarization, suckling and sleeping (see Unicef 2015 video 'Skin to Skin: Meeting Baby for the First Time' at www.babyfriendly.org.uk).

All mothers, breastfeeding or bottle feeding, should be offered the opportunity for skin-to-skin contact at birth. This simple and loving act will trigger hormonal release, calm and relax mother and baby, regulate heart rate and breathing, regulate temperature and stimulate feeding behaviour and digestion. Separation of a woman and her baby within the first hour of birth for routine procedures is unnecessary and should be avoided (NICE 2006 2013, 2015a and 2015b). The midwife also needs to ensure that the skin-to-skin process is safe by checking that the mother is alert and appropriately positioned along with the baby. The baby's position must not hamper breathing or well-being (see also Chs 42 and 43).

Midwives should ensure that they document and audit the timing and initiation of breastfeeding and the skin-to-skin contact following all births.

The mother's choice of position for feeding

Breastfeeding is a dynamic interaction between a mother and her baby. Positioning the baby at the breast and supporting effective attachment of the baby is cited as being key to successful breastfeeding (NICE 2006, 2011 and 2013). The midwife needs to provide the woman with simple, helpful information on positioning and attachment; when this goes well the mother will provide food, comfort and closeness, and the experience will be pleasurable for both. When it does not go well, the baby may not get enough milk and the mother may experience sore nipples and a cascade of challenges, including lack of self-confidence in her ability to feed and nurture her infant (Unicef UK BFI 2014b).

The mother may decide to either sit or lie down, and the midwife can help to provide an environment that enables the mother to respond to her instincts and find a position that is best for her. skin-to-skin contact aids this process, using the baby to experience touch, stimulating the neurological system and myelinization (Blackburn 2013).

Positioning the baby at the breast

Positioning is the term used to describe how a mother holds her baby to enable him or her to attach effectively.

The mother holds her baby close, in a straight line, facing her so that the baby does not have to twist the neck to feed. The baby's neck (rather than head) should be supported by the mother, enough to allow the head to extend backwards as necessary (see Fig. 44.5). The mother should then bring the baby's nose in line with her nipple and ensure the *rooting reflex* is triggered, causing the mouth to 'gape' (DH/Unicef 2015c). The CHIN acronym is an

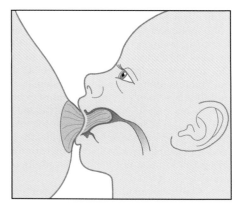

ineffective attachment

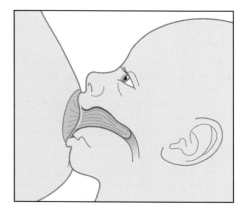

Effective attachment

Figure 44.5 Positioning and attachment of the baby at the breast. (©Start4Life leaflet DH/Unicef Baby Friendly Initiative 2015c.)

easy way to remember the principles (Harland, L, cited in Unicef UK BFI 2014b) – see Box. 44.5.

The consequences of ineffective suckling and attachment at the breast have been linked to 'failure to thrive' (Morton 1992) and early cessation of breastfeeding (Campbell 1997; Righard and Alade 1992).

Using a pacifier (dummy) may effect breastfeeding success and should be avoided in the early days. The dummy may interrupt responsive breastfeeding leading to reduced milk supply and may therefore reduce exclusive breastfeeding at 6 months (Koosha et al 2008; Righard and Alade 1992; Unicef 2013).

Attachment of the baby to the breast

With the nipple resting just below the baby's nose, he or she will begin to root. The head will tilt back as the baby gapes the mouth wide open; the tongue will move down and forward, and the baby will be able to take a big mouthful of breast; and the nipple will then slide under the top lip upwards and backwards to rest at the junction of the hard and soft palate. The baby approaches the breast leading with the chin, which enables use of the tongue and lower jaw (DH/Unicef 2015; NICE 2013).

When the baby is attached to the breast effectively, 'his mouth is wide open and he has a big mouthful of breast; his chin is touching the breast; his bottom lip is curled back' (NICE 2006).

If the baby is attached effectively there should be no friction of the tongue or gum on the nipple and no movement of the breast tissue in and out of the baby's mouth (DH/Unicef 2015).

Reflective activity 44.1
Review the animated video on attachment from available at www.unicef.org.uk/BabyFriendly/Resources/ AudioVideo/What-effective-breastfeeding-looks-like/ (Best Beginnings 2008).   How will you use this knowledge in your practice?

Signs for the midwife to assess with the mother to see if her baby is attached in the early days include the following:

- The baby has a wide open mouth and a large mouthful of breast.
- The baby's chin is firmly touching her breast.
- It does not hurt when she feeds her baby (although the first few sucks may feel strong).
- If she can see any of the areola (dark skin) around her nipple, she should see more dark skin above the baby's top lip than below the baby's bottom lip.
- The baby's cheeks stay rounded during sucking.

- The baby rhythmically takes long sucks and swallows (it is normal for the baby to pause from time to time).
- The baby finishes the feed and comes off the breast on his or her own (DH/Unicef 2015).

Assessing a breastfeed and transfer of breastmilk

Breastfeeding is an instinctive behaviour, but many women in the UK do not grow up in a breastfeeding environment and so do not learn to breastfeed from their mothers, sisters, family and friends. Therefore, it is a vitally important part of the midwife's role to provide a nurturing, kind and facilitative environment where the mother can get breastfeeding off to a good start and where she can feel safe and confident to ask for help and support 24 hours a day.

Because a mother cannot 'see' how much milk the baby is getting, she often worries that the baby is not getting enough milk; this is one of the major reasons why women stop breastfeeding before they want to (McAndrew et al 2012). The Baby-Friendly Initiative recommends that midwives should carry out two feeding assessments within the first week after birth and that the health visitor should carry out a further assessment at the new birth visit (Table 44.2). Assessing a breastfeed with the mother will help her to learn about how her baby feeds, understand how breastfeeding works and be responsive to her baby's needs.

For responsive feeding to work, mothers and babies need to stay in close contact so that they learn together and become 'tuned in' with each other. The mother will pick up on early feeding cues when her baby appears unsettled; early feeding cues include eye movements, wriggling, waving, rooting, sucking fists or blanket and making murmuring noises. Responding to her baby's needs, a mother may cuddle the baby when he or she seems lonely and just wants comfort, or when her breasts are full or when she just wants to sit down and spend time with her baby. These are all signs of a positive, growing, responsive relationship. As this takes place, oxytocin levels will rise, helping both the milk to flow and a loving bond between mother and baby to develop.

Table 44.2 Key points of a feeding assessment

Overview of an assessment of a breastfeed around day 5		Yes/No
The baby	A well-baby, content after feeds Calm and relaxed at feeds, comes off breast spontaneously 8–12 feeds in 24 hours Normal skin colour Has not lost more than 10% of birthweight	
The nappy	Wet nappies in 24 hours: Day 1–2 = 1–2 or more Day 3–4 = 3–4 or more, heavier Day 5 at least 5–6 heavy wet nappies Day 6 plus = 6 or more, heavy Stools/dirty nappies: Day 1–2 = 1 or more, meconium Day 3–4 = 2 (preferably more) changing stools Day 5 plus at least 2 dirty nappies in 24 hours, at least £2 coin size, runny and yellow, and usually more	
The mother's breasts and breastfeeding	Breasts and nipples are comfortable Nipples are same shape at the end of feed as the start The mother is responsive to the baby's need for food and comfort. There are no fewer than 8–10 feeds in 24 hours (day 1, 3–4 feeds in 24 hours).	
Weight	In the first week any weight loss greater than 7% is a warning sign that there may not be sufficient milk transfer, and the midwife should assess a full breastfeed. NICE recommends routine weighing (naked) in the first year after birth at 5 days and 10 days, then no more than fortnightly until age 2 months, then at 3, 4 and 8 to 10 months. Weight should be monitored in accordance with the 2009 UK-WHO growth charts (Wright et al 2012).	

Note: Please see full feeding assessment chart for more details at https://www.unicef.org.uk/babyfriendly/baby-friendly-resources/guidance-for-health-professionals/tools-and-forms-for-health-professionals/breastfeeding-assessment-tools/.

Box 44.5 Positioning the baby at the breast

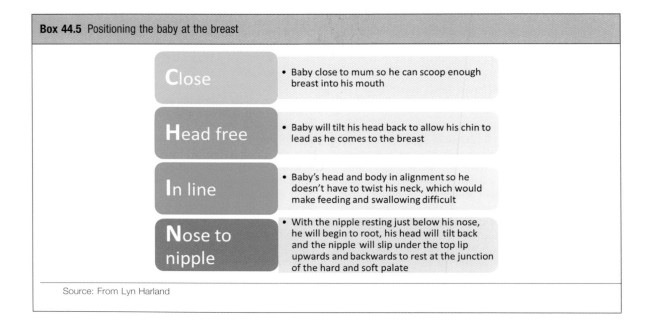

Close	• Baby close to mum so he can scoop enough breast into his mouth
Head free	• Baby will tilt his head back to allow his chin to lead as he comes to the breast
In line	• Baby's head and body in alignment so he doesn't have to twist his neck, which would make feeding and swallowing difficult
Nose to nipple	• With the nipple resting just below his nose, he will begin to root, his head will tilt back and the nipple will slip under the top lip upwards and backwards to rest at the junction of the hard and soft palate

Source: From Lyn Harland

A newborn baby cannot be spoiled by lots of attention; evidence suggests that crying is the last response of a baby to attract attention from its parents for both food and love (Gerhardt 2004).

Expression and storage of breastmilk

Women should also be shown 'how to breastfeed and maintain lactation even if they should be separated from their infants' (NICE 2006). This includes providing information on hand expression and storage of breastmilk (NICE 2006) (see Fig. 44.6).

A Cochrane review on methods of expressing breastmilk concluded there was no evidence that simultaneous pumping obtained more milk overall than sequential pumping (Becker et al 2011). However, assisting women to relax during pumping appeared to increase yield, and ensuring the woman had a choice in the method of pumping was important. The study stated that the effectiveness of the method of expressing was dependent on the reason for obtaining breastmilk, for example, if the baby was in the neonatal unit. Figure 44.6 illustrates the process of teaching a woman hand breast expression. There is further information available at www.unicef.org.uk/BabyFriendly/Resources/AudioVideo/Hand-expression/, including a video, information and leaflets.

Storage of breastmilk

A sterilized container should be used for storage. Breastmilk can be stored in the back of the refrigerator for up to 5 days at 4 °C or lower, for 2 weeks in the ice compartment of a fridge and 6 for months in a freezer. The milk can then be defrosted in the fridge and, once thawed, used straight away. Guidance for storage of breastmilk for babies in neonatal units is more stringent. For more information, see https://www.breastfeedingnetwork.org.uk/wp-content/pdfs/BFNExpressing_and_Storing.pdf and www.ukamb.org.

COMMON PROBLEMS

Many women in the UK have grown up in a bottle-feeding culture and may lack self-confidence in their ability to breastfeed and produce enough food for their baby's growth and development. The midwife is ideally placed to be able to support the mother and baby pair to learn how to breastfeed together, helping the woman to maintain her self-confidence and overcome the challenges in the early days (Entwistle et al 2010).

Insufficient milk

One of the most common reasons women give up breastfeeding is because of a perceived or actual insufficient milk supply (McAndrew et al 2012). The most common causes for insufficient milk are poor attachment, ineffective milk removal and infrequent feeding (Neifert 2004).

Lack of support and practical help from the midwife, or immediate family and friends, can undermine the woman and lead to psychological and 'iatrogenic' problems.

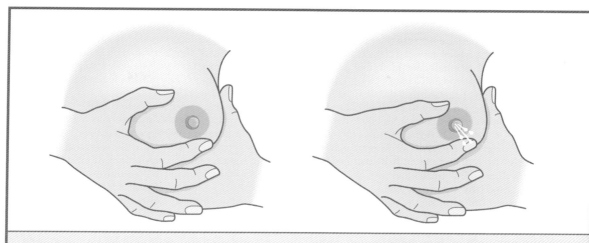

1. Begin by gently massaging the breast.

2. Cup the breast with the thumb and finger in a 'C' shape about 2-3 cm back from the base of the nipple.

3. Gently squeeze, bringing the fingers and thumb together in a rhythmic action (if no milk appears after a few minutes, move the fingers a fraction forward or back to find the right spot.

4. Continue until no more milk drops appear (avoid sliding the fingers as this can cause damage to the breast).

5. Milk can be collected in a sterile cup or bottle (or 'sucked up' in a syringe for colostrum).

6. When flow from one breast slows down, swap to the other side and repeat.

7. Breastmilk can be stored for up to five days in a fridge at 4° C or six months in a freezer.

Figure 44.6 Hand-expressing breastmilk. (©Start4Life leaflet DH/Unicef Baby Friendly Initiative 2015c.)

There are few physical causes for inadequate milk supply; midwives can help the mother to cuddle her baby, in skin-to-skin contact, so the baby is 'nuzzling' into the breast and stimulating both the physiology and breast-feeding. Some babies can be 'slow starters' as a result of such factors as the type of birth, pain relief and initial separation of mother and baby, and the midwife can help both mother and baby to get to know each other and 'catch up' on missed opportunities.

Trauma to the fetal skull during instrumental birth or difficult caesarean section can disrupt alignment of the fetal skull, cause damage to the cranial nerves and affect sucking and swallowing mechanisms (Kroeger and Smith 2004). This should gradually resolve over time.

Certain drugs reduce lactation (oral contraceptives containing oestrogen, bromocriptine, thiazide diuretics) and should therefore be avoided. Heavy smoking and alcohol consumption can reduce the milk supply (Horta et al 1997); however, Amir and Donath (2003) argue that this is more likely to be a result of psychosocial behaviours rather than physiological causes. Women at risk should be identified in the antenatal period and offered support to reduce/stop smoking and additional support to help them get breastfeeding off to a good start.

Anaemia may affect the milk supply, shorten the length of breastfeeding and lower the age of weaning (Henly et al 1995). Women who experienced postpartum haemorrhage of between 500 and 1500 mL were found to have insufficient milk supply, with infants showing failure to thrive (Willis and Livingstone 1995). Early review and treatment of such women is recommended. More recent research suggests that breastfeeding is less likely to be successful following significant blood loss, although the research notes that other factors, such as delayed maternal–newborn contact and early breastfeeding opportunities, may be hampering the success of breastfeeding, and that management and support may assist success (Thompson et al 2010; Henry and Britz 2013).

Breast surgery in which the ducts have been severed, as in breast reduction, may cause challenges if the ducts are not aligned. Surgery for breast enhancement involving silicone implants does not normally cause any complications or nerve and duct damage because the prosthesis is implanted beneath the pectoral muscle (Hale 2014). The type of surgery should normally be identified by the midwife in the antenatal period and a plan of action documented. Some work has suggested that the woman with an augmentation will be less likely to be able to successfully breastfeed exclusively (Michalopoulos 2007; Roberts et al 2015; Schiff et al 2014); however, this will vary according to the degree of surgery. The woman may be advised to attempt to feed, and the midwife will need to work with her to assess milk transfer and milk supply.

Nipple shields, especially the nonsilicone variety, may prevent the neonate from applying the stimulus required for effective milk removal from the breast and may therefore reduce the milk supply.

Medical disorders, such as hyperthyroidism or hypothyroidism, can affect milk supply. Hypopituitarism (Sheehan syndrome) affects the supply of hormones from the anterior pituitary gland and therefore prevents prolactin production. All such medical conditions require prompt referral and investigation.

Engorgement – venous/milk

Venous retention may occur because of the increase in blood and lymph circulation when the milk 'comes in', causing the breasts to feel warm, heavy and tender around days 3 to 5 (also known as breast 'fullness'). This will resolve as the baby feeds and does not normally cause any problems. However, engorgement of the breast is a pathological condition whereby oedema causes poor milk flow by constricting the milk ducts. This is caused by infrequent, ineffective milk removal and is preventable by effective breastfeeding positioning, attachment and milk transfer. Most mothers will at some time experience breast fullness and respond to their own needs to relieve the fullness by feeding their baby. Engorgement is preventable, and is often due to lack of support with breastfeeding, positioning and attachment. Every effort should be made to support effective breastfeeding to prevent the buildup of feedback inhibitor of lactation (FIL) (Unicef 2014b). It may last for 48 hours, during which time the woman will experience discomfort and a mild fever and is at risk for development of mastitis and subsequent breast abscess (WHO 2009).

Warm flannels or a hot shower or bath may improve the milk flow by increasing the blood supply around the alveoli. Gentle hand (or pump) expression will help to release the milk flow and therefore the tension around the nipple and areola so that the baby can attach more easily. If the baby is separated from the woman, then hand-expressing or a breast pump needs to be used regularly.

A Cochrane review to examine treatments used to relieve the symptoms of breast engorgement (e.g. cabbage leaves, cold packs, medication) found that although some interventions may have shown promising results, there is not sufficient evidence from well-designed trials on any intervention to justify widespread implementation (Mangesi and Dowswell 2010).

There is limited evidence surrounding the practical relief of engorgement. Midwives should help mothers to look out for symptoms so that they can help to prevent engorgement by providing support with softening the breast through massage and expression, positioning and attachment, responsive feeding and completion of suckling on one breast at a time to ensure adequate milk removal (Renfrew et al 2000). It can be helpful if women understand the normal process of milk production and why engorgement might happen.

Sore/cracked nipples

The most common cause of sore or cracked nipples is ineffective attachment (NICE 2006; RCM 2002; Renfrew et al 2000). Ineffective attachment and soreness are created as the baby compresses the end of the nipple against the hard palate, instead of taking the entire nipple in as far as the soft palate, causing damage to the nipple tissue (NICE 2006).

The psychological impact of nipple pain can cause high levels of emotional distress, and it may affect the mother–child relationship, although both will resolve once the pain is removed (NICE 2006).

Problems in the neonate, such as a short frenulum (ankyloglossia), or breast engorgement should be identified by the midwife because these may create difficulties for the neonate in attaching to the breast (NICE 2005, 2006). See 'Neonatal problems' later in the chapter.

Occasionally, the woman may suffer from a condition known as *Raynaud's phenomenon* (see chapter website resources).

Other conditions causing pain may present as eczema or psoriasis on the nipple or areola. Fungal infections, such as *Candida albicans* (thrush), can cause burning or shooting pain sensations and need to be identified swiftly and treated with the appropriate medication (Amir and Hoover 2002; Brent 2001; National Infant Feeding Network (NIFN) 2014). Midwives need to be vigilant in identifying and screening for differential diagnoses rather than assuming conservative treatment is all that is required; consultation with the infant feeding lead may be helpful.

Management

Correcting the attachment difficulty will provide immediate relief from the pain, then the nipple needs to heal; breastmilk and saliva may aid this process. Past methods of drying the nipples through exposure to air or using a hair-dryer are now known to cause scab formation and delayed healing by unnaturally drying the skin in an area that is normally moist (Inch and Fisher 2000).

Other suggested treatments using moisture, although not demonstrating significant benefits, include application of expressed breastmilk – this uses the physiological knowledge of healing through growth and repair of skin cells but may attract yeast growth from the lactose content (Renfrew et al 2000).

The effectiveness of silicone nipple shields has been demonstrated as a very last resort; in some case studies, however, they may cause a diminishing milk supply and exacerbate engorgement (Inch and Fisher 2000) and so should be treated with caution and never used as a substitute for teaching correct attachment.

Mastitis

Mastitis is an inflammatory condition of the breast that may or may not be accompanied by infection (NICE 2015c; WHO 2009). Mastitis can be incorrectly diagnosed in the first few days but is usually caused by engorgement or milk stasis producing increased pressure in the alveoli as a result of nonremoval of milk. The pressure builds up, forcing the milk out into the surrounding tissues. Mastitis most commonly occurs in the second or third week postpartum (Jones 2006).

Infective mastitis is caused by bacterial invasion, usually via a cracked nipple. *Staphylococci aureus* and streptococci are the most common organisms, and these act on the milk forced outside the alveoli into the surrounding cells.

Signs and symptoms

- Painful breast – a tender, reddened area that appears around the infected breast or segment
- Flu-like symptoms/feeling generally unwell
- Pyrexia
- May be a history of a graze or crack to the nipple

If left untreated, an abscess (or local collection of pus) may form within the breast tissue.

Management

- Provide encouragement and support for the mother – reassurance that she can continue breastfeeding.
- Provide information (Breastfeeding Network (BfN) 2009).
- Help to get the milk flowing; encourage frequent feeds, massage, and expression.
- Try changing positions.
- Analgesics/anti-inflammatories can be used to ease the pain.
- A warm compress can be used to ease discomfort.

- Antibiotics are prescribed if no improvement in 12 hours or two to three feeds (NICE 2015c; BfN 2009; Guidelines and Audit Implementation Network (GAIN) 2009).

If mastitis is untreated and the mother not helped, an *abscess* may form in the inflamed area, and drainage through needle aspiration or incision may be required to drain the pus from the infected area; therefore, urgent referral to a surgeon is required if an abscess is suspected (Jahanfar et al 2009; NICE 2015c).

Neonatal problems

Tongue tie (ankyloglossia)

A short frenulum may present the neonate with difficulty in attaching and suckling at the breast. The tongue is unable to move forward and cup the nipple and thus stimulate release of milk from the breast (NICE 2005). One of the first signs is sore nipples and poor weight gain as a result of lack of adequate milk supply, in spite of regular feeds (see chapter website resources). It is important to assess the degree of tongue tie because research suggests that frenotomy may not always be required (Cawse-Lucas et al 2015).

Cleft lip and palate

Cleft lip and palate are congenital malformations characterized by incomplete fusing of the lip and upper jaw (Wambuch and Riordan 2015). This may involve the lip or may extend to the soft and hard palate, and it may be unilateral or bilateral (see Ch. 49 and chapter website resources). This can cause the baby to have difficulty in achieving a good seal during breastfeeding, especially the baby with a cleft lip. A specially adapted teat or bottle may be required, but some babies are able to successfully breastfeed with some assistance.

Down syndrome

Down syndrome is a congenital anomaly characterized by a protruding or large tongue and hypotonicity, and often heart defects, and can be challenging for breastfeeding (see Ch. 49). Manual expressing or pumping is often required because of inadequate stimulation of the letdown reflex by the baby.

The mother will need encouragement and support for positioning the baby. Success of breastfeeding is most likely to be dictated by the severity of the cardiac abnormality, which will affect the respirations and tire the baby easily (Renfrew et al 2000).

Breastfeeding the preterm baby

Breastmilk is the optimum nutrition for the preterm infant (Henderson et al 2007). It provides additional immunity to the immature system, such as IgA, lactoferrin, lysozyme and oligosaccharides; stimulates maturation of the gastro-intestinal tract; and reduces necrotizing enterocolitis (RCM 2009). As described earlier, the breastmilk will be perfectly tailored by the mother to her individual baby. Different strategies, including expression and cup feeding, often need to be employed to support the development of breastfeeding. See the chapter website for more information and the Unicef UK Baby-Friendly Standards for neonatal units.

Twins and triplets

Mothers are able to supply breastmilk for more than one baby – the practicalities and support available may be key to success. The Multiple Births Foundation produces a booklet for professionals and parents with information on breastfeeding for multiples. (See also Ch. 57.)

Going back to work

The UK Department of Health, WHO and Unicef recommend that all babies are exclusively breastfed for 6 months (DH 2011 and 2014; WHO 2011), and thereafter with other foods until 2 years. Many women need to return to work before this time and should be encouraged and supported by the midwife to continue breastfeeding before and after work and to express either at work (dependent on facilities) or home and leave the expressed breastmilk (EBM) with the childminder or carer. It is also useful to provide information on breastfeeding support groups and counsellors (DH/Unicef 2015b; see also chapter website resources).

Unlike in other European countries where women have the right to paid breastfeeding breaks or a shorter working day, women in the UK only have some legal protection under health and safety and sex discrimination laws. Employers have legal obligations to provide health and safety protection, flexible working hours, protection from indirect sex discrimination, rest facilities and protection from harassment (www.maternityaction.org.uk).

ARTIFICIAL FEEDING

According to the UN Convention on the Rights of the Child (1989; Unicef UK 1992) every infant and child has the right to good nutrition. In the UK, children grow up in a bottle-feeding culture where only 1% of infants are breastfed exclusively until 6 months of age (35% worldwide), despite the strong evidence-based WHO and DH recommendation (Kramer and Kakuma 2006; McAndrew et al 2012; WHO 2016b).

The midwife's role is to help mothers who are partially breastfeeding to 'maximize' the amount of breastmilk the baby receives and to help mothers who are bottle feeding to do so as safely as possible, minimizing the risks. Midwives can help mothers who are bottle feeding to hold their baby close during feeds, maintain eye contact and offer the majority of feeds to their babies themselves to help enhance the mother–baby relationship.

Whatever the midwife's personal views, it is critical that a woman who chooses to artificially feed her baby is provided with clear evidence-based information, support and care in a nonjudgemental way.

Regulations surrounding infant formulae

Most infant formulae are made from modified cow's milk and manufactured to take the place of human milk in providing a sole source of nutrition for the young infant. The essential compositions of these formulae have to meet the Infant Formula and Follow–on Formula Regulations (England and Wales) of 2007, which enact the European Community Regulations 2006/141/EC. The composition of other enteral and specialist feeds must meet the Commission Directive (1999/21/EC) on Dietary Foods for Special Medical Purposes.

This means the minimum and maximum permitted levels of named ingredients, and named prohibited ingredients, are now laid down by statute. It was the view of the Scientific Advisory Committee on Nutrition (SACN) in 2007 that, 'If an ingredient is unequivocally beneficial as demonstrated by independent review of scientific data, it should be made a required ingredient of infant formula in order to reduce existing risks associated with artificial feeding' (cited in Unicef UK BFI 2014a; SACN 2008).

Midwives need to be aware of the International Code of Marketing of Breastmilk Substitutes (WHO 1981; Unicef UK BFI 2015), the aim of which is to ensure that infants receive safe and adequate nutrition through the marketing and practices surrounding breastmilk substitutes, advertising and donation of free samples or equipment directly to the general public.

The majority of infant formula brands can be divided into two groups: *whey* dominant and *casein* dominant. When whey is the dominant protein, the whey:casein ratio is closer to that of human milk, as in 'first' milks (Unicef UK BFI 2010). Casein-dominant formulae have a whey:casein ratio closer to that of cow's milk, as in 'follow-on' milks (RCM 2009; Unicef UK BFI 2014b). There is no evidence that changing from whey-based first milk to any other type of formula (second milks, follow-on milks or 'hungrier baby' milks) is necessary or beneficial – at any point. First milk is the only food bottle-fed babies need for the first 6 months of life. After this, as they start to be introduced to solid food, they can continue to receive first milk. When the baby is 1 year old, ordinary (full-fat) cow's milk can be substituted for the first milk.

Types of feed available

Analysis and further information on infant milks in the UK for infant feeding are available (RCM 2009; First Steps Nutrition 2015; see also chapter website resources).

Methods of artificial feeding

The most common method of feeding a term baby with formula milk is via the bottle. There is a range of bottles to choose from made from food-grade plastic. Teats can be made from rubber or silicone and vary in shape. There is no evidence that one teat is better than another. The milk should drip out of the upturned bottle at the rate of one drop per second.

Sterilizing equipment and preparing infant formula

The midwife needs to have a good knowledge of how to teach women to make up feeds correctly (see Table 44.3). The Start4Life 'Guide to Bottle Feeding' leaflet can be used to help mothers learn how to sterilize feeding bottles, sterilize feeding equipment and prepare infant formula feeds (DH/Unicef Baby Friendly Initiative 2015a).

Other methods

For babies who require additional help in feeding, such as babies with feeding problems and preterm babies, there is a range of strategies, including the use of syringe feeding, cup feeding and supplementary feeding. For more information, see the chapter website resources.

Table 44.3 Step-by-step guide to preparing a formula feed	
Step 1	Fill the kettle with at least 1 litre of fresh tap water (do not use water that has been boiled before).
Step 2	Boil the water. Then leave the water to cool for no more than 30 minutes, so that it remains at a temperature of at least 70°C.
Step 3	Clean and disinfect the surface you are going to use.
Step 4	It's very important that you wash your hands.
Step 5	If you are using a cold-water sterilizer, shake off any excess solution from the bottle and the teat, or rinse the bottle with cooled boiled water from the kettle (not tap water).
Step 6	Stand the bottle on a clean surface.
Step 7	Keep the teat and cap on the upturned lid of the sterilizer. Avoid putting them on the work surface.
Step 8	Follow the manufacturer's instructions and pour the amount of water you need into the bottle. Double check that the water level is correct. Always put the water in the bottle first, while it is still hot, before adding the powdered infant formula.
Step 9	Loosely fill the scoop with formula, according to the manufacturer's instructions, and level it off using either the flat edge of a clean, dry knife or the leveller provided. Different tins of formula come with different scoops. Make sure you only use the scoop that is enclosed with the powdered infant formula you are using.
Step 10	Holding the edge of the teat, put it on the bottle. Then screw the retaining ring onto the bottle.
Step 11	Cover the teat with the cap and shake the bottle until the powder is dissolved.
Step 12	It is important to cool the formula so it is not too hot to drink. Do this by holding the bottom half of the bottle under cold running water. Make sure the water does not touch the cap covering the teat.
Step 13	Test the temperature of the formula on the inside of your wrist before giving it to your baby. It should be body temperature, which means it should feel warm or cool, but not hot.
Step 14	If there is any made-up formula left after a feed, throw it away.

Source: NHS 2014

When a mother artificially feeds her baby

In the UK many women come from families where formula feeding has been the 'norm' for generations, and supporting them to make a different infant-feeding choice to their friends and families requires compassionate and sensitive conversations that keep communications open between the midwife, the mother and her family. When this is not the case, the conversation may close down and the woman ends up feeling 'pressured' or 'guilty' about her decision (Lancet 2016). Where mothers cannot or, after a sensitive conversation, choose not to breastfeed, breastmilk substitutes are available. Parents should be given information about formula milks and be advised to use 'first milks' for the 'first year' (First Steps Nutrition 2015). However, infant formula is an imperfect calculation of breastmilk, and there will always be inherent risks and significant differences between breastmilk and infant formula (Renfrew et al 2012b). Formula feeding has been described as a risk behaviour (Minchin 2015) (Box 44.6), and infants have a greater risk of several infections and disorders, creating costs not only to the NHS but also to the health and well-being of individuals and families (Renfrew et al 2009; Renfrew et al 2012b). Donor breastmilk, particularly for sick and premature infants, should be considered as a viable option (NICE 2010a).

Supporting a mother to responsively bottle feed her baby

Building a meaningful relationship with her baby is as important for a mother who is bottle feeding (formula or breastmilk) as it is for a mother who is breastfeeding; limiting the number of caregivers who feed the baby to the main caregivers – mother and partner – will help to build a relationship. Box 44.7 gives ideas for bottle feeding responsively.

It is important to discuss with the mother the importance of focusing her attention on her baby during feeds and how this helps her to respond to her baby's needs.

THE INTERNATIONAL CODE OF MARKETING OF BREASTMILK SUBSTITUTES

The International Code of Marketing of Breastmilk Substitutes (the Code) was adopted by a resolution of the World Health Assembly in 1981.

The Code requires that infant formula, follow-on formula, baby foods, bottles/teats and related equipment products should not be marketed in a way that suggests they could replace or undermine breastfeeding. The UK law is not as robust as the Code and allows companies to advertise follow-on formula.

Key points of the code

Companies may not:

- Promote their products in hospitals, in shops or to the general public

---

Box 44.6 Risks of formula feeding (Minchin 2015)

Twice as likely:
- Respiratory infection
- Otitis media
- Atopic disease: eczema or a wheeze
- Diabetes mellitus: juvenile onset of insulin-dependent diabetes mellitus (IDDM)

Five times more likely:
- Gastroenteritis
- Diarrhoea
- Urinary tract infection

Twenty times more likely:
- Necrotizing enterocolitis (preterm babies, 30–36 weeks gestation)

Box 44.7 Bottle feeding responsively

- Sit comfortably, always hold baby close, and look into the baby's eyes when feeding. This helps the baby to feel safe and loved.
- Hold the baby fairly upright, with the head supported, so that the baby can breathe and swallow.
- Brush the teat against the baby's lips; when the baby opens his or her mouth wide, allow the baby to draw in the teat.
- If the teat becomes flattened while feeding, pull gently on the corner of the baby's mouth to release the vacuum.
- Offer the baby short breaks during the feed; he or she may need to 'burp'.
- Support the baby to 'pace' the feed, she can then put her tongue over the hole to slow the flow or push the teat out of her mouth when she has had enough. Never force the baby to feed or take 'all' the milk if they do not want it.

Source: Supporting Close and Loving Relationships Unicef UK BFI, 2016

- Give free samples to mothers or free or subsidized supplies to hospitals or maternity wards
- Give gifts to health workers or mothers
- Promote their products to health workers, with any information provided by companies containing only scientific and factual material
- Promote foods or drinks for babies
- Give misleading information
- Have direct contact with mothers

For more information, see 'Working Within the International Code of Marketing of Breastmilk Substitutes: A Guide for Health Professionals' (Unicef UK BFI 2015).

(Cuthbert et al 2011). Parents are concerned about how they are going to feed their babies, and their decisions are influenced by many different events and experiences in their lives. The midwife is in a privileged position to be able to share with them information to help the mother get ready for the birth and to get breastfeeding off to a good start. The decisions mothers make at this time affect their long-term health and well-being and that of their infants. The actions and support of the midwife affect how successful the mother is in realizing her aspirations as a mother to feed and love her baby; therefore, every effort must be made to provide mother-centred, evidence-based care in relation to infant feeding and relationship building.

Reflective activity 44.2

A woman who is 36 weeks pregnant and who bottle fed her first child visits you in the antenatal clinic and asks you how she can get breastfeeding off to a good start after the baby is born. How would you help her? Here are some suggestions:

- Think about your communication skills.
- Find out what she knows.
- Use the evidence to offer her information so that she can make a birth plan.
- Give in a way that reinforces her belief in herself and her ability to breastfeed successfully.

CONCLUSION

Mothers are intuitively wired to love and nurture their infants, and they begin this loving relationship with their babies in pregnancy through touch, sound and visualization. Pregnancy is a 'magic moment' when mothers are receptive and motivated to do the best for their babies

Key Points

- Midwives are key professionals in providing information, education and support to the mother, her baby and the family regarding infant feeding and relationship building.
- Conversations should be 'mother-focused' discussions that provide evidence-based information that is accessible, supportive and nonjudgemental.
- Midwives need to be aware of their own biases and opinions regarding feeding choices to minimize the effect of both on the information and support they provide.
- Midwives should work with professional and lay colleagues within the community to provide additional support to women and their families, whatever the feeding method.
- Women who bottle feed their infant should be supported, taught the principles of correctly making up the feeds and given unbiased information about infant milks in the UK.
- Midwives should teach all parents the principles of cleaning and sterilizing feeding equipment.

References

Acta Paediatrica: [Special issue] Impact of breastfeeding on maternal and child health, *Acta Paediatr* 104(Suppl S467):1–134, 2015.

Ajetunmobi OM, et al: Breastfeeding is associated with reduced childhood hospitalization: evidence from a Scottish birth cohort (1997–2009). American Academy of Pediatrics policy statement, *Pediatrics* 115(2):496–506, 2015.

Akobeng AK, Ramanan AV, Buchan I, et al: Effect of breast feeding on risk of coeliac disease: a systematic review and meta-analysis of observational studies, *Arch Dis Child* 91:39–43, 2006.

All Party Parliamentary Group (APPG): *The 1001 critical days: the importance of the conception to age two period.* Re-launched Dec. 2015.

American Academy of Paediatrics (AAP): Policy statement: breastfeeding and the use of human milk, *Pediatrics* 129(3):e827–e841, 2012.

Amir L, Hoover K: *Candidiasis and breastfeeding*, Schaumberg, LLLI, 2002.

Amir LH, Donath SM: Does maternal smoking have a negative physiological effect on breastfeeding? The epidemiological evidence, *Breastfeed Rev* 11(2):19–29, 2003.

Arenz S, Rucket R, Koletzko B, et al: Breastfeeding and childhood obesity – a systematic review, *Int J Obes* 28:1247–1256, 2004.

Arenz S, Von Kries R: Protective effect of breastfeeding against obesity in childhood: can a meta-analysis of published observational studies help to validate the hypothesis? *Adv Exp Med Biol* 639:145–152, 2009.

Australian Health Ministers' Conference: *The Australian national breastfeeding strategy 2010–2015*, Australian Government Department of Health and Ageing, Canberra, 2009.

Bachrach VRG, Schwarz E, Bachrach LR: Breastfeeding and the risk of hospitalization for respiratory disease in infancy: a meta-analysis, *Arch Pediatr Adolesc Med* 157:237, 2003.

Ballard O, Morrow AL: Human milk composition: nutrients and bioactive factors, *Paediatr Clin North Am* 1:49–74, 2013.

Bartok C, Ventura A: Mechanisms underlying the association between breastfeeding and obesity, *Int J Pediat Obes* 4(4):196–204, 2009.

Becker GE, Cooney F, Smith HA: Methods of milk expression for lactating women, *Cochrane Database Syst Rev* 12:2011.

Bennett KE, Haggard MP: Accumulation of factors influencing children's middle ear disease: risk factor modelling on a large population cohort, *J Epidemiol Community Health* 52:786–793, 1998.

Best Beginnings: *From bump to breastfeeding* (DVD). www.bestbeginnings.info. 2008.

Blackburn ST: *Maternal, fetal and neonatal physiology – a clinical perspective*, Philadelphia, WB Saunders, 2013.

Breastfeeding Network (BfN): *Mastitis and breastfeeding* (website). www.breastfeedingnetwork.org.uk/wp-content/pdfs/BFN_Mastitis.pdf. 2009.

Brent N: Thrush in the breastfeeding dyad: results of a survey on diagnosis and treatment, *Clin Paediatr* 40:503–506, 2001.

Britton JR, Britton H, Gronwaldt V: *Breastfeeding – sensitivity and attachment* (website). www.pediatrics.aapublications.org. 2011.

Broadfoot M, Britten J, Tappin D, et al: The Baby-Friendly Hospital Initiative and breastfeeding rates in Scotland, *Arch Dis Child Fetal Neonatal Ed* 90:F114–F116, 2005.

Buccini dos Santos G, Perez-Escamilla R, Paulino LM, et al: Pacifier use and interruption of exclusive breastfeeding: Systematic review and meta-analysis, *Matern Child Nutr.* http://onlinelibrary.wiley.com/doi/10.1111/mcn.12384/abstract?campaign=wolearlyview. 2016.

Cadwell K: Latching-on and sucking of the health term neonate: breastfeeding assessment, *J Midwifery Womens Health* 52(6):638–642, 2007.

Caldeira AP, Goncalves E: Assessment of the impact of implementing the Baby-Friendly Hospital Initiative, *J Pediatr (Rio J)* 83:127–132, 2007.

Campbell CMA: Early breastfeeding failure, *Update* 55(9): 722, 724, 726–727, 1997.

Cathal MC, Layte DR: Breastfeeding and risk of overweight and obesity at nine years of age, *Social Science & Medicine* (website). www.rte.ie/news/2012/0502/growingupinrirelandobesity.pdf. 2012.

Cattaneo A, Buzzetti R: Effect on rates of breastfeeding of training for the Baby Friendly Hospital Initiative, *Br Med J* 323:1358–1362, 2001.

Cawse-Lucas J, et al: Clinical inquiry: does frenotomy help infants with tongue-tie overcome breastfeeding difficulties? *J Fam Pract* 64(2):126–127, 2015.

Chertok IR, Raz I, Shoham I, et al: Effects of early breastfeeding on neonatal glucose levels of term infants born to women with gestational diabetes, *J Hum Nutr Diet* 22(2):166–169, 2009.

Chief Nursing Officer (CNO): *England, NI, Wales and Scotland Midwifery 2020: Delivering expectations England, NI, Wales and Scotland* (website). www.gov.uk/government/uploads/system/uploads/attachment_data/file/216029/dh_119470.pdf. 2010.

Chien P, Howie P: Breast milk and the risk of opportunistic infection in infancy in industrialized and non-industrialized settings, *Adv Food Nutr Res* 10(69):2001.

Chivers P, Hands B, Parker H, et al: Body mass index, adiposity rebound and early feeding in a longitudinal cohort (Raine Study), Pediatric Highlight, *Int J Obes* 34:1169–1176, 2010.

Coad J, Dunstall M: *Anatomy and physiology for midwives*, Edinburgh, Mosby, 2011.

Colson S, Meek J, Hawdon J: Optimal positions for the release of primitive neonatal reflexes stimulating breastfeeding, *Early Hum Dev* 84:441–449, 2008.

Cuthbert C, Rayns G, Stanley K: *All babies count: prevention and protection for vulnerable babies: a review of the evidence*, NSPCC (website). www.nspcc.org.uk/Inform/resourcesforprofessionals/underones/all_babies_count_pdf_wdf85569.pdf. 2011.

Davidson R, Roberts SE, Wotton CJ, et al: Influence of maternal and perinatal factors on subsequent hospitalization for asthma in children: evidence from the Oxford record linkage study, *BMC Pulm Med* 10:14, 2010.

Davies S: *Chief Medical Officers (CMO's) annual report 2012: Our children deserve better* (website). www.gov.uk/government/publications/chief-medical-officers-annual-report-2012-our-children-deserve-better-prevention-pays. 2013.

Del Bono E, Rabe B: *The effects of breastfeeding on children, mothers and employers*, Institute for Social & Economic Research, University of Essex, Working Paper (website). www.esrc.ac.uk/my-esrc/grants/RES-062-23-1693/outputs/Read/6746ed03-2d73-4bd6-b13f-ddee4e1bb074. 2012.

Department for Health, Social Services and Public Safety (DHSSPS): *Breastfeeding – a great start: a strategy for Northern Ireland 2013–2023*, Belfast: DHSSPS, 2013.

Department of Health (DH): *The Healthy Child Programme – pregnancy and the first five years*, London, DH, 2009/2011 (2011 update available at www.dh.gov.uk/prod_consum_dh/groups/dh_digitalassets/@dh/@en/@ps/documents/digitalasset/dh_118525.pdf).

Department of Health (DH): *The Family-Nurse Partnership Programme in England: wave 1 implementation in toddlerhood and a comparison between waves 1 and 2a of implementation in pregnancy and infancy* (website). www.dh.gov.uk/prod_consum_dh/ groups/dh_digitalassets/documents/ digitalasset/dh_123366.pdf. 2011.

Department of Health (DH): *Giving all children a healthy start in life London* (website). www.gov.uk/government/ uploads/system/uploads/361660/ attachment_data/file/361660/ policy-good-example.pdf. 2014.

Department of Health (DH)/Unicef: *Guide to bottle feeding: how to prepare infant formula equipment to minimize the risks to your baby* (website). https://mypregnancy.dbh.nhs.uk/ GuidanceNotes/Start4Life-Guide-to -bottle-feeding.pdf. 2015a.

Department of Health (DH)/Unicef: *Breastfeeding after returning to work or study: information for employees and employers, students and course providers* (website). www.start4life .org.uk 2015b.

Department of Health (DH)/Unicef: *Off to the best start. Important information about feeding your baby* (leaflet), Start4Life, London, DH (website). http://www.unicef.org.uk/ Documents/Baby_Friendly/Leaflets/ otbs_leaflet.pdf. 2015c.

Dewey K, Lutter C: *Guiding principles for complementary feeding of the breastfed child*, Pan American Health Organisation, WHO (website). www.paho.com. 2001.

Duijts L, Ramadhani MK, Moll HA: Breastfeeding protects against infectious diseases during infancy in industrialized countries. A systematic review, *Matern Child Nutr* 5:199–210, 2009.

Dyson L, McCormick FM, Renfrew MJ: Interventions for promoting the initiation of breastfeeding (Review), *Cochrane Database Syst Rev* 4: 2008.

Ekstrom A, Nissen E: A mother's feelings for her infant are strengthened by excellent breastfeeding counselling and continuity of care, *Paediatrics* 118(2):309–314, 2006.

Entwistle F, Kendall S, Mead M: Breastfeeding support – the importance of self-efficacy for low-income women, *Matern Child Nutr* 6(3):228–242, 2010.

European Community Regulations 2006/141/EC, 2006.

European Community Commission Directive (1999/21/EC) on Dietary Foods for Special Medical Purposes, 1999.

Figueredo SF, Mattar MJG, Abrão ACFV: Baby-Friendly Hospital Initiative – a policy of promoting, protecting and supporting breastfeeding, *Acta Paulista de Enfermagem* 25(3):459– 463, 2012.

First Steps Nutrition: *Infant Milks Overview.* http://www. firststepsnutrition.org/newpages/ Infant_Milks/infant_milks.html. 2016.

Guidelines and Audit Implementation Network (GAIN): *Mastitis and Breastfeeding (Leaflet).* http:// www.northerntrust.hscni.net/pdf/ Mothers_Guide_to_Mastitis_and _breastfeeding.pdf. 2009.

Gerhardt S: *Why love matters: how affection shapes a baby's brain*, New York, Routledge, 2004.

Groër MW: Differences between exclusive breastfeeders, formula-feeders, and controls: a study of stress, mood, and endocrine variables, *Biol Res Nurs* 7:106–117, 2005.

Guise J-M, Austin D, Morris CD: Review of case-control studies related to breastfeeding and reduced risk of childhood leukemia, *Pediatrics* 116:e724–e731, 2005.

Gutman LM, Brown J, Akerman R: *Nurturing parenting capability: the early years*, London, Centre for Research on the Wider Benefits of Learning, The Institute of Education, 2009.

Hale T: Medications in mother's milk. Cited in *Silicone breast implants and breastfeeding*, The Breastfeeding Network (website). www.breastfeedingnetwork.org.uk/ wp-content/dibm/silicone%20 breast%20implants.pdf. 2014.

Hanson L: *Immunobiology of human milk. How breastfeeding protects babies*, Amarillo (TX), Pharmasoft, 2004.

Harder T, Bergmann R, Plagemann A, et al: Duration of breastfeeding and risk of overweight: a meta-analysis, *Am J Epidemiol* 162(5):397–403, 2005.

Heikkilä K, Sacker A, Kelly Y, et al: Breastfeeding and child behaviour in the Millennium Cohort Study, *Arch Dis Child.* doi: 10.1136/ adc.2010.201970. 2011.

Henderson A: Understanding the breast crawl: implications for nursing practice, *Nurs Womens Health* 15(4):296–307, 2011.

Henderson G, Anthony MY, McGuire W: Formula milk versus maternal breast milk for feeding preterm or low birth weight infants, *Cochrane Database Syst Rev* (4):CD002972, 2007.

Henderson G, Craig S, Brocklehurst P, et al: Enteral feeding regimens and necrotizing enterocolitis in preterm infants: a multicentre case-control study, *Arch Dis Child Fetal Neonatal Ed* 94:F120–F123, 2009.

Henly SJ, Anderson CM, Avery MD, et al: Anemia and insufficient milk in first-time mothers, *Birth* 22(2):87–92, 1995.

Henry L, Britz SP: *Loss of blood = loss of breast milk?* The effect of postpartum hemorrhage on breastfeeding success: poster describing a case study, *AWHONN, the Association of Women's Health, Obstetric and Neonatal Nurses.* doi: 10.1111/1552-6909.12198. 2013.

Henschel D, Inch S: *Breastfeeding. A guide for midwives*, Hale, Books for Midwives, 1996.

Hill PD, Humenick SS: The occurrence of breast engorgement, *J Hum Lact* 10(2):76–86, 1994.

Holmes VA, et al: Association between breast-feeding and anthropometry and CVD risk factor status in adolescence and young adulthood: the Young Hearts 2010, *Public Health Nutr* 13(6):771–778, 2010.

Horta BL, Victor CS, Menezes AM: Environmental tobacco smoke and the breastfeeding duration, *Am J Epidemiol* 146:128–133, 1997.

Horta BL, Bahl R, Martines JC, et al: *Evidence on the long-term effects on breastfeeding: systematic reviews and meta-analyses*, Geneva, WHO, 2007.

Horta BL, Victoria CG: *Long-term effects of breastfeeding: a systematic review*, Geneva, WHO, 2013.

Horvath T, Madi BC, Iuppa IM, et al: Interventions for preventing late postnatal mother-to-child transmission of HIV (Review), *The Cochrane Library* 1:2010.

Iacovou M, Sevilla-Sanz A: *The effect of breastfeeding on children's cognitive development*, Institute for Social and Economic Research, University of Essex, Working Paper 2010-40 (website). www.iser.essex.ac.uk/

publications/working-papers/
iser/2010-40.pdf. 2010.

Inch S, Fisher C: Breastfeeding: early
problems, *Pract Midwife* 3(1):12–15,
2000.

Ip S, et al: Breastfeeding and maternal
and infant health outcomes in
developed countries, Agency of
Healthcare Research and Quality,
Evid Rep Technol Assess (full Rep)
153:1–186, 2007.

Jahanfar S, Ng C-J, Teng CL: Antibiotics
for mastitis in breastfeeding women,
Cochrane Database Syst Rev
(1):CD005458, 2009.

Jaafar SH, Jahanfar S, Angolkar M, et al:
Pacifier use versus no pacifier use in
breastfeeding term infants for
increasing duration of breastfeeding
(Review), *Cochrane Database Syst Rev*
7(3):CD007202, 2011.

Jones W: *Breastfeeding and mastitis*
(website). www.breastfeeding
network.org.uk. 2006.

Kendall-Tackett KA: *Depression in new
mothers: causes, consequences, and
treatment, alternatives*, New York,
Routledge, 2009.

Kim P, et al: Breastfeeding, brain
activation to own infant cry and
maternal sensitivity, *J Child Psychol
Psychiatry* 52(8):907–915, 2011.

Koosha A, Hashemifesharaki R,
Mousavinasab N: Breastfeeding
patterns and factors determining
exclusive breastfeeding, *Singapore
Med J* 49(12):1002–1006, 2008.

Kramer MS, Aboud F, Mauchand E,
et al: Promotion of Breastfeeding
Intervention Trial (PROBIT) Study
Group. Breastfeeding and child
cognitive development: new
evidence from a large randomized
trial, *Arch Gen Psychiatry* 65(5):578–
584, 2008.

Kramer MS, et al: Promotion of
Breastfeeding Intervention Trial
(PROBIT): a randomized trial in the
Republic of Belarus, *JAMA* 285:413–
420, 2001.

Kramer MS, Kakuma R: Optimal
duration of exclusive breastfeeding,
Cochrane Database Syst Rev
(4):CD003517, 2006.

Kroeger M, Smith LJ: *Impact of birthing
practices on breastfeeding: protecting
the mother and baby continuum*,
Boston, Jones and Bartlett, 2004.

Kunz C, Rodriguez-Palmero M,
Koletzko B, et al: Nutritional and
biochemical properties of human
milk, part 1: general aspects,
proteins, and carbohydrates, *Clin
Perinatol* 26(2):307–333, 1999.

Kwan ML, Buffler PA, Abrams B, et al:
Breastfeeding and the risk of
childhood leukemia: a meta-
analysis, *Public Health Rep* 119:521–
535, 2004.

The Lancet Breastfeeding Series Group:
Breastfeeding series: The Lancet
(website). www.theLancet.com/
series/breastfeeding. 2016.

Lawrence RA, Lawrence RM:
*Breastfeeding: a guide for the medical
profession*, 8th edn, Maryland
Heights (MO), Elsevier, 2015.

Leon DA, Ronalds G: Breastfeeding
influences on later life –
cardiovascular disease, *Adv Exp Med
Biol* 639:153–166, 2009.

Lin PW, Nasr TR, Stoll BJ: Necrotizing
enterocolitis: recent scientific
advances in pathophysiology and
prevention, *Semin Perinatol*
32(2):70–82, 2008.

Lubianca Neto JF, Hemb L, Silva DB:
Systematic literature review of
modifiable risk factors for recurrent
acute otitis media in childhood,
J Pediatr 82:87–96, 2006.

Makrides M, Neumann M, Simmer K:
Are long chain polyunsaturated fatty
acids essential nutrients in infancy?
Lancet 345(8963):1463–1468, 1995.

Mangesi L, Dowswell T: Treatments for
breast engorgement during
lactation, *Cochrane Database Syst Rev*
(9):CD006946, 2010.

Marchbank T, Weaver G, Nilsen-
Hamilton M, et al: Pancreatic
secretory trypsin inhibitor is a major
motogenic and protective factor in
human breast milk, *Am J Physiol
Gastrointest Liver Physiol* 296:G697–
G703, 2009.

Mason T, Rabinovich CE, Fredrickson
DD, et al: Breastfeeding and the
development of juvenile rheumatoid
arthritis, *J Rheumatol* 22:1166–1170,
1995.

Mason F, Rawe K, Wright S: *Superfood
for babies: how overcoming barriers to
breastfeeding will save children's lives*.
Save the Children (website). www
.savethechildren.org.uk/sites/default/
files/images/Superfood_for_Babies
_UK_version.pdf. 2013.

McAndrew F, Thompson J, Fellows L,
et al: *Infant Feeding Survey 2010*,
Health and Social Care Information
Centre (website). www.ic.nhs.uk/
statistics-and-data-collections/
health-and-lifestyles-relatedsurveys/
infant-feeding-survey/infant-feeding
-survey-2010. 2012.

McCreadie RG: The Nithsdale
Schizophrenia Surveys. 16.
Breastfeeding and schizophrenia:
preliminary results and hypotheses,
Br J Psychiatry 170:334–337, 1997.

McVea KL, Turner PD, Peppler DK: The
role of breastfeeding in sudden
infant death syndrome, *J Hum Lact*
16(1):13–20, 2000.

Mead MN: Contaminants in human
milk: Weighing the risks against the
benefits of breastfeeding, *Environ
Health Perspect* 116(10):A426–A434,
2008.

Michaelsen KF, Lauritzen L, Mortensen
EL: Effects of breastfeeding on
cognitive function, *Adv Exp Med Biol*
639:199–215, 2009.

Michalopoulos K: The effects of breast
augmentation surgery on future
ability to lactate, *Breast J* 13(1):62–
67, 2007.

Mikhailov TA, Furner SE: Breastfeeding
and genetic factors in the etiology
of inflammatory bowel disease in
children, *World J Gastroenterol*
15(3):270–279, 2008.

Minchin M: *Milk matters: infant feeding
and immune disorder*, London,
BookPOD, 2015.

Ministry of Health (New Zealand): *Food
and nutrition guidelines for healthy
infants and toddlers (aged 0–2): a
background paper*, 4th edn,
Wellington, Ministry of Health,
2008 (partially revised December
2012).

Moore ER, Anderson GC, Bergman N,
et al: Early skin-to-skin contact for
mother and their healthy newborn
infants (Review), *Cochrane Database
Syst Rev* (5):CD003519, 2012.

Morton JA: Ineffective suckling: a
possible consequence of obstructive
positioning, *J Hum Lact* 8(2):83–85,
1992.

National Health Service (NHS): *Making
up infant formula* (website). www
.nhs.uk/Conditions/pregnancy-and
-baby/Pages/making-up-infant
-formula.aspx#close. 2014.

National Infant Feeding Network
(NIFN): *Statement: thrush* (website).
www.unicef.org.uk/Documents/
Baby_Friendly/Networks/NIFN_
statement_thrush_2014.pdf. 2014.

National Institute for Health and
Clinical Excellence (NICE): *Division
of ankyloglossia (tongue-tie) for
breastfeeding, Interventional Procedure
Guidance 149*, London, NICE, 2005.

National Institute for Health and Clinical Excellence (NICE): *Postnatal care: routine postnatal care of women and their babies*, Clinical Guideline 37, London, NICE, 2006.

National Institute for Health and Clinical Excellence (NICE): *Donor milk banks: the operation of donor milk bank services*, Clinical Guideline 93 (website). www.nice.org.uk/cg93. 2010a.

National Institute for Health and Clinical Excellence (NICE): *Antenatal care: routine care for the healthy pregnant woman, Clinical Guideline 62*, London, 2010b (updated; Available at www.nice.org.uk/G062).

National Institute for Health and Clinical Excellence (NICE): *Public Health Guidance 11: Improving the nutrition of pregnant and breastfeeding mothers and children in low-income households*, Quick reference guide: maternal and child nutrition (website). http://guidance.nice.org .uk/PH11. 2011 (updated).

National Institute for Health and Clinical Excellence (NICE): *Social and emotional well-being: early years, Public Health Guidance 40* (website). http:// guidance.nice.org.uk/PH40. 2012.

National Institute for Health and Care Excellence (NICE): *Postnatal care, NICE Quality Standard 37* (website). http://publications.nice.org.uk/ postnatal-care-qs37/qualitystatement-5-breastfeeding. 2013.

National Institute for Health and Care Excellence (NICE): *Nutrition: improving maternal and child nutrition, Quality Standard QS98* (website). www.nice.org.uk/ guidance/qs98. 2015a.

National Institute for Health and Care Excellence (NICE): *Intrapartum care, Quality Standard QS105* (website). www.nice.org.uk/guidance/qs105. 2015b.

National Institute for Health and Care Excellence (NICE): *Mastitis and breast abscess: clinical knowledge summaries* (website). http:// cks.nice.org.uk/mastitis-and-breast-abscess#!topicsummary. 2015c.

National Institute of Health and Care Excellence (NICE): *Contraception – natural family planning: clinical knowledge summaries*. https://cks. nice.org.uk/contraception-natural -family-planning#!topicsummary. 2016.

Neifert MR: Breastmilk transfer: positioning, latch-on and screening for problems in milk transfer, *Clin Obstet Gynaecol* 47:656–675, 2004.

Neville M: The physiology of lactation, *Clin Perinatol* 26(2):251–279, 1999.

New Zealand Ministry of Health (NZMH): *Breastfeeding is perfect for you and your baby* (website). www.health.govt.nz/your-health/ pregnancy-and-kids/first-year/ helpful-advice-during-first-year/ breastfeeding-perfect-you-and-your -baby. 2016.

Oddy WH: The long-term effects of breastfeeding on asthma and atopic disease, *Adv Exp Med Biol* 639:237–251, 2009.

Oddy WH, et al: The long-term effects of breastfeeding on adolescent mental health: a pregnancy cohort study followed for 14 years, *J Paediatr* 156(4):568–574, 2009.

Oddy W, Robinson M, Kendall G, et al: Breastfeeding and early development: a prospective cohort study, *Acta Paediatr*. doi: 10.1111/ j1651-2227.2011.02199.x. 2011.

O'Tierney PF, Barker DJ, Osmond C, et al: Duration of breastfeeding and adiposity in adult life, *J Nutr* 139(2):422S–425S, 2009.

Pisacane A, Graziano L, Mazzarella G, et al: Breastfeeding and urinary tract infection, *J Pediatr* 120(1):87–89, 1992.

Public Health England (PHE): *Rapid review to update evidence for the Healthy Child Programme 0–5* (website). www.gov.uk/government/ uploads/system/uploads/ attachment_data/file/ 429740/150520RapidReview HealthyChildProg_UPDATE_ poisons_final.pdf. 2015.

Public Health England (PHE) and Unicef: *Infant feeding: commissioning services (Summary, Parts 1, 2 & 3)*. https://www.gov.uk/government/ publications/infant-feeding -commissioning-services. 2016.

Public Health Wales: *A strategic vision for maternity services in Wales* (website). http://gov.wales/topics/ health/publications/health/ strategies/maternity/?lang=en. 2013.

Quigley MA, Cumberland P, Cowden JM, et al: How protective is breast feeding against diarrhoeal disease in infants in 1990s England? A case-control study, *Arch Dis Child* 91:245–250, 2006.

Quigley M, Hokley C, Carson C, et al: Breastfeeding is associated with improved child cognitive development: a population-based cohort study, *J Pediatr* 160:25–32, 2012.

Quigley MA, Kelly YJ, Sacker A: Breastfeeding and hospitalization for diarrheal and respiratory infection in the United Kingdom: Millennium Cohort Study, *Pediatrics* 119:e837–e842, 2007.

Ravelli ACJ, van der Meulen JHP, Osmond C, et al: Infant feeding and adult glucose tolerance, lipid profile, blood pressure and obesity, *Arch Dis Child* 82(3):248–252, 2000.

Renfrew M, Woolridge M, Ross McGill H: *Enabling women to breastfeed*, London, Stationery Office, 2000.

Renfrew MJ, et al: Breastfeeding promotion for infants in neonatal units: a systematic review and economic analysis, *Health Technol Assess* 13(40): 2009.

Renfrew MJ, McCormick FM, Wade A, et al: Support for healthy breastfeeding mothers with healthy term babies (Review), *Cochrane Database Syst Rev* (5):CD001141, 2012a.

Renfrew MJ, et al: *Preventing disease and saving resources: the potential contribution of increasing breastfeeding rates in the UK*, London, 2012b, Unicef UK BFI.

Renfrew MJ, Spiby H, D'Souza L, et al: Rethinking research in breastfeeding: a critique of the evidence base identified in a systematic review of interventions to promote and support breastfeeding, *Public Health Nutr* 10:726–732, 2007.

Righard L, Alade MO: Effect of delivery room routines on success of first breastfeed, *Lancet* 336(8723):1105–1107, 1990.

Righard L, Alade MO: Sucking technique and its effects on success of breastfeeding, *Birth* 19:185–189, 1992.

Roberts CL, Ampt AJ, Algert CS, et al: Reduced breast milk feeding subsequent to cosmetic breast augmentation surgery, *Med J Aust* 202(6):324–328, 2015.

Robertson L, Harrild K: Maternal and neonatal risk factors for childhood type 1 diabetes: a matched case-control study, *BMC Public Health* 10:281, 2010.

Rodriguez-Palmero M, Koletzko B, Kunz C, et al: Nutritional and biochemical properties of human milk: II. Lipids, micronutrients, and bioactive factors, *Clin Perinatol* 26(2):335–359, 1999.

Royal College of Midwives (RCM): *Successful breastfeeding*, 3rd edn, London, Churchill Livingstone, 2002.

Royal College of Midwives (RCM): *Infant feeding*, London, RCM, 2009.

Sacker A, Quigley M, Kelly Y: Breastfeeding and developmental delay: findings from the Millennium Cohort Study, *Pediatrics* 118:e682–e689, 2006. doi: 10.1542/peds.2005-3141.

Schiff M, Algert CS, Ampt A, et al: The impact of cosmetic breast implants on breastfeeding: a systematic review and meta-analysis, *Int Breastfeed J* 9:17, 2014.

Schore AN: Attachment and the regulation of the right brain, *Attach Hum Dev* 2(1):23–47, 2000.

Schore AN: Effects of a secure attachment relationship on right brain development, affect regulation and infant mental health, *Infant Ment Health J* 22(1–2):7–66, 2001.

Scientific Advisory Committee on Nutrition (SACN): *Update on trans fatty acids and health, position statement*, London, TSO, 2007.

Scientific Advisory Committee on Nutrition (SACN): *Infant Feeding Survey 2005: a commentary on infant feeding practices in the UK* (website). www.sacn.gov.uk/. 2008.

Scientific Advisory Committee on Nutrition (SACN): *Vitamin D and Health*. https://www.gov.uk/government/uploads/system/uploads/attachment_data/file/537616/SACN_Vitamin_D_and_Health_report.pdf. 2016.

Scott J, Ng S, Cobiac L: The relationship between breastfeeding and weight status in a national sample of Australian children and adolescents, *BMC Public Health* 12:107, 2012. www.biomedcentral.com/1471-2458/12/107.

Scottish government: *Health/infant-feeding/ improving maternal and infant nutrition: a framework for action* (website). www.isdscotland.org/Health-Topics/Child-Health/Infant-Feeding/. 2011.

Shields L, O'Callaghan M, Williams GM, et al: Breastfeeding and obesity at 14 years: a cohort study, *J Paediatr Child Health* 42(5):289–296, 2006.

Shonkoff JP, Phillips D: *From neurons to neighbourhoods: the science of early child development*, National Scientific Council on the Developing Child – Centre on the Developing Child, Harvard University, Washington DC, National Academy Press, 2000.

Silfverdal SA, Bodin L, Olc NP: Protective effect of breastfeeding: an ecologic study of *Haemophilus influenzae* meningitis and breastfeeding in a Swedish population, *Int J Epidemiol* 28(1):152–156, 1999.

Strathearn L, Iyengar U, Fonagy P, et al: Maternal oxytocin response during mother-infant interaction: Associations with adult temperament, *Hum Behav* 61:429–435, 2012.

Strathearn L, Mamun AA, Najman JM, et al: Does breastfeeding protect against substantiated child abuse and neglect? A 15-year cohort study, *Pediatrics* 123(2):483–493, 2009.

Sunderland M: *What every parent needs to know: the incredible effects of love, nurture and play on your child's development*, New York, Dorling Kindersley, 2007.

Taylor GP, et al: British HIV Association and Children's HIV Association position statement on infant feeding in the UK, *HIV Med* 12:389–393, 2011.

Thompson JF, Heal LJ, Roberts CL, et al: Women's breastfeeding experiences following a significant primary postpartum haemorrhage: a multicentre cohort study, *Int Breastfeed J* 5:5, 2010.

Unicef: *Breastfeeding on the worldwide agenda* (website). www.unicef.org/eapro/breastfeeding_on_worldwide_agenda.pdf. 2013.

Unicef UK: *UN Convention on the rights of child. Enforced in UK January 15th* (website). www.unicef.org.uk/Documents/Publication-pdfs/crcsummary.pdf?epslanguage=en. 1992.

Unicef UK Baby-Friendly Initiative (BFI): *Breastfeeding your baby*, London, Unicef UK BFI, 1998.

Unicef UK Baby-Friendly Initiative (BFI): *A guide to infant formula for parents who are bottle feeding*, London, Unicef UK BFI, 2010.

Unicef UK Baby-Friendly Initiative (BFI): *The evidence and rationale for the Unicef UK Baby-Friendly Initiative standards* (website). http://www.unicef.org.uk/Documents/Baby_Friendly/Research/baby_friendly_evidence_rationale.pdf. 2012a.

Unicef UK Baby-Friendly Initiative (BFI): *Guide to the Baby Friendly Initiative standards* (website). www.unicef.org.uk/Documents/Baby_Friendly/Guidance/Baby_Friendly_guidance_2012.pdf. 2012b.

Unicef UK Baby Friendly Initiative (BFI): *A guide to infant formula for parents who are bottle feeding: health professionals' guide* (website). www.unicef.org.uk/Documents/Baby_Friendly/Leaflets/HP_Guide_for_parents_formula_feeding.pd. 2014a.

Unicef UK Baby-Friendly Initiative (BFI): *Breastfeeding and relationship building: a workbook*, London, Unicef UK BFI, 2014b.

Unicef UK Baby-Friendly Initiative (BFI): *Working within the international code of marketing of breast-milk substitutes: a guide for health professionals* (website). www.unicef.org.uk/Documents/Baby_Friendly/Guidance/guide_int_code_health_professionals.pdf. 2015.

Unicef UK Baby Friendly Initiative (BFI): *Supporting Close and Loving Relationships*. https://353ld710iigr2n4po7k4kgvv-wpengine.netdna-ssl.com/babyfriendly/wp-content/uploads/sites/2/2016/10/Responsive-Feeding-Infosheet-Unicef-UK-Baby-Friendly-Initiative.pdf. 2016.

Unite/CPHVA: *Distinctive contribution of health visiting to public health and well-being*, Unite the Union (website). www.unitetheunion.org/pdf/HVContributionGuide4CommissionersNov08.pdf. 2008.

United Nations: *Convention on the Rights of the Child*. Adopted and opened for signature, ratification and accession by General Assembly Resolution 44/25 of 20 November 1989 entry into force 2 September 1990, in accordance with Article 49 (website). www.unicef.org.uk/Documents/Publication-pdfs/UNCRC_PRESS200910web.pdf. 1989.

United Nations: *Human Rights Office of the High Commissioner (UN) Joint* statement by the UN Special Rapporteurs on the Right to Food, Right to Health, the Working Group on Discrimination against Women in law and in practice, and the Committee on the Rights of the Child in support of increased efforts to promote, support and protect breast-feeding. http://www.ohchr.org/EN/NewsEvents/Pages/DisplayNews.aspx?NewsID=20871&LangID=E. 2016.

Uvnäs-Moberg K, Francis R: *The oxytocin factor: tapping the hormone of calm, love and healing,* Cambridge (MA), Da Capo Press, 2003.

Walker M: *Delayed lactogenesis II* (website). http://breastfeedingthegoldstandard.org/wordpress/wp-content/uploads/Delayed lactogenesisII-G4.pdf. 2015.

Wambach K, Riordan J: *Breastfeeding and human lactation,* Burlington (MA), Jones and Bartlett, 2015.

Welsh government: *Flying start* (website). http://wales.gov.uk/topics/childrenyoungpeople/parenting/help/flyingstart/?lang=en. 2010.

Welsh government: *Infant feeding guidelines from birth to 12 months* (website). www.healthchallengewales.org/sitesplus/documents/1052/Infant%20Feeding%20Guidelines%20final%20web%20may%202015.pdf Welsh Government Cardiff. 2015.

WHO Task Force on Methods for the Natural Regulation of Fertility: The World Health Organization multinational study of breastfeeding and lactational amenorrhea. III. Pregnancy during breastfeeding, *Fertil Steril* 72(3):431–440, 1999.

Widström AM, Lilja G, Aaltomaa-Michalias P, et al: Newborn behaviour to locate the breast when skin-to-skin: a possible method for enabling early self-regulation, *Acta Paediatr* 100(1):79–85, 2011.

Widström AM, Wahlberg V, Matthieson AS: Short term effects of early suckling and touch of the nipple on maternal behaviour, *Early Hum Dev* 21:153–163, 1990.

Willis CE, Livingstone V: Infant insufficient milk syndrome associated with maternal postpartum hemorrhage, *J Hum Lact* 11(2):123–126, 1995.

Wilson AC, Forsyth JS, Greene SA, et al: Relation of infant diet to childhood health: seven year follow up of cohort of children in Dundee infant feeding study, *Br Med J* 316(7124):21, 1998.

Winberg J: Mother and newborn baby: mutual regulation of physiology and behaviour – a selective review, *Dev Psychobiol* 47(3):217–229, 2005.

World Cancer Research Fund International/American Institute for Cancer Research (WCRF/AICR): *Policy and Action for cancer prevention: food, nutrition, and physical activity: a global perspective* (website). www.dietandcancerreport.org/cancer_resource_center/downloads/chapters/pr/Introductory%20pages.pdf. 2009.

World Health Organization (WHO): *International code of marketing of breastmilk substitutes,* Geneva, WHO, 1981.

World Health Organization (WHO): *Global strategy on infant and young child feeding* (website). www.who.int/nutrition/publications/infantfeeding/9241562218/en/. 2003.

World Health Organization (WHO): *Infant and young child feeding: model chapter for textbooks for medical students and allied health professionals,* Geneva, WHO, 2009.

World Health Organization (WHO): *Working with individuals, families and communities to improve maternal and newborn health* (website). http://whqlibdoc.who.int/hq/2010/WHO_MPS_09.04_eng.pdf). 2010a.

World Health Organization (WHO): *Infant and young child feeding. Fact sheet No. 342* (website). http://www.who.int/mediacentre/factsheets/fs342/en/. 2016.

World Health Organization (WHO): *Exclusive breastfeeding for six months best for babies everywhere.* Statement (website). www.who.int/mediacentre/news/statements/2011/breastfeeding_20110115/en/index.html. 2011.

World Health Organization (WHO): *Information concerning the marketing of follow up formula* (website). www.who.int/nutrition/topics/WHO_brief_fufandcode_post_17July.pdf. 2013a.

World Health Organization (WHO): *Country implementation of the International Code of Marketing of Breastmilk Substitutes: Status report 2011* (website). www.who.int/nutrition/publications/infantfeeding/statusreport2011/en/. 2013b.

World Health Organization (WHO): *Draft final report of the Commission on Ending Childhood Obesity,* Geneva, WHO, 2015.

World Health Organization/United Nations Children's Fund (WHO/Unicef): *Protecting, promoting and supporting breastfeeding: the special role of maternity services. A joint WHO/Unicef statement,* Geneva, WHO, 1989.

World Health Organization, United Nations Children's Fund (WHO/Unicef): *Acceptable medical reasons for use of breast-milk substitutes,* Geneva, WHO, 2009.

World Health Organization (WHO), UNAIDS, UNFPA, Unicef: *Guidelines on HIV and infant feeding. Principles and recommendations for infant feeding in the context of HIV and a summary of evidence,* Geneva, WHO, 2010.

Wright CM, Williams AF, Elliman D, et al: Practice pointer: Using the new UK-WHO growth charts, *BMJ* 340:c2587, 2010.

Xiao-Ming B: Nutritional management of newborn infants, *World J Gastroenterol* 14(40):6133–6139, 2008.

Zeedyk MS, Werrity I, Riach C: One year on: perceptions of the lasting benefits of involvement in a parenting support programme, *Child Soc* 22(2):99–111, 2008.

Zimmermann R, Perucchini D, Fauchere JC: Hepatitis C virus in breastmilk, *Lancet* 345(8954):928, 1995.

Resources and additional reading

Association of Breastfeeding Mothers
(ABM): www.abm.me.uk

BHIVA/CHIVA British HIV Association:
www.bhiva.org

*Bliss – for babies born too soon, too small,
too sick*: www.bliss.org.uk

Breastfeeding Network:
www.breastfeedingnetwork.org.uk

Family Planning Association: www
.fpa.org.uk

First Steps Nutrition:
www.firststepsnutrition.org/

ISIS Infant Sleep Information Source:
www.isisonline.org.uk

LactMed: *Drugs and Lactation Database/
UK Drugs and Lactation Advisory
Service*: http://bit.ly/1a8pEJY

La Leche League GB: www.laleche.org.uk

Maternity Action: www.maternityaction
.org.uk

National Childbirth Trust (NCT):
www.nct.org.uk

The Scientific Advisory Committee
on Nutrition (SACN): www.sacn.gov
.uk/

Start4Life: www.nhs.uk/start4life/

UK-WHO – growth charts: http://
bit.ly/18xAaq5

World Alliance for Breastfeeding
Action (WABA): www.waba.org.my

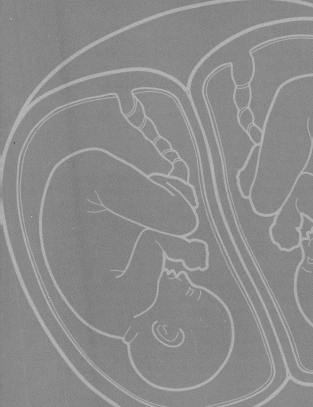

Part Eight

Women and babies with complex needs

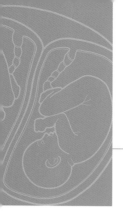

Chapter 45

The preterm baby and the small baby

Julia Petty

Learning Outcomes ?

After reading this chapter, you will be able to:

- explain the classification and definitions of babies born at early gestations and low birthweights
- understand how to assess and distinguish between babies born at low gestation and/or those with a low birthweight
- describe the common causes of preterm birth and low birthweight, the resultant problems that ensue and the implications for care
- understand the associated complications and long-term outcomes relating to preterm delivery and being born at low birthweight

INTRODUCTION

Newborn babies are classified according to their gestation, their birthweight relative to their gestational age (percentiles) and their actual birthweight. Preterm and low-birthweight (LBW) babies are discussed in this chapter, and although they are considered separately, there is certainly overlap in causes, management and long-term complications. A baby, for example, may be preterm, small for gestational age *and* LBW and needs consideration from all perspectives, as will be discussed. The midwife's role centres on the prevention of prematurity and LBW, identifying risk factors antenatally and preparing parents for a potential high-risk delivery. In the event of preterm birth, they also have a role in working with the multidisciplinary

team (MDT) to support parents in the neonatal period while their baby is cared for in transitional care (TC) or if the baby is admitted to the neonatal unit for further management.

PREMATURITY

Definitions

Preterm birth can be viewed in the context of what 'term' is, as follows:

- *Term:* Delivery at 37 to 40 completed weeks gestation.
- *Post-term:* Delivery on or after 41 weeks plus 3 days of gestation, 10 days beyond the estimated date of delivery.
- *Preterm:* Delivery at less than 37 completed weeks gestation, the group of interest in this chapter.

There are, within the preterm group, different degrees of prematurity ranging from the moderately preterm (32–37 weeks) to the very preterm (28–32 weeks) and the extremely preterm baby (less than 28 weeks). The former group most often do not pose any significant problems and will be cared for within TC for a relatively short period before discharge. The latter two preterm groups, however, are likely to need more significant care and support and will require admission to the neonatal unit for a more protracted period depending on the extent of prematurity and presenting condition. Ultimately, the aim would be to prevent preterm birth to avert this situation in the first place. Interventions to prevent preterm onset of labour are the subject of ongoing research. For more information on classification and key areas of prevention, see the chapter website resources.

Causes of prematurity

The causes of preterm onset of labour and delivery are also the subject of current research, as highlighted by the work of UK charity Tommy's (2015) and the World Health Organization (WHO 2012).

Specific events leading to prematurity are still uncertain and are likely to be a series or combination of maternal and fetal risk factors rather than a single event (Goldenberg et al 2008). They include the following:

- Pre-eclampsia
- Placental abnormalities – antepartum haemorrhage, placenta praevia
- Serious maternal diseases – acute or chronic, such as pyelonephritis, chronic nephritis or essential hypertension
- Premature prolonged rupture of membranes (PPROM)
- Intra-amniotic infection
- Cervical incompetence (history of repeated mid-trimester miscarriages)
- Maternal alcohol or substance abuse – including cigarette smoking
- Overdistension of the uterus – multiple pregnancies, polyhydramnios
- Poor obstetric history
- Lower socioeconomic status
- Unexplained reasons

Some of these problems can be identified and addressed antenatally. A crucial part of the midwife's role is in the education of women about normal pregnancy and what should be reported to them for further investigation.

Outcomes

'Outcome' refers to both mortality (survival rates) and morbidity (long-term complications). First, low gestational age at birth is a principal factor associated with perinatal mortality. Data is available to monitor trends in preterm birth and survival and to inform care. According to the latest figures by the Office for National Statistics (ONS 2015), for babies born in 2013, the majority (89%) of live births were delivered full term, 7% were preterm and 3% were post-term. Of the 7% of births that were preterm, almost 5% were extremely preterm, 11% were very preterm and 85% were moderately preterm. The infant mortality rate for babies born preterm overall in 2013 was 21.1 deaths per 1,000 live births. This was lower than the rate for preterm babies born in 2012 and 2006 (23.6 and 28.6 deaths per 1,000 live births respectively). Infant mortality was highest at the very low gestational ages. Research looking at patterns across countries and areas has also highlighted relatively higher rates in England

compared with Sweden, for example (Tambe et al 2015), and a wide variation in perinatal mortality within the UK (Manktelow et al 2015) (see chapter website resources for details).

Babies born very preterm are at particular risk of sensory, cognitive and motor dysfunction (Bolton et al 2012; Costeloe et al 2014). This is discussed later in the chapter.

Characteristics

Over the course of pregnancy, babies develop key characteristics that can be assessed through simple examination. For example, as the baby develops muscle tone, distinct posture ensues along with measurable angles of resistance in key muscle groups. In addition, the eyes transform from being fused in very premature babies to wide open when full-term. The skin and hair also give away important information in determining gestational age and a host of other characteristics, as described in the following list. These key features indicate babies are immature and form an essential part of the subjective assessment at birth and/or on admission to transitional or special care. Their appearance depends on their maturity, but some characteristic signs of prematurity are as follows:

- The head is large in proportion to the body.
- The face appears small and triangular, with a pointed chin.
- If very immature, the eyelids may be fused.
- Because of poor ossification, the cranial sutures and fontanelles are widely spaced and the skull bones soft.
- With the absence of subcutaneous fat, the skin is pinkish/red, and surface veins are prominent.
- The body is covered with varying amounts of soft downy hair in the mid-trimester – *lanugo*.
- The limbs are thin, and the more immature the baby, the greater the degree of extension.
- Muscle tone is underdeveloped.
- The nails are soft.
- The chest is small and narrow with little or no breast tissue.
- The abdomen is large, and the umbilicus appears to be low set.
- Genitalia are not fully developed:
  - The labia majora do not cover the labia minora.
  - The testes may not have descended into the scrotum.
- Suck and swallow reflexes are uncoordinated.

Assessing gestation

Antenatally, gestation and estimated date of delivery (EDD) are predicted from the date of the last menstrual period of the woman's normal menstrual cycle, early ultrasound scan measurements and uterine growth (see Chs 32 and 33). Not all mothers know their EDD; they may give birth without any antenatal care or live in a country that does not offer routine scanning; therefore, exact information about dates and gestational age may not be readily available. Moreover, practitioners must not assume gestation if the correct information is unknown about a baby on admission because this may lead to inappropriate care.

It is important to recognize the difference between a baby who is born early and one who is near term but is growth restricted/small (i.e. babies of the same weight but different gestations) to plan care most effectively. There may also be the situation where a baby is preterm but large for dates (LGA) and thus appears much older in gestation. Similarly, babies may be of similar gestations but very different weights. For example, a baby who is preterm but large in weight may look like a term baby, and thus essential potential problems associated with a preterm LGA baby may be overlooked. In addition, the survival of a baby who is extremely LBW will be influenced by the baby's gestation and maturity, and thus knowing dates will help to make decisions and plan care about what is best for that baby.

Tools exist to assess babies' gestational age – for example, the Dubowitz tool (Fig. 45.1) assesses babies on a range of criteria, including neuromuscular control, tone, presence of lanugo hair, skin appearance and many others. A similar and more recently cited tool is the Ballard Score Maturational Assessment of Gestational Age, a set of procedures developed by Dr J. L. Ballard and colleagues (Ballard et al 1991) to determine gestational age through neuromuscular and physical assessment (Fig. 45.2; see also chapter website resources).

Overall, these scoring systems require that there is a careful examination of the baby, looking at characteristics of appearance, reflexes and behaviour, and provides an indication of whether the baby is small or premature.

PROBLEMS OF THE PRETERM BABY

Initial management

The preterm baby (Fig. 45.3) is unable to perform many physiological functions adequately as a result of immaturity. Neonatal care aims to support the baby until they are able to achieve physical stability without any assistance. Preterm labour often progresses rapidly. If preterm labour is anticipated, birth should be planned in a maternity unit that can administer maternal steroids, with the appropriate level of neonatal intensive care facilities. Transfer to another hospital may be necessary and should be discussed if clinically appropriate.

Usually, preterm babies are small and fragile and require stabilization rather than active resuscitation when born. Accurate assessment of the baby's condition at birth to ensure prompt stabilization is essential. All resuscitation equipment must be checked and fully functional before the birth, including ascertaining whether it is the correct size and suitable for small babies. An experienced healthcare team, including a paediatrician or neonatologist, midwife, and neonatal nurse, must be present at birth to ensure immediate and expert stabilization. Thermal care is vital at this point because cold stress can increase mortality and morbidity in preterm babies (see Ch. 43). The radiant heater should be turned on before birth. The room temperature should be increased to $26\,°C$. Babies over 30 weeks gestation should be dried thoroughly and wrapped in a warm towel, with a hat applied. Infants under 30 weeks gestation should not be dried but should have their bodies placed immediately in a plastic occlusive wrap. This should not be covered with a towel because the radiant heater needs to be directly above the baby (UK Resuscitation Council 2015) allowing visualization of the chest and ease of access while preventing evaporative heat loss and skin damage. The preterm baby may lack surfactant, normally produced within the lungs in the last trimester of pregnancy; therefore, endogenous surfactant may be required if the condition indicates (see Ch. 46). The baby may also require ventilation support, preferably non-invasively by continuous positive airway pressure (CPAP) once a diagnosis of Respiratory Distress Syndrome (RDS) is confirmed.

Common problems of prematurity

As stated previously, preterm babies are immature and not ready to adapt to extrauterine life. The more preterm the baby, the more structurally and physiologically immature are the baby's systems. Related to this specific biology are the following conditions commonly seen in the care of the preterm baby (see chapter website resources for further information on these conditions).

Respiratory

The most common problems for preterm babies are respiratory disorders.

Respiratory distress syndrome

Respiratory distress syndrome (RDS) is a developmental deficiency in surfactant synthesis accompanied by lung immaturity. Surfactant is usually produced in larger quantities between 32 and 35 weeks gestation, and RDS is most

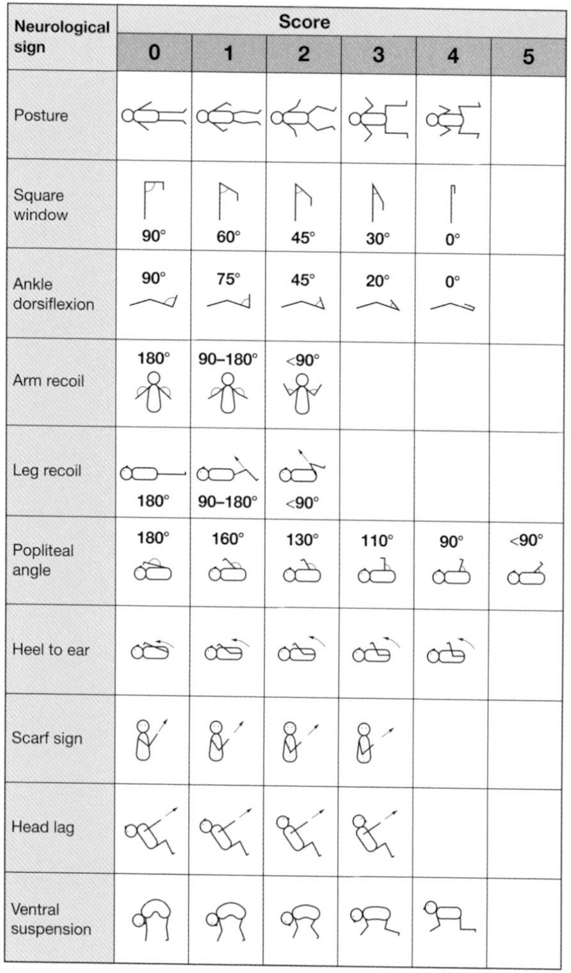

Physical (external) criteria

External sign	Score				
	0	1	2	3	4
Oedema	Obvious oedema hands and feet; pitting over tibia	No obvious oedema hands and feet; pitting over tibia	No oedema		
Skin texture	Very thin, gelatinous	Thin and smooth	Smooth, medium thickness / Rash or superficial peeling	Slight thickening / Superficial cracking and peeling, especially hands and feet	Thick and parchment-like / Superficial or deep cracking
Skin colour (infant not crying)	Dark red	Uniformly pink	Pale pink, variable over body	Pale / Only pink over ears, lips, palms or soles	
Skin opacity (trunk)	Numerous veins and venules clearly seen, especially over abdomen	Veins and tributaries seen	A few large vessels clearly seen over abdomen	A few large vessels seen indistinctly over abdomen	No blood vessels seen
Lanugo (over back)	No lanugo	Abundant, long and thick over whole back	Hair thinning, especially over lower back	Small amount of lanugo and bald areas	At least half of back devoid of lanugo
Plantar creases	No skin creases	Faint red marks over anterior half of sole	Definite red marks over more than anterior half / Indentations over more than anterior third	Indentations over more than anterior third	Definite deep indentations over more than anterior third
Nipple formation	Nipple barely visible, no areola	Nipple well defined, areola smooth and flat, diameter <0.75 cm	Areola stippled, edges not raised: diameter <0.75 cm	Areola stippled, edge raised: diameter >0.75 cm	
Breast size	No breast tissue palpable	Breast tissue on one or both sides <0.5 cm diameter	Breast tissue both sides, one or both 0.5–1.0 cm	Breast tissue both sides, one or both >1 cm	
Ear form	Pinna flat and shapeless, little or no incurving of edge	Incurving of part of edge of pinna	Partial incurving whole of upper pinna	Well-defined incurving whole of upper pinna	
Ear firmness	Pinna soft, easily folded, no recoil	Pinna soft, easily folded, slow recoil	Cartilage to edge of pinna but soft in places, ready recoil	Pinna firm, cartilage to edge, instant recoil	
Genitalia • Male	Neither testis in scrotum	At least one testis high in scrotum	At least one testis right down		
• Female (with hips half abducted)	Labia majora widely separated, labia minora protruding	Labia majora almost cover labia minora	Labia majora completely cover labia minora		

Neurological sign	Score					
	0	1	2	3	4	5
Posture						
Square window	90°	60°	45°	30°	0°	
Ankle dorsiflexion	90°	75°	45°	20°	0°	
Arm recoil	180°	90–180°	<90°			
Leg recoil	180°	90–180°	<90°			
Popliteal angle	180°	160°	130°	110°	90°	<90°
Heel to ear						
Scarf sign						
Head lag						
Ventral suspension						

Figure 45.1 The Dubowitz score: graph for reading gestational age from total score. (Dubowitz LMS, Dubowitz V, Goldberg C: Clinical assessment of gestational age in the newborn infant, J Pediatr 77(1):1–10, 1970.)

Neuromuscular maturity

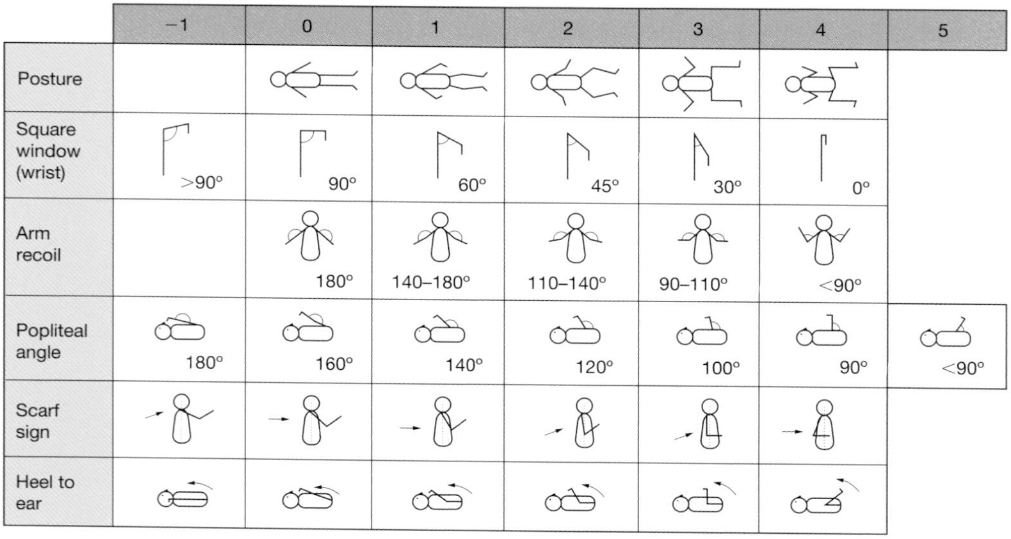

	−1	0	1	2	3	4	5
Posture							
Square window (wrist)	>90°	90°	60°	45°	30°	0°	
Arm recoil		180°	140–180°	110–140°	90–110°	<90°	
Popliteal angle	180°	160°	140°	120°	100°	90°	<90°
Scarf sign							
Heel to ear							

Physical maturity

Skin	Sticky, friable, transparent	Gelatinous, red, translucent	Smooth pink, visible veins	Superficial peeling and/or rash, few veins	Cracking, pale areas, rare veins	Parchment, deep cracking, no vessels	Leathery, cracked, wrinkled
Lanugo	None	Sparse	Abundant	Thinning	Bald areas	Mostly bald	
Plantar surface	Heel-toe 40–50 mm:−1 <40 mm:−2	>50 mm, no crease	Faint red marks	Anterior transverse crease only	Creases over anterior 2/3	Creases over entire sole	
Breast	Imperceptible	Barely perceptible	Flat areola; no bud	Stippled areola; 1- to 2-mm bud	Raised areola; 3- to 4-mm bud	Full areola; 5- to 10-mm bud	
Eye/ear	Lids fused loosely:−1 tightly:−2	Lids open; pinna flat and stays folded	Slightly curved pinna; soft; slow recoil	Well-curved pinna; soft but ready recoil	Formed and firm; instant recoil	Thick cartilage; ear stiff	
Genitals (male)	Scrotum flat, smooth	Scrotum empty; faint rugae	Testes in upper canal; rare rugae	Testes descending; few rugae	Testes down; good rugae	Testes pendulous; deep rugae	
Genitals (female)	Clitoris prominent; labia flat	Prominent clitoris; small labia minora	Prominent clitoris; enlarging labia minora	Labia majora and minora equally prominent	Labia majora large; labia minora small	Labia majora cover clitoris and labia minora	

Maturity rating

Score	Weeks
−10	20
−5	22
0	24
5	26
10	28
15	30
20	32
25	34
30	36
35	38
40	40
45	42
50	44

Figure 45.2 The Ballard score. Each of the clinical and neurological features is assessed and scored. The gestational age is determined by comparing the total score with the maturity rating grid. (Johnston PGB, Flood K, Spinks K: The newborn child, 9th edn. Edinburgh Churchill Livingstone, 2003.)

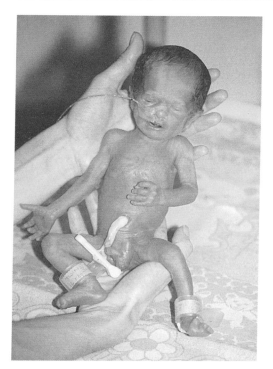

Figure 45.3 Preterm infant. (Johnston PGB, Flood K, Spinks K: The newborn child, 9th edn. Edinburgh Churchill Livingstone, 2003.)

commonly seen in babies at lower gestational age. This condition is discussed further in Chapter 46.

CPAP or ventilator management along with oxygen therapy should provide adequate respiratory support and tissue oxygenation without creating oxygen toxicity (Cherian et al 2014) or damage from excessive pressure or volume to the fragile lungs. Excessive and fluctuating quantities of oxygen are factors in the aetiology of retinopathy of prematurity (Hartnett and Penn 2012; Painter et al 2014). It is important to limit the maximum amount of oxygen given but also to ensure that sufficient qualities maintain optimum tissue oxygenation by setting appropriate pulse oximetry limits (Stenson et al 2013).

Chronic lung disease

Chronic lung disease (CLD; sometimes termed bronchopulmonary dysplasia) most commonly occurs in the preterm baby and is characterized clinically by the sustained need for oxygen supplementation after 4 weeks of age with areas of lung collapse and fibrosis shown on chest x-ray. Features of CLD include a serious disruption of lung growth. The lungs are stiff and can be difficult to ventilate,

with the need for prolonged ventilator support and oxygen, often for a significant period of time.

Apnoeas

Many preterm babies have apnoeas associated with their prematurity and require constant monitoring (Balain and Oddie 2014). Airway position is essential to reduce the potential for apnoeas caused by mechanical obstruction. Caffeine is given as a stimulant until these apnoeas of prematurity resolve (Darnell et al 2006). Apnoea monitors should be removed several days before discharge so that parents gain confidence and do not become reliant on them.

Cardiovascular/haematological

Anaemia

Anaemia is common in preterm babies. The shorter intrauterine period prevents the accumulation of an adequate iron store, and the immature gastrointestinal system does not easily digest iron supplements. The underactive bone marrow is unable to keep up sufficient red blood cell production to match the rapid rate of growth and increase in circulation. Ill babies require frequent blood tests and may have had much blood removed for sampling. Blood transfusions are often necessary, although some babies make good progress in spite of a low haemoglobin level.

Patent ductus arteriosus

In patent ductus arteriosus (PDA), the ductus arteriosus fails to close in some very preterm babies as a result of immaturity of the normal processes that would normally close it after birth. Generally, in healthy babies over 30 weeks gestation, the ductus arteriosus has closed functionally by 4 days. Only 11% of these infants have PDA, compared with 65% of infants less than 30 weeks gestation with severe respiratory distress (Clyman 2011). The presence of a PDA results in interstitial lung oedema and decreased pulmonary compliance caused by left-to-right shunting to the pulmonary circulation (Blackburn 2013). This can lead to prolonged dependence on ventilator support, which increases the risk of chronic lung disease.

Immunological

A preterm baby is more vulnerable to infection, both early (first 7 days) or late (after 7 days) onset, as a result of the following factors:

- Low maternal immunoglobulin (IgG) levels
- Thin, porous skin, which is an inefficient barrier to invading bacteria
- Limited production of tears and saliva, with fewer antibacterial factors
- Less protective stomach acid produced
- More invasive procedures and multiple contacts with hospital staff

To protect preterm babies as much as possible, standard precautions must be followed, including correct handwashing using a recommended antiseptic soap and the use of hand rub between washings. In addition, every baby should have his or her own individual equipment, which must be thoroughly cleaned daily. Ward areas should be clean and well ventilated, and soiled dressings or material should be placed in disposable bags and removed as soon as possible. All staff members, family and visitors caring for a baby must be free from any signs of infection, including coughs and sore throats. Antibiotic use is common, both prophylactically once a septic screen has been completed when infection is suspected and then specifically tailored to the individual pathogen once this is confirmed.

Fluid and electrolyte balance

Fluid imbalances, such as overload or dehydration, and electrolyte abnormalities requiring correction may result from kidney immaturity, making fluid balance challenging in the first few days of life. This is more difficult in the sick preterm baby who is ventilated. Careful titration and caution when increasing fluid requirements according to daily weight and serum electrolytes is required. Supplementation with electrolytes may be necessary.

Digestive system

If a preterm baby is too immature or unwell, there may be a risk of slow feed tolerance and absorption, milk aspiration and slow motility of the bowel. If unable to feed orally, the baby may be fed by the intravenous (IV) route initially. Total parenteral nutrition (TPN) is commenced, providing the baby with individually tailored nutrients and calories based on serum electrolyte results. Concurrently with IV fluids, tube feeding is undertaken. A naso/orogastric tube (Fig. 45.4) is used for the previously noted reasons and when the baby's suck is too weak or uncoordinated to feed by breast, cup or bottle. It is essential to check the baby's stomach acidity before feeds and to ensure the feed is slow. Non-nutritive sucking during gastric feeding has been shown to facilitate the development of sucking behaviour (Pinelli and Symington 2005); putting the baby to the breast at these times can be beneficial to the mother and baby and for the establishment of lactation (Neiva et al 2014) or a pacifier may be used for this reason, with parental agreement.

The growth requirement in preterm babies is greater than that in their mature counterparts; thus, they require a greater energy intake. Wherever possible, a mother's own fresh expressed breastmilk is preferred because it will be tailor-made to her baby's requirements, regardless of the infant's gestational age (Oras et al 2015) (see Ch. 44). The different nutritional content of preterm breastmilk compared with term breastmilk should be considered and fortification may be necessary to ensure adequate calories and additional nutrients for preterm growth (Renfrew et al 2010).

The mother should be encouraged to breastfeed, if possible, or start expressing milk, within a few hours of birth, with a minimum of six times every 24 hours. The sooner this is initiated, the greater the chance of establishing breastfeeding successfully. Midwives should teach all mothers how to express milk by hand and pump and how to store breastmilk safely (UNICEF 2013b; Nyqvist et al 2013).

Optimum nutrients are vital for the preterm baby (Embleton 2013). Along with fortification of breastmilk required to ensure this is optimum for growth, preterm babies also require additional supplementation of certain nutrients because of their limited reserves. Preterm babies have unique nutritional requirements as a result of inadequate stores at birth and the delay in red blood cell production caused by immaturity. They have small stores of fat-soluble vitamins and are at risk of vitamin deficiency. Supplementation includes protein, vitamins, iron and minerals, to achieve optimal growth and development. Supplementation has been shown to improve short-term outcomes (Kuschel and Harding 2004). Further information on feeding the preterm baby can be found on the chapter website.

Necrotizing enterocolitis

Necrotizing enterocolitis (NEC) is an inflammatory disease of the bowel thought to occur as a result of bacteria proliferating in the bowel and then penetrating the mucosal lining where there is ischaemic damage. Oedema, ulceration and haemorrhages of the bowel wall are found, which may progress to perforation or peritonitis. The condition typically develops in preterm babies who have been exposed to predisposing factors causing hypoxia and

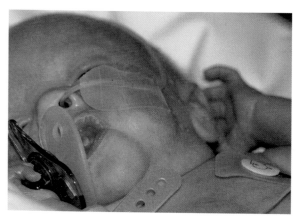

Figure 45.4 Premature baby with nasogastric tube in situ.

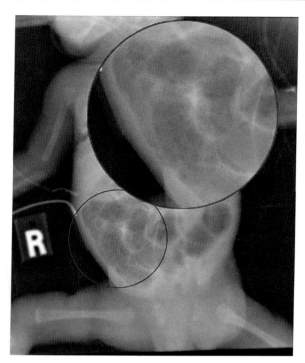

Figure 45.5 Necrotizing enterocolitis, showing dilated loops of bowel.

variations in bowel perfusion. The problem usually manifests itself within a few days of starting milk feeds because this is when colonization of the intestine is more likely (Cilieborg et al 2012).

Signs and symptoms include the following:

- Indications of sepsis
- Apnoea or septic shock
- Abdominal signs, such as distension, bile-stained vomiting/aspirate, or the passage of blood and mucus per rectum

The diagnosis is confirmed by the appearance of the bowel on radiography (Fig. 45.5) showing the presence of gas bubbles in the bowel wall. Breastmilk affords some protection against NEC, and midwives should promote breastfeeding for all babies; it is particularly important for sick, LBW and preterm babies. Appropriately screened and treated donor breastmilk may be a consideration for the preterm baby at risk of NEC.

Thermoregulation

Hypothermia

Preterm babies often have little or no brown fat stores to maintain the core temperature. The high surface area in relation to their size and their thin, porous skin facilitate rapid heat loss through evaporation. Radiant heaters may exacerbate the problem by increasing the evaporative heat loss, and their use is inappropriate for very small babies, who should be nursed in a humidified incubator for at least the first week of life. At home, following an emergency or unexpected preterm birth, if no resuscitation is required, the midwife can place the baby on the mother's abdomen or chest for skin-to-skin contact, once dried. The baby's head should be covered and the mother and baby well wrapped in dry blankets. The aim is to maintain body temperature in the thermoneutral range, at which energy requirements are reduced to a minimum and oxygen consumption is decreased (see Ch. 43).

Metabolism

Hypoglycaemia is a common problem for preterm babies in the first 48 to 72 hours. Stores of glycogen are too small to maintain blood sugar levels when energy requirements are particularly high. Because of the heat loss from their large surface area, the increased effort of breathing that accompanies respiratory difficulties and their greater rate of growth, more energy is expended compared to their term counterparts. Hypoxia, sepsis, ischaemia and hypothermia all aggravate this. Preterm babies have immature liver function, with reduced availability of liver enzymes responsible for gluconeogenesis and glycogenolysis, and are less able to produce alternative substrates such as ketone bodies.

Controversy still surrounds the clinical definition and significance of neonatal hypoglycaemia (Tin 2014), but it is generally accepted that the newborn brain can be damaged by hypoglycaemia if this is not controlled adequately in the early days of life (Simmons and Stanley 2015). Current recommendations are to maintain serum blood glucose levels above 2.6 mmol/L (Hawdon 2013; UNICEF 2013a). In at-risk babies, including preterm and LBW babies, blood sugar levels should be checked every 4 to 6 hours during the first 48 to 72 hours after birth using a glucometer.

Hepatic system

Physiological jaundice is exacerbated in preterm babies because the liver is immature, and therefore conjugation of bilirubin is further delayed (see Ch. 47). The severity of jaundice may be caused by the delayed passage of meconium in preterm babies, particularly if enteral feeds are not commenced for several days. This delay can contribute to hyperbilirubinemia because the bilirubin in meconium may be reabsorbed. The life span of red blood cells is related to gestational age and may be only 35 to 50 days in the preterm baby, who may have ongoing low-grade haemolysis. Another contributing factor is the low levels of serum albumin, which may limit extracellular binding and transport of bilirubin when concentrations are high (Smith 2013; Ives 2015). The National Institute for Health and Clinical Excellence (NICE 2010) has produced guidelines for the monitoring and care of neonatal jaundice and include gestation-specific threshold charts to record the bilirubin according to when the baby was delivered (see chapter website resources).

Liver immaturity also means the preterm baby is at higher risk of vitamin K deficiency bleeding (VKDB) (Schreiner et al 2014). Midwives need to discuss individual risk factors with parents and obtain informed consent for vitamin K administration at birth.

Neurological and sensory systems

Intraventricular haemorrhage

The preterm baby is at high risk of intraventricular haemorrhage (IVH), which emphasizes the importance of preventing perinatal and postnatal hypoxia. Fragile blood vessels and fluctuating episodes of hypotension, hypertension and/or hypoxia are all risk factors for cerebral haemorrhage. Midwives need to monitor the fetus closely during a preterm labour for early signs of any degree of compromise. In the neonatal unit, it is important to prevent instabilities of blood pressure and heart rate, through gentle handling and good pain management. Cranial ultrasound scanning is routinely performed on all preterm babies (see Fig. 45.6). Small bleeds are commonly found within a few hours of birth and are classified depending on site and severity. Major haemorrhages and/or severe hypoxia may also cause ischaemic changes in the white matter around the ventricles, resulting in periventricular cystic leukomalacia (PVL) characterized by cyst formation with major long-term neurological implications (see later discussion and chapter website resources).

Retinopathy of prematurity

Retinopathy of prematurity (ROP) is a disease of the developing retinal blood vessels and is a major complication for preterm babies surviving neonatal intensive care. One major risk factor is oxygen exposure in excessive or fluctuating quantities. This results in retinal hyperoxia, causing normal vascularization to cease, followed by a rebound retinal hypoxia that stimulates the growth of new, abnormal blood vessels in the retina extending into the vitreous body. In advanced stages, opaque, fibrous tissue forms behind the lens in the vitreous body, and retinal detachment may ensue. ROP is one of the few causes of childhood visual impairment that is largely preventable, and therefore regular screening is an essential part of the care of the preterm baby. Many extremely preterm babies will develop some degree of ROP, although this usually does not progress beyond mild disease that resolves spontaneously. Interventions that have been shown to be effective in some cases include cryotherapy and laser photocoagulation. Preventive care involves reducing the incidence of preterm and LBW babies and continuing with high-quality, controlled neonatal intensive care.

Preterm babies are also at particular risk of hearing impairment if they have experienced hypoxia, sepsis or hyperbilirubinemia or have received certain drugs (such as *gentamicin* or *furosemide*). Screening according to national recommendations is essential.

Stress, pain and developmental problems

The neonatal intensive care unit (NICU) is a busy, bright, harsh and noisy environment that could not be further from the circumstances experienced in utero. One of the aims of neonatal care is to achieve similar

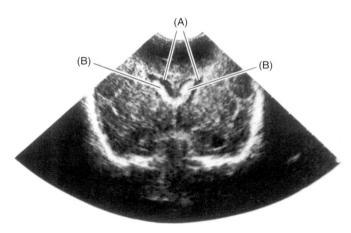

Figure 45.6 Coronal cranial ultrasound showing intraventricular haemorrhages **(B)** in dilated lateral ventricles **(A)**. (Kelnar CJH, Harvey D, Simpson C: The sick newborn baby, 3rd edn. London Baillière Tindall, 1995.)

rates of growth and development of the baby to those that would have been attained in utero, and practitioners need to be aware of the impact of surroundings, interventions, care and treatments undertaken for the baby's well-being.

Developmental care programmes are practised in many units and involve the control of external stimuli, clustering of nursing activities and careful positioning. It is important to communicate these vulnerabilities to the parents and identify strategies to support the baby in the neonatal unit (Westrup 2014). Interventions that are used to minimize the stress of babies and individualize the caregiving according to their tolerance include the following:

- Modification of the environment
- Reductions in the levels of light and noise
- Minimal handling
- Protection of sleep states
- Promotion of understanding of behavioural cues
- Promotion of relationship-based caregiving

Programmes that incorporate these areas in line with the babies' cues can be employed, such as the Newborn Individualised Developmental Care and Assessment Programme (NIDCAP) and the Brazelton Newborn Observational system. Research does appear to demonstrate some benefits of these programmes for preterm babies in terms of short-term growth, decreased respiratory support, decreased length of hospital stay and improved neurological outcomes at 2 years of corrected age (Lubbe et al 2012).

Skin

Regular skin assessment and prevention of damage or undue pressure is essential for the preterm baby because of the immaturity of the skin. Hygiene is also an important care practice to ensure the skin is kept clean and intact. If sufficiently well, the baby should have his or her face, hands, umbilical area and skin folds gently washed with warm water, when necessary. The nappy area needs particular attention because the skin is often friable and breaks down quickly when left in contact with urine or faeces. Oral hygiene is necessary for babies with an endotracheal tube in situ, for those unable to suck and for those receiving tube feeds.

Reflective activity 45.1   ><

Think of a baby you have observed or cared for who was born prematurely. How did the baby differ from a term baby?

LOW BIRTHWEIGHT

Definitions

Babies may be grouped according to their birthweight, which is especially useful when the gestation is unknown. The WHO (2004) definition of low birthweight is internationally adopted, with further subdivisions as follows:

- *Low birthweight* (LBW): lower than 2500 g at birth
- *Very low birthweight* (VLBW): lower than 1500 g at birth
- *Extremely low birthweight* (ELBW): lower than 1000 g at birth
- Large for gestational age (LGA): greater than 90th percentile
- Appropriate for gestational age (AGA): 10th to 90th percentile
- Small for gestational age (SGA): less than 10th percentile
- Intra-uterine growth restriction (IUGR): although this term often is used synonymously with SGA, IUGR specifically refers to a fetus that has not reached its growth potential because of genetic or environmental factors (Haram et al 2006; Giuliano et al 2014). Babies who are IUGR are categorized into two groups according to whether they are affected by asymmetrical or symmetrical growth restriction.

Asymmetrical growth restriction:

Growth is normal until about the third trimester of pregnancy, when complications such as pre-eclampsia develop. This adversely affects placental function, leading to reduced growth resulting from malnutrition. This is a relatively late phenomenon, and the degree of growth restriction depends on the severity of the causative condition. Head circumference and length are within normal limits for the gestational age of the baby, but birthweight is low in proportion to head circumference when plotted on a percentile chart.

Symmetrical growth restriction:

The main underlying causes of symmetrical growth restriction are early intra-uterine infections, such as *cytomegalovirus*, *rubella* or *toxoplasmosis*; maternal substance abuse, such as fetal alcohol syndrome; and other drugs taken early in the pregnancy. These have a toxic or teratogenic effect on the placenta, with fetal growth affected from the time these substances are introduced in the pregnancy. Some chromosomal anomalies and malformations also result in symmetrical SGA babies. The appearance of the baby is similar to that described previously, but the head circumference is in proportion to the overall size and weight. The prognosis for these babies is poorer than that for babies with asymmetrical growth restriction because they have been compromised for a much longer period.

All of these classifications rely on the accurate assessment of gestational age at delivery, as covered earlier in the chapter. Refer to the chapter website for further information on the LBW baby.

Causes of low birthweight

It is not uncommon for preterm babies to also be LBW/ SGA, and many of the predisposing risk factors are the same in both situations:

- Idiopathic – no cause identified
- Placental insufficiency
- Placental dysfunction (spasm of spiral arterioles reduces the intervillous blood flow and exchange of nutrients and oxygen across the placental barrier), which can result from the following conditions:
  - Pre-eclampsia
  - Maternal essential hypertension
  - Chronic renal failure
- Severe anaemia
- Sickle cell disease
- Multiple pregnancy
- Viruses – rubella, toxoplasmosis, cytomegalovirus
- Prescribed drugs, such as some steroids, anticonvulsants, antihypertensives and cytotoxics
- Maternal substance abuse – babies born to substance-abusing mothers are often growth restricted, particularly following the prolonged use of heroin, alcohol and nicotine (Diaz and Smith 2012).
- Low socioeconomic status

Outcomes

Rapid recent developments in neonatology have resulted in the survival of LBW infants above 1500 g becoming a commonplace occurrence. Birthweight, especially in the ELBW group, also has an effect on mortality and morbidity (see chapter website resources). The latest available figures for 2013 show that the overall infant mortality rate was 3.8 deaths per 1000 live births, the lowest ever recorded in England and Wales. This compares with an infant mortality rate of 3.9 deaths per 1000 live births in 2012 and 10.1 deaths per 1000 live births in 1983. In 2013, the infant mortality rates for VLBW babies (under 1500 g) and LBW babies (under 2500 g) were 164.0 and 32.4 deaths per 1000 live births, respectively (Office for National

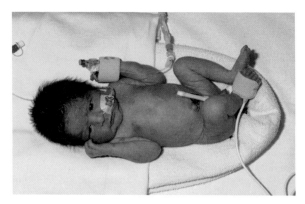

Figure 45.7 Small-for-gestational-age (SGA) baby

Statistics (ONS) 2015). Long-term morbidity is covered later in the chapter.

Characteristics

Figure 45.7 shows an SGA baby. Some of the classic characteristics are as follows:

- The head appears large in relation to the wasted appearance of the body and limbs (and lack of subcutaneous fat).
- The ribs are easily visible.
- The abdomen is hollowed.
- The skin is often dry and loose and may be peeling.
- The skin may be meconium-stained.
- The umbilical cord is thin (may also be meconium-stained).
- Baby often appears wizened and old, with an anxious, wide-awake expression.
- Muscle tone is usually good, and the baby is active.
- The baby will appear ravenously hungry and tends to suck a fist.
- Neurological responses usually correspond to gestational age.

Assessing weight

Using appropriate percentile charts, the weight, head circumference and length of the baby are plotted against gestation, and an assessment is made of the baby's growth. The percentile chart is an important part of providing a dynamic growth record and a link to neonatal management (see Ch. 42). The Royal College of Paediatrics and Child Health (RCPCH 2009) growth charts are based on measurements collected by the WHO in six different countries (Fig. 45.8; also see the chapter website resources). These describe optimal rather than average growth and set breastfeeding as the norm, illustrating how all healthy children are expected to grow.

Problems of the low-birthweight baby

Initial management

A detailed antenatal booking history is essential because this may identify risk factors associated with any type of LBW, regardless of the specific classifications discussed earlier. Careful assessment of uterine size and growth is important to enable early detection of a slow or reducing rate of growth of the fetus, possibly indicating the need for a more detailed assessment of fetal well-being. A great deal of the care required by LBW babies during the first 48 hours following birth centres around prevention and early recognition of any possible complications. In most cases, these babies can be cared for in normal postnatal wards with their mothers and do not need admission to a neonatal intensive or special care unit. Transitional care (TC) wards are an ideal place to care for those babies with minor problems, such as poor temperature control and establishment of feeding.

Labour and delivery

The growth-restricted fetus is chronically hypoxic and consequently tolerates the stresses of labour and delivery

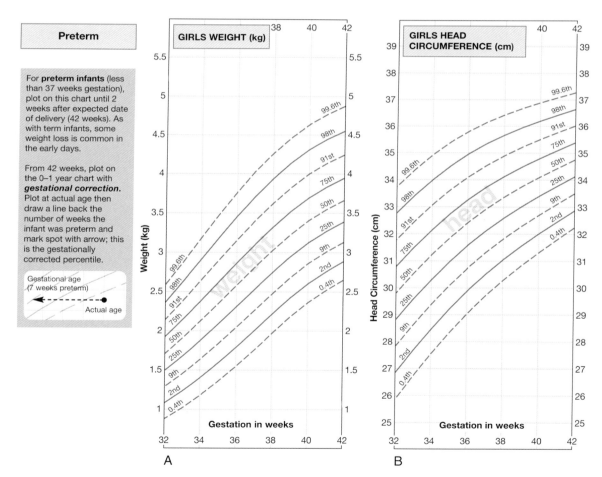

Figure 45.8 World Health Organization (WHO) growth charts, preterm infants. **A,** Weight for preterm infants less than 37 weeks (female). **B,** Girls' head circumference. (By kind permission of RCPCH/WHO/Department of Health 2009 © 2009 Royal College of Paediatrics and Child Health.)

Continued

poorly because the blood supply to the placenta is further interrupted during each contraction. The midwife should anticipate the possibility of fetal distress and perinatal asphyxia. Close fetal monitoring and observation of the liquor for meconium during labour are imperative. A paediatrician, neonatologist or advanced neonatal nurse practitioner (ANNP) should be present at the birth if the baby is known to be significantly small or compromised. Expert and urgent resuscitation is vital if required, particularly if there is meconium-stained liquor. This will prevent further hypoxia and respiratory complications that may result in long-term neurological damage.

Hypothermia

LBW babies may have only a thin layer of subcutaneous fat or be deficient in brown fat, and they have a relatively large surface area; therefore, they lose heat very rapidly.

The room temperature must be raised before birth, and the baby should be dried and wrapped in warm blankets quickly following birth. Because 80% of heat loss occurs through the head, a hat should be placed on the baby once the head is dry. The axillary temperature should be monitored carefully for the first 48 hours, and the baby may be nursed in an incubator next to the mother in the postnatal or TC ward or cared for with skin-to-skin contact with the mother to stabilize the temperature.

If the baby is well enough, early feeding is important to counter hypoglycaemia resulting from insufficient energy stores in these babies.

Hypoglycaemia

Hypoglycaemia is a common problem for LBW babies; in most cases, it can be prevented with early and regular feeding. These babies particularly benefit from

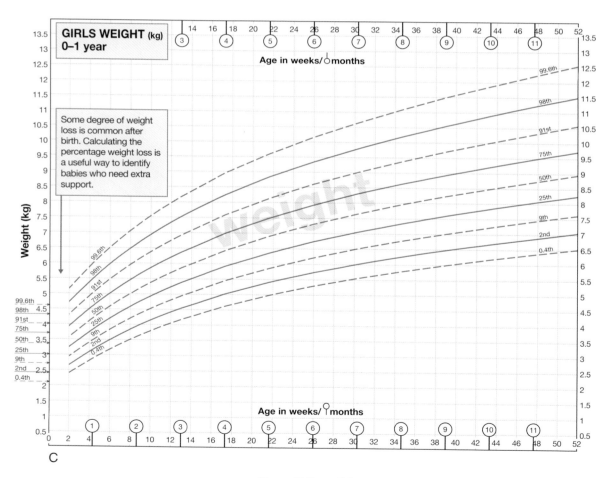

Figure 45.8, cont'd

Figure 45.8, cont'd

breastfeeding, although low-birthweight formulas are widely used and have the advantage of being more energy-dense than regular formula milk. IUGR/SGA babies have small glycogen stores, and their energy reserves are used during labour, particularly if labour is prolonged or difficult. Both hypoxia and hypothermia will exacerbate the problem of hypoglycaemia. Frequent recordings of the blood glucose level are important within the first 48 hours and should be taken at least every 4 hours until they are stable and maintained above 2.6 mmol/L.

Hypoxic ischaemic encephalopathy

A condition associated with the near-term/term baby, hypoxic ischaemic encephalopathy (HIE) can occur in IUGR/SGA babies who have limited reserves to cope with perinatal hypoxic stress and are at high risk of compromise. The midwife must facilitate close and careful monitoring during labour and early intervention to expedite birth in the event of fetal distress. Even modern methods of assessing fetal well-being are relatively insensitive, and the midwife needs to be vigilant. Mild symptoms of HIE may resolve after a few days, with little or no residual cerebral damage. More severe injuries may result in fits and cerebral palsy.

Meconium aspiration syndrome

Because small babies are unable to tolerate perinatal stress and hypoxia, this may cause relaxation of the anal sphincter, allowing meconium to be passed into the liquor and resulting in meconium aspiration syndrome (MAS). It is most common in IUGR/SGA babies with more advanced gestations. See Chapter 46 for the specific care of MAS.

Polycythaemia

Polycythaemia occurs when the venous packed cell volume is raised, and can be as high as 65%. It is a consequence of chronic intra-uterine hypoxia. To improve the oxygen-carrying capacity of the blood, the haemoglobin level may rise to more than 20 g/dL. This can result in jaundice, respiratory distress and possibly cerebral irritation. Treatment may require additional fluids and exchange plasma transfusion.

Poor feeding

Asymmetrically growth-restricted babies tend to feed eagerly and thrive from birth. Symmetrically growth-restricted babies, however, who have been starved for a prolonged period in utero, often continue the slow rate of growth postnatally and may remain small, although a degree of catch-up growth is often evident. Feeding is covered in more detail on the chapter website, under "Feeding the preterm baby" because the principles are the same for both groups of babies.

Reflective activity 45.2

Think about a baby you may have observed or cared for who was born at term or near term but was growth restricted (and thus small for gestational age). What were the potential reasons for this situation, and what did you need to consider for the newborn's initial care?

LONG-TERM COMPLICATIONS IN THE PRETERM AND LOW-BIRTH-WEIGHT BABY

As noted earlier in the chapter, extreme prematurity and ELBW can cause perinatal death, and thus it is extremely important to effectively prevent and/or reduce the occurrence whenever possible. Turning now to morbidity, babies born prematurely, at ELBW or both are at higher risk of complications in the neonatal period and for later neurodevelopmental problems (Blackburn 2013). This is supported by a significant body of research (Morsing et al 2011; Moore et al 2012; Marlow et al 2014; Boyle et al 2015; EPICure 2014; see also the chapter website resources). Antenatal and perinatal factors that influence fetal outcome include gestational age; predicted and actual fetal weight/birthweight; steroid administration; multiple pregnancy; gender; sepsis; presence and severity of any pathology; fetal growth restriction with abnormal Doppler flow studies; and fetal distress, hypoxia and/or complications at the time of birth.

Collectively, preterm and ELBW babies have an increased risk of the following compared with term babies:

- Sudden infant death syndrome (SIDS)
- Major disabilities
- Motor deficits and poorer cognitive skills

- Neurological abnormalities
- Long-term oxygen requirement
- ROP, hearing loss
- PVL leading to cerebral palsy
- Post-bleed hydrocephalus
- Chronic lung disease
- Coronary heart disease and strokes in adult life

Overall, with recent advances and developments in neonatal care, babies above 28 to 30 weeks gestation and above 1000 to 1500 g now have a much greater chance of intact survival than previously. However, for those at extremes of prematurity and/or ELBW who are discharged from the hospital, the risk of some degree of long-term morbidity needs to be considered and factored into any follow-up for the baby and family.

The paediatrician/neonatologist usually follows up preterm and LBW babies after discharge from the hospital to assess progress, development and general condition. Midwives, health visitors and general practitioners see the baby more frequently and play a crucial role in monitoring for and recognizing associated complications or deviations from normal development. Symmetrically growth-restricted and neurologically damaged babies need particularly close follow-up for several years in paediatric outpatient clinics. Other specific areas also require monitoring; for example, hearing must be carefully checked, and most neonatal units perform hearing tests routinely for preterm, sick and SGA babies. Specialist neonatal liaison nurses or midwives may be a service available to monitor these small babies in the community, offering outreach advice and support to the parents and other health professionals. This develops continuity of advice and prevents readmission to the hospital through early recognition and treatment of minor problems. Refer to the chapter website for further information on the long-term complications in these groups of babies.

Reflective activity 45.3

Consider how being born early or small, or both, can affect the baby and parents in the short and long term.

CARING FOR THE FAMILY OF THE PRETERM OR LOW-BIRTH-WEIGHT BABY

The admission of a sick or vulnerable baby to the TC ward or neonatal unit poses a significant stressor to parents. Many preterm and LBW babies are in the hospital for several weeks or months before they are ready to be discharged home. Midwives are a key part of the team providing care to these small babies and their parents, and they need to work closely with their colleagues to ensure a seamless, sensitive and high-quality service both initially and on a long-term basis. There must be good communication between the neonatal unit and the postnatal ward staff to ensure the family members receive the support they need in addition to ongoing collaboration with the MDT.

Parents must have an opportunity to see and hold their baby, however briefly, before transfer to the neonatal unit. A mother is likely to feel anxious and inadequate in a postnatal ward, especially when surrounded by other mothers who have their babies beside them. It is common for parents to display signs of grief at this time as they mourn the healthy baby they expected.

Many mothers feel extremely guilty when they give birth to a preterm or LBW baby, often blaming themselves for actions taken or omitted during the pregnancy. Midwives must offer as much support as possible during these times. Individuals react differently to stress, and midwives and neonatal staff need to learn to recognize the signs in parents and develop appropriate skills to enable families to cope during this difficult time. They must also recognize the signs of stress in themselves and in colleagues. Opportunities to share and discuss problems can be of immense benefit to all concerned. Effective personal coping strategies are therefore essential for those working with families who have preterm, sick and LBW babies.

Parents and siblings should be encouraged to become involved in their baby's care as much as possible, from the earliest days, even if the baby is being ventilated. During the time spent on the neonatal unit, the parents participate in an increasing amount of their baby's care, with support, and will gradually gain confidence. Before discharge, it is helpful for the mother/parents to stay in the hospital to care for the baby day and night on the neonatal unit or in a TC ward.

Finally, complex and difficult ethical issues arise in the care of extremely preterm and VLBW babies, especially when complications substantially increasing the risk of long-term handicap arise. During the period of care, difficult decisions arise when the baby is surviving solely because of the supportive care being given, yet the risk of handicap is known to be extremely high. Professionals and parents then need time to discuss the situation openly, and they need to be given support and guidance as early as possible (Royal College of Obstetricians and Gynaecologists 2014). Space is required to reflect on the possible consequences of continuing full intensive care for as long as it is required or of withdrawing such care to allow the baby to die in peace and dignity. This is one of the most agonizing and difficult decisions both parents and professionals have to face. Cultural factors and personal values and beliefs are deeply challenged at times like this and will influence the decisions made. Sometimes, parents

appreciate the opportunity to discuss the situation with a minister of religion or with a counsellor who is not directly involved in the care of their baby. Such help can be invaluable during this extremely stressful period (see Ch. 68). Refer to the chapter website for further information on the care of parents of preterm and LBW babies.

> **Reflective activity 45.4**
>
> What types of support do parents of babies born prematurely or small need? What support facilities are available in your locality?

CONCLUSION

Preterm and LBW babies present a range of specific problems and challenges to the MDT, within which midwives play an essential part. Care for the parents of these groups of babies starts during pregnancy and continues through labour and beyond; therefore, midwives are ideally placed to be part of the whole process, from antenatal through postnatal care and support. This chapter has discussed the definitions, outcomes, causes and specific problems of both preterm and LBW babies, identifying specific issues to each group but also acknowledging that these can overlap, and the principles of care are often the same. Finally, because these babies may present with both short- and long-term challenges, it is vital that these challenges are understood in line with the latest research. Strategies should be employed to prevent the occurrence of preterm birth and/or poor fetal and/or postnatal growth leading to LBW. However, although much research is ongoing, preterm and LBW babies continue to present to us in healthcare, and so the best care possible must be delivered in line with the evidence-based care principles outlined in this chapter.

> **Key Points**
>
> - The causes, characteristics and associated problems of the preterm and low birthweight baby are closely linked.
>
> - It is essential to be mindful of the short- and long-term health outcomes of these groups of babies and to aim to reduce the risk of complications associated with their early gestation and/or small size.
>
> - Parents who have a preterm or LBW baby will require much support from the midwife, both practical and psychological. Close liaison between the multidisciplinary team within the hospital and community staff is vital.

References

Balain M, Oddie S: Management of apnoea and bradycardia in the newborn, *Paediatr Child Health* 24(1):17–22, 2014.

Ballard JL, Khoury JC, Wedig K, et al: New Ballard score, expanded to include extremely premature infants, *J Pediatr* 119(3):417–423, 1991.

Blackburn ST: *Maternal, fetal and neonatal physiology: a clinical perspective*, 4th edn, Philadelphia, WB Saunders, 2013.

Bolton CE, et al: The EPICure study: association between hemodynamics and lung function at 11 years after extremely preterm birth, *J Pediatr* 161(4):595–601, 2012.

Boyle EM, Johnson S, Manktelow B, et al: Neonatal outcomes and delivery of care for infants born late preterm or moderately preterm: a prospective population-based study, *Arch Dis Child Fetal Neonatal Ed* (website). http://fn.bmj.com/content/early/2015/04/01/archdischild-2014-307347.full. 2015.

Cherian S, Morris I, Evans J, et al: Oxygen therapy in preterm infants, *Paediatr Respir Rev* 15(2):135–141, 2014.

Cilieborg MS, Boye M, Sangild PT: Bacterial colonization and gut development in preterm neonates, *Early Hum Dev* 88:S41–S49, 2012.

Clyman RI: Mechanisms facilitating closure of the ductus arteriosus. In Polin RA, Fox WW, Abman SH, editors: *Fetal and neonatal physiology*, 4th edn, Philadelphia, Saunders, 2011.

Costeloe KL, Hennessy EM, Haider S, et al: Short-term outcomes after extreme preterm birth in England: comparison of 2 birth cohorts in 1995 and 2006 (the EPICure Studies), *Obstetric Anesthesia Digest* 34(1):38, 2014.

Darnell RA, Ariagno RL, Kinney HC: The late preterm infant and the control of breathing, sleep and brainstem development: a review, *Clin Perinatol* 33(4):883–914, 2006.

Diaz SD, Smith LM: Drug exposure and intrauterine growth. In Preedy VR, editor: *Handbook of growth and growth monitoring in health and disease*, New York, Springer, 2012.

Dubowitz LMS, Dubowitz V, Goldberg C: Clinical assessment of gestational age in the newborn infant, *J Pediatr* 77(1):1–10, 1970.

Embleton ND: Optimal nutrition for preterm infants: putting the ESPGHAN guidelines into practice, *J Neonatal Nurs* 19(4):130–133, 2013.

EPICure: *EPICure@19* (website). www.epicure.ac.uk/epicure-1995/epicure 19. 2014.

Goldenberg RL, Culhane JF, Iams JD, et al: Epidemiology and causes of preterm birth, *Lancet* 371(9606):75–84, 2008.

Giuliano N, Annunziata ML, Tagliaferri S, et al: IUGR management: new perspectives, *J Pregnancy* (website). www.hindawi.com/journals/jp/2014/620976/. 2014.

Haram K, Softeland E, Bukowski R: Intrauterine growth restriction, *Int J Gynaecol Obstet* 93(1):5–12, 2006.

Hartnett ME, Penn JS: Mechanisms and management of retinopathy of prematurity, *N Engl J Med* 367(26):2515–2526, 2012.

Hawdon JM: Definition of neonatal hypoglycaemia: time for a rethink? *Arch Dis Child Fetal Neonatal Ed* 98(5):F382–F383, 2013.

Ives NK: Management of neonatal jaundice, *Paediatr Child Health* 25(6):276–281, 2015.

Kuschel CA, Harding JE: Multicomponent fortified human milk for promoting growth in preterm infants, *Cochrane Database Syst Rev* (1):CD000343, 2004.

Lubbe W, Van der Walt CS, Klopper HC: Integrative literature review defining evidence-based neurodevelopmental supportive care of the preterm infant, *J Perinat Neonatal Nurs* 26(3):251–259, 2012.

Manktelow BM, Smith LK, Evans TA, et al; on behalf of the MBRRACE-UK collaboration: *Perinatal mortality surveillance report UK perinatal deaths for births from January to December 2013*, Leicester, Department of Health Sciences, University of Leicester, 2015.

Marlow N: Keeping up with outcomes for infants born at extremely low gestational ages, *JAMA Pediatr* 69(3):207–208, 2015.

Marlow N, Bennett C, Draper ES, et al: Perinatal outcomes for extremely preterm babies in relation to place of birth in England: the EPICure 2 study, *Arch Dis Child Fetal Neonatal Ed* (website). http://fn.bmj.com/content/early/2014/03/06/archdischild-2013-305555.full?g=w_adc_open_tab. 2014.

Moore T, Hennessy EM, Myles J, et al: Neurological and developmental outcome in extremely preterm children born in England in 1995 and 2006: the EPICure studies, *Br Med J* 345:E7961, 2012.

Morsing E, Åsard M, Ley D, et al: Cognitive function after intrauterine growth restriction and very preterm birth, *Pediatrics* 127(4):e874–e882, 2011.

National Institute for Health and Care Excellence (NICE): *Neonatal jaundice* (website). www.nice.org.uk/guidance/cg98. 2010.

Neiva FC, Leone CR, Leone C, et al: Non-nutritive sucking evaluation in preterm newborns and the start of oral feeding: a multicenter study, *Clinics* 69(6):393–397, 2014.

Nyqvist KH, Häggkvist AP, Hansen MN, et al: Expansion of the Baby-Friendly Hospital Initiative Ten Steps to Successful Breastfeeding into Neonatal Intensive Care Expert Group recommendations, *J Hum Lact* 29(3):300–309, 2013.

Office for National Statistics (ONS): *Pregnancy and ethnic factors influencing births and infant mortality* (website). www.ons.gov.uk. 2015.

Oras P, Blomqvist YT, Nyqvist KH, et al: Breastfeeding patterns in preterm infants born at 28–33 gestational weeks, *J Hum Lact* 31(3):377–385, 2015.

Painter SL, Wilkinson AR, Desai P, et al: Incidence and treatment of retinopathy of prematurity in England between 1990 and 2011: database study, *Br J Ophthalmol* 99(6):807–811, 2014.

Pinelli J, Symington A: Non-nutritive sucking for promoting physiologic stability and nutrition in preterm infants, *Cochrane Database Syst Rev* (4):CD001071, 2005 (updated 2010).

Renfrew MJ, Dyson L, McCormick F, et al: Breastfeeding promotion for infants in neonatal units: a systematic review, *Child Care Health Dev* 36(2):165–178, 2010.

Royal College of Obstetricians and Gynaecologists: *Perinatal management of pregnant women at the threshold of infant viability – the obstetric perspective (Scientific Impact Paper No. 41)* (website). www .rcog.org.uk/en/guidelines-research -services/guidelines/sip41/. 2014.

Royal College of Paediatrics and Child Health (RCPCH): *UK-WHO growth charts – early years* (website). www.rcpch.ac.uk/Research/ UK-WHO-Growth-Charts. 2009.

Schreiner C, Suter S, Watzka M, et al: Genetic variants of the vitamin K dependent coagulation system and intraventricular hemorrhage in preterm infants, *BMC Pediatr* 14(1):219, 2014.

Simmons R, Stanley C: Neonatal hypoglycemia studies – is there a sweet story of success yet?, *N Engl J Med* 373(16):1567–1569, 2015.

Smith V: Prophylactic phototherapy for preventing jaundice in preterm or low birth weight infants, *Pract Midwife* 16(2):35–37, 2013.

Stenson BJ, Tarnow-Mordi WO, Darlow BA, et al: BOOST II United Kingdom collaborative group, BOOST II Australia collaborative group, BOOST II New Zealand collaborative group. Oxygen saturation and outcomes in preterm infants, *N Engl J Med* 368(22):2094–2104, 2013.

Tambe P, Sammons HM, Choonara I: Why do young children die in the UK? A comparison with Sweden, *Arch Dis Child* (website). http:// adc.bmj.com/content/early/2015/ 07/15/archdischild-2014308059 .short?g=w_adc_ahead_tab. 2015.

Tin W: Defining neonatal hypoglycaemia: a continuing debate, *Semin Fetal Neonatal Med* 19(1):27– 32, 2014.

Tommy's: *Premature birth statistics* (website). www.tommys.org/Page .aspx?pid=362. 2015.

UK Resuscitation Council: *Resuscitation and support of transition of babies at birth*, London, UK Resuscitation Council, 2015.

UNICEF: *Guidance on the development of policies and guidelines for the prevention and management of hypoglycaemia* (website). www .unicef.org.uk/Documents/Baby _Friendly/Guidance/hypo_policy .pdf. 2013a.

UNICEF: *Off to the best start* (website). http://www.unicef.org.uk/ BabyFriendly/Health-Professionals/. 2013b.

Westrup B: Family-centered developmentally supportive care, *Neoreviews* 15(8):e325–e335, 2014.

World Health Organization (WHO): *Low birth weight; country, regional and global estimates* (website). http://apps.who.int/iris/bitstream /10665/43184/1/9280638327.pdf. 2004.

World Health Organization (WHO): *Born too soon: the global action report on preterm birth* (website). www .who.int/pmnch/media/news/ 2012/borntoosoon_chapter2.pdf. 2012.

Resources and additional reading

Books

Boxwell G, editor: *Neonatal intensive care nursing*, 2nd edn, London, Routledge, 2010.

Gardner SL, Carter BS: *Handbook of neonatal intensive care*, 8th edn, London, Mosby, 2015.

Lissaur T, Faneroff AA: *Neonatology at a glance*, 3rd edn, Oxford, Blackwell Science Ltd, 2015.

Meeks M, Hallsworth M, Yeo H: *Nursing the neonate*, 2nd edn, Oxford, Wiley/Blackwell, 2009.

Petty J: *Bedside guide for neonatal care: learning tools to support practice*, London, Palgrave Macmillan, 2015.

Sinha SK, Miall L, Jardine L: *Essential neonatal medicine*, 5th edn, Oxford, Wiley Blackwell, 2012.

Williamson A, Crozier K: *Neonatal care: a textbook for student midwives and nurses*, Exeter, Reflect Press, 2008.

Useful websites:

Ballard assessment tool: www.ballardscore.com/.

Bamfo JE, Odibo AO: Diagnosis and management of fetal growth restriction, *J Pregnancy* (website). www.ncbi.nlm.nih.gov/pmc/articles/ PMC3087156/. 2011.

BLISS Baby Charity: www.bliss.org.uk/.

Boyle EM, Johnson S, Manktelow B, et al: Neonatal outcomes and delivery of care for infants born late preterm or moderately preterm: a prospective population-based study, *Arch Dis Child Fetal Neonatal Ed* (website). http://fn.bmj.com/ content/early/2015/04/01/ archdischild-2014-307347.full. 2015.

Campbell MK, Cartier S, Xie B, et al: Determinants of small for gestational age birth at term, *Paediatr Perinat Epidemiol* 26:525– 533 (website). doi: 10.1111/j.1365 -3016.2012.01319.x. http:// onlinelibrary.wiley.com/doi/10.1111/ j.1365-3016.2012.01319.x/full. 2012.

Crume TL, Scherzinger A, Stamm E, et al: The long-term impact of intrauterine growth restriction in a diverse US cohort of children: the EPOCH study, *Obesity (Silver Spring)* 22(2):608–615 (website). www.ncbi.nlm.nih.gov/pmc/articles/ PMC4437590/. 2014.

Furdon SA: *Prematurity treatment and management* (website). http:// emedicine.medscape.com/ article/975909-treatment. 2014.

Manktelow BM, Smith LK, Evans TA, et al; on behalf of the MBRRACE-UK collaboration: *Perinatal Mortality Surveillance Report UK Perinatal Deaths for births from January to December 2013* (website). www.npeu.ox.ac.uk/downloads/ files/mbrrace-uk/reports/ MBRRACE-UK%20Perinatal%20 Surveillance%20Report%20 2013.pdf. 2015.

Moore T, Hennessy EM, Myles J, et al: Neurological and developmental outcome in extremely preterm children born in England in 1995 and 2006: the EPICure studies, *Br Med J* 345:E7961 (website). www.bmj.com/content/345/ bmj.e7961. 2012.

Petty J: *Knowledge for neonatal nursing practice: a self-directed learning tool* (website). www.cetl.org.uk/

learning/neonatal/unit_3e/
player.html. 2012.

POPPY Study Group: *Family-centred care
in neonatal units: a summary of
research results and recommendations
from the POPPY Project* (website).
www.poppy-project.org.uk/
resources/Poppy+report+for+PRINT
.pdf. 2009.

Royal College of Paediatrics and Child
Health (RCPCH): *UK-WHO growth
charts – early years* (website).
www.rcpch.ac.uk/Research/
UK-WHO-Growth-Charts. 2015.

Royal College of Paediatrics and Child
Health (RCPCH): *Neonatal and
infant close monitoring growth chart
(NICM)* (website).

www.rcpch.ac.uk/system/files/
protected/page/NICM%20FACT%20
SHEET.pdf. 2011.

Tambe P, Sammons HM, Choonara I:
Why do young children die in the
UK? A comparison with Sweden,
Arch Dis Child (website). http://
adc.bmj.com/content/early/2015/
07/15/archdischild-2014-308059
.short?g=w_adc_ahead_tab. 2015.

Tommy's: *Explaining preterm birth*
(website). www.tommys.org/
page.aspx?pid=961. 2014.

UNICEF: *Benefits of skin to skin for
preterm babies* (website).
www.unicef.org.uk/BabyFriendly/
Health-Professionals/going-baby
-friendly/FAQs/Breastfeeding

-FAQ/Benefits-of-skin-to-skin
-contact-for-preterm-babies-/.
2010.

UNICEF: *Prevention and treatment of
hypoglycaemia in the newborn*
(website). www.unicef.org.uk/
Documents/Baby_Friendly/
Guidance/hypo_policy.pdf.
2013.

Waldron S, Mackinnon R: Neonatal
thermoregulation, *Infant* 3(3):101–
104 (website). www.neonatal
-nursing.co.uk/pdf/inf_015_nor.pdf.
2007.

World Health Organization (WHO):
Preterm birth: fact sheet (website).
www.who.int/mediacentre/
factsheets/fs363/en. 2014.

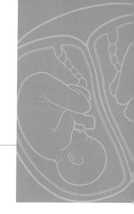

Chapter **46**

Respiratory and cardiac disorders

Julia Petty

Learning Outcomes ?

After reading this chapter, you will be able to:

- link knowledge of fetal circulation with transitional changes necessary at birth to adapt to extrauterine life
- discuss the key actions in resuscitating newborn babies who present with respiratory and/or cardiovascular compromise at birth
- relate fetal cardiac and respiratory development to the existence of related pathology in the respiratory and cardiac systems
- describe the actions that a midwife should undertake to detect and care for common respiratory and cardiac disorders

INTRODUCTION

This chapter provides an overview of fetal anatomy and physiology with a specific focus on the cardiac and respiratory systems, both normal and abnormal, relating the latter to resuscitation of the newborn. The chapter also offers an overview of some of the common respiratory and cardiac disorders midwives may encounter in practice.

Respiratory disorders comprise a significant proportion of admissions to the neonatal unit (NNU) following delivery, and congenital heart disease (CHD) is the most common serious congenital abnormality in neonates (Lawford and Tulloh 2015). Because midwives are taking on greater responsibility for the care of the newborn at birth and in the postnatal period, they need to be able to understand common conditions and to be able to respond to the challenge of resuscitating newborn babies. It is also very important for them to assess babies to confirm normality and detect abnormality and to be part of the process

of stabilizing sick babies while awaiting transfer to tertiary facilities.

NORMAL RESPIRATORY AND CARDIAC DEVELOPMENT

Midwives need to appreciate respiratory and cardiac development in utero because this facilitates understanding of normal adaptation at birth. It provides a basis for care provision in specific respiratory and cardiac disorders, as is discussed later.

Respiratory development

Fetal lungs are filled with fluid secreted by the lungs, rather than amniotic fluid. This fluid is important in facilitating the maturation and development of the fetal lungs. Approximately 300–350 mL of fetal lung fluid is produced daily by the fetus at term. In utero, it can move up the trachea, where some is swallowed by the fetus and some escapes into the amniotic fluid. At birth, a small amount of this fluid drains from the nose, but most is moved out of the alveoli into the lymphatic system with the first breaths (Greenough and Milner 2012). *Fetal breathing movements* are rapid, irregular movements, which may be seen on ultrasound as early as 10 weeks gestation. The strength and frequency of fetal breathing movements increase with gestational age (see Table 46.1). By the third trimester, breathing movements can be detected about 30% of the time, at a rate of 30 to 70 breaths per minute (bpm). It is thought that fetal breathing movements are important in enhancing lung development and growth. Fetal breathing patterns can be altered during periods of hypoxia, sometimes ceasing for several hours. Monitoring of fetal breathing movements by ultrasound is used as part of biophysical profiling to assess fetal well-being.

Table 46.1 Respiratory development in the fetus

Postconception time frame	Features of development
3–6 weeks	Fetal lungs start to develop from the foregut. The division of the foregut and the respiratory system is complete by the end of this period. Disruption at this time can lead to abnormalities such as tracheo-oesophageal fistula (Blackburn 2013).
7–16 weeks	Respiratory system continues to grow and differentiate.
16 weeks	Tracheobronchial tree is formed. Cilia and mucus-producing glands are present.
16–26 weeks	Primitive bronchioles start to develop rich vascular network required for gaseous exchange in extrauterine life.
20–24 weeks	Lung is lined with epithelium composed of *type I and type II pneumocytes*. Type II pneumocytes start to appear. Type II pneumocytes produce *surfactant,* a pulmonary lipoprotein that decreases surface tension, thus reducing the work of breathing. As gestational age increases, more surfactant is synthesized (Blackburn 2013).
24 weeks	Vascular system proliferates. Vascular system proliferation leads to thinning of the vascular epithelium, and the capillaries come into close contact with the developing airways – eventually becoming the *blood–gas barrier.*
26 weeks onwards	Terminal air sacs appear, which then develop into the alveoli. Note: Despite the lack of alveoli in babies born between 24 and 26 weeks gestation, the vascular bed is sufficient to allow some gaseous exchange, and this can, with support, sustain extrauterine life (Wert 2011).
29–35 weeks	Proliferation of alveoli starts and increases dramatically (Wert 2011). Development of alveoli continues after birth.
30 weeks onwards	Significant increase occurs in total lung surface and lung volume.
35 weeks	Fetus has sufficient surfactant and functional alveoli to support extrauterine life.

Cardiac development

The cardiovascular system is the first system to develop in the embryo. The rapidly developing embryo requires an efficient and effective way of transporting oxygen and nutrients and excreting waste products (Blackburn 2013). The heart begins to develop at around 3 weeks following conception, at first appearing like two long strands. These then undergo a process known as canalization to become two hollow endocardial tubes, which fold back on themselves and fuse to become a single tube. This becomes the *endocardium*. The tissue around the outside of the endocardial tube becomes thicker and eventually becomes the *myocardium*.

The single tube is essentially upside down at this stage, with the structures that will become the atria at the lower *(caudal)* end and the ventricular structures at the upper *(cephalic)* end. By 22 days following conception, the single cardiac tube starts to beat and blood moves from the bottom of the tube to the top. As the heart enlarges, it has to fold back on itself to be accommodated. As the tube folds from top to bottom, it twists around so that the single atrium moves to the cephalic position and the single ventricle moves to the caudal position. Between the fourth to sixth weeks following conception, septation occurs and divides the atrium and ventricle into two. During the septation process, the *foramen ovale* is formed, enabling movement of blood between the atria.

The process of cardiac development is complex, must take place in a specific sequence over a very short period of time and is controlled by cardiac genes. Alterations in the genetic material can lead to failure in development or altered growth patterns, giving rise to congenital cardiac malformations.

The fetal circulation

The placenta provides the fetus with oxygen and nutrients and also disposes of waste products. To achieve this, the fetal circulation has a number of unique features, including temporary structures to allow shunting of blood, allowing the mixing of oxygenated and deoxygenated blood, high pulmonary vascular resistance and a low systemic circulation (see Ch. 29 and chapter website resources).

The temporary structures are as follows:

- Ductus venosus
- Foramen ovale
- Ductus arteriosus
- Hypogastric arteries

Transition to extrauterine life

At birth, the newborn infant is exposed to changes in temperature and tactile stimulation, which with the hypoxic and hypercapnic changes that take place as labour progresses, stimulates the first breath. This breath inflates the lungs and forces the fetal lung fluid out into the lymphatic system (Bhutani 2012). Pulmonary vascular resistance decreases dramatically, and the pressure in the right side of the heart falls. Because gas exchange now occurs in the lungs, alveolar oxygenation concentration levels increase.

The dramatic fall in pulmonary vascular resistance and the increase in oxygen concentration facilitate the closure of the ductus arteriosus. Blood flows from the lungs to the left atrium, increasing the pressure in the left side of the heart and causing the flap-like opening of the foramen ovale to close. Blood then passes from the left atrium to the left ventricle and from there into the aorta. Clamping of the umbilical cord prevents blood flowing back into the placenta, and this increases the systemic circulatory pressure. The reduced blood flow through the umbilical cord vessels causes constriction of the ductus venosus. The changes in the temporary structures may take some time to become permanent. It is recommended that auscultation of the neonate's heart to elicit cardiac murmurs should be delayed until at least 6 hours after birth to allow for the closure of the ductus arteriosus and the foramen ovale (Onuzo 2006). Therefore, timing of cardiovascular assessment needs consideration (Carr and Foster 2014; Bedford and Lomax 2015).

Normal neonatal circulation and respiratory function

A normal term baby has a heart rate of over 100 beats per minute (bpm) (range 100–160), a respiratory rate of between 20 and 60 breaths per minute (bpm) and a mean blood pressure that equates with the baby's gestational age in weeks. Breathing is effortless and quiet. Chest movement should be equal on both sides of the chest. The mucous membranes should be pink. The expected oxygen saturation level in a newborn baby is 95–99% (Røsvik et al 2009). Infants should be well perfused and warm to touch, with adequate capillary refill and urine output (see Ch. 42 and chapter website resources).

Reflective Activity 46.1

From what you have read about normal respiratory and cardiac development in this and previous chapters, consider the key differences between *fetal* and *postnatal* circulation and lung function.

Compromised fetal cardiac and respiratory development

Having looked at the normal processes of development, it is now necessary to consider what happens during compromise of the fetus, to lead to an understanding of why resuscitation may be necessary and what conditions might be identified at birth. Fetal development can be interrupted or influenced by various adverse conditions. These comprise, for example, congenital infection, prolonged hypoxia, maternal disease, poor nutrition, radiation, drugs and other chemicals that may have a *teratogenic* effect – that is, interrupting normal fetal development.

Compromised transitional circulation at birth

The changes at birth highlighted earlier may be hindered in the adverse conditions listed previously; hence *fetal circulation* does not change over to the *neonatal circulation*, and the lungs do not start to receive blood for oxygenation. Some babies are less likely to make a successful transition to extrauterine life. Preterm infants may experience difficulty in establishing adequate lung volume or oxygenation because of poor muscle tone or lack of surfactant. Hypoxia can cause the ductus arteriosus to remain patent, particularly in preterm infants. Babies born at term by elective caesarean section are more likely to encounter problems in clearing fetal lung fluid because of the lack of stress response associated with labour. This can lead to the development of transient tachypnoea of the newborn, which is discussed shortly (Jain and Eaton 2006) along with other examples of abnormal conditions requiring specific management.

Abnormal neonatal cardiac and respiratory function

Signs of cardiac and respiratory compromise may include the following:

- Increased respiratory rate
- Apnoeic episodes
- Grunting – where the baby tries to exhale against a closed glottis to retain air in the alveoli
- Nasal flaring
- Sternal and intercostal recession – as the baby uses the accessory muscles of respiration to improve oxygenation
- Peripheral or central cyanosis
- Tachycardia or bradycardia
- Hypotension
- Poor perfusion
- Prolonged capillary refill time

    (See chapter website resources.)

Any baby showing signs of respiratory compromise should be carefully observed and monitored after transfer to a neonatal unit. For midwives working in community maternity units and birth centres, it may be necessary to care for the baby for several hours until specialist assistance arrives. Oxygen saturation monitoring should be used if available. The baby's respiratory rate should be assessed or monitored on a continual basis. To facilitate observation of the baby's respiratory function and temperature, the baby should be nursed naked in an incubator.

If the baby has a rapid respiratory rate, breastfeeding or formula feeding may be difficult and may increase the risk of aspiration. Nasogastric feeding of small volumes of milk may be possible, although a full stomach pressing on the diaphragm may cause respiratory compromise. If this occurs, enteral feeds are withheld and intravenous fluids given by an umbilical venous cannula to maintain glycaemic control.

Reflective Activity 46.2

Think about *normal* fetal circulation – then consider how this would affect the baby if the transition to postnatal life does *not* occur normally.

RESUSCITATION OF THE NEWBORN

Although *hypoxia* is a stimulus for the onset of breathing at birth, *profound hypoxia* can depress the respiratory centre in the brain and prevent or inhibit the successful transition to extrauterine life. Neonatal hypoxia may be characterized by the absence of breathing or by the presence of profound irregular gasping movements. It has been suggested that *primary apnoea* is caused by a period of acute hypoxia. During this period, breathing ceases. Initially the heart rate remains the same, but it soon falls to about 60 beats per minute (bpm). If steps are not taken to correct the hypoxia, primitive spinal centres take over and produce deep, irregular agonal gasps. Eventually the lack of oxygen causes cessation of cardiac activity, and the baby enters *terminal apnoea*. At birth it is not possible to tell which stage the baby has reached, so the approach to newborn resuscitation is the same in all of these situations.

The need for resuscitation may be anticipated in certain situations, such as intrapartum hypoxia and fetal distress, fetal cord accidents, fetal–maternal transfusion, meconium-stained or reduced liquor volume, congenital abnormalities (e.g. diaphragmatic hernia), infection, drugs (e.g. opiates) and preterm babies. However, the need for resuscitation is not always predictable; therefore, all midwives must have skills in resuscitation of the newborn following the Newborn Life Support (NLS) guidelines from the UK Resuscitation Council (UKRC 2015) – see Box 46.1 for a summary of the NLS algorithm and the chapter website resources for full details. Both outline the correct steps and further information on the central points.

As well as familiarizing oneself with the NLS algorithm, it is also important to be prepared for the need for resuscitation at any time. The necessary equipment for newborn resuscitation needs to be prepared for every birth as described in Box 46.2. See the chapter website resources for recommended home-birth equipment. When the need for complex resuscitation is anticipated, appropriate help should be summoned.

Thermal control during resuscitation is important to prevent hypothermia and any hypoxic event being exacerbated by cold stress. Babies are delivered into an environment that is considerably colder than the intra-uterine environment, they are wet and have a large surface area (see Ch. 43). This means that they cool quickly. They can lose heat through *conduction, convection, evaporation* and *radiation*. Term babies should be dried and wrapped in warm towels to prevent heat loss.

Preterm babies may be placed in a plastic bag (without drying) and placed under a radiant heat source. This method has been shown to dramatically reduce evaporative heat loss (McCall et al 2010). However, this should not be used in the community. The lack of a reliable heat source when this method is used cools the baby and increases the risk of cold stress.

Assessment is an essential part of the initial stages to guide subsequent actions. See the chapter website resources for the key questions to answer in relation to colour, tone,

Box 46.1 Newborn life support (NLS) algorithm (Courtesy of UK Resuscitation Council)

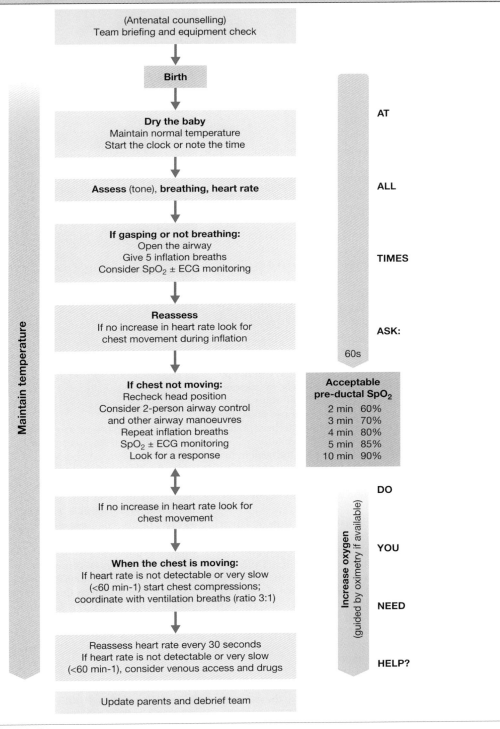

Box 46.2 Equipment for neonatal resuscitation

- Flat, stable surface
- Clock with second hand
- Stethoscope
- Light
- Heat source
- Oxygen supply
- Suction and catheters
- Towels or blankets (warmed)
- Plastic bag for preterm births (in hospital)
- 500-mL self-inflating bag with a pressure-limiting device (e.g. Laerdal)
- Oxygen reservoir attachment for self-inflating bags
- T-connector and tubing
- Size 00 and 01 masks with conformable face piece
- Guedel airways size 0, 00 and 000
- Laryngoscope – for suction under direct vision
- Endotracheal tubes 2.5, 3.0 and 3.5
- Nasogastric tubes size 8 and 10 fine gauge (FG)
- 2-mL, 5-mL and 10-mL syringes
- 21-FG and 25 FG needles

   For the recommended equipment for a home birth specifically, refer to the chapter website resources.

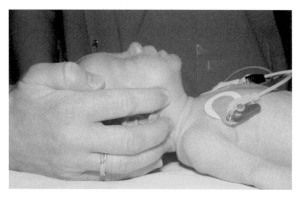

Figure 46.1 Neutral position. (Reproduced with the kind permission of the Resuscitation Council (UK).)

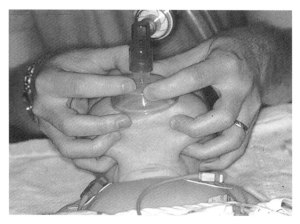

Figure 46.2 Two-person jaw thrust. (Reproduced with the kind permission of the Resuscitation Council (UK).)

breathing and heart rate. A baby who is blue and floppy with a heart rate above 100 bpm is likely to respond quickly to airway opening and minimal resuscitative measures. A baby who is pale, floppy and not breathing with a slow heart rate (<60 bpm) is likely to be seriously compromised and in need of urgent resuscitation.

Airway management is undertaken with the head in the neutral position (Fig. 46.1). Various airway-opening manoeuvres can be used, such as the *jaw thrust* with one hand or two (Fig. 46.2), suction under direct vision or the use of a Guedel airway.

Breathing is supported initially with slow inflation breaths using either a T-piece or 500-mL self-inflating bag. Current evidence suggests that resuscitation in room air is as effective as oxygen (Wang et al 2008). If a T-piece is used, the pressure limiter should be set to a maximum of 30 cmH$_2$O initially. Oxygen is administered if required according to pulse oximetry – again, see the chapter website resources for values and further details.

The baby should be reassessed after every airway manoeuvre until the chest is moving, and once this is established, ventilation breaths should continue to be delivered until regular breathing is sustained. Once the chest has been seen to move, the heart rate will normally increase. However, in some babies, the lack of oxygenated blood in the coronary circulation means that the cardiac muscle is unable to

respond to the lung inflation and the circulation of oxygenated blood. In this case, cardiac compressions may help 'bump start' the heart (Fig. 46.3). The heart rate should be assessed after 30 seconds. Once the heart rate is above 60 bpm, cardiac compressions can be stopped.

If the heart rate fails to respond despite the delivery of effective ventilation breaths and cardiac compressions, it may be necessary to consider administering drugs. In newborn babies, the umbilical vein can be cannulated easily. This route delivers drugs and fluids directly into the inferior vena cava via the *ductus venosus*. Drugs that may need to be given include *adrenaline, sodium bicarbonate, dextrose* and *0.9% sodium chloride* for volume enhancement; see the chapter website resources for further detail. *Naloxone hydrochloride* (Narcan) is not a drug of resuscitation. If a woman has been administered opiates in labour and the baby does not breathe at birth, the baby should be resuscitated first (UKRC 2010). Once effective lung inflation has been achieved, a decision may be made to

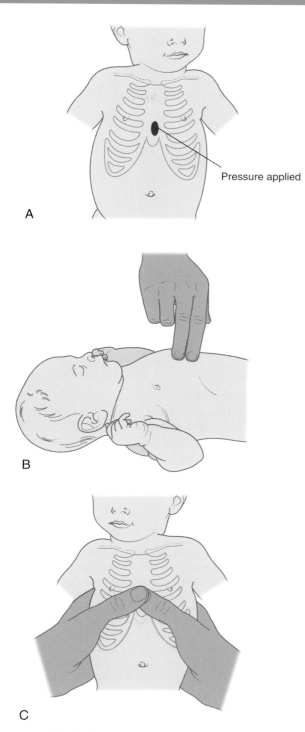

A

Pressure applied

B

C

Figure 46.3 Cardiac compression. **A,** Position for applying pressure. **B,** Using two fingers. **C,** Using two thumbs with the hands encircling the chest.

administer *naloxone hydrochloride* intramuscularly to reverse the effect of the maternal opiate. The baby's respiratory rate must be monitored closely because the effect of naloxone hydrochloride may wear off before that of the opiate. Naloxone hydrochloride should not be given to the baby of a substance-misusing woman because it can cause severe withdrawal symptoms.

Specific cases warrant particular management, such as in the presence of meconium and in the case of a preterm baby. If meconium-stained liquor is present at birth – particularly if it is thick – expert assistance should be called so that the baby can be intubated, if necessary. If expert help is unavailable, the baby should be handled gently at birth, kept warm and assessed. If the baby is breathing and crying, then no further resuscitation is needed. If the baby is unresponsive, a laryngoscope should be used to facilitate suction **under direct vision** only because routine suction has been shown to be ineffective (Wiswell et al 2000). A large-bore catheter should be used to suck out particulate matter. Suctioning should stop when all visible meconium has been aspirated or the heart rate falls below 60 bpm. If the heart rate is slow, the baby's head should be placed in the *neutral position* and inflation breaths given. Once the heart rate rises above 60 bpm, any remaining meconium may be removed with suction.

At birth, preterm babies usually manage to breathe and have a good heart rate, so the focus is stabilization rather than active, full resuscitation. They also face major challenges in maintaining their body temperature because of their comparatively large surface area. Hypothermia can cause hypoxia and hypoglycaemia and may interfere with surfactant production, leading to a worsening of respiratory distress syndrome (Petty 2010; Vilinsky and Sheridan 2014). When a preterm birth is imminent, senior help should be available. All surfaces that the baby will touch should be warmed. At birth, after the baby is placed into a plastic bag and a hat applied, the baby may need to be intubated (Fig. 46.4), and *exogenous surfactant* may be delivered via the endotracheal tube in the case of respiratory distress; see later discussion (Sweet et al 2013; Sakonidou and Dhaliwal 2014). Following stabilization, the baby is transferred to the neonatal unit for ongoing care.

Post-resuscitation care for all babies involves checking temperature and glucose and giving clear and accurate information to the parents about their baby and the subsequent plan. Objective documentation of all events is an essential part of this stage.

Reflective Activity 46.3

Can you think of a baby or babies in your care who required resuscitation or urgent attention at delivery? If so, what necessary preparation and equipment were required?

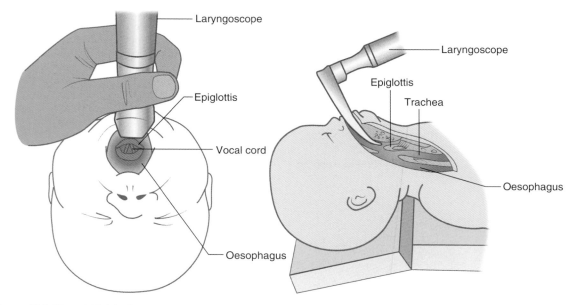

Figure 46.4 Neonatal intubation.

RESPIRATORY DISORDERS IN THE NEWBORN

Transient tachypnoea of the newborn

Transient tachypnoea of the newborn (TTN; also known as 'wet' lung') is believed to be the result of a failure to clear fetal lung fluid during transition to extrauterine life. Refer back to the earlier discussion of normal physiology to consider how fluid clearance should take place. TTN almost always affects term babies and is more common in babies born by elective caesarean section.

The baby presents with a rapid respiratory rate of 80 to 100 bpm soon after birth and intercostal and/or sternal recession. In terms of a differential diagnosis, these clinical features can also arise in other conditions, such as early onset pneumonia, although the latter may also present with grunting.

Management comprises the following:

- Infection screen to exclude or confirm pneumonia
- Prophylactic antibiotics until infection is excluded
- Chest X-ray to help confirm the diagnosis of TTN
- Care in a transitional care ward with mother sharing care
- May be nursed in neonatal unit (NNU) if continuous positive airway (CPAP) is needed

- Nursed in incubator to enable the following:
  - Close observation
  - Continuous monitoring of heart rate, respiratory rate and oxygen saturation levels
  - Warmed humidified oxygen

The treatment for TTN is supportive – the condition is self-limiting and will normally resolve within 1 to 5 days, after which the baby may be discharged home.

Meconium aspiration syndrome

Meconium-stained liquor is associated with fetal hypoxia and asphyxia and is seen primarily in term or post-term infants. It is believed that when the fetus becomes hypoxic, the anal sphincter relaxes and meconium is released into the amniotic fluid. Meconium has been found in the alveoli of stillborn infants, which suggests that aspiration may take place in utero (Mokra et al 2013). It is believed that the hypoxic fetus starts to gasp in utero, and this moves meconium-stained amniotic fluid into the fetal lungs. Of babies with meconium-stained liquor, 5% develop meconium aspiration syndrome (MAS) (Mundhra and Agarwal 2013).

The majority of babies born through meconium will be well and suffer no ill effects. It is advisable to undertake 'meconium observations' (assessing the baby's colour, tone and respiratory rate) for up to 12 hours after birth

(National Institute for Health and Care Excellence (NICE) 2014; see chapter website resources). Signs of illness in the baby include a rise in the respiratory rate (>60 bpm) and increasing cyanosis.

A baby with signs of increasing respiratory distress will need to be admitted to the NNU for continuous observation. Babies with mild respiratory distress usually respond well to the administration of warmed humidified oxygen and intravenous antibiotics may be considered. Babies with MAS who require prolonged resuscitation must be admitted to the NNU for monitoring and treatment. Traditional treatments for MAS have included intubation and ventilation using high concentrations of oxygen. However, the high pressures required to deliver the breaths (because of the high intrapulmonary pressures) can damage the lungs.

Mortality rates for severe MAS can be high as a result of pulmonary complications. Fetal hypoxia is associated with a rise in pulmonary artery pressure, and MAS is associated with an increased incidence of persistent pulmonary hypertension of the newborn (PPHN). In PPHN, the pressure in the pulmonary vasculature is elevated, causing the temporary fetal structures to remain partially open after birth, causing newborn hypoxaemia (Puthiyachirakkal and Mhanna 2013). The presence of meconium in the lung may also cause a chemical pneumonitis, which leads to inactivation of surfactant. Meconium is a viscous substance and may also cause obstruction of the airways.

Newer technologies for the management of MAS include the administration of *exogenous surfactant*. Because meconium inactivates surfactant, exogenous surfactant may reduce the need for more invasive treatments (Mok et al 2014). *Nitric oxide* is a gas that is delivered directly into the lungs via an endotracheal tube. It is a potent vasodilator and can reverse pulmonary hypertension, reducing hypoxaemia, and has been shown to be effective in treating some babies with MAS (Puthiyachirakkal and Mhanna 2013). In the most severe cases of MAS, *extracorporeal membrane oxygenation* (ECMO) may be required (Bohn 2015). ECMO is a highly invasive form of treatment during which the blood is pumped out of the body, oxygenated in an oxygenator (essentially an artificial lung) and then the oxygenated blood is returned to the baby (see chapter website resources). Few centres in the UK provide this treatment, so a baby with MAS requiring ECMO may have to be transported many miles from the 'home' unit for treatment, resulting in separation from the parents.

In relation to outcome, some survivors of severe MAS will go on to develop chronic lung disease as a consequence of the treatment for respiratory failure. A few babies with severe MAS will have neurodevelopmental delay. It is believed that this happens as a result of cerebral damage in utero, rather than as a direct consequence of meconium inhalation (Greenough and Milner 2012).

Hypoxic ischaemic encephalopathy (birth asphyxia)

Although not just a respiratory problem, hypoxic and ischaemic damage to the lungs does occur in hypoxic ischaemic encephalopathy (HIE), a multiple-system condition following prolonged distress during labour. The distressed fetus has little energy reserve should there be any interruption to the oxygen supply, and in this event the heart will not continue pumping for long, and respiratory function will be compromised. Cardiac glycogen stores allow the heart to continue in cases of asphyxia. Continued cardiac function is required to remove the accumulated lactic acid from the brain. Because glycogen stores are reduced, the capacity of the baby to withstand hypoxia is reduced.

Clinical presentation of the baby with HIE varies with severity. Six aspects of clinical presentation are assessed and may be predictive of outcome:

- Level of consciousness
- Tone and posture – neuromuscular indicator
- Primitive, complex reflexes
- Presence of seizures
- Autonomic functions
- Duration of symptoms

Treatment is aimed at minimizing further cerebral damage, alleviating symptoms and early detection of any complications, such as cerebral haemorrhage or hydrocephalus. Drugs are given to maintain cerebral perfusion and blood pressure, to reduce cerebral oedema and to control seizures. Respiratory support is usually necessitated in severe HIE until the baby is able to breathe spontaneously.

Investigations to assess the severity of damage include ultrasound, computed tomography (CT) scanning, magnetic resonance imaging (MRI) scanning and electroencephalogram (EEG) recording. Prognosis depends on the severity of the insult, but the condition may result in severe neurological damage. There is evidence that induced therapeutic cooling of babies who may have suffered a lack of oxygen at birth reduces death and disability without increasing the disability of survivors (Azzopardi et al 2008; Jacobs et al 2013).

Respiratory distress syndrome

Respiratory distress syndrome (RDS) is caused by a deficiency of surfactant (see also Ch. 45) and is inversely related to the gestational age of the baby. Referring back to the earlier discussion of fetal lung development, it can be seen that surfactant is produced by type II pneumocytes from mid-pregnancy onwards; it assists in the reduction of the surface tension of the lung and prevents complete alveolar collapse on expiration. Surfactant synthesis is reduced with hypoxaemia and acidaemia, and the hypoxic preterm baby may make such weak respiratory effort that the baby cannot release what little surfactant he or she has from the pneumocytes. Although primarily a disease affecting the lungs, the condition affects all body systems because impaired oxygenation and pulmonary hypoperfusion affect blood pressure, thus inhibiting tissue oxygenation.

Administration of a course of maternal corticosteroids (two doses) before birth reduces the incidence and severity of RDS (Roberts and Dalziel 2006; Royal College of Obstetricians and Gynaecologists (RCOG) 2010). These are most effective in reducing RDS in pregnancies that deliver 24 hours after and up to 7 days after administration of the second dose.

RDS presents soon after birth – usually within 4 hours, and is characterized by the following:

- Rapidly rising respiratory rate
- Marked sternal and intercostal recession
- Nasal flaring
- Grunting
- Arterial blood gases that usually show respiratory acidosis as a result of the trapping of carbon dioxide because the lungs are underventilated

The work of breathing is increased, and the baby quickly becomes exhausted. The baby tries to compensate by increasing the respiratory rate and pressures. In term or more mature preterm babies an *expiratory grunt* (see chapter website resources) may be audible in the baby's attempt to maintain lung volume. Intercostal and substernal recession can be quite marked, and there is a characteristic 'ground glass' appearance on chest X-ray with an air bronchogram because the air-filled airways stand out (see chapter website resources).

Onset is before 4 hours, and the pattern of the disease gets worse over the first 24 to 36 hours, then stabilizes and gradually improves. Treatment is aimed at supporting the respiratory and oxygenation status of the baby as gently as possible.

Exogenous surfactant may be required following birth to stabilize the lungs (Blennow and Bohlin 2015) and has been associated with the following:

- A dramatic fall in mortality rates from RDS and reduction in bronchopulmonary dysplasia (BPD) (Papile et al 2014)
- Reduced ventilator and oxygen requirements
- Dramatic reduction in the risk of pneumothoraces through decreased need for ventilator support

Surfactant is given via an endotracheal tube at birth – and further doses according to the baby's condition. Once stabilized, the baby may remain intubated with a ventilator delivering a mixture of air and oxygen directly using positive pressure to inflate the lungs, or, preferably, the baby may be extubated and placed on CPAP via nasal prongs, which is less invasive. CPAP allows the baby to breathe on his or her own but maintains a low pressure (about 4–6 cmH$_2$O) to prevent the lungs from collapsing between breaths (Greenough and Milner 2012). This facilitates gas exchange and also reduces damage to the surfactant-producing alveolar cells.

Babies with severe RDS are nursed in an incubator and have continuous monitoring of oxygenation, blood pressure, heart rate and respiratory rate. Their vulnerable state means that rapid fluctuations in blood pressure, arterial oxygen and carbon dioxide levels can affect the brain and kidneys, so care is directed at ensuring stability and detecting and correcting any abnormality.

RDS is not just prematurity related; surfactant deficiency can occur with hypoxia in the term baby, in babies with sepsis, in babies of diabetic mothers and in those born by elective caesarean section. The latter prevents the normal surge of catecholamines that occurs in spontaneous vaginal delivery, which play a part in surfactant release at birth. However, the majority of RDS cases are seen in preterm babies, and so the ideal scenario would be to delay premature delivery for as long as possible; refer to Chapter 45 for more information.

Very preterm babies may remain in the NNU for many months (see Ch. 45). Some go on to develop chronic lung disease (CLD), sometimes known as *bronchopulmonary dysplasia* (see chapter website resources).

Chronic lung disease

Rates of CLD vary considerably among neonatal intensive care units (NICUs). Advances over the past 20 years have included the use of antenatal corticosteroid treatment and postnatal surfactant therapy. Strategies aim to protect the lungs and include the following:

- The avoidance of intubation and limited time on full ventilation, aiming to extubate as soon as possible.
- Early use of nasal CPAP
- Minimization of the oxygen administered
- Ensuring that recommended limits are set for minimum and maximum oxygen saturation (90–95%) until the baby is ventilating in air or reaches sufficient maturity
- Adequate nutrition and calories to support the baby's growth in the period of high work of breathing and energy expenditure
- Use of diuretic therapy to limit pulmonary oedema

Many babies will be discharged from the hospital while still receiving continuous oxygen supplementation, sometimes for many months, until the proportion of new lung tissue development is adequate to sustain oxygenation without assistance. Babies with CLD will often require long-term care and follow-up. Practical and psychological support are required for parents of these babies, as is close monitoring of the baby's lung function, growth and development.

Pneumonia

Pneumonia may be acquired congenitally as a result of contamination with infective agents during labour or birth or may be of late onset – acquired after 7 days. Acquired pneumonia is most commonly seen in babies who are already intubated.

Clinical features are similar to those for TTN:

- Rapid respiratory rate soon after birth
- Intercostal and sternal recession
- Presence of respiratory grunt possible (see chapter website resources)
- Possible cyanosis
- In severe cases, group B streptococcus is associated with rapid collapse in the newborn period.

Management includes the following:

- Neonatal unit admission is required for observation and septic screening.
- Intravenous antibiotics are administered.
- Chest X-ray will help confirm the diagnosis of pneumonia.
- The baby is usually nursed in an incubator, with the following considerations:
  - Close observation
  - Continuous monitoring of heart rate, respiratory rate and oxygen saturation levels
  - Warmed humidified oxygen delivered via incubator or nasal prongs
  - May require intubation and respiratory support via a ventilator

The prognosis for term babies who contract pneumonia is good, provided the clinical features are recognized and managed promptly.

Congenital lung abnormalities

The majority of congenital abnormalities affecting the respiratory system are usually detected antenatally. Decisions about the place of birth can be made well in advance, and expert neonatal care can therefore be available at birth. Abnormalities include *congenital diaphragmatic hernia (CDH)*, *tracheo-oesophageal fistula (TOF)* and *oesophageal atresia*.

CDH can range from a small hole in the diaphragm muscle to complete agenesis, which allows the gut contents and/or liver to protrude through into the thoracic cavity in the first trimester of pregnancy. This reduces the space for lung development, and thus the lungs are hypoplastic and, in extreme cases, are incapable of supporting respiration (Leeuwen and Fitzgerald 2014). Most cases are diagnosed antenatally at the 20-week anomaly scan. Fetal surgery can be considered and offered to minimize lung damage and maximize normal lung development (Haroon and Chamberlain 2013). Overall, the prognosis for the baby depends largely on the extent of the diaphragmatic defect and the coexisting abnormalities (McBrien et al 2010). CDH may be incompatible with life if there is limited lung function.

TOF and/or oesophageal atresia are thought to occur because of abnormal separation of the primitive trachea and oesophagus in the first trimester (see Ch. 49). Oesophageal atresia may exist on its own or coexist alongside a fistula that communicates with the trachea, and many babies with this condition will have other abnormalities (Mathisen and Muniappan 2015).

Both of these congenital conditions are explained in further detail in the chapter website resources.

Reflective Activity 46.4

Think of a baby you have cared for who had a respiratory problem – how did the baby present?

CARDIAC ABNORMALITIES

The cardiovascular system is the first of the body's systems to develop and function. It is believed that the rapid development that takes place in this system makes it susceptible to teratogens. Congenital heart disease (CHD) accounts for about 30% of all reported congenital anomalies.

Causes include the following:

- Chromosomal abnormalities – about 40% of children with Down syndrome will have a cardiac malformation.
- Genetic factors – CHD is more likely if either parent or a sibling has a history of CHD.
- Teratogens – rubella or drugs, such as *phenytoin* or *warfarin*, can result in CHDs.
- Maternal disease, specifically diabetes mellitus, significantly increases the risk of a baby having CHD.
- Diagnosis of CHD comprises a combination of the following:
  - Antenatal history taking
  - Anomaly ultrasound screening (Landis et al 2013)
  - Echocardiogram for at-risk cases to increase diagnosis reliability

- Pulse oximetry, which has now been shown to be effective for postnatal screening and detection (Thangaratinam et al 2012)
- Blood pressure (Yates 2012)
- X-ray, ultrasound scan (USS), echocardiogram
- Hyperoxia test
- Examination and assessment of the newborn

For a full description and further details of diagnosis, refer to the chapter website resources.

Management

The treatment of a baby with CHD depends on the type of defect and the baby's general condition. Cardiac catheterization can be used for interventions such as widening stenosed vessels. Surgery may take place in stages. In the initial stage, treatment may be palliative and designed to alleviate symptoms. Later, as the baby grows, corrective surgery may be carried out. In complex cases, several operations may be required.

Depending on the results of the initial investigations, the baby may be referred to a specialist centre for further investigation and treatment. In some cases, even when a defect is diagnosed, it is possible for the baby to remain in the care of the parents and be referred for treatment at a later date. Whether the baby is transferred to a specialist centre or discharged, the parents need accurate information about their baby and what the future might hold. In particular, the parents of the baby who has a delayed referral require information about the clinical features of deterioration and how they should obtain assistance if they are concerned about their baby's condition.

Forms of congenital heart defects

Congenital heart disease is commonly divided into two groups: *cyanotic* and *acyanotic*. However, it must be noted that not all babies with cyanotic heart disease will be cyanosed initially.

Acyanotic heart defects

Acyanotic heart defects include patent ductus arteriosus, ventricular and atrial septal defects, pulmonary stenosis, aortic stenosis and coarctation of the aorta.

Patent ductus arteriosus

The ductus arteriosus is a temporary structure that exists to divert blood away from the lungs to the aorta in the fetal circulation (see Chs 29 and 42 and Fig. 46.5). In term babies, the ductus arteriosus normally closes within 12 to 24 hours of birth in response to the circulating high partial

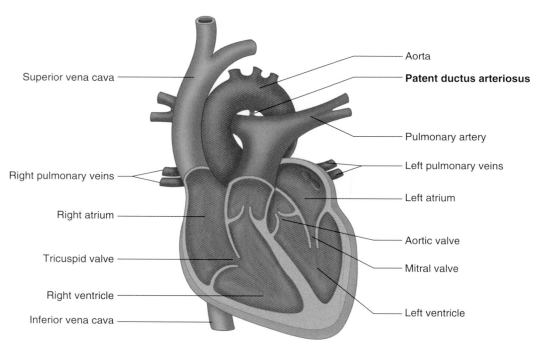

Figure 46.5 Patent ductus arteriosus.

pressure of oxygen and reduction in circulating maternal prostaglandins. Preterm babies are more likely to experience periods of hypoxia and an increase in circulating prostaglandins, which makes the ductus arteriosus more likely to remain open. Deoxygenated blood from the pulmonary arteries shunts through the ductus arteriosus into the aorta, bypassing the lungs. Preterm babies are likely to show decreasing levels of oxygenation and worsening of RDS. Term babies may be reluctant to feed and have poor growth patterns. The baby may have tachypnoea and tachycardia. On auscultation of the heart, a murmur may be heard.

Treatment includes the following:

- Oxygen as required, kept within limits
- Prevention of fluid overload
- Administration of drugs such as *indomethacin* or *ibuprofen* that have powerful antiprostaglandin action, which may be used if the baby is symptomatic, to close the ductus and avoid complications associated with it remaining open
- Surgical closure, which may be indicated if medical means fail

Atrial septal defect

Atrial septal defect (ASD) allows communication between the left and right side of the heart with mixing of oxygenated and deoxygenated blood (see Fig. 46.6). A simple ASD is a hole in the atrial septum and is rarely symptomatic. Closure is best performed before the onset of pulmonary hypertension. A complex ASD (often associated with an underlying chromosomal disorder) involves other structures, such as the mitral valve or the ventricular septum and tricuspid valve. Surgery is more complicated, and there is a higher mortality rate associated with this latter condition.

Ventricular septal defect

Ventricular septal defects (VSDs) are the most commonly occurring cardiac defect and may occur on their own or as part of a complex heart defect. The septal defect allows mixing of blood between the two ventricles. Typically, blood from the left ventricle passes through to the right ventricle during systole. The blood is then recirculated. The flow of blood from the left to the right side of the heart can lead to elevated right ventricular pressure and pulmonary hypertension. This occurs if the defect is large. The baby may show signs of respiratory distress and cyanosis and failure to thrive. Babies with a small defect may be asymptomatic, but if VSD is part of a more complex defect, then symptoms may be more obvious. Surgical correction of the defect will be carried out at an appropriate time. Small defects may close on their own.

Atrial–ventricular septal defects

Septal defects may occur in both heart chambers, making the condition more complex. There is a high association of atrial–ventricular septal defects (AVSDs) with Down

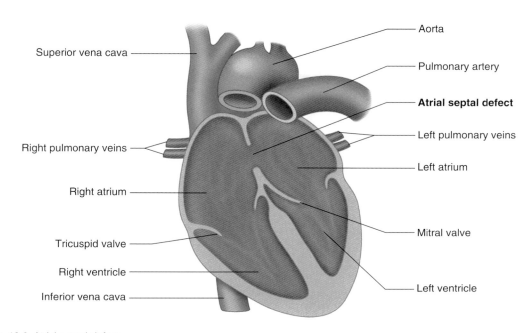

Figure 46.6 Atrial septal defect.

syndrome, and routine echocardiogram should be undertaken in all babies affected by Down syndrome.

Acyanotic, obstructive disorders

Acyanotic, obstructive disorders are 'duct dependent'; that is, the perfusion of the lower body depends on the ductus remaining open, and the baby will collapse if the ductus closes. The baby may present with RDS-type symptoms before collapse. Therefore, initial management focuses on keeping the duct open with prostaglandin prior to transfer to a tertiary centre for surgical correction of the defect and optimizing the baby's condition prior to surgery.

Coarctation of the aorta

Coarctation of the aorta is narrowing of the aorta at the point where the ductus arteriosus joins, and it may occur on its own or as part of a complex CHD (see Fig. 46.7). It is more common in males, and there is a strong association with Turner syndrome. Mild forms of the defect may be undetectable, and there may be no symptoms until the child is older. Pulses in limbs may be normal while the duct is patent. In more severe cases, femoral pulses may be weak or absent. Depending on the position of the coarctation, rapid collapse may follow closure of the ductus arteriosus as described earlier. Surgery is necessary to remove the stenosed part of the aorta, or a patch is inserted to make the narrow section of the aorta wider.

Pulmonary stenosis

Pulmonary stenosis occurs when the pulmonary valve becomes narrowed. This causes an obstruction to blood leaving the right ventricle and can lead to a reduction in blood going to the lungs. Pulmonary stenosis is also duct dependent and can show with severe cyanosis in the neonatal period. The stenosis is relieved by surgery.

Aortic stenosis

Aortic stenosis is a narrowing of the valve leading from the left ventricle into the aorta, which usually occurs alongside other heart defects. In simple cases, the baby will be asymptomatic, and there may be no sign other than a cardiac murmur. In severe cases, the baby will collapse suddenly and require urgent surgery to relieve the stenosis.

Cyanotic defects

This group of defects includes complex conditions such as transposition of the great arteries, tetralogy of Fallot and hypoplastic left heart syndrome.

Transposition of the great arteries (TGA)

In transposition of the great arteries (TGA), the major heart arteries are transposed (see Fig. 46.8). The aorta arises from the right ventricle, and the pulmonary artery arises from the left ventricle; TGA is usually associated with other cardiac defects, such as VSD. These babies

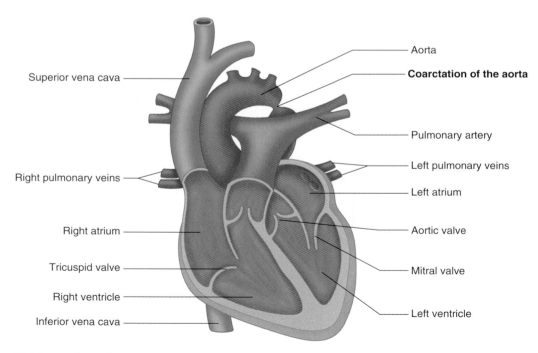

Figure 46.7 Coarctation of the aorta.

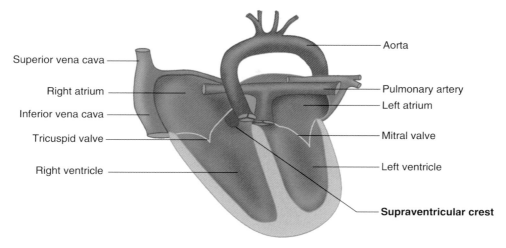

Figure 46.8 Transposition of the great arteries.

usually present within the first few hours of life – especially if there is no shunt. Cyanosis may be marked and accompanied by tachypnoea and tachycardia. Initial treatment involves an infusion of prostaglandins to open the ductus arteriosus. The foramen ovale may be surgically enlarged so that well-oxygenated blood can flow from the left ventricle into the right ventricle. Surgery to correct the defect is an arterial switch procedure.

Tetralogy of Fallot

Tetralogy of Fallot comprises four abnormalities (see Fig. 46.9):

- Ventricular septal defect
- Pulmonary stenosis
- Right ventricular hypertrophy
- Overriding of the aorta, in which the aorta is connected to the right and left ventricles and sits above the VSD

The baby develops a right-to-left shunt. There is mixing of oxygenated and deoxygenated blood at the level of the ventricles, and blood flows preferentially through the aorta, rather than the pulmonary arteries, because the pressure is lower in the larger vessel. Cyanosis may be present soon after birth or may develop in the first year of life. The baby may exhibit poor growth and failure to thrive and become breathless when engaged in any activity. The condition is treated by surgery.

Hypoplastic left heart syndrome

In hypoplastic left heart syndrome the left side of the heart is underdeveloped (hypoplastic). There is atresia of the mitral and aortic valves. The left ventricle and the aorta are underdeveloped. In contrast, the right side of the heart is

hypertrophied, and the pulmonary artery is enlarged (see Fig. 46.10). Blood passes through the ductus arteriosus into the aorta. When the ductus arteriosus closes, death follows soon afterwards. A prostaglandin infusion can be used to keep the ductus arteriosus open. Palliative surgery can be carried out so that the right ventricle is used to supply the systemic circulation. Ultimately, heart transplantation may need to be carried out to correct the problem.

Acquired cardiac problems

Acquired problems with the cardiac system can also arise, and may be secondary as a result of prolonged, chronic respiratory problems, as in the case of *cor pulmonale*, for example, or a result of cardiac failure in an acute situation, for example, cardiovascular shock in a sick baby. Assessment of the baby for compromised perfusion and cardiovascular function should be undertaken in such cases in conjunction with ongoing respiratory monitoring because the two systems work very closely together both normally and when there is a problem in one or either of them.

> **Reflective Activity 46.5**
>
> Think of a baby you have cared for who had a cardiac problem – how did the baby present?

PARENTAL CARE

The diagnosis of a serious respiratory condition or congenital cardiac defect presents major challenges for

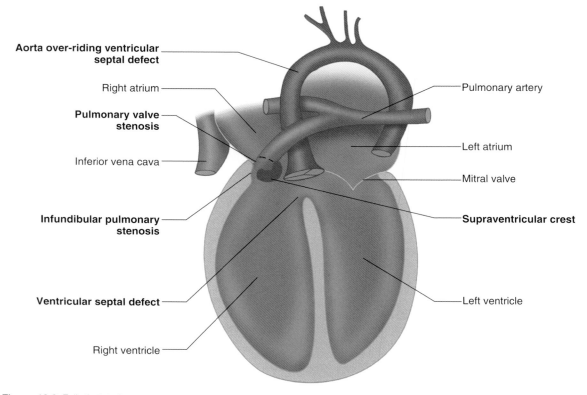

Aorta over-riding ventricular
septal defect

Right atrium

**Pulmonary valve
stenosis**

Inferior vena cava

**Infundibular pulmonary
stenosis**

Ventricular septal defect

Right ventricle

Pulmonary artery

Left atrium

Mitral valve

Supraventricular crest

Left ventricle

Figure 46.9 Fallot's tetralogy.

families. Parents will require accurate information about
the condition, any associated problems, treatment and
prognosis. A referral to a paediatric cardiologist or cardiac
surgeon may be indicated at this point. Some conditions,
as has been acknowledged, may be associated with chromosome anomalies, whereby careful antenatal counselling
of parents is required. The presence of other conditions
may well exert a strong influence on parental decision
making. If conditions are life limiting, this poses further
challenging ethical issues and difficult dilemmas for
parents. When a CHD is diagnosed antenatally, for
example, some parents may opt for termination, and some
will experience spontaneous loss of the affected fetus. If
the parents decide to continue with the pregnancy, information gained in the antenatal period will be important
in decision making about place of birth and subsequent
care. In addition, as the genetic basis of CHD is becoming
better known, the offer of antenatal counseling becomes
more important for parents who are faced with a possible
diagnosis of a serious condition in their baby.

The baby with the conditions discussed, and others not
covered, may be acutely unwell and need urgent treatment
in a specialist centre located many miles away from home.
Even after initial treatment, the baby may require many

years of follow-up, with an uncertain prognosis in relation
to both respiratory and cardiac problems. Families that
have babies with less complex defects may find themselves
coping with feelings of uncertainty as they await referral,
transfer, treatment or surgery.

Babies with CHD or chronic respiratory problems may
be difficult to feed and may exhibit poor growth, causing
further concern for the parents. Health professionals
working with parents should ensure that they receive accurate, consistent support and information. Parents of babies
with CHD and other neonatal conditions may find it
helpful to be given contact details of specialist support
groups and voluntary organizations (see chapter website
resources). Overall, parents involved in discussions about
serious illness and diagnosis in their baby and all the resultant uncertainties should have access to support services.

Reflective Activity 46.6

Reflect on the reactions and anxieties of parents who
have a baby born with a respiratory or cardiac problem.
How would you address these?

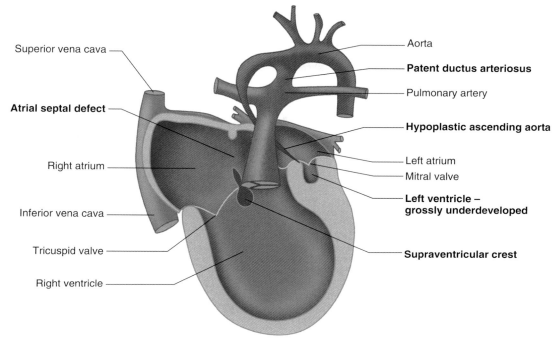

Superior vena cava

Atrial septal defect

Right atrium

Inferior vena cava

Tricuspid valve

Right ventricle

Aorta

Patent ductus arteriosus

Pulmonary artery

Hypoplastic ascending aorta

Left atrium

Mitral valve

**Left ventricle –
grossly underdeveloped**

Supraventricular crest

Figure 46.10 Hypoplastic left heart syndrome.

CONCLUSION

Respiratory and cardiac problems in the newborn arise because of failure of normal fetal and transitional lung function and circulation, which can occur for many reasons. It is vital to understand both normal and abnormal respiratory and cardiac function in the newborn to be able to assess any baby who presents with compromise as a result of hypoxia and poor perfusion.

The move towards midwife-led care means that midwives have taken on a greater responsibility for screening and detecting cardiac and respiratory disorders in the antenatal and postnatal periods. A knowledgeable and skilled midwife is able to facilitate an effective partnership with parents; the midwife should be able to provide information and support to enable parents to confirm normality in their newborn infant and to have the confidence to seek support and help if they are concerned about their baby's well-being.

Key Points

- An understanding of normal fetal and neonatal development and physiology is crucial in recognizing the transition events at birth, along with what can happen if development or transition is compromised for any reason.

- Midwives need to be alert for, and be able to recognize when there are deviations from normal in the neonate's cardiac or respiratory well-being and take the appropriate action.

- All midwives need to be skilled in resuscitation of the newborn, and those who work in out-of-hospital settings should be able to stabilize babies with respiratory and cardiac disorders while awaiting expert help.

References

Azzopardi D, Brocklehurst P, Edwards D, et al: The TOBY study. Whole body hypothermia for the treatment of perinatal asphyxial encephalopathy; a randomized controlled trial, *BMC Paediatr* 8(1):17, 2008.

Bedford CD, Lomax A: Chapter 2, Cardiovascular and respiratory assessment of the baby. In Lomax A, editor: *Examination of the newborn: an evidence-based guide*, 2nd edn, Oxford, Wiley-Blackwell, 2015.

Bhutani VK: Development of the respiratory system. In Donn SM, Sinha SK, editors: *Manual of neonatal respiratory care*, 3rd edn, New York, Springer, 2012.

Blackburn ST: *Maternal, fetal and neonatal physiology: a clinical perspective*, 4th edn, St. Louis, Saunders, 2013.

Blennow M, Bohlin K: Surfactant and noninvasive ventilation, *Neonatology* 107(4):330–336, 2015.

Bohn D: Extracorporeal membrane oxygenation in acute hypoxic respiratory failure. In Rimensberger PC, editor: *Pediatric and neonatal mechanical ventilation*, New York, Springer, 2015.

Carr N, Foster P: Examination of the newborn: the key skill. Part 2: the cardiovascular system and congenital heart disease, *Pract Midwife* 17(2):30–33, 2014.

Greenough A, Milner AD: Pulmonary disease of the newborn. In Rennie J, editor: *Roberton's textbook of neonatology*, 5th edn, Edinburgh, Elsevier, 2012.

Haroon J, Chamberlain RS: An evidence based review of the current treatment of congenital diaphragmatic hernia, *Clin Pediatr (Phila)* 52(2):115–124, 2013.

Jacobs SE, Berg M, Hunt R, et al: Cooling for newborns with hypoxic ischaemic encephalopathy, *Cochrane Database Syst Rev* (1):Art. No. CD003311, 2013.

Jain L, Eaton DC: Physiology of fetal lung fluid clearance and the effect of labor, *Semin Perinatol* 30(1):34–43, 2006.

Landis BJ, Levey A, Levasseur SM, et al: Prenatal diagnosis of congenital heart disease and birth outcomes, *Pediatr Cardiol* 34(3):597–605, 2013.

Lawford A, Tulloh RM: Cardiovascular adaptation to extra uterine life, *Paediatr Child Health* 25(1):1–6, 2015.

Leeuwen L, Fitzgerald DA: Congenital diaphragmatic hernia, *J Paediatr Child Health* 50:667–673, 2014.

Mathisen DJ, Muniappan A: Tracheo-esophageal fistula. In *Gastrointestinal surgery*, New York, Springer, pp 3–12, 2015.

McBrien A, Sands A, Craig B, et al: Impact of a regional training program in fetal echocardiography for sonographers on the antenatal detection of major congenital heart disease, *Ultrasound Obstet Gynecol* 36(3):279–284, 2010.

McCall EM, Alderdice F, Halliday HL, et al: Interventions to prevent hypothermia at birth in preterm and/or low birthweight infants, *Cochrane Database Syst Rev* (3):Art. No. CD004210, 2010.

Mok YH, Lee JH, Rehder KJ, et al: Adjunctive treatments in pediatric acute respiratory distress syndrome, *Expert Rev Respir Med* 13:1–14, 2014.

Mokra D, Mokry J, Tonhajzerova I: Anti-inflammatory treatment of meconium aspiration syndrome: benefits and risks, *Respir Physiol Neurobiol* 187(1):52–57, 2013.

Mundhra R, Agarwal M: Fetal outcome in meconium stained deliveries, *J Clin Diagn Res* 7(12):2874, 2013.

National Institute for Health and Care Excellence (NICE): *Intrapartum care: care of healthy women and their babies during childbirth* (website). www.nice.org.uk/guidance/cg190. 2014.

Onuzo OC: How effectively can clinical examination pick up congenital heart disease at birth?, *Arch Dis Child Fetal Neonatal Ed* 91(4):F236–F237, 2006.

Papile LA, Baley JE, Benitz W, et al: Respiratory support in preterm infants at birth, *Pediatrics* 133(1):171–174, 2014.

Petty J: Fact sheet: adaptation of the newborn to extra-uterine life. Part 2: thermoregulation and glucose homeostasis, *J Neonatal Nurs* 16(5):198–199, 2010.

Puthiyachirakkal M, Mhanna MJ: Pathophysiology, management, and outcome of persistent pulmonary hypertension of the newborn: a clinical review, *Front Pediatr* 2(1):23, 2013.

Roberts D, Dalziel S: Antenatal corticosteroids for accelerating fetal lung maturation for women at risk of preterm birth, *Cochrane Database Syst Rev* CD004454, 2006.

Røsvik A, Øymar K, Kvaløy JT, et al: Oxygen saturation in healthy newborns; influence of birth weight and mode of delivery, *J Perinat Med* 37(4):403–406, 2009.

Royal College of Obstetricians and Gynaecologists (RCOG): *Antenatal corticosteroids to reduce neonatal morbidity and mortality. Greentop Guideline No. 7*, London, RCOG, 2010.

Sakonidou S, Dhaliwal J: The management of neonatal respiratory distress syndrome in preterm infants (European Consensus Guidelines—2013 update), *Arch Dis Child Educ Pract Ed*. doi: 10.1136/archdischild-2014-306642. 2014.

Sweet DG, Carnielli V, Greisen G, et al: European consensus guidelines on the management of neonatal respiratory distress syndrome in preterm infants – 2013 update, *Neonatology* 103(4):353–368, 2013.

Thangaratinam S, Brown K, Zamora J, et al: Pulse oximetry screening for critical congenital heart defects in asymptomatic newborn babies: a systematic review and meta-analysis, *Lancet* 379(9835):2459–2464, 2012.

UK Resuscitation Council (UKRC): *Newborn life support*, London, UK, Resuscitation Council, 2010.

UK Resuscitation Council (UKRC): *Newborn life support*, London, UK, Resuscitation Council, 2015.

Vilinsky A, Sheridan A: Hypothermia in the newborn: An exploration of its cause, effect and prevention, *Br J Midwifery* 22(8):557–562, 2014.

Wang CL, Anderson C, Leone T, et al: Resuscitation of preterm neonates by using room air or 100% oxygen, *Pediatrics* 121(6):1083–1089, 2008.

Wert SE: Normal and abnormal structural development of the lung.

In Polin RA, Fox WW, Abman SH, editors: *Fetal and neonatal physiology*, 4th edn, Philadelphia, WB Saunders, 2011.

Wiswell TE, Gannon CM, Jacob J, et al: Delivery room management of the apparently vigorous meconium-stained neonate: results of the multicenter international collaborative trial, *Pediatrics* 105(1):1–7, 2000.

Yates RWM: Cardiovascular disease. In Rennie J, editor: *Roberton's textbook of neonatology*, 5th edn, Edinburgh, Elsevier, 2012.

Resources and additional reading

Books

Artman M, Mahoney L, Teitel DF: *Neonatal cardiology*, 2nd edn, New York, McGraw Hill, 2010.

Donn SM, Sinha SK, editors: *Manual of neonatal respiratory care*, 3rd edn, Edinburgh, Elsevier, 2012.

Lissaur T, Faneroff AA: *Neonatology at a glance*, 3rd edn, Oxford, Blackwell Science Ltd, 2015.

Meeks M, Hallsworth M, Yeo H: *Nursing the neonate*, 2nd edn, Oxford, Wiley Blackwell, 2009.

Sinha SK, Miall L, Jardine L: *Essential neonatal medicine*, 5th edn, Oxford, Wiley Blackwell, 2012.

Williamson A, Crozier K: *Neonatal care: a textbook for student midwives and nurses*, Exeter, Reflect Press, 2008.

See also the book list for Chapter 44 (in chapter website resources), which details a selection of neonatal texts, all of which have a section on respiratory and cardiac assessment, care and conditions.

Online resources

Baffa KM: *An overview of congenital cardiovascular anomalies. MSD Professional* (website). www.msdmanuals.com/en-gb/ professional/pediatrics/congenital -cardiovascular-anomalies/overview -of-congenital-cardiovascular -anomalies. 2015.

British Heart Foundation: www.bhf.org. uk/heart-health/conditions/ congenital-heart-disease

Children's Heart Federation: www.chfed .org.uk/how-we-help/information -service/heart-conditions/

Congenital Heart Defects UK: www .chd-uk.co.uk/types-of-chd-and -operations/

Hermansen CL, Lorah KN: Respiratory distress in the newborn, *Am Fam Physician* 76(7):987–994 (website). www.aafp.org/afp/2007/1001/ p987.html. 2007.

Knowledge for Neonatal Nursing Practice: *A self-directed learning tool* (website). www.cetl.org.uk/learning/ neonatal/ neonatal_care.html.

Landis BJ, Levey A, Levasseur SM, et al: Prenatal diagnosis of congenital heart disease and birth outcomes, *Pediatr Cardiol* 34(3):597–605 (website). www.ncbi.nlm.nih.gov/ pmc/articles/PMC3647457/. 2013.

Mellander M: Diagnosis and management of life-threatening cardiac malformations in the newborn, *Semin Fetal Neonatal Med* 18:302–310 (website). http://www .sfnmjournal.com/article/S1744 -165X(13)00029-2/pdf. 2013.

Stanford Newborn Nursery: *See Photo Gallery link for a range of images and audio files on respiratory and cardiac assessment.* http://newborns.stanford. edu/PhotoGallery/

Sweet DG, Carnielli V, Greisen G, et al: European consensus guidelines on the management of neonatal respiratory distress syndrome in preterm infants – 2010 update, *Neonatology* 97(4):402–417 (website). http://www.sfmp.net/ download/guidelines_2010 _neonatology.pdf. 2010.

UK Resuscitation Council: *Newborn life support guidelines; full algorithm* (website). www.resus.org.uk/ resuscitation-guidelines/. 2015.

UK Resuscitation Council: *Recommended home-birth equipment* (website). www.resus.org.uk/quality-standards/ equipment-used-in-homebirth/. 2010.

Parent resources

British Heart Foundation: *Parent page* (website). www.bhf.org.uk/ heart-health/children-and-young- people/parents

Contact a Family: www.cafamily.org.uk/ professionals/

Great Ormond Street: www.gosh.nhs .uk/medical-information/ procedures-and-treatments/helping -your-child-congenital-heart-disease -stay-healthy

UK Resuscitation Council: *Quality standards for equipment used for home birth* (website). www.resus.org.uk/ quality-standards/ equipment-used-in-homebirth/

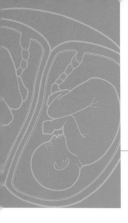

Chapter 47

Neonatal jaundice

Stephanie Michaelides

Learning Outcomes ?

After reading this chapter, you will be able to:

- explain the normal physiology of bilirubin metabolism
- identify common causes of unconjugated hyperbilirubinemia
- compare and contrast the principles of care of the jaundiced baby in all settings
- explain the role and risks of phototherapy and exchange transfusion
- recognize the clinical signs of conjugated hyperbilirubinemia
- define the acute and chronic complications of kernicterus

INTRODUCTION

Neonatal jaundice is common and occurs in a significant number of healthy full-term babies. Midwifery practice challenges include the following:

- Promoting and supporting successful breastfeeding to ensure adequate hydration of newly born babies
- Identifying those babies who are more at risk of significant hyperbilirubinemia (jaundice)
- Identifying the jaundiced baby requiring intervention and specifically those needing referral for a paediatric opinion and phototherapy (American Academy of Pediatrics (AAP) 2004; National Institute for Health and Care Excellence (NICE) 2016a)

Understanding the normal physiology of bilirubin metabolism allows recognition of why jaundice is so common in newborn babies and explains the mechanism

of jaundice in many diseases. A basic knowledge of the rare genetic diseases may also allow a greater depth of understanding of normal physiology, and these will be mentioned where appropriate.

Neonatal jaundice is extremely common, and approximately 60% of all babies develop some visible jaundice. In the majority of cases the jaundice is entirely harmless, and no treatment is required. Approximately 2% of babies need phototherapy to treat high bilirubin levels, and very few (about 10 in 100,000) develop extremely high levels with a risk of acute bilirubin encephalopathy and kernicterus (Manning et al 2007). Kernicterus should be extremely rare in a managed healthcare system because phototherapy and exchange transfusions are very effective ways of controlling bilirubin levels. The goal of management is to identify the rare baby whose bilirubin level is potentially toxic while avoiding unnecessary intervention in the remainder.

PHYSIOLOGY

The majority of bilirubin forms from the breakdown of *heme*, an iron-containing molecule, an essential component of cytochromes, myoglobin and haemoglobin. At the end of their lifespan, red blood cells are sequestered by the spleen and the haemoglobin is broken down into component parts of *heme* and *globin*. The iron molecule is then removed from the heme to be recycled and the heme molecule is oxidized to biliverdin, which is then reduced to form unconjugated bilirubin (Dennery et al 2001). Increased red cell breakdown leads to increased levels of unconjugated bilirubin. Unconjugated bilirubin is a lipid-soluble molecule that easily crosses lipid membranes, such as those within the brain. The insolubility in water means that bilirubin must be transported in the bloodstream linked to albumin. In this protein-bound state, bilirubin is not available to be filtered by the glomerulus or to enter into cell tissues (see chapter website resources).

In the liver, *unconjugated bilirubin* is transported into the cells and converted into *bilirubin diglucuronide (conjugated bilirubin)* by the enzyme *UDP glucuronosyltransferase.* Conjugated bilirubin is water-soluble and actively excreted by the liver cells into the intrahepatic bile ducts with bile salts, cholesterol and phospholipids. This bile then flows down the extrahepatic ducts and into the small intestine. Within the colon, some of the conjugated bilirubin is hydrolyzed back to unconjugated bilirubin, and the remaining is metabolized into *stercobilinogen* and *urobilinogen.* Stercobilinogen is a brown pigment that is excreted in the faeces. Urobilinogen is reabsorbed in the enterohepatic circulation to be converted back to unconjugated bilirubin. A small amount of urobilinogen is carried in the bloodstream and excreted by the kidneys.

PHYSIOLOGICAL JAUNDICE

Physiological jaundice is jaundice occurring as a consequence of the changeover from intra-uterine to extrauterine life. The fetus possesses a large number of red blood cells that contain fetal haemoglobin, which facilitates diffusion of oxygen from placental to fetal circulation. The newborn baby begins life with 6–7 million red cells per cubic millimeter, which need to reduce to the adult level of 5 million/mm^3. Fetal haemoglobin needs to be replaced by adult haemoglobin, resulting in an increase in red cell breakdown and an increased bilirubin load on the immature liver. Additionally, intestinal transit is slow until enteral feeds have been established, leading to increased reabsorption of urobilinogen via the enterohepatic circulation.

Features of physiological jaundice

- More common in breastfed babies
- Often noted at day 3 and peaks at day 5
- Not associated with anaemia
- Although not as alert as normal, the baby is usually well, and the feeding pattern is satisfactory.

Supplementing breastfeeding with water or glucose appears to have no effect on bilirubin levels in healthy newborns (Nicoll et al 1982) and should be avoided. Physiological jaundice may be exacerbated in situations that lead to increased bilirubin production (for example, polycythaemia, bruising) or decreased bilirubin excretion (poor feeding with delayed intestinal transit). In the past, it was believed that physiological jaundice could *not* lead to *kernicterus*, but unfortunately, this may not be the case, and vigilance is crucial.

EVALUATION OF JAUNDICE

The practitioner needs as much information as possible to accurately assess the risk of the baby developing jaundice, determine its significance and develop a management plan. The maternal blood group should be known and any familial predisposition to neonatal jaundice identified. Risk factors include infection during pregnancy and delivery and any bruising or perinatal trauma to the baby. Babies at high risk of developing jaundice may need to remain under hospital care for longer, and research continues into accurately identifying babies at risk (Sanpavat et al 2005).

It is important to assess the behaviour and feeding pattern of the baby – an alert baby feeding well is less of a concern than one who is sleepy and uninterested in feeding. Urine and bowel activity are also strong indicators of well-being.

Jaundice progresses from head to toe and resolves in the opposite direction, from toe to head. This is not reliable enough to be used in clinical practice, particularly in babies with dark skin tones (NICE 2016a). However, the white of the eye (the sclera) is white whatever the racial group of the baby. If the white of the eye appears yellow, the baby is certainly jaundiced, and the bilirubin level should be measured. Research is currently under way regarding whether or not a photograph of the eye with a smartphone camera could be used in the way transcutaneous bilirubin measurement (see following discussion) is currently used to estimate bilirubin.

Clinical evaluation of jaundice requires that the baby is undressed and examined in a good light, preferably natural light. Jaundice becomes clinically apparent in a pale-skinned baby when the serum bilirubin rises above 85 µmol/L (bilirubin can be measured as a concentration recorded in µmol/L or mg/dL). Attempting to estimate the serum bilirubin by 'eye' is not reliable and is not recommended by NICE (2016a). Any baby who is clinically jaundiced should have the serum bilirubin measured. Transcutaneous bilirubinometer devices have been developed that correlate well with serum bilirubin measurements, and these are suitable for use in babies more than 35 weeks gestation (NICE 2016a; NICE 2014) (see Fig. 47.1).

These devices should be used in infants over 35 weeks gestation and a postnatal age of greater than 24 hours; the devices can under-read and are not guaranteed to be accurate at high levels, so a reading greater than 250 µmol/L is an indication for serum bilirubin testing (Box 47.1; also see chapter website).

Records

To facilitate effective management, bilirubin results should be sequentially recorded. Graphs are available for preterm

Box 47.1 Taking blood for serum bilirubin measurement – preparation

To take a heel specimen correctly, the baby's foot needs to be lower than the body, and the heel needs to be warm.

It is important to recognize that this is a painful procedure. Therefore, support the baby by wrapping the baby, leaving the limb that will be used for testing free and holding the baby. It is useful to allow the baby to feed or suck on a clean finger because this can minimize the pain from the procedure being undertaken by a colleague.

and term babies, allowing bilirubin levels to be plotted against the time the blood sample was taken, enabling the measurement to be plotted against the baby's age in hours (NICE 2016a). This helps inform the practitioner about the rate of rise, and the graphs contain the recommended guideline thresholds at which level phototherapy should be commenced and when exchange transfusion may be indicated.

NICE has also developed the Bili-Wheel, which measures the bilirubin level alongside the gestation to highlight interventions required (NICE 2016a; see chapter website resources).

Reflective activity 47.1   ><

Access your local guidelines and protocols for neonatal jaundice and evaluate the following:

- Are they designed and agreed on by a multidisciplinary group?
- Are they up to date?
- Are they being used well?

UNCONJUGATED HYPERBILIRUBINEMIA

Unconjugated hyperbilirubinemia has three main causes (apart from 'physiological' jaundice), as follows:

- Increased red cell breakdown (haemolysis)
- Failure of the ability to conjugate bilirubin
- Increased enterohepatic circulation

Increased red cell breakdown

Increased red cell breakdown occurs most commonly in the neonate because of infection, bruising (for example, after ventouse or forceps delivery), polycythaemia, haemolytic disease of the newborn or, more rarely, following localized haemorrhage or thrombosis.

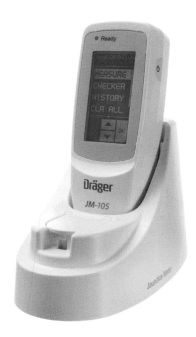

Figure 47.1 Bilirubinometer. (By kind permission of Draeger.)

Haemolytic disease of the newborn

Haemolytic disease of the newborn is the *immune-mediated red cell breakdown* that occurs in *Rhesus disease* and *ABO incompatibility* (not to be confused with *haemorrhagic disease of the newborn* – vitamin K deficiency). In haemolytic disease of the newborn, the maternal immune system has been 'immunized' against aspects of the baby's blood group (see Fig. 47.2). This 'immunization' usually occurs because of a previous pregnancy or miscarriage or following blood transfusion when fetal blood cells have passed to the maternal circulation.

Rhesus isoimmunization

Rhesus factor refers to the Rhesus C, D and E antigens expressed on red blood cells. It is the D antigen that is most likely to cause isoimmunization. An individual who is Rhesus negative does not express the D antigen and has the genotype dd. An individual who is Rhesus positive does express the D antigen and can be heterozygous (Dd) or homozygous (DD) for the Rhesus antigen D genes. Isoimmunization in a Rhesus-negative mother can occur with a heterozygous or homozygous fetus or baby, and the risk of this occurring can be predicted from a knowledge of the father's genotype as shown in Fig. 47.3.

Rhesus isoimmunization can cause a severe haemolysis that may result in fetal anaemia and a need for intrauterine blood transfusions to prevent the development of

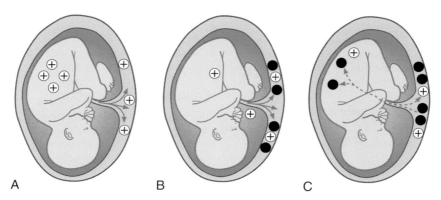

Figure 47.2 Antibody formation. **A,** The crosses represent fetal blood cells crossing over into the maternal circulation. **B,** An antibody response (black circles) is mounted by the mother. **C,** The antibodies cross into the fetal circulation, where they will break down the fetal blood cells.

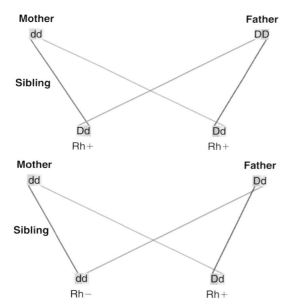

Figure 47.3 Inheritance of Rhesus factor. D represents Rhesus positivity, which is a dominant trait, and d represents Rhesus negativity. In this instance, the infant with Dd will be Rhesus positive, which may result in the Rhesus-negative mother mounting an immune response.

Box 47.2 Coombs and Kleihauer tests

Direct Coombs test: Cord blood is taken to measure the level of maternal antibodies.
  Kleihauer test: A sample of maternal blood is taken, and the number of fetal cells in the sample is estimated. A level of 50 fetal cells/50 lower-power fields is considered high.
  Blood is taken from the baby (or the cord) to measure the level of maternal antibodies. One of the complications of administering prophylactic anti-D to mothers is that this test may be positive secondary to the administered antibodies and not indicative of a spontaneous maternal production of antibodies.

hydrops fetalis (which is severe anaemia associated with significant oedema).

To prevent isoimmunization, anti-D immunoglobulin is administered to women at risk, antenatally and/or post-natally; it forms complexes with the fetal red cells to prevent the women's immune system from mounting its own immune response. Current advice from NICE is to routinely administer anti-D prophylaxis to all Rhesus-negative women antenatally at least once at 28 weeks gestation (exact regimen depends on dose used) (NICE 2008). Anti-D should also be administered at times when the women are at increased risk of isoimmunization, such as after miscarriage or after the birth of a Rhesus-positive baby. However, Anti-D should not be given prophylactically after medical management for ectopic pregnancy, to women with a threatened or complete miscarriage, or to women with a pregnancy in an unknown location (NICE 2012; NICE 2015). Women and babies at risk can be identified by taking cord and maternal blood after delivery to determine the baby's blood group and measure the presence of fetal blood cells and antibodies in the maternal system, as described in Box 47.2.

Anti-D is a blood product; therefore, before administration, informed consent must be obtained. The anti-D must be prescribed on the woman's drug chart by a medical practitioner (Nursing and Midwifery Council (NMC) 2010).

ABO incompatibility

Severe haemolysis is less common with *ABO incompatibility* than with *Rhesus D incompatibility,* but the principle of isoimmunization is the same. The ABO blood group refers to the pattern of expression of the A and B antigens on the red blood cells, as follows:

- Blood group A – genotype heterozygous AO or homozygous AA
- Blood group B – genotype heterozygous BO or homozygous BB
- Blood group AB – always heterozygous AB
- Blood group O – always homozygous OO

A mother of blood group O may develop antibodies against the A and B antigens, a mother with blood group A against the B antigen and a mother of blood group B against the A antigen. These last two examples are extremely rare, and ABO incompatibility is most common in a mother who has blood group O with a fetus that has blood group A or B.

ABO incompatibility usually manifests at less than 36 hours of age, although it may not become obvious until after 48 hours. A profile of mother's blood group being O positive should alert the midwife to this possibility.

A baby diagnosed and treated for ABO incompatibility needs to be closely observed for signs of 'late' anaemia, which may occur as a result of ongoing haemolysis by antibodies that may persist in the baby's circulation for several weeks. Symptoms include lethargy, pallor and poor feeding history. Folate and iron may be prescribed to encourage red blood cell production in the bone marrow, but it is not unusual for a baby to develop a severe anaemia requiring blood transfusion. Continuity by the midwife providing care up to 28 days can be very helpful.

Genetic causes

Biochemical or structural abnormalities of red cells may lead to a shortened lifespan with increased red cell turnover and jaundice. Examples of inherited defects of red cells are as follows:

- G6PD deficiency
  - X-linked (males affected)
  - Common in Mediterranean and Asian racial groups
  - Haemolysis can be triggered by fava beans (broad beans), mothballs or a variety of drugs and infections in babies with the deficiency (see chapter website resources)
- Spherocytosis
  - Red cells are spherical, rather than shaped as a biconcave disc
  - Red blood cells have a shortened lifespan as a result of increased sequestration within the spleen.
  - Autosomal dominant

- Pyruvate kinase deficiency
  - Autosomal recessive
  - Red blood cells have a shortened lifespan as a result of membrane defects

Failure of conjugation

The ability to conjugate bilirubin varies in individuals depending on differing levels of the enzyme *UDP glucuronosyltransferase* (secondary to individual variation in gene expression) present in the liver and the immaturity of the newborn's enzyme levels.

Prolonged *unconjugated hyperbilirubinemia* may occur in some breastfed babies as the enzyme may also be inhibited by breastmilk, as illustrated by a study of Taiwanese babies (Huang et al 2004). There is no specific test for breastmilk jaundice, and diagnosis is made when all other causes have been excluded. Management is dependent on the baby's condition: usually, the baby is active and feeds well, but jaundice is prolonged and can take up to 6 weeks to resolve.

If the baby is well and all other causes have been excluded, the management is to encourage frequent breastfeeds because 'breastfeeding jaundice' rarely requires phototherapy treatment. Previously, practitioners have advised the discontinuation of breastfeeding to confirm the diagnosis, but this can provide negative feedback to the mother regarding her ability to feed and nurture her baby and thus should be avoided.

Genetic reasons

A variety of genetic conditions affect an individual's ability to conjugate bilirubin, including the following:

- Gilbert syndrome (autosomal recessive)
- Crigler–Najjar syndrome type II (bilirubin encephalopathy/kernicterus rare) (autosomal recessive)
- Crigler–Najjar syndrome type I (bilirubin encephalopathy/kernicterus common) (autosomal recessive)

See the chapter website for more information.

Increased enterohepatic circulation

Delayed intestinal transit will increase the enterohepatic circulation of bilirubin and lead to an increased level of unconjugated bilirubin. In a normal newborn baby, intestinal peristalsis develops over the first few days as enteral feeds are established, and a delay in establishing feeds can exacerbate jaundice. The most common medical reason for delayed intestinal transit is *congenital hypothyroidism*. Babies diagnosed with congenital hypothyroidism must be commenced on thyroxine as soon as the diagnosis has been confirmed to minimize the complication of neurodevelopmental delay. Babies are normally screened for this by measuring thyroid-stimulating hormone (TSH) on the *Blood Spot Screening Card.*

The enzymes in colostrum encourage the passage of meconium (see Ch. 44), and the midwife can do much to support the woman in successful breastfeeding, thereby ensuring that the baby receives colostrum and breastmilk and avoids dehydration. The midwife also notes the passage of meconium as an important part of the baby's progress and well-being.

Complications of unconjugated hyperbilirubinemia

Kernicterus

Kernicterus describes the yellow staining of the basal ganglia seen at autopsy in babies who have had severe jaundice (Hachiya and Hayashi 2008). Abnormal signals in part of the basal ganglia (the *globus pallidus*) can be seen on magnetic resonance imaging (MRI). The term is also used to describe the chronic long-term clinical effects of severe hyperbilirubinemia.

The risk of kernicterus is influenced by such factors as the rate of rise of the bilirubin level and its maximum level. Other factors that increase an individual's susceptibility include the following:

- Young postnatal age
- Prematurity
- Hypoalbuminemia (Hulzebos et al 2008)
- Hypoxia/acidosis (both may reduce the effectiveness of the blood–brain barrier)
- Bacterial infection (Pearlman et al 1980) – for example, group B sepsis, urinary tract infections
- Medication that interferes with bilirubin binding to albumin, such as *salicylates, sulphonamides, heparin, diazepam* and *chloramphenicol*

There are also likely to be individual genetic factors that affect the risk of jaundice and the sensitivity to hyperbilirubinemia, some of which were described earlier (Hansen 2000a). The combination of *Gilbert's disease* and *G6PD deficiency* places the infant at particularly high risk. Kernicterus is rare in Europe and the United States (Dodd 1993; Newman and Maisels 1992) but may be increasing in incidence (Manning et al 2007).

Kernicterus is a lifelong severe neurological disability, and affected children have *dyskinetic cerebral palsy,* with poor movement control and involuntary movements, and sensorineural deafness. The auditory pathway appears to be particularly sensitive to damage from high bilirubin levels, and auditory spectrum neuropathy disorder can be caused by hyperbilirubinemia. Cochlear implants help some children considerably, and early referral is essential.

Table 47.1 Symptoms of acute bilirubin encephalopathy

Age	Acute symptoms
1–2 days	Poor suck, hypotonia, stupor, seizures
3–7 days	Increased tone in extensor muscles, opisthotonos, fever, seizures
>1 week	Hypertonia

Box 47.3 Risk factors for developing significant unconjugated jaundice following transfer

- Family history of neonatal jaundice
  - (e.g. genetic low levels of UDP glucuronosyltransferase, G6PD deficiency)
- Moderately preterm (35–37 weeks gestation)
- Breastfeeding
- Jaundice less than 24 hours (haemolytic disease, e.g. Rhesus/ABO)
- Asian race
- Bruising/cephalohematoma
- Infection
- Polycythaemic babies:
  - Small-for-gestational-age babies
  - Large-for-gestational-age babies (e.g. baby of diabetic mother)
  - Babies with chromosomal abnormalities (e.g. trisomy 21)
- Others:
  - Hypothyroidism

Acute symptoms may be reversible and without long-term complications if appropriately managed (Harris et al 2001) (Table 47.1). Up to 15% of babies who develop long-term complications may be asymptomatic in the acute stage (see chapter website resources).

Management of unconjugated hyperbilirubinemia

The recent trend towards home deliveries and early hospital transfer has been associated with increased readmission for jaundice and an increased reporting of babies with kernicterus. In some cases, high-risk babies can be identified (Box 47.3) and their transfer delayed. Undertaking a pre-transfer newborn bilirubin screening programme has been shown to reduce the rate of readmissions to hospital with significant jaundice (NICE 2016a). The *BiliApp* is a web-based application (app) tool that interprets newborn jaundice based on NICE guidance (Google play 2016). This app can plot the baby's jaundice levels on the appropriate chart, which facilitates evidence-based planning of follow-up and further bilirubin measurement.

In the community, there should be active breastfeeding support and careful monitoring of the jaundice by parents and community staff, with early hospital review where necessary (Bhutani and Johnson 2000). Transcutaneous bilirubinometers to screen for significant hyperbilirubinemia should also be encouraged (Engle et al 2005).

Initial assessment establishes the general condition and the most appropriate investigations and management that the baby requires. Supportive measures may include the administration of antibiotics and the correction of dehydration. These may be required in the management of unconjugated hyperbilirubinemia because meningitis and septicaemia are both more common during the first month of life than at any other time during childhood, and dehydration commonly exacerbates jaundice.

Specific treatments for unconjugated hyperbilirubinemia are *phototherapy* and *exchange transfusion*. The exact level of bilirubin that causes bilirubin encephalopathy and kernicterus and at what stage these treatments should be

Table 47.2 Consensus-based bilirubin thresholds for management of babies 38 weeks or more gestational age with hyperbilirubinemia (NICE 2016a)

Age (hours)	Bilirubin level (μmol/L) at which the following relevant action should be taken			
0			>100	>100
6	>100	>112	>125	>150
12	>100	>125	>150	>200
18	>100	>137	>175	>250
24	>100	>150	>200	>300
30	>112	>162	>212	>350
36	>125	>175	>225	>400
42	>137	>187	>237	>450
48	>150	>200	>250	>450
54	>162	>212	>262	>450
60	>175	>225	>275	>450
66	>187	>237	>287	>450
72	>200	>250	>300	>450
78		>262	>312	>450
84		>275	>325	>450
90		>287	>337	>450
≥96		>300	>350	>450
	↓	↓	↓	↓
	Repeat bilirubin measurement within 6–12 hours	Consider phototherapy (repeat bilirubin measurement within 6 hours)	Start phototherapy	Perform an exchange transfusion unless the bilirubin level falls below threshold while the treatment is being prepared

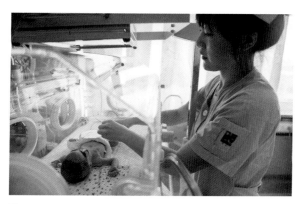
Figure 47.4 Baby receiving phototherapy. (By kind permission of Draeger.)

commenced remain contentious. Bilirubin encephalopathy is rare in full-term babies without underlying pathology, but relaxation of the treatment guidelines has led to an increase in the number of babies developing this complication (Hansen 2000b; Manning et al 2007). The aim of treatment is to identify those babies at specific risk (Bhutani and Johnson 2000) and to prevent kernicterus without exposing many more babies to unnecessary or potentially harmful treatment.

The current NICE guidelines (2016), updating the 2010 guidelines, suggest that babies should be considered within the following groups when assessing the need for phototherapy, and the aid of the BiliApp Newborn Jaundice Tool uses these risk groups:

- Low risk – well infants greater than 38 weeks
- Medium risk – well infants 35–37+ 6 weeks, or infants greater than 38 weeks with risk factors
- Higher risk – infants 35–37+ 6 weeks with risk factors.

Risk factors include G6PD deficiency, evidence of hypoxia or ischaemia, haemolytic disease, infection, lethargy, and temperature instability. Table 47.2 can be considered as a guide for babies greater than 38 weeks, but local policies and recent evidence should be consulted.

Phototherapy

The effect of light on the excretion of bilirubin has been known since the 1950s (Cremer et al 1958). Phototherapy is an artificial method that provides light of a specific wavelength to enhance bilirubin excretion. Fat-soluble unconjugated bilirubin is mainly converted into water-soluble lumirubin that can be excreted through the kidneys. The most effective light spectrum for converting the yellow bilirubin pigment to the photoisomer lumirubin is blue light, and the wavelength of blue light is in the 425 to 475 nm range.

Other factors affecting the effectiveness of phototherapy are as follows:

- Total dose of light delivered
- Energy output of light source
- Number of light sources
- Distance from infant
- Maximum skin surface area exposed to those lights

There are a number of ways of delivering phototherapy, including conventional phototherapy (see Fig. 47.4), 360-degree units, blue-light units and the fiberoptic BiliBlanket (Figs 47.5 and 47.6) (not used as first-line treatment in term babies).

Double phototherapy is the combination of two phototherapy units (*BiliBlanket* and overhead or two overheads) placed at different positions above and/or below the infant (see Fig. 47.7). This treatment can significantly increase the excretion of bilirubin (Holtrop et al 1992). There are now phototherapy units that can deliver 360 degrees of phototherapy by completely surrounding the infant within a tunnel of light.

Overhead units have incorporated or attached UV light filters designed to protect the infant from harmful rays. Manufacturer guidelines for use of different phototherapy units (such as the distance of the overhead from the infant) may vary. There have been reports of babies suffering UV burns as a direct consequence of phototherapy.

The overhead phototherapy unit requires consideration of the following aspects of care:

- May disrupt normal mother–baby interaction (BiliBlanket may be less disruptive).
- Temperature regulation – the baby's temperature must be regularly monitored (Fig. 47.8a).
- Significant increase in fluid loss from loose stools can occur because of an associated decreased intestinal transit time.
- Nutrition and hydration – it is important to continue to establish demand feeding and to prevent dehydration. Extra fluids do not need to be routinely prescribed, but the baby should be regularly assessed for signs of dehydration.
- Eye protection – the eyes must be protected as a precaution against possible damage (Fig. 47.8b).
- Maternal anxiety – it is important to ensure that the mother understands the reasons for her baby requiring treatment and its basic principles because the confidence of the mother and her enjoyment of early mothering are often affected (Brethauer and Carey 2010).

Once phototherapy has commenced, the skin is bleached, and thus transcutaneous bilirubin levels are no longer reliable. Serum bilirubin should initially be measured after 4

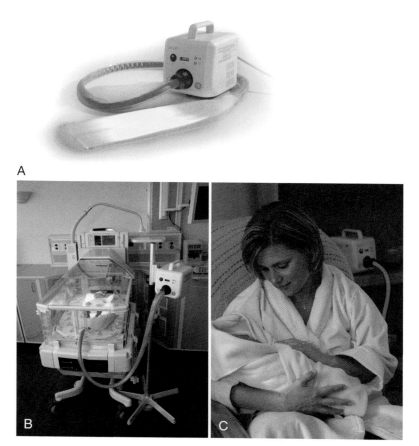

Figure 47.5 A, The Bilosoft unit. **B,** Baby receiving phototherapy with a hooded Bilisoft unit. **C,** Mother holding her baby receiving phototherapy. (Courtesy of GE Healthcare Clinical Systems UK Ltd.)

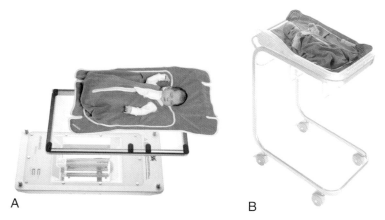

Figure 47.6 The Medela BiliBed. **A,** Phototherapy source, light-permeable support and baby in therapy blanket. **B,** Baby in crib with unit in position. (Courtesy of Medela AG.)

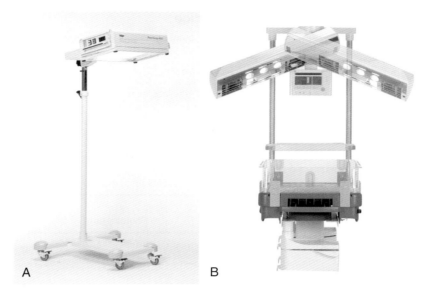

Figure 47.7 **A and B,** Phototherapy units. (Courtesy of Draeger.)

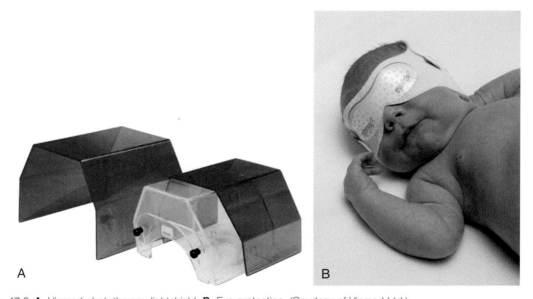

Figure 47.8 **A,** Viamed phototherapy lightshield. **B,** Eye protection. (Courtesy of Viamed Ltd.)

to 6 hours and then every 6 to 12 hours once stable or falling (NICE 2016a). After stopping phototherapy, it is important to check the serum bilirubin at 12 hours (NICE) (see Fig. 47.9) to monitor for significant rebound in hyperbilirubinemia, which may require further treatment.

Other tools have been developed to assist the team in monitoring the progress and management of jaundice (Fig. 47.10).

Exchange transfusion

Exchange transfusion involves removing the baby's blood, with maternal antibodies and bilirubin within it, and replacing it with fresh, Rhesus-negative blood. During this procedure, up to 90% of the blood may be replaced. This was the first treatment to be successfully used for severe neonatal jaundice. It is particularly useful in haemolytic

Jaundice

Treatment threshold graph for babies with neonatal jaundice

Baby's name...   Date of birth..

Hospital number...................   Time of birth...............   Direct Antiglobulin test.............   **>=38 weeks gestation**

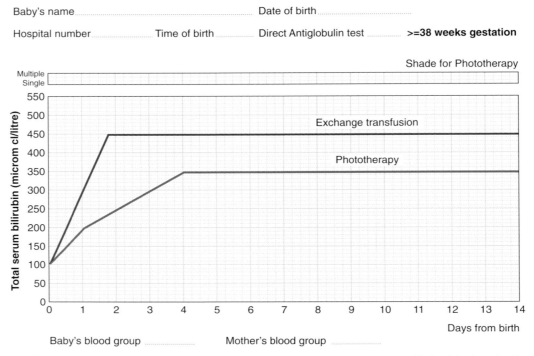

Baby's blood group ....   Mother's blood group ....

Figure 47.9 Treatment threshold for babies with neonatal jaundice over 38 weeks gestation. (National Institute for Health and Care Excellence: Adapted from CG98 Jaundice in newborn babies under 28 days (revised). Manchester, NICE 2016a. Available from https://www.nice.org.uk/guidance/cg98/evidence. Reproduced with permission. The material was accurate at the time of going to press.)

disease because both the red blood cells and the red cell antibodies causing their breakdown are removed from the neonatal circulation. Removal of the antibodies prevents late-onset anaemia.

The main indications for exchange transfusion are as follows:

- Severe haemolytic disease
- Anaemia, particularly with hydrops fetalis (high risk)
- Significant hyperbilirubinemia
- Hyperbilirubinemia uncontrolled by phototherapy
- Hyperbilirubinemia associated with polycythaemia

Exchange transfusion is sometimes carried out for other conditions, such as severe sepsis or metabolic disorders; these conditions are not within the scope of this chapter (see further reading section and chapter website).

The exact level of hyperbilirubinemia at which exchange transfusion should be performed remains difficult to define, but it is set at a level at which the risk of kernicterus outweighs the risk of the procedure (some authorities set this as 1%, although the risk of an exchange transfusion in a term baby with no other complications is less than this). It is not recommended that the ratio of bilirubin to albumin should influence the decision (NICE 2016a). Phototherapy should be continued throughout the procedure (AAP 2004; Hulzebos et al 2008).

In most cases, a two-volume exchange is performed: 160 mL/kg of the circulating blood volume is removed and replaced with transfused whole blood (commonly, packed red cells and 0.9% saline or 4.5% albumin because whole blood is difficult to obtain). The procedure must be conducted slowly under strict aseptic conditions, with precise and detailed recording of the amount of blood

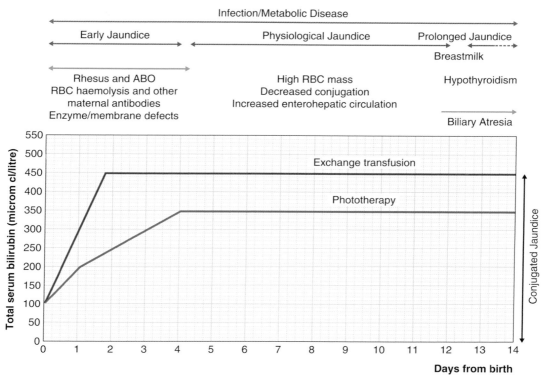

Figure 47.10 The different types of jaundice using an adaption of the NICE threshold guidelines for babies over 38 weeks gestation. RBC, red blood cell. (National Institute for Health and Care Excellence: Adapted from CG98 Jaundice in newborn babies under 28 days (revised). Manchester, NICE, 2016a. Available from https://www.nice.org.uk/guidance/cg98/evidence. Reproduced with permission. The material was accurate at the time of going to press.)

removed and amount infused. Ideally, two practitioners should undertake this to maintain high safety standards. There are two methods: single site or two site.

The preferred *two-site method* involves aspirating blood from a peripheral or umbilical artery at a similar rate to the infusion rate of a transfusion that is being delivered through a peripheral vein.

The *single-site method* involves cannulation of the umbilical vein with aspiration of 5–10 mL of blood through a three-way tap followed by infusion of the same quantity of donor blood. This may result in significant changes in central venous pressure and intravascular volume and is also associated with the complications of umbilical venous cannulation.

Once the transfusion is completed, the baby should continue to be monitored under phototherapy until the hyperbilirubinemia has begun to decrease and phototherapy is no longer needed. In most cases, an exchange transfusion followed by double phototherapy is effective;

however, some babies may require additional exchange transfusion.

Complications

Complications from exchange therapy are more common than those from phototherapy and include the following:

- Electrolyte imbalance
- Thrombocytopenia
- Infection
- Cardiac failure
- Emboli from the catheters
- Necrotizing enterocolitis

An exchange transfusion should only be performed in a baby at significant risk of kernicterus in whom the benefits of transfusion outweigh the risks of complications (Ahlfors 1994). The risks can be minimized by intensively monitoring electrolytes and platelets throughout the procedure and by reducing the changes in circulating blood volume during the procedure.

Immunoglobulin

The use of intravenous immunoglobulin to reduce ongoing haemolysis as an additional form of treatment in haemolytic jaundice has also been described, and there is now good evidence for this (NICE 2016a; Alpay et al 1999; Ergaz and Arad 1993).

PROLONGED JAUNDICE

Prolonged jaundice is jaundice after 2 weeks of age in a term and/or in a preterm baby who remains jaundiced at 3 weeks. Both situations require paediatric assessment and investigation. Investigation should normally include the following:

- Split bilirubin (direct and indirect or conjugated vs. unconjugated)
- Full blood count
- G6PD deficiency
- Urine culture (Hannam et al 2000)
- Thyroid function tests

The urgency of testing is driven by the need to consider biliary atresia because the outcome after surgery is much better if the baby is operated on before 6 weeks of age. A baby with biliary atresia may not be severely jaundiced but will have pale stools and dark urine (see following discussion).

CONJUGATED HYPERBILIRUBINEMIA

Conjugated hyperbilirubinemia is always pathological and refers to a situation where more than 15% of the total bilirubin or more than 25 µmol/L is in conjugated or 'direct reacting' form. This occurs as a direct consequence of interruption in the normal conjugation and hepatic excretion of *bilirubin diglucuronide* and results from an obstruction at any point along the pathway from the hepatocyte to the intestine. Bilirubin conjugation within the liver is often able to continue even in the presence of significant liver damage, but the excretion of the conjugated bilirubin into intrahepatic bile ducts may become obstructed. Consequently, the concentration of bilirubin diglucuronide within the hepatocytes will continue to increase, and eventually it diffuses into the bloodstream.

Conjugated jaundice can be suspected clinically in a baby with pale stools (absent stercobilinogen) and dark urine (bilirubin present). These are critical clinical features because this jaundice may initially be subtle and easily missed, and this condition always requires further assessment.

The main causes of a conjugated jaundice are as follows:

- Hepatitis with cholestasis
  - Idiopathic (unknown)
  - Prolonged total parenteral nutrition (TPN)
  - Congenital infection, such as CMV, toxoplasmosis, rubella
  - Metabolic disease – for example, alpha-1 antitrypsin deficiency
  - Galactosemia
- Bile duct abnormality
  - Biliary atresia
    - Intrahepatic – for example, Alagille syndrome (autosomal dominant)
    - Extrahepatic

In a term baby without perinatal concerns, conjugated jaundice most commonly presents as prolonged jaundice. Any term baby who remains jaundiced at 10 days to 2 weeks of age should be investigated for conjugated jaundice by examining the stools and taking blood for a 'split' bilirubin (direct and indirect bilirubin). Other recommended investigations are to ensure the baby's thyroid function was tested as part of the national screen and to consider infection. Infants with extrahepatic biliary atresia must be identified as early as possible because surgery performed at 4 to 6 weeks improves prognosis. The short-term outcome of biliary atresia has not been found to be improved by steroids (Vejchapipat et al 2007), and the long-term outcome remains guarded with regard to long-term liver disease (Hadzic et al 2003; Hartley et al 2009).

Complications

Complications may be general or specific complications of the underlying disease itself rather than direct complications of the jaundice.

General

- Deranged clotting with bleeding concerns
- Hypoglycaemia – as a result of underlying hepatic dysfunction
- Reduced absorption of fat-soluble vitamins, including vitamins A, D and K, which may require IV/IM vitamin K and appropriate vitamin preparations, such as Keto Vite

Specific

- Septicaemia
- Cataracts in galactosemia
- Microcephaly in congenital infection

Management of conjugated hyperbilirubinemia

The main objective in the management is to establish the cause of the jaundice. Phototherapy is ineffective because conjugated bilirubin is already water soluble, and the inappropriate use of phototherapy may lead to the *'bronzed baby'* syndrome. Exchange transfusion is not indicated for a conjugated hyperbilirubinemia because conjugated bilirubin is not lipid soluble in the same way as unconjugated bilirubin and will not cause kernicterus.

Signs may include the following:

- Petechiae
- Bruising
- Bleeding
- Hepatomegaly

First-line investigations should include blood glucose, liver function tests and clotting studies. Early advice should be sought from a paediatric hepatologist so that the most appropriate investigations and subsequent management can be arranged.

Transfer from hospital to home

Early transfer from home to hospital after birth is the norm for the majority of mothers and babies. However, it is crucial that the midwife is able to swiftly identify and manage babies with jaundice, and this includes knowing which babies may be at greater risk of developing pathological jaundice.

The aim of care is to identify the at-risk baby and facilitate her or his rapid return to the hospital should the bilirubin levels be found to be high or to be rising to potentially harmful levels. This requires a strategy in the National Health Service (NHS) that enables seamless teamwork across specialties (midwifery, neonatal nursing, general practice and neonatal services) to facilitate early recognition of babies with neonatal jaundice, regular monitoring of bilirubin levels and initiation of appropriate management, such as support of breastfeeding.

Before transfer from hospital/birth centre to home

It is vital that each baby is assessed by the midwife at no more than 60 minutes before leaving the unit for transfer home. This is to identify whether the baby is well enough to be transferred home and to confirm that there is an absence of jaundice.

Table 47.3 Identification of jaundice risk factors

Essential history and information	
Dates • LMP/EDD/scans – best estimate of gestation: to exclude the baby who is less than 38 weeks gestation	**Maternal history** • Maternal medical history – diabetes • Family history (general) • Family history (specific) • Previous children with jaundice • G6PD
Antenatal screening • Blood group and antibodies • VDRL/TPHA • Hepatitis B and HIV (if recorded) • Microbiological results (if done) • To identify the risk of ABO incompatibility • To identify the baby at risk of infection	**Labour and delivery** • Mode of delivery • Duration of labour, ruptured membranes • Risk factors for infection • Analgesia/trauma, which may affect breastfeeding • Cephalohematoma • Bruising • Infection

EDD, estimated delivery date; LMP, last menstrual period; TPHA, *T. pallidum* hemagglutination assay; VDRL, Venereal Disease Research Laboratory

In making this assessment, the midwife should consider the risk factors described in Table 47.3 and Box 47.4.

THE ROLE OF THE MIDWIFE WITH THE PARENTS

Parents need to be given information during the antenatal period in regard to such issues as jaundice so that they have time to assimilate the information and are prepared to receive the detail following the birth of the baby and the subsequent transfer home (NICE 2014; NICE 2016).

It is important to note that the baby is *transferred* home if the midwife providing care in the community is employed by the acute service, and thus the care and lead professional caring for that baby is the neonatologist. When the baby is *discharged*, it is normally when the midwife discharges the baby to the care of the general practitioner (GP) and health visitor. However, if the baby is going home and the community midwife is employed by the GP, then the baby is defined as being *discharged* from hospital to home, and the lead professional is the GP.

Box 47.4 A checklist to establish the need for transcutaneous bilirubin (TcB) monitoring before going home

❏ Gestation: less than 38 weeks
❏ Age of the baby less than 72 hours
❏ Check that the full assessment from head to toe has been completed and there are no deviations from normal.
❏ Overall condition: **well or not well?**
❏ Size of baby: large or small for date (exclude polycythaemia)
❏ Ethnic background of mother (Mediterranean, Pakistan, African etc.)
❏ Awake with eye-to-eye contact
❏ Muscle tone: all limbs well flexed
❏ Colour: eyes—sclera clear; mouth—gums and hard palate pink
❏ Respiratory effort: appropriate and there are no signs of respiratory distress (see Ch. 46)
❏ Temperature: baby maintaining her/his temperature (see Ch. 43)

❏ Ability to feed; absence of distended abdomen and vomiting
❏ Passed meconium and urine
❏ Review all maternal concerns: the mother's concerns must all be acted upon and excluded before the baby is transferred home.
❏ Mother has the NICE guidelines leaflet on jaundice and there has been a discussion to make sure the mother understands how to recognize jaundice and why it is important to identify jaundice to prevent the toxicity of jaundice to the brain.
❏ Inform parents that jaundice that is prolonged longer than 14 days in a baby above 37 weeks needs to be investigated to exclude liver disease and other causes.
❏ **Any concerns require referral for neonatal review.**
❏ **If the baby is fit to be transferred home, it is important to share the completed care plan with the mother and insert in the 'Red Book'. (See Ch. 42.)**

Language is very important because it provides accuracy for management and care, enabling the appropriate professionals to be involved in the care of the baby. It also provides explicit legality in interpretation of the care that will follow the baby once he or she leaves the hospital.

Reflective activity 47.2

Consider how you provide information to women and families about jaundice. What do you think are the key elements of information that they need, and how can you explain jaundice in words they will understand? You may wish to practice delivering this information with a fellow colleague.

The most important purpose of talking to parents about neonatal hyperbilirubinemia is to ensure that they understand the importance of working with the healthcare team to support the identification and management of jaundice. The mother and family need to know that there is a risk to the baby having high bilirubin levels. The priority of care is to reduce the risk to the baby of the impact of these high bilirubin levels, in particular, the risk of *kernicterus*, which, although rare, can be fatal or may cause major neurological damage, such as *cerebral palsy*. Parents also need to know what they should do and whom they should

contact if the baby's condition seems to be deteriorating or if they have any worries.

Neonatal conditions such as jaundice may require separation of the baby from his or her parents, and this is likely to create additional feelings of anxiety and fear, which may further influence how receptive the mother and father are to learning about and understanding what is happening with their baby and how much information they can retain. Therefore, as well as not 'overloading' parents with information, it is useful to ask for feedback regarding understanding before proceeding to the next part of the information (Box 47.5) whenever possible. Supportive resources, such as the NICE leaflet (NICE 2010; NICE 2016a) or locally produced information, can assist them in following and contributing to the follow-up plan of care (see Box 47.6).

FOLLOW-UP

All babies who have had significant unconjugated hyperbilirubinemia should be reviewed at least once following transfer. This enables results of investigations to be reviewed, further investigations to be arranged if appropriate, and the baby's clinical condition to be reassessed. Because one of the complications of hyperbilirubinemia is sensorineural hearing loss, these babies should have formal hearing tests (see chapter website resources).

Box 47.5 Communication example

Was what you taught what they heard?

Seek feedback to validate learning by asking the following questions:

- How can you check the skin for jaundice? (Ask for a demonstration.)
- What will you do if your baby starts to appear jaundiced at home?

Demonstration given to parents

Eyes: Show the parents what and where the sclera is and how it can be visualized.

- Inform the mother that the white part of the eyeball is called the sclera.
- Show her how to view the baby's eye if the baby is sleepy to get a good look at the sclera – this will entail that she gently pulls downward on the lower eyelid. If she notices the colour to be yellowish, it identifies that the baby is jaundiced.

Skin: Undress the baby in a warm room with natural light, for instance, by a window.

- Use the tip of the baby's nose or centre of the forehead to 'blanch' the skin.
- A pale-pink colour is normal and expected. If you notice the skin tone to be yellow, the baby may be jaundiced.

Dehydration: Parents need to understand the importance of excluding dehydration and making sure that the baby is getting an appropriately adequate amount of breastmilk. Asking the parents to record the baby's responsive feeding and how many dirty nappies the baby has in one day will enable the practitioner to identify a baby at risk.

Following completion of the demonstration, ask the mother/parents what they understood from what you have taught them.

Box 47.6 Principles of communication with parents

Communication with the mother and families must have the following characteristics:

- Provided in a simple, clear way, in language that the woman and family can understand
- Provided in manageable amounts, which may need to be repeated or rephrased to ensure understanding
- Culturally competent and sensitive (see Ch. 11)
- Based on trust and honesty between family and health service
- Based on compassion and sensitivity to the fears, anxieties and worries of the family
- Supported by appropriate written information/ leaflets (e.g. NICE factsheet 2010)

Babies with clinical evidence of acute bilirubin encephalopathy require continued neurodevelopmental follow-up and further investigations such as MRI to establish a guide to prognosis.

THE FUTURE

The importance of neonatal jaundice has been recognized in a project led by NHS England (the ATAIN project), commenced in late 2015, looking at term-newborn readmission rates to neonatal units for conditions including jaundice, hypoglycaemia, asphyxia and respiratory problems. (See chapter website resources.) Each condition is being explored by a different subgroup, which is reviewing admission data, litigation rates, treatment and management and prevention resources (human and equipment). The work of the jaundice group in particular is due to be reported in 2017 and is likely to include the development of education and training for professionals and parents, parent and user involvement and the provision of designated care bundles for jaundiced babies and their parents.

CONCLUSION

Jaundice is a common problem for the newborn baby. An understanding of the normal physiology of bilirubin metabolism enables the midwife to predict risk factors for the development of unconjugated hyperbilirubinemia and be aware of the clinical signs suggestive of a conjugated hyperbilirubinemia. The aim in dealing with unconjugated hyperbilirubinemia is to prevent babies from developing severe jaundice that may lead to bilirubin encephalopathy

Neonates who have had haemolytic jaundice require early review and regular follow-up for the first 3 months of life because the other effect of haemolysis is anaemia (especially when the treatment was phototherapy without an exchange transfusion). The baby should be seen at less than 2 weeks of age to review his or her clinical condition and to perform a full blood count. This investigation will provide information about the extent of the ongoing haemolysis (haemoglobin) and the baby's bone marrow response and ability to compensate (reticulocyte count). Some babies may require a blood transfusion at a later date.

and kernicterus. Infants with prolonged jaundice must be referred to a paediatrician to swiftly identify conjugated hyperbilirubinemia. The midwife will often be the person who will identify the jaundice and continue to provide care and support to the woman, baby and family. The midwife needs to be knowledgeable about the different aspects of care and management, be able to provide accurate and evidence-based information to the family and ensure that they feel informed and confident in the professionals providing care to the baby.

Key Points

- Jaundice is the clinical consequence of a high level of bilirubin that may be unconjugated or conjugated.

- Jaundice is common but must always be investigated when it is noted at less than 48 hours of age, is significant or is prolonged for more than 2 weeks.

- A baby with visible jaundice requires measurement of serum bilirubin level.

- A significant unconjugated hyperbilirubinemia must be treated with phototherapy or exchange transfusion to prevent the acute complications of kernicterus and long-term complications of deafness and athetoid cerebral palsy.

- It is important that midwives are knowledgeable about contemporary management of jaundice – for example, the previous management technique of sunlight is no longer recommended for the treatment of jaundice.

- A baby who is jaundiced with pale stools and dark urine requires urgent assessment and referral to a paediatric hepatologist.

References

Ahlfors CE: Criteria for exchange transfusion in jaundiced newborns, *Pediatrics* 93(3):488–494, 1994.

Alpay F, Sarici SU, Okutan V, et al: High-dose intravenous immunoglobulin therapy in neonatal immune haemolytic jaundice, *Acta Paediatr* 88(2):216–219, 1999.

American Academy of Pediatrics (AAP): Management of hyperbilirubinemia in the newborn infant 35 or more weeks of gestation, *Pediatrics* 114(1):297–316, 2004.

Bhutani VK, Johnson LH: Managing the assessment of neonatal jaundice: importance of timing, *Indian J Pediatr* 67(10):733–737, 2000.

Brethauer M, Carey L: Maternal experience with neonatal jaundice, *MCN Am J Matern Child Nurs* 35(1):8–14, 2010.

Cremer RJ, Perryman PW, Richards DH: Influence of light on the hyperbilirubinaemia of infants, *Lancet* 1094–1097, 1958.

Dennery PA, Seidman DS, Stevenson DK: Neonatal hyperbilirubinaemia, *N Engl J Med* 344(8):581–590, 2001.

Dodd KL: Neonatal jaundice – a lighter touch, *Arch Dis Child* 68(5):529–532, 1993.

Engle WD, Jackson GL, Stehel EK, et al: Evaluation of a transcutaneous jaundice meter following hospital discharge in term and near-term neonates, *J Perinatol* 25(7):486–490, 2005.

Ergaz Z, Arad I: Intravenous immunoglobulin therapy in neonatal immune hemolytic jaundice, *J Perinat Med* 21(3):183–187, 1993.

Google Play: *Bili app* (website). https://play.google.com/store/apps/details?id=com.incubateltd.biliapp&hl=en 2016.

Hachiya Y, Hayashi M: Bilirubin encephalopathy: a study of neuronal subpopulations and neurodegenerative mechanisms in 12 autopsy cases, *Brain Dev* 30(4):269–278, 2008.

Hadzic N, Davenport M, Tizzard S, et al: Long-term survival following Kasai portoenterostomy: is chronic liver disease inevitable? *J Pediatr Gastroenterol Nutr* 37(4):430–433, 2003.

Hannam S, McDonnell M, Rennie JM: Investigation of prolonged neonatal jaundice, *Acta Paediatr* 89(6):694–697, 2000.

Hansen TW: Bilirubin oxidation in brain, *Mol Genet Metab* 71(1–2):411–417, 2000a.

Hansen TW: Kernicterus in term and near-term infants – the specter walks again, *Acta Paediatr* 89(10):1155–1157, 2000b.

Harris MC, Bernbaum JC, Polin JR, et al: Developmental follow-up of breastfed term and near-term infants with marked hyperbilirubinemia, *Pediatrics* 107(5):1075–1080, 2001.

Hartley JL, Davenport M, Kelly DA: Biliary atresia, *Lancet* 374(9702):1704–1713, 2009.

Holtrop PC, Ruedisueli K, Maisels MJ: Double versus single phototherapy in low birth weight newborns, *Pediatrics* 90(5):674–677, 1992.

Huang M-J, Kua KE, Teng HC, et al: Risk factors for severe hyperbilirubinemia in neonates, *Pediatr Res* 56:682–689, 2004.

Hulzebos CV, van Imhoff DE, Bos AF, et al: Usefulness of the bilirubin/

albumin ratio for predicting bilirubin-induced neurotoxicity in premature infants, *Arch Dis Child Fetal Neonatal Ed* 93(5):F384–F388, 2008.

Manning D, Todd P, Maxwell M, et al: Prospective surveillance study of severe hyperbilirubinaemia in the newborn in the UK and Ireland, *Arch Dis Child Fetal Neonatal Ed* 92(5):F342–F346, 2007.

National Institute for Health and Clinical Excellence (NICE): *Pregnancy – routine anti-D prophylaxis for Rhesus negative women (review of TA41)* (website). http://guidance.nice.org.uk/TA156. 2008.

National Institute for Health and Clinical Excellence: *Jaundice in newborn babies: information for parents and carers (Factsheet)*, NICE, 2010.

National Institute for Health and Care Excellence: *Jaundice in newborn babies under 28 days [CG98]*. Manchester, NICE. https://www.nice.org.uk/guidance/cg98/evidence/full-guideline-245411821. 2016a.

National Institute for Health and Clinical Excellence (NICE): *Ectopic pregnancy and miscarriage: diagnosis and initial management NICE guidelines [CG154]*, London, NICE, 2012.

National Institute for Health and Care Excellence (NICE): *Jaundice in newborn babies under 28 days, NICE quality standard [QS57]*, London, NICE, 2014.

National Institute for Health and Care Excellence (NICE): *Not do recommendation: do not offer anti-D Rhesus prophylaxis to women who: receive solely medical management for an ectopic pregnancy or miscarriage or have a threatened miscarriage or have a complete miscarriage or have a pregnancy of unknown location. Interventions: Anti-D Rhesus prophylaxis*, London, NICE, 2015.

Newman TB, Maisels MJ: Evaluation and treatment of jaundice in the term newborn: a kinder, gentler approach, *Pediatrics* 89(5 Pt 1):809–818, 1992.

Nicoll A, Ginsburg R, Tripp JH: Supplementary feeding and jaundice in newborns, *Acta Paediatr Scand* 71(5):759–761, 1982.

Nursing and Midwifery Council (NMC): *Standards of medicine management*, London, 2010, NMC.

Pearlman MA, Gartner LM, Lee K, et al: The association of kernicterus with bacterial infection in the newborn, *Pediatrics* 65(1):26–29, 1980.

Sanpavat S, Nuchprayoon I, Smathakanee C, et al: Nomogram for prediction of the risk of neonatal hyperbilirubinemia, using transcutaneous bilirubin, *J Med Assoc Thai* 88(9):1187–1193, 2005.

Vejchapipat P, Passakonnirin R, Sookpotarom P, et al: High-dose steroids do not improve early outcome in biliary atresia, *J Pediatr Surg* 42(12):2102–2105, 2007.

Resources and additional reading

National Institute for Health and Care Excellence: *Jaundice in newborn babies under 28 days [CG98]*. Manchester, NICE. https://www.nice.org.uk/guidance/cg98/evidence/full-guideline-245411821. 2016a.

Excellent resource from NICE that provides the evidence supporting practice.

Royal College of Midwives (RCM): *Electronic learning programme (i-Learn): neonatal jaundice module* (website). www.rcm.org.uk. 2015.

This is an excellent free-to-members resource that includes a module on neonatal jaundice. There are also modules on examination of the newborn and thermoregulation issues for newborns.

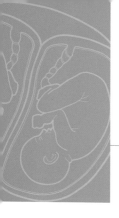

Chapter 48

Neonatal infection

Glenys Connolly

Learning Outcomes ?

After reading this chapter, you will be able to:

- explain the acquisition of infection
- describe common organisms affecting the fetus and newborn
- understand the investigation and management of the potentially infected newborn

INTRODUCTION

Infection is a major cause of neonatal morbidity and mortality worldwide. A study published in 2010 (Black et al 2010) reported that infection caused an estimated 29% of neonatal deaths worldwide, with the mortality being considerably higher in third-world and developing countries than it is in resource-rich populations.

Within the UK, the incidence of early-onset sepsis (EOS) continues to decrease as a result of improved management of premature rupture of membranes; however, the incidence of late-onset and nosocomial (hospital-acquired) sepsis is increasing, in part because of the improved survival of extremely low-birthweight babies, with their concomitant long stay in the hospital and use of parenteral nutrition via central lines (Vergnano et al 2011).

This chapter focuses on the situations midwives encounter in their day-to-day practice rather than those infants requiring more intensive management within the neonatal unit.

ACQUISITION OF INFECTION

Sepsis in the newborn period can be categorized into the following three types:

Early-onset sepsis (EOS) is variously defined as presenting at less than 24 hours to less than 72 hours; the infection is presumed to be acquired from the mother shortly before or at the time of birth.

Late-onset sepsis (LOS) presents after 72 hours as a result of community-acquired contact with family members or organisms in the environment.

Nosocomial sepsis is hospital-acquired sepsis. This most commonly affects preterm or low-birthweight infants within a neonatal unit as a result of indwelling central lines, mechanical ventilation and use of parenteral nutrition.

The mechanisms for acquisition of infection are as follows:

Transplacental: Infection is caused by organisms that can penetrate the placental barrier.
For example, viruses such as rubella can have a devastating effect on the developing fetus. *Listeria monocytogenes* can cause placentitis and lead to miscarriage or stillbirth.

Ascending: Infections most commonly acquired by this route are from the group B streptococci (GBS), *Escherichia coli* and *L. monocytogenes*, resulting in EOS.

Intrapartum: Vertically acquired infection caused by organisms in the birth canal, most commonly GBS, *E. coli*, hepatitis B virus (HBV), herpes simplex virus (HSV) and HIV, resulting in EOS or LOS.

NEWBORN IMMUNITY

Newborn infants are susceptible to infection because of the naiveté of the immune system, which has not been exposed to the organisms it encounters during and immediately following birth. Consequently, the newborn has a delayed response to invading organisms. The immune system is developing from early fetal life but does not become fully integrated until approximately 1 year of age. The newborn's skin and mucous membranes provide the initial defence, which is augmented by mucus secretions, stomach acid and skin flora. These defences may be breached by the application of scalp electrodes, fetal blood sampling, peripartum antibiotics, caesarean section and overzealous bathing, all of which disrupt host defence proteins found on the skin and in the gut flora. Similarly, both nonspecific and specific defences are diminished when white blood cell responses and cell-mediated responses are delayed.

At term, the infant does have some acquired immunity from the mother because the immunoglobulin (IgG) crosses the placenta in the third trimester and provides the infant with passive immunity to any diseases the mother has had. This lasts until approximately 2 months of age. IgM (the first-response immunoglobulin) does not cross the placenta, but the fetus synthesizes small amounts; however, adult levels of IgM are not achieved until 5 years of age. IgA is a secretory immunoglobulin found in mucous membranes and breastmilk; its predominant role is to protect the gastrointestinal tract from infection. Breastmilk has the additional benefits of lactoferrin, lysozyme, neutrophils and macrophages, bifidobacteria and cytokines, all of which serve to induce normal gut and immune development.

Pathogenesis

Pregnancy is an immunocompromised state, with the woman having reduced cell-mediated immunity responses so that she doesn't mount an immune response to the developing fetus (Isaacs 2014). This state increases susceptibility to both viral (e.g. chickenpox, HIV and influenza) and bacterial infections (e.g. *L. monocytogenes*), which can significantly affect the developing fetus because of their ability to cross the placenta to the fetus.

Generally, the fetus is protected from microorganisms in utero by the amniotic liquor, which has bactericidal and bacteriostatic properties; the intact amniotic membranes, which provide a physical barrier, and the cervical mucoid plug, which contains IgGs and antimicrobial peptides. So long as these elements remain unbreached, the fetus should not encounter any potentially harmful pathogens.

Maternal risk factors

Premature rupture of membranes (PROM) increases the risk of EOS, with the incidence steadily increasing beyond 12 hours. Maternal temperature is also implicated in EOS, with the risk increasing with a temperature greater than 38°C (Puopolo et al 2011). The National Institute for Health and Care Excellence (NICE 2012) included these factors in its published guidance regarding risk factors for newborn sepsis and the need for antibiotic therapy (Box 48.1).

Maternal antibiotic use in these situations reduces chorioamnionitis; however, with PROM, the antimicrobial used needs careful consideration. The ORACLE study

---

Box 48.1 Clinical indicators for early-onset sepsis (observed events in the infant)

- Altered behaviour or responsiveness
- Altered muscle tone (e.g. floppiness)
- Feeding difficulties (e.g. feed refusal)
- Feed intolerance, including vomiting, abdominal distension
- Abnormal heart rate (bradycardia or tachycardia)
- Signs of respiratory distress
- Hypoxia (e.g. central cyanosis or reduced oxygen saturation level)
- Jaundice within 24 hours of birth
- Apnoea
- Signs of neonatal encephalopathy
- Need for cardiopulmonary resuscitation
- Need for mechanical ventilation in a preterm baby
- Persistent fetal circulation (persistent pulmonary hypertension)
- Temperature abnormality (lower than 36°C or higher than 38°C) unexplained by environmental factors
- Unexplained excessive bleeding, thrombocytopenia or abnormal coagulation
- Oliguria persisting beyond 24 hours after birth
- Altered glucose homeostasis (hypoglycaemia or hyperglycaemia)
- Metabolic acidosis (base deficit of 10 mmol/L or greater)
- Local signs of infection (e.g. affecting the skin or eye)
- Respiratory distress starting more than 4 hours after birth
- Seizures
- Signs of shock
- Need for mechanical ventilation in a term baby

Source: NICE 2012

(Kenyon et al 2001) noted that amoxicillin-clavulanic acid (Co-amoxiclav) increased the risk of neonatal necrotizing enterocolitis more than fourfold, whereas erythromycin did not. However, although in the short term the infants of the mothers receiving erythromycin required shorter durations of respiratory support, a longer-term study showed that these infants had an increased risk of functional impairment and cerebral palsy (Bedford Russell and Steer 2008). The proposed mechanism for this is that although the erythromycin dosage may have suppressed the infection sufficiently to prolong the pregnancy, the dose was insufficient to eradicate the infection, leaving the developing fetus in a more damaging environment.

Chorioamnionitis

Clinical chorioamnionitis, which presents with signs of fever, tachycardia, and uterine tenderness, occurs in 1% to 10% of pregnancies (Tita and Andrews 2010), with membrane rupture and labour frequently ensuing. Only a relatively small proportion of newborns will develop proven sepsis following chorioamnionitis; however, the risk of cerebral palsy is significantly increased (Shatrov et al 2010).

Risk factors for early-onset sepsis

The risk factors for EOS are outlined in Box 48.2. The management is as follows: If the infant has one risk factor,

---

Box 48.2 Risk factors for early-onset neonatal sepsis

- Invasive group B streptococcal infection in a previous baby
- Maternal group B streptococcal colonization, bacteriuria or infection in the current pregnancy
- Prelabour rupture of membranes
- Preterm birth following spontaneous labour (before 37 weeks gestation)
- Suspected or confirmed rupture of membranes for more than 18 hours in a preterm birth
- Intrapartum fever higher than 38°C or confirmed or suspected chorioamnionitis
- Parenteral antibiotic treatment given to the woman for confirmed or suspected invasive bacterial infection (such as septicaemia) at any time during labour, or in the 24-hour periods before and after the birth (This does not refer to intrapartum antibiotic prophylaxis.)
- Suspected or confirmed infection in another baby in the case of a multiple pregnancy

Source: NICE 2012

---

increased surveillance should commence on the postnatal ward using a newborn early-warning chart (British Association of Perinatal Medicine (BAPM) 2015) (Fig. 48.1). If the infant has two or more risk factors, a septic screening should be undertaken, and the infant should be commenced on intravenous (IV) antibiotics until the results of the screening are received, usually 36 hours.

Infants falling into either of the red categories shown in Fig. 48.1 require screening and IV antibiotics immediately, and in most situations, they require transfer and admission to a neonatal unit.

Infants exhibiting any of the described or clinical observations in Box 48.1 need to be evaluated by a doctor or advanced neonatal nurse practitioner (ANNP). Following careful review of the history and examination of the infant, it should then be decided whether the infant needs increased surveillance using a newborn early-warning chart or screening and commencement of IV antibiotics (see Fig. 48.1).

Neonatal septic screening and antibiotic therapy

Because EOS is associated with poorer neonatal outcomes and can in certain circumstances be life threatening, the at-risk infant should be screened and treatment commenced within 1 hour of birth or recognition of risk factors. The choice of antibiotic will be dictated by local guidelines and is dependent on agreement between the neonatologists and the local microbiologist. The narrowest spectrum should be used to lessen the development of antibiotic resistance. As a general rule, a penicillin-based antibiotic will be used to cover gram-positive cocci (e.g. GBS), and an aminoglycoside such as gentamicin will be used to cover gram-negative bacilli (e.g. *E. coli*). Overuse of antibiotic therapy drives antibiotic resistance, and importantly for the newborn, it alters the colonizing microbial flora in the gut, leading to skewing of immune system development (Bedford Russell and Kumar 2015). It is for this reason that antibiotics commenced in the newborn period should stop as soon as possible, and the need for their continued use should be reviewed every 24 hours.

If a septic screening is required, it should consist of the following steps:

- Blood culture should be taken following scrupulous cleansing of the overlying skin to prevent contamination and false-positive results. The result of this should be available at 36 hours. If no organisms have been identified in the blood by this time, it is very unlikely that bloodborne sepsis is present, and the antibiotic therapy should cease. In the case of a positive culture, the antibiotics should continue for a minimum of 7 days and may have a much longer duration, depending on the organism isolated.

Newborn Early Warning and Track (NEWTT)

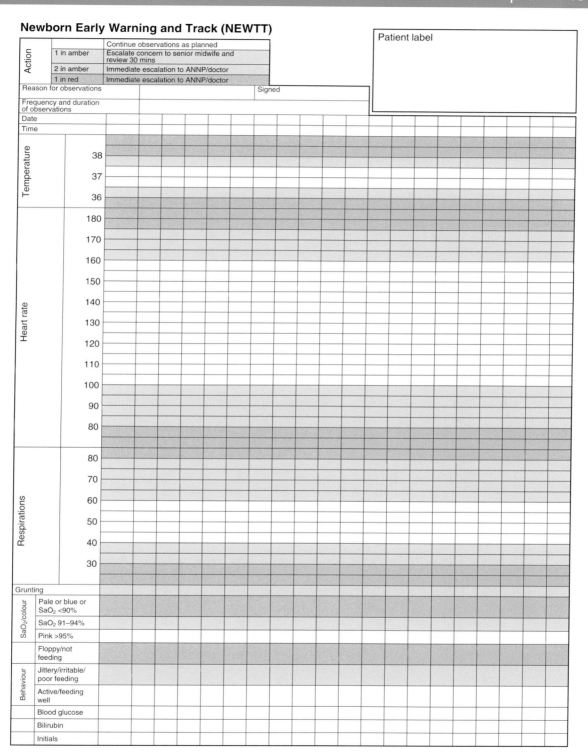

Figure 48.1 Newborn early-warning trigger and track. (Reproduced with kind permission of BAPM.)

- A full blood count should be completed to establish the white cell count, with the neutrophil count being the more reliable indicator of the presence of sepsis. Both neutropenia (less than $2–2.5 \times 10^9$) and neutrophilia (greater than 8.0×10^9) can indicate sepsis. Thrombocytopenia (low platelets) is more common in fungal infections and severe bacterial infections.

- C-reactive protein (CRP), an acute-phase protein produced by the liver, may be elevated. The CRP should be repeated 18 to 24 hours after the initial one was taken because it can be negative at first (less than 10 mmol/L) but rise significantly subsequently. Antibiotic therapy should continue in an infant with an elevated CRP even in the absence of a positive blood culture, but its use should be reviewed on a daily basis by the neonatal team and stopped as soon as possible.

- Lumbar puncture should be *considered* in the presence of an elevated CRP but *is indicated* in an infant presenting with seizures, signs of meningitis or LOS.

INFECTIONS ACQUIRED AROUND THE TIME OF BIRTH

Bacterial infections

Group B streptococcus

GBS accounts for 58% of infections in the newborn period (NICE 2014). Research suggests that it affects 0.9 per 1000 live births in the UK (Vergnano et al 2011). It can be acquired through the transplacental or vertical routes. Most cases (80%) present within hours of birth (Isaacs 2014) with respiratory distress; it can, however, present (or reoccur) as LOS up to 4 weeks of age. Infants with EOS caused by GBS are often bacteremic at birth; if left untreated, they will progress rapidly to develop meningitis (Isaacs 2014). It is for this reason that antibiotics should be commenced within an hour of the decision to screen and treat being made for any infant with suspected sepsis (NICE 2014).

Up to 40% of women in the UK have colonization of GBS within the bowel and genital tract. Women with confirmed GBS on a high vaginal swab or urine testing should have intrapartum antibiotic prophylaxis (IAP) commenced as soon as possible after the onset of labour but at least 4 hours before delivery. A Cochrane review (Ohlsson and Shah 2014) identified that IAP reduced the incidence of EOS caused by GBS compared with no treatment, but the review recommended that more robust studies need to be undertaken so that fewer women and infants are not exposed to antibiotics unnecessarily. IAP does not affect LOS caused by GBS infection. At the time of discharge from the hospital, parents of infants with proven sepsis should be given information (preferably written) regarding signs of LOS in the postnatal period (NICE 2012). This is particularly true of GBS because this infection can occur, with devastating consequences, up to 6 weeks of age.

Escherichia coli

E. coli accounts for 18% of newborn infections (NICE 2014). It can cause both EOS and LOS. *E. coli* is a major cause of neonatal urinary tract infection. Thus, a urine specimen for culture should be obtained for an infant with nonspecific signs of infection. Additionally, *E. coli* is a significant cause of neonatal meningitis.

Listeria monocytogenes

L. monocytogenes is responsible for less than 5% of EOS cases and has a more classical onset occurring at approximately 7 days of life (Isaacs 2014). It is an important infectious organism in the newborn because it carries a high morbidity and mortality rate. Maternal acquisition of *L. monocytogenes* from ingestion of undercooked meat, chicken and unpasteurized dairy products crosses the placenta and causes placentitis, which can lead to miscarriage, stillbirth and preterm labour. The midwife may suspect infection with this organism when cardiotocography (CTG) demonstrates persistent tachycardia with markedly reduced variability and shallow decelerations (Fig. 48.2). In addition, the presence of meconium-stained liquor in a fetus less than 34 weeks gestation should alert the midwife to potential listeriosis because meconium staining is very rare in infants of this gestation. Liveborn infants are often extremely unwell at birth, presenting with congenital pneumonia and hepatosplenomegaly. A pinkish-grey granulomatous rash may be present, which may be misinterpreted as petechiae. Meningitis will occur in about 30% of cases. The mortality rate is 25%, and the survivors of meningitis may develop hydrocephalus and other adverse neurological sequelae.

Viral infections

Several viruses can cause serious neonatal illness and carry a high mortality and morbidity rate. Most are acquired by vertical transmission, but some are the result of postnatal cross-infection.

Herpes viruses

Herpes simplex virus (HSV)

Neonatal HSV infections are rare but are associated with significant morbidity and mortality (Pinninti and Kimberlin, 2014). *Herpes* (Greek) means 'creeping' or 'latent', which perfectly describes the ability of the virus to lie dormant and reactivate periodically; it affects 8.4 per 100,000 live births in the UK.

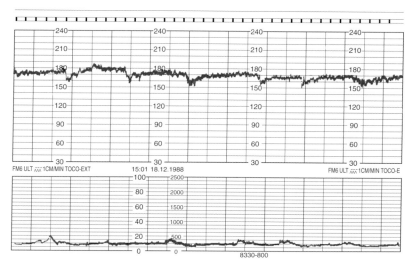

Figure 48.2 CTG suggestive of listerial infection. (This article was published in Gibb D, Arulkumaran S: Fetal monitoring in practice, ed 3, London and Edinburgh, Churchill Livingstone Elsevier, Copyright Elsevier. 2008)

HSV can be acquired transplacentally (less than 5%), vertically (85%–90%) or postnatally (5%). Transplacental acquisition may ascend even through intact membranes, with the congenitally affected infant being profoundly damaged and displaying microcephaly, chorioretinitis, skin vesicles and scarring.

HSV is more commonly acquired vertically during passage through the birth canal from maternal genital herpes. The mother may have no known history of genital herpes or be asymptomatic at the time. Primary infection during pregnancy carries an increased risk of transmission to the infant, which further increases the nearer to delivery it occurs. The Royal College of obstetrics and Gynaecology (RCOG 2014) recommends caesarean section for women with a primary herpes infection at the time of birth or within 6 weeks of the expected date of delivery. The woman may be given acyclovir during pregnancy at the time of infection and from 36 weeks gestation. Recurrent infections carry a much lower transmission rate, and women with recurrent infections may birth vaginally. The use of fetal scalp electrodes and fetal blood sampling should be avoided during labour.

Following delivery, the infant should be observed closely for signs of infection, as follows:

- Those infants born by caesarean section require normal care only and can go home after 24 hours, with parents advised to maintain scrupulous hand hygiene and to seek early medical attention should the infant show any signs of being unwell or develop lesions of the skin, eye or mouth.
- Infants born vaginally following primary infection should have conjunctival, rectal and oropharyngeal swabs for herpes polymerase chain reaction (PCR) testing taken and commence IV acyclovir three times a day empirically until results are back. Unwell infants should also have lumbar puncture and blood culture in addition to swabs.
- Infants of women who have recurrent herpes without active lesions at the time of birth should be managed as those who have been born by caesarean section.

In all cases, there should be a liaison with the neonatal team so that the postnatal plan can be activated as soon as possible.

Cytomegalovirus

Cytomegalovirus (CMV) is a herpes virus that shares many characteristics of HSV, especially the ability to cause latent infection. CMV is the most common congenital infection, and it is estimated to affect 0.3% of UK births (Williams et al 2015). CMV can be transmitted transplacentally to the fetus at any time during pregnancy, but it is most likely to cause serious harm if the mother has a primary infection during pregnancy. Congenital CMV can cause permanent impairment and disability, such as visual impairment and mental retardation, and it is the commonest non-genetic cause of sensorineural hearing loss. Approximately 10% of infants will be symptomatic at birth and present with growth restriction and microcephaly, which is associated with a poor neurological outcome (Isaacs 2014). CMV is treated with prolonged courses of IV and oral Valganciclovir, but this drug is toxic and has been shown to have equivocal results.

More asymptomatic infants are now being identified as having been exposed to CMV transmission during pregnancy when they undergo universal hearing screening. Targeted screening for CMV via salivary swab testing is currently undergoing scrutiny in the UK (Williams et al 2015) for infants who 'fail' their hearing screening because although earlier use of valganciclovir does not restore hearing loss, it does appear to prevent it from worsening.

Postnatally, CMV can be acquired by contact with infected saliva, blood, urine, genital tract secretions and breastmilk. Postnatal acquisition does not cause problems unless the infant is premature, in which case it can cause pneumonitis, enteritis and a sepsis-like syndrome; it is also linked to adverse changes in the cranial ultrasound (Nijman et al 2012).

Varicella zoster virus

Varicella zoster virus (VZV) is a herpes virus that causes varicella (chickenpox) during primary infection and causes zoster (shingles) when reactivated. Of women of child-bearing age in the UK, 95% have had varicella and are therefore immune; consequently, varicella in pregnancy is rare. If it is acquired during pregnancy, it can have devastating effects for both the woman and the developing fetus. Primary VZV in the immunosuppressed state of pregnancy can predispose the woman to life-threatening pneumonitis; depending on the gestation of the fetus (e.g. less than 20 weeks), it can lead to congenital varicella syndrome. VZV is highly teratogenic and affects 2% of fetuses exposed in early pregnancy, with effects on the brain, eye, skeleton, gastrointestinal and renal tracts. The skin may bear characteristic cutaneous scarring associated with limb defects. Women who develop the disease after 20 weeks gestation and up to 3 weeks before delivery will confer immunity to the fetus. If the woman develops VZV 5 days before or 2 days after delivery, the infant has the greatest risk for severe disease, which carries a high mortality rate (Bedford Russell and Isaacs 2012). Varicella zoster immunoglobulin (VZIG) should be administered to these infants immediately after birth; it will not prevent the disease from occurring but should lessen its severity. IV acyclovir should also be given, and the mother and infant should be nursed in isolation.

Maternal zoster infection (shingles) does not usually affect the infant. However, infants who have contracted congenital or perinatal varicella may develop shingles in the first month of life.

Other viruses/organisms

Rubella

Rubella was first described in the 18th century in Germany – hence its alternate name, German measles. If it is transmitted to the fetus in early pregnancy, less than 11 weeks, it will cause serious defects, principally congenital heart disease, severe developmental delay, deafness and cataracts. After 13 weeks it will cause deafness alone; at later than 16 weeks, there should be no defects attributable to rubella.

There is no specific treatment, but universal immunization is the most effective preventative strategy, and congenital rubella syndrome is extraordinarily rare in areas undertaking this approach. The rubella immunization (MMR) should be given to seronegative women postpartum because it is a live attenuated vaccine and is contraindicated during pregnancy.

Hepatitis B virus

Hepatitis B is a potentially life-threatening liver infection caused by the HBV and is a major global health problem. It can cause chronic infection and puts individuals at high risk of death from cirrhosis and liver cancer (World Health Organization (WHO) 2015). It is vertically transmitted by fetal exposure to maternal blood, amniotic fluid and vaginal secretions during birth. It is most common in East Asia and sub-Saharan African populations; in western Europe, the carriage rate is less than 1%. The risk of acquisition increases with the number of sexual partners and the use of IV drugs, especially if syringes and needles are shared or reused. Although all women in the UK are screened antenatally for hepatitis B surface antigen (HBsAg), only the infants of women who are antigen positive or those in the high-risk groups are offered vaccination in the postnatal period. The initial dose of vaccine should be given as soon as possible after birth (e.g. within 12 hours), with further doses at 1, 2 and 12 months (Bedford Russell and Isaacs 2012). WHO recommends universal vaccination of all infants, with the initial dose given soon after birth and the second and third doses given with the first and third 'routine' immunizations. The presence of 'e' antigen (HBeAg) in the woman's blood indicates a defective immune response to HBV, which allows its continued replication in the liver cells. This greatly increases the chance of transmission to the infant; thus, the infants of these women should also receive hepatitis B IgG.

Breastfeeding should not be discouraged because the transmission of the virus from breastmilk or blood via the nipple is negligible compared with the infant's exposure at delivery.

Hepatitis C

Hepatitis C virus (HCV) is a blood-borne virus and can be acquired during blood transfusions; it has a higher prevalence in IV drug users. It can be transmitted vertically to the infant during vaginal birth, with the transference rate being higher if the woman is also HIV positive. Vertically acquired HCV appears benign, although there are reported cases of aggressive liver disease in late childhood. If an infant is infected with HCV, prompt referral to a children's liver unit is indicated (Bedford Russell and Isaacs 2012). Breastfeeding appears to be safe.

Human immunodeficiency virus

Human immunodeficiency virus (HIV) is a retrovirus that damages the immune system and can lead to acquired immune deficiency syndrome (AIDS). The majority of infants are infected via mother-to-child transmission (MTCT) during pregnancy, birth and/or breastfeeding. In developed countries, perinatal transmission of HIV has been reduced to less than 1% by using the following combination of interventions:

- Use of maternal antenatal antiretroviral therapy (ART) from 28 weeks gestation until delivery to achieve an undetectable maternal viral load at the time of birth
- Active management of labour and birth to avoid prolonged rupture of the membranes, with avoidance of fetal sampling and instrumental delivery
- Prelabour caesarean section if the mother's viral load is detectable close to the time of birth
- Avoidance of breastfeeding (25%–40% acquisition rate)

    (Lissauer and Claydon 2012).

Women at term with negligible viral load can birth vaginally. Because the risk of gastroenteritis is potentially more harmful to the newborn in many parts of the world, breastfeeding is considered an acceptable risk, especially if ART is given as well. Following delivery, blood for HIV PCR testing should be taken from the infant (not from the cord because of potential contamination with maternal blood), with testing repeated at 1 and 3 months. The infant should receive oral ART within 6 hours of birth. Repeated blood testing is required for up to 18 months of age or until the infant can be deemed disease-free.

Parvovirus B19

Parvovirus B19 most commonly causes mild illness in children known as both 'fifth disease' and 'slapped cheek'. Infection in the mother is often asymptomatic but can cause severe anaemia in the fetus because of its effect on the fetal bone marrow, which can lead to hydrops fetalis and fetal death. Fetal anaemia may be treated by intra-uterine transfusion. Parvovirus can also lead to myocarditis, cardiomyopathy and liver disease in the newborn.

Toxoplasmosis

Toxoplasmosis occurs from exposure to *Toxoplasma gondii*, a protozoan parasite, which results from the consumption of raw or undercooked meat and from contact with the faeces of recently infected cats. Transplacental infection

may occur during a primary infection, with about 40% of fetuses becoming infected. The classic signs of congenital toxoplasmosis are hydrocephalus, seizures, cerebral calcification and chorioretinitis.

Treatment is with pyrimethamine and sulfadiazine for 1 year. Affected infants usually have long-term neurological disabilities. Asymptomatic infants remain at risk of developing chorioretinitis into adulthood.

Syphilis

Congenital syphilis is rare in the UK but is said to be increasing in developed countries (Sinha et al 2012). Penicillin is an effective treatment for both mother and fetus in cases diagnosed in the antenatal period. If treatment is given at least a month before delivery, the infant does not require postnatal treatment, unless there are concerns regarding its efficacy. Affected infants present with a number of features (see Fig. 48.3), including a characteristic rash on the soles of the feet and hands and widespread bony lesions. All women who have positive serology in pregnancy should be treated according to British Association for Sexual Health and HIV national guidelines for the management of syphilis (see www.bashh.org/guidelines).

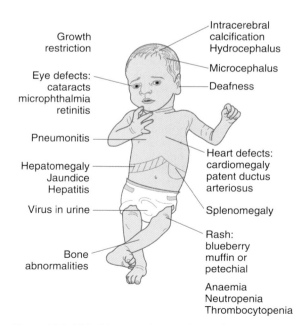

Figure 48.3 Clinical features of congenital rubella, cytomegalovirus (CMV), toxoplasmosis and syphilis. (This article was published in Lissauer T, Claydon GS: Illustrated textbook of paediatrics, 4th edn, London, Elsevier, Copyright Elsevier.)

LOCALIZED SUPERFICIAL INFECTIONS

Eye infections

Conjunctivitis in the newborn period can vary from a benign form manifesting with sticky eyes to a sight-threatening form resulting from gonococcal infection. Whereas the former will respond to cleaning with sterile saline, the latter needs aggressive management with parenteral antibiotics and saline lavages.

Organisms such as *E. coli*, *Staphylococcus aureus* and *Pseudomonas*, may cause sticky eyes in the newborn period. In otherwise clinically well infants, the eyes should be cleaned regularly with sterile saline and chloramphenicol eye drops commenced empirically until results of the swabs are available. Treatment will then be directed by the organism isolated. Severe conjunctivitis in the newborn period is often referred to as ophthalmia neonatorum, the two most serious causes of this condition are gonococcal infection and chlamydial infection.

Gonococcal infection presents classically within 24 hours of delivery with eyelid oedema and purulent discharge. Less commonly it can present immediately after birth if the infant has acquired intra-uterine gonococcal infection. Eye swabs should be taken and transported to microbiology in appropriate transport medium in an urgent manner because *Neisseria gonococci* are not well supported, even in transport medium, for more than 24 hours. The infant should have the eyes regularly lavaged with saline and receive a single dose of ceftriaxone, 25 to 50 mg/kg intravenously or intramuscularly, to a maximum dose of 125 mg (Bedford Russell and Isaacs 2012). Failure to treat this condition results in ulceration and perforation of the cornea and blindness. The mother and her sexual contacts should also be treated.

Chlamydial infection is now the commonest cause of ophthalmia neonatorum, and it presents between days 5 and 14 with a minimal to purulent discharge. The eye swabs need to be transported in specialist media; however, in many centres eye cultures have been superseded by direct fluorescent antibody testing and PCR of the eye secretions to isolate *Chlamydia trachomatis*. Chlamydial pneumonitis can develop in about 30% of infants. Treatment is with a 2-week course of oral erythromycin.

Skin and soft tissue

Omphalitis

S. aureus is the most common organism implicated in umbilical cord infection. If the cord smells offensive and is sticky, it should be cleaned and swabbed, and a course of oral flucloxacillin may be prescribed. If there is severe omphalitis with periumbilical flaring, IV flucloxacillin should be given because there is an increased

risk of organisms tracking into the cord vessels and causing septicaemia.

Rashes and abscesses

Most skin rashes in otherwise well infants are benign and usually secondary to erythema toxicum. However, *S. aureus* can cause small showers of pustules or abscesses around the nailbeds (paronychia); group A and B streptococci can also cause paronychia. If there are concerns regarding skin lesions, advice from the neonatal team should be sought. The lesions should be punctured with a sterile lancet and the pus sent for culture. IV antibiotics to cover both staphylococci and streptococci should commence while culture results are awaited. In rare situations, *S. aureus* and methicillin-resistant *S. aureus* (MRSA) can cause erythematous patches on the face and trunk, which then blister and desquamate (neonatal staphylococcal scalded skin syndrome). These infants require fluid resuscitation and IV anti-staphylococcal antibiotics.

Candidal infections can affect both the skin and oral mucosa. Oral candidiasis (thrush) is common, especially if the infant has received antibiotics. Bottle-fed infants are more susceptible than breastfed infants. Mild candidiasis causes white plaques on the tongue and buccal mucosa; more severe disease can cause painful mucosal swelling and interfere with feeding. If the mother is breastfeeding, she may develop painful candidiasis around the nipple. Unless both mother and baby are treated simultaneously, they will continue to reinfect each other.

Napkin candidal dermatitis is often associated with oral thrush and presents as an itchy red rash. The infant should always be treated with "top and tail" topical antifungal agents.

Systemic candida infection causes overwhelming septicaemia and is extremely rare in term babies. It is more commonly associated with extreme prematurity in infants with fragile skin requiring a humidified environment and those who have indwelling central lines in situ.

Prevention of these localized infections is by scrupulous attention to hygiene. Healthcare professionals need to teach the parents how to care for their infant to prevent infection. Hand hygiene is probably the most important aspect of prevention of infection, and good hand washing before and after the baby is handled cannot be overemphasized. Attention to hygiene includes the following:

- Umbilical cord care: Many parents are wary of the cord, feeling that it will hurt their baby if they touch it. Most studies do not show any benefit from active cord management in developed countries, and keeping the cord dry by not having it tucked into the napkin is usually all that is required.

- Skin care: Newborns do not require early or frequent bathing because vernix, if present, is protective. Equally, the infant needs to develop protective skin flora, so the use of baby wipes should be avoided.

Barrier creams applied to the buttocks may have a benefit in protecting against napkin dermatitis caused by prolonged contact with damp and soiled nappies.

- Eye care: Most infants do not require specific eye care, but as the face is cleaned, the eye area should be cleaned with cooled boiled water with a soaked cotton wool swab, moving from the nasal bridge area to the outer aspect in one sweep. A separate swab should be used for each eye.

- Cleaning of equipment: Although it is a fact that breastmilk and breastfeeding prevent infection, it has to be recognized that some women will choose to give formula feeds to their babies. Healthcare professionals need to support women in this choice by teaching them how to safely and effectively clean and sterilize bottles and teats to lessen the potential for oral candidiasis and gastrointestinal infections.

Reflective activity 48.1

Review local guidelines regarding antenatal screening and intra- and postpartum management of women to identify and manage infants at risk of infection.

CONCLUSION

Infection in the newborn period is a significant cause of morbidity and mortality. In increasing their knowledge of antenatal, intrapartum and postnatal factors, midwives are well placed to identify babies at a higher risk of its acquisition.

Key Points

- Antenatal, intrapartum and postnatal infection can have a devastating effect on the developing fetus or newborn baby.
- Most common infections can be effectively treated if identified early and appropriate antibiotic therapy instigated in a timely manner.
- Utilizing a newborn early warning observation system in at-risk infants increases the midwives ability to detect early and subtle signs of infection.

References

Bedford Russell A, Isaacs D: Infection in the newborn. In Rennie JM, editor: *Roberton's textbook of neonatology*, 5th edn, London, Churchill Livingstone, pp 1013–1064, 2012.

Bedford Russell AR, Kumar R: Early onset neonatal sepsis: diagnostic dilemmas and practical management, *Arch Dis Child Fetal Neonatal Ed* 100:F350–F354, 2015.

Bedford Russell A, Steer PJ: Antibiotics in labour – the ORACLE speaks, *Lancet* 372:1276–1278, 2008.

Black R, Cousens S, Johnson HL, et al: Global regional and national causes of child mortality in 2008: a systematic analysis, *Lancet* 375:1969–1987, 2010.

British Association of Perinatal Medicine (BAPM): *Newborn early warning trigger and track* (website). www.bapm.org. 2015.

Isaacs D: *Evidence-based neonatal infections*, Oxford, Wiley Blackwell, 2014.

Kenyon SL, Taylor DJ, Tarnow-Mordi W: Broad-spectrum antibiotics for

preterm, prelabour rupture of fetal membranes: the ORACLE I randomised trial, *Lancet* 31(357):979–988, 2001.

Lissauer T, Claydon GS: *Illustrated textbook of paediatrics*, 4th edn, London, Elsevier, 2012.

National Institute for Health and Care and Excellence (NICE): *Antibiotics for early-onset neonatal infection*, NICE Clinical Guideline CG 149, London, NICE, 2012.

National Institute for Health and Care and Excellence (NICE): *NICE Quality Standard QS75*, London, NICE, 2014.

Nijman J, et al: Postnatally acquired cytomegalovirus infection in preterm infants: a prospective study on risk factors and cranial ultrasound findings, *Arch Dis Child Fetal Neonatal Ed* 97:F259–F263, 2012.

Ohlsson A, Shah VS: Intrapartum antibiotics for known maternal group B streptococcal colonization, *Cochrane Database Syst Rev* (6):CD007467, 2014.

Pinninti SG, Kimberlin DW: Management of neonatal herpes simplex virus infection and exposure, *Arch Dis Child Fetal Neonatal Ed* 99:F240–F244, 2014.

Puopolo KM, Draper D, Wi S, et al: Estimating the probability of neonatal early-onset infection on the basis of maternal risk factors, *Pediatrics* 128:e1155–e1163, 2011.

Royal College of Obstetricians and Gynaecologists (RCOG): *Management of genital herpes in pregnancy* (website). www.RCOG.org. 2014.

Shatrov JG, Birch SC, Lam LT, et al: Chorioamnionitis and cerebral palsy: a meta-analysis, *Obstet Gynecol* 116:387–392, 2010.

Sinha S, Miall L, Jardine L: *Essential neonatal medicine*, 5th edn, Chichester, Wiley Blackwell, 2012.

Tita AT, Andrews WW: Diagnosis and management of clinical chorioamnionitis, *Clin Perinatol* 37:339–354, 2010.

Vergnano S, et al: Neonatal infections in England: the NeonIN surveillance network, *Arch Dis Child Fetal Neonatal Ed* 96:F9–F14, 2011.

Williams EJ, et al: First estimates of the potential cost and cost saving of

protecting childhood hearing from damage caused by congenital CMV infection, *Arch Dis Child Fetal Neonatal Ed* 100:F1–F6, 2015.

World Health Organization (WHO): *Hepatitis B. Fact Sheet No. 204*

(website). www.who.int/ mediacentre/factsheets/fs204/en/. 2015.

Useful websites:

British Association for Sexual Health and HIV: www.bashh.org/guidelines.

Chapter 49

Congenital anomalies, neonatal surgery and pain management

Glenys Connolly

Learning Outcomes ?

After reading this chapter, you will be able to:

- understand the aetiology of congenital anomalies
- describe the immediate management of common surgical conditions
- understand pain management in the newborn

INTRODUCTION

Congenital anomalies affect 2% to 3% of newborns and can be structural, biochemical, chromosomal or genetic in origin. They may have been identified antenatally in the case of structural or chromosomal abnormalities, become obvious immediately after birth or be identified later during the neonatal period.

Congenital structural *malformations* are usually as a result of incomplete embryological development or fetal insult, whereas *deformations* result from late changes to previously normal structures (e.g. talipes resulting from oligohydramnios).

Congenital anomalies are the leading cause of perinatal mortality and constitute 25% to 30% of all admissions to children's hospitals (Sinha et al 2012a); thus, they have a major financial consequence for society in addition to the anxiety for the parents and child.

Cardiac and respiratory disorders are also discussed in Chapter 45.

National registers of congenital anomalies are available, for example, the British Isles Network of Congenital Anomaly Register (BINOCAR) and European Surveillance of Congenital Anomalies (EUROCAT), the purpose of which is as follows:

- To provide essential epidemiological information on congenital anomalies in Europe

- To facilitate the early warning of new teratogenic exposures
- To evaluate the effectiveness of primary prevention
- To assess the impact of developments in prenatal screening
- To act as an information and resource centre for the population, health professionals and managers regarding clusters or exposures or risk factors of concern
- To provide a ready collaborative network and infrastructure for research related to the causes and prevention of congenital anomalies and the treatment and care of affected children
- To act as a catalyst for the setting up of registries throughout Europe to collect comparable, standardized data

(EUROCAT 2016).

Reflective activity 49.1 ><

Identify the agency that collates the congenital anomaly data in your region. Is there a high prevalence of any congenital anomalies?

AETIOLOGY

Although the cause of many abnormalities cannot be ascertained, there are several known risk factors shown in Table 49.1 (World Health Organization (WHO) 2015).

Antenatal screening by both ultrasound and blood testing (see Ch. 33) may identify anomalies, allowing for counselling of parents as to the nature of the anomaly and its prognosis. Because some anomalies are lethal, are incompatible with long-term survival or result in long-term major disability, parents may choose to terminate the

Table 49.1 Risk factors for congenital abnormalities

Associated risk	Effect
Genetic	Consanguinity increases the risk of serious genetic anomalies. Some ethnic communities also have a comparatively higher prevalence of some genetic mutations (e.g. Ashkenazi Jews and Finns).
Maternal nutritional status	Folate deficiencies can lead to neural tube defects. Poorly controlled or undiagnosed diabetes can lead to congenital heart disease.
Environmental factors	Maternal exposure to drugs, both therapeutic and recreational misuse, can have teratogenic effects. The antiepileptic medication phenytoin can lead to fetal hydantoin syndrome (cleft lip and palate, microcephaly, hypertelorism, limb deformities), cocaine causes gut and cerebral artery infarctions and alcohol causes fetal alcohol syndrome with palate, limb, ocular and cardiac malformations. Exposure to pesticides or radiation can have major teratogenic effects.
Maternal age	Advancing maternal age is associated with chromosomal defects, and younger maternal age is consistently associated with gastroschisis.
Infection	Intra-uterine viral infections (see Chs 20, 33 and 48)

pregnancy. It is for this reason that the number of babies born with spina bifida is decreasing.

Antenatal anomaly ultrasound is usually performed at 18 to 20 weeks gestation when cardiac and renal structures become discernible; this screening detects 60% to 80% of major and 35% of minor congenital malformations (Pasupathy et al 2012). Parents should be reminded that this scan is a 'snapshot' in time and that not all anomalies may be detected or be present at that time. Other screening tests are available for detection of chromosomal abnormalities, such as trisomies 21, 18 and 15 and open neural tube defects (Wolfson Institute of Preventative Medicine 2016).

In cases where the fetus is known to have a congenital malformation, the timing and mode of birth should be a joint decision between the woman/parents, obstetric team and neonatal team so that appropriately skilled personnel are present at the birth as required. Babies that require early surgical intervention should ideally be transferred to a specialist centre before birth.

FETAL SURGERY

Although many structural anomalies have a favourable outcome following postnatal surgical correction, some structural anomalies may be amenable to in-utero intervention, where the belief is that the uncorrected malformation may lead to progressive organ damage and jeopardize long-term survival.

Early attempts at fetal surgery took two forms: open surgical correction via hysterotomy or by ultrasound guided catheters. More recently, endoscopic techniques have been used.

Conditions that may benefit from in-utero intervention are those that allow for better lung growth and prevention of *pulmonary hypoplasia* caused by intrathoracic lesions or obstructive uropathies such as posterior urethral valves (PUV). In-utero intervention for PUV entails insertion of a *pigtail catheter* into the fetal bladder, allowing fetal urine to pass into the amniotic fluid and contribute to liquor volume. This may prevent *renal dysplasia* by release of back pressure on the kidney and prevent pulmonary hypoplasia, which, in the short term, allows for better postnatal survival. Longer-term follow-up from this intervention does not seem to alter long-term poor prognosis, with most children still requiring later renal transplantation. Excision of dysplastic lung tissue in cases of cystic adenomatoid malformation does appear to have increased survival in this very rare condition.

There is a growing body of experience with in-utero closure of neural tube defects, with benefits demonstrated following closure of myelomeningoceles before 25 weeks gestation (Adzick et al 2011). In this study, prenatal repair appeared to result in improved mental and motor function at 30 months of age compared with infants having surgery in the postnatal period. It did result in more premature births but did not increase mortality rates.

ABNORMALITIES OF THE ALIMENTARY TRACT

Malformations of the alimentary (digestive) tract can occur from the mouth to the anus. Some of the most commonly encountered are highlighted in this section.

Cleft lip and palate

Cleft lip and palate are the commonest anomalies in the craniofacial region and affect 1:700 live births. The face begins development at around 4 weeks, and the lip and palate should fuse around 6 weeks gestation (Moore et al 2016). Cleft lip may occur in isolation and may be unilateral (70% will be on left side) or bilateral. These defects may be detected antenatally. An isolated cleft palate (1:2000 live births) cannot be detected antenatally and may involve the soft palate only or extend further forward into the hard palate as far as the gum margin behind the front teeth (Sugarman et al 2012). In most situations the clefting will be the only defect; however, up to 15% of infants with clefting have other abnormalities associated with syndromes (see discussion later in the chapter).

Following delivery, a cleft lip will be obvious; however, cleft palate is not. Therefore, during the first examination of the infant, the midwife should visibly inspect the palate because digital examination may miss incomplete clefts. Babies with cleft palate have difficulty with suction, which can make breastfeeding difficult but not impossible. Oral feeding is usually achieved with breast or formula milk via specially adapted soft teats and bottles.

Repair of the lip is usually undertaken around 3 months of age, with palatal repair around 9 to 12 months. Despite its relatively common occurrence, cleft lip and palate are complex abnormalities that require coordinated care of a multidisciplinary team from birth to maturity so that the physical, psychological and practical needs of the infant and family are met. The outcome of surgical repair is usually very good; however, long-term problems may occur, including middle ear infections and altered dentition, speech and language. Families my benefit from contacting the Cleft Lip and Palate Association (www.clapa.com), which provides support, advice and equipment for affected families.

Pierre-Robin sequence

Pierre-Robin sequence (previously known as Pierre-Robin syndrome) is characterized by a U-shaped cleft palate with a small lower mandible (micrognathia) and a relatively large posteriorly placed tongue. Following delivery, the infant may require insertion of a Guedel airway (see Ch. 46) to hold the tongue forward and prevent airway occlusion before insertion of a nasopharyngeal airway. Airway patency is assisted by nursing the infant in the prone or side-lying positions. These babies need to be managed by the multidisciplinary cleft team and the ear nose and throat team because in some circumstances these infants may require a tracheostomy.

Intestinal obstruction

Intestinal obstruction is classified depending on the site of the blockage, either small or large intestine, and by whether the bowel is narrowed (stenosed) or blocked (atretic).

Duodenal atresia

The duodenum begins development from the fourth week of gestation. Abundant epithelial proliferation causes complete occlusion of the lumen, which should become recanalized by week 9. Partial recanalization results in "web-like" stenosis, whereas complete failure of recanalization leads to atresia (Moore et al 2016). Polyhydramnios occurs as a result of the atresia preventing passage of swallowed amniotic liquor into the intestine for reabsorption. Bilious vomiting is the most common sign of complete atresia and often occurs on the first day of life. Infants with stenosis may feed normally for the first few days of life until a milk curd sticks in the partial web and causes an obstruction, leading to vomiting. This condition is not always associated with abdominal distension because the lesion is high in the intestinal tract. Duodenal atresia is associated with trisomy 21 in one-third of cases, and a further 20% will be premature (Moore et al 2016). This condition will require surgical correction in the first few days of life.

Small bowel atresias

Small bowel atresias are thought to occur as a result of interruption of the blood supply to the fetal gut in late gestation leading to an infarcted area of bowel, which results in a jejunal or ileal atresia (Sugarman et al 2012). They can be secondary to altered developmental processes or the action of maternal use of vasoconstrictive drugs such as cocaine. Several areas within the gut may be affected. These infants are often small for gestational age, and there may be a history of polyhydramnios or dilated bowel on antenatal ultrasound. Bilious vomiting starts on day 1 to 2 of life, and the infant fails to pass normal meconium.

Treatment is by resection of the atretic areas and may result in short gut syndrome, with a need for long-term parenteral nutrition. Because there is an association of cystic fibrosis with this condition, a sweat test and DNA analysis may be undertaken (see Ch. 50).

Malrotation

Development of the midgut (small intestine, ascending colon and up to two-thirds of the transverse colon) undergoes rapid growth, with physiological herniation into the umbilical cord at around 6 weeks gestation (Moore et al 2016). At 10 to 11 weeks this loop of gut undergoes a significant counterclockwise rotation to enable it to return to the abdominal cavity, for a total rotation of 270 degrees. Once properly positioned in the abdominal cavity, these

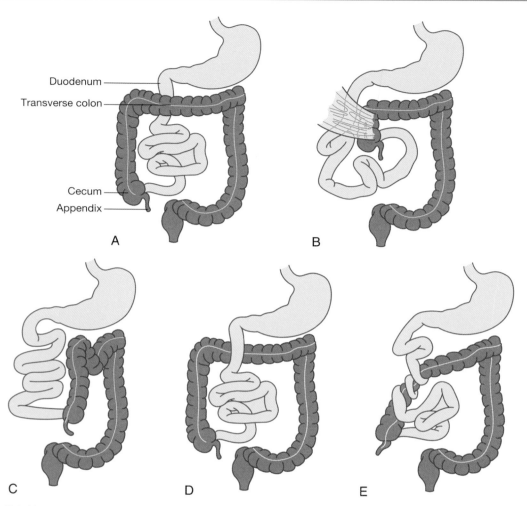

Figure 49.1 Normal and abnormal rotation. **A,** Normal Anatomy. **B,** Incomplete rotation with Ladd's bands. **C,** Non rotation. **D,** Reverse rotation (clockwise). **E,** Non fixation, leading to volvulus.

loops of gut are fixed in place by peritoneal bands to prevent them from twisting and occluding the blood supply (Fig. 49.1A). In malrotation, the midgut fails to complete its normal rotation, and the gut is malplaced and mobile, which predisposes it to twisting (volvulus) and strangulation, cutting off the gut blood flow and leading to gangrenous bowel (see Fig. 49.1). Intestinal strangulation presents with abdominal distension, rectal bleeding and bilious vomiting. This condition is a surgical emergency, and any infant presenting with bilious vomiting should have an upper gastrointestinal contrast study to exclude malrotation. Abdominal ultrasound (colour Doppler) may demonstrate abnormal positioning of the superior mesenteric artery and vein suggestive of malrotation (Sugarman et al 2012). Following confirmation of

malrotation, the infant needs urgent laparotomy and *Ladd's procedure*, whereby the gut is repositioned and fixed in place so that the blood supply is no longer compromised. This condition may present in the early neonatal period but can occur up to the first month of life.

Anorectal malformations

Anorectal malformations encompass a wide spectrum of congenital defects, from mild malposition or imperforate anus through to high rectal deformities that may involve other genito-urinary structures. Whereas the former may result in constipation and normal continence, the latter is more likely to impair continence and be associated with repeated urinary tract infections. During the midwife's early examination of the infant, the anal area should be completely examined to ensure there is a patent anal orifice that is appropriately positioned (see Ch. 42). The presence of meconium in the liquor or nappy does not confirm normality because this can be passed via a fistula before or after birth.

Hirschsprung's disease

Hirschsprung's disease occurs as a result of an absence of ganglionic cells in the submucosa of the distal bowel (aganglionosis), which prevents coordinated peristaltic activity through the bowel. It is the commonest cause of large bowel obstruction in the newborn, with an incidence of 1:5000 livebirths (Moore et al 2016). In most cases, only the rectum and sigmoid colon are affected, but it can affect much longer areas of the colon. In newborns with delayed passage of meconium (greater than 48 hours), increasing abdominal distension and bilious vomiting, Hirschsprung's disease should be suspected. Following referral, the attending clinician may undertake a digital rectal examination, which typically reveals a tightly contracted anorectum. Removal of the finger usually elicits an explosive discharge of stool and gas, which may temporarily relieve the distension. The explosive nature of the stool is caused by the back pressure proximal to the aganglionic section of affected gut being acutely released. Diagnosis is by rectal biopsy to look for the ganglionic cells. In short-segment Hirschsprung's, the baby may be managed with rectal washouts by the parents, which serve to decompress the proximal bowel. Many babies will ultimately require a two-stage operation in which a colostomy is formed in the first instance, and the aganglionic section of gut is removed; this is followed by a second operation in which the colostomy is reversed, and the two healthy ganglionic sections of gut are anastomosed.

General principles of management of infants with suspected intestinal obstruction are shown in Table 49.2.

Abdominal wall defects

Abdominal wall defects encompass the defects of **exomphalos** and **gastroschisis,** which result in infants being born with their abdominal contents outside of the abdominal cavity.

Table 49.2 General management of infants with suspected intestinal obstruction	
Bile-stained vomitus	This is never a normal finding and should not be ignored. The vomit can be described in terms of increasing colour from milk through to lemon, lime, pea, avocado and spinach. Bile in the gall bladder or duodenum is yellow, but when it refluxes and mixes with gastric juices, it turns green and indicates gastric stasis. Any single suspected bilious vomit, despite its colour, should be reported to the neonatal team because it requires immediate investigation. In-utero bilious vomiting from high obstructions can be confused with meconium-stained liquor and should be highly regarded as suspicious, especially in preterm babies.
Delayed passage of meconium	This can occur in low large bowel obstructions but can be a result of other conditions (e.g. cystic fibrosis) and thus does not necessarily indicate complete obstruction.
Abdominal distension	This may not be a feature if the obstruction is high.
Large-bore nasogastric tube	This should be passed to remove stomach contents and decompress the stomach, preventing further vomiting and reducing the risk of aspiration pneumonia.
Intravenous access	Access should be gained with fluid and electrolyte replacement to prevent dehydration, electrolyte imbalances and acid–base disturbances.
Other considerations	Some conditions (e.g. suspected malrotation – see chapter discussion) require urgent, time-critical transfer to paediatric surgical centres because failure to do so may result in strangulated obstruction of the gut, which results in gut loss and can be fatal. The transfer of infants, in these circumstances, for further urgent investigation, such as contrast studies and need for surgical review, is traumatic for the parents and further complicated if the woman has undergone caesarean section and is unable to travel with the infant. In this circumstance the father may travel with the infant; however, it has to be remembered that if the parents are not married, then only the mother can provide the consent for progression to any necessary surgical procedures (see also Chs 9 and 42).

Exomphalos is a defect resulting from the persistence of herniation of the abdominal contents into the umbilical cord (see embryology as described in the section on malrotation). It has an incidence of 1 : 5000 livebirths. The defect can contain just intestine, but in rarer situations (1 : 10,000 livebirths) the liver may also be present. Because it is a failure of complete embryonic development, it is associated with other defects (e.g. cardiac malformations and *Beckwith–Wiedemann syndrome*).

Gastroschisis differs from exomphalos in that it is herniation of the abdominal contents through a linear defect in the abdominal wall, usually to the right of the umbilicus. The umbilical cord is normally placed. As a consequence, the gut is not covered by a membrane and floats freely in the amniotic fluid. It is rarer than exomphalos, occurring in 1 in 10,000 livebirths, and has a higher incidence in younger mothers (less than 21 years). It is not generally associated with other congenital malformations, but the gut becomes thickened and matted the longer it is exposed to the amniotic fluid.

In an antenatally diagnosed abdominal wall defect, the neonatal team should be present at delivery because these infants may require significant intervention.

At delivery, the abdominal wall defects need to be protected by the use of either putting the infant, feet first, into a large polythene bag or wrapping the infant in 'cling-film'. This is especially true with gastroschisis because the exposed bowel loses masses of fluid and heat through the exposed viscera. The lesion needs to be well supported so that the blood supply is not compromised. A large-bore nasogastric tube should be inserted for gastric decompression and to prevent excessive air from getting into the gut. The infant may need significant fluid resuscitation. Long-term management is in a surgical centre and is either by staged reduction of the gut back into the abdominal cavity by use of a 'silo' (see Fig. 49.2) or by surgical replacement if the lesion is small.

Gastroschisis silo

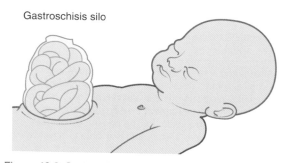

Figure 49.2 Gastroschisis silo.

DISORDERS OF THE RESPIRATORY SYSTEM

Choanal atresia

Choanal atresia affects 1 : 7000 livebirths. It results from a failure of the opening at the back of the nose and can be unilateral or bilateral and bony or membranous. It can occur as an isolated finding or as part of other craniofacial syndromes. Unilateral atresia is often an incidental finding, whereas bilateral atresias cause upper airway obstruction because babies are obligate 'nose breathers'.

The baby is pink when crying because babies draw air in through the mouth but will become cyanosed with respiratory distress when quiet. Management is by securing the airway with either a Guedel airway (see Ch. 46) or by endotracheal intubation until the infant has surgical correction, usually in the first week of life.

Congenital diaphragmatic hernia

Congenital diaphragmatic hernia (CDH) affects 1 : 2000 to 5000 births. The development of the diaphragm is complex and involves the migration of four embryonic structures. Up to the eighth week of gestation, there is communication between the pleural and peritoneal cavities. Failure of complete migration and fusion of these structures results in the abdominal contents (e.g. gut and stomach) herniating into the thoracic cavity, which impedes lung development and results in pulmonary hypoplasia and a hyperreactive pulmonary vascular bed (Badillo and Gingalewski 2014). There is a broad spectrum of severity of this condition dependent on the degree of lung hypoplasia and pulmonary hypertension. These infants are highly sensitive to hypoxaemia, acidosis and environmental stimulation.

Most cases are diagnosed by antenatal ultrasound, and these infants should be ideally delivered in a centre that provides neonatal surgery. There should be a neonatal team present at the birth because active management of these infants immediately after birth is vital to prevent hypoxaemia and acidosis. At birth, the infant should not be stimulated but should have elective intubation and a wide-bore nasogastric tube inserted into the stomach to remove any swallowed air. These combined manoeuvres prevent air from getting into the herniated gut, which would further compromise respiration. The infant needs to be sedated and given muscle relaxants, preventing swallowing of air, so that the gut continues to be decompressed throughout the early postnatal period. Surgery to repair the defect is delayed until the infant is stable on minimal ventilatory support. Infants who achieve this have a much better outcome because it confirms that there is sufficiently developed lung tissue to support respiration in the postoperative period. Rarely, infants present after 24 hours of age with respiratory symptoms (e.g. tachypnea) and increased respiratory effort. These infants have a better prognosis because this suggests that the defect is small or intermittent. CDH is associated with other congenital anomalies, including critical cardiac disease and renal malformations.

Tracheo-oesophageal fistula and oesophageal atresia

Tracheo-oesophageal fistula (TOF) occurs as a result of incomplete separation of the trachea and oesophagus at 4 weeks gestation (Moore et al 2016). Oesophageal atresia (OA) occurs as a result of incomplete canalization of the oesophagus by 8 weeks gestation. In 85% of cases, both defects occur; however, in 9% of cases, OA can occur in isolation and as an isolated H-type fistula in 4% (see Fig. 49.3). The overall incidence of these conditions is 1:3500 births. OA should be suspected when there is maternal polyhydramnios because the fetus cannot swallow the amniotic fluid, which will subsequently build up. Antenatal ultrasound may highlight the absence of a stomach bubble. At birth, the attending clinician should pass a wide-bore nasogastric to a measured length congruent to the infant's stomach position and aspirate any residual fluid. Because the stomach will contain amniotic fluid, it is not suitable for pH testing, but easy passage of the tube and the presence of several millilitres of fluid should be sufficient to confirm oesophageal patency. If resistance is encountered, the tube should be left in situ and a chest x-ray performed, which may demonstrate the tube curled up in the oesophageal pouch. Infants with undiagnosed TOF and OA present with choking and severe respiratory distress secondary to inhaled secretions that accumulate in the blind ended oesophagus or reflux of stomach acid through the fistula, leading to pneumonitis.

Management after delivery is to protect the airway by nursing the infant with head-up tilt, passage of a Replogle tube into the oesophageal pouch, which is put onto continuous low-grade suction and flushed with saline to maintain patency, and intravenous fluids to maintain hydration and glucose homeostasis. The infant should be stabilized and transferred to a neonatal surgical centre for repair of the defect. TOF and OA can occur as part of the *VACTERL* cluster, which includes Vertebral, Anal, Cardiac, Tracheal, (o)Esophageal, Renal and Limb abnormalities; thus, infants presenting with TOF and OA should undergo cardiac and renal ultrasound investigation to exclude their association.

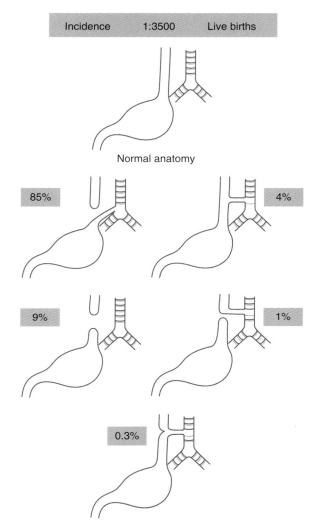

Incidence 1:3500 Live births

Normal anatomy

85%

4%

9%

1%

0.3%

Figure 49.3 Types of atresia.

DISORDERS OF THE CENTRAL NERVOUS SYSTEM

Neural tube defects

During embryological development, the central nervous system is recognizable from day 19 when it differentiates into the neural tube, which is the precursor of all of the major structures of the brain and spinal cord. A failure of this closure results in neural tube defects (NTDs). Folic acid taken preconceptually and in early pregnancy appears to be effective in reducing the incidence of NTDs because it is an important substrate necessary for neural tube development.

Anencephaly

Anencephaly occurs when the anterior neural tube fails to close, exposing a rudimentary brain with absent cerebral hemispheres. It is incompatible with long-term survival, with most affected infants dying shortly after birth. There should be an antenatal plan, agreed with the parents, that there will be no active resuscitative intervention following birth, and a compassionate care pathway will be followed. It should be determined whether the parents want to see the lesion or not. The infant should be dried and dressed with the open lesion covered with gauze and then a hat applied and given to the parents if that is their wish.

Spina bifida occulta

Spina bifida literally means 'divided spine', and this condition affects approximately 10% of the population. This defect is often an incidental finding on a spinal x-ray done for different reasons. It requires no treatment and does not pose any risk of disability or NTDs in future pregnancies. A few may have an outward sign of an underlying defect, such as a dimple or hair tuft at the base of the spine. During the newborn check, this area should be carefully examined; if a dimple is present, the base should be clearly seen to ensure that there is no sinus communicating with the spinal cord. The presence of a sinus requires referral to the paediatric neurology team.

Meningoceles

Meningoceles are a generally benign condition in which a sac containing cerebrospinal fluid (CSF) protrudes through the spinous processes. It can occur anywhere along the spine. An operation will be required to close the lesion, and the long-term prognosis is usually good.

Myelomeningoceles

Myelomeningoceles generally occur in the lumbar-sacral regions; if they are higher in the thoracolumbar region, the prognosis is poorer. Affected infants remain at a high risk of physical and developmental disabilities, including motor deficits and bladder and bowel incontinence (Hagmann and Rennie 2012); the higher the lesion, the greater is the disability. Antenatal counselling with honest information regarding the potential outcome of the condition is vital. Parents may choose to terminate the pregnancy at this time.

At delivery, any spinal lesion should be covered with cling film and the infant nursed in the prone position to avoid any trauma. Early referral to the paediatric neurology team is necessary.

Hydrocephalus

Hydrocephalus results from an imbalance between the production and absorption of CSF. It may be present in the previously described conditions, in association with another abnormality that obstructs the normal CSF pathway, such as *Arnold–Chiari* or *Dandy–Walker* malformations, or as an isolated finding. The infant head shape and size may look normal, but the fontanelle may be large and bulging, with widely separated sutures. These infants need a cranial ultrasound to assess ventricular size before referral for potential shunt insertion.

Microcephaly

Microcephaly is defined as an occipitofrontal head circumference that is 2 standard deviations (SD) below the mean for the infant's gestational age, with the head being disproportionally small in relation to the rest of the body (Sinha et al 2012b). It is an important finding in the newborn because it is reflective of impairment of brain growth. Microcephaly has multiple aetiologies, such as genetic conditions, infection or fetal alcohol syndrome, and carries a poor prognosis, including neurodevelopmental delay, motor deficits and seizures.

DISORDERS OF THE GENITOURINARY SYSTEM

Urinary tract anomalies are more commonly being detected earlier through antenatal ultrasound, which can expedite appropriate management of the condition in the neonatal period. Before this practice, many renal anomalies presented with urinary tract infections (UTIs) during childhood.

Fetal urine flow impairment can occur at any level in the urinary tract, leading to back pressure on the kidney that results in distension of the renal pelvis and *hydronephrosis*, which may affect one or both kidneys. Delayed recognition and management of some conditions of obstructed flow can lead to significant renal damage, which may ultimately result in the need for renal transplantation. When uropathy is diagnosed antenatally, it is imperative to confirm the diagnosis early in the postnatal period; most units will have a guideline on which infants need early prophylactic antibiotic therapy (to prevent UTIs) and early postnatal ultrasound examination.

Pelviureteral junction anomalies

Pelviureteral junction anomalies (PUJs) are the most common antenatally diagnosed uropathy and account for approximately half of all cases of antenatal hydronephrosis (Modi et al 2012).

The degree of antenatal hydronephrosis correlates with the severity of significant postnatal problems. Approximately 25% of infants with hydronephrosis from PUJ will require surgery in the first few years of life; however, in many infants, the condition will resolve spontaneously. Careful follow-up is required because it is not clear from the outset which category any infant will fall into.

Posterior urethral valves

PUV results from the presence of a membrane obstructing the urethra. It is the commonest cause of urinary tract obstruction and usually occurs in males. PUV should be suspected in a fetus with a thickened walled bladder. These infants may be well at birth but have marked abdominal distension and require drainage of the distended bladder with a catheter inserted via the urethra or suprapubic route. Up to 40% of infants may have renal failure at the time of birth and have significant metabolic and electrolyte derangement. Following immediate management, these infants require transfer to a specialist centre for surgical ablation of the valves and long-term follow-up. Long-term renal failure and the need for dialysis and transplantation occur in up to 50% of cases.

Hypospadias

Hypospadias occurs in 1:300 male births and is a condition whereby the urethral meatus can be found anywhere between the under surface of the glans penis, the penile shaft or the perineum. It can be associated with *chordee* and a ventral hood of the foreskin. It requires surgical correction in the first few years of life; thus, neonatal circumcision should **not** be undertaken.

Epispadias

Epispadias is a much rarer condition, occurring in 1:100,000 births, in which the urethra opens onto the dorsal surface of the penis. It is more common in males but can rarely present in females with a patulous urethra and clitoral malformation (Modi et al 2012). Its outcome is poorer than that of hypospadias, and it is often part of the more complex bladder and *cloacal exstrophy syndrome.*

> ### Reflective activity 49.2
>
> Undertake an Internet search for the phrase 'bladder and cloacal exstrophy syndrome'. What advice and resources are available for families whose baby has a diagnosis of epispadias?
>
> How can you support parents in your region?

KIDNEY DISORDERS

Renal agenesis (absence)

Renal agenesis can be unilateral or bilateral and results from the ureteric buds failing to develop or the degeneration of the ureters' primitive stalk in early intra-uterine life (Moore and Persaud 2016).

Unilateral renal agenesis occurs in 1:1000 to 1500 live births (Modi et al 2012). Although it may be associated with other urogenital anomalies, it is often an asymptomatic condition and usually an incidental finding in later life. It should be suspected in infants with a single umbilical artery.

Bilateral renal agenesis (Potter syndrome) occurs in 1:4000 births (Modi et al 2012); it is more common in males and within families, which suggests a genetic component. It is incompatible with life, with the infants who survive to birth dying shortly after birth of respiratory failure from pulmonary hypoplasia.

Cystic disease of the kidney

Congenital renal cystic diseases of the newborn are a clinically and genetically diverse group of disorders.

Autosomal-dominant polycystic kidney disease (ADPKD) occurs in 1:500 to 600 live births and seldom causes clinical problems in the newborn period.

Autosomal-recessive polycystic kidney disease (ARPKD) is much rarer, occurring in 1 in 10,000 to 40,000 births, and is variable in its expression. In the most severe cases, the infants die of pulmonary insufficiency in a Potter-like disease. Those infants who survive the newborn period develop end-stage renal failure in infancy, childhood or early adult life (Modi et al 2012).

> ### Reflective activity 49.3
>
> Review the local guidelines on the management of renal pelvic dilatation. What are the referral pathways, and who is involved in the care?

DISORDERS OF SEXUAL DEVELOPMENT

Disorders of sexual development (DSD) occur in 1:4500 livebirths. In 2006, a consensus conference suggested that the term *DSD* should replace the previous terms of *hermaphrodite, pseudohermaphrodite* and *intersex* because these terms are misleading and pejorative (Lee et al 2006). The sex should not be 'guessed' by any members of the clinical team, and the infant should be referred to with gender neutrality. Examples of the manifestation of DSDs include *clitoromegaly* and *labial fusion*, which resembles male genitalia, and *micropenis* and *bifid scrotum*, which resembles female genitalia. Following full clinical examination, the infant's sex will need to be determined by biochemical and chromosomal analysis. This condition can be very distressing for the parents and extended family, and they will require referral to a specialist multidisciplinary team for ongoing endocrine, genetic, surgical and psychological support. Until a gender is assigned, the parents cannot register the infant because this is a legal requirement within 6 weeks of birth; professional discussion with the local birth registrar may be required.

Any infant presenting with any degree of genital ambiguity must be immediately referred to the neonatal team because the commonest cause is congenital adrenal insufficiency, which is a life-threatening condition. See also Chapter 42.

CHROMOSOMAL ABNORMALITIES

Trisomy 21 (Down syndrome)

Down syndrome (DS) is the most common chromosomal abnormality among live-born infants, affecting 1:6–700 births. Its prevalence is dependent on maternal age, with very young women and women above 40 years of age being the most affected. DS is characterized by a variety of dysmorphic features, including up-slanting palpebral fissures, epicanthic folds, and brachycephaly. In addition, DS infants are hypotonic and have a protruding tongue. Diagnosis is by chromosomal analysis, with 95% of cases having a full extra chromosome 21. The remaining 5% will have either a mosaicism or a translocation affecting another chromosome, usually chromosome 14 (Caluseriu and Reardon 2012).

Trisomy 18 (Edward syndrome)

Trisomy 18 (Edward syndrome) is the second most common chromosomal abnormality, affecting approximately 1:5000 births. It has distinctive clinical features, including a prominent occiput, low-set and malformed ears, small mouth and jaw, ptosis and wide epicanthic folds and characteristic overlapping of the fingers (Pont et al 2006).

The condition is incompatible with long-term survival, with only 10% of infants surviving the first year of life. Mental retardation is severe in those infants who do survive.

Trisomy 15 (Patau syndrome)

Trisomy 15 (Patau syndrome) syndrome occurs in 1:7000 livebirths. Its features include bilateral cleft lip and palate, small triangular head and jaw, sloping forehead and malformed ears. There is a cardiac defect in 80% of cases. Survival after the first year of life is unusual.

Turner syndrome (45 XO)

Turner syndrome occurs in 1:5000 female births. The most striking features include short webbed neck with loose skin, low hairline and short stature. Lymphoedema of the hands and feet is common (Caluseriu and Reardon 2012).

Many affected infants have cardiac and renal abnormalities and should undergo renal and cardiac ultrasounds early in the neonatal period. These infants are generally of normal intelligence; they are, however, infertile and will need oestrogen therapy at the time of puberty.

Any infant presenting with *dysmorphology* or a tentative diagnosis of a genetic/chromosomal malformation must be referred to the clinical geneticist, whose role is to assist the clinical team to make a diagnosis, advise the parents of a recurrence risk and provide ongoing advice and support via a multidisciplinary team.

ABNORMALITIES OF THE SKELETAL SYSTEM

Polydactyly and syndactyly

Polydactyly describes additional digits on the hands or feet; the most common site is an extra digit on the ulnar aspect of the fifth finger. The extra digit may or may not contain bone.

Syndactyly describes fusing of the fingers or toes, which may be partial or complete (see Fig. 49.4). These conditions are often isolated but can be part of other syndromic conditions, and thus a thorough examination is required to exclude more serious conditions. Infants with these conditions should also be reviewed by the plastic surgery team.

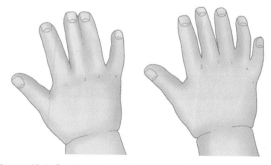

Figure 49.4 Syndactyly and polydactyly.

Limbs and feet

Foot abnormalities are relatively common and are usually associated with intra-uterine compression causing *positional talipes*. Mild cases, whereby the foot can be easily straightened to the correct position, will respond to gentle stretching exercises. More severe deformities, such as *talipes equinovarus* (clubfoot), may require physiotherapy, splinting and occasionally surgery. These infants should be referred for hip ultrasound because developmental dysplasia of the hip (see following discussion) needs to be formally excluded.

Skeletal dysplasias

Skeletal dysplasias are generally rare conditions that result in the infant having shortened limbs that are out of proportion with the rest of the body and result in dwarfism. The commonest dysplasia of this type is *achondroplasia*, which occurs in 1 : 25,000 births (Fig. 49.5). Skeletal dysplasias can be a result of genetic mutation, but they more often occur randomly. Although achondroplasia usually results in normal intelligence and independent living, some forms of dwarfism (e.g. *thanatophoric dwarfism*) are incompatible with long-term survival because they are associated with severe pulmonary hypoplasia.

Developmental dysplasia of the hip

Developmental dysplasia of the hip (DDH) occurs in 1–2 : 1000 births, the incidence of unstable hips is between 5 and 20 per 1000 births, but 60% of these will resolve spontaneously. There are well-documented risk factors for DDH such as breech presentation, macrosomic infants and oligohydramnios leading to a "crowded" intra-uterine environment. Girls are generally more affected than boys. There are also familial links, with affected parent or siblings increasing the risk by 12% and 6%, respectively. Early detection of the condition is vital to avoid long-term complications.

During the routine examination of the newborn, the Ortolani and Barlow's test should be performed (see Ch. 42) to detect unstable hips and the infant referred appropriately to undergo radiological investigation with ultrasound. Affected infants will require splinting with a *Pavlik harness* or *Van Rosen splint*. In rare cases, the infant may require management with traction or surgery.

> **Reflective activity 49.4**
>
> What is the local guidance for infants who require referral for hip ultrasound and referral pathway?

Amniotic band syndrome

Amniotic band syndrome (ABS) is a rare condition resulting from partial rupture of the amniotic sac leading to strands of amnion floating free within the amniotic fluid. These strands can encircle any part of the developing fetus and lead to digit or limb amputation. ABS can be fatal if the strands wrap around and occlude the umbilical cord, resulting in disrupted flow and fetal demise.

NEONATAL PAIN MANAGEMENT

Following birth, the newborn's nervous system is capable of perceiving and responding to painful or noxious events. Although sick and preterm infants admitted to the neonatal intensive care unit (NICU) will probably undergo many invasive and painful procedures, their pain can be effectively managed with nonpharmacological strategies (Pillai Riddell et al 2011), and when necessary infants will receive intravenous opiate analgesia to manage pain. It is

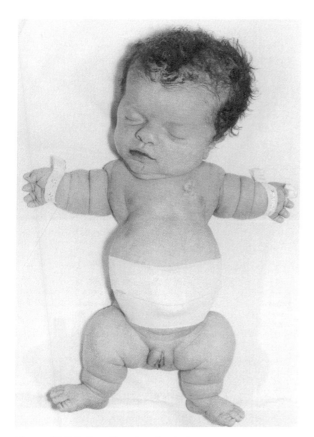

Figure 49.5 Baby with achondraplasia.

important to remember that most infants will undergo pain-inducing interventions immediately after birth and in the first week of life, for example, intramuscular vitamin K injection and heel-prick blood tests.

Because newborn infants are wholly reliant on caregivers to assess and manage their pain, midwives need to be mindful of any potential pain they may cause and use interventions to ameliorate it. Nonpharmacological strategies (with the exception of sucrose) are available in all care settings and can be used singly but are said to be better when used in combination. They include the following:

- Oral sucrose (Stevens et al 2013)
- Oral breastmilk (by breast/bottle/syringe) (Shah et al 2012)
- Non-nutritive sucking (Pillai Riddell et al 2011)
- Swaddling (Pillai Riddell et al 2011)
- Skin-to-skin/kangaroo care (Johnston et al 2014)

When undertaking capillary blood tests via heel prick, the midwife should use the appropriate size of automated lancet for a term infant (1 mm in depth by 2.5 mm in length) and sample from the lateral, medial or plantar surface of the heel because these areas are associated with less pain and reduced risk of osteomyelitis (Harling and Connolly 2010). The competent use of such devices is said to optimize blood flow and reduce pain because the incision is above the concentrated area of pain fibres. Additionally, as the blade retracts, both the operator and baby are protected from inadvertent needle-stick injury from a blade contaminated with blood.

Infants who are thought to be in pain following birth as a result of instrumental delivery leading to trauma to the scalp or difficult extraction causing fractures should be assessed and examined by a member of the neonatal team and prescribed oral analgesics accordingly. The most commonly used analgesic agent is paracetamol, which can be given as a single (loading dose) dose of 20 mg/kg (Ainsworth 2015) followed by 10- to 15-mg/kg doses every 6 to 8 hours (maximum dose should not exceed 60 mg/kg in a 24-hour period). The need for analgesia in this population should be reviewed every 24 hours because prolonged use is associated with hepatotoxicity.

CONCLUSION

Midwives have a key rol in supporting parents of a baby with a diagnosed congenital anomaly and they need to ensure that they have the necessary knowledge and skills to assist parents to reach an understanding of the short- and long-term implications of any anomaly. In dealing with an unexpected anomaly, midwives need to draw upon their counselling and caring skills to ensure that the woman and family are provided with ongoing information and support, and that long-term services are involved at the earliest stage.

Key points

- Effective history taking and identification of risk factors facilitates early effective diagnosis and care of the newborn.
- Women and families need support, counselling and preparation should an anomaly or deviation from the normal be identified.
- Bile-stained vomitus in the newborn is never a normal finding and should not be ignored. A single bile-stained vomitus should be reported to the neonatal team because it requires immediate investigation.
- Polyhydramnios should alert the midwife to potential congenital abnormalities of the gastrointestinal tract.
- Antenatal diagnosis of congenital malformations allows for counselling and support of parents and also the potential for antenatal transfer to a specialist centre with neonatal surgical facilities in infants who may require early surgical intervention.

References

Adzick NS, Thom EA, Spong CY: A randomized trial of prenatal versus postnatal repair of myelomeningocele, *N Engl J Med* 364:993–1004, 2011.

Ainsworth SB, editor: *Neonatal formulary*, 7th edn, New York, Wiley-Blackwell, 2015.

Badillo A, Gingalewski C: Congenital diaphragmatic hernia: treatment and outcomes, *Semin Perinatol* 38(2):92–96, 2014.

Caluseriu O, Reardon W: Malformation syndromes. In Rennie J, editor: *Rennie and Roberton's textbook of neonatology*, 5th edn, London, Elsevier, pp 719–817, 2012.

European Surveillance of Congenital Abnormalities (EUROCAT): *What is EUROCAT* (website). www.eurocat-network.eu/aboutus/whatiseurocat. 2016.

Hagmann C, Rennie J: Central nervous system malformations. In Rennie J, editor: *Rennie and Roberton's textbook of neonatology*, 5th edn, London, Elsevier, pp 1200–1223, 2012.

Harling E, Connolly G: Diagnostic and therapeutic procedures. In Boxwell G, editor: *Neonatal intensive care nursing*, 2nd edn, London, Routledge, pp 329–362, 2010.

Johnston C, Campbell-Yeo M, Fernandes A, et al: Skin-to-skin care for procedural pain in neonates, *Cochrane Database Syst Rev* (1):CD008435, 2014.

Lee PA, Houk CP, Ahmed SF, et al: Consensus statement on management of intersex disorders. International Consensus Conference on Intersex, *Pediatrics* 118(2):488–500, 2006.

Modi N, Smeulders N, Wilcox DT: Disorders of the kidney and urinary tract. Renal function and renal disease in the newborn. In Rennie J, editor: *Rennie and Roberton's textbook of neonatology*, 5th edn, London, Elsevier, pp 927–937, 2012.

Moore KL, Persaud TVN, Torchia MG: *The developing human. Clinically oriented embryology*, 10th edn, Oxford, Elsevier, 2016.

Pasupathy D, Denbow M, Kyle P: Antenatal diagnosis and fetal medicine. In Rennie J, editor: *Rennie and Roberton's textbook of neonatology*, 5th edn, London, Elsevier, pp 141–173, 2012.

Pillai Riddell RR, Racine NM, Turcotte K, et al: A non-pharmacological management of infant and young child procedural pain, *Cochrane Database Syst Rev* (10):CD006275, 2011.

Pont SJ, Robbins JM, Bird TM, et al: Congenital malformations among liveborn infants with trisomies 18 and 13, *Am J Med Genet* 140(16):1749–1756, 2006.

Shah PS, Herbozo C, Aliwalas LL, et al: Breastfeeding or breast milk for procedural pain in neonates, *Cochrane Database Syst Rev* (12):CD004950, 2012.

Sinha S, Maill L, Jardine L: Neonatal consequences of maternal conditions. In Sinha S, Maill L, Jardine L, editors: *Essential neonatal medicine*, 5th edn, Oxford, Wiley-Blackwell, pp 24–32, 2012a.

Sinha S, Maill L, Jardine L: Neurological disorders. In Sinha S, Maill L, Jardine L, editors: *Essential neonatal medicine*, 5th edn, Oxford, Wiley-Blackwell, pp 287–310, 2012b.

Stevens B, Yamada J, Lee GY, et al: Sucrose for analgesia in newborn infants undergoing painful procedures, *Cochrane Database Syst Rev* (1):CD001069, 2013.

Sugarman I, Stringer MD, Smyth AG: Congenital defects and surgical problems. In Rennie J, editor: *Rennie and Roberton's textbook of neonatology*, 5th edn, London, Elsevier, pp 711–738, 2012.

Wolfson Institute of Preventative Medicine: *Screening tests* (website). www.wolfson.qmul.ac.uk/epm/screening. 2016.

World Health Organization (WHO): *Congenital anomalies. Factsheet No. 370* (website). www.who.int. 2015.

Resources and additional reading

Antenatal Results and Choices: www.arc-uk.org/for-parents/links.

British and Irish Network of Congenital Anomaly Researchers: www.binocar.org/.

Cleft Lip and Palate Association: www.clapa.com.

EUROCAT: www.eurocat-network.eu.

Healthy Children: www.healthychildren.org/English/health-issues/conditions/developmental-disabilities/Pages/Congenital-Abnormalities.aspx
This U.S. website provides a wide range of information for families and practitioners.

Self-help groups for parents and families: www.self-help.org.uk/directory/birth-defects/.

Wolfson Institute of Preventative Medicine: www.wolfson.qmul.ac.uk/epm/screening.

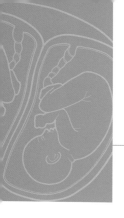

Chapter 50

Metabolic and endocrine disorders

Glenys Connolly

Learning Outcomes ?

At the end of this chapter, you will be able to:
- describe infants at risk of metabolic instability
- understand congenital and acquired metabolic disturbances
- understand the purpose and significance of newborn metabolic screening

INTRODUCTION

Metabolism comes from the Greek word *metabole* meaning 'to change'. It is, in essence, the biochemical processes occurring within living cells that are necessary for the maintenance of life. During metabolism, some substances are broken down to yield energy for cellular activity (e.g. glucose), whereas other substances necessary for life (e.g. proteins) are synthesized.

Pregnancy is primarily an anabolic (building-up) state that provides the developing fetus with adequate stores of substrate needed for the transition to a catabolic (breaking-down) state following birth.

This chapter focuses on common metabolic and endocrine problems that may affect the newborn infant.

GLUCOSE HOMEOSTASIS

During intra-uterine life, the fetus is dependent on a constant supply of transplacental glucose to provide energy for metabolic function and growth. Fetal glucose utilization at 6 mg/kg per minute is greater than the newborn's requirement of 3.5 to 5.5 mg/kg per minute, which, in turn, is almost twice the adult requirement. Fetal blood glucose levels are approximately 70% to 80% of the maternal level, which allows for the process of facilitated diffusion across the placenta. The fetus starts to store glucose in the form of glycogen from as early as 9 weeks, but the rate of deposition accelerates rapidly during the third trimester; this is probably related to the energy needs required during the process of labour and early postnatal period. Therefore, infants born before this time have a much greater risk of hypoglycaemia as a result of reduced time for deposition. During aerobic metabolism, energy in the form of adenosine triphosphate (ATP) is produced to maintain cellular function; however, during anaerobic metabolism, which occurs during labour, only one-fifteenth of ATP is produced compared with that of aerobic metabolism. Consequently, if the labour becomes prolonged or complicated, the newborn infant is at an increased risk of hypoglycaemia as a result of increased utilization of glucose. Different cells within the body have differing capacities for aerobic and anaerobic metabolism. Red blood cells are obligate glucose users but utilize glucose via an anaerobic process; thus, polycythaemic infants are at an increased risk of hypoglycaemia. Cardiac and cerebral cells, in contrast, are totally dependent on aerobic metabolism, and thus any oxygen deprivation will rapidly lead to loss of function and may result in irreversible damage. Although glucose is the major metabolic fuel for most organs, there is evidence that the newborn infant can utilize other fuel sources from lipolysis (release of fatty acids from adipose tissue stores), ketogenesis (from β-oxidation of fatty acids by the liver) and lactate (Hawdon 2012), which may offer protection to the newborn brain in healthy infants during adaptation to extrauterine life and establishment of milk feeding.

DISORDERS OF GLUCOSE BALANCE

Hypoglycaemia

The management of hypoglycaemia is by preventing it in the first case. Hypoglycaemia in the neonatal period is variously defined as levels between 1 and 4 mmol/L. The level most frequently used is greater than or equal to 2.6 mmol/L (Koh and Aynsley-Green 1998). Most newborn infants will have a low blood level if measured immediately after birth; however, as a result of the previously described compensatory mechanisms, the low level should not cause any harm. Infants who fall into a high-risk group (Table 50.1) should have early feeding as soon after birth as possible, with encouragement of skin-to-skin contact and unlimited access to breastfeeding. If the mother wishes to formula feed, then milk should be offered at 60 mL/kg per day. Feed intervals should not be greater than 3 hours, and pre-feed blood glucose monitoring should commence at 3 hours of age. If blood glucose levels fall below the recommended level, then feed volume or feed frequency should be increased. If the infant is not able to do this by mouth, then a nasogastric tube should be considered with commencement of gavage feeding. This not only ensures that the infant receives the appropriate volume but also decreases energy expenditure. This method may also prevent the need for admission to the neonatal unit for intravenous (IV) glucose, with its concomitant separation of mother and baby. Milk feeding is preferable to IV glucose because it contains other sources of energy than carbohydrate, such as fatty acids, and also stimulates gut hormones that facilitate postnatal metabolic adaptation more effectively (Lucas et al 1981).

Infants who do not fulfil 'at-risk' criteria can still develop hypoglycaemia, which has nonspecific signs and symptoms. Newborn infants have a limited repertoire of responses to illness. Lethargy, irritability poor feeding and jitteriness may be signs infection, but they are also signs of hypoglycaemia. Newborns should feed well, and if poor feeding persists, the infant should be reviewed by an experienced midwife and referred to the neonatal team as appropriate. Symptomatic hypoglycaemia (e.g. seizure activity or a blood glucose level less than 1 mmol/L) is a

Table 50.1 Infants at risk of hypoglycaemia

Infant group	Mechanism	Expected duration
Decreased stores Prematurity (Infants < 37 weeks are more at risk generally, and lower-gestation infants are further compromised.)	Decreased stores of glycogen and fat Impaired hormonal responses	Transient
Intra-uterine growth restriction	Decreased stores of glycogen and fat Impaired hormonal responses	Transient
Inborn errors of metabolism	Glycogen storage disease Enzyme deficiencies impairing utilization of stored substrate	Prolonged
Increased utilization Perinatal hypoxia	Anaerobic metabolism exhausting stores	Transient
Sepsis	Poor feeding	Transient
Hypothermia	Increased metabolic rate	Transient
Infant of diabetic mother	Increased metabolic rate and brown fat metabolism	Transient
Beckwith–Wiedemann syndrome	Hyperinsulinemia	Prolonged
Erythroblastosis fetalis	Hyperinsulinemia from islet hypertrophy	Transient
Islet cell dysplasias	Hyperinsulinemia from islet hypertrophy	Prolonged
Maternal drugs	Hyperinsulinemia Beta-blockers suppressing catecholamine responses	Transient

neonatal emergency, with the infant requiring immediate IV access and a glucose bolus (3 mL/kg) followed by IV glucose maintenance. Laboratory blood glucose levels should be sent at this time; it is ideal to also send blood for a more extensive hypoglycaemia screen, but this should not hold up the restorative therapy. It is recommended that infants who have symptomatic hypoglycaemia have early assessment with magnetic resonance imaging (MRI) as part of their follow-up because long-term neurological impairment is significant (Burns et al 2008).

Hyperglycaemia

Hyperglycaemia is not a problem for well-developed term infants and is predominantly a problem of extreme prematurity. These infants may receive increased glucose loads from IV fluids and parenteral nutrition, which they are not able to metabolize as a result of the decreased insulin responses from the immature pancreas. Hyperglycaemia from true neonatal diabetes mellitus is extraordinarily rare, occurring in 1:400,000 live births (Shield et al 1997).

DISORDERS OF ELECTROLYTE BALANCE

Hypernatremia

Hypernatremia is defined as a serum sodium level greater than or equal to 150 mmol/L (normal reference range 135–146 mmol/L) and occurs when there is a disproportionate amount of sodium in the body relative to water; it is not a result of excessive sodium intake and is more commonly a result of fluid lack. It has attracted attention in recent years predominantly because of its association with significant weight loss associated with difficulties with establishment of breastfeeding. Hypernatremic dehydration may have serious adverse consequences, such as seizures, intracranial haemorrhage, cerebral oedema and renal failure, and can result in permanent brain injury (Modi 2007). Although case reports of such complications have been described (Schroff et al 2006), they are thankfully rare, but often these infants require readmission to the hospital for controlled rehydration and may undergo multiple blood tests to monitor serum sodium levels or require septic screening and short-course antibiotic therapy as a result of the presenting signs of poor feeding, lethargy and weight loss. Management is with 'controlled rehydration', usually 100 mL/kg per day of breastmilk (if available) or formula milk rather than IV therapy because this is both safer because it is more gradual rehydration and kinder to the infant and mother because it negates the need for admission to a neonatal unit. In much rarer instances, it is the result of incorrect technique in making up formula milks.

As with hypoglycaemia, the problem of hypernatremia is one of its prevention, in which the role of the midwife and associated healthcare professionals cannot be overemphasized in supporting the establishment and success of breastfeeding and in providing education regarding the correct reconstitution of formula milks.

Hyponatraemia

Low serum sodium levels (less than 130 mmol/L) may be evident at birth as a reflection of maternal IV fluid therapy during labour. The well-developed term infant will handle this without adverse effect. Significant hyponatraemia is more likely to affect preterm infants with 'leaky kidneys' or, more frequently, the sick term infants who develop inappropriate antidiuretic hormone secretion (IADH) following hypoxic–ischemic events around the time of birth. Chronic hyponatraemia results in poor growth and is also associated with poor neurological development.

Hypocalcaemia

Symptomatic hypocalcaemia during the first few days of life occurs most commonly in preterm infants or those of diabetic mothers and those who have undergone perinatal stress. These infants may present variously with irritability, high-pitched cry, tremors, jitters, poor feeding or seizures. They require review, blood testing and correction with IV calcium if symptoms are severe (Cheetham and Schenk 2012). Intravenous calcium therapy may cause profound bradycardia and asystole and thus should be undertaken under strict electrocardiogram (ECG) control. Additionally, calcium given in this way can cause severe extravasation injury, and thus it should be given via a central line. If it is administered via a peripheral cannula, close observation of the site is mandatory (Beresford and Connolly 2010).

NEONATAL METABOLIC SCREENING

In the 1960s, Bob Guthrie, an American physician, created a simple biochemical test to detect blood phenylalanine levels; he did this by utilizing a process of bacterial inhibition. Although the newborn blood test is commonly known as the 'Guthrie test', the blood spot test has superseded the Guthrie test by tandem mass spectroscopy and can now identify a number of conditions other than just phenylketonuria (PKU). Because every infant born in the UK will undergo this test, routinely on day 5 to 6 of life, an outline of the diseases looked for in all areas of the UK follows.

Many of the diseases described are autosomal recessive (AR) in nature, which means that both parents are carriers of the defective gene but do not express the disease process themselves (see Ch. 26).

INBORN ERRORS OF METABOLISM

The majority of inborn errors of metabolism (IEMs) are AR disorders (Jones and Wraith 2012); as a category of diseases they are rare, but some are more common than others (e.g. phenylketonuria occurs in 1:10,000 to 15,000 infants, whereas isovaleric acidemia occurs in 1:155,000 infants). It is estimated that at least 600 babies are born each year in the UK with these disorders (see climb.org.uk). IEMs occur as a result of abnormalities in protein, fat or carbohydrate metabolism resulting from enzymatic deficiencies or protein transport defects that lead to a build-up of toxic metabolites. Most IEMs have no effect on the health or development of the fetus because placental perfusion removes the toxins from the fetus into the maternal circulation. As a consequence, most babies born with IEMs are of a normal birthweight and apparently healthy at birth (Jones and Wraith 2012). However, at birth, once this placental protection is removed and the infant starts to feed, there will be an accumulation of the toxic metabolites that will ultimately lead to encephalopathy, hypotonia, seizure and structural brain damage. The outcome for these infants relies on early detection, dietary manipulation and vitamin supplementation. Despite this, however, some of these rarer conditions are incompatible with long-term survival.

Phenylketonuria

The incidence of phenylketonuria (PKU) 1:10,000 to 15,000 births in the UK. PKU is caused by a deficiency of the enzyme phenylalanine hydroxylase, which is necessary to break down the amino acid phenylalanine. Phenylalanine is found in protein-rich foods. Once milk feeding commences, the infant gradually accumulates the toxic metabolite, which is neurotoxic. The newborn metabolic screening test identifies all infants with elevated blood levels of phenylalanine; therefore, early management of the condition can commence before irreparable damage occurs. Management of PKU is by restricted natural amino acid intake (sufficient for growth), with other proteins supplied in a synthetic form, leaving no excess to break down to the toxic metabolite. Over time during childhood, once brain growth is complete, the diet can be liberalized and natural protein intake increased; however, women who were diagnosed with PKU in infancy are advised to return to a restrictive diet when pregnant.

Medium-chain acyl-CoA dehydrogenase deficiency

The incidence of medium-chain acyl-CoA dehydrogenase deficiency (MCADD) is 1:8–12,000 in the UK. MCADD is a disorder of fatty acid metabolism. Fatty acids are an important source of energy and are the preferred substrate for muscle, particularly the heart (Leonard and Dezateux 2009). In normal circumstances, energy is obtained from carbohydrate; during fasting or times of illness, energy is obtained from the breakdown of fatty acids initiated by the enzyme medium-chain acyl-CoA dehydrogenase. If this process cannot be initiated, the individual becomes hypoglycaemic as a result of rapid metabolism of stored glucose and becomes encephalopathic as a result of an accumulation of the toxic metabolites, ultimately leading to acidosis and collapse. The initial episode may follow a more prolonged interval between feeds (e.g. overnight fasting) or an episode of acute illness (e.g. gastroenteritis). Management is by avoiding prolonged intervals between feeds (less than 6 hours) and meeting the energy requirements in the form of glucose during times of acute illness. For this reason, infants with this condition should have direct access to hospital admission so IV glucose can be administered during times of any illness, but especially diarrhoea and vomiting. Fats should also be avoided at this time. Older children and adults can be managed by administration of high-carbohydrate drinks (Leonard and Dezateux 2009). It has been recognized that fetal disorders of fatty acid metabolism can predispose mothers to develop acute fatty liver of pregnancy and hemolysis, elevated liver enzymes, low platelet count (HELLP syndrome).

Some areas in the UK screen for other IEMs, including glutaric aciduria type1 (incidence 1:120,000), homocystinuria (incidence 1:300,000) and isovaleric acidemia (incidence 1:155,000). This is dependent on the prevalence of the disease in different areas of the country.

Reflective activity 50.1

What information and resources do you need to perform a newborn screening blood spot test correctly to reduce the level of repeat testing as a result of incorrect technique or contamination? What information and resources are available where you practise?

Cystic fibrosis

The incidence of cystic fibrosis (CF) is 1:2500 births in the UK. CF is an AR disorder that affects pancreatic function and leads to production of viscid secretions within the respiratory and gastrointestinal tracts. Within the UK population, 1 person in 25 is a carrier of the CF mutation. Most newborns are asymptomatic, but 10% to 15%

present with meconium ileus resulting in obstruction at 48 hours of age (Newell 2012), necessitating urgent neonatal review. Screening for CF has been part of the UK metabolic screening programme since 2007, although some areas in England had introduced it much earlier. The test measures the serum immune reactive trypsin (IRT) level, which is elevated in CF. Diagnosis is then confirmed by genetic testing; there are now more than 1000 genetic mutations identified for CF, but the most common within the Caucasian population is delta F508. Early diagnosis and treatment considerably improve outcome. Breastfeeding should be encouraged because breastmilk has lipolytic and anti-infective properties. Long-term management is by pancreatic enzyme replacement therapy, high-calorie diet and chest physiotherapy.

Congenital hypothyroidism

The incidence of congenital hypothyroidism is 1 : 4000. All infants in the UK are screened for this condition. Thyroid-stimulating hormone (TSH) is measured; in those infants with a high level, the screening is repeated. All infants identified with a confirmed high level should commence thyroxine replacement as soon as possible because failure to do so will result in significant, permanent impairment of neurological function with reduced intelligence quotient and hearing and language difficulties.

Sickle-cell disease

Sickle-cell disease is a serious AR disorder of the haemoglobin molecule that causes it to distort into a crescent (sickle) shape during times of crisis (e.g. infection or low-oxygen states). This 'sickling' blocks blood vessels and results in severe pain and tissue and organ damage. It does not present in the early newborn period because fetal haemoglobin does not 'sickle' in these conditions. Although it predominantly affects infants of African or African Caribbean descent, all infants in the UK are now tested for this disorder.

Congenital adrenal hyperplasia

Congenital adrenal hyperplasia (CAH) is a generic term used to describe a series of AR disorders; up to 1 in 50 of the population carry the defect for the disorder. It is a complex disorder of adrenal steroidogenesis and is the principal cause of ambiguous genitalia (Cheetham and

Schenk 2012). CAH can lead to a salt-losing crisis as a result of inadequate production of aldosterone, which can lead to a life-threatening collapse in the newborn period. Careful examination of the external genitalia is an important facet of the newborn examination, and any newborn with bilateral undescended testis, hyperpigmented scrotum or any degree of ambiguity should be referred as a matter of urgency for senior neonatal review.

Galactosemia

The incidence of galactosemia is 1 : 45,000. This condition is not routinely screened for. It results from a lack of the enzyme galactose-1-phosphate uridyl transferase, which is necessary for the breakdown of galactose. Because galactose is found in both breast and formula milks, infants with this condition present towards the end of the first week of life with poor feeding, vomiting and jaundice. If the condition is left unchecked, the infant will develop cataracts and progressive liver damage. Management is with a galactose-free milk (e.g. soya). With time, the liver heals and the cataracts regress, but the long-term intellectual outcome is poor (Jones and Wraith 2012). Prenatal diagnosis can be made by chorionic villus sampling (CVS) at 12 weeks or amniocentesis at 16 weeks.

Reflective activity 50.2

Not all UK centres undertake the same tests. Visit https://www.gov.uk/government/collections/newborn-blood-spot-screening-programme-supporting-publications to find out what is available.

CONCLUSION

All infants, irrespective of gestational age, undergo significant metabolic changes at the time of birth. An understanding of the changes that occur and early recognition by the attending midwife may significantly improve the infant's long-term outcome.

Reflective activity 50.3

Compile a packet of information on relevant screening tests to give to women and their families.

- In the transition from intra-uterine to extrauterine life, the newborn undergoes multiple and significant metabolic changes.

- Midwives have a key role in achieving and maintaining metabolic homeostasis in the newborn by recognizing factors that put infants at risk of metabolic instability (e.g. hypoglycaemia or hypernatremia) and intervening appropriately.

- Newborn metabolic screening is part of the midwife's role, and thus midwives should have knowledge of the metabolic conditions screened for in their areas and be able to educate and support women and their families regarding these conditions.

- Inherited or acquired metabolic problems have an improved outcome if they are identified early and appropriate interventions and management strategies are commenced.

References

Beresford D, Connolly G: Fluid and electrolyte balance. In Connolly G, editor: *Neonatal intensive care nursing*, 2nd edn, London, Routledge, pp 255–278, 2010.

Burns CM, Rutherford MA, Boardman JP, et al: Patterns of cerebral injury and neurodevelopmental outcomes after symptomatic neonatal hypoglycemia, *Pediatrics* 122(1):65–74, 2008.

Cheetham T, Schenk DJ: Endocrine disorders. In Rennie J, editor: *Rennie and Roberton's textbook of neonatology*, 5th edn, London, Elsevier, pp 868–906, 2012.

Hawdon J: Disorders of metabolic homeostasis in the newborn. In Rennie J, editor: *Rennie and Roberton's textbook of neonatology*, 5th edn, London, Elsevier, pp 849–867, 2012.

Jones SA, Wraith JE: Inborn errors of metabolism in the neonate. In Rennie J, editor: *Rennie and Roberton's textbook of neonatology*, 5th edn, London, Elsevier, pp 906–920, 2012.

Koh THHG, Aynsley-Green A: Neonatal hypoglycaemia – the controversy regarding definition, *Arch Dis Child Fetal Neonatal Ed* 63:F1386–F1389, 1998.

Leonard JV, Dezateux C: Newborn screening for medium chain acyl CoA dehydrogenase deficiency, *Arch Dis Child* 94:235–238, 2009.

Lucas A, Aynsley-Green A, Bloom SR: Gut hormones and the first meals, *Clin Sci* 60:349–353, 1981.

Modi N: Avoiding hypernatraemic dehydration in healthy term infants, *Arch Dis Child Fetal Neonatal Ed* 92:F474–F475, 2007.

Newell S: Gastrointestinal disorders. In Rennie J, editor: *Rennie and Roberton's textbook of neonatology*, 5th edn, London, Elsevier, pp 706–724, 2012.

Schroff R, Hignett R, van't Hoff W: Life-threatening hypernatraemic dehydration in breastfed babies, *Arch Dis Child Fetal Neonatal Ed* 91:1025–1026, 2006.

Shield JPH, Gardner RJ, Wadsworth EKJ, et al: Aetiopathology and genetic basis of neonatal diabetes, *Arch Dis Child Fetal Neonatal Ed* 76:F39–F42, 1997.

Useful websites:

The links below are to useful UK resources on blood spot testing.

www.climb.org.uk.

www.newbornbloodspotscreening.wales.nhs.uk.

www.nsd.scot.nhs.uk/%5C%5C/services/screening/newborn screening/index.html.

www.newbornblood spot.screening.nhs.uk.

www.publichealth.hscni.net/publications/newborn-blood-spot-screening.

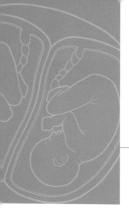

Chapter 51

Stillbirth and sudden infant death syndrome

Gail Johnson

Learning Outcomes ?

After reading this chapter, you will be able to:

- define different types of pregnancy and neonatal loss
- appreciate the incidence of pregnancy loss and perinatal and infant mortality rates
- have an understanding of the multifactorial nature of pregnancy loss, including stillbirth, neonatal death and sudden infant death syndrome (SIDS)
- appreciate the risk factors associated with perinatal, neonatal and infant death
- understand the role of the midwife and maternity service in recognizing risk factors and appropriate referral
- advise parents on modifiable behaviours to reduce risk

INTRODUCTION

In 2013, 5712 babies were stillborn or died within a few days of birth in the UK (Manktelow et al 2015). Another 249 babies died during infancy in England and Wales as a result of sudden infant death syndrome (SIDS) (Office for National Statistics (ONS) 2016). This equates to around 15 babies a day, and the effect on the family, friends and professionals is profound.

This chapter will address the variable terminology surrounding pregnancy loss and aim to explore the different types of pregnancy loss including *stillbirth, perinatal* and *neonatal and infant death, including SIDS.* The multifactorial nature related to pregnancy and risk will be addressed

alongside the role of the midwife and maternity services in recognizing risk and referring appropriately. An understanding of the public health messages and the potential benefits to behavioural change in reducing risk will be considered.

TERMINOLOGY

It remains difficult to provide a definitive terminology to describe the different types of pregnancy and neonatal loss; some terms have changed in recognition of the negative connotations for parents and families, for example, *miscarriage* rather than *spontaneous abortion.* Table 51.1 illustrates the definitions and the parameters for each loss. However, variability in terms used remains among professionals in how they refer to pregnancy loss. Nonetheless, it is essential that the professional communicates sensitively with bereaved parents and families and that the language used is clear and recognizes their grief and does not exacerbate their distress.

INCIDENCE

As highlighted in the introduction, approximately 15 babies a day die in the UK from stillbirth or neonatal death. This figure is down by approximately 1000 per year, despite a rise in the birth rate of 12%. The small decline in the mortality rate is a positive step in improving outcomes; however, the rates are less favourable compared with other similar high income countries. In 2011, *The Lancet* series on stillbirths (*The Lancet* 2011) produced a number of papers exploring the evidence around stillbirths globally. The papers identified that around 2.6 million stillbirths occur

Table 51.1 Definitions of pregnancy loss

Early miscarriage[1]	Pregnancy loss before 12 weeks gestation
Late miscarriage/late fetal loss	Pregnancy loss between 22^{+0} weeks and 23^{+6} weeks
Stillbirth	A baby born with no signs of life after 24 weeks gestation, irrespective of when the death occurred
Antepartum stillbirth	A baby born at or after 24^{+0} weeks, showing no signs of life and whose death occurred before the onset of care in labour
Intrapartum stillbirth	A baby born at or after 24^{+0} weeks, showing no signs of life and known to be alive at the onset of care in labour
Perinatal death	The death of a baby, including stillbirth and death, within the first week of life
Neonatal death (Extended perinatal death – a stillbirth or neonatal death – is the term used by MBRRACE)	Death before the age of 28 completed days after live birth *Early neonatal* is up to 7 days *Late neonatal* is from 7 to up to 28 days
Termination of pregnancy	The deliberate ending of a pregnancy, normally carried out before the fetus is capable of independent life
Infant death	Death of a baby in the first year of life
Sudden infant death syndrome	Sudden unexpected death of a previously and, apparently, healthy infant within the first year of life. If a previously undiagnosed underlying problem is found on postmortem, these cases are no longer reported as SIDS

[1]Miscarriage is used in this text, as opposed to the medical terminology of spontaneous abortion. This is in recognition of the negative connotations associated with the term abortion and the potential harm and distress to parents who experience a pregnancy loss before 24 weeks gestation (Mankletow et al 2015)

each year – more than 7300 per day. Although 98% of these deaths take place in low-income and middle-income countries, stillbirths also continue to affect wealthier nations, with around 1 in every 300 babies stillborn in high-income countries (Lawn and Kinney 2011). In the follow-up on *The Lancet* series (Lancet 2011), Heazel et al (2016) explores economic and psychosocial consequences of stillbirths. The variability in rates across and within economic status identifies that more can be done to reduce the rates and that opportunities to make a difference to stillbirth rates vary. Despite the cost analysis of reducing stillbirth, there is still no single intervention identified. However, for low-income and middle-income countries, the interventions are based around improved nutrition and recognition of risk in the antenatal period. In high-income countries, the interventions are based around recognition of risk and the implementation of evidence-based guidance. It is important to note the variations in the definition of stillbirth globally, as it can sometimes be difficult to make direct comparisons. The World Health Organisation (WHO) defines stillbirth from 28 completed weeks gestation and within *The Lancet* series, 28 weeks gestation is reported; the UK uses 24 weeks gestation, and some European countries cite 22 weeks gestation.

Qureshi et al (2015) believe that stillbirth is not adequately reported or recognized on the global health agenda and recommend having a universal definition of stillbirth to enable global comparisons. A great sadness is that many women never have access to healthcare and the devastating loss of their child goes unreported and unrecognized as significant.

The stillbirth rate in the UK remains disappointing, with the UK being ranked 21 out of 49 similar income countries. However, for the first time in 20 years, the last 5 years has seen a decline in the rate. Although there needs to be recognition that the rate is finally beginning to fall, the rates in other countries identify that the UK has more to do (The Lancet Series 2016).

INCIDENCE OF SUDDEN INFANT DEATH SYNDROME

It is difficult to determine the global occurrence of sudden infant death syndrome (SIDS); Lozano et al (2012) suggest that the number in 2010 was around 22,000 babies. This figure needs to be considered alongside the WHO global infant mortality rate – which is estimated to be 6.3 million children under the age of 5 in 2013 (WHO 2014). Like stillbirth, there are wide variations in rates, possibly resulting from reporting and data collection issues. The number of SIDS in the UK was approximately 290 in 2013, with a rate of 0.36 per 1000 births in England and Wales. There is a similar challenge with stillbirth statistics when it comes to UK and global comparisons.

Like stillbirth, the SIDS rate has declined, although there was a dramatic decline in SIDS rates after a global 'Back to Sleep' campaign, which resulted in a significant reduction of babies dying. In the UK in 2013, there was a small increase in the SIDS rate, the first rise since 2008 (ONS 2015). The reason for the increase is unclear; however, it is possible that the 'safe sleep' messages from the 1990s are not being considered as still relevant and, therefore, not being sufficiently emphasized to parents.

Reflective activity 51.1 ><

Review the Perinatal Mortality Surveillance Report – UK Perinatal Deaths for births from January through December 2013. MBRRACE-UK (Manktelow et al 2015)

How does the area in which you work compare to the units in your locality and nationally?

What are the variations and why do you think they exist?

RISK FACTORS FOR STILLBIRTH AND NEONATAL DEATH

Congenital abnormality accounts for approximately 10% of stillbirths and prematurity is a significant cause of neonatal death; however, for the majority of stillbirths and neonatal deaths, the cause is less clear and is often multifactorial and varied. A number of factors can be identified as clear risk; however, although risk factors may be present, the outcome of a baby death is not inevitable. Some women may present with a number of risk factors and have a successful outcome of pregnancy and sadly for some women, no risk factors will have been previously identified, but a stillbirth may happen. However, approximately 30% of stillbirths occur at term (37–42 weeks).

Some of the aspects known to increase the risk of stillbirth and neonatal death are highlighted in Table 51.2. Some of the elements that follow will be discussed in more detail.

The list of possible risk factors identified in Table 51.2 is not exhaustive and the issues are not particularly uncommon; therefore, midwives will meet women with one or more of these factors on a daily basis. The midwife has a clear role in identifying risk factors, supporting the woman where modifiable behaviours can reduce risk, and to advise the woman and her family on having a "safer pregnancy" (Sands 2016a).

Access to antenatal care has a positive effect on reducing mortality and morbidity for the woman, her fetus and, subsequently, her baby. The current guidelines on complex social factors in pregnancy (National Institute for Health and Care Excellence (NICE) 2010a) highlight the value of women being seen by a midwife or doctor before 12 weeks gestation and that there is an increased benefit for vulnerable women accessing care at 10 weeks gestation. If

Table 51.2 Antenatal risk factors	
Poor maternal health	Malnourishment through poor maternal diet can lead to inadequate placental perfusion and reduced fetal growth. Malnourished women may present as underweight or overweight and may also be anaemic.
Hypertensive disorders	Pre-existing hypertensive disorders or pregnancy-induced hypertension and pre-eclampsia can affect placental perfusion and add increased risk of placental abruption.
Placental dysfunction	A low lying placenta (placenta praevia) may not provide adequate fetal nutrition. Also placental insufficiency related to abruption, poor maternal nutrition or smoking/alcohol/substance use.
Pre-existing medical disorders (e.g. diabetes, cardiac disease, endocrine disorders, epilepsy)	If the medical condition is undiagnosed, poorly controlled or difficult to manage, the uterine environment may not be ideal for a developing fetus.

Table 51.2 Antenatal risk factors—cont'd

Intrahepatic cholestasis of pregnancy (ICP). (Obstetric cholestasis of pregnancy)	A disorder of pregnancy that leads to altered liver function. The woman usually presents with a relentless pruritis. Fetal morbidity and mortality is increased.
Maternal infection	Any febrile infection can make the uterine environment hostile and increase the risk of miscarriage, preterm birth and intrapartum death. Some infections may not present with a raised temperature and may go undiagnosed.
Intra-uterine growth restriction (formerly known as retardation) (IUGR)	There is increasing evidence that a growth restricted fetus is at a significantly increased risk of demise compared with a fetus of normal development. There may be a change or decrease in fetal movement in utero if the fetus becomes compromised.
Poor attendance at antenatal appointments	Women who attend after 14 weeks gestation for the first antenatal appointment and women who do not attend for regular antenatal follow-up have a higher incidence of stillbirth.
Cigarette smoking	There is significant evidence that smoking in pregnancy and passive smoking increases the risk of fetal and neonatal morbidity and mortality. Smoking has been shown to reduce placental perfusion. There are also associated risks, for example, poor diet and lifestyle.
Alcohol and substance misuse	Alcohol in pregnancy is associated with fetal alcohol spectrum disorder (FASD). The evidence to associate alcohol with stillbirth is less clear – however, it may be part of a chaotic lifestyle, and alcohol can exacerbate the risk.
Maternal obesity BMI ≥ 30	Women who begin their pregnancy with a BMI over 30 or women who rapidly gain excessive weight in pregnancy have a significant risk of developing gestational diabetes. If the woman is obese, the health professional may not be able to monitor fetal growth effectively – ultrasound equipment is less effective and midwives may not be able to palpate fetal growth abdominally.
Maternal age	Women under 20 years old and over 40 years old have a 39% higher risk.
Multiple pregnancy	One or both fetuses could be compromised through the pregnancy.
Black and minority ethnic women	Black and black British, Asian or Asian British women have a 50% higher risk.
Poverty and low-socioeconomic status	Women living in poverty have 57% higher risk.
Vulnerable women	A number of factors can make women vulnerable and less able to access and benefit from antenatal intervention.
Intrapartum risks of stillbirth and neonatal compromise	
Inappropriate care pathways	It is important that once labour begins, the woman has a full assessment to determine that she has access to the most appropriate care. Women who have been identified as *low risk* in pregnancy should still be reviewed to ensure that nothing has changed. Risk and changing circumstances need to be recognized as dynamic, and the midwife should address this at every meeting.
Assessment of fetal well-being	The progress of the labour is assessed regularly as per NICE guidance (NICE 2014). It is important to refer women who experience any deviations from the normal and to act on findings.

women are supported early in their pregnancy, they can have access to relevant information that may reduce some of the risk factors for fetal and neonatal mortality. The midwife is in a prime position to work with external agencies, where available, to provide additional and ongoing support.

If recognized, many of the risk factors can be mitigated against, and many of the interventions are relatively low cost compared with the long-term devastation of a still-birth or neonatal death and indeed the economic cost of these tragedies (Heazel et al 2016).

Obesity, malnourishment and poor diet

Obesity

Obesity is globally increasing, particularly in countries of economic wealth. In 2014, Public Health England (PHE 2016) identified that, in the UK and Ireland, 61.7% of adults are overweight or obese and that women are more likely to have an extremely high body mass index (BMI). This means midwives are seeing more overweight or obese women, who are at increased risk of gestational diabetes, pre-eclampsia, infection, congenital abnormality, preterm birth, stillbirth and neonatal death (Centre for Maternal and Child Health Enquiry (CMACE)/Royal College of Obstetricians and Gynaecologists (RCOG) 2010).

In addition to the risk to the fetus/baby, it is difficult to effectively assess fetal growth through abdominal examination/palpation, symphysis pubis fundal height measurement and ultrasound scanning. The woman may not be as aware of fetal movement and, therefore, not recognize any significant change in the pattern of fetal movements.

Malnourishment and poor diet

Women who are malnourished (see Ch. 17) can be advised on what constitutes a healthy diet and be encouraged to attend cookery classes, which are available in some children or community centres. Women who have a poor diet because of eating disorders should be referred to their GP and, where available, specialist counselling. Obese women should be advised to follow a healthy diet, which is designed to minimize weight gain in pregnancy. The Royal College of Midwives (RCM) supports the Slimming World guidance on weight management. If the midwife or doctor is in agreement that a weight management diet is appropriate, the woman can start or continue a regimen recommended by Slimming World (RCM 2016). Appropriate management of weight gain and obesity in pregnancy can reduce the incidence of gestational diabetes and make management of pre-existing diabetes easier (NICE 2010b). It can also hold significant psychological gains in terms of body image and confidence.

Reflective activity 51.2

What resources or support services are available in your region for women who are obese?

What resources do you have for testing women at risk of gestational diabetes?

Medical disorders and hypertension

Medical disorders and hypertension are covered in detail in Ch. 54. It is important the midwife recognizes the significance of pre-existing conditions and any new disorders arising in the pregnancy. Many women with an existing condition will be generally knowledgeable about their condition; however, they may not appreciate the changes that pregnancy can cause.

Smoking and substance misuse

The risks to the fetus and baby from maternal smoking and secondary (passive) smoking are well documented. NICE (2016) reviewed 24 studies and found that the risk of stillbirth was 47% higher in women who smoked. The risks increased with the more cigarettes smoked. The evidence around the benefits of stopping smoking is clear, and there is continued support for women to stop or reduce smoking in pregnancy. In 2011, approximately 13% of women were smoking at the time of birth; this equates to approximately 83,000 infants per year (Action on Smoking and Health (ASH) 2013). The overall trend for smoking in pregnancy is declining, with the rate of smoking at the time of birth down to 10.5% between April and June 2015 (Health and Social Care Information Centre (HSCIC) 2015 (England statistics)). Although the rates vary across the country, the potential risk through pregnancy, infancy and future health is significant. For some women who smoke, it is part of a "chaotic" lifestyle, which may also include other substance misuse and poor nutrition – all issues that compound the multifactorial nature of risk and poor outcomes. Smoking and substance misuse are known risk factors for placental insufficiency and fetal growth restriction, and smoking cessation support is an excellent opportunity to bring about a positive behavioural change (Flenady et al 2011), not just in that pregnancy but for the future health of the entire family.

Reflective activity 51.3

What percentage of women who give birth in your unit continue to smoke at term?

How many women accept referral to smoking cessation support?

What is your success rate once they find that support?

Intra-uterine growth restriction

There seems to be a strong correlation between intra-uterine growth restriction (IUGR) and poor pregnancy outcomes (Imdad et al 2011; Gardosi 2013; Flenady et al 2011), and the causes of IUGR are multifactorial. Around 1 in 3 term, normally formed, antepartum stillbirths are related to abnormalities in fetal growth (Draper et al 2015). Monitoring fetal growth is a key element of the antenatal assessment (NICE 2008). The midwife has a role in identifying women whose fetus may be at risk of growth restriction, for example, women who smoke, have had a previous small baby, early pregnancy loss or stillbirth. The simplest method of assessing fetal growth is through the measurement of the symphysis-fundal height (SFH) and the results plotted on a growth chart (RCOG 2014; Gardosi et al 2014). The RCOG (2014) and Gardosi et al (2014) recommend using a customized growth chart to plot fetal growth. A customized chart is designed for the individual woman and addresses maternal ethnicity, age, height and weight to provide an adjusted estimated growth chart for the fetus. The SFH is plotted on the growth chart and deviations from the normal should be reported for further investigations. Flenady et al (2011) question the effectiveness of SFH undertaken with a tape measure, although the Growth Assessment Programme (GAP) (Clifford et al 2013) suggest that measuring and plotting SFH on a customized chart can increase the detection of IUGR. After the introduction of GAP in the West Midlands, there was a regional decline in the stillbirth rates. Training for midwives on GAP has been introduced in a number of units within the UK and are currently being evaluated. The training teaches midwives how to undertake the correct measurement of the SFH and to only take the measure once. It is believed that if repeated measurements are taken, the midwife will record the result, which seems to best reflect the gestational age. In developing midwives' confidence in undertaking the measurement, it is thought that the most accurate result will be the first one. The increased detection of IUGR could be related to the midwife's heightened awareness of the link between IUGR and stillbirth and a possible increase in public awareness of what the midwife is assessing at each appointment and why. If the midwife suspects that the fetal growth is slow or slowing, it is important to refer for further review (RCOG 2014). Continuity of care from a known midwife could also help with the detection of IUGR, as it enables the woman and the midwife to develop a therapeutic relationship, which fosters open communication and reduces the ambiguity of the assessment being undertaken by different professionals.

Reflective activity 51.4

Review your unit guidelines on care for women with suspected IUGR. Do the local guidelines reflect RCOG Green-Top guidelines (No. 31)?

Reduced fetal movements

The woman will usually be aware of fetal movements from around 16 to 20 weeks gestation, with the movements increasing as the pregnancy progresses to around 32 weeks. From 32 weeks the movements tend to plateau, but should not decrease. Many women will be aware of a pattern in fetal movements and a change in the pattern, and a reduction in frequency and strength could be an indicator of fetal compromise. NICE (2008) do not recommend a formal approach to monitoring fetal movements through counting kicks, whereas, previously, women were asked to complete the *Cardiff Count to ten* chart – to record a minimum of 10 movements in a day. The evidence suggests that measuring fetal activity in this way was a poor indicator for outcomes. However, it is important that women are aware of fetal movements and, if there is a change, that they seek advice immediately (RCOG 2011). The Scottish government, Sands and Tommy's charity have invested in the AFFIRM study (Sands 2016b) to explore whether raising awareness of fetal movements among women and improving protocols (RCOG 2011 (guideline no. 57)) for health professionals in responding to women's concerns may help reduce stillbirths. The study is being conducted across the UK and is due to report in 2017. In almost half of the cases reviewed in the MBRRACE study (Draper et al 2015), reduced fetal movements had been reported and, in almost two-thirds of cases, there were additional risk factors identified; however, in many cases, women's concerns were not appropriately followed up.

Reflective activity 51.6

What advice are women given on monitoring fetal activity?
   What care/investigation is offered to women who report reduced fetal movements?

Prolonged pregnancy

The MBRRACE-UK Perinatal Confidential Enquiry into antepartum stillbirths (Manktelow et al 2015) highlighted that a third of antenatal stillbirths occurred at term. A meta-analysis demonstrated that routine induction of labour at term and post dates, reduced the incidence of perinatal death by approximately 50%. There is clearly a need to balance the risk of induction of labour and the prevention of perinatal death. However, a failure to recognize or act on known antenatal risk factors will result in a perinatal death, which could have been prevented.

HUMAN FACTORS IN STILLBIRTHS

The MBRRACE-UK report (Draper et al 2015) highlight that just over 50% of stillbirths remain 'unexplained', with the majority of deaths occurring just before the onset of labour at term, with a normally formed, singleton pregnancy. 'Unexplained' may only present part of the picture, as some deaths are being reported as a *cause unknown*, possibly because of inaccurate or inappropriate data collection. Where there is uncertainty, there may be an assumption that had labour been induced or a different plan of care introduced, the babies may well have survived with limited risk associated with induction of labour. A previous review of antenatal stillbirths, undertaken in 1996 and 1997, demonstrated similar findings to the 2015 review (Draper et al 2015) and recommended that:

- Women should be screened for gestational diabetes.
- Care of women with reduced fetal movements must be improved.
- Screening for growth restriction is poor.
- Lessons must be learnt where failures in care cause or contribute to stillbirth.

These damning findings from 1996 and 1997 were still being played out in 2013, and the pregnancy losses at term accounted for approximately a third of all stillbirths. For parents whose baby has died, it must be a difficult message to hear that for some, a different course of action could have resulted in them taking home a live baby.

The MBRRACE-UK (Manktelow et al 2015) report identified that in 60% of the stillbirths reviewed, improvements in care may have made a difference to the outcomes.

Challenges in the provision of care are multifactorial, for example, midwife shortages, inappropriate divisions in care provision and poor working relationships can contribute to a poor level of service. There may be failings from individuals but also from within the system, especially if guidelines cannot be fully implemented as a result of financial constraints. However, recognizing risk factors and acting on them could potentially save at least 600 babies every year in the UK – at least two lives every day.

A safe and collaborative work environment will provide safer and effective care for women and where professional relationships breakdown the outcomes for women and babies are poor (Kirkup 2015).

PUBLIC HEALTH MESSAGES

Understanding some of the causative and associated risks around perinatal death could bring about a reduction in the number of avoidable deaths. Parents report that if they do not know of the risks of stillbirth, they cannot make informed choices and decisions.

"As a pregnant woman, how can I contribute to the management of my own care if I don't know the risks?" Mum

(Sands 2016c)

The Sands Public Health Messaging task and finish group was set up in 2012 to work collaboratively to deliver public health messages to parents and families and to raise awareness of the risk of stillbirth. The messages are simple, and it was clear that parents needed to know what they could do to reduce their personal risk. Women did not want to hear messages about aspects that could not be changed or modified, for example, age or ethnicity. However, these remain important messages for professionals in ensuring that women are monitored appropriately (Sands 2016c).

Reflective activity 51.7

Review the *Advice for a safer pregnancy* (Sands 2016c) on the Sands website www.uk-sands.org
How does this reflect the advice and support for women in your region?

SUDDEN INFANT DEATH SYNDROME

Like stillbirth and perinatal death, the causes and associated factors are varied and multifactorial. However, a baby who has been compromised during pregnancy or birth is at increased risk of morbidity and mortality through infancy. This is a risk for many of the babies who were identified with fetal compromise but survived the birth, and it remains essential that professionals and parents are vigilant to minimize risk and further compromise.

Terminology

SIDS is sometimes referred to as sudden unexplained death in infancy or cot death. Cot death is a term frequently used by parents and the media, as it reflects the fact that the death usually occurs during sleep. The term sudden infant death syndrome was brought into common usage in the late 1960s to help bereaved parents and others to ascertain that the death was as a result of an unexplained or unintentional incident to demonstrate that the parents were not considered to be blamed for the death (Gornall 2008). A diagnosis of SIDS is reached when causes of death are excluded after a postmortem examination.

As previously mentioned, the launch of the 'Back to Sleep' campaign in 1991 saw a significant reduction in the number of SIDS cases reported (Fleming et al 2006; Moon et al 2007). The most significant reduction in the rate was seen in 1992, demonstrating the success of the 'Reduce the Risk' campaign, which encouraged parents and carers to lay babies on their back when going to sleep.

Sudden infant death occurs most commonly within the first 4 to 8 weeks of life, and boys are more likely to die than girls, at a ratio of 55 to 45 (ONS 2015). Previous data collection in the UK had put the peak of SIDS at 3 months (Centre for Maternal and Child Health Enquiry (CEMACH) 2008). However, over 6% of SIDS occurred from 12 to 24 months of age, highlighting the importance of being vigilant and keeping the baby safe (Lullaby Trust 2015).

Sleep practices and environment

Newborn babies are less able to regulate their body temperature, and overheating has been associated with SIDS (National Health Service (NHS) NHS-UK 2015); overwrapping, warm centrally heated rooms and blankets can contribute to the baby becoming too hot. It is recommended that the room the baby sleeps in is around 16°C to 18°C. In addition, babies who are lying in the prone position will be less able to lose heat through their faces (see Chs. 42 and 43). Guidance from the Lullaby Trust and the Department of Health advises that the baby's head should not be covered by blankets or a hat. In 2013 (ONS 2015), there was a rise in the incidence of SIDS during the winter and it is thought that the parents' response to the change in temperature is to wrap babies up more or to turn up the heating. The guidance also recommends that the baby is laid with the feet at the bottom of the cot or pram, 'feet-to-foot' position, to prevent the baby wriggling down under the blankets (NHS-UK 2015; Lullaby Trust 2016).

The incidence of SIDS is potentially reduced when babies sleep in the same room as their parents for the first 6 months. This is possibly because the parents are responsive to subtle changes in the baby's breathing patterns and may react to the baby's needs more quickly (Lullaby Trust 2013). However, *bed sharing* remains a risk factor for SIDS, with a significant increase in risk with cosleeping on the sofa (Fleming et al 2006; Gornall 2008; Moon et al 2007). It is important to recognize that the risk is increased if the parents smoke or have taken alcohol or drugs, which can cause drowsiness. Extreme tiredness in parents is an additional risk factor, one that most parents of a young baby will experience. A national audit carried out in 2003 and 2004 (RCM 2005) identified that women and families need clear information regarding cosleeping and recommended the development of multidisciplinary and evidence-based approaches to training and information for parents.

The Lullaby Trust advise that babies sleep on their backs in their own cot or Moses basket with the feet to the bottom of the cot, to avoid the risk of the baby wriggling under the blanket and becoming smothered or too hot (Lullaby Trust 2016).

Breastfeeding

Evidence indicates that breastfeeding could reduce the incidence of SIDS by approximately 50% (Vennemann

et al 2009), and the health benefits of breastfeeding are well reported and the link with a reduced risk of SIDS could be attributed to the IgA antibodies found in breast-milk, which fight off bacterial toxins. Discouraging bed sharing may have a detrimental effect on the duration of breastfeeding. A UNICEF statement on mother–infant bed sharing advises that parents need to understand the benefits of promoting breastfeeding and that the risks of bed sharing are increased when the mother smokes (UNICEF 2005). After the release of a new paper on the risk of bed sharing and breastfeeding, UNICEF released a further statement that continues to support their stance on ensuring that women/parents understand and appreciate the risk of bed sharing and balance that against the positive benefits of breastfeeding (UNICEF 2013).

Smoking

Smoking in pregnancy is known to increase the risk of preterm birth and low-birthweight babies, two factors that are associated with an increased incidence of SIDS. A number of studies reviewed by the Foundation for the Study of Infant Deaths (FSID) suggest that the risks of SIDS and smoking in pregnancy cannot simply be attributed to prematurity and low birthweight; smoking remains a contributory factor when other confounding variables – for example, maternal age, parity, marital status and breastfeeding – are considered (Lullaby Trust 2016). The evidence suggested that the more cigarettes smoked in pregnancy, the higher the risk of SIDS. Women who smoke in pregnancy increased the risk by two and a half to four times higher if they consumed 1 to 10 cigarettes a day. The risk increases seven to eight and a half times higher in women who smoke more than 20 cigarettes a day (Lullaby Trust 2016). The evidence highlights the benefits of encouraging women to reduce the number of cigarettes smoked in pregnancy, if they are unable to stop completely.

Smoking near or in the same room as a baby continues to pose a risk of cot death – a baby who regularly spends an hour a day in a smoky environment is twice as likely to die of SIDS as a baby in a smoke-free environment. The advice not to smoke in pregnancy and around the baby applies to parents and to the wider family environment.

Reflective activity 51.8

Review the advice for professional and parents on reducing the risk of SIDS on the Lullaby Trust website (www.lullabytrust.org.uk) and NHS Choices website (www.nhs.uk/Conditions/Sudden-infant-death-syndrome).

How does the guidance on the website reflect the advice that women receive in your area?

THE ROLE OF THE MIDWIFE IN REDUCING SIDS

Antenatal care will help improve the well-being of the mother, fetus and baby through identification of risk factors, advising on modifying behaviours and seeking medical intervention where appropriate. This role will help reduce some of the possible associated risk factors for stillbirth, perinatal death and SIDS. The midwife is in an ideal position to advise parents and the wider family on general health and raise awareness of risk. The midwife will also work in collaboration with general practitioners, health visitors and other practitioners to advise parents on modifying behaviours, for example, smoking cessation.

AFTERMATH OF A BABY DEATH

The death of a baby in pregnancy, around the time of birth or in infancy has devastating long-term consequences for the parents, wider family and health professionals.

Every unexpected neonatal or infant death is subjected to scrutiny by the coroner, and the police are required to interview the family and may take samples of clothing and bedding away as part of the in-depth review. On top of the devastating death of a child, the parents' distress is likely to be exacerbated by the intense investigations. The investigation needs to be undertaken sensitively; the parents are likely to have many questions about the death of their baby, and it is important that they are advised of any findings from the investigation.

Currently in England, Wales and Scotland, stillbirths are not subjected to review in the coroner's (procurer fiscal in Scotland) court – although in some regions, local coroners have asked for all stillbirths to be reported to them and Sands and other parent groups are calling for a change to the coroner's jurisdiction to make it possible for cases to be referred to the coroner. A ruling in Northern Ireland (NI) at the Court of Appeal (November 2013) now means that stillborn babies born in NI are reported to the coroner's office.

A number of charities have support and guidance for professionals and families after the death of a baby, whether during pregnancy or after. Sands (https://www.uk-sands.org/), Child bereavement UK (CBUK) (http://www.childbereavementuk.org/) and the Lullaby Trust (http://www.lullabytrust.org.uk/) all have excellent resources and guidance for parents and families, practitioners and service provision.

REVIEW OF PERINATAL DEATHS

Learning lessons from the death of a baby at any stage is paramount if the stillbirth, perinatal and infant death rates are to be diminished. The Each Baby Counts (EBC) project (RCOG 2016) is reviewing data from case notes where term babies (in labour) have died or have been admitted to neonatal care with *hypoxic ischemic encephalopathy* (HIE). All units in the UK have committed to share their data from case notes and identify thorough internal investigations into the death of a baby or admission to special care of a sick baby. In the EBC project data collection, to learn lessons is essential, and Morgan (2015) compares the data collection from a flight black box to what is needed after any baby death. This approach may help all units appreciate what happened and what could be done differently. Although the RCOG project is a good start, their review is of a limited population. The Sands/DH Perinatal Mortality Review Task and Finish Group in 2013 designed a data collection tool, which will collect data from all stillbirths (Sands 2013). It is anticipated that that funding to undertake the reviews will be available in 2016 (Bevan 2016 personal communication).

FOLLOW-UP CARE

After the death of a baby at any stage of pregnancy, the parents must be treated with respect and all of their questions answered as honestly as possible. The women will have access to postnatal care from the midwife, and there should be choice offered as to who visits the family. In some units, the woman will be cared for by the bereavement support team or the woman may wish to see a midwife she has known throughout her pregnancy (see Ch. 68).

The parents should be offered a postmortem on their baby and given a full explanation on the procedures and the extent of the investigations they wish to consent to (Human Tissue Authority (HTA) 2016).

FUTURE PREGNANCIES

Families who have experienced the death of a baby at any stage of pregnancy or after birth will understandably be concerned about the health of future babies, particularly if the cause of death is not ascertained. After stillbirth and neonatal death, in the next pregnancy, women are usually offered more frequent appointments and increased screening, monitoring and delivery at approximately 39 weeks gestation (Smith 2015). For parents whose baby dies in infancy, the Lullaby Trust has a programme of support, called 'Care of Next Infant' (CONI). This uses the skills and support of the paediatrician, obstetrician, family doctor, midwife, health visitor and a local CONI coordinator. The family determines the level of support, and it can include home visits to assess well-being and provide practical advice on room temperature and signs of ill health.

Reflective activity 51.9

Contact the local CONI coordinator and the midwife who is on the team to discuss their role in supporting parents.

CONCLUSION

The death of a baby is devastating for parents, the family, friends and health carers. There are approximately 22.6 million stillbirths globally per year, with approximately 5700 in the UK and 6.3 million babies dying globally before the age of 5 years, with approximately 290 SIDS deaths per year in the UK. The exact numbers are difficult to determine, but even with the conservative estimate of those previously mentioned, it is clear the numbers are too high and that many deaths could be avoided. The causes are unknown but appear to be multifactorial with further investigation and research into what is still unknown about stillbirths (Heazel et al 2015) and SIDS. Recognizing and acting on risk factors or deviations from normal in pregnancy and advising parents on modifying behaviours could help minimize the risk.

Key Points

- The midwife is a key person in identifying women and babies who might be at risk and providing information, support and referral throughout care.

- The aetiology of stillbirth and SIDS remains uncertain, although there is strong evidence that identifying and acting on risk factors in pregnancy and birth can reduce the incidence of neonatal and infant mortality and morbidity.

- Raising awareness of risk factors with parents and highlighting modifiable behaviours may reduce risk.

- Effective antenatal care and appropriate actions on deviations from normal will help improve maternal, fetal and newborn health.

- Reduction or cessation of smoking, recognition of placental insufficiency and fetal growth retardation, identification of gestational diabetes and action of reduced fetal movements will reduce the incidence of stillbirth and SIDS.

- Putting the baby on its back to sleep and avoiding overheating can reduce the risk of SIDS.

- Parents, grandparents and carers require advice on possible risk factors.

References

Action on Smoking and Health (ASH): *Smoking and reproduction fact sheet (7)* (website). http://ash.org.uk/files/documents/ASH_112.pdf. 2013.

Bevan C: *Senior Research and Prevention Officer, Sands charity*. Personal communication; *Task and Finish Group (Sands and Department of Health (DH)) Review of Perinatal Mortality Tool Kit*. 2016.

Centre for Maternal and Child Health Enquiry (CMACE) and Royal College of Obstetricians and Gynaecologists (RCOG): *Management of women with obesity in pregnancy*, March 2010.

Clifford S, Giddins S, Southam M, et al: The growth assessment protocol: a national programme to improve patient safety in maternity care, *MIDIRS Midwifery Digest* 23(4):516–523, 2013.

Confidential Enquiry into Maternal and Child Health (CEMACH): *Why Children Die: A Pilot Study 2006, England (South West, North East &* West Midland), Wales and Northern Ireland, London, CEMACH, 2008.

Court of Appeal Northern Ireland: *Court allows appeal in stillborn baby inquest case* (website). www.courtsni.gov.uk/en-GB/Judicial%20Decisions/SummaryJudgments/Documents/Court%20allows%20appeal%20in%20stillborn%20baby%20inquest%20case/j_j_Summary%20of%20judgment%20-%20In%20re%20Attorney%20General%20for%20Northern%20Ireland%20(Stillborn%20Baby%20Inquest)%2021%20Nov%2013.htm. 2013.

Draper E, Kurinczuk J, Kenyon S (editors): *On behalf of MBRRACE-UK Perinatal Confidential Enquiry: Term, Singleton, Normally Formed, Antepartum Stillbirth*. Leicester: The Infant Mortality and Morbidity Studies, Department of Health Sciences, University of Leicester, 2015.

Fleming P, Blair P, McKenna J: New knowledge, new insights, and new recommendations, *Arch Dis Child* 91(10):799–801, 2006.

Flenady V, Middleton P, Smith G, et al: Stillbirths: the way forward in high-income countries, Stillbirths 5, *The Lancet Series* 377(May 14): 2011.

Gardosi J: Maternal and fetal risk factors for stillbirth: population based study, *Br Med J* 10(3):346, f108. 2013.

Gardosi J, Giddings S, Buller S, et al: *Preventing stillbirth through improved antenatal recognition of pregnancies at risk due to fetal growth restriction conference paper, public health* (website). www.sciencedirect.com https://www.perinatal.org.uk/fetalgrowth/pdfs/PUHE2100.pdf. 2014.

Gornall J: Does cot death still exist? *Br Med J* 336(7639):302–304, 2008.

Health and Social Care Information Centre (HSCIC): *Statistics on Women's Smoking Status at the Time of Delivery, England, Quarter 2,*

2015–2016. www.hscic.gov.uk/catalogue/PUB19292. 2015.

Heazel A, Siassakos D, Blencowe H, et al: Ending Preventable stillbirths, stillbirths: economic and psychosocial consequences, *Lancet* 387(10018):604–616, 2016.

Heazel A, Whitworth M, Whitcomes J, et al: Research priorities for stillbirth: process overview and results from UK stillbirth priority setting partnership, Editorial *Ultrasound Obst Gyn* 46:641–647, 2015.

Human Tissue Authority (HTA): (website). www.hta.gov.uk/policies/sands-perinatal-post-mortem-consent-package. 2016.

Imdad A, Yakoob M, Siddiqui S, et al: Screening and triage if intrauterine growth restriction in general population and highrisk pregnancies: a systematic review with a focus on reduction of IUGR related stillbirths, *BMC Public Health* 11(Suppl 3):51, 2011.

Kirkup B: *The Report of the Morecambe Bay Investigation: An Independent Investigation into the Management, Delivery and Outcomes of Care Provided by the Maternity and Neonatal Services at the University Hospitals of Morecambe Bay NHS Foundation Trust from January 2004 to June 2013.* Stationery Office, London, 2015.

Lawn J, Kinney M: *Stillbirths: an executive summary for The Lancet's Series* (website). www.thelancet.com/pb/assets/raw/Lancet/stories/series/stillbirths/stillbirths.pdf. 2011.

Lozano R, Naghavi M, Foreman K, et al: Global and regional mortality from 235 causes of death for 20 age groups in 1990 and 2010: a systematic analysis for the Global Burden of Disease Study 2010, *Lancet* 380(9859):2095–2128, 2012.

Lullaby Trust: *Evidence Update May 2013* (website). www.lullabytrust.org.uk/document.doc?id=300. 2013.

Lullaby Trust: *SIDS Facts and Figures August 2015* (website). www.lullabytrust.org.uk/file/Facts-and-Figures-for-2013-released-2015.pdf. 2015.

Lullaby Trust: *2016 Fact Sheet 2 Smoking* (website). www.lullabytrust.org.uk/file/-----internal-documents/Fact-sheet-Smoking.pdf. 2016.

Manktelow B, Smith L, Evans T, et al; On behalf of the MBRRACE-UK

collaboration: *Perinatal Mortality Surveillance Report UK Perinatal Deaths for Births from January to December 2013*, Leicester: *The Infant Mortality and Morbidity Group*, Department of Health Sciences, University of Leicester (website). www.npeu.ox.ac.uk/downloads/files/mbrrace-uk/reports/MBRRACE-UK%20Perinatal%20Surveillance%20Report%202013.pdf. 2015.

Moon R, Horne R, Hauck F: Sudden infant death syndrome, *Lancet* 370(9598):1578–1586, 2007.

Morgan D: *Each Baby Counts Newsletter O&G November 2015* (website). www.rcog.org.uk/globalassets/documents/guidelines/research--audit/each-baby-counts-update--og-magazine-november-2015.pdf. 2015.

National Health Service (NHS) (NHS-UK): (website). www.nhs.uk/Conditions/Sudden-infant-death-syndrome/Pages/Introduction.aspx. 2015.

National Institute for Health and Care Excellence (NICE): *Antenatal care for uncomplicated pregnancies (CG62)* (website). Updated November 2014. www.nice.org.uk/guidance/cg62. 2008.

National Institute for Health and Care Excellence (NICE): *Pregnancy and complex social factors: a model for service provision for pregnant women with complex social factors* (website). www.nice.org.uk/guidance/cg110. CG110. 2010a.

National Institute for Health and Care Excellence (NICE): Weight management before, during and after pregnancy, *Public Health Guidance* 27, 2010b.

National Institute for Health and Care Excellence (NICE): *Intrapartum care for healthy women and babies* (website). www.nice.org.uk/guidance/cg190. CG190. 2014.

National Institute for Health and Care Excellence (NICE): (website) http://us8.campaign-archive2.com/?u=7864f766b10b8edd18f19aa56&id=ae7176cdaa&e=3ed52cf426. 2016.

Office for National Statistics (ONS): Unexplained deaths in infancy: England and Wales, 2013, *Eyes on Evidence* 81, February 2016.

Public Health England (PHE): *UK and Ireland Prevalence Trends* (website). www.noo.org.uk/NOO_about_

obesity/adult_obesity/UK_prevalence_and_trend. 2016.

Qureshi Z, Millum J, Blencowe H, et al: Stillbirth should be given greater priority on the global health agenda, *Br Med J* 351:2015.

Royal College of Midwives (RCM): *A Report of the Findings of the RCM UK National Bed Sharing Audit*, London, RCM, 2005.

Royal College of Midwives (RCM): *Slimming World and RCM Resources* (website). www.rcm.org.uk/slimming-world. 2016.

Royal College of Obstetricians and Gynaecologists (RCOG): *Reduced Fetal Movements; Green-Top Guidelines No. 57.* (website). www.rcog.org.uk. 2011.

Royal College of Obstetricians and Gynaecologists (RCOG): *The Investigation and Management of the Small-for Gestational-Age Fetus.* Green-top Guideline No. 31. 2nd ed. Minor revisions February 2013. (website) www.rcog.org.uk. 2014.

Royal College of Obstetricians and Gynaecologists (RCOG): *Each Baby Counts* (website). www.rcog.org.uk/en/guidelines-research-services/audit-quality-improvement/each-baby-counts/. 2016.

Sands: *Stillbirth and Neonatal Death Charity.* News Bulletin Issue 7 November 2013 (website). www.uk-sands.org/sites/default/files/Spotlight%20on%20Sands%20Issue%207%20Final.pdf. 2013.

Sands: *Stillbirth and Neonatal Death Charity* (website). www.uk-sands.org/why-babies-die/advice-for-a-safer-pregnancy. 2016a.

Sands: *Stillbirth and Neonatal Death Charity.* AFFIRM study update (website). www.uk-sands.org/research/current-projects/sands-funded-projects/affirm-%E2%80%93-can-promoting-awareness-baby%E2%80%99s-movements. 2016b.

Sands: *Stillbirth and Neonatal Death Charity. Raising Awareness of Risk* (website). www.uk-sands.org/why-babies-die/preventing-more-deaths/raising-awareness-of-risk. 2016c.

Smith GCS: Prevention of stillbirth, *Obstet Gynaec* 17:183–187, 2015.

The Lancet: *Ending preventable stillbirths* (website). www.thelancet.com/series/ending-preventable-stillbirths. 2016.

UNICEF: *Sharing a Bed with Your Baby 2005–2006* (website). www.baby friendly.org.uk/pdfs/sharingbed leaflet.pdf. 2005. Updated July 2008. 2015.

UNICEF UK: *Baby Friendly Initiative Statement on Bed Sharing Research May 2013* (website).

www.unicef.org.uk/BabyFriendly/ News-and-Research/News/ UNICEF-UK-Baby-Friendly -Initiative-statement-on-new -bed-sharing-research/. 2013.

Vennemann M, Bajanowski T, Brinkmann B, et al: Does breastfeeding reduce the risk of sudden infant death syndrome? *Pediatrics* 123(3):406–410, 2009.

World Health Organisation (WHO): *Children: Reducing Mortality Fact Sheet*, No. 178. Updated September 2014 (website). www.who.int/ mediacentre/factsheets/fs178/en/. 2014.

Resources and additional reading

The Royal College of Midwives (RCM) has an online electronic learning (RCM i-learn) module on bereavement care, which was authored by Sands and CBUK. The module is available for RCM members via https://www.rcm .org.uk/.

The RCM and Sands have developed an online network for health professionals to discuss and share good practice on the Bereavement Care Network http://bereavement-network.rcm.org.uk/.

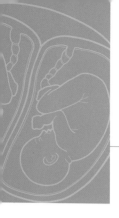

Chapter 52

Nausea and vomiting in pregnancy

Cecelia M. Bartholomew

Learning Outcomes ?

After reading this chapter, you will be able to:

- define and differentiate between physiological and pathological vomiting in pregnancy
- explain the possible consequences for mother and baby
- discuss the management and possible treatments, including self-help strategies
- plan and implement appropriate midwifery action to support the woman and family

INTRODUCTION

Nausea and vomiting in pregnancy (NVP) occurs in up to 90% of normal pregnancies such that they may be regarded as normal and presumptive symptoms of pregnancy. The conditions may range from mild to severe, which in the latter is pathological where it can become debilitating and life-threatening to the woman and her unborn baby. Although not exclusive, severe vomiting in pregnancy is strongly associated with a multiple pregnancy, the presence of a hydatidiform mole (see Ch. 53) or pre-eclampsia. Associated medical conditions such as hyperthyroidism, diabetes and gastrointestinal disorders may also be implicated.

Nausea is the feeling of impending vomiting, while *vomiting* consists of retching and forceful expulsion of stomach contents. It has been postulated that these symptoms occur when the vomiting centres in the brain are stimulated by the chemoreceptor trigger zones and vagal afferents from the gut (Lindsay et al 2012). This is despite there being no distinct anatomical vomiting centre to be located in the brain (Pleuvry 2015).

AETIOLOGY

The aetiology of the condition in pregnancy is also poorly understood, and the literature suggests a multiplicity of probable origins. The explanations that are predominantly promulgated are raising levels of hormones, including *oestrogen, progesterone, human chorionic gonadotrophin (hCG), thyroxine (T_4)* and *thyroid stimulating hormone (TSH)*. This may be compounded by physiological adaptations to pregnancy, such as reduced gastric motility or reflux oesophagitis, metabolic alterations to carbohydrate and vitamin B deficiency. A presumed anatomical positioning of a right-sided corpus luteum is thought to cause high concentrations of sex steroids in the hepatic portal system (Himoto et al 2015), inducing nausea and vomiting in pregnancy (NVP). Female fetal sex has also been shown to be associated with the symptoms (Rashid et al 2012).

Although there seems to be limited data to support the psychiatric origins, some researchers, such as Uguz et al (2012), have concluded that there is a link. However, the psychological sequelae associated with the condition may be a consequence of the physical symptoms and adverse experience of these, rather than the cause (Magtira et al 2015). It may, therefore, be premature to refute a psychological basis for NVP, as there appears to be an integration of various elements incorporating psychogenic, socio-cultural and biological factors (Buckwalter and Simpson 2002). Midwives need to be aware of the debate to ensure that they do not stereotype women and impede adequate treatment of the conditions.

There have been several theories about the theoretical function of NVP in pregnancy, but the specific role of the condition remains unknown. One hypothesis is that it may be a protective mechanism triggered by food or substances, which may contain harmful toxins and microorganisms (Mckerracher et al 2015). Flaxman and Sherman (2008) suggest that the hypothesis of prophylaxis is consistent with patterns of cravings and aversions observed in certain women and cultures.

MILD AND MODERATE NAUSEA AND VOMITING

Mild vomiting is an unpleasant but transient and self-limiting condition that commonly appears around the fifth week of pregnancy, peaks in severity at around 11 to 13 weeks and usually resolves by 22 weeks. The typical manifestation is that women feel nauseated on waking and may vomit on rising from bed. Women may report an increased sensitivity of smell, which initiates feelings of nausea that leads to aversion to some foods. Actual vomiting recedes during the day, but nausea may persist. Moderate vomiting is more serious, as the woman will vomit several times during the day, often after meals, and this may be accompanied by some weight loss and ketonuria.

HYPEREMESIS GRAVIDARUM

Hyperemesis gravidarum (HG) is a pathological condition characterized by unremitting, severe vomiting in pregnancy. It occurs in 0.3% to 2.0% of pregnancies (Ismail and Kenny 2007), is diagnosed by a process of exclusion (Kametas and Nelson-Piercy 2008) and is a leading cause of hospital admission during pregnancy.

A significant number of studies have shown that a gastric infection caused by the *Helicobacter pylori* bacterium may increase the risk of developing HG (Sandven et al 2009). However, a smaller number of investigations in populations where the infection is common could not conclude that there was a definite association between the presence of the bacteria and the likeness of developing HG (Nasir et al 2012; Boltin et al 2014). Nevertheless, where incidence of severe vomiting occurs, coinfection with the bacteria should be considered and screening for the presence of the bacteria be carried out (Clark et al 2014). The infection responds well to triple therapy and consists of *amoxicillin, metronidazole* and a *protein pump inhibitor (PPI) or H2 blocker* (Sandven et al 2009).

HG is associated with significant weight loss, ketonaemia, electrolyte imbalance and dehydration. If the persistent retching and vomiting remains uncontrolled and untreated, the woman may show signs of tachycardia, postural hypotension and muscle wasting (Boregowda et al 2013). Further complications can include considerable physical injury and pain, involving rupture of the oesophageal wall (Boehaave syndrome), diaphragmatic tears or

mucosal trauma at the junction of the stomach and oesophagus (Mallory–Weiss syndrome) (Erick 2014). Hepatic, central nervous system and renal damage (Holmgren et al 2008) or even splenic avulsion (detachment) (Nguyen et al 1995), which is rare but fatal, may result in extreme and unmanaged cases.

Wernicke's encephalopathy is a rare but serious complication that has been reported in women with severe HG. Although its presentation is that of a neuropsychiatric syndrome, it is caused by severe *thiamine* (vitamin B_1) deficiency because of the persistent vomiting (Sechi and Serra 2007). It manifests itself through symptoms of confusion, ocular abnormalities and ataxia (Chiossi et al 2006). Diagnosis is based on clinical symptoms and can be supported by an enhanced magnetic resonance imaging (MRI) scan (Kametas and Nelson-Piercy 2008). The condition responds well to treatment with thiamine (Welsh 2005).

PSYCHOSOCIAL IMPACT

Whether the condition is mild, moderate or severe, it has significant implications for the woman's physical and psychological well-being, and may well influence how she accepts and responds to her pregnancy. Extreme tiredness is common and may affect her everyday activities and family relationships (Isbir and Mete 2013). She may exhibit mounting anxiety and emotional changes that could lead to post-traumatic stress in the postnatal period (Ayyavoo et al 2014). Furthermore, unhelpful attitudes or responses from healthcare practitioners could cause her to feel that she is wasting their time, making it difficult to seek help if needed (Power et al 2010). The experience for the woman is subjective and must be dealt with showing care and compassion.

Risk to the fetus

Mild to moderate forms of NVP appear to have a protective function with favourable neonatal outcomes (Koren et al 2014). There is, however, an association between severe vomiting and miscarriages, fetuses that are small-for-gestational age and preterm delivery; but the research on the effect of severe vomiting on perinatal mortality is inconsistent (Ayyavoo et al 2014).

CARE AND MANAGEMENT OF MILD SYMPTOMS

The care and management of women with NVP depends on the intensity of the symptoms and requires a multidisciplinary approach. Even in mild cases, the woman often feels miserable and her symptoms should not be regarded as trivial. Therefore, empathic support is paramount. Her partner and family will also need reassurance and guidance on how to provide assistance during this time.

The initial assessment of the severity of the condition by the midwife is pivotal in all cases. If undiagnosed and untreated, the disease can progress from mild NVP to HG. The line of questioning should also be aimed at excluding any other conditions that may be the cause of the symptoms. There are clinical tools available internationally to evaluate the severity of the condition and its effect on the woman's quality of life, such as the *Pregnancy-Unique Quantification of Emesis/Nausea (PUQE)* index (King and Murphy 2009) or the *Hyperemesis Impact of Symptoms (HIS) tool* (Fletcher et al 2015). Although a standardized questionnaire is not commonly utilized in the UK for the initial assessment for NVP, an evaluation should be made to establish the onset, duration and frequency of the nausea and vomiting and how much food and drink are being tolerated (National Institute for Health and Care Excellence (NICE) 2013). Furthermore, it is important to establish the woman's perception of the condition, how it is affecting her mental health and well-being and her reaction to the pregnancy and the effect on her lifestyle.

In cases of mild NVP, medication is not usually required, and a change in diet and lifestyle is the initial approach to help the woman manage her symptoms. Helpful suggestions may include a milky drink at bedtime, dry toast or biscuit on waking, with frequent, small, light meals during the day and intake of higher protein and carbohydrate content with reduced fat and avoiding spicy or strong-smelling foods, unless this is what she can tolerate. Small amounts fluid may be consumed at varying periods during the day as required and should amount to about two litres (Clark et al 2014) to prevent dehydration.

Reflective activity 52.1

Contact your local hospital dietician. What dietary modifications does he/she recommend for women with nausea and vomiting in pregnancy? You may wish to discuss these with a colleague and find out what they recommend.

The woman's quality of life and day-to-day activities can be tremendously affected by NVP. She will need the support of her partner and family members to break her fast in bed and to rest as much as possible because tiredness and stress may exacerbate the vomiting. If she is employed, it can affect her ability to attend work and function effectively in her job. For that reason, she may require a letter from her general practitioner (GP) to her employer so that the appropriate adaptive changes can be negotiated. For example, she may need to change start times to avoid travelling on crowded transportation.

Alternative therapies

Complementary remedies (see Ch. 18) are often useful to treat the symptoms NVP. However, the midwife should not advise on the use of any complementary therapies, unless she has been properly trained and qualified in the field (NMC 2010). One commonly recommended treatment is the herbal medicine *ginger* for its antiemetic properties and effect on the motility of the gut (Wu et al 2008; Tiran 2012). Tiran (2012), however, advises that ginger is not suitable for all women; midwives need to be aware of the risks and benefits of this herbal medicine when advising women. Acupuncture and acupressure, using the P6 point, may also relieve vomiting in pregnancy (Lee and Saha 2011).

Pharmacological treatment

If NVP is not relieved in using conservative measures, then oral antiemetics may need to be prescribed by a GP or obstetrician. In the UK, NICE recommends an initial treatment with oral *Promethazine hydrochloride* and *Cyclizine* (NICE 2013). If after a week this is ineffective, NICE suggests switching to *Metoclopramide*, *Prochlorperazine* or *Ondansetron*. The woman needs to be reassessed for worsening of the condition, which may necessitate hospitalization for rehydration and the administration of intramuscular or intravenous antiemetics.

CARE AND MANAGEMENT OF MODERATE TO SEVERE NAUSEA AND VOMITING IN PREGNANCY

According to NICE (2013), the woman should be advised that if she begins to experience very dark urine or does not pass urine for more than 8 hours, she should seek urgent attention from her GP or local obstetric unit. She must also seek medical attention if she experiences abdominal pain, fever, haematemesis, weakness, fainting and inability to cease vomiting or keep food down for 24 hours.

A record of the woman's current weight, temperature, pulse and blood pressure is essential to assess and monitor her physical well-being and aid in the exclusion of other medical complications that may be the cause of the severe vomiting, such as thyrotoxicosis. A urinalysis is conducted for ketones, bilirubin, protein and glucose, and a midstream specimen of urine is sent for culture to exclude pyelonephritis. In addition, the fetal condition should be assessed as appropriate (depending on gestation) to establish fetal health.

If the woman reports moderate to severe NVP for more that 24 hours, despite oral antiemetic, and symptoms such as an inability to tolerate oral medication with signs of dehydration or weight loss, arrangements should be made for her to be treated in hospital. In some obstetric units, this may be managed by admitting the woman as a day case to the Early Pregnancy Assessment Unit with the aim of breaking the cycle through intravenous rehydration and intramuscular/intravenous antiemetics (Pugsley and Moore 2012).

Reflective activity 52.2

Talk to women about their experiences of nausea and vomiting in pregnancy, especially their knowledge and beliefs about its causes, duration and treatment. It will also be useful to speak to midwives who work in maternity triage or admissions department to discuss how they deal with telephone calls from women reporting symptoms.

In very severe cases, hospital admission is always required. The administration of intravenous fluids, with careful record of fluid balance is then essential to correct dehydration. *Normal saline* or *Hartmann's solution* with added potassium is commonly administered. As carbohydrate increases the demand for thiamine (Sechi and Serra 2007), fluids containing dextrose should be avoided to prevent the development of *Wernicke's encephalopathy* (Kametas and Nelson-Piercy 2008). In life-threatening cases of HG, slow-drip enteral feeding or total parenteral nutrition (TPN), supplemented by daily doses of thiamine, may be necessary (Ismail and Kenny 2007). However, such aggressive management should be a last option, as both methods carry maternal risks such as life-threatening sepsis and thrombosis (Holmgren et al 2008), requiring thromboprophylaxis (Pugsley and Moore 2012) and compliance with strict aseptic non-touch techniques (ANTT) and close observation for signs of infection.

The blood tests required at this time should assess the woman's liver, renal and thyroid function. An ultrasound scan may also be useful to eliminate *hydatidiform mole* and a multiple pregnancy as probable causes.

Moderate vomiting usually ceases quickly in most women, with those having HG experiencing relief within 2 to 3 days. Once the vomiting ceases, oral fluids and food may be gradually reintroduced, and the woman can be discharged when she is taking and tolerating a normal diet and gaining weight. In rare cases, where the vomiting is intractable, severe compromise of major organ failure may ensue; termination of the pregnancy would be considered.

Reflective activity 52.3

Locate and read your local policy for management of nausea and vomiting in pregnancy. In addition, there are a number of local policies that are available online. Take some time to peruse these documents, paying attention to when care is transferred from the community to the hospital setting.

EATING DISORDERS AND VOMITING IN PREGNANCY

Nausea and vomiting, accompanied by amenorrhoea in women of childbearing years, are not necessarily symptomatic of pregnancy but may also be features of eating disorders such as *anorexia nervosa* and *bulimia nervosa* (see Ch. 69). One study found that women with pre-existing eating disorders had a worsening of NVP (Torgersen et al 2008). An existing eating disorder accompanied by such features may not be apparent, as it may be mistaken for a normal aspect of the pregnancy. Fear for the health of the child may lead those with a known eating disorder to control or hide their symptoms, such that there is an apparent improvement in the eating disorder. There is often regression, however, to the prepregnancy state or even deterioration after giving birth (Rocco et al 2005).

Midwives need to be aware of suggestive signs of an eating disorder such as evidence of teeth decay and gum disease and over concern with body image or a prepregnancy low body mass index (BMI). Thus, the midwife must be conversant with the risks of undernutrition in pregnancy for the fetus as well as the long-term effect for the mother; an example being osteoporosis, which is consequential to endocrine changes in response to a low body weight. In pregnancy, the mother may require vitamin D supplements to improve absorption of calcium for maintaining her bone density and to prevent malformation in the skeletal system and conditions such as rickets in the newborn (see Ch. 17). For malnourished women who choose to breastfeed, this is particularly important.

Eating disorders in pregnancy also increases the risk of perinatal depression and anxiety (Micali et al 2011). A woman with an eating disorder will need individually tailored psychological intervention to address her mental health and well-being, particularly in the postnatal period (see Ch. 69 for care details on mental health in pregnancy). The healthcare professional will be required to closely monitor the pregnancy and ensure that there is adequate help for the woman and her family to attend to the condition. Thus, support should include the dietician, infant feeding specialist, the GP and community psychiatric team with the ongoing involvement of the health visitor.

Reflective activity 52.4

Look at some on the resources that are available for women with NVP and review what is available in your locality. This might include local or national groups who can provide information and support. Look critically at the information and consider which support group you would recommend.

CONCLUSION

NVP in pregnancy are common and unpleasant, but the more serious and potentially life-threatening condition of HG is fortunately rare. The cumulative and debilitating effect of these conditions may be avoided or ameliorated if the vomiting is treated promptly and effectively. The midwife should invest time in the initial assessment and identification of women who may be at risk or who present with symptoms to ensure that support with information is available to them. The midwife should be able to differentiate between physiological and pathological vomiting and manage or refer according to severity.

Key Points

- Nausea and vomiting in pregnancy are common occurrences in pregnancy, but may, on rare occasions, become pathological.
- The woman can be reassured that in mild and moderate cases, her baby is unlikely to come to any harm.
- Informed and appropriate midwifery care and advice can make the discomfort tolerable for the woman.
- The midwife must be able to distinguish between physiological and pathological vomiting and take appropriate action.
- Midwives need to be aware of suggestive signs of eating disorders in women who present with NVP.

References

Ayyavoo A, Derraik JG, Hofman PL, et al: Hyperemesis gravidarum and long-term health of the offspring, *Am J Obstet Gynaecol* 210(6):521–525, 2014.

Boltin D, Perets TT, Elheiga SA, et al: *Helicobacter pylori* infection amongst Arab Israeli women with hyperemesis gravidarum—a prospective, controlled study, *Int J Infect Dis* 29:292–295, 2014.

Boregowda G, Shehata HA: Gastrointestinal and liver disease in pregnancy, *Best Practi Res Clin Obstet Gynaecol* 27(6):835–853, 2013.

Buckwalter JG, Simpson SW: Psychological factors in the etiology and treatment of severe nausea and vomiting in pregnancy, *Am J Obstet Gynaecol* 186(5):s210–s214, 2002.

Chiossi G, Neri I, Cavazzuti M, et al: Hyperemesis gravidarum complicated by Wernicke encephalopathy: background, case report, and review of the literature, *Obstet Gynaecol Surv* 61(4):255–268, 2006.

Clark SM, Dutta E, Hankins GD: The outpatient management and special considerations of nausea and vomiting in pregnancy, *Semin Perinatol* 38(8):496–502, 2014.

Erick M: Hyperemesis gravidarum: a case of starvation and altered sensorium gestosis (ASG), *Med Hypotheses* 82(5):572–580, 2014.

Flaxman SM, Sherman PW: Morning sickness: adaptive cause or nonadaptive consequence of embryo viability?, *Am Nat* 172(1):54–62, 2008.

Fletcher SJ, Waterman H, Nelson L, et al: Holistic assessment of women with hyperemesis gravidarum: a randomised controlled trial, *International Journal of Nursing Studies* (website). http://dx.doi .org/10.1016/j.ijnurstu.2015.06.007, 2015.

Himoto Y, Kido A, Moribata Y, et al: CT and MR imaging findings of systemic complications occurring during pregnancy and puerperal period, adversely affected by natural changes, *Eur J Radiol Open* 2:101–110, 2015.

Holmgren C, Aagaard-Tillery KM, Silver RM, et al: Hyperemesis in pregnancy: an evaluation of treatment strategies with maternal and neonatal outcomes, *Am J Obstet Gynecol* 198(1):56–e1, 2008.

Isbir GG, Mete S: Experiences with nausea and vomiting during pregnancy in Turkish women based on Roy adaptation model: a content analysis, *Asian Nurs Res* 7(4):175–181, 2013.

Ismail SK, Kenny L: Review on hyperemesis gravidarum, *Best Pract Res Clin Gastroenterol* 21(5):755–769, 2007.

Kametas NA, Nelson-Piercy C: Hyperemesis gravidarum, gastrointestinal and liver disease in pregnancy, *Obstet Gynaecol Reprod Med* 18(3):69–75, 2008.

King TL, Murphy PA: Evidence-based approaches to managing nausea and vomiting in early pregnancy, *J Midwifery Women's Health* 54(6):430–444, 2009.

Koren G, Madjunkova S, Maltepe C: The protective effects of nausea and vomiting of pregnancy against adverse fetal outcome – a systematic review, *Reprod Toxicol* 47:77–80, 2014.

Lee NM, Saha S: Nausea and vomiting of pregnancy, *Gastroenterol Clin North Am* 40(2):309–334, 2011.

Lindsay J, Langmead L, Preston SL: Gastrointestinal disease. In Kumar P, Clark ML, editors: *Clinical medicine*, 8th ed, Saunders/Elsevier, 2012.

Magtira A, Paik Schoenberg F, MacGibbon K, et al: Psychiatric factors do not affect recurrence risk of hyperemesis gravidarum, *J Obstet Gynecol Res* 41(4):512–516, 2015.

Mckerracher L, Collard M, Henrich J: The expression and adaptive significance of pregnancy-related nausea, vomiting, and aversions on Yasawa Island, Fiji, *Evol Hum Behav* 36(2):95–102, 2015.

Micali N, Simonoff E, Treasure J: Pregnancy and post-partum depression and anxiety in a longitudinal general population cohort: the effect of eating disorders and past depression, *J Affect Disord* 131(1):150–157, 2011.

Nasir AA, Aboulfoutouh I, Nada A, et al: Is there an association between *Helicobacter pylori* infection and hyperemesis gravidarum among Egyptian women?, *J Evid Based Women's Health J Soc* 2(3):100–103, 2012.

National Institute for Health and Care Excellence (NICE): *Clinical knowledge summaries (CKS), nausea/vomiting in pregnancy* (website). http://cks.nice.org.uk/nauseavomiting-in-pregnancy. 2013.

Nguyen N, Deitel M, Lacy E: Splenic avulsion in a pregnant patient with vomiting, *Can J Surg* 38(5):464–465, 1995.

Nursing and Midwifery Council (NMC): *Standards for Medicines Management*, London, NMC, 2010.

Pleuvry BJ: Physiology and pharmacology of nausea and vomiting, *Anaesth Intensive Care Med* 16(9):462–466, 2015.

Power Z, Thomson AM, Waterman H: Understanding the stigma of hyperemesis gravidarum: qualitative findings from an action research study, *Birth* 37(3):237–244, 2010.

Pugsley H, Moore J: Management of early pregnancy complications, *Obstet Gynaecol Reprod Med* 22(3):76–80, 2012.

Rashid M, Rashid MH, Malik F, et al: Hyperemesis gravidarum and fetal gender: a retrospective study, *J Obstet Gynaecol* 32:475–478, 2012.

Rocco PL, Orbitello B, Perini L, et al: Effects of pregnancy on eating attitudes and disorders: a prospective study, *J Psychosom Res* 59(3):175–179, 2005.

Sandven I, Abdelnoor M, Nesheim BI, et al: *Helicobacter pylori* infection and hyperemesis gravidarum: a systematic review and meta-analysis of case–control studies, *Acta Obstet Gynecol Scand* 88(11):1190–1200, 2009.

Sechi G, Serra A: Wernicke's encephalopathy: new clinical settings and recent advances in diagnosis and management, *Lancet Neurol* 6(5):422–455, 2007.

Tiran D: Ginger to reduce nausea and vomiting during pregnancy: evidence of effectiveness is not the same as proof of safety, *Complement Ther Clin Pract* 18(1):22–25, 2012.

Torgersen L, Von Holle A, Reichborn-Kjennerud T, et al: Nausea and vomiting of pregnancy in women with bulimia nervosa and eating disorders not otherwise specified, *Int J Eat Disord* 41(8):722–727, 2008.

Uguz F, Gezginc K, Kayhan F, et al: Is hyperemesis gravidarum associated with mood, anxiety and personality disorders: a case–control study, *Gen Hosp Psychiatry* 34(4):398–402, 2012.

Welsh A: Hyperemesis, gastrointestinal and liver disorders in pregnancy, *Curr Obstet Gynaecol* 15(2):123–131, 2005.

Wu KL, Rayner CK, Chuah SK, et al: Effects of ginger on gastric emptying and motility in healthy humans, *Eur J Gastroenterol Hepatol* 20(5):436–440, 2008.

Resources and additional reading

See chapter website

Cedergren M, Brynhildsen J, Josefsson A, et al: Hyperemesis gravidarum that requires hospitalization and the use of antiemetic drugs in relation to maternal body composition, *Am J Obstet Gynecol* 198(4):412–e1, 2008.

Forbes S: Pregnancy sickness and parent-offspring conflict over thyroid function, *J Theor Biol* 355:61–67, 2014.

Golberg D, Szilagyi A, Graves L: Hyperemesis gravidarum and *Helicobacter pylori* infection. A systematic review, *Obstet Gynecol* 110(3):695–703, 2007.

Huxley R: Nausea and vomiting in early pregnancy: its role in placental development, *Obstet Gynecol* 95(5):779–782, 2000.

Indraccolo U, Gentile G, Pomili G, et al: Thiamine deficiency and beriberi features in a patient with hyperemesis gravidarum, *Nutrition* 21(9):967–968, 2005.

Kim DR, Connolly KR, Cristancho P, et al: Psychiatric consultation of patients with hyperemesis gravidarum, *Arch Womens Ment Health* 12(2):61–67, 2009.

Koren G, Boskovic R, Hard M, et al: Motherisk—PUQE (pregnancy-unique quantification of emesis and nausea) scoring system for nausea and vomiting of pregnancy, *Am J Obstet Gynecol* 186(5):S228–S231, 2002.

Lacroix R, Eason E, Melzack R: Nausea and vomiting during pregnancy: a prospective study of its frequency, intensity, and patterns of change, *Am J Obstet Gynecol* 182(4):931–937, 2000.

Wood H, McKellar LV, Lightbody M: Nausea and vomiting in pregnancy: blooming or bloomin' awful? A review of the literature, *Women Birth* 26(2):100–104, 2013.

Useful websites:

Healthtalk.org

This website provides free, reliable information about a range of health issues, by sharing people's real-life experiences. This is a unique partnership between a charity called DIPEx and The Health Experiences Research Group or 'HERG' at The University of Oxford's Nuffield Department of Primary Care.

Sickness and Hyperemesis (website). www.healthtalk.org/peoples-experiences/pregnancy-children/pregnancy/sickness-and-hyperemesis?gclid=CKv67bnOrcgCFYRl2wodp70JpA.

Motherisk.org

This is a Toronto website provided by the Hospital for Sick Children, and works as a charity. www.motherisk.org/women/morningSickness.jsp.

National Health Service (NHS) NHS Choices

The UK NHS website provides information for patients and families and includes a section on nausea and morning sickness (website). www.nhs.uk/ conditions/pregnancy-and-baby/ pages/morning-sickness-nausea.aspx#close.

Pregnancy Sickness Support (PSS)

The PSS is a registered UK charity working to improve care, treatment and support for women suffering from nausea and vomiting during pregnancy (NVP) hyperemesis gravidarum (HG) (website). www.pregnancy sicknesssupport.org.uk.

The HER (Hyperemesis Education and Research) Foundation

This is a US-based charity providing information and support for women with Hyperemesis gravidarum (website). www.helpher.org.

UpToDate® (Wolters Kluwer Health)

This website provides peer reviewed information for healthcare professionals, available through subscription. Treatment and Outcome of Nausea and Vomiting in Pregnancy (website). www.uptodate.com/ contents/treatment-and-outcome -of-nausea-and-vomiting-of -pregnancy.

Morning Sickness USA

This is a US commercial company that provides products to treat morning sickness but does have some useful information (website) www. morningsicknessusa.com. *There is also a Canadian website by the same company,* http://sosmorningsickness. org.

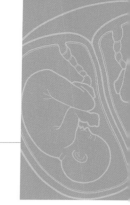

Chapter 53

Bleeding in pregnancy

Amanda Hutcherson

Learning Outcomes ?

After reading this chapter, you will be able to:

- identify the causes of vaginal bleeding in pregnancy
- discuss the midwife's role in bleeding in pregnancy both before and after the 24th week
- describe the possible implications for the health and well-being of the mother and the fetus
- discuss therapeutic termination of a pregnancy

INTRODUCTION

Vaginal bleeding during pregnancy is considered to be abnormal and should always be investigated. It may be extremely frightening for the woman and her family, so it must be managed with sensitivity, ensuring that the woman is fully informed and involved in her plan of care. It is worth noting the decision of the Supreme Court (2015) in the case of Montgomery v Lanarkshire Health Board with regard to the importance of a woman being able to make a fully informed choice about her care. An important part of the management lies within the diagnosis of the cause and in the accurate assessment and reporting of the woman's previous and present history. It is also important to recognize that medical definitions and terms, such as 'abortion', will need to be explained. This term may have a different meaning for women and families.

Bleeding from the genital tract can be divided into two categories, depending on whether it occurs before or after the 24th week of pregnancy. In UK law, fetal viability is set at 24 completed weeks of pregnancy (Parliament UK 2007), although multiple international differences can be seen (Mohangoo et al 2013), the government of the United States referring to it as a 'gray zone' of 'about 24 weeks' (USA.gov 2008). This can lead to challenging discussions when international statistics are required (Mohangoo et al 2013) or when providing care for women of non-UK nationality.

BLEEDING BEFORE THE 24TH WEEK OF PREGNANCY

Bleeding from the genital tract in early pregnancy – that is, before the 24th week – may be caused by:

- implantation bleeding
- abortion
- gestational trophoblastic disease
- ectopic pregnancy
- cervical lesions
- vaginitis
- accidental trauma
- domestic violence and abuse

IMPLANTATION BLEEDING

There may be a little bleeding when the trophoblast embeds into the endometrial lining of the uterus. The bleeding is usually bright red and of short duration. As implantation takes place 8 to 12 days after fertilization, the bleeding usually occurs just before the menstrual period is due. If mistakenly thought to be a menstrual period, this may confuse the expected date of delivery. A careful menstrual history is essential to detect probable implantation bleeding, thereby avoiding miscalculation of dates.

ABORTION

A pregnancy that ends before 24 completed weeks of gestation, and where the fetus is not alive, is termed an abortion. The classification is shown in Fig. 53.1.

Threatened abortion

Midwives should be aware that the term 'abortion' may cause confusion. Many women who have lost a wanted pregnancy find the word offensive and it should not, therefore, be used when talking to women about a pregnancy ending from natural causes. In these circumstances, the use of the word 'miscarriage' is more appropriate. A woman who has vaginal bleeding and a confirmed fetal heartbeat will be considered to have a threatened abortion (National Institute for Health and Care Excellence (NICE) 2012).

The woman should be advised that:

- if the bleeding gets worse or continues for more than 14 days, she should seek medical advice
- if the bleeding stops, she should commence or continue a recommended antenatal care schedule

Spontaneous abortion

Approximately 15% to 20% of confirmed pregnancies end in spontaneous abortion, most of these occurring before the 12th week of pregnancy.

Causes

- *Maldevelopment of the conceptus:* It has been reported that the most common cause of spontaneous abortion is a defective conceptus. Chromosomal abnormalities account for approximately 70% of defective conceptions, although spontaneous mutations may arise (Royal College of Obstetricians and Gynaecologists (RCOG) 2008; Kovacs and Briggs 2015)
- *Defective implantation* (NICE 2012; Collins et al 2013)
- *Gestational trophoblastic disease* (NICE 2012; Collins et al 2013)
- *Maternal infection:* any acute illness, particularly with a pyrexia, may cause abortion. This may be the result of the general metabolic effect of a high fever or the result of transplacental passage of viruses. Infections known to be associated include influenza, rubella, pneumonia, toxoplasmosis, cytomegalovirus, listeriosis, syphilis and brucellosis. Appendicitis in pregnancy may also be a cause (Gilo et al 2009)
- *Genital tract infection:* examples include bacterial vaginosis and vaginal mycoplasma infection (Silver and Branch 2007; McNamee et al 2014; Jakovljevic et al 2014)
- *Medical disorders:* including diabetes, thyroid disease, renal disease and hypertensive disorders (Powrie et al 2010)
- *Endocrine abnormalities:* including poor development of the corpus luteum, inadequate secretory endometrium and low serum progesterone levels (Powrie et al 2010)

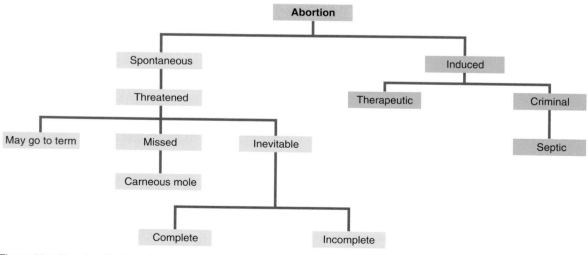

Figure 53.1 The classification of abortion.

- *Uterine abnormalities:* the majority of the female genital tract arises from the two Müllerian ducts, which form during embryonic life. Failure of development may cause structural abnormalities, such as a double uterus, unicornuate, bicornuate, septate or subseptate uterus (Kenny 2011)

- *Fibroids* (Kenny 2011)

- *Retroversion of the uterus:* this does not itself cause abortion. As the uterus enlarges, it will usually rise into the abdomen. If it fails to do so, vaginal and abdominal manipulation to correct the retroversion may cause an abortion. This situation also carries a risk of bladder damage because of urine retention. Bladder catheterization may be required until the position of the uterus changes (Kenny 2011)

- *Cervical weakness:* laceration of the cervix or undue stretching of the internal cervical os, produced by a previous abortion or childbirth, may allow the membranes to bulge through the cervical canal and rupture. This condition is often a cause of repeated pregnancy loss. Cervical cerclage (a nylon tape or suture inserted and tied around the cervix) at about the 14th week may prevent this. The tape must be removed before the onset of labour (RCOG 2011)

- *Environmental factors:* external influences may be a cause. These include environmental teratogens, such as lead and radiation, and ingested teratogenic substances, such as drugs (especially cocaine) and alcohol (Carr and Coustan 2007; Silver and Branch 2007)

- *Smoking:* exposure to tobacco smoke has been linked with spontaneous abortion, but research findings remain inconclusive (Carr and Coustan 2007)

- *Maternal age:* women in their late thirties and older have higher rates of pregnancy loss, irrespective of obstetric history (Silver and Branch 2007)

- *Stress and anxiety:* severe emotional upset may cause abortion by disrupting hypothalamic and pituitary functions; however, other factors may be implicated, as women experiencing adverse life events often have higher rates of smoking and alcohol use

- *Paternal causes:* poor sperm quality may be a factor. The father may also be the source of chromosomal abnormalities, particularly in cases of recurrent abortion (Pan et al 2010)

- *Immunological:* maternal lymphocytes with natural killer cell activity may affect trophoblast development, disrupting implantation and embryonic growth. Autoimmune diseases, such as antiphospholipid syndrome, may also cause abortion (Powrie et al 2010). Despite detailed investigations, no cause can be found in the majority of cases

Inevitable abortion

The key feature of inevitable abortion is cervical dilatation with an outcome of unavoidable pregnancy loss. The gestational sac separates from the uterine wall, and the uterus contracts to expel the conceptus. This uterine activity causes discomfort similar to that of labour contractions. Speculum examination reveals a dilating cervix, possibly with products of conception protruding through. The gestational sac may be expelled complete (*complete abortion*), or in part, usually with placental tissue retained (*incomplete abortion*).

The midwife who is called in by a woman with signs of inevitable abortion should arrange immediate care. The woman's vital signs should be recorded and an estimate of blood loss made. If the fetus has been expelled and the woman is bleeding, local policies for the management of the third stage of labour and control of postpartum bleeding should be followed. The Practical, Obstetric Multi-Professional Training (PROMPT) course manual provides contemporary information to support guideline development (Winter et al 2012). Any products of conception passed should be saved for inspection. The midwife must refer the woman for medical care either by her general practitioner (GP) or by a gynaecologist at her local hospital. If the bleeding is severe or the woman is showing signs of shock, a paramedic team from the local ambulance service should be requested. They will resuscitate the woman and stabilize her condition before transfer to a hospital. In a hospital setting, evacuation of retained products of conception (ERPC) from the uterus may be carried out and a blood transfusion may be given if blood loss has been severe.

Expectant or medical management of inevitable or incomplete abortion are both possible (NICE 2012).

Expectant management may be considered for 7 to 14 days from diagnosis of the condition, in agreement with a woman who has no history of an adverse psychological experience related to pregnancy and a low risk of haemorrhage or its effects. For example, she does not have anaemia, coagulopathies or the inability to have a blood transfusion (NICE 2012).

Medical or surgical management options should be considered in women who do not meet these criteria.

If the breasts begin to secrete, the woman could be advised to wear a well-fitting brassiere to minimize discomfort. *Cabergoline* 1 mg may be prescribed by a medical practitioner or qualified midwife prescriber to suppress lactation (NICE 2012; British National Formulary (BNF) 2015). If the woman has a Rhesus-negative blood group, anti-D immunoglobulin must be offered with full explanation and administered within 72 hours of abortion to prevent isoimmunisation and potential rhesus problems in subsequent pregnancies (Qureshi et al 2014). Women who are nonimmune to rubella can be offered rubella vaccination at this time, with the advice that pregnancy should be avoided for the next 3 months.

Missed abortion

In this condition, bleeding occurs between the gestational sac and the uterine wall, and the embryo dies. The uterus ceases to increase in size and, as the presence of the retained fetus appears to inhibit menstruation, the woman may think that her pregnancy is continuing, although other signs of pregnancy have disappeared. The bleeding from the vagina varies from nothing to a trickle of brownish discharge. As the signs of pregnancy gradually disappear, some women become aware that all is not well.

The diagnosis is confirmed by ultrasound. The uterus would eventually expel the fetus spontaneously, but this may not occur for some time. Treatment is usually to evacuate the uterus, either surgically or with *misoprostol* (Neilson et al 2013). Expectant management may be offered, with the woman given the option of returning home for a few days to await spontaneous expulsion of the fetus (Nanda et al 2012). In this case, clear instructions must be given to enable the woman and her family to observe for the potential problems of haemorrhage or septic shock. If a well-formed fetus is retained in the uterus, it can become flattened and mummified as a *fetus papyraceous* (see Fig. 53.2), rather than being reabsorbed. This is more commonly associated with a multiple pregnancy.

Recurrent abortion

This is a term used when 3 or more consecutive spontaneous abortions have occurred. Careful investigation should be undertaken to find the cause. Occasionally, the causative factors are different for each, with no clear single factor associated. However, some conditions may be implicated in recurrent pregnancy loss (Powrie et al 2010).

- *Structural abnormalities of the uterus:* these appear in up to 50% of women with recurrent abortion (for example, bicornuate uterus)

- *Weak cervix*
- *Maternal systemic disease:* diabetes and antiphospholipid antibodies
- *Genetic causes:* the incidence of chromosome disorders is considered to be around 30% in first trimester abortions (Perez-Duran et al 2015). The majority are balanced translocations. In cases of consanguineous or cousin marriage, a lethal recessive gene may cause recurrent losses
- *Uterine infection:* especially toxoplasmosis, *Mycoplasma hominis*, *Ureaplasma urealyticum* and chlamydia
- *Hormonal deficiency:* luteal phase deficits may be associated, although this theory is not universally accepted
- *Immunological factors*
- *Non-accidental injury* should also be considered

Psychological effects

Many women experience a marked grief reaction after an abortion and may require considerable counselling and support. Psychological distress may be severe and some women become clinically depressed. The grief experienced by the partner may be as intense as that of the woman, although he or she is less likely to receive support (Glasby and Tew 2015). Staff members need to treat the parents with sensitivity. The couple may wish to see their baby and staff should take account of their wishes. The guidelines written by the Miscarriage Association can provide support for this (Miscarriage Association 2015).

After the end of the 24th week of pregnancy, if born with no signs of life, the infant must be registered as a stillbirth (Home Office 2008). Many maternity hospitals offer a funeral or memorial service for previable fetuses and all must offer respectful disposal. In this situation, the hospital chaplain may be a valuable source of support and advice. Antenatal Results and Choices (ARC) can provide

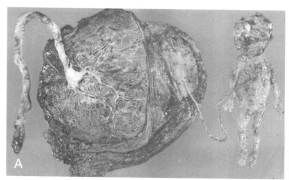
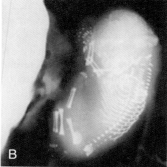

Figure 53.2 **A,** Fetus papyraceous. (Beischer N, Mackay E, Colditz P: Obstetrics and the newborn, London, WB Saunders, 1997.) **B,** Radiograph of a 13 week fetus papyraceous. (Sutkin G, Manmlock V: Fetus papyraceus. Images in clinical medicine, N Engl J Med 2004;350:1665.)

nondirective support and counselling for parents who have received high-risk antenatal screening results or diagnosis of a fetal abnormality (ARC 2015).

Reflective activity 53.1

Talk to the manager of your early pregnancy unit. What are the referral criteria?

If there is no local early pregnancy unit, identify what services are available locally, nationally and online for women with early pregnancy problems and early fetal loss.

Induced abortion

This term refers to the deliberate termination of a pregnancy. Induced abortions are classified as *therapeutic* or *criminal*.

Therapeutic abortion

Therapeutic abortion has been legal in the UK since 1967, when the Abortion Act became law (HMSO 1967) (see Ch. 9). This law does not apply to Northern Ireland. This Act allows termination of a pregnancy if two registered medical practitioners are of the opinion that continuance of the pregnancy:

1. involves risk to the life of the pregnant woman
2. involves risk of injury to her physical or mental health
3. would involve risk to the life of the pregnant woman, greater than if the pregnancy were terminated
4. that there is a substantial risk that if the child were born it would suffer from such physical or mental abnormalities as to be seriously handicapped

In current legislation, the upper gestation limit for legal termination is defined as the end of the 24th week (Dimond 2013; Human Fertilisation and Embryology Act 1990). The only circumstances in which therapeutic abortion may be carried out **after** the 24th week are:

1. if there is a risk to the woman's life
2. if there is a risk of grave permanent damage to the woman's physical or mental health

or

3. if there is a substantial risk that the child would suffer severe disability

The law also allows for selective fetal reduction in a multifetal pregnancy. Abortions after 24 weeks may only be carried out in NHS hospitals. Therapeutic abortion may be offered either as a medical or surgical procedure. Medical abortion is available to women who meet the terms of the Abortion Act by the administration of abortifacient medication. *Mifepristone* taken orally or *methotrexate* given by intramuscular or intra-uterine

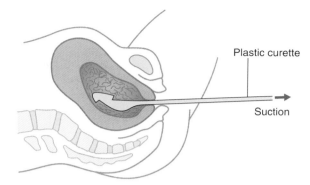

Figure 53.3 Dilatation and vacuum aspiration.

injection (BNF 2015) are in current use (2015) and must be prescribed by a doctor.

Surgical abortion is an option for women before 12 completed weeks of pregnancy (NHS Choices 2014). Carried out under sedation or general anaesthetic, it involves progressive instrumental dilatation of the cervix and gentle suction removal of the products of conception (see Fig. 53.3).

As with spontaneous abortion, anti-D immunoglobulin and rubella vaccine must be offered, as appropriate, after therapeutic abortion.

Criminal abortion

This is the termination of a pregnancy outside the terms of the Abortion Act, possibly by unauthorized and untrained persons, and is an offence punishable by law. The incidence has fallen sharply since the introduction of the UK 1967 Abortion Act. However, cases still occur: four such offences were detected in the years 2000 and 2001 (Home Department 2001) and seven in 2004 and 2005 (Home Office 2009). The crime of illegal abortion was not recorded in 2014 and 2015; however, there were seven prosecutions for the intentional destruction of a viable unborn child during this period (gov.uk 2015). The abortion may be induced either by the woman herself or by some other person, by use of drugs or instruments. Whether successful or not, the action is illegal. The methods used may cause sudden death from haemorrhage, air embolus or *vagal inhibition*. Because of lack of asepsis, infection readily occurs and may lead to chronic ill-health or salpingitis and sterility.

Septic abortion

Uterine infection may occur after spontaneous or induced abortion. It is more likely to occur after criminal abortion or spontaneous abortion where there are retained products of conception. The incidence of septic abortion has declined in countries that allow legal termination of pregnancy, but it is still a cause of maternal death by haemorrhage or sepsis (Lewis 2011). The key actions for diagnosis and management of sepsis are timely recognition, fast administration of intravenous antibiotics and quick involvement of experts – senior review is essential (Knight et al 2014). On a global level, seven million women a year in the developing world are treated in healthcare facilities for complications after an unsafe abortion (RCOG 2015).

Reflective activity 53.2

Find out what services midwives offer locally to women who have had a spontaneous abortion or second trimester termination of pregnancy.

GESTATIONAL TROPHOBLASTIC DISEASE (HYDATIDIFORM OR CARNEOUS MOLE AND CHORIOCARCINOMA)

Hydatidiform or carneous mole

This condition occurs as a result of degeneration of the chorionic villi at an early stage of pregnancy (see Fig. 53.4). Usually, the embryo is absent; occasionally, a hydatidiform mole may be found in a twin pregnancy alongside a viable fetus (NICE 2012). Molar pregnancy may be complete, with an intra-uterine multivesicular mass composed of hydropic chorionic villi, or partial – where vesicular tissue is present but less well developed,

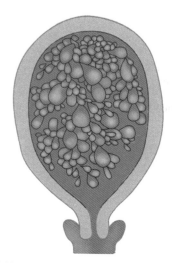

Figure 53.4 Hydatidiform mole.

along with a fetus. Vesicle formation may occur within the placenta of an apparently normal pregnancy.

Signs and symptoms

Often, the minor disorders of pregnancy, such as nausea and breast tenderness, are more severe. The woman may report intermittent bleeding per vaginam from around the 12th week of pregnancy. When the hydatidiform mole begins to abort, there may be profuse haemorrhage and grape-like cysts may be seen. Pre-eclampsia may develop even in the early weeks of pregnancy. Severe nausea and vomiting may occur. On abdominal examination, the uterus is usually large for the period of gestation and may feel soft and doughy to the examining fingers. No fetal parts are palpable and the fetal heart is absent. There may be signs of mild thyrotoxicosis because of the thyroid-stimulating hormone (TSH)-like activity of human chorionic gonadotrophin (hCG), which is secreted in large amounts by the molar vesicles. The diagnosis is suggested by the clinical findings and is confirmed by an ultrasound scan. Urinary or serum hCG levels will be high.

Treatment

Once the diagnosis of molar pregnancy is confirmed, the uterus must be completely evacuated without delay. This is achieved by careful suction curettage (see Fig. 53.3). Uterine contractions may cause molar tissue to enter the circulation via the sinuses of the placental bed. These emboli may set up metastatic disease in other sites, commonly the lungs. Medical termination should be avoided. In the absence of obstetric haemorrhage, oxytocic drugs are withheld until the uterus has been surgically emptied, a syntocinon infusion may then be used to maintain uterine contraction and haemostasis. The woman must be referred to a specialist follow-up centre (Cancer UK 2014) to facilitate early detection of malignant trophoblastic disease (choriocarcinoma). Serum beta-hCG levels will be monitored fortnightly until the values fall to within the normal range (Seckl et al 2000). It should be noted that professional opinion varies slightly on follow-up requirements, and each case is assessed on an individual basis. Avoidance of another pregnancy for an extended period of time will be strongly advised, necessitating support and careful contraceptive advice. It is important to note that the oral contraceptive pill may increase the risk of the development of invasive disease if taken while hCG levels remain elevated (Seckl et al 2013).

Choriocarcinoma

Choriocarcinoma is a malignant disease of trophoblastic tissue. It occurs after approximately 3% of complete moles (Seckl et al 2000). Levels of hCG will rise and the pregnancy test will become strongly positive again. Choriocarcinoma may occur in the next normal pregnancy an evacuation of a molar pregnancy. As the growth infiltrates the uterus and vagina, the affected woman will experience increasingly severe pain. The condition will be rapidly fatal unless treated. The disease spreads by local invasion and via the bloodstream; metastases may occur in the lungs, liver and brain.

Choriocarcinoma responds well to chemotherapy. Cytotoxic drugs, such as *methotrexate, etoposide* and *actinomycin-D*, are used singly or as combination therapy, and are nearly always completely successful. The woman should avoid another pregnancy for at least 1 year after the completion of treatment and will require hCG monitoring after any future pregnancy, as there is a risk of disease recurrence (Seckl et al 2013).

ECTOPIC OR EXTRAUTERINE GESTATION

Ectopic pregnancy occurs when the fertilized ovum implants outside the uterine cavity. In 95% of cases, the site of implantation is the uterine tube and these are known as tubal pregnancies. Occasionally, the site may be the ovary, the abdominal cavity or the cervical canal, but these are rare. The incidence of ectopic pregnancy is 1 in 150 pregnancies (NICE 2012). Ectopic pregnancy is the major cause of maternal death before 20 weeks gestation in the industrialized world, appearing to be related to pelvic infection and, in particular, chlamydia (NICE 2012).

Tubal pregnancy

Tubal pregnancy occurs when there is a delay in the transport of the zygote along the fallopian tube. This may be because of a congenital malformation of the uterine tubes or, more commonly, to tubal scarring after a pelvic infection. The ovum implants and begins to develop in the lining of the tube. The ampulla is the most common site (see Fig. 53.5).

Although tubal pregnancy may occur in the absence of any significant history, there are certain risk factors (NICE 2012):

- History of previous tubal pregnancy
- Tubal surgery
- Hormonal ovulation induction drugs used in reduced fertility and in vitro fertilization (IVF) may interfere with tubal motility
- Progesterone-releasing intra-uterine contraceptive devices (this is related to higher-dose devices)
- Tubal endometriosis
- Pelvic inflammatory disease
- Appendectomy, pelvic or abdominal surgery, which may cause adhesion formation

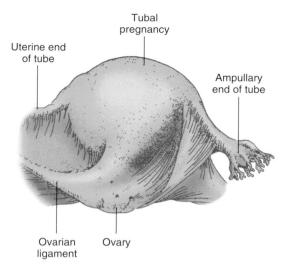

Figure 53.5 Tubal pregnancy.

- Postcoital contraception using diethylstilbestrol
- Contraceptive methods – the intra-uterine contraceptive device and the progesterone-only pill may increase the relative risk because they protect against intra-uterine pregnancy but do not prevent ovulation and fertilization

Diagnosis

NICE (2012) recommends that during clinical assessment of a woman of reproductive age, all healthcare practitioners should be aware that she may be pregnant and think about offering a pregnancy test even when symptoms are nonspecific. The signs and symptoms of ectopic pregnancy can resemble the common symptoms and signs of other conditions – for example, gastrointestinal conditions (such as appendicitis) or urinary tract infection.

Delay in diagnosis and treatment may contribute to maternal mortality and morbidity. The most accurate method currently available is a combination of serum hCG level measurement and transvaginal ultrasound scanning. Levels of hCG rise steadily in early pregnancy. Levels lower than normal or falling below the doubling time (the time in which serum levels can be expected to double) is indicative of ectopic gestation. The ultrasound scan may reveal a tubal mass or a fluid collection in the pelvis but is most useful for confirming the absence of an intra-uterine sac. As the conceptus develops and grows, the tube distends to accommodate it.

Initially, the woman will experience the usual signs of pregnancy, such as nausea and breast changes, although amenorrhoea is not always present. The uterus will soften and enlarge under the influence of the pregnancy hormones. As the tube becomes further distended, abdominal pain and some vaginal bleeding will be experienced.

If the site of implantation is the narrower proximal end of the tube, tubal rupture is likely to occur between the 5th and 7th weeks of pregnancy (see Fig. 53.6). If the pregnancy is located in the wider ampullary section, the gestation may continue until the 10th week. Occasionally, the gestational sac is expelled from the fimbriated end (see Fig. 53.7).

As the ovum separates from its attachment to the ampullary part of the tube, layers of blood clot may be deposited around the dead ovum to form a mass of blood, which may remain in the uterine tube or be expelled from the fimbriated end of the tube. When the tube ruptures, there will be severe intraperitoneal haemorrhage, and the woman will experience intense abdominal pain. There may also be referred shoulder-tip pain on lying down as blood tracks up towards the diaphragm. The woman will appear pale, shocked and nauseated and may collapse. The abdomen is tender and may be distended. Pelvic examination is usually exquisitely tender, especially on movement of the cervix. Ruptured ectopic pregnancy is an acute surgical emergency, requiring immediate treatment.

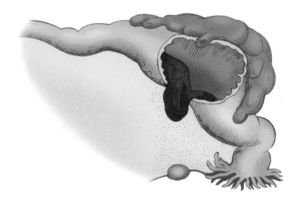

Figure 53.6 Rupture of the uterine tube.

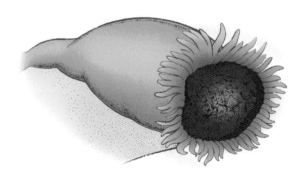

Figure 53.7 Tubal abortion.

Management

If ectopic pregnancy is suspected, a large-bore intravenous cannula (size 16 gauge) should be inserted and blood taken for cross-matching. The woman must be transferred to theatre as soon as possible. *Laparoscopic salpingotomy* may be performed unless the woman is suffering from haemorrhagic shock, when laparotomy is preferable.

If the condition is detected in the early stages, nonsurgical management may be attempted with injections of prostaglandin F_{2a} or systemic prostaglandin E_2. Medical management in the form of *methotrexate* may be offered, either intramuscularly or directly into the gestational sac. NICE recommends that systemic methotrexate can be offered as a first-line treatment to women who are able to return for follow-up and who have all of the following factors: no significant pain; an unruptured ectopic pregnancy with an adnexal mass smaller than 35 mm and no visible heartbeat; a serum hCG level less than 1500 IU/litre and no intra-uterine pregnancy (as confirmed on an ultrasound scan) (NICE 2012).

NICE (2012) recommends that surgery is offered where the use of a medical method of induced abortion is unacceptable to the woman.

Heterotopic or combined pregnancy

Heterotopic pregnancy occurs when a blastocyst from a multiple gestation implants outside the uterine cavity. It is associated with dizygotic twinning, with the extrauterine pregnancy being almost always tubal. It may follow IVF and embryo transfer. Diagnosis can be difficult and management options are limited by the presence of the intra-uterine pregnancy. The ectopic sac must be removed, but the uterus should be disturbed as little as possible and methotrexate must be avoided if the intra-uterine pregnancy is to survive (NICE 2012).

Secondary abdominal pregnancy

Very rarely, when rupture of a tubal pregnancy occurs, there may be partial extrusion of the ovum into the peritoneal cavity but with enough chorionic villi remaining attached to the tube to ensure that the embryo does not die. Chorionic villi on the surface of the ovum then become attached to the neighbouring abdominal organs, and the pregnancy continues with the fetus developing free within the abdominal cavity. The fetus is at risk of severe growth restriction because of the relatively poor placentation and may also suffer pressure deformities, as there is no protective uterine wall.

This condition is usually detected by ultrasound scanning but may be suggested by a persistently abnormal fetal lie and the fact that fetal parts are unusually easy to palpate. Delivery is by laparotomy. The placenta is usually left in situ to be absorbed, as an attempt to detach it may cause uncontrollable haemorrhage.

The rate of ectopic pregnancy in the UK is 11 per 1000 pregnancies, with a maternal mortality of 0.2 per 1000 estimated ectopic pregnancies, with about two thirds of these deaths are associated with substandard care (NICE 2012). Women who do not access medical help readily, such as women who are recent migrants, asylum seekers, refugees or women who have difficulty reading or speaking English, are at increased risk. Midwives must maintain vigilance with regard to the associated risk factors for ectopic pregnancy and seek an obstetric opinion for any woman with signs or symptoms suggestive of extrauterine gestation as an emergency procedure.

BLEEDING FROM ASSOCIATED CONDITIONS

The following conditions may cause bleeding, although, strictly speaking, they are not bleeding of early pregnancy since the bleeding is not from the site of the pregnancy.

Cervical polyp

This is a small, red, gelatinous growth attached by a pedicle to the cervix, close to the external os. It may give rise to slight irregular bleeding.

Ectropion of the cervix

A cervical erosion is formed when the columnar epithelium lining the cervical canal proliferates owing to the action of the pregnancy hormones. The ectropion forms a reddish area on the cervix, extending outwards from the external os. It may give rise to a blood-stained discharge from the vagina. No treatment is necessary and the ectropion will recede during the puerperium.

Carcinoma of the cervix

Invasive cervical carcinoma is rarely seen in pregnancy, although cervical intraepithelial neoplasia (CIN) may occasionally be discovered if a cervical smear test is taken. If the cervical cytology report suggests precancerous changes, colposcopy is performed to identify the affected areas and a small cervical biopsy may be carried out. Treatment is deferred until after delivery if the condition is not invasive.

Invasive cervical cancer is very serious, as the disease may progress quickly. On vaginal examination, the cervix is hard and irregular and bleeds when touched. There may also be a purulent vaginal discharge. If the condition is discovered in the first trimester, the pregnancy may be terminated and treatment initiated. In the third trimester, the fetus is viable and may be delivered by caesarean section. Once the infant is born, the obstetrician may carry out a radical hysterectomy (*Wertheim's hysterectomy*). Vaginal delivery is associated with a poorer prognosis for the mother, as cervical dilatation may cause dissemination of tumour cells and metastases have been reported in episiotomy sites (Cancer Research UK 2014).

A dilemma arises if the condition is discovered in the second trimester because the fetus is unlikely to survive if delivered. The woman may choose to postpone treatment for a time to allow further fetal growth; however, the delay should be no longer than 4 weeks.

Bleeding in early pregnancy may occur for a variety of reasons. It is a serious sign, and the underlying condition may be life-threatening. Any woman who reports vaginal bleeding during pregnancy must be referred to an obstetrician without delay.

BLEEDING AFTER THE 24TH WEEK – ANTEPARTUM HAEMORRHAGE

Antepartum haemorrhage is defined as bleeding from the genital tract after the 24th week of pregnancy and before the birth of the baby. Bleeding that occurs during labour is referred to as *intrapartum haemorrhage*.

Antepartum haemorrhage is a serious complication, which may result in the death of the mother or the baby.

There are two main causes of haemorrhage:

- *Placenta praevia* (unavoidable or inevitable haemorrhage) is bleeding from separation of an abnormally situated placenta. (The placenta lies partly or wholly in the lower uterine segment and bleeding is inevitable when labour begins.)
- *Abruptio placentae* (placental abruption) is bleeding from separation of a normally situated placenta.

However, extraplacental bleeding may sometimes occur. This is vaginal bleeding from some other part of the birth canal, for example, a cervical polyp, as described earlier.

PLACENTA PRAEVIA

The incidence of placenta praevia at term ranges from 0.5% to 1%. It is usually detected on ultrasound scanning in early pregnancy and may be seen in as many as one-quarter of all pregnancies in the second trimester. As the lower segment grows and stretches, the placental site appears to rise up the uterine wall, away from the internal os uteri, until at term in the majority of cases, the placenta no longer occupies the lower segment. Those cases where the placenta overlies the internal os in early pregnancy are at highest risk of haemorrhage. The classification of placenta praevia is shown in Table 53.1. The types are illustrated in Fig. 53.8.

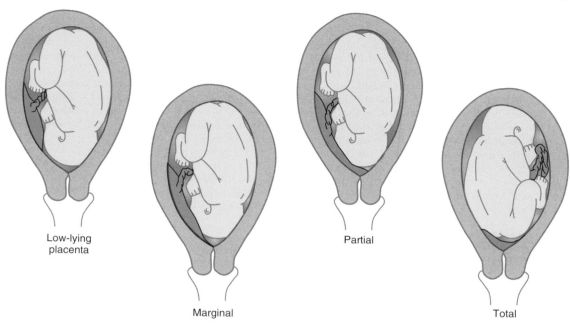

Low-lying
placenta

Partial

Marginal

Total

Figure 53.8 Placenta praevia.

Table 53.1 Classification of placenta praevia	
Low-lying placenta	Placenta mainly in the upper uterine segment but encroaching on the lower segment
Marginal	Placenta reaches to, but does not cover, the internal os
Partial	Placenta covers the internal os when closed but not completely when it is dilated
Total	Placenta completely covers the internal os

Causes

The cause of placenta praevia is unknown but the following factors are known to be associated (Kovacs and Briggs 2015):

- *Multiparity:* the increased size of the uterine cavity after repeated childbearing may predispose to placenta praevia
- *Multiple pregnancy:* the larger placental site is more likely to encroach on the lower segment of the uterus
- *Age:* risk rises with maternal age
- *Scarred uterus:* one previous caesarean section doubles the risk of placenta praevia

- *Previous myomectomy or hysterotomy*
- *Smoking:* the exact mechanism is unclear, but the relative hypoxia induced by smoking may cause enlargement of the placenta to compensate for the reduced oxygen supply
- *Placental abnormality: bipartite* and *succenturiate placentae* may cause placenta praevia. Placenta membranacea (placenta diffusa) may also be a cause (see Ch. 39). This is a rare developmental abnormality of the placenta where all the chorion is covered with functioning villi. The placenta develops as a thin membranous structure, covering an unusually large surface of the uterus. The condition may be diagnosed on ultrasound. The placenta may not separate readily in the third stage of labour, and may cause severe haemorrhage, possibly requiring hysterectomy. Fetal nutrition appears to be relatively undisturbed in cases of placenta membranacea.

Associated conditions

A low-lying placenta puts the woman and her fetus at risk of other complications. The most serious of these is *placenta accreta*. This usually occurs where the previous delivery was by caesarean section (Collins et al 2013). The combination of the relatively thin decidua in the lower segment and the presence of scar tissue increase the likelihood of trophoblastic invasion of the myometrium.

Signs and symptoms

As placenta praevia can be diagnosed on ultrasound scanning in early pregnancy, midwives will usually be aware of any woman in their care who has a low-lying placenta. However, there are women who will not have had an ultrasound scan during pregnancy, including women who choose not to do so, women who have concealed their pregnancy, women who have not accessed care or women who may have spent their antenatal period in a country where ultrasound scans are not readily available. Therefore, the midwife must be aware of the signs that indicate a possible placenta praevia:

- *Malpresentation of the fetus:* although the presentation may be cephalic, often it is not. The placenta occupies space in the pelvis and the midwife may find that the breech presents, as there is more room for the head in the fundus, or that the lie is oblique and the fetal shoulder presents.
- *Non-engagement of the presenting part:* this is especially likely with a partial or total placenta praevia.
- *Difficulty in identifying fetal parts on palpation:* an anterior placenta praevia lies between the fetus and the midwife's hand like a cushion. This makes the fetal parts relatively difficult to identify.
- *Loud maternal pulse below the umbilicus:* an anterior placenta praevia may often be detected by the presence of loud maternal arterial sounds from the placental bed. This is more easily heard with an electronic fetal heart Doppler. The fetal heart sounds may be difficult to detect, as they are muffled by the placenta, especially in a cephalic presentation.
- An *anterior placenta praevia* will cushion some of the fetal movements, and the woman may mention that she only feels fetal movement above the umbilicus.
- *Bleeding after sexual intercourse:* stimulation of the cervix during intercourse may provoke bleeding.

When this type of bleeding occurs, it usually begins after the 24th week of pregnancy, although it may occasionally occur earlier. In the third trimester of pregnancy, the lower segment is completing its development, Braxton Hicks contractions are increasing and towards the end of pregnancy, the cervix is becoming effaced. Bleeding is caused by detachment of the placenta, which cannot stretch to adapt to these changes in uterine structure. As the placenta is in the lower pole of the uterus, the blood escapes easily, thus giving rise to the classical unprovoked, fresh, painless bleeding of placenta praevia. Warning haemorrhages are associated with placenta praevia. These are small, recurrent, fresh and painless haemorrhages occurring during the third trimester. Each episode of bleeding indicates further placental detachment. If the placenta is torn, some fetal bleeding will occur, and this will further compromise the condition of the fetus. Massive obstetric haemorrhage may occur at any time but is more likely once labour begins as the cervix begins to dilate. It is impossible to predict the course of events in a case of placenta praevia and, even in the absence of bleeding, the condition is regarded as a major and life-threatening complication of pregnancy.

Management

If no serious haemorrhage has made it imperative to act, the woman will be offered the option of an elective birth at about 38 weeks gestation, aiming to avoid problems of prematurity for the infant. If the placental location is unclear, an examination may be carried out in theatre, by a senior obstetrician, with the woman suitably anaesthetized and the theatre prepared in readiness for a caesarean section. An intravenous infusion is commenced and four units of cross-matched blood must be made immediately available. With the woman in the lithotomy position, the obstetrician makes a very gentle and cautious vaginal examination, passing a finger through the cervix into the lower pole of the uterus. If the placenta is palpable, the obstetrician will immediately perform a caesarean section. If the placenta is not palpable in the lower segment, the membranes may be ruptured with the woman's consent, to encourage the start of labour. This procedure avoids unnecessary caesarean section for women in whom placenta praevia is not confirmed.

Vaginal delivery is usually possible in cases of a low-lying placenta if the fetal head is engaged. However, the presence of placental tissue within 2 cm of the internal os is a contraindication to vaginal birth (Collins et al 2013).

Active treatment

In cases where bleeding first occurs at 38 weeks or later, conservative treatment is not appropriate, as the fetus is mature. Active treatment is also necessary in cases where labour has started, if bleeding is severe or there are signs of fetal distress. An intravenous infusion is commenced, and the woman's condition is stabilized. A senior obstetrician performs an emergency caesarean section under general anaesthesia. A neonatologist should be present to attend to the baby who may be asphyxiated at birth.

Third stage

Postpartum haemorrhage may complicate the third stage of labour since there are few oblique muscle fibres to control bleeding from the placental site in the lower uterine segment.

Placenta accreta may occur in women who have had a previous caesarean section and torrential haemorrhage may result from attempts to separate the placenta. Surgical treatments, such as ligation of the internal iliac arteries and interventional radiology, may be required to control

---

Box 53.1 Key points from guidelines for the management of massive obstetric haemorrhage (Department of Health 1994; Lewis 2007; Winter et al 2012)

- Dealing with ill, bleeding women requires skilled teamwork between obstetric and anaesthetic teams, with appropriate help from other specialists, including haematologists, vascular surgeons and radiologists.
- Immediate involvement of all key staff, including senior obstetrician, anaesthetist, haematologist, blood transfusion service and portering staff.
- Minimum 20 mL sample of blood for cross-matching and coagulation studies.
- Minimum 6 units of cross-matched blood, with use of plasma expanders as necessary (not dextrans).
- Blood of the patient's own group to be used for transfusion; uncross-matched, O-negative blood to be used only if immediate transfusion is required.
- Minimum of 2 peripheral intravenous lines, using 16-gauge cannulae.
- Immediate commencement of CVP monitoring.
- Facilities for monitoring central venous and intraarterial pressure, ECG, blood gases and acid–base status should be available in consultant units.
- Rapid administration of blood and fluids (blood filtration is not necessary).
- Use of blood-warming equipment.
- Repeated estimation of haemoglobin and coagulation studies.
- Use of an early warning scoring system such as the Modified Early Obstetric Warning Scoring System (MEOWS).

Recommendations added in 2014 (Knight et al 2014) include:

- Haemoglobin levels below the normal range for pregnancy should be investigated and iron supplementation considered if indicated to optimize haemoglobin before delivery.
- Stimulating or augmenting uterine contractions should be done in accordance with current guidance and paying particular attention to avoiding uterine tachysystole or hyperstimulation.
- Fluid resuscitation and blood transfusion should not be delayed because of false reassurance from a single haemoglobin result.
- While significant haemorrhage may be apparent from observed physiological disturbances, young, fit pregnant women compensate remarkably well. A tachycardia commonly develops, but there can be a paradoxical bradycardia. Hypotension is always a very late sign; therefore, ongoing bleeding should be acted on without delay.
- In a woman who is bleeding and is likely to develop a coagulopathy or has evidence of a coagulopathy, it is prudent to give blood components before coagulation indices deteriorate.
- Early recourse to hysterectomy is recommended if simpler medical and surgical interventions prove ineffective.

---

the haemorrhage. Hysterectomy is undertaken as a last resort to save the woman's life. The midwife must be familiar with local guidelines for management of massive obstetric haemorrhage (see Box 53.1) and adequate supplies of cross-matched blood need to be available before surgery commences. The use of cell salvage in this predicted situation has proven to be successful and should be considered if the necessary equipment is available (Ralph et al 2011).

Vaginal examination in cases of placenta praevia is a high-risk procedure and should not be attempted, except with the precautions described previously.

ABRUPTIO PLACENTAE

Abruptio placentae causes bleeding by the separation of a normally situated placenta (see Fig. 53.9). It is sometimes

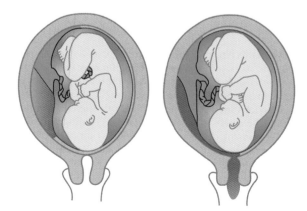

Figure 53.9 Abruptio placentae.

referred to as placental abruption or 'accidental' bleeding. Placental abruption may occur at any stage of pregnancy, or during labour, and may complicate approximately 1% of pregnancies (Collins et al 2013).

Causes

The cause of the placental separation cannot always be satisfactorily explained and in 40% of cases, no cause can be found. The following risk factors have been associated with the condition:

- Hypertensive disease: essential hypertension, pregnancy-induced hypertension (PIH) or pre-eclampsia
- Sudden decompression of the uterus: such as may follow spontaneous rupture of the membranes in cases of polyhydramnios
- Preterm prelabour: rupture of the membranes
- Previous history: placental abruption
- Trauma: for example, following external cephalic version, road traffic accident, a fall or a blow
- Smoking
- Drug abuse: for example, cocaine or marijuana
- Folate and vitamin B_{12} deficiency: although the evidence for this association is not conclusive

Maternal hypertension is the most consistent finding in cases of placental abruption.

Types

The bleeding may be revealed, concealed or partially revealed (see Fig. 53.10).

Revealed bleeding: This occurs when the site of detachment is at the placental margin. The blood dissects between the membranes and the decidua and escapes through the os uteri. With revealed placental abruption, the degree of shock is in proportion to the visible vaginal blood loss.

Concealed bleeding: This occurs when the site of detachment is close to the centre of the placenta. The blood cannot escape and a large retroplacental clot forms (see Fig. 53.9). The blood may infiltrate the myometrium, sometimes as far as the peritoneal covering, causing a marbled, petechial pattern of bleeding. This is known as a *Couvelaire uterus.* There is no visible blood loss, but the pain and shock may be severe as the intra-uterine tension rises. Increasing abdominal girth or rising fundal height are suspicious signs of concealed haemorrhage. Backache may accompany abruption in a posteriorly sited placenta.

Partially revealed bleeding: This occurs when some of the blood trickles between the membranes and the decidua to become visible as vaginal bleeding. Not all the blood escapes, and a variable amount remains concealed. In this situation, the bleeding and, thus, the degree of shock will be much more severe than the visible loss suggests.

The severity of placental abruption may be classified as mild, moderate or severe.

Mild abruptio placentae

The loss is usually slight and the bleeding may be entirely concealed, although often there is a slight trickle per vaginam. The woman may experience no more than mild abdominal pain, the uterus is not tender and the fetus is alive. There is no sign of maternal shock.

Moderate abruptio placentae

The blood loss is heavier, the abdominal pain is more severe and, on palpation, the uterus may be tender and

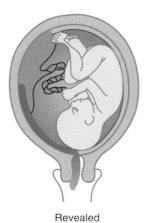 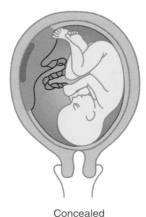 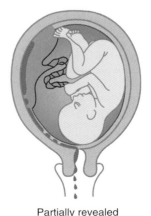

| Revealed | Concealed | Partially revealed |

Figure 53.10 Types of abruptio placentae.

firm. The mother may be hypotensive and have a tachy-cardia, and usually there are signs of fetal distress.

Severe abruptio placentae

This is an obstetric emergency. More than half the placenta will have separated, the blood loss will exceed 1 L, and the mother will display signs of haemorrhagic shock. Abdominal pain will be severe. On palpation, the uterus may be hard and tender (sometimes described as feeling 'woody' to the touch), and on auscultation, fetal heart sounds will not be heard. There is an increased risk of coagulation disorders. It is essential to remember that the amount of bleeding from the vagina is no guide to the degree of placental separation.

VASA PRAEVIA

This unusual condition may result in vaginal bleeding. It is associated with velamentous insertion of the cord (see Ch. 39). One of the fetal vessels traverses the membranes in the region of the internal os, in front of the presenting part. Occlusion of the vessel may occur as the presenting part compresses the membranes. When the membranes rupture, the vessel can be torn and severe fetal bleeding occurs, which may appear to be vaginal bleeding. The perinatal mortality associated with this condition is high (Collins et al 2013). Diagnosis is difficult, but a pulsating vessel may be felt on vaginal examination. Velamentous insertion can often be detected on routine ultrasound examination from the second trimester of pregnancy and vasa praevia can be confirmed by transvaginal colour Doppler scanning.

If vasa praevia is suspected, the midwife should leave the membranes intact and inform the obstetrician. The midwife should be aware that there may be a higher risk of vasa praevia in placenta praevia where there is a succenturiate lobe and in IVF pregnancies.

Outcome

If there is minor detachment of the placenta and the mother and fetus are in good condition, the woman will be advised to stay in the hospital setting for observation. If the bleeding ceases and all appears well, she may be discharged. The pregnancy will be closely monitored with ultrasound scans and regular cardiotocography to assess fetal growth and well-being. There is an increased risk of poor fetal growth and preterm birth after an episode of placental abruption.

In a case of moderate or severe abruptio placentae, the most important treatment is to empty the uterus. If fetal condition permits, labour is induced by rupturing the membranes and an oxytocic infusion is commenced. Vaginal delivery may be possible.

If the fetus is in poor condition, delivery will be by caesarean section unless the woman is already in the second stage of labour, when a forceps delivery will be performed. *Ergometrine* 500 µg is given intravenously at delivery to control haemorrhage in the third stage of labour. It is usual to continue a *syntocinon infusion* for some hours after delivery to maintain uterine contraction. The increased risk of haemorrhage requires prebirth preparation of cross-matched blood (six to eight units to be available). The most effective treatment for severe haemorrhage and defective coagulation is the transfusion of fresh blood. If fresh blood is not available, fresh frozen plasma should be given, as this contains fibrinogen, platelets and clotting factors III, V and VIII.

Major haemorrhage and its resulting hypotension may lead to avascular necrosis of the pituitary gland (Sheehan's syndrome), the clinical features of which include failure of lactation and persistent amenorrhoea, leading to secondary infertility (Collins et al 2013).

Reflective activity 53.3

Locate and read your unit/hospital policy for management of bleeding in later pregnancy.

MANAGEMENT OF ANTEPARTUM HAEMORRHAGE AND THE MIDWIFE'S ROLE

At home

If called by a woman with bleeding, the midwife must ascertain the amount of bleeding and organize immediate care. If the reported bleeding is heavy, the midwife should ask a paramedic team from the local ambulance service to attend to avoid delay in transfer to a hospital.

The woman is encouraged to lie on her side or with a pillow or towel wedged under the right hip to achieve a slight pelvic tilt and avoid supine hypotensive syndrome. Blood pressure, pulse rate and temperature will be recorded at regular, frequent intervals. A modified, early obstetric warning (MEOWS) chart (Lewis 2011, see Box 53.1) will be helpful to keep track of these observations. The blood loss needs to be measured, and sanitary pads and any soiled clothing, sheets and pads should be retained to allow detailed estimation of blood lost. The presence of pain is suggestive of abruptio placentae, while painless, bright bleeding may indicate placenta praevia. The on call obstetric consultant at the nearest maternity unit must be contacted, as the woman will require admission for appropriate ongoing care. The midwife should inform the obstetrician of the severity of the bleeding, colour of the blood (fresh or dark), nature and location of pain, if present, and the woman's general condition. If the initial loss is small, the woman's blood pressure and pulse rate will be normal and she will appear well. The assessment of blood pressure should be treated with caution, with reference to the woman's medical record if possible. A normal blood pressure may falsely represent a low blood pressure in women with a history of hypertension. In these cases, the pulse and respiration rate may be more indicative of bleeding. If the loss is severe, the woman will present the typical picture of a haemorrhagic shock with symptoms of pallor, sweating, restlessness, thirst, a rising pulse rate, rising respiration rate and falling blood pressure. In this case emergency assistance is needed, and a paramedic team from the ambulance service should be called. An intravenous infusion is started and group O Rhesus-negative blood may be given if available. Plasma expanders, such as *Haemacel, Gelofusine* or *hetastarch* (*Hespan*) preparations, may be used.

When assessing a woman who is bleeding, **no vaginal examination** should be made. If this is a case of placenta praevia, a vaginal examination could precipitate a disastrous haemorrhage. Rectal examinations are similarly dangerous. Abdominal examination should be avoided if possible, as this may provoke Braxton Hicks contractions, which may accelerate bleeding.

In the hospital

The woman is admitted to the delivery suite/labour ward, and the attendance of a senior obstetrician is requested. If there are signs of severe haemorrhage, a senior anaesthetist and haematologist should also be in attendance.

Until the diagnosis is clear, she must be treated as having a potential placenta praevia, although there may be some features that help in making a diagnosis (see Table 53.2). Often the distinction is not clear; it is particularly difficult if the mother has had a small revealed abruption but no pain, no apparent cause for the bleeding and no signs of pre-eclampsia.

If bleeding has been severe, the treatment must be swift, as the woman's condition will deteriorate rapidly. The aim is to restore normal blood volume and, thus, improve the mother's general condition, deliver the baby if necessary,

Table 53.2 Differential diagnosis – placenta praevia and abruptio placentae

Clinical sign	Placenta praevia	Abruptio placentae
Pain	No pain	Abdominal pain Uterine pain, may be severe; backache if placenta is posterior
Colour of blood loss	Usually bright red; fresh	May be a darker colour
'Warning' haemorrhages	Yes	No
Onset of bleeding	Possibly following coitus; otherwise, unexpected Usually no clots	May follow trauma, exertion Clots may be present
Degree of shock	In proportion to visible loss May be lower blood pressure and raised pulse and respiratory rate	May be more severe than visible loss suggests Raised pulse and respiratory rate and lowered blood pressure
Consistency of uterus	Soft, nontender	Increased uterine tone, may be tense, rigid, 'woody'
Palpation	Fetus usually fairly easy to palpate	Tense uterus makes palpation difficult
Presentation	May be a malpresentation	Probably cephalic
Engagement	Not engaged	May be engaged
Fetal heartbeat	Probably present	May be absent or compromised
Abdominal girth	Equivalent to gestation	May increase because of concealed haemorrhage
History/ultrasound (USS)	USS may have suggested low lying placenta	May show normally situated placenta, but USS will show abruption and clots

and avoid the dangerous complications of renal failure and blood coagulation disorders. Two intravenous cannulae (16 FG gauge) are inserted, blood is taken for grouping and cross-matching, and at least six units of blood cross-matched. The duty haematologist and blood bank must be informed if large quantities of blood are likely to be needed. Other blood tests include full blood count – essential for haemoglobin estimation and platelet count – urea and electrolytes, clotting studies and fibrin degradation products.

Temperature, pulse, blood pressure, fetal heart and vaginal loss should be observed. The pulse and blood pressure are recorded as frequently as the woman's condition dictates: every 5 minutes if the bleeding is continuous. Maternal oxygen saturation should be observed using a pulse oximeter. Oxygen may be given by facemask if required. The fetal heart should be continuously monitored by external cardiotocography while the bleeding persists. Gentle pressure should be used so as not to stimulate further bleeding or uterine activity. Placing a mark on the abdomen during the first assessment of the fetal heart may reduce the need for excessive palpation. A Foley indwelling urinary catheter is inserted, and the urinary output is closely monitored, a marked decrease being a grave sign. The urine is tested for protein. The midwife records an estimate of the blood loss, observing for the appearance of blood clotting: blood with normal clotting factors will clot in room air; if this fails to happen, deranged clotting should be suspected. Analgesia, such as *morphine*, may be required if the woman is in pain. An intravenous infusion of saline 0.9% or Hartmann's solution (Ringer's lactate) will be commenced. Blood transfusion may be required, and several units of blood or packed cells may be needed if the haemorrhage has been substantial. In such cases, central venous pressure (CVP) should be monitored to avoid the dangers of over or under transfusion.

The abdominal girth can be measured and recorded to observe for concealed haemorrhage. Meticulous observation and recording of vital signs, blood loss and fluid balance are essential to assess the woman's condition and plan her care. Ongoing management of the situation is governed by the condition of the mother and fetus. The midwife may need to involve the social worker if there are other children at home for whom care arrangements need to be made. The needs of the partner, which include support and information, should also be addressed.

If the haemorrhage is not severe and urgent delivery is not indicated, the woman may be transferred to the antenatal ward once the bleeding settles and her condition is stable. In the absence of pain or active bleeding, the woman should not be confined to her bed and can be encouraged to wear her usual clothes during the day. In cases of placenta praevia, at least two units of cross-matched blood should always be available; local policy will dictate the regularity of sample update (and this is usually weekly). This enables cross-match of fresh blood

and ensures ready availability of blood should haemorrhage occur. If the bleeding is caused by placenta praevia, the woman may be advised to remain in the hospital until delivery. The midwife must ensure that the woman and her partner are fully informed about her condition and likely management.

After an antepartum haemorrhage, tests to assess fetal well-being will be carried out because premature separation of the placenta may result in impaired placental function. Fetal growth will be assessed by ultrasound, and periodic, continuous fetal heart monitoring will be performed. Women who have a Rhesus-negative blood group should be offered anti-D Immunoglobulin in line with local policy, after each episode of bleeding.

COMPLICATIONS

Blood coagulation disorders (see Ch. 67): When tissue damage occurs, there is a release of thromboplastin from the local cells. Thromboplastin activates the clotting mechanism, and this results in the conversion of fibrinogen into fibrin. The sticky web of fibrin traps the cellular components of the blood and a clot forms, sealing off the bleeding point. The clot is later dispersed by plasmin, which is the active product of the fibrinolytic system. When a clot is broken down, fibrin degradation products (FDPs) are formed. Clot dispersal is a protective mechanism to prevent capillary blockage.

The system of initial clot formation followed by fibrinolysis is normally delicately balanced. If the coagulation system fails, bleeding will persist; if the fibrinolytic system fails, clotting will persist.

Occasionally, tissue damage is so severe or widespread that there is a massive release of thromboplastin into the general circulation. Widespread clotting will then occur throughout the body. This condition is known as *disseminated intravascular coagulation* (DIC). This is extremely dangerous, as the microthrombi generated by the thromboplastin will occlude small blood vessels. This results in ischaemic tissue damage within the body organs: the damaged tissue releases thromboplastin, which stimulates further clotting. Thus, a chain reaction of tissue damage and uncontrolled clotting occurs. Any body organ may be affected: renal damage will result in oliguria or anuria; liver damage will lead to jaundice. If the lungs are affected, dyspnoea and cyanosis will occur; convulsions or coma indicate cerebral involvement. Microthrombi in the retina may cause blindness; if the pituitary gland is affected, Sheehan's syndrome, a condition that may have serious long-term effects on the mother's health and her future fertility, may occur. Eventually, the available circulating platelets are depleted. Clotting factors, such as prothrombin (factor II), thromboplastin (factor III), proaccelerin (factor V), antihaemophilic factor (factor VIII) and fibrinogen (factor I), are exhausted. No further coagulation can take place and bleeding becomes apparent. This may take the form of oozing from venipuncture sites, mucous membrane bleeding, petechiae and uncontrollable uterine haemorrhage.

DIC is always a secondary event, occurring as a result of massive tissue damage and thromboplastin release. It may complicate conditions such as severe pre-eclampsia, septicaemia or amniotic fluid embolism. It may also occur after abruptio placentae, when thromboplastin is released from the damaged placental, decidual and myometrial tissue. Unless DIC is recognized and treated promptly, the condition may become uncontrollable, with death an inevitable outcome. The midwife must be aware of any woman who is at risk of DIC and be alert for the signs of coagulation failure. All maternity units should have an emergency protocol for dealing with such cases. Any woman with abruptio placentae should have screening tests for coagulation defects. These tests include:

- partial thromboplastin time (normally 35–45 seconds)
- prothrombin time (normally 10–14 seconds)
- thrombin time (normally 10–15 seconds)
- fibrinogen levels (2.5–4 g/L)
- fibrin degradation products
- whole blood film and platelet count

Fresh frozen plasma, packed cells and platelets are used in the treatment of DIC. Heparin is rarely used, as it may exacerbate the haemorrhage, especially if the uterus is not empty.

Acute renal failure: This may occur after severe shock in cases of antepartum haemorrhage.

Postpartum haemorrhage: After severe abruptio placentae, postpartum haemorrhage is most likely to be caused by a blood coagulation disorder, whereas after placenta praevia, it is caused by the inability of the lower uterine segment to contract effectively. Aortic compression may be necessary to control cases of intractable haemorrhage.

Infection: Sepsis is likely owing to the woman's lowered resistance after a state of severe shock, a large blood transfusion, increased intervention in labour and anaemia.

Anaemia: The haemoglobin must be checked and anaemia corrected in the puerperium.

Psychological disturbances/psychoses: Psychological disorders after childbirth are more likely after complications of pregnancy and labour, and may be caused by ensuing anaemia or post-traumatic stress (PTS) syndrome (see Ch. 69).

CONCLUSION

Bleeding in pregnancy remains a major cause of maternal morbidity and mortality (Knight et al 2014). The midwife must be familiar with local policy for management of bleeding in pregnancy and regular emergency drills should be held in maternity units to ensure that the obstetric team can respond to haemorrhage quickly and appropriately. Midwives must be familiar with the recommended guidelines for the management of massive obstetric haemorrhage.

The importance of training for midwives and obstetricians in identifying women who might be at risk is clear, and closely linked to speedy appropriate referral. Clear information and support for the woman and her family throughout the process will help reduce psychological sequelae. Ideally, the midwife will be the person providing continuity during the woman's pregnancy, facilitating holistic, sensitive and appropriate care to the woman, her baby and family.

Key Points

- Vaginal bleeding at any stage of pregnancy is always abnormal and may be indicative of a serious complication.
- Midwives need to educate the woman and her family regarding deviations from normal, and ensure that they are aware of what action should be taken and with whom they should communicate.
- Midwives must be aware of the possible causes of bleeding in pregnancy.
- A prompt and appropriate response may prevent the loss of the fetus and may save the mother's life.
- Midwives must be aware of the possible emotional, social and psychological effect of bleeding or pregnancy loss for the woman and her partner.

References

Antenatal Results and Choices (ARC): (website). www.arc-org.uk. 2015.

British National Formulary (BNF): (website). www.medicines complete.com/mc/bnf/current/. 2015.

Cancer Research UK: (website). www .cancerresearchuk.org/about-cancer/ type/cervical-cancer/treatment/ cervical-cancer-and-pregnancy. 2014.

Carr R, Coustan D: Nonprescription drugs and alcohol: abuse and effects in pregnancy. In Reece EA, Hobbins JC, editors: *Clinical obstetrics: the fetus & mother*, 3rd edn, Oxford, Wiley-Blackwell, 2007.

Collins S, Arulkumaran A, Hayes K, et al: *Oxford handbook of obstetrics and gynaecology*, Oxford, OUP, 2013.

Department of Health England: *Report on Confidential Enquiry into Maternal Deaths in the United Kingdom 1988–1990*. London, HMSO, 1994.

Dimond B: *Legal aspects of midwifery*, 4th edn, London, Quay Books, 2013.

Gilo NB, Dennis A, Landy HJ: Appendicitis and cholecystitis in pregnancy, *Clin Obstet Gynecol* 52(4):586–596, 2009.

Glasby J, Tew J: *Mental health policy and practice*, 3rd edn, London, Palgrave, 2015.

Gov.UK: *Statistics, Historical Crime Data* (website). www.gov.uk/government/ statistics/historical-crime-data. 2015.

HMSO: Abortion Act (website). www .legislation.gov.uk/ukpga/1967/87/ contents. 1967.

Home Department: *Criminal Statistics England and Wales 2000*, London, The Stationery Office, 2001.

Home Office: *Identity and Passport Service, General Registrar Office, Official Information on Births, Deaths and Marriages* (website). www.gro.gov.uk/gro/content. 2008.

Home Office: *Crime Statistics* (website). http://webarchive.national archives.gov.uk/20130128103514/ http://homeoffice.gov.uk/science-research/research-statistics/. 2009.

Human Fertilisation and Embryology Act, London: *Office of Public Sector Information* (website). www. legislation.gov.uk/ukpga/1990/37/ contents. 1990.

Jakovljevic A, Bogavac M, Nikolic A, et al: The influence of bacterial vaginosis on gestational week of the completion of delivery and biochemical markers of inflammation in the serum, *Vojnosanit Pregl* 71(10):931–935, 2014.

Kenny C: Antenatal obstetric complications. In Baker PN, Kenny C, editors: *Obstetrics by ten teachers*, 19th edn, Boca Raton, CRC Press, 2011.

Knight M, Kenyon S, Brocklehurst P, et al; On behalf of MBRRACE-UK, editors: *Saving Lives, Improving Mothers' Care – Lessons Learned to Inform Future Maternity Care from the UK and Ireland Confidential Enquiries into Maternal Deaths and Morbidity 2009–2012*, University of Oxford, Oxford: National Perinatal Epidemiology Unit, 2014.

Kovacs J, Briggs P: *Lectures in obstetrics, gynaecology and women's health*, London, Springer, 2015.

Lewis G, editor: *Saving Mothers' Lives: Reviewing Maternal Deaths to Make Motherhood Safer – 2003–2005*, The Seventh Report on Confidential Enquiries into Maternal Deaths in the United Kingdom. London, CEMACH, 2007.

Lewis G: Saving Mothers' Lives Reviewing maternal deaths to make motherhood safer: 2006–2008, *Br J Obstet Gynaecol* 118(1), 2011.

McNamee KM, Dawood F, Farquharson RG: Mid-trimester pregnancy loss, *Obstet Gynecol Clin North Am* 41(1):87–102, 2014.

Miscarriage Association: *Management of miscarriage: your options* (website). www.miscarriageassociation.org .uk/wp/wp-content/leaflets/ Management-of-miscarriage.pdf. 2015.

Mohangoo AD, Blondel M, Gissler M, et al: *The Euro-Peristat Scientific Committee, 2013. International Comparisons of Fetal and Neonatal Mortality Rates in High-Income Countries: Should Exclusion Thresholds Be Based on Birth Weight or Gestational Age?* (website). Available in Open Access. http://journals.plos .org/plosone/article?id=10.1371/ journal.pone.0024727. 2013.

Nanda K, Lopez LM, Grimes DA, et al: *Cochrane Pregnancy and Childbirth Group Cochrane Database of Systematic Reviews*. 2012.

National Health Service (NHS) NHS Choices: *Abortion* (website). www.nhs.uk/conditions/Abortion/ Pages/Introduction.aspx. 2014.

National Institute for Health and Care Excellence (NICE): *Ectopic Pregnancy and Miscarriage: Diagnosis and Initial Management in Early Pregnancy of Ectopic Pregnancy and Miscarriage* (website). www.nice.org.uk/ guidance/qs69. 2012.

Neilson JP, Hickey M, Vazquez J: Medical treatment for early fetal death (less than 24 weeks), *Cochrane Database Syst Rev* 2013.

Pan F, Zhang AX, Pan LJ: Male factors in repeated spontaneous abortion, *Zhong Hua Nan Ke Xue* 16(6):542–546, 2010.

Parliament UK: *Defining Viability*. (website). www.publications .parliament.uk/pa/cm200607/ cmselect/cmsctech/1045/104505 .htm. 2007.

Perez-Duran J, Najera Z, Trujillo-Cabrera Y, et al: 2015 Aneusomy detection with Karyolite-Bac on Beads® is a cost-efficient and high throughput strategy in the molecular analyses of the early pregnancy conception losses (website). *Mol Cytogenet* 8:63. Published online 2015 Aug 12. doi: 10.1186/s13039-015-0168-x. 2015.

Powrie RO, Greene MF, Camann W, editors: *De Swiet's medical disorders in pregnancy*, Oxford, Wiley-Blackwell, 2010.

Qureshi H, Massey E, Kirwin D, et al: BCSH guideline for the use of anti-D immunoglobulin for the prevention of haemolytic disease of the fetus and newborn, *Transfus Med* 24(1):8–20, 2014.

Ralph CJ, Sulivan I, Faulds J: Intraoperative cell salvaged blood as part of a blood conservation strategy in caesarean section: is fetal red cell contamination important? *Br J Anaesth* (website). doi: 10.1093/ bja/aer168, 2011.

Royal College of Obstetricians and Gynaecologists (RCOG): *Early Miscarriage Information* (website). www.rcog.org.uk/globalassets/ documents/patients/patient -information-leaflets/pregnancy/ early-miscarriage.pdf. 2008.

Royal College of Obstetricians and Gynaecologists (RCOG): *Cervical Cerclage. Green–top Guideline No. 60.* RCOG https://www.rcog.org.uk/globalassets/documents/guidelines/gtg_60.pdf, 2011.

Royal College of Obstetricians and Gynaecologists (RCOG): *The Global Cost of Unsafe Abortion* (website). www.rcog.org.uk/en/news/bjog-release-the-global-cost-of-unsafe-abortion/. 2015.

Seckl MJ, Fisher R, Salwerno G, et al: Choriocarcinoma and partial hydatidiform moles, *Lancet* 356(9223):36–39, 2000.

Seckl MJ, Sebire NJ, Fisher R, et al; On behalf of the ESMO Guidelines Working Group*: Gestational trophoblastic disease: ESMO Clinical Practice Guidelines for diagnosis, treatment and follow-up, *Ann Oncol* 24(Suppl 6):vi39:1–vi39:12, 2013.

Silver R, Branch D: Sporadic and recurrent pregnancy loss. In Reece EA, Hobbins JC, editors: *Clinical obstetrics: the fetus & mother*, 3rd edn, London, Blackwell, 2007.

Supreme Court: Judgement Montgomery (Appellant) v Lanarkshire Health Board (Respondent) (Scotland) (website). www.supremecourt.uk/cases/docs/uksc-2013-0136-judgment.pdf. 2015.

Sutkin G, Manmlock V: Fetus papyraceus. Images in clinical medicine, *N Engl J Med* 350:1665, 2004.

USA.gov: *Limits of Viability: Definition of the Gray Zone* (website). www.ncbi.nlm.nih.gov/pubmed/18446176. 2008.

Winter C, Crofts J, Laxton C, et al: *PROMT, Practical Obstetric Multi-Professional Training Course Manual*, 2nd edn, Cambridge University Press, 2012.

Resources and additional reading

Please refer to the chapter website resources.

MBRRACE-UK: Mothers and Babies: Reducing Risk through Audits and Confidential Enquiries across the UK https://www.npeu.ox.ac.uk/mbrrace-uk

This is an important resource for those working in the maternity services to access. The site includes investigation into causes of maternal deaths, stillbirths and infant deaths, which provides robust national information to support the delivery of safe, equitable, high quality, patient-centred maternal, newborn and infant health services.

Resources for women:

Miscarriage Association: http://www.miscarriageassociation.org.uk/information/signs-and-symptoms/pain-bleeding-or-spotting/?gclid=CLiA-ebW4tMCFYi97Qodpr0Adw - *useful information for women and families*

Tommy's Charity: https://www.tommys.org/pregnancy-information/symptom-checker/i-am-bleeding-pregnancy?gclid=CMzJ8v_W4tMCFeq17Qodji0BCA

Molar Pregnancy Online community: http://www.molarpregnancy.co.uk/info.html

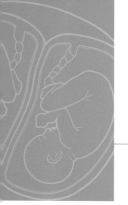

Chapter 54

Hypertensive and medical disorders in pregnancy

Judy Bothamley and Maureen Boyle

Learning Outcomes

After reading this chapter, you will be able to:

- identify the different types of hypertensive disorders in pregnancy
- recognize the features of pre-eclampsia
- understand the key principles of care for women with a range of medical disorders
- acknowledge the need for women with medical disorders to be supported by midwives with a knowledge of their condition
- appreciate the need for women with hypertensive and medical conditions to be supported for both their physical and psychological needs

INTRODUCTION

Women with complex medical conditions require knowledgeable, supportive midwifery care that will address not only the physical aspects of their condition but also offer a connection with the reality of pregnancy as a normal and exciting life event for each individual woman and her family. Obesity, older maternal age, advances in the care of medical conditions, such as cardiac disease, and the complex medical problems of women born outside the UK has contributed to an increase in women with complicated disorders using maternity services. The midwife requires good skills of observation and assessment built on a knowledge base that considers the underlying disorder and the implications of that for the woman, her pregnancy and the fetus. Recurring themes in relation to medical conditions and hypertensive disorders includes the need for women to use preconception (see Ch. 27) services before pregnancy, optimize their health and have access to appropriate specialist multidisciplinary services that include midwifery care.

HYPERTENSIVE DISORDERS

Hypertensive disorders complicate 10% to 15% of pregnancies, making them the most common medical condition affecting pregnancy (Nelson-Piercy 2015). They are generally classified into 3 types: chronic or pre-existing hypertension, gestational hypertension and pre-eclampsia (PET).

Pre-eclampsia, the most significant of the range of hypertensive disorders in pregnancy, contributes to increased maternal and perinatal morbidity and mortality. Much of antenatal care in the second and third trimester centres on the early detection of this unique complication of pregnancy.

Measurement of blood pressure and assessment of proteinuria underpin diagnosis in hypertensive disorders, although it is important to remember that PET is a multi-system disorder that can present initially with normal blood pressure. A detailed knowledge of the pathophysiology of PET and other hypertensive disorders will help midwives make effective assessments of women and enable timely recognition and referral.

Blood pressure

The physiological changes of pregnancy cause the blood pressure (BP) to drop in early pregnancy until around 18 weeks gestation and then to slowly rise towards term. Obtaining a baseline blood pressure reading in the first trimester aids management.

A reading of 140/90 mmHg is regarded as the upper limit of normal (see Box 54.1 for classification of BP ranges). The confidential enquiry into maternal deaths and morbidity (Harding et al 2016) recommends that a systolic pressure of 150 mmHg or above requires investigation and effective treatment with antihypertensive medication (see Box 54.2). A systolic measurement above 180 mmHg should be considered a medical emergency and urgent referral for effective antihypertensive medication is required (Harding et al 2016). A cerebral haemorrhage (cerebrovascular accident) (CVA or stroke) has been noted to occur when the blood pressure rises above 155 mm Hg systolic (Nathan et al 2015). It is important to note that blood pressure needs to be taken and interpreted in context with signs and symptoms.

Accurate measurement of blood pressure is essential. The diastolic measurement is taken at stage V (five) of the Korotkoff sounds (absence of sound). The woman should be in a sitting or semireclining position, so that her arm and the sphygmomanometer cuff are at the same level as the heart. Large-size cuffs should be available for women who have an arm circumference greater than 32 cm (Nathan et al 2015). The cuff should be inflated to 20 to 30 mmHg above the estimated systolic blood pressure and then deflated slowly at a rate of 2 mm Hg per second. Readings should be recorded to the nearest 2 mmHg (NICE 2014). It is acknowledged that fluctuations in BP will occur because of physiological reasons, including anxiety (white coat syndrome), exercise, a full bladder and smoking. Midwives are advised to take a few readings, allowing time to rest in between to exclude physiological reasons for a high blood pressure, although they should be careful not to "explain away" a high blood pressure as simply caused by anxiety or exercise but rather to gain an objective accurate assessment. Automated blood pressure devices are useful, as they provide a more objective measurement and are convenient for serial measurements of BP that allow trends to be observed. However, they may underestimate blood pressure, particularly in pre-eclampsia and, therefore, need to be checked by a manual reading periodically. The use of blood pressure equipment, validated for use in pregnancy that is regularly maintained, is essential.

Box 54.1 Definitions for ranges of hypertension

Mild hypertension Diastolic 90–99 mmHg, systolic 140–149 mmHg

Moderate hypertension Diastolic 100–109 mmHg, systolic 150–159 mmHg

Severe hypertension Diastolic ≥ 110 mmHg, systolic ≥ 160 mmHg

Source: NICE 2011a

Box 54.2 Antihypertensive medication in pregnancy*

Labetalol is the first-line oral antihypertensive advised by NICE (2011a) for pregnancy, provided the woman is not asthmatic; it should be used with caution in diabetics. It can also be given in severe pre-eclampsia as an intravenous infusion (NICE 2011a).

Methyldopa and *nifedipine* are recommended as second-line alternative medications to labetalol (NICE 2011a).

Hydralazine is used as an infusion for the treatment of acute severe hypertension. It can cause a sudden, profound maternal hypotension with fetal consequences because of poor placental perfusion. Frequent monitoring of blood pressure and continuous cardiotocograph (CTG) recording is indicated.

Magnesium sulphate: although magnesium sulphate is primarily an anticonvulsive, it also has a strong hypotensive effect and further antihypertensive medication may not be necessary. It is recommended as a first-line treatment of eclampsia and to prevent eclampsia in those at high risk.

ACE inhibitors are considered unsuitable for use during pregnancy, as they have adverse fetal and neonatal effects but may be prescribed in the postnatal period.

Source: Bramham et al 2013a; Jordan 2010; NICE 2011a; Nelson-Piercy 2015

---

*Antihypertensive medication needs to be prescribed by a medical practitioner. Midwives should refer to local guidelines for medication protocols, consult with the prescribing doctor and follow regulations for medicines administration (NMC 2008).

Reflective activity 54.1   ✕

How does your technique of taking blood pressure compare with the manner described?

How could you improve your technique to increase the accuracy?

Urinalysis

In the clinical setting, it is convenient to use a 'dipstick' test for urine. This will provide an estimation of protein in the urine and findings of 1 + and above are considered significant. Visual reading of the dipstick is the most widely and cost-effective method used, although use of automated reading of the stick may improve accuracy. Protein in the urine may indicate damage to the endothelial lining of the glomerular, which allows leaking of protein out of the capillaries into the urine, a feature of PET and other renal complications. Other explanations for proteinuria are contamination of the sample or the presence of a urinary tract infection (UTI). To minimize contamination, the woman should use a clean specimen jar, wipe away any excess vaginal discharge with some wet tissue, hold the specimen jar away from the body and collect just the middle section of the stream of urine. Presence of a UTI may or may not be accompanied with symptoms of cystitis (see renal disorders later in chapter). A positive finding on a 'dip stick' test should, therefore, be followed up with further laboratory testing. A 24-hour urine collection remains the 'gold standard' for quantification of protein, and a level of more than 300 mg in 24 hours is considered abnormal. However, this test is time consuming and the collection may be incomplete. Protein creatinine ratio (PCR) on a specimen of urine has been found to be helpful in diagnosing significant proteinuria. A PCR level of greater than or equal to 30 mg/mmol is considered as significant proteinuria in a singleton pregnancy (NICE 2011a).

Oedema

Although 85% of women with pre-eclampsia develop oedema, it is no longer considered a cardinal sign because it is a feature of normotensive and hypertensive pregnancies. Pathological oedema associated with pre-eclampsia occurs in the pretibial area, hands, face and abdomen, and does not resolve with rest and elevation. Excessive weight gain may be because of occult oedema. As part of the assessment for PET, the midwife should ask the woman or her partner whether a substantial or rapid increase in oedema has been noticed.

PRE–EXISTING (CHRONIC) HYPERTENSION

Pre-existing (chronic) hypertension is hypertension that predates pregnancy. It is recognized as either a high BP identified before 20 weeks gestation or if the woman has a normal BP but has been taking antihypertensive medication before pregnancy.

Most pre-existing hypertension is termed *'essential'* hypertension. This is when there is no identifiable direct disorder that causes the hypertension but arises from a combination of genetic and environmental factors. It is more common in black women (indicating a genetic predisposition), and the incidence increases with age, raised BMI, increased salt intake and physical inactivity. *Secondary* hypertension is pre-existing hypertension, arising as a consequence of disorders such as renal disease (see section later in chapter), cardiac disease, thyroid or adrenal gland abnormalities. Any woman noted to have hypertension in early pregnancy needs referral for a medical review to establish any cause for the high blood pressure and to start effective treatment (Nelson-Piercy 2015).

Management

Before pregnancy, women with chronic hypertension will require a review of their medication as some types of antihypertensive medication is not suitable in pregnancy. They should aim to keep their dietary salt intake low (NICE 2011a). Women will be advised to aim to be a healthy weight before pregnancy and should be given support for smoking cessation as indicated.

Women with chronic hypertension will require antenatal care from a consultant obstetrician, physician and a midwife. Antihypertensive drugs may be prescribed if the diastolic blood pressure exceeds 150/100 mmHg (NICE 2011a). Although many women with chronic hypertension will have a relatively normal pregnancy, a number of complications may occur. Women with pre-existing hypertension from whatever cause are at increased risk of superimposed pre-eclampsia and, therefore, more frequent antenatal visits to screen for features of PET (see next section) and clear information for the woman and her family on recognizing the symptoms of PET is required. Complications of severe hypertension are renal failure, heart failure and cerebral haemorrhage (stroke). Frequent BP monitoring and use of antihypertensive medication may be required to keep blood pressure at a safer level.

The fetus is at risk because the placental circulation may be poor; hence, fetal hypoxia, intra-uterine growth restriction (IUGR) and/or placental abruption may occur. Enhanced surveillance of fetal well-being is indicated and where fetal compromise or concern for the mother's well-being is identified, induction of labour (IOL) will be recommended. Frequent monitoring of maternal BP and continuous CTG is indicated during labour. Where the danger is more acute or arises earlier in pregnancy, caesarean section (CS) may be indicated.

Postnatally, women will require monitoring of their BP and will generally continue on their antenatal medication for the first 2 weeks. At that point, a review of longer-term antihypertensive medication will be made with further follow-up at 6 weeks after birth (NICE 2011a).

GESTATIONAL HYPERTENSION

Gestational hypertension (also known as pregnancy-induced hypertension (PIH)) is new hypertension, presenting after 20 weeks gestation without significant proteinuria or any other features of PET (NICE 2011a). Women who acquire hypertension in the second half of pregnancy may go on to develop pre-eclampsia. A third of women who have gestational hypertension before 34 weeks go on to develop PET over the next 5 weeks (Magee et al 2015), whereas only 7% of those who develop hypertension for the first time in the last few weeks of

Box 54.3 Risk factors for PET

- First pregnancy
- Pre-eclampsia in a previous pregnancy
- 10 years since a previous pregnancy
- Age 40 years or more
- Body mass index (BMI) of 35 or more
- Family history of pre-eclampsia (in mother or sister)
- Booking diastolic blood pressure of 80 mm Hg or more
- Booking proteinuria of 1 + or more, on more than one occasion, or quantified at >0.3 g/24 hours in the absence of infection
- Multiple pregnancy
- Underlying pre-existing medical conditions such as diabetes, hypertension, renal disease, antiphospholipid antibodies

Source: Milne et al 2005; NICE 2011a

Box 54.4 Pre-eclampsia (PET) bloods

Full blood count (FBC)

Renal function tests: Raised serum uric acid and/or raised serum creatinine may indicate reduced renal clearance of these waste products of metabolism because of renal impairment in PET. A low serum albumin reflects loss of protein through 'leaky' glomerular.

Liver function tests (LFTs): Serial measurements of *liver enzymes*, particularly alanine amino transferase (ALT) or aspartate amino transferase (AST), are performed. Transaminase concentrations increase in liver impairment and are a feature of HELLP syndrome (a complication of pre-eclampsia).

Clotting studies: Performed when the platelet count $< 100 \times 10^9$ L as disseminated intravascular coagulation (DIC) disorder may develop.

pregnancy show features of PET. PET is associated with worse outcomes for mother and baby than gestational hypertension and, therefore, the assessment by the midwife of any women with hypertension will be geared towards early detection, referral and education of the woman regarding PET (see section PET).

Women with gestational hypertension will be referred for medical and obstetric assessment, normally to a day assessment unit. They will be assessed for risk factors for PET (Box 54.3), have regular measurement of blood pressure, urine tested for proteinuria, monitoring of the fetal heart and have a range of blood tests (see Box 54.4). Admission to hospital is indicated if BP exceeds 160/110 mmHg. Antihypertensive medication that aims to keep BP within safe limits may be prescribed. IOL may be indicated to improve maternal and fetal well-being.

After delivery, women should continue any prescribed medications and have their BP reviewed at least daily initially and more often as clinically indicated. There should be a plan of care made for transfer to community that will include: who will provide follow-up care and when, frequency of blood pressure monitoring needed and the thresholds for reducing or stopping treatment (NICE 2011a).

PRE-ECLAMPSIA

The International Society for the Study of Hypertension in Pregnancy (ISSHP) agreed a revised definition of pre-eclampsia in 2014. They defined pre-eclampsia as

hypertension developing after 20 weeks gestation and the co-existence of one or more of the following new onset conditions: proteinuria, other maternal organ dysfunction (renal, liver, neurological, haematological complications) or uteroplacental dysfunction (fetal growth restriction) (Tranquilli et al 2014).

This revised international definition acknowledges PET as a multisystem disorder. Although high BP and proteinuria are frequent features of PET, they are not the only ones. The midwife needs to be familiar with the symptoms of PET and recognize these in woman with or without high BP or proteinuria. Follow-up examination, blood and urine tests will aim to determine the presence of any of the signs of PET. Box 54.5 lists signs and symptoms associated with PET.

Pathophysiology

PET is a multisystem disorder with a complex aetiology that is unique to pregnancy. The changes seen in PET appear to be caused by a complex interplay of abnormal genetic, immunological and placental factors. Despite much research, the cause of pre-eclampsia and HELLP syndrome is uncertain and recent research has centred on finding ways to identify it early to allow more frequent monitoring of pregnancies at risk. Early changes in the way the placenta embeds in the uterus is a strong predisposing factor in the development of PET, but it is the generalized response in the maternal endothelial system that leads to the widespread inflammation, platelet aggregation and vasoconstriction that underlies multi-organ dysfunction. (See Figure 54.1.)

Box 54.5 Signs and symptoms of PET

Symptoms

- Headache – severe, persistent, not resolved by mild analgesic medication
- Visual disturbances – may include dim or blurred vision, difficulty reading, spots or flashes of light
- Nausea and/or vomiting
- Rapid increase in swelling of the face, hands and feet
- Severe pain just below the ribs

Signs

- Hypertension
- Proteinuria
- Rapidly progressing oedema
- Liver involvement (elevated liver function tests and/or epigastric/right upper quadrant tenderness)
- Neurological complications, including eclampsia, altered mental status, stroke, hyperreflexia, severe headaches
- Visual disturbances – loss of field of vision, blindness
- Renal insufficiency (creatinine > 90 µmol/L)
- Oliguria (< 30 mL urine/hour)
- Haematological complications (thrombocytopenia, DIC, haemolysis)
- Fetal growth restriction
- Placental abruption

   Note: Not all women with severe pre-eclampsia present with all these symptoms and signs. Indeed any one symptom, with or without hypertension and proteinuria, is sufficient to indicate that the condition is worsening.

   Source: Tranquilli et al 2014; Nelson-Piercy 2015

Box 54.6 Assessments that may be performed in the DAU

BP profile: 3 blood pressure recordings at least 10 minutes apart

Urinalysis: Dipstick urine. An automated reader may be used. Send off urine sample for PCR (possible 24-hr urine collection) (see discussion urinalysis)

Clinical assessment of maternal symptoms related to PET

Clinical assessment of fetal size and well-being: measurement of symphysis – fundal height, enquiries regarding fetal movements, fetal heart auscultation and CTG as indicated

Ultrasound scan for assessment of fetal growth, liquor measurement and umbilical artery Doppler

PET bloods (see Box 54.4)

Medical review by senior doctor

Allocate the woman to a consultant-led pathway as indicated

Identification and diagnosis of PET

Midwives will be screening for PET at each antenatal visit. This includes identifying any risk factors for PET, taking an accurate blood pressure reading, testing urine for protein, assessing for significant non-dependent oedema, measurement of fundal height and assessing any other symptoms. Women who have additional symptoms such as headache, visual disturbances, epigastric pain or are generally feeling unwell must have their blood pressure measured and urine tested for protein. They should be referred for further assessment and medical review, even if the blood pressure is not significantly raised. Step up assessment is normally organized at a day assessment unit (DAU) where the woman can have access to a range of tests and be seen by the obstetrician so a diagnosis can be established, any treatment commenced and plan of care made (see Box 54.6). Same day referral is recommended for women with moderate and severe hypertension and/

or for those with characteristic symptoms. Transfer by ambulance from a community setting will be indicated where the woman has severe hypertension and/or significant symptoms of PET. Women will need a full explanation of the implications of any abnormal findings during the routine antenatal assessment backed up with written information. Women with PET often feel well and without knowledge of the implications of PET, will not be able to make a fully informed choice regarding their care. Understandably, this may be an anxious time for the woman and her family; therefore, clear, accurate information and active involvement in decisions and opportunities to answer questions is vital for psychological well-being.

   Depending on the results of the DAU assessment, the woman may be transferred back into routine antenatal care in the community, be advised to have more frequent assessment at the DAU or be admitted to a hospital. Those women who are not admitted will require detailed information about the symptoms of PET, knowledge of the potential dangers of fulminating PET and most importantly how to contact the unit if she notices any signs herself. Arrangements for follow-up should be clear and information about how she will receive any outstanding test results given.

Reflective activity 54.2   ><

Visit a maternity day assessment unit and find out what tests are carried out to assess the progress of pre-eclampsia. List what the normal test results should be and keep these in your personal record/resource book.

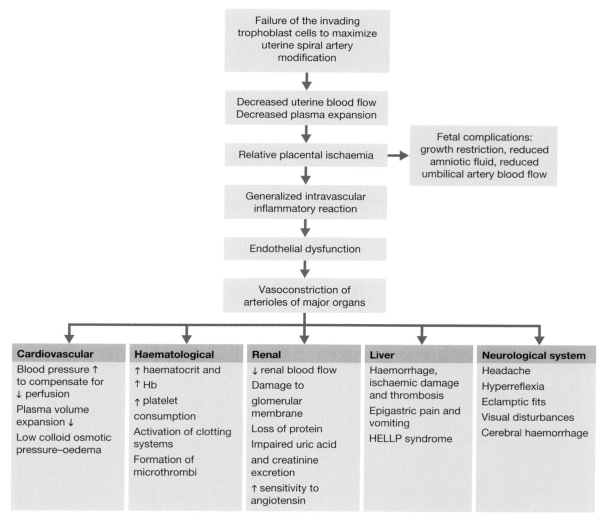

Figure 54.1 Pathogenesis and features of pre-eclampsia. (Bothamley J, Boyle M: Medical conditions affecting pregnancy and childbirth. Oxford, Radcliffe, 2009.)

Management of severe PET

Women with severe PET have a high mortality and morbidity rate and, therefore, management in a high dependency unit setting and consultation with a multidisciplinary team (MDT) that includes a senior obstetrician, neonatologist, obstetric anaesthetist, midwives, haematologist and possibly the critical care outreach team is needed. Table 54.1 lists complications of severe PET. Delivery of the baby (and placenta) is the only effective way to stop the progression of PET, but the decision to deliver will be balanced against

'expectant' management that will allow time for further fetal growth and administration of corticosteroids that will aid fetal lung maturity. Management priorities will include frequent maternal and fetal assessment, controlling the blood pressure, reducing the risk of seizure with the use of magnesium sulphate, fluid restriction and monitoring of fluid balance, preventing thromboembolism and determining the timing of delivery. Although the priorities for physical care will be great, the need for psychological support by the midwife for the woman and her family cannot be underestimated.

Table 54.1 Complications of severe PET

Complication	Features	Key points of care
Eclampsia	Uncontrolled seizures in association with features of PET. May occur before, during or after labour.	Urgent anaesthetic, obstetric and critical care referral. See guidance for management of tonic-clonic seizure in epilepsy section. Use of magnesium sulphate is recommended for management of eclamptic seizure.
Pulmonary oedema	Indicated by deteriorating respiratory function. Increased respiratory rate, reduced oxygen saturation and 'wheezing'. Caused by fluid overload.	Urgent anaesthetic, obstetric and critical care referral. Oxygen therapy. Fluid restriction, strict monitoring of fluid balance. Support of respiratory function.
Disseminated intravascular coagulation (DIC)	Recognized by abnormal tests of coagulation and/or uncontrolled bleeding.	Urgent anaesthetic, obstetric, haematology and critical care referral. Blood product replacement.
Placental abruption	See Ch. 53.	
HELLP **H**aemolysis **E**levated **L**iver enzymes **L**ow **P**latelets	Diagnosed by a combination of laboratory findings and clinical signs and symptoms such as epigastric (right upper quadrant) pain, nausea, malaise and other features of PET.	Urgent anaesthetic, obstetric, haematology and critical care referral. Care as per management of severe PET. Care to manage the potential for haemorrhage.
Cerebral haemorrhage/stroke Hypertension, pre-eclampsia and eclampsia are significant risk factors for stroke	Severe headache, impaired consciousness and raised systolic BP often accompany neurological deficit.	Urgent anaesthetic, neurological, obstetric and critical care referral.
Acute renal failure	See section on renal disorders.	
Acute fatty liver of pregnancy (AFLP); rare but potentially fatal	Vomiting, abdominal pain, jaundice. Abnormal liver function tests, hypoglycaemia, renal impairment, coagulation disorder.	Urgent anaesthetic, obstetric, haematology and critical care referral. Liver specialist required to direct care.

Source: Crovetto et al 2013

Maternal and fetal assessment

Women who are admitted with severe PET will require frequent (up to every 5 min) observations of vital signs with particular attention paid to blood pressure, respirations, oxygen saturation readings, pulse and level of consciousness. A modified early obstetric warning system (MEOWS) chart and a high dependency unit (HDU) chart that records observations, fluid balance, medications and results will be commenced. An automated BP device may be used to allow frequent serial measurement of BP. Assessment of fetal well-being may include continuous CTG monitoring. Observation for any deteriorating features such as headache, epigastric pain, and neurological impairment should be noted and requires prompt referral.

Control of blood pressure

A significant rise in blood pressure must be treated regardless of other signs and symptoms of PET to reduce the risk of maternal intracranial haemorrhage. Most doctors will prescribe antihypertensive medication when the systolic blood pressure is greater than 140 to 170 mmHg or diastolic pressure greater than 90 to 110 mmHg. Treatment is mandatory for severe hypertension when the blood pressure is greater than 170/110 mmHg. It will be important not to lower the blood pressure too low or too rapidly, as this may lead to placental hypoperfusion and this will compromise the fetus. Women with severe PET have reduced circulating plasma volume, and this makes them be very sensitive to relatively small doses of antihypertensive agents that may cause an abrupt drop in BP.

It is also important to note that even when the blood pressure is controlled, this does not halt the progression of the disease – only delivery can do this, but it can reduce the incidence of complications such as cerebral haemorrhage.

Fluid restriction and fluid balance

Women with severe PET are very sensitive to fluid overload and are at risk of developing pulmonary oedema. Accurate monitoring of fluid intake (which normally includes restriction of fluids to approximately 80 mL/hour) and hourly urinary output is essential.

Magnesium sulphate

Magnesium sulphate is recommended as part of the treatment of women with severe PET, as it has a hypotensive effect but also is known to reduce the incidence of eclamptic seizures (Duley et al 2010). Midwives should follow a written protocol for administration. Complications of magnesium sulphate include sudden hypotension. Toxic levels may occur if there is renal impairment reducing the drug clearance. Signs and symptoms of magnesium sulphate toxicity would include loss of deep tendon reflexes, depressed respiratory rate, double vision, slurred speech, flushing, weakness, drowsiness or a reduced urine output. Magnesium sulphate toxicity can be treated with calcium gluconate IV, and the midwife should ensure this is easily available.

Labour care

Care and assessment of maternal and fetal well-being will continue as for other labouring women but with increased observations. Labour may be induced or a caesarean section indicated. An epidural may be advised because of the benefits it provides in terms of lowering of the blood pressure, although a pre-load fluid is normally omitted. Tests of coagulation are important in relation to siting and removal of epidural catheter and for any surgical intervention. Syntocinon should be given for third stage delivery because ergometrine causes a rise in blood pressure. A paediatrician or practitioner skilled in neonatal resuscitation must be present at the birth.

Emotional care

The woman must be kept informed and involved in all aspects of care, using information that is accessible and evidence-based. It is also important to include, if possible, a visit to the neonatal unit (NNU). Women and their families may be extremely anxious, and information, sensitive care and full involvement in decision-making are crucial for them.

Postnatal care

Frequent monitoring of maternal well-being will continue post-delivery and although delivery of the baby is seen as contributing to the resolution of PET, symptoms and complications persist into the initial postnatal period. The care outlined earlier will continue. Prophylaxis for venous thromboembolism is indicated (see Ch. 41).

The baby may have been delivered preterm and/or have complications related to IUGR. The challenge for the midwife will be to support mother-baby adaptation between an unwell mother and an unwell baby. Where possible, mother and baby should have some skin-to-skin contact before the baby is transferred to the neonatal unit. The midwife should facilitate good lines of communication between the NNU staff and the parents, ensuring they are kept informed regarding the care and the condition of the baby. A photograph of the baby for the mother to have with her is helpful. Expression of colostrum and breastmilk is a practical way the mother can contribute to the baby's well-being.

Follow-up

Women may be transferred into community care when their blood pressure is controlled, their symptoms have resolved and blood tests are within normal parameters. They may need to continue antihypertensive medication, and a plan of care should include how frequently their blood pressure needs to be measured and when their medication reviewed. Women will need information regarding the need to contact medical and/or midwifery care if symptoms reappear. Women who have had hypertension in pregnancy have an increased risk of developing hypertension and/or PET in subsequent pregnancies. The risk is increased (up to 1 in 4) where women have had severe complications of PET and birth before 34 weeks. For women who have severe PET with delivery before 28 weeks gestation, the risk of recurrence is even greater (up to 1 in 2). There is also an increased risk of developing hypertension in later life. Women are advised to aim to maintain their weight within a normal range BMI. The use of a prescribed daily dose of 75 mg of aspirin from 12 weeks gestation in subsequent pregnancies has been shown to reduce the incidence of PET in at risk pregnancies (Bujold et al 2010; NICE 2011a).

ANAEMIA

Anaemia is a deficiency in the quantity or quality of red blood cells (RBCs). It is estimated that 40% of pregnant women worldwide are anaemic (WHO 2008). Haemoglobin (Hb) is the protein structure in RBCs that carries oxygen to cells throughout the body. A woman is considered to be anaemic if she has an Hb less then 110 g/L in the first trimester, although a level of less than 105 g/L is more widely adopted in the second trimester when the physiological haemodilution of pregnancy is at its greatest. Postpartum anaemia is defined as Hb level less than 100 g/L (Pavord et al 2011).

Iron deficiency is the most common cause of anaemia in pregnancy but other nutritional deficiencies can affect RBC production, including a lack of folate and vitamin B_{12}. Excessive blood loss, particularly related to the third stage of labour, may leave women vulnerable to the effects of anaemia in the postnatal period. Box 54.7 lists the signs and symptoms of anaemia. The effect of anaemia on the woman and her infant can be significant, giving rise to a range of complications that can affect her sense of well-being and her ability to adapt to parenthood (see

Box 54.8). Other causes of anaemia include inherited or acquired disorders that affect Hb synthesis, red blood cell production or red blood cell survival (Bothamley and Boyle 2009). Sickle cell disease is a genetically inherited disorder that affects the structure of the Hb. Malaria and hookworm infestation are common causes of anaemia in resource-poor settings (Goonewardene et al 2012).

Investigations

The assessment and investigation of anaemia should aim to determine the underlying cause of the anaemia and direct treatment. The midwife should gather information such as general health, diet, blood loss, presence of infection and any other pre-existing conditions associated with anaemia. In the UK, it is recommended that the level of Hb is measured, as part of a full blood count (FBC), with the "booking" blood tests and repeated at 28 weeks gestation (NICE 2014). The Hb level is not the only test to consider in the diagnosis. Investigations will include measuring the mean cell volume (MCV), mean cell haemoglobin (MCH) and, most importantly, the serum ferritin level that reflects the woman's iron stores. Screening for haemoglobinopathies should be done at the same time. Postpartum women with an estimated blood loss over 500 mL, antenatal anaemia (unresolved) and any symptoms of anaemia should have their haemoglobin level checked within 48 hours of delivery.

Iron-deficiency anaemia

The requirement for iron increases significantly in pregnancy and although iron absorption from the gastrointestinal tract improves, women may not be able to

---

Box 54.7 Signs and symptoms of anaemia
Fatigue
Pallour of mucous membranes
Headaches
Irritability
Dizziness, fainting and weakness
Breathlessness on exertion
Palpitations
Digestive upsets and loss of appetite
Feeling colder than normal
Pica – craving for non-food items, such as ice and dirt

Box 54.8 Complications of anaemia in pregnancy and childbirth
Maternal complications
Preterm delivery
Placental abruption
Increased postpartum blood loss (secondary to impaired uterine muscle function)
Lower tolerance to blood loss
Increased susceptibility to infection
Poor work capacity and performance
Disturbances of postpartum cognition and emotion
Fetus and infant
Low birthweight
Iron deficiency in first 3 months of life
Impaired psychomotor and/or mental development
Source: Pavord 2011

consume adequate iron from dietary sources alone. Low iron stores before pregnancy are associated with an increased risk of anaemia during the latter half of pregnancy when demand for iron is greatest (Goonewardene et al 2012). The main risk factors for having low iron stores include poor intake of iron, poor absorption of iron and heavy blood loss from frequent menstruation and after birth.

Changes in diet to improve iron stores include consuming haem iron (iron derived from red meat, fish and poultry), increasing vitamin C (known to help absorption of iron) and avoiding tea and coffee with meals (known to interfere with absorption). Information regarding dietary sources of iron should be given verbally and backed up with written information in an appropriate language for the woman. However, despite these measures and depending on the iron stores before pregnancy, many women will require oral iron supplementation. Routine supplementation with iron is not recommended in the UK, although may be advocated in resource-poor settings where women are likely to have poor iron stores (Goonewardene et al 2012).

Management

Where anaemia is diagnosed, treatment with daily oral iron, commonly ferrous sulphate, is recommended. Women are advised to take their iron tablets with orange juice and on an empty stomach to maximize absorption. They should take care to keep their medication out of reach of young children. Women often find taking iron tablets unpleasant and report stomach upset, black stools and constipation. Iron tablets may be better tolerated if taken at night. Increasing the dose gradually or recommending a tablet with a smaller amount of iron may improve symptoms. Advice regarding avoiding constipation should be given (Jordan 2010).

Investigations for other causes of anaemia, including haemoglobinopathies, should be considered, and midwives should refer all cases where there are significant symptoms, severe anaemia (Hb less than 70 g/L) in late pregnancy or where there is failure to improve with oral treatment. Where oral iron treatment proves unsuitable, iron can be given intramuscularly, although this is rare, as the injection is very painful and may discolour the skin (Jordan 2010). Intravenous iron may be considered from the second trimester onwards in those women who do not respond to oral treatment. However, this route is associated with complications including anaphylaxis and, therefore, requires trained personnel to administer this (Pavord 2011). Blood transfusion is also used to treat severe anaemia, particularly after major obstetric haemorrhage.

Folic acid deficiency anaemia

Folic acid is essential for DNA synthesis and cell duplication. Folate requirements increase threefold in pregnancy and a deficiency can arise due to a poor diet or from conditions such as coeliac disease that causes malabsorption of nutrients from the gastrointestinal tract (Bothamley and Boyle 2009). Folic acid deficiency gives rise to megaloblastic anaemia whereby the RBCs are larger, misshapen and have a shorter survival time in the bloodstream.

Dietary sources of folate are lightly cooked green leafy vegetables, such as broccoli and spinach, fruit and nuts. After the demonstrated link between neural tube defects and intake of folic acid, all pregnant women, and those intending to become pregnant, are advised to take 400 micrograms folic acid daily (NICE 2014). A higher dose may be prescribed in those at risk (Jordan 2010).

HAEMOGLOBINOPATHIES

Haemoglobinopathies are inherited conditions in which one or more abnormal globin chain structures wholly or partly replace normal adult haemoglobin (HbA). Antenatal screening aims to identify women with haemoglobinopathies who will require specialist care in pregnancy and to offer couples who are carriers of the genetic variant, options for fetal screening. The main haemoglobinopathies that complicate pregnancy are sickle cell disease and thalassaemia.

Sickle cell disorders

When reviewing the inheritance for sickle cell disease, an abnormal allele is denoted S (sickle haemoglobin) and a healthy allele is denoted A (adult haemoglobin). An individual inherits two alleles for each gene, one from each parent. The most serious combination relevant to pregnancy is sickle cell disease (HbSS), but the sickle allele can combine with other Hb variants (see Ch. 26). When a person is sickle cell trait (HbAS), they are healthy but can pass the abnormal gene to their offspring. Box 54.9 lists some of the possible combinations. Sickle cell variants have their origins in sub-Saharan Africa and the Middle East. Sickle cell trait is thought to provide some protection against malaria. Because of population migration, the variant is increasingly found in European populations.

Sickle cell disease results in life-long complications, linked to premature destruction of red blood cells and sickling crises. Features of pregnancy predispose to an increase in sickling crises associated with childbirth. Box 54.10 lists both the long-term and pregnancy-related complications of sickle cell disease. Box 54.11 lists triggers to sickling crises relevant to pregnancy.

Box 54.9 Possible genetic combinations of haemoglobin with reference to sickle cell disorders

HbAA	Normal adult haemoglobin
HbAS	Sickle cell trait – normally healthy, although they need to avoid significant dehydration, may have an increased incidence of urinary tract infection and a slightly higher risk of thromboembolism in pregnancy. May pass on abnormal allele to offspring and, therefore, partner testing advised.
HbSS	Sickle cell anaemia – chronic condition featuring painful sickling crisis, complications and anaemia
Hb SC	Haemoglobin SC disease
Hb S β Thal	Sickle beta thalassaemia

Source: Bothamley and Boyle 2009

Box 54.10 Complications of sickle cell disease

Long-term (women may have these before pregnancy and assessment in the preconception period is advised)

- Chronic anaemia
- Damage to the spleen, increasing vulnerability to infection
- Gallstone formation
- Joint damage
- Renal, liver, cardiac and respiratory disorders
- Cerebrovascular accidents (stroke)

Pregnancy-related

- Increased risk of vascular complications, including increased sickling crisis
- Urinary tract infection
- Acute chest syndrome
- Blood transfusion
- Admission to critical care unit
- Higher incidence of placental abruption and placenta praevia
- Higher incidence of hypertension and pre-eclampsia
- Higher incidence of venous thromboembolism
- Maternal anaemia, leading to fetal/newborn anaemia
- Hypoperfusion of the placental circulation as a result of sickling in the uterine placental decidua, leading to fetal hypoxia and IUGR
- Preterm and operative delivery more likely

Source: Oteng-Ntim et al 2015; Howard and Oteng-Ntim 2012

Box 54.11 Triggers to sickling crises in pregnancy and childbirth

- Infection
- Sudden change in temperature – cold or hot
- Dehydration – related to nausea and vomiting in early pregnancy and labour
- Physical exertion
- Hypoxia – related to illness and anaemia
- Psychological stress

Management

Preconception and antenatal care

The best possible outcome for women with sickle cell disease will be when a specialist multidisciplinary team, including a haematologist, a specialist haemoglobinopathies nurse, an obstetrician and a midwife liaise effectively to provide care. Box 54.12 lists some of the key features to be considered in both the preconception period and during antenatal care. Midwives will be involved with supporting the woman through a complex pregnancy, assisting in surveillance of maternal and fetal well-being and responding promptly to incidences of critical ill health. Box 54.13 identifies the key points of care during a sickling crisis.

Reflective activity 54.3

Consider the midwives' responsibilities when a woman with sickle cell is admitted with a sickling crisis in pregnancy. Think of the immediate response to her physical care and psychological support.

Labour and postnatal care

The tenets of care in labour centre around the need for good psychological support and maximizing care to avoid triggers to crises. The will include promoting hydration, encouraging mobilization, maintaining good aseptic techniques to avoid infection, preventing excess blood loss and promoting a vaginal birth.

There is a higher risk for thrombosis in the postpartum period, so early mobilization, effective pain relief, hydration and thromboprophylaxis are important. Women will be high risk for complications and the midwife will need to maintain regular observations and refer as indicated. Breastfeeding should be encouraged. Couples may be offered early Hb electrophoresis testing of the newborn, although the newborn blood spot sample will also provide information regarding the infant's Hb status. Contraception should be discussed.

Box 54.12 Key features to be considered in the preconception period and antenatal care

- Advice to women about the challenges of pregnancy to her own health and fetal well-being
- Implications for the genetic inheritance for her offspring – offer partner testing
- Need for investigations of existing or developing organ damage to the renal, liver, cardiac and respiratory systems
- Screen for pre-eclampsia
- Retinal screening
- Monitoring of fetal growth and well-being
- Review of anaemia and need for prescribed folic acid therapy. Avoid iron overload
- Blood tests for red blood cell antibodies and plans for obtaining cross-matched blood, should the need arise
- Review need for exchange blood transfusions
- Risk assessment for thromboprophylaxis
- Review of any medications to ensure suitability for pregnancy and breastfeeding
- Review of antibiotic prophylaxis and screening for common infections, including urinary tract infections
- Vaccinations, avoiding live attenuated vaccines in pregnancy
- Psychological support

Source: Royal College of Obstetricians and Gynaecologists (RCOG) 2011a; Oteng-Ntim et al 2012

Thalassaemia

Thalassaemia refers to a number of genetic conditions, common in people of Mediterranean and Asian origin, that cause abnormal Hb development. A defect in the alpha-globin chain (alpha-thalassaemia) or beta-globin chains (beta-thalassaemia) result in thin, short-lived red blood cells, often misshapen and deficient in Hb, causing anaemia. In the UK, all women are screened for thalassaemia at booking and partner testing offered for those found to be carrying an abnormal Hb variant.

In pregnancy, for those with alpha-thalassaemia trait, normal antenatal care is usually sufficient, whereas those with beta-thalassaemia trait may need extra iron supplements if they are iron deficient. Closer surveillance of fetal growth and well-being is advised. Beta-thalassaemia major is a chronic condition requiring repeated blood transfusions, regular drug therapy, and women with this will require significant specialist care (RCOG 2014).

Box 54.13 Key points of care during a sickling crisis

- Prompt involvement of specialist MDT
- Prompt pain management
- Assessment and treatment of any underling cause or complications of the crises
- Frequent monitoring of maternal and fetal well-being. Use of a MEOWS chart and including frequent assessment for pain
- Oxygen saturation monitoring and facial oxygen as required
- Careful fluid balance, avoiding dehydration
- Ensure stable temperature
- Thromboprophylaxis

CARDIAC DISORDERS

Cardiac disease remains the largest single cause of maternal deaths, with 51 women dying of cardiac causes in the period from 2012–2014 (Nair and Knight 2016). A wide range of conditions affect the heart in a mild, moderate or severe way, and conditions may be generally divided into conditions that are congenital (existing at birth) or acquired (secondary to complications such as infection or obesity). Some women with severe cardiac disease are counselled to avoid pregnancy. The physiological changes in pregnancy that include increased plasma volume, increased cardiac output, increased stroke volume, increased heart rate and enhanced coagulation pose considerable threat to women with significant pre-existing heart disease. However, many women who have had congenital heart defects corrected as a child are now embarking on successful pregnancies, particularly when their care is managed by joint expert specialist cardiac and obstetric service. More recently, some of the poorest outcomes in relation to cardiac disease in pregnancy have involved women who have structurally normal hearts but died from myocardial infarction and ischaemic heart disease linked to lifestyle factors such as increased maternal age, obesity and smoking. Table 54.2 outlines some cardiac conditions affecting pregnant women.

Midwives need to be aware that women may present with previously undiagnosed cardiac disease. Some degree of breathlessness can be normal in pregnancy but could be a sign of a cardiac disorder. Box 54.14 lists signs and symptoms that may indicate cardiac disease. Referral to appropriate medical help is required.

Preconception assessment

All women with known heart disease are recommended to have preconception care with a specialist cardiac obstetric team. For some women, this assessment will result in advice against pregnancy. Adjustments before pregnancy

Table 54.2 Cardiac conditions affecting pregnant women

Rheumatic heart disease (RHD)	May affect woman born outside UK Damages heart valves
Valve disorders Mitral stenosis	Congenitally acquired or from RHD
Aortic regurgitation Aortic stenosis Mitral valve prolapse	Prosthetic valves – vulnerable to thrombosis in pregnancy
Infective endocarditis	Those who have had previous cardiac surgery vulnerable
Marfan syndrome	Genetic disorder of connective tissue Prone to mitral prolapse, mitral or aortic regurgitation and aortic dissection/rupture
Congenital heart disease • Atrial septal defects • Ventricular septal defects • Patent ductus arteriosus • Tetralogy of Fallot • Aortic coarctation • Pulmonary stenosis • Transposition of great arteries	Many conditions are now successfully treated in childhood Require assessment before pregnancy Genetic disposition; assessment of fetus advised
Eisenmenger's syndrome and *pulmonary hypertension*	Arise from untreated congenital defects High mortality rate and pregnancy usually not advised
Cardiomyopathy • Ventricular dysfunction • Peripartum cardiomyopathy	May be caused by thickening or dilation of muscle walls in heart Rare and serious complication of pregnancy
Ischaemic heart disease • Coronary arterial disease • Myocardial infarction	Associated with diabetes, obesity, smoking, high cholesterol, advanced maternal age and family history

Source: Bothamley and Boyle 2009 (b) originally published in Midwives August/September 2009 issue. Reprinted with permission.

Box 54.14 Signs and symptoms that may indicate cardiac disease

- Breathlessness of sudden onset
- Breathlessness associated with chest pain
- Breathlessness when lying down or during the night
- Increased respiratory rate
- Unexplained tachycardia
- Hypotension
- Chest pain
- Palpitations associated with symptoms such as collapse or fainting

Sources: Vause et al 2016; Bothamley and Boyle 2009b

---

may include surgical correction and valve replacement (Windram et al 2014). Changes to medication may be required to avoid drugs, such as warfarin, which are harmful to the developing fetus (Mohan and Nelson-Piercy 2014a).

Antenatal care

The multidisciplinary team in pregnancy should include a cardiologist, an obstetrician, an anaesthetist, a fetal-medicine specialist, a haematologist, a neonatologist, a specialist midwife and a cardiac nurse. If the woman has not had preconception care, the midwife needs to arrange referral to specialist care promptly. The team should document a clear plan of care, as provision for women with cardiac disease will vary.

Assessment of a woman's cardiac health may include a regular assessment of her heart rhythm, auscultation of the heart sounds, listening to lung bases, measurement of cardiac enzymes (Troponin), and the use of technology such as echocardiograms, computed tomographic pulmonary angiograms (CTPAs) or electrocardiograms (ECGs).

The medical team will evaluate the woman's drug regimen throughout the antenatal period. Risk of venous thromboembolism is increased for woman with cardiac conditions in pregnancy and the need for thromboprophylaxis will require ongoing consideration.

Midwives should perform assessment of blood pressure, heart rate, respiratory rate, temperature and oxygen saturations at each antenatal visit and more regularly as indicated, especially if admitted to hospital. Most cardiac conditions carry an increased risk of pre-eclampsia and IUGR (Windram et al 2014); therefore, regular antenatal midwifery assessment is required. Prompt referral to senior medical staff is needed should the midwife identify any signs and symptoms of deteriorating cardiac health, such as dyspnoea, cough or chest pain.

Psychological support provided by the midwife that acknowledges the normal aspects of her pregnancy and the anticipation of parenthood is fundamental. Women and their partners need help, information and easy access to services during what may be a particularly anxious time. Weight control is important, as excessive weight gain places extra strain on the heart. Infection needs to be identified early and treated with antibiotics to reduce the risk of bacterial endocarditis; dental work, which may be a potential source of infection, should be carried out early in pregnancy.

Tests to screen for fetal cardiac anomalies should be discussed with the woman. There may be a risk to the fetus of inherited cardiac conditions, and some drugs taken by women with cardiac disease also carry a possibility of teratogenicity. Tests may include nuchal translucency, fetal echocardiography, regular assessment of fetal growth and Doppler examinations (Swan 2014).

Labour care

Most women with heart diseases are able to have a normal vaginal birth, although plans for birth in an obstetric-led unit are strongly advised because of the increased cardiac demands of labour (Windram et al 2014). Women with more complex conditions are likely to need the time of birth planned or elective CS may be recommended. For woman on therapeutic anticoagulants, timing of medication requires close monitoring (McLintock 2014). Epidural analgesia is recommended but with caution in regard to hypotension and the degree of anticoagulation. Table 54.3 lists some key elements of management to consider when caring for a woman with cardiac disease in labour.

The time immediately after the birth of the baby is the time of most significant haemodynamic instability. Despite blood loss at delivery, cardiac output remains significantly elevated above pregnancy levels for 1 to 2 hours postpartum with peak cardiac output occurring immediately after birth (Blackburn 2013). Postpartum haemorrhage, with potential

for substantial loss of blood volume, can compromise cardiac function. Oxytocic drugs have major haemodynamic effects and need to be used with caution (Mohan and Nelson-Piercy 2014a). Pulmonary oedema can develop in women with pre-eclampsia and/or fluid overload. Close monitoring in an HDU area should continue after delivery, although the midwife should encourage skin-to-skin contact early by feeding the baby. The demands of the mother's physical care should not exclude her experience of the normal joys of parenting.

Postnatal care

Continuing close observation of vital signs is necessary, as complications may occur in the first few days postnatally. Measures to prevent thromboembolism, including effective pain relief to ensure early mobilization, adequate hydration and thromboprophylaxis are important aspects of postnatal care.

The risk of congenital heart disease in the baby is increased and, therefore, careful examination of the baby and early paediatric referral is essential.

Careful plans should be made for transfer to the community. Women need practical help to enable them to rest and cope with the demands of the baby. An appointment should be made with the cardiologist 4 to 6 weeks postnatally to assess cardiac function. The combined oestrogen-progesterone contraceptive pill is associated with increased risk of VTE and hypertension for some women with cardiac disease; therefore, a discussion regarding contraception, planning of pregnancies and a reminder of the benefit for preconception counselling is required (Mohan and Nelson-Piercy 2014a).

THYROID DISORDERS

At least 2% to 3% of women are affected by thyroid dysfunction so the midwife is likely to encounter women with disorders of the thyroid in pregnancy (Girling and Sykes 2013). Thyroid hormones triiodothyronine (T3) and thyroxine (T4) control metabolism and have a key role in growth and development. By 4 to 6 weeks gestation, there is an increase in the production of thyroid hormones. The thyroid gland enlarges and iodine requirements increase threefold. Untreated thyroid disorders are associated with infertility, increased early pregnancy loss and adverse pregnancy and neonatal outcomes. Fetal neurological development depends on adequate thyroid hormone in the first 12 weeks gestation (Jefferys et al 2015).

There are numerous causes of thyroid disorders and they are categorized into low levels of thyroid hormone (hypothyroid) or high levels (hyperthyroid). Table 54.4 lists some of the features of thyroid disorders and possible signs and symptoms in untreated individuals.

Table 54.3 Key elements of the management of a woman with cardiac disease in labour

Analgesia and anaesthesia	Regional anaesthesia normally recommended to ease the exertion and pain of labour Caution: fluid shift, anticoagulation
Position	Avoid aortocaval compression Upright left lateral is best
Fluid balance	Vital importance to maintain strict fluid balance Use fluid pumps for greater accuracy
Monitoring maternal well-being	Regular frequent assessment of BP, pulse, respiratory rate and oxygen saturations May require central venous pressure (CVP) monitoring, arterial line (BP and blood gases) and ECG
Fetal monitoring	Continuous CTG
Shortened second stage	Avoid Valsalva manoeuvre – elective instrumental delivery may be indicated
Oxytocic agents should be used with caution. The medical team present should prescribe the medication required for the management of the third stage	Slow infusion of diluted oxytocin is recommended as an alternative to a bolus dose. Ergometrine and carboprost are contraindicated (Mohan and Nelson-Piercy 2014a)
Strict aseptic technique	
Risk assessment for antibiotic cover	According to the agreed care plan, based on the risk of endocarditis
Antiembolism stockings	

Hyperthyroidism

Gestational thyrotoxicosis is the most common cause of hyperthyroidism in the first trimester. It just occurs for a short time because of high levels of HCG and is noted in women with hyperemesis gravidarum and multiple pregnancies. Treatment is supportive with hydration and antiemetics until symptoms resolve when HCG levels fall around 12 weeks gestation (Pearce 2015).

Graves' disease usually predates pregnancy but may arise for the first time in the first or early second trimester. If untreated, there is an increased risk of complications (see Table 54.4). In women who are poorly controlled, there is a risk of a thyroid crisis, or 'storm', with hyperpyrexia, palpitations, chest pain and tachycardia, which may lead to heart failure (Sullivan and Goodier 2013).

An endocrine specialist should direct treatment with antithyroid drugs, such as *carbimazole* or *propylthiouracil* (PTU). Both drugs cross the placenta (PTU less so) and may cause fetal hypothyroidism and/or goitre. The aim of treatment is to control maternal symptoms on the lowest possible dose of antithyroid medication. A specialist should discuss the implications of the medication on fetal development and the effect on the fetus if maternal hyperthyroidism is not controlled. Full thyroid function tests should be taken before conception, when pregnancy is confirmed at booking, at least monthly during pregnancy and in the postnatal period. In a third of women, Graves' disease goes into remission in pregnancy and the antithyroid drugs can be discontinued (Pearce 2015).

During the antenatal period, assessment of maternal heart rate, weight gain and experience of nausea and vomiting should be carried out. Clinical assessment of the fetus includes listening to the fetal heart, monitoring for IUGR and may include serial ultrasound scans to assess growth and to detect goitre (Pearce 2015). Breastfeeding is usually recommended but where medication is prescribed, these need to be reviewed for safety. Monitoring of the infant's development and thyroid function is advised (Jordan 2010).

Table 54.4 Thyroid disorders

	Hyperthyroidism (↑T3 and T4) Increased basal metabolic rate	Hypothyroidism (↓T3 and T4) Decreased metabolic rate

Causes	Autoimmune – Graves' disease (most common)
	Transient gestational hyperthyroidism
	Toxic adenoma
	Iatrogenic – caused by treatment with
	  thyroxine medication
		Autoimmune – Hashimoto's disease (most common)
		Iodine deficiency
		Previous thyroidectomy
		After surgery or radioactive iodine treatment for
		  hyperthyroidism

Signs and
  Symptoms
	Weight loss with good appetite. Fatigue
	Anxiety, physical restlessness, nervousness,
	  excessively emotional
	Hair loss
	Fast pulse, heart palpitations, breathlessness
	Intolerance to heat; warm, sweaty skin
	
	Diarrhoea
	Exophthalmos (protrusion of the eyes) in
	  Graves' disease
	Oligomenorrhoea or amenorrhoea
		Weight gain and poor appetite. Fatigue
		Mental sluggishness, depression, lethargy, psychosis
		
		Dry skin, brittle hair
		Slow, weak pulse
		Dry, cold skin; poor tolerance to cold. Puffy
		  appearance on face hands and feet
		Constipation
		
		Anovulation

Treatment	Thionamides (antithyroid medication) Radioactive iodine – contraindicated in pregnancy Surgery – unusual in pregnancy	Thyroxine
Complications in pregnancy	Miscarriage IUGR Preterm delivery Preeclampisa Fetal thyrotoxicosis Thyroid storm and heart failure	Miscarriage Hypertension Preterm delivery Stillbirth Decreased child intelligence

Source: Blackburn 2013; Bothamley and Boyle 2009; Girling and Sykes 2013

Hypothyroidism

Hypothyroidism occurs in about 3% of pregnancies and is most commonly caused by an autoimmune condition known as *Hashimoto's thyroiditis*. Women who have symptoms and/or are not on treatment are at risk of adverse outcomes (see Table 54.4).

Treatment is by thyroxine supplementation, and when well controlled, there are no adverse effects on pregnancy. Medication is particularly important during the first 12 weeks gestation, a crucial time for fetal neurological development. Thyroid function is normally checked at booking and measured again with routine tests at 28 weeks gestation. Alterations to the dose of medication is not normally required in pregnancy and they can continue with their medication while breastfeeding. Some women, for example, those who have had a thyroidectomy for thyroid cancer, may require dose adjustment in pregnancy.

Thyroxine absorption is reduced by iron and calcium so should be taken separate to other supplements (Girling and Sykes 2013).

RENAL DISORDERS

Marked changes to the physiology and anatomy of the renal system are required to support the physiological demands of pregnancy (Box 54.15). The most common complications of the renal system are urinary tract infections (UTI) and renal stones. *E coli* (a normal commensal organism of the rectum) causes UTI in up to 90% of cases. Preterm labour and sepsis are serious yet preventable consequences of a UTI in pregnancy. Table 54.5 lists types of UTI and the implications of these infections and renal stones in pregnancy and recommended

Table 54.5 Urinary tract infections and renal stones

	Features	Implications for pregnancy	Management
Asymptomatic bacteriuria (ASB) Clinically significant numbers of bacteria but no clinical symptoms Affects 4%–7% of pregnancies	No symptoms Only identified with routine screening	Increased risk of pyelonephritis Preterm birth	Send midstream urine sample for microscopy, culture and sensitivity (MC&S) at booking Antibiotic treatment for 5–7 days if diagnosed. Ensure adequate fluid intake Follow-up urine samples to ensure initial cure and to identify any recurrence
Cystitis Significant bacteriuria with symptoms. Affects 1% of pregnancies	Symptoms: dysuria, urinary frequency, urgency, haematuria	Increased risk of pyelonephritis Preterm birth	Send midstream urine sample for MC&S to confirm diagnosis, although the presence of nitrates and leucocytes on dipstick, accompanied with classical symptoms, will usually be enough to initiate treatment Antibiotic treatment. Ensure adequate fluid intake Follow-up urine samples to ensure initial cure and to identify any recurrence
Pyelonephritis Significant bacteriuria with systemic illness and symptoms	Symptoms: abdominal or flank pain, urinary symptoms	Increased risk of preterm labour Preterm rupture of membranes Low birthweight Sepsis Acute respiratory syndrome	Admission for IV antibiotics within 1 hour of being assessed Urine and blood cultures Sepsis bundle as indicated IV fluids Paracetamol Ultrasound to identify any underlying cause Follow-up urine samples to ensure initial cure and to identify any recurrence Recurrence rate 10%–18%
Urolithiasis (renal stones) Around 1 in 250 pregnancies	Signs and symptoms: colicky flank pain and haematuria. Other symptoms: include fever, nausea and vomiting and signs of UTI	Preterm labour May cause UTI, which can lead to pyelonephritis and reduced renal function	Up to 80% renal stones are passed spontaneously with analgesia, hydration and antibiotics for any infective complications Urine dipstick and culture is useful to investigate for infective complications of a stone but is not diagnostic Multidisciplinary input from urology specialists

Source: Cox and Reid (2015)

Box 54.15 Changes related to the urinary system in pregnancy

- Marked dilation of ureters and renal calyces that increases urinary stasis
- Pressure from enlarging uterus and displacement of bladder
- Increased glomerular filtration rate (GFR)
- Changes to tubular handling of certain substances
- Increased potential for bladder damage and urinary tract infection

Box 54.16 Conditions that may cause chronic renal disease

- Glomerulonephritis (acute or chronic)
- Polycystic renal disease
- Chronic pyelonephritis
- Diabetic nephropathy
- Systemic lupus erythematosus
- Congenital abnormality of the lower urinary tract
- Solitary kidney
- Nephrotic syndrome

Source: Piccoli et al 2015

Box 54.17 Complications associated with renal disease in pregnancy

Maternal
- Deterioration of renal function
- Increased thrombosis
- Increased risk of ascending UTI, leading to pyelonephritis and sepsis
- Hypertension
- Pre-eclampsia

Fetus/newborn
- Prematurity
- Fetal IUGR
- Inheritance of maternal renal disorders
- Side effects of maternal medication/treatment

Source: Piccoli et al 2015; Hall and Brunskill 2013

Box 54.18 Midwifery care for women with renal disorders

- Information given on how to collect an accurate MSU and 24-hour urine collection.
- Equipment and instructions for home assessment for protein as appropriate, although a protein–creatinine ratio commonly used.
- Information concerning a healthy diet and lifestyle to improve immunity, avoid infections and prevent anaemia.
- Hygiene technique – wiping front to back after using the toilet to prevent faecal contamination of urethra.
- Keep adequately hydrated – advice to limit fluids may apply in some situations, including PET.
- Maintenance of accurate fluid balance in appropriate situations.
- Ensure women have information regarding symptoms of PET and signs of premature labour, and who to contact if any concerns arise.
- Avoidance of catheterization and impeccable technique if necessary.
- Risk assessment and advice about preventing thromboembolism.
- Psychological support and recognition of the normal aspects of her pregnancy and the anticipation of parenthood.
- Advice and referral regarding follow-up, future pregnancies, contraception and need for preconception care.

Source: Bothamley and Boyle 2009

management. Box 54.16 lists chronic renal conditions. Successful pregnancy for woman with chronic renal disease will depend on prepregnancy renal function. Common complications include hypertension, pre-eclampsia, preterm delivery and a worsening on their renal function (see Box 54.17). Box 54.18 discusses some key principles of midwifery care for women with renal conditions.

Chronic renal disorders

Pregnancy, for women with renal disease, may be detrimental to their health, causing deterioration of their renal function and a poor pregnancy outcome (see Box 54.17). Those women with declining renal impairment (defined by serum creatinine levels), hypertension and proteinuria before pregnancy are more at risk. As with all chronic conditions, preconception care should be available to ensure these women have their condition assessed, medications reviewed and health optimized before becoming pregnant.

Antenatal care

Women will require frequent assessment at a multidisciplinary specialist clinic. Renal function should be closely monitored with regular blood and urine tests. Urine testing may involve a 24-hour urine collection, although this has largely been replaced by measurement of protein: creatinine ratio (PCR) on a single specimen. Women may be taught to test their own urine in between antenatal visits.

The midwife should remain involved in the woman's care as an important source of psychological support and advice about the general aspects of pregnancy. The midwife will carry out regular screening for urinary tract infections, blood pressure monitoring, early identification of any signs and symptoms of pre-eclampsia and fetal assessment. The classical features of pre-eclampsia; hypertension and proteinuria may be pre-existing in women with renal disease, making it more difficult to distinguish the development of superimposed pre-eclampsia (Piccoli et al 2015). The midwife can give information to the woman about recognizing pre-eclampsia and signs of early labour, including whom to contact if concerns arise.

As the renal system is responsible for production of erythropoietin (necessary for haemoglobin), anaemia is screened regularly.

Medications that may be prescribed include antihypertensive drugs, prophylactic antibiotics, low-dose aspirin and low molecular weight heparin thromboprophylaxis (Lightstone 2011).

Increased fetal surveillance, including regular growth scans and Doppler studies, is indicated.

If renal function declines to the stage where dialysis is required, the woman may be offered the choice of terminating the pregnancy, but her renal function may continue to decline even after the pregnancy is stopped. Dialysis is possible during pregnancy but it is a very high-risk process (Hall and Brunskill 2013).

Labour care

As a result of compromised renal function, fluid overload can occur at any time for the woman with renal disease; however, this is much more likely in labour when intravenous fluids are commonly used. This may increase hypertension and ultimately lead to pulmonary oedema. Observation for respiratory signs and symptoms (shortness of breath, raising respiratory rate, decreased oxygen saturation levels, frothy sputum and crackles heard during lung auscultation) is necessary. Strict fluid balance must be observed and documented clearly. Fluid restriction may be applied.

Regular assessment using a MEOWS chart is indicated. Cardiac monitoring may be undertaken during labour, depending on the woman's condition, and abnormalities may represent increasing serum potassium that will need to be speedily reversed. Arterial blood gas analysis may indicate metabolic acidosis, and this may also need rapid treatment.

Postnatal care

As with all medical conditions, breastfeeding is encouraged but a review of any medication being taken must be undertaken first – and this should have been done during pregnancy to enable feeding to commence immediately after birth.

Renal assessment will continue as necessary, and the midwife should ensure that appropriate follow-up is organized. Contraception should be discussed.

Renal transplant

Growing numbers of women are embarking on pregnancy after organ transplant (Bramham et al 2013b). After successful transplant fertility improves and contraception is recommended initially. Women are advised to delay pregnancy until 1 to 2 years after transplant when their health is optimum, blood pressure is normal, suppressive medication is at maintenance levels and there is no sign of graft rejection. Information about the possible effect of any pregnancy on their health, the graft and their offspring needs to be discussed fully with the woman and her family. A recent review of the pregnancies of women after renal transplant concluded that most pregnancies are successful, but the rate of maternal and neonatal complications are relatively high, with 77% (n = 81) of women having a good outcome, which was defined as a live birth after 32 weeks gestation. For the remaining 23% (n = 24) of women with poor outcomes, including first or second trimester loss, neonatal death and congenital abnormalities were reported (Bramham et al 2013b). Box 54.19 lists the complications for mother and her offspring based on this UK study. Poorer outcomes occurred in women who had more than one previous transplant, a serum creatinine > 125 µmol/L in the first trimester and a raised diastolic BP.

Box 54.19   Complications of pregnancy after renal transplant

Complications of pregnancy after a renal transplant for mother and her offspring based on UKOSS study are as follows:

- Preterm birth (50%)
- Caesarean delivery (72%)
- Pre-eclampsia (24%)
- New hypertension in pregnancy (16%)
- Admission to HDU/ITU (20%)
- Small for gestation age (24%)

Bramham et al 2013b

A nephrologist, an obstetrician and a member of the transplant team should direct the care for the woman; however, the woman still requires midwifery care and support. The detail regarding care will be similar to that given to women with chronic renal disorders (as discussed under the section *chronic renal disorders*) with additional concerns related to increased risks (Box 54.19), problems associated with immunosuppressive medication and monitoring for graft rejection.

Immunosuppressive medication increases the risk of infection and may increase the development of gestational diabetes (Deshpande et al 2011). The midwife should assess the woman and seek to prevent all types of infection through hand washing, strict asepsis when indicated, regular assessment and clinical evaluation of any relevant signs and symptoms. Prophylactic antibiotics would be considered.

Normal vaginal birth is possible although rates of CS are high. A lower segment CS may be more difficult because of the position of the transplanted ureter (Hall and Brunskill 2013).

Neonatal problems include those associated with prematurity. The safety of breastfeeding while on immunosuppressive medication is unknown and individual assessment of medication needs to be made and discussed with the woman (Lightstone 2011).

Acute renal failure

Acute renal failure (ARF) is an abrupt reduction in renal function and is usually associated with persistent, diminished, urine output of less than 30 mL per hour and less than 400 mL per day. It can occur in those with known renal compromise, in women with serious illness, in conjunction with another pregnancy complication, such as haemorrhage and pre-eclampsia or because of obstruction/damage to the renal system. Monitoring urinary output is part of routine care, particularly in a woman who is unwell or after surgery, so any deviation from normal urine output should be identified early and appropriate referral made (Bothamley and Boyle 2009). Serum screening (electrolytes and renal function tests) and possibly renal ultrasound, if obstruction is suspected, will establish the diagnosis. Management depends on the cause, which may be prerenal (e.g. hypovolaemia) or renal (tubular or cortical necrosis). Emphasis is on avoiding and/or treating raised levels of urea and other waste products in the blood, acidosis, hyperkalaemia and fluid overload. Central venous pressure (CVP) will be required to guide fluid balance and prevent fluid overload. Renal dialysis may be needed.

DIABETES

Diabetes is a disorder of glucose metabolism. In diabetes, a lack of insulin or an increase in insulin resistance means that body cells are unable to utilize glucose, thus depriving them of energy and causing a rise in blood sugar levels. In the UK, 5% of pregnancies are complicated by diabetes and there are 3 main types that affect women of childbearing age (see Box 54.20) (NICE 2015). Women may embark on pregnancy with pre-existing type 1 or type

---

Box 54.20 Types of diabetes

Type 1 diabetes (T1DM)

This occurs mainly in young adults and the onset is usually sudden. There is a complete lack of insulin that is thought to arise from the autoimmune destruction of the insulin-producing beta cells in the pancreas. A lack of insulin leads to hyperglycaemia (high blood sugar). Classic symptoms of untreated T1DM includes glycosuria (glucose in the urine), polyuria (increased urine output), polydipsia (increased thirst), increased hunger, ketosis and weight loss. Untreated, or poorly controlled T1DM, can lead to metabolic acidosis, coma and death. Long-term multisystem, microvascular complications caused by the high levels of blood glucose include hypertension, retinopathy (causing problems with vision), nephropathy (causing deterioration in renal function) and neuropathy.

Type 2 diabetes (T2DM)

T2DM is characterized by hyperglycaemia (high blood sugar) in the context of insulin resistance and a relative lack of insulin. In the past, it developed mostly in older age but more recently is associated with obesity in the younger population. Some ethnic groups (for example south Asian, African, Afro-Caribbean) are more likely to develop T2DM, indicating a genetic predisposition. Symptoms may be thirst, hunger and frequent urination, although the condition develops slowly and the diagnosis is, therefore, frequently delayed. Diet changes, weight loss and an increase in exercise may be enough to control blood sugar levels within a normal range. Women with T2DM should check their blood sugars regularly and may require oral hypoglycaemic agents, such as metformin, or, if further deterioration occurs, insulin injections may be needed.

Gestational diabetes

Gestational diabetes is hyperglycaemia that is first recognized during pregnancy. The risk factors for developing gestational diabetes are the same as type 2 diabetes and include raised BMI, family history of diabetes, certain ethnic groups and a previous macrocosmic baby. Screening is recommended to identify women with gestational diabetes (see section *Testing for gestational diabetes*).

2 diabetes but the majority of diabetes in pregnancy (87.5%) is gestational diabetes (NICE 2015). This is when women with an underlying predisposition to developing diabetes acquire a level of carbohydrate intolerance and/or features of diabetes in pregnancy. Considerable changes to carbohydrate metabolism, driven by placental hormones, occur in pregnancy. These changes help the woman's body prepare for labour and breastfeeding by laying down fat stores in the first trimester and aid fetal growth in the second and third trimester. Essentially, pregnancy acts like a 'stress test' for diabetes. Most women adapt to these changes but others develop a degree of carbohydrate intolerance measured as raised blood sugars on an oral glucose tolerance test (OGTT). These physiological changes will also pose challenges to those women with pre-existing diabetes that will affect their diet, activity and medication.

Lifestyle factors, including changes in diet and a reduction in activity, has led to increased levels of obesity in the general population and has contributed to a rise in the number of women of childbearing age developing type 2 diabetes and gestational diabetes. Diabetes may cause complications for both mother and fetus/newborn (see Box 54.21), although these can be minimized by optimum diabetic control and specialist care before and during pregnancy.

Testing for gestational diabetes

An oral glucose tolerance test (OGTT) involves instructing a woman to fast overnight (water is permitted). A blood test is taken in the morning to measure the fasting blood sugar. After the ingestion of a measured 75 g glucose drink or food, another blood test is taken 2 hours later. Box 54.22 lists the indications for an OGTT. The test may be done soon after booking and/or repeated at 24 to 28 weeks pregnancy when the effect of the pregnancy related changes are higher.

Gestational diabetes is confirmed if the woman has either a fasting blood glucose level of 5.6 mmol/L or above or a 2-hour blood glucose level of 7.8 mmol/L or above (NICE 2015). Women diagnosed with gestational diabetes will require referral to the diabetic clinic within 1 week. They will need referral to a dietician, support and instruction in measuring their blood sugar levels, increasing exercise and review of the need for medication.

Management of diabetes

Preconception care

Ideally, a multidisciplinary team, including obstetricians, endocrinologists, diabetic specialist nurses, specialist midwives and a dietician will be involved in the care of diabetic woman before and during pregnancy. Although long recognized as an important part of a successful pregnancy, preconception counselling is received by only about one-third of diabetic women (CEMACH 2007; Murphy et al 2011).

Box 54.21 Complications of diabetes in pregnancy

Maternal complications

- Miscarriage
- Maternal hypoglycaemia (in T1DM in early pregnancy)
- Infection
- Diabetic ketoacidosis (DKA)
- Pre-eclampsia
- Polyhydramnios
- Preterm labour
- Deterioration of diabetic retinopathy, nephropathy
- Operative delivery

Fetal/newborn complications

- Congenital abnormality
- Stillbirth
- Macrosomia
- Those related to preterm birth
- Birth injury (related to shoulder dystocia)
- Neonatal hypoglycaemia
- Polycythaemia
- Respiratory distress syndrome
- Increased perinatal mortality

Source: McCance 2015; Hawthorne 2011

Box 54.22 Indications for an OGTT

- Previous large baby weighing 4.5 kg or more
- History of diabetes in first-degree relatives, i.e. mother, father or siblings
- Body mass index (BMI) of 30 kg/m^2 or above
- Previous gestational diabetes (testing required as soon as possible after booking and repeated 24 to 28 weeks)
- Ethnic origin (black Caribbean, South Asian and Middle Eastern and any other high-risk ethnic groups)
- Glycosuria 1 + on two or more occasions or 2 + on one occasion

Source: NICE 2015

The aims of preconception care include supporting the woman to optimize blood sugar levels, with the aim to achieve Hb A1c less than 6.5% (NICE 2015), although less than 7% may be a more realistic level for those on insulin (International Diabetes Federation (IDF) 2009). HbA1c (glycosylated haemoglobin) is a blood test that gives an indication of the levels to which the red cells have been exposed to glucose over the last 2 months and, as such, is a guide to the effectiveness of measures to control blood sugar levels. Studies have shown a link between higher HbA1c levels around the time of conception and poor pregnancy outcome, including increased risk of miscarriage, congenital malformation, stillbirth and neonatal death (McCance 2015; Bell et al 2012). The sensitive period for fetal development in relation to blood sugars appears to be in the period from conception up until 7 weeks gestation. Box 54.23 lists other key elements of preconception care. Opportunities for recommending and referring women of childbearing age to seek timely preconception care need to be taken by GPs, midwives in the postnatal period (planning for future pregnancies), specialist nurses and endocrinologists. Use of multimedia and Internet sources may help disseminate this information (Diabetes UK 2015; Spence et al 2013). NICE (2015) provides detailed evidence-based guidance of preconception care and the reader is recommended to access this online.

Antenatal care

Care is best provided in a specialist diabetic clinic where the woman can access members of the MDT, including the midwife. Pregnancy will be a challenging time for both newly diagnosed and those with pre-existing diabetes. The midwife should aim to provide support, continuity, ease of access and information that will acknowledge the normal aspects of pregnancy and anticipation of parenthood. The woman will need support, motivation and empowerment in adjusting to the demands of monitoring blood sugars, tailoring medication and diet requirements. Pregnancy changes make this more difficult. Target blood sugar levels are as follows: fasting 5.3 mmol/L, 1 hour after meals; 7.8 mmol/L, 2 hours after meals; 6.4 mmol/L (NICE 2015). The desire to keep blood sugars tightly controlled can lead to hypoglycaemia, particularly in early pregnancy when there is an increased sensitivity to insulin and other factors such as nausea and vomiting that affect carbohydrate metabolism. As pregnancy progresses for women with type 1 diabetes, the insulin dose to maintain normoglycaemia may increase threefold over the period of pregnancy. Women with type 2 diabetes who have previously achieved control of blood sugar with diet, exercise or oral hypoglycemic agents are likely to require insulin (McCance 2015).

In addition to the regular requirements of antenatal care, woman with diabetes will need more frequent visits and assessment. The NICE (2015) guidelines for diabetes in pregnancy set out detailed plans for antenatal care and the reader is recommended to consult these. Box 54.24 summarizes some of the key recommendations of these guidelines. Guidelines relevant to the care of woman with a raised BMI should be considered as indicated for some women with gestational diabetes and T2DM (CMACE/RCOG 2010; NICE 2010).

Box 54.23 Key elements of preconception care

- Discuss the importance of a planned pregnancy and consider appropriate contraception until optimal glycaemic control has been achieved
- Information and education regarding diabetes in pregnancy
- Aim for a HbA1c < 6.5% before conception
- Monitor blood sugar levels with increased frequency to achieve target levels without risk of hypoglycaemia
- Women should carry dextrose tablets and their families instructed in use of glucagon because of increased risk of hypoglycaemia
- Discuss the risk of maternal and fetal complications of a diabetic pregnancy and provide access to information and support
- Promote lifestyle modifications such as weight loss (very important in type 2 diabetes), smoking and alcohol cessation
- Increased folic acid supplements (5 mg/day) from the preconception period until 12 weeks gestation. These will need to be prescribed
- Review medications
- Retinal and renal assessment before pregnancy to determine baseline and review treatment for any hypertension
- Offer women with type 1 diabetes blood ketone testing strips and a meter. They need to test for ketonaemia if they become hyperglycaemic or unwell

Source Patel et al 2014; McCance 2015; NICE 2015

Reflective activity 54.4

Attend a maternity diabetic clinic and take the opportunity to talk to women about their experiences of diabetes in pregnancy.

Box 54.24 Summary of the key recommendations of NICE (2015) guidelines for care of diabetes in pregnancy

Antenatal

- Early "booking" with a midwife and MDT and increased frequency of visits
- Continue relevant elements listed in Box 54.23, which ideally will have commenced preconception
- Review of diabetic-related complications, including regular retinal assessment, renal assessment and BP monitoring
- Education and midwifery assessment for signs and symptoms of pre-eclampsia
- Detection and treatment of any infection such as a UTI
- Review for signs of ketoacidosis if the woman is hyperglycaemic or becomes unwell
- Preventive medication, including low-dose aspirin (to prevent PET) and thromboprophylaxis (to prevent VTE) considered
- Fetal assessment – this includes review for structural congenital abnormality (including fetal heart) and regular assessment of growth, amniotic fluid volume and well-being. The midwife will assess fetal well-being with measurement of fundal height, assessment of fetal movements and auscultation at each visit

Labour care

Birth in a labour ward with access to senior obstetric support and neonatal care is advised. Women with T1DM and T2DM will be offered IOL/CS at around 38 weeks gestation (NICE 2015). Those with uncomplicated gestational diabetes may await spontaneous labour, but pregnancy is not recommended to go beyond 40 weeks gestation.

Capillary blood glucose testing should be carried out every hour during labour, and IV dextrose and insulin infusions may be required to maintain blood sugars between 4 and 7 mmol/L (NICE 2015). Electronic fetal monitoring should be continuous because of the increased risks of fetal hypoxia during labour.

Women with a raised BMI will require care according to a specific care pathway with factors such as mobility, specialist equipment, anaesthetic review, risk of shoulder dystocia, risk of PPH and need for thromboprophylaxis to be considered (CMACE/RCOG 2010).

Neonatal care

The aim in the neonatal period will be to keep mother and baby together where easy access to advanced level neonatal support and early neonatologist review is possible. These babies are particularly prone to respiratory distress syndrome, jaundice and hypoglycaemia, so require close observation. In intra-uterine life, the fetal cells in the islets of Langerhans produce more insulin than normal in response to the high maternal blood sugar levels. After birth, the pancreas continues to produce excess insulin initially, but the continuous glucose supply via the placenta is now cut off so the baby becomes hypoglycaemic. To prevent this, early feeding within 30 minutes of birth, then 2 to 3 hourly, is essential and the baby's blood glucose levels are measured 2 to 4 hours after birth, or earlier if there are signs of hypoglycaemia (NICE 2015).

Postnatal care

The pregnancy physiological changes to carbohydrate metabolism revert back to normal with the delivery of the placenta. Women with insulin-treated diabetes should reduce the amount of insulin injected immediately after birth. They normally revert to prepregnancy doses but should review their blood sugars frequently to establish optimum normoglycaemic levels (Bothamley and Boyle 2009). Women with gestational diabetes should stop medication after the birth and receive information about weight control, exercise, diet and how to recognize hyperglycaemia. The midwife should ensure women with gestational diabetes have a postnatal OGTT test arranged. Regular follow-up is required, as they have an increased risk of developing T2DM. It is also possible that women with gestational diabetes actually have T2DM that was previously undiagnosed.

Breastfeeding is encouraged, although women with T1DM may need an extra snack or meal at the time of feeding to avoid hypoglycaemia. Women with type 2 diabetes can resume oral hypoglycaemics, but only *metformin* and *glibenclamide*, if they are breastfeeding (NICE 2015).

Measures to reduce thromboembolism are indicated and slow wound healing may complicate postnatal recovery (Bothamley and Boyle 2009).

RESPIRATORY DISORDERS

Asthma

Asthma is a chronic inflammatory disorder of the respiratory system that is characterized by episodic breathlessness, wheezing, shortness of breath, excessive production of mucus, cough and a sensation of tightness in the chest. Symptoms are often worse at night. Acute exacerbations (asthma attacks) are triggered by a range of factors (see Box 54.25) and cause inflammation, narrowing of the airways, and contraction of the smooth muscle of the airway walls (bronchospasm). It is a preventable cause of maternal death linked to smoking and lack of education about the need to continue regular medication when pregnant (Nelson-Piercy et al 2014).

There is a complex link between pregnancy and asthma. Some pregnant women experience fewer asthmatic attacks, possibly owing to the increased production of corticosteroids

---

Box 54.25 Known triggers in asthma attacks

- Allergens, such as pollen, animals, house dust mites
- Smoking
- Certain foods/medicines, nut, milk and egg allergies, alcohol, preservatives, colouring agents
- Hyperventilation
- Environmental factors, such as dust, pollution, chemicals, cigarette smoke
- Exercise
- Cold or dry air
- Upper respiratory tract viral infections
- Omitting regular prescribed asthma medication

Box 54.26 Areas with high prevalence of tuberculosis

- Sub-Saharan Africa
- Indian subcontinent
- South Asia
- Eastern Europe and Baltic states
- Russian Federation and former Soviet Union states

Source: WHO 2013

---

in pregnancy, some may stay the same, but a few may have more frequent exacerbations, particularly those who have severe asthma before pregnancy. Links have been shown between poor control of asthma and poor pregnancy outcomes, including premature labour, pre-eclampsia and low birthweight (Nelson-Piercy 2015). Respiratory viral infections are the most frequent cause of exacerbations of asthma in pregnancy, although poor adherence to inhaled corticosteroid therapy has also been identified as a common cause for serious asthma attacks. Complications are less likely to arise where asthma is controlled well (Nelson-Piercy 2015), so it is important to encourage women to maintain their drug therapy. Smoking cessation is also very important. Regular assessment of peak expiratory flow rates (PEFR) and a review of inhaler technique is good practice.

Drug therapy is by inhaled anti-inflammatory agents, beta-agonists ("relievers") or steroids ("preventers"). These are safe during pregnancy and midwives should assure women of this. As Goldie and Brightling (2013) point out, poorly controlled asthma carries greater risks for the fetus than do the drugs used to treat it. Medication to control asthma and treatment for severe asthma exacerbations is the same in pregnancy as for non-pregnancy and clinicians are advised to follow recognized guidelines (British Thoracic Society (BTS) Scottish Intercollegiate Guidelines Network (SIGN) 2014). Management will include urgent admission to a hospital, nebulized bronchodilators, high flow oxygen, IV and oral corticosteroids, other medication as per guidelines, enhanced observations of the woman, continuous CTG monitoring of the fetus and involvement of senior staff and the critical care team (Nelson-Piercy 2015).

Exacerbations rarely occur in labour, and women should continue to take their regular medication. Salbutamol inhalers should be available in labour wards in case women leave their own at home (Jordan 2010). Those taking regular oral steroids will need parental hydrocortisone during labour (BTS/SIGN 2014). A plan for suitable medications in labour should be documented in the antenatal period. Medications that cause bronchospasm, such as haemobate and ergometrine, should be used with caution (Nelson-Piercy 2015) and, in some cases, non–steroidal anti-inflammatory medications (NSAIDs), such as aspirin and diclofenac, are contraindicated (Goldie and Brightling 2013). Opiates for pain relief should be used with caution (Nelson-Piercy 2015).

Breastfeeding is recommended and may protect the baby from developing atopic asthma (Nelson-Piercy 2015). Women should continue their regular medication in the postnatal period (BTS/SIGN 2014).

Tuberculosis (TB)

TB is an infectious disease caused by the bacterium *Mycobacterium tuberculosis*. It is a major cause of morbidity and death worldwide. TB is transmitted by coughing and, therefore, is more easily spread where there is overcrowding, poor natural light and poor ventilation (Public Health England (PHE) 2013; Bothamley 2012). Babies and young children are most at risk of serious complications of TB, including TB meningitis, and midwives may be involved with the newborn Bacillus Calmette–Guérin (BCG) vaccination programme (NICE 2011b; Bothamley 2006).

Midwives have a role in identifying features of TB in pregnant women, although symptoms of pregnancy, such as fatigue, may mask some of the characteristic features of TB and delays in diagnosis may occur.

Box 54.26 lists countries of high prevalence and Box 54.27 lists the common symptoms of TB. About 50% of pregnant women with TB have extrapulmonary TB (TB of lymph nodes, kidney, spine), which will feature atypical symptoms (Knight et al 2009; Kothari et al 2006)

Diagnostic tests for TB include microscopy and culture of sputum, a chest x-ray (safe in pregnancy if uterus is shielded (Knight et al 2009) and a tuberculin skin test. A new blood test (QuantiFERON-TB Gold; T-SPOT.*TB*) that provides faster results is also now available.

A respiratory physician will direct treatment with support from TB nurses. Good outcomes for mother and baby can be expected if anti-tuberculosis treatment regimens are followed (Bothamley 2006; Bothamley and Boyle 2015).

Box 54.27 Symptoms of active tuberculosis

- Fever – most often at night and can result in drenching night sweats
- Unexplained weight loss or poor weight gain in pregnancy
- Poor appetite
- Unusual tiredness

In pulmonary TB:
- Persistent productive cough that gets progressively worse over several weeks
- Coughing up blood

There is reassuring evidence that the most commonly used drug treatments for TB – rifampicin, isoniazid, pyrazinamide and ethambutol – are suitable for use in pregnancy and breastfeeding (Bothamley 2001). There can be some complications of treatment and close monitoring of liver function and supplements of pyridoxine (vitamin B_6) are recommended. The usual treatment for TB requires a 6-month course of medication and completion of the full course of drug treatment is the key to optimum outcomes for mother and baby. A woman-centred approach, free of stigmatization, supported by motivated health professionals, including TB nurses and continuity of midwifery care, will build the trust and understanding required to support the woman to complete her treatment (Bothamley 2006; Bothamley and Boyle 2015).

Multidrug-resistant tuberculosis (MDR TB) and extensively drug-resistant TB complicate the effectiveness of antituberculosis treatment and pose considerable threat to the spread of and the ability to treat TB. HIV infection increases the risk and severity of TB. Conversely, TB accelerates the progression of HIV disease (Pratt 2007).

Summary of care of pregnant woman with tuberculosis

Preconception care

Pregnancy should be avoided while the woman is being treated for TB. However, for those receiving standard medication regimens, pregnancy is not contraindicated and women should continue taking their medication. Oral contraception may be affected by TB medication and barrier methods of contraception are advised. HIV testing should be offered (Bothamley and Boyle 2015).

Antenatal care

A coordinated multidisciplinary team service, including a respiratory physician, TB nurse and the infection control team alongside the maternity care team, is required. Women may be vulnerable, wary of health professionals and face language and social barriers to antenatal care (Bothamley 2006; Bothamley and Boyle 2015). Liaison with the wider multidisciplinary team with regard to contact tracing, adherence to treatment, monitoring side effects of treatment and education to reduce the spread of TB is fundamental. There is a risk of infection of the newborn through other family contacts who may have TB and are not being treated. Antenatal care will best be provided away from other pregnant women if the woman has just started treatment, when adherence to treatment is questionable, or when the woman has MDR TB (Bothamley and Boyle 2015).

Labour care

Most women with TB will have been diagnosed antenatally and have completed at least 2 weeks of treatment, making them non-infectious. However, labour will be a high-risk time for aerosol spread and, therefore, if a negative-pressure room is available, it should be used; otherwise, care in a single room with an open window is advised. Advice should be sought from the hospital infection control team (Bothamley and Boyle 2015).

Postnatal care

Separation of mother and baby is not normally required and should be avoided. Breastfeeding is considered safe for those on standard TB medications and is recommended. The respiratory physician and TB nurses should be informed of the birth and will provide specialist advice on preventative treatment for the baby in consultation with the neonatologists (Bothamley and Boyle 2015).

Reflective activity 54.5

Look up your local policy regarding infection control measures when caring for a woman with a respiratory infection.

EPILEPSY

Epilepsy is a relatively common neurological condition, affecting around 1 in 200 women attending antenatal clinics (Mohan and Nelson-Piercy 2014b). The term 'epilepsy' refers to a sudden abnormal discharge of electrical energy from cerebral neurones, which causes a seizure. For most, the cause of epilepsy is unknown but may be a genetic disposition to a lower threshold for seizure or from a brain injury. Epilepsy affects each woman differently with a range of symptoms and causes and with varying degrees of severity. It is important that the midwife documents the specific features and triggers for epilepsy for an individual woman. Box 54.28 lists some of the triggers for seizure activity. It can be seen from this list that triggers for seizures correspond with common pregnancy symptoms, including tiredness, constipation and anxiety.

Although, in general, a woman with epilepsy can expect good outcomes, her pregnancy is not without risk with an increase in seizures reported in up to a third of women. Seven maternal deaths between 2010 and 2013 were attributed to epilepsy (Nair and Knight 2015). Maternal deaths related to epilepsy in pregnancy are often classified as sudden unexpected death in epilepsy (SUDEP) (Knight et al 2014). It is suggested that maternal concerns regarding the effect of their antiepileptic treatment on the baby may result in them discontinuing their medication, placing them at substantial risk of seizures and SUDEP. There is an emphasis on the need for opportunistic preconception care and ongoing involvement of a liaison epilepsy nurse integrated into antenatal care to provide continued support as part of a coordinated specialist MDT (Kelso and Wills 2014).

Seizures

Seizures vary from a brief lapse of attention (*absence seizures* (previously known as petit mal)), which can almost go unnoticed to severe and prolonged convulsions involving the whole body (*tonic–clonic seizures*). *Myoclonic* seizures involve sudden jerky movements of whole body or of arms or legs, and focal seizures have variable symptoms, depending on the networks of the brain affected. Seizures can vary in frequency from less than one a year to several a day (Mohan and Nelson-Piercy 2014b).

Tonic-clonic seizures (previously known as grand mal) involve initial stiffening of the body (tonic phase) and the woman falls to the ground. The jaw muscles contract and she may bite her tongue. Breathing stops momentarily and cyanosis may be evident. Incontinence of urine and faeces may occur. This tonic phase may last for a minute or more. The clonic phase starts immediately afterwards and involves rhythmically jerking movements, lasting several seconds to minutes. After the clonic phase, a period of recovery known as the postictal phase where consciousness gradually returns, occurs. The woman may remain drowsy and disorientated for some time and usually has painful muscles, a bad headache and a sore tongue. This kind of seizure is associated with a variable period of fetal hypoxia and puts the woman at greatest risk of SUDEP. Severe injury and drowning (dependent on where she is) may occur. The psychological effect is significant. Up to 4% of women with epilepsy can experience a tonic–clonic seizure during labour or within the first 24 hours after birth (NICE 2012). Box 54.29 summarizes the care for a seizure.

Antiepileptic medication

Antiepileptic drugs (AEDs) work by acting on neurons at the synaptic membrane or by modulating the neurotransmitters to slow down the tendency for action potential, thus inhibiting the explosive bursts of electrical activity that cause seizures. AEDs will control seizures in up to 80% of epileptic patients with most requiring only one drug (monotherapy). The physiological changes that occur in pregnancy influence the distribution, availability and metabolism of AEDs (Adab and Chadwick 2006). It is important that the woman be referred to specialist neurology care for assessment of her medication before pregnancy. The aim will be to achieve good seizure control, preferably on a single medication with a better safety profile in pregnancy, and on the lowest possible dosage. A systematic review that analysed data from 59 studies estimated that the highest incidence of congenital malformation was linked to use of sodium valproate and/or when more than one medication was required to control seizures (Meador et al 2008). An analysis of data from an international register of AEDs in pregnancy found that the lowest rates of malformation were observed in single therapy, lower doses of lamotrigine and carbamazepine (Tomson et al 2011). A full discussion with regard to AEDs will be based on balancing risks of uncontrolled convulsive seizures against possible risks to the fetus both from taking medication and not taking it. Some AEDs interfere with combined oral contraception and other side effects include an increased risk of depression (Jordan 2010).

Preconception care

The main aim of preconception care is to optimize seizure control on a medication regimen that the woman is motivated to continue (see earlier section). The risks of SUDEP and practical considerations of safety should be reviewed. It will be recommended that 5 mg of folic acid be commenced 3 months before conception and continued throughout pregnancy. Inherited risks of epilepsy can also be discussed (Mohan and Nelson-Piercy 2014b). There is a poor record of women with epilepsy accessing preconception services and health professionals need to explore innovative ways to provide opportunistic information to women of childbearing age with epilepsy.

Antenatal care

MDT care will include an obstetrician, a neurologist, an epilepsy specialist nurse and a midwife. The regular pattern of antenatal care will be followed with extra attention given to adherence to medication, nausea and vomiting that may affect medication blood levels and triggers such as sleep deprivation and anxiety. Monitoring of blood levels of some types of AEDs may be indicated and adjustment to medication made as pregnancy progresses (Mohan and Nelson-Piercy 2014b).

Enhanced fetal screening will include a detailed anomaly scan at 18 to 20 weeks and fetal echocardiography (NICE 2012). Maternal oral vitamin K supplementation is required from 36 weeks gestation for women taking certain AEDs (Mohan and Nelson-Piercy 2014b). Continuity of midwifery care will provide essential support to normalise the woman's pregnancy experience.

Labour care

Most women with epilepsy will have a normal vaginal birth, although delivery in a consultant-led unit is recommended. There is a 4% increased risk of seizures during labour and for the 24 hours after (Thomas et al 2012).

AEDs should be continued and, if not tolerated, orally given by IV or rectal route. One-to-one midwifery care is essential and the woman should not be left alone and precautions taken, such as not locking toilet doors. Most forms of pain relief are acceptable, although pethidine should be avoided. Labouring in water will be particularly hazardous and generally is not recommended (Epilepsy Action 2014). However, for a woman who has been seizure-free for a long time and does not require AEDs, an individual choice may be made to labour in water (RCOG 2016). Hoisting equipment should be at hand. Effective pain relief with an epidural may help to prevent seizures by minimizing triggers such as tiredness, pain and hyperventilation. The newborn should receive the standard 1 mg IM dose of vitamin K (Mohan and Nelson-Piercy 2014b).

Postnatal care

Sleep deprivation and missing a dose of AEDs because of upheaval in routines may contribute to an increased risk of seizures in the postnatal period. Breastfeeding is recommended, although AEDs do cross into breastmilk (albeit mostly in small amounts) so an individual review of medication and safety in breastfeeding is required (Mohan and Nelson-Piercy 2014b). Box 54.30 lists safety measures for mother and baby. Charity organizations, such as Epilepsy Action, provide detailed information, guidance and support for women with epilepsy (Epilepsy Action 2014). Medication may need review and gradually revert to pre-pregnancy regimens. Planning advice for future pregnancies and effective contraception needs to be discussed (NICE 2012). Women with epilepsy are at increased risk of depression in the postpartum period. Support and

---

Box 54.30 Some examples of safety information for the mother with epilepsy

- The mother should not be left alone in the first days after the birth, as she is at higher risk of seizures.
- Sleep deprivation needs to be avoided so she will need help at night. Expressing breastmilk during the day will allow delegation of feeding at night.
- Women should only bath with someone else around, or in very shallow water, or shower.
- The baby can be changed or dressed on the floor.
- A brake can be fitted to the pram/pushchair, which will operate if the mother lets go.
- The baby can be fed and cuddled when the mother is propped up comfortably against the wall on the floor.
- The baby could be bathed when someone else is there or washed with a cloth instead of bathing.
- Hot drinks should be kept away from the baby.

Source: Epilepsy Action (2014); Bothamley and Boyle 2009

education that seeks to empower the woman in the many positive aspects of her parenting and timely referral to specialist help will improve the woman's psychosocial experiences of parenthood.

INTRAHEPATIC CHOLESTASIS OF PREGNANCY

Intrahepatic cholestasis of pregnancy (ICP) (also known as *obstetric cholestasis*) is a disease arising in the third trimester, which is normally characterised by intense pruritus (itching) without a rash (often palms of hands, soles of feet), abnormal liver function tests (LFTs) and elevated maternal bile acid levels. Serum bile acids levels greater than 40 µmol/L are associated with an increased rate of preterm delivery (iatrogenic and spontaneous), admission to NNU and stillbirth (Geenes et al 2014). Other complications include meconium-stained liquor and disordered coagulation, relating to poor absorption of vitamin K (a fat-soluble vitamin) and, thus, increasing the risk of PPH (RCOG 2011b).

The cause of ICP is unknown but may arise from genetic, hormonal or environmental factors. Women are more likely to get ICP if their mother or sister has ICP, and it is likely to recur in subsequent pregnancies and is more common in multiple pregnancies. It occurs in 0.7% of pregnancies in multiethnic populations, with a higher incidence (1.2%–1.5%) in women of Indian-Asian or Pakistani-Asian origin (RCOG 2011b).

Women presenting with severe or characteristic itching should be referred to an obstetrician for investigation and diagnosis. Older studies showed an increase in rate of stillbirth after 37 weeks gestation and, therefore, many obstetricians will offer an IOL around this time, although complications of prematurity need to be considered with this approach. Fetal assessment has limited predictive value in identifying fetal demise but is offered for reassurance (Geenes and Williamson 2015). Ursodeoxycholic acid (UDCA) medication has been shown to relieve itching for some but not all women, although results are equivocal for benefits in reducing rates of stillbirth (Gurung et al 2013). Other strategies for managing the distressing effect of itching include topical applications of calamine lotion or aqueous cream. Antihistamines may be prescribed, as they may help promote sleep (Chambers and Tuson 2012).

The psychological effect of the condition should not be underestimated. Intense physical discomfort, lack of sleep and heightened anxiety over concern for affect on the baby will have a considerable effect on well-being (Steele 2012; Chambers and Tuson 2012). Additional support by the midwife, information and referral to organizations, such as 'ICP Support' (Tuson and Chambers 2013), are recommended.

Because the condition is related to oestrogen, women should avoid oral contraceptives containing oestrogen (Nelson-Piercy 2015).

CONCLUSION

Midwives will encounter women with complex medical disorders in everyday maternity care. These women will benefit from the support of a midwife who is knowledgeable with regard to their medical condition and is able to be vigilant in the assessment of the woman and the fetus/baby through pregnancy, birth and the postnatal period.

Whilst pre-conception planning and assessment is highly recommended for women with medical conditions the midwife will encounter many women in early pregnancy who will have not benefited from this and will thus require prompt and efficient referral to the relevant medical/obstetric practitioner.

A multidisciplinary approach with regular assessment aided by clear lines of communication and documentation will enable optimum care and a fulfilling experience of childbirth for women with medical conditions.

Key Points

- Preconception assessment that aims to optimize health, adjust medication and make plans for care is recommended for women with hypertensive and medical conditions.

- The initial 'booking' assessment offers the opportunity for the midwife to record key features, take accurate baseline assessments, order appropriate tests, ensure referral to the multidisciplinary team and plan out a schedule of care that is individualized to best meet the needs of women with hypertensive and medical conditions in pregnancy.

- The well-being of mother and fetus should be accurately assessed by the midwife at each stage of the childbearing process. This assessment should take account of risk factors and include an understanding of the underlying medical condition. Early recognition and prompt and appropriate referral is essential.

- Good teamwork with the multidisciplinary team is essential, aided by clear written and verbal communication.

- The focus of care should not just include the medical aspects of her condition but seek to encourage a positive journey for women and their families as they anticipate parenthood.

References

Adab N, Chadwick D: Management of women with epilepsy during pregnancy, *Obstet Gynaecol* 8(1):20–25, 2006.

Bell R, Glinianaia S, Tennant P, et al: Peri-conception hyperglycaemia and nephropathy are associated with risk of congenital anomaly in women with pre-existing diabetes: a population-based cohort study, *Diabetologia* 55:936–947, 2012.

Blackburn ST: *Maternal, fetal and neonatal physiology*, 4th edn, Philadelphia, Saunders Elsevier, 2013.

Bothamley G: Drug treatment for tuberculosis during pregnancy: safety considerations, *Drug Saf* 24(7):553–565, 2001.

Bothamley J: Tuberculosis in pregnancy: the role for midwives in diagnosis and treatment, *Br J Midwifery* 14(4):182–185, 2006.

Bothamley J, Boyle M: *Medical conditions affecting pregnancy and childbirth*, Oxford, Radcliffe, 2009.

Bothamley J, Boyle M: Cardiac disorders in pregnancy, *Midwives* 12(4):34–36, 2009b.

Bothamley G: Screening for tuberculosis in pregnancy, *Expert Rev Obstet Gynecol* 7(4):387–395, 2012.

Bothamley J, Boyle M: *Infections affecting pregnancy and childbirth*, London, Radcliffe Publishing, 2015.

Bramham K, Nelson-Piercy C, Brown MJ, et al: Postpartum management of hypertension, *Br Med J* 346:30–34, 2013a.

Bramham K, Nelson-Piercy C, Gao H, et al: Pregnancy in renal transplant recipients: a UK national cohort study, *Clin J Am Soc Nephrol* 8(2):290–298, 2013b.

British Thoracic Society. Scottish Intercollegiate Guidelines Network: *British Guideline on the Management of Asthma* (website). www.brit-thoracic.org.uk/document-library/clinical-information/asthma/btssign-asthma-guideline-quick-reference-guide-2014/. 2014.

Bujold E, Roberge S, Lacasse Y, et al: Prevention of preeclampsia and intrauterine growth restriction with aspirin started in early pregnancy: a meta-analysis, *Obstet Gynecol* 116(2):402–414, 2010.

Centre for Maternal and Child Enquiries and the Royal College of Obstetricians and Gynaecologists: *CMACE/RCOG Joint Guideline: Management of Women with Obesity in Pregnancy*. London, CMACE/RCOG, 2010.

Chambers J, Tuson A: Obstetric cholestasis, *Pract Midwife* 10(9):26–29, 2012.

Confidential Enquiry into Maternal and Child Health (CEMACH): *Diabetes in Pregnancy: Are we providing the best care?* Findings of a National Enquiry: England, Wales and Northern Ireland, London, CEMACH, 2007.

Cox S, Reid F: Urogynaecological complications in pregnancy: an overview, *Obstet Gynaecol Reprod Med* 25(5):123–127, 2015.

Crawford PM, Marshall F: *Coping with epilepsy*, 3rd edn, London, Sheldon Press, 2013.

Crovetto F, Somigliana E, Peguero A, et al: Stroke during pregnancy and pre-eclampsia, *Curr Opin Obstet Gynecol* 25(6):425–432, 2013.

Deshpande NA, James NT, Kucirka LM, et al: Pregnancy outcomes in kidney transplant recipients: a systematic review and meta-analysis, *Am J Transplant* 11:2388–2404, 2011.

Diabetes UK: *Pregnancy and diabetes* (website). www.diabetes.org.uk/Guide-to-diabetes/Living_with_diabetes/Pregnancy/. 2015.

Duley L, Gülmezoglu AM, Henderson, Smart DJ, et al: Magnesium sulphate and other anticonvulsants for women with pre-eclampsia, *Cochrane Database Syst Rev* (11):2010.

Epilepsy Action: *Epilepsy and having a baby* (website). www.epilepsy.org.uk/sites/epilepsy/files/info/references/Epilepsy%20and%20having%20a%20baby%20B112.pdf. 2014.

Geenes V, Chappell LC, Seed PT, et al: Association of severe intrahepatic cholestasis of pregnancy with adverse pregnancy outcomes: a prospective population-based case-control study, *Hepatology* 59(4):1482–1491, 2014.

Geenes V, Williamson C: Liver disease in pregnancy, *Best Pract Res Clin Obstet Gynaecol* 29(5):612–624, 2015.

Girling J, Sykes L: Thyroid disorders and other endocrinological disorders in pregnancy, *Obstet Gynaecol Reprod Med* 23(6):171–179, 2013.

Goldie MH, Brightling CE: Asthma in pregnancy, *Obstet Gynaecol* 15:241–245, 2013.

Goonewardene M, Shehata M, Hamad A: Anaemia in pregnancy, *Best Pract Res Clin Obstet Gynaecol* 26:3–24, 2012.

Gurung V, Middleton P, Milan SJ, et al: Interventions for treating cholestasis in pregnancy, *Cochrane Database Syst Rev* (6):CD000493, 2013.

Hall M, Brunskill NJ: Renal disease in pregnancy, *Obstet Gynaecol Reprod Med* 23(2):31–37, 2013.

Harding K, Redmond P, Tuffnell D, on behalf of the MBRRACE-UK Hypertensive disorders of pregnancy chapter writing group: Caring for women with hypertensive disorders of pregnancy. In Knight M, Nair M, Tuffnell D, et al; on behalf of MBRRACE-UK, editors: *Saving Lives, Improving Mothers' Care – Surveillance of Maternal Deaths in the UK 2012–14 and Lessons Learned to Inform Maternity Care from the UK and Ireland Confidential Enquiries into Maternal Deaths and Morbidity 2009–14*. Oxford: National Perinatal Epidemiology Unit, University of Oxford, pp 69–75, 2016.

Hawthorne G: Maternal complications in diabetic pregnancy, *Best Pract Res Clin Obstet Gynaecol* 25(1):77–90, 2011.

Howard J, Oteng-Ntim E: The obstetric management of sickle cell disease, *Best Pract Res Clin Obstet Gynaecol* 26:25–36, 2012.

International Diabetes Federation (IDF): *Global Guideline on Pregnancy and Diabetes* (website). www.idf.org/guidelines/pregnancy-and-diabetes. 2009.

Jefferys A, Vanderpump M, Yasmin E: Thyroid dysfunction and reproductive health, *Obstet Gynaecol* 17:39–45, 2015.

Jordan S: *Pharmacology for midwives: the evidence base for safe practice*, 2nd edn, Basingstoke, Palgrave Macmillan, 2010.

Kelso A, Wills A, on behalf of the MBRRACE-UK Neurology Writing

Group: Learning from Neurological Complications. In Knight M, Kenyon S, Brocklehurst P, et al; on behalf of MBRRACE-UK, editors: *Saving Lives, Improving Mothers' Care – Lessons Learned to Inform Future Maternity Care from the UK and Ireland Confidential Enquiries into Maternal Deaths and Morbidity 2009–2012*, Oxford, National Perinatal Epidemiology Unit, University of Oxford, 2014.

Knight M, Kurinczuk JJ, Nelson-Piercy C, et al; UK Obstetric Surveillance System: Tuberculosis in pregnancy in the UK, *Br J Obstet Gynaecol* 116(4):584–588, 2009.

Knight M, Nair M, Shah A, et al; on behalf of the MBRRACE-UK: Surveillance and Epidemiology Chapter Writing Group. Maternal Mortality and Morbidity in the UK 2009–2012: Surveillance and Epidemiology. In Knight M, Kenyon S, Brocklehurst P, on behalf of MBRRACE-UK, editors: *Saving Lives, Improving Mothers' Care – Lessons learned to inform future maternity care from the UK and Ireland Confidential Enquiries into Maternal Deaths and Morbidity 2009–2012*, Oxford, National Perinatal Epidemiology Unit, University of Oxford, 2014.

Kothari A, Mahadevan N, Girling J: Tuberculosis and pregnancy: results of a study in a high prevalence area in London, *Eur J Obstet Gynecol Reprod Biol* 126(1):48–55, 2006.

Lightstone L: Renal disease in pregnancy, *Medicine (Baltimore)* 39(8):497–501, 2011.

Magee LA, Pels A, Helewa M, et al: The hypertensive disorders of pregnancy, *Best Pract Res Clin Obstet Gynaecol* (29):643–657, 2015.

McCance DR: Diabetes in pregnancy, *Best Pract Res Clin Obstet Gynaecol* 29(5):685–689, 2015.

McLintock C: Thromboembolism in pregnancy: challenges and controversies in the prevention of pregnancy-associated venous thromboembolisation and management of anticoagulation in women with prosthetic heart valves, *Best Pract Res Clin Obstet Gynaecol* 28:519–536, 2014.

Meador K, Reynolds MW, Crean S, et al: Pregnancy outcomes in women with epilepsy: as systematic review and meta-analysis of published pregnancy registers and cohorts, *Epilepsy Res* 81:1–13, 2008.

Milne F, Redman C, Walker J, et al: The pre-eclampsia community guideline (PRECOG): how to screen for and detect onset of pre-eclampsia in the community, *Br Med J* 330:576–580, 2005.

Mohan A, Nelson-Piercy C: Drugs and therapeutics, including contraception for women with heart disease, *Best Pract Res Clin Obstet Gynaecol* 28(4):471–482, 2014a.

Mohan AR: Nelson-Piercy C: Neurological disease in pregnancy, *Obstet Gynaecol Reprod Med* 24(10):303–308, 2014b.

Murphy HR, Roland JM, Skinner TC, et al: Effectiveness of a regional pre pregnancy care programme in women with type 1 and type 2 diabetes, *Diabetes Care* 33:2514–2520, 2011.

Nair M, Knight M: Maternal Mortality in the UK 2012–2014. In Knight M, Nair M, Tuffnell D, et al; on behalf of MBRRACE-UK, editors: *Saving Lives, Improving Mothers' Care – Surveillance of Maternal Deaths in the UK 2012–14 and Lessons Learned to Inform Maternity Care from the UK and Ireland Confidential Enquiries into Maternal Deaths and Morbidity 2009–14*. Oxford: National Perinatal Epidemiology Unit, University of Oxford, pp 11–32, 2016.

Nair M, Knight M, Shah A: Maternal mortality and morbidity in the UK 2011-2013: Surveillance and Epidemiology. In Knight M, Tuffnell D, Kenyon S, et al; on behalf of MBRRACE-UK, editors: *Saving Lives, Improving Mothers' Care – Surveillance of maternal deaths in the UK 2011–2013 and lessons learned to inform maternity care from the UK and Ireland Confidential Enquiries into Maternal Deaths and Morbidity 2009–13*, Oxford, National Perinatal Epidemiology Unit, University of Oxford, pp 7–21, 2015.

Nathan HL, Duhig K, Hezelgrave NL, et al: Blood pressure measurement in pregnancy, *Obstet Gynaecol* 17:91–98, 2015.

National Institute for Health and Care Excellence (NICE): *Weight management before, during and after pregnancy. NICE public health guidance 27*. London, NICE, 2010.

National Institute for Health and Care Excellence (NICE): *Tuberculosis: Clinical Diagnosis and Management of Tuberculosis, and Measures for Its Prevention and Control*. London, NICE, 2011b.

National Institute for Health and Care Excellence (NICE): *Antenatal Care: NICE Clinical Guideline 62* (website). www.nice.org.uk/guidance/cg62/resources/guidance-antenatal-care-pdf. 2014.

National Institute for Health and Care Excellence (NICE): *Diabetes in Pregnancy: Management of Diabetes and Its Complications from Preconception to the Postnatal Period: NICE Guideline 3* (website). www.nice.org.uk/guidance/ng3/resources/diabetes-in-pregnancy-management-of-diabetes-and-its-complications-from-preconception-to-the-postnatal-period-51038446021. 2015.

National Institute for Health and Clinical Excellence (NICE): *Hypertension in Pregnancy. The Management of Hypertensive Disorders During Pregnancy*. [CG 107]. London, NICE, 2011a.

National Institute for Health and Clinical Excellence (NICE): *The Epilepsies: The Diagnosis and Management of the Epilepsies in Adults and Children in Primary and Secondary Care*. [CG 137], London, NICE, 2012.

Nelson-Piercy C: *Handbook of obstetric medicine*, 5th edn, Boca Raton, CRC Press Taylor and Francis Group, 2015.

Nelson-Piercy C, MacKillop L, Williamson C, Griffiths M, on behalf of the MBRRACE-UK medical complications chapter writing group: Caring for women with other medical complications. In Knight M, Kenyon S, Brocklehurst P, et al; on behalf of MBRRACE-UK, editors. *Saving Lives, Improving Mothers' Care – Lessons Learned to Inform Future Maternity Ccare from the UK and Ireland Confidential Enquiries into Maternal Deaths and Morbidity 2009–12*. Oxford: National Perinatal Epidemiology Unit, University of Oxford, pp 81–87, 2014.

Nursing and Midwifery Council (NMC): *Standards for medicines management*, NMC, 2008.

Oteng-Ntim E, Ayensah B, Knight M, et al: Pregnancy outcome in patients with sickle cell disease in the UK – a national cohort comparing sickle cell anaemia HbSS with HbSC, *Br J Haematol* 169(1):129–137, 2015.

Oteng-Ntim E, Nazir S, Singhal.T, et al: Sickle cell disease in pregnancy, *Obstet Gynaecol Reprod Med* 22(9):254–262, 2012.

Patel N, Hameed A, Banerjee A: Pre–existing type 1 and type 11 diabetes in pregnancy, *Obstet Gynaecol Reprod Med* 24(5):129–134, 2014.

Pavord S, Myers B, Robinson S, et al: *UK Guidelines on the Management of Iron Deficiency in Pregnancy: British Committee for Standards in Haematology* (website). www.bcshgui delines.com/documents/UK _Guidelines_iron_deficiency_in _pregnancy.pdf. 2011.

Pearce EN: Thyroid disorders during pregnancy and postpartum, *Best Pract Res Clin Obstet Gynaecol* 29(5):700–706, 2015.

Piccoli G, Caiddu G, Atttini R, et al: Pregnancy in chronic kidney disease: questions and answers in a changing panorama, *Best Pract Res Clin Obstet Gynaecol* 29(5):625–642, 2015.

Pratt RJ: Examining tuberculosis trends in the UK, *Nurs Times* 103(38):52–54, 2007.

Public Health England (PHE): *Tuberculosis in the UK: 2013 Report* (website). www.hpa.org.uk/webc/ HPAwebFile/HPAweb_C/1317139 689583. 2013.

Royal College of Obstetricians and Gynaecologists (RCOG): *Green-top Guideline 43. Obstetric Cholestasis* (website). www.rcog.org.uk/ globalassets/documents/ guidelines/gtg_43.pdf. 2011b.

Royal College of Obstetrics and Gynaecology (RCOG): *Management of Sickle Cell Disease in Pregnancy:*

Green-top Guideline 61 (website). www.rcog.org.uk/globalassets/ documents/guidelines/gtg_61.pdf. 2011a.

Royal College of Obstetrics and Gynaecology (RCOG): *Management of Beta Thalassaemia in pregnancy: Green-top Guideline 66* (website). www.rcog.org.uk/globalassets/ documents/guidelines/gtg_66 _thalassaemia.pdf. 2014.

Royal College of Obstetricians and Gynaecologists (RCOG): *Green-top Guideline 68. Epilepsy in Pregnancy* (website). https://www.rcog.org.uk/ globalassets/documents/guidelines/ green-top-guidelines/gtg68_epilepsy. pdf. 2016.

Spence M, Harper R, Mc Cance D, et al: The systematic development of an innovative DVD to raise awareness of preconception care, *Eur Diab Nurs* 10(1):7–12b, 2013.

Steele G: Reflections on a pregnancy complicated by obstetric cholestasis, *Pract Midwife* 10(9):30–32, 2012.

Sullivan SA, Goodier C: Endocrine emergencies, *Obstet Gynecol Clin North Am* 40:121–135, 2013.

Swan L: Congenital heart disease in pregnancy, *Best Pract Res Clin Obstet Gynaecol* 28(4):495–506, 2014.

Thomas SV, Syam U, Devi JS: Predictors of seizures during pregnancy in women with epilepsy, *Epilepsia* 53:e85–e88, 2012.

Tomson T, Battinao D, Bonizzoni E, et al; EURAP study group: Dose – dependant risk of malformations with antiepileptic drugs: an analysis of data form EURAP epilepsy and

pregnancy registry, *Lancet Neurol* 10:609–617, 2011.

Tranquilli AL, Dekker G, Magee L, et al: The classification, diagnosis and management of the hypertensive disorders of pregnancy: a revised statement from the ISSHP, *Pregnancy Hypertens* 4(2):97–104, 2014.

Tuson A, Chambers J: Top ten things to know about intrahepatic cholestasis of pregnancy (ICP), *Ess MIDIRS* 4(10):27–30, 2013.

Vause S, Clarke B, Thorne S, et al, on behalf of the MBRRACE-UK cardiovascular chapter writing group: Lessons on cardiovascular disease. In Knight M, Nair M, Tuffnell D, et al; on behalf of MBRRACE-UK, editors: *Saving Lives, Improving Mothers' Care – Surveillance of Maternal Deaths in the UK 2012–14 and Lessons Learned to Inform Maternity Care from the UK and Ireland Confidential Enquiries into Maternal Deaths and Morbidity 2009–14.* Oxford: National Perinatal Epidemiology Unit, University of Oxford, pp 33–68, 2016.

Windram J, Colman J, Wald R, et al: Valvular heart diseases in pregnancy, *Best Pract Res Clin Obstet Gynaecol* 28(4):507–518, 2014.

World Health Organization (WHO) *Global Tuberculosis Report 2013* (website). www.who.int/tb/ publications/global_report/en/. 2013.

World Health Organisation (WHO): *Worldwide Prevalence of Anaemia 1993–2005* (website). http:// whqlibdoc.who.int/publications/ 2008/9789241596657_eng.pdf. 2008.

Further Reading

Bothamley J, Boyle M: *Medical Conditions affecting Pregnancy and childbirth*. Oxford, Radcliffe, 2009.

A comprehensive review of a range of medical conditions and the impact they have on the woman and her pregnancy. Each chapter begins with a review of the physiological changes to the relevant body system in pregnancy. The management is divided into pre-conception, antenatal, labour and postnatal care. It includes a focus on the midwifery care alongside care by the multidisciplinary team and emphasizes that women with complex medical conditions need knowledgeable midwifery support.

Nelson-Piercy C: *Handbook of Obstetric Medicine*, 5th edn. Boco Raton, CRC Press Taylor and Francis Group, 2015.

A concise, up to date handbook in a readable, quick reference format. Although intended for medical students and doctors, the background information is useful for student midwives and midwives. Whilst not referenced, each chapter has recommended further reading.

Knight M, Nair M, Tuffnell D, et al, on behalf of MBRRACE-UK: *Saving Lives, Improving Mothers' Care – Surveillance of maternal deaths in the UK 2012–14 and lessons learned to inform maternity care from the UK and Ireland Confidential Enquiries into Maternal Deaths and Morbidity 2009–14*. Oxford, National Perinatal Epidemiology Unit, University of Oxford, 2016.

Each year MBRRACE publishes data and recommendations for improvements in care based on an audit of maternal deaths and morbidity. In each publication they focus on a few areas in more detail. This report features, amongst other things, a review of cardiac disease and hypertensive disorders.

Jordan S: *Pharmacology for Midwives: The evidence base for safe practice*, 2nd edn. Basingstoke, Palgrave Macmillan, 2010.

A comprehensive pharmacology textbook that includes a range of background information on medical conditions. It includes midwifery responsibilities in relation to pharmacology management. It should be read in conjunction with hospital protocols as the specifics may change, but a very useful guide.

Useful organisations

Diabetes UK: https://www.diabetes.org.uk/

Diabetes UK is a charity that provides an excellent range of resources to support people with diabetes. The breadth of information on their website is also useful for professionals and includes specific information on diabetes in pregnancy.

Sickle cell Society: http://sicklecellsociety.org

Provides advice and support to those with sickle cell disease and their families.

Epilepsy Action: https://www.epilepsy.org.uk

Extensive resources for women, their families and health professionals.

Royal College of Obstetrics and Gynaecology: https://www.rcog.org.uk

Offers a range of publications including information sheets for women. The green-top guidelines provide a useful review on evidenced recommendations for care for a range of medical conditions as well as obstetric complications.

British Thoracic Society: https://www.brit-thoracic.org.uk/document-library/clinical-information/asthma/btssign-asthma-guideline-quick-reference-guide-2014/

Useful guide on management of asthma.

Action on Pre–eclampsia (APEC): http://action-on-pre-eclampsia.org.uk

Provides information and support for women affected by pre–eclampsia. Has a range of resources including E-learning and study days for midwives.

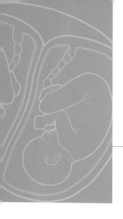

Chapter 55

Sexually transmitted infections

Jo Bates

INTRODUCTION

This chapter addresses the most common STI, HBV and HIV infections, including modes of transmission, signs and symptoms of infection, screening and treatment in the woman and the neonate. The role of the midwife in treatment and management will be outlined. Ethical principles guiding midwifery practice will also be considered and applied to this important aspect of the midwives' role.

Public Health England (PHE) reported that in 2013 there were 450,000 STI diagnoses in England (PHE 2014a). In Scotland in 2013, there was a slight decrease in cases of chlamydia, but an increase in genital herpes and 354 newly diagnosed cases of HIV (Health Protection Scotland 2014). Public Health Wales (2015) also reported an increase in chlamydia, warts, herpes, gonorrhoea, HIV and syphilis. Northern Ireland reported an increase in

diagnoses of chlamydia, gonorrhoea, genital herpes and syphilis, but a decrease in genital warts and 6000 new cases of HIV during 2013 (HSC Public Health Agency 2014a and 2014b).

HIV new diagnoses for both men and women in the United Kingdom (UK) in 2013 totaled 6000, bringing the overall number of individuals diagnosed with HIV to 133,767 (PHE 2014a). These figures, overall, are steadily increasing, which may be partly because of increased rates of screening with more individuals accessing services but also because of increasing prevalence of these conditions.

STIs occur in all age groups in both men and women from teenage years to 60s and beyond; however, young people are disproportionately affected by STIs (PHE 2014a). Many STIs occur in women of childbearing years of which a significant proportion will become clients of midwifery services. This highlights a key role of midwives in identifying those at risk and offering screening for STIs and HIV. Furthermore, midwives are able to utilize their health promotion skills and knowledge to educate women and men to have a positive and proactive approach to staying sexually healthy.

STIs are transmitted via penetrative sexual activity, oral sex, and close sexual contact with an infected person or by the sharing of sex toys between infected person(s). They can be categorized according to their cause, which are bacteria, viruses and parasites. There are at least 25 STIs that have been identified (AVERT (Averting HIV and AIDS) 2015). The most common STIs include chlamydia, gonorrhoea, genital warts (human papilloma virus (HPV)), genital herpes simplex virus (HSV), syphilis, HIV, HBV and trichomoniasis. There are, however, other infections, which can be linked to sexual activity but are not necessarily sexually transmitted, such as vaginal candidiasis and bacterial vaginosis (BV). Furthermore, scabies and pubic lice can be transmitted by close bodily contact, which does not need to be sexual (Woodward and Robinson 2011). Pregnant women, with the exception of some, who have

| Box 55.1 | Signs and symptoms of some STIs

Box 55.1 Signs and symptoms of some STIs

Many STIs have similar signs and symptoms, such as discharge, abdominal pain or discomfort and discomfort on irritation.

In women, STIs can go unnoticed, which highlights the importance of the midwife helping women identify their individual risk.

Women may experience vaginal discharge and possibly intermenstrual bleeding

Men may have signs and symptoms, which include urethral discharge, rashes or ulceration on the penis and sometimes testicular discomfort.

undergone assisted reproductive technology (ART) or possibly those in a same-sex relationship, will all have had penetrative sex and, therefore, all are potentially at risk of contracting an STI or HIV. For many women, the risk will be low, as they are likely to be in a long-term monogamous relationship. For others, however, the risk may be significantly higher. This may be because of the woman having unprotected sex with more than one partner who may have an infection or the woman's partner having sex with others who may have an STI or HIV. The midwife has a role to play in helping women determine their risk level and to offer information, screening, treatment and referral to Contraceptive and Sexual Health Services (CASH) as appropriate. (See Box 55.1.)

The midwife has a duty to recognize potential risk of infection in the neonate and to refer to the paediatric team (Nursing and Midwifery Council (NMC) 2012). The midwife must then work as part of a multidisciplinary team to ensure that the neonate is treated in a timely and appropriate way. The midwife is the health professional who is most likely to have a strong, trusting relationship with the mother (and her partner) and who is, therefore, key to ensuring that good communication between the multidisciplinary team and the mother is maintained to facilitate a positive outcome for mother and neonate (NMC 2012; NMC 2015).

Reflective activity 55.1

Before reading any further, reflect upon your current knowledge of STIs to identify gaps in your knowledge.

CHLAMYDIA

Chlamydia is the most commonly diagnosed STI, especially in 15 to 24 year olds (PHE 2015a; National Chlamydia Screening Programme (NCSP) 2013). It is caused by

the bacteria *Chlamydia trachomatis*, which, if left undiagnosed and untreated, can cause long-term health consequences, such as pelvic inflammatory disease (PID), ectopic pregnancy and tubal infertility (NCSP 2013). In men, the infection can cause urethritis, epididymitis or epididymo-orchitis and, over time, can affect fertility (Richens 2011; NHS Choices 2015). Genital chlamydia can be asymptomatic in up to 70% of women and 50% to 70% of men. The most common signs and symptoms in women include dysuria, unusual vaginal discharge, bleeding during or after sex, lower abdominal pain or discomfort, intermenstrual bleeding and heavier periods compared with usual (Family Planning Association (FPA) 2015a; NHS Choices 2015). During pregnancy, chlamydia infection can spread from the lower genital tract to the uterus, which can cause chorioamnionitis and this, in turn, may cause premature rupture of the membranes (PROM), preterm delivery and postnatal infection (Wilson 2011).

Chlamydia is transmitted through sexual contact, although individuals do not need to have penetrative sex for transmission to occur. Bacteria can be transferred from one mucous membrane to another, for example, to the eyes, throat, anus, vagina, cervix or urethra. Incubation period in women is unknown (Richens 2011) but is at least 2 weeks after the last exposure (British Association for Sexual Health and HIV (BASHH 2008) Clinical Effectiveness Group (CEG) 2008). In men, the incubation period is less than 4 weeks (Richens 2011).

It is important to remember that STIs in pregnancy can be asymptomatic; therefore, a risk assessment should be completed as part of routine antenatal care.

Chlamydia in pregnancy and in the neonate

Chlamydia infection in pregnancy can cause PROM, preterm delivery, chorioamnionitis and postnatal infection (endometritis) (Wilson 2011). Infection transmission to the neonate can be as high as 50% to 70% according to Wilson (2011) if the infection in the mother is untreated. Although intra-uterine transmission can occur, the most risky time is during vaginal birth as the fetus passes through the infected lower genital tract and cervix (Medforth et al 2011). The main presentation in the neonate is conjunctivitis between 5 to 12 days (Wilson 2011), although others report the incubation period in the neonate as between 10 to 14 days (Medforth et al 2011). The infection is known as *Chlamydia neonatorum*, with between 30% and 40% of neonates developing this. A further 10% to 20% of neonates will develop pneumonia, which is particularly serious in preterm neonates, potentially causing respiratory distress and apnoea. If the infection is not treated, it can lead to chronic pulmonary disease and asthma (Pellowe and Pratt 2006; Medforth et al 2011). Most STIs can be treated and harm to the neonate prevented especially if the infections are detected and treated early.

Conjunctivitis in the neonate often appears in one eye and then affects the other eye after 2 to 7 days. Oedema and erythema of the eyelids is often present along with a discharge from the eyes, which is watery initially and then becomes purulent (Pellowe and Pratt 2006), often referred to as 'sticky eye'. Swabs should be taken and sent to the laboratory for culture and sensitivity and antibiotic treatment, which is usually in the form of eye drops administered.

Otitis media can occur because of infection of the nasopharynx and pneumonia may develop between 4 to 12 weeks; therefore, it is imperative that neonates with chlamydia infection are diagnosed and promptly treated with systemic antibiotics (Medforth et al 2011). In female infants, vaginal infection may also occur (Wilson 2011) (see Ch. 48).

GONORRHOEA

Gonorrhoea is caused by the bacteria *Neisseria gonorrhoeae* and is caused by transmission of infected secretions from one mucous membrane to another. Gonorrhoea can be transmitted to the urethra, endocervix, rectum, pharynx and conjunctiva (BASHH 2015). It is the second most common bacterial STI in the UK after chlamydia (NHS Wales 2014). The incubation period is 2 to 5 days; however, it can be asymptomatic in as many as 50% of women and 1 in 10 men. The most common presenting symptom in women is increased and/or change in vaginal discharge. Lower abdominal pain may be a feature of infection, as may dysuria but not frequency of micturition. Infection of the endocervix is asymptomatic in as many as 50% of women. In men, urethral discharge and dysuria are the most common presenting symptoms (Bignell and FitzGerald 2011). Untreated gonorrhoea has potentially serious consequences, such as pelvic inflammatory disease (PID), in women and epididymo-orchitis or prostatits in men.

In recent years, gonorrhoea has become increasingly resistant to antibiotics. The treatment was subsequently changed in 2011 to a dual combination of ceftriaxone and azithromycin, which has had some effect in slowing resistance. In 2013, resistance to both of these antibiotics was detected (PHE 2014b). This underlines the growing problem of antibiotic resistance for the treatment of bacterial infections. Furthermore, in the case of STIs, the midwife has a role to play in imparting the safer sex message as part of their public health role. Midwives should keep in mind that STIs often coexist, for example, gonorrhoea may be detected alongside chlamydia and/or *Trichomonas vaginalis* and/or *Candida albicans* (Bignell and FitzGerald 2011).

Gonorrhoea in pregnancy and in the neonate

Gonorrhoea in pregnancy can be asymptomatic; however, the infection may ascend to the uterine cavity and cause chorioamnionitis, PROM, preterm delivery, low birth-weight and postnatal endometritis (Wilson 2011). Treatment with antibiotics can be given during pregnancy according to local or national guidelines.

Transmission rate to the neonate is around 40% if the mother is untreated (Wilson 2011). The main feature is conjunctivitis, which presents as 'sticky eye' at 2 to 5 days after birth. There is usually a purulent discharge and swelling of the eyelids and, if left untreated, this may lead to permanent damage to the eyes caused by corneal ulceration and perforation, which can cause blindness (Wilson 2011). Swabs should be taken from each affected eye and sent to the laboratory for culture and sensitivity. Treatment is usually with antibiotic eye drops (see Ch. 48).

SYPHILIS

Syphilis is a bacterial infection caused by the spirochete bacterium, *Treponema pallidum*. It can be transmitted sexually or from mother to child in pregnancy (French 2011). Syphilis continues to be a serious infection with potentially (but rarely in developed countries) fatal consequences if left undetected and untreated. Syphilis has several stages of progression: primary, secondary, early latent and late latent (sometimes called tertiary).

Transmission is through direct contact with a person who has an infected lesion known as a chancre. A chancre is usually a single (but can be multiple), painless, firm, round ulceration with defined edges. This is the first stage of syphilis, with symptoms appearing usually between 9 to 90 days with most cases appearing between 14 to 21 days after the initial infection French (2011). As the chancre usually occurs in places of the body which are difficult to see, such as the vagina, and that the lesion is painless, this stage of the infection can be unnoticed. The chancre is usually present for around 3 to 6 weeks (sometimes up to 10 weeks) and, during this time, the lesion is teeming with spirochetes and is highly infectious.

The symptoms of secondary syphilis usually appear around 4 to 8 weeks after the initial infection. These often appear as a skin rash that is not itchy and found on the trunk, arms, legs, palms of the hands, soles of the feet and sometimes on the face (French 2011). The individual may also have swollen glands, sore throat, headaches, weight loss, aching muscles and fatigue (Centres for Disease Control and Prevention (CDC) 2014). These symptoms will disappear with or without treatment; however, without treatment, the infection will progress to the next stage.

The early latent stage is when the infection has been present for less than 2 years, and late latent stage, when it has been present for more than 2 years (French 2011). Although the individual has had no signs of infection, syphilis remains in their body and can manifest many years later (10 to 20) in some cases (CDC 2014). The infection can affect many systems of the body, including the nervous and cardiovascular systems, the brain, bones and soft tissues and the eyes. If untreated, this can lead to death.

Syphilis in pregnancy and in the neonate

Although rates of syphilis in pregnant women in the UK remains very low, PHE (2014b) state that there has been a steady increase in the number of women diagnosed with infectious syphilis who are of childbearing age. PHE (2013) report that most cases of congenital syphilis were seen in the infants of women who were unable to access health services for reasons that were multifactorial. These included women who experienced cultural barriers, socio-economic deprivation or who had chaotic lifestyles. This highlights the importance of identifying women at risk of infection and facilitating attendance at antenatal clinics, which requires a multiagency, multiprofessional approach (PHE 2013).

Syphilis has potentially serious consequences in pregnancy, as it can cause spontaneous abortion, intra-uterine growth restriction, intra-uterine death, stillbirth, congenital syphilis and perinatal death (Medforth et al 2011). It can be transferred to the fetus via the placenta throughout pregnancy; however, the risk of congenital syphilis is determined by the stage of the infection in the mother (Wilson 2011). Antenatal screening for syphilis is well established in the UK with women being routinely offered screening usually at or around the time of the first booking visit by the midwife. PHE (2014b) report that there is 96% coverage in screening within England. However, with cases of congenital syphilis still being reported in the UK, it is evident that there are some gaps in the provision of screening, treatment and intervention strategies. The midwife has a key role in offering screening, information and education to women and their partners and to refer on to the appropriate health professionals when necessary (NMC 2012).

Women can be treated for syphilis in pregnancy and the earlier treatment is administered, the more effective it is likely to be in preventing congenital syphilis. Treatment is usually with a course of intramuscular (IM) procaine penicillin.

Congenital syphilis is defined as early congenital, which occurs before the infant is 2 years old and late congenital, which is after 2 years of age.

At birth, many infants are asymptomatic, but signs of early congenital syphilis are a copper-coloured rash, hepatosplenomegaly, blood stained or mucopurulent nasal discharge, causing snuffles. Osteochondritis can occur, especially in the long bones and the ribs. Some infants may develop meningitis, hydrocephalus and seizures (Caserta 2013).

Late congenital syphilis presents with gummatous lesions often on the nose, hard palate and periosteal lesions. Eyes may be affected, deafness can occur and neurosyphilis may develop (Caserta 2013). (see Ch. 48.)

Treatment is most effective if given to the mother before the birth, as this also treats the fetus. However, penicillin can be administered to the infant or child to clear the infection, but damage that has already occurred cannot be reversed. Partner notification is a crucial component of the prevention of onward transmission of STIs. Genitourinary medicine clinics (GUM) and CASH clinics have staff who are trained in Partner Notification and who can provide this service.

Reflective activity 55.2

Check in your area of work whether resources are available for women in regard to STIs and contraception, for example, written information and leaflets.

HERPES

Herpes is caused by the herpes simplex virus (HSV) and is the most common cause of sexually acquired genital ulceration in the UK (Patel and Gupta 2011). There are 2 subtypes of the virus:

Type 1 (Herpes Simplex Virus 1 (HSV1)) causes cold sores (oral herpes) but can cause genital infection.

Type 2 (Herpes Simplex Virus 2 (HSV2)) is historically associated with genital infection. This type is more likely to cause recurrent anogenital symptoms.

In the past, most HSV1 infections occurred in children and presented as oral blisters and painful ulcers commonly known as 'cold sores'. Infection with HSV1 during childhood reduced symptoms of HSV2 infection in adulthood in the event of the individual coming into sexual contact with another person with the infection. Currently, fewer children are contracting HSV1 and so are theoretically more susceptible to infection when they start to become sexually active. HSV1 is now the most common cause of genital herpes in the UK (Patel et al 2014).

HSV is transmitted via sexual contact with an infected person. It can also be transmitted via oral sex with a person who has a cold sore, via sharing of sex toys, by close skin-to-skin contact during sex and it can be transmitted on the hands. Some individuals who have the virus can transmit the infection even though they have no symptoms; this is known as asymptomatic shedding. The risk of transmission in this way is low but is highest in the first year after the person initially contracted the virus. As outbreaks become less frequent, the risk of asymptomatic shedding reduces (FPA 2014b). The incubation period for HSV infection is between 5 to 14 days; however, according to Patel and Gupta (2011), less than half of those who contract HSV develop signs or symptoms at the time of the first infection. Features of infection at first episode, which can occur sometime after the initial infection was acquired, include formation of blisters on the mucous membranes in the anogenital area. These develop into extremely painful ulcers. The individual may also feel generally unwell and report lack of energy, fatigue, muscle aches and headaches.

After the individual has recovered from the initial infection, the virus becomes dormant in the local sensory ganglia. Recurrent episodes can occur throughout life when the individual is exposed to certain triggers such as stress, being unwell, exposure to UV light, such as from the sun and sunbeds, drinking excess alcohol and immunosuppression (such as occurs in pregnancy). Outbreaks tend to reoccur most frequently in the first year after the initial infection and become less frequent and milder over time.

Herpes in pregnancy and the neonate

If the mother acquires HSV for the first time up to 27 + 6 weeks of pregnancy, she should be referred to GUM for confirmation of the diagnosis and treatment commenced according to local policy and guidelines. Acyclovir is usually the drug of choice, either orally or intravenously (BASHH 2015; RCOG 2014). Obstetric review is also required. Providing the woman does not go into premature labour within 6 weeks she can be expected to proceed to a normal vaginal birth. If initial infection occurs at or after 28 weeks of pregnancy, treatment should be commenced as soon as possible, usually with acyclovir, either orally or intravenously, depending on clinical presentation. Delivery by caesarean section is usually recommended, especially if the initial infection occurred with 6 weeks of expected delivery, as the risk of neonatal transmission is as high as 41% (BASHH and RCOG 2014). Congenital herpes is a serious infection because of transfer of the virus in utero; however, this is rare (BASHH and RCOG 2014).

If a woman has a recurrence of HSV during pregnancy or at the time of birth, the risk of transmission to the neonate is low. This means that in the absence of other factors, a normal vaginal delivery can be anticipated for these women. Treatment with oral acyclovir may be recommended from 36 weeks onwards, as it reduces the risk of asymptomatic shedding and, therefore, the need for

caesarean section. However, Patel and Gupta (2011) point out that invasive monitoring, such as fetal scalp electrode and fetal blood sampling, should be avoided because this could increase the risk of transmission of the virus to the neonate. BASSH and RCOG (2014) state that there is no increased risk of congenital abnormalities, PROM, premature labour and fetal growth restriction in women who test seropositive for HSV.

The greatest risk of infection for the fetus is if the mother contracts HSV for the first time in the third trimester of pregnancy, especially within 6 weeks of delivery. This is because the neonate is likely to be born before passive immunity from the mother has occurred. In these cases, caesarean section is recommended to minimize the risk of infection to the fetus/neonate.

For women who have a recurrent episode of HSV at the time of delivery, the risk of transmission to the neonate is low, at approximately 0% to 3% for a vaginal delivery (BASHH and RCOG 2014). Caesarean section may be considered if there are other risk factors present.

HSV1 and HSV2 infection in the neonate is low in the UK (1:60,000 live births) (Wilson 2011). Nevertheless, HSV infection in the neonate is extremely serious and can prove to be fatal. Infection is usually via direct contact with maternal secretions; however, BASHH and RCOG (2014) state that in 25% of cases, postnatal infection occurred. Oral herpes can be transmitted to the neonate, and this is an area where the midwife can educate the parents about protecting their baby from exposure to the infection. For women who are co-infected with HSV and HIV, recurrent episodes of HSV are likely to be more frequent and more severe. They may also be more at risk of asymptomatic shedding of HSV.

HSV infection is classified according to where the site of the infection occurred:

- Skin, eye or mouth
- Central nervous system, presenting as encephalitis
- Disseminated infection where multiple organs are involved. This has the worst prognosis and is more common in preterm neonates

(Wilson 2011; BASHH and RCOG 2014).

Prognosis for the neonate is improved the sooner the infection is diagnosed and treatment commenced.

GENITAL WARTS – HUMAN PAPILLOMA VIRUS

Genital warts are the most common viral sexually transmitted infection and are caused by human papilloma virus (HPV) with 70,612 cases diagnosed in 2014 in England alone (PHE 2015b). There are over a 100 genotypes of HPV, which have been identified, with 40 of these infecting the genital area. Some of these are classed as low risk or high risk, depending on the degree of risk they present in causing or contributing to the cause of cervical cancer. Most genital warts are caused by the low risk types, HSV 6 and HSV 11; however, HPV 16 and HPV 18 are more high-risk genotypes and are known to have caused at least 70% of cervical cancers (World Health Organisation (WHO) 2015). Genital warts are transmitted by direct skin-to-skin contact; penetrative sex does not have to occur and they can be transmitted whether condoms are used or not, as condoms do not always cover the area (skin) where genital warts may be present. The incubation period is anywhere between 2 weeks to 9 months. Once a person is infected, they will always have the virus; however, many may never develop visible warts, but, nevertheless, they can still transmit the virus (Woodward and Robinson 2011). Warts usually appear as either a single, fleshy, painless lump in the genital area or in clusters. There are various treatments available, including topical preparations, cryotherapy, laser and excision. It is important that an accurate diagnosis is sought so that the most appropriate treatment can be commenced; therefore, referral to GUM is advised. Treatment, however, will not eradicate the virus and future outbreaks may or may not occur. Some people only ever have one episode of visible warts, others may have many episodes. Infection with HPV can be very distressing for some people, and these individuals may require counselling and ongoing support.

Genital warts in pregnancy and the neonate

Genital warts may appear for the first time during pregnancy or may reappear even though the woman has not had an episode for a long period of time. This is because of the immunosuppressive effect of pregnancy. Warts may sometimes be treated during pregnancy; however, a medical review will be required to ensure the safest treatment is prescribed, usually treatment is delayed until after delivery (Medforth et al 2011). Occasionally, warts may be removed if they are obstructing the vaginal outlet and very occasionally a caesarean section may be required, although this is uncommon. HPV can be transmitted to the neonate during vaginal birth but the risk is small. Infection in the neonate can result in conjunctivitis or laryngeal papillomatosis, which is when warts develop on the voice box, although the risk of this is very small. The midwife has an important role in ensuring the woman is aware of the importance of attending routine cervical screening. A national immunization programme was introduced in 2008 to protect girls aged 11 to 14 from HPV 16 and 18; therefore, it is anticipated that the incidence of cervical cancer will significantly reduce in the future (Cancer Research UK 2014).

Reflective activity 55.3 ><

Consider how, as a midwife, you can discuss sexual health with women in your care.

HEPATITIS B VIRUS

Hepatitis B virus (HBV) replicates in the liver and is present in large amounts in the blood of infected individuals and is also present in other body fluids, such as vaginal fluid, semen and saliva (PHE 2014c). HBV is able to survive outside of the body for at least a week and only small amounts of the virus need be present in the blood of the infected person for it to be passed on to others (British Liver Trust (BLT) 2012). HBV can be transmitted via sexual activity, sharing of contaminated needles (drug use or tattoos), mother-to-child transmission (MTCT), needlestick injury, body piercing or via transfusion of infected blood products in countries where blood donor and blood donations are not tested (PHE 2014c). Incubation period is 40 to 160 days. Infection with HBV can be acute or chronic. Acute infection may cause flulike illness with symptoms of fatigue, joint pain, abdominal pain, nausea and vomiting and loss of appetite. More severe symptoms can be diarrhoea, pale-coloured stools, dark urine and jaundice. Acute infection usually last for less than 6 months and is self- limiting. Most people clear the virus, meaning that they are no longer infectious; however, blood tests will show hepatitis B antibodies (BLT 2012). Chronic infection may occur in some individuals (10%) who have had an acute infection acquired in adulthood; however, most people will have acquired the infection during childhood. There are usually no symptoms with chronic infection but the individual will be infectious to others. Chronic infection is determined as infection present for longer than 6 months. Around 25% of those with a chronic infection will develop chronic liver disease and a few of those may go on to develop liver cancer (BLT 2012; PHE 2014c).

The incidence of acute hepatitis in England in 2014 was 0.91 per 100,000 population (488 cases). There were more men than women with the condition, which is partly attributed to men who have sex with men (MSM), although heterosexual transmission also was recorded in both men and women (PHE 2014c). Acute infectious hepatitis is a notifiable disease in England and Wales.

Hepatitis B in pregnancy and the neonate

Hepatitis B is screened for in early pregnancy for HBV surface antigen (HBsAg). If this is positive, then a further blood sample will be obtained to repeat the test and confirm diagnosis. Women who are classed as highly infectious have a 70% to 90% chance of transmitting the virus to their infant. In women who are classed as infected but not highly infectious the risk of transmission to the infant is 10%. Of the infants who become infected, around 90% will develop chronic infection and will be at risk of developing liver disease in later life; however, immunization can prevent this in 90% of cases (Department of Health (DH) 2011). The National Institute for Health and Care Excellence (NICE) (2013) states that women who test positive for the HBsAg should be referred to a hepatologist or gastroenterologist who has an interest in hepatology within 6 weeks of receiving the result. Treatment can be offered to women in the third trimester to reduce the risk of transmission of HBV to the infant.

The infant should be vaccinated according to DH guidelines (2011) as follows:

- 1 dose at birth
- 1 month after the first dose
- 2 months after the first dose
- 12 months after the first dose plus a blood test to check the immunity status of the child

It is essential that the full course of vaccinations is completed, as even with complete compliance and with the full vaccination programme, 10% of individuals will go onto develop chronic infection (DH 2011). A further booster dose is given at around 5 years in children who are at continued risk.

HUMAN IMMUNODEFICIENCY VIRUS

Human immunodeficiency virus (HIV) is a retrovirus, meaning that the genome of HIV contains an enzyme known as reverse transcriptase. This enzyme allows the virus to make copies of itself by transcribing RNA into DNA within the host cell such as the CD4 'helper' lymphocyte. The DNA of HIV becomes combined into the genome of the host cell (Williams et al 2011). This means HIV is able to replicate itself within host cells of the immune system. There are different strains, types, groups and subgroups of HIV, as the virus is able to mutate readily. There are two types of HIV, HIV 1 and HIV 2. Both of these can be transmitted via sex, through blood and mother to child (AVERT 2015). HIV 1 is the predominant virus worldwide. HIV 2 appears to be less easily transmitted and has a longer period of time between initial infection and illness (AVERT 2015).

HIV can be transmitted via unprotected sex, sharing of needles with an infected person, mother to child during pregnancy, via breastfeeding and through infected blood products. HIV can also be transmitted via oral sex, although this carries less risk of infection.

There are four different stages of infection: primary, clinically asymptomatic, symptomatic HIV and progression from HIV to AIDS. The primary stage occurs at the time of initial infection and lasts for a few weeks. The person may experience mild flu-like symptoms with a fever (96% of people), swollen glands (74%), pharyngitis (70%) and an erythematous rash (70%) (Tenant-Flowers and Mindel 2012). However, the infection may be missed at this stage because symptoms may be attributed to a cold or flu and not linked to possible HIV infection. Stage 2 is clinically asymptomatic and lasts on average for 10 years during which the person has no symptoms but may on occasion have swollen glands. They are, however, infectious to others, although levels of the virus in the blood remain low. HIV replicates at a slow rate during this stage but does not stop. Stage 3 is symptomatic of HIV, with symptoms starting to occur usually in the form of opportunistic infections. The body is less able to deal with infections as the immune system has become damaged. Some examples of infections that may occur are recurrent pneumonia, candidiasis of bronchi, trachea, lungs or oesophagus, herpes simplex with ulcers present for greater than 1 month, herpes zoster, cytomegalovirus and tuberculosis. Cervical dysplasia and invasive cervical cancer may occur and other conditions, such as lymphoma and Kaposi's sarcoma, may develop (AVERT 2015). Progression from HIV to AIDS occurs as the immune system becomes increasingly damaged. Some individuals may have co-infections. For example, 9% of people who are HIV positive are also infected with hepatitis C (National Aids Trust (NAT) 2012); hepatitis B and tuberculosis are also conditions which can co-infect individuals who have HIV.

Globally, there were 35 million people living with HIV; however, there have been around 78 million individuals infected with the virus since the start of the epidemic. Thirty-nine million people have died from acquired immune deficiency syndrome (AIDS) related illnesses (UNAIDS 2014). In the UK, there were an estimated 107,800 people living with HIV in 2013 – around a quarter of these individuals were unaware of their infection, thereby potentially putting others at risk if they were to have sex without the protection of a condom. Six thousand individuals were diagnosed with HIV in the UK in 2013 and a further 320 people were diagnosed with AIDS (PHE 2014d). In 2012, 675,800 women were screened for HIV during pregnancy, which is an uptake rate of 98%. Of these, 0.19% (1310) tested positive and 0.04% (1 in 2500) were new diagnoses. Mother-to-child transmission rate was less than 1% in children whose mothers were known to have HIV (PHE 2014d).

HIV in pregnancy and the neonate

Antenatal screening for HIV is now well established in the UK and operates on an opt-out rather than opt-in basis.

In other words, women are routinely offered HIV screening unless they state they want to opt out. There is a small chance that women may become infected with HIV during pregnancy, so, therefore, those women at high risk or those who develop seroconversion symptoms should be retested during pregnancy. Without interventions, mother-to-child transmission (MTCT) of HIV in breastfeeding women is 20% to 30%. With interventions, however, MTCT is reduced to around 1% (Wilkinson and Mercey 2012). Women found to be HIV positive in pregnancy must be referred to the multidisciplinary team, including an HIV specialist, specialist midwife, obstetrician and paediatrician; however, other health and social care workers may need to be involved, such as the social work team, health visitor, GP and others (NMC 2012; Wilkinson and Mercey 2012).

INTERVENTIONS DURING PREGNANCY

If the woman's health is good and she does not require treatment for herself during pregnancy, she has two options regarding management:

Zidovudine monotherapy with a caesarean section if the viral load (how much virus is detectable in the blood) is consistently low.

or

A short course of combination therapy, starting after the first trimester with an option of vaginal delivery if the viral load is undetectable.

Some women who are HIV positive will require drug treatment for their own health. In these cases women should be commenced on combination antiretroviral therapy (cART) as soon as is practical (Wilkinson and Mercey 2012).

Women who are HIV positive are more at risk of developing infections and other conditions during pregnancy, which the midwife should be aware of. HIV infection increases the risk of CIN and cervical cancer. Therefore, women who are over 25 years old who have not had cervical screening within the last 12 months should be offered this test and thereafter on an annual basis. Genital infections, such as herpes or genital warts (HPV), may reoccur during pregnancy and may be more severe and persistent than in women who are not HIV positive. In some cases, prophylactic treatment may be required along with referral to specialist services (Wilkinson and Mercey 2012).

Breastfeeding is not recommended because of the risk of HIV transmission via breastmilk (BHIVA 2014; BHIVA and Children's HIV Association (CHIVA) 2010); however, some women may choose to breastfeed because of cultural norms or personal choice. It is imperative that the woman fully understands the risks of breastfeeding and is able to make a fully informed decision in choosing not to bottle feed. An interpreter may be necessary if there is a language barrier and, in the event of the woman choosing to breastfeed, the midwife must ensure that the paediatrician, health visitor, social worker and supervisor of midwives are informed. BHIVA and CHIVA (2010) do not endorse automatic referral to safeguarding teams when a mother who is on effective drug therapy and has a repeatedly undetectable viral load chooses to breastfeed; however, close monitoring of the mother's drug treatment, which should continue until 1 week after breastfeeding has ended, is strongly recommended.

The midwife can help reduce the risk of transmission of HIV to the neonate by ensuring good attachment at the breast to prevent nipple trauma and preventing the development of mastitis. Exclusive breastfeeding is advised with early discontinuation onto infant formula or solid foods before 6 months (BHIVA and CHIVA 2010).

Infants born to mothers who are HIV positive will have maternal HIV antibodies detectable within their blood for up to 18 months. The infant will be commenced on antiretroviral treatment soon after birth. Guidelines published in 2014 by BHIVA state that infants should be tested for HIV during the first 48 hours after birth and before discharge from hospital. Testing should be repeated 2 weeks after prophylactic drugs have stopped at the age of 6 weeks and again at 12 weeks of age. If the infant is at additional risk, then testing should be further repeated at 18 months of age. With access to and avoidance of breastfeeding MTCT of HIV is almost eliminated (McMaster and Stokes 2012); however, for those infants who do test positive less than 1 year of age, treatment should be commenced as soon as possible

---

Reflective activity 55.4

Consider what additional support and information an HIV-positive pregnant woman may need during pregnancy.

Find out what services there are to support the woman and her family in your area.

Reflective activity 55.5

There is ongoing data collection around the incidence of HIV and STIs. Undertake an Internet search for "HIV and STI surveillance" and identify the latest data.

The Centre for Infectious Disease Surveillance (CIDSC) is part of Public Health England.

ETHICAL PRINCIPLES FOR MIDWIVES RELATING TO STI AND HIV SCREENING AND TREATMENT

Confidentiality is paramount within midwifery practice and this is especially true within sexual health. In the UK, sexual health records are held separately and not shared with others (e.g. in shared NHS records). This means that STI testing and treatment is not included in shared records unless there is consent for those attending sexual health clinics or services (BASHH 2015). Midwives work within the rules of confidentiality on a daily basis and are bound by the NMC Code (2015).

Non-maleficence is a term that many are familiar with, as it means that first and foremost, one should do no harm to another (Beauchamp and Childress 2013). This means both direct harm such as not to cause pain or suffering and unintentional harm such as (perhaps) neglect or by omission. Indeed one must not only do no harm but also be proactive in preventing harm (Foster and Lasser 2011). Within midwifery practice, this applies to sexual health and HIV screening, as the consequences of undiagnosed infection can be immense and result in long-term illness and morbidity, even death for affected individuals. Furthermore, an undiagnosed infection can be passed onto an intimate partner and also to the fetus or infant during pregnancy or birth, thereby causing distress and harm to others. Midwives also have a role to play in administering treatment to women and referring them to a sexual health or HIV specialist and other appropriate professionals, such as social workers or counsellors, that an infection is appropriately managed and that the woman has the best care possible for physical and emotional needs. This not only fulfils the ethical principle of non-maleficence but is a professional requirement, as stated in the NMC Rules (2012). (See Ch. 8.)

Beneficence is an ethical principle that means that one has a moral obligation to act for the benefit of others (Foster and Lasser 2011). However, Beauchamp and Childress (2013) suggest that although there is a moral obligation to do no harm to individuals, it may not always have an obligation to do good for others or act beneficently towards others. Midwives, however, are not only acting for a good outcome of care for the mother but also the fetus and neonate, thereby striving for the benefit of others. This, again, applies to sexual health and HIV screening, as already discussed, and prompt diagnosis, referral and treatment is crucial for optimum outcome for mother and infant.

Justice within midwifery practice applies to inequalities in access to services and the right for individuals to be treated fairly. Furthermore, each person should have the same opportunity (for treatment, for example) and be treated with respect free from discrimination (Foster and Lasser 2011). This principle can also be applied more broadly in terms of the fair distribution and allocation of services and resources. When applying this principle to sexual health and HIV within midwifery practice, justice is achieved by ensuring that all women are offered HIV screening and that all women who are identified as having risk factors for an STI are offered screening and treatment regardless of their age, social status or place of residence.

Autonomy is the right of individuals to hold their own views and to be able to make choices and decisions based on their own values and beliefs (Beauchamp and Childress 2013). In broader terms, this is also associated with respect for and dignity of others (Foster and Lasser 2011). Within midwifery practice, this is linked to informed consent and the right of the woman to make decisions that she feels are right for her and her infant based on full knowledge of risk and benefit in regards to screening, treatment, management and referral where appropriate.

CONCLUSION

This chapter has discussed STIs and HIV and linked this to the role of the midwife in caring for the mother, fetus and neonate. Ethical principles have also been linked to the sexual health role of the midwife when offering screening, management and treatment for women and infants in the midwife's care. STIs and HIV can result in serious health problems for mother, fetus and infant. Most STIs can be diagnosed easily and treatment is extremely effective in most individuals, resulting in improved short- and long-term outcomes for mother and infant. The midwife has a pivotal role to play in sexual health not only by offering screening to women but also by ensuring correct treatment is initiated and appropriate referral is made. Crucially, however, the main role of the midwife within this aspect of her role is education of women and their partners in her care.

Key Points

- STIs in pregnancy can be asymptomatic; therefore, a risk assessment should be completed as part of routine antenatal care.
- Most STIs can be treated and harm to the neonate prevented, especially if the infections are detected and treated early.
- STIs often coexist; therefore, it is important that if one STI is present, then there may be others present as well.
- The presence of an STI can facilitate the transmission of HIV.
- Partner notification is a crucial component of the prevention of onward transmission of STIs. Genitourinary medicine clinics (GUM) and CASH clinics have staff who are trained in Partner Notification who can provide this service.

References

AVERT (Averting HIV and AIDS): *What is HIV?* (website). www.avert.org/hiv.htm. 2015.

Beauchamp TL, Childress JF: *Principles of biomedical ethics*, 7th edn, Oxford, Oxford University Press, 2013.

Bignell C, FitzGerald M: *UK National Guideline for the Management of Gonorrhoea in Adults. British Association of Sexual Heath and HIV* (website). www.bhiva.org. 2011.

British Association of Sexual Health and HIV (BASHH) Clinical Effectiveness Group: *Testing for chlamydia – the "window period".* (website). www.bashh.org. 2008.

British Association of Sexual Health and HIV & Royal College of Obstetricians and Gynaecologists: *Management of Genital Herpes in Pregnancy* (website). www.bashh.org. 2014.

British Association of Sexual Health and HIV (BASHH): *Patient confidentiality within sexual health services* (website). www.bashh.org. 2015.

British HIV Association: British HIV Association guidelines for the management of HIV infection in pregnant women 2012. Updated May 2014, *HIV Med* 15(Suppl 4):1–77, 2014.

British HIV Association & Children's HIV Association: *Position Statement on Infant Feeding in the UK* (website). www.bhiva.org. 2010.

British Liver Trust: *Hepatitis B* (website) www.britishlivertrust.org.uk/. 2012.

Cancer Research UK: *HPV vaccines* (website). www.cancerresearchuk.org. 2014.

Caserta MT: *Congenital Syphilis. MSD Manual Professional Version* (website). www.msdmanuals.com. 2013.

Centre for Disease Control and Prevention (CDC): *Syphilis; CDC Fact Sheet* (website). www.cdc.gov. 2014.

Department of Health (DH) (Immunisation Group): *Hepatitis B Antenatal Screening and Newborn Immunisation Programme. Best Practice Guidance.* London, Crown Copyright, 2011.

Family Planning Association (a): *Chlamydia* (website). www.fpa.org.uk. 2015.

Family Planning Association (b): *Genital herpes* (website). www.fpa.org.uk/. 2014.

Foster IR, Lasser J: *Professional ethics in midwifery practice*, Sudbury, Jones & Bartlett Publishers, 2011.

French P: Syphilis: Clinical Features, Diagnosis and Management. In Rogstad KE, editor: *ABC of Sexually Transmitted Infections*, 6th edn, Chichester, Sussex, Wiley-Blackwell, 2011.

Health Protection Scotland: *Scotland's Sexual Health Information 2013* (website). www.hps.scot.nhs.uk/. 2014.

HSC Public Health Agency: *HIV Surveillance in Northern Ireland 2014: An Analysis of Date for Calendar Year 2013* (website). www.publichealth.hscni.net/. 2014a.

HSC Public Health Agency: *Sexually Transmitted Infection Surveillance in Northern Ireland 2014: An Analysis of Data for Calendar Year 2013* (website). www.publichealth.hscni.net/. 2014b.

McMaster P, Stokes S: Adler MW, Edwards SG, Miller RR, et al, editors: *ABC of HIV and AIDS*, 6th edn, Chichester, Wiley-Blackwell, BMJ Books, 2012.

Medforth J, Battersby S, Evans S, et al, editors: *Oxford handbook of midwifery*, Oxford, Oxford University Press, 2011.

National Aids Trust: *Hepatitis C and HIV Co-Infection* (website). http://nat.org.uk. 2012.

National Chlamydia Screening Programme: *Genital Chlamydia Trachomatis* (website). www.chlamydiascreening.nhs.uk/. 2013.

National Health Service (NHS) Choices: *Chlamydia complications* (website). http://www.nhs.uk. 2015.

National Health Service (NHS) Wales: *Gonorrhoea* (website). http://nhsdirect.wales.nhs.uk. 2014.

National Institute for Health and Care Excellence (NICE): *Hepatitis B (Chronic): Diagnosis and Management.* NICE Guidelines CG165. London, NICE, 2013.

Nursing and Midwifery Council (NMC): *Midwives rules and standards 2012*, London, NMC, 2012.

Nursing and Midwifery Council (NMC): *The Code: professional Standards of Practice and Behaviour for Nurses and Midwives*, London, NMC, 2015.

Patel R, Gupta N: Genital ulcer disease. In Rogstad KE, editor: *ABC of sexually transmitted infections*, 6th edn, Chichester, Sussex, Wiley-Blackwell, 2011.

Patel R, Green J, Clarke E, et al: 2014 UK national guideline for the management of anogenital herpes, *Int J STD AIDS*, SAGE, April 2015 (website). www.bashh.org. 2014.

Pellowe C, Pratt RJ: Neonatal conjunctivitis and pneumonia due to chlamydia infection, *Infant* 2(1):16–17, 2006.

Public Health England (PHE): Recent epidemiology of infectious syphilis in England, *Infection reports* 7(44):2013 (website). www.gov.uk. 2013.

Public Health England (PHE): *HIV in the United Kingdom: 2014 Report* (website). www.gov.uk. 2014a.

Public Health England (PHE): *Elimination of Congenital Syphilis in the United Kingdom: The End of a Public Health Problem?* (website). www.gov.uk. 2014b.

Public Health England (PHE): *Hepatitis B: Clinical and Public Health Management. Information for Health Professionals on the Diagnosis, Prevention and Treatment of Hepatitis B* (website). https://www.gov.uk. 2014c.

Public Health England (PHE): *National HIV Surveillance Data Tables* (website). www.gov.uk. 2014d.

Public Health England (PHE): *Health Protection Report* (Vol 9, No 22) (website). www.gov.uk. 2015a.

Public Health England (PHE): *New STI Figures Show Rapid Increases Among Gay Men* (website). https://www.gov.uk. 2015b.

Public Health Wales, Communicable Disease Surveillance Centre: *Sexual Health in Wales Surveillance Scheme. Quarterly Report* (website). www.wales.nhs.uk/sites3/page.cfm?orgId=457&. 2015.

Richens J: Main presentations of sexually transmitted infections in male patients. In Rogstad KE, editor: *ABC of sexually transmitted infections*, 6th edn, Chichester, Sussex, Wiley-Blackwell, 2011.

Tenant-Flowers M, Mindel A: Clinical staging and natural history of untreated hiv infection. In Adler

MW, Edwards SG, Miller RR, et al, editors: *ABC of HIV and AIDS*, 6th edn, Chichester, Wiley-Blackwell, BMJ Books, 2012.

UNAIDS: *Fact sheet 2014* (website). www.unaids.org>douments>factsheet. 2014.

Wilkinson C, Mercey D: Women and HIV. In Adler MW, Edwards SG, Miller RR, et al, editors: *ABC of HIV and AIDS*, 6th edn, Chichester, Wiley-Blackwell, BMJ Books, 2012.

Williams I, Daniels D, Gedela K, et al: HIV. In Rogstad KE, editor: *ABC of sexually transmitted infections*, 6th edn, Chichester, Sussex, Wiley-Blackwell, 2011.

Wilson J: Sexually transmitted infections and HIV in pregnancy. In Rogstad KE, editor: *ABC of sexually transmitted infections*, 6th edn, Chichester, Sussex, Wiley-Blackwell, 2011.

Woodward CLN, Robinson AJ: Genital growths and infestation. In Rogstad KE, editor: *ABC of sexually transmitted infections*, 6th edn, Chichester, Sussex, Wiley-Blackwell, 2011.

World Health Organisation (WHO): *Human Papilloma Virus and Cervical Cancer. Fact Sheet* (No. 380) (website). http://who.int/media centre/factsheets/fs380/en/. 2015.

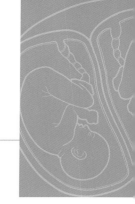

Chapter 56

Abnormalities of the genital tract

Lindsey Rose

Learning Outcomes ?

After reading this chapter, you will be able to:

- understand the major anomalies of the female genital tract and their origin
- explain the effect of anomalies on fertility, pregnancy, labour and the puerperium
- describe three main types of uterine displacement and their affect on labour
- understand the implications of female genital mutilation
- know the role of the midwife in the care of a woman with a genital tract anomaly

INTRODUCTION

The true incidence of reproductive tract anomalies is uncertain and their role in reproductive difficulties is unclear (Saravelos et al 2008; Shulman 2008). Although structural abnormalities of the uterus must be considered during pregnancy and labour, other conditions such as fibroids or uterine displacements may also present difficulties. Female genital mutilation (sometimes referred to as female circumcision or cutting) also presents health risks for mother and baby. The midwife must be able to give appropriate and safe care for any woman presenting with a genital tract anomaly.

DEVELOPMENTAL ANOMALIES

Most of the female genital tract arises from the Müllerian ducts (see Ch. 29), which form during embryonic life and which fuse by the 12th week after fertilization. The median septum then breaks down, thus forming a single uterus. Should this process fail, abnormalities such as *double uterus* (with or without a double cervix and vagina), *bicornuate uterus* or *subseptate uterus* will occur (Fig. 56.1) (Narayan 2015). As the Müllerian ducts and Wolffian ducts (see Ch. 29) develop close together, genital tract anomalies may be accompanied by malformations of the kidney and ureters. Therefore, care should include assessment of the urinary system (Edmunds 2011).

Diethylstilbestrol

Diethylstilbestrol (DES) is a synthetic nonsteroidal oestrogen used between 1948 and 1971 as a method of treating various complications in pregnancy, such as recurrent pregnancy loss and threatened abortion (Goodman et al 2011). Girls who have been exposed to DES in utero have an unusually high incidence of uncommon anomalies. These include an increased incidence of:

- cervical anomalies
- uterine malformations, such as hypoplastic and T-shaped uteri
- cervical cancer

Reproductive function can also be impaired, leading to difficulties in conception or infertility. Ectopic pregnancy, preterm birth and spontaneous abortion are more common problems associated with DES (Royal College of Obstetricians and Gynaecologists (RCOG) 2002; Jurkovic 2011)

Unicornuate uterus

A unicornuate uterus accounts for 2.4% to 13% of all Müllerian anomalies (Caserta et al 2014). This abnormality arises from failure of development of one of the Müllerian ducts, resulting in a uterus with one horn. There is a higher rate of spontaneous abortion, breech

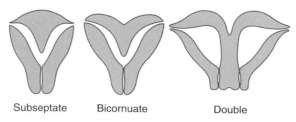

Subseptate   Bicornuate   Double

Figure 56.1 Uterine malformations.

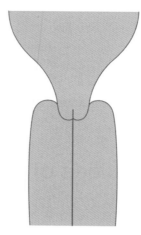

Figure 56.2 Longitudinal vaginal septum.

presentation, fetal growth restriction and preterm labour, possibly because of the limited space in the uterine cavity (Caserta 2014). Caesarean delivery is, therefore, more likely. If the pregnancy develops in a rudimentary horn, the outcome is usually a spontaneous abortion or occasionally rupture of the rudimentary horn, as the myometrium becomes rapidly stretched.

Double uterus (uterus didelphys)

Complete failure of the medial fusion of the Müllerian ducts may result in a duplication of the uterus and cervix (Bhattacharya 2010; Narayan 2015). This may be accompanied by a double vagina or a longitudinal vaginal septum (Tahlan et al 2014). The incidence is unknown, as it often remains asymptomatic, and women with this condition usually require fertility treatment. As the pregnancy progresses, the midwife will notice that the fundus is abnormal in shape and may feel unusually wide. The non-pregnant uterus will enlarge under the influence of the pregnancy hormones and may occupy space in the pelvis, thus, obstructing labour. Multiple pregnancies are rare with this condition (Bhattacharya 2010), although it has been recorded (Nanda et al 2009); however, breech presentation is common (Arulkumaran 2011).

Subseptate and bicornuate uterus

This is caused by the partial or complete failure of the Müllerian duct septum to resorb. A complete septate extends into the internal cervical os and the uterus has two cavities. A partial septate does not extend to the internal os. The abdomen will appear outwardly normal.

There are varying degrees of a bicornuate uterus. A complete bicornuate uterus has two separate uterine cavities and one cervix; in the case of a partial bicornuate uterus, the septum affects only the fundus and is outwardly distinguishable on abdominal palpation by the heart-shaped fundus (Fig. 56.1).

These anomalies do not usually cause difficulties in conception or in early pregnancy. However, they are associated with transverse lie and breech presentation, as the abnormal uterine structure hinders the normal process

of spontaneous version between 30 and 34 weeks gestation. External cephalic version of the fetus in this case, is generally unsuccessful.

The midwife should consider the possibility of structural abnormality of the uterus in any woman with a history of recurrent malpresentation. The progress of the first and second stage of labour is usually normal where there is a subseptate or bicornuate uterus. However, retained placenta may occur in the third stage, due to the shape of the uterus. Congenital abnormalities of the uterus, such as a bicornuate uterus, are also predisposing factors for uterine inversion (Francois and Foley 2012; Kroll and Lyne 2006).

Vaginal septum

A vaginal septum (Fig. 56.2) may be longitudinal or transverse, complete or partial. It is associated with dyspareunia, dysmenorrhea, primary amenorrhea and infertility. A longitudinal vaginal septum is associated with uterine anomalies, such as a septate uterus or uterus didelphys. It may present clinically as a difficulty in inserting tampons, persistent bleeding despite the presence of a tampon, or dyspareunia. It may also be asymptomatic (Neto et al 2014).

Associated problems

The presence of a uterine malformation is associated with an increased risk of recurrent spontaneous miscarriage and preterm birth (Mackay et al 2008; Narayan 2015)

The midwife should refer the woman to an obstetrician so that appropriate care may be planned, as there is a higher likelihood of the need for intervention during labour. Women should be fully informed of the potential obstetric complications, which may include malpresentations, IUGR, cord prolapse, abruption, postpartum haemorrhage and an increased risk of a caesarean section (Narayan 2015).

Reflective activity 56.1

Think about the potential needs of a woman with a double uterus. What factors would you discuss with her? What would you include in her care plan?

DISPLACEMENTS OF THE UTERUS

Retroversion of the gravid uterus

Retroversion of the uterus, which is when the pregnant uterus falls back into the hollow of the sacrum (Fig. 56.3), is normally of little clinical significance (Mackay et al 2008). During pregnancy, the condition usually resolves spontaneously as the uterus grows and rises into the abdomen around the 12th week (Mukhopadhyay and Arulkumaran 2010).

Rarely, however, the retroversion fails to resolve and the uterus becomes fixed or incarcerated in the pelvis between the sacral promontory and symphysis pubis. Between the 12th and 16th week of pregnancy, the retroverted pregnant uterus fills the pelvis and the cervix is drawn up towards the pelvic brim. The anterior vaginal wall and the urethra become stretched, the urethra narrows and, as a result, the woman is unable to pass urine (Kent and Barton-Smith 2006).

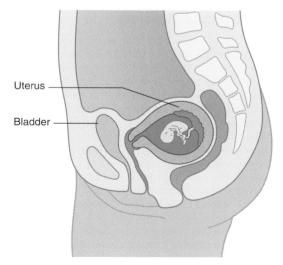

Uterus

Bladder

Figure 56.3 Incarceration of the gravid uterus.

Diagnosis

The woman will initially report pelvic pressure and difficulty in micturition and later of complete inability to pass urine. The bladder becomes more distended and, if unrelieved, overflow incontinence will occur.

The woman will experience severe abdominal pain. On abdominal examination, there is a soft swelling (the bladder) above the pubis, which may extend to the umbilicus and may be mistaken for the uterus. The fundus is not palpable at the brim of the pelvis. A pelvic ultrasound scan will assist the diagnosis (Mukhopadhyay and Arulkumaran 2010).

Treatment

The bladder is emptied with an indwelling catheter and is then kept empty until bladder tone returns. Once the bladder is empty, the uterus usually corrects its malposition spontaneously. This may be assisted if the mother lies in the semiprone or Sims position. The retroversion will not recur because the uterus will, in a few days, be too big to fall back into the pelvis. Persistent retroversion has been reported but is rare (Hamoda et al 2002).

Risks

- *Urinary tract infection,* owing to stasis of urine in the over-distended bladder. A catheter specimen of urine should be sent for microscopy and any infection must be treated promptly.
- *Sloughing of the bladder,* which may cause rupture
- *Spontaneous abortion*
- *Persistent incarceration,* which may cause sacculation of the anterior uterine wall. The pregnancy will then enlarge into the abdomen and this may confuse the diagnosis. Delivery will be by caesarean section.

Anteversion of the gravid uterus (pendulous abdomen)

This rare condition (Fig. 56.4) may occur in multiparous women whose abdominal muscles have been weakened by repeated pregnancies or those who have a midline abdominal wall hernia, possibly associated with an old scar (Gupta 2011; Saha et al 2006). Separation of the rectus abdominis muscle allows the uterus to fall forwards and, in extreme cases, the fundus may lie below the symphysis pubis. As the uterus becomes heavier, the woman experiences backache and abdominal pain. The presenting part will not engage and dystocia is likely because the long axis of the uterus is at an angle to the pelvic brim. An abdominal binder may bring relief (Gupta 2011; Saha et al 2006). This should be worn during labour to facilitate engagement and descent of the fetus. The 'all-fours' delivery position should be avoided.

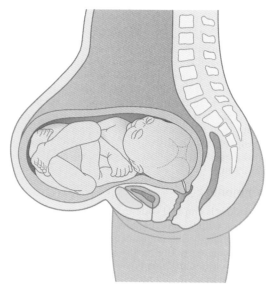

Figure 56.4 Pendulous abdomen.

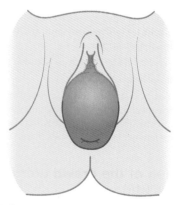

Figure 56.5 Complete uterine prolapse (uterine procidentia), non-pregnant uterus.

Prolapse of the gravid uterus

Uterine prolapse is rare in pregnancy (Fig. 56.5). Laxness of the uterovaginal supports allows the uterus to descend so that the cervix is found at or just behind the vaginal introitus. The condition mainly affects the first trimester of pregnancy, as the uterus increases in size and weight and the ligaments soften and relax. A ring pessary can be used to support the cervix and uterus and may relieve the prolapse. As the uterus grows into the abdomen, the

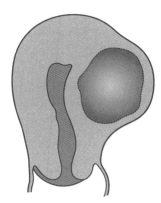

Figure 56.6 Uterine fibroid.

condition improves, although it may recur later in pregnancy. Caesarean section may be recommended to prevent further damage to the uterovaginal supports (Mukhopadhyay and Arulkumaran 2010).

> **Reflective activity 56.2**
>
> What information and advice would you give a woman who (at 8 weeks gestation) has been told that she has a retroverted uterus?

PELVIC MASSES

Fibromyomata (fibroids)

Fibroids (leiomyomas) are the most common pelvic tumours, occurring in 20% to 40% of women of childbearing age (Narayan 2015). They are more common in older women and in young West Indian and West African women. The presence of fibroids increases the risk of complications, such as threatened abortion, antepartum haemorrhage, breech presentation and caesarean birth (Mukhopadhyay and Arulkumaran 2010).

On uterine palpation, one or more swellings may be felt, continuous with the uterine wall (Fig. 56.6). A large fibroid may be mistaken for the fetal head. In pregnancy, hypertrophy of the myometrial fibres and increased vascularity and oedema cause the fibroid to enlarge and soften.

Red degeneration or impaction of a fibroid, usually during the second trimester, may cause acute pain and vomiting in pregnancy. This usually resolves within a few days without surgical intervention (Monga and Dobbs 2011). Torsion of a pedunculated fibroid, however, may require myomectomy but is rare and only considered when conservative management (bed rest, hydration and analgesics) fails (Simms-Stewart and Fletcher 2012; Narayan 2015). Most fibroids are found in the body of the uterus and do not affect the course of labour. Rarely, one may occur in the lower segment beneath the presenting part. This may prevent fetal descent into the pelvis and may obstruct labour. Postpartum haemorrhage is a risk in the third stage of labour (Simms-Stewart and Fletcher 2012).

Pregnancy complicated by fibroids is considered high risk and the labour and birth should take place in a hospital setting in case difficulty should arise. During the puerperium, fibroids regress and become smaller, as autolysis reduces the myometrial mass (Mukhopadhyay and Arulkumaran 2010).

The midwife should refer any woman with a history of treatment for fibroids before pregnancy for an ultrasound scan to assess the size, location and number of fibroids (Narayan 2015). Myomectomy involves incisions on the uterus and this may pose a risk of scar rupture. Selective embolization of fibroids is often the preferred treatment but is contraindicated in pregnancy and in women wishing to become pregnant (Narayan 2015).

Ovarian cyst

Ovarian cysts are relatively common and, in isolation, may not cause any pain. Corpus luteum cysts occur after ovulation and may cause pain if they haemorrhage or rupture. Theca luteal cysts are more common in pregnancy, particularly in multiple pregnancies. They are usually diagnosed on ultrasound scan and most resolve spontaneously (Monga and Dobbs 2011). The cyst may be in the abdomen or in the pelvis (Fig. 56.7). There is a risk of malignancy or torsion, the risk of malignancy rising with increasing age. Torsion is most likely during the second trimester or in the puerperium (Mukhopadhyay and Arulkumaran 2010). Simple nonmalignant cysts can be successfully

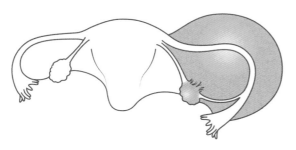

Figure 56.7 A uterus with a simple serous cyst.

removed during pregnancy, although conservative management is also an option (Siew-Fei et al 2014).

FEMALE GENITAL MUTILATION

Female genital mutilation (FGM) is the removal of all or part of the external female genitalia or causes injury to the female genitalia for non-medical reasons (World Health Organisation (WHO) 2014). The custom still persists among some groups, particularly those from Nigeria, Ethiopia, Sudan and Egypt. FGM may be viewed as a rite of passage into adult status within the community. It is usually performed before the age of 15 (WHO 2014).

WHO (2008 and 2014) classifies FGM as follows:

- *Type 1: clitoridectomy* – partial or total removal of the clitoris and/or the prepuce (Fig. 56.8)
- *Type 2: partial or total excision of the clitoris and labia minora* with or without excision of the labia majora (Fig. 56.8)
- *Type 3: infibulation* – narrowing of the vaginal opening, excision of part or all of the external genitalia and stitching/narrowing of the vaginal opening (also called *pharaonic circumcision*) (Figs 56.8 and 56.9)
- *Type 4: any other harmful procedure carried out for non-medical reasons.* This includes pricking, piercing, scraping, incising or cauterizing of the female genitalia (Department of Health (DH) 2015; RCOG 2015).

FGM is illegal in the UK and many other countries and is considered to be a violation of human rights (Royal College of Nursing (RCN) 2015; Female Genital Mutilation Act 2003). It carries a significant immediate mortality from haemorrhage and sepsis. Lifelong morbidity from urinary infection, pelvic inflammatory disease, endometriosis and renal damage may follow.

Infibulation presents particular problems in childbearing. In pregnancy, urinary tract infection is more common. The rates of caesarean section, postpartum haemorrhage and perinatal death are increased in women who have undergone FGM (WHO 2014). Deinfibulation is best performed around 20 weeks gestation to avoid having to cut the scar tissue in labour and the risk of causing further damage (RCN 2015). When attending the woman in childbirth, the midwife must be prepared to support the registrar to perform an anterior episiotomy (unless they have had specific training), separating the labial remnants (Fig. 56.10), and the perineum must be meticulously repaired. Repair of the labia in such a way as to restore the infibulated state is illegal (RCOG 2015).

If the infant is a girl, the midwife must be aware that the family may wish to have the child circumcised. Under the terms of the Female Genital Mutilation Act 2003 (as

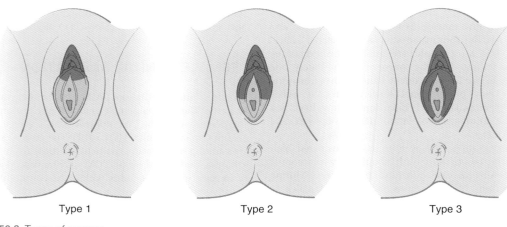

Type 1   Type 2   Type 3

Figure 56.8 Types of surgery.

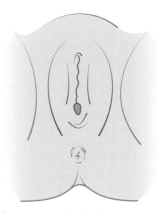

Figure 56.9 Appearance after healing of type 3 (infibulation).

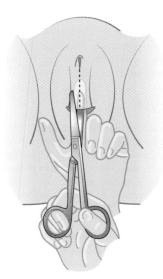

Figure 56.10 Direction of anterior episiotomy for type 3 (infibulation).

amended by the Serious Crime Act 2015 Part 5), it is illegal to have this carried out in the UK or abroad under the principle of 'extraterritoriality'. Midwives should initiate their local Safeguarding protocol if they feel that a female child is at risk (DH 2014).

At the first antenatal visit, the midwife should identify whether the woman has undergone genital mutilation. Skillful communication is essential and the words used should reflect a well-informed, nonjudgemental and sensitive approach. If the woman and the midwife do not speak the same language, an interpreter must be used – this should *not* be a family member. A careful history must be taken; details of any previous births must be recorded, including any surgical interventions required, and the condition of the infant and the woman's health since the birth. A physical examination should be carried out, with consent. Minor degrees of genital mutilation will probably

require no special attention, apart from ascertaining the woman's wishes regarding her labour and birth care. Section 5B of the 2003 Act (through the Serious Crime Act 2015) introduces a mandatory-reporting duty. This requires all regulated health and social care professionals and teachers in England and Wales to report to the police, known cases of FGM in under 18 year olds, identified in the course of their professional duties. The RCOG has also provided guidance for clinicians in the care of women who have undergone FGM or are considered at risk (RCOG 2015). The Department of Health, along with other professional bodies, has provided resources for professionals to support them with this sensitive area of work and information for the families that they are dealing with (DH 2015).

Infibulation, however, may present problems. Detailed information about previous pregnancies and births will help inform the current management. The woman's beliefs and knowledge about the effect of her surgery on childbirth must be assessed. Her wishes for this pregnancy and birth should be discussed, but the midwife must make it clear that reinfibulation after the birth is not permitted by law. The possibility of the need for episiotomy should be raised. Advice regarding hygiene in pregnancy is essential, especially the need to reduce the risk of urinary tract infection.

Defibulation services should be available to women who request it. Ideally, this procedure should be performed before pregnancy or around 20 weeks gestation (RCOG 2015). The midwife should refer the woman to an obstetrician. In all her communication, the midwife must be aware of the social implications of her advice and actions.

The Foundation for Women's Health, Research and Development (FORWARD) website contains information on FGM, including potential sequelae such as obstetric fistula formation.

general health and enquire about the information and advice that may have been given by other health professionals. Lower abdominal or periumbilical scars suggest gynaecological surgery and the midwife should enquire about the procedure. If there is a history of reproductive problems or gynaecological surgery, the woman should be referred to an obstetrician for an opinion on management of the pregnancy and labour.

Psychological support is essential. The midwife must be sensitive in ascertaining the history and giving advice and care during pregnancy. Working in partnership with the woman may ameliorate some of the psychological effects by focusing on normality, as far as is practical within the circumstances. Anxiety may be reduced and feelings of control and satisfaction enhanced if the woman is an informed and equal partner.

The midwife may be the first healthcare practitioner that the woman comes into contact with, and may pave the way not just for this pregnancy, but also for interactions with other practitioners within the health services. A sensitive, respectful and caring approach ensures that the woman's experience of healthcare is positive and will also contribute to the health of the woman, her baby and family.

> **Reflective activity 56.3**
>
> Review your unit policy on the care of a woman with type 3 genital mutilation. If no policy is available, how would you get one written? What issues would you include?

CONCLUSION

The true incidence of genital tract anomaly is unknown. The diagnosis may be made only after investigations for reproductive problems, such as recurrent pregnancy loss, pain or infertility.

A thorough but tactful history must be taken, with particular attention to ensuring dignity and privacy during the consultation. The midwife should assess the woman's

> **Key Points**
>
> - The true incidence of anomalies is unknown but may have significant implications for fertility and childbearing.
> - Midwives must be able to identify women at risk of related problems and implement appropriate care.
> - Midwives should be aware of different cultural practices in their own practice areas and be knowledgeable about the effect of such practices on the reproductive health of the woman and on her baby.
> - The legal and ethical difficulties that may present in this area must be considered, while maintaining respect and sensitivity for the views and beliefs of others.

References

Arulkumaran S: Malpresentation, malposition, cephalopelvic disproportion and obstetric procedures. In Edmunds DK, editor: *Dewhurst's textbook of obstetrics and gynaecology*, 8th edn, Chichester, Wiley Blackwell, 2011.

Bhattacharya S, Mistri PK: *Twin pregnancy in a woman with uterus didelphys, OJHAS* 9(4):24 (website). <www.ojhas.org/issues36/2010-4-24.htm>. 2010.

Caserta D, Mallozzi M, Meldolesi C, et al: Pregnancy in a unicornuate uterus: a case report, *J Med Case Rep* 8:130, 2014.

Department of Health (DH): *Safeguarding children and young people* (website). www.gov.uk/government/publications/safeguarding-children-and-young-people/safeguarding-children-and-young-people. 2014.

Department of Health (DH): FGM: Mandatory Reporting in Healthcare (website). www.gov.uk/government/publications/fgm-

mandatory-reporting-in
-healthcare. 2015.

Edmunds DK: Normal and abnormal
development of the genital tract. In
Edmunds DK, editor: *Dewhurst's
textbook of obstetrics and gynaecology*,
8th edn, Chichester, Wiley
Blackwell, 2011.

Female Genital Mutilation Act 2003
(website). www.legislation.gov.uk/
ukpga/2003/31/pdfs/ukpga
_20030031_en.pdf. 2003.

Francois KE, Foley MR: Antepartum and
postpartum hemorrhage. In Gabbe S,
Niebyl JR, Galan HL, et al, editors:
*Obstetrics: normal and problem
pregnancies*, 6th edn, Philadelphia,
Elsevier Saunders, 2012.

Goodman A, Schorge J, Greene M: The
long-term effects if in utero
exposures: the DES story, *N Engl J
Med* 362:2082–2084, 2011.

Gupta S: *A comprehensive textbook of
obstetrics & gynecology*, New Delhi,
Jaypee Brothers Medical Publishers,
2011.

Hamoda H, Chamberlain P, Moore N,
et al: Conservative treatment of
incarcerated gravid uterus, *Br J
Obstet Gynaecol* 109(9):1074–1075,
2002.

Jurkovic D: Ectopic pregnancy. In
Edmunds DK, editor: *Dewhurst's
textbook of obstetrics and gynaecology*,
8th edn, Chichester, Wiley
Blackwell, 2011.

Kent A, Barton-Smith P: Asymptomatic
incarcerated retroverted uterus with
anterior sacculation at term, *Int J
Gynecol Obstet* 96(2):128, 2006.

Kroll D, Lyne M: Uterine inversion and
uterine rupture. In Boyle M, editor:
*Emergencies around childbirth: a
handbook for midwives*, Abingdon,
Radcliffe Medical Press Ltd, 2006.

Mackay Hart D, Norman J: *Gynaecology
illustrated*, 5th edn, London,
Churchill Livingstone, 2008.

Monga A, Dobbs S, editors: *Gynaecology
by ten teachers*, 19th edn, London,
CRC Press, 2011.

Mukhopadhyay S, Arulkumaran S:
Gynecological disorders in
pregnancy. In Arulkumaran S,
Sivanesaratnam V, Chatterjee A,
et al, editors: *Essentials of obstetrics*,
Anshan, Tunbridge Wells, 2010.

Nanda S, Dahiya K, Sharma N, et al:
Successful twin pregnancy in an
unicornuate uterus with one fetus in
the non-communication
rudimentary horn, *Arch Gynecol
Obstet* 280(6):993–995, 2009.

Narayan H: *Compendium for the
antenatal care of high-risk pregnancies*,
Oxford, Oxford University Press,
2015.

Neto A, Nóbrega B, Filho JÓT, et al:
Intrapartum diagnosis and
treatment of longitudinal vaginal
septum. Case reports in obstetrics
and gynecology. Anglia Ruskin
University Library (website). http://
libweb.anglia.ac.uk. 2014.

Royal College of Nursing (RCN),
Female Genital Mutilation: An RCN
Resource for Nursing and Midwifery
Practice (2nd ed.). (website). www
.rcn.org.uk/__data/assets/pdf
_file/0010/608914/RCNguidance
_FGM_WEB2.pdf. 2015.

Royal College of Obstetricians and
Gynaecologists (RCOG): *Fetal and
Maternal Risks of Diethylstilboestrol
Exposure in Pregnancy*, London,
RCOG, 2002.

Royal College of Obstetricians and
Gynaecologists (RCOG): *Female
Genital Mutilation and Its
Management (Green-top Guideline No.
53)*, London, RCOG, 2015.

Saha P, Rohilla M, Prasad GR, et al:
Herniation of gravid uterus: report
of 2 cases and review of literature,
MedGenMed 8(4):14, 2006.

Saravelos S, Cocksedge K, Li T-C:
Prevalence and diagnosis of
congenital uterine anomalies in
women with reproductive failure: a
critical appraisal, *Hum Reprod
Update* 14(5):415–429, 2008.

Shulman L: Müllerian anomalies,
Clin Obstet Gynecol 51(1):214–222,
2008.

Siew-Fei N, Cheung V, Ting-Chung P:
Surgical management of adnexal
masses in pregnancy, *JSLS* 18(1):71–
75, 2014.

Simms-Stewart D, Fletcher H:
Counselling patients with uterine
fibroids: a review of the
management and complications,
Obstet Gynaecol Int (website)
www.hindawi.com/journals/
ogi/2012/539365/. 2012.

Tahlan S, Agarwal K, Gandhi G: Vaginal
delivery in a case of longitudinal
vaginal septum: a case report, *J Clin
Biomed Sci* 2014.

World Health Organization (WHO):
Female genital mutilation and
obstetric outcome: WHO
collaborative prospective study in
six African countries, *Lancet*
367(9525):1835–1841, 2006.

World Health Organization (WHO):
Female Genital Mutilation *(Fact
Sheet No. 241) Updated 2014*
(website). www.who.int. 2014.

Resources and additional reading

Foundation for Women's Health,
Research and Development
(FORWARD): Female Genital
Mutilation (website). www.forwar
duk.org.uk/key-issues/fgm. 2015.

Home Office: Introducing Mandatory
Reporting for Female Genital
Mutilation. A Consultation
(website). www.gov.uk/government/
publications/2010-to-2015
-government-policy-violence
-against-women-and-girls. 2014.

Home Office training on FGM: https://
www.fgmelearning.co.uk/

Home Office FGM resource pack, 2016.
https://www.gov.uk/government/
publications/female-genital
-mutilation-resource-pack/female
-genital-mutilation-resource-pack

Chapter 57

Multiple pregnancy

Jane Denton and Wendy O'Brien

Learning Outcomes   ?

After reading this chapter, you will be able to:
- describe the incidence of multiple births
- understand how twins arise and the importance of determination of chorionicity and zygosity
- explain the additional information and support required to prepare women to care for two or more babies
- describe the management of pregnancy and birth
- explain postnatal care
- describe how to support and care for bereaved parents

THE INCIDENCE OF MULTIPLE BIRTHS

The incidence of multiple births continues to rise, mainly because of the increased availability of treatments for infertility (Kurinczuk 2006) but also because of women delaying childbearing (Cleary-Goldman et al 2005). In the UK, the multiple birth rate in 2014 was 15.9 per thousand (Fig. 57.1) and a total of 12,049 pairs of twins and 163 sets of triplets were born (Figs 57.2 and 57.3).

Multiple pregnancies carry higher risks for the mothers and babies (National Institute for Health and Care Excellence (NICE) 2011) and can impose a greater burden practically, financially and emotionally on the parents (Jenkins and Coker 2010; Botting et al 1990) and also on neonatal services (Ledger 2006; Collins and Graves 2000).

The rate of conception of multiple pregnancies is almost certainly higher than the recorded data suggests. Early ultrasound scans have shown that although there may be two or more fetal sacs in the first few weeks, some fetuses may die during the first trimester. This is described as 'the vanishing twin syndrome' (Bryan 2005; Landy and Keith 2005). If a multiple birth occurs before 24 weeks gestation and includes both live births and dead fetuses, the fetal deaths are not registerable.

If a dead fetus is delivered with a live birth after 24 weeks gestation, it should be registered as a stillbirth even if death occurred much earlier in the pregnancy (Royal College of Obstetricians and Gynaecologists (RCOG) 2005).

FACTS ABOUT MULTIPLES

How twins arise

There are two types of twins: monozygotic and dizygotic.

- *Monozygotic* ('identical', MZ, monozygous, uniovular) twins arise when a fertilized egg (zygote) divides into two identical halves during the first 14 days after fertilization. They will have the same genetic makeup and will therefore be of the same sex, apart from the rare case of an XO/XY chromosomal anomaly (Perlman et al 1990).
- *Dizygotic* ('non-identical', DZ, dizygous, fraternal or binovular) twins result from the fertilization of two separate ova (eggs) by two separate sperm. They may be of the same or of different sex and are no more genetically alike than any other siblings.

Causes of twinning

The cause of monozygotic twinning is unknown, but recent reports suggest that slightly more are born after the use of drugs to stimulate ovulation and assisted conception procedures. The incidence of MZ twins throughout

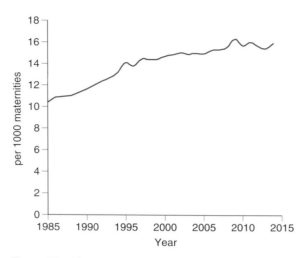

Figure 57.1 Multiple-birth rate, UK.

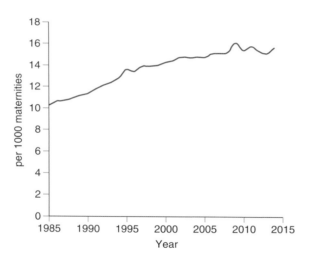

Figure 57.2 Twinning rate, UK.

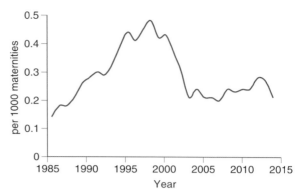

Figure 57.3 Triplet rate, UK.

the world was approximately 3.5 to 4 per 1000 until the recent slight rise, which may be associated with fertility treatments (Nakasuji et al 2014).

Dizygotic twinning is different because there are several known associated factors (Chitayat et al 2006): maternal age, parity, race, maternal height and weight and infertility treatments.

DETERMINATION OF ZYGOSITY

Zygosity determination refers to finding out whether or not twins, triplets or more are dizygotic (non-identical) or monozygotic (identical). Midwives should understand the importance of this for the clinical care of the mothers and babies so that it is not incorrectly assumed that if the babies are the same sex and dichorionic, they are necessarily dizygotic (non-identical) (Fig. 57.4). Accurate information about zygosity and how it can be determined should be provided as soon as a multiple pregnancy is diagnosed (Cutler et al 2015). Figure 57.5 provides a flowchart for determining zygosity.

Placentation

Chorionicity is the number of chorionic (outer) membranes that surround babies in a multiple pregnancy.

Amnionicity is the number of amnions (inner membranes) that surround babies in a multiple pregnancy.

Dichorionic diamniotic (DCDA) – two chorions and two amnions. These twins (or triplets or more) can be dizygotic or monozygotic. All dizygous twins have dichorionic (two chorions) and diamniotic (two amnions) placentas. Approximately one-third of monozygous twins also have DCDA placentas; this arises if the embryo divides within the first 3 or 4 days after fertilization, before implanting in the uterus.

Monochorionic diamniotic (MCDA) – one chorion and two amnions. These twins are monozygotic. In approximately two-thirds of cases, the division of the embryo occurs between 4 and 8 days after fertilization and the placenta will be MCDA.

Monochorionic monoamniotic (MCMA) – one chorion and one amnion. These twins are monozygotic twins. MCMA occurs in about 1% of cases and arises when the embryo divides later, between 9 and 12 days.

Figure 57.6 shows these types of placentation.

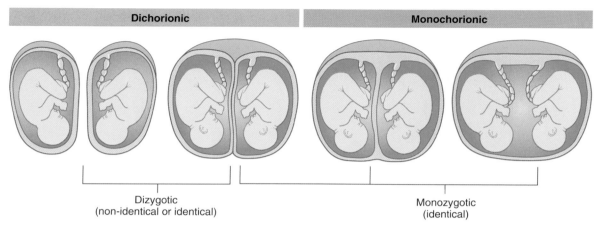

| Dichorionic | Monochorionic |

Dizygotic
(non-identical or identical)

Monozygotic
(identical)

Figure 57.4 Relationship between zygosity and chorionicity.

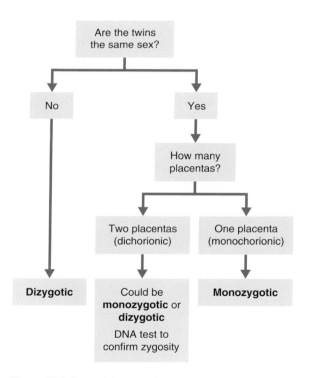

Figure 57.5 Determining zygosity.

It is essential to label twins antenatally using orientation and to record the labelling clearly in the notes. The fetuses should not be labelled 'Twin 1' and 'Twin 2' based on the gestational sac nearest to the cervix because this can cause confusion. Dias et al (2011) state that this method will only be accurate in 10% of cases and that in the 90% of pregnancies that have a left/right (vertical) orientation there is a switch in presentation. This does not apply in the case of monoamniotic twins where the lack of an intertwin membrane exists.

Importance of chorionicity

When a twin pregnancy is diagnosed on ultrasound scan, an assessment of the chorionicity should be made (preferably during the first trimester) by measuring the thickness of the dividing membranes (NICE 2011). Nearly all monochorionic placentas have blood vessels linking the placenta together. As long as the blood flow can pass in both directions, there will not be a problem; however, if anastomoses occur between an artery and a vein, causing the blood to flow in one direction only, *twin-to-twin transfusion syndrome* is likely to occur. This happens in approximately 15% of MCDA twins (RCOG 2016).

Zygosity determination after birth

DNA testing

Currently, the most accurate method of zygosity determination is to compare DNA (see the Multiple Births Foundation website: www.multiplebirths.org.uk).

Monozygotic or dizygotic		Monozygotic	
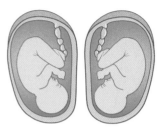	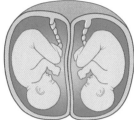	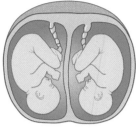	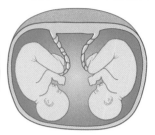
Separate placenta 2 chorions 2 amnions	Fused placenta 2 chorions 2 amnions	Single placenta 1 chorions 2 amnions	Single placenta 1 chorions 2 amnions

Figure 57.6 Placentation of twins.

DIAGNOSIS OF A MULTIPLE PREGNANCY

Ultrasound examination

Ultrasound examination in early pregnancy is recommended to provide accurate dating and early detection of multiple pregnancy. Bricker (2014) and NICE (2011) recommend that this should be undertaken at a gestation of approximately 11 weeks 0 days to 13 weeks 6 days. This is desirable for several reasons. First, it allows accurate chorionicity determination, which in turn allows appropriate planning of care, including discussion about screening for aneuploidy and other fetal complications such as twin-to-twin transfusion syndrome and fetal growth restriction. Second, it allows labelling of each fetus to enable consistent assessment when ultrasound scanning is undertaken and screening and diagnostic tests are being interpreted. Finally, it enables discussion about the risks of higher-order multiple pregnancy and the possibility of fetal reduction in settings where this is acceptable (Bricker 2014).

Abdominal examination

Inspection

In settings where ultrasound scanning is not available or has not been undertaken, a midwife must always be alert to the possibility of twins if, on inspection, the uterus looks larger than expected for the gestation, especially after 20 weeks, and fetal movements are seen over a wide area, although the diagnosis need not always be of twins. A history of twins in the family should also be taken into account.

Palpation

On abdominal palpation, the fundal height may be greater than expected for the period of gestation. If two fetal poles (head or breech) are felt in the fundus of the uterus and multiple fetal limbs are palpable, this may be indicative of a multiple pregnancy. A smaller-than-expected head for the size of the uterus may suggest that the fetus is small and that there may be more than one present. Location of three poles is diagnostic of at least two fetuses.

Auscultation

Hearing two fetal heart rates is not diagnostic of a twin pregnancy because one heart rate can be heard over a wide area. The use of 'Sonicaid' machines in the monitoring of fetal heartbeats has improved detection of more than one fetal heart rate, but heartbeats must be listened to simultaneously for at least 1 minute. If the two heartbeats have a variation of more than 10 beats per minute, almost certainly twin infants are present.

ANTENATAL SCREENING

The UK National Screening Committee (NSC) current standard for screening in multiple pregnancy in the first trimester is combined screening, which is a measurement of nuchal translucency (NT) in combination with maternal serum biochemistry. Biochemical screening alone should not be used. In the second trimester, results for the serum screening can be given only for the pregnancy and not for the baby. Second-trimester biochemical screening should not be used for triplet pregnancies (NICE 2011). The advent of non-invasive prenatal testing (NIPT), also known as cell-free DNA, holds great promise, but its application to twin pregnancy is still in the early stages of development. Aneuploidy screening in multiple pregnancy is complex for the following reasons: there is a higher risk of aneuploidy, the sensitivity of the screening tests is lower, the false-positive rate is higher and the likelihood of needing invasive diagnostic testing is higher, as is the risk of complications. In the event of one affected fetus, the option of selective termination can affect the normal fetus/fetuses (Bricker 2014).

Chorionic villus sampling (CVS) can be performed from the 11th week of gestation and has a 3% to 4% risk of miscarriage in a multiple pregnancy. Amniocentesis can also be performed in twin pregnancies, usually between 15 and 20 weeks. The risk of miscarriage is about 2.5%. Both tests should be performed in a specialist fetal medicine centre.

ANTENATAL PREPARATION

Early diagnosis of multiple pregnancy and chorionicity is extremely important so that parents have the additional specialist support and advice they need (Bryan et al 1997).

At whatever stage parents are told, it is essential that whoever shares the news is aware of the effect the revelation may have. Although some mothers and fathers are delighted to know that more than one baby is expected, there are reactions of shock and disbelief in many cases. It is important that an obstetrician or midwife is available to answer questions and give appropriate counselling at this time (NICE 2011). It is helpful if the mother can be put in touch with other parents of twins who can understand and provide reassurance. Contact numbers for local twins groups and information about other relevant support organizations can be a great source of reassurance (see chapter website resources).

Parent education

The news that two or more babies are expected can come as a considerable shock to some families, and the woman should be immediately referred to a midwife with a special interest or lead in multiple pregnancies, where available, or to an obstetrician and a named midwife to give the opportunity to discuss any concerns (Leonard and Denton 2006).

As soon as a multiple pregnancy is diagnosed, written information should be given containing contact numbers of the specialist midwife, the parent education department at the local hospital, and national twin organizations, such as the Multiple Births Foundation (MBF) and Tamba (Twins and Multiple Births Association) and local twins clubs. The MBF and Tamba provide classes and meetings to prepare for parenting multiples and a range of publications.

Parenting education classes should be booked as early as possible; ideally, the woman should commence these at 24 weeks gestation, which is earlier than for a singleton pregnancy, or specialist multiple pregnancy classes at 28 weeks. Specialist classes should include information about

diet; risks, signs and symptoms of preterm labour; timing and mode of delivery; breastfeeding; and planning for how to cope practically and emotionally with caring for two or more babies, including sources of help (NICE 2011).

When planning classes, contact with the local twins club can provide a very useful source of practical information. Mothers from twins clubs are usually delighted to participate and offer practical information for example about feeding, equipment and clothes (Leonard and Denton 2006).

Midwives should always be aware of the higher risk of antenatal and postnatal depression with a multiple pregnancy (Fisher 2006; Thorpe 1991).

Midwives must be aware of the enhanced role of fathers in the care of multiples, and their cooperation in the mother's care should be sought from the start.

Reflective activity 57.2

Find out what types of information and education are provided for parents specific to multiple births in your local area.

Preparation for breastfeeding

Mothers expecting twins or triplets will inevitably give a lot of thought to how they are going to feed their babies, not only from the nutritional aspect but also from the practical one because feeding will take up a large part of the first months. Mothers should be reassured that breastfeeding is not only possible for two babies and in some cases three (MBF 2011), but can be a very rewarding experience for all. Breastmilk is ideal for all babies and especially important because twins, and more so triplets, tend to be born prematurely and have low birthweights.

Early in the pregnancy, the mother should be given information about breastfeeding and local classes and the contact numbers for breastfeeding organizations. Both parents should have the chance to talk through any issues with a midwife; a good idea is to suggest they meet with another mother who has successfully breastfed twins.

COMPLICATIONS ASSOCIATED WITH A MULTIPLE PREGNANCY

When the pregnancy is multiple, minor disturbances are likely to be exaggerated. Morning sickness is often severe and prolonged. Heartburn can be persistent. Increased abdominal pressure may cause oedema of the ankles and varicose veins in the legs and vulva. As the pregnancy progresses, dyspnoea, backache and exhaustion are common.

Anaemia: Two or more fetuses make greater demands on the woman's stores of iron and folic acid. Women with twin and triplet pregnancies should be given the same advice about diet, lifestyle and nutritional supplements as for those with singleton pregnancies; however, because there is a higher incidence of anaemia, a full blood count (FBC) at 20 to 24 weeks should be taken and repeated at 28 weeks. If needed, iron and folic acid should be prescribed (NICE 2011).

More serious complications

Women with a multiple pregnancy have two to three times higher risk of developing hypertensive disorders in pregnancy (Ch. 54). In addition, if it occurs, it is more likely to occur earlier than in a singleton pregnancy and to be more severe; therefore, urinalysis and blood pressure monitoring should be performed at each antenatal contact. If another moderate risk factor for hypertension exists (of which multiple pregnancy is one), low-dose aspirin (75 mg) should be considered from 12 weeks gestation (Bricker 2014; NICE 2010).

Almost all other complications of pregnancy are increased in multiple pregnancy, such as intrahepatic obstetric cholestasis (ICP) and antepartum haemorrhage (including placenta praevia because of the larger placental site). The management of these complications is the same as that of singleton pregnancy.

- *Acute polyhydramnios* can occur as early as 16 weeks. It may be associated with fetal abnormalities, but with monochorionic twin pregnancies, it is more likely to be attributable to twin-to-twin transfusion syndrome (see following discussion). The midwife should always be alert for the woman who complains of a rapid increase in her abdominal girth in the second trimester or a uterus that is continuously hard. This is a result of the rapid increase in amniotic fluid (polyhydramnios). Urgent obstetric intervention is required to prevent premature labour and possible fetal demise.
- *Twin-to-twin transfusion syndrome* (TTTS) can be acute or chronic and occurs in approximately 15% of monochorionic diamniotic twin pregnancies (RCOG 2016). It arises because of unequal blood flow through placental anastomoses from one fetus to the other. The donor twin transfuses blood via arteriovenous anastomoses of the placenta to the recipient twin. This results in growth restriction, oligohydramnios and anaemia in the donor twin ('stuck twin') and hyperperfusion, hypervolemia and congestive heart failure in the recipient twin. It may develop at any time in gestation, but the risk is highest at 16 to 24 weeks. D'Antonio and Bhide (2014) and NICE (2011) recommend that monitoring for feto-fetal transfusion should not begin in the first trimester but that monitoring with ultrasound, including identification of membrane folding, should

be carried out fortnightly until 24 weeks. These complications of monochorionic twins are responsible for a high early fetal loss rate (Dias and Akolekar 2014). Laser coagulation of connecting placental vessels may prolong the pregnancy until the fetuses are viable.

- *Preterm labour* is a major risk with multiple pregnancy. More than 50% of twins and almost all triplets are born before 37 weeks, and approximately 15% to 20% of admissions to neonatal units (NNUs) are associated with preterm twin and triplet pregnancies. Birth before 28 weeks also occurs frequently in these pregnancies (NICE 2011). If labour does begin prematurely when the chances of survival are not good, the mother may be given drugs to inhibit uterine activity. Oral nifedipine and intravenous atosiban are the tocolytic drugs commonly used in the management of preterm labour, with nifedipine being the preferred choice (NICE 2015) (see Ch. 58). However, an association with the use of nifedipine in multiple pregnancy and pulmonary oedema suggests that atosiban may be preferable to nifedipine in this context (RCOG 2011). NICE (2015) recommends the use of magnesium sulphate for neuroprotection of the baby; it is given to women between 24 and 29 +6 weeks of pregnancy who are in established labour or having a planned birth within 24 hours. NICE also recommends consideration of its use between 30 and 33 +6 following the same criteria. The cause of preterm labour is said to be multifactorial, and optimal methods for prediction and prevention remain the subject of ongoing debate (Bricker 2014).

It is well known that antenatal corticosteroids reduce neonatal complications in preterm infants, and although these are considered less effective in multiple pregnancies (Bricker 2014), NICE (2011) recommends that women with twin and triplet pregnancies should be informed of the benefits of targeted corticosteroids because of the increased risk of preterm birth.

FETAL ABNORMALITIES ASSOCIATED WITH MONOZYGOTIC TWINS

Conjoined twins: This results from the incomplete monozygotic division of the fertilized ovum after 12 days of conception, therefore resulting in different degrees of fusion between the two fetuses. It is extremely rare, occurring in 1.47 per 100,000 births (Mutchinick et al 2011). Delivery has to be by caesarean section; separation of the babies is sometimes possible, depending on which internal organs are involved.

Acardiac twins (twin reversed arterial perfusion, TRAP): In acardia, one twin presents without a well-defined cardiac structure and is only kept alive through placental anastomoses to the circulatory system of the healthy (pump) co-twin (RCOG 2016). Early diagnosis is needed so that intra-fetal laser therapy can be performed before 16 weeks to attempt to reduce the risk of an adverse outcome (D'Antonio and Bhide 2014).

ANTENATAL CARE

Although antenatal monitoring is mainly targeted at early detection of specific complications, such as those resulting from TTTS, it is recognized that MCDA twins have a higher rate of birth discordance, growth restriction and prematurity. Therefore, relatively uncomplicated MCDA twin pregnancy warrants close antenatal follow-up and planned delivery at an optimal gestation (Nair and Kumar 2009). NICE (2011) recommends that clinical care for women with multiple pregnancies should be provided by a dedicated multidisciplinary team consisting of a core team of specialist obstetricians, midwives and ultrasonographers, all of whom have experience managing twin and triplet pregnancies. NICE also recommends an enhanced team for referrals, which should include a perinatal mental health professional, a woman's health physiotherapist, an infant feeding specialist and a dietician. Referrals to the enhanced team would be dependent on the individual woman's needs. Antenatal care should include screening for aneuploidy; screening for structural abnormalities, particularly cardiac abnormalities because these are more common in twin and higher-order pregnancies (Bricker 2014); and monitoring for feto-fetal transfusion syndrome, intra-uterine growth restriction, maternal complications and preterm birth.

INTRAPARTUM CARE

It is advisable that all mothers expecting a multiple birth be booked for delivery in a consultant unit. Ideally, in the case of triplets and higher-order births, this should be a hospital that can offer intensive neonatal care facilities, for example, a regional referral unit.

Timing of birth

The stillbirth rate of singletons at 42 weeks is equivalent to that of twins at 38 weeks. Dias and Akolekar (2014) therefore recommend expectant management for uncomplicated dichorionic twins up to 38 weeks. The current recommendation for monochorionic twins is to offer women an elective birth from 36 weeks gestation unless there are complications indicating that an earlier delivery should be discussed (RCOG 2016).

Complications during labour and birth

The risks during labour for mothers and babies are much greater in a multiple pregnancy. In addition to preterm delivery, other complications are more common, including the following:

Malpresentation: Although malpresentations can occur more frequently than with singleton births, in about half of twin pregnancies, both babies are cephalic presentations; in three-quarters of cases, the first baby presents by the vertex.

Cord prolapse: This is a particular risk in cases of premature rupture of the membranes, malpresentation and polyhydramnios and in the interval between the births of the first and second twin.

Prolonged labour: The length of the first stage of labour is usually similar to that of a singleton birth. However, because of the overdistension of the uterus and abdominal muscles, there may be uterine inertia in some women.

Monoamniotic twins: Because monoamniotic twins share the same sac, there is the risk of cord entanglement. Delivery is recommended between 32 and 34 weeks gestation by caesarean section (RCOG 2016).

Deferred delivery of the second twin: In the last few years there have been cases reported where the first twin has been born, often very prematurely, and then labour has stopped. Labour in some instances has not recommenced again for a period of time; pregnancies have been recorded with a gap of 30 days or more (van Eyck et al 2005). This can be beneficial to the second twin because corticosteroids can be administered to help mature the lungs. Throughout this period, the mother will need an enormous amount of support from midwives. She will be concerned about the twin who has been born, still being pregnant and the unborn twin. The woman will need close monitoring for signs of infection.

Onset of labour

The average gestational duration of multiple pregnancies with two, three and four babies are as follows:

- Twins: 37 weeks
- Triplets: 34 weeks
- Quadruplets: 32 weeks.

Care in labour

When a woman expecting a multiple birth is admitted in labour, the team who will be present at the birth should be informed. In addition to midwives and the obstetrician(s), an anaesthetist and neonatologist should be available. All those in attendance should be introduced to the parents, with their presence and role explained. If students and other observers are included, the woman's permission must be sought; ideally, this should take place before labour commencement, and the number of observers should be kept to a minimum to maintain privacy and dignity.

First stage

The first stage of labour is conducted as for a singleton labour, although a multiple pregnancy is considered high risk. For this reason, comprehensive handover is essential and must ensure that experienced or well-supported staff are allocated to provide care and that two midwives are available at critical points of care, such as siting of epidural and the actual birth. It is also necessary to ensure intravenous access is secured and blood taken for a FBC and group-and-save in established labour.

Continuous electronic fetal monitoring of each baby must be observed using a twin monitor if available so that both fetal hearts maybe monitored simultaneously. Two external transducers can achieve this. If any difficulty or concerns arise, once the membranes are ruptured, a scalp electrode can be placed on the presenting twin and the external monitor on the second twin. Uterine activity must be monitored at the same time. When using a twin monitor, it is very important to respond accordingly to signals and not to ignore any alarms or questions it may generate. It is crucial to ensure that each twin's fetal heart is identified and recorded and that a 3-way check is undertaken to establish this and repeated whenever monitoring is commenced or recommenced, for example, following insertion of epidural anaesthesia, changes in position or repositioning of transducers (Patel 2016, personal communication). It also very important to be clear about which transducer is monitoring which twin. Inadvertently recording maternal heart rate as opposed to fetal heart rate is widely reported in multiple births (Hanson 2010). Any concerns regarding the fetal heart rate or distinguishing this from maternal pulse should be escalated immediately to an obstetrician and a portable ultrasound scan performed if possible.

3-way check:

Maternal pulse compared with Twin 1

Maternal pulse compared with Twin 2

Twin 1 compared with Twin 2

Epidural anaesthesia is the pain relief of choice offered to women giving birth to multiples. This form of pain relief has the added advantage that if such manoeuvres as internal version, forceps delivery, ventouse extraction and emergency caesarean section are needed, adequate pain relief is in situ.

It is widely accepted that the risk to the second-born infant is significantly higher (Smith et al 2002).

If there are any signs of fetal compromise at any time during the first stage of labour to either baby, an emergency caesarean section must be performed.

Second stage

An obstetrician, anaesthetist and neonatologist should be present together with the midwife because of the risk of complications. The delivery room should be closely located to an operating theatre and big enough to accommodate two sets of resuscitation equipment and a transport incubator. The delivery trolley should include the requirements for amniotomy and assisted delivery and extra cord clamps. An oxytocin infusion is prepared in case of uterine inertia following the birth of the first twin (Dodd and Crowther 2005).

The second stage is conducted as is usual for the birth of a singleton baby. The cord should be firmly clamped in two places and cut between the clamps. Extra cord clamps may be needed if blood gases are to be taken; local unit policy should be followed for this. If the maternal side is not secure, the second baby, in the case of monochorionic twins, may suffer exsanguination. When the first twin is born, the time of delivery must be noted. The first infant and the cord should be clearly labelled 'Twin 1' or with the parents' chosen name, if known. The baby should be shown to the mother if the condition is satisfactory, or the parents should be constantly informed of progress if resuscitation is required. When the baby's condition is satisfactory, the suckling of the baby's breastfeeding will stimulate uterine activity.

The lie, presentation and position of the second fetus must be ascertained by abdominal palpation and confirmed by vaginal examination. If transverse or oblique, this must be corrected by external version to a longitudinal lie. If this is not possible, an emergency caesarean section is performed. The fetal heart rate and the mother's pulse rate must be checked after each procedure; this should also be confirmed by portable ultrasound scan if available. When it has been confirmed that there is no cord presentation, the second sac of membranes is ruptured following the initial contraction after the birth of the first twin when the presenting part has descended into the pelvis. Once again the fetal heart is checked; if there are any concerns, a scalp electrode is applied, and a further check is made to make sure that the cord has not prolapsed. If contractions do not resume very soon after the birth of the first twin, an oxytocin infusion may be needed. The birth is conducted in the normal way, taking care to note the time and label the baby 'Twin 2', and the same for the cord. The interval between the births varies considerably. It has been suggested that 30 minutes should be the maximum time (Barrett 2006). Depending on gestation and individual circumstances, delayed delivery may be considered, but this is not usual practice. If more than two babies are expected, the delivery is usually by caesarean section (see following discussion).

Undiagnosed twins

It is unusual in economically developed countries for a multiple pregnancy to remain undiagnosed at the time of delivery. However, where ultrasonography is not available or not used routinely for all expectant mothers, or in the case of an 'unbooked' woman, this can still occur, particularly if women are new to the country and not aware of antenatal care. In this situation, uterotonic preparations for third-stage management should not be administered until after the birth of the baby so that there is no risk to a possible twin of severe anoxia, which may lead to death or precipitate delivery of a possibly brain-damaged infant. Rupture of the uterus is also a risk. If drugs have been administered, the second baby requires immediate delivery. In such a situation, an appreciation of the gravity of there being two babies should be appreciated by midwives and appropriate support given.

Third stage

Following birth, there is an increased risk of postpartum haemorrhage from the large placental site and overdistended uterine muscles, which may also contribute because the abdominal muscles are more relaxed. Active management of the third stage varies in different units as to whether to give an injection of Syntocinon 10 IU intramuscularly after the birth of the last baby, before the cord is clamped and cut (NICE 2014), or an intramuscular injection of Syntometrine 1 mL. When the uterus is felt to contract, controlled cord traction is applied to both/all cords at the same time.

Examination of placenta and membranes

The midwife must make the usual examination to ensure completeness and detect any deviation from normal. If the babies are of different sex, then they must be dizygotic twins, with either two separate placentas or one that has fused together, but each will have its own set of membranes, that is, amnion and chorion. When the babies are of the same sex, they may be monozygotic or dizygotic. The placenta should be sent for histological examination

Delivery of triplets and higher-order births

The greatest risk for triplet and higher-order births is preterm delivery; 75% of triplet pregnancies result in spontaneous birth before 35 weeks (NICE 2011). The recommended method of delivery of triplets and

higher-order births is caesarean section. Elective birth is planned from 35 weeks after a course of antenatal corticosteroids has been offered. The delivery of triplets or more is a major event for all staff and the parents. As much information as possible should be given to the parents about the increased risk of admission to a special care baby unit (NICE 2011). The parents should be informed of the procedure and the roles of the many personnel in the obstetric theatre. It is crucial that the neonatal team is briefed in advance of the delivery and that each baby has its own designated team.

Regardless of the number of infants involved, the parents should be shown their babies as soon as possible after birth. If it is necessary to transfer some or all of the infants to the NNU, photographs should be taken and brought to the mother as soon as possible. Ideally, the babies should be photographed together so that the realities of the multiple birth are established. However, if this is not possible, the pictures should be clearly labelled with the birth order of the babies.

POSTNATAL CARE

The immediate postnatal care for a mother who has given birth to twins or more is the same as that for a singleton mother, but with special attention to her blood loss and the involution of the uterus. Because the babies are likely to be smaller and preterm, it is more difficult for them to maintain their body temperature, so they must be kept warm. Delivery by caesarean section is more common, and women may feel grief and disappointment about not experiencing a normal birth (Fisher 2006).

Following delivery, the mother is likely to be very tired. She has probably suffered from a sleep deficit over several months, and a more complicated birth or caesarean section may compound her exhaustion. The lochia in the first few days is often heavier than after a singleton delivery, and the woman is more likely to complain of afterpains.

In addition, the woman has two or more babies for whom she must care. Her anxieties may be increased if her babies are preterm. One, both, or, in the case of triplets or more, all, may be nursed in the NNU. Parents of twins admitted to a neonatal intensive care unit (NICU) experience even greater stress than those with one baby (Pector and Smith-Levitin 2002). The mother will need additional support and help if she has one baby on the postnatal ward with her and one in the NNU. She may feel more inclined to stay with the healthy baby on the ward; however, if the long-term outcome is uncertain, she should be encouraged to spend as much time as possible with the sick baby.

Some units have established transitional care wards where small, well babies can remain with their mothers with the aid of specially trained midwives or nurses who are available to support, assist and advise them on the care and specialized feeding the babies need.

Sadly, it is not uncommon for very sick babies to be transferred, sometimes without their mother, from the delivery hospital to a regional referral unit where intensive neonatal nursing care can be offered. This situation is traumatic for all of the family. Midwifery staff must strive to reunite the family as soon as the condition of the babies allows. Regular communication during the separation is vital. The splitting up of the family group is often avoided if the babies are transferred to the regional referral unit in utero.

Feeding multiples

During the first few weeks, the woman is going to need a lot of extra support and advice to help her establish breastfeeding (MBF 2011). The parents should be advised that it can take at least 4 to 6 weeks to get into a routine with feeding and caring for their babies. Twins can breast-feed separately or together; if fed together, the feeds will only take a little longer than with a single baby. The breastfeeding woman will have more quality time with her babies because she has no bottles to sterilize or feeds to make up (see Ch. 44).

While in the hospital, help should be available at every feed until the woman feels confident. It is advisable in the first few days for her to feed her babies separately; this gives her a chance to get to know each baby as an individual and to feel confident in handling and putting the baby to the breast. It can be overwhelming for the mother in her first pregnancy to achieve perfect feeding of two babies together right from the start. Once breastfeeding is established, some mothers prefer to feed both infants together, thus saving time; others prefer to feed separately but wake the second to feed immediately after the first so that the routine is maintained. There is no one right way; it has to be the mother's preference and what fits in with her family, developing the mother's confidence and ability to cope. The main causes of nipple soreness and backache are incorrect positioning of both babies at the breast and the mother's sitting position while feeding. It is very important for mothers to be taught right from the start to use plenty of pillows to support their backs and also to take the weight of the babies for feeding. The pillows should bring the babies up to nipple level so the mother can sit with her back straight and not lean forward over the babies. Because the weight of the babies is taken by the pillows, the mother's hands are free to reposition a baby should either of them come off the breast and to lift one baby up for winding purposes. There are a variety of positions in which the mother can hold her babies for feeding. The most usual one for newborns is the underarm hold (Fig. 57.7).

Some mothers will choose to wholly or partially give formula feeds to their babies, and partners, family and friends are then able to help with feeding routines.

Whatever the mother's choice of feeding method, the midwife should support her in that choice.

Going home from the hospital

Because more multiples are born preterm, it is more common for the woman to go home several days or weeks before her babies. If the babies are preterm and admitted to a NNU, every effort is made to discharge them together, but this is not always possible. One baby may be fit to go

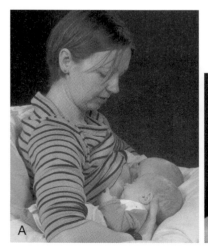
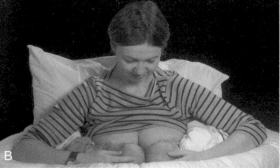

Figure 57.7 Mother well positioned and successfully breastfeeding.

home, but the other may require neonatal care for longer. This will put added strain on the parents, who have to care for one baby at home while finding time to visit the sick one in hospital. Mothers of premature twins may feel less prepared to cope at home and less effective as parents (Boivin et al 2005); it is vital for NNU staff, midwives and health visitors in the community to ensure continuity of care and support. Arranging for the mother to stay on the NNU will help her to gain confidence in caring for the babies before discharge. This transition will be smoother if the mother has adequate help at home for the first few weeks after discharge.

Sources of help

There is no statutory help routinely available for mothers of twins, triplets or more in the UK. If there are concerns about the family circumstances and the parents' ability to cope, then social services should be contacted before the babies are born. Parents may be reluctant to accept or ask for help from family and friends, but this can be invaluable and should be encouraged (Beck 2002).

Family relationships

A woman may find it more difficult to relate to both/all of her babies at the beginning.

A strong preference may develop for one of the babies in the early days. The mother should be reassured that this is not unusual with multiples; in time, a close relationship with the other baby or babies will develop. However, midwives should always be alert to signs that could indicate depression, which is more common with multiple births.

Becoming overtired and feeling overwhelmed with the immensity of their task is also a risk for both parents. There may also be problems with other children in the family, especially toddlers. It is hard enough for an older sibling to accept one new baby; when two or more arrive simultaneously, there may be real difficulties. Single older children may see their parents as a pair and the twins as a pair and themselves on their own, so it is helpful for the parents to arrange for a special friend to spend time with the older child. It is usual for the new babies to give a present to their older sibling; it is a good idea for the older child to choose a small different gift for each twin. Bringing the first gifts the twins receive can make the sibling feel very special.

Individuality and identity

Most parents of twins appreciate the importance of their children developing their own identities. This should be discussed in the antenatal period, and parents of twins are encouraged to treat their children as individuals, giving them the same opportunities as a single-born child.

Ways in which they can emphasize their individuality should be discussed in parent education classes. These include choosing names that do not sound the same or rhyme and commence with a different first letter and dressing the children in different-coloured clothes (Bryan and Hallett 2001).

Postnatal depression

In view of all the possible complications, increased risk of surgical intervention and the other stresses involved in having a multiple birth, it is perhaps not surprising that there is an increased risk of depression (Choi et al 2009; Thorpe et al 1991).

The health professionals caring for the mother should recognize the signs that depression is developing. It is helpful if there is continuity of care by a known midwife and a health visitor who has been introduced to the family before the babies are born. If the babies are still in the hospital, it is still important for the mother to receive visits from her midwife and health visitor at home.

Bereavement

Mortality rates for multiple births have long been established as significantly higher than those of singletons, with twins about five times, and triplets about 10 times, more likely to die within the first year of life (Fig. 57.8).

The higher incidence of preterm delivery and the associated complications are the main reasons for the increased death rates. The loss of all of the babies in a multiple pregnancy is tragic, and the grief of the parents is usually fully recognized, but the situation is more complex when one twin or triplet dies, leaving parents to cope with

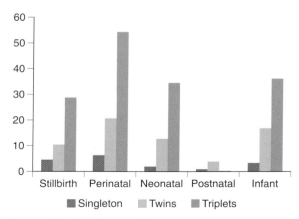

Figure 57.8 Mortality in multiple births.

grieving for the dead baby (or babies if two triplets die) at the same time as caring for the survivor (Richards et al. 2015). Professionals, family and friends can fail to realize that the grief is just as great when one baby dies, and the joy of having a healthy child will not diminish the depth of the emotions or compensate for the loss. Parents may be regarded as ungrateful for the survivor, particularly if one twin dies during pregnancy or delivery or shortly after birth. They may need help to fully acknowledge their feelings and should be given information and support and offered counselling, which should be ongoing, as soon as the death is confirmed. The loss of status of being parents of twins, triplets or more must not be underestimated. They will continue to be parents of however many children are born, and this should always be acknowledged (Bryan 2005).

Encouragement should be given to the parents to talk about the confusing, contradictory feelings they may have and to think and talk about their dead baby because this will allow the mourning process to take place (Hayes et al 2015; Lewis and Bryan 1988) (see Ch. 68).

If the babies are dichorionic, same-sex twins (or triplets), the parents should be given the option for DNA testing so they will know the zygosity of their babies.

Each case must be treated individually, and the information and care required will vary in some ways depending on when the baby died. The different situations and recommendations for the care of these families are given in detail in the section on bereavement in the *Guidelines for Professionals* of the MBF (Bryan and Hallett 1997).

Reflective activity 57.3

Find out what services are available nationally and locally to support bereaved parents of twins or more (see Ch. 68 on grief and loss).

Disability

The risk of disability is greater with multiple births. The chance of a triplet pregnancy resulting in a baby with cerebral palsy is 47 times greater, and for a twin pregnancy it is 8 times greater, than that of a singleton pregnancy (Petterson et al 1990). Caring for one child with a disability and another who is healthy brings many challenges, especially with twins. Often, the healthy child has just as many problems and may imagine that he or she caused the problem or resent the attention paid to the other child. Many potential emotional and behavioural problems may be avoided if the family is supported and advised appropriately as early as possible.

Multifetal pregnancy reduction

Multifetal pregnancy reduction may be offered to parents who conceive triplets or more on the basis that reduction to two or even one fetus provides a better chance of the healthy survival of each baby. The procedure is usually carried out between the 10th and 12th weeks of pregnancy; the most common method is to inject potassium chloride into the fetal thorax. When parents are presented with this immensely difficult decision, they must be provided with information about the risks and consequences of the procedure and offered counselling so that they consider the implications fully before making a final choice (see Ch. 28).

Selective feticide

If one of the babies in a multiple pregnancy has a serious abnormality, the same clinical procedure as described for multifetal pregnancy reduction may be used. Again, the parents will need very detailed information about the risks and counselling before making their final decision. Because the dead baby will remain in the uterus until the delivery, the midwife has an important role to play in acknowledging the bereavement and supporting the mother through this very emotional time before and after the birth.

Planning ahead

It is important that good family planning advice is offered to the parents following a multiple birth. Genetic counselling may be needed for those who have lost a baby. Follow-up of survivors should be arranged, especially when the infants are monozygous or have experienced neonatal complications.

Key Points

- Multiple-birth families have special needs, and midwives should be prepared for the additional and different management, information and support needed to ensure the best outcomes for the whole family.
- The incidence of multiple births is increasing because of the wider availability of infertility treatments and an aging pregnant population.
- It is important to determine chorionicity and zygosity accurately.
- Risk management is an important part of care.
- Obtaining adequate support throughout childbirth and beyond is essential.
- Established voluntary networks are an important source of support.

References

Barrett JFR: Management of labour in multiple pregnancies. In Kilby M, Baker P, Critchley H, et al, editors: *Multiple pregnancy*, London, RCOG, pp 223–233, 2006.

Beck CT: Mothering multiples: a meta-synthesis of qualitative research, *MCN Am J Matern Child Nurs* 27(94):214–221, 2002.

Boivin M, Perusse D, Dionne G, et al: The genetic-environmental etiology of parents' perceptions and self-assessed behaviors toward their 5-month-old infants in a large twin and singleton sample, *J Child Psychol Psychiatry* 46(6):612–630, 2005.

Botting BJ, Macfarlane AJ, Price FV, et al: *Early days. Three, four and more: a study of triplets and higher order births*, London, HMSO, 1990.

Bricker L: Optimal antenatal care for twin and triplet pregnancy: the evidence base, *Best Pract Res Clin Obstet Gynaecol* 28:305–317, 2014.

Bryan E: Psychological aspects of prenatal diagnosis and its implications in multiple pregnancies, *Prenat Diagn* 25(9):827–834, 2005.

Bryan EM, Denton J, Hallett F: *Guidelines for professionals: multiple pregnancy*, London, Multiple Births Foundation, 1997.

Bryan EM, Hallett F: *Guidelines for professionals: bereavement*, London, Multiple Births Foundation, 1997.

Bryan EM, Hallett F: *Guidelines for professionals: twins and triplets: the first five years and beyond*, London, Multiple Births Foundation, 2001.

Chitayat D, Hall J: Genetic aspects of twinning. In Kilby M, Baker P, Critchley H, et al, editors: *Multiple pregnancy*, London, RCOG, pp 89–94, 2006.

Choi Y, Bishai D, Minkovitz MD: Multiple births are a risk factor for postpartum maternal depressive symptoms, *Pediatrics* 123(4):1147–1154, 2009.

Cleary-Goldman J, D'Alton ME, Berkowitz RL: Prenatal diagnosis and multiple pregnancy, *Semin Perinatol* 29(5):312–320, 2005.

Collins J, Graves G: The economic consequences of multiple gestation pregnancy in assisted conception cycles, *Hum Fertil* 3(4):275–283, 2000.

Cutler TL, Murphy K, Hopper J, et al: Why accurate knowledge of zygosity is important to twins, *Twin Res Hum Genet* 18(3):298–305, 2015.

D'Antonio F, Bhide A: Early pregnancy assessment in multiple pregnancies, *Best Pract Res Clin Obstet Gynaecol* 28:201–214, 2014.

Dias T, Akolekar R: Timing of birth in multiple pregnancy, *Best Pract Res Clin Obstet Gynaecol* 28:319–326, 2014.

Dias T, Ladd S, Mahsud-Dornan S: Systematic labeling of twin pregnancies on ultrasound, *Ultrasound Obstet Gynecol* 38:130–133, 2011.

Dodd JM, Crowther CA: Evidence-based care of women with a multiple pregnancy, *Best Pract Res Clin Obstet Gynaecol* 19(1):131–153, 2005.

Fisher J: Psychological and social implications of multiple gestation and birth, *Aust N Z J Obstet Gynaecol* 46(Suppl 1):S29–S37, 2006.

Hanson L: Risk management in intrapartum fetal monitoring, *J Perinat Neonatal Nurs* 24(1):7–9, 2010.

Hayes L, Richards J, Crowe L, et al: Development of guidelines for health professionals supporting parents who have lost a baby from a multiple pregnancy, *Infant* 11(5):164–166, 2015.

Jenkins DA, Coker R: Coping with triplets: perspectives of parents during the first four years, *Health Soc Work* 35(3):169–180, 2010.

Kurinczuk J: Epidemiology of multiple pregnancy: changing effects of assisted conception. In Kilby M, Baker P, Critchley H, et al, editors: *Multiple pregnancy*, London, RCOG, pp 121–137, 2006.

Landy HJ, Keith LG: The vanishing fetus. In Blickstein I, Keith L, editors: *Multiple pregnancy, epidemiology, gestation, and perinatal outcome*, London, Taylor & Francis, pp 108–118, 2005.

Ledger WL: The cost to the NHS of multiple births after IVF treatment in the UK, *Br J Obstet Gynaecol* 113:21–25, 2006.

Leonard LG, Denton J: Preparation for parenting multiple birth children,

Early Hum Dev 82(6):371–378, 2006.

Lewis E, Bryan EM: Management of perinatal loss of a twin, *Br Med J* 297(6659):1321–1323, 1988.

Multiple Births Foundation (MBF): *Guidance for health professionals on feeding twins, triplets and higher order multiples*, London, MBF, 2011.

Mutchinick OM, et al: Conjoined twins: a worldwide collaborative epidemiological study of the International Clearinghouse for Birth Defects Surveillance and Research, *Am J Med Genet C Semin Med Genet* 157(4):274–287, 2011.

Nair M, Kumar G: Uncomplicated monochorionic diamniotic twin pregnancy, *J Obstet Gynaecol* 29(2):90–93, 2009.

Nakasuji T, Saito H, Araki R, et al: The incidence of monozygotic twinning in assisted reproductive technology: analysis based on results from the 2010 Japanese ART national registry, *J Assist Reprod Genet* 31(7):803–807, 2014.

National Institute for Health and Care Excellence (NICE): *Hypertension in pregnancy: diagnosis and management*, London, NICE, 2010.

National Institute for Health and Care Excellence (NICE): *Multiple pregnancy: The management of twin and triplet pregnancies in the antenatal period. Clinical Guidance 129*, London, NICE, 2011.

National Institute for Health and Care Excellence (NICE): *Intrapartum care for healthy women and babies*, London, NICE, 2014.

National Institute for Health and Care Excellence (NICE): *Preterm labour and birth*, London, NICE, 2015.

Patel, A: *Personal communication on teaching care of twins in labour*. Practice Development Midwife, Northern Devon Healthcare NHS Trust, 2016.

Pector EA, Smith-Levitin M: Mourning and psychological issues in multiple birth loss, *Semin Neonatol* 7(3):247–256, 2002.

Perlman EJ, Stetton G, Tuckmuller CM, et al: Sexual discordance in monozygotic twins, *Am J Med Genet* 37(4):551–557, 1990.

Petterson B, Stanley F, Henderson D: Cerebral palsy in multiple births in Western Australia: genetic aspects, *Am J Med Genet* 37(3):346–351, 1990.

Richards J, Graham R, Embleton N, et al: Mothers' perspective on the perinatal loss of a co-twin: a qualitative study, *BMC Pregnancy Childbirth* 15:143, 2015.

Royal College of Obstetricians and Gynaecologists (RCOG): *Registration of stillbirths and certification for pregnancy loss before 24 weeks of gestation. Good Practice No. 4,* London, RCOG, 2005.

Royal College of Obstetricians and Gynaecologists (RCOG): *Tocolysis for women in preterm labour. Greentop Guideline No. 1b,* London, RCOG, 2011.

Royal College of Obstetricians and Gynaecologists (RCOG): *Management of monochorionic twin pregnancy. Greentop guideline,* London, RCOG, 2016.

Smith GC, Pell JP, Dobbie R: Birth order, gestational age and risk of delivery related perinatal death in twins; retrospective cohort study, *Br Med J* 325:1004, 2002.

Thorpe K, Golding J, Macgillivray I, et al: Comparison of prevalence of depression in mothers of twins and mothers of singletons, *Br Med J* 302(6781):875–878, 1991.

Van Eyck J, Arabin B, van Lingen RA: Delayed-interval delivery. In Blickstein I, Keith L, editors: *Multiple pregnancy, epidemiology, gestation, and perinatal outcome,* London, Taylor & Francis, pp 640–644, 2005.

Resources and additional reading

Multiple Births Foundation: www.multiplebirths.org.uk.

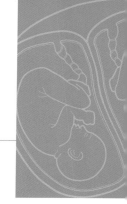

Chapter 58

Preterm labour

Sima Hay

Learning Outcomes ?

After reading this chapter, you will be able to:
- identify the risk factors for preterm labour, preterm prelabour rupture of membranes and preterm birth
- critically discuss prophylactic and preventive measures to reduce the risks of preterm labour and birth
- review recommended drugs for preterm labour (tocolytics)
- critically explore the management of preterm labour and birth
- discuss implications of preterm labour and preterm birth for the baby and the family

INTRODUCTION

The definition of spontaneous preterm labour (PTL) is labour resulting in preterm birth (PTB) before 37 completed weeks and after 24 weeks gestational age, with the onset of regular uterine contractions associated with effacement and progressive cervical dilatation. There may or not be rupture of membranes, and in some cases, it may present with only accompanied abdominal pain or backache.

There are three subcategories of PTB, based on gestational age (World Health Organization (WHO) 2012):

- Extremely preterm (less than 28 weeks; the gestation for the extremely preterm designation in the UK is 24 weeks)
- Very preterm (28 to less than 32 weeks)
- Moderate to late preterm (32 to greater than 37 weeks)

PTB is a major cause of neonatal morbidity and mortality and has long-term adverse consequences on health. Long-term morbidity includes cerebral palsy, neurodevelopmental delay and chronic lung disease. The neonatal outcome is dependent on the gestational age at birth and associated features such as infection. The lower the gestational age, the higher is the risk of mortality and morbidity (Platt 2014).

EPIDEMIOLOGY

The estimated incidence of PTB is between 5% and 12% in most developed countries, and 25% in developing countries. In England and Wales in 2012, 7% of live births were preterm. Out of this 7%, almost 5% were extremely preterm (between 24 and 27 weeks), 11% were preterm (between 28 and 31 weeks) and 84% were moderately preterm (32–36 weeks) (ONS 2012).

This rate has not changed despite advancing knowledge of risk factors related to preterm labour (PTL) and the introduction of many public health and medical interventions, such as tocolytic drugs, designed to delayed preterm birth. The rates of preterm birth are increasing in some developing countries, possibly as a result of increasing maternal age and underlying conditions such as diabetes and hypertensive disorders (Steer 2005).

In half of the cases of PTL, the membranes are intact at presentation. P-PROM with subsequent PTL accounts for around 20% of cases, although it is thought to have a different pathophysiology, mainly related to infection (Goldenberg et al 2000).

The precise aetiologies of PTL are not fully understood; often, no cause is found. Some consider that it is a syndrome, a multifactorial disorder with many causes

(Piso et al 2014). On the basis of the clinical presentation, PTB can be classified as follows:

1. Spontaneous PTB, when PTL onsets spontaneously, occurring in 45% of all PTB
2. PTB following P-PROMs, occurring in 15% of all PTB
3. Iatrogenic PTB, when delivery is indicated (either elective/emergency) for pregnancy complications associated with maternal disease, such as hypertensive or renal disease, or developing fetal distress, accounting for 30% of all births

Reflective activity 58.1

Review the incidence of preterm birth in your unit. How does the rate compare with the rate England and Wales? Has the rate changed in the past 10 years?

Risk factors

PTL may arise from different pathological processes that activate the onset of labour leading to PTB (Voltolini et al 2013). Although a precise cause cannot be established in most cases, there are a number of associated predisposing risk factors, which may also be interrelated. The risk factors for spontaneous PTL can be divided into maternal characteristics, pregnancy complications and obstetric history (Hamilton and Tower 2013) (see Table 58.1).

There is a genetic influence on the rates of PTL across ethnic groups. Black women are three times more likely to have PTL than women of any other ethnicity (Goldenberg et al 2000). This disparity remains unchanged and unexplained.

Maternal factors such as smoking; substance/drug abuse, especially cocaine use and alcohol consumption; poor nutritional status; low body mass index (BMI); low socioeconomic status; low and high maternal age; and

stress and depression are all associated with increased risk of PTL.

Corticotropin-releasing hormone (CRH) may be a link between maternal psychological stress and PTL (Vendittelli and Lachcar 2002). CRH is known to determine the duration of pregnancy, with levels rising just before birth. In PTL, it is suggested that CRH levels may rise as a result of stress (Piso et al 2014).

Local infections arising from the urinary and genital tract and systemic infection such as malaria are strongly associated with PTB (Goldenberg et al 2000; Steer 2005).

Intra-uterine infections can lead to PTL, which is related to activation of the innate immune system. The microorganisms most commonly identified are genital mycoplasmas, which are linked to bacterial vaginosis (BV).

BV is characterized by an overgrowth of anaerobic bacteria in the vagina, which can predispose the woman to preterm delivery. The mechanism is not entirely understood, but it is thought to be through an ascending infection before or during early pregnancy (Hay et al 1994). For women with a history of PTB or late mid-trimester miscarriage, detecting and treating BV early in pregnancy may prevent a proportion of these women from having a further episode of PTB (Ugwumadu et al 2003). Sexually transmitted infections, including *Chlamydia trachomatis* and *Neisseria gonorrhoea*, should also be considered as possible causes of infections that have a role in PTL. Other pregnancy-related risk factors include excessive or impaired uterine distension, such as in multiple pregnancy, polyhydramnios and uterine anomaly.

The recurrence risk in women with a previous PTL and birth ranges from 3% to over 40%, depending on the number and gestational age of previous PTBs. Short cervical length as measured with the use of transvaginal ultrasonography at 18 to 24 weeks gestation is a consistent predictor of an increased risk of preterm delivery (Hibbard et al 2000).

Table 58.1 Risk factors for preterm labour

Maternal characteristics	Current pregnancy complications	Obstetric history
Race	Multiple pregnancy	Shortened cervix
Low BMI (< 19)	Polyhydramnios	Cervical surgery
Poor nutrition	Hypertensive disease	1 previous PTL = 3%–21% risk
Periodontal disease	Infection: UTI, pyelonephritis,	2 previous PTL = 42% risk
Psychological stress	genital tract infection (e.g. bacterial vaginosis, GBS)	Previous second-trimester loss
Depression	Bleeding < 24 weeks	Repeat history of TOP
Smoking		
Drug/alcohol abuse		
Low socioeconomic status		
Age less than 18 or over 40		

BMI, body mass index; GBS, group B streptococcus; TOP, termination of pregnancy; UTI, urinary tract infection. (Adapted from Hamilton and Tower 2013.)

PREDICTION AND PREVENTION OF PRETERM LABOUR

Currently, there is no single test that can reliably identify and predict women who may have a premature labour. The two most promising markers currently used to identify women at risk are transvaginal ultrasound assessment of cervical length and measurement of the cervicovaginal fetal fibronectin levels (Iams 2014).

Cervicovaginal fetal fibronectin

Fetal fibronectin (fFn) is a protein found in amniotic fluid, placental tissue and the extracellular substance of the decidua basalis next to the intervillous space. By 22 weeks gestation, following the fusion of the chorion and the decidua, fFn secretion stops. Before onset of labour, the separation of the chorion from the decidua releases secretion of fFn, which then can be detected in vaginal secretions (Lockwood and Kuczynski 1999). Therefore, if the test is positive, it is a powerful biochemical PTB predictor.

Transvaginal ultrasound

Transvaginal ultrasound to measure cervical length and funnelling has been studied as a screening test for PTL. It has been shown to be safe and acceptable to women (Iams et al 1996). The normal mean range of cervical length at 24 weeks is 35.2 mm +/− 8.3 mm. In normal low-risk pregnancies, the length of the cervix remains constant until the third trimester. Iams et al's (1996) study demonstrated that cervical length and incidence of PTB had an inverse relationship. Less than 15 mm is a sensitive predictor of severe prematurity, and it is associated with a 50% risk of PTL before 32 weeks gestation.

Socioeconomic status

Low socioeconomic status is associated with significantly increased risk of PTB (Messer et al 2010). There is growing evidence that social policy may have an impact on reducing the risk of PTB. In 2012, WHO commissioned a report on PTB titled 'Born Too Soon'. This Global Action Report outlined comprehensive measures of prevention.

The recommended measures start from preconception and continue throughout the pregnancy. Preconception care initiatives include education on smoking cessation, better family planning and interpregnancy spacing, economic empowerment programs that alleviate poverty, community-based interventions (e.g. teenage human papillomavirus (HPV) vaccination), micronutrient food supplementation and partner education to reduce domestic violence (Messer et al 2010). Smoking cessation is one preventive measure that has been implemented with encouraging results, whereas many of the other measures have yet to be globally put into action. However, in 2013, the UK program '1001 Critical Days' (Parent Infant Partnership (PIP) 2013) was launched as a national initiative highlighting the importance of providing a seamless provision of services between conception to age 2, with the aim of enhancing the outcomes for all children. Midwives have endorsed this manifesto and play a pivotal role in the provision of services described.

Prophylactic treatments

Vaginal progesterone and cervical cerclage are two prophylactic treatments that should be considered and offered as a choice to women to reduce their risk of PTB (National Institute for Health and Care Excellence (NICE) 2015).

Vaginal progesterone

Progesterone inhibits uterine contractions and cervical ripening, promoting pregnancy (Meis et al 2003). Several studies have suggested that the prophylactic use of progesterone reduces the rates of PTB in women with a singleton pregnancy and a history of spontaneous preterm birth (Fonseca et al 2003; Meis et al 2003) or a short cervix identified on transvaginal ultrasound between 19 and 25 weeks gestation (Fonseca et al 2007; Hassan et al 2011).

A Cochrane review (Dodd et al 2013) summarized the effects of progesterone in women with a prior history of preterm birth based on 11 randomized controlled trials (RCTs) that included 1899 women. Progesterone was associated with a reduced risk of preterm birth at less than 34 weeks (relative risk (RR) 0.31, 95% confidence interval (CI) 0.14–0.69) and perinatal mortality (RR 0.50, 95% CI 0.33–0.75). There were also decreased rates of infants with a low birthweight of less than 2500 g, necrotizing enterocolitis, admission to a neonatal intensive care unit and neonatal death. The benefits of vaginal progesterone for women with signs of cervical shortening or funnelling are compelling in reducing their risk for PTB.

Cervical cerclage

Cerclage, an encircling suture placed around the cervix before or during pregnancy to correct structural weakness or defects, has been a controversial treatment for a short cervix (Iams 2014). The clinical presentations for which prophylactic cervical cerclage has been shown to be of greatest benefit in reducing the risk of PTL are, first, maternal history of PTB or mid-trimester loss between 16 and 34 weeks and, second, in women who have had either a P-PROM or history of cervical surgery or trauma and transvaginal ultrasound between 16 and 24 weeks of pregnancy identifies a short cervix (i.e. less than 25 mm) (NICE 2015).

In a meta-analysis of the effectiveness of cervical cerclage, real benefit was seen when cerclage was performed in women with three previous preterm deliveries. For women with two or fewer previous preterm deliveries, cervical cerclage offered no significant benefit (Berghella et al 2010). Women with multiple pregnancies, however, even in the presence of a short cervix, do not seem to benefit from cerclage, and there is evidence that it may even increase perinatal mortality by increasing preterm deliveries and miscarriage (Rafael et al 2014).

PRETERM PRELABOUR RUPTURE OF THE MEMBRANES

Preterm prelabour rupture of the membranes (P-PROM) is defined as rupture of the membranes before the onset of labour in women at less than 37 weeks gestation. It occurs in only 2% of pregnancies but is associated with 40% of preterm deliveries and with intra-uterine infection, which almost always results in premature birth. P-PROM is a major risk factor for intra-uterine infection/ chorioamnionitis, which causes maternal sepsis, a leading direct cause of maternal death, and is a major contributor to neonatal morbidity (e.g. pneumonia) and neonatal mortality (Merenstein and Weisman 1996).

The link between ascending infection from the lower genital tract and P-PROM has been recognized. Increasing evidence confirms that infection and inflammation are primary causes of a significant proportion of P-PROM cases, with further evidence that bacteria have the ability to cross the intact membranes (Hay et al 1994). Bacterial infection causing overt neonatal sepsis is most commonly attributable to group B streptococcus (GBS) (Heath and Schuchat 2007) (see Ch. 48). The primary source of GBS infection is vertical transmission of maternal genitourinary or gastrointestinal GBS colonization. The time between rupture of membranes and delivery is a known risk factor for increased risk of neonatal GBS sepsis.

The risk factors for P-PROM are similar to those of PTL in that it can be divided into maternal factors and utero-placental risk factors (see Table 58.2).

Diagnosing P-PROM

The diagnosis can usually be confirmed clinically by maternal history, clinical examination and laboratory evaluation. The most common symptom is leaking or a gush of watery fluid from the vagina or continuing involuntary loss per vaginam.

In the absence of uterine contractions, a visual inspection of the cervix with a sterile speculum will reveal a pool of watery fluid in the posterior blade of the speculum.

If the pooling of amniotic fluid is observed, the recommendation by NICE (2015) is not to perform any further diagnostic testing for confirmation of P-PROM, such as the widely used Nitrazine test, which detects pH change in the lost vaginal fluid. Amnicator, which is one brand of Nitrazine test, has a sensitivity of 90%, but false-positive results occur as a result of contamination with fluids such as urine, blood or semen.

However, to diagnose the possible source of potential infection, during the speculum examination, low vaginal swabs for infections such as BV, *C. trachomatis* and *N. gonorrhoea*, and GBS should be considered.

Digital examination should be avoided because this can shorten latency and has been shown to increase the risk

Table 58.2 Risk factors for preterm premature rupture of the membranes (P-PROM)

Maternal risk factors	Utero-placental risk factors
Antepartum vaginal bleeding	Uterine anomalies (such as uterine septum)
Direct abdominal trauma	Placental abruption (may account for 10%–15% of P-PROM)
Previous preterm birth	Advanced cervical dilatation (cervical insufficiency)
Cigarette smoking or illicit drug use (e.g. cocaine raises blood pressure)	Prior cervical surgery
Anaemia and nutritional deficiencies of copper and ascorbic acid	Cervical shortening in the second trimester (< 2.5 cm)
Low body mass index (BMI < 19.8 kg/m^2)	Uterine overdistension (polyhydramnios, multiple pregnancy)
Low socioeconomic status	Amniotic infection (chorioamnionitis)
Unmarried status	Multiple bimanual vaginal examinations (but not sterile speculum or transvaginal ultrasound examinations)

of infection in some studies (Alexander et al 2000). The cervix may be assessed digitally only if there is evidence of cervical dilation on visual inspection of the cervix and/or regular contractions.

If there is no evidence of amniotic fluid pooling during speculum examination or if it is equivocal, then to aid the diagnosis, NICE (2015) recommends that either one of the following two minimally invasive tests are used, for which fetal membrane rupture dipstick vaginal swab tests should be taken. Both tests have been shown to be a suitable marker in P-PROM diagnosis, the tests can be performed with a low vaginal swab without use of a speculum and diagnosis of P-PROM can be made with the aid of a diagnostic machine within 10 minutes, with an estimated sensitivity of 99% (Caughey 2008; Khooshideh 2015). The two tests are as follows:

Option 1 test: detects insulin-like growth factor binding protein-1 (lGBP-1), which is a protein in amniotic fluid that accumulates at high concentrations when the membranes are ruptured

Option 2 test: identifies trace amounts of PAMG-1, a placental glycoprotein that is abundant in amniotic fluid and is rarely found in blood and vaginal secretions (Caughey 2008; Khooshideh 2015)

Early and accurate diagnosis of P-PROM is essential for gestational age-specific obstetric interventions designed to optimize perinatal outcome and minimize serious complications, such as cord prolapse and infectious morbidity (chorioamnionitis, neonatal sepsis).

NICE (2015) gives clear recommendations on the management of the woman with a possible presentation of P-PROM, depending on the gestation and the results of either of the previously described P-PROM tests.

If the test for P-PROM is negative, and no further amniotic fluid is observed, then antenatal prophylactic antibiotics are not recommended, and the woman should be given the information that it is unlikely that she has P-PROM, but if any further signs suggestive of P-PROM or PTL develop, she should return to labour ward. The woman would also be advised to continue to be aware of fetal movements and to report any change immediately.

If the test for P-PROM is positive, assessment of the woman's clinical condition, medical and obstetric history, and gestational age should all form part of the decision making regarding the care offered to the woman.

Extremely preterm presentation, less than 23 weeks gestation, requires a difficult decision that must be made jointly with the woman, her family and the neonatal team. Clear information on the possible outcomes is crucial in the decision-making process. Perinatal survival is estimated at 13% compared with 50% if P-PROM occurs at 24 to 26 weeks of pregnancy, and the risk of pulmonary hypoplasia is approximately 50% if P-PROM is at 19 weeks, falling to 10% at 25 weeks of pregnancy.

If gestation is between 23 and 24 weeks, admission to a hospital with tertiary services for the first 7 days is recommended, including liaison with the neonatal team. Maternal assessment includes observation of her vital signs, abdominal examination and confirmation of the gestation of pregnancy and vaginal loss. Because ascending infection from the lower genital tract is commonly present in P-PROM, the midwife must observe the women for signs of clinical chorioamnionitis or fever, fetal/maternal tachycardia, decreased fetal movements, discoloration of liquor and uterine tenderness. It is not necessary to do weekly high vaginal swabs, full blood count (FBC) or C-reactive protein because the sensitivity of these tests in the detection of intra-uterine infection is low (NICE 2015).

Other antenatal investigations include cardiotocography, which may be useful because fetal tachycardia is used in the definition of clinical chorioamnionitis. Also, biophysical profile score and Doppler velocimetry may be carried out; these tests are of limited value in predicting fetal infection, but they are useful for assessing growth.

The antibiotic of choice following a diagnosis of P-PROM is erythromycin 250 mg four times a day for a maximum of 10 days or until the woman is in established labour, whichever is sooner (NICE 2015). Kenyon et al (2013) found in 222 trials involving over 6000 women with P-PROM before 37 weeks gestation that the use of antibiotics following P-PROM is associated with a statistically significant reduction in chorioamnionitis and neonatal infection. If the woman is known to be GBS positive, conservative management is with intravenous (IV) penicillin G 3 g stat then 1.5 g every 6 hours for 5 days, repeated after 5 weeks, if still undelivered.

Antenatal corticosteroids should be considered routine for a woman with P-PROM between 24 and 34 weeks gestation because there is strong evidence that use of a single course of antenatal corticosteroids will accelerate fetal lung maturation in women at risk of preterm birth. Further information is required concerning optimal dose to delivery interval, optimal corticosteroid use and effects in multiple pregnancies (Murphy et al 2009) (see following discussion under 'Management of Preterm Labour').

If the gestation is 34 to 36 weeks and chorioamnionitis has been excluded, then induction of labour with intrapartum antibiotic prophylaxis should be considered.

There appears to be no consensus within fetal medicine on the optimal timing of delivery of women with P-PROM between 34 and 37 weeks. When considering the optimal timing, it is important to recognize the three significant causes of neonatal death associated with P-PROM, which are prematurity, sepsis and pulmonary hypoplasia. Mortality is four times higher in those with sepsis than those without sepsis. In addition, there are maternal risks associated with chorioamnionitis (Goldenberg et al 2000).

The essential part of the care for the expectant mother and her family is support with an appropriate level of information (NICE 2015) (see the following section on information and support for women at increased risk of PTL).

There is insufficient data to make clear recommendations for home versus outpatient monitoring rather than continued hospital admission in women with P-PROM. Hospital admission is recommended for at least 5 to 7 days before a decision is made to allow women with P-PROM to go home. Clear written and oral advice on self-monitoring of pulse and temperature at home every 4 to 8 hours should be given because those with subclinical intra-uterine infection deliver earlier than non-infected women. Information on signs and symptoms of labour or any alterations in the vaginal loss and further advice to avoid sexual intercourse, protected or not, should be given. Follow-up attendance in a day assessment unit twice per week is advised.

Diagnostic criteria of preterm birth

PTL may be challenging to recognize, but regular uterine activity with a contraction frequency of at least one every 10 minutes is indicative when occurring with one of the following: ruptured membranes, evidence of progressive cervical change on repeat vaginal examinations or if any change by the same examiner, level of presenting part. In a nulliparous woman, findings acceptable for a diagnosis of PTL are cervical dilatation of 2 cm or more or partial effacement (to a length of 1 cm or less).

The diagnosis remains clinical, with a careful history and speculum examination being important components. Digital examination should be avoided if there is any suggestion of P-PROM (Table 58.3).

MANAGEMENT OF PRETERM LABOUR

The outcome for babies delivered between 34 and 37 weeks gestation is generally good, and labour is normally allowed to proceed at this gestation. However, communication and support for the woman and her family are still paramount, and a holistic approach of the midwife and the rest of the team is essential. The woman and her family are likely to be anxious; therefore, reassurance and empathy when giving explanations and information, both written and oral, to support her are recommended (NICE 2015). The information should be given as early as possible, taking into account the likelihood of preterm birth and the status of labour. Providing the opportunity to speak to the neonatal team and a neonatologist on the likelihood of the baby surviving and other outcomes, including long-term morbidities and risks for the baby, is important. Preparing the woman for the neonatal care of the preterm infant, including the location and a tour of the unit, if possible, and explaining the immediate problems that can arise in a preterm infant is vital.

Table 58.3 Initial investigations for preterm labour

Investigations	Rationale
Urinalysis	For proteinuria and Nephur test
MSU	Culture
HVS	Culture, *Chlamydia*, bacterial vaginitis
Insert IV; take blood	FBC, U&Es, glucose
Ultrasound assessment	Asap practical for presentation, weight estimate (especially if < 32 weeks) Liquor volume (by amniotic fluid index) Umbilical artery Doppler
Consider:	
Kleihauer	Rh-negative mother
Urine	Drug screen
Blood	Listeria culture C-reactive protein

FBC, full blood count; HVS, high vaginal swab; MSU, mid stream urine; U&Es, urea and electrolytes.

If an extremely premature birth is predicted, opportunities to talk about and state their wishes on resuscitation and an opportunity to tour the neonatal unit is highly recommended.

Anticipating the need for in utero transfer should be considered early; if the maternity unit is not a tertiary centre or not able to admit a premature infant, an in utero transfer has better clinical outcomes for the woman and the infant than transfer after birth (Fowlie et al 2008).

TREATMENT OF PRETERM LABOUR

Tocolysis

Tocolytic therapy can prolong pregnancy for up to 48 hours in approximately 80% of cases, which is beneficial in allowing time for administration of corticosteroids and in utero transfer to occur, which may possibly improve the neonatal outcome (Voltolini et al 2013).

Before commencing tocolysis, several factors should be considered to determine whether the woman would benefit from drug therapy, such as availability of neonatal care, need to transfer to another unit, preference of the woman and other clinical signs that may contraindicate the stopping of the labour (e.g. infection/bleeding) (NICE 2015).

The main tocolytics used are calcium channel blockers such as nifedipine, which inhibits the reflux of calcium ions across the cell membrane, thereby decreasing the tone in the smooth muscular tone (Sanborn 1995). Nifedipine is the first-line drug of choice. It is associated with maternal side effects such as flushing, headache, palpitations and hypotension. In particular, nifedipine should be avoided in women with cardiac disease, and care should be taken in women with diabetes or multiple pregnancy because there are reports of pulmonary oedema (Voltolini et al 2013).

Advantages of nifedipine are that it can be given orally 20 mg, followed by 10 to 20 mg three to four times per day for up to 48 hours. This can be adjusted in response to observed uterine activity. Total doses higher than 60 mg are associated with an increased risk of side effects.

Nifedipine may be offered to women between 24 and 25 weeks of pregnancy who have intact membranes and are suspected PTL or between 26 and 33 weeks of pregnancy who have intact membranes and are suspected or diagnosed PTL.

If nifedipine is contraindicated, oxytocin receptor antagonists such as atosiban may be offered. This is the only drug licensed for treatment of threatened PTL. It is given as an initial bolus of 6.75 mg over 1 minute, followed by an infusion of 18 mg/hour for 3 hours then reduced to 6 mg/hour for up to 45 hours. Similar to nifedipine, it should only be continued for 48 hours (NICE 2015).

Emergency cervical sutures ('rescue sutures')

Emergency cervical sutures are performed when the cervix is objectively open and the membranes are at or below the external os before 26 weeks gestation (Hamilton and Tower 2013). Cervical cerclage reduces the incidence of preterm birth in women at risk of recurrent PTB without statistically significant reduction in perinatal mortality or neonatal morbidity (Alfirevic et al 2012).

Compared with expectant management, a rescue suture may increase the length of the pregnancy by 4 to 5 weeks. Indicators of poor outcome are membranes below the external os, cervical dilatation over 4 cm, signs of infection (raised C-reactive protein or white blood cell count) and continued vaginal bleeding. Failure of the suture is closely associated with post-birth chorioamnionitis. Rescue sutures must be based on clinical presentation, cervical dilatation and uterine activity. It should not be offered to women with any signs of infection, vaginal bleeding or uterine contractions (NICE 2015).

Antibiotics

Extreme PTB is usually associated with infection, most commonly ascending infection from the vagina, and

several studies have assessed antibiotic use in the prevention of PTB. The largest study to date was the ORACLE II study (Kenyon et al 2008), which investigated women presenting with symptoms of spontaneous PTL with intact membranes. The primary outcome was a reduction in neonatal death with the use of antibiotics. The routine prescribing of antibiotics to women in spontaneous PTB did not reduce neonatal death, but it did reduce the risk of maternal infection. Further follow-up of the participants in the ORACLE II study at 7 years found an increased risk of cerebral palsy in the children who received antibiotics (odds ratio 1.93; 95% CI (1.21e3.09) for erythromycin and 1.69 (1.07e2.67) for coamoxiclav). When antibiotics were combined, risks were higher still than with erythromycin alone (4.55% vs. 2.29%). It has been suggested that the use of antibiotics could be masking a subclinical infection and keeping a baby within a hostile environment longer, thus increasing the risk of cerebral palsy. Therefore, routine prescription of antibiotics is not recommended in the presence of intact membranes and should be restricted to specific clinical indications such as chorioamnionitis, GBS and P-PROM (Kenyon et al 2013).

Corticosteroids

Corticosteroids are used in PTL to increase fetal surfactant and accelerate fetal lung maturity. They have been shown to be beneficial in reducing neonatal death, respiratory distress syndrome (RDS), necrotizing enterocolitis, cerebrovascular haemorrhage and neonatal intensive care admissions. The optimum time between administration of steroids and delivery is from 24 hours to 7 days, although there has been a trend towards benefit following 7 days (Roberts and Dalziel 2006).

A single course of corticosteroids, two intramuscular injections of 12 mg betamethasone 24 hours apart, is given. Every effort should be made to administer steroids to all women at risk of PTL between 24 and 36 weeks gestation.

The effectiveness of the repeat doses of corticosteroids in women who have not delivered within 7 days, who remain at risk of delivery, is debated (Hamilton and Tower 2013). The routine offer of repeat courses of maternal corticosteroids should not be made, but the interval since the end of the last course, gestational age and the likelihood of birth within 48 hours should all be taken into account (NICE 2015).

Magnesium sulphate for neuroprotection

There are high rates of cerebral palsy in preterm infants, with 14.6% being reported at less than 28 weeks gestation and 6.2% between 28 and 31 weeks (Hamilton and Tower 2013). Magnesium sulphate ($MgSO_4$) is widely used as a treatment for seizure prophylaxis in pre-eclampsia and the treatment of eclampsia. Although it is not recommended as a tocolytic agent, there is evidence suggesting that maternal administration of magnesium sulphate may reduce the risks of cerebral palsy in the preterm neonate (Hamilton and Tower 2013). A Cochrane review (Doyle et al 2009) reported that magnesium sulphate was associated with a lower RR of cerebral palsy and lower RR of gross motor dysfunction.

The recommended dosing regimen (NICE 2015) is as follows:

- Women between 30 and 33 weeks of pregnancy are given a 4-g IV bolus of magnesium sulphate over 15 minutes, followed by an infusion of 1 g per hour until birth or over 24 hours, whichever is sooner.

The dose may have to be reduced, and careful monitoring for clinical signs of magnesium toxicity, at least every 4 hours, is necessary. This includes recording and close observation of maternal vital signs – pulse, blood pressure, respiratory rate – and deep tendon and patellar reflexes. Also, regular monitoring of urinary output should be carried out to observe for developing signs of oliguria or other signs of renal failure.

During labour and delivery, the method of fetal monitoring will depend on the gestation and should be discussed with the woman, taking her wishes into consideration (NICE 2015). The midwife plays an important part in discussing the option of continuous monitoring versus intermittent auscultation with the woman. There is a dearth of evidence that for a woman with no other risk factor than PTL one method of fetal assessment improves outcome for the baby over the other (NICE 2015). Although a normal cardiotocography trace is reassuring and may indicate that the fetus is coping well with the labour, an abnormal trace does not always indicate that fetal hypoxia or acidosis is present. The use of fetal scalp electrodes for fetal heart rate monitoring is not recommended if the woman is fewer than 34 weeks pregnant unless the benefits outweigh the potential risks (NICE 2015). Also, fetal blood sampling is not advised for the same reason in women below 34 weeks pregnant, although it may be considered between 34 and 36 weeks of pregnancy.

The mode of delivery and the risks and benefits of the options of vaginal birth versus caesarean section should be discussed with the woman and her family. Vaginal birth should be carefully controlled and nontraumatic, assisted by an experienced midwife and obstetrician. Artificial rupture of the membranes should be avoided because this leads to the cervix closing down and compounding presentation. Episiotomy may be considered because it will prevent bruising to the preterm infant. The neonatologist should be kept informed of the progress of labour and should be present with the neonatal team should resuscitation be required (NICE 2015).

The role of the midwife in the care of the woman is important in enabling and facilitating the woman to optimize her experience and care. It is also vital that the midwife is able to ensure the woman is part of the decision making between the teams (Hodnett et al 2011).

Delayed cord clamping

Delayed cord clamping after preterm birth may be associated with improved neonatal outcomes. Delaying clamping for between 30 and 120 seconds improves placental perfusion and increases the infant's blood volume at birth by approximately 30%. In a Cochrane review, Rabe et al (2012) suggested that it reduced the need for blood transfusion and reduced the risks of necrotizing enterocolitis and intraventricular haemorrhage.

The recommended timing of the cord clamping for preterm babies born vaginally or by caesarean section is to wait 30 seconds but no longer than 3 minutes before clamping the cord, positioning the baby at or below the level of placenta before clamping (providing the mother and baby are stable). If the baby needs urgent resuscitation or there is significant maternal bleeding, the midwife should consider milking the cord and clamp as soon as possible (NICE 2015).

EFFECT ON FAMILIES FOLLOWING PRETERM BIRTH AND THE ROLE OF COMMUNITY MIDWIFE

The birth of the preterm baby is undoubtedly an acutely stressful event for both parents. Following the birth, mothers experience significant psychological distress during their infant's hospitalization (Singer et al 1999). Also, the loss of the expectant or anticipated role as a result of the infant separation is a major source of stress.

Despite more open access to intensive care units and improved communication, mothers of premature infants are likely to experience significant levels of stress. Evidence suggests that some of the sources of stress for parents include the fragile appearance of infant, fear regarding the infant's survival and alteration of parental role and the separation from their infant brought about by admission to the neonatal unit (Davis et al 2003). This increased stress and uncertainty surrounding a premature birth increases the need for support while the mother adjusts to her new role. Supportive care has been related to less maternal depression and greater parental competence (Davis et al 2003).

The woman is likely to be discharged home before the baby, so the role of both the midwife and the community midwife during this postnatal period is multifaceted. The midwife has a vital role in providing the appropriate postnatal care, in preparing and supporting the mother and her family to cope with the emotional and physical demands of caring for a preterm baby and in developing a positive bond with their baby. The midwife also provides guidance on and further support with breastfeeding, encouraging expressing of colostrum as soon as possible, and guidance on maintaining lactation, which has a significant benefit to the preterm baby and the mother (Menon and Williams 2013). Communication and information-giving are important aspects of supporting the mother to adapt in this transitional phase of parenthood.

CONCLUSION

The management of preterm birth has seen major advances because of the prevention strategies that are currently available for asymptomatic women at risk of preterm birth, including progesterone and cervical cerclage. There is a shift in the focus of antenatal treatment, with the use of prenatal magnesium sulphate and corticosteroids, to reduce neonatal intensive care admissions and longer-term disabilities associated with preterm birth, consequently relieving emotional consequences for the woman and her family. The role of the midwife throughout the pregnancy journey and following birth in providing support and appropriate care is vital in assuring the woman and her family's experience remains a positive one.

Key points

- Preterm labour complicates approximately 7% of UK pregnancies.
- The aetiology of PTL is multifactorial; PTL leads to PTB, which greatly affects neonatal morbidity and mortality.
- Prophylactic cervical cerclage and the use of progesterone for the prevention of PTL in women at risk may prolong pregnancy.
- Antenatal corticosteroids are the only drug proven to improve neonatal outcome in PTL.
- Delayed cord clamping has the potential to improve some neonatal outcomes.
- Magnesium sulphate can, at best, delay PTL for long enough for the maximum benefit of steroids and possible in utero transfer to occur.
- Provision of appropriate information and support to the woman and her family is a vital part of the management of PTL.

References

Alexander JM, Mercer BM, Miodovnik M, et al: The impact of digital cervical examination on expectantly managed preterm rupture of membranes, *Am J Obstet Gynecol* 183:1000–1007, 2000.

Alfirevic Z, Stampalija T, Roberts D, et al: Cervical stitch (cerclage) for preventing preterm birth in singleton pregnancy, *Cochrane Database Syst Rev* (4):CD008991, 2012.

Berghella V, Keeler SM, To MS, et al: Effectiveness of cerclage according to severity of cervical length shortening: a meta-analysis, *Ultrasound Obstet Gynecol* 35:468–473, 2010.

Caughey A, Robinson J, Norwitz E: Contemporary diagnosis and management of preterm premature rupture of membranes, *Rev Obstet Gynecol* 1(1):11–22, 2008.

Davis L, Edwards H, Mohay H, et al: The impact of very premature birth on the psychological health of mothers, *Early Hum Dev* 73(1–2):61–70, 2003.

Dodd JM, Jones L, Flenady V, et al: Prenatal administration of progesterone for preventing preterm birth in women considered to be at risk of preterm birth, *Cochrane Database Syst Rev* (7):CD004947, 2013.

Doyle LW, Crowther CA, Middleton P, et al: Magnesium sulphate for women at risk of preterm birth for neuroprotection of the fetus, *Cochrane Database Syst Rev* (1):CD004661, 2009.

Fonseca EB, Bittar RE, Carvalho MH, et al: Prophylactic administration of progesterone by vaginal suppository to reduce the incidence of spontaneous preterm birth in women at increased risk: a randomized placebo-controlled double-blind study, *Am J Obstet Gynecol* 188:419–424, 2003.

Fonseca EB, Celik E, Parra M, et al: Progesterone and the risk of preterm birth among women with a short cervix, *N Engl J Med* 357:462–469, 2007.

Fowlie P, Booth P, Skeoch C: Moving the preterm infant. In McGuire W, Fowlie P, editors: *ABC of preterm birth (ABC Series)*, London, Blackwell Publishing, 2008.

Goldenberg RL, Hauth JC, Andrews WW: Intrauterine infection and preterm delivery, *N Engl J Med* 342(20):1500–1507, 2000.

Hamilton S, Tower C: Management of preterm labour, *Obstet Gynaecol Reprod Med* 23:4, 2013.

Hassan SS, Romero R, Vidyadhari D, et al; PREGNANT Trial: Vaginal progesterone reduces the rate of preterm birth in women with a sonographic short cervix: a multicenter, randomized, double-blind, placebo-controlled trial, *Ultrasound Obstet Gynecol* 38:18–31, 2011.

Hay PE, Lamont RF, Taylor-Robinson D, et al: Abnormal bacterial colonisation of the genital tract and subsequent preterm delivery and late miscarriage, *Br Med J* 308(6924):295–298, 1994.

Heath P, Schuchat A: Perinatal group B streptococcal disease, *Best Pract Res Clin Obstet Gynaecol* 21(3):411–424, 2007.

Hibbard JU, Tart M, Moawad AH: Cervical length at 16-22 weeks' gestation and risk for preterm delivery, *Obstet Gynecol* 96:972–978, 2000.

Hodnett E, Gates S, Hofmeyr G, et al: Continuous support for women during childbirth, *Cochrane Database Syst Rev* (2):CD003766, 2011.

Iams JD: Prevention of preterm parturition, *N Engl J Med* 370:254–261, 2014.

Iams JD, Goldenberg RL, Meis PJ, et al: The length of the cervix and the risk of spontaneous premature delivery, *N Engl J Med* 334:567–572, 1996.

Kenyon S, Boulvain M, Neilson JP: Antibiotics for preterm rupture of membranes, *Cochrane Database Syst Rev* (2):CD001058, 2013.

Kenyon S, Pike K, Jones DR, et al: Childhood outcomes after prescription of antibiotics to pregnant women with preterm rupture of the membranes: 7-year follow-up of the ORACLE I trial, *Lancet* 372(9646):1310–1318, 2008.

Khooshideh M, Radi V, Hosseini R, et al: The accuracy of placental alpha-microglobuline-1 test in diagnosis of premature rupture of the membranes, *Iran J Reprod Med* 13(6):355–360, 2015.

Lockwood CJ, Kuczynski E: Markers of risk for preterm delivery, *J Perinat Med* 27(1):5–20, 1999.

Meis PJ, Klebanoff M, Thom E, et al: National Institute of Child Health and Human Development Maternal-Fetal Medicine Units Network: prevention of recurrent preterm delivery by 17 alpha-hydroxyprogesterone caproate, *N Engl J Med* 348:2379–23-85, 2003.

Menon G, Williams TC: Human milk for preterm infants: why, what, when and how? *Arch Dis Child Fetal Neonatal Ed* 98(6):F559–F562, 2013.

Merenstein GB, Weisman LE: Premature rupture of the membranes: neonatal consequences, *Semin Perinatol* 20:375–380, 1996.

Messer LC, Oakes JM, Mason S: Effects of socioeconomic and racial residential segregation on preterm birth: a cautionary tale of structural confounding, *Am J Epidemiol* 171(6):664–673, 2010.

Murphy K, Hannah M, Willan A, et al: Multiple courses of antenatal corticosteroids for preterm birth (MACS): a randomised controlled trial, *Lancet* 372(9656):2143–2151, 2009.

National Institute for Health and Care Excellence (NICE): *Preterm labour and birth [NG 25]* (website). www.nice.org.uk/guidance/ng25. 2015.

Office for National Statistics (ONS): *Statistical bulletin*. Gestation-specific infant mortality in England and Wales, 2012 (website). www.statistics.gov.uk. 2012.

Parent Infant Partnership (PIP): *1001 critical days manifesto* (website). www.1001criticaldays.co.uk/the_manifesto.php. 2013.

Piso B, Zechmeister-Koss I, Winkler R: Antenatal intervention to reduce preterm birth: an overview of Cochrane reviews, *BMC Res Notes* 7:265, 2014.

Platt MJ: Outcomes in preterm infants, *Public Health* 128(5):399–403, 2014.

Rabe H, Diaz-Rossello JL, Duley L, et al: Effect of timing of umbilical cord clamping and other strategies to influence placental transfusion at preterm birth on maternal and infant outcomes, *Cochrane Database Syst Rev* (8):CD003248, 2012.

Rafael TJ, Berghella V, Alfirevic Z: Cervical stitch (cerclage) for preventing preterm birth in multiple pregnancy, *Cochrane Database Syst Rev* (9):CD009166, 2014.

Roberts D, Dalziel SR: Antenatal corticosteroids for accelerating fetal lung maturation for women at risk of preterm birth, *Cochrane Database Syst Rev* (3):CD004454, 2006.

Sanborn BM: Ion channels and the control of myometrial electrical activity, *Semin Perinatol* 19(1):31–40, 1995.

Singer LT, Salvator A, Guo S, et al: Maternal psychological distress and parenting stress after the birth of a very low-birth-weight infant, *J Am Med Assoc* 281:799–805, 1999.

Steer P: The epidemiology of preterm labour, *Br J Obstet Gynaecol* 112(Suppl 1):1–3, 2005.

Ugwumadu A, Manyonda I, Reid F, et al: Effect of early oral clindamycin on late miscarriage and preterm delivery in asymptomatic women with abnormal vaginal flora and bacterial vaginosis: a randomised controlled trial, *Lancet* 361(9362):983–988, 2003.

Vendittelli F, Lachcar P: Threat of premature labor, stress, psychosocial support and psychotherapy: a review of the literature, *Gynécol Obstét Fertil* 30(6):503–513, 2002.

Voltolini C, Torricelli M, Conti N, et al: Understanding spontaneous preterm birth: from underlying mechanisms to predictive and preventive interventions, *Reprod Sci* 20(11):1274–1292, 2013.

World Health Organization (WHO): *Born too soon*. The global action report on preterm birth (website). www.who.int/pmnch/media/news/2012/preterm_birth_report/en/index1.html. 2012.

Resources and additional reading

Royal College of Obstetricians and Gynaecologists (RCOG): *Green-top Guideline No. 44. Preterm prelabour rupture of membranes* (website). www.rcog.org.uk/womens-health/clinical-guidance/preterm-prelabour-rupture-membranes-green-top-44. 2006.

Royal College of Obstetricians and Gynaecologists (RCOG): *Scientific Impact Paper No. 29. Magnesium sulfate to prevent cerebral palsy following preterm birth*, London, RCOG, 2010.

Royal College of Obstetricians and Gynaecologists (RCOG): *Greentop Guideline No. 60.*

Cervical cerclage, London, RCOG, 2011.

Royal College of Obstetricians and Gynaecologists (RCOG): *Greentop Guideline. No. 7. Antenatal corticosteroids to reduce neonatal morbidity and mortality*, London, RCOG, 2011.

Useful websites:

Bliss: www.bliss.org.uk/

Bliss is a charity that is concerned with parents of premature or sick babies in the UK. Bliss exists to ensure that all babies born too soon, too small or too sick in the UK have the best possible chance of survival and of reaching their full potential.

Group B Strep support: http://gbss .org.uk/health-professionals/guidelines/

This charity supports parents and professional in preventing GBS infection in newborn babies.

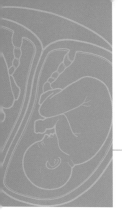

Chapter 59

Obstetric interventions

Sam Bassett

Learning Outcomes ?

After reading this chapter, you will be able to:

- reflect upon your own practice to assess any aspects that may influence operative delivery rates
- explore local protocols, policies and guidelines that may have the potential to reduce the increasing operative delivery rates
- examine the information given to women regarding their choices in labour and delivery
- ensure that appropriate and effective care is provided for women experiencing instrumental and operative deliveries
- ensure that the most appropriate and relevant postdelivery care is provided for both mother and baby
- consider the emotional and physical impact of birth requiring intervention, and ensure a compassionate and empathic approach to women and their families

INTRODUCTION

Although it is universally accepted that the best way for a baby to enter the world is through spontaneous vaginal delivery, normal birth rates have continued to fall. Of the 646,904 deliveries that took place within National Health Service (NHS) hospitals in England in 2012–2013, only 60.9% were spontaneous vaginal deliveries; 26.2% were caesarean section births, and 12.9% were instrumental births (Health and Social Care Information (HSIC) 2015).

This chapter explores the possible rationale for this increasing trend towards operative delivery and the role of the midwife within this trend, beginning with instrumental births and concluding with births by caesarean section. The discussion includes an exploration of the indications, contraindications, possible complications and the midwife's role within the procedures.

OPERATIVE VAGINAL DELIVERIES

The history of forceps and ventouse

Many myths and claims have been put forward regarding the origins of obstetric forceps, from wall carvings in the temple of Kom Ombo in 250 BC to the works of Hippocrates in 400 BC. However, their use at this time is likely to have been as instruments for sacrificial or destructive purposes. It was not until the Chamberlen family in the 16th century invested in and used these instruments to assist in delivery that forceps took shape, although at that time, it did not necessarily mean that a live birth might be achieved (Fig. 59.1) (see also Ch. 2). At a time when childbirth proved to be a lucrative and notable business for doctors, the family then kept their nature a secret for nearly a century. However, over the centuries, knowledge of forceps grew, and they were developed further by leading obstetricians of the time, including Simpson, Barnes and Keilland, and despite the subsequent development of ventouse-assisted delivery and the increasing use of caesarean section (CS) for difficult deliveries, forceps still remain an integral part of obstetric practice.

Ventouse extraction developed in the 18th century, derived initially from a technique known as 'cupping' with a glass attached to an air pump. However, designing the vacuum-based instrument as used today proved difficult because of the difficulty in obtaining and maintaining a seal, and it was not until Malmström introduced his

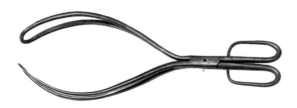

Figure 59.1 Original Chamberlen forceps, 1680. (Courtesy of Wellcome Library, London.)

revolutionary stainless steel cup in 1956 that ventouse extraction became increasingly popular. In the early 1980s the soft vacuum cup was first introduced, followed by the disposable soft-cup extractors and handheld vacuum pumps used today. Once the sole remit of obstetricians, there are now midwives who have extended their scope of practice by undertaking further training to become *midwifery ventouse practitioners*, and although data is not robust at present, initial studies have demonstrated comparable outcomes to that of obstetricians (Alexander et al 2002; Murray et al 2014).

Forceps versus ventouse

A Cochrane review of 32 studies (6597 women) comparing the choice of instruments concluded that although forceps are a better instrument for achieving a successful vaginal delivery, their use is associated with increased risk of escalation to a caesarean section, more third and fourth degree perineal tears (with or without episiotomy), increased requirements for pain relief, flatus incontinence and facial injury to the baby. Ventouse delivery is associated with less perineal/genital injury and less perineal pain in the short and long term but more *cephalhematoma* and *retinal haemorrhage* in babies (O'Mahony et al 2010). However, a 5-year follow-up of a randomized controlled trial (RCT) showed no significant differences in long-term outcome between the two instruments for either the mother or the child (Johanson et al 1999). This led the Royal College of Obstetricians and Gynaecologists (RCOG 2011) to state that both instruments are safe and that their choice must be based on the obstetrician's assessment of the clinical situation at that time and the obstetrician's level of skill.

Can an assisted birth be avoided?

A Cochrane review of 23 trials (over 15,000 women) covering a wide range of maternity settings identified that continuous support in labour increases the chance of a spontaneous vaginal birth (Hodnett et al 2013). This support may entail support of emotional and physical needs, informed choice and advocacy, all of which have been shown to increase the woman's feelings of control and competence, thus enhancing physiological labour processes and reducing the need for obstetric intervention. In addition, women were less likely to require analgesia, reported higher satisfaction ratings and had slightly shorter labours, and their babies had higher Apgar scores at 5 minutes. The effect of this support is enhanced even further if the care provided to the woman is from a midwife she knows and trusts (Sandall et al 2015).

Appropriate use of electronic fetal monitoring (EFM) is an important issue to consider, with continuous fetal monitoring being significantly associated with an increase in the number of instrumental vaginal births and caesarean sections (Alfirevic et al 2013). Maternal upright or lateral positions in labour, especially during the second stage, have also been found to have a significant association with a reduction in assisted deliveries as opposed to supine or lithotomy (Gupta et al 2012). The use of epidural analgesia will also increase a woman's risk of an instrumental delivery (Anim-Somuah et al 2011) (see Ch. 38). However, there is no evidence to support the hypothesis that discontinuing an epidural reduces this incidence, and in contrast, it can result in an increase of inadequate pain relief for the woman (Torvaldsen et al 2004). Alternatively, there is more evidence to support delayed pushing with an epidural, with a recent Cochrane review of 13 trials (287 women) concluding that although this can lead to an increase in the length of the second stage of around 54 minutes, it reduces maternal pushing by 20 minutes and slightly increases the spontaneous vaginal delivery rate (Lemos et al 2015).

> **Reflective activity 59.1**
>
> What is the intervention rate in your maternity unit? How does it compare with the national rates? What factors do you think are responsible for the rate?

Indications for an instrumental delivery

The following short list is not absolute but meant to give a general idea of the most common indications for the use of forceps or vacuum extraction during the second stage of labour:

- Prolonged second stage of labour as a result of maternal exhaustion, epidural analgesia, soft tissue resistance of the perineum, or an occipito-posterior position of the fetus
- Fetal distress necessitating immediate delivery
- Nonreassuring cardiotocography (CTG) tracing

- To avoid the increase in maternal cardiac output witnessed in pushing with women with medically significant conditions, such as cardiopulmonary or vascular conditions

Contraindications for an instrumental delivery

- Malpresentation (i.e. face or brow presentation)
- Unengaged head
- Incomplete cervical dilatation
- Inability to define position
- Any suspicion of cephalo-pelvic disproportion
- Inexperienced operator
- Ventouse – should not be performed in gestations under 34 weeks; should be used with caution between 34 and 36 weeks

Place of delivery

Any instrumental delivery with a high risk of failure should be considered a trial and ideally be undertaken in an operating theatre to facilitate timely delivery by caesarean section, if required, and should be performed by a senior obstetrician. Higher rates of failure are associated with the following:

- Maternal body mass index (BMI) over 30
- Estimated fetal weight over 4000 g or clinically big baby
- Occipito-posterior position
- Midcavity delivery or when one-fifth of the head is palpable per abdomen

If an instrumental delivery is necessary

The woman and her companion are likely to be extremely apprehensive once the need for an instrumental delivery is recommended. When the midwife has summoned the appropriate personnel, which will preferably include a senior obstetrician, a neonatologist and another person who can assist with assembling equipment, there is likely to be several strangers in the room. Midwives then have to prioritize the care they give and, where possible, involve other members of the team to assist the doctors or ventouse practitioner, rather than leave the woman's side. Midwives must remember that they remain the woman's advocate and must be present to explain all the procedures, provide support and encouragement and ensure that there is a respectful environment within the delivery room. There should be little discussion in the room that does not include the woman.

Procedure

Before the procedure, consent must be obtained from the woman. This will require a full but simple explanation and rationale of the procedures being provided to the woman, which may require the presence of a translator.

An abdominal examination is performed to check lie, presentation, position and descent of the fetus and that uterine contractions are satisfactory.

Adequate analgesia/anaesthesia must be considered.

Before the delivery, the mother is usually helped into the lithotomy position. If the woman has a history of *symphysis pubis dysfunction* (SPD), care must be taken to lift both legs together, keeping within the pain-free range of hip movement. The midwife must ensure that the woman is covered with a sheet as much as possible and for as long as possible to protect her dignity and privacy. Both legs are flexed simultaneously and gently onto the abdomen, and the feet are moved to the outer sides of the supports and placed in the leg rests or stirrups together to avoid sacro-iliac strain. To prevent obstruction of venous return and possible thrombosis by pressure, care is taken to ensure that the legs are fully abducted. Once the mother is correctly positioned, the foot part of the bed is lowered, and the mother's buttocks are lifted to the edge of the bed. The operator can now proceed.

The bladder is emptied by means of a catheter. If an indwelling catheter is already present, it should be removed or the balloon deflated to prevent potential damage to the urethra.

A vaginal examination is performed to ensure that the cervix is fully dilated and that the membranes are ruptured, the position and station of the fetal head are defined and the degree of moulding is ascertained, and there is a final check that there is no indication of cephalopelvic disproportion.

Checks are made that necessary equipment for the instrumental delivery is present, correct and in good working condition. The delivery can then proceed. An episiotomy may be performed, although it is less likely to be used for a vacuum extraction delivery (see Ch. 40).

Forceps delivery

Forceps may be used in two ways: *to exert traction without rotation* and to correct malposition, for example, occipito-posterior position, *by rotation before traction*. Rotation is rarely performed now because of the trauma to the mother and the baby (see Figs 59.2 and 59.3). There are definitive texts available (see chapter website resources) that outline the procedures for forceps delivery, but here it is more pertinent to discuss certain principles for all types of delivery.

Ventouse/vacuum extraction

The vacuum extractor or ventouse consists of a cup made of metal or soft material, such as silicone rubber, a traction

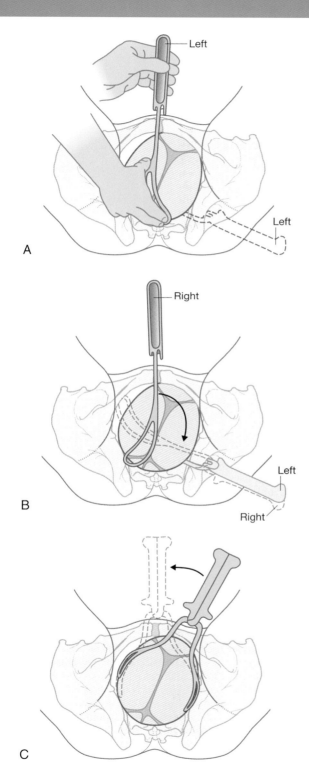

A

B

C

Figure 59.2 **A–C,** Forceps application. (Lindow and Hayashi 2010.)

device and a vacuum system providing negative pressure, by which the cup is attached to the fetal scalp. For equipment and procedure, see Fig. 59.4 (also see the chapter website resources).

The cups were originally metal, but the softer caps that have been available since the early 1980s are proving more popular. Previously, the metal cup formed a 'chignon', but now the soft cup relies on covering a larger surface area to develop sufficient traction, and this has led to less scalp trauma.

A neonatologist/paediatrician may be in attendance for the delivery, if not, a practitioner skilled in neonatal resuscitation. Checks are made that neonatal resuscitation equipment is available, clean and in good working order (see Ch. 46). The Resuscitaire, including the overhead heater, should be switched on, and the equipment should be laid out.

Reflective activity 59.2

Reflect on the last instrumental delivery you were present for – whether you were assisting or supporting the woman and partner. Think about the following:

Were the equipment, resources and personnel all appropriate and well prepared?

Were the woman and her partner sufficiently prepared and supported?

If in the same situation again, what would you do differently?

Neonatal complications

Depending on the reason for the instrumental delivery, the baby may suffer *hypoxia*, have lower Apgar scores and require appropriate resuscitation. Facial or scalp bruising is also common. A *cephalhematoma* can occur after a ventouse delivery as a result of the suction of the ventouse cup; if large enough, this can result in jaundice caused by excess bilirubin, a substance produced by the breakdown of blood as the cephalhematoma is resolving (see Chs 30, 42 and 47).

Overall, the risks of birth trauma using the ventouse and/or forceps are fortunately now relatively rare, and they are usually associated with inexperienced operators, duration of application of the instrument, station of the fetal head at the start of the delivery, difficulty of the delivery and the condition of the baby at the start of the procedure.

As discussed, *retinal haemorrhages* are more common in ventouse deliveries, but these are often superficial and resolve quickly. With forceps, a facial palsy may occur as a result of the compression of the facial nerve that runs anteriorly to the ear caused by the forceps blade; however, this is usually temporary. Rare complications that may

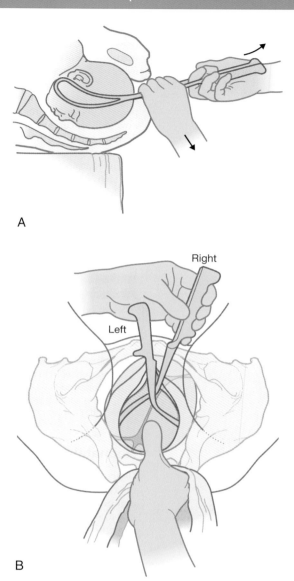

A

Right

Left

B

Figure 59.3 **A, B,** Traction and removal of forceps. (Lindow and Hayashi 2010.)

occur include *lacerations to the scalp, intracranial haemorrhage* in ventouse and *skull fractures* from forceps. The most serious complication that can occur is *subgaleal haemorrhage,* which is more common in ventouse and midcavity forceps deliveries (see Ch. 30) (Swanson et al 2012).

By far, the biggest reason for malpractice litigation in this area results from failure to abandon the procedure at an appropriate time; thus, prolonged, repeated or excessive traction with no progress should be avoided. The risks to the baby also increase dramatically when both ventouse and forceps are used, so this should only be undertaken by an experienced obstetrician practitioner. Overall, though, these risks need to be balanced with the increased risk of major *obstetric haemorrhage,* increased hospital stay and neonatal admission to the special care neonatal unit associated with a CS in the second stage of labour (Murphy et al 2001). It is also worth noting that the rates of serious neonatal complications in instrumental deliveries are actually comparable with those of caesarean sections undertaken at full dilatation (Walsh et al 2013).

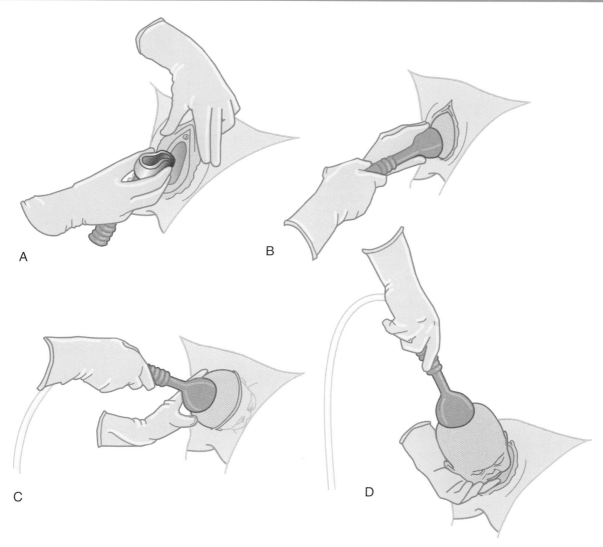

Figure 59.4 Application and delivery with ventouse. (Lindow and Hayashi 2010.)

Maternal complications

The most common maternal injuries from instrumental deliveries are to the genital tract, including cervical, vaginal and perineal tears; haematomas, rectal lacerations (see Ch. 40); and an increased risk of haemorrhage. Bladder or urethral injury may also occur, causing urinary retention and, on rare occasion, the formation of a fistula. Perineal pain as a result of bruising, oedema, trauma and episiotomy is common and can cause short- and long-term pain and discomfort and affect infant feeding and return to sexual activity. Pelvic floor disorders and long-term pelvic

floor morbidity have also been strongly associated with instrumental delivery (Handa et al 2012). The psychological effects of instrumental delivery should never be underestimated, with operative deliveries positively associated with psychological trauma and post-traumatic stress disorder (Gamble and Creedy 2005).

Postnatal care

At delivery, if the baby's condition permits, he or she should be given to the mother immediately. If resuscitation is required, then as soon as the condition is satisfactory, the baby should be given to the mother, with a relevant explanation for any necessary procedures that were undertaken. If the baby is transferred to the neonatal intensive care unit, then the parents must be kept informed of the baby's condition and taken to visit as soon as possible. Once the doctors have left, the midwife should ensure that the parents have a quiet and protected time to recover and develop a relationship with their baby (see Ch. 42).

Postnatal observations will be as for any birth, but particular attention should be paid to pain from perineal trauma, urinary output in case any damage has occurred to the bladder and signs of postpartum haemorrhage as a result of uterine atony and trauma. Particular requirements may include analgesia and assistance with feeding because of discomfort. It is also important to observe the neonate for any signs of trauma and ensure that a thorough, careful examination is carried out, with appropriate referral should any deviations from the normal be noted. Because of the possible link discussed earlier with acute trauma symptoms and post-traumatic stress disorder, there must be an opportunity for the midwife to review the woman's experience with her and discuss any concerns regarding the intervention and the procedure with the parents. It is also an appropriate time to ensure that the woman is assured that she did not 'fail' in the birth process in any way. The midwife might, at this point, identify whether further counselling and/or support may be required and refer to these services should this be required.

CAESAREAN SECTION

Caesarean section (CS) is the delivery of the fetus, placenta and membranes through a surgical incision in the abdominal wall and uterus. There are two types of caesarean section, lower segment and classical.

A *lower-segment caesarean section (LSCS)* was traditionally performed through a transverse Pfannenstiel incision, a curved incision 2 cm above the symphysis pubis, but it is now recommended that these be performed through a transverse incision known as the Joel-Cohen incision, a straight incision 3 cm above the symphysis pubis (see Fig. 59.5), because evidence has shown that this type of incision is associated with shorter operating times and reduced postoperative febrile morbidity (National Institute for Health and Clinical Excellence (NICE 2011)).

A *Classical Caesarean Section* involves a long vertical incision being made in the midline of the abdomen and uterus and is rarely performed because of the higher risk of scar rupture in a subsequent pregnancy (incidence of 2%–9%) (Guise et al 2010). It may also be used in the case of placenta praevia, cervical carcinoma, or lower-segment uterine myomas and for the delivery of preterm infants before the 28th week when the lower uterine segment has not fully formed.

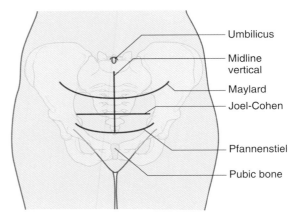

Figure 59.5 Types of caesarean section incisions.

Classification of caesarean section

Caesarean sections are currently classified into four categories based on their degree of urgency (NICE 2011):

1. Immediate threat to the life of the woman or fetus

2. Maternal or fetal compromise that is not immediately life-threatening

3. No maternal or fetal compromise but needs early delivery

4. Delivery timed to suit woman or staff

Although obstetric units have auditable standards set for 30-minute decision-to-delivery intervals for *category 1* and 75 minutes for a *category 2 CS*, there is always the inherent dilemma between timely delivery of the baby and the potential risk of injuring mother, baby or both as a result of undue haste. Therefore, the decision-to-delivery interval for both category 1 and 2 is recommended to be 'as quickly as possible'.

Indications for caesarean section

A CS is medically indicated where there is a significant risk of adverse outcome for mother or baby. In general, these indications can usually be classified into two categories: (1) *a planned CS* in which the procedure is performed as a result of a problem known in advance, or (2) as a result of an unexpected complication that has suddenly arisen during the antenatal or intrapartum period and therefore can be classed as unplanned (Table 59.1).

There has been much debate within the media concerning the right of a mother to choose a CS despite there being no medical indication. Despite the media portraying mothers choosing this option to enable them to fit childbirth into their social calendars, this is often far from the truth. Many women choose this option because of a fear of childbirth (*tocophobia*) or because of a previous

Table 59.1 Indications for caesarean section (CS)

Planned CS	Unplanned (emergency) CS
Malpresentation, such as breech, brow or shoulder presentation (However, a breech presentation may be delivered vaginally if there is no suspected cephalopelvic disproportion or other contraindications)	Fetal distress/nonreassuring cardiotocography (CTG) trace
Twin pregnancy where the presenting twin is not cephalic	Umbilical cord prolapse in the first stage of labour
Placenta praevia/known morbidly adherent placenta	Placental abruption
HIV-positive women who are not receiving any retroviral treatment with a high viral load despite taking antiretroviral therapy Women with Hepatitis C	Slow progress in labour despite interventions to accelerate
An outbreak of primary genital herpes simplex virus (HSV) in the third trimester of pregnancy	Maternal medical complications such as pre-eclampsia/eclampsia
Previous complication/condition that may indicate a repeat caesarean section, such as shoulder dystocia, third or fourth degree perineal tear, cephalopelvic disproportion, fibroids, repeated previous caesarean sections	Undelivered shoulder dystocia despite repeated manoeuvres to facilitate delivery (see Ch. 64)
Where the neonate is likely to be severely compromised by the stress of labour, such as severe intra-uterine growth restriction or severe rhesus isoimmunization	
Fetal abnormality, such as hydrocephalus, gastroschisis or macrosomia	

traumatic birth experience (*secondary tocophobia*) (Nama and Wilcock 2011). For this reason, pregnant women who request a CS because of anxiety regarding childbirth should be referred to a healthcare professional with expertise in perinatal mental health support (NICE 2011).

If a woman still requests a CS after such interventions, an obstetrician is duty bound to explore, discuss and record the specific reasons for this request and ensure that her final decision is fully informed, with all risks and benefits of CS versus vaginal birth discussed and recorded. After this, an obstetrician can still decline a woman's request; if this is the case, the obstetrician must refer her to an obstetrician who will be willing to perform the operation.

Risks of a caesarean section to the mother

CS is a major surgical procedure that, undoubtedly, can save both neonatal and maternal lives in a small number of cases. Nevertheless, CS rates have significantly increased, with an incidence of 26.2% in 2014 (HSIC 2015); in comparison, maternal and neonatal mortality rates do not appear to be decreasing.

In the short term, although a CS may reduce the risk of perineal and abdominal pain during birth and within the first 3 days postpartum, injury to the vagina, early postpartum haemorrhage and obstetric shock, it also lengthens

hospital stay and may increase the risk of hysterectomy as a result of postpartum haemorrhage and cardiac arrest. Although not robust, there is conflicting evidence linking CS with *deep vein thrombosis* (DVT), hysterectomy, anaesthetic injury, blood transfusion, infection and even maternal death (NICE 2011).

Risks of caesarean section to the fetus

Because of maternal cardiovascular changes, infants born by CS are more likely to have low Apgar scores; for this reason, a practitioner skilled in neonatal resuscitation should always be present when the CS is performed.

Later, respiratory distress may develop, which is usually caused by transient *tachypnea of the newborn* (see Chs 42 and 46). This is more apparent in babies delivered by elective caesarean section (ELCS) than in those who are delivered vaginally as a result of the lack of catecholamines being produced by the mother in labour; these would normally cross the placenta and 'switch off' the production of lung fluid by the fetal lung pneumocytes, thus preparing the baby for birth and extrauterine life. However, this risk is reduced significantly after 39 weeks. Therefore, ELCS should not routinely be performed before 39 weeks gestation. Although rare, there is also a small 2% chance that the surgeon's knife may lacerate the fetus during the operation (NICE 2011).

Can a caesarean section be avoided?

Many of the points previously discussed in relation to reducing the incidence of an instrumental delivery also apply here, with continuous support in labour and appropriate use of EFM remaining key to midwifery practice. Other factors related to midwifery practice that are thought to have an effect on reducing the incidence of CS include admission only once in established labour, admission to a standalone midwifery-led unit and unrestricted eating during labour, although further RCTs are needed to fully substantiate these. Factors that have been found to reduce the likelihood of a CS include the involvement of a consultant obstetrician in the decision-making process, induction of labour after 41 weeks gestation and the use of a partogram with a 4-hour action line once in established labour.

Factors that have been found to have no influence on the likelihood of a CS (although they may affect other outcomes) include walking in labour, nonsupine positions in the second stage, immersion in water, epidural analgesia in labour and the use of raspberry leaves. The use of complementary therapies also remains debatable, with no properly evaluated trials to substantiate their use. The use of active management in labour and early amniotomy in preventing a CS for failure to progress is also no longer recommended.

The midwife's role before surgery

Most hospitals will have a preoperative checklist for the midwife to complete before surgery, and this will generally include the points discussed here. Whether the CS is planned or unplanned, the midwife needs to ensure that the woman understands the reasons for surgery and that a consent form has been signed and obtained before the operation.

If currently taking thromboprophylactic low-molecular-weight heparin (LMWH) and regional anaesthesia is planned, ideally the last dose should have been administered at least 12 hours before surgery (RCOG 2015a). If the nature of the CS prevents this, ensure the anaesthetist and obstetrician have been informed. Because a CS increases the risk of a venous thromboembolic event (VTE), antiembolism stockings are usually applied to all women either pre- or postoperatively.

Attention needs to be given to removing any pubic hair that may cover the potential incision site. If performed on the day of surgery electric clippers with a single-use head should be used. Using ordinary razors for hair removal will increase the risk of surgical site infection (Tanner et al 2011). If preferred, women may choose to use a depilatory cream at home before admission.

At a minimum, a sample of venous blood should have been collected for haemoglobin assessment, with the results previously obtained. If warranted by the maternal severity of illness of the case in question, this may also include *group-and-save/crossmatch and clotting*.

Documentation of when the woman last ate and drank is recorded along with confirmation that any prescribed antacid therapy such as *ranitidine* has been administered.

Vital signs such as respiratory rate, temperature, pulse, blood pressure, urinalysis and presence or absence of oedema should be taken and recorded; an abdominal examination completed; and fetal heart auscultation undertaken to confirm fetal well-being. CTG is not usually required unless previously indicated.

The woman should be dressed in a theatre gown and wearing appropriate identification labels.

Women are usually advised not to wear any makeup or false nails and/or nail varnish to ensure that the anaesthetist can observe her colour.

Ideally, all jewellery should be removed for safety reasons because of the use of diathermy during the procedure, but if this is not possible, it should be covered with surgical tape.

Because of the position of the bladder, the woman will need to be catheterized before the incision. Some women will prefer to have this procedure performed before entering the operating theatre because a greater degree of privacy can be maintained. However because the procedure can be an uncomfortable experience, some will choose to be catheterized once the regional anaesthesia has been inserted. The pros and cons of both will need to be discussed for the woman to make an informed choice.

The midwife will also have a large role in supporting the woman's partner because unless it is a category 1 caesarean section, the partner will be given the option to attend. Operating theatres can be unfamiliar and frightening places to be in, especially if the CS is being undertaken for an emergency situation.

Choice of anaesthesia

General anaesthesia

Use of general anaesthesia (GA) in obstetric women is fraught with difficulties. For this reason, it is usually only performed for category 1 caesarean sections, where time is of the essence, or at the women's request after discussion of all the risk factors.

For pregnant women, by far the biggest risks are *airway complications* because advanced pregnancy reduces a woman's functional residual volume, the volume of air in the lungs at the end of normal passive expiration, by up to 500 mL. This means that if not breathing spontaneously, the woman will become hypoxic much more quickly because she has less oxygen left in her lungs to use as a reserve. In practice, this equates to an anaesthetist having approximately 30 seconds to intubate successfully.

Although this time frame usually is not problematic in the general adult population, pregnant women are also prone to weight gain and retention of fluid around their larynxes, further complicating intubation.

Another complication that may occur is acid aspiration syndrome (*Mendelson syndrome*), which pregnant women are more prone to because of delayed gastric emptying and increased intra-abdominal and intra-gastric pressures, exacerbated further when associated with the use of narcotics and/or GA. However, this may be reduced through the application of cricoid pressure during intubation, which is therefore recommended before a GA caesarean section.

Regional anaesthesia – spinal and epidural blocks

For the reasons detailed previously, epidurals or spinal blocks are usually the anaesthesia of choice for CS rather than GA. An epidural is usually the method of choice if already in situ because this is easy to 'top up' with a stronger local anaesthetic solution. Alternatively, a spinal block can be used because this is quick to administer, is only required for a relatively short period of time and requires only a small amount of anaesthesia.

Although the mother is numb from the waist down with both approaches, she is awake and able to see and hold her baby at birth, thus facilitating the establishment of early mother-to-baby bonding. The partner may also be present to provide support to the mother and share in the experience.

It is beyond the scope of this chapter to provide a full discussion of either epidural or spinal anaesthesia, and the reader is recommended to visit other sources of evidence to explore the technicalities further.

In theatre

Operating theatres by their nature create busy environments, often a complete contrast for a birthing woman who, until this point, may have had only one midwife in attendance. Therefore, it is important for the midwife to brief the woman and her partner that usually there will be an obstetrician who will perform the surgery, the obstetrician's assistant, an anaesthetist, an operating department practitioner (ODP), a scrub nurse/midwife, one or two theatre nurses and two midwives, one to care for the woman and her partner and the other to care for the baby. If the CS is a category 1 or 2, a neonatologist/paediatrician will also need to be present.

If a regional anaesthesia is being used, the woman will usually adopt a lateral or sitting position on the operating table for insertion, before being laid flat. However, because pregnant women are prone to *aortocaval occlusion* if the supine position is employed for too long, the operating table is tilted laterally until the infant is delivered to minimize the risk of supine hypotensive syndrome.

Intermittent pneumatic compression boots may also be applied while the woman is on the operating table to reduce the risk of venous thrombosis. In addition, prophylactic antibiotics (not *co-amoxiclav/Augmentin*) are usually administered before skin incision because there is a greater reduction of the risk of maternal infection compared with offering prophylaxis after the incision, with no effect observed on the infant.

During the birth, the woman's preferences should still be accommodated wherever possible, such as the playing of music, the lowering of the screen to facilitate the mother witnessing the birth or silence so that the mother's voice is the first thing the newborn infant hears outside of the uterus.

Care of the infant in theatres

Once delivered from the mother's abdomen, if no resuscitative measures are required, then as per a vaginal birth, it is optimal if the cord is not clamped earlier than a minute from the birth (NICE 2014). If the mother is awake and the baby appears well at birth, the baby should be given to the mother immediately; wherever possible, skin-to-skin contact and early breastfeeding should be actively encouraged.

However, it is important that the midwife considers the temperature of the theatre. Theatres tend to have cold environments, so measures to keep the baby warm, such as drying, covering with a warmed towel and placing a hat on the baby, are recommended (see Ch. 43).

A preterm or ill baby will more than likely be admitted to the neonatal unit for special or intensive care. In such cases, it is important that an umbilical artery pH is taken to assess fetal well-being and guide any ongoing care for the baby. The parents will naturally be very anxious, and they should be encouraged to visit the baby as soon as possible in the unit. However, if this is not possible because of the severity of maternal illness, then ensure that the neonatal unit staff members take photographs of the baby for the mother to view.

Although currently not supported by robust evidence, there is an emerging interest in the role of the human *microbiome* and how a CS may affect this. Microbiomes are comprised of the trillions of commensal microbiota that colonize the skin, gut and mucosal surfaces of the human body. Once considered to be irrelevant, they are now thought to have a major role in the human immune system. As the baby passes through the birth canal in a vaginal birth, it is colonized by friendly maternal vaginal and faecal bacteria such as *Lactobacillus*, *Prevotella* and *Sneathia*. In contrast, a baby born by CS is colonized by bacteria in the hospital environment and maternal skin – predominately *Staphylococcus* and *Clostridium difficile*. This difference in the microbiome 'seeding' is thought to form a possible rationale for why babies born by CS may be more prone to an increased risk of particular diseases

(Azad et al 2013). As a result, some women may want to perform a vaginal seeding, in which gauze soaked in normal saline is folded up like a tampon and inserted into the mother's vagina for at least an hour. It is removed before surgery and kept in a sterile container; once the baby is born, the swab is applied to the mouth, face, and the rest of the body. Until backed up by more robust evidence, the midwife's role within this process is likely to be minimal, although the midwife will need to be aware in case a mother wants to follow this procedure.

Immediate postoperative care

In the immediate postoperative recovery period, regardless of the method of anaesthesia, observations of respirations, pulse, blood pressure, oxygen saturations, level of consciousness, vaginal loss, wound dressing and, if applicable, any wound drainage system need to be recorded, as per hospital guidelines.

An accurate *fluid balance* chart will also be essential, with any inputs via intravenous therapy and outputs such as via the urinary catheter recorded. Many hospitals will now provide women with analgesia via a *patient-controlled analgesia (PCA) pump*, but if not, pain levels need to be closely monitored and analgesia administered if appropriate.

When the woman's postoperative condition is satisfactory, the anaesthetist will give permission for her to be discharged to the care of the postnatal ward staff. Instructions and details of the surgery and anaesthetic should be recorded in the notes, and an accurate verbal handover of these should be given to the receiving midwife.

Observations on return to postnatal ward

There is a high risk of postpartum haemorrhage, adding to the amount of blood lost during the operation. The uterus may not contract effectively, and there is the very serious complication of the unsuspected continuation of intra-peritoneal bleeding after the operation. The following observations and care routines are guidelines only, but they denote safe and best practice:

- *Respiratory rate, heart rate, blood pressure, sedation and pain:* After recovery from the anaesthesia, these should be checked every half hour for the next 2 hours, and hourly thereafter until stable or satisfactory. In practice, the frequency of observations is reduced after 6 hours, but observations should be continued, at a minimum, every 4 hours up to 48 hours.
    - Women who have had intrathecal (spinal) opioids should have hourly observations of respirations, sedation and pain scores for at least 12 hours for diamorphine and 24 hours for morphine.
    - For women with a PCA or who have had epidural opioids should have hourly monitoring of

respiratory rate, sedation and pain scores throughout treatment and continued for 2 hours after discontinuation of PCA.

- *Temperature:* At a minimum, temperature should be monitored every 4 hours for up to 48 hours. However, the midwife should be constantly alert for any signs or symptoms of a possible infection, such as increased respiratory rate, tachycardia, pyrexia, vomiting, offensive lochia and abdominal pain and distension.
- *Intravenous infusion lines:* Check that these are patent and running as per regime – these are usually discontinued once the woman is eating and drinking.
- *Bleeding:* Inspect wound dressing and sanitary pad for blood loss every time observations are recorded.
- *Caesarean wound:* The dressing is usually removed 24 hours after surgery. Assess the wound regularly for signs of infection (such as increasing pain, redness or discharge), separation or dehiscence. If required, removal of sutures or clips is usually undertaken around day 5.
- *Pain relief:* Ensure adequate analgesia is prescribed and administered. Initially, as discussed, this may be administered in the form of a PCA pump, or in the form of intramuscular opiates. Provided there are no contraindications, nonsteroidal anti-inflammatory drugs are usually also offered because these can reduce the need for opioids.
- *Nutritional intake:* As soon as the woman feels hungry or thirsty, she can eat or drink. Occasionally, if the surgeon is worried that the bowel was handled excessively during surgery, the surgeon may request that food is withheld until bowel sounds are heard. This ensures that the serious condition of paralytic ileus, an obstruction of the intestine resulting from paralysis of the intestinal muscle, has not developed.
- *Urinary catheter:* This is usually removed once the woman is mobile, and a trial without catheter (TWOC) is undertaken to ensure the woman can pass urine and empty her bladder. However, if an epidural was used and 'topped up', removal of the catheter should be no sooner than 12 hours after the 'top up'.
- *Thromboprophylaxis:* Because a caesarean section increases the risk of developing a deep vein thrombosis, antiembolic stockings, hydration, early mobilization and active and passive leg exercises are encouraged for all women. If a woman has already been on prophylactic LMWH antenatally and regional anaesthesia has been used, her next dose should not be administered until at least 4 hours following the spinal block or after the epidural catheter has been removed, and the catheter should not be removed within 12 hours of the most recent injection

(RCOG 2015b). If the caesarean section has been performed under general anaesthesia, LMWH should be administered as soon after the operation as possible, provided there is no evidence of postpartum haemorrhage. Although rare, there is also always a possibility of pulmonary embolism developing; thus, any unexplained shortness of breath and/or chest pain warrants urgent investigation.

- *Hygiene:* The psychological benefits of a bed bath and vulval toilet for women following a caesarean section should not be underestimated; at a minimum, all women should have an opportunity to wash their face, clean their teeth and put on fresh clothing in the hours following their caesarean section. When mobile, women are then recommended to shower daily, keeping the wound clean and dry.

- *Positioning:* With a painful abdominal wound, women may initially find it difficult to rise from a lying to a sitting and/or standing position; thus, moving slowly, supporting the abdomen and analgesia if required can all prove advantageous. A woman will also require help in finding a comfortable position in which to breastfeed her baby, and suggestions such as lying on her side in bed with her baby alongside her or on a pillow tucked under her arm, with the baby's trunk and feet under her arm, rather than lying across her abdomen, can help.

- *Transfer home:* Following caesarean section, if recovering well and apyrexial, women can now be offered early discharge home after 24 hours (NICE 2011). However, most women tend to stay on average 2 to 3 days before discharge. Where possible, they are advised to have support available to them once at home.

- *Contraception:* Women can resume sexual intercourse at any point when they feel comfortable; they will require the same contraceptive advice as any other postnatal woman (see Ch. 27).

- *Driving:* Women are usually advised to refrain from driving for at least 6 weeks and to check with their insurance company before resuming.

- *Psychological support:* Although a caesarean section does not automatically put a woman at increased risk of depression or post-traumatic stress disorder, each case will need careful consideration, and the midwife must be alert for any possible developing signs and symptoms. Discussion regarding the reasons for the operation and the procedure is recommended and can be undertaken by both the midwife and obstetrician.

Vaginal birth after caesarean section

With rising CS rates, the counselling of women and management of birth after CS remain important issues. Many women will request a vaginal birth after caesarean section (VBAC), and they can be reassured that success rates of a planned VBAC are around 72% to 75%, rising to 85% to 95% if the woman has had a previous vaginal birth (RCOG 2015c). However, there are risks and benefits of a VBAC versus a repeat caesarean section, which will need to be explained in full.

A successful VBAC carries by far the fewest complications and therefore is usually recommended, although a review of the previous indication for CS and current pregnancy would be needed to identify any possible contraindications. These would include previous uterine rupture, classical caesarean scar and other absolute contraindications such as in the case of major placenta praevia.

Because the integrity of the uterus has been weakened, there is potentially a small risk (0.5%) of uterine rupture with VBAC (Guise et al 2010). Historically, an increasing number of caesarean sections were thought to increase the risk of rupture, but a National Institute of Child Health and Human Development (NICHD) study has since proved that there is no significant difference between one, two or more previous caesarean sections (Landon et al 2006). However, it is worth noting that a short interdelivery interval (less than 12 months) can potentially increase this risk. Clinical features associated with rupture can include the following:

- Abnormal CTG/ fetal heart rate – especially acute bradycardia
- Severe abdominal pain, often persisting between contractions
- Acute onset of scar tenderness
- Abnormal vaginal bleeding
- Haematuria
- Cessation of uterine contractions, especially if they have been good up to this point
- Signs of shock in the mother, such as increased respirations, tachycardia, hypotension and loss of consciousness
- Loss of station of the presenting part
- Change in shape of mother's uterus and an inability to pick up the fetal heart in the same/expected site

Women can be reassured that their risk of an adverse outcome with VBAC is similar to that of nulliparous women. With a repeat elective caesarean section, there is a risk of placenta praevia and/or accreta in future pregnancies because the fertilized egg prefers to implant on unscarred tissue, and the associated pelvic adhesions with repeated caesarean sections may become problematic in any future abdominal/pelvic surgery.

Women who request a VBAC are usually advised to birth in an obstetric unit to allow access to continuous fetal monitoring, intravenous access and the facilities for an immediate CS and advanced neonatal resuscitation if required. Wherever possible, labour induction or augmentation is best avoided because of the two- to threefold increased risk of rupture compared with a spontaneous VBAC labour. If indicated, the involvement of a senior obstetrician is warranted, with induction preferred via the means of an amniotomy over that of traditional prostaglandins.

individual woman, no matter the mode of birth. Midwives need to be aware of potential interventions that may negate the need for operative delivery. However, if women do require an operative-style delivery, they – perhaps more than usual – require the midwife's unique skills and understanding to bring a degree of normalcy to a potentially overmedicalized event.

Reflective activity 59.3

How do you think you can contribute to ensuring that the mother's and family members' experience of intervention can be viewed as positively as possible, and how can the maternal–newborn relationship be enhanced after the birth?

CONCLUSION

The numbers of normal physiological births are decreasing in the UK, and the figures for caesarean section and instrumental deliveries are rising. Although this may appear as a dichotomy to the midwife's normal role in physiological birth, it is imperative that midwives can provide appropriate and relevant care tailored to each

---

Key Points

- The potential morbidity and mortality risk to the woman and the neonate of any operative delivery needs to be balanced by the value of these procedures in bringing the woman and baby at risk to a safe birth.

- There are several aspects of the care provided by midwives and their colleagues that may reduce the need for intervention and augmentation, such as positioning, nutrition and the presence of a supportive person.

- It is important that midwives are familiar with both the evidence and procedures associated with operative delivery so they can provide optimal care for women and their partners through the antenatal, intrapartum and postnatal periods, thus ensuring that women feel positive, empowered and supported throughout.

References

Alexander J, Anderson T, Cunningham S: An evaluation by focus group and survey of a course for midwifery ventouse practitioners, *Midwifery* 18:165–172, 2002.

Alfirevic Z, Devane D, Gyte GML: Continuous cardiotocography (CTG) as a form of electronic fetal monitoring (EFM) for fetal assessment during labour, *Cochrane Database Syst Rev* (5):CD006066, 2013.

Anim-Somuah M, Smyth RM, Jones L: Epidural versus non-epidural or no analgesia in labour, *Cochrane Database Syst Rev* (12):CD000331, 2011.

Azad M, Konya T, Maughan H, et al: Gut microbiota of healthy Canadian infants: profiles by mode of delivery and infant diet at 4 months, *Can Med Assoc J* 185(5):385–389, 2013.

Gamble J, Creedy D: Psychological trauma symptoms of operative birth, *B J Midwifery* 13(4):218–224, 2005.

Guise JM, Eden K, Emeis C, et al: *Vaginal birth after cesarean: new insights.* Evidence Reports/ Technology Assessments, No. 191, Rockville (MD), Agency for Healthcare Research and Quality, 2010.

Gupta JK, Hofmeyr GJ, Shehmar M: Position in the second stage of labour for women without epidural analgesia, *Cochrane Database Syst Rev* (16):CD002006, 2012.

Handa VL, Blomquist JL, McDermott KC, et al: Pelvic floor disorders after vaginal birth: effect of episiotomy, perineal laceration, and operative birth, *Obstet Gynecol* 119(2):233–239, 2012.

Health & Social Care Information (HSIC): *Maternity and children data set* (website). www.hscic.gov .uk/maternityandchildren. 2015.

Hodnett ED, Gates S, Hofmeyr G, et al: Continuous support for women during childbirth, *Cochrane Database Syst Rev* (7):CD003766, 2013.

Johanson RB, Heycock E, Carter J, et al: Maternal and child health after assisted vaginal delivery: five-year follow up of a randomised controlled study comparing forceps and ventouse, *Br J Obstet Gynaecol* 106:544–549, 1999.

Landon MB, Spong CY, Thom E, et al: National Institute of Child Health and Human Development Maternal-Fetal Medicine Units Network. Risk of uterine rupture in a trial of labour with women with multiple and single prior caesarean section, *Obste Gynaecol* 108:12–20, 2006.

Lemos A, Amorim MMR, Dornelas de Andrade A, et al: Pushing/bearing down methods for the second stage of labour, *Cochrane Database Syst Rev* (10):CD009124, 2015.

Lindow SW, Hayashi R: Assisted vaginal delivery. In James DK, Steer PJ, Weiner CP, et al, editors: *High risk pregnancy: management options* (expert consult – online and print), 4th edn, London, Saunders, 2010.

Murphy DJ, Liebling RE, Patel R, et al: Early maternal and neonatal morbidity associated with operative delivery in second stage of labour: a cohort study, *Lancet* 358(9289):1203–1207, 2001.

Murray S, Whitaker L, Rendall L, et al: Comparison of instrumental vaginal births by assisted birth practitioner midwives and medical practitioners, *B J Midwifery* 22(10):700–705, 2014.

Nama V, Wilcock F: Caesarean section on maternal request: is justification necessary? *The Obstetrician & Gynaecologist* 13:263–269, 2011.

National Institute for Health and Clinical Excellence (NICE): *Caesarean section. Clinical guideline 132* (website). www.nice.org.uk/guidance/cg132, 2011.

National Institute for Health and Care Excellence (NICE): *Intrapartum care for healthy women and babies* (website). www.nice.org.uk/guidance/cg190, 2014.

O'Mahony F, Hofmeyr GJ, Menon V: Choice of instruments for assisted vaginal delivery, *Cochrane Database Syst Rev* (11):CD005455, 2010.

Royal College of Obstetricians and Gynaecologists (RCOG): *Operative vaginal delivery. Greentop Guideline No. 26* (website). www.rcog.org.uk/globalassets/documents/guidelines/gtg_26.pdf. 2011.

Royal College of Obstetricians and Gynaecologists (RCOG): *Thrombosis and embolism during pregnancy and the puerperium, reducing the risk. Greentop Guideline No. 37a* (website). www.rcog.org.uk/en/guidelines-research-services/guidelines/gtg37a/. 2015a.

Royal College of Obstetricians and Gynaecologiests (RCOG): *Thrombosis and Embolism during Pregnancy and the Puerperium: the acute management of. Green-top Guideline No. 37b* (website). https://www.rcog.org.uk/en/guidelines-research-services/guidelines/gtg37b. 2015b.

Royal College of Obstetricians and Gynaecologists (RCOG): *Birth after previous caesarean birth. Greentop Guideline No. 45* (website). www.rcog.org.uk/en/guidelines-research-services/guidelines/gtg45/. 2015c.

Sandall J, Soltani H, Gates S, et al: Midwife-led continuity models versus other models of care for childbearing women, *Cochrane Database Syst Rev* (9):CD004667, 2015.

Swanson AE, Veldman A, Wallace EM, et al: Subgaleal hemorrhage: risk factors and outcomes, *Acta Obstet Gynecol Scand* 912:260–263, 2012.

Tanner J, Norrie P, Melen K: Preoperative hair removal to reduce surgical site infection, *Cochrane Database Syst Rev* (11):CD004122, 2011.

Torvaldsen S, Roberts C, Bell JC, et al: Discontinuation of epidural analgesia late in labour for reducing the adverse delivery outcomes associated with epidural analgesia, *Cochrane Database Syst Rev* (4):CD004457, 2004.

Walsh CA, Robson M, McAuliffe FM: Mode of delivery at term and adverse neonatal outcomes, *Obstet Gynecol* 121(1):122–128, 2013.

Additional reading and resources

Please refer to the chapter website resources.

National Health Service (NHS) Choices: http://www.nhs.uk/conditions/pregnancy-and-baby/pages/ventouse-forceps-delivery.aspx

Source of information for women and families.

National Institute for Health and Care Excellence (NICE): *Intrapartum care for healthy women and babies*, CG190, 2014: https://www.nice.org.uk/guidance/cg190/resources/intrapartum-care-for-healthy-women-and-babies-35109866447557

This is a source of the clinical guidelines and the evidence underpinning the guidelines, plus resources for professionals and patients.

Royal College of Midwives (RCM), 2012: www.rcm.org.uk

This website has useful information and news on midwifery and maternity care. It has several resources including RCM i-learn (electronic learning menu, including care of the newborn) and evidence-based guidelines for midwifery-led care in labour: https://www.rcm.org.uk/clinical-practice-and-guidance/evidence-based-guidelines

This online publication includes guidelines around nutrition, pain relief and care of the newborn.

Royal College of Obstetricians and Gynaecologists (RCOG): www.rcog.org.uk

Good website with materials including downloadable 'Green Top Guidelines', leaflets and information for women and families. The Royal College of Midwives library is also housed at the RCOG, and there are a range of records, artifacts and materials of historical interest.

Scottish Intercollegiate Guidelines Network (SIGN): http://www.sign.ac.uk/guidelines/published/index.html

This site also holds a range of resources and guidelines for health care, based on good evidence.

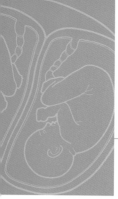

Chapter 60

Induction of labour and prolonged pregnancy

Alison Brodrick

Learning Outcomes ?

After reading this chapter, you will be able to:

- discuss the indications, contraindications and implications for induction of labour
- evaluate the common reasons/pregnancy conditions that may indicate induction
- review the efficacy of the common induction methods used
- evaluate the management of prolonged pregnancy

INDUCTION OF LABOUR

Induction of labour (IOL) is the generic term used for artificially initiating labour before spontaneous labour onset occurs. The process of IOL and the method used will depend on the clinical scenario. In England, the incidence of IOL has increased steadily over the last decade and for 2013–2014 was reported to be 25% (HSCIS 2015). Although current guidance advises that IOL should only be used when the risks of continuing the pregnancy outweigh intervention (National Institute for Health and Clinical Excellence (NICE) 2008), as many as 50% of labours are induced without a medical indication (Stock et al 2012). This has added to a growing debate about the risks and timing of IOL compared with waiting for spontaneous labour.

There is currently considerable debate as to whether IOL actually increases the risk of caesarean section (CS). When compared directly with a sample group of women in spontaneous labour, CS rates will be higher in the induced group (Jonsson et al 2013; Ehrenthal et al 2010). However, when an IOL is being discussed, the alternative is *expectant management* (awaiting spontaneous labour to occur). In the expectant group, some women will not labour spontaneously, and some may develop problems, requiring induction. Research using these two groups as comparators has shown that the CS rate is unaffected or reduced in the IOL group (Stock et al 2012; Gülmezoglu 2012).

ASSESSING THE NEED FOR INDUCTION

The decision to induce is based on an assessment of the clinical picture and with full discussion with the woman, respecting her wishes. Women need adequate information to understand the risks of induction, the risks of continuing the pregnancy, the method of induction and the implications for intrapartum care. Induction of labour has a significant effect on the health of the fetus and baby, and it is associated with a longer, more painful labour and a negative birth experience (Shetty et al 2005). There is also a risk of the procedure failing, resulting in delivery by CS.

Medical indications for IOL mainly relate to increased risk of fetal and/or maternal compromise if delivery is delayed. There should be clear evidence that the induction is beneficial to the mother and/or fetus.

Maternal indications

Hypertension: Hypertensive disorders are one of the principal indications for induction, and timely intervention may become necessary to avoid serious maternal morbidity and perinatal compromise (see Ch. 54).

Diabetes: Women with type 1 or type 2 diabetes and no other complications are advised to have an induction of labour or, if indicated, a caesarean section between 37 +0 weeks and 38 +6 weeks of pregnancy. For women with gestational diabetes, it is recommended that IOL is considered before 40 +6 if spontaneous labour has not ensued (NICE 2015).

Cholestasis: For women with cholestasis, close monitoring of blood chemistry will usually determine when induction is necessary to outweigh the risks of stillbirth if the pregnancy continues. IOL after 37 weeks should be discussed with the woman (Royal College of Obstetricians and Gynaecologists (RCOG) 2011).

Advanced maternal age: Unexplained antenatal and intrapartum stillbirths increase with advancing maternal age and increasing length of pregnancy in both primigravid and multigravid women. Following publication of a scientific paper (RCOG 2013), the recommendation is to offer IOL between 39 and 40 weeks. This will inevitably reduce the incidence of stillbirth, but the longer-term consequences of such a policy have yet to be evaluated.

Maternal request: Induction of labour may be requested by women for social or emotional reasons – for example, a partner being posted abroad with the armed services or increased anxiety or stress that may or may not be directly associated with the pregnancy. Induction should not be routinely offered, but in exceptional circumstances, it may be considered at or after 40 weeks (NICE 2008).

Poor obstetric history: Induction is sometimes undertaken to alleviate the anxiety and stress associated with subsequent pregnancies following previous adverse outcome, although it may have no clinical relevance to the current pregnancy.

Fetal indications

Fetal growth restriction: Induction may be indicated if there is evidence of diminished fetal well-being caused by uteroplacental insufficiency, which is often characterized by intra-uterine growth restriction, abnormal fetal movements and/or abnormal fetal umbilical blood flow detected by Doppler ultrasound. If the fetus is severely growth restricted, a caesarean section is the preferred method of elective delivery because of the risk of further fetal compromise during labour (NICE 2008).

Macrosomia: Many women worry about their baby being too big, and in the past, suspected macrosomia was an indication for induction in an attempt to avoid a difficult delivery and, in particular, shoulder dystocia. However, accurate diagnosis of estimated fetal weight remains problematic, and randomized controlled trials (RCTs) demonstrate no effect on the rates of caesarean birth, instrumental birth or spontaneous birth compared with expectant management. Suspected macrosomia that is not complicated by diabetes is not an indication for induction (NICE 2008).

Fetal death: When fetal death has occurred, a plan should be made with the parents regarding timing and method of induction. If the membranes have ruptured or if there is evidence of infection or bleeding, then immediate induction is indicated (NICE 2008). National guidelines for this situation have been recommended (Draper et al 2015).

Rhesus isoimmunization: Rhesus isoimmunization is still the most common cause of fetal anaemia. Regular surveillance during pregnancy will determine when an intra-uterine fetal blood transfusion is necessary and also the optimal time for IOL (Santiago et al 2010).

Fetal anomaly: Labour may be induced to terminate pregnancy if the fetus has a lethal abnormality or a malformation likely to result in significant handicap. It may also be indicated when the baby would benefit from planned early surgery.

Contraindications

Absolute contraindications for induction of labour are the same as for vaginal delivery, and include the following:

- **Placenta praevia:** When the placenta is partially or completely covering the os, there is potential for massive haemorrhage.

- **Oblique or transverse lie:** These positions carry risks of cord prolapse and obstruction.

- **Breech:** Current guidance states that IOL can be considered for carefully selected breech cases (RCOG 2006). However, in the UK there is a very cautious view taken, and IOL is generally not recommended; this also applies to augmentation of labour. In some European countries IOL may be considered more acceptable.

- **Severe fetal compromise:** In this situation, the fetus is unlikely to tolerate the stress of labour, and a caesarean section is indicated.

Induction of labour in specific circumstances

Previous caesarean section: IOL is contraindicated if there is a classical incision (i.e. a midline longitudinal incision) on the uterus or if there was extension of uterine tears during a previous caesarean. Unless there are other medical/obstetric complications, women with one previous transverse caesarean section should be informed of the risks and benefits of expectant management versus IOL and supported in an informed decision. For women with two or more previous caesarean sections, IOL is generally not recommended because of the risk of uterine rupture.

History of precipitate birth: Women can find a precipitate labour very frightening; however, there is no evidence to suggest IOL is beneficial, and it may actually incur unnecessary risk (NICE 2008) (see Ch. 61). Where possible, other solutions that address the woman's fears should be discussed, including offering planned home birth if appropriate.

Fetal macrosomia: In the absence of diabetes and with no other indication, IOL to prevent a prolonged pregnancy offers no benefit (NICE 2014a).

Maternal request: There are many circumstances when women may request an IOL. Often, women find the pregnancy physically or psychologically difficult and see IOL as a way of ending the pregnancy. Some women may make requests based on personal circumstances, for instance, availability of partner or family for support. Women need appropriate information to understand the process of IOL and its risks. IOL should only be offered for a medical need. However, such requests are dealt with on an individual basis, and an IOL at/over 40 weeks may be indicated (NICE 2008).

If the woman cannot have a safe vaginal delivery, induction of labour should not be considered.

Methods of induction

Induction is usually timed for when it will be most successful, that is, near the onset of spontaneous labour. But,

as discussed previously, there are situations when it will be necessary to intervene before term to reduce the risk of fetal and/or maternal compromise.

The method of induction and preferred pharmacological products will be influenced primarily by cervical and membrane status, parity and provider preference. When IOL is being considered, it is important to complete an assessment of the cervix to aid the decision making around timing and method of IOL. The success of induction and subsequent length of labour are primarily determined by how favourable the cervix is at the time of induction.

Cervical assessment

The cervix is assessed using the *Bishop score*, which has been in use since the 1960s (Bishop 1964). The Bishop score gives a numerical score based on the assessment of five qualities (see Table 60.1):

- Cervical dilatation
- Cervical consistency
- Length of cervix
- Position of the cervix
- Station of the presenting part

When the total score is greater than 8, the cervix is said to be 'ripe' or favourable and more likely to respond positively to labour being induced (NICE 2008). If the cervix is unfavourable, there is a higher chance of the IOL failing.

Membrane sweeping

Before carrying out an assessment of the cervix and before starting a formal IOL process, all women should be offered membrane sweeping (NICE 2008).

Sweeping or stripping the membranes from the lower uterine segment involves the practitioner undertaking a vaginal examination, then placing a finger inside the cervix and making a circular, sweeping action to separate the membranes from the cervix. The theory behind this method is that localized *prostaglandin* production is

Table 60.1 Modified Bishop's scoring system				
Feature for assessment	**Score**			
	0	**1**	**2**	**3**
Dilatation of cervix (cm)	<1	1–2	2–4	>4
Consistency of cervix	Firm	Medium	Soft	–
Length of cervix (cm)	4	2–4	1–2	<1
Position of cervix	Posterior	Mid	Anterior	–
Station in cm relative to ischial spines	−3	−2	−1/0	+1/+2

increased (Mitchell et al 1977). In a Cochrane systematic review, sweeping the membranes was found to be associated with an increase in spontaneous labour onset and reduction in the need for formal IOL methods (Boulvain et al 2005). There was no increase in maternal or neonatal infection or premature rupture of the membranes, but one trial (Boulvain et al 1998) reported increased maternal discomfort during and after the procedure, with both vaginal bleeding and painful contractions not leading to the onset of labour during the 24 hours following the intervention. It should be noted that the trials on membrane sweeping have been small, and more research is needed, including the benefit of repeat sweeping, which has not been adequately evaluated. The process of membrane sweeping can be very uncomfortable for the woman, and a full explanation and consent must be gained before the procedure.

Pharmacological methods of induction

Prostaglandins

In the UK, vaginal prostaglandin *E2 (PGE2)* is the preferred method unless there is a clinical reason not to use it. It is available in gel, tablet and slow-release pessary; all of these preparations have similar efficacy. PGE2 is used for cervical ripening and is the first step in inducing labour; it should not be attempted unless the aim is to bring pregnancy to an end. The product should be inserted into the *posterior vaginal fornix*, avoiding administration into the cervical canal because this may cause hyperstimulation (see Fig. 60.1).

Vaginal PGE2 is associated with improved cervical status and reduced need for oxytocin augmentation, the recommended regime (NICE 2008) is as follows:

- One cycle of vaginal PGE2 tablets or gel: one dose, followed by a second dose after 6 hours if labour is not established (up to a maximum of two doses)
- One cycle of vaginal PGE2 controlled-release pessary: one dose over 24 hours

Contraindications to PGE2 are presented in Table 60.2.

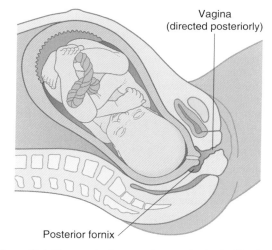

Figure 60.1 Placement of pessary in posterior fornix. (Reprinted with permission from Marshall J, Raynor M, editors: Myles Textbook for Midwives, London, Churchill Livingstone, Elsevier, 2014.)

Table 60.2 Contraindications to vaginal PGE2

Fetal	Pregnancy	Maternal
Severe IUGR	Placenta praevia	Previous hysterotomy, classical caesarean section, cervical tear
Absent or reversed end diastolic flow on Doppler	Vasa praevia	History of myomectomy or other full-thickness uterine incision
Abnormal CTG	Undiagnosed vaginal bleeding in pregnancy	Pelvic structural abnormality
Presenting part above pelvic inlet	Prior use of CRB or prostaglandin gel	Active cardiac, pulmonary, renal or hepatic disease
Cephalo-pelvic disproportion	Any contraindication to labour induction	Active genital herpes
Transverse lie		Invasive cervical cancer
Oblique lie		Untreated severe maternal hypertension
		Hypersensitivity to prostaglandins

CRB, cervical ripening balloon; CTG, cardiotocograph; IUGR, intra-uterine growth restriction

Before the insertion of PGE2, an abdominal examination should be carried out to confirm presentation, position and station of the fetus; a cardiotocograph (CTG) trace should then be completed to establish fetal well-being. Following administration, the woman is advised to remain recumbent for at least 30 minutes, during which time continuous electronic fetal monitoring is recommenced to assess fetal reaction to the induction process. After this time, the woman is able to move and mobilize as normal. Once contractions begin, a CTG trace should be recommenced.

The main complication associated with prostaglandin administration is *uterine hyperstimulation* with or without fetal heart-rate abnormalities (Enkin et al 2000); for this reason, it may be contraindicated for some women (see Table 60.2). Iatrogenic uterine hyperstimulation and *fetal heart-rate abnormalities* during the cervical ripening period can lead to a need for emergency CS and its associated morbidity. Failure to produce any significant change in cervical favourability may also lead to delivery by CS. Other less common effects include the following:

- Maternal gastrointestinal side effects
- Maternal pyrexia from the effect on the thermoregulating centre in the brain
- Intra-uterine infection

Oxytocin

Artificial oxytocin, usually in the form of *Syntocinon*, diluted with normal saline, is given via intravenous infusion to either augment or induce labour. It is used after cervical ripening has occurred and in the presence of ruptured membranes.

The dose is titrated and increased slowly using a volumetric pump until regular strong contractions are maintained and to avoid hyperstimulation or prolonged contractions (*hypertonus*), which can cause fetal hypoxia as a result of compromised placental circulation. Hyperstimulation can also result in uterine rupture (see Ch. 63), and the consequences of inappropriate oxytocin use are highlighted in a recent MBRRACE report (Knight et al 2014). The drug has a short half-life, so stopping the infusion should suffice if hyperstimulation occurs; the use of tocolytics may also be required (NICE 2008).

The use of artificial oxytocin requires continuous fetal monitoring and close observation; if there is a suspicion of fetal compromise, the oxytocin infusion is stopped. Depending on the assessment of fetal well-being, the infusion may be restarted, usually at a half dose. If a CS is necessary, the infusion must remain stopped.

The antidiuretic effect of oxytocin can lead to water retention and hyponatraemia, with serious associated maternal sequelae, although this is rare and preventable with strict fluid management and minimal infusion volume. Therefore, careful assessment of fluid balance must be maintained and recorded on the partogram and labour notes.

Antiprogesterones

In the UK, *mifepristone* is used only when fetal death has occurred and is used as a priming agent before the use of prostaglandin *E1-misoprostol (PGE1)*. Given vaginally, PGE1 results in very strong contractions, and birth is likely to ensue much quicker compared with PGE2 use. It is also strongly associated with hyperstimulation; thus, it is only used when fetal well-being is not a concern.

Mechanical methods of induction

Artificial rupture of the membranes (ARM) should only be considered if the cervix is already favourable or if there is a contraindication to PGE2 (see Table 60.2).

Following discussion with and consent of the woman, the clinician must first perform an abdominal palpation to ensure the presenting part is cephalic and engaged. After this, a vaginal examination is performed, and the cervical os and membranes are digitally examined. Using a specially designed plastic 'Amnihook' (EMS Medical Group), the forewaters are pierced. Less commonly, surgical steel forceps or a fetal scalp electrode is used. If the fetal head is high, there is an increased risk of cord prolapse. In these cases, a *controlled* ARM may be needed; this is usually done in theatre and involves stabilizing the head abdominally while the membranes are ruptured.

A CTG trace should be commenced after amniotomy to ensure fetal well-being. If the CTG trace is reassuring, the woman is normally advised to mobilize. For some women, especially multigravid women, this procedure will be enough to stimulate labour. If contractions do not ensue, then an oxytocin infusion is commenced.

Potential hazards of amniotomy include the following:

- Ascending intra-uterine infection, including mother-to-child vertical transmission of HIV infection
- Early decelerations of the fetal heart rate
- Umbilical cord prolapse
- Bleeding from the cervix, the fetal vessels in the membranes (vasa praevia) or the placental site

A *balloon catheter* can be used to induce labour by applying pressure to the cervix. It can be a single- or double-balloon catheter. A double-balloon catheter is considered more beneficial because it applies pressure to the internal and external os. Studies comparing balloon catheters with vaginal prostaglandins report an increase in vaginal birth rates (Cromi et al 2012). Other studies, however, have shown no difference in vaginal birth rates but a reduced risk of hyperstimulation (Du et al 2015). Although not recommended by NICE (2008) as an effective method, some maternity units in the UK favour this method when managing an IOL for women with a previous CS because the risk of hyperstimulation and therefore uterine rupture will be lower.

Other methods for inducing labour

Natural methods of cervical ripening and IOL that allow women to have greater control over the induction process are inexpensive and are perceived as being less medicalized.

There is evidence that *breast/nipple stimulation*, which results in the production of oxytocin, can stimulate contractions, and studies have shown the ability of this method to induce labour (Kavanagh et al 2005). Similarly, *sexual intercourse* may stimulate uterine contractions, and the addition of semen, which is believed to contain prostaglandin concentrate, may have a role (Kavanagh et al 2001). However, further robust research is needed to prove efficacy.

Studies looking at *acupuncture* to induce cervical ripening and oxytocin release have reported some success (Smith et al 2008), but further research is needed.

There is also some evidence that *reflex zone therapy* can have therapeutic value in stimulating labour (Tiran 2009). Also, the properties contained in certain essential oils can increase contractions; with the addition of massage, they can reduce anxiety and balance oxytocin levels (Evans 2009). *Shiatsu* and *aromatherapy* have been used individually in some maternity units to increase the numbers of women experiencing spontaneous labour, with some success (Ingram et al 2005; Tillett and Ames 2010).

Although research has been unable to prove the efficacy of the use of one complementary therapy in inducing labour, there may be benefit in offering a package of therapies. Some maternity units in the UK have therefore set up a 'post-dates clinic' that includes aromatherapy, reflex zone therapy and a membrane sweep. This type of clinic is only suitable for healthy, low-risk women who are post-dates. The results, based on local audit data, show some positive effects, including a reduction in post-dates' induction (Weston and Grabowska 2013). A large research trial is needed, and midwives need to remember their limitations and accountability when advising or supporting women using complementary therapies (see Ch. 18).

Location and timing of induction of labour

It is recommended that planned IOL in an inpatient setting should be carried out in the morning because of increased maternal satisfaction (Dodd et al 2006) and the potential to reduce the length of stay in the hospital (NICE 2008).

More recently, there has been a trend in developed countries to offer uncomplicated post-dates IOL in an outpatient setting. National guidance supports induction in an outpatient setting provided that there are safety and support procedures in place and continuous auditing of outcomes (NICE 2008). There is growing evidence that this service achieves greater satisfaction for women (Reid et al 2011; O'Brien et al 2013) without compromising safety. Oster et al (2011) reported that women who received outpatient cervical priming and returned home were better able to relax and were better prepared for labour and birth.

Care during induction of labour

Before IOL is carried out, there should be a full discussion with the woman and her partner regarding the reasons for induction and the subsequent plan. This also includes discussion of the risks and benefits and the likely expected duration of the process. It is also important that women understand that an induced labour is likely to be more painful than a spontaneous labour. However, just because the woman is being induced, the midwife should not assume that pharmacological pain relief is necessary; each woman should be treated as an individual with the same access to non-pharmacological pain relief and mobility as women in spontaneous labour (see Ch. 38). It is also important that midwives support women who are being induced to feel confident in their ability to birth.

The process of induction includes the following steps:

- History taking, including assessment of fetal movements

- Assessment and recording of maternal temperature, pulse, blood pressure and respiration

- Abdominal palpation to assess fetal lie, presenting part, descent and fetal growth

- Assessment of fetal well-being via 20-minute CTG trace

- After consent, a vaginal examination to assess the Bishop score

- If needed, PGE is administered, and the woman is advised to lie down for 30 to 60 minutes to aid absorption. During this time, the CTG is usually continued.

After this, women can move freely and should be informed to report when contractions start.

When contractions begin, fetal well-being should be assessed with continuous electronic fetal monitoring. Once the CTG is confirmed as normal, intermittent auscultation may be appropriate, depending on the reason for IOL; see the NICE (2014b) *Intrapartum Care: care of healthy women and their babies during childbirth* guideline.

If the fetal heart rate is abnormal after administration of vaginal PGE2, the recommendations on management of fetal compromise in the *Intrapartum Care* guideline (NICE 2014b) should be followed.

The Bishop score should be reassessed 6 hours after vaginal PGE2 tablet or gel insertion, or 24 hours after vaginal PGE2 controlled-release pessary insertion, to monitor progress.

If a woman returns home after insertion of vaginal PGE2 tablet or gel, she should be asked to contact her obstetrician/midwife in the following circumstances:

• When contractions begin, or

• If she has had no contractions after 6 hours.

Once active labour is established, maternal and fetal monitoring should be carried out as described in *Intrapartum Care* (NICE 2014b).

If labour does not occur, it may be appropriate to offer further prostaglandins; if the cervix has 'ripened', it may be possible to artificially rupture the membranes, which is usually carried out on the labour ward and will include the addition of an oxytocin infusion if needed.

It is important that the midwife is aware that some women may be fearful and anxious at this time, and the midwife should ensure that the women and partner know how they can contact the midwife; midwives should emphasize their availability for emotional and practical support (NICE 2014b; Care Quality Commission (CQC) 2015).

INTERNATIONAL PERSPECTIVES

In high-income countries such as the United States and Australia, IOL is commonplace and comparative to UK rates. Across Europe there is more variation. According to the European Perinatal Health Report (Euro-peristat 2013), the rates in 2010 ranged from 6.8% in Lithuania to over 27% in Brussels, Malta and Northern Ireland. However, there is also variation in the definitions of IOL, with some countries including ARM and others including only the use of cervical ripening and oxytocin.

In developing countries, access to IOL plays an important part in realizing the Millennium Development Goals (MDGs) (see Ch. 1). With the highest perinatal mortality rate of 56 per 1000 live births, Africa also has the lowest IOL rate at 4.4% (Vogel et al 2013). In a secondary analysis of the *WHO Global Survey on Maternal Neonatal Health 2004–2005* (Bukola et al 2012), the differences in perinatal mortality rates among women in Africa who were induced versus not induced was shown to be stark: 31.7 per 1000 deliveries versus 87.7 per 1000 deliveries, respectively. In many low-income countries, the decision to induce is compounded by challenges in availability of drugs, appropriate healthcare staffing, fetal monitoring facilities and access to safe CS (Vogel et al 2013).

Interestingly, this debate is not confined solely to developing countries; in some high-income countries, a differing rate of IOL and neonatal/maternal outcomes is evident when comparing access to public versus private healthcare, with adverse perinatal outcomes higher in public hospitals (Robson et al 2009).

PROLONGED PREGNANCY

Prolonged, post-term and *post-dates* are terms that are often used interchangeably to mean a pregnancy that has continued beyond a duration that is considered normal. The widely accepted definition is a pregnancy continuing for more than 42 weeks or greater than 294 days (International Federation of Gynaecology and Obstetrics (FIGO) 1980). The term *post-mature* refers to the neonate and a set of clinical features exhibited when pregnancy has become pathologically long; this is not exclusive to prolonged labour and can be displayed in neonates born at 39 to 40 weeks. In developed countries, IOL procedures are usually commenced for post-dates between 41 and 42 weeks to prevent the risks associated with prolonged pregnancy.

The reported incidence of prolonged pregnancy (over 42 weeks) is between 5% and 10% (Olesen et al 2003). The most common cause is inaccurate dating. Dating by ultrasound scan alone has been shown to be a more accurate predictor of the birth date than dating by the last menstrual period (LMP) calculation alone or with a 14, 10 or 7 day adjustment 'rule' (Mongelli et al 1996). With more accurate assessment of gestational age using ultrasound and with IOL policies for post-dates, the incidence of prolonged pregnancy is decreasing, with some countries reporting figures as low as 0.4% (Simpson and Stanley 2011). Current guidance recommends early ultrasound scanning to assess gestational age to ensure consistency of approach and reduce the number of inductions of labour for perceived post-dates (NICE 2008). In women who have had one prolonged pregnancy, there is a 20% risk of reoccurrence; this drops to 15% if it is a different partner (Simpson and Stanley 2011). Prolonged pregnancy is noted to be associated with primigravity and maternal obesity. The fetus is known to play a role in labour onset, and any hormonal imbalance can cause pregnancy prolongation (see Ch. 35). Major abnormalities that affect the fetal central nervous system or endocrine system, such as *anencephaly* and *adrenal hypoplasia*, are also associated with prolonged pregnancy, as is carrying a male fetus.

Risks of prolonged pregnancy

Fetal

Epidemiological studies indicate an increase in perinatal risks when pregnancy progresses beyond 40 weeks

(Gülmezoglu et al 2006). After adjusting for congenital abnormalities, the incidence of perinatal death is lower when labour is induced from 41 weeks compared with expectant management; the overall risk, however, remains small at 2 to 3:1000 (NICE 2008).

Studies have shown a gradual deterioration in placental function after 40 weeks and an increased risk of chronic progressive uteroplacental insufficiency (Battaglia et al 1995). In a prolonged pregnancy, uteroplacental insufficiency is one reason for the rise in risk to the fetus because it is associated with reduced fetal growth, oligohydramnios, passage of meconium, asphyxia and, ultimately, stillbirth. However, some placentas will continue functioning as normal. In the absence of uteroplacental insufficiency, fetal growth therefore continues, although at a reduced rate after 38 weeks gestation (Boyd et al 1988). In this group, babies born at 42 completed weeks are three to seven times more likely to weigh over 4000 g than those delivered before 41 completed weeks (Fabre et al 1998). Macrosomia increases the risk of dysfunctional labour, shoulder dystocia, brachial plexus injury and clavicular fracture in the baby.

Other perinatal risks include the following:

- Meconium aspiration
- Birth asphyxia
- Admission to neonatal unit (NNU)

Maternal

The main risk to the mother is prolonged labour and operative delivery, which is more common in both induced and spontaneous labour. Other risks include the following:

- Postpartum haemorrhage
- Genital tract trauma
- Chorioamnionitis

Post-maturity syndrome

Gibb (1985) first described the features of the post-mature infant. Such infants are alert and appear mature, but they have a decreased amount of soft tissue mass, particularly subcutaneous fat; their body length is increased in relation to body weight; and the skin may hang loosely on the extremities and is often dry and peeling. There is an absence of vernix and lanugo, although they often have abundant scalp hair. The fingernails and toenails are long. The nails and umbilical cord may be stained with meconium passed in utero.

Post-maturity syndrome is also associated with oligohydramnios (Clement et al 1987), with features similar to those seen in the growth-restricted infant. Knox Ritchie (1992) describes this syndrome as an expression of chronic fetal malnutrition, which is not confined to post-term

pregnancy. As few as 10% of prolonged pregnancies are complicated by this syndrome (Resnik 1994).

Management of prolonged pregnancy

In most developed countries, management is started with 'post-dates' with the aim of preventing prolonged pregnancy; this usually begins with membrane sweeping from 40 weeks, considered by NICE (2008) to be an integral part of prevention. Elective induction is then scheduled between 41 and 42 weeks.

It is important, however, that consent to elective induction involves appropriate information and discussion between the midwife and the woman. This includes discussing the risks, benefits and alternatives to induction. In one study, as many as 48% of women wanted more information about induction (Singh and Newburn 2000).

After a full discussion, some women may decide to await spontaneous labour (*expectant management*). For these women, it is important that they understand the significance of fetal activity and report any changes. It would also be prudent to remind women about reporting any vaginal loss or feeling of being generally unwell. An ultrasound estimation of maximum amniotic pool depth is considered useful, and NICE (2008) also recommend twice-weekly CTG, although this has limited accuracy in determining fetal well-being and a tendency to provide false reassurance (Pattison and McCowan 1999). Maintaining a positive relationship with women who decide on expectant management is important. Women need to be assured that they can seek advice if there are any subtle changes and be confident that their midwife will be an advocate for their informed choice.

Women and their partners are likely to experience a range of emotions when faced with IOL. However, involving the woman and her partner in decision making is likely to increase their feelings of control over what happens. An individual plan of care can then be made and documented in the woman's notes. For normal, healthy women choosing expectant management, the lead professional usually changes to an obstetrician at 42 weeks, and further informed discussion around suitability of choice of place of birth needs to take place.

Economic analysis

Gülmezoglu et al (2006) conclude that a policy of routine IOL after 41 weeks reduces the risk of perinatal death and meconium aspiration syndrome in normally formed babies while having comparable other maternal and fetal outcomes. A cost–benefit analysis of IOL versus expectant management concludes that offering IOL from 41 weeks is the most cost-effective and beneficial strategy (NICE 2008) and outweighs any associated costs/risks. In developed countries, offering elective induction between 41 and 42 weeks is now the norm. There is also evidence that women prefer IOL to expectant management when pregnancy is prolonged (Roberts and Young 1991; Westfall and Benoit 2004). Redshaw et al (2007) found that although 30% of women did not feel they had had a say in their labour being induced, they believed it to be necessary for the health and well-being of themselves and the baby. This normalization of elective induction to prevent prolonged pregnancy may explain why some women view it positively.

CONCLUSION

It is important that midwives are highly knowledgeable and skilled in providing balanced and evidence-based information to women and their families in preparing for induction of labour, and ensure that sufficient time is allowed for questions and discussion. Many women have prepared psychologically for a normal labour, needing sensitive care to support them through the experience of induction and to feel that their views and wishes are respected. This can be assisted by the woman, midwife and other members of the multidisciplinary team working together to design and agree a plan of care which is individualized, culturally sensitive and appropriate to the needs of the woman and her family.

Key Points

- Accurate dating of pregnancy is essential to avoid unnecessary induction of labour and attendant risks to the woman and baby.
- Women need appropriate information and support regarding induction of labour and must be involved in the decision making.
- Expectant management and induction of labour are both valid options for management of post-term pregnancy.
- All women should be offered membrane sweeping from 40 weeks onward.
- Pharmacological methods of induction require careful management to ensure fetal and maternal well-being.
- During labour, women need to feel supported to maintain some mobility and be supported with a strategy for coping with pain.

References

Battaglia C, Artini PG, Ballestri M, et al: Hemodynamic, hematological and hemorrheological evaluation of post-term pregnancy, *Acta Obstet Gynecol Scand* 74(5):336–340, 1995.

Bishop EH: Pelvic scoring for elective induction, *Obstet Gynecol* 24:266–268, 1964.

Boulvain M, Fraser W, Marcoux S, et al: Does sweeping of the membranes reduce the need for formal induction of labour? A randomised controlled trial, *Br J Obstet Gynaecology* 105(1):34–40, 1998.

Boulvain M, Stan C, Irion O: Membrane sweeping for induction of labour, *Cochrane Database Syst Rev* (1):CD000451, 2005.

Boyd ME, Usher RH, McClean FH, et al: Obstetric consequences of postmaturity, *Am J Obstet Gynecol* 158(2):343–348, 1988.

Bukola F, et al: Unmet need for induction of labor in Africa: secondary analysis from the 2004–2005 WHO Global Maternal and Perinatal Health Survey (a cross-sectional survey), *BMC Public Health* 12:722, 2012.

Care Quality Commission (CQC): *Maternity services survey 2015* (website). www.cqc.org.uk/content/maternity-services-survey-2015. 2015.

Clement D, Schifrin BS, Kates RB: Acute oligohydramnios in postdate pregnancy, *Am J Obstet Gynecol* 157(4 Pt 1):884–886, 1987.

Cromi A, Ghezzi F, Uccella S, et al: A randomized trial of preinduction cervical ripening: dinoprostone vaginal insert versus double-balloon catheter, *Am J Obstet Gynecol* 207:121–125, 2012.

Dodd JM, Crowther CA, Robinson JS: Morning compared with evening induction of labor: a nested randomized controlled trial, *Obstet Gynecol* 108(2):350–360, 2006.

Draper ES, Kenyon S, editors, on behalf of MBRRACE-UK: *EMBRACE-UK perinatal confidential enquiry: term, singleton, normally formed, antepartum stillbirth*, The Infant Mortality and Morbidity Studies, Leicester, Department of Health Sciences, University of Leicester, 2015.

Du C, Liu Y, Liu Y, et al: Double-balloon catheter vs. dinoprostone vaginal insert for induction of labor with an unfavorable cervix, *Arch Gynecol Obstet* 291(6):1221–1227, 2015.

Ehrenthal DB, Jiang X, Strobino DM: Labor induction and the risk of a cesarean delivery among nulliparous women at term, *Obstet Gynecol* 116:35–42, 2010.

Enkin M, Keirse MJNC, Neilson J, et al: *A guide to effective care in pregnancy and childbirth*, 3rd ed, Oxford, Oxford University Press, 2000.

Euro-peristat: European perinatal health report: The health and care of pregnant women and their babies in 2010 (website). www.europeristat.com. 2013.

Evans M: Post dates pregnancy and complementary therapies,

Complement Ther Clin Pract 15(4):220–224, 2009.

Fabre E, Gonzalez de Aguero R, de Augustin JL, et al: Macrosomia: concept and epidemiology. In Kurjak A, editor: *Textbook of perinatal medicine*, vol 2, London, Parthenon, pp 1273–1289, 1998.

Gibb D: Prolonged pregnancy. In Studd J, editor: *The management of labour*, London, Blackwell Scientific, 1985.

Gülmezoglu AM, Crowther CA, Middleton P: Induction of labour for improving birth outcomes for women at or beyond term, *Cochrane Database Syst Rev* (4):CD004945, 2006.

Gülmezoglu AM, Crowther CA, Middleton P, et al: Induction of labour for improving birth outcomes for women at or beyond term, *Cochrane Database Syst Rev* (6):CD004945, 2012.

Health and Social Care Information Centre (HSCIS): *Hospital episode statistics. NHS Maternity Statistics – England 2013–14, V2* (website). www.hscic.gov.uk/catalogue/ PUB16725. 2015.

Ingram J, Domagala C, Yates S: The effects of shiatsu on post-term pregnancy, *Complement Ther Med* 13(1):11–15, 2005.

International Federation of Gynecology and Obstetrics (FIGO): International classification of disease update, *International Journal of Gynecology and Obstetrics* 17:634–640, 1980.

Jonsson M, Cnattingius S, Wikstroem AK: Elective induction of labor and the risk of cesarean section in low-risk parous women: a cohort study, *Acta Obstet Gynecol Scand* 92:198–203, 2013.

Kavanagh J, Kelly AJ, Thomas J: Sexual intercourse for cervical ripening and induction of labour, *Cochrane Database Syst Rev* (2):CD003093, 2001.

Kavanagh J, Kelly AJ, Thomas J: Breast stimulation for cervical ripening and induction of labour, *Cochrane Database Syst Rev* (3):CD003392, 2005.

Knight M, Kenyon S, Brocklehurst P, et al, editors, on behalf of MBRRACE-UK: *Saving lives, improving mothers' care – lessons learned to inform future maternity care from the UK and Ireland. Confidential Enquiries into Maternal Deaths and Morbidity 2009–12*, Oxford, National Perinatal Epidemiology Unit, University of Oxford, 2014.

Knox Ritchie JW: Obstetrics for the neonatologist. In Roberton NRC, editor: *Textbook of neonatology*, 2nd ed, London, Churchill Livingstone, pp 83–119, 1992.

Mitchell MD, Klint APF, Bibby J, et al: Rapid increases in plasma prostaglandin concentrations after vaginal examination and amniotomy, *Br Med J* 2(6096):1183–1185, 1977.

Mongelli M, Wilcox M, Gardosi J: Estimating the date of confinement: ultrasonographic biometry versus certain menstrual dates, *Am J Obstet Gynecol* 174(1):278–281, 1996.

National Institute for Health and Clinical Excellence (NICE): *Induction of labour. CG70*, London, NICE, 2008.

National Institute for Health and Care Excellence (NICE): *Intrapartum care: care of healthy women and their babies during childbirth. CG190*, London, NICE, 2014a.

National Institute for Health and Care Excellence (NICE): Induction of labour. NICE Pathway (website). http://pathways.nice.org.uk/ pathways/induction-of-labour. 2014b.

National Institute for Health and Care Excellence (NICE): *Diabetes in pregnancy: management of diabetes and its complications from preconception to the postnatal period. NG3*, London, NICE, 2015.

O'Brien E, Rauf Z, Alfirevic Z, et al: Women's experiences of outpatient induction of labour with remote continuous monitoring, *Midwifery* 29(4):325–331, 2013.

Olesen AW, Westergaard JG, Olsen J: Perinatal and maternal complications related to post-term delivery: a national register-based study, 1978–1993, *Am J Obstet Gynecol* 189(1):222–227, 2003.

Oster C, Adelso PL, Wilkinson C, et al: Inpatient versus outpatient cervical priming for induction of labour: therapeutic landscapes and women's preferences, *Health Place* 17(1):379–385, 2011.

Pattison N, McCowan L: Cardiotocography for antepartum fetal assessment, *Cochrane Database Syst Rev* (1):CD001068, 1999.

Redshaw M, Rowe R, Hockley C, et al: *Recorded delivery: a national survey of women's experience of maternity care 2006*, Oxford, National Perinatal Epidemiology Unit, University of Oxford, 2007.

Reid M, Norman JE, Bollapragada SS, et al: The home as an appropriate setting for women undertaking cervical ripening before the induction of labour, *Midwifery* 27:30–35, 2011.

Resnik R: Post-term pregnancy. In Creasy RK, Resnik R, editors: *Maternal-fetal medicine: principles and practice*, 3rd edn, London, WB Saunders, pp 521–526, 1994.

Roberts LJ, Young KR: The management of prolonged pregnancy – an analysis of women's attitudes before and after term, *Br J Obstet Gynaecol* 98(11):1102–1106, 1991.

Robson SJ, Laws P, Sullivan EA: Adverse outcomes of labour in public and private hospitals in Australia: a population-based descriptive study, *Med J Aust* 190(9):474–477, 2009.

Royal College of Obstetricians and Gynaecologists (RCOG): *Breech Presentation, Management (Green-top Guideline No. 20b)*, London, RCOG, 2006.

Royal College of Obstetricians and Gynaecologists (RCOG): *Obstetric cholestasis (Green Top Guideline No. 43)*, London, RCOG, 2011.

Royal College of Obstetricians and Gynaecologists (RCOG): *Induction of labour at term in older mothers (Scientific Impact Paper No. 34)*, London, 2013, RCOG.

Santiago MD, Lima Rezende CA, Cabral ACV, et al: Determining the volume of blood required for the correction of fetal anaemia by intrauterine transfusion during pregnancies of Rh isoimmunised women, *Blood Transfus* 8(4), 2010.

Shetty A, Burt R, Rice P, et al: Women's perceptions, expectations and satisfaction with induced labour – a questionnaire based study, *Eur J Obstet Gynecol Reprod Biol* 123:56–61, 2005.

Simpson P, Stanley K: Prolonged pregnancy, *Obstetrics, Gynaecology and Reproductive Medicine* 21(9):257–262, 2011.

Singh D, Newburn M: *Access to maternity information and support*, London, NCT Publications, 2000.

Smith CA, Crowther CA, Collins CT, et al: Acupuncture to induce labour: a randomized controlled trial, *Obstet Gynaecol* 112(5):1067–1074, 2008.

Stock SJ, Ferguson E, Duffy A, et al: Outcomes of elective induction of labour compared with expectant management: population based study, *Br Med J* 344:e2838, 2012.

Tillett J, Ames D: The uses of aromatherapy in women's health, *J Perinat Neonatal Nurs* 24(3):238–245, 2010.

Tiran D: Structural reflex zone therapy in pregnancy and childbirth: a new approach, *Complement Ther Clin Pract* 15(4):234–238, 2009.

Vogel JP, Souza JP, Gulmezoglu AM: Patterns and outcomes of induction of labour in Africa and Asia: a secondary analysis of the WHO Global Survey on Maternal and Neonatal Health, *PLoS One* 8(6):e65612, 2013.

Westfall RE, Benoit C: The rhetoric of 'natural' in natural childbirth: childbearing women's perspectives on prolonged pregnancy and induction of labour, *Soc Sci Med* 59(7):1397–1408, 2004.

Weston M, Grabowska C: Complementary therapy for induction of labour, *Pract Midwife* 16(8):16S–18S, 2013.

Resources and additional reading

Cheyne H, Purva A, Williams B: Elective induction of labour: The problem of interpretation and communication of risks, *Midwifery* 28(4):412–415, 2012.

The European Perinatal Health Report: *Health and care of pregnant women and babies in Europe in 2010* (website). www.europeristat.com/reports/european-perinatal-health-report-2010.html. 2010.

World Health Organization (WHO): *Global survey maternal and perinatal health* (website). www.who.int/reproductivehealth/topics/maternal_perinatal/globalsurvey/en/. 2010.

World Health Organization (WHO): *Recommendations for induction of labour* (website). http://www.ncbi.nlm.nih.gov/books/NBK131963/. 2011.

Useful websites:

NHS Choices: www.nhs.uk/conditions/pregnancy-and-baby/pages/induction-labour.aspx#.

This site offers useful IOL information for women.

Chapter 61

Rhythmic variations of labour

Dr Sarah Church and Tracey Barnfather

Learning Outcomes ?

After reading this chapter, you will be able to:

- recognize altered patterns of uterine action and understand how these patterns may contribute to a prolonged or precipitate labour
- discuss the midwife's role in the prevention, care and management of altered patterns of uterine action
- critically review how promoting normality (regardless of labour pattern) can influence a positive progression/outcome

INTRODUCTION

This chapter explores the issues that surround altered uterine action, including prevention, diagnosis, management and associated problems. To maximize learning, it is anticipated that the reader has a working knowledge of the interrelationship between the physiology and psychology associated with labour and how the midwife can proactively support the woman during normal labour (see Chs 35, 36 and 37).

In normal labour, the uterine contractions become progressively longer and stronger, and they increase in frequency, causing the complete effacement and progressive dilatation of the os uteri in the first stage of labour, steady delivery of the baby in the second stage and expulsion of the placenta and membranes and control of haemorrhage in the third stage (Chs 35, 36 and 37).

Altered uterine action can occur at any stage of labour and is often attributed to an abnormal pattern of uterine contractility, resulting in slow or rapid progress. Vigilant observation and assessment of a woman in labour is therefore paramount in the prevention, detection and diagnosis of altered uterine action. Unfortunately, there is no way to predict the kind of labour progression (in terms

of dilatation and descent) that a given contractile pattern will produce – that is, the quality of contractions can give little information about the course of labour. In this context, the value of antenatal education in preparing the woman and her partner for labour and the possibility of a 'non-perfect' labour is important. Accurate diagnosis of *active* as opposed to *preactive labour* is essential because this directs future decisions and actions (Neal and Lowe 2014). Because abnormal uterine action may be *inefficient* or *overefficient*, a tool often used to assess the progress of labour is the partogram.

The partogram

The partogram is an observation chart that may be used to facilitate assessment of the progress of labour, including maternal and fetal well-being (Ch. 36).

Historically, progress is measured by linear progression along a prescribed time scale, whereby a curve of cervical dilatation is measured in centimetres plotted against time in hours (Friedman 1955) and descent of the head abdominally. Over the years, modifications to the partogram have occurred, resulting in the introduction of *alert* and *action* lines (Fig. 61.1). Once labour is confirmed as being in the active phase, cervical dilatation is expected to progress at less than 2 cm dilatation in 4 hours (National Institute for Health and Care Excellence (NICE) 2014). Some countries, for example, Germany (Petersen et al 2011) and Brazil (de Azevedo Aguiar et al 2013), do not use partograms as a routine procedure. Studies have reported that applying an action line in these practice environments result in an increase of intervention. Conversely, when the World Health Organization (WHO) modified partogram was introduced in India, for example, the findings demonstrated a significant improvement in maternal and fetal well-being (Penumadu and Hariharan 2014). Clearly, this demonstrates that partograms are only a tool, and the progress of labour should not be assessed

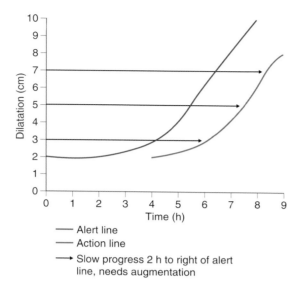

Figure 61.1 Normogram/partogram. (Reproduced from Studd J: Partograms and normograms of cervical dilatation in management of primigravid labour, Br Med J 4(5890):451–455, 1973, with permission from BMJ Publishing Group Ltd.)

upon cervical effacement and dilation alone without the assessment of the descent of the presenting part abdominally and the woman's emotional well-being. A woman's behaviour or the recognition of the 'purple line' (originally described by Hobbs in 1998) can also contribute towards assessment of progress (Shepherd et al 2010). McDonald (2010) advocates not using partograms for 'low-risk' women and emphasizes the importance of listening to the woman. This discussion illustrates that a partogram can be both an aid and a hindrance, and its validity can be questioned. A Cochrane review (Lavender et al 2012) concluded that the evidence did not support the routine use of a partogram. The review stated that the challenge would be removing a document that has informed clinical practice for over 70 years and concluded that use of a partogram is left to the discretion of local policy.

Reflective activity 61.1   ✕❮

Access five partograms from archived records of women whom you have cared for. Using the NICE guidance, conduct an audit of your records.

Write a short reflective piece for your professional portfolio and identify how this evidence could support your Nursing and Midwifery Council (NMC) 2015a revalidation and/or your professional portfolio.

PROLONGED LABOUR

Predominately, the diagnosis is the length of active labour, which is dependent on the actual time at which labour is presumed to have begun; therefore, accurate history is essential because it is recognized that if admitted to a birthing room in the latent phase, this may prevent the woman from following her own labour pattern and increase the rate of intervention and iatrogenic injury (Chuma et al 2014).

Prolonged labour is described as a clinical presentation of labour that has exceeded the expected time limits. This is the result of an alteration in uterine contractility that is considered to interfere with the normal progress of labour. Delay is confirmed when the progress of active labour falls into the action lines on a partogram. The NICE guidance for intrapartum care was reviewed in 2014. Although recommendations for prolonged labour have remained unchanged, they do suggest that parity and the woman's emotional state should be taken into consideration along with uterine activity, effacement and dilatation of the cervix, lack of descent or rotation and the position of the presenting part.

Maternal fatigue directly influences uterine efficiency; therefore, compassionate care supported by nutrition is key to preventing this from occurring. There is an increase of prolonged labour with nulliparous women because the birth of the first child alters the birth canal; therefore, subsequent deliveries are usually easier. Furthermore, if the previous delivery was normal, the mother has the benefits of experience and belief in herself.

Considering the debate, it is clear the midwife must be skilled in assessing physical and psychological well-being; however, the midwife must also be mindful of cultural influences. For example, in a study conducted in Pakistan, women reported the belief that if a labour is prolonged, it is attributable to the will of Allah, and therefore they accept this as the norm (Chesney and Davies 2005). Clearly, this could have implications if intervention is believed to be warranted for maternal and fetal well-being. In Palestine, primigravidas are viewed as 'high risk', regardless of their medical and social background (Hassan et al 2013); therefore, education and guidance for women and healthcare workers who migrate to the UK could make a positive difference in these women's expectations and birth experience.

Causes of prolonged labour

- Inefficient uterine action
- Cephalopelvic disproportion
- Occipitoposterior position
- Asynclitism

- Malpresentation of the fetus
- Macrosomia
- Cervical resistance, dystocia or previous surgery
- Maternal obesity
- Maternal mental well-being influenced by place of birth, those present
- Victims of rape; cognitive experience that may result in a prolonged second stage (Nerum et al 2009)

The provision of appropriate midwifery care is crucial to the early diagnosis of underlying problems, which, if undetected, may create potential hazards to the mother and fetus. Midwifery care should be focused on the following areas:

- *Prevention of maternal dehydration* to prevent ketosis and excessive tiredness (Hall Moran and Dykes 2006).
- *Regular emptying of bladder and/or rectum.* A full bladder and/or rectum can impede progress by delaying descent and cause potential damage to maternal structures.
- *Maternal position* to maximize gravity and increase the woman's comfort can make a positive difference to uterine activity and fetal well-being (Gizzo et al 2014).

Potential risks to the mother

- Risk of intra-uterine infection
- An obstructed labour
- Ruptured uterus
- Increased risk of operative intervention, anaesthesia and postpartum haemorrhage
- Psychological trauma caused by the cumulative effects of feeling loss of control and increased intervention
- Nulliparous women have a seven-fold increase of levator ani avulsion – disconnection of the insertion of the muscle to the inferior pubic ramus and/or pelvic side wall, causing urinary incontinence (Gartland et al 2012).

Whatever the outcome, if a prolonged birth occurs, it is important that women understand why and feel that they are part of the decision-making process (Elmir et al 2010) because it can have lifelong implications for the woman (Nystedt and Hildingsson 2014).

Risks to the fetus

Prolonged labour is associated with fetal acidosis, intra-uterine hypoxia and infection (Chs 46 and 48). Other risks are those associated with assisted birth and the mother's birth experience because this may negatively affect their relationship (Nystedt and Hildingsson 2014).

Principles of midwifery management

With careful and vigilant care and attention, the midwife should be alerted to the development of a prolonged labour and, therefore, be in a position to support the woman with any subsequent action necessary. The following points are particularly relevant:

- Careful assessment of the woman's physical and psychological condition should be undertaken throughout labour, reporting (and recording) any deviations from normal to an obstetrician (NMC 2012).
- Continuous fetal heart monitoring may be required if oxytocin is used (NICE 2014); however, where only an amniotomy has been performed, intermittent auscultation may be appropriate to encourage the woman to remain mobile.
- Continuous one-to-one support for the woman and her partner is crucial to facilitate high-quality care (NICE 2015), in which assessment of progress, provision of good communication and informed consent can be enhanced.
- Midwives should provide supportive and compassionate care for women and their partners/supporters during labour, addressing their emotional needs and displaying an empathetic and caring attitude.
- The provision of adequate and appropriate pain relief should be discussed with the woman and her partner; this is a key aspect of the midwife's role. Non-pharmacological approaches may incorporate the use of coping strategies, including breathing and relaxation. Women should be encouraged and supported to adopt different positions and use water when appropriate (Harper 2014).
- Preventing maternal fatigue and encouraging women to eat and drink limits the effect of starvation (Singata et al 2013) and avoids the use of medical intervention to treat nonexistent dystocia.
- Providing emotional support may limit maternal anxiety; it is known that high levels of anxiety interfere with normal uterine activity (Lowe 2007).
- The midwife should act as an advocate for the woman as required and work collaboratively with members of the multidisciplinary team (NMC 2015b).

Principles of the active management of labour

A package of care intervention referred to as the *Active Management of Labour* (AML) was introduced by O'Driscoll in 1968 as a means to promote the continuance of regular effective contractions. AML has the following components: one-to-one continuous support; strict definition of established labour; early routine amniotomy; vaginal examination every 2 hours; use of oxytocin if labour is slow in nulliparous women with singleton pregnancies at term, with the aim of shortening labour and reducing the rate of caesarean section (O'Driscoll et al 2003). Although some studies have attempted to evaluate these combined interventions (Brown et al 2008), the evidence reviewed does not indicate that the caesarean section rate is reduced. For this reason, the NICE *Intrapartum Care* guidelines (NICE 2014) discourage routine use of the active management just described, instead offering a more measured approach to relevant interventions that include amniotomy and use of oxytocin.

Amniotomy

Amniotomy is a procedure in which the amniotic membranes are ruptured artificially. Although amniotomy is considered a common procedure in accelerating labour, it is important to remember that amniotomy is not a part of physiological labour (Royal College of Midwives (RCM) 2012). In a recent systematic review of 15 studies involving a total of 5583 women, Smyth et al (2013) concluded that the use of amniotomy did not shorten the length of the first stage of labour, and their findings suggested a possible increase in the rate of caesarean section. This calls into question the belief that rupturing the amniotic membranes accelerates labour. On this basis, the possible impact of this procedure on the nature, experience and efficiency of uterine contractions remains unclear, and as a result, NICE (2014) suggests that amniotomy should not be routinely performed in labour where labour is progressing normally. Where a delay in established labour for women with intact membranes occurs, the evidence suggests that an amniotomy followed by a vaginal examination 2 hours later should be considered (NICE 2014).

Although Smyth et al (2013) note that none of the studies reviewed evaluated whether the use of amniotomy increased women's pain in labour, recent NICE guidance (NICE 2014) suggests that women are advised that labour may be shortened by an hour and that contractions may become stronger and more painful. Midwives should discuss this with the women so that they can make informed decisions and maintain control of their labour; otherwise, the increase in the intensity of pain may be difficult to cope with, leading to feelings of failure, lower levels of satisfaction and decrease in self-efficacy (Quartana et al 2009). Accurate assessment of established labour and justification for performing amniotomy must be carefully addressed and documented.

In situations where there is a concern about fetal wellbeing, performing an amniotomy may be considered necessary to assess the colour of the amniotic fluid and the possible application of a fetal scalp electrode for the continuous monitoring of fetal well-being. Where there is no concern about fetal well-being, there are benefits of maintaining intact membranes: the maintenance of an even hydrostatic pressure to the whole fetal surface during labour causes a reduced likelihood of infection and fetal hypoxia.

Augmentation with oxytocin

A synthetic form of the hormone oxytocin known as Syntocinon has been used for many years for the augmentation of labour where a delay in progress has been determined by an obstetrician. Before this decision is made, a full assessment of the labour must be undertaken and documented. An assessment of cervical dilatation, descent and rotation of the occiput and changes in the strength, duration and frequency of uterine contractions should be undertaken (NICE 2014).

In a systematic review (Bugg et al 2011) of eight trials involving 1338 low-risk women in studies where oxytocin, no treatment or delayed treatment for slow progress in labour were assessed, it was found that although the use of oxytocin showed a shortening of labour by 2 hours, there was no difference in the rate of caesarean section. When augmentation with oxytocin is required, vigilant midwifery care is essential. The physiological effect of contractions is well tolerated by the healthy fetus at term; however, the administration of an oxytocin infusion may lead to the development of uterine hyperstimulation, resulting in fetal compromise (Simpson and James 2008; WHO 2014). Although it is rare for a primigravid uterus to rupture, in a multigravida, oxytocin should be used with extreme caution after obstructed labour has been excluded. In these situations, a multidisciplinary approach to care is required. Jonsson et al (2007) in a study of disciplinary actions in obstetric malpractice noted that injudicious use of oxytocin was common and a primary reason for disciplinary action in 33% of the cases.

Use of oxytocin

- It is essential that a full discussion of the need for oxytocin is undertaken with the woman and her partner and that informed consent is obtained.

- The woman and her partner will be informed that the frequency and strength of contractions will increase, and for this reason, it may be appropriate to arrange an epidural (if appropriate) before the oxytocin infusion is commenced (NICE 2014).

- Oxytocin should be prescribed by an obstetrician (who has undertaken a full assessment) and administered intravenously using an infusion pump that is titrated according to local policies.

- The midwife needs to follow local drug administration policies in the preparation of the oxytocin infusion; the midwife must place a completed sticker on the infusion bag and in the woman's notes. It will be prescribed on the woman's prescription chart and on an intravenous infusion chart. NICE (2014) recommends that the oxytocin infusion should be increased every 30 minutes, until uterine contractions at the rate of 4 to 5 every 10 minutes can be palpated.

- A management plan and the timing of next assessment will be written clearly in the woman's notes. The midwife should monitor blood pressure and pulse every hour or as directed in the management plan. Input and output should be assessed every 4 hours.

- Continuous electronic fetal monitoring (EFM) will be used to monitor fetal well-being.

- The midwife carefully observes uterine action by palpation of the abdomen and by observing the woman's response to contractions. The midwife should not rely on the visual representation of uterine contractions on the cardiotocograph strip as evidence of efficient uterine activity. The midwife should ensure that the uterus relaxes adequately between contractions and that there are no signs of hyperstimulation or fetal distress.

- If uterine hyperstimulation or fetal distress occurs, the oxytocin infusion must be turned off immediately and the obstetrician informed (NMC 2012). The woman should be encouraged to adopt the left lateral position, with vigilant observation of the fetal heart rate. Maternal facial oxygen is not recommended as part of fetal resuscitation because hyperoxia in the mother can cause hypoxia in the fetus (NICE 2014).

- If women develop any additional risk factors that increase the possibility of caesarean section, or have received opioids, then a histamine (H_2) receptor antagonist or antacid should be administered.

- After delivery, the infusion should not be stopped abruptly but reduced gradually based on the woman's condition to reduce the risk of postpartum haemorrhage; specifically, the contractile state of the uterus and the blood loss must be assessed and documented.

Table 61.1 Causes of prolonged second stage of labour

Causes	
Maternal	**Fetal**
• Inefficient uterine action • Maternal obesity • Full bladder or rectum • Rigid perineum • A contracted pelvic outlet	• Persistent occipitoposterior position • Deep transverse arrest • Malpresentations • Fetal macrosomia • Fetal abnormality

Management of a prolonged second stage of labour

It is important to consider that prolonged labour can occur at any stage, and the progress of the first stage may influence the management of the second and third stages (see Table 61.1). Historically, time limits have been imposed on the length of the second stage: current NICE guidance (2014) defines delay in the *active second stage* as 2 hours for nulliparous women and 1 hour for multiparous women. The midwife must be confident of accurate assessment of the active and passive phases of labour to prevent unnecessary intervention. Throughout, the midwife must remain vigilant and assess each woman on an individual basis. If maternal and/or fetal observations occur outside the normal ranges, then relevant referral is required.

If progress is slow, adoption of an upright maternal position is believed to enhance direct pressure of the presenting part against the posterior wall of the vagina that stimulates the release of oxytocin (*Ferguson's reflex;* see Ch. 37) and thereby enhances the urge to bear down. In a nulliparous woman, if there is no progress after an hour of active second stage, she should be offered an amniotomy if the membranes are intact; the same plan of action applies for multiparous women, but after 30 minutes (NICE 2014). Once delay is confirmed, the woman should be reviewed by an obstetrician, and a plan of care should be agreed on with the woman.

Management of a prolonged third stage of labour

A diagnosis of 'prolonged' third stage of labour is defined in minutes depending on management approach: 60 if passive and 30 if active (NICE 2014). If problems have occurred during the labour, active management of the third stage is recommended because of the associated risks (e.g. atonic uterus). Women at greater risk of complications of prolonged third stage are those who have had inadequate contractions earlier in this labour, developed a constriction ring, have a full bladder or have a morbidly adhered placenta.

In addition to active management of the third stage of labour with oxytocic drugs, heightened vigilance is essential (observing for signs of shock and/or haemorrhage); the midwife must ensure the bladder is empty and avoid 'fiddling' with the uterus. Encouraging adoption of an upright maternal position maximizes any benefit from gravity. Promoting skin-to-skin contact between mother and infant may stimulate the uterus to contract by the release of oxytocin (Saxton et al 2014). In some instances, oxytocin may have to be administered intravenously by infusion, such as in cases where contractions are inadequate or absent or the previous management has failed.

The psychological aspects of prolonged labour

The psychological and emotional needs of women who experience a prolonged or augmented labour focus on the intensity of pain experienced (Nystedt et al 2006). Often this results in the woman feeling out of control, accompanied by fear and a sense of vulnerability (Johnson and Slade 2003). With increased intervention and the knowledge of an associated risk of an emergency caesarean section or instrumental delivery, women are more likely to appraise their birth experience negatively. The midwife should provide clear communication as part of one-to-one support in labour to allay unnecessary anxiety and enhance the women's understanding of proposed intervention, thereby supporting informed decisions.

It is important that women have an opportunity to discuss their labour experience with midwives at a suitable time in which the events of labour can be discussed and rationalized. A detailed assessment of a woman's physical and emotional state and social situation should take place before the woman returns home; this facilitates postnatal health and well-being. Appropriate help and support should be put in place to facilitate her physical recovery and her transition to motherhood; experience of a prolonged labour is considered comparable to those recovering from an acute or sudden illness (Nystedt et al 2008). This may be a useful opportunity to identify women who may need more specialized counselling to which the midwife can refer.

OVEREFFICIENT UTERINE ACTION (PRECIPITATE LABOUR)

A precipitous labour is usually defined as a rapid labour where labour and delivery occur within 2 hours. The first stage of labour may occur almost without pain, and only when the vertex is about to be born does the woman become aware of it. Alternatively, contractions may feel almost continuous, accompanied by intense pain. The labour is associated with placental abruption, lacerations of the cervix and perineum and an increased risk of post-partum haemorrhage and retained placenta. Fetal complications include hypoxia as a result of intense and frequent contractions, and intracranial haemorrhage may occur as a result of rapid descent through the birth canal. Other dangers include injuries sustained as a result of being delivered in an unsuitable place or falling to the ground. Although there is limited data available, it is more common in multiparous woman and may be aided by a minimal resistance of the maternal soft tissues.

If the woman has a history of precipitate birth, it is important that the midwife discusses the potential reoccurrence with her and offers her information and support. A delivery pack needs to be provided for the home, and midwives within the practice area should be made aware of her history and address. In the event of a rapid onset of contractions, the woman is advised to call for medical assistance and to lie on her side in a safe place to reduce the urge to push, thus aiming to reduce maternal and neonatal trauma from a rapid delivery.

TONIC UTERINE ACTION

Definition

Tonic uterine action is a state of *hypertonicity* in which the uterus maintains a contraction lasting more than 2 minutes. It is a rare condition in which the uterus increases powerful contractions to overcome an obstruction. It is synonymous with severe acute pain accompanied by rapid deterioration in maternal condition, prolonged cord compression and placental abruption resulting in intra-uterine death as a result of the cessation of oxygen delivery to the fetus.

Midwifery management

The midwife's role is to summon emergency medical and midwifery aid to resuscitate the mother because immediate delivery is required to prevent a ruptured uterus. The management usually includes birth by caesarean section. Caution must be taken not to confuse tonic uterine action with *tetanic uterine action*, which occurs as a result of uterine hyperstimulation, usually caused by the incautious use of oxytocics. If oxytocin is being administered intravenously, the infusion must be stopped immediately. Encourage the woman to adopt the left lateral position to enhance uteroplacental blood flow, and inform the obstetrician.

CERVICAL DYSTOCIA

In cervical dystocia, the uterus contracts normally, but the cervix fails to dilate. Its occurrence is rare, but diagnosis is important to prevent maternal and fetal distress. The cervix might efface but fails to dilate; the woman may present with a history of cervical surgery or congenital abnormality of the cervix. It is important that this condition is excluded before the use of oxytocin because of the associated risk of uterine rupture. Vaginal delivery is therefore impossible, and a caesarean section is performed.

CONCLUSION

Good midwifery care, including the accurate diagnosis of established labour, maintenance of a positive care environment and prevention of maternal dehydration and fatigue, may prevent the development of prolonged labour and will certainly aid fast diagnosis and management. Promoting self-efficacy is essential, supported by good communication skills and an empathetic, compassionate approach to care. However, if prolonged labour occurs, the midwife needs to remember the importance of vigilance and accurate record keeping. Working in partnership with the woman and liaising with relevant healthcare professionals is crucial.

Sensitive and empathetic midwifery care is essential to support women experiencing precipitate delivery and in the careful planning of future births. In either situation, the midwife should recognize the potential need for an opportunity for the woman to discuss her labour experiences.

Key Points ⚷

- An accurate assessment of the onset of labour should be made to minimize the introduction of unnecessary interventions.
- Collaboration and cooperation between the woman, midwife and obstetrician are essential.
- The midwife must remain vigilant throughout labour and recognize that prolonged labour can occur at any stage of labour.

References

Brown HC, Paranjothy S, Dowswell T, et al: Package of care for active management in labour for reducing caesarean section rates in low-risk women, *Cochrane Database Syst Rev* (4):CD004907, 2008.

Bugg GJ, Siddiqui F, Thornton JG: Oxytocin versus no treatment or delayed treatment for slow progress in the first stage of spontaneous labour, *Cochrane Database Syst Rev* (7):CD007123, 2011.

Chesney M, Davies S: Women's birth experiences in Pakistan—the importance of the Dai, *Evidence-Based Midwifery* 3(1):26–32, 2005.

Chuma C, Kihunrwa A, Matovelo D, et al: Labour management and obstetric outcomes among pregnant women admitted in latent phase compared to active phase of labour at Bugando Medical Centre in Tanzania, *BMC Pregnancy Childbirth* 14:84, 2014.

de Azevedo Aguiar C, Gonvalves R, d'Andretta Tanaka A: Use of the partogram in labor: analysis of its application in different care models, *Open J Obstet Gynecol* 3(9A):1–8, 2013.

Elmir R, Schmeid V, Wilkes L, et al: Women's perceptions and experiences of a traumatic birth: a meta-ethnography, *J Adv Nurs* 66(10):2142–2153, 2010.

Friedman EA: Primigravid labor – a graphicostatistical analysis, *Obstet Gynecol* 6:567–589, 1955.

Gartland D, Donath S, Macarthur C, et al: The onset, recurrence and associated obstetric risk factors for urinary incontinence in the first 18 months after a first birth: an Australian nulliparous cohort study, *Br J Obstet Gynaecol* 119:1361–1369, 2012.

Gizzo S, Di Gangi S, Novena N, et al: Women's choice of positions during labour: return to the past of a modern way to give birth? A cohort study in Italy, *Biomed Res Int* doi: 10.1155/2014/638093, 2014.

Hall Moran V, Dykes F: *Maternal and infant nutrition and nurture: controversies and challenges*, London, Quay, 2006.

Harper B: Birth, bath, and beyond: the science and safety of water immersion during labor and birth, *J Perinat Educ* 23(3):124–134, 2014.

Hassan SJ, Sundby J, Husseini A, et al: Translating evidence into practice in childbirth: a case from the Occupied Palestinian Territory, *Women and Birth* 26(2):e82–e89, doi: 10.1016/j.wombi.2012.12.002, 2013.

Hobbs L: Assessing cervical dilatation without VEs. Watching the purple line, *Pract Midwife* 1(11):34–35, 1998.

Johnson RC, Slade P: Obstetric complications and anxiety during pregnancy: is there a relationship? *J Psychosom Obstet Gynaecol* 24:1–14, 2003.

Jonsson M, Nordens SL, Hanson U: Analysis of malpractice claims with a focus on oxytocin use in labour, *Acta Obstet Gynecol Scand* 86(3):315–319, 2007.

Lavender T, Hart A, Smyth R: Effect of partogram use on outcomes for women in spontaneous labour at term, *Cochrane Database Syst Rev* (8):CD005461, 2012.

Lowe N: A review of factors associated with dystocia and caesarean section in nulliparous women, *J Midwifery Womens Health* 52:216–228, 2007.

McDonald G: Diagnosing the latent phase of labour: use of the partogram, *Br J Midwifery* 18(10):630–637, 2010.

National Institute for Health and Care Excellence (NICE): *Intrapartum care. NICE Guideline CG190*, London, NICE, 2014.

National Institute for Health and Care Excellence (NICE): *Safe midwifery staffing for maternity settings. NG4*, London, NICE, 2015.

Neal J, Lowe N: Outcomes of nulliparous women with spontaneous labor onset admitted to hospitals in preactive versus active labor, *J Midwifery Womens Health* 59(1):28–33, 2014.

Nerum H, Halvorsen L, Øian P, et al: Birth outcomes in primiparous women who were raped as adults: a matched controlled study, *Br J Obstet Gynaecol* 117(3), 2009.

Nursing and Midwifery Council (NMC): *Midwives rules and standards*, London, NMC, 2012.

Nursing and Midwifery Council (NMC): *How to revalidate with the NMC. Requirements for renewing your registration and demonstrating your continuing fitness to practise* (website).

www.nmc.org.uk/globalassets/sitedocuments/revalidation/how-to-revalidate-final-draft.pdf. 2015a.

Nursing and Midwifery Council (NMC): *The Code: professional standards of practice and behaviour for nurses and midwives* (website). www.nmc.org.uk/globalassets/sitedocuments/nmc-publications/revised-new-nmc-code.pdf. 2015b.

Nystedt A, Hildingsson I: Diverse definitions of prolonged labour and its consequences with sometimes subsequent inappropriate treatment, *BMC Pregnancy Childbirth* 14(233), 2014.

Nystedt A, Högberg U, Lundman B: Some Swedish women's experiences of prolonged labour, *Midwifery* 22:56–65, 2006.

Nystedt A, Högberg U, Lundman B: Women's experiences of becoming a mother after prolonged labour, *J Adv Nurs* 63(3):250–258, 2008.

O'Driscoll K, Meagher D, Robson M: *Active management of labour*, 4th edn, London, Mosby, 2003.

Penumadu K, Hariharan C: Role of partogram in the management of spontaneous labour in primigravida and multigravida, *Int J Reprod Contracept Obstet Gynecol* 3(4):1043–1049, 2014.

Petersen A, Ayerle G, Fromke C, et al: The timing of interventions during labour: descriptive results of a longitudinal study, *Midwifery* 27(6):e267–e273, 2011.

Quartana PJ, Campbell CM, Edwards PR: Pain catastrophizing: a critical review, *Expert Rev Neurother* 9(5):745–758, 2009.

Royal College of Midwives (RCM): *Evidence-based guidelines for midwifery-led care in labour*, London, RCM, 2012.

Saxton A, Fahy K, Hastie C: Effects of skin-to-skin contact and breastfeeding on the incidence of PPH: a physiologically based theory, *Women and Birth* 27(4):250–253, 2014.

Shepherd A, Cheyne H, Kennedy S, et al: The purple line as a measure of labour progress: a longitudinal study, *BMC Pregnancy Childbirth* 10:54, 2010.

Simpson KR, James DC: Effects of oxytocin-induced uterine hyperstimulation during labor on fetal oxygen status and fetal heart rate patterns, *Am J Obstet Gynecol* 199:34.e1–34.e5, 2008.

Singata M, Tranmer J, Gyte GML: Restricting oral fluid and food intake during labour, *Cochrane Database Syst Rev* (8):CD003930, 2013.

Smyth RMD, Markham C, Dowswell T: Amniotomy for shortening spontaneous labour, *Cochrane Database Syst Rev* (6):CD006167, 2013.

World Health Organization (WHO): *WHO recommendations for augmentation of labour*, Geneva, WHO, 2014.

Resources and Additional Reading

Ängeby K, Wilde-Larsson B, Hildingsson I, et al: Primiparous women's preferences for care during a prolonged latent phase of labour, *Sex Reprod Healthc* 6(3):145–150, 2015.

Kither A: Samangaya: abnormal labour, *Obstet Gynaecol Reprod Med* 23(4):121–125, 2013.

Lavender T, Hart A, Smyth RMD: Effect of partogram use on outcomes for women in spontaneous labour at term, *Cochrane Database Syst Rev* (7):CD005461, 2013.

Magowan B, Owen P, Thompson A: *Clinical obstetrics and gynaecology*, 3rd edn, London, Saunders, 2014.

Useful websites:

Western Australia Department of Health – intrapartum care guidelines: www.kemh.health.wa.gov.au/

development/manuals/O&G_guidelines/sectionb/5/b5.8.2.pdf.

WHO Reproductive Health Library – effect of partogram use on outcomes for women in spontaneous labour: http://apps.who.int/rhl/pregnancy_childbirth/childbirth/routine_care/cd005461/en/.

Chapter 62

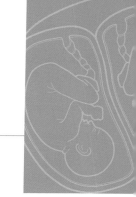

Malpositions and malpresentations

Terri Coates

INTRODUCTION

This chapter considers the recognition, management and care of the mother and fetus when the presentation is an occipitoposterior (OP) position, breech, face or brow and when an oblique or transverse lie results in a shoulder presentation. Compound presentation is also discussed.

Malposition and malpresentations of the fetus can occur in both pregnancy and labour. The midwife has a key role in identifying these, using best evidence to inform and support the mother and using effective skills to undertake safe management and care. With associated higher rates of maternal and perinatal morbidity and mortality, it is essential that careful attention is given to the diagnosis of malposition and malpresentations to maximize good fetal outcomes (Akmal and Patterson Brown 2009; Gardberg et al 2011; Simkin 2010).

Although primarily a practitioner of the 'normal', the midwife must be fully conversant with the problems and practicalities that both malposition and malpresentations can present. In such circumstances, skills are often tested to the limit, and the midwife's ability to gain the confidence of the woman and to work effectively and cooperatively with the wider healthcare team is paramount in achieving a safe and successful outcome for both mother and baby. In dealing with malpositions and malpresentations of the fetus, the midwife needs to be knowledgeable about the latest evidence or lack of it. Time should be taken to help to inform the woman regarding decisions in relation to her care and provide her with the options available (Evans 2007; Munro and Jokinen 2012; Nursing and Midwifery Council (NMC) 2015).

In spite of the evidence, some women may choose a path, for personal, cultural or religious reasons, that is not in keeping with the recommended evidence or accepted institutional practices. Nevertheless, it is a woman's right to choose for herself, and the midwife needs to ensure that in such circumstances, the woman continues to receive the relevant information, advice and support necessary. In achieving this, the midwife should consult with her supervisor of midwives and, with the woman's permission, share the proposed plan of care with her and the lead obstetrician (NMC 2015). All discussions with the woman must be clearly documented in her maternity notes and accurately reflect the advice given, the options available and choices she has made and any further plans.

IDENTIFYING MALPOSITIONS AND MALPRESENTATIONS OF THE FETUS

Midwives must be able to employ a range of skills to assist them in identifying the fetus in malpositions and malpresentations, which include the following:

Malpositions

- A position other than occipitoanterior in a fetus with a vertex presentation.

Malpresentations (any presentation other than vertex)

- Face
- Brow
- Breech presentation
- Shoulder presentation/oblique lie

INCIDENCE

The incidence of malpositions and malpresentations varies according to gestation and parity and the condition of the mother and fetus. The midwife needs to consider the likelihood and the reasons why these presentations might occur as part of the assessment, diagnosis and plan of the woman's care.

A malposition is the commonest cause of non-engagement of the fetal head at term in a primigravida; it is also the commonest cause of prolonged labour and mechanical difficulties associated with the birth. Women should be reassured that more than 76% of the OP labours end in a spontaneous birth of the baby (Desbriere et al 2013).

CLINICAL ASSESSMENT

In identifying malpositions or malpresentations, the midwife should take into account the gestational age of the fetus, the woman's parity, and any history that might suggest the likelihood of such anomalies or abnormalities. The clinical skills of abdominal and vaginal assessment that the midwife may perform as part of a woman's antenatal and intrapartum care are central to the recognition of the presentation, engagement, attitude, lie and position of the fetus.

Underlying this is the need to be fully conversant with the anatomy of the maternal pelvis, the engaging diameter of the fetal presentations and subsequent implications for the process of birth.

Above all, the midwife must be able to draw the findings together and make a diagnosis upon which discussions with the woman and clinical decisions will be based.

Failure to identify the position of the fetus with accuracy will affect the ability of the midwife to offer appropriate advice and care. Ultrasound is now advised as the most reliable method of confirming fetal position (Peregrine et al 2007; Munro and Jokinen 2012).

Reflective activity 62.1

Using a doll and pelvis model, check your knowledge of the anatomy of the pelvis and the fetal skull and normal mechanisms of labour (see Chs 36 and 37).

MALPOSITION OF THE OCCIPUT

The fetus is in an occipitoposterior position (OPP) when the fetal occiput lies adjacent to the sacroiliac joint and occupies either the left or right posterior quadrants of the mother's pelvis with the brow directed anteriorly.

Occipitoposterior positions occur in approximately 10% to 25% of pregnancies during the early stage of labour and in 10% to 15% during the active phase, most of which end normally (Gardberg and Tuppurainen 1994a; Desbriere et al 2013).

Causes of OPP include the following:

- *Android pelvis:* The narrow forepelvis forces the fetal head to adjust and take up a posterior position to enter the pelvic brim.
- *Anthropoid pelvis* may also lead to a persistent OPP.
- *Pendulous abdomen or a flat sacrum*
- *Anterior placenta* is also associated with an OPP towards term (Gardberg and Tuppurainen 1994b).
- *High maternal body mass index (BMI)* has been associated with (Desbriere et al 2013), although this should be confirmed by other studies
- *Malrotation from an occipitoanterior position:* Malrotation to an OPP can occur in up to two-thirds of those who go on to deliver as OPP (Gardberg et al 1998; Peregrine et al 2007).

Fetal positioning

There has been much interest in various methods of fetal positioning the last few years within the midwifery community. It is believed by some that a modern lifestyle of less physical activity and poor posture may have increased the risk of OPP and that changes in maternal position or movements can persuade the fetus to change position in pregnancy or during labour. Midwives need to consider that maternal positioning has been unsupported by reliable research and relies upon personal beliefs and empirical practice (Stremler et al 2005; Hunter et al 2007; Simkin 2010; Desbriere et al 2013).

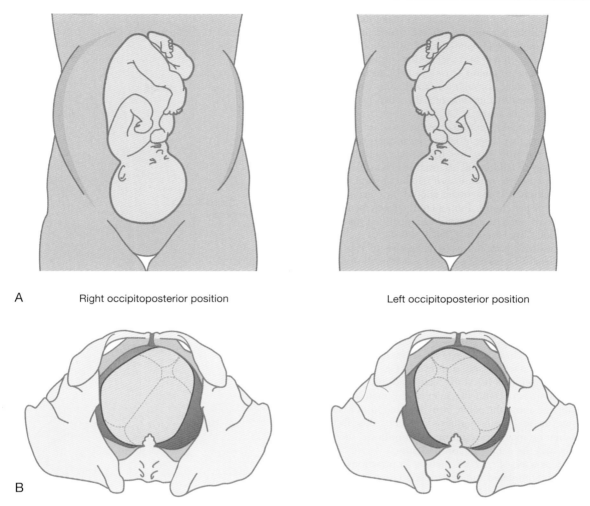

A   Right occipitoposterior position   Left occipitoposterior position

B

Figure 62.1 Occipitoposterior positions. **A,** Abdominal findings – the anterior shoulders are well out from the midline, or fetal limbs are easily palpable. This may cause a misdiagnosis of multiple pregnancy. **B,** Vaginal findings – on vaginal examination, the anterior fontanelle is easily felt and recognized by its shape and size.

The practices are not in themselves harmful; if women find the positions comfortable during pregnancy or as part of an active labour, then they should not be discouraged. However, some midwives have reported discontinued use of these approaches because of concerns about women experiencing anxiety and voicing feelings of failure if rotation of their baby did not occur (Walmsley 2000).

Occipitoposterior positions (Fig. 62.1) place a heavy responsibility on the midwife. Where the labour is progressing satisfactorily, the outcome is likely to be spontaneous rotation to an anterior position followed by a normal vertex delivery, although the labour may be long and tiring. In caring for a woman in prolonged labour, the midwife has the exacting task of maintaining a close watch on the progress she is making, attending to her physical care and providing the encouragement, reassurance and emotional support that the woman needs.

Although malpositions can and do resolve, the midwife should be aware of the potential for delay and the possibility adverse outcomes that may arise when the labour is prolonged or slow or OPP persists. Midwives must be alert to the possibility of abnormal labour, and they must be vigilant to recognize any complications promptly and call for appropriate assistance.

Kind, supportive midwifery care will take into account all of the mother's requirements and maintain a positive attitude throughout a potentially difficult labour. Comfort measures, breathing and relaxation techniques and encouragement to remain active can help. As the levels of discomfort change throughout labour, the woman may choose a variety of methods of pain relief. (Methods of pain relief are discussed in Ch. 38.)

Having a spinal or epidural analgesia is not associated with a longer first stage of labour or an increased chance of a caesarean birth. However, it is associated with a longer second stage of labour and an increased chance of vaginal instrumental birth, regardless of whether or not the fetus is malpositioned. The woman should have access to the analgesia of her choice, and an epidural may be required in the latent phase if pain is severe (National Institute of Health and Care Excellence (NICE) 2014).

The midwife also needs to be aware of the altered mechanism of a fetus in a posterior position, during which the fetus tends to be in a deflexed attitude, with the anterior fontanelle immediately over the internal cervical os. The fetal spine is towards the forward curve of the maternal lumbar spine so that the fetus finds it difficult or impossible to adopt a flexed position. As the fetal spine straightens, the fetus tends to 'square' the shoulders and raise the chin from the chest, resulting in a deflexed, erect 'military' attitude of the fetal head, as shown in Fig. 62.2.

Such movements bring the fetal head into a more difficult relationship with the inlet of the maternal pelvis. Misaligned above the pelvic brim, the fetal head is slow to engage as its larger diameters present. This ill-fitting presentation may also result in early rupture of the membranes and the danger of cord prolapse.

There is a *loss of fetal axis pressure*, contractions are not effectively stimulated and descent is delayed. This can lead to slow, uneven cervical dilatation and prolonged labour. In the process of birth, the engaging diameter of the fetal head is reduced, with that at right angles being elongated. In an occipitoposterior position, the fetal head is compressed in unfavourable diameters, resulting in 'sugar loaf' moulding, creating a greater risk of damage to the tentorium cerebelli and the likelihood of intracranial haemorrhage (see Ch. 30). With a persistent occipitoposterior position, these wider diameters may also result in increased trauma to the woman's vagina and perineum.

Diagnosis of the occipitoposterior position

During pregnancy

The diagnosis is often made by abdominal examination using Leopold manoeuvres (see resources list and chapter website). On inspection, the abdomen appears flattened, or slightly depressed, below the umbilicus (see Fig. 62.3).

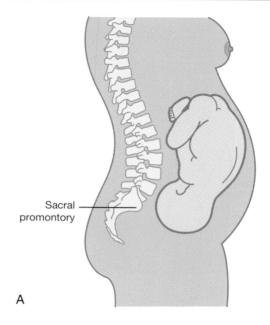

Sacral promontory

A

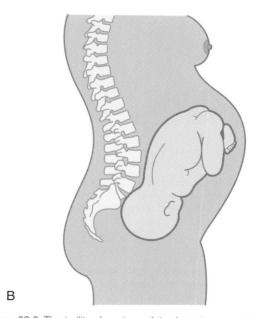

B

Figure 62.2 The 'military' posture of the fetus in an occipitoposterior position. **A,** Well-flexed fetus. **B,** OP position. Deflexed with straight spine and wider engaging diameter.

These observations rely upon the woman being relatively lean and the volume of liquor being normal. On palpation, the fetal head is commonly high. If the fetus is almost occipitolateral, the deflexed head may feel large because the occipitofrontal diameter is palpated.

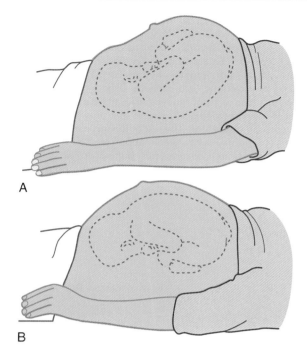

Figure 62.3 Abdominal contour when the fetus is in the occipitoposterior position **(A)**, compared with the more rounded contour of the occipitoanterior position **(B)**.

The occiput and brow may be felt at the same level at the pelvic inlet, whereas the fetal back can be palpated out in the flank. If the occiput is markedly posterior, the high head feels small as the bitemporal diameter is palpated; movements of the fetal limbs can often be seen or easily felt, and it may be impossible to feel the back (see Fig. 62.1). The fetal heart sounds can be heard in the midline just below the umbilicus. If the heart sounds are audible in one flank, it suggests that the fetal back is directed towards that side. However, the location of fetal heart sounds is not a reliable sign of determining how or where the fetus is located (Simkin 2010).

Midwifery advice must be based on the best available evidence and practice, and the use of an ultrasound scan is more accurate than abdominal examination and vaginal examination in determining fetal position (Peregrine et al 2007; Munro and Jokinen 2012).

During labour

The diagnosis may be made by abdominal examination, although as labour advances, the head may become flexed and engaged. The cephalic prominence of the sinciput can be felt above the pubic bone and on the opposite side to the fetal back. The midwife should be alert whenever the cephalic prominence is felt on the same side as the fetal

back and should consider the possibility of a face or brow presentation and seek to exclude these. A deflexed head before or in the process of engagement in the maternal pelvis can become extended to a brow presentation or hyperextended to a face presentation. 'Coupling' of contractions is associated with occipitoposterior positions. The midwife may identify this phenomenon when she palpates the mother's abdomen or on the tocograph tracing if electronic fetal monitoring is in progress.

On vaginal examination, the findings depend on the degree of flexion of the fetal head. Palpation of the anterior fontanelle is usually diagnostic of an occipitoposterior position. When the head is partially or well flexed, the anterior fontanelle is felt towards the front of the pelvis, whereas occasionally the posterior fontanelle is just within reach at the back. With a deflexed head, the anterior fontanelle is almost central and, unless obscured by caput, easily recognizable by its size and shape.

Intrapartum sonography is becoming more common to assist in accurate diagnosis of malpositions and malpresentations because it is more reliably accurate than information gained from abdominal examination and vaginal examination combined.

Progress in labour

The progress of labour will depend on the regularity and strength of uterine contractions and the *degree of flexion* of the fetal head. The shape of the maternal pelvis and the maternal position may be significant in determining how the fetus negotiates the pelvic inlet, cavity and outlet.

Flexion of the fetal head

If the head is flexed, labour will probably be completely normal. The engaging diameter is the suboccipitofrontal (10 cm). The occiput reaches the pelvic floor and rotates anteriorly through three-eighths of a circle, and the baby is born with the occiput anteriorly (Fig. 62.4).

When the head remains deflexed, it tends to remain high or is slow to engage. Labour is slow to become established, with hypotonic and irregular uterine contractions. However, flexion may improve, and once the head becomes flexed, labour usually accelerates and continues normally, with a long internal rotation and an occipitoanterior birth (Fig. 62.4a).

Deflexion of the fetal head

The midwife needs to be fully conversant with the mechanism of the persistent OPP and how this translates into what the woman experiences. If the head remains deflexed, labour is likely to be prolonged and painful. Although backache may be a common characteristic, it should not be considered diagnostic of OPP, and absence of backache does not indicate an anteriorly positioned fetus (Simkin 2010). The outcome of labour is dependent on the size, shape and dimensions of the pelvis in relation to those of the fetal skull and the efficiency of uterine contractions.

Persistent occipitoposterior position

The mechanism of persistent occipitoposterior position (POP) is that the lie is longitudinal, presentation vertex and attitude deflexed – the engaging diameter is the occipitofrontal and measures 11.5 cm. The position may be either right or left occipitoposterior, and the presenting part is the anterior aspect of the right (ROP) or left (LOP) parietal bone. Descent takes place with deficient flexion, and the biparietal diameter of the fetal head is held up on the sacrocotyloid diameter of the maternal

pelvis (see Ch. 24), so that the sinciput becomes the leading part. When the sinciput meets the resistance of the pelvic floor, it rotates forward one-eighth of a circle (Fig. 62.4c). The sinciput passes under the pubic arch and the occiput into the hollow of the sacrum. With good contractions, spontaneous delivery ensues; with flexion, the occiput sweeps the maternal perineum; then, once the glabella is visible, the brow and face are delivered by extension. The rest of the mechanism follows that of a normal vertex presentation (see Ch. 37). This is called *persistent occipitoposterior position* or *'face-to-pubes'* delivery and is often associated with an anthropoid pelvis (Fig. 62.4c).

A   Flexion – 'Long rotation'

Onset of labour	Descent and flexion	Internal rotation: ROT to ROA

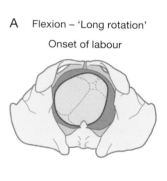   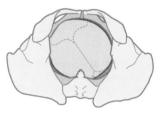

Internal rotation: ROA to OA

Extension complete: birth of head

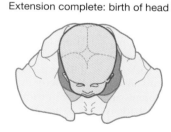

B   Slight flexion – Arrest in the transverse

Onset of labour	Descent and flexion	Internal rotation to ROT – Deep Transverse Arrest

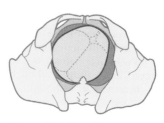   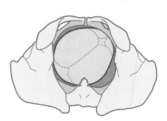   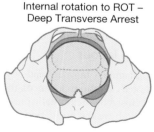

Figure 62.4 Possible outcomes of an occipitoposterior position. The fetal head enters the pelvis with the occiput posteriorly.

C **No flexion**, 'military position' – 'short rotation'

Onset of labour occipito posterior

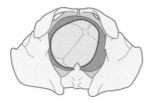

Descent

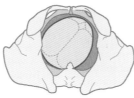

Internal rotation: ROP to direct OP

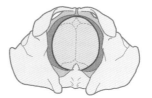

OP: birth of head

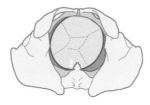

OP: crowning

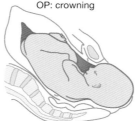

OP: flexion complete

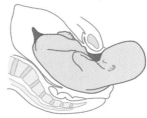

Persistent occipitoposterior
position – 'face to pubes'

D Slight flexion – Brow presentation

No mechanism for delivery

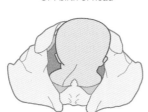

E Extension – face presentation

LMA: onset of labour

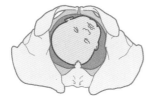

Extension and descent

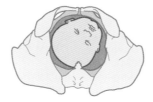

Internal rotation: LMA to MA

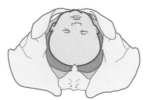

Flexion: head delivered

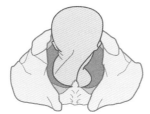

Extension: head delivered

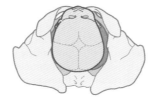

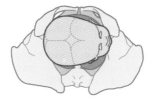

Figure 62.4, cont'd Possible outcomes of an occipitoposterior position. The fetal head enters the pelvis with the occiput posteriorly.

Deep transverse arrest

Deep transverse arrest (DTA) (Fig. 62.4b) may occur if the head remains deflexed. The fetal head may attempt a long rotation, but because of wider diameters and prominence of the ischial spines, it can become caught in the transverse diameter of the obstetric outlet, between the ischial spines.

The midwife should explain the situation to the woman, obtaining informed consent (see chapter website resources) for the necessary procedures (NMC 2015).

DTA should be suspected if there is delay in the second stage of labour or any fetal distress; the midwife must not delay summoning appropriate assistance (NMC 2012).

On vaginal examination, the sagittal suture is found in the transverse diameter of the pelvis with a fontanelle at each end, close to the ischial spines.

Digital or manual rotation of the occiput should be considered to correct the position of the fetal head. There are two techniques that can be undertaken by an obstetrician or an appropriately trained and experienced midwife. Both methods require the woman to give consent and have adequate analgesia, an empty bladder and a fully dilated cervix.

The tips of the index and middle fingers are placed along a suture line, preferably where there is overlap of the bones (e.g. the parietal bone overlapping the occipital bone). Pressure is exerted upwards with the tips of fingers to rotating the posterior fontanelle towards the symphysis pubis. Or, the whole hand is inserted and the thumb and fingers are positioned under the anterior and posterior parietal bones (Phipps et al 2014). Rotation can be performed between or during contractions. The rotation may take two or three contractions to complete; the head may be held in place for another couple of contractions as the woman pushes to ensure that the position is maintained.

Manual rotation can reduce the operative delivery rate, reduce obstetric and neonatal complications and may have a significant effects in low-income countries where the risks of maternal morbidity and mortality are higher (Lumbiganon et al 2010; Graham et al 2014; Phipps et al 2014).

Vacuum extraction (ventouse) can be used to complete the delivery (Ch. 59); a posterior cup must be used. Once the posterior cup is applied, the head is pulled downwards and rotates spontaneously to an OA position. The head is never rotated using a ventouse cup because this would cause sheering injuries to the fetal scalp. Delivery using rotational forceps, by an experienced obstetrician, has similar outcomes for the neonate and results in fewer cases of severe haemorrhage than emergency caesarean section (Aitken et al 2015).

Caesarean section is sometimes necessary to deliver the fetus in an occipitoposterior position. This is likely when complications such as cord prolapse and fetal distress occur or when true cephalopelvic disproportion is diagnosed.

Extension of the fetal head

It is possible that the fetal head may either be in a slightly extended position or may adopt this as labour progresses, resulting in a *brow* presentation (Fig. 62.4d). Unless the fetus is particularly small or preterm, then it is unlikely that it will be born vaginally. Full extension of the fetal head may lead to a face presentation, which, if mento-anterior, may deliver vaginally (Fig. 62.4e).

Complications of OPP

Midwives need to consider complications that might arise (Table 62.1) and be fully aware of what action should be taken. Vigilant care can minimize the risk of complications.

Care in labour

Kind, compassionate and woman-centred care is expected for every labour. For those women whose baby is malpositioned, the following aspects of care are also paramount:

- Communication and support
- One-to-one care
- General comfort and pain relief
- Encouragement to maintain ambulation
- Assessment of progress using most appropriate methods
- Effective assessment of maternal and fetal well-being
- Being alert to the signs of possible obstructed labour
- Appropriate confident clinical decisions
- Prompt referral when necessary
- Accurate and detailed record keeping
- Allowing time for discussion in the postnatal period and referral for psychological debriefing if required

MALPRESENTATIONS OF THE FETUS

Malpresentation refers to the orientation of the fetus and may be diagnosed during pregnancy or in labour. Any presentation other than vertex is termed a malpresentation, and this therefore includes *breech*, *face*, *brow* and *shoulder*. When midwives encounter a malpresentation of the fetus, they will draw upon similar knowledge and many of the skills they use in the care and management of women whose babies were in an occipitoposterior position.

In all malpresentations, there is commonly an ill-fitting presenting part, often associated with early rupture of the membranes because of uneven pressure on the bag of forewaters. This results in an increased risk of cord prolapse. An ill-fitting presenting part is also associated with

Table 62.1 Complications of occipitoposterior (OP) position

Complication	Reason
Prolonged latent phase (more than 8 hours)	A larger presenting diameter fails to stimulate the cervix and initiate labour.
Early rupture of the membranes	Poorly fitting presenting part and uneven pressure on the forewaters lead to less chance of spontaneous labour after prelabour rupture of membranes.
Cord prolapse	As with any ill-fitting presenting part, the membranes tend to rupture early, and the cord may prolapse.
Prolonged labour	This is associated with a deflexed head, poorly fitting presenting part and misaligned fetal axis pressure. A slightly contracted pelvis may compound this. Hypotonic and inefficient or overefficient uterine contractions may result. In such circumstances, the development of either fetal or maternal distress is more likely, and operative intervention and anaesthesia are often necessary. Postpartum haemorrhage is therefore an added risk.
Retention of urine	Pressure on the urethra that results from the wider diameters of the OP position.
Premature expulsive effort	The wider diameter of the OP position results in pressure on the sacral nerves, and the woman may feel the need to push before full dilatation of the cervix. This may cause cervical oedema or cervical trauma. Early dilatation of the anus can also occur while the head is still high.
Infection	This is more likely because of early rupture of the membranes, especially if labour is prolonged, and can be compounded by an increased number of vaginal assessments.
Trauma to the mother's soft tissues	The risk of trauma is increased with the wider diameter of the OP position. When this is persistent, the biparietal diameter and large occiput distend the maternal perineum. Instrumental delivery may also increase the risk of maternal trauma.
Posttraumatic stress disorder or postnatal depression	Prolonged, difficult, painful and traumatic labour might result in mental ill-health. This can be exacerbated when the mother has no control over events and is not involved in decision making. This, together with maternal exhaustion and an unsettled baby, may lead to difficulty in maternal–infant bonding.
Maternal exhaustion	From prolonged labour
Unsettled or difficult-to-feed infant	An OP position and a prolonged labour with an assisted delivery will baby's result in discomfort and pain for both mother and baby. This can impede early attempts to breastfeed, and extra support should be offered.
Fetal intracranial haemorrhage	Upward moulding of the fetal skull may lead to stretching and damage of the tentorium cerebelli and consequent tearing of the great vein of Galen, resulting in haemorrhage and intracranial damage.
Increased perinatal mortality and morbidity	This might result from cord prolapse, prolonged labour, instrumental delivery, infection and intracranial haemorrhage and is increased because of hypoxia and birth trauma.

poor uterine action and slower cervical dilatation, and therefore labour may be prolonged with the concomitant risk of infection and operative intervention.

Breech presentation

A breech presentation occurs when the fetal buttocks lie lowermost in the maternal uterus and the fetal head occupies the fundus. The lie is longitudinal, the denominator is the sacrum and the presenting diameter is the bitrochanteric, which measures 10 cm.

Breech presentation is common before 37 weeks gestation, with a suggested incidence of 15% at 29 to 32 weeks gestation, reducing to 3% to 4% at term (Hannah et al 2000). One fetus in four will present by the breech at some stage in pregnancy. In preterm labour it is not surprising to find the breech presentation, and these infants comprise a quarter of all babies born by breech. However, by the 34th week of pregnancy, the majority will have turned to a vertex presentation.

Types

Four types of breech presentation are described (Fig. 62.5a–d). They are determined by the way in which the fetal legs are flexed or extended, and these have implications for the birth.

- *Flexed* or *complete* breech: The fetus sits with the thighs and knees flexed with the feet close to the buttocks. This is more common in multigravidas.

- *Extended* or *frank* breech: The fetal thighs are flexed; the legs are extended at the knees and lie alongside the trunk, with the feet near the fetal head. This is the commonest type of breech presentation and occurs most frequently in primigravidas towards term. This is because their usually firm uterine and abdominal muscles allow only limited fetal movement, and the fetus is therefore unable to flex its legs and turn to a cephalic presentation.

- *Footling presentation:* One or both feet present below the fetal buttocks, with hips and knees extended. This relatively rare type of breech presentation is more likely to occur when the fetus is preterm. A foot may occasionally be felt at the level of the buttocks and might be confused with a footling presentation. Usually, as labour advances, it slips behind the buttocks, returning to an obvious flexed breech position.

- *Knee presentation:* One or both knees present below the fetal buttocks, with one or both hips extended and the knees flexed. This is the least common of all types of breech presentation.

There is a higher perinatal mortality and morbidity rate with breech presentation, which is largely a result of prematurity and congenital abnormalities of the fetus, in addition to birth asphyxia and birth trauma (Hannah et al 2000). The clinical setting, failure to respond to delay in progress and lack of clinical experience may also contribute to poorer outcomes (Kotaska et al 2009).

In providing care, the midwife must be conversant with the latest developments surrounding the management and optimal mode of delivery. Although the outcomes of the *UK Term Breech Trial* have dominated the discourse around the mode and management of breech births (Hannah et al 2000) and significantly influenced practice in the UK and abroad, the evidence is at best uncertain, conflicting and contradictory (Glezerman 2006; Goffinet et al 2006; Hofmeyr et al 2015a; Kotaska 2004; Kotaska et al 2009; Van Idderkinge 2007; Waites 2003). Although vaginal breech delivery remains controversial, a recent review has shown low absolute risk for vaginal breech births (Berhan and Haileamlak 2015).

The need to provide expertise in vaginal breech delivery will not disappear, and therefore practitioners need to understand the mechanisms and skills around breech birth. Some women present too late or arrive in labour with an unexpected breech presentation. Even where a policy of planned caesarean section is in place, some women will reject the choice of a planned caesarean section and choose to have a vaginal breech birth in the hospital or home setting because of personal, cultural or religious reasons.

Causes

The fetus may adopt the breech position for a variety of reasons, although the true cause is often unknown. In most cases, no single cause can be identified, and it is a random occurrence. The most common cause is likely to be an error of orientation without an identifiable cause or any obvious abnormalities. Causes include the following:

- Abnormal size and shape of the pelvis

- Uterine anomalies

- Placenta or fibroids occupying the lower uterine segment

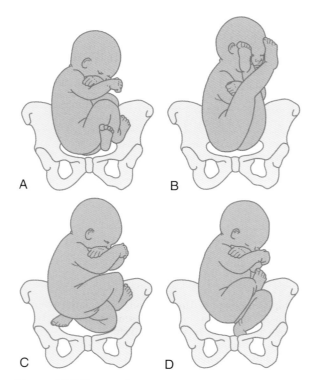

Figure 62.5 Types of breech presentation. **A,** Flexed. **B,** Extended. **C,** Knee. **D,** Footling.

- Abnormal liquor volume
- Multiple pregnancy
- Maternal conditions or fetal abnormalities resulting in poor postural tone
- Congenital anomalies: incidence known to be two to three times higher in those fetuses presenting by breech (see Table 62.2)

Diagnosis during pregnancy

The midwife needs to be alert to the gestational age of the fetus but should not be unduly concerned before 36 weeks gestation. A history of a previous breech presentation may be significant, and if the breech persists, then referral to an obstetrician should be made and the likely cause identified.

The woman may give a history of discomfort under the ribs as a result of the presence of the hard fetal head or describe fetal movements in the lower pole of the uterus. Her description of her baby's movements and how she feels can be valuable elements in the diagnosis of a breech presentation.

Abdominal examination may be difficult to distinguish between a breech and a vertex presentation, and a high index of suspicion is an asset for diagnosis. Abdominal palpation skills do vary, and approximately 25% of breech presentations are missed in late pregnancy, resulting in approximately 1 : 100 women with undiagnosed breech presentations at the start of labour (Walker and Sabrosa 2014).

The method of conducting the abdominal examination may have consequences for detecting a breech presentation or finding a ballottable fetal head in the uterine fundus.

Although inspection of the maternal abdomen usually reveals nothing that indicates a breech presentation,

Table 62.2 Causes of breech presentation	
Primigravida	Firm abdominal and uterine muscles may prevent flexion of the fetal legs, especially when they are already extended.
Uterine anomalies	Bicornuate uterus may restrict fetal movement. Previous breech birth may also be strongly associated with a uterine anomaly.
Oligohydramnios	Reduced liquor volume restricts the ability of the fetus to turn in the uterus. The condition may also be associated with fetal anomalies and fetal compromise.
Placental location	Placenta praevia may prevent the fetal head from fitting into the lower uterine segment and entering the pelvis. A placenta situated in one or other cornua of the uterus reduces the breadth of space in the upper segment and can lead to a breech presentation.
Uterine fibroids	These can interfere with fetal activity or, when situated in the lower uterine segment, can prevent the fetal head from entering the lower pole of the uterus.
A contracted pelvis	The fetal head is unable to enter the pelvic brim.
Fetal anomalies such as trisomy 21 and hydrocephalus	These can cause fetal hypotonia. Reduced or restricted fetal activity makes it difficult for the fetus to turn. Hydrocephalus can prevent the fetal head engaging in the pelvis.
Multiple pregnancy	There is usually insufficient space to turn.
Maternal alcohol or drug abuse	May lead to fetal hypotonia, in which the lack of movement or reduced or restricted fetal activity makes it difficult for the fetus to turn.
Grande multiparity	Lax abdominal and uterine muscles allow movement and may lead to an unstable lie.
Polyhydramnios	Overdistension of the uterus enables the fetus to be more mobile.
Prematurity	Increased incidence at earlier gestation; smaller fetus with greater space within the uterus to adopt a breech position
Impaired fetal growth, short umbilical cord and fetal death	Compromised fetus may result in decreased fetal activity. May be associated with fetal or maternal conditions having an adverse effect on the fetus, which results in reduced or restricted fetal mobility.

occasionally fetal movements can be seen in the lower pole. On palpation, the presenting part feels firm but less hard and less rounded than the head. The diagnosis is usually made by feeling the hard, round and ballottable head in the fundus of the uterus.

Over time, the sequence in which *Leopold manoeuvres* (see resources section and chapter website) have been applied during abdominal palpation has changed, with identification of the lie often taking place before palpation of the presenting part. In such circumstances, especially at term, the uterus might be stimulated, increasing tone or even stimulating a contraction. This will result in the presenting part feeling hard, and the fetal head, if in the uterine fundus, becomes fixed and more difficult to ballot. As a consequence, breech presentations can be missed.

A primigravida with an extended breech may simulate a cephalic presentation. The woman's firm abdominal muscles brace the extended legs and compress the breech, allowing it to enter deep into the pelvis. The presenting part may be out of reach of the midwife's palpating fingers and can be mistaken for the deeply engaged head. The baby's feet, lying under the chin, make ballottement more difficult. If the placenta is situated on the anterior uterine wall, identification of the fetal head is further obscured.

Fetal heart sounds, classically heard above the umbilicus in breech presentations, may be heard at maximum intensity in an extended breech where the heart sounds are commonly heard in a vertex presentation: halfway between the superior anterior iliac spine and the maternal umbilicus.

Ultrasound imaging is helpful for the following:

- Confirmation of presentation
- Identification of fetal attitude
- Estimation of fetal weight and liquor volume
- Confirmation or ruling out of abnormalities
- Confirmation of those women with breech presentation after 36 weeks gestation, for which external cephalic version (ECV) should be offered (Royal College of Obstetricians and Gynaecologists (RCOG) 2006b).

Vaginal examination may be carried out by the midwife or obstetrician to exclude a deeply engaged head and confirm breech presentation. If the head is deeply engaged, the shoulders palpate just above the pelvic brim and are sometimes difficult to distinguish from the breech. On vaginal examination, an extended breech has a hard, compressed presenting part similar to a cephalic presentation, and the cleft of the buttocks may imitate the line of the sagittal suture.

Midwives should be aware of these deceptive findings, and, unless certain that the presentation is vertex, need to be cautious. If in doubt or if convinced that the presentation is breech after 36 weeks gestation, confirmation by ultrasound examination should be sought, and the woman should be informed of the findings. Where a breech presentation exists, the midwife should discuss the evidence and implications and, as appropriate, refer promptly to a senior obstetric colleague.

Diagnosis during labour

During labour, the presenting part may initially be high. On vaginal examination, the breech feels soft and irregular. The hard sacrum and the anus should be felt, and it is important to distinguish the breech from a face presentation.

The midwife will note that in a breech presentation the landmarks of the fetal ischial tuberosities are on either side of the fetal anus and form a straight line. This differs from a face presentation, in which the fetal mouth and malar prominences form a triangle.

Fresh, 'toothpaste like', thick meconium may be found on the examining finger and is diagnostic of a breech presentation. The fetal genitalia are soft and not easily recognized because they become oedematous during labour.

In a flexed breech, the feet may be palpable alongside the buttocks, but these usually fall back behind the presenting part as labour advances. On vaginal examination, the features of the foot that distinguish it from a hand are as follows: shorter digits, larger size but limited range of movements of the big toe, the presence of a heel.

Associated risks

Breech presentation carries increased risks to a healthy mother and fetus from either a complicated vaginal delivery or caesarean section (Kotaska et al 2009; Van Idderkinge 2007). Poorer outcomes following vaginal breech delivery, therefore, might result from some underlying condition causing breech presentation rather than damage during delivery (Hofmeyr et al 2015b). A study following up the UK's Term Breech Trial found no differences in long-term neonatal morbidity between babies born by vaginal birth and those born by caesarean section (Whyte et al 2004; Rielberg et al 2005).

Care and management – pregnancy

The midwife who diagnoses a breech presentation should, depending on the woman's preferences, either refer her to a senior obstetrician or discuss the case with his or her supervisor of midwives. The midwife must inform the woman as to her options of care, and these, together with the mother's choices, should be clearly documented in her maternity record.

The four options she will need to consider are as follows:

- Planned external cephalic version (ECV)
- Spontaneous or assisted vaginal breech birth
- Planned induction of labour
- Planned caesarean section

Spontaneous cephalic version of the breech

Although the vast majority of breech presentations will have turned to the vertex by term, it occurs with diminishing frequency as pregnancy advances.

The use of alternative approaches and techniques to promote spontaneous cephalic version has been widely reported, although the effectiveness of these has yet to be confirmed. There is insufficient evidence from well-controlled trials to support the use of postural management in converting breech to cephalic presentations (Hofmeyr and Kulier 2012). *Moxibustion* is used in traditional Chinese medicine to encourage fetal activity and version of the fetus in breech presentations. A systematic review (Coyle et al 2012) found limited evidence to support the use of moxibustion for correcting breech presentation, and more evidence is needed concerning the benefits and safety of moxibustion.

External cephalic version (ECV) is strongly advocated (RCOG 2006a) and well evaluated (Collins et al 2007; Hofmeyr et al 2015b; Hutton et al 2015) (see chapter website resources). The procedure is considered both safe and effective, reducing the chance for breech presentation at birth and caesarean section. Tocolysis is also associated with fewer failures of ECV (Hofmeyr and Kulier 2012). ECV should be offered to all women with an uncomplicated breech presentation at term (Hofmeyr et al 2015a). This role could be undertaken by appropriately trained and supported midwives and obstetric colleagues and could significantly reduce the incidence of breech presentation (Walker and Sabrosa 2014).

Mechanism of vaginal breech delivery

Although caesarean section is increasingly considered as the optimal mode of delivery for the breech presentation (Hannah et al 2000), women may still choose to have a vaginal breech birth or may present in advanced labour with an undiagnosed breech. Midwives must be fully conversant with the management and mechanisms of breech presentation and be able to orientate themselves to the position that the mother adopts in labour.

There are six positions in breech presentation. The denominator is the sacrum, and its relationship to the maternal pelvis determines the position. The positions are the same as the vertex presentations, substituting the sacrum for the occiput (Fig. 62.6):

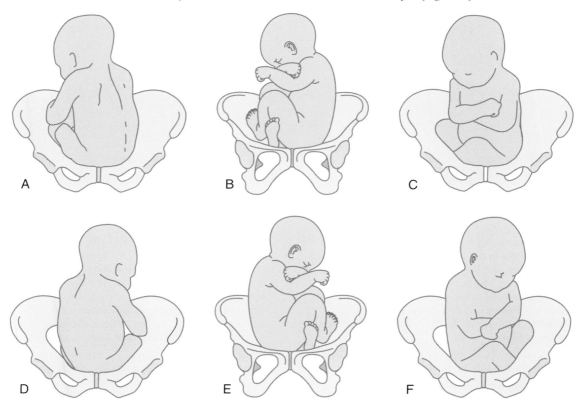

Figure 62.6 Breech positions. **A,** Left sacroanterior (LSA). **B,** Left sacrolateral (LSL). **C,** Left sacroposterior (LSP). **D,** Right sacroanterior (RSA). **E,** Right sacrolateral (RSL). **F,** Right sacroposterior (RSP).

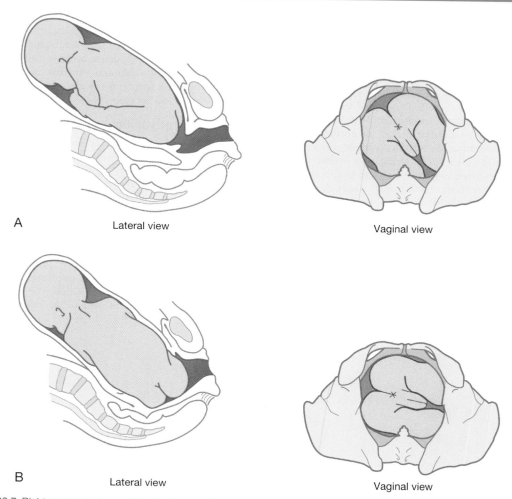

A   Lateral view   Vaginal view

B   Lateral view   Vaginal view

Figure 62.7 Right sacroanterior position. **A,** Onset of labour. **B,** Descent and internal rotation of the buttocks.

1. *Left sacroanterior position (LSA) (Fig. 62.6a):* The sacrum points to the left iliopectineal eminence, and the abdomen and legs are directed towards the right sacroiliac joint. The left buttock is anterior and the bitrochanteric diameter is in the left oblique diameter. The natal cleft is in the right oblique diameter. A caput may form on the left buttock and on the genitals.

2. *Left sacrolateral (LSL) (Fig. 62.6b):* The sacrum is towards the left side of the pelvis.

3. *Left sacroposterior (LSP) (Fig. 62.6c):* The sacrum points to the left sacroiliac joint, and the abdomen towards the right iliopectineal eminence.

4. *Right sacroanterior position (RSA) (Fig. 62.6d):* The sacrum points to the right iliopectineal eminence, and the abdomen is directed towards the left sacroiliac joint. The right buttock is anterior and the bitrochanteric diameter is in the right oblique diameter. The natal cleft is in the left oblique diameter. A caput may form on the right buttock and on the genitals.

5. *Right sacrolateral (RSL) (Fig. 62.6e):* The sacrum is towards the right side of the pelvis.

6. *Right sacroposterior (RSP) (Fig. 62.6f):* The sacrum points to the right sacroiliac joint, and the abdomen towards the left iliopectineal eminence.

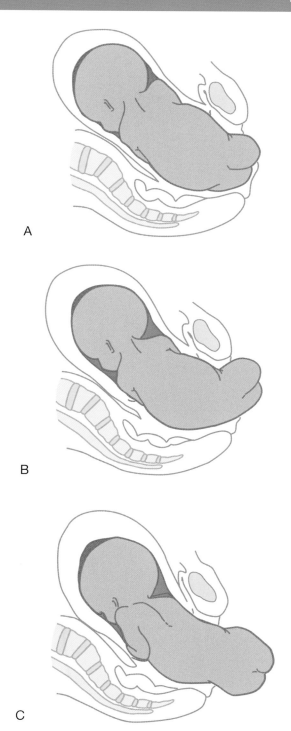

A

B

C

Figure 62.8 Birth of the buttocks. **A,** Breech crowning or 'rumping'. **B,** Birth of posterior buttock. **C,** Birth of anterior buttock.

The fetus may be positioned in a direct anterior or posterior position.

With the breech in either the left or right sacroanterior position and good contractions, there is descent. The mechanism of the right sacroanterior position is illustrated in Fig. 62.7a and b. The fetus engages with the bitrochanteric diameter (10 cm) in the right oblique diameter of the pelvic brim and descends into the pelvic cavity.

With further contractions, the anterior buttock meets the resistance of the pelvic floor and rotates forwards through one-eighth of a circle (45 degrees) and comes to lie behind the symphysis pubis. The bitrochanteric diameter now lies in the anteroposterior diameter of the outlet. Lateral flexion of the trunk allows the continued descent of the buttocks along the curve of the birth canal (Fig. 62.8a–c). The anterior buttock normally passes under the symphysis pubis and 'rumps', followed by the posterior buttock, which sweeps over the perineum.

With the birth of the buttocks the shoulders descend into the pelvis with the bisacromial diameter (11 cm) in the right oblique diameter of the brim. Internal rotation of the shoulders through one-eighth of a circle brings the anterior shoulder behind the symphysis. The right (anterior) shoulder and arm escape under the symphysis and the left (posterior) shoulder and arm pass over the perineum (Fig. 62.9a–c).

The flexed head engages with the suboccipitobregmatic (9.5 cm) or suboccipitofrontal diameter (10 cm) lying in the right oblique or transverse diameter of the brim. Internal rotation of the head carries the occiput behind the symphysis. The face now lies in the hollow of the sacrum. External rotation of the buttocks and shoulders is produced by the internal rotation of the head. The back of the baby's head and body now face in the same direction as the mother's abdomen.

It is essential that the back of the fetus orientates in the same direction as the mother's abdomen, and if it does not, it is gently assisted to do so. The chin, face, vertex and occiput are born over the perineum by a movement of flexion to complete the delivery (Fig. 62.10a–c).

Management of breech labour

When a woman chooses to have a vaginal breech birth, the midwife needs to ensure that she does so from an informed position (Marshall 2010). A careful history should be taken to ensure that there are no medical or obstetric contraindications for vaginal breech birth and that both woman and baby are in good health.

If possible, a detailed ultrasound scan should be carried out for the following reasons:

- Confirm a singleton pregnancy
- Exclude obvious fetal abnormality
- Estimate fetal weight and attitude

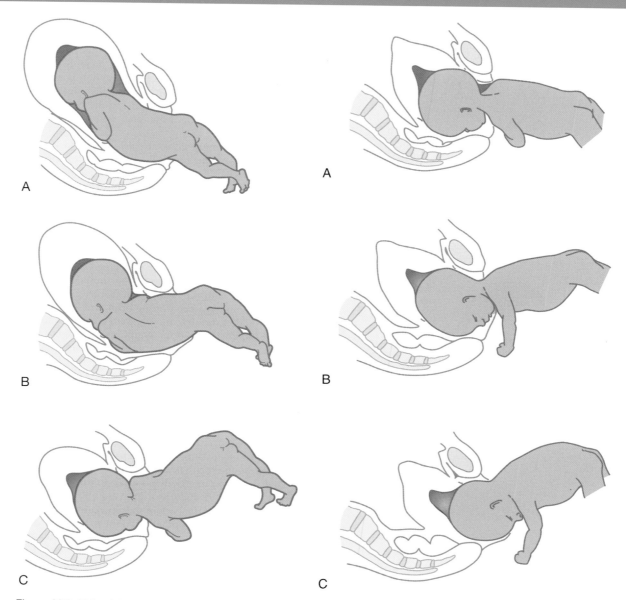

Figure 62.9 Birth of the shoulders. **A,** Feet born, shoulders engaging. **B,** Descent and internal rotation of shoulders. **C,** Posterior shoulder born; head has entered the pelvis.

Figure 62.10 Birth of the head. **A,** Anterior shoulder born; descent of the head. **B,** Internal rotation and beginning flexion of the head. **C,** Flexion of the head complete.

- Determine placental position
- Assess liquor volume

A thorough clinical assessment of pelvic capacity should be performed. Currently, pelvimetry to measure maternal pelvic diameters for safe delivery is deemed unnecessary,

with good progress in labour being indicative of adequate fetal–pelvic proportions (Kotaska et al 2009).

Even when labour is established, consideration should be given to performing an ECV in an attempt to alter the presentation of the fetus from breech to cephalic. Although it is preferable for a vaginal breech labour to be conducted in hospital and under the supervision of an experienced obstetrician or midwife, this may not always be possible; maternal choice and unexpected and rapid delivery sometimes prevent transfer to hospital. Supervisors of midwives also have a role in facilitating the woman's admission to hospital and in supporting those midwives with the relevant skill to accompany her if requested to do so by the mother. Midwives must ensure that they have up to date knowledge and skills to cope with an emergency breech birth (NMC 2012 and 2015).

First stage of labour

The first stage of labour in a breech presentation differs little from that of normal labour. If the breech is not engaged, as is probable in a flexed breech, there is a risk of early rupture of the membranes and prolapse of the umbilical cord. The midwife must be vigilant and immediately exclude the possibility of cord prolapse when the membranes rupture. Where the breech is engaged, the legs are probably extended, and the risk of cord prolapse is reduced.

The value of upright positions, ambulation and support in labour are equally pertinent to women labouring with a breech presentation. The midwife provides continued support and continuity, carefully monitoring the progress of labour and the condition of the woman and fetus. A close working relationship with the wider maternity care team is also essential, and although the experienced midwife may conduct the breech delivery, the support of a senior obstetrician should be readily available if necessary.

Because of the associated risk in breech presentation, continuous monitoring of the fetal heart should be offered and recommended in breech labour (RCOG 2006b). Some women who pursue a vaginal birth may reject this and opt for intermittent monitoring. In such circumstances, observations on the maternal condition and progress in labour should be carried out in keeping with the recommended guidelines for intermittent monitoring (NICE 2014).

In most cases, the first stage of labour progresses normally. Augmentation may be required should uterine action be hypotonic. This must be done with extreme caution – in some units, breech presentation may be considered a contraindication for augmentation. There is no evidence that epidural anaesthesia is essential, and its use depends on the wishes and needs of the woman.

Occasionally, the breech may begin to descend through the cervix before the cervical os is fully dilated and this gives the woman a desire to push. Although uncommon, the buttocks may then descend easily, but the larger head cannot pass through the incompletely dilated cervix, and dangerous delay results. The use of epidural anaesthesia makes this less likely because the woman does not experience the premature urge to push.

Second stage of labour

When full dilatation of the cervical os has been confirmed, the mother may adopt a semirecumbent, all-fours, upright or supported squatting position to aid expulsive efforts and the descent of the fetus.

Standing positions for the birth should be treated with caution because of an association with premature separation of the placenta. Midwives experienced in the management of breech birth advocate women adopting a kneeling position for the birth of the body and a forward-leaning 'prayer position' for the birth of the head (Cronk 2005; Evans 2005).

Where an obstetrician is conducting the delivery, the woman is usually in the lithotomy position. The woman may remain upright before the onset of the active second stage to advance the breech and lithotomy can be delayed until the breech is visible.

The midwife should ensure that appropriate and experienced help is at hand and that a paediatrician and senior obstetrician are present or readily available and that an anaesthetist can be quickly in attendance in case operative intervention suddenly becomes necessary.

If the fetal breech and body descend well, then it is likely that spontaneous breech birth will occur with little assistance from the midwife or obstetrician. This is more common in multigravidas or when the fetus is small and preterm.

Assisted breech delivery

A medically managed vaginal breech birth employs techniques to assist the delivery with the woman predominantly in the lithotomy position. The bladder is emptied before delivery. When the posterior buttock distends the perineum, the perineum is infiltrated with local anaesthetic (unless an epidural anaesthetic or a pudendal block is employed), and an episiotomy may be performed. The posterior buttock then emerges, and the breech advances more quickly.

As the trunk descends, the back will rotate anteriorly, allowing the fetal shoulder to enter the maternal pelvis in the transverse or oblique diameter of the inlet. Traction on the fetus **is not a part** of British practice because this can give rise to extension of the head and nuchal displacement of the arms. There should be no interference and, increasingly, obstetricians, like midwives, apply the rule of *'hands off the breech'* and will try to avoid unnecessary manipulations.

Once the umbilicus is visible, previous practice dictated gently pulling down a loop of the umbilical cord to relieve any tension. However, this is *no longer* advocated. At this stage, compression of the cord is likely, and time is an imperative.

From the complete delivery of the buttocks, some authorities advocate that the baby should be delivered within 15 minutes. Some believe that in vaginal breech birth, there may be benefits from rapid delivery of the baby to prevent progressive acidosis. This needs to be weighed against the potential trauma of a quick delivery. To date, there is insufficient evidence to evaluate the effects of expedited vaginal breech birth (Hofmeyr et al 2015c).

If the fetal legs do not deliver spontaneously, inserting the index finger behind the thigh to flex the knee and abduct the leg may gently disengage them. However, if the practitioner is prepared to wait, they will usually deliver as the trunk descends.

With the next contraction, the shoulder blades appear; the arms, which are normally flexed across the chest, will usually slip out on their own and the shoulders are born in the anteroposterior diameter of the pelvic outlet. The head at this stage is entering the transverse or oblique diameter of the pelvic inlet. Some authorities advocate that from complete delivery of the baby's body until full delivery of the head, no more than 5 minutes should elapse.

At this stage, a number of manoeuvres may be used to facilitate the delivery of the head. If all is proceeding well, spontaneous, but controlled, delivery may be used when the head is at the pelvic outlet. Midwives who assist women to give birth using a forward-leaning position use the analogy of 'getting the woman to move from a Christian prayer position to a Muslim prayer position' because this aids release of the head, facilitating its delivery. It has been observed that when the fetus begins to draw up its knees, the fetal head also flexes. If the woman then moves forward as described previously, her pelvis rotates over the fetal head, causing its spontaneous release Alternatively, the *Mauriceau–Smellie–Veit* or *Burns–Marshall manoeuvre* may be used.

Mauriceau–Smellie–Veit manoeuvre is an effective method of delivering the fetal head, and the underlying principle is that of 'flexion before traction' (Fig. 62.11). It offers good control of the head and may also be used when there is delay in the descent of the head.

The manoeuvre involves a combination of jaw flexion and shoulder traction and can be used for any breech delivery, but it is of particular value when the fetal head is extended and forceps may be difficult to apply.

The practitioner supports the baby with the legs straddling his or her left arm (Fig. 62.11); three fingers slide into the vagina, feeling for the baby's cheekbones (malar bones). Originally, the middle finger was inserted into the baby's mouth to maximize traction, but this is not recommended because it could result in dislocation of the jaw. Instead, the ring and index fingers rest on the cheekbones while the middle finger applies pressure to the chin.

The index and ring fingers of the practitioner's right hand are hooked over the baby's shoulders, to apply traction, while the middle finger presses on the occiput to

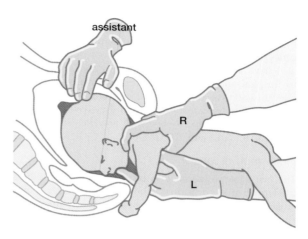

Figure 62.11 Mauriceau–Smellie–Veit manoeuvre.

aid flexion. An assistant may apply suprapubic pressure if needed.

As gently as possible, the baby's head is flexed and aided through the pelvic cavity to the outlet, after which the trunk is raised to bring the mouth into view. The air passages are then cleared, and the birth of the head is completed in the usual way.

Burns–Marshall manoeuvre is considered a medical procedure. Once the body is born, the baby is allowed to hang by his or her own weight for a few moments to facilitate descent and flexion of the head. When the nape of the neck and hairline come into view, the head is ready to be delivered (Fig. 62.12). Grasping the baby by the ankles and using slight traction, the practitioner directs the trunk upwards in a wide arc over the woman's abdomen.

The perineum should then be depressed with the fingers to expose the mouth of the fetus and allow it to be cleared of any blood or mucus, enabling the baby to breathe freely.

The birth of the head then proceeds very slowly to avoid any sudden release of pressure that might give rise to an intracranial haemorrhage. To avoid this danger, Wrigley's or Neville–Barnes forceps may be applied to the aftercoming head, which allows careful control of the speed with which the head is born.

Reflective activity 62.2

Using a manikin or doll and pelvis model, rehearse the mechanisms of a breech presentation, and the different manoeuvres that can be used (e.g. Mauriceau–Smellie–Veit and Lövset's manoeuvres).

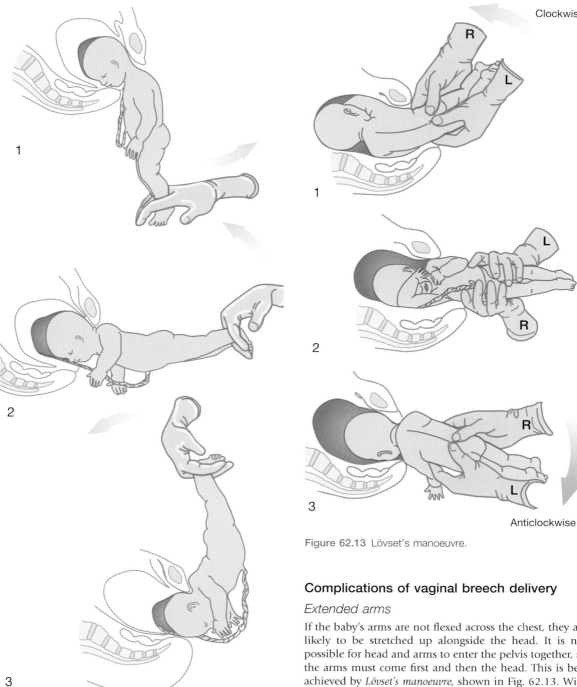

Clockwise

1

2

3

Anticlockwise

Figure 62.13 Lövset's manoeuvre.

1

2

3

Figure 62.12 Burns–Marshall manoeuvre.

Complications of vaginal breech delivery

Extended arms

If the baby's arms are not flexed across the chest, they are likely to be stretched up alongside the head. It is not possible for head and arms to enter the pelvis together, so the arms must come first and then the head. This is best achieved by *Lövset's manoeuvre*, shown in Fig. 62.13. With the baby in a right sacrolateral position, the manoeuvre depends on the fact that the posterior shoulder is below the sacral promontory and anterior shoulder above the symphysis pubis.

The practitioner grasps the baby's thighs with thumbs over the sacrum, and, being careful to avoid pressure above the pelvic girdle, which could cause abdominal injury, pulls the baby gently downwards, at the same time turning the baby, back upwards, through a half circle (180 degrees). The former posterior shoulder now becomes anterior and is released under the symphysis pubis, while at the same time, the other shoulder is brought into the pelvic cavity. The baby is then turned back through a half circle in the opposite direction, and the other arm is released in the same way.

This procedure does not require an anaesthetic, can be carried out by a midwife and, correctly performed, is safe and successful, even in cases where the baby has one arm at the back of the neck (nuchal displacement).

Extended head

After the birth of the shoulders, the baby is allowed to hang from the vagina to facilitate descent and flexion of the head. If the neck and hairline are not visible within a few seconds, the most likely reason is extension of the head. The head may be delivered by the *Mauriceau-Smellie-Veit manoeuvre*, described previously.

Entrapment of the fetal head

Entrapment of the fetal head is an extremely rare but dangerous situation in the term breech. It occurs when the breech is delivered and the cervix is not fully dilated and traps the fetal head. In this situation, the midwife must call for urgent medical assistance. The obstetrician will try to release the head from the cervix, but mortality and morbidity rates are high.

Although more commonly used in shoulder dystocia, *McRobert's manoeuvre* (see Ch. 64) has been used as a means to facilitate release of the fetal head where the occiput is held up on the symphysis pubis (Shushan and Younis 1992).

It is possible, for a variety of reasons, for a midwife to be faced with an unexpected and emergency breech delivery. In community practice, the midwife should, with the mother's consent, make every effort to transfer her into hospital. When labour is not advancing very quickly, this is usually possible.

If the labour is progressing rapidly, however, delivery may be imminent, and the risks of transfer may be considerable. If the contractions are strong and effective, there is every chance that the breech will deliver easily, although the midwife should call for skilled help because unexpected complications may still occur. The midwife's management of the breech birth is as described previously.

Face presentation

Face presentation occurs when the head and neck are hyperextended but the limbs flexed, so that the fetus lies

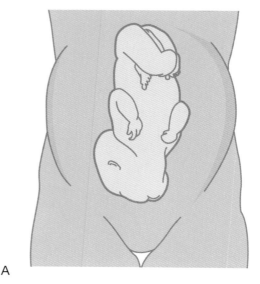

A

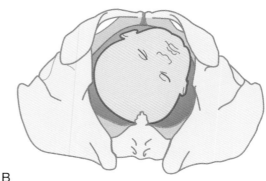

B

Figure 62.14 Anterior face presentation. **A,** Abdominal view. **B,** Vaginal view.

in the uterus in a curious S-shaped attitude with the occiput against the shoulder blades and the face directly over the internal os (Fig. 62.14). The presenting portion is between the orbital ridges and the chin, with the latter being the denominator (Marino 2016). Face presentation is uncommon and occurs in 1 of every 600 to 800 live births, averaging about 0.2% of live births.

Primary face presentation is present before the onset of labour, and causative factors are similar to those leading to general malpresentation and those that prevent head flexion or favour extension (Marino 2016), including the following:

- Birthweight over 4000 g (Tapisiz et al 2014)

- *Anencephaly* – where there is no vertex to present

- Tumours of the fetal neck preventing flexion of the head

Table 62.3 Complications that may occur with a face presentation

Complication	Reason
Cord prolapse	Ill-fitting presenting part and early rupture of the membranes
Obstructed labour	The face does not mould and therefore cannot overcome minor degrees of cephalopelvic disproportion. A persistent posterior face presentation leads to obstructed labour.
Emergency operative delivery	As a result of obstructive labour or fetal distress
Severe perineal trauma	Wider diameters: although the presenting diameter is the submentobregmatic at 9.5 cm, it is the submentovertical of 11.5 cm that distends the vagina and perineum. Risk of operative delivery
Intracranial haemorrhage	Anoxia and abnormal moulding of the fetal skull
Facial bruising and oedema	The inability of the face to mould and injury to the soft tissue

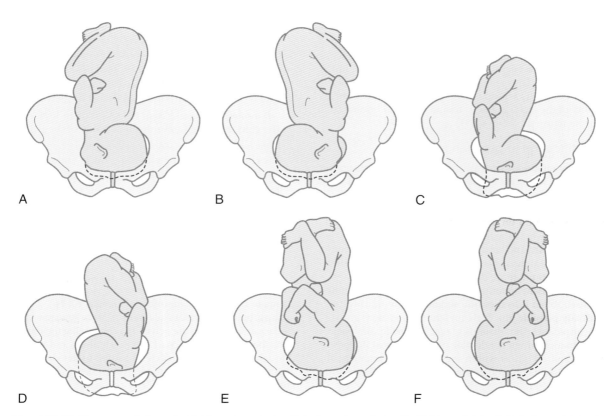

Figure 62.15 Face presentations. **A,** Right mentoposterior. **B,** Left mentoposterior. **C,** Right mentolateral. **D,** Left mentolateral. **E,** Right mentoanterior. **F,** Left mentoanterior.

- Excessive tone in the fetal extensor muscles that may cause extended attitude, then face presentation (may persist for a few days after birth)

Secondary face presentations that develop in labour. Causes include the following:

- deflexed occipitoposterior position – the biparietal diameter has difficulty in passing the sacrocotyloid diameter of the maternal pelvis; the bitemporal diameter descends more quickly, the head extends, and the face presents.
- uterine obliquity (uterus tilted sideways) – the force of uterine contractions may be directed towards the front of the head, so that the head extends as it enters the pelvis.
- More likely to occur in a flat pelvis
- Uterus laxity
- Prematurity
- Polyhydramnios
- Multiple pregnancy
- No obvious reason

The presenting diameters of the face presentation are to some degree favourable (i.e. 9.5 cm); however, the initial reason for the fetus adopting this position, the risk of the fetus being in a mentoposterior position and the reduced ability of the facial bones to mould create additional risks for the fetus (see Table 62.3).

Identification in pregnancy

Face presentation is not easily diagnosed in pregnancy but should be suspected if on abdominal palpation a deep groove is felt between the fetal head and back and the cephalic prominence and fetal back are on the same side.

If heart sounds are heard through the anterior chest wall on the side where the limbs are palpated, these may seem unusually loud and clear when the position is mentoanterior (MA). In mentoposterior (MP) positions, the fetal heart sounds are more difficult to hear.

When face presentation is suspected, ultrasound should be used to confirm the clinical diagnosis.

During labour, the high presenting part may give rise to suspicion. The diagnosis can be made on vaginal examination, when gentle palpation will reveal the orbital ridges and the gums within the mouth. Occasionally, the fetus will further help the diagnosis by sucking the examining finger.

Once a face presentation is diagnosed, it is essential to determine the position of the chin, whether it is anterior or posterior. A *posterior face presentation*, unless it rotates to an anterior position, will lead to obstructed labour. When the midwife diagnoses a face presentation, a senior obstetrician should be informed as soon as possible. If the chin is lateral or posterior, the urgency of the situation must be stressed.

As labour progresses, it becomes increasingly difficult to distinguish facial landmarks on vaginal examination because the face becomes oedematous. Vaginal examinations must be carried out with great care to avoid trauma to the eyes. Ultrasound may be utilized to assess progress.

Mechanisms

The lie is longitudinal, the presentation is the face, the denominator is the chin and the attitude is hyperextended. The engaging diameter is submentobregmatic (9.5 cm). There are six positions in which the face may present (Fig. 62.15).

1. *Right mentoposterior* (RMP) is an extension of an LOA. The chin points to the right sacroiliac joint.
2. *Left mentoposterior* (LMP) is an extension of an ROA. The chin points to the left sacroiliac joint.
3. *Right mentolateral* (RML) is an extension of an LOL. The chin is directed towards the right side of the pelvis.
4. *Left mentolateral* (LML) is an extension of an ROL. The chin is directed towards the left side of the pelvis.
5. *Right mentoanterior* (RMA) is an extension of an LOP. The chin points to the right iliopectineal eminence.
6. *Left mentoanterior* (LMA) is an extension of an ROP. The chin points to the left iliopectineal eminence.

Face presentation develops before the head is engaged in the pelvis. The mentum is anterior in 60% to 80% of cases, transverse in 10% to 12%, and posterior in 20% to 25%, with most rotating to the anterior (Marino 2016).

In a mentoanterior position, the extended head enters the brim of the pelvis with the face presenting. The chin points to the iliopectineal eminence, and the sinciput points to the opposite sacroiliac joint (Fig. 62.16).

The submentobregmatic diameter (9.5 cm) engages, and the face descends into the pelvis. The chin, being the lowest part, meets the resistance of the pelvic floor and rotates through one-eighth of a circle to escape under the pubic arch. The face appears at the vulval outlet (Fig. 62.17). Further uterine contractions drive the vertex and occiput over the perineum, and thus, by a movement of flexion, the head is born. Restitution and external rotation take place.

A face presentation can only be born spontaneously if the chin is anterior. There is no mechanism by which the chin can be born when it lies at the back of the pelvis. The neck is too short to span the length of the sacrum and is already at the point of maximum extension, and obstructed labour

labour will usually progress normally, with a vaginal delivery rate of 60% to 70%. However, in spite of this, in developed countries in the 21st century there is a lower threshold to move to caesarean section when face presentation is identified.

Management

In a mentoanterior position, labour often proceeds normally, although, as in any malpresentation, the membranes may rupture early, prolapse of the cord is possible and labour is sometimes prolonged. In the second stage, normal delivery is anticipated, aided by an episiotomy, because although the submentobregmatic diameter is only 9.5 cm, it is the submentovertical of 11.5 cm that distends the perineum at the time of delivery.

If there is delay in the second stage, the obstetrician will apply forceps. If normal delivery occurs, extension is maintained by applying pressure on the sinciput until the chin has escaped under the symphysis pubis; the head is then flexed to allow the vertex and occiput to sweep the perineum.

At birth, the baby is usually in good condition, although the eyelids and lips will be grossly oedematous and the face congested. The bruising and unsightly appearance can cause the mother and her partner considerable alarm and anxiety. The midwife should warn them what to expect and describe how the baby might look. The mother should be reassured that the bruising and oedema will subside within a few days and suckling, which at first may be difficult, is usually normal in 48 hours.

Brow presentation

Brow presentation (Fig. 62.19) is the least common of malpresentations. The head is midway between flexion and extension, with the mentovertical diameter of 13.5 cm attempting unsuccessfully to enter the transverse diameter of the pelvic brim. A small head might enter a large pelvis only to be arrested in the cavity.

The incidence varies from 1 in 500 to 1 in 1400 deliveries. Brow presentation may be encountered early in labour but is usually a transitional state and converts to a vertex presentation after the fetal neck flexes. Occasionally, further extension may occur, resulting in a face presentation.

The causes are, with the exception of anencephaly, the same as in face presentation, and include (Marino 2016) the following:

- Cephalopelvic disproportion
- Fetal prematurity
- Increasing parity

These account for more than 60% of cases of persistent brow presentation.

Brow presentation, undiscovered and untreated, will lead to obstructed labour, uterine rupture, and raised perinatal and maternal morbidity and mortality.

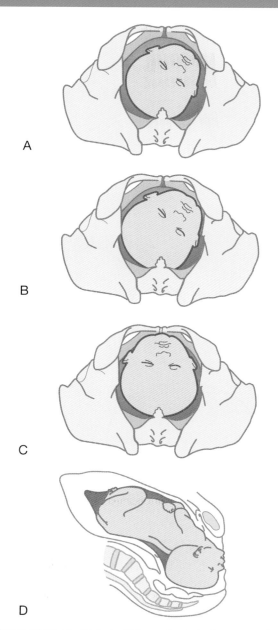

Figure 62.16 Mechanism of labour of anterior face presentation. **A,** LMA – onset of labour. **B,** Extension and descent. **C,** Vaginal view. **D,** Lateral view.

occurs (see Fig. 62.18). Spontaneous rotation of the head from the mentolateral or mentoposterior to the mentoanterior position can, and occasionally does, take place, and spontaneous delivery may then occur.

In a face presentation with the chin to the front, an adequate pelvis, a healthy fetus and good contractions, the

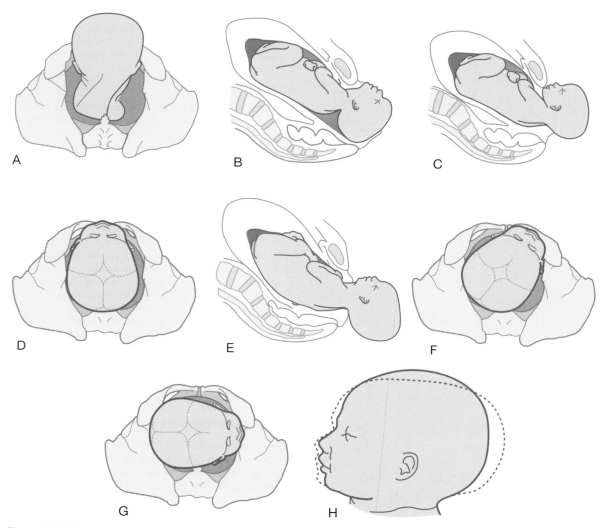

Figure 62.17 Mechanism of labour of anterior face presentation – birth of the face. **A,** Flexion. **B,** Flexion beginning. **C,** Flexion complete. **D,** Vaginal view. **E,** Lateral view. **F,** Restitution – MA to LMA. **G,** External rotation – LMA to LMT. **H,** Moulding.

Identification

On abdominal examination, the head is high, and the presenting diameter is unusually large. As with face presentation, a groove may be felt between the occiput and the back, and the cephalic prominence will be on the same side as the fetal back.

On vaginal examination, the presenting part may be too high to identify. If the brow is within reach, the orbital ridges may be felt on one side and the anterior fontanelle on the other. The diagnosis should be confirmed by ultrasound.

Management

In brow presentation, three outcomes are possible. The brow may do the following:

- convert to a vertex presentation
- convert to a face presentation, or
- remain as a persistent brow presentation.

The midwife must immediately call an obstetrician if a brow presentation is suspected or diagnosed in labour, and a woman at home should be alerted to the situation and its dangers and transferred into hospital.

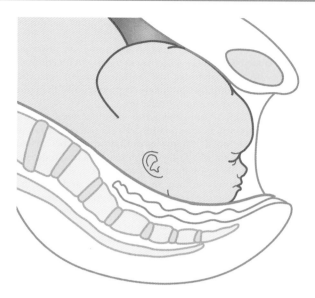

Figure 62.18 Obstructed labour with fetus in the mentoposterior position.

As in all malpresentations, the membranes are likely to rupture early, and there is a risk of cord prolapse; thus, to exclude this, a vaginal examination should be made as soon as the membranes rupture.

If a brow presentation is diagnosed early in labour, it may convert to a face presentation, becoming fully extended, or it may flex to a vertex presentation and deliver normally. If the brow presentation persists, however, and the fetus is a normal size, it will be impossible to deliver vaginally, and a caesarean section will be performed. There are few reports of brow presentations delivering vaginally (Hakmi 2008).

Oblique and transverse lie leading to shoulder presentation

A shoulder presentation occurs as a result of a transverse or an oblique lie (Fig. 62.20). Shoulder presentation is not uncommon and is only problematic if the fetus is not cephalic by 36 weeks gestation. At term, an unstable or transverse lie presents a considerable risk to both mother and fetus, with cord prolapse being more common than with a flexed vertex presentation. If uncorrected, shoulder presentation will result in obstructed labour, and unless the lie is corrected, a caesarean section is the only mode of delivery.

Causes of an unstable lie and shoulder presentation are as follows:

- Laxity of the uterine and abdominal muscles (most frequent with high parity)

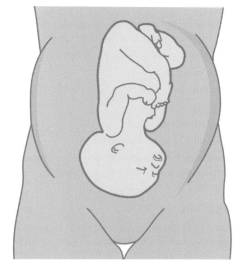

A

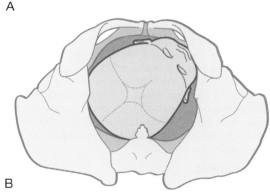

B

Figure 62.19 Brow presentation. **A,** Abdominal view. **B,** Vaginal view.

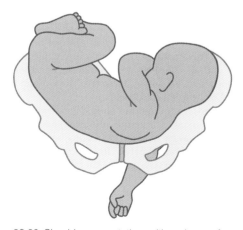

Figure 62.20 Shoulder presentation, with prolapse of one arm.

- Placenta praevia (if a woman has a persistent oblique lie, even without sentinel bleeding, placenta praevia should be considered as a possible cause).

Contributory factors include the following:

- Multiple pregnancy
- Polyhydramnios
- Uterine abnormality
- Contracted pelvis
- Occasionally, a large uterine fibroid
- An overdistended bladder, which may displace the presenting part and cause a transient oblique lie

Identification

Abdominal examination and continuity are key to making the diagnosis of an oblique, transverse or unstable lie and therefore the presence of a shoulder presentation. The abnormal lie is easily diagnosed in pregnancy from the shape of the uterus, which appears too broad, with the fetal poles felt on either side of the abdomen, whereas the fundus is unusually low. Palpation will reveal the fetal head on one side and the breech on the other and no presenting part within the pelvis.

In an oblique lie, the fetal head, or breech, is found in one or the other iliac fossa. If a nonlongitudinal lie is found after the 36th to 37th week of pregnancy, an obstetrician must be informed. Ultrasound may be used to confirm the diagnosis, identify the presentation and detect the possible cause.

Management

As pregnancy advances, a nonlongitudinal lie tends to revert to longitudinal and stabilize; however, if this does not occur, after 36 weeks gestation, the obstetrician will attempt to correct the lie by external version to a longitudinal lie and cephalic presentation. At term, labour may then be induced while the lie remains longitudinal and the presentation cephalic.

The likelihood of reversion to an oblique or transverse lie is high. The attendant risk is that the membranes may rupture and the cord or arm prolapse; or labour may commence before the lie is corrected. The woman may be admitted to hospital for observation.

Ultrasound examination should exclude placenta praevia and fetal or uterine abnormalities. A vaginal examination may be made to detect any pelvic abnormality such as a contracted pelvis. In labour, the lie is closely monitored; if necessary, gentle lateral pressure may be applied to the uterus to help maintain a longitudinal lie.

Once labour is established and the fetal head enters the pelvis, the membranes can be ruptured. Labour should then progress normally. In cases where the woman has a poor obstetric history, or if complications occur in labour,

there is likely to be early recourse to caesarean section as the safest mode of delivery.

If undetected or inadequately monitored, an unstable lie in labour is a serious obstetric emergency. With contractions, the fetal shoulder will be forced down into the pelvis, the membranes are likely to rupture, and the cord and/or the fetal arm may prolapse.

The midwife should recognize shoulder presentation during abdominal examination. Once placenta praevia has been excluded, vaginal examination can be carried out, and the fetal ribs or the hand may be felt. On detecting an unstable lie or shoulder presentation, the midwife must immediately inform an obstetrician, and if in the community, rapidly transfer the woman to hospital. Turning the woman onto all fours in an exaggerated Simms position or, alternatively, to a knee chest position is of value in displacing the shoulder and reducing the mother's urge to push. Where an arm or cord prolapses, this manoeuvre is **essential** (see Ch. 65). If the lie is uncorrected, caesarean section will be necessary, and it may well be the safest mode of delivery even when the fetus has died.

Compound presentation

Compound presentation is a presentation in which a hand or foot lies alongside the head. Very rarely, both a hand and a foot come down. This tends to occur when the fetus is small and the pelvis large or when there is any condition preventing the descent of the head into the pelvis. Lower abdominal pain and a lack of fundal dominance is often noted. The pain experienced by the mother is best dealt with through non-pharmacological means such as effleurage, where the birth partner or midwife applies light circular stroking movements to massage the mother's lower abdomen.

Compound presentation is only of significance in advanced labour when the membranes have ruptured. Usually, the limb recedes as the presenting part descends. A fetal hand may withdraw spontaneously from a gentle touch of the midwife's examining fingers. When the compound presentation persists, labour usually ends in a normal or a low instrumental delivery, with an increased risk to the mother of vaginal and perineal trauma.

POSTNATAL AND NEONATAL IMPLICATIONS

Where labour has been complicated by a malposition or malpresentation, the mother's plans and expectations for the early postnatal period may have to be revised.

Every new mother deserves kind empathetic care. The midwife should take time to document an individualized postnatal care plan as soon as possible after the birth. When drawing up a postnatal plan of care, the mother needs to be given an opportunity to talk about her needs and expectations. The conversation and ensuring management and care need to be carefully documented. A full description of postnatal care can be found in Chapter 41. Handheld notes can be used to document information given and can help the mother understand physical changes in the postnatal period, promoting her own and the baby's well-being.

Immediate care of the mother must include adequate analgesia. When analgesia is adequate the mother will be better able to mobilize and care for her baby, and the risks of remaining in bed will be reduced.

A complicated labour and birth increase the risk of puerperal complications for both mother and baby. Close liaison with the neonatal unit must be maintained if the baby requires specialist care, and the parents must be given appropriate support (see Ch. 46).

The midwife must discuss with the mother and document significant signs of illness, specifically, signs of infection and thromboembolism (Ch. 66). Following a difficult birth, especially when there may have been a period of separation from the baby, the midwife must ensure the parents recognize the infant's feeding cues and signs that the baby is feeding well (Ch. 44). Midwives must also provide verbal and written information for parents to recognize signs of illness in the newborn (Ch. 42).

A complicated birth is never planned and rarely anticipated, and the mother should be given time in the postnatal period to discuss her labour and birth when she is ready to do so. If debriefing is required, then the midwife should make appropriate referrals.

CONCLUSION

It is important that the midwife is knowledgeable about contemporary care and management of malpositions and malpresentations and is able to impart this information to the woman in a clear, realistic and accessible manner. Good preparation for labour and birth and the different strategies that might be required should be discussed before labour if possible, and a plan should be agreed on and documented, involving the whole maternity care team.

The midwife's primary role is to monitor, support and enhance the experience of the pregnancy and birth, and where there are deviations from normal, make quick and appropriate referral. Midwives should be familiar with the mechanisms of malpositions and malpresentation and the manoeuvres that they may use in facilitating birth.

It is important to inspire confidence in the mother, but midwives must also have confidence in themselves and in their ability to support the woman in her choice of birth and to manage this effectively when a malposition or malpresentation occurs.

Key Points

- Malpositions and malpresentations of the fetus may increase the risks of maternal and neonatal morbidity and mortality.

- The midwife should be able to identify women and babies at risk of malpositions and malpresentations through effective clinical assessment and take appropriate and timely action.

- The midwife should ensure that the woman and her partner feel prepared, supported and enabled to make informed choices.

- Effective communication and teamwork are crucial in the provision of safe and appropriate care to women and their babies.

- Manoeuvres and other skills based on anatomical, physiological and evidence-based principles should be practised on a regular basis by those providing care to women and their babies.

References

Aitken AR, Aitken CE, Alberry MS, et al: Management of fetal malposition in the second stage of labor: a propensity score analysis, *Am J Obstet Gynecol* 212(355):1–7, 2015.

Akmal S, Paterson-Brown S: Malpositions and malpresentations of the fetal head, *Obstetrics, Gynaecology, and Reproductive Medicine* 19(9):240–246, 2009.

Berhan Y, Haileamlak A: The risks of planned vaginal breech delivery versus planned caesarean section for term breech birth: a meta-analysis including observational studies, *Br J Obstet Gynaecol* 123(1):49–57, 2015.

Collins S, Ellaway P, Harrington D, et al: The complications of external cephalic version: results from 805 consecutive attempts, *Br J Obstet Gynaecol* 114(5):636–638, 2007.

Coyle ME, Smith CA, Peat B: Cephalic version by moxibustion for breech presentation, *Cochrane Database Syst Rev* (5):CD003928, 2012.

Cronk M: Hands off that breech! *Aims Journal* 17(1):3–4, 2005.

Desbriere R, Blanc J, Le Dû R, et al: Is maternal posturing during labor efficient in preventing persistent occiput posterior position? A randomized controlled trial,

Am J Obstet Gynecol 208(60):1–8, 2013.

Evans J: *Breech birth: what are my options?* London, AIMS Publications, 2005.

Evans J: First do no harm, *Pract Midwife* 10(8):22–23, 2007.

Gardberg M, Tuppurainen M: Persistent occiput posterior presentation – a clinical problem, *Acta Obstetrica Gynecologica Scandinavia* 73(1):45–47, 1994a.

Gardberg M, Tuppurainen M: Anterior placental location predisposes for occiput posterior presentation near term, *Acta Obstet Gynecol Scand* 73(2):151–152, 1994b.

Gardberg M, Laakkonen E, Salevaara M: Intrapartum sonography and persistent occiput posterior position: a study of 408 deliveries, *Obstet Gynecol* 91(5 Pt 1):746–749, 1998.

Gardberg M, Leonova Y, Laakkonen E: Malpresentations – impact upon mode of delivery, *Acta Obstet Gynecol Scand* 90(5):540–542, 2011.

Glezerman M: Five years to the term breech trial: the rise and fall of a randomized controlled trial, *Am J Obstet Gynecol* 194(1):20–25, 2006.

Goffinet F, Carayol M, Foidart JM, et al: Is planned vaginal delivery for breech presentation at term still an option? Results of an observational prospective study in France and Belgium, *Am J Obstet Gynecol* 194(4):1002–1011, 2006.

Graham K, Phipps H, Hyett JA, et al: Persistent occiput posterior: outcomes following digital rotation: A pilot randomized controlled trial, *Aust N Z J Obstet Gynaecol* 54:268–274, 2014.

Hakmi A: Brow presentation does not mean cesarean section, *J Obstet Gynaecol* 28(2):255–256, 2008.

Hannah ME, Hannah WJ, Hewson SA, et al: Term Breech Trial Collaborative Group: planned caesarean section versus planned vaginal birth for breech presentation at term: a randomised multicentre trial, *The Lancet* 356(9239):1375–1383, 2000.

Hofmeyr GJ, Kulier R: Cephalic version by postural management for breech presentation, *Cochrane Database Syst Rev* (10):CD000051, 2012.

Hofmeyr G, Hannah M, Lawrie TA: Planned caesarean section for term breech delivery, *Cochrane Database Syst Rev* (7):CD000166, 2015a.

Hofmeyr G, Kulier R, West HM: External cephalic version for breech presentation at term, *Cochrane Database Syst Rev* (4):CD000083, 2015b.

Hofmeyr G, Kulier R, West HM: Expedited versus conservative approaches for vaginal delivery in breech presentation, *Cochrane Database Syst Rev* (7):CD000082, 2015c.

Hunter S, Hofmeyr GJ, Kulier R: Hands and knees posture in late pregnancy or labour for fetal malposition (lateral or posterior), *Cochrane Database Syst Rev* (4):CD001063, 2007.

Hutton EK, Hofmeyr G, Dowswell T: External cephalic version for breech presentation before term, *Cochrane Database Syst Rev* (7):CD000084, 2015.

Kotaska A: Inappropriate use of randomised trials to evaluate complex phenomena: case study of vaginal breech delivery, *Br Med J* 329:1039–1042, 2004.

Kotaska A, Menticoglou S, Gagnon R, et al: Maternal Fetal Medicine Committee, Society of Obstetricians and Gynaecologists of Canada: vaginal delivery of breech presentation, *J Obstet Gynaecol Can* 31(6):557–566, 2009.

Lumbiganon P, Laopaiboon M, Gulmezoglu AM, et al: Method of delivery and pregnancy outcomes in Asia: the WHO global survey on maternal and perinatal health 2007-2008, *Lancet* 375:490–499, 2010.

Marino T: Face and brow presentation. http://emedicine.medscape.com/article/262341-overview#a1. 2016.

Marshall JE: Facilitating vaginal breech at term. In Marshall JE, Raynor MD, editors: *Advancing skills in midwifery practice*, Edinburgh, Churchill Livingstone/Elsevier, pp 89–102, 2010.

Munro J, Jokinen M: *Persistent lateral and posterior fetal positions at the onset of labour in evidence based guidelines for midwifery-led care in labour*. Royal College of Midwives Trust (website). www.rcm.org.uk/sites/default/files/Persistent%20Lateral%20and%20Posterior%20Fetal%20Positions%20%20at%20

the%20Onset%20of%20Labour.pdf. 2012.

National Institute for Health and Care Excellence (NICE): *NICE guidelines [CG190]. Intrapartum care: care of healthy women and their babies during childbirth* (website). www.nice.org.uk/guidance/cg190/chapter/1-recommendations#pain-relief-in-labour-regional-analgesia. 2014.

Nursing and Midwifery Council (NMC): Midwives rules and standards 2012 (website). www.nmc.org.uk/globalassets/siteDocuments/NMC-publications/Midwives-Rules-and-Standards-2012.pdf. 2012.

Nursing and Midwifery Council (NMC): *The Code: professional standards of practice and behaviour for nurses and midwives* (website). www.nmc.org.uk/standards/code/www.nmc-uk.org/code. 2015.

Peregrine E, O'Brien P, Jauniaux E: Impact on delivery of ultrasonographic fetal head position prior to induction of labour, *Obstet Gynecol* 109(3): 618–625, 2007.

Phipps H, de Vries B, Hyett J: Prophylactic manual rotation for fetal malposition to reduce operative delivery, *Cochrane Database Syst Rev* (12):CD009298, 2014.

Rielberg CCT, Elferink-Stinkens PM, Visser GHA: The effect of the Term Breech Trial on medical intervention behaviour and neonatal outcome in the Netherlands: an analysis of 35,453 term breech infants, *Br J Obstet Gynaecol* 112:205–209, 2005.

Royal College of Obstetricians and Gynaecologists (RCOG): External cephalic version and reducing the incidence of breech presentation (Greentop Guideline No. 20b. reviewed 2010) (website). www.rcog.org.uk/files/rcog-corp/uploaded-files/GT20aExternal Cephalica2006.pdf. 2006a.

Royal College of Obstetricians and Gynaecologists (RCOG): The management of breech presentation (Greentop Guideline No. 20b) (website). www.rcog.org.uk/files/rcog-corp/uploaded-files/GT20bManagement_ofBreechPresentation.pdf. 2006b.

Shushan A, Younis JS: McRoberts manoeuvre for the management of the aftercoming head in breech delivery, *Gynecol Obstet Invest* 34(3):188–189, 1992.

Simkin P: The fetal occiput posterior position: state of the science and a new perspective, *Birth* 37(1):61–71, 2010.

Stremler R, Hodnett E, Petryshen P, et al: Randomised controlled trial of hands and knees positioning for occipitoposterior position in labour, *Birth* 32:243–251, 2005.

Tapisiz OL, Aytan H, Altinbas SK, et al: Face presentation at term:

a forgotten issue, *J Obstet Gynaecol Res* 40(6):1573–1577, 2014.

Van Idderkinge B: Planned vaginal breech delivery: should this be the mode of choice? *Obstetrics and Gynaecology* 9(3):171–176, 2007.

Waites B: *Breech birth*, London, Free Association Books, pp 67–78, 2003.

Walker S, Sabrosa R: Assessment of fetal presentation: exploring a woman-centred approach, *Br J Midwifery* 22(4):240–244, 2014.

Walmsley K: Managing the OP labour, *MIDIRS Midwifery Digest* 10:61–62, 2000.

Whyte H, Hannah M, Saigal S: Outcomes of children at two years after planned cesarean birth vs planned vaginal birth for breech presentation at term: the international randomised Term Breech Trial, *Am J Obstet Gynecol* 191(3):864–871, 2004.

Resources and additional reading

See also the chapter website for more information.

General issues

Permezel M, Walker S, Kyprianou K: *Beischer and Mackay's obstetrics, gynaecology and the newborn*, 4th edn, London, Elsevier, 2015.

A useful illustrated textbook from Australia-based obstetricians.

Antenatal examination of the abdomen

https://www.youtube.com/watch?v=xb12IkpbfTQ.

This is a UK-based video clip of the abdominal examination from Kings/ Guys and St. Thomas that includes preparation for objective structured clinical examinations (OSCEs).

www.youtube.com/watch?v=nIog3oizP8A.

This U.S.-based video clip provides a systematic examination, including the Leopold manoeuvres.

Posterior fetal positions

Royal College of Midwives (RCM): Royal College of Midwives evidence based guidelines for midwifery-led care in labour (website). www.rcm.org.uk/clinical-practice -and-guidance/evidence-based -guidelines. 2012.

Includes a range of issues, including positions for labour and birth and persistent lateral and posterior fetal positions at the onset of labour.

National Institute for Health and Care Excellence (NICE) – evidence search: https://www.evidence.nhs.uk.

Useful source of evidence-based information; updated on a regular basis.

Vaginal delivery after manual rotation (query bank) www.rcog.org.uk.

The query bank is a useful resource on the RCOG website often giving answers to clinical queries not given elsewhere.

'Spinning Babies'

http://spinningbabies.com.

Although 'spinning babies' seems to be popular there is no evidence to suggest that this is any more than normal rotation in action and may be misinforming both midwives and mothers.

Breech

Royal College of Obstetricians and Gynaecologists (RCOG): A breech baby at the end of pregnancy (website). www.rcog.org.uk/ globalassets/documents/patients/ patient-information-leaflets/ pregnancy/a-breech-baby-at-the-end -of-pregnancy.pdf. 2008.

Useful and very clear leaflet for women on breech presentation at the end of pregnancy.

National Childbirth Trust (NCT): *Breech babies and birth* (website). www.nct .org.uk/birth/breech-birth. 2015.

Useful and comprehensive information on breech birth for women and their families.

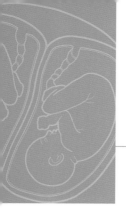

Chapter 63

Obstructed labour and uterine rupture

Alison Brodrick

Learning Outcomes ?

By the end of this chapter, you will be able to:

- understand the consequences of obstructed labour
- describe the risk factors associated with ruptured uterus
- recognize signs of obstructed labour
- articulate the different types of uterine rupture
- describe the incidence rates of uterine rupture

INTRODUCTION

Obstructed labour occurs when the fetus is unable to descend through the birth canal despite the presence of good uterine contractions.

In the developed world, which has good antenatal and intrapartum care and access to skilled practitioners, an obstructed labour is usually identified promptly, and appropriate, timely intervention is taken. In developing countries, however, it is often a very different scenario. With limited access to healthcare, poor nutrition and poverty, higher rates of obstructed labour lead to significant maternal morbidity and mortality (Oyston et al 2014). In addition, it is a significant contributor to perinatal morbidity and mortality.

It is important to distinguish between slow progress or delay in labour and obstructed labour. When cervical dilatation and descent slows, the most likely cause is ineffective uterine contractions – when good contractions resume, dilation and descent will also resume. In obstructed labour, the fetus cannot descend through the pelvis in spite of effective uterine contractions. In obstructed labour, vaginal birth is mechanically impossible.

Morbidity and mortality associated with obstructed labour

Estimation of rates and sequelae of prolonged labour is difficult because it relies on each country maintaining consistent data and epidemiological studies using the same definition of prolonged labour. Also, without access to healthcare, women in obstructed labour die from haemorrhage, sepsis or uterine rupture, all terminal conditions that may be listed as the cause of death. Hence the actual numbers of women dying as a result of obstructed labour may be higher (Oyston et al 2014).

In 2013, obstructed labour accounted for 18,789 deaths worldwide, with huge variation from country to country. Almost 62% of these deaths occurred in western sub-Saharan Africa (n = 7099) and South Asia (n = 4521), whereas in Australasia just two deaths occurred from obstructed labour (Kassebaum et al 2014).

When obstructed labour is prolonged, the presenting part is impacted against the soft tissues of the pelvis, causing ischaemic vascular injury, tissue necrosis and formation of an obstetric fistula.

An obstetric fistula is an abnormal channel between the rectum and vagina (rectovaginal fistula) or the bladder and vagina (vesicovaginal fistula). According to the United Nations Population Fund (UNFPA), as many as 3 million women are believed to suffer from obstetric fistula, and another 30,000 to 130,000 cases develop each year in Africa alone (Wall 2006).

Women suffering obstetric fistula live physically challenging lives with limited or no access to treatment; there are also huge social ramifications, with victims being banned from their homes and shunned by their communities (World Health Organization (WHO) 2005).

Through timely diagnosis and treatment of obstructed labour, maternal death and obstetric fistula can be prevented, but this requires access to emergency obstetric care, something that remains unavailable to most mothers in developing countries (Paxton et al 2006).

OBSTRUCTED LABOUR

Causes

Cephalopelvic disproportion occurs when there is an anatomical disproportion between the fetal head and the maternal pelvis. This occurs because the pelvis is too small or is abnormal in shape or because the fetus is abnormal or too large for the pelvis through which it has to pass.

The head is the largest part of the fetus; once it has passed through the brim of the pelvis, the rest of the fetus should pass through without difficulty. The probability is that the cavity and outlet are also of adequate dimensions to accommodate the passage of a normal fetus. However, in practice, there can be cephalopelvic disproportion at the cavity or outlet of the pelvis too. It is important to appreciate and recognize the different types of pelves and how these may influence the way the fetal head negotiates its passage through the bony canal.

Problems associated with the anatomical shape of the pelvis are rare; however, such problems should be considered if the following uncommon conditions present:

- Medical conditions, such as rickets or osteomalacia, that could adversely affect the size and shape of the pelvis
- Spinal deformities such as scoliosis
- Pelvic fractures or injuries that may have altered the normal shape and dimensions of the pelvis

It is well documented that poor childhood nutrition and subsequent compromised growth in females may result in contracted pelvic dimensions and elevated risk of cephalopelvic disproportion (Kirk 2011). This may apply to migrant populations from poorer countries that settle in the UK, although this has not yet been highlighted as a problem in the literature.

The size of the fetus can also have an effect. A baby over the 97th percentile may be too large to pass through the pelvis. This may be a result of high parity, prolonged pregnancy or diabetes. Women who are overweight and obese are also more likely to produce a baby over the 97th percentile (Heslehurst et al 2008).

The issue of increased maternal body mass index (BMI) is important to consider because obesity levels worldwide continue to increase. In obese women, myometrial contractibility is reduced, often leading to prolonged labour and higher deposits of pelvic fat that can obstruct the birth canal and lead to obstructed labour (Zhang et al 2007).

Cephalopelvic disproportion should not be confused with disproportion attributable to malposition, with a deflexed head and asynclitism presenting with a larger diameter (e.g. occipitoposterior position). Good uterine contractions with judicious use of Syntocinon if needed can remedy a relative disproportion because the contractions cause flexion and rotation.

Skilled assessment and observation are needed to diagnose genuine cephalopelvic disproportion when the vertex is in the occipitoanterior position and unable to descend, causing relative disproportion as a result of deflexion and malposition of the head.

Other rarer causes of obstructed labour include the following:

- Malpresentations, such as shoulder, brow and persistent mentoposterior face presentations
- The available space in the pelvis being occupied by a large tumour, for example, a fibroid or an ovarian cyst
- An unusually large or abnormal fetus with a condition such as hydrocephalus

Identifying obstructed labour

In normal labour, effective uterine contractions aid descent of the presenting part and dilatation of the cervix. Descent of the presenting part is an important sign of normal labour progress; in obstructed labour, the presenting part remains high or descends initially and then is unable to descend any further. This results in a poorly applied presenting part at the cervix, and the cervix can be slow to dilate or may dilate initially and then arrest.

If the condition is allowed to continue, the contractions become longer, stronger and more frequent in an effort to overcome the obstruction, until, eventually, tonic contractions occur. Uterine exhaustion may occur, especially in the primigravida, when the contractions cease for a while and then restart with renewed vigour.

Table 63.1 provides the clinical indications of obstructed labor.

In advanced obstructed labour, an oblique ridge may actually be seen running across the abdomen. This is Bandl's retraction ring and denotes a marked difference in thickness between the tonically retracted upper uterine segment and the dangerously thinned lower segment (Fig. 63.1). The continuous retraction cuts off the fetal oxygen supply, resulting in fetal demise. At this stage there is a high risk of uterine rupture and maternal death unless timely intervention is available.

Management

Most cases of definite obstructed labour will occur in the first stage of labour, and a caesarean section will be indicated. In the second stage of labour, early recognition of conditions such as deep transverse arrest is essential so that a rotation may be possible and a vaginal birth achieved.

In developing countries, where a woman can be in obstructed labour for a number of days, resulting in sepsis and maternal exhaustion, there is still a place for procedures such as symphysiotomy, which can be life-saving

Table 63.1 Clinical indications of obstructed labour

Maternal signs	Tachycardia Pyrexia Oliguria Haematuria Maternal exhaustion Severe and continual pain
Abdominal examination	Presenting part remains high Absence of liquor Uterus is closely moulded around the baby Uterus feels hard
Vaginal examination	Vagina is hot and dry Increased caput and moulding Oedematous cervix Slow or no progress in cervical dilatation
Fetal signs	Early and variable decelerations suggestive of head compression

Source: El-Hamamy and Arulkumaran 2005

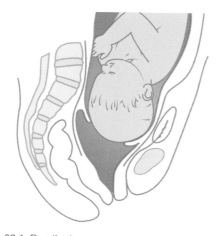

Figure 63.1 Band's ring.

interventions (Wykes et al 2003). Symphysiotomy also carries less risk than performing a caesarean section if access to such facilities is available. If the fetus is already dead, destructive practices such as craniotomy and cleidotomy may be required to save the mother (Maharaj and Moodley 2002).

Prevention

Labour is a dynamic process, and there are many causes of slow progress or delay in labour, including environmental and maternal psychological factors (Walsh and Devane 2012; see also Ch. 36). As discussed earlier, true definite obstructed labour is rare and is very difficult to predict in a primigravida before the onset of labour. The most reliable assessment of pelvic ability is the previous uncomplicated labour and birth of a baby of similar weight.

Over the years, efforts have been made to identify women at risk of obstructed labour; these have included assessing maternal height and shoe size (Mahmood et al 1988), fetal weight and maternal age (Dahan and Dahan 2005) and measuring maternal pelvic dimensions using radiological pelvimetry (Pattinson 2000). All of these parameters have been proven to be unsatisfactory in predicting obstructed labour and pelvic competence; therefore, the only valid method to diagnose cephalopelvic disproportion is a retrospective assessment of the labour outcome (Korhonen et al 2015).

Use of the partogram has been shown to play an important role in some resource-poor countries (Kavya Mahesh and Hariharan 2014), enabling early recognition of obstructed labour and a timely transfer to the tertiary unit. The aim is to prevent the negative sequelae associated with obstructed labour. Although the partogram is endorsed by WHO (1988) and adopted worldwide as an integral component of intrapartum care, in the developed world its primary aim of preventing obstructed labour has been questioned (Lavender et al 2008).

In the developing world, it is hoped that actualization of the Millennium Development Goals will result in a reduction in the morbidity and mortality associated with obstructed labour. This is a difficult task because of the lack of infrastructure, equipment and knowledge in addition to geographical, sociocultural and political barriers (Oyston et al 2014).

Reflective activity 63.1

Marie is 36 years of age; she is a primigravida with a BMI of 39. You have just taken over her care, and you notice Marie is tired and tearful. She is very worried because everyone has been telling her that her baby is big, and her mother had three caesareans. On palpation, you notice that the head is not engaged in the pelvis. On examination, the cervix is loosely applied, and the dilatation has stayed the same at 8 cm. What other observations might you now look for? What would your initial management involve?

UTERINE RUPTURE

Rupture of the uterus is a serious complication of labour resulting in high rates of fetal and maternal death. It is more prevalent and severe in developing countries, where the majority of uterine ruptures are a result of obstructed labour and rates as high as 75% have been reported in women with an unscarred uterus (Hofmeyr et al 2005). In the developed world, uterine rupture is rare and is usually associated with dehiscence and extension of a uterine scar.

Types of uterine rupture

It is important to understand and differentiate between the different types of uterine rupture:

Complete or true rupture: This involves the full thickness of the uterine wall and pelvic peritoneum, with extrusion of fetal parts and intraamniotic contents into the peritoneal cavity (Ofir et al 2004).

Incomplete rupture: This involves the myometrium but not the pelvic peritoneum, which remains intact. It is sometimes called occult or silent rupture, and commonly it is called dehiscence; this is more common than a complete rupture. Incomplete rupture is more frequently associated with a previous lower-segment caesarean section scar and tends to present with less violent and dramatic signs and symptoms, possibly because of the avascular nature of the scar tissue.

The true incidence and risk factors for ruptured uterus can be difficult to determine from the medical literature because studies have used different interpretations of what constitutes a ruptured uterus (Hofmeyr et al 2005). Some only include a complete rupture, whereas others do not distinguish between complete and incomplete ruptures.

The UK's largest national population-based case-control study using the UK Obstetric Surveillance System (UKOSS) has reported the incidence rate and features of complete uterine rupture in the UK, excluding incidental asymptomatic uterine dehiscence. For all maternities the rate is reported at 0.2 per 1000. For women aiming for a vaginal birth after one caesarean, the risk is quoted as 2.1 per 1000 compared with 0.3 for women planning a repeat caesarean (Fitzpatrick et al 2012). In the MBRRACE UK report (2009–2012), four women were reported as having died as a result of uterine rupture; none had a scar on the uterus, and three of the cases involved oxytocic drug use to augment or induce labour (Knight et al 2014).

Risk factors

In the developed world, the main risk factor for uterine rupture is still a scarred uterus, and this is particularly relevant given the global rise in primary caesarean section rates. However, rates of rupture will vary according to a variety of associated risk factors, including pregnancy planning interval and uterine closure technique (Roberge et al 2011).

Rupture in a scarred uterus

The most common reason for rupture in a scarred uterus is rupture of a previous lower-segment caesarean scar, although any other surgery to the uterus or investigations such as hysteroscopy can also cause damage to the uterus. During these procedures, trauma or perforation, which is not always recognized, may lead to a scarred uterus, which can result in rupture in a subsequent pregnancy, usually at the fundus (Hockstein 2000).

Although it is rarely seen in the UK, the risk of rupture in women with a classical scar (a longitudinal scar in the body of the uterus) is increased, and an elective caesarean section is usually advised in a subsequent pregnancy at approximately 38 weeks gestation. The evidence regarding rupture rates after two or more caesareans is conflicting. This is mainly a result of the small numbers of women having two or more caesareans in the Western world and the resultant difficulty of being able to sufficiently power a large study.

It is generally accepted, however, that the rate increases with each caesarean section (Guise 2005). In the UK, women who choose to labour after two or more caesareans should be supported in their decision, provided they have been counselled regarding the increased risk of rupture, hysterectomy and blood transfusion (Royal College of Obstetricians and Gynaecologists (RCOG) 2015). Shared decision making in these cases is paramount, looking at the full clinical picture, considering maternal characteristics (Guise 2005) and listening to the mother's wishes.

Rupture in an unscarred uterus

In an unscarred uterus the rupture is often more traumatic in nature and associated with an increase in morbidity and mortality for the mother and newborn (Lao and Leung 1987).

A traumatic rupture of an unscarred uterus is often caused by the following:

- Misuse of oxytocic drugs and prostaglandins
- Use of instruments
- Intra-uterine manipulations

The misuse of oxytocic drugs and uterine stimulants is a dominant predisposing risk factor for ruptured uterus (Knight et al 2014; Grossetti et al 2007; Kayani and Alfirevic 2005). Great care must be exercised in the use of oxytocic drugs for inducing or augmenting labour, especially in multiparous women because hypertonic contractions are more easily stimulated. There is also an increased risk of uterine rupture in women with an intra-uterine fetal death. When there is no concern for fetal well-being, higher levels of oxytocic drugs, which are often needed to induce the labour, may be administered without the same degree of caution exercised with a live fetus.

An association is also observed with cephalopelvic disproportion, malpresentation, and delivery of a macrosomic fetus (Ofir et al 2004; Miller et al 1997; Sweeten et al 1995).

Less common is a spontaneous rupture in an unscarred uterus; this may occur as a result of very strong uterine contractions (not induced or augmented by the use of oxytocic drugs) and tends to be associated with grand multiparity. Abruptio placentae can increase the risk because of disruption and distension of the uterine wall. Some cases of spontaneous rupture in a primigravida with an unscarred uterus have been discussed by authors (Shreya et al 2014), but this is a rare occurrence.

The exact cause is not always clear, and although other risk factors such as advanced maternal age (Shipp et al 2002) have been discussed, the infrequency of uterine rupture can make it difficult to draw robust conclusions.

When rupture occurs in an unscarred uterus, it tends to be longitudinal tears. Cases in the literature describe a cervical tear that extends longitudinally into the lower uterine segment, either anteriorly or posteriorly, resulting in serious haemorrhage because of the poor retraction (Eden et al 1986; Golan et al 1980). Tears may further extend into the vascular upper uterine segment, thereby increasing morbidity and mortality. In some cases, a rupture may occur in the upper uterine segment only.

Signs and symptoms

Complete rupture of the uterus often presents as an acute event with dramatic maternal collapse. An incomplete rupture is far less dramatic and often difficult to diagnose. Sometimes it is diagnosed after the birth or at caesarean section.

Table 63.2 lists the commonly reported clinical signs of uterine rupture. This is not meant as a definitive list; women will often present in different ways and with varying symptoms.

The most significant marker for diagnosing obstructed labour is considered to be a non-reassuring fetal heart-rate tracing, typically with significant variable decelerations and/or bradycardia (Fitzpatrick et al 2012). Using continuous fetal heart monitoring is therefore recommended for all women labouring with a previous scar.

Management

The initial management will depend on the maternal and fetal condition. If the mother is already compromised, her airway, breathing and circulation will need to be assessed and fluid resuscitation commenced. Immediate preparation for surgery, either caesarean section or, if the rupture is suspected after delivery, laparotomy. Once the baby is delivered and the obstetrician has identified the type,

Table 63.2	Uterine rupture signs and symptoms
Complete rupture	**Incomplete rupture**
Constant abdominal pain	Scar tenderness*
Reduction or cessation of contractions	Reduction or cessation of contractions
Fetal distress	Maternal tachycardia
Fetus may be palpated in the abdomen	Vaginal bleeding
Maternal collapse	Shoulder pain
	Anxiety
	Restlessness
	Dizziness
	Fetal distress
	Maternal collapse

*Although abdominal pain and scar tenderness are regarded as classical signs, these symptoms do not present in many cases

location and extent of the rupture, the following surgical options usually apply:

- Simple repair of the rupture – the treatment of choice whenever possible (Lim et al 2005; Mesleh et al 1999)

- Uterine and internal hypogastric artery ligation to control haemorrhage

- Hysterectomy may be necessary

Aftercare

It is essential that women and their families be provided with a clear explanation of the events and the implications for future pregnancies. Depending on the severity of the incident, the family may need to talk at different time points in their postnatal journey. The psychological impact for the mother and her partner should not be underestimated; Souza et al (2009) examined women's experience of a 'near miss' emergency in pregnancy and childbirth and found that women experienced a feeling of fear, grief, and imminence of death. It is important that any psychological morbidity does not go unrecognized because it can have long-term consequences for the mother (Ayers et al 2006). Appropriate communication between maternity services and primary care providers is essential to ensure ongoing assessment and treatment.

Reflective activity 63.2

How would you present the evidence to enable a woman to make an informed choice about mode and place of birth after one caesarean section?

CONCLUSION

Globally, many women die as a result of obstructed labour and the lack of available emergency care. In the developed world, the morbidity and mortality that can be associated with obstructed labour are usually avoided by timely intervention. Complete uterine rupture, which can result from an obstructed labour, is also a rare event in the UK. For women who have had a caesarean section, it is important that appropriate and accurate data are used to support informed decisions regarding mode of birth in subsequent pregnancies.

Key Points

- Obstructed labour requires early recognition and management; in developing countries, it is a major contributor to maternal morbidity and mortality.

- In developing countries, using a partogram can aid early recognition of obstructed labour. In developed countries, the widespread adoption of partograms is of unproven benefit.

- There are no proven techniques for diagnosing cephalopelvic disproportion during pregnancy.

- During labour, appropriate monitoring of descent and progress should ensure timely diagnosis of cephalopelvic disproportion.

- In the UK, the rate of complete rupture associated with previous caesarean scar is reported to be 1:500.

- Any scar on the uterus may rupture during labour, and the likelihood increases when oxytocin and prostaglandins are used.

- Women may need psychological support following an unexpected traumatic event.

References

Ayers S, Eagle A, Waring H: The effects of childbirth-related post-traumatic stress disorder on women and their relationships: a qualitative study, *Psychol Health Med* 11(4):389–398, 2006.

Dahan MH, Dahan S: Fetal weight, maternal age and height are poor predictors of the need for caesarean section for arrest of labor, *Arch Gynecol Obstet* 273(1):20–25, 2005.

Eden RD, Parker RT, Gall SA: Rupture of the pregnant uterus: a 53-year review, *Obstet Gynecol* 68(5):671–674, 1986.

El-Hamamy E, Arulkumaran E: Poor progress of labour, *Curr Obstet Gynaecol* 15(1):1–8, 2005.

Fitzpatrick KE, Kurinczuk JJ, Alfirevic ZP, et al: Uterine rupture by intended mode of delivery in the UK: a national case-control study, *PLoS Med* 9(3):e1001184, 2012.

Golan A, Sandbank O, Rubin A: Rupture of the pregnant uterus, *Obstet Gynecol* 56(5):549–554, 1980.

Grossetti E, Vardon D, Creveuil C, et al: Rupture of the scarred uterus, *Acta Obstet Gynecol Scand* 86(5):572–578, 2007.

Guise J: Evidence-based vaginal birth after caesarean section, *Best Pract Res Clin Obstet Gynaecol* 19(1):117–130, 2005.

Heslehurst N, Simpson H, Ells LJ, et al: The impact of maternal BMI status on pregnancy outcomes with immediate short-term obstetric resource implications: a meta-analysis, *Obes Rev* 9:635–683, 2008.

Hockstein S: Spontaneous uterine rupture in the early third trimester after laparoscopically assisted myomectomy, *J Reprod Med* 45(2):139–141, 2000.

Hofmeyr GJ, Say L, Gülmezoglu AM: WHO systematic review of maternal mortality and morbidity: the prevalence of uterine rupture, *Br J Obstet Gynaecol* 112(9):1221, 2005.

Kassebaum NJ, et al: Global, regional, and national levels and causes of maternal mortality during

1990–2013: a systematic analysis for the Global Burden of Disease Study 2013, *Lancet* 384(9947):980–1004, 2014.

Kavya Mahesh P, Hariharan C: Role of partogram in the management of spontaneous labour in primigravida and multigravida, *International Journal of Reproduction* 3(4):1043, 2014.

Kayani SI, Alfirevic Z: Uterine rupture after induction of labour in women with previous caesarean section, *Br J Obstet Gynaecol* 112(4):451–455, 2005.

Kirk H: Compromised skeletal growth? Small body size and clinical contraction thresholds for the female pelvic canal, *International Journal of Paleopathology* 3–4(1):138–149, 2011.

Knight M, Kenyon S, Brocklehurst P, et al on behalf of MBRRACE-UK, editors: *Saving lives, improving mothers' care – lessons learned to inform future maternity care from the UK and Ireland Confidential Enquiries into Maternal Deaths and Morbidity*

2009–12, Oxford, National Perinatal Epidemiology Unit, University of Oxford, 2014.

Korhonen U, Taipale P, Heinonen S: Fetal pelvic index to predict cephalopelvic disproportion – a retrospective clinical cohort study, *Acta Obstet Gynecol Scand* 94(6):615–621, 2015.

Lao TT, Leung BFH: Rupture of the gravid uterus, *Eur J Obstet Gynecol* 25(3):175–180, 1987.

Lavender T, Tsekiri E, Baker L: Recording labour: a national survey of partogram use, *Br J Midwifery* 16(6):359–362, 2008.

Lim AC, Kwee A, Bruinse HW: Pregnancy after uterine rupture – a report of 5 cases and a review of the literature, *Obstet Gynecol Surv* 60(9):613–617, 2005.

Maharaj D, Moodley J: Symphysiotomy and fetal destructive operations, *Best Pract Res Clin Obstet Gynaecol* 16(1):117–131, 2002.

Mahmood TA, Campbell DM, Wilson AW: Maternal height, shoe size, and outcome of labour in white primigravidas: a prospective anthropometric study, *Br Med J* 297(6647):515, 1988.

Mesleh R, Kurdi A, Algwiser A, et al: Intrapartum rupture of the gravid uterus, *Saudi Med J* 20(7):531–535, 1999.

Miller AD, Goodwin MT, Gherman BR, et al: Intrapartum rupture of the unscarred uterus, *Obstet Gynecol* 89(5):671–673, 1997.

Ofir K, Sheiner E, Levy A, et al: Uterine rupture: differences between a scarred and an unscarred uterus, *Am J Obstet Gynecol* 191(2):425–429, 2004.

Oyston C, Rueda-Clausen CF, Baker PN: Current challenges in pregnancy-related mortality, *Obstetrics, Gynaecology and Reproductive Medicine* 24(6):162–169, 2014.

Pattinson RC: Pelvimetry for fetal cephalic presentations at term, *Cochrane Database Syst Rev* (2):CD000161, 2000.

Paxton A, Bailey P, Lobis S, et al: Global patterns in availability of emergency obstetric care, *Int J Gynaecol Obstet* 93(3):300–307, 2006.

Roberge S, Chaillet N, Boutin A, et al: Single- versus double-layer closure of the hysterotomy incision during cesarean delivery and risk of uterine rupture, *Int J Gynecol Obstet* 115(1):5–10, 2011.

Royal College Obstetricians and Gynaecologists (RCOG): *Birth after previous caesarean birth*, Greentop Guideline No. 45, London, RCOG, 2015.

Shipp TD, Zelop C, Repke JT, et al: The association of maternal age and symptomatic uterine rupture during a trial of labor after prior cesarean delivery, *Obstet Gynecol* 99(4):58, 2002.

Shreya T, Anjali R, Uma P, et al: Spontaneous unscarred fundal rupture after normal vaginal delivery, *International Journal of Reproduction* 3(3):780, 2014.

Souza JP, Cecatti JG, Parpinelli MA, et al: An emerging "maternal near-miss syndrome": narratives of women who almost died during pregnancy and childbirth, *Birth* 36(2):149–158, 2009.

Sweeten KM, Graves WK, Athanassiou A: Spontaneous rupture of the unscarred uterus, *Am J Obstet Gynecol* 172(6):1851–1856, 1995.

Wall LL: Obstetric vesicovaginal fistula as an international public-health problem, *Lancet* 368:1201–1209, 2006.

Walsh D, Devane DA: Metasynthesis of midwife-led care, *Qual Health Res* 22(7):897–910, 2012.

World Health Organization (WHO): The partograph: a managerial tool for the prevention of prolonged labour. In WHO, editor: *Section 1: The principle and strategy. WHO Document No. WHO/MCH/88.3*, Geneva, WHO, 1988.

World Health Organization (WHO): Lerberghe WV, editor: *The world health report 2005: make every mother and child count*, Geneva, WHO, 2005.

Wykes CB, Johnston TA, Paterson-Brown S, et al: Symphysiotomy: a lifesaving procedure, *Br J Obstet Gynaecol* 110(2):219–221, 2003.

Zhang J, Bricker L, Wray S, et al: Poor uterine contractility in obese women, *Br J Obstet Gynaecol* 114(3):343–348, 2007.

Resources and additional reading

World Health Organization (WHO): *Recommended interventions for improving maternal and newborn health* (website). www.who.int/maternal_child_adolescent/documents/who_mps_0705/en/.

WHO's list of the interventions that are the desirable standard and should be available to all women during pregnancy, delivery and postpartum.

Chapter 64

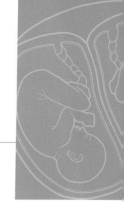

Shoulder dystocia

Terri Coates

Learning Outcomes ?

After reading this chapter, you will be able to:

- identify risk factors for shoulder dystocia
- describe shoulder dystocia
- describe the signs that would be diagnostic for shoulder dystocia
- demonstrate manoeuvres that are likely to be effective and identify which manoeuvres are not likely to be effective in this emergency situation
- state which manoeuvres are likely to cause harm if undertaken
- perform or participate in a locally agreed on drill or procedure for shoulder dystocia
- anticipate the immediate consequences of shoulder dystocia for the mother and the infant
- describe the longer-term consequences of associated neonatal injuries
- provide support and information to women and their families during and after a case of shoulder dystocia

INTRODUCTION

Shoulder dystocia is an obstetric emergency with a potentially catastrophic outcome. It refers to deliveries where manoeuvres other than normal gentle axial traction are needed to complete the delivery of the anterior shoulder (Resnik 1980; Royal College of Obstetricians and Gynaecologists (RCOG) 2012). (Axial traction is traction in line with the fetal spine, i.e. without lateral deviation (RCOG 2012).)

MECHANISM

In a normal labour the shoulders enter the pelvic brim in the oblique or transverse diameter. (For a complete description of the normal mechanism of labour, see Ch. 37.) In shoulder dystocia there is an arrest of the normal mechanism of labour as the shoulders attempt to enter the pelvis in the anteroposterior (smallest) diameter of the pelvic brim and become trapped. The diameter of the fetal shoulders or bisacromial diameter is 12.4 cm and should fit comfortably through the widest diameter of the pelvic brim. Shoulders are sufficiently flexible to allow those of even of a large baby to negotiate the pelvis, and thus shoulder dystocia is a failure of the shoulders to spontaneously traverse the pelvis after the fetal head has been delivered.

Some or all of the following will alert midwives to suspect that shoulder dystocia has occurred:

- Crowning is extremely slow.
- Difficulty is encountered with delivery of the face and chin.
- The head remains tightly applied to the vulva or even retracts (*turtle sign*).
- Restitution does not occur.
- The shoulders fail to descend.
- The interval between the birth of the head and the body is greater than 60 seconds, and gentle axial traction does not complete delivery (RCOG 2012).

The *turtle sign* is caused by reverse traction from the shoulders. The anterior shoulder is wedged onto the symphysis pubis, and the posterior shoulder may still be above the pelvic brim (Fig. 64.1). Gentle axial traction, that is, traction in line with the fetal spine, is diagnostic because it does not complete the delivery. Pulling or

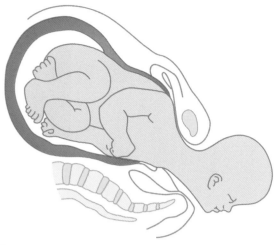

Figure 64.1 Shoulder dystocia.

traction in any other direction to deliver the anterior shoulder is likely to impede delivery by wedging the infant's anterior shoulder more firmly onto the symphysis pubis and can cause damage to the brachial plexus (see Fig. 64.10).

Initial actions

The midwife must recognize shoulder dystocia and summon help immediately from midwifery, obstetric, paediatric and anaesthetist colleagues because the outcome for both mother and infant is potentially very serious. The midwife must not wait for assistance but should utilize the manoeuvres most likely to result in successful delivery (Spain et al 2015). At home the community midwife should summon help and anticipate the need for resuscitation of both mother and baby. Wherever the birth is taking place, resuscitation equipment should have been previously prepared.

The mother should be discouraged from pushing because this may result in the shoulders being further impacted on the symphysis pubis.

The midwife should remain calm and in control of the situation, maintaining clear communication with the mother and her partner. Anxiety is likely to be communicated to the mother even if little is said.

When help arrives, clear diagnosis of shoulder dystocia must be given.

INCIDENCE AND RISK

The incidence of shoulder dystocia is around 0.58% at term, but the risk increases to 1.3% by 42 weeks gestation (Johnstone and Meyerscough 1998; RCOG 2012). However, a lack of agreement over the definition affects the number of cases reported (Johnstone and Myerscough 1998).

The risk of shoulder dystocia rises with increasing birthweight and length of gestation, birth order and maternal age (Acker et al 1986; Gross et al 1987; Johnstone and Myerscough 1998; Overland et al 2012). Johnstone and Myerscough (1998) point out that half of all babies with shoulder dystocia weigh less than 4 kg and are not considered to be large, and only 4% of large babies suffer shoulder dystocia.

Any difficulty with the birth of the shoulders that requires the midwife to employ additional manoeuvres should be classified as shoulder dystocia (Resnik 1980; RCOG 2012).

Identification of risk factors

Ideally, all potential cases of shoulder dystocia would be identified antenatally; the associated maternal and neonatal morbidity and mortality could then be prevented. The sensitivity of single predictive risk factors is poor. At present, midwives and obstetricians can do no more than anticipate the problem by identifying those factors that give a strong index of suspicion.

Maternal obesity is a frequently occurring factor associated with shoulder dystocia (maternal body mass index (BMI) > 30 at booking, or weight at delivery greater than 90 kg). The greater the maternal weight, the higher the risk (Athukorala et al 2007).

Maternal diabetes and gestational diabetes are associated with asymmetrical fetal growth. The body and particularly the shoulders are larger than in babies of mothers who are not diabetic (Acker et al 1985; RCOG 2012).

Spellacy et al (1985) studied the data from 33,545 deliveries and concluded that women with either insulin-dependent or gestational diabetes are more likely to deliver a macrosomic infant and are therefore at a higher risk of a delivery complicated by shoulder dystocia.

Fetal macrosomia is the strongest independent risk factor for shoulder dystocia (Athukorala et al 2007). Infants of non-diabetic mothers who have birthweights of 4000 to 4449 g have a 10% risk of shoulder dystocia, whereas infants of the same weight born to diabetic mothers have a 31% risk of developing shoulder dystocia, because of their asymmetrical growth (Acker et al 1985; Spellacy et al 1985). It is equally important that midwives should remember that approximately 48% of births complicated by shoulder dystocia occur with infants who weigh less than 4000 g (RCOG 2012).

A previous delivery complicated by shoulder dystocia is a predictive risk factor, with a recurrence rate of around 10% for subsequent deliveries (Olugbile and Mascarenhas 2000; Smith et al 1994; Usta et al 2008). However, this may be an underestimation because women may opt for a caesarean section for the next pregnancy.

Use of ultrasound to predict the macrosomic fetus

Ultrasonic estimation of fetal weight is widely used because it is objective and can be reproduced (Combs et al 1993). However, Chauhan et al (1992) suggest that ultrasonic diagnosis of the large infant is generally no more accurate than clinical estimation and that if a woman has had a baby before, her own estimate is likely to be as good as an ultrasound measurement. Ultrasound estimation of fetal weight is most accurate at term but still has a +/– 10% margin of error (Francis et al 2011). Elective induction for infants diagnosed as macrosomic on ultrasound scan increases the risk of caesarean section and does not prevent shoulder dystocia (Hall 1996; RCOG 2012).

Ultrasound estimation of fetal weight can be therefore used with clinical judgement to assess the safest method of delivery, especially for the post-mature, large-for-gestational age or suspected macrosomic fetus.

Prediction of impending shoulder dystocia

Most labours preceding shoulder dystocia are normal (McFarland et al 1995). In some cases, the first hint of trouble the midwife may experience during a delivery is the slow extension of the baby's head and then the chin remaining tight against the mother's perineum (Coates 1995). In spite of current technology, shoulder dystocia usually occurs unexpectedly (RCOG 2012).

Unfortunately, the absence of risk factors cannot be relied upon to exclude the possibility of shoulder dystocia. It is therefore important that the midwife has a sound knowledge of the interaction between the physiology and mechanism of labour and the manoeuvres that may be used to complete the delivery in the shortest time possible. This is to ensure the best outcome for the mother and her infant. All members of the labour ward team must be familiar with the agreed protocol, and 'drills' should be practised on a regular basis by all grades of staff (Draycott et al 2008; Maternal and Child Health Research Consortium (MCHRC) 1998).

MANOEUVRES FOR MANAGEMENT OF SHOULDER DYSTOCIA

The following descriptions of manoeuvres are arranged from the simple, requiring only movement of the mother, to the complex, where direct manipulation of the baby is required. These manoeuvres cannot really be learned or fully understood by reading alone, and it is suggested that the reader should work through the manoeuvres using a doll and pelvis model or phantom in addition to attending skills drills (RCOG 2012). Manoeuvres most likely to result in a successful delivery should be utilized first (Spain et al 2015).

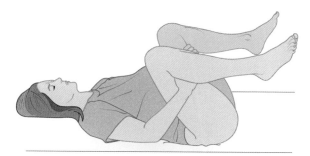

Figure 64.2 McRoberts manoeuvre.

McRoberts manoeuvre

McRoberts manoeuvre is the first choice of manoeuvre in most circumstances because it has been proven to be safe and effective. The manoeuvre (Fig. 64.2) requires the mother to lie flat on her back (or with a slight lateral tilt to prevent supine hypotension), and then she is assisted into an exaggerated knee–chest position (Gonik et al 1983).

Once the mother has adopted this position, the midwife should be able to proceed with a normal delivery of the shoulders. Smeltzer (1986) suggests that this manoeuvre has the following effects:

1. Rotates the symphysis pubis superiorly by approximately 8 cm
2. Elevates the anterior shoulder
3. Pushes the posterior shoulder over the sacrum
4. Flexes the fetal spine
5. Straightens maternal lordosis
6. Opens the pelvic inlet to its maximum
7. Brings the inlet perpendicular to the maximum expulsive force
8. Removes weight-bearing forces from the sacrum
9. Removes the sacral promontory as a point of obstruction (Figs 64.3 and 64.4).

This was supported by later radiological studies (Gherman et al 2000).

Maternal and fetal models were used by Gonik et al (1989) to assess the forces used to extract the fetal shoulders. The McRoberts manoeuvre was compared with the lithotomy position and was found to consistently require less force to remove the shoulders.

The RCOG (2012) advocates the use of the McRoberts manoeuvre as a first step if shoulder dystocia is diagnosed; if the manoeuvre is unsuccessful at the first attempt, the RCOG recommends a second attempt before attempting other manoeuvres.

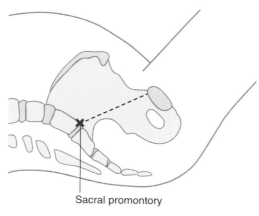

Figure 64.3 Brim of pelvis in dorsal position.

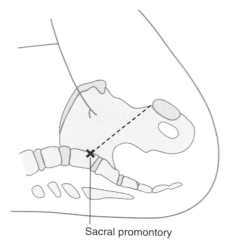

Figure 64.4 Brim of pelvis in McRoberts position.

All-fours position

When there is a minor degree of shoulder dystocia, movement of the mother can dislodge the obstruction so the shoulders can negotiate the pelvis normally; assisting the mother into an *all-fours position* can work in this way. The all-fours position (Fig. 64.5) also can be used to optimize the space in the sacral curve for the midwife to undertake the direct or rotational manoeuvres as described in this chapter. Generally, this position, which acts as an 'upside-down McRoberts position' carries the same positive effects as those previously described and will allow the posterior shoulder to deliver first (Macdonald and Day-Stirk 1995).

If a mother is already on all fours and shoulder dystocia is encountered, then the midwife should assist her to

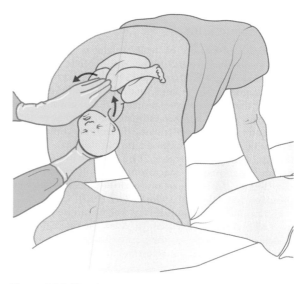

Figure 64.5 Woods' manoeuvre with the woman in the all-fours position.

move into the McRoberts position. If this is not possible, then direct manoeuvres can be undertaken while the all-fours position is maintained.

The all-fours position can only be used if the woman is willing and able to manoeuvre onto her knees, and it is not suitable for women who have a dense epidural block. It is difficult to maintain eye contact while the woman is in the all-fours position, and the midwife must ensure that good clear verbal contact is maintained. It is a useful position for a larger or overweight woman, who may find it difficult to adopt the McRoberts position.

Reflective activity 64.1

Role-play with a colleague, with one of you playing the woman and one the midwife, and try the following scenarios:

- Assisting a woman from the lithotomy position into:
  - the McRoberts position
  - the all-fours position
- Assisting a woman from a semirecumbent position into:
  - the McRoberts position.
- Assisting a woman out of a birthing pool after diagnosing shoulder dystocia

Practise the instructions that you might have to give to a mother regarding moving from one position to another. Consider how easy/difficult it was getting into these different positions and how you could prepare women antenatally for such an emergency.

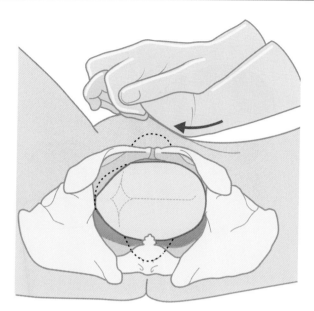

Figure 64.6 Use and direction of suprapubic pressure when the back is on the woman's left.

Suprapubic pressure

The application of suprapubic pressure is intended to displace the anterior shoulder and allow it to enter the pelvis in an oblique diameter (Fig. 64.6). Pressure is applied by either the midwife or assistant (using both hands locked, elbows straight, as for cardiac massage) on the mother's abdomen against the baby's back. Pressure is exerted in the direction that the baby is facing.

Suprapubic pressure can be used on its own or with other non-invasive manoeuvres, such as the McRoberts manoeuver. It may also be used effectively with the rotational manoeuvres described later in the chapter.

Non-invasive procedures have been shown to be effective in up to 69/76 (91%) of cases of shoulder dystocia (Luria et al 1994). However, if the non-invasive manoeuvres described have been unsuccessful, then direct rotational manoeuvres are required. It is at this stage that extra analgesia or anaesthesia may be required. Meanwhile, the midwife should not delay attempting to complete the delivery.

Episiotomy

Shoulder dystocia is a bony dystocia and as such is not greatly affected by soft tissue. An episiotomy may prevent injury to the mother's pelvic floor and perineum during any direct manipulation of the fetus and/or accommodate the midwife's or obstetrician's hand while undertaking direct rotational manoeuvres. It is extremely difficult to perform an episiotomy with the baby's chin firmly pressed against the woman's perineum.

Rotational manoeuvres

Abduction and adduction

To rotate the fetal shoulders, the midwife has to insert a hand into the vagina and locate the fetal back or the fetal chest; the shoulders can rotate in either direction.

Rotation by *abduction* involves putting pressure on the chest approximately below the clavicle so that the shoulder and arm are moved *away* from the chest.

Rotation by *adduction* requires the midwife's hand to be positioned over the fetal back and exert pressure on the posterior shoulder, pushing the shoulder *towards* the chest.

The baby might only rotate in one direction; therefore, knowledge of both methods is required. A more complete description of the rotational manoeuvres follows.

To undertake a rotational manoeuvre, the midwife should assist the woman into the McRoberts or lithotomy position with her buttocks well over the edge of the bed so that there is no restriction to the sacrum or coccyx during the manoeuvre. In a home setting, the McRoberts or all-fours position should be used. These are practical positions for undertaking further manoeuvres and removing restrictions to the sacrum and coccyx that are present when the mother is in the dorsal or semirecumbent position.

Woods' manoeuvre

The method Woods (1943) used to relieve shoulder dystocia involves inserting as much of the hand as is necessary into the vagina to locate the anterior surface of the posterior shoulder (clavicle). The shoulder is then rotated through 180 degrees in the direction of the fetal back (see Fig. 64.5), which actually causes an abduction of the fetal shoulders (see chapter website resources).

This rotation may dislodge the anterior shoulder and enable the posterior shoulder to enter the pelvic brim. The posterior shoulder becomes the anterior following the rotation and may be delivered by normal axial traction and the delivery completed. There is some interest in the *reverse wood screw* manoeuvre in which the hand is inserted and applies pressure to the back of the shoulder, rotating in the opposite direction (Hinshaw 2003).

Rubin manoeuvre

Rubin (1964) emphasized the importance of having both of the infant's shoulders adducted and presented measurements to demonstrate that in this position, the circumference of the baby's body is less than if the shoulders were abducted. To achieve the Rubin manoeuvre, a hand must be inserted into the vagina as far as is necessary to locate

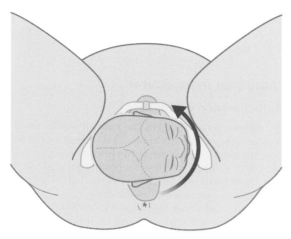

Figure 64.7 Rubin manoeuvre: the shoulders are adducted as the shoulder is rotated anteriorly.

a shoulder. The shoulders are pushed into the oblique diameter with the aid of suprapubic pressure over the fetal back (see chapter website resources). Once the shoulders are in the oblique diameter and free of the symphysis pubis, the delivery can be completed (see Fig. 64.7).

O'Leary (2009) suggested that both the Woods' and Rubin manoeuvres may be more successful if they are used in conjunction with gentle but firm suprapubic pressure in the direction that facilitates the vaginal rotation (see Fig. 64.6).

Delivery of the posterior arm

The technique is to insert a hand into the vagina along the curve of the sacrum and locate the posterior arm or hand. The fetal arm should then be swept over the chest and delivered (Fig. 64.8).

If this manoeuvre fails once the posterior arm has been delivered, the fetus may be rotated using either the Woods' or Rubin manoeuvre so that the shoulder and arm that have been delivered are rotated to the anterior position, thus unlocking the obstruction (this is similar to the Burns–Marshall manoeuvre as described in Ch. 62).

Zavanelli manoeuvre

The Zavanelli manoeuvre is a revolutionary concept (Sandberg 1985). Unlike the other manoeuvres described, it reverses the whole mechanism of delivery. Cephalic replacement is followed by a caesarean section. Although it is unlikely that a midwife would ever need to undertake this manoeuvre, it may be a last resort if practising in a remote area away from immediate obstetric support.

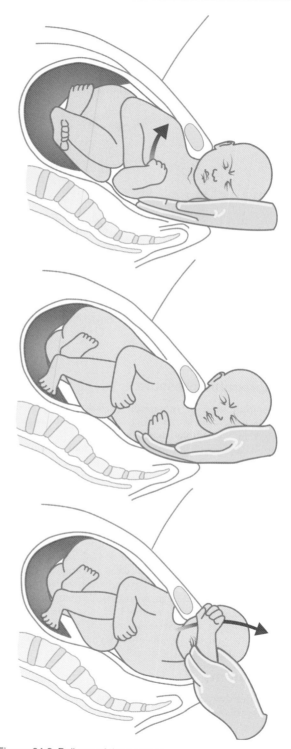

Figure 64.8 Delivery of the posterior arm.

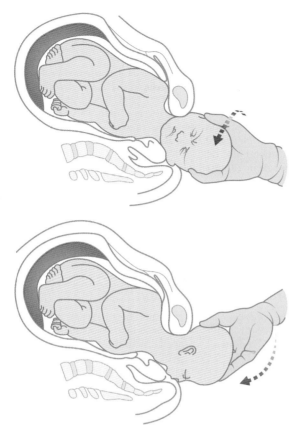

Figure 64.9 Zavanelli manoeuvre.

OTHER PROCEDURES

Symphysiotomy

Surgical separation of the symphysis pubis to enlarge the pelvis for delivery has been proven clinically useful for cephalopelvic disproportion but is associated with high maternal morbidity. Although symphysiotomy has been used for the relief of shoulder dystocia, the few cases reported reveal high maternal morbidity (Broekman et al 1994).

Cleidotomy

A clavicle can fracture spontaneously during a normal delivery of a normal-weight infant or a delivery complicated by shoulder dystocia. Deliberate fracture of the clavicle is a difficult procedure, especially in a large, mature fetus. O'Leary (2009: 78) points out that although clavicular fracture is often mentioned, 'its use has never been substantiated' to resolve shoulder dystocia.

Fundal pressure

Fundal pressure together with traction provides the worst outcome for brachial plexus injury (Gross et al 1987). Fundal pressure will result in the shoulder or shoulders being further impacted and impede progress, can damage the brachial plexus and has also been associated with uterine rupture and maternal death (O'Leary 2009). It is therefore a practice that **should not** be used (RCOG 2012).

MATERNAL OUTCOMES

Shoulder dystocia is associated with a higher risk of physical and psychological morbidity and mortality for mother and baby, including the following:

- Potential for physical and psychological trauma to mother

To carry out the manoeuvre, the fetal head is returned to the prerestitution position of either direct occipitoanterior or direct occipitoposterior. The head is then manually flexed and returned to the vagina (Sandberg 1985) (Fig. 64.9). Delivery is then completed by caesarean section.

The role of the midwife in such circumstances would normally be to support the mother, monitor and record the condition of both the mother and the fetus and ensure that all the personnel necessary are called to deal with this obstetric emergency.

Sandberg (1985: 482) suggests that the Zavanelli manoeuvre 'must occupy the bottom priority until its virtue and applicability … can be confirmed'. The Zavanelli manoeuvre must remain the last resort; however, it has proved to be a life-saving procedure. Midwives should understand the mechanisms of the Zavanelli manoeuvre and hope that they will never need to use it.

- Possibility of uterine rupture from fundal pressure
- Postpartum haemorrhage (PPH) and/or shock
- Soft tissue damage – cervix, vagina and perineum
- Infection
- Postnatal depression
- Post-traumatic stress disorder
- The loss of the 'perfect birth' and the 'perfect baby'
- Possible problems with maternal–infant interaction

Uterine rupture

Maternal deaths associated with shoulder dystocia have been caused by the use of fundal pressure resulting in uterine rupture and from haemorrhage during delivery or immediately postpartum (RCOG 2012).

Postpartum haemorrhage and/or shock

Benedetti and Gabbe (1978) described maternal morbidity from shoulder dystocia as considerable: in their study, 68% of cases had an estimated blood loss of more than 1000 mL. Others have recorded extensive vaginal, cervical and perineal lacerations; uterine rupture; and vaginal haematoma as sequelae to shoulder dystocia (Gross et al 1987; RCOG 2012).

It is wise to anticipate postpartum haemorrhage if shoulder dystocia is encountered.

Soft tissue damage – cervix and vagina

Soft tissue damage may include *vulval haematoma* and minor and major lacerations. Because these may cause a significant degree of blood loss, the midwife should examine the cervix, vagina and labia very carefully following delivery to diagnose any lacerations and take appropriate action (see Ch. 40).

Infection

Increased vaginal examinations and manoeuvres are likely to increase the risk of infection for the woman. This may be exacerbated by soft tissue damage and blood loss.

The loss of the 'perfect birth' and the 'perfect baby'

Women will have had plans and expectations for the birth of the baby. It may be difficult for the woman to come to terms with the reality of a shoulder dystocia birth and its sequelae. Following any traumatic birth experience, the mother and her partner may wish to discuss the events and understand what happened. The midwife caring for the woman should be aware of signs of post-traumatic stress disorder (PTSD); this is discussed further in Chapter 69.

Midwifery, obstetric and support staff attending a traumatic delivery are also vulnerable to PTSD and may wish to seek help.

BIRTH INJURY AND FETAL OUTCOMES

The most obvious and immediate consequence for the infant whose birth has been complicated by shoulder dystocia is asphyxia (MCHRC 1998; RCOG 2012).

Airway protective reflexes are reduced by asphyxia. Midwives should therefore prepare for the reception of an asphyxiated baby and must call for a paediatrician to attend the delivery (Box 64.1). Cord blood should be taken. (Resuscitation of the newborn is described in Ch. 46.)

Careful examination of the newborn is always important but is imperative following a traumatic delivery (see also Ch. 42). The most commonly reported injuries following deliveries complicated by shoulder dystocia involve the brachial plexus, and therefore the newborn must be assessed by an experienced senior clinician.

Brachial plexus injury

The prevalence of congenital brachial palsy (CBP) is 1 : 2300 of all live births; 60% of CBP is associated with shoulder dystocia, compared with the normal population risk of 0.2% to 1% (Royal College of Paediatrics and Child Health (RCPCH) 2000; Evans-Jones et al 2003). Although many brachial plexus injuries are associated with shoulder dystocia, high birthweight and assisted delivery, around 7.5% of cases have no associated risks reported (RCPCH 2000). There is no reliable method of predicting risk of either shoulder dystocia or brachial plexus injuries (Evans-Jones et al 2003).

Erb's palsy is the most commonly reported brachial plexus injury following shoulder dystocia, although there may be a proportion of cases in which the brachial plexus is damaged before birth (Doumouchtsis and Arulkumaran 2009). This is the result of damage to the nerve roots C5–C6 (Fig. 64.10). The arm on the affected side lies in the classical 'waiter's tip' position (Fig. 64.11).

Klumpke's palsy is damage to the lower plexus that results in a paralysis of the forearm and hand, resulting in a "claw hand," in which the forearm is supinated and the wrist and fingers are hyperextended. Klumpke's palsy

---

Box 64.1 Calling for help (hospital)

- Senior midwifery colleagues
- Senior obstetrician
- Senior paediatrician/neonatologist
- Anaesthetist

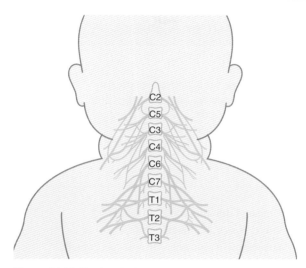

Figure 64.10 The brachial plexus of the neonate.

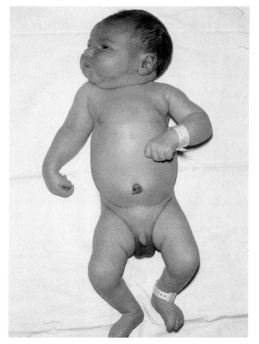

Figure 64.11 Erb's palsy. (Permezel M, Walker S, Kyprianou K: *Beischer and Mackay's obstetrics, gynaecology and the newborn*, 4th edn, London, Elsevier, 2015.)

may be associated with Horner's syndrome (see chapter website resources).

Following delivery, if the baby has a flaccid arm or an unequal Moro reflex (see Ch. 42), then the midwife must suspect a brachial plexus injury and inform a senior

paediatrician. Serious conditions are associated with congenital brachial plexus injury, such as cervical cord injury and cerebral injury, and these will require urgent treatment.

There are four degrees of injury to the brachial plexus:

1. *Stretch injury.* Injury depends on the degree of stretch. Further damage is caused by compression resulting from swelling and bruising. This is the least severe injury; recovery may be complete within 6 to 18 months.

2. *Rupture.* The nerve is torn, perhaps in several places, and may require surgery to restore function.

3. *Neuroma.* Scar tissue that develops following injury.

4. *Avulsion.* Nerves are pulled or torn from the spinal cord. This is the most severe injury and is likely to require several stages of surgery to restore nerves; it may require muscle graft and tendon transfer.

Diagnosis may be complex because there may be a combination of injuries.

Treatment for congenital brachial plexus injury

The baby will be referred to a paediatric physiotherapist, and the parents will be taught how to maintain the affected arm in a natural position until any bruising or swelling resolves. The physiotherapist will then teach the parents a series of exercises for the affected arm.

Physiotherapy is used to maximize the use of the arm to prevent muscle contracture. Motion exercises develop strength and flexibility, and tactile stimulation is used to improve sensory awareness. It is important to keep the joints supple for the best outcome. However, these exercises are time consuming, and parents will require support and encouragement in addition to as much information as is available concerning their baby's condition. Parents should be referred to support groups (see chapter website for contact addresses).

Some congenital brachial plexus injuries resolve within months; those that have not resolved may need surgery to improve function. The midwife is not in a position to estimate recovery and should not give any reassurance of a specific time frame.

Bony injury

Shoulder dystocia and high birthweight are considered risk factors for clavicular fractures. Clavicular fractures can also be unpredictable and unavoidable, and may occur in 0.4% to 4% of normal births internationally (Roberts et al 1995; Paul and Williamson 2013; Lurie et al 2011). The baby may be in considerable pain, and an irregularity may be felt over the site of the fracture on examination. However, if the fracture is not displaced, an irregularity may only be felt over the site of the fracture several days after birth as a callus forms as part of the healing process.

Box 64.2 Injuries associated with shoulder dystocia

- Sternomastoid tumour
- Congenital brachial palsy (CBP)
- Horner's syndrome
- Paralyzed hemidiaphragm
- Facial palsy
- Phrenic nerve palsy
- Fractured clavicle
- Fractured humerus
- Shoulder dislocation
- Bruising
- Cerebral palsy

Box 64.3 The HELPERR mnemonic

H	Help – call for help
E	Episiotomy
L	Legs hyperflexed (McRoberts position)
P	Pressure suprapubically
E	Enter the vagina
R	Remove the posterior arm
R	Roll the woman onto her hands and knees

Source: ALSO 2000

The callus will resolve within a couple of months. If a midwife suspects that a clavicle has been fractured, a paediatrician must examine the baby. The paediatrician may order x-rays to confirm the diagnosis and to rule out other bony injury. An analgesic, such as paracetamol in a paediatric dosage, may be prescribed if the baby appears to be suffering any discomfort.

The humerus may have also been damaged following shoulder dystocia, especially if the posterior arm has to be delivered to release the impaction. Both arms should be examined carefully after delivery and in the first weeks following delivery to exclude bony injury and monitor the degree of congenital brachial plexus injury.

Careful examination of the newborn must be undertaken following any delivery, with special attention taken following a traumatic delivery, to exclude any injury not immediately apparent (see Box 64.2).

NOTES AND RECORD KEEPING

There are many events in midwifery that happen with alarming rapidity (Nursing and Midwifery Council (NMC) 2015) and as such are difficult to record contemporaneously. Accurate records are vital for all deliveries and especially following any emergency situation. Upon arrival of a resuscitation team, one person should be allocated to act as scribe and record the personnel present, the timing of the manoeuvres and the outcome of each attempt in chronological order. The important or main events in a case of shoulder dystocia are as follows:

- Time of delivery of the head
- Position(s) of the woman before and during birth
- Time assistance was summoned
- Time assistance arrived
- Time and duration each manoeuvre

- Time and duration of axial traction
- Effect of each manoeuvre
- Episiotomy if and when this was performed
- Position the baby's head faces after restitution
- Position of the fetal back
- Time of delivery of the body
- Apgar score and resuscitation of the baby
- Cord blood results
- Results of the examination following birth
- Information provided to parents at and after the birth
- Completion of risk management processes (RCM 2000)

EDUCATION, TRAINING AND DEVELOPMENT

Regular scenario training or 'drills' and thorough knowledge of local procedure for shoulder dystocia are recommended (Draycott et al 2008; MCHRC 1998; RCOG 2012). Most maternity units have instituted such educational and development strategies and have demonstrated improved staff performance and outcome with the PROMPT course (Winter et al 2012) (Fig. 64.12) (Draycott et al 2008; RCOG 2012) using an algorithm, compared with training where a mnemonic is used.

The Advanced Life Support in Obstetrics (ALSO) has also been a useful means of gathering multidisciplinary groups together to practise emergency skills in a safe environment. Where a mnemonic such as HELPERR (Sokol et al 2003) (see Box 64.3) is in use, it must be underpinned by a clear evidence-based rationale and should be clearly understood by the whole team.

The nature of shoulder dystocia as a comparatively rare but serious emergency means that some practitioners may never have the experience of dealing with it or may never observe a case before they have to deal with

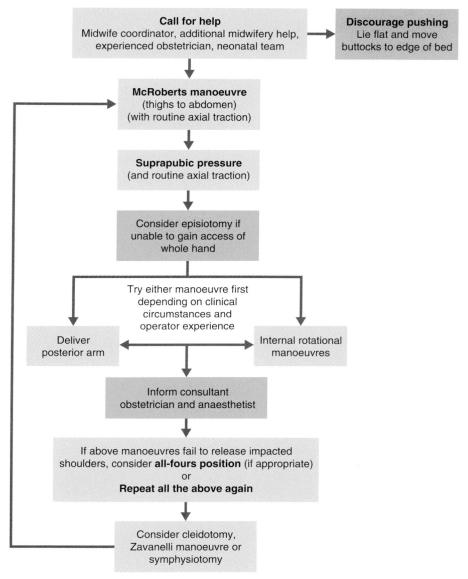

Call for help
Midwife coordinator, additional midwifery help, experienced obstetrician, neonatal team

Discourage pushing
Lie flat and move buttocks to edge of bed

McRoberts manoeuvre
(thighs to abdomen)
(with routine axial traction)

Suprapubic pressure
(and routine axial traction)

Consider episiotomy if unable to gain access of whole hand

Try either manoeuvre first depending on clinical circumstances and operator experience

Deliver posterior arm

Internal rotational manoeuvres

Inform consultant obstetrician and anaesthetist

If above manoeuvres fail to release impacted shoulders, consider **all-fours position** (if appropriate)
or
Repeat all the above again

Consider cleidotomy, Zavanelli manoeuvre or symphysiotomy

Baby to be reviewed by midwife/neonatologist after birth and referred for consultant neonatal review if any concerns

Figure 64.12 Algorithm for the management of shoulder dystocia. (Winter C, Crofts J, Laxton C, Barnfield S, Draycott T, editors: PROMPT: PRactical Obstetric Multi-Professional Training. Practical locally based training for obstetric emergencies. Course Manual, 2nd edn, Cambridge, 2012, Cambridge University Press, pp 169–178.)

it as lead practitioner. It is therefore vital that following an incident of shoulder dystocia (and any other emergency), there is a forum to discuss the individual case and its management in a systematic and critically reflective way. This will highlight elements of learning, good practice and communication and identify areas that require additional attention. This forum should be multidisciplinary and should at its heart have a non-blame and development principle (Department of Health 2000; Draycott et al 2008).

Reflective activity 64.3

Review your local protocols and clinical guidelines. Are these up to date and evidence based? Is there a regular shoulder dystocia drill carried out locally? If not, you may wish to work with colleagues to plan a regular drill, as recommended by CESDI (MCHRC 1998) and the RCOG (2012), involving a range of colleagues to practise the manoeuvres and management. Ensure that there is an opportunity to reflect together after the sessions.

CONCLUSION

Shoulder dystocia is a rare but serious complication of labour. Midwives should commit to memory a series of manoeuvres that have been proven to be effective and be aware of those manoeuvres that are ineffective or dangerous. Current knowledge of labour ward protocol or procedure is necessary for all members of the labour ward staff. All members of staff who may be involved in such an emergency should take part in practice 'drills' on the labour ward (MCHRC 1998; RCOG 2012; RCM 2000).

Permanent damage is rare. Babies who do suffer brachial plexus injury must be swiftly referred to a specialist centre

for surgical assessment, and parents should be provided with appropriate support and information to help them care for their child. The psychological impact of such a traumatic birth should be considered by the care team, and opportunities should be provided for talking, debriefing and further counselling, should this be necessary.

Key Points

- Shoulder dystocia is an emergency, and midwives should prepare for the unexpected, be involved in 'drills' and ensure that local procedures are manageable.

- If shoulder dystocia occurs, help should be summoned immediately.

- The most simple and non-invasive manoeuvres should be attempted, progressing to the direct and rotational manoeuvres as needed.

- Careful examination of the newborn must be carried out to exclude injuries not immediately obvious at birth. Any deviations from the norm should be investigated and specialist referral organized promptly, ensuring parents are fully informed throughout.

- Full and accurate records must be maintained.

- Reflection and discussion with the mother and partner and all those involved in the delivery are essential.

References

Acker DB, Sachs BP, Friedman EA: Risk factors for shoulder dystocia, *Obstet Gynecol* 66(6):762–768, 1985.

Acker DB, Sachs BP, Friedman EA: Risk factors for shoulder dystocia in the average weight infant, *Obstet Gynecol* 67(5):614–618, 1986.

Advanced Life Support in Obstetrics (ALSO): *Advanced Life Support in Obstetrics provider course syllabus*, 4th edn, Leawood (KS), American Academy of Family Physicians, 2000.

Athukorala C, Crowther CA, Willson K, et al: Women with gestational diabetes mellitus in the ACHOSIS trial: risk factors for shoulder dystocia, *Aust N Z J Obstet Gynaecol* 47(1):37–41, 2007.

Benedetti TJ, Gabbe SG: Shoulder dystocia a complication of fetal

macrosomia and prolonged second stage of labour with mid pelvic operative delivery, *Obstet Gynecol* 52(5):526–529, 1978.

Broekman AMW, Smith YG, van Dessel T: Shoulder dystocia and symphysiotomy: a case report, *Eur J Obstet Gynecol Reprod Biol* 53(2):142–143, 1994.

Chauhan SP, Lutton PM, Bailey KJ, et al: Intrapartum clinical, sonographic, and parous patients' estimates of newborn birth weight, *Obstet Gynecol* 79(6):956–958, 1992.

Coates T: Shoulder dystocia. In Alexander J, Levy V, Roch S, editors: *Midwifery practice*, vol 5, London, Macmillan, 1995.

Combs AC, Singh NB, Khoury JS: Elective induction versus spontaneous labour after sonographic diagnosis of fetal

macrosomia, *Obstet Gynecol* 81(4):492–496, 1993. 2000.

Department of Health (DH): *An organisation with a memory: report of an expert group on learning from adverse events in the NHS*, London, DH, 2000.

Doumouchtsis SK, Arulkumaran S: Are all brachial plexus injuries caused by shoulder dystocia?, *Obstet Gynecol Surv* 64(9):615–623, 2009.

Draycott TJ, Crofts JF, Ash JP, et al: Improving neonatal outcome through practical shoulder dystocia training, *Obstet Gynecol* 112(1):14–20, 2008.

Evans-Jones G, Kay SP, Weindling AM, et al: Congenital brachial plexus injury: incidence, causes and outcome in the UK and Republic of Ireland, *Arch Dis Child Fetal Neonatal Ed* 88:F185–F189, 2003.

Francis A, Tonks A, Gardosi J: Accuracy of ultrasound estimation of fetal weight at term, *Arch Dis Child Fetal Neonatal Ed* 96(Suppl):Fa61, 2011.

Gherman RB, Tramont J, Muffley P, et al: Analysis of McRoberts' manoeuvre by X-ray pelvimetry, *Obstet Gynecol* 95(1):43–47, 2000.

Gonik B, Stringer CA, Held B: An alternate manoeuvre for management of shoulder dystocia, *Am J Obstet Gynecol* 145(7):882–883, 1983.

Gonik B, Allen R, Sorab J: Objective evaluation of the shoulder dystocia phenomenon: effect of maternal pelvic orientation on force reduction, *Obstet Gynecol* 74(1):44–48, 1989.

Gross SJ, Shime J, Forrine D: Shoulder dystocia: predictors and outcome. A five-year review, *Am J Obstet Gynecol* 56(2):336–344, 1987.

Hall MH: Guessing the weight of the baby, *Br J Obstet Gynaecol* 103(8):734–736, 1996.

Hinshaw K: *The 'enter' manoeuvres for shoulder dystocia clarified (using 'LOT' position as an example). ALSO* (website). www.also.org.uk/download/shoulder%20dystocia%20-%20explanation.pdf. 2003.

Johnstone FD, Myerscough PR: Shoulder dystocia, *Br J Obstet Gynaecol* 105(8):811–815, 1998.

Luria S, BenArie A, Hagay Z: The ABC of shoulder dystocia management, *Asia Oceania J Obstet Gynaecol* 20(2):195–197, 1994.

Lurie S, Wand S, Golan A, et al: Risk factors for fractured clavicle in the newborn, *Journal of Obstetrics and Gynaecology Research* 37(11):1572–1574, 2011.

Macdonald SE, Day-Stirk F: A midwife's perspective (shoulder dystocia), *Clinical Risk* 1(2):61–65, 1995.

McFarland M, Hod M, Piper JM, et al: Are labor abnormalities more common in shoulder dystocia?, *Am J Obstet Gynecol* 173(4):1211–1214, 1995.

Maternal and Child Health Research Consortium (MCHRC): *Confidential Enquiry into Stillbirth and Deaths in Infancy: 5th annual report*, London, MCHRC, 1998.

Nursing and Midwifery Council (NMC): The Code: professional standards of practice and behaviour for nurses and midwives (website). www.nmc-uk.org. 2015.

O'Leary JA, editor: *Shoulder dystocia and birth injury: prevention and treatment*, New Jersey, Humana Press, 2009.

Olugbile A, Mascarenhas L: Review of shoulder dystocia at the Birmingham Women's Hospital, *J Obstet Gynaecol* 20(3):267–270, 2000.

Overland EA, Vatten LJ, Eskild A: Risk of shoulder dystocia: associations with parity and offspring birthweight. A population study of 1,914,544 deliveries, *Acta Obstet Gynecol Scand* 91(4):483–488, 2012.

Paul S, Williamson D: *Clavicle fractures in newborns*, Journal of Family Health (website). www.jfhc.co.uk/clavicle_fractures_in_newborns_30227.aspx. 2013.

Permezel M, Walker S, Kyprianou K: *Beischer and Mackay's obstetrics, gynaecology and the newborn*, 4th edn, London, Elsevier, 2015.

Resnik R: Management of shoulder girdle dystocia, *Clin Obstet Gynecol* 23(2):559–564, 1980.

Roberts SW, Hernandez C, Maberry MC, et al: Obstetric clavicular fracture: the enigma of normal birth, *Obstet Gynecol* 86(6):978–981, 1995.

Royal College of Midwives (RCM): Clinical risk management. Paper 2: Shoulder dystocia, *RCM Midwives J* 3(11):348–351, 2000.

Royal College of Obstetricians and Gynaecologists (RCOG): *Shoulder dystocia. RCOG Guideline No. 42* (2nd ed.) (website). www.rcog.org.uk/guidelines. 2012.

Royal College of Paediatrics and Child Health (RCPCH): *British Paediatric Surveillance Unit (BPSU) 14th annual report 1999–2000*, London, BPSU, 2000.

Rubin A: Management of shoulder dystocia, *J Am Med Assoc* 189(11):835–837, 1964.

Sandberg EC: The Zavanelli maneuver: a potentially revolutionary method for the resolution of shoulder dystocia, *Am J Obstet Gynecol* 152(4):479–484, 1985.

Smeltzer JS: Prevention and management of shoulder dystocia, *Clin Obstet Gynecol* 29(2):299–308, 1986.

Smith RB, Lane C, Pearson JF: Shoulder dystocia: what happens at the next delivery?, *Br J Obstet Gynaecol* 101(8):713–715, 1994.

Sokol RJ, Blackwell SC: American College of Obstetricians and Gynecologists (ACOG) Committee on Practice Bulletins-Gynecology, ACOG practice bulletin: shoulder dystocia. Number 40, November 2002, *Int J Gynecol Obstet* 80(1):87–92, 2003.

Spain JE, Frey HA, Tuuli MG, et al: Neonatal morbidity associated with shoulder dystocia maneuvers, *Am J Obstet Gynecol* 212(3):353.e1–353.e5, 2015.

Spellacy WN, Miller S, Winegar A, et al: Macrosomia, maternal characteristics and infant complications, *Obstet Gynecol* 66(2):158–161, 1985.

Usta IM, Hayek S, Yahya F, et al: Shoulder dystocia: what is the risk of recurrence?, *Acta Obstetrica Gynecologica Scandinavica* 87(10):992–997, 2008.

Winter C, Crofts J, Laxton C, et al, editors: *PROMPT: PRactical Obstetric Multi-Professional Training. Practical locally based training for obstetric emergencies. Course manual*, 2nd edn, Cambridge, Cambridge University Press, pp 169–178, 2012.

Woods CE: A principle of physics as applicable to shoulder delivery, *Am J Obstet Gynecol* 45:796–805, 1943.

Resources and additional reading

Permezel M, Walker S, Kyprianou K:
*Beischer and Mackay's obstetrics,
gynaecology and the newborn*, 4th
edn, Elsevier, 2015.

*A useful illustrated textbook from
Australian obstetricians.*

Useful websites:

American Congress of Obstetricians
and Gynaecologists (ACOG):
www.acog.org.

*American Academy of Family Physicians
(AAFP)– one article in a series on
Advanced Life Support in Obstetrics
(ALSO®): Available from
www.aafp.org.*

Erb's Palsy Group:
www.**erbspalsy**group.co.uk/.

*Although we all hope that we never have
need of the Erb's Palsy Group, this is a
useful support group for families with
an affected child. The group also holds
annual study days for midwives and
physiotherapists.*

Midwife Thinking: **midwifethinking**.
com/2010/12/03/**shoulder-dystocia**-
the-real-story/.

*Midwifery blog with an informative and
balanced discussion about shoulder
dystocia. Some useful links to other
sites.*

*Royal College of Obstetricians and
Gynaecologists (RCOG) – Guideline
No. 42 on shoulder dystocia:*
www.rcog.org.uk/globalassets/
documents/guidelines/
gtg42_25112013.pdf.

*Royal College of Obstetricians and
Gynaecologists (RCOG) – patient
guidelines on shoulder dystocia:* www.
rcog.org.uk/globalassets/documents/
patients/patient-information-
leaflets/pregnancy/pi-shoulder-
dystocia.pdf.

Chapter 65

Presentation and prolapse of the umbilical cord

Lyn Jones

Learning Outcomes ?

After reading this chapter, you will be able to:

- differentiate between presentation and prolapse of the umbilical cord
- identify predisposing factors for cord presentation or prolapse
- discuss the midwifery management of cord presentation and prolapse
- discuss the possible consequences to the woman and the fetus/neonate
- be aware of the statutory responsibilities of the midwife in relation to emergency care

INTRODUCTION

Cord prolapse is an obstetric emergency that has a high risk of perinatal mortality and consistently features in perinatal mortality enquiries (Royal College of Obstetricians and Gynaecologists (RCOG) 2014).

In emergency situations, midwives must act within the limits of their knowledge and competence but have a duty to ensure that they maintain the knowledge and skills for safe and effective practice (Nursing and Midwifery Council (NMC) 2015). Clinical governance frameworks recommend that all staff receive training in the management of obstetric emergencies, including cord prolapse (RCOG 2014).

Cord prolapse can be defined as the descent of the umbilical cord through the cervix alongside (occult) or past the presenting part (overt) in the presence of ruptured membranes (RCOG 2014). (See Fig. 65.1).

Cord presentation can be defined as the presence of the umbilical cord between the fetal presenting part and cervix with or without ruptured membranes (RCOG 2014).

The incidence of the umbilical cord descending below the presenting part is approximately 0.1% to 0.6%, increasing to 1% with breech presentation (RCOG 2014).

Cord prolapse of any type can potentially compromise fetal circulation, as perinatal hypoxia can occur as a result of intermittent or prolonged compression and mechanical occlusion of the prolapsed cord or vasospasm as a result of the relatively lower temperature in the vagina and vulval introitus (Goonwardene 2012).

CAUSES

Anything that will prevent either the well-fitting application of the presenting part into the lower uterine segment or its descent into the pelvis, thus making descent of the umbilical cord alongside or past the presenting part more likely.

PREDISPOSING FACTORS

These can be subdivided into different categories, which may aid the midwife in highlighting women at risk.

General

- An unusually long umbilical cord
- Congenital anomaly such as anencephaly or hydrocephaly
- Prematurity or low birthweight of <2500 g
- Breech presentation
- Multiparity
- Transverse, oblique and unstable lie, particularly after 37 weeks gestation
- Polyhydramnios

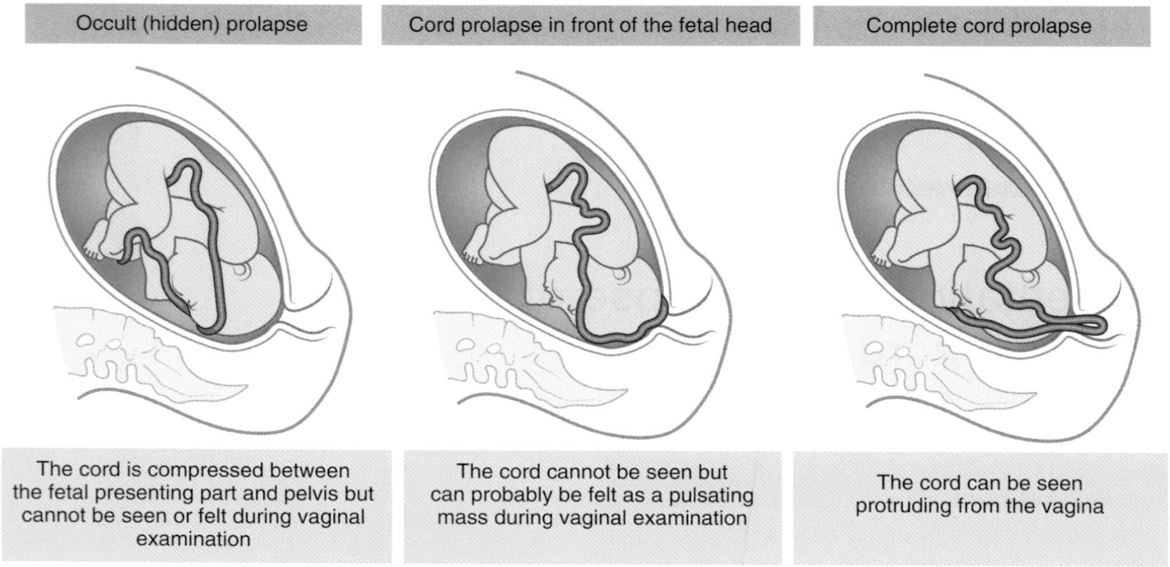

Occult (hidden) prolapse	Cord prolapse in front of the fetal head	Complete cord prolapse
The cord is compressed between the fetal presenting part and pelvis but cannot be seen or felt during vaginal examination	The cord cannot be seen but can probably be felt as a pulsating mass during vaginal examination	The cord can be seen protruding from the vagina

Figure 65.1 Variation of cord prolapse/presentation. (McKinney et al 2013.)

- Uterine fibroids
- Low-lying placenta/placenta praevia
- Second twin
- Contracted or pelvic abnormalities
- Premature rupture of membranes before engagement of the presenting part

Clinician – iatrogenesis

- Artificial rupture of membranes (ARM), particularly with a high presenting part
- Vaginal manipulation of the fetus with ruptured membranes
- External cephalic version (during procedure)
- Internal podalic version
- Stabilizing induction of labour before ARM
- Insertion of intra-uterine pressure transducer
- Large balloon catheter induction of labour

(Cox et al 2009; Hinshaw et al 2010; Yamada et al 2013; RCOG 2014)

DIAGNOSIS

It is important that a thorough, detailed history and assessment of the woman is taken, which should alert the midwife to any pre-existing risk factors (Hinshaw et al 2010). Cord presentation and prolapse may occur without outward physical signs and with a normal fetal heart rate pattern, and it might be first diagnosed at routine vaginal examination in labour (RCOG 2014). It is, therefore, vital that cord prolapse is excluded at every vaginal examination (RCOG 2014). If a midwife is faced with a situation of unexplained fetal distress, cord compression should be considered (Chakravarti et al 2004).

In most cases, there are three ways in which the midwife may detect cord prolapse or presentation:

'See it'

Overt cord prolapse is likely to reveal itself upon rupture of the membranes; therefore, vaginal examination at the point the membranes rupture is prudent, particularly in the presence of risk factors (RCOG 2014).

'Hear it'

Occult (hidden) cord prolapse (Fig. 65.1) is often based on suspicion related to changes in the fetal heart rate. This could be subtle in nature and may be more readily obvious when interpreting the CTG, highlighting the need for the midwife to remain vigilant in the monitoring of both maternal and fetal well-being, particularly when intermittent auscultation is used (NMC 2015; NMC 2012). In addition to national guidance in respect of fetal heart rate monitoring, auscultation of the fetal heart is recommended after a vaginal examination and after a spontaneous rupture of membranes (RCOG 2014).

'Feel it'

Cord presentation or prolapse may be palpated while undertaking a vaginal examination. Pulsation of the cord will be felt by the examiner's fingers and would be synchronous with the fetal heart rate. Conversely, uterine arterial pulsation may be felt in the vaginal fornices but is synchronous with the maternal heart rate. This highlights the necessity for the midwife to undertake fetal heart rate auscultation simultaneously with maternal pulse to differentiate the two (RCOG 2014).

> **Box 65.1** Actions in the management of cord prolapse
>
> - Call medical assistance with urgency.
> - Remain with the woman.
> - Relieve pressure on the cord.
> - Improve fetal oxygenation.
> - Monitor fetal heart rate as appropriate.
> - Expedite delivery.
> - Keep clear, accurate and contemporaneous records.

MANAGEMENT OF CORD PRESENTATION

If cord presentation is suspected, the midwife must aim to keep the membranes intact and attempt to relieve any potential compression and call for medical assistance (NMC 2015; NMC 2012). While in left lateral, the mother's hips and buttocks are raised using either a pillow or wedge. This is known as exaggerated Sims' position.

This is particularly useful within the home setting where medical assistance will not be readily available. This position serves to elevate the maternal pelvis, which may encourage the umbilical cord to move; however, if it does not, delivery is likely to be by caesarean section.

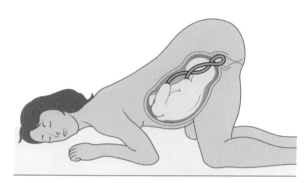

Figure 65.2 Knee chest position. (Goonwardene 2012.)

MANAGEMENT OF CORD PROLAPSE

Overt cord prolapse is a time-critical emergency requiring rapid management (Box 65.1). Transport and treatment happen simultaneously. In a home setting, this requires 'blue light' paramedic ambulance. Management will be dependent on the stage of labour and whether the fetus is dead or alive.

Within the hospital environment, the midwife can be relatively confident that pulling an emergency bell will summon assistance in a timely manner, settings outside of the hospital will be more challenging. Tchabo (1988) suggested that up to 25% of umbilical cord prolapses occur outside of the hospital setting. This highlights not only the need for all midwifery practitioners to keep updated in the management of obstetric emergencies, but also to remain calm and professional while dealing with the emergency (RCOG 2014; NMC 2012; NMC 2015).

Absence of both cord pulsation and fetal heart rate are suggestive of fetal death, but this must be confirmed by ultrasound scan. If fetal death is confirmed, labour is likely to proceed without intervention. This can be extremely distressing for both parents and the remaining family who often cannot understand the rationale for not undertaking a caesarean section. If the fetus is known or suspected to be alive, the management is immediate delivery. The midwife must attempt to keep the fetus in good condition until delivery is effected (Goonwardene 2012; RCOG 2014).

Minimal handling of any loops of cord is recommended to reduce the risk of vasospasm and subsequent fetal hypoxic acidosis (RCOG 2014). However, there is insufficient evidence to recommend the practice of umbilical cord replacement (funic reduction) in managing cord prolapse (RCOG 2014).

The midwife should assess cervical dilatation and the descent of the presenting part. If the cervix is found to be fully dilated and the presenting part is low, vaginal or instrumental birth may be appropriate; however, the midwife should anticipate the need for neonatal resuscitation (Goonwardene 2012). If this is not the case, the most urgent intervention is to elevate the presenting part above the pelvic inlet to relieve the cord compression. Traditionally, the knee–chest position with buttocks raised (see Fig. 65.2), in conjunction with digital pressure, has been recommended in hospital settings (Hinshaw et al 2010). This is impractical and unsafe during transfer to the ambulance and transportation from the home settings (Hinshaw et al 2010). As a result, exaggerated Sims' position (see Fig. 65.3) and lowering of the head end of the

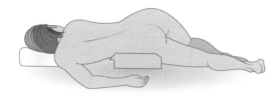

Figure 65.3 Exaggerated Sims' position. (Squire 2002.)

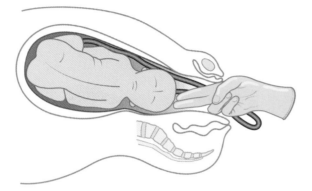

Figure 65.4 Displacement of presenting part away from pelvic inlet. (Goonwardene 2012.)

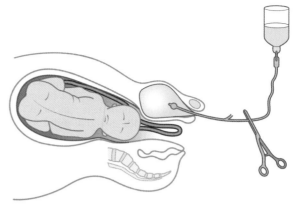

Figure 65.5 Filling the bladder. (Goonwardene 2012.)

Reflective activity 65.1   ✕❮

Access your hospital/unit guideline on management of cord prolapse and reflect on how the guidelines are applied in practice.
      Consider the emergency training within your area.

Key Points in Relation to Reflective Activity 65.1   ⌗❍

• Do your unit guidelines reflect current evidence?
• Is the training in your unit effective in preparing practitioners to deal with this emergency in all settings?
• If not, what can you do to improve this?
• Do community midwives in your Trust carry equipment to fill the bladder?

ambulance trolley below the level of the pelvis is preferable (Hinshaw et al 2010).
      Digital pressure to relieve cord compression is achieved by insertion of a gloved hand into the vagina and pushing forcibly upward, elevating the presenting part out of the pelvis to protect the cord from occlusion (see Fig. 65.4). This digital pressure should be maintained either until ambulance transfer or in theatre at caesarean section.

Bladder filling

An alternative to digital pressure, which has been shown to be beneficial, particularly if a delay in delivery is anticipated, is bladder filling (Caspi et al 1983; Chetty and Moodley 1980; Houghton 2006; RCOG 2014). This raises the presenting part for an extended period of time. A 16-gauge self-retaining (Foley) catheter is inserted. Sterile saline (0.9%) is instilled via a giving set, attached to the catheter and the catheter clamped to retain the fluid. A dose of 500 mL to 750 mL has been shown to elevate the presenting part sufficiently to eliminate the need for digital pressure (Goonwardene 2012; RCOG 2014) (see Fig. 65.5), providing this can be done quickly, and it is particularly useful when transferring in from home-birth settings (Hinshaw et al 2010). The midwife should be mindful in ensuring that the bladder is emptied before delivery of the baby (RCOG 2014).

Psychological care

Midwives should recognize that any obstetric emergency is likely to be traumatic for both the parents and the midwife and has implications for informed consent. Good communication skills can help the midwife gain not only the cooperation of the mother but also help her achieve a sense of choice and control, both of which will be affected in these circumstances (NMC 2012; NMC 2015). Even if the outcome is good, there may be feelings of anger or resentment. Time to discuss the events with the couple post birth must be facilitated to ensure that any questions they have may be addressed. The midwife should not underestimate the impact that emergency situations can have on both them and the team, particularly if the outcome is poor. Care should be taken to ensure all team members have an opportunity to debrief, including student midwives who, dependent on their level of training, may have less understanding of what has just happened.

Long-term outcomes for the mother may include:

- Sepsis due to the invasive nature of the interventions
- Complications of operative procedures, such as Mendleson's syndrome (pulmonary acid aspiration syndrome), particularly if general anaesthesia is used
- Postpartum haemorrhage
- Post-traumatic stress disorder
- Bereavement if the fetus/neonate dies or has suffered hypoxic brain injury
- Separation, bonding and feeding issues, particularly if baby is admitted to neonatal intensive care unit (NICU).

For the fetus/neonate:

Cord pH drops by 0.04 per minute (Cox et al 2009); therefore, prompt recognition and management will have a direct impact on fetal outcome, which may include:

- Separation from parents
- Admission to NICU – with associated risk of infection as a result of invasive procedures
- Hypoxic brain injury (hypoxic ischemic enecphalopathy (HIE))
- Intrapartum or perinatal death

CONCLUSION

Cord prolapse is a potentially life-threatening emergency for the fetus and carries with it a significant risk of neonatal morbidity. The midwife is a key professional who needs to be alert to risk factors and to undertake prompt urgent action when cord prolapse is suspected or confirmed.

The psychological support the woman and her family needs is an important aspect of postnatal care and also in preparation for any future pregnancies. This will call on the communication skills of the midwife and others involved in the care.

The midwife needs to develop skills and competencies in managing cord prolapse, be aware of the potential psychological distress that the emergency can cause to the individuals involved in care, and seek appropriate help and support.

The safe management of this emergency demands a high level of clinical knowledge and excellent interpersonal skills.

Reflective activity 65.2

You are a community midwife and you are called to a planned home birth at 06.00 hours of a woman called Marion, who has had three children.

This will be her third home birth, and she is 38+1/40 gestation. When you arrive, she is in obvious labour. At her last antenatal visit yesterday, the presenting part was five-fifths palpable.

Marion's husband, Jeff, lets you in and you find Marion leaning over the kitchen sink with contractions occurring four times in 10 minutes. As you are saying 'hello' to her, Marion has the urge to bear down and her membranes rupture. Copious amounts of clear liquor are draining, and she informs you that something warm is dangling from her vagina. On inspection, the cord is clearly visible.
How would you proceed?

Key Points in Relation to Reflective activity 65.2

- Consider the midwives responsibility and accountability. What are your priorities?
- Can the husband assist in any way?
- What information would you give the emergency service operator?
- Can you employ bladder filling if you are on your own?

Key Points

- Cord prolapse and presentation are relatively rare occurrences.
- This is a life-threatening emergency for the fetus.
- It is often the midwife who makes the diagnosis.
- Help must be summoned as a priority.
- Prompt recognition and action can improve perinatal outcomes.
- Good record keeping is vital, particularly in relation to timing of events (NMC 2015).
- Midwives need to be alert to those risk factors that may predispose to cord prolapse or presentation.
- Regular multidisciplinary training is recommended for all birth settings.
- Parents and staff need to have the opportunity to 'debrief'.

References

Caspi E, Lotan Y, Schreyer P: Prolapse of the cord: reduction of perinatal mortality by bladder instillation and caesarean section, *Isr J Med Sci* 19:541–545, 1983.

Chakravarti S, Gupta K, Datta S: Malposition, malpresentations and cord prolapse. In Arulkumaran S, Sivanesaratnam V, Chatterjee A, et al, editors: *Essentials of obstetrics*, Tunbridge Wells, Anshan, 2004.

Chetty RM, Moodley J: Umbilical cord prolapse, *S Afr Med J* 57(4):128–129, 1980.

Cox C, Grady K, Howell C, editors: *Managing Obstetric Emergencies and Trauma: The MOET Course Manual*, 2nd edn, London, Royal College of Obstetricians and Gynaecologists (RCOG) Press, 2009.

Goonwardene M: Umbilical cord prolapse. In Chandraharan E, Arulkumaran S, editors: *Obstetric and intrapartum emergencies*, Cambridge, Cambridge University Press, 2012.

Hinshaw K, Simpson H, Wieteska S, et al: *Pre-hospital obstetric emergency training*, Sussex, Wiley-Blackwell, 2010.

Houghton G: Bladder filling: an effective technique for managing cord prolapse, *Br J Midwifery* 14(2):88–89, 2006.

McKinney ES, Murray SS, James SR, et al: *Maternal child nursing*, 4th edn, Elsevier, 2013.

Nursing and Midwifery Council (NMC): *Midwives Rules and Standards*, London, NMC, 2012.

Nursing and Midwifery Council (NMC): *The Code: Professional Standards of Practice and Behaviour for Nurses and Midwives*, London, NMC, 2015.

Royal College of Obstetricians and Gynaecologists (RCOG): *Umbilical Cord Prolapse – Green Top Guideline No. 50*, London, Royal College of Obstetricians and Gynaecologists (RCOG), 2014.

Squire C: Shoulder dystocia and umbilical cord prolapse. In Boyle M, editor: *Emergencies around childbirth*, Oxford, Radcliffe Medical, 2002.

Tchabo JG: The use of the contact hysteroscope in the diagnosis of cord prolapse. In Cox C, Grady K, Howell C, editors: *Managing Obstetric Emergencies and Trauma: The MOET Course Manual*, 2nd edn, London, Royal College of Obstetricians and Gynaecologists (RCOG) Press, 1988.

Yamada T, Kataoka S, Takeda M, et al: Umbilical cord presentation after use of a trans-cervical balloon catheter, *J Obstet Gynaecol Res* 39:658–662, Wiley, 2013.

Resources and additional reading

Gibbons C, O'Herlihy C, Murphy JF: Umbilical cord prolapse: changing patterns and improved outcomes, *Br J Obstet Gynaecol* 121:1705–1709, 2014.

Chapter 66

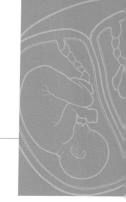

Maternal morbidity following childbirth

Professor Mary Steen

Learning Outcomes ?

After reading this chapter, you will be able to:

- gain knowledge and understanding of physical health problems following pregnancy and childbirth
- identify risk factors that predispose mothers to morbidity
- understand the midwife's role in identifying and referring any deviations from what is considered to be normal physiology when a mother's body is reverting back to non-pregnant status
- consider the possible effects on women's physical, emotional and psychological well-being if these are not recognized and managed

INTRODUCTION

Globally, after birth, a recuperation period of around 40 days is traditionally viewed as the puerperium and there is an expectation a woman's body will have recovered sufficiently and return to a non-pregnant status of health (Waugh 2011). The concept of postnatal care is one that aims to assist the mother, her baby and family towards attaining an optimum health status (Steen and Wray 2014). However, maternal morbidity after childbirth is an important aspect of postnatal care that needs consideration. The World Health Organisation (WHO) (2010) has reported that returning to a non-pregnant state of health can take much longer, as many new mothers can experience health and well-being issues. Wray and Bick (2012) have highlighted that, for some mothers, returning to a good state of health can take up to a year after birth.

The postnatal period is defined as 'a period after the end of labour during which the attendance of a midwife upon a woman and baby is required, being not less than 10 days and for such longer period as the midwife considers necessary' (Nursing and Midwifery Council (NMC) 2012). Providing individualized postnatal care to mothers and babies is underpinned by the NMC (2012) Midwives Rules and Standards, and professional care by the NMC Code (NMC 2015). The National Institute for Health and Care Excellence (NICE 2006 and 2014) have recommended a postnatal care pathway and defined core care to be provided for mothers and babies during the first few days and then weeks following birth.

NICE (2006 and 2014) postnatal care is divided into three time periods:

- The first 24 hours after birth
- The first 2 to 7 days
- The period from day 8 to around 6 to 8 weeks

During the postnatal period, mothers go through a transitional period of physiological and emotional/psychological change that is also influenced by cultural and sociological factors. In the UK, the majority of postnatal care is given in the mother's own home or in a relative's home. Occasionally, a mother may be in a hostel or a mother and baby home. Providing effective and individualized postnatal care to a diverse population of mothers needs to be considered. A woman-centred approach tailored to meet individual needs will promote good standards of care (NICE 2006 and 2014). Various levels of support will be required by mothers. For example, it is likely that a first-time mother and a mother who has had birth complications will be more likely to need extra support than a second-time mother who has experienced a straightforward birth.

Adopting a flexible approach to caring for mother and babies, which includes the engagement of their families and communities after birth, will help meet individual health needs and ultimately this will promote many benefits (Redshaw and Heikkila 2010; Steen and Wray 2014). The quality of postnatal care provided to mothers, babies and families in the first few weeks after birth can have a positive effect and assist mothers and families during the transition to parenthood (National Childbirth Trust (NCT) 2012). A partnership approach for postnatal care where a trusting relationship can develop is recommended (Wray and Bick 2012). This is to enable a woman to openly discuss how she genuinely feels both physically and emotionally.

ROLE OF MIDWIFE

It is essential that a midwife is familiar with a mother's medical and obstetric history and her well-being status when assessing whether or not she is recuperating as expected following childbirth (Redshaw et al 2007). During the postnatal period, the midwife needs to advise the mother about some possible health problems she can be at risk of developing and how to recognize signs and symptoms (NICE 2006 and 2014). This will require educating the woman about what she should be expecting during the puerperium, what is normal, and what would be a deviation. How to seek advice and help needs to be discussed with mothers, partners and family members. Contact numbers and regular reminders to seek help is an important message to convey if a mother is feeling unwell or she has any concerns.

It is also important that midwives have the knowledge and skills to determine when to be proactive and undertake specific observations when there are indications to do so. Therefore, the midwife needs to be able to acknowledge and recognize what are normal expected outcomes following birth and also be able to identify signs of what is not normal and when to instigate care that will involve further investigation, tests and the support of other health professionals (NICE 2006 and 2014).

To assist the midwife to assess degrees of urgency, a status level of 'Emergency', 'Urgent' and 'Non-Urgent' has been recommended by NICE (2006 and 2014).

An **emergency status** is classified as:

- When a life-threatening or potential life-threatening situation is identified

An **urgent status** is classified:

- When there is a potentially serious situation, which needs appropriate action

A **non–urgent status** is classified:

- When there is a need to continue to monitor and assess

Where a pregnancy or a birth has involved a medical or obstetric complication, a mother's care is likely to differ from those mothers whose pregnancy and birth has had no complications. Interestingly, it has been highlighted that some women still want to be 'checked over' (physically), regardless of complications, as a means of obtaining contact and feedback from the midwife about their bodies and recovery, separate from their baby (Wray 2011).

To reduce the risk of maternal morbidity happening within disadvantaged mothers, more intense postnatal care will be required and addressing public health targets to promote healthy lifestyles to the mother, her partner and family during the postnatal period is an essential aspect of this care. Working alongside other professionals, services and local communities will assist to meet individual needs of susceptible mothers.

RECOGNIZING MATERNAL MORBIDITY

A midwife will consider the health of newly birthed mothers from a viewpoint of confirming normality. An assessment of the mother's physical appearance will assist in the overall management of her postnatal care and will guide in the decision making of whether there is a need to consider any further investigations or referrals. In general, the accumulation of a number of clinical signs will assist the midwife in making decisions about the presence or potential for morbidity. In addition, consideration must be given to the potential that mothers are susceptible to common illnesses as well, for example, a common cold or gastric problems. Mothers are also susceptible to influenza, demonstrated by the evidence of 1 in 11 women who died from influenza (CMACE 2011). Increasing immunization rates in pregnancy against seasonal influenza provides some protection in the postnatal period.

Life-threatening health problems

In high resource countries, newly birthed mothers are at very low risk of mortality if there have been no antenatal complications or previous serious medical history (Lewis 2007; Knight et al 2014; UNICEF 2015).

UNICEF (2015) states that 'The lifetime risk of maternal death in industrialized countries is 1 in 4000, versus 1 in 51 in countries classified as "least developed"'.

This clearly highlights that some mothers can die during the postnatal period in developed countries mainly as a result of haemorrhage, thromboembolism, infection and eclampsia. The leading cause of direct maternal deaths in the triennium 2006–2008 was reported to be infection (CMACE 2011). See Table 66.1 , which illustrates potential life-threatening conditions and urgency status.

It is important that verbal communication is on-going throughout emergency situations, as the mother may still

Table 66.1 Potential life-threatening conditions and urgency status

Sign and symptoms	Evaluate for	Action
Sudden or profuse blood loss, or blood loss and signs/symptoms of shock, including tachycardia, hypotension, hypoperfusion, change in consciousness	**Haemorrhage** Post-partum haemorrhage (PPH)	Emergency action
Offensive/excessive vaginal loss, tender abdomen or fever. If no obstetric cause, consider other causes	PPH, sepsis/other pathology	Urgent action
Unilateral calf pain, redness or swelling	**Thromboembolism** Deep Vein Thrombosis (DVT)	Emergency action
Shortness of breath or chest pain	Pulmonary Embolism (PE)	Emergency action
Fever, shivering, rigours, abdominal pain and/or offensive vaginal loss If temperature exceeds 38°C, repeat in 4–6 hours. If temperature still high or other symptoms and measurable signs, evaluate further	**Infection** Infection – genital tract sepsis	Emergency action
Severe or persistent headache	**Eclampsia**	Emergency action
Diastolic BP is greater than 90 mmHg and accompanied by another sign/symptom of pre-eclampsia	Pre-eclampsia Eclampsia	Emergency action
Diastolic BP is greater than 90 mmHg and no other sign/symptom, repeat BP within 4 hours. If it remains above 90 mmHg after 4 hours, evaluate	Pre-eclampsia Eclampsia	Emergency action

Adapted from NICE guidelines (NICE 2006)

be able to hear and also it will assist to calm her partner or any relatives if they are present.

It is noteworthy that most maternal deaths in countries classified as 'least developed' by UNICEF are preventable. It is well recognized that most maternal deaths occur in the first month after birth and nearly half of these cases occur within the first 24 hours and approximately two-thirds occur during the first week (Renfrew et al 2014; ten Hoope-Bender 2014; Nour 2008).

WHO (2010) recommends that low- to middle-resourced countries provide postnatal care in the first 24 hours to all mothers and a clinical examination should be undertaken within 1 hour of birth. If birth has taken place at home, then the first postnatal contact should be as early as possible within this time frame and, if possible, extra contact between 24 to 48 hours is desirable. In addition, mobile phone-based postnatal care contacts between mothers and the health facility may be helpful in between visits. Ideally, four postnatal contacts are recommended.

Improvements in nutritional status, prevention of anaemia (a major contributing factor to the risk of post-partum haemorrhage), increasing awareness of cleanliness (importance of washing hands) to prevent infections developing, access to health care facilities, including family planning services, the presence of skilled birth attendants and availability of emergency obstetric care can

assist to reduce maternal mortality rates in developing countries (United Nations 2013; WHO 2014).

Engaging and educating girls is vital to improve maternal health and well-being in low-resourced countries. It is well recognized that the risk of maternal mortality is higher among women with no education, and also has an impact on women who have received 1 to 6 years of education when compared with women who received 12 years of education (United Nations 2013; see also The Girl Effect, 2008, in *Resources and Additional Reading*).

Haemorrhage

Primary postpartum haemorrhage (PPH) is a potentially life-threatening condition that can occur immediately after birth or within 24 hours of delivery of the placenta and membranes. This condition presents as a sudden and excessive vaginal blood loss. After 24 hours and up to 6 weeks postnatally, *a secondary PPH* can occur and a mother may have excessive or prolonged vaginal loss (Cunningham et al 2005a; Steen and Gibbon 2012). Commonly, the placental site is the source of both a primary or secondary PPH. Retained products of conception and placental tissue can prevent uterine involution and this then can be complicated with an infection, i.e. sepsis (Lewis 2007). Sometimes genital tract trauma might be the cause of a primary postpartum haemorrhage and this trauma will need to be identified and repaired as soon as possible (Steen 2010). The causes of a PPH are often referred to as the *four Ts: tone, trauma, tissue and thrombin* (Anderson and Etches 2007).

NICE (2006 and 2014) has reported that there is insufficient evidence to recommend routine measurement of fundal height, as the process of involution is highly variable between individual women. However, it is recommended that an abdominal palpation should be undertaken if a mother feels unwell, has some abdominal pain, a marked change in her vaginal loss, which can be heavier or offensive, or is passing clots. Uterine involution, in combination with other observations such as a high or low temperature reading, rapid pulse or any abdominal tenderness and offensive lochia, can help to identify maternal morbidity (Lewis 2011).

Subinvolution of the uterus may be suspected where the uterus fails to follow the expected progressive reduction in size. On palpation, the mother's uterus may feel what is commonly referred to as being 'boggy', which may indicate that there is an infection, or sometimes the cause may be retained products of conception. Antibiotics and oxytocic drugs may be prescribed and, in some cases, an evacuation of the uterus – usually under general anaesthesia – is advocated, which is commonly referred to as an Evacuation of Retained Products of Conception (ERPC).

Thromboembolism

Many mothers experience oedema of ankles and feet after birth but this should resolve steadily over the first few days as normal levels of activity are resumed. However, oedema in ankles and feet should be bilateral and not accompanied by pain and inflammation. If a mother complains of any localized pain and there are visible signs of inflammation in one calf, this may indicate a deep vein thrombosis (DVT) and needs urgent referral. A DVT is when a blood clot forms in one of the deep veins in the leg, normally in the calf. This may remain localized and may cause an obstruction in the blood flow and, more dangerously, the clot may detach and may move to another area such as the lungs as an embolus.

If a mother collapses and there are no obvious signs of haemorrhage, then other reasons need to be considered, for example *thromboembolism*. The midwife needs to ensure that emergency assistance is called for as soon as possible and that the mother is safe, maintains her airway and any basic circulatory needs are addressed. The midwife should also administrator oxygen to the mother. The midwife needs to be alert to women who are at increased risk of developing a thromboembolism, as described in Box 66.1.

Prophylactic precautions for women who undergo an elective or emergency caesarean section include using thromboembolitic (TED) stockings and heparin to be prescribed as recommended by NICE (2006 and 2014) and Royal College of Obstetricians and Gynaecologists (RCOG 2015a and 2015b). Early ambulation is also helpful.

Box 66.1 Risk factors for DVT/thromboembolism

Obesity

Smoking

Age (older than 35 years)

History of superficial thrombosis

Previous VTE and thrombophilia

Prolonged bed rest

Multiparty

Gross varicose veins

Paraplegia

Caesarean section and instrumental delivery

Stillbirth

Preterm birth

Dehydration

Has also been associated with long air journeys

(RCOG 2015a)

Infection

It is not necessary to undertake a mother's temperature routinely if she appears physically well but if a mother complains of feeling unwell, describes 'flu-like symptoms or there are signs or symptoms of possible infection, then the midwife needs to undertake and record a temperature reading. Where there is a rise in temperature above 38 °C, it is usual for this to be considered a deviation from normal and of clinical significance (NICE 2006 and 2014). Assessing the mother's pulse rate, for a full minute, can assist to indicate whether there is a deviation from normal. The midwife needs to observe the respiratory rate and a number of other signs of being healthy, such as general appearance, colour, skin and body temperature and any unpleasant body odour. It is essential to listen very closely to exactly what the mother says to gain an insight into any health problems emerging. Any deviations from normal must be acted upon, and any referrals or treatment clearly recorded.

Eclampsia

Routine observations of a mother's blood pressure without any clinical reasons are not required if the baseline recording has been recorded within a normal range (NICE 2006 and 2014). If there has been a previous history of hypertension or pre-eclampsia, then the mother's blood pressure and any treatment will be assessed according to her individual care needs assessment. Although rare, some mothers can develop pre-eclampsia and eclampsia postnatally, with no previous history during the antenatal period. It is important that a midwife is aware of the possibility of pre-eclampsia happening and alert to signs and symptoms. If a mother complains of, for example, having headaches, visual disturbances, and/or any epigastric pain, then taking a blood pressure reading, urine sample and referring her to the obstetrician while in the hospital, or her family doctor if she has returned home, is advocated. She will need to be followed up with observations of her blood pressure and antihypertensive treatment (NICE 2010).

COMMON HEALTH PROBLEMS

Breast problems

It is essential that midwives offer support and advice on common breast and breastfeeding problems. Sometimes a mildly raised temperature may be related to the increasing production of breastmilk (Stables and Rankin 2010). Physical problems such as engorgement, cracked or bleeding nipples, mastitis and signs of *Candida albicans* (thrush) are some of the common problems a mother may experience. Engorgement on postnatal day 3 and 4 is a common problem for all women (Stables and Rankin 2010). If a mother is breastfeeding or formula feeding, she needs to be advised to wear a well-fitting brassiere and may need analgesia. If a mother is breastfeeding and she has some engorgement, it is important that she feeds her baby on demand and is aware of ways she can alleviate the engorgement, i.e. performing breast massage (from under her axilla towards the nipple), use of hot and cold compresses and how to hand express. If not breastfeeding, she should avoid touching the breasts, take analgesia and be reassured that the engorgement will subside (see Ch. 44).

Vaginal blood loss

Most women can clearly identify colour and consistency of vaginal loss if asked and will be able to describe any changes (Marchant et al 2002). It is important for a midwife to ask direct questions about the woman's vaginal loss – whether this is more or less, lighter or darker than previously and whether the woman has any concerns. It is of particular importance to record any clots passed and when these occurred. Clots can be associated with future episodes of excessive or prolonged postpartum bleeding.

Assessment that attempts to quantify the amount of loss or the size of a clot is problematic. However, the use of descriptions that are common to both the woman and a midwife can improve accuracy in these physical assessments, for example, asking the mother how often she has to change her maternity pad and describing her blood loss in her own words.

Urinary

Soon after giving birth, a woman's body has to reabsorb excess fluid and then void large amounts of urine (Cunningham et al 2005b) – see also Chapter 35. A woman's urine output should resolve within the first few days of giving birth. Bladder care is important and sometimes, an involuting uterus may be palpated to one side and this may indicate a full bladder. The mother will be asked to pass urine and then her uterus will be palpated again. If a woman has difficulty in trying to pass urine, then doing this in a warm bath and/or running a tap and hearing water running may gently help a woman to void, especially if she has some vulval swelling (Steen 2013). If the mother is unable to pass urine within 6 hours of birth, then urinary retention must be considered (NICE 2013). Retention of urine is more likely to occur after epidural analgesia, prolonged labour and an instrumental delivery because of trauma and possible loss of sensation (Stables and Rankin 2010). Catheterization of the bladder in these circumstances may be indicated.

It is important that a midwife recognizes urinary retention, as an overfull bladder can lead to denervation, an atonic bladder and the risk of irreversible damage to the detrusor muscle and parasympathetic nerves. Bladder damage can predispose a mother to urinary incontinence and infections in the short and long term (Steen 2013).

Urinary stress, urge incontinence, uterovaginal prolapse and cystocele are associated with pelvic floor damage (Stables and Rankin 2010). NICE (2006 and 2014) has recommended that pelvic floor muscle exercises should be taught as first-line treatment for urinary incontinence and a systematic review has confirmed that pelvic floor exercises undertaken during pregnancy and postnatally can prevent urinary incontinence (Mørkved and Bø 2014). It is important that women are given opportunities to discuss any urinary incontinence, as this is often a taboo subject and many women will not disclose (Steen 2013). If urinary incontinence does not resolve, a referral to a specialist must be undertaken (Gerrard and Hove 2013).

Bowel

Bowel problems, such as constipation and haemorrhoids, can be a common problem for some newly birthed mothers. Some women will have had bowel problems during pregnancy and a prolonged labour or difficult birth can exacerbate the problem. A prolonged labour and difficult birth can also predispose some mothers to suffer from these ailments. Approximately 44% of mothers have been reported to suffer from constipation (Derbyshire et al 2007). It is also estimated that around 20% of mothers can suffer from haemorrhoids, which can be very painful but usually improve within a few days of giving birth (Abramowitz et al 2002). However, the prevalence of these bowel problems may be underestimated, as many mothers will find it difficult and often embarrassing to confide in a health professional (Steen 2013). Being constipated and straining when attempting to have a bowel movement can lead to an anal fissure, which may be painful and problematic to heal.

Faecal incontinence can sometimes occur, and this may involve the involuntary loss of faeces but can include faecal urgency and flatus incontinence (Bick et al 2009). It has been reported that around 3% to 10% of mothers will experience faecal problems, and mothers who have urinary incontinence problems appear to be at increased risk (Meschia et al 2002). Faecal incontinence is associated with third and fourth degree tears and instrumental deliveries (RCOG 2015c). Prophylactic antibiotics can be helpful in preventing infection and breakdown of sutured third or fourth degree tears and reducing the risk of faecal incontinence (Duggal et al 2008).

A diet high in fluids and fibre is recommended, and the use of prophylactic laxatives that are non-irritant to the bowel and fibre supplements can be prescribed to alleviate constipation (Eogan et al 2007). To alleviate painful haemorrhoids, a high fibre diet and plenty of fluids, and sometimes laxatives to soften stools are recommended. Local application of hydrocortisone ointment may be advised to reduce inflammation and pain (NICE 2007). Mothers who have perineal sutures may need extra reassurance that when they need to open their bowels that any stitches will not disrupt (Steen 2012).

Perineal problems

Morbidity associated with perineal trauma that can be naturally occurring (tears) or surgically induced (episiotomy) is a major women's health problem (Steen 2012). There has been an increase in Obstetric Anal Sphincter Injuries (OASIS) reported (RCOG 2015c). The need to follow-up women who have sustained anal sphincter injuries to identify any on-going problems, receive physiotherapy and a consultation with an obstetrician is recommended (see Ch. 40).

It is well recognized that perineal trauma can have both short- and long-term negative health and well-being consequences, which can also lead to social problems (RCOG 2004). Perineal pain and discomfort affects the majority of women to some degree and the associated inflammation caused by perineal trauma exacerbates the severity (East et al 2012). Alleviating perineal pain and discomfort is a high priority after birth. Bick and Bassett (2013) have recommended that all women should be asked if they have any perineal pain or discomfort. If a woman reports that she has no perineal pain or discomfort, then it is not essential for the midwife to examine her perineum. However, if a midwife has any concerns that the woman is declining because she may be embarrassed or afraid, the

midwife may need to explore this concern and reassure her that perineal pain and discomfort affects many women and healing of the perineum needs to be assessed (Steen 2007a). When reviewing the evidence to alleviate perineal pain and discomfort, both systemic and localized treatments may be necessary to achieve adequate pain relief to meet individual women's needs (Steen and Roberts 2011). A combination of oral analgesia, bathing, *diclofenac* suppositories (first 24 hours) and localized cooling can help alleviate perineal pain and discomfort.

Caesarean section wounds

A caesarean section is a major operation that involves the surgical cutting of major abdominal muscles, soft tissues and skin. Palpation of the abdomen after this surgical intervention is likely to be painful for the woman in the first few postnatal days. Around postnatal day 3 or 4, when the mother's abdomen is less tender, uterine involution may be assessed by performing an abdominal palpation if there is a clinical indication to do so. The caesarean section wound needs to be observed for healing and any signs of infection. Prior to a caesarean section being performed, women are routinely prescribed antibiotics, as there is evidence to show that the incidence of subsequent wound infection and endometritis is significantly reduced (Smaill and Hofmeyr 2000). A wound dressing is applied for the first 24 hours and then removed, as this aids healing and reduces infection. The midwife will need to advise the mother how to take care of her wound and discuss signs and symptoms of a wound infection. Obese women are more at risk of a wound infection because of abdominal skin folds being present, which can create an ideal warm and moist environment for an infection to occur. A dry dressing or a negative wound pressure dressing over the suture line might be advocated. It is important to consider that mothers who have had a caesarean section will need time to recover from this operation and sufficient time given to promote healing of the wound as well as emotional/psychological adjustment to the birth (Mander 2007).

A wound that is inflamed and tender and an accompanying pyrexia is indicative of an infection and a wound swab should be taken for microorganism culture. Medical advice must be sought and antibiotics may be prescribed. A midwife needs to be alert to the possibility that a haematoma or an abscess can also form underneath the wound. It is, therefore, vitally important for a midwife to ask the mother if she has increased pain and pressure around the wound.

Musculoskeletal

During the postnatal period, many women continue to suffer from musculoskeletal problems. The effects of progesterone and relaxin during the first 6 months contribute to this as a mother gradually returns to her non-pregnant status and changing posture (Steen 2007b). Backache can be a common problem for some mothers and associated pain can affect everyday living activities. Pelvic girdle and symphysis pubic pain can also be a continuing problem. If there are any musculoskeletal issues that persist, then a referral can be made for the mother to attend physiotherapy clinic (Aslan and Fynes 2007).

Anaemia

Anaemia is a common problem after childbirth. Many women have iron-deficiency during their pregnancy and even though this has been identified and iron supplementation commenced, anaemia can continue to be a health issue for some women (Wray and Steen 2014). A rapid pulse rate in an otherwise well woman might suggest that she is anaemic. A large blood loss after birth and haemorrhage requires a review of a mother's blood profile, i.e. red blood cell count, volume, haemoglobin and ferritin levels. Depending of the severity of iron deficiency and any pre-existing haemoglobinopathies will guide whether iron supplements, an infusion or a blood transfusion will be advocated as treatment (Bhandal and Russel 2006).

Tiredness and fatigue

Most women will report tiredness and fatigue during the first few weeks after birth, and lack of sleep at the end of pregnancy, giving birth and establishing feeding can take its toll. It is, therefore, vitally important that a newly birthed mother is advised to consciously make time to rest and sleep during the postpartum period. For example, she should be advised to take the opportunity to have a 'nap' during the day when her baby is sleeping and not to feel guilty about doing this. A midwife may need to reassure a mother that household chores can wait and it takes time to adjust to caring for a newborn. Tiredness and fatigue can have an adverse effect on a mother's health and well-being status. Being tired and fatigued will inevitably have a negative effect on a woman's ability to care for her newborn (Troy and Dalgas-Pelish 2003). Tiredness and fatigue can lead to maternal exhaustion and has been associated with maternal depression (Taylor and Johnson 2010). In addition, maternal depletion of nutrients has been recognized and this can contribute to mothers feeling tired and becoming exhausted and depressed (King 2003). Women should be encouraged to maintain a healthy balanced diet and drink plenty of fluids (DH 2007; Steen 2007a) – see Chapter 17. Midwives can play a vital role in supporting a woman to have realistic expectations about life after birth and advising her to nurture herself and on the importance of finding time to rest and recuperate.

Headaches

Postnatally, some women are susceptible to headaches and these are associated with tiredness and stress. A midwife should ask the mother about the severity, duration and how often she suffers from the headache, if and what medication has been taken and whether this helped to alleviate the symptoms. Further exploration about fluid intake, diet, lack of sleep and any worries should be considered as these can trigger headaches.

It is important that the mother's blood pressure is monitored to exclude hypertension or pre-eclampsia as a cause. Sometimes following an epidural, a mother can report severe headache, especially upon standing, and this is caused by a *dural tap* and the leakage of a small amount of cerebral spinal fluid (see Ch. 38). To resolve the headache, the insertion of 10 to 20 mL of blood into the epidural space (a blood patch) is required (NICE 2006 and 2014).

LONGER TERM IMPLICATIONS

Postnatal care is often referred to as being the 'Cinderella' of maternity services (Steen and Wray 2014; Lewis 2007). It has been reported that some mothers feel poorly supported and are often disappointed with the care they receive (Wray 2006; WHO 2010). Bhavnani and Newburn (2010) highlighted that some mothers who had an instrumental or caesarean section were the least satisfied with their postnatal care. This information needs to be considered when postnatal care is being given, and it is more likely that mothers who have had birth interventions will need additional support and care.

Health promotion is important and opportunities to advise mothers and other family members, if available, about healthy lifestyles should be undertaken. There is cumulative evidence that being active and undertaking exercise postnatally is beneficial (Goodwin et al 2000; Clapp et al 2002; Berk 2004; Steen 2007b). Exploring a mother's level of activity, motivation to exercise, her diet, how well she is able to have some rest and what her sleeping patterns are will help a midwife gain an overall picture of how well the mother is. Maternal well-being and resilience are important aspects to consider, as these will reduce the risk of maternal morbidity and illness. The link between mental and physical health is well recognized (Drake 2013). Anxiety and stress are associated with cognitive, behavioural and autonomic symptoms, and this can include headaches, dizziness, palpations, restlessness, insomnia, gastric problems, muscular aches and/or urinary frequency (Woods 2012).

It is also recognized that maternal mental health problems can have a negative impact upon the health and well-being of infants, which can contribute to bonding and attachment issues (Steen et al 2013). This can then in turn have long-term consequences for children and adolescents emotional, behavioural, cognitive and social skills (Halligan et al 2007). Therefore, it is important for midwives to consider if there are any underlying mental health problems that may be associated with physical symptoms (Steen and Steen 2014).

CULTURALLY AND LINGUISTICALLY DIVERSE CONSIDERATIONS

It is vitally important to consider mothers from culturally and linguistically diverse (CALD) backgrounds, as these mothers are at increased risk of mental health problems (Steen et al 2015; Steen and Green 2016). Midwives need to be aware of the increased susceptibility for mental health problems and communication difficulties if a newly birthed mother is a recent immigrant or refugee. An Australian report identified communication as the most significant challenge to address when caring for these mothers (Each Social and Community Health (EACH) Report 2011). There is good evidence that professional accredited interpreters can improve clinical outcomes for immigrant women who speak limited English (Karliner et al 2007). Offering an interpreting service and using an interpreter for postnatal contact visits will improve communication and help break down language barriers. This will ensure that women are informed and supported and able to report deviations from normal or problems so these can be addressed appropriately, thus reducing morbidity.

Benefits of befriending have been shown to help new mothers adjust and develop coping and resilience skills during the transition to motherhood (Darcy et al 2011; Johnson et al 2000; Molloy 2007; Steen 2007b). Psychological therapies have also helped some mothers to alleviate their anxiety and stress, and addressed post traumatic distress disorder (PTSD) symptoms after a traumatic birth and depression (Steen et al 2013).

Fertility and contraceptive advice is also within the sphere of practice of a midwife. Midwives need to keep themselves up to date with current evidence and be aware of the sexual health needs of individual mothers (see Chs 13 and 27).

Influences of family and community

Providing midwifery care that adopts a woman-focused and family-included approach has many benefits, such as optimal bonding and maternal infant attachment to take place and an increase in self-esteem and confidence.

There is evidence that many fathers feel excluded, unsure and fearful (Steen et al 2012). Reaching out

---

Reflective activity 66.1

A young first-time mother who had an emergency caesarean section for failure to progress, is from a CALD background, living in a socially deprived urban area with limited social support, is now 4 days' postnatal, feels generally unwell and has a low grade fever.

- What immediate observations and actions does the midwife need to undertake?
- What follow-up care will the midwife provide to this disadvantaged young mother?
- What support and advice can a midwife provide to this vulnerable young mother about her health and well-being?
- What local and community support can be accessed to help this young mother to remain healthy?

– involving fathers in maternity care (Royal College of Midwives (RCM) 2011), highlighted that fathers need to be supported, involved and prepared to enable them to support the mother and baby. It is, therefore, important that fathers and also other family members are included in postnatal care and support.

The emphasis that 'it takes a village to bring a child up' has been recently promoted by the Family Included Global Alliance (FIGA) 2015. It is also important to consider that some mothers may be in abusive relationships and need additional support and advice to assist them to manage their own individual circumstances and needs (Steen and Keeling 2012).

CONCLUSION

There has been increasing awareness that it is important to promote good health and well-being of newly birthed mothers and babies throughout the world, as this has implications for population health and healthcare costs. Postnatal care aims to assist the mother, her baby and family towards attaining an optimum health status. Providing postnatal care to a diverse population of mothers needs to be taken into consideration. A postnatal care pathway and defined core care for mothers and babies during the first few days and weeks after birth is recommended. It is important that a midwife offers mothers advice about some possible health problems she can be at risk of developing and how to recognize signs and symptoms. The early identification of maternal morbidity and referral for medical assistance when there is any cause for concern is paramount. It is important that a midwife reviews a woman's vital signs when there is an indication of an abnormality and illness. In addition, a status level of urgency, **'Emergency'**, **'Urgent'** and **'Non-Urgent'** is helpful when determining what actions a midwife needs to take to assessing maternal morbidity. In high resource countries, mothers are at very low risk of mortality when there is no history of antenatal complications or previous serious medical or obstetric problems. However, there are some mothers who can die during the postnatal period. Haemorrhage, thromboembolism, infection and eclampsia are the main causes of maternal mortality and the leading cause of direct maternal deaths has been reported to be infection.

In addition, a postnatal care pathway and defined core care for mothers and babies during the first few days and then weeks after birth is recommended. Therefore, it is important that a mother and her baby receive continuous care whenever possible and that a trusting relationship is developed with a midwife. Engaging with family and local communities will also help a midwife to support mothers during the postnatal period, which will reduce their ongoing risk of morbidity and assist with the transition to motherhood.

Key Points

- Maternal morbidity after childbirth is an important aspect of postnatal care that needs serious consideration.

- A postnatal care pathway and defined core care for mothers and babies during the first few days and then weeks after birth is recommended.

- It is important that mothers are advised about health problems they may be at risk of developing and how to recognize signs and symptoms.

- It is crucial that the midwife is aware of communication and other cultural challenges when giving postnatal care.

- A midwife needs to review a woman's vital signs when there is an indication of an abnormality and/or illness.

- A status level of urgency **'Emergency'**, **'Urgent'** and **'Non-Urgent'** is helpful when determining what actions a midwife needs to take when assessing maternal morbidity.

References

Abramowitz L, Sobhani I, Benifla JL, et al: Anal fissure and thrombosed external haemorrhoids before and after delivery, *Dis Colon Rectum* 45(5):650–655, 2002.

Anderson JM, Etches D: Prevention and management of postpartum hemorrhage, *Am Fam Physician* 75:875–882, 2007.

Aslan E, Fynes M: Symphysial pelvic dysfunction, *Curr Opin Obstet Gynecol* 19(2):133–139, 2007.

Berk B: Recommending exercise during and after pregnancy: what the evidence says, *Int Childbirth Educ* 19(2):18–22, 2004.

Bhandal N, Russell R: Intravenous versus oral iron therapy for postpartum anaemia, *Br J Obstet Gynaecol* 113(11):1248–1252, 2006.

Bhavnani V, Newburn M: *Left to your own devices: the postnatal care experiences of 1260 first time mothers.* NCT, London, 2010.

Bick D, Bassett S: How to provide postnatal perineal care, *Midwives* (2):2013 (website). www.rcm.org .uk/news-views-and-analysis/ analysis/how-to-provide-postnatal -perineal-care. 2013.

Bick D, MacArthur C, Knowles H, et al: *Postnatal care: evidence and guidelines for management*, 2nd edn, Edinburgh, Churchill Livingstone, 2009.

Centre for Maternal and Child Enquiries (CMACE): Saving Mothers' Lives: reviewing maternal deaths to make motherhood safer: 2006–2008. The Eighth Report on Confidential Enquiries into Maternal Deaths in the United Kingdom, *Br J Obstet Gynaecol* 118(Suppl 1):1–203, 2011.

Clapp JE, Kim H, Burciu B, et al: Continuing regular exercise during pregnancy: effect of exercise volume on fetoplacental growth, *Am J Obstet Gynecol* 2002(186):142–147, 2002.

Cunningham FG, Leveno KJ, Bloom S, et al, editors: Puerperal infection. In *Williams obstetrics*, 22nd edn, New York, McGraw Hill Medical, 2005a.

Cunningham FG, Leveno KJ, Bloom S, et al, editors: Maternal physiology. In *Williams obstetrics*, 22nd edn, New York, McGraw Hill Medical, 2005b.

Darcy JM, Grzywacz JG, Stephens RL, et al: Maternal depressive symptomatology: 16-month follow-up of infant and maternal health-related quality of life, *J Am Board Fam Med* 24(3): 249–257, 2011.

Department of Health (DH): *Maternity Matters: choice, Access and Continuity of Care in a Safe Service*, London, DH, 2007.

Derbyshire EJ, Davies J, Detmar P: Changes in bowel function: pregnancy and the puerperium, *Dig Dis Sci* 52(2):324–328, 2007.

Drake M: The physical health needs of individuals with mental health problems – setting the scene. In Collins E, Drake M, Deacon M, editors: *The physical care of people with mental health problems: a guide for best practice*, London, Sage Publications Ltd, 2013.

Duggal N, Mercado C, Daniels K, et al: Antibiotic prophylaxis can prevent postpartum perineal wound complications, *Obstet Gynecol* 111(6):1268–1273, 2008.

Each Social and Community Health Report (EACH Report): *The Pregnancy and Post Birth Experience of Women from Refugee Backgrounds*

Living in the Outer East of Melbourne. Australia, 2011.

East CE, Sherburn M, Nagle C, et al: Perineal pain following childbirth: prevalence, effects on postnatal recovery and analgesia usage, *Midwifery* 28(1):93–97, 2012.

Eogan M, Daly L, Behan M, et al: Randomised clinical trial of a laxative alone versus a laxative and a bulking agent after primary repair of obstetric anal sphincter injury, *Br J Obstet Gynaecol* 114(6):736–740, 2007.

Family Included Global Alliance, (FIGA) (website). www.family included.com. 2015.

Gerrard J, Hove RI: RCM/CSP Joint Statement on Pelvic Floor Muscle Exercise: improving Health Outcomes for Women Following Pregnancy and Birth, *Royal College of Midwives* (website). www.rcm.org .uk/sites/default/files/CSP-000924 _RCM.PDF. 2013.

Goodwin A, Astbury J, McKeen J: Body image and psychological well-being in pregnancy: a comparison of exercisers and non-exercisers, *Aust N Z J Obstet Gynaecol* 40(4):442–447, 2000.

Halligan SL, Murray L, Martins C, et al: Maternal depression and psychiatric outcomes in adolescent offspring: a 13-year longitudinal study, *J Affect Disord* 97(1–3):145–154, 2007.

ten Hoope-Bender P, et al: Improvement of maternal and newborn health through midwifery, *Lancet* 384(9949):1226–1235, 2014.

Johnson Z, Molloy B, Scallan E, et al: Community Mothers Programme – seven year follow up of a randomised controlled trial of non-professional intervention in parenting, *J Public Health Med* 22(3):337–342, 2000.

Karliner LS, Jacobs EA, Chen AH, et al: Do professional interpreters improve clinical care for patients with limited English proficiency? A systematic review of the literature, *Health Serv Res* 42(2):727–754, 2007.

King JC: The risk of maternal nutritional depletion and poor outcomes increases in early or closely spaced pregnancies, *J Nutr* 133(5):1732S–1736S, 2003.

Knight M, Kenyon S, Brocklehurst P, et al. On behalf of MBRRACE-UK (eds.). On behalf of MBRRACE-UK: *Saving Lives, Improving Mothers' Care – Lessons Learned to Inform Future Maternity Care from the UK and Ireland Confidential Enquiries into Maternal Deaths and Morbidity 2009–2012.* Oxford: National Perinatal Epidemiology Unit, University of Oxford, 2014.

Lewis G, editor: The Confidential Enquiry into Maternal and Child Health (CEMACH). *Saving Mothers' Lives: Reviewing Maternal Deaths to Make Motherhood Safer 2003–2005. The Seventh Report on Confidential Enquiries into Maternal Deaths in the United Kingdom.* CEMACH, London, 2007.

Lewis G, editor: On behalf of centre for maternal and child enquiries (CMACE): Saving Mothers' Lives: reviewing maternal death to make motherhood safe 2006–2008. The Eighth Report on the confidential Enquires into Maternal Deaths in the UK, *Br J Obstet Gynaecol* 118(1):1–203, 2011.

Mander R: *Caesarean: just another way of birth?*, London, Routledge, 2007.

Marchant S, Alexander J, Garcia J: Postnatal vaginal bleeding problems and general practice, *Midwifery* 18:21–24, 2002.

Meschia M, Buonaguidi A, Pifarotti P, et al: Prevalence of anal incontinence in women with symptoms of urinary incontinence and genital prolapse, *Obstet Gynecol* 100(4):719–723, 2002.

Molloy M: Volunteering as a community mother: a pathway to lifelong learning, *Community Pract* 80(5):28–32, 2007.

Mørkved S, Bø K: Effect of pelvic floor muscle training during pregnancy and after childbirth on prevention and treatment of urinary incontinence: a systematic review, *Br J Sports Med* 48:299–310, 2014.

National Childbirth Trust (NCT): Postnatal Care. NCT, Alexandra House, Oldham Terrace, London, W3 6NH (website). www.nct.org.uk/ professional/research/pregnancy -birth-and-postnatal-care/postnatal -care. 2012.

National Institute for Health and Care Excellence (NICE): *Routine Postnatal Care of Women and Their Babies.* NICE, London (website). www.nice .org.uk/guidance/cg37. 2006; 2014.

National Institute for Health and Clinical Excellence (NICE): *Antenatal and Postnatal Mental Health: Clinical Management and Service Guidance.* NICE, London, 2007.

National Institute for Health and Clinical Excellence (NICE): *Hypertension in Pregnancy: The Management of Hypertensive Disorders During Pregnancy*, Guidelines CG107, NICE, London (website). www.nice.org.uk/ guidance/cg107. 2010.

National Institute for Health and Care Excellence (NICE): *Urinary Incontinence: The Management of Urinary Incontinence in Women.* Guidelines CG171, NICE, London (website). www.nice.org.uk/ guidance/cg171. 2013.

National Institute for Health and Care Excellence (NICE): *Intrapartum care: care of healthy women and their babies during childbirth*, Guidelines CG190, NICE, London (website). www.nice .org.uk/guidance/cg190. 2014.

Nour N: An introduction to maternal mortality, *Rev Obstet Gynecol* 1(2):77–81, 2008.

Nursing and Midwifery Council (NMC): *Midwives Rules and Standards*, NMC, London, 2012.

Nursing and Midwifery Council (NMC): *The Code: professional Standards of Practice and Behaviour for Nurses and Midwives*, NMC, London, 2015.

Redshaw M, Heikkila K: *Delivered with Care.* Oxford NPEU, UK, 2010.

Redshaw M, Rowe R, Hockley C, et al: *Recorded Delivery: A National Survey of Women's Experience of Maternity Care.* National Perinatal Epidemiology Unit, Oxford, 2007.

Renfrew MJ, et al: Midwifery and quality care: findings from a new evidence-informed framework for maternal and newborn care, *Lancet* 384(9948):1129–1145, 2014.

Royal College of Midwives (RCM): *Reaching Out: Involving Fathers in Maternity Care.* RCM, London, 2011.

Royal College of Obstetricians and Gynaecologists (RCOG): *Methods and Materials Used in Perineal Repair.* RCOG Guideline No. 23. Royal College of Obstetricians & Gynaecologists, London, 2004.

Royal College of Obstetricians and Gynaecologists (RCOG): *Reducing the Risk of Venous Thromboembolism during Pregnancy and the Puerperium.*

Green-top Clinical Guideline No. 37a, RCOG, London, 2015a.

Royal College of Obstetricians and Gynaecologists (RCOG): *Thrombosis and Embolism During Pregnancy and the Puerperium, the Acute Management.* Green-top Guideline No. 37b, RCOG, London, 2015b.

Royal College of Obstetricians and Gynaecologists (RCOG): *The Management of Third- and Fourth-Degree Perineal Tears.* Clinical Guideline No. 29, RCOG, London, 2015c.

Smaill F, Hofmeyr GJ: *Antibiotic prophylaxis for caesarean section, Cochrane Review,* The Cochrane Library, Issue 3. Update Software, Oxford, 2000.

Stables D, Rankin J: The puerperium. In Stables D, Rankin J, editors: *Physiology in childbearing with anatomy and related biosciences,* 3rd edn, London, Bailliere Tindall/ Elsevier, 2010.

Steen M: Perineal tears and episiotomy: how do wounds heal?, *Br J Midwifery* 15(5):273–274, 276–280, 2007a.

Steen M: Well-being & beyond, *Midwives* 10(3):116–119, 2007b.

Steen M: Care and consequences of perineal trauma, *Br J Midwifery* 18(6):358–362, 2010.

Steen M: Risk, recognition and repair of perineal trauma, *Br J Midwifery* 20(11):768–772, 2012.

Steen M: Promoting continence in women following childbirth, *Nurs Stand* 28(1):49–57, 2013.

Steen M, Downe S, Bamford N, et al: Not-patient and not-visitor: a metasynthesis fathers' encounters with pregnancy, birth and maternity care, *Midwifery* 28(4):422–431, 2012.

Steen M, Gibbon K: Abnormal labour and emergencies. In Steen M, editor: *Supporting women to give birth at home: a practical guide for midwives,* London, Routledge, Taylor & Francis Group, 2012.

Steen M, Green B: Mental health in pregnancy and early parenthood. In Steen M, Thomas M, editors: *Mental health across the life span,* Routledge. Taylor Francis, Oxford, 2016.

Steen M, Jones A, Woodworth B: Anxiety, bonding and attachment during pregnancy, the transition to parenthood and psychotherapy, *Br J Midwifery* 21(12):844–850, 2013.

Steen M, Keeling J: STOP! Silent screams, *Pract Midwife* 15(2):28–30, 2012.

Steen M, Roberts T: The consequences of pregnancy and birth for the pelvic floor, *Br J Midwifery* 19(1):692–698, 2011.

Steen M, Robinson M, Robertson S, et al: Pre and post survey findings from the Mind 'Building resilience programme for better mental health: pregnant women and new mothers, *EBM* 13(3):92–99, 2015.

Steen M, Steen S: Striving for better maternal mental health, *Pract Midwife* 17(3):11–14, 2014.

Steen M, Wray J: Physiology and care during the puerperium. In Marshall J, Raynor M, editors: *Myles textbook for midwives,* London, Churchill Livingstone, Elsevier, 2014.

Taylor J, Johnson M: How women manage fatigue after childbirth, *Midwifery* 26(3):367–375, 2010.

Troy NA, Dalgas-Pelish P: The effectiveness of a self care intervention for the management of postpartum fatigue, *Appl Nurs Res* 16(1):38–45, 2003.

UNICEF: *Maternal Mortality Has Declined Steadily Since 1990, but Not Quickly Enough to Meet the MDG Target* (website). http://data .unicef.org/maternal-health/ maternal-mortality#sthash .65hRm2wE.dpuf. 2015.

United Nations: *We Can End Poverty. Millennium Development Goals and Beyond 2015.* Department of Public Information, Fact Sheet (website). http://www.un.org/millennium goals/pdf/Goal_5_fs.pdf. 2013.

Waugh LJ: Beliefs associated with Mexican immigrant families' practice of la cuarentena during postpartum recovery, *J Obstet Gynecol Neonatal Nurs* 40(6):732–741, 2011.

Woods L: Psychological interventions in anxiety and depression. In Smith G, editor: *Psychological interventions in mental health nursing,* Maidenhead, UK, Open University Press/McGraw Hill Education, 2012.

World Health Organization (WHO): *WHO technical consultation on postpartum and postnatal care.* WHO Document Production Services, Geneva (website). http:// whqlibdoc.who.int/hq/2010/ WHO_MPS_10.03_eng.pdf. 2010.

World Health Organisation (WHO): Recommendations on postnatal care of the mother and newborn. WHO library cataloguing publications data (website). http://www.who.int/ maternal_child_adolescent/ documents/postnatal-care -recommendations/en. 2014.

Wray J: Seeking to explore what matters to women about postnatal care, *Br J Midwifery* 14(5):246–254, 2006.

Wray J: Feeling cooped up after childbirth – the need to go out and about, *Pract Midwife* 14(2):2011.

Wray J, Bick D: Is there a future for universal midwifery postnatal care in the UK?, *MIDIRS Midwifery Digest* 22(4):495–498, 2012.

Wray J, Steen M: Physical health problems and complications in the puerperium. In Marshall J, Raynor M, editors: *Myles textbook for midwives,* London, Churchill Livingstone, Elsevier, 2014.

Resources and additional reading

Bhavnani VN, Newburn M: *Left to Your Own Devices: The Postnatal Care Experiences of 1260 First-Time Mothers*: NCT research into women's experiences of postnatal care, London, NCT, 2010.

Each Social & Community Health Report (EACH Report): The Pregnancy and Post Birth Experience of Women from Refugee Backgrounds Living in the Outer East of Melbourne. Australia (website). www.each.com.au/health-promotion/images/uploads/EACH_HMHB_Report_VR5_24-11-11.pdf. 2011.

Every newborn, an executive summary for The Lancet's Series (website). http://www.thelancet.com/series/everynewborn. *Lancet* 2014.

Knight M, Kenyon S, Brocklehurst P, et al; On behalf of MBRRACE-UK (eds). On behalf of MBRRACE-UK, Saving Lives, Improving Mothers' Care – Lessons Learned to Inform Future Maternity Care from the UK and Ireland Confidential Enquiries into Maternal Deaths and Morbidity 2009–12. National Perinatal Epidemiology Unit, University of Oxford Oxford, 2014 (website). www.npeu.ox.ac.uk/downloads/files/mbrrace-uk/reports/Saving%20Lives%20Improving%20Mothers%20Care%20report%202014%20Full.pdf.

Delivered with care NPEU Report (website). www.npeu.ox.ac.uk/research/nms-2010-2012.

National Maternity Survey: Women's Experience of Maternity Care: a National Maternity Survey, undertaken by the NPEU in 2010.

NHMRC: *Cultural Competency in Health: a Guide for Policy, Partnerships and Participation*, Canberra, Australia, National Health and Medical Research Council, 2006.

WHO recommendations on postnatal care of the mother and newborn (website). www.who.int/maternal_child_adolescent/documents/postnatal-care-recommendations/en/.

WHO – Postnatal care for mothers and Newborns. Highlights from WHO guidelines 2013 (website). http://www.who.int/maternal_child_adolescent/publications/WHO-MCA-PNC-2014-Briefer_A4.pdf?ua=1. 2013.

Multi-Cultural Health: A Guide for Health Professionals – Cultural Dimensions of Pregnancy, Birth and Post-Natal Care (website). www.health.qld.gov.au/multicultural/health_workers/cultdiver_guide.asp.

The Girl Effect: The Clock is Ticking (website). https://www.youtube.com/watch?v=1e8xgF0JtVg.

The girl effect is about leveraging the unique potential of adolescent girls to end poverty for themselves, their families, their communities, their countries and the world. This short clip provides a very clear message about the need for girls to have access to education.

Chapter 67

Complications related to the third stage of labour

Luisa Acosta and Andrea Aras-Payne

Learning Outcomes ?

After reading this chapter, you will be able to:

- understand why the period immediately after the birth of the baby may result in complications during and after the third stage of labour and what the implications are for women and their families
- recognize risk factors, signs and symptoms
- demonstrate evidence-based knowledge of the midwife's role in managing emergency situations in this period
- outline how the multidisciplinary team can further treat and manage emergency situations as necessary

INTRODUCTION

Although the third stage of labour is usually uneventful, significant complications may occur because of the rapid change in physiology at this time. These complications and the related risks may continue for some period after delivery of the placenta. The most common complication associated with the third stage of labour is postpartum haemorrhage (PPH). This chapter will essentially examine PPH and other complications related to the third stage of labour. Further complications occurring immediately after childbirth, which may not necessarily be related to the third stage, are also discussed in this chapter.

POSTPARTUM HAEMORRHAGE

A postpartum haemorrhage (PPH) is a common emergency, which may happen swiftly and without warning.

For the majority of births, the midwife is likely to be the only healthcare professional in attendance and, therefore, it is essential that they have a thorough understanding of the complication. A midwife's prompt recognition and action may spare the woman dangerous blood loss and save her life.

Obstetric haemorrhage, which includes abnormal bleeding in the antepartum, intrapartum and postpartum period, is a significant cause of maternal mortality and morbidity. Worldwide, it is the leading cause of maternal mortality, attributing to 27% of maternal deaths with some regions in Northern Africa and Asia reporting figures above 50% (Say et al 2014). Primary PPH, the most common type of obstetric haemorrhage, accounts for two-thirds of these numbers. The incidence is notably lower in higher income countries. In the UK, haemorrhage is the third leading cause of direct maternal death. Paterson-Brown and Bamber (on behalf of the MBRRACE-UK haemorrhage writing group 2014) reported that between 2009 and 2012, there were 14 deaths attributed to PPH.

Although the incidence of PPH varies widely and depends on the definitions used, there appears to be a rising trend in the occurrence (Knight et al 2009; Lutomski et al 2012; Kramer et al 2013). In England, the incidence has risen from 7% to 13% in the past decade (Health and Social Care Information Centre 2015).

In high income countries, many maternal deaths from haemorrhage are associated with substandard care (Paterson-Brown and Bamber 2014). Following recommendations from Confidential Enquiry (Centre for Maternal and Child Enquiries 2011) reports and Royal College of Obstetric and Gynaecology (RCOG 2009) guidelines, all maternity services now have a policy for managing haemorrhage and run regular skills drills and simulation training so that all members of the multidisciplinary team are able to work together effectively to improve the outcome for the women in their care.

Definition

PPH is defined as excessive bleeding from the genital tract occurring any time from the birth of the baby to the end of the puerperium.

- *Primary PPH* is when excessive bleeding occurs in the first 24 hours after the birth.

- *Secondary PPH* is when abnormal or excessive bleeding occurs between 24 hours and 12 weeks postnatally. It is a significant contributor of maternal death in developing countries and affects approximately 2% of births in developed countries (Alexander et al 2009; Dossou et al 2015). Most studies report peak incidence at 1 to 2 weeks after the birth (Dossou et al 2015). The most common cause is subinvolution of the uterus, secondary to retained products and/or infection.

Primary PPH

Primary PPH is often defined by using the estimated blood loss (EBL) and, traditionally, a loss of 500 mL or more has been regarded as a PPH (WHO 1990). For women undergoing a caesarean section, a PPH is defined as a blood loss greater than 1000 mL (Mukherjee and Arulku-maran 2009). Yet this amount may also be considered as a normal physiological blood loss in women who are healthy. However, for women who are anaemic or who have a low body mass index, this amount or less may cause severe compromise (Moore and Chandraharan 2010).

Using the EBL to define PPH is notoriously difficult. In addition to the varying clinical impact the blood loss may have on individual women, it is also likely to be inaccurate (Bose et al 2006; Lilley et al 2015), incorrectly recorded (Briley et al 2014) or it may be concealed.

With consideration of the variables in estimating blood loss, the RCOG (2009) guidelines advocate that when estimating blood loss to define PPH – if blood loss is estimated as 500 mL to 1000 mL and there are no clinical signs of maternal compromise – staff should be alerted to monitor the woman and be ready for possible action. This is a categorized as a minor PPH and certain fundamental measures need to be undertaken. Should the EBL be above 1000 mL or the woman shows any sign of compromise no matter what the blood loss is, it is categorized as a major PPH and a full protocol of measures must be initiated and prompt action taken to resuscitate and arrest bleeding.

A major PPH can be further subdivided into moderate (1000–2000 mL of blood loss) and severe (over 2000 mL of blood loss).

Causes

PPH may arise from the placental site or from a genital tract laceration, and usually falls into four categories commonly known as the '4 Ts' (see Table 67.1).

Table 67.1 Causes of PPH – the 4 'Ts'

Tone	Uterine atony: Excessive bleeding from the placental site when the uterus fails to contract and retract adequately. As there is a placental circulation of 500 to 600 mL/min at term (Blackburn 2013), if uterine arteries are not ligated by the muscle fibres surrounding them, blood loss can be rapid and dangerous. 70% to 90% of PPH cases are from uterine atony (Winter et al 2012).
Tissue	Any tissue that hinders uterine contraction (as above): retained or adherent placenta, placental/membrane fragments and blood clots.
Trauma	Genital tract lacerations, episiotomy, haematomas, ruptured or inverted uterus.
Thrombin	Blood coagulation disorders: These include pre-existing disorders, e.g. von Willebrand's syndrome, disseminated intravascular coagulopathy, HELLP syndrome and anticoagulant therapy.

Risk factors

The risk factors are listed in this section. However, midwives must note that PPH can occur in women who have no identifiable risks:

- Previous PPH or retained placenta.

- Multiple pregnancy, polyhydramnios and fetal macrosomia: All may cause uterine over-distension, leading to poor retraction. In multiple pregnancy, there is a larger placental site, which is more likely to encroach upon the poorly retractile lower uterine segment, thus increasing the risk of haemorrhage.

- Anaemia affects the ability to withstand haemorrhage.

- Antepartum haemorrhage from placenta praevia, placental abruption or any unclassified antepartum bleeding may subsequently result in PPH. With placenta praevia, the retractile ability of the lower uterine segment is deficient and, therefore, control of bleeding from the placental site is poor. A Couvelaire uterus may occur in severe, concealed placental abruption and the damaged muscle fibres fail to contract and retract effectively (Fig. 67.1). Women who have had an antepartum haemorrhage may also be anaemic, increasing the threat from PPH.

- Prolonged labour: If contractions were weak or uncoordinated during labour, it may continue into the third stage. The uterus will fail to contract and

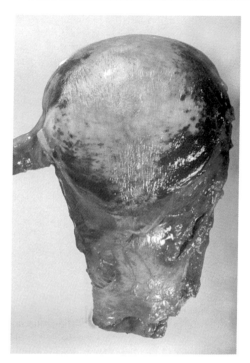

Figure 67.1 Couvelaire uterus. (This article was published in Beischer N, Mackay E, and Colditz P: Obstetrics and the newborn, London, Baillière Tindall, London, Copyright Elsevier, 1997)

retract effectively. Occasionally, prolonged labour, because of mechanical difficulty, may lead to uterine exhaustion and atony.

- Previous caesarean section and caesarean section: Surgery and scarring of the uterus is a risk factor for placenta praevia and accrete – see further details discussed later in this chapter.

- Pre-eclampsia/hypertensive disease in pregnancy: Both increase the risk of induction and operative deliveries. Coagulopathy is also a potential complication of hypertensive disease. Some drugs used to prevent seizures may contribute to uterine atony.

- General anaesthesia: Uterine atony may occur if anaesthesia is prolonged, and is especially likely if halogenated anaesthetic agents are used.

- Fibroids: Interfere with efficient contraction and retraction.

- Mismanagement of the third stage of labour: Unnecessary massaging, squeezing or otherwise 'fiddling' with the uterus can disrupt the rhythm of myometrial activity, causing only partial separation of the placenta.

- Retained placenta and blood clots: Unless the uterus is empty, it cannot retract completely.

- Tocolytic drugs: Drugs given to suppress uterine activity in preterm labour may cause atony in the third stage should labour progress.

- Induced or augmented labours: Uterine inefficiency necessitating the use of oxytocics may contribute to PPH.

- Inversion of the uterus: Any degree of uterine inversion will interfere with efficient contraction and retraction.

- Chorioamnionitis: This will impair uterine contraction. Chorioamnionitis will impair contractions during labour causing the labour to become prolonged, further exacerbating the risk of PPH.

- Disseminated intravascular coagulation may occur secondarily to other major problems (discussed later in this chapter).

- Medical disorders such as idiopathic thrombocytopenia and inherited coagulopathies increase the risk of PPH.

Prevention

During pregnancy

Preventing PPH begins at the initial 'booking' interview when midwives will identify women at higher risk. Any woman whose history suggests that she is at risk should be booked for a hospital birth where immediate and effective treatment can be provided. Conditions such as anaemia should be treated with iron and folic acid supplements. In severe cases, intramuscular iron or even blood transfusion may be required to raise the haemoglobin levels prior to delivery (RCOG 2015).

For women who are expecting to undergo an elective caesarean section and who are at increased risk of haemorrhage or who refuse blood products, intraoperative blood cell salvage should be offered (RCOG 2015).

Labour

During labour, careful management may reduce the likelihood of PPH and some precautions can minimize the severity of the bleed.

For women at risk:

- Insert a wide bore intravenous cannula (16G or larger)

- Take blood samples to establish haemoglobin levels and have blood group confirmed.

- Ensure the serum is saved, thereby speeding up the process of cross-matching donor blood, should it become necessary.

- Monitor the progress of labour and avoid dehydration, ketoacidosis and exhaustion.

- Prompt referral to an obstetrician if there are signs of prolonged labour.

- An oxytocin infusion may be required and should be maintained for at least 1 hour after the end of the third stage.
- The bladder should be kept empty, as a full bladder may impede efficient uterine action.

Third stage

Correct management is essential. The midwife should discuss the management of the third stage with the woman, preferably before labour commences. An actively managed third stage with routine prophylactic administration of oxytocics (Begley et al 2011) (see also Ch. 39) and controlled cord traction will reduce the frequency and severity of PPH (WHO 2012). Once the placenta is delivered, the uterus must be palpated to ensure that it is well contracted. If the uterus is atonic, fundal massage (rubbing up a contraction) should be commenced by using one hand to cup the fundus and firmly massage in a rotational movement until the uterus starts to become firm (Crafter 2016) (see Fig. 67.2). Breastfeeding or nipple stimulation may also help the uterus to contract but it is not an effective treatment for PPH.

Accurate estimation of blood loss

There is still significant emphasis on the assessment of blood loss volume. Many methods to estimate blood loss

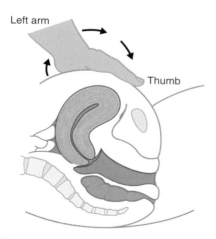

The left hand is cupped over the uterus ( ) and massages it with a firm circular motion in a clockwise direction

Figure 67.2 'Rubbing up' a contraction. The left hand is cupped over the uterus and massages it with a firm circular motion in a clockwise direction. (Boyle M: Emergencies around childbirth: a handbook for midwives, Oxford, Radcliffe Publishing, 2002. Reproduced with permission of Radcliffe Publishers.)

have been used: visual estimation, weighing of swabs and incontinent sheets and the use of drapes to collect blood loss. Blood loss is usually underestimated (Bose et al 2006; Al-Kadri et al 2014), although recently there are reports of overestimation as well (Lilley et al 2015). The trend is that the more the blood loss, the greater the inaccuracy. Regular clinical simulations and education may improve blood loss estimation (Al-Kadri et al 2014).

Inaccurate detection of blood loss volume may delay treatment of a PPH; therefore, even though estimating blood loss volume remains an important tool for diagnosing PPH, practitioners should be placing more emphasis on clinical decisions based on the woman's risk, rate of blood flow and observations (Weeks 2015). This will enable early detection and prompt treatment.

Managing PPH

The principles of management

A multidisciplinary approach is essential at every stage of management. It must be noted that maternity units vary in the management of PPH, especially with pharmacological protocols. Midwives should follow their hospital guidelines as appropriate. Management of bleeding before the delivery of the placenta, minor PPH and major PPH will be examined separately.

Bleeding before the delivery of the placenta

Before the delivery of the placenta, there may be excessive bleeding from the placental site when the placenta is partially detached or wholly detached but undelivered. The bleeding should alert the midwife to take action. Skilled medical assistance should be summoned immediately, while the midwife must remain with the woman for support and to commence treatment. The placenta must be delivered as soon as possible and, if at home, the midwife should do this, if possible, before transferring the woman to hospital.

If the woman has not received an oxytocic drug for the third stage, this now should be administered. This drug is usually oxytocin 5 to 10 IU by intramuscular injection, causing the uterus to contract within 2.5 minutes. The

---

Box 67.1 The principles of management

- Communication and escalation
- Resuscitation of the mother
- Arrest the bleeding
- Fluid replacement
- Monitoring and investigation
- Documentation

placenta is then delivered by controlled cord traction. If the uterus remains soft, a further dose may be given. If Syntometrine (oxytocin 5 IU and ergometrine 500 µg/1 mL) was given for third stage management, the placenta needs to be delivered before the ergometrine takes effect, as this may cause the placenta to become trapped (Belfort and Dildy 2011) and exacerbate the bleeding. Fundal stimulation must be avoided, as this too can lead to placental entrapment.

The bladder should be empty before another attempt is made to deliver the placenta with controlled cord traction. Once the placenta is delivered, an intravenous Syntocinon infusion is recommended and the genital tract should be inspected to exclude traumatic haemorrhage (discussed later in this chapter).

If the placenta cannot be delivered, prepare for the obstetrician to perform a manual removal of the placenta and membranes under anaesthetic. The midwife may also perform this procedure in an emergency situation (NMC 2012). Retained placenta is discussed later in this chapter.

Managing a minor PPH

The following actions should be taken when a minor PPH is diagnosed. The order in which the actions are to be taken may vary and, where possible, actions should be taken simultaneously:

- *Call for assistance*: Alert the senior midwife, obstetrician and anaesthetist. Ask for a second midwife to help in the room if in the maternity unit, or ask for a second midwife to come to the home immediately to assist while waiting for the emergency services to arrive. Do not leave the woman alone.

- *'Rub up' a contraction*: This must be done as soon as possible. Massaging the uterus will usually stimulate a contraction and expel any blood clots (Fig. 67.2).

- *Gain intravenous access:* Insert 2 wide-bore cannulas. This is to obtain blood samples, administer drugs and commence fluid replacement with a crystalloid infusion.

- *Establish the cause* (Paterson-Brown and Howell 2014):
  - Check that the uterus is well contracted.
  - Ensure placenta has been delivered and that it is complete.
  - Examine the cervix, vagina and external genitalia for lacerations. If found, pressure should be applied and suturing performed.
  - Observe for signs of clotting disorders, such as abnormal clotting of blood or oozing from wounds and cannula sites. Review notes to establish if there is a history of coagulation disorders or predisposing factors.

- *Give first-line oxytocic drug for uterine atony*: Drug protocols vary, but the following may be considered:
  - Intramuscular Syntometrine (oxytocin 5 IU and ergometrine 500 µg/1 mL) if it has not already been given for the management of the third stage. May be repeated after 2 to 4 hours (Belfort and Dildy 2011).
  - If an oxytocic has been given, a second dose of oxytocin 5 to 10 IU may be given by intramuscular injection or 5 IU slow intravenous injection. Caution is needed with bolus doses of oxytocics, as they may exacerbate maternal hypotension.
  - This may be followed by ergometrine 250 to 500 µg. Ergometrine may be given intramuscularly or, cautiously, intravenously in the absence of hypertension (Joint Formulary Committee 2015).

- An intravenous infusion of 40 IU of oxytocin in 500 mL of normal saline over 4 hours should be commenced. This is to maintain the tone of the uterus.

- *Ensure the bladder is empty* by passing an indwelling catheter, as a full bladder can impede uterine contraction and retraction.

- *Assessment of maternal condition:* Respirations, pulse, blood pressure and oxygen saturations should be undertaken every 15 minutes, and the temperature hourly.

- *Estimating blood loss* can be done by observation and weighing of swabs and incontinence pads. Do not dispose of these until the woman's condition is stabilized.

It is essential that these steps are taken as soon as the midwife suspects that the uterus is failing to contract, the woman is showing signs of compromise or if bleeding is unusually heavy. In most cases these are effective if used in good time. Delay will result in further blood loss and the woman's condition will deteriorate rapidly in which case a full emergency protocol must be initiated.

If the placenta and membranes are not complete, an exploration and evacuation of the uterus is carried out by an obstetrician under anaesthesia.

The midwife should ensure that her documentation is complete and that she has commenced a Modified Early Obstetric Warning Score (MEOWS) and fluid balance chart. Clear and appropriate communication with the multidisciplinary team and the woman is essential at all times.

> **Reflective activity 67.1**
>
> Review how emergency transfer of a woman from her home to hospital is managed in your area.

Major obstetric haemorrhage

This is a life-threatening event that may take place in the antenatal, intrapartum or postnatal period, and is characterized by severe maternal compromise. The incidence is approximately 5.8 per 1000 maternities (Lennox and Marr 2014). Major PPH accounts for most cases of major obstetric haemorrhage, although the cause is often related to problems occurring in the antepartum and intrapartum period (Weeks 2015). It has been estimated that the incidence of major PPH is approximately 1.8 to 4.2 per 1000 births (Carroli et al 2008; Kramer et al 2013).

Managing a major PPH

A major PPH is a blood loss of 1000 mL or more, or any lesser amount that causes maternal compromise (RCOG 2009). In addition to the measures taken above for a minor PPH, as soon as the emergency is recognized, the following should be undertaken immediately and all actions should be taken simultaneously where possible:

- Call for help: Pull the emergency bell or dial '999' if at home. The full multidisciplinary protocol for managing massive obstetric haemorrhage must be initiated. The team should include the midwife who is caring for the woman plus other key staff including:

- *Rub up a contraction:* Continue as described previously (see Fig. 67.2).

- *Delegation of responsibilities:* One member of staff should take the lead. This may be the midwife, although once the multidisciplinary team is involved, it will usually be the anaesthetist or obstetrician. A scribe is needed to document all events, actions taken and treatment given.

- *Maternal resuscitation*: Place the bed flat and assess the woman's airway, breathing and circulation. Oxygen therapy is to be commenced (10–15 L/min). Ensure the airway is kept patent, to allow adequate ventilation and lung expansion. Intubation may be necessary. Look for signs of cyanosis.

Box 67.2 Call for help

- Senior midwife (and midwife in charge)
- Senior obstetrician (and consultant obstetrician)
- Senior anaesthetist
- Additional support staff
- Haematologist, blood bank and theatre staff are to be alerted
- Portering staff should be ready to transfer of specimens for laboratory analysis.

- *Intravenous access:* If not already done, two large-bore cannulas (14 g or follow local guidelines) should be inserted.

- *Blood samples:* Full blood count, cross-matching and clotting studies (4–6 cross-matched units of blood must be requested). Some maternity units will request screening of urea and electrolytes.

- *Fluid replacement:* Two litres of crystalloid may initially be infused, as these are known as good short-term intravascular volume expanders (Schorn and Phillippi 2014). This may be followed by 1.5 litres of colloid if blood products are not available. Colloids are more efficient in expanding the intravascular volume (Paterson-Brown and Howell 2014). However, caution is needed, as there is controversy about the amount, timing and nature of clear fluids to be used, as large amounts can interfere with coagulation and, more rarely, colloids have been known to cause an anaphylactic reaction (Karri et al 2009). Fluids should be warmed to prevent hypothermia (RCOG 2009).

- *Blood transfusion*: Blood transfusion should be commenced as soon as possible when there is the need. All maternity units keep at least two units of emergency group O Rhesus-negative blood in the blood refrigerator. This may be used while awaiting cross-matched supplies. Blood should be passed through a warming device and a pressure bag should be used to ensure that it is infused as rapidly as possible. A filter should not be used because this will slow the infusion. Other blood products will be administered on instruction of the haematologist. These include fresh frozen plasma, platelets and cryoprecipitate.

- *Second-line drugs:* In addition to oxytocin and ergometrine (as described in the management of a minor PPH section), the following drugs may be considered (under doctor's instruction) if the uterus remains atonic:

  - Carboprost (Hemabate) 250 µg may be administered by deep intramuscular injection and can be repeated every 15 minutes, up to eight doses (Joint Formulary Committee 2015). It also may be injected directly into the myometrium by the obstetrician but must not be given intravenously.

  - Misoprostol (1000 mgc) may be given rectally as a one-off dose.

- *Bimanual compression of the uterus:* To be undertaken if the measures mentioned previously do not stop the bleeding. (Fig. 67.3 and Box 67.3). Aortic compression also may be carried out. See the next section for technique for these procedures (Fig. 67.4 and Box 67.4).

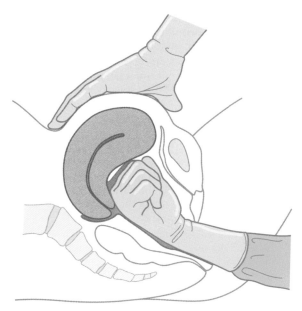

Figure 67.3 Internal bimanual compression of the uterus.

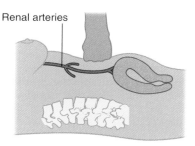

Figure 67.4 Abdominal aortic compression.

Box 67.4 Abdominal aortic compression

This has been used as a short-term emergency measure to control severe haemorrhage while awaiting emergency assistance. The midwife places a fist above the fundus and the umbilicus and pushes down to compress the aorta against the spine and reduce blood flow to the uterus. Adequacy of compression can be assessed by checking for the absence of femoral pulses (Winter et al 2012; Keogh and Tsokos 1997).

Box 67.3 Internal bimanual compression

- Using cone shaped fingers insert one hand gently into the anterior fornix of the vagina.
- Form a fist and apply pressure to the anterior wall of the uterus.
- The external hand dips down behind the uterus and pulls it forwards towards the symphysis. The hands are pushed together, compressing the uterus and placental site.
- Continue the pressure until the haemorrhage is under control.
- This is a highly invasive and painful procedure and should be used with discretion.
- The woman and her partner should be informed about what to expect prior to undertaking it. External bimanual compression may also be done by squeezing the uterus between the hands.

- *Ongoing assessment of maternal condition and blood loss*: Respirations, pulse, blood pressure and oxygen saturations should be monitored continuously and temperature should be taken every 15 minutes, as the woman is likely to become hypothermic; therefore, measures need to be taken to keep her warm.
- *Hourly urine measurements*: a drainage bag with a urometer is to be attached to the indwelling catheter. This is to assess renal function.

- *Prepare for early transfer to theatre.*
- Documentation: All observations must be accurately recorded on a MEOWS chart. This should alert staff to abnormal trends, prompting them to take immediate action. Alongside this, the fluid balance needs to be recorded. Clear contemporaneous records need to be made noting the staff in attendance, time and sequence of events, details of drug, blood and fluid administration and the condition of the mother. Most maternity units use a structured proforma to aid accurate record keeping. An incident form must also be completed.
- *Communication*: Ongoing communication with the multidisciplinary team and sensitive discussion and explanation of events with mother and partner at an appropriate time.

Additional management of major obstetric haemorrhage

An anti-shock garment may be useful to shunt blood from the extremities to the vital organs while the woman is awaiting surgical procedures (WHO 2012). This is particularly useful in low resource settings. The woman's legs may be elevated to alleviate signs of shock (Winter et al 2012), although this should be used with care, as this may cause pooling of blood in the uterine cavity, which may impede uterine contraction.

A central venous line is used for closer monitoring of fluid replacement and to avoid fluid overload. Arterial blood will be taken to measure blood gases.

The midwife must watch carefully for any signs of deterioration and shock.

Hypothermia may occur because of shock and the rapid infusion of fluids. This may exacerbate shock and coagulopathy (Hess 2007). The woman must be kept warm and dry.

Reflective activity 67.2   ><

Visit your local maternity unit and obstetric theatres and find out where the drugs and intravenous fluids required for management of haemorrhage and shock are kept.

Surgical procedures

- *Uterine tamponade*: This is to be attempted prior to laparotomy. The hydrostatic balloon catheter is now known to be more effective, safer and easier to insert than uterine packing (Weeks 2015). The balloon is inflated with sterile normal saline, taking the shape of the uterus and applying pressure to the placental site.

- *Compression sutures*: These are absorbable sutures, which are inserted through the thickness of both uterine walls to compress the uterus. An example of this is the B-Lynch suture (B-Lynch et al 1997). (See Fig. 67.5.)

- *Pelvic vessel ligation*: If other methods fail, arterial ligation will be necessary. This may involve the internal iliac artery, ovarian artery or uterine artery.

- *Hysterectomy*: Every attempt to conserve the uterus will be made, but if these measures fail to control the bleeding, a hysterectomy is necessary to save the woman's life.

Radiological procedures

- *Uterine artery embolization*: This can be performed before laparotomy if the woman is stable enough and facilities for interventional radiology are present. The procedure is done by femoral artery puncture, where the catheter is guided to the site and the vessel is embolized with gelatin sponge.

- *Internal iliac balloon catheter*: These can be inserted via the femoral artery for women who are at high risk. Should haemorrhage occur, the balloon can be inflated to control bleeding.

Traumatic PPH

Although uterine atony is the most common cause of PPH, traumatic PPH needs to be considered when the uterus appears to be well contracted but vaginal bleeding is observed (Winter et al 2012; RCOG 2009). Approximately 10% of cases of PPH are from laceration of the genital tract, with 7 maternal deaths from haemorrhage

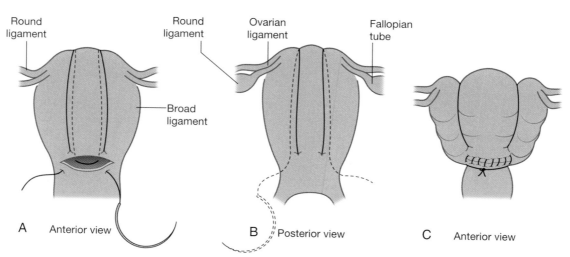

Figure 67.5 B-Lynch suture in the uterus: **A,** anterior and **B,** posterior views showing the application of the suture; **C,** the anatomical appearance after competent application. (Reprinted with permission from B-Lynch C, Coker A, Lawal A, et al: The B-Lynch surgical technique for the control of massive postpartum haemorrhage: an alternative to hysterectomy? Five cases reported, Br J Obstet Gynaecol 104(3):372–375, 1997. Illustrations by Mr Philip Wilson FMAA RMIP.)

associated with genital tract trauma reported in a recent UK and Ireland Confidential Enquiries Report (Paterson-Brown and Bamber 2014).

Trauma can include lacerations to the external genitalia: labia, clitoris and perineum (episiotomy or tears), which often bleed freely. It also includes deeper lacerations of the vaginal walls, cervix and the lower uterine segment, which will cause severe haemorrhage. Traumatic PPH is likely to complicate a difficult instrumental birth or may follow a rapid labour. Haemorrhage from uterine rupture may occur in obstructed labour or if a scar ruptures.

Superficial bleeding points can be easily seen and treated by direct pressure. For further investigation to identify the bleeding point, a woman will need to be positioned in lithotomy under a direct light source. A laceration of the cervix is suspected if the bleeding begins immediately after the birth and continues steadily, although the uterus is well contracted. Speculum examination will help visualize the trauma and bleeding may be temporarily controlled by digital pressure or by applying a sponge or arterial pressure forceps before suturing the laceration. An obstetrician must be summoned and the laceration sutured as soon as possible. Delay in attending to the bleeding inevitably causes greater blood loss. Tears to the upper part of the vagina, the cervix or the uterus are sutured under anaesthesia. In cases of severe haemorrhage from a ruptured uterus, it may be necessary to perform a hysterectomy.

A vulval haematoma may cause a PPH. This can occur after perineal repair with inadequate haemostasis, where there has been damage to vulval varicosities or when there is no obvious trauma and the perineum is intact. It appears as a localized swelling, usually one-sided, which looks tense and shiny. The pain may be severe and there may be signs of shock. A surprisingly large amount of blood may be present. The midwife must call for medical assistance and intravenous access must be secured, as replacement fluids may be needed. The haematoma should be drained under anaesthesia and an indwelling drain may remain after surgery. Because of the risk of infection, attention to perineal hygiene as well as pain relief are essential.

As with other causes of PPH, prompt recognition and early intervention are required to minimize blood loss and the consequent complications.

Care following PPH

The woman will need to be cared for in a high dependency setting or may be transferred to intensive care. The woman's general condition is assessed continuously and it is important to palpate the fundus repeatedly to ensure that it remains well contracted and to observe the amount and nature of the blood loss. Her respirations, pulse, blood pressure and oxygen saturations must be recorded every 15 minutes until her condition is satisfactory and MEOWS and fluid balance charts are to be maintained. Central venous pressure should be measured when it is

necessary to give large volumes of fluid intravenously to avoid overtransfusion.

Sedation may be required and the woman needs to be kept dry, warm and comfortable.

Use of the SBAR (Situation-Background-Assessment-Recommendation) tool (NHS Institute for Innovation and Improvement 2008) will aid with communication when handing over care between practitioners and between wards.

Complications following PPH

The woman is at risk of thromboembolism because of immobility and the effect of fluid and blood transfusion. Therefore, well-fitting antiembolism stockings must be worn. Thromboprophylaxis will be commenced once coagulation parameters return to normal (Nama and Chandraharan 2013).

The woman is likely to suffer from chronic iron-deficiency anaemia unless adequate treatment is instituted during the puerperium. She is also susceptible to developing puerperal sepsis and in severe and prolonged shock, she may develop anuria because of tubular necrosis.

A more rare but serious complication is postpartum hypopituitary (Sheehan's) syndrome. The pituitary gland, which is larger during pregnancy, is prone to infarction as a result of hypovolaemia. The damage can vary and may lead to an inability to lactate because of deficient prolactin secretion, amenorrhoea, hypothyroidism and adrenal cortex failure. Eventual atrophy of the breasts and genital organs will also occur (Belfort 2015). This syndrome can appear immediately postpartum or later in life.

HYPOVOLAEMIC SHOCK

Shock is a condition in which the circulatory system cannot maintain sufficient perfusion to the vital organs (WHO 2003). Cellular oxygen and nutritional requirements are not met and metabolic waste cannot be removed. The ensuing hypotension and reduced tissue perfusion will result in cell starvation, leading to cell death and irreversible organ damage or death.

Hypovolaemic shock occurs when the circulating blood volume is too low to meet tissue requirements. It is associated with severe obstetric haemorrhage and may follow coagulopathy, such as that associated with amniotic fluid embolism. It may also occur due to vasodilation. For example, as a result of epidural anaesthesia (Paterson-Brown and Howell 2014).

Signs of deterioration/recognition of hypovolaemic shock

Most childbearing women are healthy and unlikely to show signs of deterioration provided that blood loss does not exceed the physiological volume expansion that occurs in pregnancy. A woman can lose up to 15% of her blood volume without showing the signs of shock (Paterson-Brown and Howell 2014). After this, clinical signs of hypovolaemia will start to appear. These signs are difficult to detect at first and, therefore, midwives must be alert for any subtle changes in the condition of the woman in her care.

The following signs indicate deepening shock, which will affect all body organs and systems:

- *Heart rate*: In the early stages of shock, the pulse will remain normal. As the heart rate rises, the volume grows weaker until the rapid, thready pulse of severe haemorrhage is noted. Tachycardia reflects the cardiac response to underperfusion of the vital organs. Above 100 beats per minute is considered abnormal. However, even though most women become tachycardiac, a paradoxical bradycardia can occur, which may be misleading (Paterson-Brown and Howell 2014).

- *Blood pressure*: Although the mother is losing blood, for some time the compensatory mechanisms in her body will keep her blood pressure normal. Peripheral, splanchnic and renal vasoconstriction ensure that vital organs, such as the heart and brain, continue to be perfused. Once 30% to 40% of the blood volume is lost, the blood pressure will fall (Cockings and Waldmann 2006). If the systolic pressure falls below 90 mmHg or it falls by 30 mmHg, there is cause for concern and by this time, the woman will already be in the late stages of shock.

- *Increasing pallor of the skin*: The skin becomes cold and sweaty. The lips become bluish and mucous membranes blanched. Perfusion of the skin decreases (Baskett et al 2007). Capillary refill time is prolonged.

- *Temperature*: Falls to a subnormal level.

- *Respiration*: Initially tachypnoea occurs, but as the shock deepens, breathing becomes deep and sighing.

- *Urinary output*: Output decreases, followed by anuria.

- *Altered mental state*: In early shock, restlessness and anxiety may occur. The woman may experience thirst, nausea or faintness. Later, as perfusion of the brain decreases, she may become confused and finally lose consciousness after 50% of her blood volume has been lost (Baskett et al 2007).

- *Metabolic acidosis*: A late sign occurring after cellular metabolism becomes deranged, following reduced tissue perfusion and cellular hypoxia. Cell death is irreversible and the woman will be close to death at this stage (Baskett et al 2007).

Aids for recognizing shock:

Capillary refill time is assessed by pressing a fingernail for 5 seconds. The colour should return in 2 seconds.

The Rule of 30 (Nama and Chandraharan 2013): Rise in pulse greater than 30/minute, drop in systolic blood pressure by 30 mmHg, increased respiratory rate to greater than 30/minute; at least 30% blood loss (drop in haematocrit by 30%).

Shock Index (SI): This is a simple tool that can predict adverse clinical outcomes. The heart rate is divided by the systolic blood pressure. The normal value is 0.5 to 0.7 (Mukherjee and Arulkumaran 2009). An SI of greater than 0.9 indicates that intervention or referral to a higher level facility is necessary and an SI of 1.7 means that urgent action is needed (Nathan et al 2015).

Disseminated intravascular coagulation

Disseminated intravascular coagulation (DIC) is a coagulopathy that results in steady, persistent oozing of blood even though there is adequate uterine contraction and retraction. Blood does not clot, venipuncture sites may ooze, bleeding from the mouth or nose may be evident, haematuria may be present and petechiae may also appear. DIC is never a primary phenomenon, but secondary when supplies of circulating fibrinogen and other blood clotting factors become depleted and the coagulation system fails. Hypoxia that accompanies major haemorrhage may cause the local release of thromboplastin from the damaged tissue, triggering the formation of microthrombi around the body. This further exhausts the circulating coagulation factors. The thrombi will block capillaries, thus causing more tissue damage and release of thromboplastin.

As the condition worsens, blood levels of fibrin degradation products (FDPs) rise. These are toxic to the myometrium and will interfere with efficient uterine contraction and retraction, thus exacerbating haemorrhage. If DIC is allowed to progress, the condition will become uncontrollable and maternal death may ensue.

At every delivery, the midwife should note whether the blood is clotting and whether the clot is firm or friable. Absent or unstable clot formation along with results from clotting studies are an indication of DIC. Treatment must be prompt and the midwife should call for medical assistance and the on-call haematologist immediately. Frequent and accurate observations of the maternal vital signs, blood loss and fluid balance will need to take place. Central venous pressure and/or arterial line may be required.

Once the underlying cause and hypovolaemia are treated, blood products such as red cells, fresh frozen plasma and platelets are used to replace clotting factors. In some cases, *cryoprecipitate* is administered. NICE (2014) recommends the use of intravenous *tranexamic acid* and rarely *recombinant factor VIIa* if clotting factors are normal, but only under the direction of a consultant haematologist.

PROLONGED THIRD STAGE AND RETAINED PLACENTA

The third stage is considered prolonged when it exceeds 30 minutes with active management, and up to 1 hour with physiological management (NICE 2014). The risk of PPH is linked with a prolonged third stage of labour and significantly increases with time. Women whose third stage exceeds 30 minutes are 6 times more likely to have a PPH (Magann et al 2005).

The incidence of retained placenta is approximately 3% (Cheung et al 2011). A retained placenta may be completely detached but trapped in the cervix or lower uterine segment, be partially separated or be completely adherent when no separation has occurred at all. There may be evidence of bleeding from the placental site; however, in cases where the placenta is completely adherent to the uterine wall, there may be no obvious bleeding.

Causes

The following may cause delay in the third stage by interfering with the descent and expulsion of a separated placenta:

- *Full bladder* (emptying of the bladder should be initiated when there is a delay in the delivery of a placenta)
- *Constriction ring* (a localized spasm of uterine muscle just above the lower segment) and reforming of the cervix

Other associated risks for retained placenta:

- Uterine atony
- Uterine abnormality (e.g. fibroids, bicornuate or subseptate uterus) or uterine scar (previous uterine surgery or caesarean section)
- Older maternal age
- Induced labour
- Preterm labour
- Previous retained placenta
- Previous miscarriages or abortion
- Pre-eclampsia, small-for-gestational age, stillbirth (defective placental disorders)
- Mismanagement of the third stage, and fundal 'fiddling'

(Belachew et al 2014; Endler et al 2014; Endler et al 2012; Nikolajsen et al 2013; Magann et al 2008; Weeks 2008; Adelusi et al 1997).

The management of a retained placenta is determined by the clinical situation and the amount of blood lost. The midwife will need to make the appropriate referral in the identified timeframes if the placenta is not delivered, or earlier if excessive bleeding is observed. If the woman is not in an obstetric unit, a transfer will need to be organized. An indwelling urinary catheter will need to be inserted, intravenous access secured and blood taken for cross matching. Breastfeeding or nipple stimulation also can be considered to help with the release of oxytocin. Adequate analgesia should be offered prior to any vaginal examination and anaesthesia is required for any uterine exploration or manual removal of placenta. Intravenous oxytocic drugs should not be given routinely to deliver a retained placenta; however, they can be considered if the woman is bleeding excessively (NICE 2014). Umbilical vein oxytocin has been shown to have little or no effect, and is therefore not a recommended treatment (NICE 2014; Nardin et al 2011). Routine use of prostaglandins needs further investigation (Grillo-Ardila et al 2014). Sublingual nitroglycerin (for a trapped placenta) can be effective but further research is required to establish the role of tocolytic drugs in the management of retained placenta as well as the use of ultrasound scanning to help identify the type of retained placenta (Abel-Aleem et al 2011). The woman will need to be transferred to theatre as soon as possible, and a further examination to see if the placenta has separated should be undertaken prior to anaesthesia. Preparations for significant blood loss should be put in place (Paterson-Brown and Howell 2014). Although the activities of a midwife include the manual removal of placenta in an emergency (NMC 2012) (see Fig. 67.6), in high-income countries it is unlikely that the midwife would be required to undertake this. The midwife must carefully monitor the woman's condition in the postnatal period and refer her for medical attention if signs of uterine infection appear. A single dose of antibiotics is recommended after the procedure (Chongsomchai et al 2014; WHO 2009). The woman should be advised to have future births in a hospital, as the risk of recurrence is high.

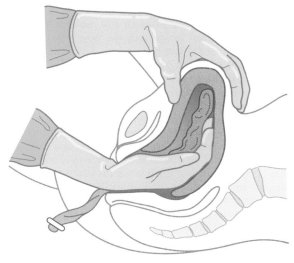

Figure 67.6 Manual removal of placenta.

Box 67.5 Types of morbidly adherent placenta

Placenta accreta	The decidua basalis is deficient and the chorionic villi adhere to the myometrium.
Placenta increta	The villi deeply invade the myometrium.
Placenta percreta	The villi have penetrated the myometrium as far as the serous coat of the uterus. Involvement of adjacent structures may occur. This type is very rare.

Morbid adherence of the placenta

This occurs when the placental villi penetrate more deeply than normal beyond the decidua basalis. The incidence of morbidly adherent placentae is thought to be rising and has been attributed to the increase in caesarean births. A combination of previous caesarean section and current placenta praevia are high-risk factors for abnormal trophoblastic penetration and the more caesarean births a woman has had, the more likely she is to have this condition (Silver et al 2015). The condition carries with it an increased risk of major obstetric haemorrhage and the associated complications, including hysterectomy and in some cases death (Patterson-Brown and Bamber 2014). There are three types of abnormally adherent placenta:

Fitzpatrick et al (2015) reported from their UK-based study that of those women diagnosed with placenta accreta, increta or percreta (1.7 per 10 000 maternities), half were suspected in the antenatal period. Although colour doppler ultrasound and or magnetic resonance imaging have shown to help identify some potential cases (Fitzpatrick et al 2015; D'Antonio et al 2013), it is suggested that high-risk women, such as those who have had a previous caesarean section and also now have placenta praevia, are treated as though they have a morbidly adherent placenta. Pre-birth preparations should be put in place (Fitzpatrick et al 2015; RCOG 2009). Preparations can help improve outcomes and reduce complications such as excessive haemorrhage and the need for a blood transfusion. As these women are at high risk of needing a hysterectomy preparation for surgery and pre-birth counselling can be arranged, timing of delivery and management will depend on clinical needs. The area of adherence may be focal, partial or total. When the placenta does not separate and has not been disturbed, there may be an opportunity to facilitate conservative management (leave the placenta in situ to reabsorb) or elective hysterectomy, which are both associated with less blood loss. If the placenta is partially separated, adherent portions can be left in place while those partially separated need to be delivered. In these situations, there is likely to be extensive

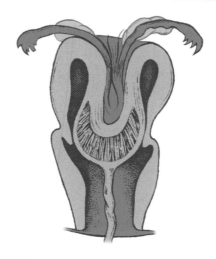

Figure 67.7 Inversion of the gravid uterus.

Box 67.6 Degrees of uterine inversion

- First degree inversion: The fundus is inverted but does not pass through the cervix.
- Second degree inversion: The inverted fundus protrudes through the cervix and lies in the vagina.
- Third degree inversion: The uterus is completely inverted and the fundus appears outside the vaginal introitus.
- Fourth degree inversion: Both the uterus and vagina are inverted and visible beyond the vaginal introitus. This is termed total inversion.

blood loss and high risk of hysterectomy (Paterson-Brown and Howell 2014; RCOG 2011a).

ACUTE UTERINE INVERSION

This is a rare but serious complication of the third stage of labour, where the uterus is partly or completely turned inside out (Fig. 67.7). The condition is associated with severe and profound shock and may be associated with haemorrhage if the placenta has become separated from the uterus. Incidence of uterine inversion have been reported as 1 in 20,000 births (Witteveen et al 2013).

Degrees of inversion are described as:

Acute inversion occurs within 24 hours of birth, subacute within 30 days and chronic, which is rare, after 30 days.

Causes include:

- *Mismanagement of the third stage of labour*: Results from either excessive pressure on the fundus or from excessive traction on the cord when the uterus is relaxed. It is particularly likely to occur when the placenta is situated in the uterine fundus.
- *Short umbilical cord*
- *Manual removal of the placenta*: Inversion of the uterus may occur if the operator's hand is quickly withdrawn from the uterus while the other hand is still applying fundal pressure.
- *Precipitate delivery*: Especially if the woman is in an upright position.
- *Macrosomia*
- *Morbidly adherent placenta*
- *Spontaneous inversion*: Occasionally, the cause is unknown. It may result from uterine atony and a sudden increase in the intra-abdominal pressure, such as occurs during coughing or straining.
- *Congenital abnormalities of the uterus*

However, inversion of the uterus is unpredictable and in around 50% of cases, there are no risk factors or mismanagement of the third stage (Bhalla et al 2009).

Diagnosis

Minor degrees of uterine inversion may not be recognized if there is only a slight indentation of the fundus. The woman may report pain, and lochia is likely to be heavy.

If the inversion is more serious, the woman will report severe pain and, on palpation, a hollow will be felt in the fundus of the uterus. Haemorrhage will occur if the placenta has separated.

If there is a complete inversion, the uterus will not be palpable in the abdomen and the inverted fundus will be visible at the vulva. The woman will report severe lower abdominal pain and may report a sensation of prolapse or 'something coming down'. Initially neurogenic shock occurs, owing to traction on the infundibulopelvic and round ligaments and compression of the ovaries. As severe blood loss ensues, hypovolemic shock will develop (Senanayake et al 2013).

Management

This must be swift and the emergency help of a multidisciplinary team must be summoned immediately. Uterine replacement and treatment for shock need to be managed concurrently. Uterotonic drugs, if in progress, must be stopped so as to relax the uterus prior to reinsertion and, where possible, the uterus should be replaced immediately. Replacement is more likely to be successful the earlier the uterus is repositioned; over time, maternal shock will increase and may become irreversible. If delayed, vascular congestion and oedema of the uterus may also occur making replacement more difficult. If immediate replacement is not possible and the uterus is outside the vulva, it should be gently placed back inside the vagina. Rough or prolonged digital manipulation will increase the accompanying vasovagal shock. The foot of the bed should be raised to alleviate shock by reducing traction on the infundibulopelvic ligaments. Intravenous access is required for full blood count, cross-matching and clotting studies; intravenous fluid replacement needs to commence as well as the administration of IV drugs. Oxygen therapy should be initiated and vital signs continuously monitored. Urinary catheterization is needed and appropriate analgesia given. If the placenta is still attached, it **must not** be removed, as torrential haemorrhage may result. The woman must be transferred to theatre immediately (Paterson-Brown and Howell 2014).

In theatre, the uterus is replaced either manually or by the hydrostatic method, preferably under general anaesthetic. To assist with the replacement of the uterus, drugs may be given to relax the cervical ring. In a manual replacement, the part of the uterus which inverted last is replaced first, meaning the fundus returns last. A hand is placed on the abdomen to give counter pressure; otherwise, the uterus may be pushed up too high. The hand is not removed from the uterus until intravenous oxytocics are given and the uterus contracts. Only then should the manual removal of the placenta take place.

If unsuccessful, the hydrostatic method, as described by O'Sullivan (1945), can be carried out; however, uterine rupture needs to be excluded before this procedure. Once the obstetrician replaces the uterus in the vagina, warm normal saline is infused into the vagina via a rubber tube. This is held in place and the introitus sealed by the other hand. A ventouse cup, attached to a giving set, may also improve the seal. This technique, however, can prove to be difficult and impractical (Belfort and Dildy 2011). A better seal is produced when the woman lies with her legs together. The pressure exerted by the fluid distends the vagina and effects replacement of the uterus without aggravating the shock. Recently, the use of a Bakri postpartum balloon has shown to not only reduce uterine inversion but also prevent its recurrence (Ida et al 2015). If other interventions fail, surgical correction via laparotomy is performed.

Further treatment for shock and haemorrhage may then be required; care in a high-dependency area is advisable. As the risk of puerperal sepsis is high, antibiotic cover is required.

In the recovery period, the midwife should encourage the woman to carry out her postnatal pelvic floor exercises; referral to an obstetric physiotherapist may be helpful if the abdominal and pelvic floor muscle tone is particularly poor. The woman should be seen by the obstetrician 6 to 8 weeks after birth to exclude chronic uterine inversion.

As this condition may recur, the woman should be advised to give birth in a hospital if she becomes pregnant again (Winter et al 2012).

AMNIOTIC FLUID EMBOLISM

Amniotic fluid embolism (AFE), a rare condition unique to pregnancy, is still a leading cause of maternal mortality (Harper and Wilson 2014; McDonnell et al 2013). The reported incidence of AFE varies, and comparison between countries can be difficult because of variations in definition, data collection and reporting mechanisms (Tuffnell and Slemeck 2014). In the UK, all cases of AFE are reported to the United Kingdom Obstetric Surveillance System (UKOSS).

The total incidence of AFE is estimated at 1.7 per 100,000 UK maternities with a mortality rate of 0.3 per 100,000 (19% of reported cases). Of the women who survive AFE, 7% endure permanent neurological injury and another 17% experience other major morbidities. Perinatal mortality and morbidity rates are also significantly higher for women who experience AFE (Fitzpatrick et al 2015).

AFE presents with a sudden and dramatic change in the either maternal or, if still pregnant, the fetal condition, is more likely closer to term and tends to occur during labour, birth or soon after birth (usually within 30 minutes) but may also arise after an amniocentesis or uterine evacuation (Tuffnell and Slemeck 2014).

The underlying pathophysiology of AFE is still unclear. AFE is thought to be an acute anaphylactic-type response to amniotic fluid, fetal hair, meconium and/or debris entering the maternal circulation rather than the fluid itself, causing an obstruction. In some women, the presence of amniotic fluid within the maternal circulatory system appears to trigger devastating systemic dysfunction involving the respiratory, cardiovascular and haematological systems (Tuffnell and Slemeck 2014). This can be in two phases, initially seen as an anaphylactic response, where the signs are hypotension, difficulty in breathing, chest pain, altered mental state, fetal compromise and maternal collapse. Secondary phase includes severe haemorrhage and coagulation disorders (Tuffnell and Chipeta 2013).

Risk factors include maternal age over 35 years, multiple pregnancy, macrosomia, artificial rupture of membranes, augmentation and induction of labour, meconium, placental abruption, placenta praevia, uterine rupture, instrumental delivery and caesarean section (Fitzpatrick et al 2015; O'Connor et al 2015; McDonnell et al 2013; Conde-Agudelo and Romero 2009). For amniotic fluid to enter the maternal circulation, physical barriers between the maternal circulation systems and amniotic fluid need

to be broken. It is proposed that small tears in the lower uterine segment and veins in the endocervix allow for entry during labour and delivery, with an osmotic gradient helping transfer of fluid (Tuffnell and Slemeck 2014). This appears to be supported by the identified risk factors above where breaches to the utero-placental barriers may occur and where the intra-amniotic pressure is increased and amniotic fluid may be forced into the maternal circulation (McDonnell et al 2013).

Diagnosis can be difficult, but agreed UK case definition recommends the following criteria must be present for a diagnosis to be made (Fitzpatrick et al 2015):

If a previously healthy asymptomatic woman presents with cardiac or respiratory failure during labour, at caesarean section or immediately after birth, AFE should always be suspected (Boyle 2016).

Management of AFE will depend on clinical circumstances, the focus being on oxygenation, circulatory system support and correction of coagulopathy (Tuffnell and Slemeck 2014). The midwife must immediately call for medical assistance and commence cardiopulmonary resuscitation. High concentrations of oxygen should be administered; intubation and mechanical ventilation are likely to be needed. Intravenous access needs to be gained, an infusion commenced and a urinary catheter inserted; careful measurement of fluid balance is required so as to

---

Box 67.7 Criteria for diagnosis of AFE

Either

Acute maternal collapse (in the absence of any other clear cause) with one or more of the following features:

- Cardiac arrest
- Cardiac arrhythmias
- Acute hypotension
- Acute hypoxia
- Coagulopathy/haemorrhage (excluding women with maternal haemorrhage as the first presenting feature in whom there was no evidence of early coagulopathy or cardio-respiratory compromise)
- Premonitory symptoms, e.g. restlessness, numbness, agitation, tingling
- Seizures
- Shortness of breath
- Acute fetal compromise

Or

Postmortem diagnosis where fetal squames or hair were present in the maternal lungs

However, these are not found in every case, and women who have fetal material in their circulatory system do not necessarily develop AFE.

avoid fluid overload. Pulse oximetry and ECG will help monitor maternal condition; a pulmonary artery catheter may also need to be considered. Correction of coagulopathy and uterine atony requires immediate and urgent attention; a hysterectomy may be required (Boyle 2016; Patterson-Brown and Howell 2014; Tuffnell and Slemeck 2014). If the woman is still pregnant, continuous CTG needs to be in place. In the case of a cardiac arrest, a caesarean section will need to be performed as quickly as possible (within 5 minutes). Although the outcomes for the fetus are better when the time interval from collapse to birth is short, a caesarean section is carried out for the benefit of the woman, as adequate and effective resuscitation is better achieved when the uterus is empty (RCOG 2011b). Once a decision to perform a perimortem caesarean section has taken place, the massive obstetric haemorrhage protocol will need to be triggered (Harper and Wilson 2014).

Reflective activity 67.3

If you attend a woman after a major complication in the third stage of labour, talk to her afterwards about her perception of the experience.

PSYCHOLOGICAL CONSIDERATIONS

The sudden nature of the emergency often means that explanations given while it is happening are brief and hurried. The midwife and obstetricians involved in her care should find an appropriate time to discuss the event with the woman and her partner. She must be given the opportunity to ask questions and information needs to be provided about what happened, why this occurred, potential risks and how future births may be managed (Thompson et al 2011). Emotional sequelae must be given due attention, as women who have had difficult births may be

more susceptible to post traumatic stress disorder and postnatal depression (Hallewell 2016). The mother may feel more vulnerable because of separation from her baby during and after the event. It is also likely that she will have breastfeeding difficulties and, therefore, the midwife will need to provide breastfeeding support and ensure that the mother gets sufficient opportunity to bond with her baby. Information and advice about her physical recovery and day-to-day strategies for coping with her new baby should be given. She will need postnatal follow-up after discharge from a hospital.

CONCLUSION

The third stage is the most dangerous part of the childbirth continuum. Complications can arise with little warning. As the senior professional present at the majority of births in the UK, it is usually the midwife who has the responsibility for identifying the complication and beginning emergency treatment. Midwives must be aware of risk factors, observe for signs of deterioration and know how to respond appropriately. Prompt referral, good communication and accurate documentation are essential for the safety of the woman. The long-term consequences of complications arising in the third stage may be both physical or psychological.

Key Points

- PPH is a major cause of maternal mortality and morbidity worldwide.
- Complications may arise without warning and the woman's condition can deteriorate rapidly.
- Prompt recognition and management of blood loss and shock is critical.
- The midwife needs to be able to monitor the woman's condition, refer appropriately and work collaboratively, to ensure safe and effective care at this time.

References

Abel-Aleem H, Abdel-Aleem MA, Shaahan OM: Tocolysis for management of retained placenta, *Cochrane Database Syst Rev* (1):Art. No.CD007708, 2011.

Adelusi B, Soltan M, Chowdhury N, et al: Risk of retained placenta: multivariate approach, *Acta Obstet Gynecol Scand* 76(5):414–418, 1997.

Alexander J, Thomas P, Sanghera J: Treatments for secondary postpartum haemorrhage (Systematic Review), *Cochrane Database Syst Rev* (4):CD 002867, 2009.

Al-Kadri H, Dahlawi H, Al Airan M, et al: Effect of education and clinical assessment on the accuracy of post partum blood loss estimation, *BMC Pregnancy Childbirth* 14:110, (website). www.biomedcentral.com/1471-2393/14/110. 2014.

Baskett TF, Calder AA, Arulkumaran S: *Munro: Kerr's operative obstetrics*, 11th edn, London, Elsevier, 2007.

Begley CM, Gyte GM, Devane D, et al: Active versus expectant management of the third stage of labour, *Cochrane Database Syst Rev* (9):CD007412, 2011.

Beischer N, Mackay E, Colditz P: *Obstetrics and the newborn*, London, Baillière Tindall, 1997.

Belachew J, Cnattingius S, Mulic-Lutvica A, et al: Risk of retained placenta in women previously delivered by caesarean section: a population-based cohort study, *Br J Obstet Gynaecol* 121:224–229, 2014.

Belfort MA: *Overview of postpartum haemorrhage*, Up-To-Date (website). www.uptodate.com/contents/overview-of-postpartum-hemorrhage. 2015.

Belfort MA, Dildy A: Postpartum haemorrhage and other problems of the third stage. In James DK, Steer PJ, Weiner CP, et al, editors: *High risk pregnancy: management options*, 3rd edn, Philadelphia, Saunders Elsevier, 2011.

Bhalla R, Wuntakal R, Odejinmi F, et al: Acute inversion of the uterus, *The Obstetrician & Gynaecologist* 11:13–18, 2009.

Blackburn ST: *Maternal, fetal and neonatal physiology. A clinical perspective*, 4th edn, Philadelphia, Elsevier Saunders, 2013.

B-Lynch C, Coker A, Lawal A, et al: The B-Lynch surgical technique for the control of massive postpartum haemorrhage: an alternative to hysterectomy? Five cases reported, *Br J Obstet Gynaecol* 104(3):372–375, 1997.

Bose P, Regan F, Paterson-Brown S: Improving the accuracy of estimated blood loss at obstetric haemorrhage using clinical reconstructions, *Br J Obstet Gynaecol* 113(8):919–924, 2006.

Boyle M: Amniotic fluid embolism (anaphylactoid syndrome of pregnancy), Chapter 11. In Boyle M, editor: *Emergencies around childbirth: a textbook for midwives*, 3rd edn, Boca Raton, CRC Press, 2016.

Briley A, Seed PT, Tydeman G, et al: Reporting errors, incidence and risk factors for postpartum haemorrhage and progression to severe PPH: a prospective observational study, *Br J Obstet Gynaecol* 121(7):876–888, 2014.

Carroli G, Cuesta C, Abalos E, et al: Epidemiology of postpartum haemorrhage: a systematic review, *Best Pract Res Obstet Gynaecol* 22(6):999–1012, 2008.

Centre for Maternal and Child Enquiries: Saving mothers' lives: reviewing maternal deaths to make motherhood safer: 2006–2008. The Eighth Report of the Confidential Enquiries into Maternal Deaths in the United Kingdom, *Br J Obstet Gynaecol* 118(Suppl 1):1–203, 2011.

Cheung W, Hawkes A, Ibish S, et al: The retained placenta: historical and geographical rate variations, *J Obstet Gynaecol* 1:37–42, 2011.

Chongsomchai C, Lumbiganon P, Laopaiboon M: Prophylactic antibiotics for manual removal of retained placenta in vaginal birth, *Cochrane Database Syst Rev* (10):CD004904, 2014.

Cockings JGL, Waldemann CS: Assessing and replenishing lost volume. In B-Lynch C, Keith LG, Lalonde Ab, et al, editors: *A textbook of postpartum hemorrhage: a comprehensive guide to evaluation, management and surgical intervention*, Duncow, Sapiens, 2006.

Conde-Agudelo A, Romero R: Amniotic fluid embolism: an evidenced-based

review, *Am J Obstet Gynecol* 201(5):445, e1–13, 2009.

Crafter H: Intrapartum and primary postpartum haemorrhage, Chapter 10. In Boyle M, editor: *Emergencies around childbirth: a handbook for midwives*, 3rd edn, Boca Raton, CRC Press, 2016.

D'Antonio F, Iacovella C, Bhide A: Prenatal identification of invasive placentation using ultrasound: systematic review and meta-analysis, *Ultrasound Obstet Gynecol* 42:509–517, 2013.

Dossou M, Debost-Legrand A, Déchelotte P, (Didier Lémery Françoise Vendittelli), et al: Severe secondary postpartum hemorrhage: a historical cohort, *Birth* 42(2):149–155, 2015.

Endler M, Saltvedt S, Cnattingius S, et al: Retained placenta is associated with pre-eclampsia, stillbirth, giving birth to a small-for-gestational age infant, and spontaneously preterm birth: a national register-based study, *Br J Obstet Gynaecol* 121:1462–1470, 2014.

Endler M, Grunewald C, Saltvedt S: Epidemiology of retained placenta, *Obstet Gynecol* 119(4):801–809, 2012.

Fitzpatrick KE, Tuffnell D, Kurinczuk JJ, et al: Incidence, risk factors, management and outcomes of amniotic-fluid embolism: a population-based cohort and nested case-control study, *Br J Obstet Gynaecol* doi: 10.1111/1471-0528.13300, 2015.

Grillo-Ardila CF, Ruiz-Parra AI, Gaitan HG, et al: Prostaglandins for management of retained placenta, *Cochrane Database Syst Rev* (5):CD010312, 2014.

Harper A, Wilson R, On behalf of the MBRRACE-UK Amniotic Fluid Embolism chapter writing group: Caring for Women with Amniotic Fluid Embolism. In Knight M, Kenyon S, Brocklehurst P, et al, On behalf of MBRRACE-UK, editors: *Saving Lives, Improving Mothers' Care – Lessons Learned to Inform Future Maternity Care from the UK and Ireland Confidential Enquiries into Maternal Deaths and Morbidity 2009–12*, Oxford, National Perinatal Epidemiology Unit, University of Oxford, 2014.

Hallewell L: Psychological considerations for emergencies around childbirth, Chapter 14. In Boyle M, editor: *Emergencies around childbirth: a handbook for midwives*, 3rd edn, Boca Raton, CRC Press, 2016.

Health and Social Care Information Centre (HSCIC): *Compendium of Maternity Statistics – England 2013-2014* (website). www.hscic.gov.uk/catalogue/PUB16725. 2015.

Hess JR: Blood and coagulation support in trauma care, *Hematology Am Soc Hematol Educ Program* 187–191, doi: 10.1182/asheducation-2007.1.187, 2007.

ASH Education Book January 1, 2007 vol. 2007 no. 1.

Ida A, Ito K, Kubota Y, et al: Successful reduction of acute puerperal uterine inversion with the use of a Bakri postpartum balloon, *Case Rep Obstet Gynecol*. Article ID 424891, 2015.

Joint Formulary Committee: *British National Formulary*, London, BMJ Group and Pharmaceutical Press (website). www.medicinescomplete.com. 2015.

Karri K, Raghavan R, Shahid J: Severe anaphylaxis to Volplex, a colloid solution during cesarean section: a case report and review, *Obstet Gynaecol Int* 374791, PMCID: PMC2778838. doi: 10.1155/2009/374791, 2009.

Kramer MS, Berg C, Abenhaim H, et al: Incidence, risk factors, and temporal trends in severe postpartum hemorrhage, *Am J Obstet Gynecol* 209(5):449.e1–449.e7, doi: 10.1016/j.ajog.2013.07.007, 2013.

Lennox C, Marr L: *Scottish Confidential Audit of Severe Maternal Mortality. 10th Annual Report. Health Improvement Scotland* (website). www.healthcareimprovementscotland.org/our_work/reproductive,_maternal_child/programme_resources/scasmm.aspx. 2014.

Lilley G, Burkett-St Laurent E, Precious D, et al: Measurement of blood loss during postpartum haemorrhage, *Int J Obstet Anesth* 14(1):8–14, doi: 10.1016/j.ijoa.2014.07.009, 2015.

Lutomski J, Byrne B, Devane D, et al: Increasing trends in atonic postpartum haemorrhage in Ireland: an 11-year population-based cohort study, *Br J Obstet Gynaecol* 119(3):306–314, doi: 10.1111/j.1471-0528.2011.03198, 2012.

Keogh J, Tsokos N: Aortic compression in massive postpartum haemorrhage – an old but lifesaving technique, *Aust N Z J Obstet Gynaecol* 37(2):237–238, 1997.

Knight M, Callaghan WM, Berg C, et al: Trends in postpartum hemorrhage in high resource countries: a review and recommendations from the International Postpartum Hemorrhage Collaborative Group, *BMC Pregnancy Childbirth* 9:55, doi: 10.1186/1471-2393-9-55 (website). www.biomedcentral.com/1471-2393/9/55, 2009.

Magann EF, Evans F, Chauhan SP, et al: The length of the third stage of labor and the risk of postpartum hemorrhage, *Obstet Gynecol* 105(2):290–293, 2005.

Magann EF, Doherty DA, Briery CM, et al: Obstetric characteristics for a prolonged third stage of labor and risk for postpartum hemorrhage, *Gynecol Obstet Invest* 65(3):201–205, 2008.

McDonnell N, Percival V, Paech M: Amniotic fluid embolism: a leading cause of maternal death yet still a medical conundrum, *Int J Obstet Anesth* 22:329–336, 2013.

Moore J, Chandraharan E: Management of massive postpartum haemorrhage and coagulopathy, *Obstet Gynaecol Reprod Med* 20(6):174–180, 2010.

Mukherjee S, Arulkumaran S: Post-partum haemorrhage, *Obstet Gynaecol Reprod Med* 19(5):121–126, 2009.

Nama V, Chandraharan E: Massive obstetric haemorrhage. In Chandraharan E, Arulkumaran S, editors: *Obstetric and intrapartum emergencies: a practical guide to management*, Cambridge, Cambridge University Press, 2013.

Nardin JM, Weeks A, Carroli G: Umbilical vein injection for management of retained placenta, *Cochrane Database Syst Rev* (5):2011.

Nathan HI, El Ayadi A, Hezelgrave NL, et al: Shock index: an effective predictor of outcome in postpartum haemorrhage, *Br J Obstet Gynaecol* 122:268–275, 2015.

National Institute for Health and Clinical Excellence (NICE): *Intrapartum Care. Care of Healthy Women and Their Babies During Childbirth*. Clinical Guideline CG 190, London, NICE, 2014.

NHS Institute for Innovation and Improvement: *SBAR – Situation – Background – Assessment – Recommendation*, Coventry, NHS Institute (website). www.institute.nhs.uk/quality_and_service_improvement_tools/quality_and_service_improvement_tools/sbar_-_situation_-_background_-_assessment_-_recommendation.html. 2008.

Nikolajsen S, Lokkegaard ECL, Bergholt T: Reoccurrence of retained placenta at vaginal delivery: an observational study, *Acta Obstet Gynecol Scand* 92:421–425, 2013.

Nursing and Midwifery Council (NMC): *Midwives rules and standards*, London, NMC, 2012.

Paterson-Brown S, Bamber J, On behalf of the MBRRACE-UK haemorrhage writing group: Prevention and Treatment of Haemorrhage. In Knight M, Kenyon S, Brocklehurst P, et al, On behalf of MBRRACE-UK, editors: *Saving Lives, Improving Mothers' Care – Lessons learned to inform future maternity care from the UK and Ireland Confidential Enquiries into Maternal Deaths and Morbidity 2009–12*, Oxford, National Perinatal Epidemiology Unit, University of Oxford, 2014.

Paterson-Brown S, Howell C: *Managing obstetric emergencies and trauma*, 3rd edn, Cambridge, Cambridge University Press, 2014.

O'Connor M, Smith A, Nair M, et al: *UKOSS Annual Report*, Oxford, National Perinatal Epidemiology, 2015.

O'Sullivan JV: Acute inversion of the uterus, *Br Med J* 2(1):282–283, 1945.

Royal College of Obstetricians and Gynaecologists (RCOG): *Prevention and Management of Postpartum Haemorrhage*, Green-top guideline No. 52. London, Royal College of Obstetricians and Gynaecologists, 2009.

Royal College of Obstetricians and Gynaecologists (RCOG): *Placenta Praevia, Placenta Praevia Accreta and Vasa Praevia: Diagnosis and Management*, Green-top guideline No. 27. London, Royal College of Obstetricians and Gynaecologists, 2011a.

Royal College of Obstetricians and Gynaecologists (RCOG): *Maternal Collapse in Pregnancy and the Puerperium*, Green-top guideline

No.56. London, Royal College of Obstetricians and Gynaecologists, 2011b.

Royal College of Obstetricians and Gynaecologists (RCOG): *Blood Transfusion in Obstetrics*, Green-top guideline No.47. London, Royal College of Obstetricians and Gynaecologists, 2015.

Say L, Chou D, Gemmill A, et al: Global causes of maternal death: a WHO systematic analysis, *Lancet Glob Health* 2(6):e323–e333, DOI http://dx.doi.org/10.1016/S2214-109X(14)70227-X, 2014.

Schorn NM, Phillippi JC: Volume replacement following severe postpartum hemorrhage, *J Midwifery Women's Health* 59(3):336–343, 2014.

Senanayake H, Ranaweera P, Rishard M: Acute puerperal uterine inversion. In Chandraharan E, Arulkumaran S, editors: *Obstetric and intrapartum emergencies*, Cambridge, Cambridge University Press, 2013.

Silver R, Fox K, Barton J, et al: Center of excellence for placenta accrete, *Am J Obstet Gynecol* 561–568, 2015.

Thompson JF, Ford JB, Raynes-Greenow CH, et al: Women's experiences of care and their concerns and needs following a significant primary postpartum hemorrhage, *Birth* 38(4):327–335, 2011.

Tuffnell D, Chipeta H: Amniotic fluid embolus. In Chandraharan E, Arulkumaran S, editors: *Obstetric and intrapartum emergencies*, Cambridge, Cambridge University Press, 2013.

Tuffnell D, Slemeck E: Amniotic fluid embolism, *Obstetrics, Gynaecology and Reproductive Medicine* 24(5):148–152, 2014.

Weeks AD: The retained placenta, *Best Pract Res Clin Obstet Gynaecol* 22(6):1103–1117, 2008.

Weeks A: The prevention and treatment of postpartum haemorrhage: what do we know, and where do we go next?, *Br J Obstet Gynaecol* 122:202–212, 2015.

Winter C, Crofts J, Laxton C, et al, editors: Major obstetric haemorrhage, module 6. *Practical obstetric multiple professional training course manual*, 2nd edn, Cambridge, Cambridge University Press, 2012.

Witteveen T, van Stralen G, Zwart J, et al: Puerperal uterine inversion in the Netherlands: a nationwide cohort study, *Acta Obstet Gynecol Scand* 92:334–337, 2013.

World Health Organization (WHO): *The prevention and management of postpartum haemorrhage*. Report of a Technical Working Group, Geneva 3–6, July 6, 1989, Geneva, WHO, 1990.

World Health Organization (WHO): *Shock. Managing complications in pregnancy and childbirth. A guide for midwives and doctors (MCPC)*, Geneva, WHO, 2003.

World Health Organisation (WHO): *WHO guidelines for the management of postpartum haemorrhage and retained placenta*, Geneva, WHO, 2009.

World Health Organisation (WHO): *Recommendations for the prevention and treatment of Postpartum Haemorrhage*, Geneva, WHO, 2012.

Chapter 68

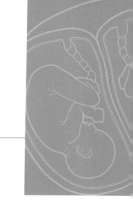

Pregnancy loss and the death of a baby: grief and bereavement care

Cheryl Titherly

Learning Outcomes ?

After reading this chapter, you will be able to:

- identify the unique impact of grief in relation to pregnancy loss and the death of a baby and the complexities of the grieving process
- consider the individual needs of women, their partners and families who experience a pregnancy loss or the death of a baby, including around memory making
- understand the key elements of communicating sensitively and effectively with bereaved parents
- recognize the importance of on-going support for bereaved parents and the potential impact of their loss on all subsequent pregnancies
- identify the impact of loss of healthcare professionals. Explore and identify your own support needs and know how to access support locally

INTRODUCTION

One in four women experiences a pregnancy loss or the death of a baby before, during or shortly after birth (Tommy's Charity 2015).

In the UK in 2013:

- Miscarriage occurred in an estimated one in five recognized pregnancies (Tommy's Charity 2015)
- There were 2732 terminations of pregnancy for fetal anomaly (Department of Health (DH) 2014)
- One in 216 births was a stillbirth. This is around 10 babies a day (Office for National Statistics 2015).
- One in 370 babies died in the neonatal period (the first 28 days of life) (Office for National Statistics 2015) (see also Ch. 16).

Pregnancy loss and the death of a baby before, during or shortly after birth are not rare occurrences, happening more often than most people realize. Bereavement care and supporting parents whose baby has died is a significant part of midwifery and a part that when done well can have a lasting positive impact on the parents. In this chapter, the role of the midwife in supporting women and families after the death of a baby is discussed, and strategies for developing skills, resources and services for bereaved parents is included.

'I feel we were extremely well looked after during the whole time. It was the worst time of our whole lives, but all of the staff who looked after us were exceptionally professional and amazing' – Parent.

(Redshaw et al 2014)

When the grieving process is complicated by insensitive care, there can be short-term and lifelong repercussions for the parents (Lewis and Bourne 1989). Appropriate bereavement care and support throughout are essential. 'Sensitive, supportive care cannot take away pain; it cannot even soften grief. But it changes the way loss is felt, and it can make grieving *easier*' (Henley and Kohner 2001). Recognizing and responding to the parents' feelings, understanding their individual needs and supporting them to make informed choices are key elements of good care for professionals involved in supporting these parents before, during and after the birth of their baby (Schott et al 2007; NMC 2015).

There is no right or wrong way to grieve or to experience a pregnancy loss or the death of a baby. Each parent is individual with different circumstances and needs, and the death of that baby will be experienced differently (CBUK 2013a).

There are some key elements of good care that will help many parents, but it is for the midwife caring for each individual parent to work with them to provide sensitive, empathic and individualized care.

The death of a baby before, during, or shortly after birth because of miscarriage, termination of pregnancy for fetal anomaly, stillbirth or neonatal death is often unexpected and feels against the natural order of things. It is unique, incomprehensible and unlike any other death. When an adult or a child dies, family members have memories to draw upon and a life to remember, but when a baby dies, parents grieve the hoped for future with their child. There are few tangible memories. When a pregnancy is confirmed, many parents will conceptualize the full-term healthy baby they are expecting. Many will begin to plan for their future with this baby, and hopes and dreams will begin to form around themselves as parents or as a larger family. Plans are often made for where the baby will sleep, maternity leave, the baby's name and for the future together. All of these hopes and dreams can be lost at the point of diagnosis, whether of fetal anomaly, miscarriage, stillbirth or neonatal death.

For most parents, the death of a baby is a significant and painful experience, regardless of the cause or gestational age. Parents depend on healthcare professionals, including midwives, to sensitively care for them and offer relevant and accurate information to support them in the choices they face in this difficult time.

UNDERSTANDING LOSS AND GRIEF

'If bereavement is what's happened to you, grief is how you feel, and mourning is what you do'.

(Dr Richard Wilson, Consultant Paediatrician)

There are many theories explaining the grieving process, including Bowlby's (1980) attachment theory; Kubler-Ross's stages of grief (denial, anger, bargaining, depression, acceptance), developed in the late 60s (Kubler-Ross 2014); Parkes' (1972) phases of grief; and Worden's (2009) *'tasks of mourning'* developed in 1991, which we will look at further in this chapter. The main criticism of many of these theories is that they can feel too simplistic and linear. Grief is not neat and tidy. Grief can be messy and unpredictable. The dual process model (Stroebe and Schut 1999) highlights the complexity and variability of grief. It describes how a griever will oscillate between loss-orientated and restoration-orientated tasks and that normal grief will be experienced as a back and forth between confronting and avoiding the loss (see Fig. 68.1).

Grief is exhausting, emotionally and physically, and can be very isolating and lonely.

'An odd by-product of loss is that I'm aware of being an embarrassment to everyone I meet. At work, at the club, in the street, I see people, as they approach me, trying to make up their minds whether they'll 'say something about it' or not. I hate it if they do, and if they don't…R has been avoiding me for a week'.

(C.S. Lewis 1961)

Worden's four tasks of mourning (Box 68.1) acknowledge the flexible phases of grief that hopefully result in the individual modifying their relationship with the deceased in a way that enables them to move forwards, while maintaining a bond.

This theory can appear very linear, but Worden does recognize that those grieving may move between these stages and revisit ones already 'completed' as their grief work continues. These stages can be helpful for recognizing emotions and reactions you may have witnessed in practice.

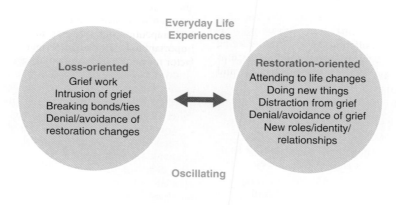

Figure 68.1 A dual process model of coping with loss. (From Stroebe MS, Schut H: The dual process model of coping with bereavement: rationale and descriptions, Death Studies 23(3):197–224, 1999.)

Box 68.1 Worden's tasks of mourning

This includes four key stages:
1. To accept the reality of the loss
2. To work through to the pain of grief
3. To adjust to an environment in which the deceased is missing
4. To find an enduring connection in the midst of embarking on a new life (originally emotionally relocating the deceased)

Worden 2009

Worden's tasks of mourning:
1. Accepting the reality of the loss

Initially, the parents may not believe the bad news and may be in a state of shock and denial, even when a death has been anticipated. Some bereaved parents cry uncontrollably, become hysterical or collapse, whereas others feel faint or numb and can display few signs of emotion, appearing very controlled, calm and detached. The initial shock may last for hours or several days. This natural reaction is a form of emotional protection that disappears as parents gradually take in the full impact of events. Each experience of grief is unique and previous losses may complicate the reaction to this current bereavement.

Parents may initially be unable to acknowledge what has happened and may temporarily manage by denying the reality. These parents need time and help to do what is right for them. It is not helpful for professionals to collude with denial and unreality, for example, by avoiding talking about the baby who has died, somehow making the baby's death seem less important or not fully acknowledging its significance.

Midwives can help enable parents to gradually face reality. Being sensitive to parents' needs, discussing what other parents have valued, offering choices, such as seeing and holding their dead baby, being involved as much as they feel able in the preparations for the funeral, and observing rituals and traditions, all can help make what has happened real. Families from different faiths may need support for the mourning rituals appropriate to their culture (Thomas 2001; Schott et al 2007). Please see the Spiritual needs section for more on this.

Worden's tasks of mourning:
2. Working through to the pain of grief

As denial and numbness gradually subside, the bereaved parents usually experience the full impact of what has happened. Intensely painful feelings may last many weeks or months. This normal reaction to an extraordinary event can be overwhelming as they think about what could have been and what the future now holds. Bereaved parents are often incapable of thinking about anything or anybody else and are consumed with thoughts of their baby, themselves and how they feel. Painful reminders are all around them. Innocent comments may be misinterpreted and cause distress. Susan Hill (1990), a writer and bereaved mother, eloquently described her extreme sensitivity after the death of her baby Imogen as 'like having one skin less', and appreciated the professionals who treated her gently.

It is normal to feel extremely sad, guilty, angry and resentful. Many parents struggle with feelings of guilt about some aspect of their baby's death. Parents may think about their behaviours or actions that they may blame for causing the death of their baby, such as painting the nursery or carrying heavy shopping. These punishing thoughts can intrude into all aspects of their life.

Feelings of anger are often unexpected and hard to manage. The parents may feel anger for the loss of control that death brings. Their anger can be directed at the medical and midwifery team for not recognizing a problem sooner or for not keeping their baby alive, and anger can be directed at a God who allowed it to happen and possibly towards their baby for not living and leaving them. Sometimes, unexpected resentment towards a family member or their partner adds to this exhausting and painful time.

Grief is a normal response to loss. Grief is not a mental illness, although sleeplessness, anxiety, fear, anger and a preoccupation with self can all add up to a feeling of 'going mad'. These feelings are normal, and when experienced and expressed, slowly become less intrusive. Talking or writing about difficult experiences with someone who is interested and willing to listen is one of the healing ways to express grief. Attempts to cut short these emotions rarely help in the long term and may cause deep-seated problems in the years ahead. If grief is denied, or anger and guilt persist to the exclusion of other feelings over a number of months, specialist help may be required from a therapeutic counsellor or mental health team. It is important to be aware that perinatal death is a known risk factor for poor maternal mental health outcomes.

Worden's tasks of mourning:
3. Adjusting to an environment in which the deceased is missing

However short a time the parents had to get to know their baby, both during pregnancy and/or after the birth, facing a future without this child in the family is a difficult and painful process. Nothing can fill the void their baby has left and each day can bring reminders of their baby's absence – the empty nursery, unopened Babygros or the pregnant friend. The future seems uncertain and frightening.

It may take many months before the mother, particularly, is able to focus less on the sad events surrounding the baby's death and regain some of her interest in life. Parents may also revisit the feelings of loss at what would have been significant milestones in their baby's life, such as expected date of birth, anniversaries and birthdays.

Worden's tasks of mourning: 4. To find an enduring connection in the midst of embarking on a new life

This involves learning to live with what has happened. Parents grow to accept a different and new way of life without their baby, while remembering and holding on to precious memories. This makes it crucial to help parents who choose to to create memories during the short time they may have with their baby. It is a process of reinvesting in life again alongside the knowledge that their baby will not be forgotten. This can often feel like a betrayal and is perhaps more difficult than generally recognized.

When parents are able to look to the future while recalling memories of their baby, they may find comfort and pleasure in these memories. It is a way of making life meaningful again and gaining back some control so that the bereaved parents are not continually ambushed by memories of the death and painful feelings.

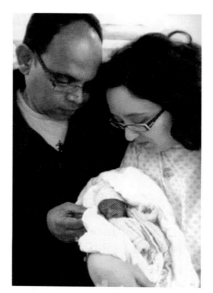

Figure 68.2 Lisa and Shelly with their baby Leo, stillborn at 25+1 weeks due to severe pre-eclampsia. (This image provided courtesy of the parents. Further reproduction or distribution is not permitted.)

> ### Reflective activity 68.1 ><
>
> Think about different types of childbearing losses and the different circumstances that may surround each death, including cause, gestation and the parents' personal circumstances.
>
> Think about:
> - how this may influence the support and care parents receive;
> - whether the care offered on your unit changes, depending on gestation or cause;
>   - If it does, why does it?
> - How might this impact the parent's experience of bereavement care and their grieving process?
>
> Write down a description of what good bereavement care means to you.

The importance of the loss

When a baby lives only a short time or dies before birth because of miscarriage, termination of pregnancy for fetal anomaly or stillbirth, it can be assumed that the loss is not as significant as the death of an adult. Pregnancy is a time of anticipation and many parents develop a strong bond with their baby long before it is born (Fig. 68.2).

When a baby dies, parents grieve for all they had hoped for and the lost opportunity of parenting their child in the future they had planned together.

A Stillbirth and Neonatal Death Society (Sands) teardrop sticker placed on the mother's notes (with her consent) after a baby's death, alerts all professionals to the parents' immediate and long-term need for sensitive, empathic care. At initial booking, it is important for the midwife to identify women who have had previous losses – miscarriage, termination, stillbirth or neonatal death – and discuss the implications for the current pregnancy. This may mean opening up a potentially painful conversation. The midwife must also be aware that the parent may want to talk about their baby who died. It may be a long time since anyone spoke about the baby with the parent. Friends and family may feel uncomfortable and avoid talking about the baby who died, not appreciating some parents' need to talk or not seeing the parents' grief as being as legitimate as that for other losses (Crawley et al 2013). Some parents may not want or be able to think about or discuss a previous loss during a subsequent pregnancy for fear of the same thing happening again.

The midwife can help prepare the parents for reactions and feelings that they might experience during the pregnancy and birth of a subsequent baby, which might include mixed feelings and high levels of anxiety concerning the baby's well-being and survival (Caelli et al 1999;

Hunfeld et al 1997). The healthcare team can be alert to this mother's needs, and ensure that support systems are available during the pregnancy and puerperium (Thomas 2001; Schott et al 2007).

DIFFERENT PARENTAL RESPONSES IN BEREAVEMENT

Even when a couple is grieving, each parent can feel alone in their grief, and normal patterns in relationships may become disrupted. As a mother's and partner's needs are different, they may find they are unable to communicate with one another and to express the complexity of their feelings. Each will have experienced the pregnancy and baby differently. It is normal then that they might grieve differently and from different perspectives.

The mother may be more *loss-oriented* and focus on the emotions they are experiencing. She may feel a strong need to make memories and to frequently recall and be reminded of and talk about her baby who has died. Partners can be generally more *restoration-oriented* – wanting things to return to normal and prefer to look to the future. Although they feel the loss, it is a loss not to be acknowledged (Puddifoot and Johnson 1997), and this response may be interpreted by their partner and others as being uncaring and less interested in their baby. It is important to remember, however, that the experience of grief is influenced and mediated by a great many factors and that men and women may react in many different ways. It should never be presumed that a mother or father will think or react in a certain way because of gender.

The midwife can assist the couple to understand the different perspectives and ways of working with their grief with open communication so that they are able to support each other.

SUPPORTING PARENTS

'Professionals in hospitals and in the community have only one chance to provide care that fosters the clinical, emotional, practical and psychosocial well-being of parents who have experienced stillbirth. By ensuring that parents receive care that is clinically skilled, emotionally intelligent [and] consistent and authentically caring, there is the best chance that, even in the midst of a difficult situation, they will have the healthiest experience possible, as well as the best chance of achieving optimum well-being in the longer term'.

(Downe et al 2013)

Communication and listening

Good communication is an essential element of bereavement care. What constitutes good communication will depend on the individual parent and their needs. However, most parents appreciate being listened to, being given time, receiving clear and honest information and receiving sensitive, empathic and individualized care.

Although parents need support and information, it should be remembered that it can be difficult for distressed parents to absorb and understand all of the information they are given at this time. It is useful to check understanding and gently ask parents to explain to you what they have understood about what they have been told. Appropriate written information should also be given to parents. Midwives should remember that the parent will most likely have to repeat a lot of what they are told to partners, family members and friends over the coming days and weeks. Information may need to be given more than once and in small amounts. Parents may not want the information you have to give them but may want more information about their baby's condition or to know more about the reason for their baby's death. Any help the midwife can provide in obtaining this information will be welcomed (Schott et al 2007). It might be that there are not any answers or a further explanation you can offer. It is best to be honest about this. It is acceptable to admit your own limitations and explain that you do not know but that you will arrange where possible and appropriate for them to see someone who might be able to help – a genetic counsellor or consultant obstetrician, for example.

Parents appreciate healthcare professionals who offer them empathy and understanding, are able to show they care and are not afraid to express their own emotions. In expressing feelings, professionals act as role models and tears are unlikely to be viewed negatively if genuinely felt. However, parents need support and should not have to be concerned about their midwife's feelings or experiences of grief.

Parents remember when you refer to their baby by name and acknowledge the significance of their baby's death. Not all parents name their baby though, so it is important to follow the parent's lead.

Parents need the opportunity to talk about how they feel with someone they trust and, if possible, to be able to express their emotions openly. It is not helpful for parents to be told how they feel; only they can know.

'Although the medical care was excellent, we really felt that there was a lack in emotional support. No one to talk to. I so desperately wanted and needed to talk to somebody, a professional, about what we were going through, and the decisions we had to make'.

(Bereaved Mother, (Redshaw et al 2014: 17))

Midwives can spend time with a couple talking about everyday things. Offering opportunities for normal conversation can be useful as well as being quiet and recognizing that just being there and being available to the parents is valuable. Do allow silences. Self-aware midwives can be intuitive and trust their own instincts when interacting with parents; listening carefully is the key. Active listening involves verbal and nonverbal communication, from the parents and the healthcare professionals. Being aware of any mannerisms you may have that may communicate something you do not intend, for example, checking your watch or tapping your foot, may be interpreted as you not having time or being in a rush. This will not encourage communication from the parents.

Touching is the most basic form of comfort and communication. This may be a hand on the arm, or an arm around the parent's shoulder. Not all parents will want this, so the practitioner needs to use their communication skills and own judgement here.

It is important to talk to both parents and acknowledge that both parents are grieving. It is helpful to provide information to parents who may want to do the practical things that have to be done, together.

All staff – hospital and community based – need to adopt a team approach with everyone being aware of the procedures to follow when a death occurs. Good multidisciplinary team relationships are essential to provide the best possible care to bereaved parents.

BREAKING BAD NEWS

'The worst bit for me was knowing something was going wrong but no one actually told me'.

(Bereaved mother)

Whether their baby's death is anticipated or occurs unexpectedly, parents value the support of caring, professional staff. It is often at the point of receiving bad news that parents will begin grieving the healthy baby they had hoped and planned for. Parents remember the way they are told bad or difficult news, and the words, actions and attitudes of the professionals involved. This can place a heavy burden on the professional who has the responsibility of giving parents the news. Explaining bad news involves both parents together whenever possible and appropriate, and should take place in a private and appropriate room. Parents appreciate honesty and a genuinely caring approach by the professional in this situation. Clear, unambiguous information needs to be sensitively communicated in a way that uses language the parents understand. An interpreter needs to be present when parents do not speak or understand English. Children and other family members should not be used to translate or convey information to parents.

Information may have to be repeated more than once. Questions should be answered as honestly as possible and allowances should be made for parents to respond in their own time. Offering time and actively listening to what they have to say avoids parents being left with confusing information.

When breaking bad news, it is important to prepare the parents for what is coming. Starting a sentence with *'I'm sorry…'* or *'I'm afraid…'* gives the parents an indication of what is coming. Give time and acknowledge any emotions, including shock. Parents will then need to know three key pieces of information: 1) what has been diagnosed; 2) what the diagnosis means for the pregnancy and the mother and 3) what happens next. Always ensure the parents are given the opportunity to ask questions then and there and given a named healthcare professional they can contact with any questions later on.

THE SCAN – THE DIAGNOSIS

Unless attending because of concerns about the pregnancy, many parents view a scan as an opportunity to meet the baby and to get a picture to share with friends and family. However, often the sonographer will be the first person to suggest or confirm that something is wrong. When an appointment is made for a scan, the parents need to be clearly told and understand that the scan is being performed to identify any anomaly that their baby may have and that if something is seen, they will be told. A partner or friend may accompany the mother.

When the scan reveals an anomaly or that their baby has died, it can be a huge shock for the parents and this needs to be recognized. The sonographer needs to communicate and follow the principles of breaking bad news discussed above. These situations require the presence of a doctor as soon as possible to confirm a possible diagnosis and to discuss what happens next. The mother and partner should be offered an opportunity to see the image of their baby while the doctor explains honestly and sensitively what has been seen on the scan. All staff members need to be familiar with the care pathways and unit policies to be followed in such circumstances. When further tests are necessary, these need to be consented and carried out as soon as possible while allowing parents time to consider their options. The reliability of these tests and any risks involved must be carefully explained to the parents.

Parents are likely to be in shock and need privacy and time to absorb what they have been told and to consider their options. It is important though that the parents do not feel abandoned at this time. If the parents decline a scan image of their baby, ask them if they would like a scan image kept in a sealed and clearly labelled envelope in the mother's notes in case they change their mind and want the image later on. It is the responsibility of the midwife looking after these parents to inform them about what can happen next and that the community team and their general practitioner (GP) will receive all the relevant information. This liaison between the hospital and the community is vital for parents when leaving the hospital.

Reflective activity 68.2

What system does your maternity unit/service have in place to ensure effective communication when managing a pregnancy loss or the death of a baby?

How do **you** personally ensure that a death has been appropriately communicated to colleagues in the community, including midwives, GPs and health visitors?

MISCARRIAGE

Miscarriage is the loss of a pregnancy before 24 weeks gestation. For many people, the miscarriage of their baby at any gestation in pregnancy is a devastating experience. Pregnancy and the feelings associated with becoming parents are unique. Expectations and the hopes and dreams of the future together with their baby are all lost with a miscarriage, as well as the physical baby and potentially the parents' self-image as parents-to-be.

Women who have not announced their pregnancy may find grieving after a miscarriage isolating and may struggle to speak about their miscarriage and seek support (Higson 2015).

'Some women will receive adequate support and permission to grieve for their baby, while other women may be subjected to chastisement by relatives or other individuals for seeking to grieve over that perceived as a non-entity, and as such denied support and compassion'.

(Kenworthy and Kirkham 2011)

There is not a standard way of caring for all women at this time; midwives need to recognize and respond to parents' very varied feelings, trying to understand what each individual needs. If this is unclear, it is important to feel able to ask. It is crucial to bear in mind that there may be a lack of support for the parents around their miscarriage, possibly because of no one else knowing about the pregnancy or possibly because of a difficulty that many people experience in talking about pregnancy loss and the death of a baby. Midwives should inform parents of the

support available to them through the hospital and support groups, such as the Miscarriage Association and the Stillbirth and Neonatal Death Society (Sands).

Parents can find medical terminology used by professionals such as *'blighted ovum'*, *'missed abortion'* or *'non-viable fetus'* unhelpful, meaningless and hurtful. Midwives need to use sensitive language to communicate effectively with parents and support them while avoiding jargon and remaining clear and honest.

Sands offers a template certificate acknowledging the birth of a baby before 24 weeks gestation when the baby is born with no signs of life. This certificate acknowledges the baby's birth and should be offered to parents. Some parents will want to keep this as a memento. The certificate can be adapted for each hospital and is downloadable from the Sands website.

TERMINATION OF PREGNANCY FOR FETAL ANOMALY

Jane Fisher, Director of Antenatal Results and Choices (ARC), a support organization that supports women through antenatal screening and its aftermath, including when the very difficult decision to end a wanted pregnancy is made, says 'Nothing can take away the pain and sadness but we hear consistently how much women and their partners value compassionate, nonjudgemental care through what is often a traumatic experience. It can be important in their recovery that they can look back and remember being treated sensitively by confident competent staff' (Fisher 2015).

Parents who make the very difficult decision to end a wanted pregnancy often want the healthcare professionals caring for them to acknowledge the difficulty associated with termination of pregnancy for fetal anomaly (TOPFA) and to recognize that the baby was wanted. Using medical terminology such as 'product of conception' to describe the dead baby can be hurtful for parents, as it can seem to invalidate the baby.

Parents need clear, unbiased information, in understandable language, about their baby's diagnosis and the options available to them, including information about choice of method of termination. Providing written information before any decisions are made is crucial. ARC provides support leaflets around TOPFA and continuing with a pregnancy with a prenatal diagnosis.

'At a time of crisis, information gives strength and understanding, whereas to be deprived of information is disempowering and adds to parents' distress. They need information about what may happen, is happening, or has happened, to them and to their baby. They need to know about what choices they have, and how to make those choices. And they need

information about practical matters, procedures and arrangements'.

(Kohner and Leftwich 1995)

It is crucial to recognize the importance of choice. 'Most women greatly valued being given choices, including whether to have the termination or not, the method of termination, the types and levels of analgesia, whether to spend time with the baby or not, and what to do with the baby's remains' (Fisher and Lafarge 2014). Parents will need to be supported through the decision-making process, as in this context choice carries a lot of responsibility and burden.

Some decide to continue with their pregnancy and need support to do what is right for them. Whichever decision is made, their choice will involve grieving for the healthy baby they had been expecting.

When parents have made a decision to end the pregnancy, they may not feel able to experience or express any attachment to their baby. The grief of these parents can be complicated by feelings of guilt, as they have had to make a decision no one expects to have to make. It is hugely important that healthcare professionals are non-judgemental and offer as much emotional support as is needed. For parents facing TOPFA, fear of being judged is a huge challenge. Parents are grateful for and value non-judgemental care from healthcare professionals and others, including faith leaders.

'Possibly the most influential element in women's experience was healthcare professionals' ability to care for them in an empathetic way…it was healthcare professionals' kindness that women were most grateful for'.

(Fisher and Lafarge 2014)

It is important to ensure seamless care where women are referred to tertiary units or the independent sector for care. On-going bereavement care after TOPFA must be offered to parents (Lyus et al 2013). Parents should also be told about the support organizations offering on-going bereavement support, such as ARC and Sands.

Women with a multiple pregnancy may be offered a fetal reduction to reduce the overall risk for the pregnancy or because one or more of the babies has been diagnosed with a fetal anomaly. Parents should be supported in making the decision that feels most manageable for them. They must be given time, accurate information and sensitive care (Fraser 2010).

LABOUR WHEN A BABY HAS DIED DUE TO MISCARRIAGE OR TOPFA

Hospitals can be impersonal, frightening places and the sensitive care offered by a midwife is crucial. Providing an atmosphere in which parents are able to trust the professional caring for them is enhanced by having a suitable, comfortable and private bereavement room. The entire team needs to know when bereaved parents are admitted to the unit.

On meeting these parents, the midwife needs to acknowledge the situation and then spend time listening to parents, building a relationship and responding to their varied needs and feelings. Not all parents realize that the labour and birth of their baby will need to be physically the same as giving birth to a live baby. This realization may be hard to comprehend and may cause anger and disbelief.

'To find myself carrying death and, even worse, being told I had to give birth to death, was the most horrific scenario'.

(Bereaved Mother)

PRACTICAL CONSIDERATIONS OF BIRTH

'The silence in the delivery room was deafening. This was the reality – this was death at birth'.

(Bereaved Mother)

A mother who is expecting a stillbirth, TOPFA or late miscarriage requires significant emotional support. The Sands Tool (Sands 2014a) for maternity services is a useful resource for maternity services, and states that every woman should have an experienced midwife to look after her throughout her labour and birth. It is also important that the labour environment is appropriate for the mother. Ideally, a separate bereavement room or suite should be provided away from crying babies, with private facilities and space for a partner or supporter to stay with the mother (see Figs 68.3a and b). If this is impossible, the mother's preference should be respected around delivering on a labour ward or gynaecology ward, depending on what feels most manageable for them – bearing in mind the practicalities of physical care.

The principles of care during labour for this woman are similar to those for a woman expecting a live birth (see Box 68.2). It is important that healthcare professionals discuss pain relief with women. Opiate-based pain relief is available to women in labour with a baby that has died. The woman may want to think carefully about any side effects of strong pain relief. Some women will experience nausea, dizziness and a feeling of being outside of themselves. Women who want to be aware at the time of their baby's birth and want to remember those moments may decline opiate-based pain relief.

Discussing birth preferences and having some control in a situation where parents can feel powerless may be

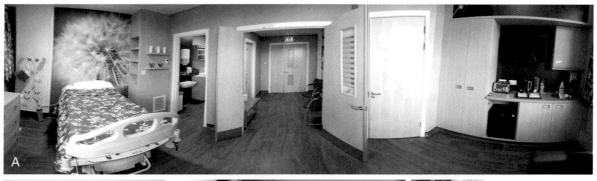

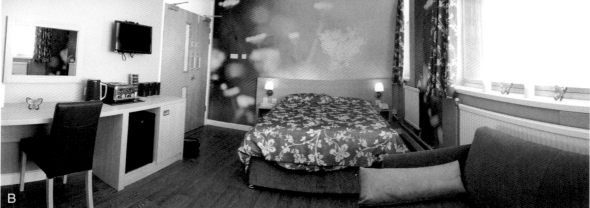

Figure 68.3 Two of the bereavement rooms/suites at Leicester Royal Infirmary.

Box 68.2 Bereavement care – best practice points

1. Actively listen, give honest and clear information and gently check understanding, include partners where possible
2. Care for bereaved parents in an appropriate environment, a dedicated bereavement room or suite should be available
3. Give written information where possible, including a named contact with contact details and support literature
4. Support parents' individual choices, including around making memories
5. Ensure staff have access to a bereavement midwife, support and bereavement care training

---

psychologically valuable. To avoid later regrets about how the birth was managed and experienced, 'parents should be given time to make decisions that are right for them' (Boden et al 2015). These choices may provide important memories on which to focus in the process of grieving.

'I didn't have any control over the situation at all and I don't think either of us really knew what was happening until well after'.

(Bereaved Mother)

The woman may be in a state of shock and, therefore, it is preferable to provide good continuity of care, and the midwife providing that care should be aware of the possibility that information may not be as easily understood and that this information needs to be simple and accessible, and may need to be repeated.

The midwife needs to be aware that the woman is often so immersed in her grief that she may pay little attention to what she is physically experiencing. The mother should be fully informed about what is happening and have all choices communicated to her clearly and sensitively. If a decision has to be made during labour, it is important for the woman to understand what is happening and what may happen. Some decisions might be time pressured, and this needs to be explained to the mother.

'I felt I could have been informed better of what was happening and why…'

(Bereaved Parent) (Redshaw et al 2014: 29)

If healthcare professionals are entering the room that the mother does not know, where possible, they should be introduced and the reason for them being there should be explained.

'I felt too many professionals were in the room. I couldn't take in what was being said to me'.

(Bereaved Mother) (Redshaw et al 2014: 16)

It is also important to acknowledge the partner or support person and to be aware of what they are witnessing or experiencing. 85% of fathers or partners who experienced the stillbirth of their baby felt positive about the way they were treated during labour. However, 37% did not feel listened to or only 'to some extent', 33% did not feel as though their concerns were taken seriously and 39% felt that their needs were not acknowledged. With regards to decision making, 36% of fathers or partners reported they did not feel fully informed (Redshaw et al 2014).

Respecting parents

As soon as possible after their baby's death, a visit from a senior doctor, with the midwife, is valuable for parents and provides acknowledgement of the significance of their baby's death. They will need time with a designated person who can help them with the practical arrangements, to understand what steps to take, legal requirements, what the hospital can and cannot arrange and choices about a postmortem and funeral. Providing written information to support verbal explanation, devised in consultation with families, is useful so parents can refer back to it as needed while in the hospital and also at home.

Making memories

Parents should be supported in seeing and holding their baby if they decide to. Not all parents will want to see their baby and this decision must be respected and supported. For those that do, this provides the parents with an opportunity to make precious memories with their baby. Some parents will need you to talk through what the baby may look like or to describe particular aspects of the baby's appearance before they feel able to see their baby. For some parents, this will be their first experience of death, and they may be frightened of what their baby will look or feel like. It can be useful for the midwife to explain to the parents what other parents have done and found useful, as this can normalize their own feelings and can be a gentle way to make suggestions. It is important that parents are prepared and supported in making informed choices at this crucial time and that it is recognized that the decisions made will be individual to each parent.

These hours after the birth are immensely valuable. Nothing in life can prepare parents for such a tragedy and observing the staff's tenderness and interactions with their baby can remain with the parents for a lifetime.

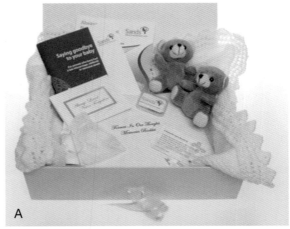

A

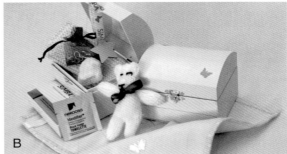

B

Figure 68.4 **A,** Sands Memory Box. **B,** SIMBA memory box.

The importance of memories

Midwifery and neonatal staff who help parents get to know and parent their baby in the brief time they have together provide a source of precious memories, which can be vitally important in the months ahead (Sands 2014b). Many units offer parents a memory box, which can be used to store any special mementoes of their baby, and these can be supplied from organizations such as Sands; Simpsons Memory Box Appeal (SIMBA); 4Louis; and the LilyMae Foundation (see Figs 68.4a and b). Momentos can include photographs, their baby's name-band, foot and hand prints, a lock of hair, a page where words can be written by anyone who knew the parents and baby, a blessing or naming card, letters and perhaps the clothes the baby wore, a blanket the baby has been wrapped in and the anniversary cards and gifts that people choose to collect and keep for the future. Sharing these memories with other people has been shown to have a positive impact on maternal mental health following stillbirth (Crawley et al 2013).

Spiritual needs

Different cultures have varying rituals and traditions that are followed around death; they can provide an opportunity to honour the importance of what has happened and help them face reality. When religions and cultures are different from our own, a lack of knowledge and understanding of specific spiritual needs may leave professionals feeling helpless and families dissatisfied (Arshad et al 2003). Asking parents what they would like and offering them time to explore what is important for them can be invaluable. It is important that assumptions are not made about what a parent may want based on their cultural or religious background. Individuals from within the same religious or ethnic groups may make different choices. Each individual must have all of their options explained to them. If a parent wishes to speak with a spiritual leader about the requirements for their baby's funeral according to their religion this should be supported. Wherever possible, the personal, cultural or religious needs of parents should be met (HTA 2014).

Many hospitals keep a Book of Remembrance in which parents may make an entry, either soon after the birth or at a later date.

It is best for the midwife and others to refrain from talking about their personal beliefs with bereaved families but to be open to what may be appropriate for them. This illustrates the need for the midwife to be knowledgeable about different cultures and religions and their rituals but never make assumptions about what parents from a particular group will wish to do after a bereavement (Schott et al 2007; Child Bereavement UK (CBUK) 2013a).

Washing and dressing the baby after death

This may be the one opportunity parents have to choose clothes for their child and may be one of the few opportunities for parents to parent their baby (see Fig. 68.5). Staff can make a difference by providing information, enabling parents to make choices, including:

- Would the parents like to wash and dress their baby themselves?
- Would they prefer to watch their baby being washed and dressed by a member of staff?
- Do they have clothes they would like to dress their baby in?

It is important for the midwife to be gently present at this point, so that if the parents are anxious, they can be supported.

It should be unit policy to have a selection of new baby clothes from which parents can choose to dress their baby and later keep when they return home. These clothes and anything else associated with the baby can be treasured by the family if they are taken home. Clothes their baby has

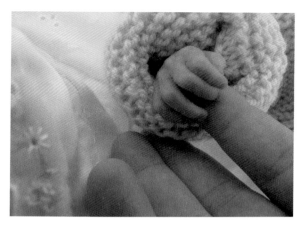

Figure 68.5 Catherine with her baby Jack, stillborn at 26 weeks due to placental abruption, wearing his knitted blue cardigan. (This image provided courtesy of the parents. Further reproduction or distribution is not permitted.)

worn are best left unwashed, as initially the smell of baby on the clothes will provide parents with a tangible reminder of their baby. Parents may choose not to see and hold, wash or dress their baby and this decision needs to be respected and supported.

The value of photographs

For many people, scan images and camera or mobile phone photographs of their baby who has died, are immensely important. These parents will be interested in what their baby looked like and will value pictures that clearly show details their baby's profile, their hands and feet, and perhaps sensitively taken photographs of their baby naked. These photographs can bring comfort and help validate parents' feelings of grief when they return home without their baby. Midwives should not assume that parents will not want photographs if their baby's appearance has deteriorated or if there is a visible anomaly. Sometimes seeing the anomaly can help parents come to terms with what has happened. Parents may like to know they can have a photograph of themselves holding their baby (see Fig. 68.2), a family picture with their other children (see Fig. 68.6), a photo with one parent (see Fig. 68.7) or the grandparents or with midwives who cared for them. Some parents may prefer to have close-up images of their baby's feet or hands or images taken of their baby with a teddy or blanket they can then keep (see Fig. 68.8). When a twin dies, taking care and time to photograph the live twin and the dead twin together is something parents may not naturally consider and yet may so value in what can be a complicated grief process in the years ahead.

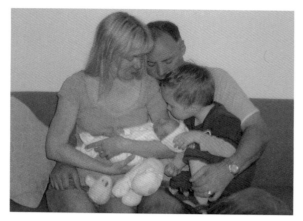

Figure 68.6 Lyne and Peter with son Travis and baby Jude, stillborn in 2006. (This image provided courtesy of the parents. Further reproduction or distribution is not permitted.)

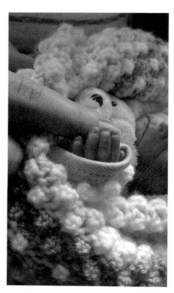

Figure 68.8 Christina with her baby Evelyn Ann, who was stillborn at 26 weeks in 2014. (This image provided courtesy of the parents. Further reproduction or distribution is not permitted.)

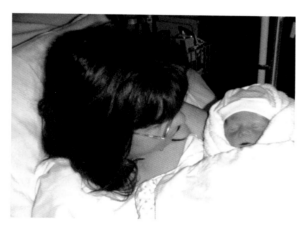

Figure 68.7 Carolyn with her baby Rebecca, stillborn at 38+2 weeks in 2002 due to placental abruption. (This image provided courtesy of the parents. Further reproduction or distribution is not permitted.)

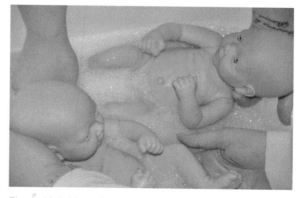

Figure 68.9 Memorial photography training image from a Gifts of Remembrance workshop with midwives.

Later in life, the surviving twin may be interested to know about the sibling who died and to know that his or her twin was acknowledged and mourned – parents in multiple birth and death situations have a great deal to manage and can find this image helpful. Some parents may not feel able to look at scan images or photographs of their baby straight away. It can help to put any images taken (with consent from the parents) into a sealed and clearly labeled envelope in the mother's notes in case the parents change their mind later on.

There are training workshops healthcare professionals can attend in memorial photography, and it is useful if midwives can gain skills in achieving a good photograph. *Gifts of Remembrance* run practical training sessions for midwives in memorial photography (see Fig. 68.9).

INVOLVING BROTHERS AND SISTERS

When a baby dies, parents may be reluctant to involve their other children. They themselves are grieving and may feel helpless and overwhelmed and possibly uncertain about their own ability to manage their children's grief. It is natural for them to want to protect their children from painful situations and it can be helpful if they are told this is a normal reaction. However, this may leave siblings scared, unprotected from their own fantasies about what has happened and unsupported in their feelings.

Whenever possible, it is helpful if parents prepare their other children when their baby sibling is not expected to live, giving honest information appropriate to their children's age (Sands 2014c). Children need to understand that most babies who are sick in the hospital get better and go home, but sadly sometimes babies die. It is important not to overwhelm children with information but to be guided by them and to answer their questions honestly and clearly without using euphemisms that might be misinterpreted.

Most children who have been sensitively prepared and have chosen to see their dead baby brother or sister are not afraid and generally gain an understanding of death and what has happened (see Fig. 68.6). What children do not know or are not told about, they often make up and their fantasies can be worse than the reality.

Sometimes they experience feelings of guilt, especially if they were not looking forward to having a new sibling. They need to be reassured that the baby's death had nothing to do with their thoughts or actions, and that their parents love them. It is also important to reassure children, where possible, that they and their parents are alright (ARC 2004).

Parents may be concerned that frightening memories of a dead baby will leave their children with upsetting images – this is unlikely, especially when the children have been prepared for what to expect (see Fig. 68.10). Children respond well to factual explanations of death and having information such as 'When people die it means their body doesn't work any more'. It is useful to explain that the baby may feel cold to touch and that the skin may be mottled and the baby's lips or skin may be blue. It is not helpful to liken death to sleeping because people who are asleep are not dead and their bodies work very well (CBUK 2013b; CBUK 2013c; CBUK 2016a). The sibling may also become frightened of falling asleep themselves.

It is important for staff to make a direct offer of help to families and ensure there is time to discuss parents' worries and anxieties. However, parents are individuals and not all of them will feel able to involve their children directly or tell them about the death immediately. Different cultures will have different ways of dealing with death, and sensitivity is paramount when offering parents information so that they can make informed choices, for example, a photograph to take home to the children of their brother or sister who has died. It is helpful for staff to explain to parents that they may meet resistance from

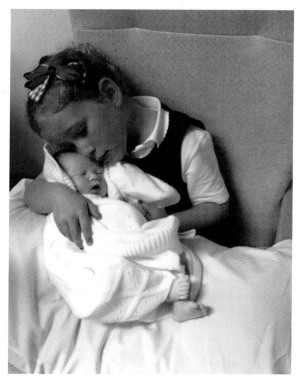

Figure 68.10 Big sister Harriet with Baby Beatrice, who died in 2013 from a fetal-maternal haemorrhage at 38 weeks. (This image provided courtesy of the parents. Further reproduction or distribution is not permitted.)

grandparents and others who did not receive this type of care years ago.

Professionals can suggest children might like to have something special for themselves – perhaps a footprint on coloured paper they have chosen or a photograph of them with their baby brother or sister. Children can be helped if they are allowed to share in and create memories.

Communicating with siblings: The decision is not whether or not to talk to children, but who will do the talking and when and how, as it is impossible for parents not to communicate with children. They read body language, overhear conversations and notice changes in routine. Children quickly sense when something serious is happening. They require clear, simple, truthful and often repeated, but brief explanations about what has happened and what may happen next.

Children do not need protecting from their feelings, but support in them. Young siblings will not grieve in the same way as older children and often express themselves through play, drawing or with friends.

Children's reactions and understanding: Children have a shorter concentration span than adults and cannot tolerate intense emotions for very long. This does not mean that they are not sometimes upset and sad. Few children under the age of 5 will understand the permanance of death. They think in literal, concrete terms and therefore metaphors or euphemisms such as 'lost' or 'gone away' are confusing. Children need adults to say the words 'has died' or 'is dead'. By 6 years of age, most children begin to understand death as permanent and that it can happen to them.

FAMILY AND FRIENDS

Grandparents and members of the wider family and friends can also be affected by the death of a baby. Often they will grieve for their grandchild/niece/nephew and for the sadness of the parents. They may be a main source of support for the grieving parents in the months ahead and may also need support themselves.

Involvement of a close family friend can also be supportive, particularly if a parent faces bereavement on their own without a partner. It can be important for the parent to have a support person to share the memories and experience of their baby and to help with decisions such as funeral arrangements. Not all parents will want to have a funeral for their baby, but some of those that do will invite the midwives who cared for them and their baby.

ORGAN DONATION

Parents will not necessarily consider asking about heart valve or other tissue or organ donation. They will rely on – and appreciate – the professionals who care for them to provide them with information to make informed choices; it is, therefore, important that information is given considering the individual circumstances of each parent when organ donation is possible. Parents who are not asked may wonder why and later may even resent this lack of information.

Parents need to have clear information and explanations from the donor team in their particular region, and would need to be aware that heart valve donation (usually referred to as tissue donation), carried out up to 48 hours after the death of a term baby, may require a large part of the heart to be retained. If a donation from their baby is to be used, blood samples will need to be taken from the mother, father and baby to test for HIV, hepatitis B and C and syphilis.

POSTMORTEM EXAMINATION (AUTOPSY)

All staff should receive appropriate training in how to sensitively discuss consent for a hospital postmortem with parents. Although a doctor may request and provide information for postmortem consent, it is often the midwife that the parents turn to, to ask for further information, clarification and support, and all midwives must understand the ethical, legal and emotional responsibilities involved (HTA 2006 and 2014; CBUK 2016b). Obtaining parents' consent should be seen as a continuing process, not limited to the signing of a form. Sands have a Post Mortem Consent Pack to help healthcare professionals with this, available on the Sands and HTA websites (Sands 2014b).

A postmortem may provide helpful information (Sands 2014b), such as:

- It may confirm the cause of the baby's death.
- It can confirm or change an existing clinical diagnosis.
- It may identify conditions that might not have been diagnosed otherwise.
- It can exclude some causes of death or possible factors such as infection.
- It can help assess the chances of problems recurring in a future pregnancy.
- For some families, it can help them resolve specific questions and may help them come to terms with what happened and facilitate emotional closure (Heazell et al 2012).
- In the case of genetic conditions, a postmortem may also indicate the need for other members of the family to be offered investigation.

A postmortem can also inform the parents of the sex of their baby if this is unknown. Some parents will not want this information, but others will find it helpful during the grieving process.

Parents will want different levels of detail about the postmortem (Sands has a useful leaflet for parents). Graphic details about the postmortem examination may be too overwhelming for some parents, and they need to be offered the opportunity to choose how much or how little information they would like and given time to consider their decision and ask any questions. Sensitive and caring communication is essential in this situation to ensure consent is a process and is properly sought. It is important that parents feel in control, understand what they are consenting to (if anything) and have the right to say what happens during and after the postmortem examination.

Many parents want to know where their baby will be (the baby may be transferred to a different hospital for the postmortem) and that they will be cared for respectfully throughout. It is also important to inform parents that they can see the baby again after a postmortem if they wish.

If parents consent to a postmortem, it is important that the consultant involved after the baby's death meets with the parents and discusses the findings of the postmortem as soon as possible after the death. Many parents value an opportunity to talk to the pathologist before or after the examination. Opting for a postmortem does not exclude the option of taking baby home or out of the hospital if parents choose this.

Coroner's postmortem

The coroner or procurator fiscal may or may not decide that a postmortem should be carried out to try to establish the cause of death.

In the event of a sudden or unexplained death, a coroner's postmortem is legally required and in this situation the parents' permission is not requested. The parents' need for time, information and sensitive support is vital. The coroner is responsible for informing parents if organs and/or tissue have been retained to ascertain the cause of death. The length of time an organ will be retained and when it will be returned to the body before burial or cremation should be discussed. It is crucial that parents are informed that, with their consent, tissue blocks and slides may be kept as part of the medical record. Parents need to understand that while enquiries into the cause of their baby's death are underway, the death cannot be registered and so final funeral arrangements cannot be made. Often, however, when an inquest is required, it is held very soon after the death and the funeral need not be delayed. Information regarding a coroner's postmortem and whether an inquest is needed should be available for parents in written format.

RESPECTFUL DISPOSAL

Parents of babies born dead before 24 weeks gestation who choose to arrange a burial or cremation for their baby themselves, may need help with planning a ceremony, which can be held in the hospital, in a church, at the crematorium or cemetery or at a different place of the parents' choice. Parents do not generally know about how to manage this and may welcome information and support (RCN 2015). Some parents may prefer not to be involved in the arrangements themselves but may want to know the decisions made on their behalf in the months to come, making good record keeping essential.

All parents need information about the options available to them, and there will be regional and country variations, such as that incineration is not an option in Scotland (RCN 2015). An information sheet clearly explaining all options with the relevant costs, if any, and considerations can be valuable. Parents must know they have time to make these decisions and discuss any restrictions, ensuring parents are not rushed and are able to make informed choices (RCN 2015).

TAKING A BABY HOME

Some parents choose to take their baby home or out of the hospital to a place of special meaning for them. There is no legal reason this cannot happen unless the death has been referred to the coroner or procurator fiscal. Where possible, parents need information about the option of taking their baby home or out of the hospital (CBUK 2016c). Some parents will want to spend time with their baby outside of a clinical environment. Some will use this as an opportunity to introduce baby to family members, including siblings, grandparents and aunties and uncles. Friends may also be invited to see the baby. This time can be precious and used to make many memories in the home environment.

Where baby is taken home, support must be offered to the parents, particularly if there is a history of mental health problems. Parents must be informed about how to care for their baby's body at home, especially if a postmortem will be completed. A cuddle cot can be very helpful here. Where the parents do not feel able to take baby home, they should be offered an extended stay in hospital in a bereavement room or suite, with the baby. Although it is not legally required, to prevent misunderstandings, Sands offers a certificate for hospitals to complete to document that the body of the baby has been released to the parents. This is for the parents to have with them when they leave the hospital with the baby's body. When there is a coroner's postmortem, permission must be sought from the coroner (Sands 2014b).

Leaving the hospital

When parents leave the hospital, where possible, a member of staff should walk with them out to their car or taxi. It is crucial that community staff members are aware of the baby's death and parents know who to contact once at home. Hospital policies need to be clear and enhance liaison between hospital and home services to provide continuity of care for bereaved parents.

Making an appointment for the parents to visit the consultant again and perhaps the midwife who cared for them for a follow-up bereavement visit is useful. They can share again what happened at their baby's death or maybe have explained anything they did not understand at the time. This may also be an opportunity to discuss any results of a postmortem or other investigations carried out after the baby's death. This time can be a valuable way of finding out what support the parents have or may need.

REGISTRATION OF THE DEATH

Legally, when a baby is born dead before 24 weeks gestation, there is no legal requirement or option for registration. However, if the parents choose to have their baby buried or cremated, they will need written confirmation of the birth from the doctor or midwife attending the delivery. Some units issue a form/certificate to record that the parents are taking their baby's body, and this is formally recommended as best practice. This certificate can also serve to acknowledge the birth of the baby and can become an important memento.

After 24 weeks gestation, when a baby is stillborn, the doctor or midwife who attended the delivery gives the parents a *Medical Certificate of Stillbirth* and should explain that the stillbirth of their baby must be registered by either or both parents at the registry office within 42 days in England and Wales, 21 days in Scotland and within a year in Northern Ireland.

When a baby is born alive, *regardless of gestational age*, and dies within 28 days of birth, a doctor, by law, must confirm the death and provide a medical certificate to enable both the birth and death to be registered within 5 days of the death.

When parents are married, either or both can register, but when parents are unmarried, the registration needs to be done by the mother. The mother's partner should accompany her if they wish for their name to appear on their baby's certificate.

Follow-up appointment and the postnatal period

The mother requires a high standard of postnatal care, including emotional support, physical assessment, and information, ensuring she understands the normal physiological process of the puerperium and what can be considered normal including pain, bleeding and lactation.

Wherever the woman is cared for, the environment must feel appropriate to them in their circumstances. Continuity of carer must be an aim and the same principles of keeping information simple and accessible should be retained. Bereaved mothers can find it especially hard when their breasts fill with milk, which is a tangible reminder that there is no baby to feed. Some women will want to suppress lactation, others may decide to donate their milk. All options should be discussed with the mother. During the postnatal period, the woman still requires midwifery care to ensure that she is physically recovering from the birth, and any physical wounds are healing. It is also an opportunity for the midwife to assess the woman's psychological progress, and provide information and guidance on other services and support that would be useful.

RETURN VISIT TO THE HOSPITAL UNIT

Some parents want to come back to the unit to see the midwife in the antenatal clinic or to see the person who cared for them and their baby. The opportunity to talk through what happened at the time of their baby's death, particularly if the mother had a general anaesthetic, can be very valuable. Ideally, a time should be arranged so that when parents arrive on the unit, someone expects them and they have a clear idea how long the member of staff can spend with them. The parent may want to talk through any test results. This information will need to be clear and also given in written form for the parent to take home and digest. Parents should be offered the option of contacting a known healthcare professional with any questions that arise once they are home. Some parents will want to be seen outside of a maternity care setting. This should be facilitated where possible.

AFTERCARE AND THE MONTHS AHEAD

It is important that parents are offered aftercare once they have returned home when their baby has died. When parents leave hospital, they should be given the name and contact details of a healthcare professional, preferably a known bereavement midwife. Parents should also be offered a telephone call from a healthcare professional and a home visit at a time that best suits them. Not everyone will want a home visit from a midwife when their baby has died, but those who accept will most likely value the opportunity to speak about what has happened, ask questions and check they are physically well. It is also vital that the woman receive the same level of postnatal examination and care.

Some parents may decline the initial offer, but realize once they are home, they do need the support. They should be told they can change their mind about accepting/declining aftercare when the offer is made. It is important to look at what your unit offers and make sure that all women experiencing the death of a baby are offered the same support, with a minimum of an offer of a telephone call and/or a home visit, a named contact (midwife) and written information about where they can access further support if needed, such as through local support groups like Sands.

Appropriate care needs to be available in the months after the death of a baby. Parents need to know how to access support no matter how long it is since their baby has died (Jennings 2001).

In a busy unit, it is not always possible for healthcare professionals to give parents as much time as they need, both at the time of the death and afterwards. A designated bereavement midwife can be key in offering appropriate, on-going support to parents once they have returned home, and can work as a link between hospital- and community-based healthcare professionals to make sure everyone who needs to know what has happened does know. This helps ensure the best possible care for the parents. Parents say that just knowing that support is available can help them to manage their feelings and relationships.

The death of a baby can be a very lonely experience, with many parents saying they feel isolated when they return home and their healthcare team no longer contacts them. Community midwives, health visitors and GPs must be informed about the death of a baby (unless otherwise requested by the parent).

HOW PROFESSIONALS CAN HELP

Although some midwives feel that there is little they can do to help bereaved parents, simply listening is often very helpful. It is important that staff are able to actively listen to parents' stories with openness and without taking a defensive position (Kenworthy and Kirkham 2011). Listening can be very difficult, particularly if the parents are angry or blame the healthcare professionals for the death of their baby. It can be helpful if the midwife who delivered the baby or cared for the parent(s) is available to listen to parents, answer their questions and where possible contribute to their memories of what happened (Redshaw et al 2014; Kenworthy and Kirkham 2011). This can help parents develop their story of what happened and why.

Giving time to parents when they experience the death of their baby has many potential benefits for the parents, both in the short and longer term (Crawley et al 2013; Kenworthy and Kirkham 2011; Swanson KM 1999; Moulder 1998: 222). Staff should give parents as much time as possible. Giving parents' time, providing individualized care and supporting parents in their decision making, being honest and acknowledging the impact of the death of their baby will benefit many parents at the time their baby dies and in the weeks and months that follow.

All staff need support and adequate training in providing bereavement care and communication skills, including ancillary staff.

THERAPEUTIC USE OF OURSELVES

When a baby dies, the exposure to the parents' grief, sadness and pain may remind midwives of their own previous bereavements (Thomas and Chalmers 2005). Midwives themselves may have experienced pregnancy loss or had difficulty in becoming pregnant, and this can impact their feelings and experience of caring for women and families who also experience the death of a baby (Bewley 2010).

The process of helping is an active one, requiring a willingness to become involved and show empathy but remain separate, enabling the provision of sensitive and compassionate care. This requires a high degree of self-awareness and recognition of your own feelings. As care givers, if you are able to acknowledge and appropriately express your own anger, fear, sadness and embarrassment, other people's emotions can be accepted more easily.

Interactions with people who are profoundly distressed can engender feelings of inadequacy and helplessness, and this is in contrast to the normal healthcare role of helping 'make people feel better and remove pain'. In bereavement, people cannot be made better – but they can be helped through their grief with good care, providing positive memories at a difficult time.

When caring for bereaved families, the caregiver's feelings often mirror those of the family – anger, sadness, confusion, a sense of failure. Management that recognizes and acknowledges the value of staff's contributions in this work and their need for support helps build individuals' self-esteem in times of stress. Having access to a professional offering support or counselling based in the hospital can be as valuable for staff as it is for parents. Midwives must receive appropriate training in bereavement care.

Looking after ourselves as professionals

Emotions can be felt physically in different parts of the body – tension can be felt in the muscles of the shoulder, grief and sadness perhaps in the muscles around the neck, heart and stomach. Knowing which parts of our body are affected in times of stress, enables identification of ways of releasing these trapped emotions. Relaxation, exercise, listening to music or watching a favourite programme on television and seeking support are all possible therapeutic outlets.

When people feel unable to manage their own emotions, they can develop protective strategies, such as distancing themselves from other people's emotions, appearing unaffected and detached or conversely becoming very busy to avoid their emotional pain. They may develop negative feelings about themselves and their work and see themselves as failures. This can manifest itself as anger or resentment, which can affect family and professional relationships. Some of the warning signs of feeling depleted include experiencing chronic exhaustion; frequently feeling upset; difficulties in eating or sleeping or engaging with people; developing headaches or backaches; having nightmares; feeling worthless and pessimistic; avoiding contact with others; arriving late for work and leaving early. It is important for healthcare professionals to take the time to care for themselves and get to know what helps them too.

SUPPORT AND TRAINING FOR MIDWIVES WORKING IN PARTNERSHIP WITH FAMILIES

Caring for distressed parents can be difficult and demanding, and requires staff to work in an environment that considers their needs and values them as individuals. Where appropriate, support mechanisms should be in place and training in bereavement care should be provided. Bereaved parents are deeply grateful for good bereavement care and remember the care they received for the rest of their lives. Midwives themselves will find that where they have been able to give that level of care, they themselves can be enriched.

Bereavement care training and support should be an intrinsic part of maternity care, whatever the setting (Schott et al 2007). Using counselling and listening skills is an essential part of the professional's role and requires training, enabling midwives to care effectively when managing the death of a baby (Thomas and Chalmers 2005) (see Box 68.3).

It is important that the midwife is knowledgeable about the:

- legal framework around loss and bereavement;
- policies relevant to different areas of care;
- different choices available for parents;
- local and national support and information sources for parents;
- supporting and developing student midwives' and junior staff's skills in bereavement;
- need for different members of staff to be involved in providing bereavement care (this includes other professional staff and ancillary colleagues);
- psychological and professional needs of themselves and colleagues;
- value of debriefing/reflective sessions, as a support, development and sharing good practice process;
- support available to midwives.

Box 68.3 Sands principles of bereavement care (Sands 2016)

Parents' perspectives and collaborative working with healthcare professionals have informed these principles of bereavement care.

1. Care should be individualized so that it is parent led and caters for their personal, cultural or religious needs. Parents should always be treated with respect and dignity. Sensitive, empathetic care is crucial and may involve spending time with parents. This should be recognized by managers and staff.

2. Clear communication with parents is key and it should be sensitive, honest and tailored to meet the individual needs of parents. Childbearing losses can involve periods of uncertainty and staff should avoid giving assurances that may turn out to be false. Trained interpreters and signers should be available for parents who need them.

3. In any situation where there is a choice to be made, parents should be listened to and given the information and support they need to make their own decisions about what happens to them and their baby.

4. No assumptions should be made about the intensity and duration of grief that a parent will experience. It is important that staff accept and acknowledge the feelings that individual parents may experience.

5. Women and their partners should always be looked after by staff members who are specifically trained in bereavement care and in an environment that the parent feels is appropriate to their circumstances. In

addition to good emotional support, women should receive excellent physical care during and after a loss.

6. A partner's grief can be as profound as that of the mother's; their need for support should be recognized and met.

7. All staff members who care for bereaved parents before, during or after the death of a baby should have opportunities to develop and update their knowledge and skills. In addition, they should have access to good support for themselves.

8. All parents whose babies die should be offered opportunities to create memories. Their individual wishes and needs should be respected.

9. The bodies of babies and fetal remains should be treated with respect at all times. Options around sensitive disposal should be discussed and respectful funerals should be offered.

10. Good communication between staff and healthcare teams is crucial in ensuring that staff members are aware of parents' preferences and decisions; therefore, parents do not need to repeatedly explain their situation. This includes the handover of care from hospital to primary care staff, which should ensure that support and care for parents is seamless. Ongoing support is an essential part of care and should be available to all those who want it and should continue to be made available to all women and their partners during a subsequent pregnancy and after the birth of another baby.

When healthcare professionals do take the time to talk about their needs, their feelings, their reactions to situations and to understand their strengths and limitations, then working with bereaved families can be special and rewarding.

Support agencies

There are a number of support organizations that offer on-going support to bereaved families. Support is offered in the form of helplines, face-to-face support groups, online forums and support booklets and mobile 'apps'. Most parents will appreciate information about the local and national support groups. National agencies, such as the Stillbirth and Neonatal Death Society (Sands), Antenatal Results and Choices (ARC) and The Miscarriage Association offer information and support for parents, and also provide literature and resources to help and support healthcare professionals.

CONCLUSION

Midwives working with bereaved families must give sensitive and empathic care; respect parents' wishes and feelings whatever they may be; offer them as much time as they need to talk about what has happened; actively listen to what they have to say; ensure they have as much information as is available and that they have understood it; answer parents' questions honestly; give time and make sure parents have a named health professional contact for support in the future.

The MBRRACE-UK reports (Draper et al 2015) and Homer and others in The Lancet series (2016) have highlighted the need for good bereavement care when a baby dies and also highlight the need for bereavement care training and specialist bereavement midwives. Sands has developed an audit tool for maternity services to monitor and evaluate their bereavement services (Sands 2014a), available on the Sands website.

Midwives have to balance caring for the complex needs that the mother and her family have, which must include a consideration for physical, social, psychological and spiritual needs, at a time when she requires a high level of sensitive and skilled care (Thomas 2001). This balance requires significant self-knowledge and an ability to be truly with the parents through their pain and sadness, in order to support and guide them through this period. An awareness of their own needs and those of their healthcare colleagues is also imperative in ensuring a strong and supportive team.

Working with bereaved parents can be difficult and emotionally exhausting, but knowing that bereaved parents have been helped through one of the worst periods of their lives, by your good care, can be immensely rewarding.

References

Antenatal Results and Choices (ARC): *Talking to Children (2nd ed)*. 2004.

Arshad M, Horsfall A, Yasin R: Pregnancy loss and the Holy Qu'ran, *B J Midwifery* 12(8):481–484, 2003.

Bewley C: Midwives and failed motherhood: working with midwives who have experienced their own reproductive or pregnancy related loss, *MIDIRS* 20(1):7–10, 2010.

Boden, et al: Caring for parents, *AIMS* 27(3):5, 2015.

Bowlby J: *Attachment and Loss* (vol 3), Loss, Sadness and Depression, Harmondsworth, Penguin, 1980.

Caelli K, Downie J, Knox M: Through grief to healthy parenthood: facilitating the journey through a family pregnancy support programme, *Birth Issues* 8(3):85–90, 1999.

Child Bereavement UK (CBUK) authored by Adams J: *When Your Baby Dies – A Particular Sort of Grief* (website). www.childbereavementuk .org. 2013a.

Child Bereavement UK (CBUK) authored by Adams J: *When a newborn dies – explaining to young children* (website). http:// childbereavementuk.org/wp -content/uploads/2016/05/1.1- When-a-newborn-dies-explaining-to -young-children-Feb-2014.pdf? noredir=true. 2013b.

Child Bereavement UK (CBUK): *Explaining miscarriage or stillbirth to young children* (website). http://childbereavementuk.org/ wp-content/uploads/2016/05/ 1.1-Explaining-miscarriage -and-stillbirth-Feb-2014.pdf?noredir =true. 2013c.

Child Bereavement UK CBUK: *How Children and Young People Grieve*. Information Sheet. Child Bereavement UK (website). http:// www.childbereavementuk.org/files/ 5414/0868/5878/How_Children _and_Young_People_Grieve.pdf. 2016a.

Child Bereavement UK (CBUK): *Post Mortem Examination, High Wycombe* (website). http://childbereavementuk .org/for-families/death-of -a-baby-or-child/post-mortem -examination/. 2016b.

Child Bereavement UK (CBUK) authored by Chalmers A, Adams J: *Saying Goodbye to Your Baby or Child* (website). www.childbereavementuk .org. 2016c.

Crawley R, Lomax S, Ayers S: Recovering from stillbirth: the effects of making and sharing memories on maternal mental health, *J Reprod Infant Psychol* 31:195–207, 2013.

Department of Health (DH): *Report on abortion statistics in England and Wales for 2013* (website). https:// www.gov.uk/government/uploads/ system/uploads/attachment_data/ file/319460/Abortion_Statistics _England_and_Wales_2013.pdf. 2014.

Downe S, Schmidt E, Kingdon C, et al: Bereaved parents' experience of stillbirth in UK hospitals: a qualitative interview study, *BMJ Open* 3:e002237, 2013.

Draper ES, Kurinczuk JJ, Kenyon S: *MBRRACE-UK Perinatal Confidential Enquiry: Term, Singleton, Normally Formed, Antepartum Stillbirth. Leicester: The Infant Mortality and Morbidity Studies* (website). https:// www.npeu.ox.ac.uk/downloads/ files/mbrrace-uk/reports/ MBRRACE-UK%20Perinatal%20 Report%202015.pdf. 2015.

Fisher J: *Care for women after termination for fetal abnormality* (verbal correspondence). 2015.

Fisher J, Lafarge C: Women's experience of care when undergoing termination of pregnancy for fetal anomaly in England, *J Reprod Infant Psychol* doi: 10.1080/02646838 .2014.970149, 2014.

Fraser E: *Tamba Bereavement Support Group booklet for parents who have lost one or more babies from a multiple birth*, Guildford, TAMBA BSG, 2010.

Heazell A, McLaughlin M-J, Schmidt E, et al: A difficult conversation? The views and experiences of parents and professionals on the consent process for perinatal postmortem after stillbirth, *Br J Obstet Gynecol* 119:987–997, 2012.

Henley A, Kohner N: *When A baby dies: the experience of late miscarriage, stillbirth and neonatal death*, London, Routledge, 2001.

Higson N: Support for loss, *AIMS J* 27:3(17):2015.

Hill S: *Family*, London, Penguin, 1990.

Homer CSE, Malata A, ten Hoope- Bender P: *Supporting women, families, and care providers after stillbirths*, The Lancet – Ending Preventable Stillbirths, A Series by The Lancet (website). http://www.thelancet.com/series/ ending-preventable-stillbirths. 2016.

Human Tissue Authority (HTA): *Code of Practice – Post Mortem Examination* (website). www.hta.gov .uk/guidance/codes_of_practice.cfm. 2006.

Human Tissue Authority (HTA): *2014 for review 2016* Code of Practice 5: Disposal of Human Tissue (website). https://www.hta.gov.uk/ sites/default/files/Code_of_practice _5_-_Disposal_of_human_tissue.pdf. 2014.

Hunfeld JAM, Taselaar-Kloos AKG, Agterberg G, et al: Trait anxiety, negative emotions, and the mothers' adaptation to an infant born subsequent to late pregnancy loss: a case-control study, *Prenat Diagn* 17(9):843–851, 1997.

Jennings P: *The First Two Years Experience of Child Bereavement Support Posts. Evaluation of the Department of Health Project, High Wycombe*, CBT, 2001.

Kenworthy D, Kirkham M: *Midwives coping with loss and grief: stillbirth, professional and personal losses*, London, Radcliffe Publishing Ltd, 2011.

Kohner N, Leftwich A: *Training Pack: Pregnancy Loss and the Death of a Baby: National Extension College in Association with SANDS, SATFA and the Miscarriage Association*. ISBN 1 85356 609 8, 1995.

Kubler-Ross E: *On death and dying*, London, Routledge, 2014.

Lewis CS: *Grief observed*, New York, Seabury Press, 1961.

Lewis E, Bourne S: Perinatal death, *Baillieres Clin Obstet Gynaecol* 3(4):935–953, 1989.

Lyus R, Robson S, Parsons J, et al: Second trimester abortion for fetal abnormality, *Br J Med* 347:f4165, doi: 10.1136/bmj.f4165, 2013.

Moulder C: *Understanding pregnancy loss: perspectives and issues in care*, London, Macmillan, 1998.

Nursing and Midwifery Council (NMC): *The Code: Professional standards of practice and behaviour for nurses and midwives*, NMC, 2015.

Office for National Statistics (ONS): *Child Mortality Statistics* (website). www.ons.gov.uk. 2015.

Parkes CM: *Bereavement: studies of grief in adult life*, Harmondsworth, Penguin, 1972.

Puddifoot JE, Johnson MP: The legitimacy of grieving: the partner's experience at miscarriage, *Soc Sci Med* 45(6):837–845, 1997.

Redshaw M, Rowe R, Henderson J: *Listening to Parents: The Experience of Women and Their Partners After Stillbirth or the Death of Their Baby After Birth*. National Perinatal Epidemiology Unit, Oxford (website). www.npeu.ox.ac.uk/downloads/les/listeningtoparents/report/Listening%20to%20Parents%20Report%20-%20March%202014%20-%20FINAL%20-%20PROTECTED.pdf, 2014.

Royal College of Nursing (RCN): *Managing the Disposal of Pregnancy Remains*, RCN Guidance for Nursing and Midwifery Practice, RCN London (website). https://www.rcn.org.uk/-/media/royal-college-of.../2015/.../005347.pdf. 2015.

Schott J, Henley A, Kohner N: *Pregnancy loss and the death of a baby: guidelines for professionals*, 3rd edn, London, Stillbirth and Neonatal Death Society (SANDS), 2007.

Stillbirth and neonatal death charity (Sands): *Audit Tool for Maternity Services: Caring for Parents Whose Baby has Died* (website). https://www.uk-sands.org/sites/default/files/SANDS%20Audit%20Tool%20MARCH%202011%20w%20DEC%202014%20INSERT.pdf. 2014a.

Stillbirth and neonatal death charity (Sands): *Saying Goodbye to Your Baby* (website). https://www.uk-sands.org/sites/default/files/AW%20SAYING%20GOODBYE%20TO%20YOUR%20BABY%20LR%20SS%20LR%20final-April%202014.pdf. 2014b.

Stillbirth & Neonatal Death Charity (Sands): *Supporting Children When A Baby Has Died* (website). https://www.uk-sands.org/sites/default/files/%E2%80%A2AW%20SUPPORTING%20CHILDREN%20211113%20LR%20SP%20LINKED.pdf. 2014c.

Stillbirth & Neonatal Death Charity (Sands): *Sands Principles of Good Bereavement Care* (website). www.sands.org. 2016.

Stroebe MS, Schut H: The dual process model of coping with bereavement: rationale and descriptions, *Death Stud* 23(3):197–224, 1999.

Swanson KM: Effects of caring, measurement, and time on miscarriage impact and women's well-being, *Nurs Res* 48:288–298, 1999.

Thomas J: The death of a baby: guidance for professionals in hospital and community, *J Neonatal Nurs* 7(5):167–170, 2001.

Thomas J, Chalmers A: Working with families and loss: the therapeutic use of ourselves, *Infant* 1(6):182, 2005.

Tommy's Charity: *Miscarriage and Ectopic Pregnancy Statistics* (website). http://www.tommys.org/Page.aspx?pid=383. 2015.

Wilson R: Personal communication with Thomas J, quoted p955 in Ch. 70 Grief and Bereavement in Macdonald SE, Magill-Cuerden, J: Mayes Midwifery, London, Edinburgh, Balliere Tindall, 2011.

Worden JW: *Grief counselling and grief therapy*, 4th edn, London, Routledge, 2009.

Resources and additional reading

Antenatal Results & Choices (ARC): www.arc-uk.org.
Provides nondirective support and information to expectant and bereaved parents throughout antenatal screening and its aftermath.

Child Bereavement UK (CBUK): www.childbereavement.org.uk.
Supports families when a baby or child of any age dies or is dying, or when a child is facing bereavement.

Schott J, Henley A: After a stillbirth – offering choices, creating memories, *Br J Midwifery* 17(12):798–800, 2009.

Stillbirth and Neonatal Death Society (SANDS): www.uk-sands.org.
Support for anyone when a baby dies during pregnancy, during or shortly after birth. Runs support groups throughout the UK. Provides bereavement care training for professionals. Includes a range of leaflets and information for parents and professionals.

The Miscarriage Association: www.miscarriageassociation.org.uk.
Support for parents after miscarriage.

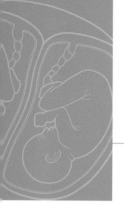

Chapter 69

Maternal mental health and psychological issues

Kathryn Gutteridge

Learning Outcomes

After reading this chapter, you will be able to:

- appreciate the global context of women's mental health across all cultures and economies
- understand the range of mental health problems that present during pregnancy and childbirth
- be aware of the short- and long-term effects and implications of mental health problems on the mother, baby and family
- appreciate the impact of pregnancy, childbirth and transition to parenting on women's mental health and psychological well-being
- understand the importance of early detection of mental illness, and know how to contribute effectively to treatment and management of minor and major disorders
- appreciate the value of working collaboratively within the wider multidisciplinary team within each professional boundary
- confidently offer advice and support to women and be aware of the sources of help and support available locally and nationally

INTRODUCTION

This chapter offers a comprehensive overview of the mental and psychological problems that pregnant and childbearing women encounter. Pregnancy is considered a time associated with joy, happiness and fulfilment. The reality, however, is that for many women, pregnancy will, in fact, cause a recurrence of impaired mental health, increase otherwise controlled anxiety problems or be the precursor of a primary illness (Raphael-Leff 1993). In clinical settings, pregnancy is more often described as a life crisis and a time where there is a huge shift in the emotional and psychological equilibria in a woman's life. In some ways the emotional ebb and flow masks the real issues that women are trying to deal with and society often considers these emotional changes as the pregnancy norm.

There is recognition that despite improvements in the understanding, detection and treatment of pregnancy-related mental health disorders, many women do not seek help and consequently try to cope with their illness, hiding their unhappiness from their caregivers and family (Association for Postnatal Illness 2015). Women still fear discrimination and long-term repercussions if they reveal a previous emotional imbalance or psychiatric illness, and to compound this issue, MIND, the mental health charity, has found 'shocking gaps in services' across the United Kingdom (MIND 2015). Up to 50% of all women are thought to have suffered some form of emotional disturbance during their lifetime and the risk is much higher among women who are socially excluded (Hogg 2013; MIND 2014).

It is also crucial to be aware that there may be significant short- and long-term effects of mental illness, affecting both the mother and her baby (Scottish Intercollegiate Guidelines Network (SIGN) 2012; Murray and Cooper 1997, Teixeira et al 1999). To further this, a report commissioned by the Centre for Mental Health (Bauer et al 2014) discovered that inadequate service provision for women with perinatal mental health illnesses costs society approximately £8.1 billion for each year of births in the UK. This burden is unacceptable and the Maternal Mental Health Alliance (MMHA), a coalition of professional support organizations and families, has come together to lobby for better service provision, education and support (Hogg 2013; MMHA, NSPCC, Royal College of Midwives (RCM) 2014).

A GLOBAL PERSPECTIVE OF WOMEN'S MENTAL HEALTH

In Western society, there is greater awareness of mental well-being and illness; however, it remains a poorly understood aspect of healthcare with health professionals receiving little training in their education.

Depression is a serious public health issue and it is estimated by the World Health Organisation (WHO) that it will be the greatest burden of disease and cause of premature death worldwide by 2020 (WHO 2000). In an authoritative report, WHO state women are twice as likely as men to be diagnosed with depression and that violence and self-inflicted injuries will also feature as a characteristic of women's mental health.

Saltman (1991) identified that one of the reasons for the high rates of women's psychological and mental morbidity is the focus on mortality. While mortality overall is reduced, there has been little progress in understanding and redressing factors that contribute to mental illness. Another primary concern in understanding the mental well-being of women is suicide and its determinants (Department of Health (DH) 1999; 2003). In global studies of women in their peak reproductive years, ages 15 to 44, it was shown that suicide was second only to tuberculosis as a cause of death (WHO 2000). Murray and Lopez (1996) found that in 1990, 180,000 women in China committed suicide and 87,000 women in India died by self-immolation.

From an international perspective, minority groups in the US, such as black and Hispanic mothers, have a higher prevalence of depressive symptoms compared with non-Hispanic white mothers (Lund et al 2010), while Swedish studies indicate that incidence of depression in pregnant women range from 13.7% to 29.2% (Melville et al 2010). Other international research shows that women in Brazil, Pakistan, India and Japan are just as likely to encounter women who are either depressed in the ante or postnatal period (Rich-Edwards et al 2006; Kitamura et al 2006; Tannous et al 2008; Klainin and Arthur 2009). The Australian National Health and Medical Research Council (NHMRC) published a series of reports in May 2011 that outlined the extent of maternal mental illness, showing the effect on women and families and, in particular, the transgenerational impact on children (Austin and Highet 2011).

Further research has shown that there are strong inverse relationships with poverty, social position, ethnic background, marital support and access to healthcare (Shrivastava et al 2015; Bartley and Owen 1996). Being a participant in decisions about healthcare and life choices has a significant impact on psychological and mental well-being during and outside of pregnancy and a sense of control is critical to wellness.

Health and social behaviours may have an impact on well-being, with tobacco and drug/alcohol misuse being common in women with anxiety and depressive disorders (DH 2003). Understanding the dependency that such behaviours engender is critical for midwives to support positive pregnancy outcomes.

A misconception in the Western world is that there are higher stress levels and, therefore, a comparatively higher percentage of those suffering mental health disorders; however, there is substantial evidence that developing societies are also at risk. The most common cause in developing nations is the impact of unstable governments and social structures giving rise to conflict and violence. This is of increasing concern, given the current status of refugee- and asylum-seeking behaviours and the movement of vulnerable women and children across the globe. The latter decade has seen shifting numbers of human trafficking and women and children seeking refuge across Europe. Kelly (2000) states that the 'strongest flows now are taking place within Europe – a shift from the picture in previous decades, where trafficked women came primarily from Asia and South America'. Certainly, since the opening of European borders and migrant movement, there has been a notable rise in young women associated with the sex industry, seeking a place of safety and claims of entrapment (Home Office and Immigration Control 2011).

VIOLENCE AGAINST WOMEN

Whether by their intimate partners or women/men not known to them, violence is probably the most prevalent and certainly the most representative gender-based cause of depression in women. In studies of the effect on women in war-torn communities, it was revealed that rape, torture and murder were by far the most common weapon in the entrapment and subjugation of women and their children (WHO 2000). The impact of these crimes leads to a range of mental health illnesses; depression, self-harm and trauma. Violence and abuse of women consistently features in mental health and physical morbidity. Abusive behaviour, particularly in an intimate relationship, has a detrimental impact on the woman; fear, lack of freedom, humiliation and threat of harm all contribute to deny women's human rights (WHO 1997).

A joint report by the Home Office into sexual offending (2013) confirmed yet again that women were 16 times more likely to experience a sexual crime compared with men of a similar age. Around 1 in 20 women aged 16 to 59 reported a sexual crime of a serious nature and, if including crimes such as unwanted touching, then the number increases to 1 in 5 women (Ministry of Justice, Home Office and Office of National Statistics 2013).

Women are more likely than men to suffer abuse throughout their lifetime, particularly rape, sexual assault and child sexual abuse (Itzin et al 2010). Research has consistently shown that between 20% and 30% of women have been sexually abused as a child, compared with 10% of male children (DH 2003). A later UK DH (2013) publication cites 'annual incidence of sexual violence reported to the Police at just under 55,000 lies between that for strokes (60,000) and coronary heart disease (46,000) in women in the UK' (DH 2013). This report indicates that 1 in 10 women have experienced some form of sexual victimization, including rape, and that 'strangers' are only responsible for 8% of rapes. Sexual abuse, particularly experienced as a child, has considerable significance for childbearing women, physically during the birth and psychologically throughout childbirth and parenting (Gutteridge 2009 and 2001).

Over the latter years, there has been a surge in reported cases of historical sexual abuse. These cases that were once dismissed by legal authorities are now given the time and precedence that they deserve. In fact, the UK Home Secretary Theresa May appointed New Zealand judge Lowell Goddard to lead on a public enquiry into allegations of high profile and public figures and historic sexual abuse. Besides this, a public enquiry into Jimmy Savile (a deceased high profile perpetrator) jointly conducted by the police and the National Society for the Prevention of Cruelty to Children (NSPCC), Giving Victims a Voice, was published on 11 January 2013 (Gray and Watt 2013). Savile was reported to have conducted multiple acts of sexual abuse over a period of 50 years with victims ranging between the age of 8 and 60 years old, with much of these assaults taking place within NHS and Crown establishments.

Society is familiar with media exposures of celebrity acts of abuse and legal systems more responsive to victims with historical cases being presented through legal processes.

It would appear that societal influences, largely gender based, have negative influences on the psychological/mental well-being of women, particularly where powerful influences such as politics and powerful status preside. It is clear, however, that mental health cannot be explained through biomedical determinants alone and it is naive to see women's mental health only through a framework of reproductive perspective.

PREGNANCY, CHILDBIRTH AND MENTAL HEALTH

There is an increased risk of mental illness associated with childbirth, mostly in the postpartum period, but problems may also be present before or during pregnancy. Many factors associated with postnatal mental illness are present during pregnancy, for example, a lack of a confiding relationship, lack of support, marital tension, socioeconomic problems and a previous psychiatric history (O'Hara and Zekoski 1988; Romito 1989; O'Hara 2009), and so depression may occur both in pregnancy and in the postpartum period (Evans et al 2001; Green and Murray 1994; Watson et al 1984; SIGN 2012). There appears to be a positive correlation between women who lack positive maternal role models and the development of anxiety-based depressive disorders during pregnancy and the postnatal period (Gutteridge 1998).

While there is deepening awareness of postnatal depression and psychotic illness after childbirth, there is latterly more published work on the incidence of, and morbidity associated with, *antenatal* depression. A notably depressed mood in pregnancy has been associated with poor attendance at antenatal clinics, substance misuse, low birthweight and preterm labour (Hedegaard et al 1993; Pagel et al 1990). Whereas it was once thought that pregnancy was a protective factor against depression, Watson et al (1984) found that in 24% of cases of detected postnatal depression, symptoms were present during pregnancy.

There is now clear evidence that psychopathological symptoms in pregnancy have physiological consequences for the fetus (Teixeira et al 1999). A cohort study of depressed mood during pregnancy and after childbirth concluded that research and clinical efforts towards recognizing and treating antenatal depression must be improved (Evans et al 2001). The Confidential Enquiry into Maternal Deaths (Lewis 2004) recommends better detection and management of psychiatric disorders antenatally to reduce the mortality rate. Services must be designed to meet the needs of all women, and a crucial part of the service should address the mental health needs of women. Since this report and in subsequent reports covering psychiatric deaths, suicide remains under detected because of reporting mechanisms (Lewis 2007; Oates and Cantwell 2011).

WHO IS 'AT RISK'?

Many women experience mixed reactions to their pregnancy, with transient feelings of anxiety and fear; they should be reassured that this is normal and be encouraged to discuss these feelings openly (Musters et al 2008) (see Ch. 12). The incidence of detected mental illness in the first trimester of pregnancy is thought to be as high as 15%, with only 5% of these women having suffered from previous episodes of mental illness. In the second and third trimesters of pregnancy, the incidence of new episodes of mental illness is less, at only about 5% (Redshaw and Henderson 2013).

The majority of episodes of new mental illness during pregnancy are minor conditions or neuroses. The most common condition is depressive neurosis with anxiety, but phobic anxiety states and obsessive–compulsive disorders may also occur. In most cases, these neurotic mental illnesses resolve by the second trimester of pregnancy and there seems to be no added risk of these women developing postnatal depression. The outlook is different for those women who begin their pregnancies with chronic neurotic conditions. Their illness is likely to continue throughout pregnancy and may be exacerbated during the third trimester into the puerperium.

Minor mental illness is more likely to occur in the first trimester of pregnancy in women who have marked neurotic traits in the premorbid personality. It also tends to occur in women who have a history of neurotic disorders and in those with social problems, such as marital tension. Other predisposing factors include a history of previous abortion and the possibility of the present pregnancy being terminated (Wilson et al 1996). Women with a poor obstetric history or those who have undergone extensive infertility treatment may also exhibit signs of increased anxiety in early pregnancy.

The onset of minor mental illness later in pregnancy, usually during the third trimester, is less common than in the first trimester. When it occurs at this stage in pregnancy, however, the risk of the woman developing postnatal depression is increased (Forman et al 2000).

Major mental illnesses include bipolar disorder, severe depression and schizophrenia. The risk of a woman developing a new episode of mental illness in pregnancy is lower than at other times in her life. When women with a history of major mental illness become pregnant, there is no particular increase in the risk of a relapse during pregnancy if they are well stabilized and their illness is in remission. Although the risk of major mental illness is reduced in pregnancy, it is greatly increased in the first 3 months after the birth (National Institute for Health and Care Excellence (NICE) 2014a).

THE MIDWIFE'S ROLE IN THE ANTENATAL PERIOD

There is growing emphasis on the development of the public health role of the midwife, with promotion of mental well-being representing an area where the midwife can make a valuable contribution (DH 2007). The midwife has a responsibility to provide holistic care, meeting the physical, psychological and emotional needs of all women. Ideally, all women should be treated with sensitivity during pregnancy and enabled during meetings with the midwife to discuss any issues that may predispose them to impaired mental health.

A midwife has a special relationship in a woman's lifetime; s/he has a privileged position in which s/he is able to ask direct and intrusive questions regarding a woman's fertility and sexual history. This is a trusting and a confiding relationship in which the midwife begins to feature strongly in a woman's life history (see Ch. 12), entrusting her body to the midwife and allowing her to care for her developing fetus.

Kirkham (2000) acknowledges the exclusivity of this relationship and identifies themes such as trust, friendship, purpose and the place of self within this dynamic context (see Ch. 12). In no other professional relationship is there such a potential for influencing change than between midwife and childbearing woman. In Midwifery 2020, a report by the Chief Nurses for England Wales, Scotland and Northern Ireland stated that 'Midwives will embrace a greater public health role' (DH 2010), which affirms that for the future, midwives will be more involved in this aspect of healthcare.

Some women will live within a culture where there is no recognition of minor depressive illness or anxiety states (Wilson et al 1996). Any attempt to enquire whether the woman is symptomatic may be restricted by family members who associate mental illness with shame and stigma (Oates 2001). The midwife should recognize that presentations of ongoing minor physical disorders and concerns about the pregnancy may be the only way women can express feelings. To ensure that all women receive adequate support and help, independent, trained interpreters should be available for women whose first language is not English and every attempt must be made to see the woman unaccompanied.

Overall, the midwife should form an integral part of a team, providing support, advice and continuing care. Referral to other health professionals should not end midwifery input but should enhance the care pathway.

Assessment

Taking a comprehensive history at the beginning of pregnancy is vital to assess risk, review and plan care around any deterioration of mental and psychological health. Emotional lability during pregnancy is expected; however, the midwife and the maternity care team should make ongoing assessments throughout. (NICE 2014a; RCOG 2011), a universal and continuous enquiry approach (see Box 69.1) and both SIGN (2012) and the RCOG (2011) recommend the use of a detailed plan for those women at high risk of major mental illnesses.

Assessment tools should only be used as part of a subsequent evaluation for the routine monitoring of outcomes and only by appropriately trained health professionals (NICE 2014a; CG192 2014; Buist et al 2002).

It is essential that an accurate history is taken and any reported current or past mental illness is adequately investigated and assessed. This should be done with extreme sensitivity to eradicate any fears the woman may have of discrimination (Robinson 2002). If the woman is under the care of a GP, psychiatrist, community psychiatric nurse or psychologist, attempts should be made to work

Box 69.1 Mental health assessment

First health contact visit

At a woman's first contact with services in both the antenatal and postnatal periods, healthcare professionals (including midwives, obstetricians, health visitors and GPs) need to ask questions about:

- past or present severe mental illness, including schizophrenia, bipolar disorder, psychosis in the postnatal period and severe depression
- previous treatment by a psychiatrist/specialist mental health team, including inpatient care
- family history of perinatal mental illness

Other specific predictors, such as poor relationships with her partner, should not be used for the routine prediction of the development of a mental disorder.

Ongoing screening

At a woman's first contact with primary care, during her 'booking' visit or initial first visit and postnatally (usually at 4 to 6 weeks and 3 to 4 months), healthcare professionals (including midwives, obstetricians, health visitors and GPs) should ask two questions to identify possible depression.

Also consider asking about anxiety using the 2-item Generalized Anxiety Disorder scale (GAD-2):

- Over the last 2 weeks, how often have you been bothered by feeling nervous, anxious or on edge?
- Over the last 2 weeks, how often have you been bothered by not being able to stop or control worrying?

(NICE 2014a)

---

collaboratively within this team to ensure the woman's whole needs are met.

The majority of minor illnesses will resolve spontaneously by the second trimester of pregnancy. The woman will require support, counselling, reassurance and information communicated in a caring, intelligible way. Psychotropic drugs are rarely necessary or prescribed at this stage of pregnancy; instead, therapy to help the woman relax and reduce anxiety seems to be effective. Midwives may be involved in counselling and supporting these women and teaching relaxation techniques. Sometimes a social worker is also required to help tackle social issues that may be the cause of the problem.

Women with a history of single episodes of major mental illness in the past but who have been well for some time are usually advised by their psychiatrist to stop their medication before conception and remain off the medication particularly in the first trimester (NICE 2014a). However, an assessment should be made by a specialist service, usually consisting of a perinatal psychiatrist and

specialist midwife/mental health nurse before discontinuing any psychotropic medication, as withdrawal may be detrimental to the woman.

Reflective activity 69.1

You are meeting a 16-year-old young woman who is booking her pregnancy with you; she seems nervous and ill at ease. You start to ask her routine questions, and you sense that she is feeling uncomfortable. Her answers show an unremarkable medical history; however, when you ask her if she has a partner, she becomes evasive. You notice that her body language is closed and she is reluctant to share eye contact.

What are your thoughts and what challenges do you feel this young woman encounters through her pregnancy?

While there is no significant risk of relapse during pregnancy for this group of women, there is a marked risk of developing puerperal psychosis during the first 3 months after delivery (Cox 1986). Measures should be put in place to monitor and assess for deterioration postnatally (Bick et al 2002). This should be in collaboration with specialist perinatal psychiatric services.

RISK OF SUICIDE

The Confidential Enquiry into Maternal Deaths (Lewis 2004 and 2007; Knight et al 2016), using the Office for National Statistics (ONS) linkage data, indicates that suicide remains the leading cause of maternal death (indirect category). There is misconception that women who live within socially deprived situations suffer a greater risk of mental health problems; in contrast, CEMACH highlighted that the following characteristics were risk indicators:

- white, older woman
- married and living in comfortable circumstances
- second or subsequent pregnancy
- generally well educated
- working in the caring or health industry
- has a history of a mental health disorder
- has a baby under 3 months old
- is in contact with or receiving treatment from psychiatric services
- likely to die violently

Therefore, the suicide profile of childbearing women is significantly disparate to that of the non-pregnant population. The risk of deterioration is significantly elevated in the last trimester of pregnancy and the first 12 weeks postpartum when the risks of both suicide and infanticide should be considered. Although rare, most cases of infanticide where there is evidence of serious maternal mental illness will be associated with a suicide attempt or successful suicide (Marks and Kumar 1993). In contrast women who die from substance misuse are generally young, unsupported, living alone and often unemployed (Oates and Cantwell, 2011).

MBRRACE-UK (formerly CEMACE and CEMACH) recommend that women with a history of severe depression or psychotic disorder be referred to a specialist perinatal mental health team and an appropriate care plan developed, aiming to support women through pregnancy and minimize the risk of severe postnatal disorder (Royal College of Psychiatrists 2000; Knight et al 2016). Where a woman is under the care of a psychiatrist when pregnancy is diagnosed, there should be careful liaison between the obstetrician, midwife and mental health team to ensure that the woman's care is seamless and holistic, and that appropriate management plans are made to maximize the outcome for mother and baby. This is especially relevant when deciding on the woman's ongoing and future drug regimen. Additionally, Oates (in RCP 2001) recommends care is best delivered under the auspices of a managed network approach, whereby those women who are at greatest risk of relapse receive care from specialist service providers.

COMMON MATERNAL MENTAL HEALTH DISORDERS

Generalized anxiety disorder

Generalized anxiety disorder (GAD) is a condition where excessive anxiety is experienced on most days. Symptoms are described as a fast heart rate, palpitations, feeling sick, tremor, sweating, dry mouth, chest pain, headaches, nausea and tachypnoea. GAD develops in about 1 in 50 people at some stage in life. Slightly more women are affected than men, and usually it first develops in the early 20s. The most effective treatment is considered to be cognitive behavioural therapy (CBT). (See NICE CG192 2014a.)

Advice and care

- Referral to general practitioner (GP) and/or mental health services if anxiety is affecting daily life.
- May stop medication and referral to commence CBT.
- May need to change to a safer drug, if the decision is to maintain medication.

Panic disorder

This is an anxiety disorder and is characterized by unexpected and repeated episodes of intense fear accompanied by physical symptoms that may include chest pain, heart palpitations, shortness of breath, dizziness or abdominal distress.

Advice and care

- Refer to GP or mental health services.
- If symptoms are managed by medication, may stop medication and start CBT.
- May switch to a safer drug, if the decision is to maintain medication.

Obsessive–compulsive disorder

Obsessive–compulsive disorder (OCD) is a common mental health condition that affects 2% of the population. It is characterized by obsessive thoughts that cause anxiety. This leads to rituals or repetitive actions. Examples of compulsions include excessive hand washing, cleaning, counting, checking, touching, arranging, hoarding, measuring, excessive neatness and repeating tasks or actions (NICE CG31, 2005).

OCD has two main features:

- experiencing frequent, disturbing, unwanted thoughts that result in fears and compulsions
- acts or rituals carried out in response to fears caused by the obsessions

Advice and care

- Refer to specialist mental health services for management of symptoms.
- If taking medication alone, may stop the medication and start psychological therapy.
- If not taking medication, psychological therapy should be considered before drug treatment.

Posttraumatic stress disorder (PTSD)

This is a normal reaction to an extraordinary event where the individual experiences intense terror and fears for his or her life (see NICE CG26, 2006). It is reported from survivors of road/air accidents, military combat, physical, emotional and sexual abuse, terrorist attacks, hostage situations and being diagnosed with a life-threatening illness. Childbirth is now recognized as a situation that may trigger a PTSD response and this might not have been recognized from past pregnancies but may present in a subsequent pregnancy. PTSD symptoms include flashbacks and nightmares, avoidance, numbing of emotions and hyperarousal.

Advice and care

- Recognize that childbirth has the potential to induce trauma symptoms.
- There is no convincing evidence for drug treatments for PTSD in any patients, so psychological treatments

are preferred. The favoured therapies in this situation are NLP (neuro-linguistic programming) and EMDR (eye movement desensitization and reprocessing).

Bipolar disorder

(See NICE CG192, 2014a)

The prevalence of bipolar disorder at the onset of pregnancy is similar to a non-pregnant population as just over 4% (Sharma and Pope 2012). Estimates would suggest that it is likely that approximately 2 per 1000 pregnancies occur in women with chronic schizophrenia, and approximately the same number in women with pre-existing bipolar disorder. These women are likely to be in contact with secondary psychiatric services (Wilson et al 1996).

There are a growing number of women with pre-existing psychotic and affective disorders who will suffer a relapse in their illness during or after pregnancy. It is estimated that 2 per 1000 live births will fall into this category (Wilson et al 1996).

Advice and care

- Early referral to specialist perinatal mental health services.
- If a woman with bipolar disorder has an unplanned pregnancy and is stopping lithium as prophylactic medication, an antipsychotic should be offered.
- If a pregnant woman with bipolar disorder is stable on an antipsychotic drug and likely to relapse without medication, she should be maintained on the antipsychotic and monitored for weight gain and diabetes.
- If a pregnant woman who is not taking medication develops acute mania, medication is considered. The dose should be kept as low as possible and monitored carefully.
- If moderate-to-severe depressive symptoms occur in pregnant women with bipolar disorder, psychological treatment (CBT) should be considered.
- Use combined medication and structured psychological treatments for severe depressive symptoms.
- A multi-professional approach should be used to manage the complex symptoms, treatment programmes and achieve best outcomes.
- Fetal medicine obstetric services and neonatology should be involved with fetal screening and management of the baby after birth.

Schizophrenia

There is no data for the prevalence of schizophrenia in women of a reproductive age group. General figures suggests that around 1 in every 100 people are affected. It affects men and women equally and seems to be more common in city areas and in some minority ethnic groups. It is rare before the age of 15, but can start at any time after this, most often between the ages of 15 and 35. Estimates would suggest it is likely that approximately 2 per 1000 pregnancies occur in women with chronic schizophrenia. Schizophrenia is characterized by hallucinations, hearing voices, delusions, loss of insight and depression. Suicide is common in people diagnosed with schizophrenia.

Advice and care

- Early referral to specialist perinatal mental health services.
- Use of a detailed plan (SIGN 2012).
- Women with schizophrenia who are planning a pregnancy or who are pregnant should be treated according to the NICE clinical guideline on schizophrenia (NICE CG 178, 2014b).
- If the woman is taking an atypical antipsychotic drug, consideration should be given to switching to a low-dose typical antipsychotic.
- If breastfeeding, treat according to clinical guidance for schizophrenia, except that women receiving depot medication should be advised that their infants may show extrapyramidal symptoms several months after administration of the depot. These are usually self-limiting.
- A multi-professional approach should be used to manage these complex symptoms, treatment programmes and achieve best outcomes.
- Fetal medicine obstetric services and neonatology should be involved with fetal screening and management of the baby after birth.
- Child protection and social service support may be required to support parenting.

Self-harm

(See NICE CG113, 2014c)

Self-harm, also known as self-injury, is a common behaviour and is more likely to affect young women than men; up to 10% of 14- to 16-year-olds have self-harmed themselves. Prevalence is noted among young ethnic females and other discriminated groups. It is a way of coping with extreme emotional distress and is secretive in its manifestation. Some expressions of self-harm are cutting, gouging, burning, scratching, purging, eating disorders and hair pulling.

Advice and care

- Referral to specialist mental health services.
- Identification of the type of self-harm and risk assessment of current frequency of self-harming behaviours.

- Offer support throughout pregnancy.
- Consider child protection and social service support if self-injury escalates.

Eating disorders

These are characterized by a fear of being fat and out of control with food, which ultimately has a detrimental impact on the health of the individual. Girls and women are 10 times more likely than boys and men to suffer from anorexia or bulimia. Prevalence is estimated to be about 1 in 150 girls. Women with bulimia nervosa are prone to unplanned pregnancy, in part because vomiting reduces the efficacy of oral contraceptives. Some of the effects of eating disorders are:

- reduced stomach capacity
- tiredness, weakness and temperature changes
- metabolism slows down
- constipation
- stunted height
- brittle bones (which break easily)
- failure to get pregnant
- liver damage
- dental problems, particularly in bulimia
- hair loss
- death in extreme cases – anorexia nervosa has the highest death rate of any psychological disorder

Advice and care

- A woman with anorexia nervosa who is planning a pregnancy or has an unplanned pregnancy or is breastfeeding should be treated in reference to guidance (NICE CG 9, 2004).
- If a woman who is taking medication for bulimia nervosa is planning a pregnancy or is pregnant, healthcare professionals should consider gradually stopping the medication.
- Referral for specialist treatment should be considered.
- Midwifery support and education about dietary needs should be provided throughout pregnancy.
- Refer to consultant obstetrician if BMI is below 19.
- Referral to nutritionist or dietician.

Substance misuse

It is increasingly evident since the global growth of social drug consumption and the incidence of substance abuse that the general mental health of the population has suffered. Mental diagnoses such as bipolar disorder and personality disorders are increasing; theories suggest that social drug use is one of the main reasons and, therefore,

this factor will increase the number of women at risk presenting during pregnancy (NICE CG110, 2010).

There is good evidence to suggest that during the postnatal period all women are at increased risk of developing a mental illness and for those women who are already diagnosed with a severe mental illness, rates of relapse increase profoundly and they will, therefore, require specialist services (Lewis 2007).

Advice and care

- Initial assessment 'booking' history should enquire about all drug and alcohol usage.
- If there is illicit drug usage, refer to specialist drug and alcohol team.
- Refer to social services and consider child protection programme of support.
- Maintain close contact and work as part of the multidisciplinary team.
- If drug usage is controlled, a plan of care for birth and immediate postnatal care should be shared with the team.
- If drug usage is uncontrolled and dismissed, then a child protection plan should be initiated and baby will need observation for neonatal abstinence syndrome.
- Breastfeeding is not necessarily excluded and may be the best form of managing neonatal abstinence programmes.

These conditions are not exclusive and constitute a range of problems with which women may present when pregnant. The midwife's role must be to recognize the problems, and risk assess the woman's current mental well-being and refer to the appropriate health professional or specialist service. The midwife must continue to work within the multidisciplinary team while continuing to offer support and guidance to the woman so that she receives normal midwifery care throughout her childbearing experience.

Reflective activity 69.2

Consider how you might respond when a woman with bipolar disorder books early in her pregnancy at your antenatal clinic. (See chapter website resources for points you may consider.)

FEAR AND TRAUMA IN LABOUR AND BIRTH

Some women find childbirth a fulfiling experience, but for others, it is the most traumatic experience of their life

(Niven 1992). The anticipation and unpredictability of birth can cause women anxiety and in some cases extreme distress. In most cases apprehension is normal; however, if the worry is all-consuming and the woman overwhelmed by these emotions, she is more likely to experience heightened pain levels and discomfort. Current estimates of women who report fear around childbirth are between 24% and 31% with nulliparous women at the higher end of the range (Toohill et al 2014; Storksen et al 2012).

The experiences of labour and birth for those women who have longstanding fear of hospitals and associated procedures, such as needle phobia, are likely to be more difficult. In these situations, it is important that the midwife understands and helps the woman plan her care around these anxieties to avoid further trauma.

Women who have experienced traumatic life events are much more likely to have issues with control and pain. Examples of this are women who were abused as children, survivors of rape/sexual abuse, and women who have experienced violent relationships (Gutteridge 2009 and 2001).

There is a significant difference between women who profess to be worried or frightened of some aspect of childbirth and those women who are morbidly terrified of pregnancy and birth known as 'tokophobia'. Tokophobia was originally documented by Hofberg and Brockington in 2000 who found these definitive commonalities with these women:

- the fear had originated during adolescence
- contraception, including sterilization, was used to avoid/delay pregnancy
- avoidance of pregnant women or situations associated with pregnancy
- secondary tokophobia occurred as a result of a previous unsatisfactory/traumatic birth
- were likely to be depressed and anxious during pregnancy
- may demand a method of delivery

There is increasing awareness that events around the time of birth can seriously affect a woman's mental and pyschopathological well-being (Storksen et al 2012; Laing 2001; Pantlen and Rohde 2001). Women have reported experiencing intense fear, helplessness and a loss of control when recalling their birth experiences. One study found that women who suffered an adverse birth experience were likely to develop trauma symptoms associated with post-traumatic stress disorder (Creedy et al 2000), described as 'extreme psychological distress following exposure to a traumatic and threatening experience' (Lyons 1998).

Midwife's role

A detailed history should be taken for all women and risks identified in relation to pre-existing mental health problems and psychological disorders. Monitoring of mood and anxiety levels throughout pregnancy can be achieved through the use of the questions recommended by NICE (2014a). A discussion should take place with the woman to identify the source of her concerns and a plan formulated for the birth that should be acceptable to her. This must be communicated to the maternity team and documented clearly so that when a woman comes into hospital she does not have to negotiate with her caregivers (Bloom 2002). Problems may arise where there is doubt about a woman's capacity to consent to or refuse treatment. Where a woman's capacity is questioned, a supervisor of midwives should be involved and appropriate legal advice should be sought (see Ch. 9). The primary aim should always be to act in the woman's best interests and as her advocate if required.

Support during labour is vital; this could be the woman's birthing partner but should also consist of continuous midwifery input and support. Women who disclose fears around certain procedures during childbirth should have clear plans to help the caregiver and reduce any anxiety with the woman.

Throughout the birth it is important that the woman understands and is kept informed; she should be asked for consent prior to any procedures. After the birth, it is important to consider the woman's reaction to the event and any signs of emotional distress noted and documented. Postnatal debriefing after a 'difficult' birth is generally discouraged, although explanations about procedures and events may be a natural part of the woman's way of coming to terms with the birth (NICE 2014a). However, there is a growing body of opinion that women would benefit from a form of postnatal debriefing to help reduce the psychological morbidity experienced by many women after pregnancy and childbirth (Lavender and Walkinshaw 1998; Pantlen and Rohde 2001).

If the woman's reaction and anxieties appear to be severe, she should be referred to specialist psychiatric services for an assessment and possible treatment. It is important that the midwife works together with any other health professionals in supporting the woman and her baby during recovery (Tuohy and McVey, 2008).

Reflective activity 69.3

A primparous woman attends the maternity unit with suspected rupture of membranes at 38 weeks gestation; she is 39 years old. She is supported by her partner and doula and seems agitated. The midwife performs the normal baseline observations; she then seeks consent to perform a speculum examination to confirm if there is liquor visible. The woman immediately declines and says she wishes to leave as she is planning a homebirth.

How would you approach this situation, and what are the possible causes of her anxiety and behaviour?

POSTNATAL PERIOD

The reported incidence of depression in women after childbirth is between 10% and 15% (Cox et al 1993; Kumar and Robson 1984), but when questioned, many midwives and women report a higher incidence. The actual cause of depressive illness after childbirth is unknown but is thought to be multifactorial, a combination of biological, psychological and social factors. Rarer forms of psychiatric illness, such as psychoses, affect even fewer women but are dramatic in effect and impact.

Biological reasons include genetic make-up, gynaecological and obstetric problems (Stein et al 1989), parity and maternal age, the hormonal changes which occur in the early puerperium, and the appearance and behaviour of the baby. The mother may experience a reactive depression if her baby dies or is born with a congenital abnormality, particularly if previously undiagnosed. Psychological factors may include the woman's early relationship with her parents, personality development, acceptance of her sexuality and the ability to accept dependence (Raphael-Leff 2005; Cox 1986). Women who display anxious or obsessional traits in their personality, or appear controlling and compliant, have a greater risk of developing postnatal depression. Another symptom is anomie, which is a painful feeling of the inability to experience love or pleasure. These mothers often feel that they do not, or cannot love their babies, but usually their baby is obviously lovingly handled and cared for by the mother.

Detection and recognition

The previous psychiatric history of the woman (and her family) has been found to be a risk factor in many cases. The consistent finding of epidemiological studies carried out to date is that the major factors of aetiological importance are psychosocial in nature (Murray and Cooper 1997). The occurrence of stressful life events and lack of personal support from family, partner or friends have consistently been found to raise the risk of postnatal depression (Levy and Kline 1994; Stein et al 1989).

The midwife has the opportunity to assess mood changes and adaptation to parenthood, which will be facilitated if she has gotten to know the woman before the birth. This relationship is vital and the information the midwife is often the first step in identifying a problem. There are tools that may assist in confirming the presence of depressive and anxiety symptoms that may be used to confirm the midwife's suspicions. Using questions recommended by NICE (2014a) at every contact visit is important. If the midwife has confidence in her skills to use other assessment tools, there are several commonly used.

Edinburgh Postnatal Depression Scale

The Edinburgh Postnatal Depression Scale (EDPS) has been developed for the diagnosis of postnatal depression (Cox and Holden 1994) (see chapter website resources). It is a simple, self-rating, 10-item scale that was designed to be used at about 6 weeks postpartum but can also be used at other times, including the antenatal period for high-risk women (Clement 1995). Scores for individual items range from 0 to 3, according to severity, and the total score is the sum of the scores for the individual items. Women who score 12 or more on the scale are likely to be suffering from depressive illness. Referral for further assessment and treatment should then be offered. Initially, the midwife's responsibility is to detect the symptoms, and refer the woman for specialist support.

Because of the difficulties associated with detecting postnatal depression within other cultures, a Punjabi version of the EPDS has also been developed, which has proved to be successful in trials to date (Clifford et al 1999).

Where midwives have been trained to deliver evidence-based postnatal advice and support, based on the woman's description of symptoms, rates of postnatal depression have been shown to be reduced (MacArthur et al 2002). Women at risk of postnatal depression will require particularly close observation in the postnatal period.

Generalized Anxiety Disorder 7-item (GAD-7) scale

This screening tool is an easy self-assessment that is universally used within healthcare settings. It was developed by Spitzer et al (2006) and is simple and effective in detecting this variant.

PHQ-9 (Patient Health Questionnaire)

This screening tool focuses on detecting generalized depression and has a sensibility of over 90% and is easy to use. Many doctors in primary care use this assessment tool to detect depression with reliable rates of self-reporting.

W-DEQ (Wijma Delivery Expectancy/ Experience Questionnaire)

This tool was developed in 1998 by Wijma and Wijma to identify women who expressed a fear of birth. Previously, it was difficult to detect these women and more specifically to assess the degree of their fear; however, this Scandinavian tool was validated after research and trials. The W-DEQ has also been trialled in Italian, British and Australian women with research validating its sensitivity.

Postnatal conditions

Emotional changes during childbirth

Pregnancy is a time that both women and health professionals accept as emotionally labile. The change of hormones in early pregnancy and again after the birth gives way to emotional ebb and flow, with some women more prone than others. However, it is fair to say that some degree of emotional instability is normal and should be explained as such to women and their families. Usually, this condition is self-limiting and resolves with support.

Advice and care

- Ensure adequate rest and good nutrition.
- Reassurance and support through family and friends or external measures, such as family support worker, *Homestart* or other new parent support groups.
- Antenatal support from Parent Education, National Childbirth Trust and local women's support groups.
- Provision of information about different services and support networks within the woman's area.

Postpartum 'blues' or 'baby blues'

It is important to distinguish between the normal mood and emotional changes that occur after the birth, known as 'baby blues', which is a period of tearfulness and mood lability. This transition lasts a matter of days and affects more than 50% to 80% of all women, especially primigravida (Romito 1989). The condition typically presents between 2 and 4 days after birth and symptoms include tearfulness, irritability, mood instability, headache, tiredness and oversensitivity (Hannah et al 1992). The woman needs the opportunity to talk about her feelings and her physical discomfort, which should reduce, as the condition frequently coincides with breast discomfort. In most cases, the condition is self-limiting, but studies have found that women who suffer from this condition are more likely to go on to develop postnatal depression (Beck et al 1992; O'Hara and Zekoski 1988; O'Hara et al 1991).

Advice and care

- Rest and extra support
- Generally requires no treatment but reassurance and support
- Meeting other new mothers is often helpful
- Distinguish between transient mood changes and clinical signs of puerperal psychosis

Postnatal depression

This is considered to be any non-psychotic depressive illness of mild to moderate severity within the first year after childbirth. Prevalence rates range between 10% and 28%, and it affects women from all cultures, ethnic backgrounds and socioeconomic groups. However, for many women (up to 75%), their illness will begin in the antenatal period and may go undetected. Causes include past history of psychopathology and psychological disturbance

during pregnancy; poor or lack of partnership relationship; lack of social support, the parents' perceptions of their own upbringing; and possibly their own lack of role models from their own parents; antenatal parental stress; stresses such as unemployment; unplanned pregnancy; or delay in pregnancy such as through IVF (see Ch. 28); not breastfeeding; depression of the father, and having more than two children (SIGN 2012).

Some features of postnatal depression are low mood, poor sleep pattern, loss of appetite, tearfulness, anxiety, a sense of failure, guilt, shame and isolation. The most common time for detection is around 4 to 6 weeks postnatally (Cox et al 1993). Early recognition is critical for effective intervention measures and reducing morbidity (Hatloy 2013). The response to treatment and prognosis is good if detection and support is initiated early.

Advice and care

- Treatment may consist of pharmacological methods, such as antidepressants, depending upon presenting symptoms and other medication.
- Other forms of psychotherapeutic treatments may be appropriate, such as cognitive behavioural therapy, interpersonal psychotherapy, guided self-help and nondirective counselling in the woman's home.
- Exercise and other forms of positive self-nurture, such as yoga and relaxation, are also helpful.
- Social services intervention and child protection referral may be necessary if illness is severe with risk to self and baby.

Posttraumatic stress disorder

Posttraumatic stress disorder (PTSD) is an adjustment, anxiety or dissociative disorder after exposure to a traumatic event, either as a victim or witness (real or perceived). While PTSD in the general population is better acknowledged, there remains some scepticism around its incidence and childbirth.

Although it is difficult to imagine that such an extreme reaction can be caused by childbirth, which is described as a normal life event, it is the perception of the woman that is the critical denominator. Some of the triggers that may precipitate a stress reaction have been identified as:

- vaginal examination
- catheterization
- assisted birth – forceps or ventouse delivery
- theatre delivery
- separation – baby taken to NICU
- breastfeeding
- unkind or unsympathetic caregiver

The trauma experienced during childbirth has many causative factors that are entirely perceptual for the individual woman; however, the work of Kendall-Tackett and Kaufman-Kantor (1993) identified that there are significant outcomes that will occur:

- Physical trauma: performing an episiotomy or other invasive procedure may result in physical harm/ trauma and, therefore, the woman's perception could be feelings of mutilation.
- Stigma: the woman feels blemished or marked in some way because of an aspect of her birth experience – this might be a scar of some sort or indwelling catheter.
- Betrayal: the woman perceives herself to have been let down or abused by the health professionals associated with her delivery.
- Powerlessness: maternal perceptions relating to lack of, or loss of control, which often is central to birth-related trauma.

The ICD-10 classification of mental and behavioural disorders (WHO 1992) stipulates that trauma symptoms should include re-experiencing of the event(s) by flash-backs and/or nightmares. The individual may also be hypervigilant and experience physical and emotional 'numbing'; avoidance of triggers that may cause distress is common. Symptoms generally become apparent after 6 to 12 weeks and may persist for years, if not recognized and treated, after by depression and suicide attempts.

Advice and care

- Early recognition of symptoms and behaviours after birth
- Allow woman to talk about her experiences
- Refer to specialist services if symptoms are intrusive and limiting
- Information about support – Birth Trauma Association; local support groups
- Provide ongoing multidisciplinary support
- Social services intervention and child protection referral may be necessary if illness is severe with risk to self and baby

Puerperal psychosis

This is regarded as a serious mental illness during the perinatal period, consistently affecting 2 in 1000 women. It is a psychotic illness and requires immediate psychiatric intervention and expert support. Severe episodes of 'baby blues' may lead to postnatal depression and, if untreated, depression may develop into a major depressive psychosis (Cox 1986).

Characteristics of the illness are rapid onset (usually within the first postnatal week), hallucinations, mood swings, loss of contact with reality, intrusive thought processes and loss of inhibitions (Kendall et al 1987).

One explanation for the development of puerperal psychosis is the major change that occurs in the levels of the steroid hormones at this time, especially the drop in oestrogen (Wieck 1989). It is thought that high-risk patients develop a hypersensitivity of the central D2 recep-tors and that this may be related to the effect of the drop in the oestrogen level on the dopamine system. Another theory is that the condition is related to the fall in proges-terone levels that occur after delivery (Dalton 1985).

Psychosocial and obstetric factors are also thought to be possible causes of puerperal psychosis. Those who appear to be at higher risk include:

- first and second degree relative with a history of puerperal psychosis
- primiparae who have had major obstetric problems, including caesarean section
- women from the higher socioeconomic groups
- women who are older than average at the birth of their first child, are married, and have a relatively long interval from marriage to the birth of their first child
- those who have had a major life event such as bereavement of a close family member shortly before or after the birth of their child

Advice and care

- Antenatal risk assessment is critical; any family history of perinatal mental illness increases the risk.
- Risk of suicide and infanticide is high, so a careful and timely response is critical to best outcomes.
- Need to exclude organic illness, such as sepsis (which could make the woman febrile and confused).
- Referral to specialist perinatal mental health service for immediate assessment (within 4 hours of recognition).
- Treatment consists of medication, hospitalization with baby into specialist mother and baby services and, sometimes although rarely now, electroconvulsive treatment.
- Prognosis is usually good, with complete recovery; however, risk of recurrence is increased in future pregnancies.
- Social services intervention and child protection referral may be necessary if illness is severe with risk to self and baby.
- Ongoing support may be necessary from specialist services after hospital discharge to monitor well-being.

1141

Reflective activity 69.4

A 14-day postnatal woman attends your clinic; she was discharged from midwifery care 3 days ago. The woman had a ventouse delivery for fetal distress in the second stage and the baby initially required resuscitative measures. After a short postnatal stay in hospital, both woman and baby were discharged home to community care. She goes home to her husband; he is a police inspector and works long hours. The couple moved to this area after his promotion 6 months ago.

The woman is tearful and is obviously distressed; she tells you she can't cope and is worried about her baby's feeding.

What are your immediate thoughts and what are your plans for the woman and her baby?

MEDICATION DURING PREGNANCY AND BREASTFEEDING

To minimize the risk of harm to the fetus or infant, all drugs should be prescribed judiciously for women who are planning a pregnancy, currently pregnant or breastfeeding. As a result, the thresholds for non-drug treatments, particularly psychological treatments, are likely to be lower than those set in the NICE clinical guidelines on specific mental disorders, and prompt and timely access to treatments should be ensured if they are to be of benefit.

Discussions about treatment options for a woman with a mental disorder who is pregnant or breastfeeding should include:

- the risk of relapse or deterioration in symptoms and the woman's ability to cope with untreated or sub-threshold symptoms

- severity of previous episodes, response to treatment, and the woman's preference

- the possibility that stopping a drug with known teratogenic risk after pregnancy has been confirmed but may not remove the risk of malformations

- the risks and the benefits from stopping medication abruptly are clear

- the need for prompt treatment because of the potential impact of an untreated mental disorder on the women and/or fetus or infant

- the increased risk of harm associated with drug treatments during pregnancy and the postnatal period, including the risk in overdose

- treatment options that enable the woman to breastfeed if she wishes, rather than recommending she does not breastfeed

When prescribing a drug for a woman with a mental disorder who is planning a pregnancy, pregnant or breastfeeding, prescribers should:

- choose drugs with lower risk profiles for the woman and the fetus or infant

- start at the lowest effective dose, and slowly increase it; this is particularly important where the risks may be dose related

- use monotherapy in preference to combination pharmacological treatments

- consider additional precautions for preterm, low birthweight or sick infants

Stopping any medication that is prescribed for a mental illness must be managed by a medical practitioner and preferably a perinatal psychiatrist; the risk to the woman may outweigh any fetal benefit. Acute withdrawal and rapid deterioration is likely with tragic consequences (NICE 2014).

COORDINATED MATERNITY CARE

The last decade has seen greater awareness and attention given to women's mental health during childbearing; this is largely due to the realization that not only is it detrimental to women and their families but also to wider society. Roles such as *Health Midwives* have developed, and these practitioners can act as a source of expertise to the team, and additional support to the woman and her family (Maternal Mental Health Alliance, NSPCC, Royal College of Midwives 2014). Women who have a mental illness in the postnatal period are less likely to return to work when they expect and to have ongoing interventions that are both pharmacological and therapeutic (Tsivos et al 2015). When looking at low to middle income countries, it would appear that the effects of perinatal mental health illnesses are just as likely with more severe consequences for the woman and her baby but also her family (Lund et al 2010).

Other studies have shown more subtle effects of depressed women when caring for their infants suggested to cause:

- mother and infant malattunement

- delayed infant cognitive development

- delayed speech development

- infant nutritional deficit

- poorer psychosocial functioning

While these determinants are important, it is vital that an understanding develops where these variants are more likely to occur. For example, if a woman lives in a low income country where nutrition for herself is poor and she has a limited understanding of baby care, then it is understandable that her baby is likely to fall into a higher risk for growth and development delay.

In Gerhardt's book, 'Why Love Matters', she outlines that if the woman's affect is low, then her interactions with her baby will be suppressed. She goes further to warn that women who have disharmony with their babies' needs and moods can promote production of cortisols, which, under prolonged periods, may go on to predict that the baby in adulthood will have less ability to cope with stressful situations (Gerhardt 2015).

The consequences of perinatal mental illness are evident and, therefore, service provision and interventions must be coordinated and comprehensive. NICE guidance recommends that clinical networks are established for perinatal mental health services, managed by a coordinating board of healthcare professionals, commissioners, managers, and service users and carers (NICE 2014a).

These networks should provide a specialist multidisciplinary perinatal service in each locality, which provides direct services, consultation and advice to maternity services and other mental health services and community services; in areas of high morbidity these services may be provided by separate specialist perinatal team access to specialist expert advice on the risks and benefits of psychotropic medication during pregnancy and breastfeeding.

There should be clear referral and management protocols for services across all levels of the existing frameworks for mental health problems, to ensure effective transfer of information and continuity of care for service users, with defined roles and competencies for all professional groups involved.

To support these recommendations in the future, NICE plans to publish standards to assist commissioners and providers in establishing services and pathways of care. It has never been more important for midwives to work in collaboration with all service providers and to enable women and their babies to receive high quality care that reduces the impact of perinatal mental health.

CONCLUSION

All women must be cared for with sensitivity, and encouraged to explore their own feelings in a safe and supported way. They should be confident that their care will be non-prejudiced and that there will be no stigma associated with disclosure of previous mental illness. Adequate resources must be made available to ensure the woman receives the care appropriate to her needs. There is growing recognition among midwives of the value of self-reflection. Midwives caring for women with profound emotional disturbances may reflect on their own life experiences, identifying a personal need for support.

Initially midwives should be encouraged to discuss any areas of difficulty with their supervisor of midwives, but ultimately they will only be able to offer holistic, woman-centred care if they are emotionally well themselves (see Ch. 12). It is essential that employers recognize the potential stress midwives may be under when caring for women with profound problems and ensure that an adequate level of nonjudgemental support exists for staff as well as for women using the service (Hammett 1997).

Key Points

- It is important that midwives assess and monitor women's mental health during pregnancy and childbirth.
- Mental health problems may be experienced before, during or after the physiological and socio-psychological impact of pregnancy and childbirth.
- Midwives can support and prepare women should they experience minor or major mental health problems.
- Collaborative working and effective referral are crucial in supporting and managing women who experience mental health difficulties and their families.
- Midwives need to be aware of the potential impact of mental health problems on the family and wider society.

References

Association for Postnatal Illness (APNI): *Association for Postnatal Illness* (website). APNI: http://apni.org/. 2015.

Austin MP, Highet N: *Guidelines Expert Advisory Committee. Clinical practice guidelines for depression and related disorders – anxiety, bipolar disorder and puerperal psychosis – in the perinatal period. A guideline for primary care professionals.* Melbourne,

Beyondblue: the national depression initiative, 2011.

Bartley M, Owen C: Relation between socioeconomic status, employment and health during economic change, *Br Med J* 313(7055):445–449, 1996.

Bauer A, Parsonage M, Knapp M, et al: *Costs of perinatal mental health problems,* London School of Economics and Political Science, London, 2014.

Beck C, Reynolds MA, Rutowski P: Maternity blues and postpartum depression, *J Obstet Gynecol Neonatal Nurs* 21(4):287–293, 1992.

Bick D, MacArthur C, Knowles H, et al: *Postnatal care: evidence and guidelines for management,* Edinburgh, Churchill Livingstone, 2002.

Bloom J: Midwifery and perinatal mental health care provision, *Br J Midwifery* 9(6):385–388, 2002.

Buist AE, Barnett BE, Milgrom J: To screen or not to screen – that is the question in perinatal depression, *Med J Aust* 177:101–105, 2002.

Clement S: 'Listening visits' in pregnancy: a strategy for preventing postnatal depression? *Midwifery* 11(2):75–80, 1995.

Clifford C, Day A, Cox J: A cross-cultural analysis of the use of the Edinburgh Post-natal Depression Scale (EPDS) in health visiting practice, *J Adv Nurs* 30(3):655–664, 1999.

Cox JL, Holden JM, editors: *Perinatal psychiatry: use and misuse of the Edinburgh postnatal depression scale*, London, Gaskell, 1994.

Cox JL: *Postnatal depression. A guide for health professionals*, Edinburgh, Churchill Livingstone, 1986.

Cox J, Murray D, Chapman G: A controlled study of the onset, duration and prevalence of postnatal depression, *Br J Psychiatry* 163(1):27–31, 1993.

Creedy DK, Shochet IM, Horsfall J: Childbirth and the development of acute trauma symptoms: incidence and contributing factors, *Birth* 27(1):104–108, 2000.

Dalton K: Progesterone prophylaxis used successfully in postnatal depression, *Practitioner* 229:507–508, 1985.

Department of Health (DH): *National Service Framework for Mental Health: Modern Standards and Service Models for Mental Health.* London, Department of Health, 1999.

Department of Health (DH): *Mainstreaming Gender and Women's Mental Health: Implementation Guidance.* London, Department of Health, 2003.

Department of Health (DH): *Maternity Matters: Choice, Access and Continuity of Care.* London, Department of Health, 2007.

Department of Health (DH): *Midwifery 2020, Delivering Expectations.* Department of Health, Cambridge, Jill Rogers Associates, 2010.

Department of Health (DH): *NHS England Public Health Functions to be Exercised by NHS England Service Specification No. 30: Sexual Assault Service.* Department of Health. 2013.

Evans J, Heron J, Francomb H, et al: Cohort study of depressed mood during pregnancy and after childbirth, *Br Med J* 323:257–260, 2001.

Forman DN, Videbech P, Hedegaard MD: Postpartum depression: identification of women at risk, *Br J Obstet Gynaecol* 107(10):1210–1217, 2000.

Gerhardt S: *Why love matters: how affection shapes a baby's brain*, 2nd edn, London, Routledge, 2015.

Gray DPW, Watt P: 'Giving Victims a Voice': *A joint MPS and NSPCC report into allegations of sexual abuse made against Jimmy Savile under Operation Yewtree.* NSPCC and Metropolitan Police, 2013.

Green JM, Murray D: The use of the Edinburgh Postnatal Depression Scale in research to explore the relationship between antenatal and postnatal dysphoria. In Cox JL, Holden JM, editors: *Perinatal psychiatry: use and misuse of the Edinburgh Postnatal Depression Scale*, London, Gaskin, 1994.

Gutteridge KE: *'From Me to Mother; the Psychodynamic Journey Women Make in Adaption to Motherhood'*. Birmingham, MSc dissertation, University of Central England, 1998.

Gutteridge KE: Failing women: the impact of sexual abuse on childbirth, *Br J Midwifery* 3(5):312–315, 2001.

Gutteridge KE: From the deep. Surviving child sexual abuse into adulthood: consequences and implications for maternity services, *MIDIRS: Midwifery Digest* 19(1):125–129, 2009.

Hammett PL: Midwives and debriefing. In Kirkham MJ, Perkins ER, editors: *Reflections on midwifery*, London, Baillière Tindal, 1997.

Hannah P, Adams D, Lee A, et al: Links between early post-partum mood and post-natal depression, *Br J Psychiatry* 160(6):777–780, 1992.

Hatloy I: *MIND: Postnatal Depression* (website). www.mind.org.uk/ information-support/types-of-mental-health-problems/postnatal-depression/#.VffeUdJVhHw. 2013.

Hedegaard M, Henriksen TB, Sabroe S, et al: Psychological distress in pregnancy and preterm delivery, *Br Med J* 307(6898):234–239, 1993.

Hofberg K, Brockington I: Tokophobia: an unreasoning dread of childbirth. a series of 26 cases, *Br J Psychiatry* 176:83–85, 2000.

Hogg S: *Prevention in Mind.* NSPCC. http://www.nspcc.org.uk/Inform/ resourcesforprofessionals/ underones/spotlight-mental-health_wdf96656.pdf. 2013.

Home Office: *Human trafficking: the government's strategy*, Home Office Publications, 2011.

Itzin C, Taket A, Barter-Godfrey S: *Domestic and sexual violence and abuse: tackling the health and mental health effects*, London, Routledge, 2010.

Kelly L, Regan L: *Stopping taffic: exploring the extent of, and responses to, trafficking in women for sexual exploitation in the U.K.* Home Office; Police Research Series Paper 125, 2000.

Kendall RE, Chalmers JC, Platz C: Epidemiology of puerperal psychoses, *Br J Psychiatry* 150:662–673, 1987.

Kendall-Tackett K, Kauffman-Kantor G: *Postpartum depression: a comprehensive approach for nurses*, California, Sage, 1993.

Kirkham M: *The mother-midwife relationship*. Hampshire, Palgrave MacMilllan, 2000.

Kitamura T, Yoshida K, Okano T, et al: Multicentre prospective study of perinatal depression in Japan: incidence and correlates of antenatal and postnatal depression, *Arch Womens Ment Health* 9(3):121–130, 2006.

Klainin P, Arthur DG: Postpartum depression in Asian cultures: a literature review, *Int J Nurs Stud* 46:1355–1373, 2009.

Knight M, Nair M, Tuffnell D, et al, editors: *On behalf of MBRRACE-UK. Saving Lives, Improving Mothers' Care – Surveillance of maternal deaths in the UK 2012–14 and lessons learned to inform maternity care from the UK and Ireland Confidential Enquiries into Maternal Deaths and Morbidity 2009–14*, Oxford, National Perinatal Epidemiology Unit, University of Oxford, 2016.

Kumar R, Robson K: A prospective study of emotional disorders in childbearing women, *Br J Psychiatry* 144(1):35–47, 1984.

Laing KG: Post-traumatic stress disorder: myth or reality? *Br J Midwifery* 9(7):447–451, 2001.

Lavender T, Walkinshaw SA: Can midwives reduce postpartum psychological morbidity? A randomized trial, *Birth* 25(4):215–219, 1998.

Levy V, Kline P: Perinatal depression: a factor analysis, *Br J Midwifery* 2(4):154–159, 1994.

Lewis G: *The Confidential Enquiry into Maternal and Child Health (CEMACH). Saving Mothers Lives; Reviewing Maternal Deaths to make Motherhood Safer 2003-05. The Seventh Report of the United Kingdom Confidential Enquiries into Maternal Deaths*. London, CEMACH, 2007.

Lewis GE: *Confidential Enquiries into Maternal Deaths (CEMACH); Why Mothers Die. 2002-2004. The Sixth Report on Confidential Enquiries into Maternal Deaths in the United Kingdom*. London, Royal College of Obstetricians and Gynaecologists, 2004.

Lund C, Breen A, Flisher AJ, et al: Poverty and common mental disorders in low and middle income countries: a systematic review, *Soc Sci Med* 71:517–528, 2010.

Lyons S: A prospective study of post-traumatic stress symptoms one month following childbirth in a group of 42 first-time mothers, *J Infant Reprod Psychol* 16(2/3):91–95, 1998.

MacArthur C, Winter HR, Bick DE, et al: Effects of redesigned community postnatal care on womens' health 4 months after birth: a cluster randomised controlled trial, *Lancet* 359(9304):378–385, 2002.

Marks MN, Kumar R: Infanticide in England and Wales, *Med Sci Law* 33(4):329–339, 1993.

Maternal Mental Health Alliance, NSPCC, Royal College of Midwives (2014 Specialist) Mental Health Midwives: *What They Do and Why They Matter* (website). www.nspcc.org.uk/Inform/resourcesfor professionals/underones/mental-health-midwives- pdf_wdf99836.pdf. 2014.

Melville JL, Gavin A, Guo Y, et al: Depressive disorders during pregnancy: prevalence and risk factors in a large urban sample, *Obstet Gynaecol* 116:1064–1070, 2010.

MIND: *Attitudes to mental illness 2013 research report: prepared for time to change* (website). http://www.mind.org.uk/. MIND, February 2014.

MIND: *MIND: Postnatal Depression*. www.mind.org.uk/information-support/types-of-mental-health-problems/postnatal

-depression/#.Vfgnd9JVhHw. 2015.

Ministry of Justice, Home Office and Office of National Statistics: *An Overview of Sexual Offending in England and Wales*. Crown Publications, 2013.

Murray L, Cooper PJ: Effects of postnatal depression on infant development, *Arch Dis Child* 77(2):99–101, 1997.

Murray JL, Lopez AD: *The Global Burden of Disease: A Comprehensive Assessment of Mortality and Disability from Diseases, Injuries and Risk Factors in 1990 and Projected to 2020*. Harvard School of Public Health, Boston, World Health Organisation (WHO), 1996.

Musters C, McDonald E, Jones L: Management of postnatal depression, *Br Med J* 337:399–403, 2008.

National Institute for Clinical Excellence (NICE): *NICE CGC09. Eating Disorders: Core Interventions in the Treatment and Management of Anorexia Nervosa, Bulimia Nervosa and Related Eating Disorders CG09*. London, UK: NICE Publications, 2004.

National Institute for Health and Clinical Excellence (NICE): *NICE CG 31. Obsessive-Compulsive Disorder: Core Interventions in the Treatment of Obsessive-Compulsive Disorder and Body Dysmorphic Disorder*. NICE, UK, 2005.

National Institute for Health and Clinical Excellence (NICE): *NICE CG26. Post-Traumatic Stress Disorder (PTSD): The Management of PTSD in Adults and Children in Primary and Secondary Care*. NICE, UK, 2006.

National Institute for Health and Clinical Excellence (NICE): *NICE CG 110. Pregnancy and Complex Social Factors: A Model for Service Provision for Pregnant Women with Complex Social Factors*. London UK, NICE, 2010.

National Institute for Health and Care Excellence (NICE): *NICE CG192. Antenatal and Postnatal Mental Health: Clinical Management and Service Guidance*. UK, NICE, 2014a.

National Institute for Health and Care Excellence (NICE): *Psychosis and schizophrenia in adults: treatment and management*. NICE guidelines. (CG178). London, UK, NICE, 2014b.

National Institute for Health and Care Excellence (NICE): *NICE CG113.

Self-Harm: Longer Term Management CG113*. London, UK, NICE publications. 2014c.

NICE 2014: *National Institute of Clinical Excellence (UK) Antenatal and postnatal mental health: clinical management and service guidance*. http://www.nice.org.uk/CG192. 2014.

Niven C: *Psychological care for families; before, during and after birth*, Oxford, Butterworth-Heinmann, 1992.

Oates, M in Royal College of Psychiatrists. CR88: *Perinatal mental health services. Recommendations for provision of services for childbearing women*, London, Royal College of Psychiatrists, 2001.

Oates M, Cantwell R: Chapter 11: Deaths from psychiatric causes in *Saving Mothers' Lives. Reviewing Maternal Deaths to Make Motherhood Safer 2006–2008*. Reviewing maternal deaths to make motherhood safer 2006–2008. The Eighth Report of the Confidential Enquiries into Maternal Deaths, (CMACE), 118:Suppl1. London, United Kingdom: *British Journal of Obstetrics and Gynaecology*. 2011.

O'Hara MW: Postpartum depression: what we know, *J Clin Psychol* 65:1258–1269, 2009.

O'Hara MW, Schlechte JA, Lewis DA, et al: Controlled prospective study of postpartum mood disorders: psychological, environmental, and hormonal variables, *J Abnorm Psychol* 100(1):63–73, 1991.

O'Hara MW, Zekowski EM: Postpartum depression: a comprehensive review. In Kumar R, Brockington IF, editors: *Motherhood and mental illness* (vol 2), Causes and Consequences, London, Wright, pp 17–63, 1988.

Pagel MD, Smilkstein G, Regen H, et al: Psychosocial influences on new born outcomes: a controlled prospective study, *Soc Sci Med* 30:597–604, 1990.

Pantlen A, Rohde A: Psychologic effects of traumatic live deliveries, *Zentralbl Gynakol* 123(1):42–47, German. PMID: 11385911, 2001.

Raphael-Leff J: *The psychological processes of childbearing*, 4th edn, London, Chapman and Hall, Anna Freud Centre, 2005.

Raphael-Leff J: *Pregnancy – the inside story*. London, Karnac. New York, Other Press, 2001, 1993.

Redshaw M, Henderson J: From antenatal to postnatal depression:

associated factors and mitigating influences, *J Womens Health* 22(6):518–525, 2013.

Rich-Edwards JW, Kleinman K, Abrams A, et al: Sociodemographic predictors of antenatal and postpartum depressive symptoms among women in a medical group practice, *J Epidemiol Community Health* 60(3):221–227, 2006.

Robinson J: The perils of psychiatric records, *Br J Midwifery* 10(3):173, 2002.

Romito P: Unhappiness after childbirth. In Chalmers I, Enkin M, Keirse MJ, editors: *Effective care in pregnancy and childbirth* (vol 2), Childbirth, Oxford, Oxford University Press, 1989.

Royal College of Obstetricians and Gynaecologists (RCOG): *Management of Women with Mental Health Issues During Pregnancy in the Postnatal Period: Good Practice No 14*, London, RCOG (website). www.rcog.org.uk/files/rcog-corp/ManagementWomenMentalHealthGoodPractice14.pdf. 2011.

Royal College of Psychiatrists (RCP): *Perinatal Mental Health Services* (Council Report CR88). Royal College of Psychiatrists, London, 2000.

Royal College of Psychiatrists (RCP): *Perinatal mental health services. recommendations for provision of services for childbearing women.* (Council Report CR88), Royal Colleges of Psychiatrists, London, 2001.

Saltman D: *Women and health: an introduction.* Sydney, Harcourt Brace Jovanovich. 1991.

Scottish Intercollegiate Guidelines Network (SIGN): *Management of Perinatal Mood Disorders.* Edinburgh, SIGN. (SIGN publication no. 127) (website). www.sign.ac.uk. 2012.

Sharma V, Pope CJ: Pregnancy and bipolar disorder: a systematic review, *J Clin Psychiatry* 73:1447–1455, 2012.

Shrivastava SR, Shrivastava PS, Ramasamy J: Antenatal and postnatal depression: a public health perspective, *J Neurosci Rural Pract* 6(1):116–119, 2015.

Spitzer RL, Kroenke K, Williams JBW, et al: A brief measure for assessing generalised anxiety disorder, *Arch Intern Med* 166:1092–1097, 2006.

Stein A, Cooper PJ, Campbell EA, et al: Social adversity and perinatal complications: their relation to postnatal depression, *Br Med J* 171(29):1073–1074, 1989.

Storksen HT, Eberhard-Gran M, Garthus-Niegel S, et al: Fear of childbirth; the relation to anxiety and depression, *Acta Obstet Gynecol Scand* 91:237–242, 2012.

Tannous L, Gigante LP, Fuchs SC, et al: Postnatal depression in southern Brazil: prevalence and its demographic and socioeconomic determinants, *BMC Psychiatry* 8:1, 2008.

Teixeira JM, Fisk NM, Glover V: Association between maternal anxiety in pregnancy and increased uterine artery resistance index: cohort based study, *Br Med J* 318(7177):153–157, 1999.

Toohill J, Fenwick J, Gamble J, et al: Psycho-social predictors of childbirth fear in pregnant women: an Australian study, *Open J Obstet*

Gynecol 4(9):531–543, http://dx.doi.org/10.4236/ojog.2014.49075. 2014.

Tsivos ZL, Calam R, Sanders MR, et al: Interventions for postnatal depression assessing the mother-infant relationship and child developmental outcomes: a systematic review, *Int J Womens Health* 23(7):429–447, 2015.

Tuohy A, McVey C: Experience of pregnancy and delivery as predictors of postpartum depression, *Psychol Health Med* 13:43–47, 2008.

Watson JP, Elliott SA, Rugg AJ, et al: Psychiatric disorder in pregnancy and the first postnatal year, *Br J Psychiatry* 144(5):453–462, 1984.

Wieck A: Endocrine aspects of postnatal mental disorders, *Clin Obstet Gynaecol* 3(4):857–877, 1989.

Wijma KL, Wijma B, Zar M: Psychometric aspects of the W-DEQ; a new questionnaire for the measurement of fear of childbirth, *J Psychosom Obstet Gynecol* 19(2):84–97, 1998.

Wilson LM, Reid AJ, Midmer DK, et al: Antenatal psychosocial risk factors associated with adverse family outcomes, *CMAJ* 154(6):785–799, 1996.

World Health Organisation (WHO): *Violence Against Women: A Priority Health issue*, Geneva, WHO, 1997.

World Health Organisation (WHO): *The ICD-10 Classification of Mental and Behavioural Disorders*, Geneva, WHO, 1992.

World Health Organisation (WHO): *Women's Mental Health – An Evidence Based Review*, Geneva, WHO, 2000.

Resources and additional reading

Everyone's Business. This is the Maternal Mental Health Alliance's new campaign – Everyone's Business – calls for all women throughout the UK who experience perinatal mental health problems to receive the care they and their families need, wherever and whenever they need it.

(website). http://everyonesbusiness.org.uk/.

Royal College of Midwives (RCM): *Specialist Mental Health Midwives: What They Do and Why They Matter* (website). www.rcm.org.uk/sites/default/files/MMHA%20SMHMs%20Nov%2013.pdf. 2014.

Royal College of Obstetricians and Gynaecologists (RCOG): *Management of Women with Mental Health Issues During Pregnancy in the*

Postnatal Period: Good Practice No 14. London, RCOG (website). www.rcog.org.uk/files/rcog-corp/ManagementWomenMentalHealthGoodPractice14.pdf. 2011.

NHS Scotland: *The knowledge Network.* 2015 Maternal Mental Health e-learning resource – 2 modules available online: Module 1: Understanding maternal mental health; an introduction to information on mental illnesses that may affect women during pregnancy and postnatal periods. Module 2: maternal mental health and professional roles including through preconception care, pregnancy and the postnatal period (website). www.knowledge.scot.nhs.uk/ maternalhealth/learning/maternal-mental-health.aspx.

Scottish Intercollegiate Guidelines Network (SIGN): *Management of perinatal mood disorders*, Edinburgh, SIGN. (SIGN publication no. 127) (website). www.sign.ac.uk/pdf/ sign127.pdf. 2012.

Royal College of Obstetricians and Gynaecology (RCOG): *Good Practice No 14. Management of Women with Mental Health Issues During Pregnancy and the Postnatal Period*, 2011.

Support for Women and Professional Information

Specialist Mental Health Midwives: *What they do and why they matter* (website). www.baspcan.org.uk/files/ MMHA%20SMHMs%20Report.pdf.

Mothers for mothers (website). www.mothersformothers.co.uk/

Pandas Foundation

www.pandasfoundation.org.uk

Pandas Foundation vision is to support every individual with pre- or postnatal depression (PND) in England. We campaign to change the law, provide Pandas Help Line, offer advice to all and much more.

The Association for Postnatal Illness – www.apni.org

Provides a telephone helpline, information leaflets for sufferers and healthcare professionals and a network of volunteers who have themselves experienced postnatal illness.

Action on Postpartum Psychosis

http://app-network.healthunlocked.com

Postnatal Illness Support

Formerly Veritee's postnatal illness website: www.pni.org.uk

MIND

Information for all matters relating to mental health:

www.mind.org.uk

Birth Trauma Association

This Website offers information and support to mothers who have had a traumatic birth experience or who are suffering from post-birth traumatic syndrome.

www.birthtraumaassociation.org.uk

Fatherhood Institute

A fatherhood think-and-do-tank (website). www.fatherhoodinstitute.org.

Fathers Reaching Out

A support network for men whose wives or partners are suffering from postnatal depression (PND).

www.fathersreachingout.com

Ante–Natal Depression

www.depression-in-pregnancy.org

Resources

My Wellbeing Plan – from Tommys charity

www.tommys.org/file/Wellbeingplan.pdf

Edinburgh Postnatal Depression Scale – (Cox L, Cox JM, Holden R Sagovsky: Detection of postnatal depression: development of the 10-item Edinburgh Postnatal Depression Scale, *Br J Psychiatry* 150:782–786, 1987 (website). https://psychology-tools.com/epds/

PHQ-9

GAD Anxiety Tool

Tokophobia Tool aid for assessment

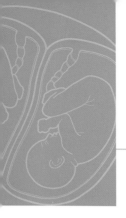

Chapter 70

Midwifery for the future...where next?

Gail Johnson and Sue Macdonald

INTRODUCTION

Midwifery has evolved over thousands of years, with many changes being introduced as knowledge, skills and technology define the care and societies needs and expectations change. The scope of the midwife's role in the 21st century is unrecognizable to that outlined in the 1902 Midwives Act. Yet the core of the midwife's role remains the same: to support the woman through pregnancy, birth and the puerperium with care, ensuring the safe birth of the baby and enabling a positive transition to motherhood. It is important to recognize that midwifery practitioners include midwives engaged in research, midwifery education, management and clinical practice. All have a particular contribution to the development of the profession and to the care provided to women, their babies and families.

Since the 14th edition of *Mayes' Midwifery*, there has been a plethora of research, professional guidance papers and policy documents and reports, which impact on midwives and maternity services. Some reports have challenged current health service delivery, and the professionals' approach to care has also been questioned, with an acknowledgement that most women and families are satisfied with the quality of care they receive (House of Commons Committee of Public Accounts 2014; CQC 2015) and the degree of information, support and care from midwives (Redshaw et al 2007; Redshaw and Henderson 2015).

The Francis Report (2013) into care at Mid Staffordshire Hospital, although not focused on the maternity services, has important messages for those within the NHS. The investigation found that care was system driven rather than patient centred. Leadership across the service was unsatisfactory and outcomes for patients at the hospital were poor with a higher than expected number of deaths. An equally damning report, specifically into maternity services at Morecambe Bay Hospitals (Kirkup 2015), demonstrated similar findings: a lack of leadership, poor professional relationships and systems failures, which led to the avoidable deaths of babies and women. Given these distressing reports on the evidence of poor care in health services, midwifery practice needs to continue to evolve. Regular

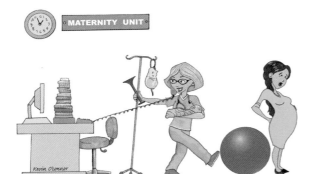

Figure 70.1 A midwife of today?

changes in the political milieu and their influences impact on services, which can be seen as unsure of its true direction. Other research has pointed to a lack of attention or less perceived time allocated to certain aspects of maternity care, including the postnatal period (Bhavnani and Newburn 2010; Redshaw and Henderson 2015). What is clear is that maternity services need to be flexible, adaptable, open, honest and safe, based on tenets of care and compassion, with a clear model focused on the woman and her baby.

This text highlights the complexity and challenges in midwifery practice (see Fig. 70.1). The midwife in the 21st century is required to work in multiple settings with an ever increasing network of professionals and more knowledgeable women and families with their own expectations of care. In addition, the changing political climate both at home and abroad bring about demographic vagaries and variabilities in the needs of women. This final chapter will briefly address challenges that may face midwives in the 21st century to maintain their roles within the midwifery profession and maternity service.

THE FUTURE

What the future of the midwifery profession holds is in many ways reassuringly the same, with the woman and her baby being at the heart of care (National Maternity Review, NHSE (England) 2016; Lancet Series 2014: Renfrew et al 2014). How care is delivered and what the woman's needs will be will continue to provide a degree of uncertainty and challenge. Women themselves value midwifery care, and when this is reduced or insufficient can feel less supported and under confident in their transition to motherhood (Bhavnani and Newburn 2010; CQC 2015).

Nonetheless, with so many reports seeming to undermine the profession and the changes in regulation and supervision, the midwife now and in the future needs to be knowledgeable, competent, confident and able to

work as part of a team, and above all be resilient (Hunter and Warren 2014).

If midwives are to have their role properly recognized, they must be clear of what their role is and its professional boundaries. Where shared responsibilities are required in caring for women and families within the multiprofessional environment, agreeing distinct pathways and responsibilities for different practitioners roles is essential. Where multiple providers are offering support and care in health and social care, then, ideally, a choice should be made on who is best to lead and who can build the best relationship. The essential element is to ensure good channels of communication between all healthcare and other providers. In many cases, the midwife is most likely to provide continuity to the woman during the pregnancy and childbirth period.

In responding to the increasing complexities in women's health needs and changes in society and public expectations, it is opportune to consider how midwives may work flexibly and broaden their remit within the public health agenda to meet the needs of society (DH/PHE 2013; DH/PHE/RCM/NHSE 2016). Altering economic climates demand new ways of working to provide an effective and efficient midwifery service that utilizes support where necessary.

Although many resources for this book and the website have drawn upon midwifery in UK literature, messages for midwives working with women throughout the world are similar. In countries where the midwifery profession is established, women have optimum opportunity to birth in ways that suit them. In countries without strong midwifery presence, the aim should be to develop this, as research and evidence show that where there is a strong, well-educated and regulated midwifery profession, maternal and perinatal mortality and morbidity are lower (see Ch. 1). The aim must be to provide educated midwives for all women all over the world, as this is proven to impact on quality of maternity care, and reduction in maternal and perinatal mortality and morbidity (WHO 2004).

Clinical care

Within this textbook, the depth and breadth of the midwife's role in clinical care has been addressed. New technologies, services and choices mean that midwives will work in different settings and with an ever increasing stakeholder network. Women and families also have access to more information, have greater understanding of their own wishes and are generally more confident in presenting their needs. For women who are less confident, midwives have a role in providing accessible, unbiased information and encouraging them to fully participate in their choices.

This is also balanced alongside societal changes, a shrinking world and an increasing number of women who were not born in the UK accessing maternity services. For women born outside of the UK, access to clinical care may be challenging, leaving these women vulnerable and isolated. For all of these women, midwives need to ensure that their voices are heard and their particular wishes and needs are respected.

The midwife of the future is likely to find their practice in different settings: in the acute hospital, midwifery-led birth centres, community centres and in the woman's home. With womens' roles in society changing, they are likely to demand a service that fits in better with **their** lives, for example, more evening and weekend services, and more access through different media, including video conferencing, e-mail and instant messaging. This is likely to require speedy response, and a confidence and competence with accessing different media for this purpose. There is already evidence that midwives are committed to using alternative media to link with different groups of women (Redshaw and Henderson 2015; Mander 2011) and the development of applications (apps) such as the 'Babybuddy' (Best Beginnings 2016) are used by midwives as resources for women and their families.

Providing women with choices and enabling families to make decisions in their care is government policy in the UK (NICE 2014; DH 2007a; Birthrights 2013; Which? 2016). A recent review of women's maternity care experiences demonstrates diversity in experiences that women receive in the UK; however, the report notes that midwives are in a powerful position to influence the care that women receive (CQC 2015; Jomeen and Redshaw 2013). Women's voices and views need to be heard antenatally, in labour, and during the postnatal and neonatal care periods so that clinical care takes place in non-threatening spaces, and always with the ability to respond to emergencies. In many services, investment has developed better spaces with more 'user friendly' areas and better décor, but this needs also to take account of the human and other resources to enable an appropriate practice environment (see Box 70.1).

Working with women

The 1960s and 1970s saw a move from home to hospital birth and a further shift of power from the woman to professionals. The medicalization of birth placed the woman in a role as a compliant recipient of care (see Ch. 2). Women in the 21st century rightly want to be the core of the service and to have a choice in their care (see Ch. 34). The Maternity Review (NHSE 2016 (England)) clearly emphasizes continuity of carer as key, and this has been supported by research and evidence (Sandall et al 2016; Renfrew et al 2014; Devane et al 2010). This review is more than a revisit to Changing Childbirth (DH 1993), it moves the woman's care away from risk to an individualized plan of care and suggests a greater degree of power, illustrated

---

> **Box 70.1** Features of practice environments
>
> The environment needs to include:
>
> - Provision of unbiased and equitable information, tailored to meet the needs of the individual
> - Sufficient time and staff for appointments and examinations with adequate time for discussion and decision making
> - Knowledge sharing in partnership through communication with women to promote their decision making
> - Promotion of better birth experience irrespective of complexities, working with women to accomplish as positive a birth as possible (RCM Better Births Initiative 2016)
> - Ready access to information and evidence for women and staff
> - Direct communication with and referral between multidisciplinary teams
> - Pathways for rapid access to emergency care, to medical facilities and other interventions as necessary
> - Development for all midwives of their leadership qualities to articulate for women in their care, recognizing their individual wishes
> - Education and training of midwives to develop knowledge and skills to practise with autonomy and recognize when to liaise with other agencies (NMC 2015)

---

by a recommendation that the woman has control of how her care is commissioned.

Women want clear, unbiased advice, offered in simple lay terms, that does not indicate a professional's individual view, but gives the options and implications of a choice of action to tailor to their individual circumstances. This is not an easy task for each professional who has a mantle of their own prejudices and biases that need to be set aside. The Darzi report (DH 2007b) indicates that professionals must provide a personalized service that gives control to women and families.

Building partnerships with women and working with their organizations, such as the Association for Improvement of the Maternity Services (AIMS) and the National Childbirth Trust (NCT), and local user groups, will assist in providing a service where their needs are met.

The influence of a qualified midwife present at birth has been shown to effect a reduced morbidity and mortality rate for both mother and baby (WHO 2004; Save the Children 2015) (see Ch. 1). In this century, an aim would be to see education, training and registration for midwives in all countries of the world. The caveat is that, as midwives become qualified, the costs of maternity services rises, thus presenting service providers and policy makers with a dilemma and a perceived need to employ non-qualified staff who can undertake other duties – including maternity support workers, nursery nurses and other ancillary staff. Clear parameters and boundaries are crucial to ensure that it is midwives who provide skilled care and information to women through the pregnancy and childbirth continuum. Their responsibility is to be knowledgeable, know their limitations and how to harness appropriate multi-professional help when needed to ensure a safer birth. To see a fulfilment of this aim and to reduce inequalities in birth means continuing training and lifelong learning for all midwives, including professional updating that recognizes the value of normalization of birth where possible (see Ch. 5). The need to change behaviours and attitudes that have become reliant on interventions, however minor, also should be addressed.

The care continuum

Traditionally, in the UK, the midwives remit has been the provision of care through pregnancy, labour and postnatal periods. This has made the midwife the recognized expert of the normal within this continuum, both for women with a low- and high-risk pregnancy, as they make the transition to motherhood. As care provision costs have increased alongside a rising birth rate and insufficient numbers of midwives (RCM 2015a, b, c), there have been a number of initiatives to provide women and babies with care, and this has included delegating other personnel to providing care to women, especially within the postnatal period. Two challenges are here – the first is to question whether the task/role should be delegated and the second is to ensure that the person delegated to is appropriate. An example has been that there has been a reduction in the postnatal role of midwives, which appears to have been accepted sometimes uncritically. Midwives do need to challenge what this loss of one significant aspect of care means for the women and babies, and equally importantly for midwives and midwifery itself both in the short and long term.

A multi-social and multicultural society

In 2013, 26.5% of babies were born in the UK to women who themselves were born outside of the UK (ONS 2014). International economic hardship, civil and political unrest leads to more families seeking asylum and safety. The multicultural nature of the UK can present challenges to the delivery of maternity services. Women whose native language is not English may have difficulty accessing relevant services or even be unaware of their entitlement. Racial prejudice and a lack of understanding of needs can leave some women vulnerable, and the midwife needs to be culturally sensitive and competent in providing care

and supporting women and families (see Ch. 11). Many of the larger cities in the UK are hosting women from a number of different countries and where many different languages are spoken. For example, London has 3.1 million people born outside of the UK (NPI 2015) and the 2011 census (The Migration Observatory 2013) highlights that around 100 different languages are spoken. Where there are larger populations of women from a particular group, it is often easier to provide care tailored to their needs. However, where women find themselves in smaller communities, it is likely that they will be more isolated, less well understood and unsupported.

Research evidence and policy highlight that vulnerable women and women from black and minority populations (BME) have poorer pregnancy outcomes (Manktelow et al 2015; West et al 2015). This remains the case for BME women who are second and third generations in the UK. The midwife has a clear remit in identifying women who may be isolated, and in delivering care that meets the individual needs of all women, and this often demands that vulnerable and BME women have access to increased levels of support (see Ch. 23).

Inevitably, because of changes in living styles and social family structures, economic uncertainty and varied cultures in our society, the demands are for professionals to adapt and manage change in caring for women and families with diverse needs while ensuring equality of provision (DH 2008).

While there have always been people who have lived by travelling, now, with easier modes of travel enabling crossing of national boundaries, different populations and societies are migrating, some willingly, for their own interests and economics, but others enforced, as political migrants, with an emergence of a varied multicultural society. Depending on the reasons for relocation, these people may require high levels of health interventions and may lack the language and knowledge to seek their own health needs. The first health encounter for many is the maternity service; therefore, the midwife may be the first person to identify those in different groups at risk of special needs, and has an opportunity for taking a broad health review to identify health concerns (see Box 70.2). A social and health needs assessment may divulge specific problems for subsequent care.

Whatever circumstances women face, a midwife will need to identify their individual choices for care and overcome any language problems with advice for appropriate actions. It is the midwife who becomes a mediator and pivot between the health agencies in providing flexibility and continuity in care.

Governance

While clinical governance and its structures are discussed in Chapter 4, midwives have a responsibility to determine

- Teenagers and vulnerable women who are unsupported
- Families where young men are to become fathers
- Adoptive parents and those who have had fertility treatment (see Ch. 23)
- Women seeking care outside health service expectations – such as women planning a 'freebirth'
- Families with members with disabilities
- Asylum seekers and refugee women
- Homeless women
- Those with alternative lifestyles or those who are socially deprived
- Those with mental health problems
- Those dependent upon drugs, alcohol or smoking
- Women who seek pregnancy outside normal expectations of fertility or with complex medical conditions

their own governance to meet women's needs. This includes their involvement in decision making for themselves and collaborating with women and in their maternity services policy development to influence the way in which they are governed. In essence, midwives need to be political at local levels and able to translate national policy and research to local needs. For example, it is good practice to discuss national publications multi-professionally and to collaborate and communicate through structures in the maternity service at ward and community service levels (RCOG/RCA/RCM/RCP 2007; RCOG 2008) before decisions for implementation.

In the UK, midwives are governed by the Nursing and Midwifery Council (NMC), the regulatory body which sets the standards for education and maintains the register of eligible practitioners. In addition, midwives were supported in practice by a supervisor of midwives, a midwife whose key role was protecting the public through ensuring that maternity services and midwifery practices were safe. Following the ombudsman review of midwifery supervision (PHSO 2013), a change in statute means that midwifery supervision will no longer be a legal requirement (see Ch. 3).

From April 2016, nurses and midwives will have to demonstrate that they meet the NMC requirements to stay on the NMC register through *Revalidation*. Revalidation is not significantly different for midwives than meeting the previous PREP requirements. However, there is a need to write reflective accounts and to reflect on feedback from practice to demonstrate learning. The process is more

formalized and requires the midwife to collect evidence throughout the 3 years before revalidation. Once the evidence is collected, there needs to be a meeting with a professional colleague to review the evidence and once it is completed, a confirmer can sign to state that the practitioner has met the NMC requirements (NMC 2016) (see Ch. 5).

Management structures meeting the needs of women

A management structure for a maternity unit must be planned so that efficient services deliver quality effectively and meet the needs of women and their babies (RCM 2009). Services must be accessible and equitable. Quality is measured by criteria and standards but may also be perceived in different ways by those who receive care. Strategy development is a measure of quality of a maternity service and is a multi-professional activity requiring involvement of all the teams involved (RCOG 2008). Furthermore, involving women in a maternity unit decision making assists in creating a culture where women-centred care is recognized (Proctor 1998).

It is critical that both midwives and users are meaningfully involved in the management of services, and able to adapt and develop them so that the service is flexible, responsive and centred on the needs of women, their babies and families.

Midwives as leaders

Key leaders within the profession promote midwifery and maternity services within national and local organizations (DH 2002; Warwick 2015). These people negotiate on behalf of midwifery and the maternity services, but each midwife requires demonstrable leadership skills. These skills enable the midwife to understand the components of health and maternity care; how the service is run and managed; their place within it; and have the tools to influence how the service is provided and developed. Leadership can be utilized at all levels of the service and will influence care (Knight et al 2015) and also the workforce well-being addressing issues, including bullying, inequality and racism (West et al 2015) and professional development of the team.

It is also important that there are midwives in senior and influential positions within maternity and health service; therefore, midwives need to grasp this leadership challenge and work towards having midwives at all levels and be supportive of their midwife managers in their role (Divall 2015) (see Ch. 7).

Midwives need the confidence to:

- act as role models for students and others in the service

- practise within a changing environment, recognizing when to be flexible to meet service needs, and contribute to change themselves

- effectively assess and determine, then articulate the needs of women and families, influencing the wider women's health agenda

- ensure a healthy and supportive working climate

- challenge poor practice, undermining or bullying behavior

- actively contribute to organizations' standard-setting, policy-making and development of guidelines

- access, use, and promote best evidence appropriately, tailoring it to the individual needs of women and families

- take a lead on key activities that promote high quality midwifery care for women, their babies and families

The lessons from the impact of poor leadership (Francis 2013; Kirkup 2015) need to be translated into high quality leadership in healthcare and in maternity services.

THE IMAGE OF THE MIDWIFE

It is important for midwives to be aware of their public image and how they can contribute to ensuring that this is positive and realistic. Some images in the media can provide a positive image (e.g. *Call the midwife* TV drama (Sanghani 2014)), and some are less positive, as in some American 'soap operas' (Kline 2007) and these dramas may be seen and inform women's understanding of what a midwife is.

People are generally very interested in the work of midwives, and increasingly, midwives are asked to comment on care, and on research and policy on television, radio and newspapers. This provides a valuable opportunity to promote maternity care, to demonstrate the role of the midwife, and to inform women and families; however, it is important to have some preparation and ideally some training in presentation skills so that the interview conveys the right messages, and that the midwife presents well and confidently. There are some available guidelines online (Walker 2013), and if you are being interviewed on behalf of an organization, a press officer will usually provide some guidance and support at the time.

Education and continuing professional development

Midwifery pre-registration education in the UK is embedded in higher education institutes (HEI), and recent changes proposed, makes it unclear what impact the proposed funding changes will have on the recruitment and retention of new students.

Generally, midwives are now responsible for the organization and funding of their own continuing professional development (CPD), although some maternity services support some activities, and this includes mandatory training, including sessions on moving and handling and resuscitation. This can disadvantage many midwives who are not in a position to fund their own development or cannot be freed from family commitments to find time to attend. This has meant that for many midwives their 'development' is based on mandatory training, which meets the needs of the unit but not necessarily the professional development needs of the midwife.

The health service environment needs to promote an organization of learning which is responsive to the needs of its clients. This environment is one that actively supports multi-professional education and training sessions and has an effective review system for staff that actively develops its staff. It learns from critical review and involves staff and women in the process (see Ch. 5).

Midwives need to be able to:

- learn from incidents, mistakes and also from incidents of good practice (DH 2000)

- lack defensiveness, reflecting and permitting people to see where there is a fault

- regularly commit to education, training and development through active reflection

- use technology competently to share information with women

- question the status quo to create new ways of caring for women

- contribute through innovation and creativity to developing a dynamic and appropriate maternity service

Communication and relationships

The role of the midwife as an autonomous practitioner is well established in statute and in practice. However, the diverse and complex nature of women and maternity care means that midwives must not work in isolation. Many reports, including CEMACH (2007) and the Kings Fund (2008), have previously highlighted the importance of good inter-professional communication and working. More recently, the Kirkup Report (2015) demonstrated what can happen when midwives work in isolation; the harm caused where professional relationships were weak or absent; in the poor maternal and perinatal outcomes. Unfortunately, within some maternity services, there is a criticism of the relationships between midwives and doctors and that bullying and undermining behaviours are frequently reported in maternity care. Where professional relationships break down and there is a culture of bullying – professionals feel undervalued, perform poorly and the outcomes for women and babies are harmful. Where strong professional relationships are established, there is a culture of respect and understanding and a commitment to providing the best care for women and their babies.

Continuity and continued care from the midwife has beneficial effects for women and/or their babies with complex health needs (see Ch. 59).

To overcome the breakdown in relationships and to foster a culture of collaboration, professionals need to understand their roles and how they impact on each other and on women. Working and training together is identified as an efficient way of developing a shared culture and a common understanding that the woman is central in the care.

Quality enhancement structures

The prime concern for women and families is the outcome of a healthy mother and child. The effects of childbirth on families are little researched and the impact of long-term effects of maternity care on family relationships requires exploration. There is little knowledge of the long-term impact of interventions and minor trauma on the mother/child relationships and family dynamics. Therefore, reducing any risk of complications or problems is important in providing care. Being prepared for any eventuality and possible emergencies and ensuring systems to reduce delays and efficient management are in place are essential. This includes midwives being aware of their own limitations and having an intuitive sense of situations. In view of this, corporate maternity unit policies need to be in place for risk reduction for maternal and infant mortality and morbidity. Risk management includes reducing mortality and morbidity through risk reduction, reporting analysis and statistical analysis of outcome figures in maternity care. Good interdisciplinary communication and teamwork are also key factors (Knight et al 2015).

The institutional figures may be compared with those at a national level, but the implications for individual midwives are that they need to constantly undertake reflection and self-review of their own engagement with areas of risk and reduction of safety at birth to improve practices. A balance needs to be set between women's choices and perceived risks by a professional, as we all have different views of what is meant by the term 'risk'. While the concept of risk may be considered a measurement of safety, each person has different notions of what is acceptable to them. It is also critical to be knowledgeable with the systems in place for dealing with problems and, in particular, complaints (see Ch. 4). Making a sincere apology and directing the woman and family to the correct processes is important (NHS Litigation Authority (NHSLA) 2014).

TECHNOLOGY AND HEALTH

New technologies and the miniaturization of computers mean that the cost of technologies is reducing and access is increasing. Often women have access to information about health and lifestyles that can help them be more prepared for their childbirth experience. However, accessing unmonitored information can increase anxiety and potentially cause harm.

Handheld scanners and dopplers can enable women to be cared for away from the acute setting – for example, keeping women in rural communities at home for longer. However, it is important that all new technologies are introduced with caution and that their value is appropriately assessed. It is also crucial that any machinery used is carefully calibrated and in good working condition.

> ### Reflective activity 70.1
>
> What kind of technology would you wish to see implemented in the postnatal period? What could make a difference to the outcomes for women or babies?

The midwife needs to see the increased use of technology as a servant rather than master, ensuring that skills in using the technology are appropriately updated and the machinery and its limitations and advantages clearly explained to women and families.

THE MIDWIFE WITH GLOBAL VISION

In the *14th edition*, The Millennium Development Goals (MDGs) were the main target for addressing world health, and Chapter 1 has highlighted the need to now work towards the Sustainable Development Goals (SDG), Global Strategy Women's, Children's and Adolescent's Health (GS2) and other global mandates to improve health and well-being internationally, having reached the end of the MDG agenda (WHO 2015a,b; Women and Children First UK 2016; Ki-moon 2010).

The impact of midwifery care on the health of a nation is little understood. Recognizing the work of a midwife in all countries of the world was a WHO priority in the Safe Motherhood Initiative (Women and Children First UK 2016; WHO 2004), and it is recognized that where a midwifery system is in place, maternal and perinatal mortality and morbidity are significantly lowered. Midwives now have opportunities to learn from each other in different countries to discover how midwifery may be adapted to the needs of women in differing societies, for example, through organizations such as the International Confederation of Midwives (ICM 2016) and through working on initiatives such as the RCM Global Twinning project (RCM 2016). Preventing morbidity and mortality are key objectives. Unless current trends of mortalities are reduced, women and families will continue to be at risk. In all countries, reducing morbidity from the effects of childbirth is equally important.

Everyone has a responsibility in the changes taking place within the environment, and promoting normal birth is one way of conserving naturalness in society. An active approach towards reducing *climate change* that affects the many lives of vulnerable societies requires a new way of thinking in all maternity units to conserve and reduce energy consumption. The MDGs were aspirational and perhaps retrospectively unachievable. Nonetheless, much has been done to improve the lives of woman, their babies and families globally (UN 2008 and 2015).

Reflective activity 70.2

Think of one aspect of midwifery care where you could implement a measure to reduce the carbon footprint in the maternity unit and make savings for the environment.

CONCLUSION

The vision of the future of midwifery is in the hands of midwives. It is they who will articulate their views for themselves and for women to policy makers. Midwives need to listen to women and work with organizations for women and cultural groups who act on behalf of women. Social divides between rich and poor will make it essential that midwives hone their skills to recognize those most at risk, using preventive action to mitigate the risks that are life-endangering. A global economy, with global information technology (IT) and increasing advances in digital technology, means new modes of working and ways of communicating with women internationally, especially in building on evidence. Midwifery will always link between fundamentals of practice using a sound knowledge base and practical skills and advances in new forms of care.

Thus, in the 21st century, midwives in all parts of the world will become increasingly skilled through their own professional development. In retaining separateness as a profession but engaging with other professions collaboratively and exploiting advantages in technology to support essential midwifery practice, strength, vision, integrity and flexibility will be essential attributes for all in readiness to face the future.

Key Points

- Midwives, in conjunction with women, need to create their own vision of their role and the midwifery services.

- Each midwife needs to develop leadership skills, to articulate for women and to ensure that midwifery education, research and practice responds to societal needs.

- Midwifery needs to be socially and culturally responsive to ensure that the psychological, social and physical individual needs of women, their babies and families are met.

- Midwives must recognize the governance agenda and professional responsibility and ensure accountability in actions when practising autonomously.

- Collaboration and partnership with women and multi-professionals and agencies in all aspects of care, identifying a lead professional is essential to provide comprehensive maternity care.

- Utilization of technology and digitization has the propensity to transform communication in all parts of the world and thus the ways in which midwives practise. This needs to be incorporated into providing care that retains normality but supports improved care for those at risk.

- The Sustainable Development Goals (SDGs), Global Strategy Women's, Children's and Adolescent's Health (GS2) pertain to all countries of the world and thus midwives have a responsibility to be aware of their international role in caring for women and children (WHO 2015c).

References

Best Beginnings: *Baby Buddy App* (website). www.bestbeginnings .org.uk/baby-buddy. 2016.

Bhavnani V, Newburn M: *Left to your own devices: the postnatal care experiences of 1260 first-time mothers.* London, 2010.

Birthrights 2013 Human Rights in Maternity Care Fact Sheet (website). www.birthrights.org.uk/library/ factsheets/Human-Rights-in -Maternity-Care.pdf. 2013.

Care Quality Commission (CQC) (website). www.cqc.org.uk/content/ maternity-services-survey-2015. 2015.

Confidential Enquiry into Maternal and Child Health (CEMACH): *Saving Mothers' Lives: Reviewing Maternal Deaths to Make Motherhood Safer – 2003-2005. The Seventh Report of the Confidential Enquiries into Maternal Deaths in the United Kingdom,* 2007.

Department of Health (DH): *Changing Childbirth: Report of expert maternity group; part 1,* 1993.

Department of Health (DH): *An Organisation with a Memory: Report of an Expert Group on Learning from Adverse Events in the NHS.* Department of Health, London, 2000.

Department of Health (DH): *Shifting the Balance of Power: The Next Steps.* Department of Health, London, 2002.

Department of Health (DH): *Maternity Matters: Choice Access and Continuity of Care in a Safe Service.* Department of Health, London, 2007a.

Department of Health (DH): *Our NHS Our Future (The Darzi Report).* Department of Health, London, 2007b.

Department of Health (DH): *Making the Difference: The Pacesetters Beginner's Guide to Service Improvement for Diversity and Equality and Diversity in the NHS.* Department of Health, London, 2008.

Department of Health (DH); Public Health England (PHE): *Nursing and Midwifery Action at the Three Levels of Public Health Practice* (website). www.gov.uk/government/uploads/ system/uploads/attachment_data/ file/208814/3_Levels.pdf. 2013.

Department of Health (DH); Public Health England (PHE); Royal College of Midwives (RCM); NHS England (NHSE): *Midwifery Public Health Contribution to Compassion in Practice through Maximising Wellbeing and Improving Health in Women, Babies and Families* (website). www.gov.uk/government/uploads/ system/uploads/attachment_data/ file/208824/Midwifery_strategy_ visual_B.pdf. 2016.

Devane DBM, Begley C, Clarke M, et al: *Socio-Economic Value of the Midwife: a Systematic Review, Meta-Analysis, Meta-Synthesis and Economic Analysis of Midwife-Led Models of Care,* London, Royal College of Midwives (RCM), 2010.

Divall B: Negotiating competing discourses in narratives of midwifery leadership in the English, *Midwifery* 31(11):1060–1066, 2015.

Francis R: *Report of the Mid Staffordshire NHS Foundation Trust Public Inquiry* (website). www.gov.uk/government/ uploads/system/uploads/attachment _data/file/279124/0947.pdf. 2013.

House of Commons Committee of Public Accounts: *Maternity Services in England Fortieth Report of Session 2013–14 Report (chaired by Rt Hon Margaret Hodge).* House of Commons Select Committee, London, 2014.

Hunter B, Warren L: Midwives' experiences of workplace resilience, *Midwifery* 30(8):926–934, 2014.

International Confederation of Midwives (website). www.internationalmidwives .org. 2016.

Jomeen J, Redshaw M: Ethnic minority women's experience of maternity services in England, *Ethn Health* 18(3):280–296, 2013.

Ki-moon B: *Global strategy for women's and children's health,* New York, United Nations, 2010.

Kings Fund: *Safe Births: Everybody's Business* (website). www.kingsfund .org.uk/sites/files/kf/field/field_ publication_file/safe-births -everybodys-business-onora-oneill -february-2008.pdf. 2008.

Kirkup B: *The Report of the Morecambe Bay Investigation: An Independent Investigation into the Management, Delivery and Outcomes of Care Provided by the Maternity and Neonatal Services at the University Hospitals of Morecambe Bay NHS Foundation Trust from January 2004 to June 2013* (website). www.gov.uk/

government/publications. Stationery Office, London, 2015.

Kline KN: Midwife attended births in prime-time television: craziness, controlling bitches, and ultimate capitulation, *Women and Language* 30(1):20–29, 2007.

Knight M, Tuffnell TD, Kenyon S, et al (eds.): On behalf of MBRRACE-UK, *Saving Lives, Improving Mothers' Care – Surveillance of Maternal Deaths in the UK 2011–13 and Lessons Learned to Inform Maternity Care from the UK and Ireland Confidential Enquiries into Maternal Deaths and Morbidity 2009–13* (website). www.npeu.ox.ac .uk/downloads/files/mbrrace-uk/ reports/MBRRACE-UK%20Maternal %20Report%202015.pdf.National Perinatal Epidemiology Unit, University of Oxford, Oxford, 2015.

Mander J: *Worcestershire Website for Expectant and New Families Kidderminster Shuttle.* www.kidderm instershuttle.co.uk/news/local/ 8907960.Worcestershire_website _for_expectant_and_new_families/. 2011.

Manktelow B, Smith L, Evans T, et al On behalf of the MBRRACE-UK collaboration. *Perinatal Mortality Surveillance Report UK Perinatal Deaths for Births from January to December 2013.* Leicester: The Infant Mortality and Morbidity Group, Department of Health Sciences, University of Leicester, 2015.

National Health Service Litigation Authority (NHSLA): '*Saying Sorry – Information Leaflet* (website). www.nhsla.com/claims/Documents/ Saying%20Sorry%20-%20 Leaflet.pdf. 2014.

National Institute for Health and Care Excellence (NICE): *Intrapartum Care: Care of Healthy Women and Their Babies During Childbirth* (website). www.nice.org.uk/guidance/cg190. 2014.

New Policy Institute (NPI): *London's Population by Country of Birth* (website). http://www.london spovertyprofile.org.uk/indicators/ topics/londons-geography- population/londons-population-by- country-of-birth/. 2015.

NHS England (NHSE): *National Maternity Review: Better Births; Improving Outcomes and Maternity Services in England. A 5 year Forward*

View for Maternity Care (website). www.england.nhs.uk/wp-content/ uploads/2016/02/national-maternity-review-report.pdf. 2016.

Nursing and Midwifery Council (NMC): *The Code: professional Standards of Practice and Behaviour for Nurses and Midwives*, London, Nursing and Midwifery Council, 2015.

Nursing and Midwifery Council (NMC): *Revalidation* (website). http://revalidation.nmc.org.uk/. 2016.

Office for National Statistics (ONS): *Births in England and Wales by Parents' Country of Birth: 2013; Annual Statistics on Live Births*. 2014.

Parliamentary and Health Service Ombudsman (PHSO): *Midwifery Supervision and Regulation: recommendations for Change*, London, House of Commons. The Stationery Office, 2013.

Proctor S: What determines quality in maternity care: comparing perception of childbearing women and midwives, *Birth* 25(2):85–93, 1998.

Redshaw M, Henderson J: *Safely Delivered: a National Survey of Women's Experience of Maternity Care 2014*, National Perinatal Epidemiology Unit, Oxford, University of Oxford, 2015.

Redshaw MR, Hockley R, Brocklehurst CP: *Recorded delivery: a national survey of women's experience of maternity care 2006*, Oxford, National Perinatal Epidemiology Unit (NPEU), 2007.

Renfrew MJ, McFadden A, Bastos MH, et al: Midwifery and quality care: findings from a new evidence-informed framework for maternal and newborn care, *Lancet* 384(9948):1129–1145, 2014.

Royal College of Midwives (RCM): *Guidance Paper: Staffing Standard in Midwifery Services* (website). www.rcm.org.uk/college/standards-and-practice/guidance-papers/. 2009.

Royal College of Midwives (RCM): *State of Maternity Services Report 2015*. Royal College of Midwives (RCM), London, 2015a.

Royal College of Midwives (RCM): (website). www.rcm.org.uk/news-views-and-analysis/news/the-rcm -welcomes-nice-report-on-safe -staffing-in-midwifery. 2015b.

Royal College of Midwives (RCM): *Position Statement: Safe Staffing* (website). www.rcm.org.uk/sites/ default/files/Safe%20Midwife%20 Staffing_final.pdf. 2015c.

Royal College of Midwives (RCM): *The Global Twinning Project* (website). www.rcm.org.uk/ global-midwifery -twinning-project. 2016.

Royal College of Midwives (RCM): *Better Births Initiative* (website). www.rcm.org.uk/better-births-initiative. 2016.

Royal College of Obstetricians and Gynaecologists (RCOG), Royal College of Anaesthetists (RCA), Royal College of Midwives (RCM), Royal College of Paediatrics and Child Health (RCP): *Safer Childbirth: minimum Standards for the Organisation and Delivery of Care in Labour*, London, RCOG, 2007.

Royal College of Obstetricians and Gynaecologists (RCOG): *Standards for Maternity Care*, London, RCOG, 2008.

Sandall J, Soltani H, Shennan A, et al: Midwife led models of midwifery care for childbearing women and other models of care for childbearing women, *Cochrane Database Syst Rev* (8):Art. No.CD004667, 2016.

Sanghani R: *What is It Actually Like to be a Midwife Today? The Telegraph Online* (website). www.telegraph.co.uk/women/ mother-tongue/10668429/ What-is-it-actually-like-to-be-a-midwife-today.html. 2014.

Save the Children: *The Urban Disadvantage: State of the World's Mothers Report 2015*. Save the Children UK and USA, 2015.

The Migration Observatory: *London Census Profile 2011* (website). www.migrationobservatory.ox.ac.uk/ briefings/london-census-profile. 2013.

United Nations (UN): *United Nations Millennium Development Goals* (website). www.un.org/millennium goals. 2008.

United Nations (UN): *The Millennium Development Goals Report 2015* (website). www.un.org/ millenniumgoals/2015_MDG_ Report/pdf/MDG%202015%20 rev%20(July%201).pdf. 2015.

Walker K: *Media training: five tips for a great interview, The Guardian* (website). www.theguardian.com/ women-in-leadership/2013/jul/24/ top-tips-media-training-interviews. 2013.

Warwick C: *Leadership in maternity services, The Health Foundation* (website). http://patientsafety.health .org.uk/sites/default/files/ resources/6.leadership_in _maternity_services-v2.pdf. 2015.

West M, Dawson J, Kaur M: *Making the difference: diversity and inclusion in the NHS*, London, Kings Fund, 2015.

Which? *Birth Choice* (website). www.which.co.uk/birth-choice/. 2016.

Women and Children First (UK): *Safe Motherhood* (website). https://www .womenandchildrenfirst.org.uk/ impact/key-issues/safe-motherhood. 2016.

World Health Organization (WHO): *Making pregnancy safer: the critical role of the skilled attendant: a joint statement by WHO, ICM and FIGO*. Geneva, WHO Regional Office, 2004.

World Health Organization (WHO): *Strategies Towards Ending Preventable Maternal Mortality (EPMM)*, Geneva, World Health Organization (website). http://www.everywoman everychild.org/resources/ publications, 2015a.

World Health Organization (WHO):*Health in 2015: From MDGs, Millennium Development Goals to SDGs, Sustainable Development Goals* (website).http://apps.who.int/iris/ bitstream/10665/200009/1 /9789241565110_eng.pdf?ua=1. 2015b.

World Health Organization (WHO): *Nurses and Midwives: A Force for Enhancing Health and Strengthening Health Systems*. WHO Geneva (website). www.euro .who.int/__data/assets/ pdf_file/0004/287356/NURSES-AND-MIDWIVES-A-Vital -Resource-for-Health-Compendium.pdf. 2015c.

Resources and additional reading

Association for Improvement of the Maternity Services (AIMS).

http://www.aims.org.uk/).

This is a voluntary pressure group who campaign for better services for childbearing women, and support midwives in providing care. The (website) has a range of useful resources and links.

Byrom S, Downe S: *The roar behind the silence: why kindness, compassion and respect matter in maternity care,* London, Pinter and Martin, 2015.

This book is focused on kindness and compassion and includes chapters from leading midwives and researchers in maternity care.

National Childbirth Trust.

https://www.nct.org.uk.

One of the largest charities and pressure groups for parents. The NCT provides local classes and information for women and their families.

Royal College of Midwives.

www.rcm.org.uk.

Good source of national and international news and resources on midwifery and access to the RCM electronic learning programme and portfolio (i-learn and i-folio).

The Lancet series on Midwifery.

http://www.thelancet.com/series/ midwifery.

Published in 2014, this series is a wide ranging, evidence-based resource, examining international midwifery, reviewing clinical, policy and health system perspectives.

World Health Organization (WHO): *Nurses and midwives: A force for enhancing health and strengthening health systems.* WHO, Geneva (website). www.euro.who.int/__ data/assets/pdf_file/0004/287356/ NURSES-AND-MIDWIVES-A-Vital-Resource-for-Health-Compendium.pdf. 2015c.

This is a compendium of good practices in nursing and midwifery that illustrates the fundamental importance of these healthcare professionals to public health and well-being. Its 55 case studies from 18 countries provide examples of how nurses and midwives enhance health and are working towards achieving Sustainable Development Goal 3: Ensure healthy lives and promoting well-being for all at all ages.

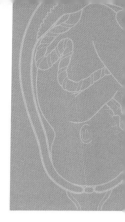

Index

Page numbers followed by "*f*" indicate figures, "*t*" indicate tables, and "*b*" indicate boxes.

A

A National Health Service Trust v. D Lloyd, 141
Abdomen, physical assessment of, 726–727
Abdominal aortic compression, 1097*b*, 1097*f*
Abdominal examination
  antenatal, 521–528
  auscultation in, 527
  in breech presentation, 1033
  findings throughout pregnancy, 527–528
  in labour, 598
  observation in, 521–522
  palpation in, 522–527, 522*f*
    attitude in, 524, 524*f*
    engagement of the fetal head in, 523, 524*f*, 528
    fetal lie in, 523*f*
    fundal, 526*f*, 527
    lateral, 526*f*, 527
    pelvic, 525–527, 526*f*
    presentation in, 523*f*
Abdominal muscle exercises, 335–336
Abdominal wall defects, 861–862, 862*f*
Abdominal wall muscles, 333, 334*f*
Abduction, in shoulder dystocia, 1063
ABO blood grouping, 538
ABO incompatibility, 717, 830, 832
Abortion, 413, 896–900, 896*f*
  fetal anomaly, 1115
  induced, 899
    criminal, 899
    therapeutic, 899, 899*f*
  and maternal death, 6*t*

missed, 898
  ultrasound screening for, 543
recurrent, 898
septic, 899–900
spontaneous, 896–899
  see also Miscarriage
Abortion Act 1967, 152, 152*b*, 899
Abruptio placentae, 903, 906–908, 906*f*
  causes of, 907
  differential diagnosis of, 909*t*
  types of, 907–908
  in uterine rupture, 1056
Abscess, mastitis and, 777
Absorption, 160–163
Abuse, 296–297
  children, 226, 226*b*
  denial of, 297–298
  domestic violence and, 344–346
  sexual, 202–203, 203*b*, 1132
Academic gaming, 99
Academics, influence of, 211
Acardiac twins, 971
Accoucheurs, 30
Accountability, 132
Accreditation of prior experiential learning (APEL), 88–89
Accreditation of prior learning (APL), 88–89
ACE inhibitors, 915*b*
Acetabulum, 359*f*–360*f*
Achondroplasia, 402, 867, 867*f*
Acid aspiration syndrome, 999
Acquired cardiac problems, 823, 823*b*
Acquired immunodeficiency syndrome (AIDS). *see* HIV/AIDS
Acrocyanosis, 711–712, 719
Acrosomal exocytosis, 444
Acrosome reaction, 444

Act-utilitarianism, 132
ACTH. *see* Adrenocorticotrophic hormone (ACTH)
Actinomycin-D, choriocarcinoma and, 901
Action on Smoking and Health (ASH), 880
'Active childbirth' movements, 37–38
Active management, third stage of labour, 652–653
  versus expectant management, 653–656
  history of, 652–653
  principles of, 655–656
Activist, 90
Acts and omissions, 132
Acts of Government
  Abortion Act 1967, 152, 152*b*, 899
  Adoption and Children Act 2002, 220
  Apprenticeships, Skills, Children and Learning Act 2009, 220
  Children Act 1989. *see* Children Act 1989
  Children Act 2004, 136
  Children and Adoption Act 2006, 220
  Children and Young Persons Act 2008, 220
  Children (Leaving Care) Act 2000, 220
  Congenital Disabilities (Civil Liability) Act 1976, 155
  Control of Substances Hazardous to Health Regulations 2002, 153
  Data Protection Act 1998, 153

1159